SEVENTH EDITION

ORTHOPEDIC PHYSICAL ASSESSMENT

David J. Magee, PhD, BPT, CM

Professor Emeritus
Department of Physical Therapy
Faculty of Rehabilitation Medicine
University of Alberta
Edmonton, Alberta, Canada

Robert C. Manske, PT, DPT, MEd, SCS, ATC, CSCS

Professor
Wichita State University
Department of Physical Therapy
Via Christi Ascension Orthopedic and Sports Physical Therapy
Wichita, Kansas, United States

ELSEVIER

Elsevier
3251 Riverport Lane
St. Louis, Missouri 63043

ORTHOPEDIC PHYSICAL ASSESSMENT, SEVENTH EDITION   ISBN: 978-0-323-52299-1

Notice

Practitioners and researchers must always rely on their own experience and knowledge in evaluating and using any information, methods, compounds or experiments described herein. Because of rapid advances in the medical sciences, in particular, independent verification of diagnoses and drug dosages should be made. To the fullest extent of the law, no responsibility is assumed by Elsevier, authors, editors or contributors for any injury and/or damage to persons or property as a matter of products liability, negligence or otherwise, or from any use or operation of any methods, products, instructions, or ideas contained in the material herein.

Previous editions copyrighted 2014, 2008, 2006, 1997, 1992, and 1987.

Library of Congress Control Number: 2020931964

Senior Content Strategist: Lauren Willis
Senior Content Development Manager: Luke Held
Senior Content Development Specialist: Sarah Vora
Publishing Services Manager: Julie Eddy
Senior Project Manager: Rachel E. McMullen

Printed in Canada

Last digit is the print number: 9 8 7 6 5 4 3 2 1

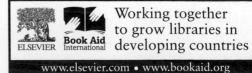

Dedication

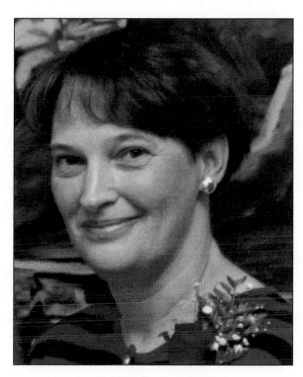

Bernice Sharon Magee
1945–2019
"My Rock and the Family's Glue"

Preface to the Seventh Edition

In 2014, when I completed the 6th edition of *Orthopedic Physical Assessment,* I thought it would be the last revision that I would do. Fortunately, I have been given an opportunity by Elsevier to do a 7th edition of the book and to work with the individual who will take over as author/editor of *Orthopedic Physical Assessment*–Dr. Robert Manske, who will work with my irreplaceable developmental editor, Bev Evjen, on any future editions. With the support of Elsevier, I believe the book is in good hands.

I remember when the first edition was printed and Elsevier told me they were going to print a first run of 8000 copies. All I could think about was "how long would it take to sell 8000 copies when I only taught 40 physical therapy students a year?" The book went through three printings in the first year and the rest, as they say, "is history!" To do something in your life and have it succeed well beyond all of one's expectations, hopes, and dreams has been very gratifying and hugely rewarding. The support of people who have provided input and constructive criticism is greatly appreciated and their input has contributed greatly to the book. The support of these people, my models for the photos in the book, my students, and my family are greatly appreciated.

When the first edition was published in 1987, I hoped at that time that I would be able to develop a series of books that would meet the needs of rehabilitation clinicians in the area of musculoskeletal conditions. With the assistance of the other editors, James Zachazewski, Sandy Quillen, and Rob Manske, and with a number of experts in their respective fields, my dream became a reality with the **Musculoskeletal Rehabilitation Series,** with *Orthopedic Physical Assessment* being the cornerstone of the book series.

In this edition of *Orthopedic Physical Assessment,* information has been updated in all of the chapters with several new tests and figures, especially in the area of concussions and assessment of the hip. The tables on the reliability and validity of many of the special tests and the examples of many functional tests have been moved to the Student Consult website, where they are available electronically for those who want them. Reliability studies for testing show variability in their outcomes, so key tests are highlighted using different icons because the value of the tests have been demonstrated clinically and/or statistically that they contribute to determining what the problem is. Hopefully, this will help students and clinicians determine which tests could be effective depending on the pathology being presented. These special tests do not replace a good history or examination.

This book, as the title suggests, is about assessing for musculoskeletal pathology. It is not a pathology textbook. As part of the Musculoskeletal Rehabilitation Series, the companion book to *Orthopedic Physical Assessment* is ***Pathology and Interventions in Musculoskeletal Rehabilitation,*** which goes into much greater detail on pathological conditions and their treatment. As "bookends" to these two books, ***Scientific Foundations and Principles of Practice in Musculoskeletal Rehabilitation*** provides information on healing of different tissue types, pain and aging, and the principles of different types of practice to treat different musculoskeletal tissue types; while ***Athletic and Sport Issues in Musculoskeletal Rehabilitation*** deals with more acute injuries and issues related to the more active individual, specific groups, and specific activities as they relate to sport.

David J. Magee, PhD, BPT, CM
2020

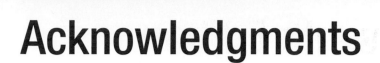

Acknowledgments

The writing of a book such as this, although undertaken by two people, is, in reality, the bringing together of ideas, concepts, and teachings developed and put forward by colleagues, friends, clinicians, and experts in the field of musculoskeletal assessment. When the book was first published in 1987, I had no idea of how successful it would be. It has succeeded in becoming more than I could have ever imagined in seven languages.

In particular, for this edition, I would like to thank the following people:

My family, especially my wife, Bernice, for putting up with my moods and idiosyncrasies, especially at 4 a.m.!

Bev Evjen, our irreplaceable developmental editor and friend. Without her help, encouragement, persistence, and eye for detail, this edition, as with previous editions and in fact the whole Musculoskeletal Rehabilitation Series, would not be what it is.

Rob Manske, who has agreed to author *Orthopedic Physical Assessment* going forward. I believe the book is in good hands and will be well looked after in the future.

Judy Chepeha, who has acted as the clinician model through five editions of the book. Her support and willingness to be part of the book has greatly enhanced it and added consistency to the book.

Our undergraduate, graduate, and postgraduate students from Canada, the United States, Brazil, Chile, and Japan, who provided us with many ideas for revisions, collected many of the articles used as references, and helped us with many of the tables.

The many **authors and publishers,** who were kind enough to allow us to use their photographs, drawings, and tables in the text so that explanations could be clearer and more easily understood. Without these additions, the book would not be what we hoped for.

Ted Huff and **Jodie Bernard,** our medical illustrators, whose skills and attention to detail have made a significant contribution to the success of *Orthopedic Physical Assessment*.

Our photographer, **Brian Gavriloff,** whose photographic talents added immeasurably to the book.

Dr. Andrew Porter for many of the radiographic images he provided for the diagnostic imaging portions of the book.

Our models, **Tanya Beasley, Paul Caines, Lee-Anne Clayholt, Carolyn Crowell, Michelle Cuthbert, Vanessa de Oliveira Furino, Devon Fraser, Ian Hallworth, Nathaniel Hay, Sarah Kazmir, Megan Lange, Tysen LeBlanc, Dolly Magee, Shawn Magee, Theo Magee, Tommy Magee, Harry Magee, Henry Magee, Nicole Nieberding, Judy Sara, Paula Shoemaker, Holly Stevens, Ben Stout, Brandon Thome, Veronica Toy, Joan Matthews-White,** and **Yung Yung Wong,** whose patience and agreement to be models for the many explanatory photographs and videos is very much appreciated.

Brent Davis, Luke Kriley, and **Jameson Fay,** who researched and updated the tables of psychometric properties of the Special Tests for this edition.

My colleagues, who contributed ideas, suggestions, radiographs, and photographs, and who typed and reviewed the manuscripts.

The **people at WB Saunders (Elsevier),** especially **Kathy Falk** who has guided me and supported me through several editions and **Lauren Willis, Sarah Vora,** and **Rachel McMullen** for their ideas, suggestions, assistance, and patience for this edition.

My teachers, colleagues, and mentors, who encouraged me to pursue my chosen career.

To these people and many others—thank you for your help, ideas, and encouragement. Your support played a large part in the success and completion of this book.

David J. Magee, PhD, BPT, CM
2020

Acknowledgments

I would first and foremost like to thank **David Magee** for allowing me to help with this 7th edition of *Orthopedic Physical Assessment*. I commonly refer to this text as the "Orthopedic Bible." I feel extremely blessed to have David mentor me through the process of revising a book of this magnitude and significance. Despite many unexpected events during this revision, David has always been gracious, kind, and patient with me through this process. It is never easy to give up control. However, he has slowly and patiently handed me pieces of rope, bit by bit, making sure that he did not give me enough to hang myself. He has taught me so much more than he will ever realize—things like taking pride in your work, overall work ethic, attention to detail, dependability, fairness, honesty, integrity, and humility to name just a few. The 7th edition of *Orthopedic Physical Assessment* with David and Bev will probably be one of my proudest work accomplishments.

Secondly, I want to thank **Bev Evjen.** David told me many years ago when we worked on our *Athletic and Sport Issues* book, how important Bev is to *Orthopedic Physical Assessment* and the whole Musculoskeletal Rehabilitation Series. That was a complete understatement. This process would not work without Bev's unyielding friendship, attention to detail, persistence, and amazing organizational skills. She is an amazingly, wonderful person who is always looking out for our best interests. Thank you, Bev!

Thirdly, I would like to thank the **faculty, staff, and students** at Wichita State University where I have worked for the last 23 years, **all of my many colleagues** I have worked with at various Via Christi–Ascension locations in Wichita over the last 25 years, and **past and present patients** who allow me to use the various tests from this book to help determine their orthopedic issues. They all drive me to continue to enhance my education and become not only a better teacher, but more importantly a better clinician. You are all incredibly talented therapists and staff and your friendship means so much to me.

Finally, thank you to **my beautiful wife, Julie, and our unbelievable children, Rachael, Halle, and Tyler**. Thank you for adding so much to my life.

Robert C. Manske, PT, DPT, MEd, SCS, ATC, CSCS
2020

Contents

Video Contents

The following video clips are available online at https://studentconsult.inkling.com using the pin code provided in this textbook.

6   Elbow

7   Forearm, Wrist, and Hand

CHAPTER 1

Principles and Concepts

A musculoskeletal assessment requires a proper and thorough systematic examination of the patient. A correct diagnosis depends on a knowledge of functional anatomy, an accurate patient history, diligent observation, and a thorough examination. The differential diagnosis process involves the use of clinical signs and symptoms, physical examination, a knowledge of pathology and mechanisms of injury, provocative and palpation (motion) tests, and laboratory and diagnostic imaging techniques. It is only through a complete and systematic assessment that an accurate diagnosis can be made. The purpose of the assessment should be to fully and clearly understand the patient's problems, from the patient's perspective as well as the clinician's, and the physical basis for the symptoms that have caused the patient to complain. As James Cyriax stated, "Diagnosis is only a matter of applying one's anatomy."[1]

One of the more common assessment recording techniques is the problem-oriented medical records method, which uses "SOAP" notes.[2] SOAP stands for the four parts of the assessment: Subjective, Objective, Assessment, and Plan. This method is especially useful in helping the examiner to solve a problem. In this book, the subjective portion of the assessment is covered under the heading Patient History, objective under Observation, and assessment under Examination.

Although the text deals primarily with musculoskeletal physical assessment on an outpatient basis, it can easily be adapted to evaluate inpatients. The primary difference is in adapting the assessment to the needs of a bedridden patient. Often, an inpatient's diagnosis has been made previously, and any continuing assessment is modified to determine how the patient's condition is responding to treatment. Likewise, an outpatient is assessed continually during treatment, and the assessment is modified to reflect the patient's response to treatment.

Regardless of which system is selected for assessment, the examiner should establish a **sequential method** to ensure that nothing is overlooked. The assessment must be organized, comprehensive, and reproducible. In general, the examiner compares one side of the body, which is assumed to be normal, with the other side of the body, which is abnormal or injured. For this reason, the examiner must come to understand and know the wide variability in what is considered normal. In addition, the examiner should focus attention on only one aspect of the assessment at a time, for example, ensuring a thorough history is taken before completing the examination component. When assessing an individual joint, the examiner must look at the joint and injury in the context of how the injury may affect other joints in the kinetic chain. These other joints may demonstrate changes as they try to compensate for the injured joint.

Each chapter ends with a summary, or précis, of the assessment procedures identified in that chapter. This section enables the examiner to quickly review the pertinent steps of assessment for the joint or structure being assessed. For further information, the examiner can refer to the more detailed sections of the chapter.

Total Musculoskeletal Assessment

- Patient history
- Observation
- Examination of movement
- Special tests
- Reflexes and cutaneous distribution
- Joint play movements
- Palpation
- Diagnostic imaging

Patient History

Ideally, the environment for the assessment should be private and as free of distractions as possible. The examiner should always introduce himself or herself to the patient and then sit beside or in front of the patient to enhance the notion that the examiner is focused on the patient. Showing kindness and respect help to create an environment that facilitates the exchange of information.[3]

A complete medical and injury history should be taken and written to ensure reliability. This requires effective and efficient communication on the part of the examiner and the ability to develop a good rapport with the patient and, in some cases, family members and other members of the health care team. This includes speaking at a level and using terms the patient will understand (common sense questions); taking the time to listen; and being empathic, interested, caring, and professional.[4] Naturally, emphasis in taking the history should be placed on the portion of the assessment that has the greatest clinical relevance. Often the examiner can make the diagnosis by simply *listening to the patient.*[5,6] This really means the patient, with the appropriate prompting, will tell the clinician about the complex symptoms that leads the clinician to make the appropriate diagnosis.[6] No subject areas should be skipped. Repetition helps the examiner to become familiar with the characteristic history of the patient's complaints so that unusual deviation, which often indicates problems, is noticed immediately. Even if the diagnosis is obvious, the history provides valuable information about the disorder, its present state, its prognosis, and the appropriate treatment. The history also enables the examiner to determine the type of person the patient is, his or her language and cognitive ability, the patient's ability to articulate, any treatment the patient has received, and the behavior of the injury. In addition to the history of the present illness or injury, the examiner should note relevant past history, treatment, and results. Past medical history should include any major illnesses, surgery, accidents, or allergies. In some cases, it may be necessary to delve into the social and family histories of the patient if they appear relevant. Lifestyle habit patterns, including sleep patterns, stress, workload, and recreational pursuits, should also be noted.

It is important that the examiner politely but firmly keeps the patient focused and discourages irrelevant information. Questions and answers should provide practical information about the problem. In addition, the examiner should listen for any potential **red flag** signs and symptoms (Table 1.1) that would indicate the problem is not a musculoskeletal one or could be more serious pathology that should be referred to the appropriate health care professional.[7-9] Serious systemic pathology may be indicated by sweating, pallor/flushing, sallow/jaundiced complexion, tremors/shaking, increased body temperature, and altered blood pressure. A lone red flag would not necessarily indicate serious pathology. It should be considered in the context of the individual's history and the findings of assessment.[9] **Yellow flag** signs and symptoms are also important for the examiner to note as they denote problems that may be more severe or may involve more than one area requiring a more extensive examination, or they may relate to cautions and contraindications to treatment that the examiner might have to consider, or they may indicate overlying psychosocial issues that may affect treatment.[10]

The patient's history is usually taken in an orderly sequence. It offers the patient an opportunity to describe the problem and the limitations caused by the problem as he or she perceives them. To achieve a good functional outcome, it is essential that the clinician heed to the patient's concerns and expectations for treatment. After all, the history is the patient's report of his or her own condition. Sometimes, patients' reported outcomes are included as part of the history. These outcomes give the status of the patient's health and problems and are given directly by the patient and how the problem(s)

▼ **TABLE 1.1**

Red Flag Findings in Patient History That Indicate Need for Referral to Physician

Cancer	• Persistent pain at night • Constant pain anywhere in the body • Unexplained weight loss (e.g., 4.5–6.8 kg [10–15 lbs] in 2 weeks or less) (5% or more in 4 weeks) • Loss of appetite • Unusual lumps or growths • Unwarranted fatigue • Change in bowel or bladder habits • Sores that will not heal • Unusual bleeding or discharge • Obvious change in wart or mole • Nagging cough or hoarseness
Cardiovascular	• Shortness of breath • Dizziness • Pain or a feeling of heaviness in the chest • Pulsating pain anywhere in the body • Constant and severe pain in lower leg (calf) or arm • Discolored or painful feet • Swelling (no history of injury)
Gastrointestinal/ Genitourinary	• Frequent or severe abdominal pain • Frequent heartburn or indigestion • Frequent nausea or vomiting • Change in or problems with bowel and/or bladder function (e.g., urinary tract infection), incontinence • Unusual menstrual irregularities
Miscellaneous	• Fever or night sweats • Recent severe emotional disturbances • Swelling or redness in any joint with no history of injury • Pregnancy
Neurological	• Changes in hearing • Frequent or severe headaches with no history of injury • Problems with swallowing or changes in speech • Changes in vision (e.g., blurriness or loss of sight) • Problems with balance, coordination, or falling • Fainting spells (drop attacks) • Sudden weakness • Bilateral pins and needles

Adapted from Stith JS, Sahrmann SA, Dixon KK, et al: Curriculum to prepare diagnosticians in physical therapy, *J Phys Ther Educ* 9:50, 1995.

affects the patient's quality of life.[11] The clinician should ask questions that are easy to understand and should not lead the patient. For example, the examiner should not say, "Does this increase your pain?" It would be better to say, "Does this alter your pain in any way?" The examiner should ask one question at a time and receive an answer to each question before proceeding with another

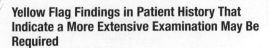

Yellow Flag Findings in Patient History That Indicate a More Extensive Examination May Be Required

- Abnormal signs and symptoms (unusual patterns of complaint)
- Bilateral symptoms
- Symptoms peripheralizing
- Neurological symptoms (nerve root or peripheral nerve)
- Multiple nerve root involvement
- Abnormal sensation patterns (do not follow dermatome or peripheral nerve patterns)
- Saddle anesthesia
- Upper motor neuron symptoms (spinal cord) signs
- Fainting
- Drop attacks
- Vertigo
- Autonomic nervous system symptoms
- Progressive weakness
- Progressive gait disturbances
- Multiple inflamed joints
- Psychosocial stresses
- Circulatory or skin changes

question. Open-ended questions ask for narrative information; closed or direct questions ask for specific information. Direct questions are often used to fill in details of information given in open-ended questions, and they frequently require only a one-word answer, such as yes or no. In any musculoskeletal assessment, the examiner should seek answers to the following pertinent questions.

1. *What is the patient's age and sex?* Many conditions occur within certain age ranges. For example, various growth disorders, such as Legg-Perthes disease or Scheuermann disease, are seen in adolescents or teenagers. Degenerative conditions, such as osteoarthritis and osteoporosis, are more likely to be seen in an older population. Shoulder impingement in young people (15 to 35 years) is more likely to result from muscle weakness, primarily in the muscles controlling the scapula, whereas the condition in older people (40+ years) is more likely to be the result of degenerative changes in the shoulder complex. Some conditions show sex and even race differences. For example, some cancers are more prevalent in men (e.g., prostate, bladder), whereas others occur more frequently in women (e.g., cervical, breast), yet still others are more common in white people.

2. *What is the patient's occupation?* What does the patient do at work? What is the working environment like? What are the demands and postures assumed?[12] For example, a laborer probably has stronger muscles than a sedentary worker and may be less likely to suffer a muscle strain. However, laborers are more susceptible to injury because of the types of jobs they have. Because sedentary workers usually have no need for high levels of muscle strength, they may overstress their muscles or joints on weekends because of overactivity or participation in activity that they are not used to. Habitual postures and repetitive strain caused by some occupations may indicate the location or source of the problem.

3. *Why has the patient come for help?* This is often referred to as the **history of the present illness** or **chief complaint.**[3] This part of the history provides an opportunity for patients to describe in their own words what is bothering them and the extent to which it bothers them. It is important for the clinician to determine what the patient wants to be able to do functionally and what the patient is unable to do functionally. In other words, is there a functional limitation? It is often this functional limitation that leads the patient to seek help. It is also essential to ensure that the clinician knows what is important to the patient in terms of outcome, whether the patient's expectations for the following treatment are realistic, and what direction functional treatment should take to ensure the patient can, if at all possible, return to his or her previous level of activity or realize his or her expected outcome.[13]

4. *Was there any inciting trauma (macrotrauma) or repetitive activity (microtrauma)?* In other words, what was the **mechanism of injury,** and were there any predisposing factors? If the patient was in a motor vehicle accident, for example, was the patient the driver or the passenger? Was he or she the cause of the accident? What part of the car was hit? How fast were the cars going? Was the patient wearing a seat belt? When asking questions about the mechanism(s) of injury, the examiner must try to determine the direction and magnitude of the injuring force and how the force was applied. By carefully listening to the patient, the examiner can often determine which structures were injured and how severely by knowing the force and mechanism of injury. For example, anterior dislocations of the shoulder usually occur when the arm is abducted and laterally rotated beyond the normal range of motion (ROM), and the "terrible triad" injury to the knee (i.e., medial collateral ligament, anterior cruciate ligament, and medial meniscus injury) usually results from a blow to the lateral side of the knee while the knee is flexed, the full weight of the patient is on the knee, and the foot is fixed. Likewise, the examiner should determine whether there were any predisposing, unusual, or new factors (e.g., sustained postures or repetitive activities, general health, or familial or genetic problems) that may have led to the problem.[14]

5. *Was the onset of the problem slow or sudden?* Did the condition start as an insidious, mild ache and then progress to continuous pain, or was there a specific episode in which the body part was injured? If inciting trauma has occurred, it is often relatively easy to determine the location of the problem. Does the pain get worse as the day progresses? Was the sudden onset caused by trauma, or was it sudden with locking because of muscle spasm (spasm lock) or

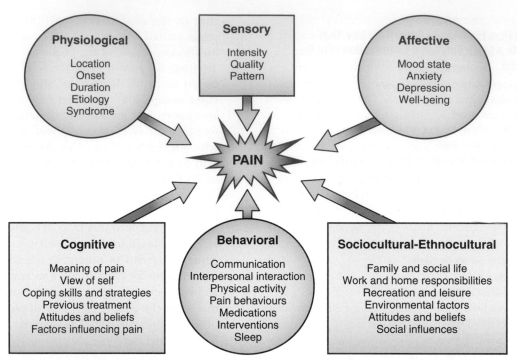

Fig. 1.1 The dimensions of pain. (Redrawn from Petty NJ, Moore AP: *Neuromuscular examination and assessment: a handbook for therapists*, London, 1998, Churchill-Livingstone, p 8.)

pain? Is there anything that relieves the symptoms? Knowledge of these facts helps the examiner to make a differential diagnosis.

6. *Where are the symptoms that bother the patient?* If possible, have the patient point to the area. Does the patient point to a specific structure or a more general area? The latter may indicate a more severe condition or referral of symptoms **(yellow flag).** The way in which the patient describes the symptoms often helps to delineate problems. Has the dominant or nondominant side been injured? Injury to the dominant side may lead to greater functional limitations. Are the problems local (e.g., a sprain) or systemic (e.g., rheumatoid arthritis)?

7. *Where was the pain or other symptoms when the patient first had the complaint?* Pain is subjective, and its manifestations are unique to each individual. It is a complex experience involving several dimensions (Fig. 1.1).[15,16] If the intensity of the pain or symptoms is such that the patient is unable to move in a certain direction or hold a particular posture because of the symptoms, the symptoms are said to be severe. If the symptoms or pain become progressively worse with movement or the longer a position is held, the symptoms are said to be irritable.[17,18] **Acute pain** is new pain that is often severe, continuous, and perhaps disabling and is of sufficient quality or duration that the patient seeks help. Acute injuries tend to be more irritable resulting in pain earlier in the movement, or minimal activity will bring on symptoms, and often the pain will remain after movement has stopped.[4]

Chronic pain is more aggravating, is not as intense, and has been experienced before, and in many cases, the patient knows how to deal with it. Acute pain is more often accompanied by anxiety, whereas chronic pain is associated with depression.[19] When tissue has been damaged, substances are released leading to inflammation and **peripheral sensitization** of the nociceptors (also called **primary hyperalgesia**) resulting in localized pain. If the injury does not follow a normal healing pathway and becomes chronic, **central sensitization** (also called **secondary hyperalgesia**) may occur. Peripheral sensitization is a local phenomenon, whereas central sensitization is a more central process involving the spinal cord and brain. Central sensitization manifests itself as widespread hypersensitivity to such physical, mental, and emotional stressors as touch, mechanical pressure, noise, bright light, temperature, and medication.[20,21]

Has the pain moved or spread? The location and spread of pain may be marked on a body chart, which is part of the assessment sheet (eAppendix 1.1). The examiner should ask the patient to point to exactly where the pain was and where it is now. Are trigger points present? **Trigger points** are localized areas of hyperirritability within the tissues; they are tender to compression, are often accompanied by tight bands of tissue, and, if sufficiently hypersensitive, may give rise to referred pain that is steady, deep, and aching. These trigger points can lead to a diagnosis, because pressure on them reproduces the patient's symptoms. Trigger points are not found in normal muscles.[22]

In general, the area of pain enlarges or becomes more distal as the lesion worsens and becomes smaller or more localized as it improves. Some examiners call the former **peripheralization of symptoms** and the latter, **centralization of symptoms**.[23–25] The more distal and superficial the problem, the more accurately the patient can determine the location of the pain. In the case of referred pain, the patient usually points out a general area; with a localized lesion, the patient points to a specific location. **Referred pain** tends to be felt deeply; its boundaries are indistinct, and it radiates segmentally without crossing the midline. The term *referred pain* means that the pain is felt at a site other than the injured tissue because the same or adjacent neural segments supply the referred site. Pain also may shift as the lesion shifts. For example, with an internal derangement of the knee, pain may occur in flexion one time and in extension another time if it is caused by a loose body within the joint. The examiner must clearly understand where the patient feels the pain. For example, does the pain occur only at the end of the ROM, in part of the range, or throughout the ROM?[14]

8. *What are the exact movements or activities that cause pain?* At this stage, the examiner should not ask the patient to do the movements or activities; this will take place during the examination. However, the examiner should remember which movements the patient says are painful so that when the examination is carried out, the patient can do these movements last to avoid an overflow of painful symptoms. With cessation of the activity, does the pain stay the same, or how long does it take for the pain to return to its previous level? Are there any other factors that aggravate or help to relieve the pain? Do these activities alter the intensity of the pain? The answers to these questions give the examiner some idea of the irritability of the joint. They also help the examiner to differentiate between musculoskeletal or mechanical pain and systemic pain, which is pain arising from one of the body's systems other than the musculoskeletal system (Table 1.2).[24] Functionally, pain can be divided into different levels, especially for repetitive stress conditions.

Pain and Its Relation to Severity of Repetitive Stress Activity

- Level 1: Pain after specific activity
- Level 2: Pain at start of activity resolving with warm-up
- Level 3: Pain during and after specific activity that does not affect performance
- Level 4: Pain during and after specific activity that does affect performance
- Level 5: Pain with activities of daily living
- Level 6: Constant dull aching pain at rest that does not disturb sleep
- Level 7: Dull aching pain that does disturb sleep

Note: Level 7 indicates highest level of severity.

TABLE **1.2**

Differentiation of Systemic and Musculoskeletal Pain

Systemic	Musculoskeletal
<ul><li>Disturbs sleep</li><li>Deep aching or throbbing</li><li>Reduced by pressure</li><li>Constant or waves of pain and spasm</li><li>Is not aggravated by mechanical stress</li><li>Associated with the following:<ul><li>Jaundice</li><li>Migratory arthralgias</li><li>Skin rash</li><li>Fatigue</li><li>Weight loss</li><li>Low-grade fever</li><li>Generalized weakness</li><li>Cyclic and progressive symptoms</li><li>Tumors</li><li>History of infection</li></ul></li></ul>	<ul><li>Generally lessens at night</li><li>Sharp or superficial ache</li><li>Usually decreases with cessation of activity</li><li>Usually continuous or intermittent</li><li>Is aggravated by mechanical stress</li></ul>

From Meadows JT: *Orthopedic differential diagnosis in physical therapy—a case study approach*, New York, 1999, McGraw Hill, p 100. Reproduced with permission of the McGraw-Hill Companies.

9. *How long has the problem existed?* What are the duration and frequency of the symptoms? Answers to these questions help the examiner to determine whether the condition is acute, subacute, chronic, or acute on chronic and to develop some understanding of the patient's tolerance to pain. In general, **acute conditions** are those that have been present for 7 to 10 days, **subacute conditions** have been present for 10 days to 7 weeks, and **chronic conditions** or symptoms have been present for longer than 7 weeks. In **acute on chronic** cases, the injured tissues usually have been reinjured. This knowledge is also beneficial in terms of how vigorously the patient can be examined. For example, the more acute the condition, the less stress the examiner is able to apply to the joints and tissues during the assessment. A full examination may not be possible in very acute conditions. In that case, the examiner must select those procedures of assessment that will give the greatest amount of information with the least stress to the patient. Does the patient protect or support the injured part? If so, this behavior signifies discomfort and fear of pain if the part moves, usually indicating a more acute condition.

10. *Has the condition occurred before?* If so, what was the onset like the first time? Where was the site of the original condition, and has there been any radiation (spread) of the symptoms? If the patient

is feeling better, how long did the recovery take? Did any treatment relieve symptoms? Does the current problem appear to be the same as the previous problem, or is it different? If it is different, how is it different? Answers to these questions help the examiner to determine the location and severity of the injury.

11. *Has there been an injury to another part of the kinetic chain as well?* For example, foot problems can lead to knee, hip, pelvic, and/or spinal problems; elbow problems may contribute to shoulder problems; and hip problems can contribute to knee problems.

12. *Are the intensity, duration, or frequency of pain or other symptoms increasing?* These changes usually mean the condition is getting worse. A decrease in pain or other symptoms usually means the condition is improving. Is the pain static? If so, how long has it been that way? This question may help the examiner to determine the present state of the problem. These factors may become important in treatment and may help to determine whether a treatment is helping. Are pain or other symptoms associated with other physiological functions? For example, is the pain worse with menstruation? If so, when did the patient last have a pelvic examination? Questions such as these may give the examiner an indication of what is causing the problem or what factors may affect the problem. It is often worthwhile to give the patient a pain questionnaire, visual analog scale (VAS), numeric rating scale, box scale, or verbal rating scale that can be completed while the patient is waiting to be assessed.[26–30] It has been shown that a reduction of approximately 30% change or 2 points (i.e., 2 cm) on a VAS from one test period to the next represents a clinically important difference.[28,31] It is also important to realize that a 1 point intensity change from 8 to 9 represents a greater subjective increase than does an increase from 2 to 3.[31] The McGill-Melzack pain questionnaire and its short form (eTools 1.1 and 1.2)[32–34] provide the patient with three major classes of word descriptors—sensory, affective, and evaluative—to describe their pain experience. These designations are used to differentiate patients who have a true sensory pain experience from those who think they have experienced pain (affective pain state). Other pain-rating scales allow the patient to visually gauge the amount of pain along a solid 10-cm line (VAS) (Fig. 1.2) or on a thermometer-type scale (Fig. 1.3).[35] It has been shown that an examiner should consistently use the same pain scales when assessing or reassessing patients to increase consistent results.[36–39] The examiner can use the completed questionnaire or scale as an indication of the pain as described or perceived by the patient. Alternatively, a self-report pain drawing (see eAppendix 1.1), which (with the training and guidelines of the raters) has been shown to have reliability, can be used for the same purpose.[40]

13. *Is the pain constant, periodic, episodic (occurring with certain activities), or occasional?* Does the condition bother the patient at that exact moment? If the patient is not bothered at that exact moment, the pain is not constant. **Constant pain** suggests chemical irritation, tumors, or possibly visceral lesions.[24] It is always there, although its intensity may vary. If **periodic** or **occasional pain** is present, the examiner should try to determine the activity, position, or posture that irritates or brings on the symptoms, because

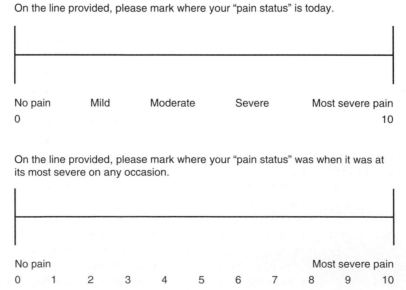

Fig. 1.2 Visual analog scales for pain. Examples only. Note: For an actual examination, the lines would be 10 cm long divided into 1 cm sections.

Pain Rating Scale

Instructions:
 Below is a thermometer with various grades of pain on it from "No pain at all" to "The pain is almost unbearable." Put an X by the words that describe your pain best. Mark how bad your pain is **at this moment in time.**

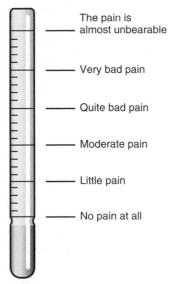

—— The pain is almost unbearable

—— Very bad pain

—— Quite bad pain

—— Moderate pain

—— Little pain

—— No pain at all

Fig. 1.3 "Thermometer" pain rating scale. (Redrawn from Brodie DJ, Burnett JV, Walker JM, et al: Evaluation of low back pain by patient questionnaires and therapist assessment, *J Orthop Sports Phys Ther* 11[11].528, 1990.)

The Roles-Maudsley Satisfaction Score[a]

Grade 1	Excellent—no symptoms, no pain, full movement and activity (no symptoms following treatment)
Grade 2	Good—occasional discomfort, full movement and activity (significant improvement from treatment)
Grade 3	Fair—some discomfort after prolonged activity (somewhat improved after treatment)
Grade 4	Poor—pain limits activities (symptoms unchanged or worse after treatment)

[a]Posttreatment scores of patient satisfaction.

this may help to determine what tissues are at fault. This type of pain is more likely to be mechanical and related to movement and stress.[24] **Episodic pain** is related to specific activities. At the same time, the examiner should be observing the patient. Does the patient appear to be in constant pain? Does the patient appear to be lacking sleep because of pain? Does the patient move around a great deal in an attempt to find a comfortable position?

14. *Is the pain associated with rest? Activity? Certain postures? Visceral function? Time of day?* Pain on activity that decreases with rest usually indicates a mechanical problem interfering with movement, such as adhesions. Morning pain with stiffness that improves with activity usually indicates chronic inflammation and edema, which decrease with motion. Pain or aching as the day progresses usually indicates increased congestion in a joint. Pain at rest and pain that is worse at the beginning of activity than at the end implies acute inflammation. Pain that is not affected by rest or activity usually indicates bone pain or could be related to organic or systemic disorders, such as cancer or diseases of the viscera. The **Roles-Maudsley Score** is sometimes used as a 4-point assessment of pain and limitations of activity.

Chronic pain is often associated with multiple factors, such as fatigue or certain postures or activities. If the pain occurs at night, how does the patient lie in bed: supine, on the side, or prone? Does sleeping alter the pain, or does the patient wake when he or she changes position? Intractable pain at night may indicate serious pathology (e.g., a tumor). Movement seldom affects visceral pain unless the movement compresses or stretches the structure.[17] Symptoms of peripheral nerve entrapment (e.g., carpal tunnel syndrome) and thoracic outlet syndromes tend to be worse at night. Pain and cramping with prolonged walking may indicate lumbar spinal stenosis (neurogenic intermittent claudication) or vascular problems (circulatory or vascular intermittent claudication). Intervertebral disc pain is aggravated by sitting and bending forward. Facet joint pain is often relieved by sitting and bending forward and is aggravated by extension and rotation. What type of mattress and pillow does the patient use? Foam pillows often cause more problems for persons with cervical disorders because these pillows have more "bounce" to them than do feather or buckwheat pillows. Too many pillows, pillows improperly positioned, or too soft a mattress may also cause problems.

15. *What type or quality of pain is exhibited?* **Nerve pain** tends to be sharp (lancinating), bright, and burning and also tends to run in the distribution of specific nerves. Thus the examiner must have detailed knowledge of the sensory distribution of nerve roots (dermatomes) and peripheral nerves because the different distributions may tell where the pathology or problem is if the nerve is involved. **Bone pain** tends to be deep, boring, and localized. **Vascular pain** tends to be diffuse, aching, and poorly localized and may be referred to other areas of the body. **Muscle pain** is usually hard to localize, is dull and aching, is often aggravated by injury, and may be referred to other areas (Table 1.3). If a muscle is injured, when the muscle contracts or is stretched, the pain will increase. Inert tissue, such as ligaments, joint capsules, and bursa, tends to exhibit pain similar to muscle pain and may be indistinguishable from muscle pain in the resting state (e.g., when the examiner is taking the history);

TABLE **1.3**

Pain Descriptions and Related Structures

Type of Pain	Structure
Cramping, dull, aching	Muscle
Dull, aching	Ligament, joint capsule
Sharp, shooting	Nerve root
Sharp, bright, lightning-like	Nerve
Burning, pressure-like, stinging, aching	Sympathetic nerve
Deep, nagging, dull	Bone
Sharp, severe, intolerable	Fracture
Throbbing, diffuse	Vasculature

however, pain in inert tissue is increased when the structures are stretched or pinched. Each of these specific tissue pains is sometimes grouped as **neuropathic pain** and follows specific anatomic pathways and affect specific anatomic structures.[24] The Leeds Assessment of Neuropathic Symptoms and Signs (LANSS) Pain Scale (eTool 1.3) has been developed to determine if neuropathic causes dominate the pain experience.[41] In contrast, **somatic pain** is a severe chronic or aching pain that is inconsistent with injury or pathology to specific anatomic structures and cannot be explained by any physical cause because the sensory input can come from so many different structures supplied by the same nerve root.[18] Superficial somatic pain may be localized, but deep somatic pain is more diffuse and may be referred.[42] On examination, somatic pain may be reproduced, but visceral pain is not reproduced by movement.[42]

16. *What types of sensations does the patient feel, and where are these abnormal sensations?* If the problem is in bone, there usually is very little radiation of pain. If pressure is applied to a nerve root, radicular pain (radiating pain) results from pressure on the dura mater, which is the outermost covering of the spinal cord. If there is pressure on the nerve trunk, no pain occurs, but there is paresthesia, or an abnormal sensation, such as a "pins and needles" feeling or tingling. Paresthesia is an unpleasant sensation that occurs without an apparent stimulus or cause (to the patient). Autonomic pain is more likely to be a burning type of pain. If the nerve itself is affected, regardless of where the irritation occurs along the nerve, the brain perceives the pain as coming from the periphery. This is an example of **referred pain.**

17. *Does a joint exhibit locking, unlocking, twinges, instability, or giving way?* Seldom does locking mean that the joint will not move at all. **Locking** may mean that the joint cannot be fully extended, as is the case with a meniscal tear in the knee, or it may mean that it does not extend one time and does not flex the next time

(**pseudolocking**), as in the case of a loose body moving within the joint. Locking may mean that the joint cannot be put through a full ROM because of muscle spasm or because the movement was too fast; this is sometimes referred to as **spasm locking. Giving way** is often caused by reflex inhibition or weakness of the muscles, and so the patient feels that the limb will buckle if weight is placed on it or the pain will be too great. Inhibition may be caused by anticipated pain or instability.

In nonpathological states, excessive ROM in a joint is called **laxity** or **hypermobility.** Laxity implies the patient has excessive ROM but can control movement in that range and no pathology is present. It is a function of the ligaments and joint capsule resistance.[43] This differs from flexibility, which is the ROM available in one or more joints and is a function of contractile tissue resistance primarily as well as ligament and joint capsule resistance.[43] Gleim and McHugh[43] describe flexibility in two parts: static and dynamic. Static flexibility is related to the ROM available in one or more joints; dynamic flexibility is related to stiffness and ease of movement. Laxity may be caused by familial factors or may be job or activity (e.g., sports) related. In any case, laxity, when found, should be considered normal (Fig. 1.4). If symptoms occur, then laxity is considered to be hypermobility and has a pathological component, which commonly indicates the patient's inability to control the joint during

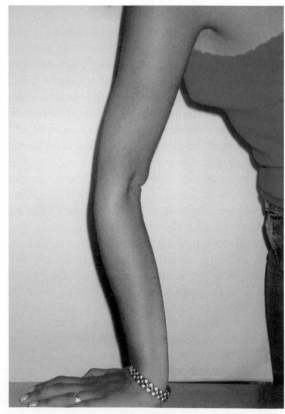

Fig. 1.4 Congenital laxity at the elbow leading to hyperextension. This may also be called *nonpathological hypermobility.*

movement, especially at end range, which implies instability of the joint. Instability can cover a wide range of pathological hypermobility from a loss of control of arthrokinematic joint movements to anatomic instability where subluxation or dislocation is imminent or has occurred. For assessment purposes, instability can be divided into translational (loss of arthrokinematic control) and anatomic (dislocation or subluxation) instability.[44] **Translational instability** (also called *pathological* or *mechanical instability*) refers to loss of control of the small, arthrokinematic joint movements (e.g., spin, slide, roll, translation) that occur when the patient attempts to stabilize (statically or dynamically) the joint during movement. **Anatomic instability** (also called *clinical* or *gross instability,* or *pathological hypermobility*) refers to excessive or gross physiological movement in a joint where the patient becomes apprehensive at the end of the ROM because a subluxation or dislocation is imminent. It should be noted that there is confusion in the application of the terms used to describe the two types of instability. For example, mechanical instability is sometimes used to mean anatomic instability because of anatomic or pathological dysfunction. **Functional instability** may mean either or both types of instability and implies an inability to control either arthrokinematic or osteokinematic movement in the available ROM either consciously or unconsciously during functional movement. These instabilities are more likely to be evident during high-speed or loaded movements. Both types of instability can cause symptoms, and treatment centers on teaching the patient to develop muscular control of the joint and to improve reaction time and proprioceptive control. Both types of instability may be voluntary or involuntary. **Voluntary instability** is initiated by muscle contraction, and **involuntary instability** is the result of positioning. Another concept worth remembering during assessment for instability is the **circle concept of instability**, which was originally developed from shoulder studies[45,46] but is equally applicable to other joints. This concept states that injury to structures on one side of a joint leading to instability can, at the same time, cause injury to structures on the other side or other parts of the joint. Thus an anterior shoulder dislocation can lead to injury of the posterior capsule. Similarly, anterolateral rotary instability of the knee leads to injury to posterior structures (e.g., arcuate-popliteus complex, posterior capsule) as well as anterior (e.g., anterior cruciate ligament) and lateral (e.g., lateral collateral ligament) structures. Thus the examiner must be aware of potential injuries on the opposite side of the joint even if symptoms are predominantly on one side, especially when the mechanism of injury is trauma.

18. *Has the patient experienced any bilateral spinal cord symptoms, fainting, or drop attacks?* Is bladder function normal? Is there any "saddle" involvement (abnormal sensation in the perianal region, buttocks, and superior aspect of the posterior thighs) or vertigo? "Vertigo" and "dizziness" are terms often used synonymously, although vertigo usually indicates more severe symptoms. The terms describe a swaying, spinning sensation accompanied by feelings of unsteadiness and loss of balance. These symptoms indicate severe neurological problems, such as cervical myelopathy, which must be dealt with carefully and can (e.g., in cases of altered bladder function) be emergency conditions potentially requiring surgery. Drop attacks occur when the patient suddenly falls without warning or provocation but remains conscious.[24] It is caused by neurological dysfunction, especially in the brain.

19. *Are there any changes in the color of the limb?* Ischemic changes resulting from circulatory problems may include white, brittle skin; loss of hair; and abnormal nails on the foot or hand. Conditions such as reflex sympathetic dystrophy, which is an autonomic nerve response to trauma, however minor, can cause these symptoms, as can circulatory problems such as Raynaud disease.

20. *Has the patient been experiencing any life or economic stresses?* These psychological stressors are sometimes considered to be **yellow flags** that alter both the assessment and subsequent treatment.[47,48] Divorce, marital problems, financial problems, or job stress or insecurity can contribute to increasing the pain or symptoms because of psychological stress. What support systems and resources are available? Are there any cultural issues one should be aware of? Does the patient have an easily accessible living environment? Each of these issues may increase stress to the patient. Pain is often accentuated in patients with anxiety, depression, or hysteria, or patients may exaggerate their symptoms (**symptom magnification**) in the absence of objective signs, which may be called **psychogenic pain**.[4,49,50] Thus psychosocial aspects can play a significant role with injury.[51–54] Because of the importance of these psychosocial aspects related to movement such as anxiety, questionnaires such as the Fear-Avoidance Beliefs Questionnaire (FABQ)[55] (eTool 1.4) and the Tampa Scale for Kinesiophobia (eTool 1.5)[56–61] have been developed.[56,62–64] Most of the studies related to the psychosocial aspects of injury have been related to the low back but could be used for other joints. The focus of these questionnaires is on the patient's beliefs about how physical activity and work affect his or her injury and pain.[52,65,66] Fig. 1.5 outlines the different pathways normally followed after injury and the pathway followed in a patient who fears movement will increase the pain or cause reinjury.[55] Table 1.4 outlines some of the psychological processes affecting pain.[52] These processes have been divided into different colored "flags" (Table 1.5), but it is important to note that these psychological flags, other than the red flag, are

different from pathological "flags" previously mentioned.[54] Waddell and Main[47] consider illness behavior normal with patients who are exhibiting both a physical problem and varying degrees of illness behavior (Table 1.6). In these cases, it may be beneficial to determine the level of psychological stress or to refer the patient to another appropriate health care professional.[48] When symptoms (such as pain) appear to be exaggerated, the examiner must also consider the possibility that the patient is malingering. Malingering implies trying to obtain a particular gain by a conscious effort to deceive.[67]

Reactions to Stress

- Aches and pains
- Anxiety
- Changed appetite
- Chronic fatigue
- Difficulty concentrating
- Difficulty sleeping
- Irritability and impatience
- Loss of interest and enjoyment in life
- Muscle tension (headaches)
- Sweaty hands
- Trembling
- Withdrawal

---

21. *Does the patient have any chronic or serious systemic illnesses or adverse social habits (e.g., smoking, drinking) that may influence the course of the pathology or the treatment?* In some cases, the examiner may use a medical history screening form (eTool 1.6) or a health status questionnaire[68–70] to determine the presence of conditions that may affect treatment or require referral to another health care professional.

22. *Is there anything in the family or developmental history that may be related, such as tumors, arthritis, heart disease, diabetes, allergies, and congenital anomalies?* Some disease processes and pathologies have a familial incidence.

23. *Has the patient undergone an x-ray examination or other imaging techniques?* If so, x-ray overexposure must be considered; if not, an x-ray examination may help to yield a diagnosis.

24. *Has the patient been receiving analgesic, steroid, or any other medication? If so, for how long?* High dosages of steroids taken for long periods may lead to problems, such as osteoporosis. Has the patient been taking any other medication that is pertinent? Anticoagulants (e.g., aspirin or anticoagulant therapy) increase the chance of bruising or hemarthrosis because the clotting mechanism is altered. Does the patient know why he or she was given a particular medication? Often, patients do not know and should be encouraged to keep an up-to-date list of the medications they are taking. Patients may not regard over-the-counter formulations, birth control pills, and so on as medications. If such medications have been taken for a long period, their use may not seem pertinent to the patient. How long has the patient been taking the medication? When did he or she last take the medication? Did the medication help?[71] It is also important to determine whether medication is being taken for the condition under review. If analgesics or antiinflammatories were taken just before the patient's visit for the assessment, some symptoms may be masked.

25. *Does the patient have a history of surgery or past/present illness?* If so, when was the surgery performed, what

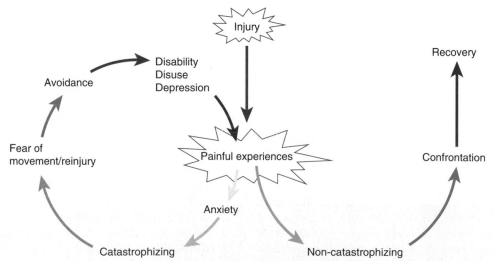

Fig. 1.5 Pathways normally followed after injury *(right)* and pathways followed by patient who fears movement will increase pain or cause reinjury *(left)*. (Modified from Waddell G, Newton M, Henderson I, et al: A fear-avoidance beliefs questionnaire [FABQ] and the role of fear-avoidance beliefs in chronic low back pain and disability, *Pain* 52:157–168, 1993.)

TABLE **1.4**

Summary of Psychological Processes

Factor	Description	Possible Effect on Pain and Disability	Example of Treatment Strategy
Attention	Pain demands our attention	• Vigilance may increase pain intensity • Distraction may decrease its pain intensity	• Distraction techniques • Interceptive exposure
Cognitions	How we think about our pain may influence it	• Interpretations and beliefs may increase pain and disability • Catastrophizing (irrational thoughts that something is far worse than it is) may increase pain • Negative thoughts and beliefs may increase pain and disability • Expectations may influence pain and disability • Cognitive sets may reduce flexibility in dealing with pain and disability	• Cognitive restructuring • Behavioral experiments designed, for example, to disconfirm unrealistic expectations and catastrophizing
Emotions and emotion regulation	Pain often generates negative feelings; these negative feelings may influence the pain as well as fuel cognitions, attention, and overt behaviors	• Fear may increase avoidance behavior and disability • Anxiety may increase pain disability • Depression may increase pain disability • Distress, in general, fuels negative cognitions and pain disability • Positive emotions might decrease pain	• Cognitive-behavioral therapy programs for anxiety and depression • Activation (to increase positive emotion) • Relaxation • Positive psychology techniques that promote well-being and positive emotions
Overt behavior	What we do to cope with our pain influences our perception of pain	• Avoidance behavior may increase disability • Unlimited activity (overactivity) may provoke pain • Pain behaviors communicate pain	• Operant, graded activity-training • Exposure in vivo • Coping strategies training

Modified from Linton SJ, Shaw WS: Impact of psychological factors in the experience of pain, *Phys Ther* 91:703, 2011.

TABLE **1.5**

Summary of Different Types of Psychological Flags

Flag	Nature	Examples
Red	Signs of serious pathology	• Cauda equina syndrome, fracture, tumor
Orange	Psychiatric symptoms	• Clinical depression, personality disorder
Yellow	Beliefs, appraisals, and judgments	• Unhelpful beliefs about pain; indication of injury as uncontrollable or likely to worsen • Expectations of poor treatment outcome, delayed return to work
	Emotional responses	• Distress not meeting criteria for diagnosis of mental disorder • Worry, fears, anxiety
	Pain behavior (including pain coping strategies)	• Avoidance of activities due to expectations of pain and possible reinjury • Over-reliance on passive treatments (e.g., hot packs, cold packs, analgesics)
Blue	Perceptions about the relationship between work and health	• Belief that work is too onerous and likely to cause further injury • Belief that workplace supervisor and workmates are unsupportive
Black	System or contextual obstacles	• Legislation restricting options for return to work • Conflict with insurance staff over injury claim • Overly solicitous family and health care providers • Heavy work, with little opportunity to modify duties

From Nicholas MK, Linton SJ, Watson PJ, et al: Early identification and management of psychological risk factors (yellow flags) in patients with low back pain: a reappraisal, *Phys Ther* 91:739, 2011.

TABLE **1.6**

Spectrum of Clinical Symptoms and Signs

	Physical Disease	Illness Behavior
Pain		
Pain drawing	Localized Anatomic	Nonanatomic Regional Magnified
Pain adjectives	Sensory	Emotional
Symptoms		
Pain	Musculoskeletal or neurological distribution	Whole leg pain Pain at the tip of the tailbone
Numbness	Dermatomal	Whole leg numbness
Weakness	Myotomal	Whole leg giving way
Time pattern	Varies with time and activity	Never free of pain
Response to treatment	Variable benefit	Intolerance of treatments Emergency hospitalization
Signs		
Tenderness	Musculoskeletal distribution	Superficial Nonanatomic
Axial loading	Neck pain	Low back pain
Simulated rotation	Nerve root pain	Low back pain
Straight leg raising	Limited on formal examination No improvement on distraction	Marked improvement with distraction
Motor	Myotomal	Regional, jerky, giving way
Sensory	Dermatomal	Regional

From Waddell G, Main CJ: Illness behavior. In Waddell G, editor: *The back pain revolution*, Edinburgh, 1998, Churchill Livingstone, p 162.

was the site of operation, and what condition was being treated? Sometimes, the condition the examiner is asked to treat is the result of the surgery. Has the patient ever been hospitalized? If so, why? Health conditions such as high blood pressure, heart and circulatory problems, and systemic diseases (e.g., diabetes) should be noted because of their effect on healing, exercise prescription, and functional activities.[4]

Taking an accurate, detailed history is very important. ***Listen to the patient—he or she is telling you what is wrong!***[6] While taking the history, the examiner, with experience, will commonly be generating a differential diagnosis in his or her mind and allows the patient's answers to direct any logical follow-up questions. As the history taking proceeds, the list of probable diagnoses is narrowed down until there are one or two possibilities which will then direct the rest of the assessment.[3] With experience, the examiner should be able to make a **preliminary "working" diagnosis** from the history alone. The observation and examination phases of the assessment are then used to confirm, alter, or refute the possible diagnoses. What an examiner looks for in observation and tests for in examination is often related to what she or he has found when taking a history.

Observation

In an assessment, observation is the "looking" or inspection phase. Its purpose is to gain information on visible defects, functional deficits, and abnormalities of alignment. Much of the observation phase involves assessment of **normal standing posture** (see Chapter 15). Normal posture covers a wide range, and asymmetric findings are common. The key is to determine whether these findings are related to the pathology being presented. The examiner should note the patient's way of moving as well as the general posture, manner, attitude, willingness to cooperate, and any signs of overt pain behavior.[72] Observation may begin in the waiting room or as the patient is being taken to the assessment area. Often the patient is unaware that observation is occurring at this stage and may present a different picture. The patient must be adequately undressed in a private assessment area to be observed properly. Male patients should wear only shorts, and female patients should wear a bra or halter top and shorts. Because the patient is in a state of undress, it is essential for the examiner to explain that observation and detailed looking at the patient are integral parts of the assessment. This explanation may prevent a potentially embarrassing situation that can have legal ramifications.

Overt Pain Behavior[72]

- *Guarding*—Abnormally stiff, interrupted or rigid movement while moving the joint or body from one position to another
- *Bracing*—A stationary position in which a fully extended limb supports and maintains an abnormal distribution of weight
- *Rubbing*—Any contact between hand and injured area (i.e., touching, rubbing, or holding the painful area)
- *Grimacing*—Obvious facial expression of pain that may include furrowed brow, narrowed eyes, tightened lips, corners of mouth pulled back and clenched teeth
- *Sighing*—Obvious exaggerated exhalation of air usually accompanied by the shoulders first rising and then falling; patients may expand their cheeks first

As the patient enters the assessment area, the examiner should observe his or her gait (see Chapter 14). This initial gait assessment is only a cursory one; however, problems, such as Trendelenburg sign or drop foot, are easily noticed. If there appears to be an abnormality, the gait may be checked in greater detail after the patient has undressed.

The examiner should be positioned so that the dominant eye is used, and both sides of the patient should be compared simultaneously. During the observation stage, the examiner is looking only at the patient and does not ask the patient to move; the examiner usually does not palpate, except possibly to learn whether an area is warm or hot or to find specific landmarks.

After the patient has undressed, the examiner should observe the posture, looking for asymmetries and determining whether the asymmetries are significant or applicable to the problem being assessed. In doing so, the examiner should attempt to answer the following questions often by comparing both sides:

1. What is the normal body alignment? Anteriorly, the nose, xiphisternum, and umbilicus should be in a straight line. From the side, the tip of the ear, the tip of the acromion, the high point of the iliac crest, and the lateral malleolus (anterior aspect) should be in a straight line.
2. Is there any obvious deformity? Deformities may take the form of restricted ROM (e.g., flexion deformity), malalignment (e.g., genu varum), alteration in the shape of a bone (e.g., fracture), or alteration in the relationship of two articulating structures (e.g., subluxation, dislocation). **Structural deformities** are present even at rest; examples include torticollis, fractures, scoliosis, and kyphosis. **Functional deformities** are the result of assumed postures and disappear when posture is changed. For example, a scoliosis due to a short leg seen in an upright posture disappears on forward flexion. A pes planus (flatfoot) on weight bearing may disappear on non–weight bearing. **Dynamic deformities** are caused by muscle

action and are present when muscles contract or joints move. Therefore they are not usually evident when the muscles are relaxed. Dynamic deformities are more likely to be seen during the examination phase.
3. Are the bony contours of the body normal and symmetric, or is there an obvious deviation? The body is not perfectly symmetric, and deviation may have no clinical implications. For example, many people have a lower shoulder on the dominant side or demonstrate a slight scoliosis of the spine adjacent to the heart. However, any deviation should be noted because it may contribute to a more accurate diagnosis.
4. Are the soft-tissue contours (e.g., muscle, skin, fat) normal and symmetric? Is there any obvious muscle wasting?
5. Are the limb positions equal and symmetric? The examiner should compare limb size, shape, position, any atrophy, color, and temperature.
6. Because pelvic position plays such an important role in correct posture of the whole body, the examiner should determine if the patient can position the pelvis in the **"neutral pelvis" position.** This dynamic position is such that the anterior superior iliac spines are one-to-two finger widths lower than the posterior superior iliac spines on the same side in normal standing. When looking for the "neutral pelvis" position, the examiner must be able to answer three questions in the affirmative. If not, there are probably hypomobile and/or hypermobile structures affecting the pelvic position. The three questions are:
   (1) Can the patient get into the "neutral pelvis" position? (If not, why not?)
   (2) Can the patient hold the "neutral pelvis" position while doing distal dynamic movement? (If not, why not?)
   (3) Can the patient control the dynamic "neutral pelvis" while doing dynamic movement (e.g., walking, running, jumping)?
   If the answer to any of these questions is "no," the examiner should consider adding pelvic "core muscle" control activities to any treatment protocol.
7. Are the color and texture of the skin normal? Does the appearance of the skin differ in the area of pain or symptoms, compared with other areas of the body? Ecchymosis or bruising indicates bleeding under the skin from injury to tissues (Fig. 1.6). In some cases, this ecchymosis may track away from the injury site because of gravity. Trophic changes in the skin resulting from peripheral nerve lesions include loss of skin elasticity, shiny skin, hair loss on the skin, and skin that breaks down easily and heals slowly. The nails may become brittle and ridged. Skin disorders (e.g., psoriasis) may affect joints (e.g., psoriatic arthritis). Cyanosis, or a bluish color

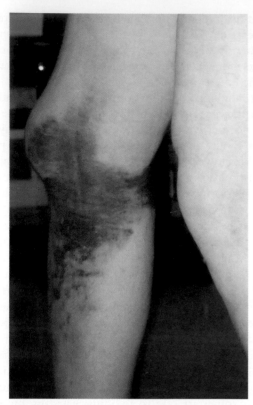

Fig. 1.6 Ecchymosis around the knee following rupture of the quadriceps and dislocation of the patella. Note how the ecchymosis is tracking distally toward the foot because of gravity from the leg hanging dependent.

to the skin, is usually an indication of poor blood perfusion. Redness indicates increased blood flow or inflammation.

8. Are there any scars that indicate recent injury or surgery? Recent scars are red because they are still healing and contain capillaries; older scars are white and primarily avascular. Fibers of the dermis (skin) tend to run in one direction, along so-called cleavage or tension lines. Lacerations or surgical cuts along these lines produce less scarring. Cuts across joint flexion lines frequently produce excessive (hypertrophic) scarring. Some individuals are also prone to keloid (excessive) or hypertrophic scarring. Hypertrophic scars are scars that have excessive scar tissue but stay within the margins of the wound. Keloid scars expand beyond the margins of the wound. Are there any callosities, blisters, or inflamed bursae, indicative of excessive pressure or friction to the skin? Are there any sinuses that may indicate infection? If so, are the sinuses draining or dry?

9. Is there any crepitus, snapping, or abnormal sound in the joints when the patient moves them? Sounds, by themselves, do not necessarily indicate pathology. Sounds on movement become significant only when they are related to the patient's symptoms. Crepitus may vary from a loud grinding noise to a squeaking noise. Snapping, especially if not painful, may be caused by a tendon moving over a bony protuberance. Clicking is sometimes heard in the temporomandibular joint and may be an indication of early nonsymptomatic pathology.

10. Is there any heat, swelling, or redness in the area being observed? All of these signs along with pain and loss of function are indications of inflammation or an active inflammatory condition.

11. What attitude does the patient appear to have toward the condition or toward the examiner? Is the patient apprehensive, restless, resentful, or depressed? These questions give the examiner some indication of the patient's psychological state and how he or she will respond to the examination and treatment.

12. What is the patient's facial expression? Does the patient appear to be apprehensive, in discomfort, or lacking sleep?

13. Is the patient willing to move? Do the joints move as they normally should? Are patterns of movement normal? If not, how are they abnormal? Any alteration should be noted and included in the observation portion of the assessment.

On completion of the observation phase of the assessment, the examiner should return to the original preliminary working diagnosis made at the end of the history to see if any alteration in the diagnosis should be made with the additional information found in this phase.

Examination

Principles

Because the examination portion of the assessment involves touching the patient and may, in some cases, cause the patient discomfort, the examiner must obtain a valid consent to perform the examination before it begins. A valid consent must be voluntary, must cover the procedures to be done (informed consent), and the patient must be legally competent to give the consent (eAppendix 1.2).[73,74]

The examination is used to confirm or refute the suspected diagnosis, which is based on the history and observation. The examination must be performed systematically with the examiner looking for a consistent pattern of signs and symptoms that leads to a differential diagnosis. Special care must be taken if the condition of the joint is irritable or acute. This is especially true if the area is in severe spasm or if the patient complains of severe unremitting pain that is not affected by position or medication, severe night pain, severe pain with no history of injury, or nonmechanical behavior of the joint.

Red Flags in Examination Indicating the Need for Medical Consultation[75]

- Severe unremitting pain
- Pain unaffected by medication or position
- Severe night pain
- Severe pain with no history of injury
- Severe spasm
- Inability to urinate or hold urine
- Elevated temperature (especially if prolonged)
- Psychological overlay

In the examination portion of the assessment, a number of principles must be followed.

1. Unless bilateral movement is required, the normal side is tested first. Testing the normal side first allows the examiner to establish a baseline for normal movement for the joint being tested[76] and shows the patient what to expect, resulting in increased patient confidence and less patient apprehension when the injured side is tested.

2. The patient does active movements before the examiner does passive movements. Passive movements are followed by resisted isometric movements (see later discussion). In this way, the examiner has a better idea of what the patient thinks he or she can do before the structures are fully tested.

3. Any movements that are painful are done last, if possible, to prevent an overflow of painful symptoms to the next movement that, in reality, may be symptom free.

4. If active range of motion (AROM) is not full, overpressure is applied only with extreme care to prevent the exacerbation of symptoms.

5. During AROM, if the ROM is full, overpressure may be carefully applied to determine the end feel of the joint. This often negates the need to do passive movements.

6. Each active, passive, or resisted isometric movement may be repeated several times or held (sustained) for a certain amount of time to see whether symptoms increase or decrease, whether a different pattern of movement results, whether there is increased weakness, or whether there is possible vascular insufficiency. This repetitive or sustained activity is especially important if the patient has complained that repetitive movement or sustained postures alter symptoms.

7. Resisted isometric movements are done with the joint in a neutral or resting position so that stress on the inert tissues is minimal. Any symptoms produced by the movement are then more likely to be caused by problems with contractile tissue.

8. For passive range of motion (PROM) or ligamentous tests, it is not only the degree (i.e., the amount) of the opening but also the quality (i.e., the end feel) of the opening that is important.

9. When the examiner is testing the ligaments, the appropriate stress is applied gently and repeated several times. The stress is increased up to but not beyond the point of pain, thereby demonstrating maximum instability without causing muscle spasm.

10. When testing **myotomes** (groups of muscles supplied by a single nerve root), each contraction is held for a minimum of **5 seconds** to see whether weakness becomes evident. Myotomal weakness takes time to develop.

11. At the completion of an assessment, because a good examination commonly involves stressing different tissues, the examiner must warn the patient that symptoms may exacerbate as a result of the assessment. This will prevent the patient from thinking any initial treatment may have made the patient worse and thus be hesitant to return for further treatments.

12. If, at the conclusion of the examination, the examiner has found that the patient has shown unusual signs and symptoms or if the condition appears to be beyond his or her scope of practice, the examiner should not hesitate to refer the patient to another appropriate health care professional.

Principles of Examination

- Tell the patient what you are doing (informing)
- Test the normal (uninvolved) side first
- Do active movements first, then passive movements, and then resisted isometric movements
- Do painful movements last
- Apply overpressure with care to test end feel
- Repeat movements or sustain certain postures or positions if history indicates
- Do resisted isometric movements in a resting position
- Remember that with passive movements and ligamentous testing, both the degree and quality (end feel) of opening are important
- With ligamentous testing, repeat with increasing stress
- With myotome testing, make sure that contractions are held for 5 seconds
- Warn the patient of possible exacerbations
- Maintain the patient's dignity
- Refer if necessary

Vital Signs

In some cases, the examiner may want to begin the examination by taking the patient's vital signs to establish the patient's baseline physiological parameters and vital signs (Table 1.7) and review the medical history screening card (see eTool 1.6). Ideally, the patient should sit for approximately 5 minutes before vital signs are taken so that the values are not affected by exertion.[77] These include the pulse (most commonly the

TABLE **1.7**

Vital Sign Normal Ranges

Age Group	Respiratory Rate	Heart Rate	Diastolic Blood Pressure	Systolic Blood Pressure	Temperature	Weight (kg)	Weight (lbs)
Newborn	30–50	120–160	Varies	50–70	97.7°F (36.5°C)	2–3	4.5–7
Infant (1–12 months)	20–30	80–140	Varies	70–100	98.6°F (37.0°C)[a]	4–10	9–22
Toddler (1–3 years)	20–30	80–130	48–80	80–110	98.6°F (37.0°C)[a]	10–14	22–31
Preschooler (3–5 years)	20–30	80–120	48–80	80–110	98.6°F (37.0°C)[a]	14–18	31–40
School age (6–12 years)	20–30	70–110	50–90	80–120	98.6°F (37.0°C)[a]	20–42	41–92
Adolescent (13–17 years)	12–20	55–105	60–92	110–120	98.6°F (37.0°C)[a]	>50	>110
Adults (18+ years)	18–20	60–100	<85	<130	98.6°F (37.0°C)[a]	Varies	Depends on body size

[a]Range from 97.7°F to 99.5°F (36.5°C to 37.5°C).
Remember these points:
- The patient's normal range should always be taken into consideration.
- Heart rate, blood pressure, and respiratory rate are expected to increase during times of fever or stress.
- Respiratory rate for infants should be counted for a full 60 seconds.

radial pulse at the wrist is used), blood pressure, respiratory rate, temperature (98.6°F or 37°C is normal, but it may range from 97.7°F [36.5°C] to 99.5°F [37.5°C]), and weight. Table 1.8 outlines guidelines for blood pressure measurement. High blood pressure values should be checked several times at 15- to 30-minute intervals with the patient resting in between to determine whether a high reading is accurate or is being caused by anxiety ("white coat syndrome") or some similar reason. If three consecutive readings are high, the patient is said to have high blood pressure (hypertension) (Table 1.9). If the readings remain high, further investigation may be warranted.[78–80]

Scanning Examination

The examination described in this book emphasizes the joints of the body, their movement, and their stability. It is necessary to examine all appropriate tissues to delineate the affected area, which can then be examined in detail. Application of tension, stretch, or isometric contraction to specific tissues produces either a normal or an appropriate abnormal response. This action enables the examiner to determine the nature and site of the present symptoms and the patient's response to these symptoms. The examination shows whether certain activities provoke or change the patient's pain; in this way, the examiner can focus on the subjective response (i.e., the patient's feelings or opinions) as well as the test findings. The patient must be clear about his or her side of the examination. For instance, the patient must not confuse questions about movement-associated pain ("Does the movement make any difference to the pain?" "Does the movement bring on or change the pain?") with questions about already existing pain. In addition, the examiner attempts to see whether patient responses are measurably abnormal. Do the movements cause any abnormalities in function? A loss of movement or weakness in muscles can be measured and therefore is an objective response. Throughout the assessment, the examiner looks for two sets of data: (1) what the patient feels (subjective) and (2) responses that can be measured or are found by the examiner (objective).

To ensure that all possible sources of pathology are assessed, the examination must be extensive. This is especially true if there are symptoms when no history of trauma is present. In this case, a scanning or screening examination is performed to rule out the possibility of referral of symptoms, especially from the spine. Similarly, if there is any doubt about where the pathology is located, the scanning examination is essential to ensure a correct diagnosis. The scanning examination is a "quick look" or scan of a part of the body involving the spine and extremities. It is used to rule out symptoms, which may be referred from one part of the body to another. It is divided into two scans: the upper limb scan and the lower limb scan.

TABLE **1.8**

Guidelines for Measurement of Blood Pressure

Posture	Blood pressure obtained in the sitting position is recommended. The subject should sit quietly for 5 min, with the back supported and the arm supported at the level of the heart, before blood pressure is recorded.
Circumstances	No caffeine during the hour preceding the reading. No smoking during the 30 min preceding the reading. A quiet, warm setting.
Equipment	**Cuff size:** The bladder should encircle and cover two thirds of the length of the arm; if it does not, place the bladder over the brachial artery. If bladder is too short, misleading high readings may result. **Manometer:** Aneroid gauges should be calibrated every 6 months against a mercury manometer.
Technique	**Number of readings:** • On each occasion, take at least two readings, separated by as much time as is practical. If readings vary by more than 5 mm Hg, take additional readings until two consecutive readings are close. • If the initial values are elevated, obtain two other sets of readings at least 1 week apart. • Initially, take pressure in both arms; if the pressures differ, use the arm with the higher pressure. • If the arm pressure is elevated, take the pressure in one leg (particularly in patients younger than 30 years of age). **Performance:** • Inflate the bladder quickly to a pressure 20 mm Hg greater than the systolic pressure, as recognized by disappearance of the radial pulse. • Deflate the bladder by 3 mm Hg every second. • Record the Korotkoff phase V (disappearance), except in children, in whom use of phase IV (muffling) may be preferable if disappearance of the sounds is not perceived. • If the Korotkoff sounds are weak, have the patient raise the arm and open and close the hand 5–10 times, and then reinflate the bladder quickly.
Recordings	Blood pressure, patient position, arm and cuff size.

From Kaplan NM, Deveraux RB, Miller HS: Systemic hyperextension, *Med Sci Sports Exerc* 26:S269, 1994.

TABLE **1.9**

Classification of Hypertension by Age

	MAGNITUDE OF HYPERTENSION				
	Normal	Mild, Stage 1	Moderate, Stage 2	Severe, Stage 3	Very Severe, Stage 4
Child (6–9 years)					
Systolic	80–120	120–124	125–129	130–139	≥140
Diastolic	50–75	75–79	80–84	85–89	≥90
Child (10–12 years)					
Systolic	80–120	125–129	130–134	135–144	≥145
Diastolic	50–80	80–84	85–89	90–94	≥95
Adolescent (13–15 years)					
Systolic	110–120	135–139	140–149	150–159	≥160
Diastolic	60–85	85–89	90–94	95–99	≥100
Adolescent (16–18 years)					
Systolic	110–120	140–149	150–159	160–179	≥180
Diastolic	60–90	90–94	95–99	100–109	≥110
Adult (>18 years)					
Systolic	110–130	140–159	160–179	180–209	≥210
Diastolic	80–90	90–99	100–109	110–119	≥120

Reprinted by permission, from McGrew CA: Clinical implications of the AHA preparticipation cardiovascular screening guidelines, *Athletic Ther Today* 5(4):55, 2000.

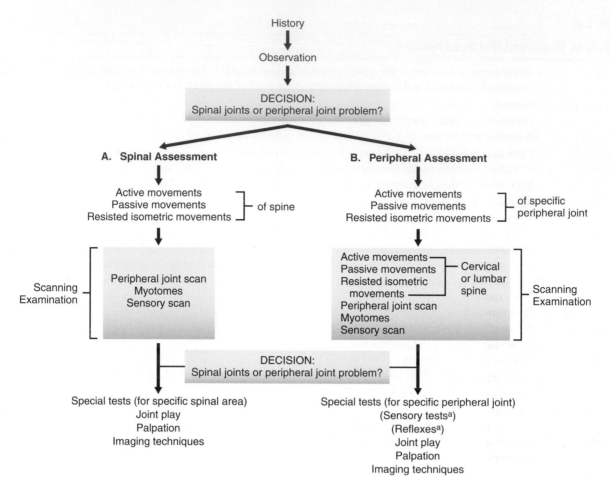

Fig. 1.7 The scanning examination used to rule out referral of symptoms from the spine. (A) Spinal assessment (i.e., based on the history, the clinician feels the problem is in the spine). (B) Peripheral joint assessment (i.e., based on the history, the clinician feels the problem is in a peripheral joint). ([a]These are done if scanning examination is not done.)

It is part of the examination that is used, where necessary, along with a detailed and focused examination of one or more of the joints.

When to Use the Scanning Examination

- There is no history of trauma
- There are radicular signs
- There is trauma with radicular signs
- There is altered sensation in the limb
- There are spinal cord ("long track") signs
- The patient presents with abnormal patterns
- There is suspected psychogenic pain

As with all assessments, the use of a scanning examination depends on what the examiner found in the history and observation. For assessment of the spine, the scanning examination is integrated into the examination as a regular part of the cervical or lumbar assessment (Fig. 1.7A) and includes a peripheral joint scan,

myotome testing, and a sensory scan. If, when assessing the peripheral joints, the examiner suspects a problem is being referred from the spine, the scanning examination is "inserted" into the examination of that joint (Fig. 1.7B). For the scanning examination, the peripheral joints are "scanned," with the patient doing only a few key movements at each joint. The movements should include those that may be expected to exacerbate symptoms that are derived from the history. The examiner then tests the upper or lower limb myotomes (key muscles representing a specific nerve root). After these tests, a sensory scanning examination (sensory scan) can be performed that may include the appropriate reflexes, the sensory distributions of the dermatomes and peripheral nerve distribution, and selected neurodynamic tests (e.g., upper limb tension test, slump test) if the examiner suspects some neurological involvement. At this point, the examiner makes a decision or an "educated guess" as to whether the problem is in the cervical spine, lumbar spine, or the peripheral joint, based on the information gained. Once the decision is made, the examiner either completes the spinal assessment (in the case of a suspected spinal problem) or turns instead to completing the assessment of the appropriate peripheral joint (see Fig. 1.7). The scanning examination should add no more than 5 or 10 minutes to the assessment.

The idea of the scanning examination was developed by James Cyriax,[1] who also, more than any other author, originated the concepts of "contractile" and "inert" tissue, "end feel," and "capsular patterns" and contributed greatly to development of a comprehensive and systematic physical examination of the moving parts of the body. Although several of his constructs and paradigms have been questioned,[81–83] the basic principles of ensuring that all tissues are tested remains sound.

Spinal Cord and Nerve Roots

To further comprehend and ensure the value of the scanning examination, the examiner must have a clear understanding of signs and symptoms arising from the spinal cord and nerve roots of the body and those arising from peripheral nerves. The scanning examination helps to determine whether the pathology is caused by tissues innervated by a nerve root or peripheral nerve that is referring symptoms distally.

The nerve root is that portion of a peripheral nerve that "connects" the nerve to the spinal cord. Nerve roots arise from each level of the spinal cord (e.g., C3, C4), and many, but not all, intermingle in a plexus (brachial, lumbar, or lumbosacral) to form different peripheral nerves (Fig. 1.8). This arrangement can result in a single nerve root supplying more than one peripheral nerve. For example, the median nerve is derived from the C6, C7, C8, and T1 nerve roots, whereas the ulnar nerve is derived from C7, C8, and T1 (Table 1.10). For this reason, if pressure is applied to the nerve root, the distribution of the sensation or motor function is often felt or exhibited in more than one peripheral nerve distribution (Table 1.11). Therefore, although the symptoms seen in a nerve root lesion (e.g., paresthesia, pain, muscle weakness) may be similar to those seen in peripheral nerves, the signs (e.g., area of paresthesia, where pain occurs, which muscles are weak) are commonly different. The examiner must be able to differentiate a dermatome (nerve root) from the sensory distribution of a peripheral nerve, and a myotome (nerve root) from muscles supplied by a specific peripheral nerve. In addition, neurological signs and symptoms, such as paresthesia and pain, may result from inflammation or irritation of tissues, such as facet joints and interspinous ligaments or other tissues supplied by the nerve roots, and they may be demonstrated in the dermatome, myotome, or sclerotome supplied by that nerve root. This irritation can contribute to the referred pain (see later discussion).

Nerve roots are made up of anterior (ventral) and posterior (dorsal) portions that unite near or in the

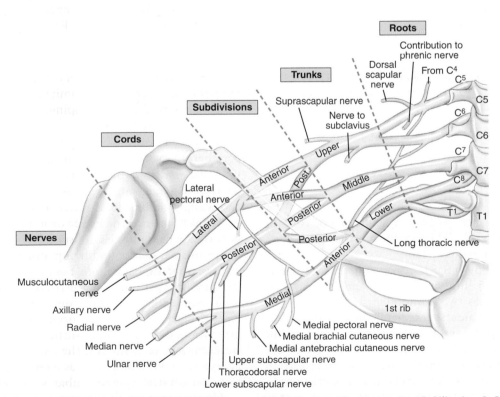

Fig. 1.8 The brachial plexus. (From Neuman DA: *Kinesiology of the musculoskeletal system—foundations for rehabilitation*, St Louis, 2010, Mosby Elsevier, p 150.)

TABLE **1.10**

Common Peripheral Nerves and Their Nerve Root Derivation

Peripheral Nerve	Nerve Root Derivation
Axillary	C5, C6
Supraclavicular	C3, C4
Suprascapular	C5, C6
Subscapular	C5, C6
Long thoracic	C5, C6, C7
Musculocutaneous	C5, C6, C7
Medial cutaneous nerve of forearm	C8, T1
Lateral cutaneous nerve of forearm	C5, C6
Posterior cutaneous nerve of forearm	C5, C6, C7, C8
Radial	C5, C6, C7, C8, T1
Median	C6, C7, C8, T1
Ulnar	C(7)8, T1
Pudendal	S2, S3, S4
Lateral cutaneous nerve of thigh	L2, L3
Medial cutaneous nerve of thigh	L2, L3
Intermediate cutaneous nerve of thigh	L2, L3
Posterior cutaneous nerve of thigh	S1, S2, S3
Femoral	L2, L3, L4
Obturator	L2, L3, L4
Sciatic	L4, L5, S1, S2, S3
Tibial	L4, L5, S1, S2, S3
Common peroneal	L4, L5, S1, S2
Superficial peroneal	L4, L5, S1
Deep peroneal	L4, L5, S1, S2
Lateral cutaneous nerve of leg (calf)	L4, L5, S1, S2
Saphenous	L3, L4
Sural	S1, S2
Medial plantar	L4, L5
Lateral plantar	S1, S2

intervertebral foramen to form a single **nerve root** or **spinal nerve** (Fig. 1.9). They are the most proximal parts of the peripheral nervous system.

The human body has 31 nerve root pairs: 8 cervical, 12 thoracic, 5 lumbar, 5 sacral, and 1 coccygeal. Each nerve root has two components: a **somatic** portion, which innervates the skeletal muscles and provides sensory input from the skin, fascia, muscles, and joints, and a **visceral** component, which is part of the autonomic nervous system.[84] The autonomic system supplies the blood vessels, dura mater, periosteum, ligaments, and intervertebral discs, among many other structures.

Examples of Autonomic Nervous System Involvement (Yellow Flags)

- Ringing in the ears
- Dizziness
- Blurred vision
- Photophobia (sensitivity to light)
- Rhinorrhea (runny nose)
- Sweating
- Lacrimation (tearing)
- Generalized loss of muscle strength
- Increase in heart rate
- Flushing (vasodilatation)

The sensory distribution of each nerve root is called the **dermatome**. A dermatome is defined as the area of skin supplied by a single nerve root. The area innervated by a nerve root is larger than that innervated by a peripheral nerve.[85] The descriptions of dermatomes in the following chapters should be considered as examples only, because slight differences and variabilities occur with each patient and dermatomes also exhibit a great deal of overlap.[86,87] The variability in dermatomes was aptly demonstrated by Keegan and Garrett in 1948 (Fig. 1.10).[88] The overlap may be demonstrated by the fact that, in the thoracic spine, the loss of one dermatome often goes unnoticed because of the overlap of the adjacent dermatomes.

Spinal nerve roots have a poorly developed epineurium and lack a perineurium. This development makes the nerve root more susceptible to compressive forces, tensile deformation, chemical irritants (e.g., alcohol, lead, arsenic), and metabolic abnormalities. For example, compression of the nerve root could occur with a posterolateral intervertebral disc herniation, a "burner" or stretching of the nerve roots or the brachial plexus in a football player or alcoholic neuritis in an alcoholic. Pressure on nerve roots leads to loss of muscle tone and mass, but the loss is often not as obvious as when pressure is applied to a peripheral nerve. Because the peripheral nerve that innervates the muscle is usually supplied by more than one nerve root, more muscle fibers are likely to be affected and wasting or atrophy is more evident if the peripheral nerve itself is damaged. In addition, the pattern of weakness (i.e., which muscles are affected) is different for an injury to a nerve root and to a peripheral nerve, because a nerve root supplies more than one peripheral nerve. Pressure on a peripheral nerve resulting in a neuropraxia leads to temporary nonfunction of the nerve. With this type of injury, there is primarily motor involvement, with little sensory or autonomic involvement, and although weakness may be demonstrated, muscle atrophy may not be evident. With more severe peripheral nerve lesions (e.g., axonotmesis and neurotmesis), atrophy is evident.

Myotomes are defined as groups of muscles supplied by a single nerve root. A lesion of a single nerve root is

TABLE **1.11**

Nerve Root Dermatomes, Myotomes, Reflexes, and Paresthetic Areas

Nerve Root	Dermatome[a]	Muscle Weakness (Myotome)	Reflexes Affected	Paresthesias
C1	Vertex of skull	None	None	None
C2	Temple, forehead, occiput	Longus colli, sternocleidomastoid, rectus capitis	None	None
C3	Entire neck, posterior cheek, temporal area, prolongation forward under mandible	Trapezius, splenius capitis	None	Cheek, side of neck
C4	Shoulder area, clavicular area, upper scapular area	Trapezius, levator scapulae	None	Horizontal band along clavicle and upper scapula
C5	Deltoid area, anterior aspect of entire arm to base of thumb	Supraspinatus, infraspinatus, deltoid, biceps	Biceps, brachioradialis	None
C6	Anterior arm, radial side of hand to thumb and index finger	Biceps, supinator, wrist extensors	Biceps, brachioradialis	Thumb and index finger
C7	Lateral arm and forearm to index, long, and ring fingers	Triceps, wrist flexors (rarely, wrist extensors)	Triceps	Index, long, and ring fingers
C8	Medial arm and forearm to long, ring, and little fingers	Ulnar deviators, thumb extensors, thumb adductors (rarely, triceps)	Triceps	Little finger alone or with two adjacent fingers; *not* ring or long fingers, alone or together (C7)
T1	Medial side of forearm to base of little finger	Disc lesions at upper two thoracic levels do not appear to give rise to root weakness. Weakness of intrinsic muscles of the hand is due to other pathology (e.g., thoracic outlet pressure, neoplasm of lung, and ulnar nerve lesion). Dural and nerve root stress has T1 elbow flexion with arm horizontal. T1 and T2 scapulae forward and backward on chest wall. Neck flexion at any thoracic level.		
T2	Medial side of upper arm to medial elbow, pectoral and midscapular areas			
T3–T12	T3–T6, upper thorax; T5–T7, costal margin: T8–T12, abdomen and lumbar region	Articular and dural signs and root pain are common. Root signs (cutaneous analgesia) are rare and have such indefinite area that they have little localizing value. Weakness is not detectable.		
L1	Back, over trochanter and groin	None	None	Groin; after holding posture, which causes pain
L2	Back, front of thigh to knee	Psoas, hip adductors	None	Occasionally anterior thigh
L3	Back, upper buttock, anterior thigh and knee, medial lower leg	Psoas, quadriceps, thigh atrophy	Knee jerk sluggish, PKB positive, pain on full SLR	Medial knee, anterior lower leg

Continued

TABLE **1.11**

Nerve Root Dermatomes, Myotomes, Reflexes, and Paresthetic Areas—cont'd

Nerve Root	Dermatomeᵃ	Muscle Weakness (Myotome)	Reflexes Affected	Paresthesias
L4	Medial buttock, lateral thigh, medial leg, dorsum of foot, big toe	Tibialis anterior, extensor hallucis	SLR limited, neck flexion pain, weak or absent knee jerk, side flexion limited	Medial aspect of calf and ankle
L5	Buttock, posterior and lateral thigh, lateral aspect of leg, dorsum of foot, medial half of sole, first, second, and third toes	Extensor hallucis, peroneals, gluteus medius, dorsiflexors, hamstring and calf atrophy	SLR limited one side, neck flexion painful, ankle decreased, cross leg raising—pain	Lateral aspect of leg, medial three toes
S1	Buttock, thigh, and leg posterior	Calf and hamstring, wasting of gluteals, peroneals, plantar flexors	SLR limited, Achilles reflex weak or absent	Lateral two toes, lateral foot, lateral leg to knee, plantar aspect of foot
S2	Same as S1	Same as S1 except peroneals	Same as S1	Lateral leg, knee, and heel
S3	Groin, medial thigh to knee	None	None	None
S4	Perineum, genitals, lower sacrum	Bladder, rectum	None	Saddle area, genitals, anus, impotence, massive posterior herniation

ᵃIn any part of which pain may be felt.
PKB, Prone knee bending; *SLR,* straight leg raising.

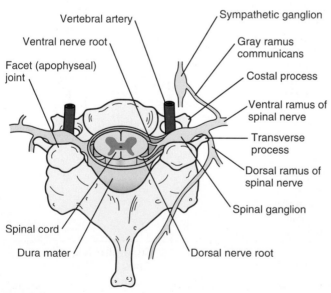

Fig. 1.9 Spinal cord, nerve root portions, and spinal nerve in the cervical spine and their relation to the vertebra and vertebral artery.

usually associated with paresis (incomplete paralysis) of the myotome (muscles) supplied by that nerve root. It therefore takes time for any weakness to become evident on resisted isometric or myotome testing, and for this reason, the isometric testing of myotomes is held for *at*

least 5 seconds. On the other hand, a lesion of a peripheral nerve leads to complete paralysis of the muscles supplied by that nerve, especially if the injury results in an axonotmesis or neurotmesis, and the weakness therefore is evident right away. Differences in the amount of resulting paralysis arise from the fact that more than one myotome contributes to the formation of a muscle embryologically.

A **sclerotome** is an area of bone or fascia supplied by a single nerve root (Fig. 1.11). As with dermatomes, sclerotomes can show a great deal of variability among individuals.

It is the complex nature of the dermatomes, myotomes, and sclerotomes supplied by the nerve root that can lead to referred pain, which is pain felt in a part of the body that is usually a considerable distance from the tissues that have caused it. Referred pain is explained as an error in perception on the part of the brain. Usually, pain can be referred into the appropriate myotome, dermatome, or sclerotome from any somatic or visceral tissue innervated by a nerve root, but, confusingly, it sometimes is not referred according to a specific pattern.[89] It is not understood why this occurs, but clinically it has been found to be so.

Many theories of the mechanism of referred pain have been developed, but none has been proven conclusively.

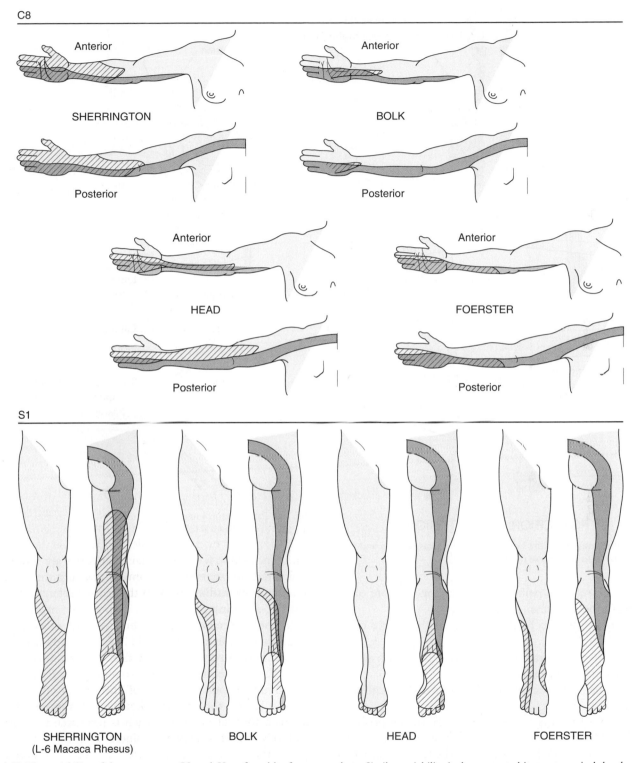

Fig. 1.10 The variability of dermatomes at C8 and S1 as found by four researchers. Similar variability is demonstrated in most cervical, lumbar, and sacral vertebrae. (Redrawn from Keegan JJ, Garrett FD: The segmental distribution of the cutaneous nerves in the limbs of man, *Anat Rec* 101:430, 433, 1948. Copyright © 1948. This material is used by permission of Wiley-Liss, a subsidiary of John Wiley & Sons.)

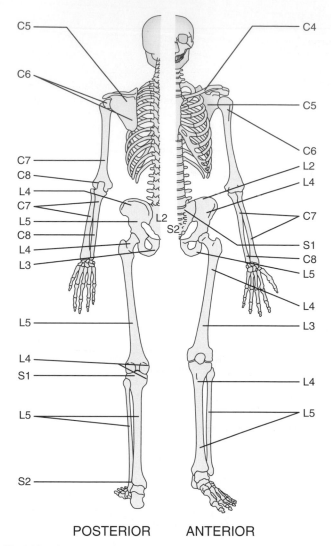

C5
C6
C7
C8
L4
C7
L5
C8
L4
L3
L5
L4
S1
L5
S2
L2
S2

C4
C5
C6
L2
L4
C7
S1
C8
L5
L4
L3
L4
L5

POSTERIOR   **ANTERIOR**

Fig. 1.11 Sclerotomes of the body. Lines show areas of bone and fascia supplied by individual nerve roots.

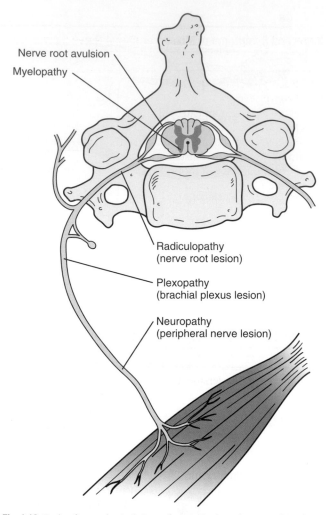

Nerve root avulsion
Myelopathy

Radiculopathy
(nerve root lesion)

Plexopathy
(brachial plexus lesion)

Neuropathy
(peripheral nerve lesion)

Fig. 1.12 Path of neurological tissue from spinal cord to muscles, showing sites of neurological lesions.

In general, referred pain may involve one or more of the following mechanisms:

1. Misinterpretation by the brain as to the source of the painful impulses
2. Inability of the brain to interpret a summation of noxious stimuli from various sources
3. Disturbance of the internuncial pool by afferent nerve impulses.

Referral of pain is a common occurrence in problems associated with the musculoskeletal system. Pain is often felt at points remote from the site of the lesion. The site to which pain is referred is an indicator of the segment that is at fault: it indicates that one of the structures innervated by a specific nerve root is causing signs and symptoms in other tissues supplied by that same nerve root. For example, pain in the L5 dermatome could arise from irritation around the L5 nerve root, from an L5 disc causing pressure on the L5 nerve root, from facet joint involvement at L4–L5 causing irritation of the L5 nerve root, from any muscle supplied by the L5 nerve root, or from any visceral structures having L5 innervation. Referred

pain tends to be felt deeply; its boundaries are indistinct, and it radiates segmentally without crossing the midline. **Radicular** or **radiating pain,** a form of referred pain, is a sharp, shooting pain felt in a dermatome, myotome, or sclerotome because of direct involvement of or damage to a spinal nerve or nerve root.[71] A **radiculopathy** refers to radiating paresthesia, numbness or weakness but not pain.[90] A **myelopathy** is a neurogenic disorder involving the spinal cord or brain and resulting in an upper motor neuron lesion; the patterns of pain or symptoms are different from that of radicular pain, and often both upper and lower limbs are affected (Fig. 1.12).

Peripheral Nerves

Peripheral nerves are a unique type of "inert" tissue (see the later discussion) in that they are not contractile tissue, but they are necessary for the normal functioning of voluntary muscle. The examiner must be aware of potential injury to nervous tissue when examining both contractile and inert tissue. Table 1.12 shows some of the tissue changes that result when a peripheral nerve lesion occurs.

In peripheral nerves, the epineurium consists of a loose areolar connective tissue matrix surrounding the nerve

TABLE **1.12**

Signs and Symptoms of Mixed Peripheral Nerve (Lower Motor Neuron) Lesions[a]

Motor	Sensory	Sympathetic
• Flaccid paralysis • Loss of reflexes • Muscle wasting and atrophy • Lost synergic action of muscles • Fibrosis, contractures, and adhesions • Joint weakness and instability • Decreased range of motion and stiffness • Disuse osteoporosis of bone • Growth affected	• Loss of or abnormal sensation • Loss of vasomotor tone: warm flushed (early); cold, white (later) • Skin may be scaly (early); thin, smooth, and shiny (later) • Shallower skin creases • Nail changes (striations, ridges, dry, brittle, abnormal curving, luster lost) • Ulceration	• Loss of sweat glands (dryness) • Loss of pilomotor response

[a]Primarily axonotmesis and neurotmesis.

TABLE **1.13**

Classification of Nerve Injuries According to Seddon

Grade of Injury	Definition	Signs and Symptoms
Neuropraxia (Sunderland 1°)	A transient physiological block caused by ischemia from pressure or stretch of the nerve with no Wallerian degeneration	• Pain • No or minimal muscle wasting • Muscle weakness • Numbness • Proprioception affected • Recovery time: minutes to days
Axonotmesis (Sunderland 2° and 3°)	Internal architecture of nerve preserved, but axons are so badly damaged that Wallerian degeneration occurs	• Pain • Muscle wasting evident • Complete motor, sensory and sympathetic functions lost (see Table 1.12) • Recovery time: months (axon regenerates at rate of 1 inch/month, or 1 mm/day) • Sensation is restored before motor function
Neurotmesis (Sunderland 3°, 4°, and 5°)	Structure of nerve is destroyed by cutting, severe scarring, or prolonged severe compression	• No pain (anesthesia) • Muscle wasting • Complete motor, sensory, and sympathetic functions lost (see Table 1.12) • Recovery time: months and only with surgery

Data from Seddon HJ: Three types of nerve injury, *Brain* 66:17–28, 1943.

fiber. It allows changes in growth length of the bundled nerve fibers (funiculi) without allowing the bundles to be strained. The perineurium protects the nerve bundles by acting as a diffusion barrier to irritants and provides tensile strength and elasticity to the nerve. Peripheral nerves therefore are most commonly affected by pressure, traction, friction, anoxia, or cutting. Examples include pressure on the median nerve in the carpal tunnel, traction to the common peroneal nerve at the head of the fibula during a lateral ankle sprain, friction to the ulnar nerve in the cubital tunnel, anoxia of the anterior tibial nerve in a compartment

syndrome, and cutting of the radial nerve with a fracture of the humeral shaft. Cooling, freezing, and thermal or electrical injury may also affect peripheral nerves.

Nerve injuries are usually classified by the systems of Seddon[91] or Sunderland.[92] Seddon, whose system is most commonly used, classified nerve injuries into neuropraxia (most common), axonotmesis, and neurotmesis (Table 1.13). Sunderland followed a similar system but divided axonotmesis and neurotmesis into different levels or degrees (Table 1.14). Any examination of a joint must include a thorough peripheral nerve examination, especially if there are neurological signs and symptoms. The examiner must be able not only to differentiate inert tissue lesions from contractile tissue lesions but also to determine whether a contractile tissue malfunction is the result of the contractile tissue itself or a peripheral nerve lesion or a nerve root lesion.

Sensory loss combined with motor loss should alert the examiner to lesions of nervous tissue.[93–95] Injury to a single peripheral nerve (e.g., the median nerve) is referred to as a **mononeuropathy**. Systemic diseases (e.g., diabetes) may affect more than one peripheral nerve. In this case, the pathology is referred to as a **polyneuropathy**. Careful mapping of the area of sensory loss and testing of the muscles affected by the motor loss allow the examiner to differentiate between a peripheral nerve lesion and a nerve root lesion. (An example is shown in Table 1.15.) If electromyographic studies are to be used to determine the grade of nerve injury, denervation cannot be evaluated for at least 3 weeks after injury to allow Wallerian degeneration to occur and to allow regeneration (if any) to begin.[96–98] Muscle wasting usually becomes obvious after 4 to 6 weeks and progresses to reach its maximum by approximately 12 weeks following injury. Circulatory changes after nerve injury vary with time. In the initial or early stages, the skin is warm, but after approximately 3 weeks, the skin becomes cooler as a result of decreased circulation. Because of the decreased circulation and altered cell metabolism, trophic changes occur to the skin and nails.

When assessing a patient, the examiner must also be aware of what has been called the **double-crush syndrome** or double-entrapment neuropathy.[99–102] The theory of this lesion (which has not yet been proved but has clinical supporting evidence) is that, although compression or pathology at one point along a peripheral nerve or nerve root may not be sufficient to cause signs and symptoms, compression or pathology at two or more points may lead to a cumulative effect that results in apparent signs and symptoms.[103] Because of this cumulative effect, signs and symptoms may indicate one area of involvement (e.g., the carpal tunnel), whereas other areas (e.g., cervical spine, brachial plexus, thoracic outlet) may be contributing to the problem. Similarly, cervical lesions may be involved in tennis elbow (lateral epicondylitis) syndromes. Upton and McComas[99] believed that

TABLE **1.14**

Correlation of Seddon and Sunderland Classification of Nerve Injuries

	SUNDERLAND (DEGREE)				
Seddon	First	Second	Third	Fourth	Fifth
Neuropraxia	███				
Axonotmesis		████			
Neurotmesis			████	████	

Shaded areas indicate equivalent terms.
From Morrey BF, editor: *The elbow and its disorders*, ed 2, Philadelphia, 1993, WB Saunders, p 814.

TABLE **1.15**

Comparison of Signs and Symptoms for C7 Nerve Root Lesion and Median Nerve Lesion at Elbow

	C7 Nerve Root	Median Nerve
Sensory alteration	Lateral arm and forearm to index, long, and ring fingers on palmar and dorsal aspect	Palmar aspect of thumb, index, middle, and half of ring finger Dorsal aspect of index, middle, and possibly half of ring finger
Motor alteration	Triceps Wrist flexors Wrist extensors (rarely)	Pronator teres Wrist flexors (lateral half of flexor digitorum profundus) Palmaris longus Pronator quadratus Flexor pollicis longus and brevis Abductor pollicis brevis Opponens pollicis Lateral two lumbricals
Reflex alteration	Triceps may be affected	None[a]
Paresthesia	Index, long and ring fingers on palmar and dorsal aspect	Same as sensory alteration

[a]No "common" reflexes are affected; if the examiner tested the tendon reflexes of the muscles listed, they would be affected.

compression proximally on the nerve trunk could increase the vulnerability of the peripheral nerves or nerve roots at distal points along their paths because axonal transport would be disrupted. In addition, diseased nerves are more susceptible to injury; thus the presence of systemic disease (e.g., diabetes, thyroid dysfunction) may make the nerve more susceptible to compression somewhere along its path.[94] Finally, the signs and symptoms could potentially be arising from both a nerve root lesion and a peripheral nerve lesion. Only with meticulous assessment can the clinician delineate where the true problems lie, which may be due to trauma, degeneration, or anatomic anomalies.

Similarly, the loss of extensibility of the nervous tissue at one site may produce increasing tensile loads when the peripheral nerve or nerve root is stretched, leading to mechanical dysfunction.[104] This is the principle behind the **neural tension** or **neurodynamic tests**, such as the straight leg raise, slump test, and upper limb tension test,[104–106] and may provide a partial explanation for lesions, such as cervical spine lesions mimicking tennis elbow and carpal tunnel syndrome. These tests put neural tissue (e.g., neuraxis of the central nervous system [CNS], meninges, nerve roots, peripheral nerves) under tension when they are performed and may duplicate symptoms that result during functional activity.[104,106,107] For example, sitting in a car is closely mimicked by the action of the slump test and straight leg raising. However, they often do not, by themselves, indicate where the problem lies. Further testing (e.g., nerve conduction tests, electromyography) may be needed to determine the exact site of the problem.

Neural tissue moves toward the joint at which elongation is initiated. Thus, if cervical flexion is initiated, the nerve roots, even those in the lumbar spine, move toward the cervical spine. Likewise, flexion of the whole spine causes movement toward the lumbar spine, and extension of the knee or dorsiflexion of the foot causes neural movement toward the knee or ankle.[104,106,107] These "tension points" can potentially help to determine where the restriction to movement is occurring. Normally, tension tests are not painful, although the patient is often aware of increased tension or discomfort in the spine or the limb. Because tension tests indicate neural mobility and sensitivity to mechanical stresses, they are considered positive only if they reproduce the patient's symptoms, if the patient's response is altered by movement of a body part distal to where the symptoms are felt (e.g., foot dorsiflexion causing symptoms in the lumbar spine), or if there is asymmetry in the response.[104] When doing tension tests, the examiner should note the angle or position at which the restriction occurs and what the resistance feels like. With irritable conditions, only those parts of the test that are needed to cause positive results should be performed. For example, in the slump test, if neck flexion and slumping cause positive signs, there is no need to cause further discomfort to the patient by doing knee extension and foot dorsiflexion.

In the examination, testing of neurological tissue occurs during active, passive, and resisted isometric movement, as well as during functional testing, specific tests, reflexes, and cutaneous distribution and palpation.

Examination of Specific Joints

The examiner should use an unchanging, systematic approach to the examination that varies only slightly to elaborate certain clues given by the history or by asymmetric responses. For example, if the history is characteristic of a disc lesion, the examination should be a detailed one of all the tissues that may be affected by the disc and a brief one of all the other joints to exclude contradictory signs. If the history suggests arthritis of the hip, the examination should be a detailed one of the hip and a brief one of the other joints—again, to exclude contradictory signs. As the movements are tested, the examiner is looking sometimes for the patient's subjective responses and sometimes for clinical objective findings. For example, if examination of the cervical spine shows clear signs of a disc problem, as the examination is continued down the arm, the examiner looks more for muscle weakness (objective) rather than for elicitation of pain (subjective). In contrast, if the history suggests a muscle lesion, pain will probably be provoked when the arm is examined. In either case, the structures expected to be normal are not omitted from the examination. There are only a few situations in which deviation from this systematic routine should occur: when there is uncertainty about where the pathology lies (in which case, a scanning examination must be performed with combined assessment of the spine and one or more peripheral joints); when there is no history of trauma or indication of pathology in a specific joint yet the patient complains of pain in that joint (again, a scanning examination is performed); or when the joint to be assessed is too acutely injured or irritable to do the total systematic examination.

If there is an organic lesion, some active, passive, or resisted isometric movements will be abnormal or painful, and others will not. Negative findings must balance positive ones, and the examination must be extensive enough to allow characteristic patterns to emerge. Determination of the problem is not made on the strength of the first positive finding; it is made only after it is clear that there are no other contradictory signs. Movements may be repeated several times quickly to rule out any problem, such as vascular insufficiency, or if the patient has indicated in the history that repetitive movements increase the symptoms. Likewise, sustained postures may be held for several seconds or combined movements may be performed if the history indicates increased symptoms with those postures or movements.

Contractile tissues may have tension placed on them by stretching or contraction.[1] These structures include the muscles, their tendons, and their attachments into

TABLE **1.16**

Differential Diagnosis of Muscle Strains, Tendon Injury, and Ligament Sprains

	1° Strain	2° Strain	3° Strain (Rupture)	Paratenonitis* Tendinosis†	1° Sprain	2° Sprain	3° Sprain
Definition	Few fibers of muscle torn	About half of muscle fibers torn	All muscle fibers torn (rupture)	*Inflammation of tendon †Intratendinous degeneration	Few fibers of ligament torn	About half of ligament torn	All fibers of ligament torn
Mechanism of Injury	Overstretch Overload	Overstretch Overload Crushing	Overstretch Overload	Overuse Overstretch Overload †Aging	Overload Overstretch	Overload Overstretch	Overload Overstretch
Onset	Acute	Acute	Acute	Chronic Acute	Acute	Acute	Acute
Weakness	Minor	Moderate to major (reflex inhibition)	Moderate to major	Minor to moderate	Minor	Minor to moderate	Minor to moderate
Disability	Minor	Moderate	Major	Minor to major	Minor	Moderate	Moderate to major
Muscle Spasm	Minor	Moderate to major	Moderate	Minor	Minor	Minor	Minor
Swelling	Minor	Moderate to major	Moderate to major	*Minor to major (thickening) †No	Minor	Moderate	Moderate to major
Loss of Function	Minor	Moderate to major	Major (reflex inhibition)	Minor to major	Minor	Moderate to major	Moderate to major (instability)
Pain on Isometric Contraction	Minor	Moderate to major	No to minor	Minor to major	No	No	No
Pain on Stretch	Yes	Yes	No[a]	Yes	Yes	Yes	No[a]
Joint Play	Normal	Normal	Normal	Normal	Normal	Normal	Normal to excessive
Palpable Defect	No	No	Yes (if early)	†May have palpable module	No	No	Yes (if early)
Crepitus	No	No	No	Possible	No	No	No
ROM	Decreased	Decreased	May increase or decrease depending on swelling	Decreased	Decreased	Decreased	May increase or decrease depending on swelling Dislocation or subluxation possible

[a]Not if it is the only tissue injured; however, often with 3° injuries, other structures will suffer 1° or 2° injuries and be painful.
ROM, Range of motion.

the bone. **Nervous tissues** and their associated sheaths also have tension put on them by stretching and pinching, as do **inert tissues.** Inert tissues include all structures that would not be considered contractile or neurological, such as joint capsules, ligaments, bursae, blood vessels, cartilage, and dura mater. Table 1.16 demonstrates differential diagnosis of injuries to contractile tissue (strains and paratenonitis) and inert tissue (sprains). Some examiners separate vascular tissues from the other inert tissues; however, for the most part, when doing a musculoskeletal examination, they can be grouped with the other inert tissues with the understanding that they do present their own unique signs and symptoms.

When doing movement testing, the examiner should note whether pain or restriction predominate. If pain predominates, the condition is more acute, and gentler assessment and treatment are required. If restriction predominates, the condition is subacute, or chronic, and more vigorous assessment and treatment can be performed.

Active Movements

Active movements (AROM) are "actively" performed by the patient's voluntary muscles and have their own special value in that they combine tests of joint range, control, muscle power, and the patient's willingness to perform the movement. These movements are sometimes referred to as **physiological movements.** The end of active movement is sometimes referred to as the **physiological barrier.** Contractile, nervous, and inert tissues are involved or moved during active movements. When active movements occur, one or more rigid structures (bones) move, and such movement results in movement of all structures that attach to or are in close proximity to that bone. Although active movements are usually the first movements done, they either are not performed at all or are performed with caution during fracture healing or if the movement could put stress on newly repaired soft tissues. The examiner should note which movements, if any, cause pain or other symptoms and the amount and quality of pain that results. For example, small, unguarded movements causing intense pain indicate an acute, irritable joint. If the condition is very irritable or acute, it may not be possible to elicit all the movements desired. In this case, only those movements that provide the most useful information should be performed. The examiner should note the rhythm of movement along with any pain, limitation, or unusual (e.g., instability jog) or trick movements that occur. Trick movements are modified movements that the patient consciously or unconsciously uses to accomplish what the examiner has asked the patient to do. For example, in the presence of deltoid paralysis, if the examiner asks the patient to abduct the arm, the patient can accomplish this movement by laterally rotating the shoulder and using the biceps muscle to abduct the arm.

Active movement may be abnormal for several reasons, and the examiner must try to differentiate the cause. Pain is a common cause for abnormal movement as is muscle weakness, paralysis, or spasm. Other causes include tight or shortened tissues, altered length-tension relationships, modified neuromuscular factors, and joint-muscle interaction. In some cases, the patient may not be able to actively move the joint through the available ROM because of weakness, pain, or tight structures. This inability to move through the available ROM is sometimes called a **lag.** The most common example of this is a quadriceps lag in which the quadriceps is not able to actively take the knee

into full extension even if full passive extension is possible. (This is commonly seen after surgery.) It is important to remember that a lag may also be caused by tightness of tissues acting in the opposite direction (e.g., in the knee, tight posterior capsule, tight hamstrings, or scarring).

The active movement component of the examination is a functional test of the anatomic and dynamic aspects of the body and joints while demonstrating correct or incorrect motor function, which is the ability to demonstrate skillful and efficient movement patterns while maintaining control of voluntary postures.[12,108] The examiner should ensure the movement is performed at a smooth constant speed in the desired direction using the most efficient pathway through full ROM.[109,110] This will involve the integration and synchronization of prime movers and synergists through the whole or part of the kinetic chain involved in the movement.

When testing active movements, the examiner should note where in the arc of movement the symptoms occur. For example, pain occurs during abduction of the shoulder between 60° and 120° if there is impingement under the acromion process or coracoacromial ligament. Any increase in intensity and quality of pain should also be noted. This information helps the examiner to determine the particular tissue at fault. For example, bone pain, except in the case of a fracture or tumor, often is not altered with movement. By observing the patient's reaction to pain, the examiner can get some idea of how much the condition is affecting the patient and the patient's pain threshold. By noting the pattern of movement, the quality and rhythm of the movement, the movements in other joints, and the observable restriction, the examiner can tell if the patient is "cheating" (using accessory muscles or muscle substitution) to do the movement and what tissues are affected. For example, "shoulder hiking" may indicate a capsular pattern of the shoulder or incorrect sequential firing of different muscles.

Examiner Observations During Active Movement

- When and where during each of the movements the onset of pain occurs
- Whether the movement increases the intensity and quality of the pain
- The reaction of the patient to pain
- The amount of observable restriction and its nature
- The pattern of movement
- The rhythm and quality of movement
- The movement of associated joints
- The willingness of the patient to move the part

In general, active movements are performed once or twice in each desired direction while the examiner notes the pattern of movement and any discrepancies or cheating/substitution movements. If the patient has noted pain or difficulty with any particular movements, these movements should be done last to ensure no overflow of symptoms to other movements. If the patient has complained that certain repetitive movements or sustained postures are the problem, the examiner should ensure that the movements are repeated (5 to 10 times) or sustained (usually 5 to 20 seconds but may depend on history) until the symptoms are demonstrated.

There are standard movements for each joint, and these movements tend to follow cardinal planes (i.e., they are single plane movements). However, if the patient complains of problems outside these standard movements or if symptoms are more likely to be elicited by combined movements (i.e., movements in multiple planes or around combined axes), repeated movements, movements with speed, or movements under compression, then these should be performed.[111-113] McKenzie has reported that repeated movements increase symptoms in irritable acute tissues or in internal derangements,[23] whereas postural dysfunctions change little with repeated movements.

In some cases, especially if the joints are not too reactive or irritable, overpressure may carefully be applied at the end of the AROM. If the overpressure does not produce symptoms and the end feel is normal, the movement is considered normal and the examiner may decide that passive movements are unnecessary.

Passive Movements

Passive movements (PROM) are primarily performed to determine the available anatomic ROM and end feel. The PROM may be within normal limits, hypermobile (see the Patient History section) or hypomobile. Palpation of measurement points can play a major role when using palpable landmarks for goniometry.[114] With passive movement, the examiner puts the joint through its ROM while the patient is relaxed. These movements may also be referred to as **anatomic movements.** The end of passive movement is sometimes referred to as the **anatomic barrier.** Normally, the physiological barrier (active movement) occurs before the anatomic barrier (passive movement) so that passive movement is always slightly greater than active movement. The movement must proceed through as full of a range as possible and should, if possible, involve the same motions as were performed actively. Positioning the patient (e.g., sitting, lying supine) may have an effect on AROM and PROM, so the examiner must consider positioning. Differences in ROM between active and passive movements may be caused by muscle contraction or spasm, muscle deficiency, neurological deficit, contractures, or pain. AROM and PROM may be measured by goniometer, inclinometer, examiner estimation ("eyeballing"), or a similar measure.[115,116] With most of these methods, it is difficult to show consistent differences of less than 5°.[117,118] Goniometry is especially useful

for measuring and recording joint or fracture deformities and has been shown to have a satisfactory level of intratester reliability,[118-120] although this may depend on the motion measured.[120] Measurements at different times show progression or regression of the deformity. Although there are sources that describe ROMs for various joints, the values given are averages and do not necessarily constitute the ROM needed to do specific activities or the ROM that is present in a specific patient. Normal mobility is relative. For example, gymnasts tend to be classed as lax (nonpathological hypermobility) in most joints, whereas elderly persons tend to be classed as hypomobile. However, for these individual populations, the available ROM may be considered normal. In reality, the important question is, does the patient have the ROM available to do what he or she wants to do functionally? Certain pathological states, such as Ehlers-Danlos syndrome, may also affect ROM. For example, if several joints demonstrate excessive ROM, a condition referred to as **benign joint hypermobility syndrome** may exist.[121] The **Beighton Hypermobility Index** for this condition is a modification of the Carter and Wilkinson Scoring Criteria (see Chapter 17). This index used in isolation, if positive, means the individual has widespread joint hypermobility. Generalized joint hypermobility is said to be present when a score of 4 or more is found on the Beighton test.[122-124]

Examiner Observations During Passive Movement

- When and where during each of the movements the pain begins
- Whether the movement increases the intensity and quality of pain
- The pattern of limitation of movement
- The end feel of movement
- The movement of associated joints
- The range of motion available

Beighton Hypermobility Index Scoring Criteria[125,126]

- Patient can bend and place hands flat on floor without bending knees (1 point)
- Knee(s) can hyperextend past 0° (1 point for each knee)
- Elbow(s) can hyperextend past 0° (1 point for each elbow)
- Thumb can be bent backward to touch forearm (1 point for each thumb)
- Little finger can be bent backward beyond 90° (1 point for each little finger)

Note: Maximum score = 9.

Likewise, the **Brighton Diagnostic Criteria,** which is not widely used in orthopedics, measures joint mobility and skin abnormalities.[121,125] Using these criteria, the patient must have two major criteria, one major and two minor criteria, or four minor criteria to be diagnosed with benign joint hypermobility syndrome.

Each movement must be compared with the same movement in the opposite joint or, secondarily, with accepted norms. Although passive movement must be gentle, the examiner must determine whether there is any limitation of range (**hypomobility**) or excess of range (**hypermobility** or **laxity**) and, if so, whether it is painful. Hypermobile joints tend to be more susceptible to ligament sprains, joint effusion, chronic pain, recurrent injury, paratenonitis resulting from lack of control (instability), and early osteoarthritis. Hypomobile joints are more susceptible to muscle strains, pinched nerve syndromes, and paratenonitis resulting from overstress.[127,128] **Myofascial hypomobility** results from adaptive shortening or hypertonicity of the muscles or from posttraumatic adhesions or scarring. **Pericapsular hypomobility** has a capsular or ligamentous origin and may result from adhesions, scarring, arthritis, arthrosis, fibrosis, or tissue adaptation. Restriction may be in all directions but not the same amount in each direction (e.g., capsular pattern). **Pathomechanical hypomobility** occurs as a result of joint trauma (micro or macro) leading to restriction in one or more directions.[24] Hypermobility is not the same as instability. Instability covers a wide range of pathological hypermobility. Although there are tests to demonstrate general hypermobility, these tests should be interpreted with caution because patients demonstrate a wide range of variability between joints and within joints.[129,130] With careful assessment, one often finds that a joint may be hypermobile in one direction and hypomobile in another direction. It must also be remembered that

evidence of hypomobility or hypermobility does not necessarily indicate a pathological state in the person being assessed. The examiner should attempt to determine the cause of the limitation (e.g., pain, spasm, adhesions, compression) or hypermobility (e.g., injury, occupational, genetic, disease) and the quality of the movement (e.g., lead pipe, cogwheel).

End Feel.[1] When assessing passive movement, the examiner should apply overpressure at the end of the ROM to determine the quality of end feel (the sensation the examiner "feels" in the joint as it reaches the end of the ROM) of each passive movement (Table 1.17). However, care must be taken when testing end feel, to be sure that severe symptoms are not provoked. If the patient is able to hold a position at the end of the physiological ROM (end range of active movement) without provoking symptoms or if the symptoms ease quickly after returning to the resting position, then the end feel can be tested. Pain with pathological end feels is common.[82] However, if the patient has severe pain at end range, end feel should only be tested with extreme care. A proper evaluation of end feel can help the examiner to assess the type of pathology present, determine a prognosis for the condition, and learn the severity or stage of the problem. By determining if pain or restriction is the main problem, the examiner can determine if a more gentle treatment should be given (pain predominating) or a more vigorous treatment (restriction predominantly). The end feel sensations that the examiner experiences are subjective, so intrarater reliability tends to be good, whereas interrater reliability is poor.[81] Many clinicians develop their own

TABLE 1.17

Normal and Abnormal End Feels

End Feel	Example
Normal	
Bone to bone	Elbow extension
Soft-tissue approximation	Knee flexion
Tissue stretch	Ankle dorsiflexion, shoulder lateral rotation, finger extension
Abnormal	
Early muscle spasm	Protective spasm following injury
Late muscle spasm	Spasm due to instability or pain
"Mushy" tissue stretch	Tight muscle
Spasticity	Upper motor neuron lesion
Hard capsular	Frozen shoulder
Soft capsular	Synovitis, soft-tissue edema
Bone to bone	Osteophyte formation
Empty	Acute subacromial bursitis
Springy block	Meniscus tear

classification, with the most common ones used[82] developed by Cyriax,[1] Kaltenborn,[111] and Paris.[131]

Cyriax described three classic **normal end feels:**[1]

- *Bone-to-Bone.* This is a "hard," unyielding sensation that is painless. An example of normal bone-to-bone end feel is elbow extension.
- *Soft-Tissue Approximation.* With this type of end feel, there is a yielding compression (mushy feel) that stops further movement. Examples are elbow and knee flexion, in which movement is stopped by compression of the soft tissues, primarily the muscles. In a particularly slim person with little muscle bulk, the end feel of elbow flexion may be bone-to-bone.
- *Tissue Stretch.* There is a hard or firm (springy) type of movement with a slight give. Toward the end of ROM, there is a feeling of springy or elastic resistance. The normal tissue stretch end feel has a feeling of "rising tension or stiffness." This changing tension has led to this end feel sometimes being divided into two types: **elastic (soft)** and **capsular (hard).** This feeling depends on the thickness and type of tissue being stretched, and it may be very elastic, as in the Achilles tendon stretch, slightly elastic, as in wrist flexion (tissue stretch), or hard, as in knee extension. A hard end feel is firm with a definite stopping point, whereas soft end feel implies a softer end feel without a definite stopping place.[132] Tissue stretch is the most common type of normal end feel; it is found when the capsule and ligaments are the primary restraints to movement. Examples are lateral rotation of the shoulder, knee extension, and metacarpophalangeal joint extension.

In addition to the three normal types of end feel, Cyriax described five classic **abnormal end feels,** several of which have subdivisions and each of which is commonly associated with some degree of pain or restricted movement.[1,133]

- *Muscle Spasm.* This end feel is invoked by movement, with a sudden dramatic arrest of movement often accompanied by pain. The end feel is sudden and hard. Cyriax called this a "vibrant twang."[1] Some examiners divide muscle spasm into different parts. **Early muscle spasm** occurs early in the ROM, almost as soon as movement starts; this type of muscle spasm is associated with inflammation and is seen in more acute conditions. **Late muscle spasm** occurs at or near the end of the ROM. It is usually caused by instability and the resulting irritability caused by movement. An example is muscle spasm occurring during the apprehension test for anterior dislocation of the shoulder. Both types of muscle spasm are the result of the subconscious efforts of the body to protect the injured joint or structure, and their occurrence may be related to how quickly the examiner does the movement. **Spasticity** is slightly different and is seen with upper motor neuron lesions.[134] It is a form of muscle hypertonicity that offers increased resistance to stretch involving primarily the flexors in

the upper limb and extensors in the lower limb and may be associated with muscle weakness. The **Modified Ashworth Scale** is sometimes used to measure spasticity and resistance to passive movement, but its reliability has been questioned.[135–137] Some clinicians use the **Tardien Scale.**[138,139] Both of these scales are more commonly used when assessing neurological conditions and upper motor lesion problems rather than musculoskeletal conditions. A **tight muscle** may give its own unique end feel. This is similar to normal tissue stretch, but it does not have as great an elastic feel.

Modified Ashworth Scale for Muscle Tone Measurement[137]

0 = Normal tone, no increase in tone

1 = Slight increase in muscle tone, manifested by a catch and release or minimal resistance at the end of the range of motion (ROM) when the affected part(s) is moved in flexion or extension

1+= Slight increase in muscle tone, manifested by a catch, followed by minimal resistance throughout the remainder (less than half) of the ROM

2 = More marked increase in muscle tone through most of the ROM, but affected part(s) easily moved

3 = Considerable increase in muscle tone, passive movement difficult

4 = Affected part(s) rigid in flexion or extension

From Bohannon R, Smith M: Interrater reliability of a modified Ashworth scale of muscle spasticity, *Phys Ther* 67(2):206, 1987.

- *Capsular.* Although this end feel is similar to tissue stretch, it does not occur where one would expect (i.e., it occurs earlier in the ROM), and it tends to have a thicker feel to it. ROM is obviously reduced, and the capsule can be postulated to be at fault. Muscle spasm usually does not occur in conjunction with the capsular type of end feel except if the movement is fast and the joint acute. Some examiners divide this end feel into **hard capsular,** in which the end feel has a thicker stretching quality to it, and **soft capsular** (boggy), which is similar to normal tissue stretch end feel but with a restricted ROM. The hard capsular end feel is seen in more chronic conditions or in full-blown capsular patterns. The limitation comes on rather abruptly after a smooth, friction-free movement. The soft capsular end feel is more often seen in acute conditions with stiffness occurring early in the range and increasing until the end of range is reached. Maitland calls this "resistance through range."[140] Some authors interpret this soft, boggy end feel as being the result of synovitis, soft-tissue edema, or hemarthrosis.[141] Major injury to ligaments and the capsule often causes a **soft end feel** until the tension is taken up by other structures.[142]
- *Bone-to-Bone.* This abnormal end feel is similar to the normal bone-to-bone type, but the restriction occurs before the end of ROM would normally occur or where a bone-to-bone end feel would not be expected.

An example is a bone-to-bone end feel in the cervical spine resulting from osteophyte formation.

- *Empty.* The empty end feel is detected when movement produces considerable pain. The movement cannot be performed or stops because of the pain, although no real mechanical resistance is being detected. Examples include an acute subacromial bursitis or a tumor. Patients often have difficulty describing the empty end feel, and there is no muscle spasm involved.
- *Springy Block.* Similar to a tissue stretch, this occurs where one would not expect it to occur; it tends to be found in joints with menisci. There is a rebound effect with a thick stretching feel although it is not as stretchy as a hard capsular end feel, and it usually indicates an internal derangement within the joint. A springy block end feel may be found with a torn meniscus of a knee when it is locked or unable to go into full extension.

Capsular Patterns.[1] With passive movement, a full ROM must be carried out in several directions. A short, too-soft movement in the midrange does not achieve the proper results or elicit potential findings. In addition to evaluating the end feel, the examiner must look at the **pattern of limitation or restriction**. If the capsule of the joint is affected, the pattern of limitation is the feature that indicates the presence of a **capsular pattern** in the joint. This pattern is the result of a total joint reaction, with muscle spasm, capsular contraction (the most common cause), and generalized osteophyte formation being possible mechanisms at fault. Each joint has a characteristic pattern of limitation. The presence of this capsular pattern does not indicate the type of joint involvement; only an analysis of the end feel can do that. Only joints that are controlled by muscles have a capsular pattern; joints, such as the sacroiliac and distal tibiofibular joints, do not exhibit a capsular pattern. Dutton pointed out that capsular patterns are based on empirical findings rather than research, and this may be the reason capsular patterns may be different or inconsistent.[4] In fact, Hayes et al.[81] felt the pattern of limitation was useful but the proportional limitation concept should not be used. Table 1.18 illustrates some of the common capsular patterns seen in joints.

Noncapsular Patterns.[1] The examiner must also be aware of **noncapsular patterns,** for example, a limitation that exists but does not correspond to the classic capsular pattern for that joint. In the shoulder, abduction may be restricted but with very little rotational restriction (e.g., subacromial bursitis). Although a total capsular reaction is absent, there are other possibilities, such as ligamentous adhesions, in which only part of a capsule or the accessory ligaments are involved. There may be a local restriction in one direction, often accompanied by pain, and full, pain-free ROM in all other directions. A second possibility is **internal derangement,** which commonly affects only certain joints, such as the knee, ankle, and elbow. Intracapsular fragments may interfere with the normal sequence of motion. Movements causing impingement of the fragments will be limited, whereas other motions will be free. In the knee, for example, a torn meniscus may cause a blocking of extension, but flexion is usually free. Loose bodies cause limitation when they are caught between articular surfaces. A third possibility is **extra-articular lesions.** These lesions are revealed by disproportionate limitation, extra-articular adhesions, or an acutely inflamed structure limiting movement in a particular direction. For example, limited straight leg raising in the lumbar disc syndrome is referred to as a **constant length phenomenon.** This phenomenon results when the limitation of movement in one joint depends on the position in which another joint is held. The restricted tissue (in this case, the sciatic nerve) must lie outside the joint or joints (in this case, hip and knee) being tested. The constant length phenomenon may also result from muscle adhesions that cause restriction of motion.

Inert Tissue.[1] After the active and passive movements are completed, the examiner should be able to determine whether there are problems with any of the **inert tissues.** The examiner makes such a determination by judging the degree of pain and the limitation of movement within the joint. For lesions of inert tissue, the examiner may find that active and passive movements are painful in the same direction. Usually pain occurs as the limitation of motion approaches. Resisted isometric movements (discussed later) are not usually painful unless some compression is occurring. During the examination, inert tissues are tested or stressed during active and passive movements, functional testing, selected special tests, joint play testing, and palpation.

Inert tissue refers to all tissue that is not considered contractile or neurological. Four classic patterns may be seen in lesions of inert issue, according to the ROM available (or restriction present) and the amount of pain produced.[1]

Patterns of Inert Tissue Lesions

- Pain-free, full range of motion (ROM)
- Pain and limited ROM in every direction
- Pain and excessive or limited ROM in some directions
- Pain-free, limited ROM

---

1. If the *range of movement is full and there is no pain,* there is no lesion of the inert tissues being tested by that passive movement; however, there may be lesions of inert tissue in other directions or around other joints.
2. The next possible pattern is one of *pain and limitation of movement in every direction.* In this pattern, the entire joint is affected, indicating arthritis or capsulitis. Each joint has its own capsular pattern (see Table 1.18), and the amount of limitation is not

TABLE **1.18**

Common Capsular Patterns of Joints

Joint	Restriction[a]
Temporomandibular	Limitation of mouth opening
Atlanto-occipital	Extension, side flexion equally limited
Cervical spine	Side flexion and rotation equally limited, extension
Glenohumeral	Lateral rotation, abduction, medial rotation
Sternoclavicular	Pain at extreme of range of movement, especially horizontal adduction and full elevation
Acromioclavicular	Pain at extreme of range of movement, especially horizontal adduction and full elevation
Ulnohumeral (elbow)	Flexion, extension
Radiohumeral	Flexion, extension, supination, pronation
Proximal (superior) radioulnar	Supination, pronation equally limited
Distal radioulnar	Full range of movement, pain at extremes of rotation
Radiocarpal (wrist)	Flexion and extension equally limited
Intercarpal	None
Midcarpal	Equal limitation of flexion and extension
Carpometacarpal (thumb)	Abduction, extension
Carpometacarpal (fingers)	Equal limitation in all directions
Trapeziometacarpal	Abduction, extension
Metacarpophalangeal and interphalangeal	Flexion, extension
Thoracic spine	Side flexion and rotation equally limited, extension
Lumbar spine	Side flexion and rotation equally limited, extension
Sacroiliac, symphysis pubis, and sacrococcygeal	Pain when joints are stressed
Hip[b]	Flexion, abduction, medial rotation (but in some cases medial rotation is most limited)
Knee (tibiofemoral)	Flexion, extension
Distal tibiofibular	Pain when joint stressed
Talocrural	Plantar flexion, dorsiflexion
Talocalcaneal (subtalar)	Limitation of range of movement (varus, valgus)
Midtarsal	Dorsiflexion, plantar flexion, adduction, medial rotation
Tarsometatarsal	None
First metatarsophalangeal (big toe)	Extension, flexion
Second to fifth metatarsophalangeal	Variable
Interphalangeal	Flexion, extension

[a]Movements are listed in order of restriction.
[b]For the hip, flexion, abduction, and medial rotation are always the movements most limited in a capsular pattern. However, the order of restriction may vary.

usually the same in each direction; however, although there is a set pattern for each joint, other directions may also be affected. All movements of the joint may be affected, but the motions described for the capsular pattern usually occur in the particular order listed. For example, the capsular pattern of the shoulder is lateral rotation most limited, followed by abduction and medial rotation. In early capsular patterns, only one movement may be restricted; this movement is usually the one that has the potential for the greatest restriction. For example, in an early capsular pattern of the shoulder, only lateral rotation may be limited, and the limitation may be slight.

3. A patient with a lesion of inert tissue may experience *pain and limitation or excessive movement in some directions but not in others,* as in a ligament sprain or local capsular adhesion. In other words, a noncapsular pattern is presented. Movements that stretch,

pinch, or move the affected structure cause the pain. Internal derangement that results in the blocking of a joint is another example of a lesion of inert tissue that produces a variable pattern. Extra-articular limitation occurs when a lesion outside the joint affects the movement of that joint. Because these movements pinch or stretch the involved structure (e.g., bursitis in the buttock, acute subacromial bursitis), pain and limitation of movement occur on stretch or compression of these structures. If a structure such as a ligament has been torn, the ROM may increase if swelling is minimal, especially right after injury, indicating instability (pathological hypermobility) of the joint and can be seen in spinal or peripheral joints. Swelling often masks instability because it puts the tissues under tension. Pathological hypermobility, if present, results in greater than normal movement at the joint, causes pain, puts neurogenic structures at risk, and can result in progressive deformity and degeneration.[143]

4. The final inert tissue pattern is *limited movement that is pain free.* The end feel for this type of condition is often of the abnormal bone-to-bone type, and it usually indicates a symptomless osteoarthritis—that is, osteophytes are present and restrict movement, but they are not pinching or compressing any sensitive structures. If this situation is encountered, it should be left alone because it is not causing the patient any problem other than restricted ROM and attempts at treatment could lead to further problems.

Resisted Isometric Movements

Resisted isometric movements are the movements tested last in the examination of the joints. This type of movement consists of a strong, static (isometric), voluntary muscle contraction, and it is used primarily to determine whether the contractile tissue is the tissue at fault, although the nerve supplying the muscle is also tested. If the muscle, its tendon, or the bone into which they insert is at fault, pain and weakness result; the amount of pain and weakness is related to the degree of injury and the patient's pain threshold. If movement is allowed to occur at the joint, inert tissue around the joint will also move, and it will not be clear whether any resulting pain arises from contractile or inert tissues. Therefore the joint is put in a neutral or resting position (see Table 1.34 later) so that minimal tension is placed on the inert tissue. The patient is asked to contract the muscle as strongly as possible while the examiner resists to prevent any movement from occurring and to ensure that the patient is using maximum effort. To keep movement to a minimum, it is best for the examiner to position the joint properly in the resting position and then to say to the patient, "Don't let me move you." In this way, the examiner can ensure that the contraction is isometric and can control the amount of force exerted. Movement cannot

be completely eliminated, but this method minimizes it. Some compression of the inert tissues (e.g., cartilage) occurs with the contraction, and there may be some joint shear as well, but it will be minimal if done as described.

Examiner Observations During Resisted Isometric Movement

- Whether the contraction causes pain and, if it does, the pain's intensity and quality
- Strength of the contraction
- Type of contraction causing problem (e.g., concentric, isometric, eccentric, econcentric)

If, as advocated, this isometric hold method is used, then movement against this resistance would require muscle strength of grade 3 to 5 on the muscle test grading scale (Table 1.19).[144] If the muscle strength is less than grade 3, then the methods advocated in muscle testing manuals could be used.[140,145,146] When using manual muscle testing, repeated testing should be done by the same person to decrease the variability that occurs when different people measure muscle strength.[146] If the examiner is having difficulty differentiating between grade 4 and grade 5, an eccentric break method of muscle testing may be used. This method starts as an isometric contraction, but then the examiner applies sufficient force to cause an eccentric contraction

TABLE **1.19**

Muscle Test Grading (Modified Oxford Scale)

Grade	Value	Movement Grade
5+	Normal (100%)	Complete ROM against gravity with maximal resistance
4	Good (75%)	Complete ROM against gravity with some (moderate) resistance
3+	Fair+	Complete ROM against gravity with minimal resistance
3	Fair (50%)	Complete ROM against gravity
3−	Fair−	Some but not complete ROM against gravity
2+	Poor+	Initiates motion against gravity
2	Poor (25%)	Complete ROM with gravity eliminated
2−	Poor−	Initiates motion if gravity is eliminated
1	Trace	Evidence of slight contractility but no joint motion
0	Zero	No contraction palpated

ROM, Range of motion.

or a "break" in the patient's isometric contraction. This method provides a more recognizable threshold for maximum isometric contraction.[144] However, it must be recognized that all three methods are subjective for normal and good values. When a muscle is tested in the resting position, it is usually being tested in its position of optimum length so that maximum force, if necessary, can be elicited. However, in some cases, a muscle, because of pathology, may become lengthened or shortened leading to weakness when tested in the normal resting position. Testing a muscle in the fully lengthened position tightens the inert components of muscle and puts more stress on the contractile tissues, whereas testing it in a shortened position puts it in its weakest position. For example, Kendall et al.[147] called muscle weakness that results from muscle lengthening **stretch weakness** or **positional weakness**. Thus, if the examiner has found ROM to be limited or excessive during passive movement testing, consideration should be given to performing the isometric tests in different positions of the ROM to see if the problem is not one of strength but of muscle length. This action will also help to differentiate between weakness throughout the ROM (**pathological weakness**) from weakness only in certain positions (positional weakness). If, in the history, the patient has complained of symptoms in a different position than those commonly tested, the examiner may modify the isometric test position to try to elicit the symptoms. If the patient has complained that a concentric, eccentric, or econcentric contraction has caused the problem, the examiner may include these movements, with or without load, in the examination, but only after the isometric tests have been completed. Econcentric or pseudoisometric contraction involves two-joint muscles in which the muscle is acting concentrically at one joint and eccentrically at the other joint, the result being minimal or no change in muscle length. Two-joint muscles are among the most frequently injured muscles (e.g., hamstrings, biceps, gastrocnemius) often because of the different actions occurring over the two joints at the same time.

In some cases, machines may be used to measure muscle strength, but care should be taken because these tests are often not isometric and they are often not performed in functional positions nor at functional speeds. However, they do provide a comparison or ratio between right and left and between different movements.

Muscle weakness, if elicited, may be caused by an upper motor neuron lesion, injury to a peripheral nerve, pathology at the neuromuscular junction, a nerve root lesion, or a lesion or disease (myopathy) of the muscle, its tendons, or the bony insertions themselves. For the first four of these causes, the system of muscle test grading may be used. For nerve root lesions, myotome testing is the method of choice. When testing for muscle lesions, it is more appropriate to test the resisted

movements isometrically first, to determine which movements are painful, then perform individual muscle tests, as advocated in texts such as that of Daniels and Worthingham,[145] to determine exactly which muscle is at fault.

Signs and Symptoms of Upper Motor Neuron Lesions

- Spasticity
- Hypertonicity
- Hyperreflexia (deep tendon reflexes)
- Positive pathological reflexes (e.g., Babinski, Hoffman)
- Absent or reduced superficial reflexes
- Extensor plantar response (bilateral)

Signs and Symptoms of Myopathy (Muscle Disease)[85]

- Difficulty lifting
- Difficulty walking
- Myotonia (inability of muscle to relax)
- Cramps
- Pain (myalgia)
- Progressive weakness
- Myoglobinuria

Causes of Muscle Weakness

- Muscle strain
- Pain/reflex inhibition
- Peripheral nerve injury
- Nerve root lesion (myotome)
- Upper motor neuron lesion (even when muscle shows increased tone)
- Tendon pathology
- Avulsion
- Psychological overlay

If the contraction appears weak, the examiner must make sure that the weakness is not caused by pain or by the patient's fear, unwillingness, or malingering. The examiner can often resolve such a finding by having the patient make a contraction on the good side first, which normally will not cause pain. Weakness that is not associated with pain or disuse is a positive neurological sign indicating that a nerve root, peripheral nerve, or upper motor neuron lesion is at least part of the problem.

Contractile Tissue.[1] With resisted isometric testing, the examiner is looking for problems of **contractile tissue,** which consists of muscles, their tendons, attachments (e.g., bone), and the nervous tissue supplying the contractile tissue. Both active movements and resisted isometric testing demonstrate symptoms if contractile tissue is affected. Other parts of the examination, which will test contractile tissue, include passive movement, functional testing, specific special tests, and palpation. Usually, passive movements are normal (i.e., passive movements are full and pain free), although pain may be exhibited at the end of the ROM when the contractile or nervous tissue is stretched. If contractile tissue has been injured, active movement is painful in one direction (contraction) and passive movement, if painful, is painful in the opposite direction (stretch). Resisted isometric testing is painful in the same direction as active movement. If the muscles are tested as previously described, not all movements will be found to be affected, except in patients with psychogenic pain and sometimes in patients with an acute joint lesion, in which even a small amount of tension on the muscles around the joint provokes pain. However, if the joint lesion is acutely severe, passive movements (when tested) will be markedly affected, and there will be no confusion as to where the lesion lies. As with inert tissue, four classic patterns have been identified with lesions of contractile and nervous tissue.[1] (However, in this case, one is dealing with pain and strength rather than pain and altered ROM.)

Patterns of Contractile Tissue and Nervous Tissue Lesions

- No pain, and movement is strong
- Pain, and movement is relatively strong (but not as strong as it should be)
- Pain, and movement is weak
- No pain, and movement is weak

---

1. Movement that is *strong and pain free* indicates that there is no lesion of the contractile unit being tested or the nervous tissue supplying that contractile unit, regardless of how tender the muscles may be when touched. The muscles and nerves function painlessly and are not the source of the patient's discomfort.

2. Movement that is *strong and painful* indicates a local lesion of the muscle or tendon. Such a lesion could be a first- or second-degree muscle strain. The amount of strength is usually determined by the amount of pain the patient feels on contraction, which results from reflex inhibition that leads to weakness or cogwheel contractions. A second-degree strain produces greater weakness and more pain than a first-degree strain. Similarly, tendinosis, tendinitis, paratenonitis, or paratenonitis with tendinosis (Table 1.20) all may lead to contractions that are strong (relative) and painful, but one that is not usually as strong as on the good side; and the pain is in or around the tendon, not the muscle.[148,149] If there is a partial avulsion fracture, again, the movement will be strong and painful. However, if the avulsion is complete, the movement will be weak and painful (see later discussion). Typically, there is no primary limitation of passive movement when contractile tissue is injured, although end range may be painful (stretch), except, for example, in the case of a gross muscle tear with hematoma where the muscle, which is often in spasm, is being stretched. In this case, the patient may develop joint stiffness secondary to disuse. This is often caused by protective muscle spasm of adjacent muscles that allow, for example, some joint

---

TABLE **1.20**

Bonar's Modification of Clancy's Classification of Tendinopathies

Pathological Diagnosis	Concept (Macroscopic Pathology)	Histological Appearance
Tendinosis	Intratendinous degeneration (commonly caused by aging, microtrauma, and vascular compromise)	Collagen disorientation, disorganization, and fiber separation with an increase in mucoid ground substance, increased prominence of cells and vascular spaces with or without neovascularization, and focal necrosis or calcification
Tendinitis/partial rupture	Symptomatic degeneration of the tendon with vascular disruption and inflammatory repair response	Degenerative changes as noted above with superimposed evidence of tear, including fibroblastic and myofibroblasts proliferation, hemorrhage and organizing granulation tissue
Paratenonitis	Inflammation of the outer layer of the tendon (paratenon) alone, regardless of whether the paratenon is lined by synovium	Mucoid degeneration in the areolar tissue is seen. A scattered mild mononuclear infiltrate with or without focal fibrin deposition and fibrinous exudate is also seen
Paratenonitis with tendinosis	Paratenonitis associated with intratendinous degeneration	Degenerative changes as noted for tendinosis with mucoid degeneration with or without fibrosis and scattered inflammatory cells in the paratenon alveolar tissue

From Khan KM, Cook JL, Bonar F, et al: Histopathology of common tendinopathies—update and implications for clinical management, *Sports Med* 27:399, 1999.

contracture to be superimposed on the muscle lesion. This stiffness then takes precedence in the treatment. One should always remember that it is easier to maintain physiological function than it is to restore it.

3. Movement that is *weak and painful* indicates a severe lesion around that joint, such as a fracture. The weakness that results is usually caused by reflex inhibition of the muscles around the joint, secondary to pain.

4. Movement that is *weak and pain free* indicates a rupture of a muscle (third-degree strain) or its tendon or involvement of the peripheral nerve or nerve root supplying that muscle. If the movement is weak and pain free, neurological involvement or a tendon rupture should be suspected first. With neurological involvement, the examiner must be able to differentiate between the muscle innervation of a nerve root (myotome) and the muscle innervation of a peripheral nerve (see Table 1.15 as an example). In addition, the examiner should be able to differentiate between upper and lower motor neuron lesions (see Table 1.12). Third-degree strains are sometimes masked because, if the force is great enough to cause a complete tear of a muscle, the surrounding muscles, which assisted the movement, may also be injured (first- or second-degree strain). The pain from these secondary muscles can mask the third-degree strain to the primary mover. However, the tested weakness would be greater with the third-degree strain (and its lack of pain). Although significant pain can occur at the time of the third-degree injury, this pain usually quickly subsides to a dull ache, even when the muscle is contracting, because there is no tension on the muscle, which no longer has two attachment (origin and insertion) points. For this reason, a gap or hole in the muscle may be palpated. When the third-degree injured muscle does contract, the muscle may bunch up or bulge, giving an obvious deformity (Fig. 1.13).

If all movements around a joint appear painful, the pain is often a result of fatigue, emotional hypersensitivity, or emotional problems. Patients may equate effort with discomfort, and they must be told that they are not necessarily the same.

Janda put forth an interesting concept by dividing muscles into two groups: postural and phasic.[150] He believed that **postural** or **tonic muscles**, which are the muscles responsible for maintaining upright posture, have a tendency to become tight and hypertonic with pathology and to develop contractures but are less likely to atrophy, whereas **phasic muscles**, which include almost all other muscles, tend to become weak and inhibited with pathology. The examiner must be careful to note the type of muscle affected and the ROM available (active movements) as well as the strength and production of pain (resisted isometric movements) when testing contractile tissue. Table 1.21 shows the muscles that are postural and

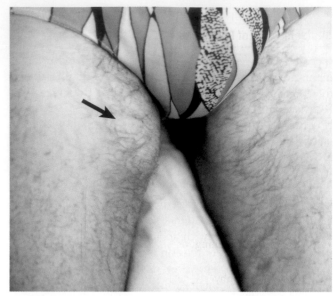

Fig. 1.13 Rupture (3° strain) of right adductor muscle. Note the bulge *(arrow)* in the muscle caused when the patient is asked to contract the muscle.

TABLE **1.21**

Functional Division of Muscle Groups[a]

Muscles Prone to Tightness (Postural Muscles)	Muscles Prone to Weakness (Phasic Muscles)
• Gastrocnemius and soleus • Tibialis posterior • Short hip adductors • Hamstrings • Rectus femoris • Iliopsoas • Tensor fasciae latae • Piriformis • Erector spinae (especially lumbar, thoracolumbar, and cervical portions) • Quadratus lumborum • Pectoralis major • Upper portion of trapezius • Levator scapulae • Sternocleidomastoid • Scalenes • Flexors of the upper limb	• Peronei • Tibialis anterior • Vastus medialis and lateralis • Gluteus maximus, medius, and minimus • Rectus abdominis • External oblique • Serratus anterior • Rhomboids • Lower portion of trapezius • Short cervical flexors • Extensors of upper limb

[a]Janda considers all other muscles neutral.
Modified from Jull G, Janda V: Muscles and motor control in low back pain. In Twomey LT, Taylor JR, editors: *Physical therapy for the low back: clinics in physical therapy*, New York, 1987, Churchill Livingstone, p 258.

prone to tightness and those that are phasic and prone to weakness. Table 1.22 shows the characteristics of postural and phasic muscles. If a muscle imbalance is present, the tight muscles must first be stretched to their normal length and tone before strength can be equalized.[151,152]

TABLE **1.22**

Characteristics of Postural and Phasic Muscle Groups

Muscles Prone to Tightness (Postural Muscles)	Muscles Prone to Weakness (Phasic Muscles)
Predominantly postural function	Primarily phasic function
Associated with flexor reflexes	Associated with extensor reflexes
Primarily two-joint muscles	Primarily one-joint muscles
Readily activated with movement (shorter chronaxie)	Not readily activated with movement (longer chronaxie)
Tendency to tightness, hypertonia, shortening, or contractures	Tendency to hypotonia, inhibition, or weakness
Resistance to atrophy	Atrophy occurs easily

Modified from Jull G, Janda V: Muscles and motor control in low back pain. In Twomey LT, Taylor JR, editors: *Physical therapy for the low back: clinics in physical therapy*, New York, 1987, Churchill Livingstone.

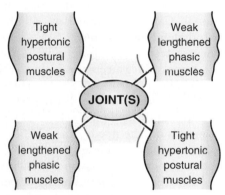

Fig. 1.14 Postural and phasic muscle response to pathology producing "crossed syndromes."

Janda and his associates further expanded this concept with the "upper crossed syndrome" and "pelvic crossed syndrome," which show muscles (primarily postural) on one diagonal at a joint to be tight and hypertonic, whereas muscles on the other diagonal are weak and lengthened (Fig. 1.14).[152,153] This concept of tight and hypertonic muscles in one aspect of a joint with weak lengthened muscles in the opposite aspect is one that examiners should remember for all joints, especially when looking at chronic joint injuries as both types of muscles tend to be present and require different treatment approaches.

In addition, the examiner should always consider the action of **force couples** surrounding a joint. Force couples are counteracting groups of muscles functioning either by cocontraction to stabilize a joint or by one group acting concentrically and the opposing group

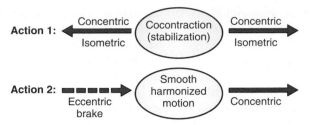

Fig. 1.15 Force couple action.

acting eccentrically to cause a controlled joint motion that is smooth and harmonized (Fig. 1.15).[154] Pathology to one of the force couple muscles or to one of the force couples acting about a joint can lead to muscle imbalance, instability, and loss of smooth coordinated movement.

Other Findings During Movement Testing

When carrying out the examination of the joints, the examiner must be aware of other findings that may become evident and may help to determine the nature and location of the problem. For example, it should be noted whether there is excessive ROM (hypermobility or laxity) within the joints. Comparison of the normal side with the involved side of the body gives some indication as to whether the findings on the affected side would be considered normal. For example, an apparently excessive range (laxity) may just be the normal ROM for that patient. It must also be remembered that joints on the nondominant side tend to be more flexible than those on the dominant side.

It is also important to note whether a **painful arc** is present; this finding indicates that an internal structure is being squeezed or pinched in part of the ROM. Sounds (e.g., crepitus, clicking, or snapping) should be noted. However, to be pathologically significant, these sounds must be related to the patient's symptoms. They may be caused by structures slipping over one another (e.g., tendons slipping over bone), loose bodies or arthritic changes in the joint, abnormal movement of structures (e.g., meniscus click on opening or closing of the temporomandibular joint), or a tear in a structure (e.g., a tear in the triangular cartilaginous disc of the wrist). **Pain at the extreme of ROM** may be caused by squeezing or stretching of structures around the joint or even in the joint, especially if the movement takes the joint into its close packed position.

Functional Assessment

Functional assessment plays an important role in the evaluation of the patient.[155] It is different from the analysis of specific movement patterns of active, passive, and resisted isometric movements used to differentiate between inert, neurological, and contractile tissue. Functional assessment may involve task analysis, observation of certain patient activities, or a detailed evaluation of the effect of the injury or disability on the patient's ability to function in everyday life. Reiman and Manske[156] have organized functional tests into different levels of difficulty for assessment purposes (Table 1.23). Determining what the patient hopes is an appropriate functional outcome, and determining what the patient can and cannot do functionally can be extremely important in the choice of treatments that will be successful. Primarily, functional assessment helps the examiner to establish what is important to the patient and the patient's expectations. It commonly represents a measurement of a **whole-body task performance ability,** as opposed to isolated examination of a joint. That being said, Paxton et al.[157] recommend that functional assessment should involve joint-specific questions and activity level questions along with general health questions. These may be in one questionnaire or in several instruments. Because it is part of each individual joint assessed, the functional testing should demonstrate whether an isolated impairment affects the patient's ability to perform everyday activities.

The examiner should attempt to establish what functional factors are important to the patient. For example, functional testing may include movements under different loads to determine the patient's ability to work or play. Likewise, repeated movements and sustained postures may be necessary for work, recreational, or social activities. In some cases, movements at different speeds or under different loads may be necessary to determine pathology.[113] For example, a traumatic shoulder instability may not be evident in a swimmer except when he or she is actually doing the activity at the speed and load at which the activity is done in the water.

Because functional testing relates to the effect of the injury on the patient's life, those activities that cause symptoms, those that are restricted by symptoms, and the factors (e.g., strength, power, flexibility) that are needed to perform the activities must be considered. For example, if the patient is seated normally while a history is taken, the examiner knows the patient has the functional ROM (agility) for sitting with 90° of hip and knee flexion. Table 1.24 lists some functional outcome measures that should be considered. The activities should be simple, patient-oriented, and based on coordinated functional movement of the joints, and they should be activities the patient wants to do. Although most functional outcomes or tests are subjective, this does not make them any less effective.[158]

The functional assessment is important to determine the effect of the condition or injury on the patient's daily life, including his or her sex life. Functional impairment may be slightly annoying or completely disabling for the patient. Functional activities that should be tested, if appropriate, include self-care activities, such as walking, dressing, daily hygiene (e.g., washing, bathing, shaving, combing hair), eating, and going to the bathroom; recreational activities, such as reading, sewing, watching television, gardening, and playing a musical instrument; and other activities, such as driving, dialing a telephone, getting groceries, preparing meals, and hanging clothes. Goldstein nicely divided activities of human function into four broad areas, which are then broken down into more discrete levels (eTable 1.1).[159] The examiner should consider which of these are important to the patient and ensure that they are considered in the assessment. eTool 1.7 shows some of the daily living skills and mobility questions that may be of concern to both the examiner and the patient. The Short Musculoskeletal Function Assessment (SMFA) helps to determine how much the patient is bothered by functional problems (eTool 1.8).[160] Other functional assessment tool (FAT) examples that are available include the Functional Capacity Evaluation (FCE),[159] the Functional Independence Measure (FIM),[161] the physical performance test,[162] the functional status test,[163] the Arthritis Impact Measurement Scale (AIMS) 2,[164] the FAT,[165] the Short-Form-36 (SF-36) Health Status Survey,[166,167] the Sickness Impact Profile,[168] the SMFA Questionnaire,[169] and the Sock Test.[170] The particular tool used depends on the needs of the patient and the presenting pathological problem.

Part of this functional assessment occurs during the history when the examiner asks the patient which activities can be done easily, which can be done with some difficulty, and which cannot be done at all. During the observation, the examiner notes what the patient can and cannot do within the confines of the assessment area. Finally, during the examination, functional testing or a work analysis may be performed. For example, when examining the hand, the examiner notes the power and dexterity exhibited during performance of fundamental maneuvers, such as gripping and pinching. The following is an example of a work activity analysis, which may be evaluated if the patient is hoping to return to that activity and to do it successfully.[171] Regardless of which functional test is used, the examiner must understand the purpose of the test. A functional test should not be done just because it is available. It should not be used in isolation but rather in conjunction with the overall assessment so that a complete assessment picture of the patient can be developed.

TABLE **1.23**

Levels That Can Be Used for Assessment of Function in an Individual

Levels for the Assessment of Function	Assessment Examples
Level I	
Assessment primarily at the level of subjective report (patient and clinician)	• Self-report measures most indicative of dysfunction • Biopsychosocial measures relevant to dysfunction • Self-report of activity rating scales (patient interpretation on specific requirements of his/her necessary activity level to return to previous level of function) • Clinician analysis of specific sport/occupation/ADLs with respect to requirements (e.g., specific type of movements, energy system involvement)
Level II	
Assessment primarily at the level of impairment	• Anthropometric measurements (e.g., body mass index, girth and height measurements) • Muscle length • Manual muscle testing • ROM • Sensation • Joint play
Level III	
Assessment primarily at the level of static observation/posture/balance	• Static posture • Static balance (bilateral and single-leg balance static assessment)
Level IV	
Assessment primarily at the level of dynamic posture, general movement patterns, and single plane dynamic balance	• Dynamic posture (i.e., posture of individual as he or she performs movements required) • General movement patterns (e.g., walking, transfer movements) • Dynamic balance predominantly in one plane of movement without quality assessment (e.g., functional reach test, tandem walking)
Level V	
Assessment primarily at the level of movement patterns encountered during higher level tasks and/or multiplanar dynamic balance	• Assessment of movement patterns the individual performs with his or her primary tasks (e.g., specific sport, occupational, and other tasks) • Four square step
Level VI	
Assessment primarily at the level of specific movement patterns	• Functional movement screen • Movement impairment syndrome assessment
Level VII	
Assessment of the individual primarily at the level of PPM occurring predominantly in one plane of movement	• 1RM testing • Trunk endurance • Sit-up endurance • Supine bridge • Loaded forward reach • Lunge • Flexed arm hang • Step-down • Single-leg squat • Single-leg inclined squat on total gym
Level VIII	

Assessment primarily at the level of PPM occurring predominantly in one plane of movement, but requiring one or more of the following:
• Limited base of support
• Multiple joint involvement
• Multiple muscle group involvement
• Explosive movement
	• Aerobic endurance testing one or more of the following:
	  ◦ 1-mile walk
	  ◦ Rockport walk
	  ◦ 1- to 5-mile run
	  ◦ 12-min run
	  ◦ 20-meter shuttle run
	• Wingate anaerobic power
	• Star excursion balance test
	• Knee bending in 30 seconds
	• Single jump and hop testing in one plane of movement for one or more of the following:
	  ◦ Standing long jump
	  ◦ Single-hop for distance
	  ◦ Vertical jump
	• Seated chest pass
	• Seated shot put throw

Continued

TABLE **1.23**

Levels That Can Be Used for Assessment of Function in an Individual—cont'd

Levels for the Assessment of Function	Assessment Examples

Level IX
 	
Assessment primarily at the level of PPM occurring predominantly in multiple planes of movement and/or requiring explosive movement
	• Jump and hop testing in multiple planes of movement or requiring multiple jumps or hops for one or more of the following:
	  ◦ Side-hop
	  ◦ One-legged cyclic hop
	  ◦ Hexagon jump
	  ◦ Modified hexagon hop
	  ◦ Figure-eight hop
	  ◦ Carioca drill
	  ◦ 6-meter timed hop
	  ◦ Triple jump for distance
	  ◦ Triple hop for distance
	  ◦ Single-leg crossover hop for distance
	  ◦ Hop testing after fatigue
	• Shuttle run
	• Bosco test
	• Running-based anaerobic sprint test
	• Lower extremity functional test
	• Speed and agility testing for one or more of the following:
	  ◦ Edgren side-step
	  ◦ Illinois agility
	  ◦ Pro agility (5-10-5)
	  ◦ Three-cone drill
	  ◦ T-test
	  ◦ Zigzag run
	• Sidearm medicine ball throw
	• Underkoffler softball throw for distance

Level X Assessment primarily at the level of PPM in multiple planes and/or explosive type of movement with the quality of the performance also assessed	• Balance error scoring system • Functional throwing performance index • Multiple single-leg hop stabilization • Tinetti assessment tool
Level XI Assessment primarily at the level of replication of the specific tasks performed during the individual's sport/occupation/daily activity and/or clustering of PPM that replicate component(s) of the sport/occupation/daily activity	• Functional capacity evaluation • Firefighting "ability test" • BEAST90 • Functional abilities test
Level XII Cumulative assessment (FPT) including performance assessment (quantitative and qualitative) with self-report and biopsychosocial measures	Assessment forward and backward along the functional continuum using each parameter of function (i.e., impairment, performance measures, and self-report measures) as necessary

1RM, One repetition maximum; *ADL,* activities of daily living, *BEAST90,* ball-sport endurance and sprint test; *FPT,* functional performance testing; *PPM,* performance-based measures; *ROM,* range of motion.

Modified from Reiman MP, Manske RC: The assessment of function how is it measured? A clinical perspective, *J Man Manip Ther* 19:95–97, 2011.

Example of an Analysis of Work Activity

Job title: *Packer*
Essential function: Packing individual cobbler cups for shipping

STEPS

1. Select a box
2. Place the box on the conveyor side rack
3. Pick up one cobbler cup in each hand
4. Place the cups into the packing box
5. Repeat steps 3 and 4 until 36 cups are in a box
6. Place the filled box on the "sealing table"
7. Fold the short flaps of the box lid
8. Fold the longer flaps of the box lid
9. Tape down the long flaps of the box using the manual taping machine
10. Place the sealed box on the pallet

From Ellexson MT: Analyzing an industry: job analysis for treatment, prevention, and placement, *Orthop Phys Ther Clin* 1:17, 1992.

Numerical scoring systems are often used as part of the functional assessment and often play a role in **clinical prediction rules** (also called **clinical decision rules** or **risk scores**) that quantify different parts of the history, physical examination, and laboratory results in making a diagnosis or prognosis.[172–176] By combining the different clinical findings, it is felt that a clinician's diagnostic accuracy is increased.[8,155,172,177–180] Clinical prediction rules, which are usually based on 3 to 5 clinical characteristics, should not be used in isolation and are not designed to replace clinical judgement.[181] They are adjuncts to the assessment process identifying a set of predictors that will correctly classify a patient's current status or future state.[180,182] They aid in the process of making a diagnosis, help to establish a likely prognosis, and help to select an appropriate intervention.[182] Proper utilization of the rules is determined by how similar the characteristics of the patient or target population is to the cohort that provided the developmental data.[18,155,182,183] The Ottawa Ankle and Foot Rules and the Pittsburgh Knee Rules are examples of clinical prediction rules.[114,181]

The numeric scoring systems are often more related to function as it applies to a specific joint and often a specific activity rather than to the whole body (eTool 1.9),[184] and for many, functional assessment plays only a small part. With these numeric systems, the clinician must ensure that the scoring systems really measure what they say they measure. To be effective, a numeric scoring system must demonstrate universality, practicality, reliability, reproducibility, effectiveness, and inclusiveness, and it must have been validated.[185] The terminology and methods must be described precisely; the criteria should be related to functional outcome (what the patient desires) rather than clinical outcome (what the clinician desires), and the measures must be sensitive enough to show a difference.[186] eTool 1.10 shows a functional assessment involving the entire upper limb.[187] Table 1.25 demonstrates tests that could be used in an examination of simulated activities of daily living (ADLs).[188] Similar charts can and have been developed for almost all joints of the body. However, many of these numeric scoring systems have been developed from the clinician's perspective rather than from what the patient thinks is important.

Functional tests may also be used as provocative tests to bring on the symptoms the patient has complained of or to determine how the patient is progressing or whether he or she is ready to return to activity. Examples of these tests include the hop test and disco test for the knee. These tests, in reality, could be used for all the weight-bearing (lower limb) joints. However, it must be remembered that many of these provocative or stress tests are designed for very active persons and are not suitable for all populations.

Special (Diagnostic) Tests

After the examiner has completed the history, observation, and evaluation of movement, special tests may be performed for the involved joint. Many special tests are available for each joint to determine whether a particular type of disease, condition, or injury is present. They are sometimes called *clinical accessory, provocative, motion, palpation,* or *structural tests.* These tests, although strongly suggestive of a particular disease or condition when they yield positive results, do not necessarily rule out the disease or condition when they yield negative results. This will depend on the sensitivity and specificity of each test, as well as the skill and experience of the clinician.

Special tests should seldom be used in isolation or as "stand-alone" tests. They should be considered only as part of an overall clinical assessment that includes history, observation, and the rest of the examination.[189,190] One of the problems with special tests is that many clinicians, especially those with less experience, hope that any special tests they

TABLE **1.24**

Examples of Functional and Clinical Outcomes

Clinical Outcomes	Functional Outcomes
• Strength	• Power
• Range of motion	• Agility
• Proprioception	• Kinesthetic awareness
• Endurance (muscular)	• Endurance (muscular and cardiovascular)
• Swelling	• Speed
• Pain	• Activity specificity
• Psychological overlay	• Pain
	• Skill level required for activity
	• Psychological preparedness
	• Daily living skills

TABLE **1.25**

Summary Description of Tests in Simulated Activities of Daily Living Examination (SADLE)

Test	Measure	Units	Instrumentation
Two-leg standing, eyes open	Maximum time of three 30-second trials	Seconds	Stopwatch
One-leg standing, eyes open	Maximum time of three 30-second trials	Seconds	Stopwatch
Two-leg standing, eyes closed	Maximum time of three 30-second trials	Seconds	Stopwatch
One-leg standing, eyes closed	Maximum time of three 30-second trials	Seconds	Stopwatch
Tandem walking with supports	Time to take 10 heel-to-toe steps	Steps/second	Stopwatch and parallel bars
Tandem walking without supports	Time to take 10 heel-to-toe steps	Steps/second	Stopwatch and parallel bars
Putting on a shirt	Average time of two trials	Seconds	Stopwatch and shirt
Managing three visible buttons	Average time of two trials	Seconds	Stopwatch and cloth with three buttons mounted on a board
Zipping a garment	Average time of two trials	Seconds	Stopwatch and cloth with zipper mounted on a board
Putting on gloves	Average time of two trials	Seconds	Stopwatch and two garden gloves
Dialing a telephone	Average time of two trials	Seconds	Stopwatch and telephone
Tying a bow	Average time of two trials	Seconds	Stopwatch and large shoelaces mounted on a board
Manipulating safety pins	Average time of two trials	Seconds	Stopwatch and two safety pins
Picking up coins	Average time of two trials	Seconds	Stopwatch and four coins placed on a plastic sheet
Threading a needle	Average time of two trials	Seconds	Stopwatch, thread, and large-eyed needle
Unwrapping a Band-Aid	Time for one trial	Seconds	Stopwatch and one Band-Aid
Squeezing toothpaste	Average time of two trials	Seconds	Stopwatch, tube of toothpaste, and a board
Cutting with a knife	Average time of two trials	Seconds	Stopwatch, plate, fork, knife, and Permoplast
Using a fork	Average time of two trials	Seconds	Stopwatch, plate, fork, and Permoplast

Modified from Potvin AR, Tourtellotte WW, Dailey JS, et al: Simulated activities of daily living examination, *Arch Phys Med Rehab* 53:478, 1972.

use will give them a definitive answer as to what is wrong.[191] Although a special test may give a definitive answer, more commonly it does not, but combined with the other information from the assessment, a clearer picture of the problem arises. No physical test is 100% reliable, valid, sensitive, or specific. In this book, the author has highlighted key tests that the clinician should practice, become comfortable with, and become confident in their use because the value of these tests has been demonstrated clinically (via examiner experience) and/or statistically to show that they contribute to determining what the problem is. It is better to learn one or two tests well and to be confident and proficient in their use rather than learning all the possible tests used to confirm a certain pathology. The "Key to Classifying Special Tests" has been developed to give an indication whether the author feels it is worthwhile to learn to do the test based on present evidence and the clinician's experience. That being said, even the tests with an ✓ icon will or can be ineffective if the conditions outlined in the "Key for Classifying Special Tests" box are not met. Without these conditions being met, even the best test may fail to confirm the diagnosis regardless of its utility score, Quality Assessment of Diagnostic Accuracy Studies (QUADUS) score, or reliability or validity value.[192,193] The research on the tests is important but so is the experience of the clinician and the "state" of the patient. The ✓ icon does not imply the tests are infallible. It means they are useful along with the history and the rest of the examination in making a diagnosis.

Key for Classifying Special Tests

The following is based on the authors' clinical experience and review of the literature:

☑ Implies that the test has moderate to strong statistical (research) and clinical (examiner experience) support, or the authors have found the test useful along with the history and examination in making a clinical diagnosis

⚠ Implies that the test has minimal statistical (research) and some clinical (examiner experience) support, or the authors have found the test helpful along with the history and examination in making a clinical diagnosis

❓ Implies that the test has insufficient statistical (research) evidence, but it may demonstrate clinical support for its use in the hands of an experienced examiner along with the history and examination in making a clinical diagnosis

Special Test Considerations

Any special test, regardless of its classification, can be positively or negatively affected by the:
- Patient's ability to relax
- Presence of pain and the patient's perception of the pain
- Presence of patient apprehension
- Skill of the clinician
- Ability and confidence of the clinician

When deciding to use these diagnostic tests or grouping or clustering them in clinical prediction rules, the examiner must determine if the test will give reliable and useful information that will help in the diagnosis and subsequent treatment.[194,195] To be useful, a diagnostic test must give reliable data (i.e., consistent results regardless of who does the test), must be valid (i.e., test what it says it tests), and must be accurate to maximize patient outcomes.[194,196] As previously stated, care must be taken considering the usefulness of a special test, because the test is influenced by both the patient and the clinician. One single study reporting on the reliability, validity, or other measures of test usefulness gives a good indication that the test can be useful in certain circumstances (in this case, those circumstances used to test the test), but research studies always involve compromises in terms of what is controlled and what is not controlled when doing the study. For example, many tests are confirmed during surgery when the patient is unconscious. Looking at the analysis of one test by different authors shows the wide variability in outcomes.[197,198] Given all these factors, it is easy to see that special tests, although they have an important role to play, should not be used in isolation, nor should they be the single deciding factor in making a diagnosis.

Reliability may be affected by cooperation of the patient, which may be influenced by the patient's ability to relax, tolerate pain, describe apprehension, and show

TABLE **1.26**

Benchmark Intraclass Correlation Coefficient Values

Value	Description
<0.75	Poor to moderate agreement
>0.75	Good agreement
>90	Reasonable agreement for clinical measurements

Data from Portney LG, Walkins MP: *Foundations of clinical research—applications to practice*, Upper Saddle River, NJ, 2000, Prentice-Hall, p 565.

sincerity; it may be affected by the skill of the clinician, which may be influenced by experience, his or her ability to relax, and to confidently do the test; and it may be affected by the calibration of equipment.[194] Several methods are used to determine reliability, but the intraclass correlation coefficient (ICC) is the preferred index because it reflects both agreement and correlation among ratings.[199] It is calculated through analysis of variance (ANOVA) using variance estimates.[199] Table 1.26 shows ICC agreement values that are illustrative for diagnostic tests. With nominal data, the kappa statistic (κ) is applied after the percentage agreement between testers has been determined.[199]

When performing a test, it is also useful, in terms of reliability, to know the standard error of measurement (SEM).[199] The SEM reflects the reliability of the response when the test is performed many times. It is an indication of how much change there might be when a test is repeated. If the SEM is small, then the test is stable with minimal variability between tests.[199]

Diagnostic tests should be evaluated on their diagnostic accuracy or ability to determine which people have the condition or disease and those who do not as this will have an impact on subsequent treatment and patient outcomes.[200] The most useful methods of determining whether a test is a good test for the pathology under consideration are sensitivity, specificity, and likelihood ratios.[194–196,199–208] Sensitivity implies the ability of a test to identify people who have a particular condition, dysfunction, or disease when they do (i.e., a true-positive).[194,196,199,205,208] Specificity, on the other hand, is used to determine which people do not have a particular condition, dysfunction, or disease (i.e., a true-negative).[194,196,198,204,208] Sensitivity and specificity values for tests are usually based on a "gold standard," or reference test (e.g., diagnostic imaging, what was found at surgery).[208,209] If the clinician is unsure that the patient has a particular condition, dysfunction or disease, then the examiner would want to use a test of exclusion or discovery that has a high sensitivity as it will rule out those people who do not have the problem, provided the test's specificity is equal to or higher than another test testing for the same thing.[203] On the other hand, if the examiner has a high level of suspicion (based on the preceding history, observation, and examination) that the problem is present and wants to confirm that decision (confirmation test), then the examiner would want a test with higher specificity to "rule in" those people who do have the problem, provided the test's sensitivity is equal to or higher than another test testing for the same thing.[196,203] This is especially true if further evaluation or treatment is expensive or dangerous. To prevent healthy people from receiving unnecessary expensive or dangerous treatment, high specificity is desired.[204] In an ideal world, one would want a test that has both high sensitivity and high specificity. To try to solve these differences in levels of sensitivity and specificity, likelihood ratios are often recommended as determinants of the usefulness of a test.[194,196,200,203,205,210] Likelihood ratios are based on determining the odds that a condition, dysfunction, or disease is present by combining sensitivity and specificity to indicate whether the test will raise or lower the probability of the patient having the condition, dysfunction, or disease.[194,205] The higher the likelihood ratio, the greater is the likelihood that the patient has the problem.

There are two other issues that the clinician should be aware of when considering special or diagnostic tests. Although beyond the scope of this book, clinicians should also consider responsiveness, which is the ability of a test to detect a clinically important change, and the minimal clinically important difference (MCID), which is the smallest difference in the result of a test that the clinician perceives as beneficial or significant in the context that it may result in a particular treatment or change in treatment.[201,202,211,212]

Tests can be more accurately performed right after injury (during the period of tissue shock—5 to 10 minutes after injury), under anesthesia, or in chronic conditions where pain may be less of a factor. Each examiner tends to use those tests he or she has found to be clinically effective. Under no circumstances should special tests be used in isolation, nor is it necessary to learn all of the special tests. They should be viewed as an integral part of a total examination.[213] They should be considered as tests to confirm a tentative diagnosis, to make a differential diagnosis, to differentiate between structures, to understand unusual signs, or to unravel difficult signs and symptoms.[112]

Special Test Uses[112]

- To confirm a tentative diagnosis
- To make a differential diagnosis
- To differentiate between structures
- To understand unusual signs
- To unravel difficult signs and symptoms

Note: Special tests should NOT be used in isolation.

For each joint examination described in this book, specific tests are mentioned for specific conditions. The tests can be used to differentiate contractile, inert, and neurological pathology.

Currently, most clinicians want to use only tests that are highly reliable and have good sensitivity and specificity. Although this goal is highly desirable, it is not always possible. Several books have quantified the value of some of these tests, and in reviewing these books it will be seen that for many of the tests their utility is questioned.[197,198] Thus, as previously mentioned, these tests should not be used in isolation but as part of a much larger assessment. In this book, the author has included many special tests—more like an encyclopedia of tests, rather than only the ones that have shown good reliability, sensitivity, or specificity. This has been done for three reasons: (1) to provide a source for different tests, (2) to provide test examples for individuals who may want to test the reliability, specificity, and sensitivity of the tests where this has not been done before, and (3) to show that test results depend on the state of the patient and the ability and experience of the clinician. Tests that the author has found to be particularly effective and have provided useful and reliable information have been highlighted in boxes, and the author recommends that the students learn *these* tests. Many of the tests are similar and show similar results; the choice of which ones to use depends on which ones give the best results for the individual examiner and which tests provide the most useful and reliable information to the examiner.[214] For example, both the Lachman test and anterior drawer test may be used to test the anterior cruciate ligament, although the literature indicates the Lachman test is more sensitive.[215,216]

If desired, the examiner can design his or her own special tests or modify the described tests. Sometimes, the examiner can reproduce the same movement that the patient described as the mechanism of injury, which may provoke the symptoms. However, the addition of too many special tests only makes the picture more confusing and the diagnosis more difficult. In addition, care should be taken when performing these tests, because they are usually provocative tests and will provoke signs and symptoms, including pain and apprehension. Thus special tests should be done with caution and may be contraindicated in the presence of severe pain, acute and irritable conditions of the joints, instability, osteoporosis, pathological bone diseases, active disease processes, unusual signs and symptoms, major neurological signs, and patient apprehension.

In addition to the special tests, the examiner may also make use of **laboratory tests** ordered by a physician for specific conditions. With osteomyelitis, for example, a positive blood culture is likely to be obtained, the white blood cell count will be elevated, and the erythrocyte sedimentation rate will be increased. If a physician is the examiner, he or she may decide to draw fluid out of a joint

TABLE 1.27

Normal Laboratory Values Used in Orthopedic Medicine[a]

Laboratory Test	Normal Range
White blood cell (WBC) count	$4–9 \times 10^9/L$
Red blood cell (RBC) count	$4.3–5.4 \times 10^{12}/L$ (male) $3.8–5.2 \times 10^{12}/L$ (female)
Hematocrit (HCT)	38%–50% (male) 34%–46% (female)
Hemoglobin (Hgb)	130–170 g/L (male) 115–160 g/L (female)
Erythrocyte sedimentation rate (ESR)	0–10 mm/hour (male) 0–15 mm/hour (female) 0–10 mm/hour (children)
Myoglobin (Mb)	30–90 ng/mL
Ferritin	25–465 µg/mL (male) 15–200 µg/mL (female)
Platelet count	140,000–350,000/mm³
Calcium	8.5–10.5 mg/dL
Ionized calcium	4.2–5.4 mg/dL
Alkaline phosphatase	25–92 U/L
Antinuclear antibodies screen	Negative
Uric acid	3.5–7.2 mg/dL (male) 2.6–6.0 mg/dL (female)
Rheumatoid arthritis factor	<1.20

[a]Values may vary slightly depending on equipment used.

(aspirate) with a hypodermic needle to view the synovial fluid. Tables 1.27 to 1.29 present normal laboratory values, laboratory findings in some bone diseases, and a classification of synovial fluid as examples of laboratory tests and values.

Reflexes and Cutaneous Distribution

After the special tests, the examiner can test the superficial, deep tendon, or pathological reflexes to obtain an indication of the state of the nerve or nerve roots supplying the reflex. If the neurological system is thought to be normal, there is no need to test the reflexes or cutaneous distribution. However, if the examiner is unsure whether there is neurological involvement, both reflexes and sensation should be tested to clarify the problem and where the problem actually is.

Most often, the deep tendon reflexes (sometimes referred to as *muscle stretch reflexes*)[41] are tested with a reflex hammer. A deep tendon reflex can be elicited from almost any tendon with practice. The more common deep tendon reflexes tested are shown in Table 1.30. Tables 1.31 and 1.32 demonstrate superficial and pathological

reflexes. Superficial reflexes are provoked by superficial stroking, usually with a sharp object. A pathological reflex is not normally present, except in the very young (<5 to 7 months) in whom the cerebrum is not fully developed.[42] If it is present in adults and children, it often signals a pathological condition.

With a loss or abnormality of nerve conduction, there is a diminution (hyporeflexia) or loss (areflexia) of the stretch reflex. Aging also causes a decreased response. Upper motor neuron lesions produce findings of spasticity, hyperreflexia, hypertonicity, extensor plantar responses, reduced or absent superficial reflexes, and weakness of muscles distal to the lesion. Lower motor neuron lesions involving nerve roots or peripheral nerves produce findings of flaccidity, hyporeflexia or areflexia, hypotonicity, fasciculation, fibrillations, and weakness and atrophy of the involved muscles (see Table 1.12).[217]

Deep tendon reflexes are performed to test the integrity of the spinal reflex, which has a sensory (afferent) and motor (efferent) component.[17] Abnormal deep tendon reflexes are not clinically relevant unless they are found with sensory or motor abnormalities. To properly test the deep tendon reflexes, the patient must be relaxed and the examiner must ensure that the muscle of the tendon to be tested is relaxed. The tendon to be tested is put on slight stretch, and an adequate stimulus is applied by dropping the reflex hammer onto the tendon. The examiner should tap the tendon five or six times to uncover any fading reflex response, indicative of developing nerve root signs. If the deep tendon reflexes are difficult to elicit, the reflexes often can be enhanced by having the patient clench the teeth or squeeze the hands together (**Jendrassik maneuver**) when testing the lower limb or squeeze the legs together when testing the upper limb. These activities increase the facilitative activity of the spinal cord and thereby accentuate minimally active reflexes.[218]

Superficial reflexes are tested by stroking the skin with a moderately sharp object that does not break the skin. The expected responses are shown in Table 1.31. A great deal of practice is needed to become proficient in testing the superficial reflexes.

Pathological reflexes, which are not usually evident because they are suppressed by the cerebrum at the brain stem or spinal cord level (see Table 1.32), may indicate upper motor neuron lesions if present on both sides or lower motor neuron lesions if present on only one side.[42] Improper stimulation (e.g., too much pressure) may lead to voluntary withdrawal in normal subjects, and the examiner must take care not to confuse this reaction with the pathological response. The two most commonly tested pathological reflexes are the Babinski reflex (lower limb) and the Hoffman reflex (upper limb).

To be of clinical significance, findings must show asymmetry between bilateral reflexes unless there is a central lesion. The eliciting of reflexes often depends on the skill of the examiner. The examiner should not be overly

TABLE **1.28**

Laboratory Findings in Bone Disease

Condition	Calcium	Inorganic Phosphorus	Alkaline Phosphatase	Calcium	Phosphorus
Hyperparathyroidism, primary	↑	↓	↑	↑	↑
Hyperparathyroidism, secondary	N-↓	↑	R↑	↑	↑
Hyperthyroidism, marked	N	N	↑	↑	↑
Hypothyroidism	N	N	N	N	N
Senile osteoporosis	N	N-O↓	N	N	N
Rickets (child)	↓	↓	↑	N	N
Osteomalacia (adult)	N-↓	↓	↑	N	N
Paget disease	R↑	R↓	↑	N	N
Multiple myeloma	↑	N-↑	R↑	↑	↑

N, Normal; *O*, occasionally; *R*, rarely; ↑, increased; ↓, decreased.
Adapted from Quinn J: Introduction to the musculoskeletal system. In Meschan I, editor: *Synopsis of analysis of roentgen signs in general radiology*, Philadelphia, 1976, W.B. Saunders Co., p 27.

TABLE **1.29**

Classification of Synovial Fluid

Fluid Type	Appearance	Total WBC Count/mm³	%PMNs
Normal	Clear, viscous, pale yellow	0 to 200	<10%
Group 1 (noninflammatory)	Clear to slightly turbid	200 to 2000	<20%
Group 2 (inflammatory)	Slightly turbid (cloudy)	2000 to 50,000	20% to 75%
Group 3 (pyarthrosis)	Turbid to very turbid, purulent	>50,000 to 100,000	>75%
Group 4 (crystal induced)	White, cloudy, turbid	500 to 200,000	>90%
Group 5 (hemorrhagic)	Red	200 to 2000	50% to 75%

Modified from Spender RT: Arthrocentesis and synovial fluid analysis. In West SG: *Rheumatology secrets,* ed 3, Philadelphia, 2015, Elsevier.

TABLE **1.30**

Common Deep Tendon Reflexes

Reflex	Site of Stimulus	Normal Response	Pertinent Central Nervous System Segment
Jaw	Mandible	Mouth closes	Cranial nerve V
Biceps	Biceps tendon	Biceps contraction	C5–C6
Brachioradialis	Brachioradialis tendon or just distal to the musculotendinous junction	Flexion of elbow and/or pronation of forearm	C5–C6
Triceps	Distal triceps tendon above the olecranon process	Elbow extension/muscle contraction	C7–C8
Patella	Patellar tendon	Leg extension	L3–L4
Medial hamstrings	Semimembranosus tendon	Knee flexion/muscle contraction	L5, S1
Lateral hamstrings	Biceps femoris tendon	Knee flexion/muscle contraction	S1–S2
Tibialis posterior	Tibialis posterior tendon behind medial malleolus	Plantar flexion of foot with inversion	L4–L5
Achilles	Achilles tendon	Plantar flexion of foot	S1–S2

concerned if the reflexes are absent, diminished, or excessive on both sides, especially in young people, unless a central lesion is suspected. Exercise just before testing or patient anxiety or tenseness may lead to accentuated tendon reflexes.[106] Hyporeflexia or areflexia indicates a lesion of a peripheral nerve or spinal nerve root as a result of impingement, entrapment, or injury. Examples would be nerve root compression, cauda equina syndrome, or peripheral neuropathy. Hyporeflexia or areflexia may be seen in the absence of muscle weakness or atrophy because of the involvement of the efferent loop of the reflex arc in the reflex. Hyperactive or exaggerated reflexes (hyperreflexia) indicate upper motor neuron lesions as seen in neurological disease and cerebral or brain stem impairment. If a disc herniation and compression occur above the cervical enlargement in the cervical spine, the reflexes of the upper extremity are exaggerated. If the cervical enlargement is involved (which is more commonly the case), then some reflexes are exaggerated and some are decreased.[219]

TABLE **1.31**

Superficial Reflexes

Reflex	Normal Response	Pertinent Central Nervous System Segment
Upper abdominal	Umbilicus moves up and toward area being stroked	T7–T9
Lower abdominal	Umbilicus moves down and toward area being stroked	T11–T12
Cremasteric	Scrotum elevates	T12, L1
Plantar	Flexion of toes	S1–S2
Gluteal	Skin tenses in gluteal area	L4–L5, S1–S3
Anal	Contraction of anal sphincter muscles	S2–S4

Deep Tendon Reflex Grading

0—Absent (areflexia)
1—Diminished (hyporeflexia)
2—Average (normal)
3—Exaggerated (brisk)
4—Clonus, very brisk (hyperreflexia)

At the same time, the examiner can perform a **sensory scanning examination** by checking the cutaneous distribution of the various peripheral nerves and the dermatomes around the joint being examined. The sensory

TABLE **1.32**

Pathological Reflexes[a]

Reflex	Elicitation	Positive Response	Pathology
Babinski[b]	Stroking of lateral aspect of sole of foot	Extension of big toe and fanning of four small toes Normal reaction in newborns	Pyramidal tract lesion Organic hemiplegia
Chaddock	Stroking of lateral side of foot beneath lateral malleolus	Same response as above	Pyramidal tract lesion
Oppenheim	Stroking of anteromedial tibial surface	Same response as above	Pyramidal tract lesion
Gordon	Squeezing of calf muscles firmly	Same response as above	Pyramidal tract lesion
Piotrowski	Percussion of tibialis anterior muscle	Dorsiflexion and supination of foot	Organic disease of central nervous system
Brudzinski	Passive flexion of one lower limb	Similar movement occurs in opposite limb	Meningitis
Hoffman (Digital)[c]	"Flicking" of terminal phalanx of index, middle, or ring finger	Reflex flexion of distal phalanx of thumb and of distal phalanx of index or middle finger (whichever one was not "flicked")	Increased irritability of sensory nerves in tetany Pyramidal tract lesion
Rossolimo	Tapping of the plantar surface of toes	Plantar flexion of toes	Pyramidal tract lesion
Schaeffer	Pinching of Achilles tendon in middle third	Flexion of foot and toes	Organic hemiplegia

[a]Bilateral positive response indicates an upper motor neuron lesion. Unilateral positive response may indicate a lower motor neuron lesion.
[b]Test most commonly performed in lower limb.
[c]Test most commonly performed in upper limb.

examination is performed for several reasons. First, it is used to determine the extent of sensory loss, whether that loss is caused by nerve root lesions, peripheral nerve lesions, or compressive tunnel syndromes. Second, because function is often tied to sensation, it is used to determine the degree of functional impairment. Third, because sensory function returns before motor function, it can be used to determine nerve recovery after injury or repair as well as when reeducation can commence. In addition, if sensory function remains after injury to the spinal cord, it is a good indication that some motor function, at least, will be restored.[220] Finally, it is part of the total assessment and is often necessary for medicolegal reasons. Although the sensory distribution of peripheral nerves may vary from person to person, they tend to be more consistent than dermatomes.[88,221] The examiner must be able to differentiate between sensory loss involving a nerve root (dermatome) and that involving a peripheral nerve (see Table 1.15 for an example).

The sensory examination begins with a quick scan of sensation. To do this, the examiner runs his or her relaxed hands relatively firmly over the skin to be tested bilaterally and asks the patient whether there are any differences in sensation. The patient's eyes may be open for the scan. If the patient notes any differences in sensation between the affected and unaffected sides, then a more detailed sensory assessment is performed. The examiner should note the patient's ability to perceive the sensation being tested and the difference, if any, between the two sides of the body. In addition, distal and proximal sensitivities should be compared for each form of sensation tested. During the detailed sensory testing, the patient should keep his or her eyes closed so that the results will indicate the patient's perception and interpretation of the stimuli, not what the patient sees happening. With the detailed sensory testing, the examiner marks out, or delineates, the specific area of altered sensation and then correlates the area with the known dermatome and peripheral nerve distribution. However, the examiner must be aware that the abnormal sensation does not necessarily come from the indicated nerve root or peripheral nerve; because of referred pain, it may come from any structure supplied by that nerve root. In some cases, the paresthesia may involve no specific pattern, or it may involve the entire circumference of a limb. This **"opera glove"** or **"stocking" paresthesia** or anesthesia may result from vascular insufficiency or systemic disease.

Superficial tactile (light touch) sensation, which is commonly the first sensation affected, can be tested with a wisp of cotton, soft hairbrush, or small paint or makeup brush. Superficial pain can be tested with a flagged pin (holding a piece of tape attached to a pin), pinwheel, or other sharp object. Only light tapping should be used. Approximately 2 seconds should elapse between each stimulus to avoid summation. It is the group II afferent fibers (Table 1.33) that are being tested. Perception to pinprick may range from absence of awareness, through

TABLE **1.33**

Nerve Fiber Classification

Sensory Axons	Axon Diameter (μm)	Conduction Velocity (m/sec)	Innervation
Ia (Aα)	12–22	65–130	Muscle spindles (annulospiral endings)
Ib (Aα)	12–22	65–130	Golgi tendon organs
II (Aβ)	5–15	20–90	Pressure, touch, vibration (flower spray endings)
III (Aδ)	2–10	6–45	Temperature, fast pain
IV (C)	0.2–1.5	0.2–2.0	Slow pain, visceral, temperature, crude touch

pressure sensation, hyperanalgesia with or without radiation, localization, and sensation of sharpness, to normal perception.

If desired, the examiner may also test other sensations. Two test tubes (one with hot water, one with cold) are used to assess sensitivity to temperature (lateral spinothalamic tract and group III fibers), one containing hot water and one containing cold water. A normal response to this test does not necessarily mean that the patient has normal temperature sensation. Rather, the patient can distinguish between hot and cold, each at one level in the range, but not necessarily between different degrees of hot and cold. Sensitivity to vibration (i.e., how long until vibration stops) may be tested by holding a tuning fork (usually 30- or 256-cps tuning forks are used) against bony prominences; this tests the integrity of group II fibers and the dorsal column and medial lemniscal systems. Deep pressure pain (group II Aβ fibers) can be tested by squeezing the Achilles tendon, the trapezius muscle, or the web space between the thumb and index finger or by applying a knuckle to the sternum. To test proprioception and motion (i.e., the skin and joint receptors, muscle spindles, dorsal column and medial lemniscal systems, and group I and II fibers), the patient's fingers or toes are passively moved, and the patient is asked to indicate the direction of movement and final position while keeping the eyes closed. To ensure that pressure on the patient's skin cannot be used as a clue to direction of movement, the test digit should be grasped between the examiner's thumb and index finger.

Cortical and discriminatory sensations may be tested by two-point discrimination, point localization, texture discrimination, stereognostic function (i.e., identification of familiar objects held in the hand), and graphesthesia (i.e., recognition of letters or numbers written with a blunt object on the patient's palms or other body parts). These techniques also test the integrity of the dorsal column and lemniscal systems.

Joint Play Movements

All synovial and secondary cartilaginous joints, to some extent, are capable of an AROM, termed "voluntary movement" (also called *active physiological movement*) through the action of muscles crossing over the joint. In addition, there is a small ROM that can be obtained only passively by the examiner; this movement is called **joint play** or **accessory movement.** These accessory movements are not under voluntary control; however, they are necessary, for full painless function of the joint and full ROM of the joint. **Joint dysfunction** signifies a loss of joint play movement.

The existence of joint play movement is necessary for full, pain-free voluntary movement to occur. An essential part of the detailed assessment of any joint includes an examination of its joint play movements. If any joint play movement is found to be absent or decreased, this movement must be restored before the patient can regain functional voluntary movement. In most joints, this movement is normally less than 4 mm in any one direction.

Mennell's Rules for Joint Play Testing[222]

- The patient should be relaxed and fully supported
- The examiner should be relaxed and should use a firm but comfortable grasp
- One joint should be examined at a time
- One movement should be examined at a time
- The unaffected side should be tested first
- One articular surface is stabilized, while the other surface is moved
- Movements must be normal and not forced
- Movements should not cause undue discomfort

In some cases, joint play movements may be similar to or the same as movements tested during passive movements or ligamentous testing. This is most obvious in joints that have minimal movement and in joints that do not have muscles acting directly on them, such as the sacroiliac joints and superior tibiofibular joints.

Loose Packed (Resting) Position

To test joint play movement, the examiner places the joint in its resting position, which is the position in its ROM at which the joint is under the least amount of stress; it is also the position in which the joint capsule has its greatest capacity.[223] The resting position (sometimes called the *loose packed* or *maximum loose packed position*) is one of minimal congruency between the articular surfaces and the joint capsule with the ligaments being in the position of greatest laxity and passive separation of the joint surfaces being the greatest. This position may be the anatomic resting position, which is usually considered in the midrange, or it may be just outside the range of pain and spasm. The advantage of the loose packed position is that the joint surface contact areas are reduced and are always

changing to decrease friction and erosion in the joints. The position also provides proper joint lubrication and allows the arthrokinematic movements of spin, slide, and roll. It is therefore the most common position used for treatment using joint play mobilizations. Examples of resting positions are shown in Table 1.34.

Close Packed (Synarthrodial) Position

The close packed position should be avoided as much as possible during an assessment except to stabilize an adjacent joint, because in this position, the majority of joint structures are under maximum tension. In this position, the two joint surfaces fit together precisely (i.e., they are fully congruent). The joint surfaces are tightly compressed; the ligaments and capsule of the joint are maximally tight; and the joint surfaces cannot be separated by distractive forces. It is the position of maximum joint stability. Thus this position is commonly used during treatment to stabilize the joint, if an adjacent joint is being treated. Ligaments, bone, or other joint structures, if injured, become more painful as the close packed position is approached. If a joint is swollen, the close packed position cannot be achieved.[142] In the close packed position, no accessory movement is possible. Examples of the close packed positions of most joints are shown in Table 1.35.

Palpation

Initially, palpation for tenderness plays no part in the assessment because referred tenderness is real and can be misleading. Only after the tissue at fault has been identified is palpation for tenderness used to determine the exact extent of the lesion within that tissue, and then palpation is done only if the tissue lies superficially and within easy reach of the fingers. Palpation is an important assessment technique that must be practiced if it is to be used effectively.[224–227] Tenderness often does enable the examiner to name the affected ligament or the specific section or exact point of the tearing or bruising.

To palpate properly, the examiner must ensure that the area to be palpated is as relaxed as possible. For this to be done, the body part must be supported as much as possible. As the ability to perform palpation develops, the examiner should be able to accomplish the following:

Examiner Observations When Palpating a Patient

- Differences in tissue tension and texture
- Differences in tissue thickness
- Abnormalities
- Tenderness
- Temperature variation
- Pulses, tremors, and fasciculations
- Pathological state of tissues
- Dryness or excessive moisture
- Abnormal sensation

TABLE 1.34

Resting (Loose Packed) Position of Joints

Joint	Position
Facet (cervical, thoracic, and lumbar spine)	Midway between flexion and extension
Temporomandibular	Mouth slightly open (freeway space), lips together, teeth not in contact
Glenohumeral	40° to 55° abduction, 30° horizontal adduction (scapular plane)
Acromioclavicular	Arm resting by side in normal physiological position
Sternoclavicular	Arm resting by side in normal physiological position
Ulnohumeral (elbow)	70° flexion, 10° supination
Radiohumeral	Full extension, full supination
Proximal (superior) radioulnar	70° flexion, 35° supination
Distal (inferior) radioulnar	10° supination
Radiocarpal (wrist)	Neutral with slight ulnar deviation
Intercarpal	Neutral or slight flexion
Midcarpal	Neutral or slight flexion with ulnar deviation
Carpometacarpal (thumb)	Midway between abduction-adduction and flexion-extension
Carpometacarpal (fingers)	Midway between flexion and extension
Metacarpophalangeal	Slight flexion
Interphalangeal	Slight flexion
Sacroiliac (resting)	Neutral pelvis
Sacroiliac (loose pack)	Counternutation
Hip	30° flexion, 30° abduction, slight lateral rotation
Knee (tibiofemoral)	25° flexion
Distal tibiofibular	Plantar flexion
Talocrural (ankle)	10° plantar flexion, midway between maximum inversion and eversion
Subtalar (talocalcaneal)	Midway between extremes of range of movement
Midtarsal	Midway between extremes of range of movement
Tarsometatarsal	Midway between extremes of range of movement
Metatarsophalangeal	10° extension
Interphalangeal	Slight flexion

TABLE 1.35

Close Packed Position of Joints

Joint	Position
Facet (cervical, thoracic, and lumbar spine)	Full extension
Temporomandibular	Clenched teeth
Glenohumeral	Full abduction and lateral rotation
Acromioclavicular	Arm abducted to 90°
Sternoclavicular	Maximum shoulder elevation and protraction
Ulnohumeral (elbow)	Extension with supination
Radiohumeral	Elbow flexed 90°, forearm supinated 5°
Proximal radioulnar	5° supination
Distal radioulnar	5° supination
Radiocarpal (wrist)	Extension with radial deviation
Intercarpal	Extension
Midcarpal	Extension with ulnar deviation
Carpometacarpal (thumb)	Full opposition
Carpometacarpal (fingers)	Full flexion
Metacarpophalangeal (fingers)	Full flexion
Metacarpophalangeal (thumb)	Full opposition
Interphalangeal	Full extension
Sacroiliac	Nutation
Hip	Full extension, medial rotation, abduction
Knee (tibiofemoral)	Full extension, lateral rotation of tibia
Distal tibiofibular	Maximum dorsiflexion
Talocrural (ankle)	Maximum dorsiflexion
Subtalar	Supination
Midtarsal	Supination
Tarsometatarsal	Supination
Metatarsophalangeal	Full extension
Interphalangeal	Full extension

1. Discriminate differences in tissue tension (e.g., effusion, spasm) and muscle tone (i.e., spasticity, rigidity, flaccidity). **Spasticity** refers to muscle tonus in which there may be a collapse of muscle tone during testing. It is the result of hypersensitivity of the reflex arc and changes in the CNS resulting in overactivity of muscles and is a component of an upper motor neuron lesion.[134] **Rigidity** refers to involuntary

resistance being maintained during passive movement and without collapse of the muscle. It is the result of hypertonia seen in extrapyramidal lesions.[134] **Flaccidity** means there is no muscle tone.

2. Distinguish differences in tissue texture. For example, the examiner can, in some cases, palpate the direction of fibers or presence of fibrous bands.
3. Identify shapes, structures, and tissue type and thereby detect abnormalities. For example, bone deformities (e.g., myositis ossificans) may be palpated.
4. Determine tissue thickness and texture and determine whether it is pliable, soft, and resilient. Is there any obvious swelling? Edema is an abnormal accumulation of fluid in the intercellular spaces; in contrast, swelling is the abnormal enlargement of a body part. It may be the result of bone thickening, synovial membrane thickening, or fluid accumulation in and around the joint. It may be intracellular or extracellular (edema), intracapsular or extracapsular. Swelling may be localized (encapsulated), which may indicate intra-articular swelling, a cyst, or a swollen bursa. Visualization of swelling depends on the depth of the tissue (a swollen olecranon bursa is more obvious than a swollen psoas bursa) and the looseness of the tissues (swelling is more evident on the dorsum of the hand than on the palmar aspect because the dorsal tissues are not "held down" to adjacent tissue). Swelling that develops immediately or within 2 to 4 hours of injury is probably caused by blood extravasation into the tissues (ecchymosis) or joint. Swelling that becomes evident after 8 to 24 hours is caused by inflammation and, in a joint, by synovial swelling. Bony or hard swelling may be caused by osteophytes or new bone formation (e.g., in myositis ossificans). Soft-tissue swelling such as edematous synovium produces a boggy, spongy feeling (like soft sponge rubber), whereas fluid swelling is a softer and more mobile, fluctuating feeling. Blood swelling is usually a harder, thick, gel-like feeling, and the overlying skin is usually warmer. Pus is thick and less fluctuant; the overlying skin is warm, and the temperature is usually elevated. Older, longstanding soft-tissue swelling (e.g., a skin callus) feels like tough, dry leather. Synovial hypertrophy has a hard, thick feeling to it with little give. The more leathery the thickening feels, the more likely it is to be chronic and caused by local symptoms. Softer thickenings tend to be more acute and associated with recent symptoms.[140] Pitting edema is thick and slow moving, leaving an indentation after pressure is applied and removed. It is commonly caused by circulatory stasis and is most commonly seen in the distal extremities. Long-lasting swelling may cause reflex inhibition of the muscles around the joint, leading to atrophy and weakness. Blood swelling within a joint is usually aspirated because of the irritating and damaging effect it has on the joint cartilage.

Swelling

- Comes on soon after injury → blood
- Comes on after 8–24 hours → synovial
- Boggy, spongy feeling → synovial
- Harder, tense feeling with warmth → blood
- Tough, dry → callus
- Leathery thickening → chronic
- Soft, fluctuating → acute
- Hard → bone
- Thick, slow-moving → pitting edema

5. Feel variations in temperature. This determination is usually best done by using the back of the examiner's hand or fingers and comparing both sides. Joints tend to be warm in the acute phase, in the presence of infection, with blood swelling, after exercise, or if they have been covered (e.g., with an elastic bandage).
6. Determine joint tenderness by applying firm pressure to the joint. The pressure should always be applied with care, especially in the acute phase.

Grading Tenderness When Palpating

- Grade I—Patient complains of pain
- Grade II—Patient complains of pain and winces
- Grade III—Patient winces and withdraws the joint
- Grade IV—Patient will not allow palpation of the joint

7. Feel pulses, tremors, and fasciculations. Fasciculations result from contraction of a number of muscle cells innervated by a single motor axon. The contractions are localized, are usually subconscious, and do not involve the whole muscle. Tremors are involuntary movements in which agonist and antagonist muscle groups contract to cause rhythmic movements of a joint. Pulses indicate circulatory sufficiency and should be tested for rhythm and strength if circulatory problems are suspected. Table 1.36 indicates the more commonly palpated pulses that may be used to determine circulatory sufficiency and location.
8. Determine the pathological state of the tissues in and around the joint. The examiner should note any tenderness, tissue thickening, or other signs or symptoms that would indicate pathology. Painful scars or neuromas may be diagnosed using the **thumbnail test.** This test involves running the dorsum of the thumbnail over the scar. If this action elicits a sharp pain, it is a possible indication of a neuroma within the scar. Diffuse sensitivity may suggest complex regional pain syndrome (reflex sympathetic dystrophy).

TABLE **1.36**

Common Circulatory Pulse Locations

Artery	Location
Carotid	Anterior to sternocleidomastoid muscle
Brachial	Medial aspect of arm midway between shoulder and elbow
Radial	At wrist, lateral to flexor carpi radialis tendon
Ulnar	At wrist, between flexor digitorum superficialis and flexor carpi ulnaris tendons
Femoral	In femoral triangle (sartorius, adductor longus, and inguinal ligament)
Popliteal	Posterior aspect of knee (deep and hard to palpate)
Posterior tibial	Posterior aspect of medial malleolus
Dorsalis pedis	Between first and second metatarsal bones on superior aspect

9. Feel dryness or excessive moisture of the skin. For example, acute gouty joints tend to be dry, whereas septic joints tend to be moist. Nervous patients usually demonstrate increased moisture (sweating) in the hands.

10. Note any abnormal sensation, such as dysesthesia (diminished sensation), hyperesthesia (increased sensation), anesthesia (absence of sensation), or crepitus. Soft, fine crepitus may indicate roughening of the articular cartilage, whereas coarse grating may indicate badly damaged articular cartilage or bone. A creaking, leathery crepitus (snowball crepitation) is sometimes felt in tendons and indicates pathology. Tendons may "snap" over one another or over a bony prominence. Loud, snapping, pain-free noises in joints are usually caused by cavitation, in which gas bubbles form suddenly and transiently owing to negative pressure in the joint.

Palpation of a joint and surrounding area must be carried out in a systematic fashion to ensure that all structures are examined. This procedure involves having a starting point and working from that point to adjacent tissues to assess their normality or the possibility of pathological involvement. The examiner must work slowly and carefully, applying light pressure initially and working into a deeper pressure of palpation, then "feeling" for pathological conditions or changes in tissue tension.[224] The uninvolved side should be palpated first so that the patient has some idea of what to expect and to enable the examiner to know what "normal" feels like. Any differences or abnormalities should be noted and contribute to the diagnosis.

Diagnostic Imaging

Although it is important, the diagnostic imaging portion of the examination is usually used only to confirm a clinical opinion and must be interpreted within the context of the whole examination.[228,229] As with special tests, diagnostic imaging should be viewed as one part of the assessment to be used when it will help to confirm or establish a diagnosis.[230] In some cases, clinical decision rules have been developed (e.g., Ottawa ankle and foot rules). These rules increase the accuracy of diagnostic assessments, but the examiner should be aware that the rules apply primarily to acute, first-time injuries.[228] Although this book has examples of diagnostic imaging in each chapter, the reader is advised to consult more detailed texts on the subject for more in-depth knowledge.[231–234]

Reasons for Ordering Diagnostic Imaging

- To confirm a diagnosis
- To establish a diagnosis
- To determine the severity of injury
- To determine the progression of a disease
- To determine the stage of healing
- To enhance patient treatment
- To determine anatomic alignment

Plain Film Radiography

Conventional plain film radiography (also called *x-rays,* although this term is technically incorrect; they should be called x-ray films[233]) is the primary means of diagnostic imaging for musculoskeletal problems. It offers the advantages of being readily available, being relatively cheap, and providing good anatomic resolution. On the negative side, it does expose the patient to radiation, and it offers poor differentiation of soft-tissue structures and is not sensitive to subtle pathology.[228] Radiographs are not taken indiscriminately. Because x-rays have the potential for causing cell damage, there should be a clear indication of need before a radiograph is taken, and the process should not be considered routine.[235]

Radiographs are viewed as though the patient was standing in front of the viewer in the anatomic position.[233] For example, using an anteroposterior (AP) x-ray film of a patient's right lower limb would be viewed with the fibula on the viewer's left-hand side regardless of the position of the anatomic side marker.[233]

Normally, the clinician orders a minimum of two projections at a 90° orientation to each other—most commonly, AP and lateral projections. Two views are necessary because x-rays take planar images; so all structures in the path of the x-ray beam are

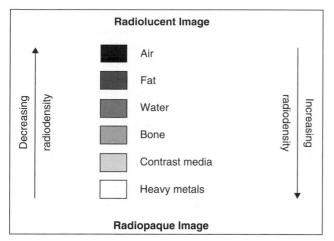

Radiolucent Image

Decreasing radiodensity →

Increasing radiodensity ↓

- Air
- Fat
- Water
- Bone
- Contrast media
- Heavy metals

Radiopaque Image

Fig. 1.16 Radiographic density *(shades of gray)* as related to object radiodensity. Note that the shade may vary depending on thickness of tissue. (From Richardson JK, Iglarsh ZA: *Clinical orthopaedic physical therapy*, Philadelphia, 1995, WB Saunders, p 630.)

superimposed on each other, and abnormalities may be difficult to evaluate with only one view. Two views give information concerning the dimensions of a structure, whether foreign bodies or lesions are present and their location, and to determine the alignment of fractures.[233] Other views may be obtained, depending on clinical circumstances and specific needs.[235–238] In the lumbar spine, AP, lateral, and oblique views are commonly taken.

X-rays are part of the electromagnetic spectrum and have the ability to penetrate tissue to varying degrees. X-ray imaging is based on the principle that different tissues have different densities and produce images in different shades of gray.[239] The greater the density of the tissue, the less penetration of x-rays there is and the whiter its image appears on the film (Fig. 1.16). In order of descending degree of density are the following structures: metal, bone, soft tissue, water, fat, and air. These differences give the six basic densities on the x-ray plate.

When viewing the x-rays, the examiner must identify the film, noting the name, age, date, and sex of the patient, and the examiner must identify the type of projection taken (e.g., AP, lateral, tunnel, skyline, weight bearing, stress type). Rules that should be kept in mind to minimize diagnostic errors when taking radiographs are outlined in the following box.

Rules to Minimize Errors When Taking X-Rays[240]

1. If possible, the patient should be awake
2. The x-ray beam must be perpendicular to the anatomic region being examined
3. The x-ray source should be the farthest possible distance from the region being examined (minimal distance: 2.75 m)

The x-ray plates that are developed after exposure to the roentgen rays enables the examiner to see any fractures, dislocations, foreign bodies, or radiopaque substances that may be present. The main function of plain x-ray examination is to rule out or exclude fractures or serious disease such as infection (osteomyelitis), ankylosing spondylitis, or tumors and structural body abnormalities such as developmental anomalies, arthritis, and metabolic bone diseases. Thus the main purpose of x-ray films is to determine the state of bone and its surrounding soft tissue. Bone remodeling (the taking up [osteoblastic action] and removal [osteoclastic action] of bone) goes on continuously in the body with the rate of change being the result of several factors, such as disuse, aging, or disease. If removal occurs quicker than uptake, then **osteoporosis** (decrease in bone mass) results. Remodeling is related to **Wolff's law**, which states that changes in form and function of bone is followed by changes in its internal structure or that bone responds (like any tissue) to the stress and strain placed on it. For x-ray films, osteoporosis (similar to other conditions such as osteomalacia) results in an increase in radiolucency. This increased radiolucency is called **osteopenia**.

Uses of Plain Film Radiography[231]

- Fractures
- Arthritis
- Bone tumors
- Skeletal dysplasia

Commonly, an **ABCDs search pattern** is used when looking at radiological images (Table 1.37).[233] With soft-tissue injuries, clinical findings should take precedence over x-ray findings. It is desirable to know whether an x-ray has been taken so that the examiner can obtain the films if necessary. The examiner should be aware of obvious and unusual x-ray findings that distract attention from other tissue that is actually the cause of the pain; such x-ray abnormalities are significant only if clinical examination bears out their relevance. With experience, the examiner becomes able to detect many important soft-tissue changes on x-ray examination, such as effusion in joints, tendinous calcifications, ectopic bone in muscle, tissue displaced by tumor, and the presence of air or foreign body material in the tissues. Radiographs may also be used to indicate bone loss. For osteoporosis to be evident on x-ray, approximately 30% to 35% of the bone must be lost (Fig. 1.17). **Cortical thickness** can be used to determine bone loss. The most common place for measuring cortical thickness is the midpoint of the second or third metacarpal shaft (Fig. 1.18). Normally, the sum should be one half of the total bone diameter.

Examiner Observations When Viewing an X-Ray Film

- Overall size and shape of bone
- Local size and shape of bone
- Number of bones
- Alignment of bones
- Thickness of the cortex
- Trabecular pattern of the bone
- General density of the entire bone
- Local density change
- Margins of local lesions
- Any break in continuity of the bone
- Any periosteal change
- Any soft-tissue change (e.g., gross swelling, periosteal elevation, visibility of fat pads)
- Relation among bones
- Thickness of the cartilage (cartilage space within joints)
- Width and symmetry of joint space
- Contour and density of subchondral bone

The examiner should keep in mind the maturity of the patient when viewing films. Skeletal changes occur with age,[241] and the appearance and fusion of the epiphyses, for example, may be important in interpreting the pathology of the condition seen. Soft-tissue structures and bone can be seen, provided there is something to outline them. For example, the joint capsule may be silhouetted by the pericapsular fat, or air in the lungs may silhouette a cardiac shadow. Anatomic variations and anomalies must be ruled out before pathology can be ruled in; for example, accessory navicular, bipartite patella, and os trigonum may be confused with fractures by the unsuspecting examiner. The fabella is often confused with a loose body in the knee in the AP projection x-ray film.

Radiographs may also be used to determine the maturity index of a patient. A special film of the wrist is taken to assess skeletal maturity (Fig. 1.19). These films can be compared with established films in a bone

TABLE **1.37**

ABCDs Search Pattern for Radiologic Image Interpretation

Division	Evaluates	LOOK FOR Normal Findings	LOOK FOR Variations/Abnormalities
A: Alignment	General skeletal architecture	Gross normal size of bones Normal number of bones	Supernumerary (extra) bones Absent bones Congenital deformities Developmental deformities Cortical fractures
	General contour of bone	Smooth and continuous cortical outlines	Avulsion fractures Impaction fractures Spurs Breaks in cortex continuity
	Alignment of bones to adjacent bones	Normal joint articulations Normal spatial relationships	Markings of past surgical sites Fracture Joint subluxation Joint dislocation
B: Bone density	General bone density	Sufficient contrast between soft-tissue shade of gray and bone shade of gray	General loss of bone density resulting in poor contrast between soft tissues and bone
		Sufficient contrast within each bone, between cortical shell and cancellous center	Thinning or absence of cortical margins
	Texture abnormalities	Normal trabecular architecture	Appearance of trabeculae altered; may look thin, delicate, lacy, coarsened, smudged, fluffy
	Local bone density changes	Sclerosis at areas of increased stress, such as weight-bearing surfaces or sites of ligamentous, muscular, or tendinous attachments	Excessive sclerosis (increase in bone density) Reactive sclerosis that walls off a lesion (e.g., tumor) Osteophytes

TABLE **1.37**

ABCDs Search Pattern for Radiologic Image Interpretation—cont'd

Division	Evaluates	LOOK FOR	
		Normal Findings	Variations/Abnormalities
C: Cartilage spaces	Joint space width	Well-preserved joint spaces imply normal cartilage or disc thickness	Decreased joint spaces imply degenerative or traumatic conditions
	Subchondral bone	Smooth surface	Excessive sclerosis as seen in degenerative joint disease Erosions as seen in the inflammatory arthritides
	Epiphyseal plates	Normal size relative to epiphysis and skeletal age	Compare contralaterally for changes in thickness that may be related to abnormal conditions or trauma
D: Soft tissues	Muscles	Normal size of soft-tissue image	Gross wasting
	Fat pads and fat lines	Radiolucent crescent parallel to bone Radiolucent lines parallel to length of muscle	Gross swelling Displacement of fat pads from bony fossae into soft tissues indicates joint effusion Elevation or blurring of fat planes indicates swelling of nearby tissues
	Joint capsules	Normally indistinct	Observe whether effusion or hemorrhage distends capsule
	Periosteum	Normally indistinct Solid periosteal reaction is normal in fracture healing	Observe periosteal reactions: solid, laminated or onionskin, spiculated or sunburst, Codman triangle
	Miscellaneous soft tissue findings	Soft tissues normally exhibit a water-density shade of gray	Foreign bodies evidenced by radiodensity Gas bubbles appear radiolucent Calcifications/ossification appear radiopaque

Modified from McKinnis LN: *Fundamentals of musculoskeletal imaging*, Philadelphia, 2005, F.A. Davis.

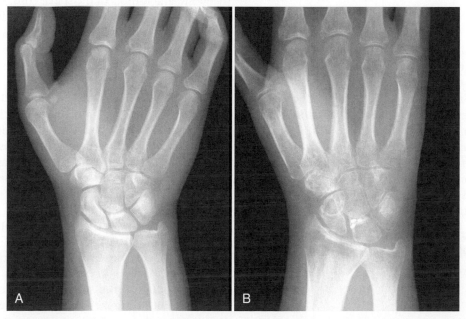

Fig. 1.17 Osteoporosis of immobilization and disuse. Radiographs obtained immediately before wrist ligament reconstruction (A) and 2 months later (B) are shown. (B) Observe the extent of the osteopenia. (From Resnick D, Kransdorf MJ: *Bone and joint imaging*, Philadelphia, 2005, Elsevier, p 547.)

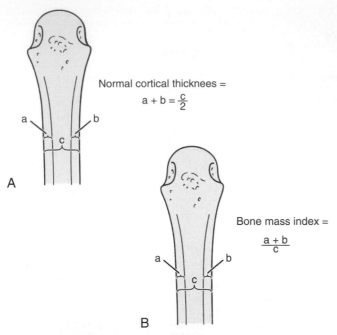

Normal cortical thicknees =

$$a + b = \frac{c}{2}$$

Bone mass index =

$$\frac{a + b}{c}$$

Fig. 1.18 (A) Cortical thickness measurements are usually based on the cortices at the midshaft of the second or third metacarpal. Normally, the sum of the two cortices should equal approximately one half the overall diameter of the shaft. (B) Cortical thickness may also be expressed as an index of bone mass, which is the sum of the cortices divided by diameter.

atlas such as that compiled by Gruelich and Pyle.[241] For the spine, Sanders et al.[242] have advocated the use of the simplified Tanner-Whitehouse-III Skeletal Maturity Assessment (Table 1.38). This is often done before epiphysiodesis and leg-lengthening procedures to ensure that the child is of a suitable skeletal age to do the procedure.

Arthrography

Arthrography is an invasive technique in which air, a water-soluble contrast material containing iodine, or a combination of the two (double contrast) is injected into a joint space, and a radiograph is taken of the joint. The air or contrast material outlines the structures within the joint or communicating with the joint (Fig. 1.20). It is especially useful in detecting abnormal joint and bursal communications, synovial abnormalities, articular cartilage lesions, and the extent of or pathology to the capsule.[233] It is used primarily in the hip, knee, ankle, shoulder, elbow, and wrist.[235]

Uses of Arthrography[231]

- Steroid injections
- Aspirations
- Joint kinematics

Computed Arthrography (Computed Tomography Arthrography)

This technique combines arthrography and computed tomography (CT) to image joints. This method provides a three-dimensional definition of the joint, and the dye helps to delineate articular surfaces and joint margins. It is usually reserved for those cases in which conventional CT scanning has not provided adequate anatomic detail (e.g., shoulder instability).[44,235,238]

Uses of Computed Tomography Arthrograms[231]

- Loose bodies
- Joint surfaces

Venogram and Arteriogram

With a venogram or an arteriogram, radiopaque dye is injected into specific vessels to outline abnormal conditions (Fig. 1.21). This technique may be used to diagnose arteriosclerosis, investigate tumors, and demonstrate blockage after traumatic injury.

Myelography

Myelography is an invasive imaging technique that is used to visualize the soft tissues within the spine. A water-soluble radiopaque dye is injected into the epidural space by spinal puncture and allowed to flow to different levels of the spinal cord, outlining the contour of the thecal sac, nerve roots, and spinal cord. A plain x-ray film is then taken of the spine (Figs. 1.22 and 1.23). In many cases nowadays, CT scans and magnetic resonance imaging (MRI) scans have taken the place of myelograms.[235] This technique is used to detect disc disease, disc herniation, nerve root entrapment, spinal stenosis, and tumors of the spinal cord. The clinician should be aware that myelograms can have adverse side effects. Grainger[243] reported that 20% to 30% of patients receiving myelograms complained of headache, dizziness, nausea, vomiting, and seizures.[239]

Tomography and Computed Tomography

Tomography has become a common imaging technique for musculoskeletal disorders, especially when computer enhanced (CT scan). It produces cross-sectional images of the tissues. Conventional tomography, which is also called *thin-section radiography* or *linear tomography*, tends to show one small area or plane in focus with other areas or planes appearing fuzzy or blurred. The conventional tomogram is seldom used today except when subtle bone density alterations are sought.

The CT scan involves the same thin cross sections or "slices" taken at specific levels (Fig. 1.24). CT scans produce cross-sectional images based on x-ray attenuation. Because of computer enhancement, CT

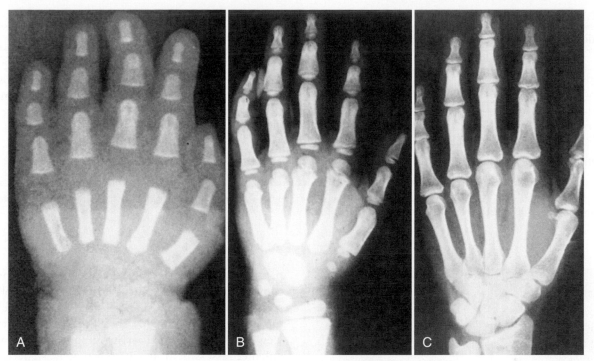

Fig. 1.19 X-ray films showing skeletal maturity. (A) Male, newborn. (B) Male, 5 years old. (C) Female, 17 years old.

TABLE **1.38**

Key Findings of the Simplified Tanner-Whitehouse-III Skeletal Maturity Assessment

Stage	Key Features	Tanner-Whitehouse-III Stage	Greulich and Pyle Reference	Related Maturity Signs
1. Juvenile slow	Digital epiphyses are not covered	Some digits are at stage E or less	• Female: 8 years and 10 months • Male: 12 years and 6 months (note fifth middle phalanx)	Tanner stage 1
2. Preadolescent slow	All digital epiphyses are covered	All digits arc at stage F	• Female: 10 years • Male: 13 years	Tanner stage 2, starting growth spurt
3. Adolescent rapid—early	The preponderance of digits is capped. The second through fifth metacarpal epiphyses are wider than their metaphyses	All digits are at stage G	• Female: 11 and 12 years • Male: 13 years and 6 months and 14 years	Peak height velocity, Risser stage 0, open pelvic triradiate cartilage
4. Adolescent rapid—late	Any of distal phalangeal physes are clearly beginning to close	Any distal phalanges are at stage H	• Female: 13 years (digits 2, 3, and 4) • Male: 15 years (digits 4 and 5)	Girls typically in Tanner stage 3, Risser stage 0, open triradiate cartilage
5. Adolescent steady—early	All distal phalangeal physes arc closed. Others are open	All distal phalanges and thumb metacarpal are at stage I. Others remain at stage G	• Female: 13 years and 6 months • Male: 15 years and 6 months	Risser stage 0, triradiate cartilage closed: menarche only occasionally starts earlier than this

Continued

TABLE **1.38**

Key Findings of the Simplified Tanner-Whitehouse-III Skeletal Maturity Assessment—cont'd

Stage	Key Features	Tanner-Whitehouse-III Stage	Greulich and Pyle Reference	Related Maturity Signs
6. Adolescent steady—late			• Female: 14 years • Male: 16 years (late)	Risser sign positive (stage 1 or more)
7. Early mature	Only distal radial physis is open. Metacarpal physeal scars may be present	All digits are at stage I. The distal radial physis is at stage G or H	• Female: 15 years • Male: 17 years	Risser stage 4
8. Mature	Distal radial physis is completely closed	All digits are at stage I	• Female: 17 years • Male: 19 years	Risser stage 5

From Sanders JO, Khoury JG, Kishan S, et al: Predicting scoliosis progression from skeletal maturity: a simplified classification during adolescence, *J Bone Joint Surg Am* 90(3):541, 2008.

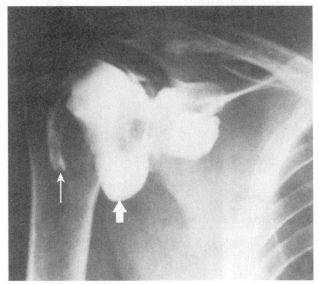

Fig. 1.20 Normal arthrogram, shoulder in lateral rotation. Note the good dependent fold *(wide arrow)* and the outline of the bicipital tendon *(narrow arrow)*. (From Neviaser TJ: Arthrography of the shoulder, *Orthop Clin North Am* 11:209, 1980.)

produces superior tissue contrast resolution compared with conventional x-rays, thus enabling greater details of subtle bone pathology.[228,244] CT provides excellent bony architecture detail and has good resolution of soft-tissue structures.[234] Its disadvantages include limited scanning plane, cost, exposure to radiation (dosage similar to or greater than that of plain x-rays), alteration of the image by artifacts, and degradation of soft-tissue resolution in obese people.[44,235] The CT scan, or computed axial tomography (CAT) scan, is a radiological technique that may be used to assess for disc protrusions, facet disease, or spinal stenosis.[245] The technique may also be used to assess complex fractures, especially those involving joints, dislocations, patellofemoral alignment and tracking, osteonecrosis, tumors, and osteomyelitis. Because only a small cross-sectional area in one plane is viewed with each scan, multiple images or scans are taken to get a complete view of the area.[44] CT arthrography may be used to enhance assessment of intra-articular structures and may be used for patients who cannot tolerate conventional MRI.

Single-photon emission computed tomography (SPECT) scanning is a specialized type of CT scanning used in orthopedics primarily to detect spondylolysis.[234]

Uses of Computed Tomography Scans[231]

- Complex fractures
- Comminuted fractures
- Intra-articular fragments
- Fracture healing (e.g., nonunion)
- Bone tumors

Radionuclide Scanning (Scintigraphy)[246]

With bone scans (osteoscintigraphy), chemicals labeled with radioactive isotopes (radioactive tracers) such as technetium 99m–labeled methyl diphosphonate complexes are intravenously injected several hours before the scan to localize specific organs that concentrate the particular chemical. The isotope is then localized where there is a high level of metabolic activity (e.g., bone turnover) relative to the rest of the bone. The radiograph reveals a "hot spot" (Fig. 1.25) indicating areas of increased mineral turnover.[233] Although plain film radiographs do not show bone disease or stress fractures until there is 30% to 50% bone loss, bone scans show bone disease or stress fractures with as little as 4% to 7% bone loss (Fig. 1.26).[245] Because the isotope is excreted

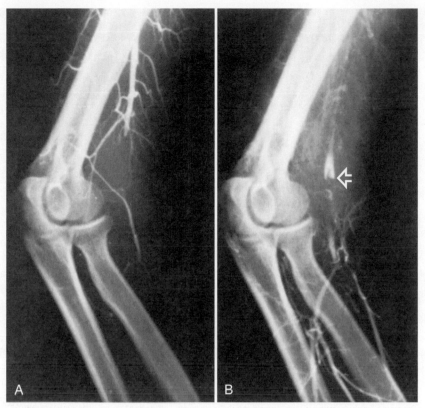

Fig. 1.21 Occlusion of brachial artery. (A) Arteriogram of a young man with a previously reduced elbow dislocation and an ischemic hand shows an occluded brachial artery. (B) A later film shows fresh clot *(arrow)* in the brachial artery and reconstituted radial and ulnar arteries. Primary repair and thrombectomy treated the ischemic symptoms. (From McLean G, Frieman DB: Angiography of skeletal disease, *Orthop Clin North Am* 14:267, 1983.)

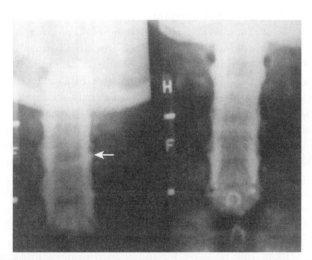

Fig. 1.22 Myelogram of cervical spine. Note how radiopaque dye fills root sheaths *(arrow)*.

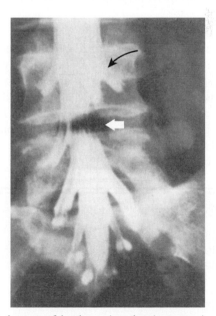

Fig. 1.23 Myelogram of lumbar spine showing extrusion of nucleus pulposus of L4–L5 *(large arrow)*. Note how radiopaque dye fills dural recesses *(small arrow)*. (From Selby DK, Meril AJ, Wagner KJ, et al: Water-soluble myelography, *Orthop Clin North Am* 8[1]:82, 1977.)

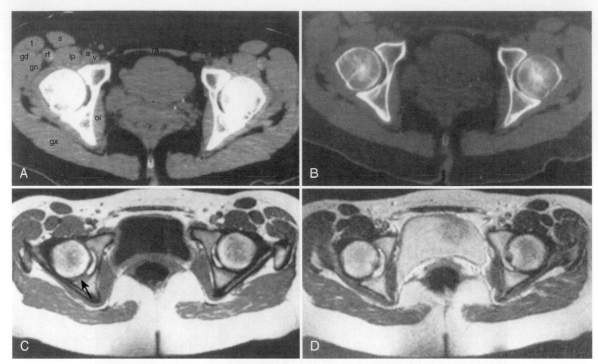

Fig. 1.24 (A) Normal computed tomography (CT) image at the level of the mid acetabulum obtained with soft-tissue window settings shows the homogeneous, intermediate signal of musculature. *a,* Common femoral artery; *gd,* gluteus medius; *gn,* gluteus minimus; *gx,* gluteus maximus; *ip,* iliopsoas; *oi,* obturator internus; *ra,* rectus abdominis; *rf,* rectus femoris; *s,* sartorius; *t,* tensor fascia lata; *v,* common femoral vein. (B) Axial CT at bone window settings reveals improved delineation of cortical and medullary osseous detail. Note anterior and posterior semilunar acetabular articular surfaces and the central nonarticular acetabular fossa. (C) Normal midacetabular T1-weighted axial 0.4-T magnetic resonance image (MRI) (*TR,* 600 ms; *TE,* 20 ms) of a different patient shows a normal, high-signal-intensity image of fatty marrow (adult pattern) and subcutaneous tissue, low-signal-intensity image of muscle, and absence of signal in the cortical bone. The thin articular hyaline cartilage is of intermediate signal intensity *(arrow).* (D) T2-weighted MRI (*TR,* 2000 ms; *TE,* 80 ms) shows decreasing high signal intensity in fatty marrow and subcutaneous tissue with increased signal intensity in the fluid-filled urinary bladder. (From Pitt MJ, Lund PJ, Speer DP: Imaging of the pelvis and hip, *Orthop Clin North Am* 21[3]:553, 1990.)

by the kidneys, the kidneys and bladder are often visible in bone scans. Bone scans are used for lytic (bone-loss) diseases, infection, fractures, and tumors. They are highly sensitive to bone abnormalities but do not tell what the abnormality is (low specificity). The whole body may be imaged, and a gamma camera picks up the tracer.[245] High-resolution MRI and CT scans are replacing bone scans in some cases.[247]

Uses of Scintigraphy

- Skeletal metastases
- Stress fractures
- Osteomyelitis

Discography

The technique of discography involves injecting a small amount of radiopaque dye into the nucleus pulposus of an intervertebral disc (Fig. 1.27) under radiographic guidance. It is not a commonly used technique but may be used to determine disruptions in the nucleus pulposus or the annular fibrosus and is sometimes used as a provocative test to see whether injection into the disc brings on the patient's symptoms.[245]

Magnetic Resonance Imaging

MRI is a noninvasive, painless imaging technique with high contrast resolution that uses exposure to magnetic fields, not ionizing radiation, to obtain an image of bone and soft tissue. MRI is based on the effect of a strong magnetic field on hydrogen atoms. T1 images show good anatomic detail of soft tissues (Fig. 1.28), whereas T2 images are used to demonstrate soft-tissue pathology that alters tissue water content.[44,243] MRI offers excellent tissue contrast, is multiplanar (i.e., can image in any plane), and has no known adverse effects. In some patients, claustrophobia is a problem, and artifacts may result if the patient does not remain still.[241] For musculoskeletal conditions, plane film radiographs are commonly taken and viewed to determine if an MRI is necessary.[229]

MRI is used to assess for spinal cord tumors, intracranial disease, and some types of CNS diseases (e.g., multiple sclerosis); it largely replaced myelography in the evaluation of disc pathology. It also aids in the diagnosis of muscle, meniscal and ligamentous tears, synovial pathology,

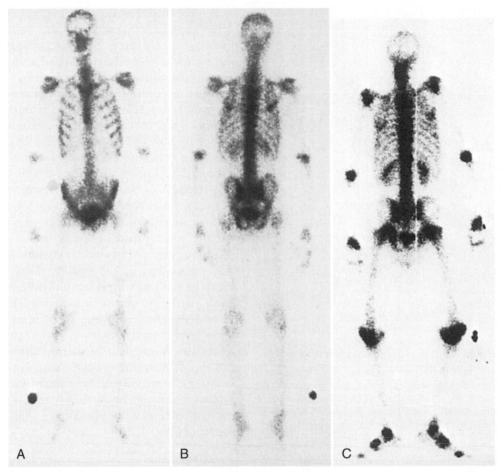

Fig. 1.25 Whole-body bone scans. (A) Normal adult anterior scan. (B) Normal adult posterior scan. (C) Posterior scan showing joint involvement of rheumatoid arthritis. (From Goldstein HA: Bone scintigraphy, *Orthop Clin North Am* 14:244, 250, 1983.)

abnormal patellofemoral tracking, joint pathology, cartilage, bone marrow pathology, osteonecrosis, stress fractures, and osteochondral lesions.[44,231,248]

Uses of Magnetic Resonance Imaging[230]

- Intra-articular structures (e.g., meniscus, loose bodies)
- Musculotendinous injury
- Joint instability
- Osteomyelitis
- Fractures
- Stress injury
- Disc disease
- Soft-tissue tumors
- Skeletal malformations
- Bone bruises

On the negative side, MRI is expensive, and specificity of pathology (e.g., tendon strain versus tendinitis) may not be possible with its use, and there is a high prevalence of positive findings in asymptomatic patients.[249,250] The presence of some metallic objects (e.g., cardiac pacemakers) may make its use contraindicated because of the magnetic pull, especially if the objects are not solidly fixed to bone. It has been reported that MRI is safe with prosthetic joints and internal fixation devices, provided that they are stable.[235]

MR arthrography may enhance assessment of intra-articular structures, such as shoulder instability, ankle impingement, labral tears, wrist ligament tears, and loose bodies.[231,251]

Fluoroscopy

Fluoroscopy is a technique that is used to show motion in joints through x-ray imaging; it also may be used as a guidance technique for injections (e.g., in discography). It is only rarely used because of the amount of radiation exposure. It is sometimes used to position fracture fragments and to demonstrate abnormal motion.

Diagnostic Ultrasound Imaging

Diagnostic ultrasound imaging (DUSI) is a useful adjunct that is used clinically for assessment of a wide variety of musculoskeletal conditions.[252] Diagnostic ultrasound (US) is very different from therapeutic US, which is performed at very high frequencies of 8,000,000 Hz or greater to stimulate tissues beneath

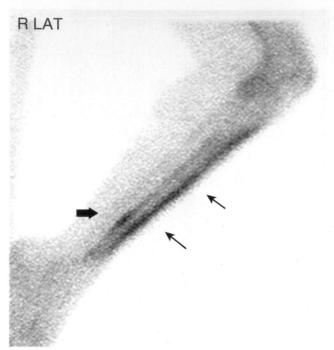

R LAT

Fig. 1.26 Stress fracture of the tibia and anterior shin splint. A short fusiform area of increased uptake in the posterior aspect of the distal shaft of the tibia represents a stress fracture *(large arrow).* A long longitudinal area of increased uptake in the anterior aspect of the tibial shaft is consistent with a shin splint *(small arrows).* (From Resnick D, Kransdorf MJ: *Bone and joint imaging,* Philadelphia, 2005, Elsevier, p 103.)

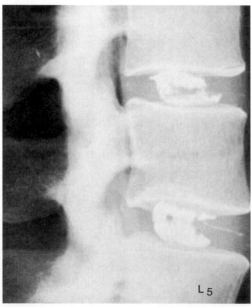

L 5

Fig. 1.27 Normal discogram shown with barium paste. (From Farfan HF: *Mechanical disorders of the low back,* Philadelphia, 1973, Lea & Febiger, p 96.)

the skin's surface to promote healing for a variety of musculoskeletal injuries. Diagnostic US offers several unique strengths over other imaging techniques. It allows both static and dynamic assessment, which can

be helpful in differentiating various injuries. The clinician can also interact with the patient while doing the imaging, allowing the clinician to obtain a relevant history to help guide the DUSI examination and to identify the cause of the complaints.[253] Prices for US units are becoming more reasonable, which is allowing more clinicians to use an examination tool that visualizes the tissues under the skin and is absent of radiation, has widespread availability, and can even allow dynamic visualization of soft-tissue structures. Increased technologies allow imaging at frequencies of 10 to 15 MHz.[254] Higher-frequency transducers (between 12 and 18 MHz) allow for improved imaging and visualization of muscles, tendons, ligaments, and the joint capsule. Sound waves are transmitted into tissues by a transducer through a coupling agent with calculation of the time it takes for the echo to return to the transducer from different interfaces. The depth of the structure is determined, and an image is formed. The lower the frequency, the deeper the tissue penetration, however, the lower the resolution of details. A greater frequency allows better visualization of more superficial structures. Newer, more compact US machines are currently no larger than a notebook and can be carried from room to room with much greater ease of portability than previous larger machines (Fig. 1.29).

Uses of Diagnostic Ultrasound Imaging[230]

- Hip dysplasia in children
- Joint effusion
- Tendon pathology
- Ligament tears
- Soft-tissue tumors
- Vascular disease

Transducer application to an exposed area is gentle pressure so as not to cause pain or significantly distort the soft tissues. A gel coupling medium or gel pads help to improve image resolution. Acoustic waves are emitted by the US and are transmitted and dissipated as the result of molecular vibrations and intertissue collisions.[255] Tissues such as tendon and bones can be described as **hyperechoic** (i.e., a brighter or stronger than normal image) or **isoechoic** (i.e., producing US images equal to normal tissues), muscle is **hypoechoic** (i.e., darker), and fluid is **anechoic** (i.e., absent of an echo). Veins, arteries, nerves, and some tendons are round or oval. Veins compress easily, arteries compress less and may pulsate, and nerves compress the least of the three. Tendons do not compress. Nerves can be a mixture of hypoechoic and hyperechoic.[256] Bone is usually hyperechoic and visualized as the

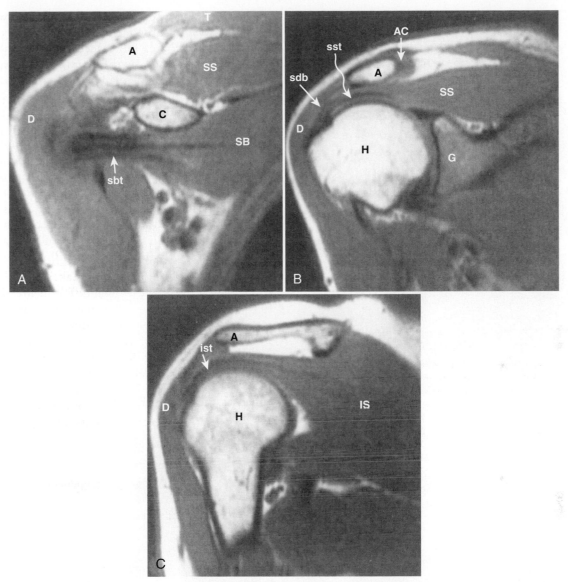

Fig. 1.28 Magnetic resonance T1-weighted coronal oblique images from anterior (A) to posterior (C). *A*, Acromion; *AC*, acromioclavicular joint; *C*, coracoid; *D*, deltoid muscle; *G*, glenoid of scapula; *H*, humerus; *IS*, infraspinatus muscle; *ist*, infraspinatus tendon; *SB*, subscapularis muscle; *sbt*, subscapularis tendon; *sdb*, subdeltoid-subacromial bursa; *SS*, supraspinatus muscle; *sst*, supraspinatus tendon; *T*, trapezius muscle. (From Mayer SJ, Dalinka MK: Magnetic resonance imaging of the shoulder, *Orthop Clin North Am* 21:500, 1990.)

outer cortical surface. Underneath the cortical bone, the cancellous bone may be black due to the sound waves not penetrating deep enough for accurate visualization. Anechoic structures, such as fluid, are black because they are much less dense and the sound waves pass completely through them.

The best DUSI visualization is when the sound beam is directed with the incident beam at an angle of 90° to the structures being visualized. With a decreased angle, anisotropy can occur and a loss of image quality occurs. **Anisotropy** is the appearance of a false hypoechoic area (i.e., an artifact) with the US. With anisotropy, the returning sound echoes make the structural fibers appear to be pathological when they may not be. Therefore use

of **toggling** (i.e., side to side) and the **heel-toe maneuver** (i.e., forward-backward movement) of the transducer may optimize beam reflectivity. Transducer type is important because different sizes and shapes are used for different structures. A flat transducer can enhance structures that are relatively close to the surface. Other transducers are rounded and are for a larger field of view or deeper viewing. Smaller transducers are used on the hand, wrist, and foot.

US views should be performed in at least two different angles. The longitudinal or long axis view, and the transverse or short axis view are most commonly used. In a long axis view, the clinician can see the length of the tendon running parallel. The short axis view is taken as a

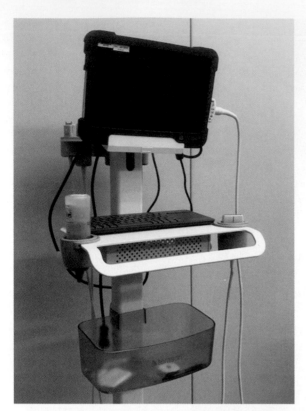

Fig. 1.29 Modern diagnostic ultrasound imaging device.

view in the transverse plane. Each have their own specific uses, described in subsequent chapters.

As DUSI becomes more accepted in rehabilitation, its use is increasing. In the hands of an experienced operator, DUSI can provide good image detail and cross-sectional images in different planes. No radiation is used, and no harmful biological effects have been reported. It also has the advantage of providing dynamic (moving) real-time images because tissue can be examined as they move. The primary limitation to the use of DUSI is that it is operator dependent and requires proper training and experience for accurate image acquisition and interpretation.[253] Learning how to correctly use and interpret DUSI is an art and takes practice and skill. An understanding of basic anatomy is essential. Correctly interpreting findings between normal and pathological anatomy is critical. With practice, any clinician can become increasingly skilled at the use of DUSI.

Xeroradiography

Xeroradiography is a technique in which a xeroradiographic plate replaces the normal x-ray film. On the plate, there is a thin layer of a photoconductor material, which enhances the image (Fig. 1.30). This technique is used

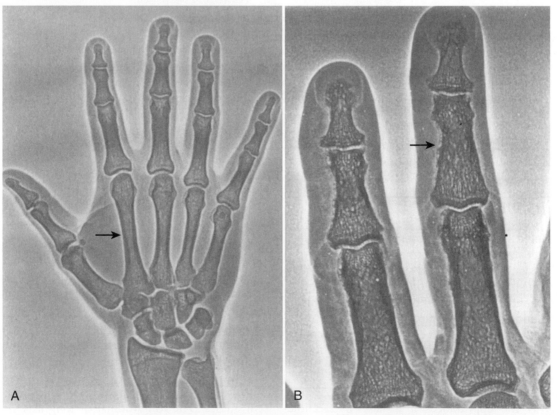

Fig. 1.30 Xeroradiography. (A) Normal examination. Note the ability to demonstrate both soft tissues and bony structures on a single examination. The halo effect *(arrow)* around the bony cortices is an example of edge enhancement. (B) Hyperparathyroid bone changes shown on xeroradiography. The subperiosteal bone resorption *(arrow)* and distal tuft erosion are well shown. (A, From Weissman BN, Sledge CB: *Orthopedic radiology*, Philadelphia, 1986, WB Saunders, p 11. B, From Seltzer SE, Weissman BN, Finberg HJ, et al: Improved diagnostic imaging in joint diseases, *Semin Arthritis Rheum* 11[3]:315, 1982.)

when the margins between areas of different densities need to be exaggerated.[239,257]

Précis

Each chapter ends with a précis of the assessment to serve as a quick reference. The précis does not follow the text description exactly but is laid out so that each assessment involves minimal movement of the patient to decrease patient discomfort. For example, all aspects of the examination that are performed with the patient standing are done first, followed by those done with the patient sitting, and so on.

Case Studies

Case studies are provided as written exercises to help the examiner develop skills in assessment. Based on the presented case study, the reader should develop a list of appropriate questions to ask in the history based on the pathology of the conditions, what should especially be noted in observation, and what part of the examination is essential to make a definitive diagnosis. Where appropriate, example diagnoses are given in parentheses at the end of each question. At the end of the case study, the reader can develop a table showing the differential diagnosis for the case described. Tables 1.39 and 1.40 illustrate such differential diagnosis charts.

TABLE **1.39**

Differential Diagnosis of Claudication and Spinal Stenosis

Vascular Claudication	Neurogenic Claudication	Spinal Stenosis
Pain[a] is usually bilateral	Pain is usually bilateral but may be unilateral	Usually bilateral pain
Occurs in the calf (foot, thigh, hip, or buttocks)	Occurs in back, buttocks, thighs, calves, and feet	Occurs in back, buttocks, thighs, calves, and feet
Pain consistent in all spinal positions	Pain decreased in spinal flexion Pain increased in spinal extension	Pain decreased in spinal flexion Pain increased in spinal extension
Pain brought on by physical exertion (e.g., walking)	Pain increased with walking	Pain increased with walking
Pain relieved promptly by rest (1–5 min)	Pain decreased by recumbency	Pain relieved with prolonged rest (may persist hours after resting)
Pain increased by walking uphill		Pain decreased when walking uphill
No burning or dysesthesia	Burning and dysesthesia from the back to buttocks and leg or legs	Burning and numbness present in lower extremities
Decreased or absent pulses in lower extremities	Normal pulses	Normal pulses
Color and skin changes in feet—cold, numb, dry, or scaly skin; poor nail and hair growth	Good skin nutrition	Good skin nutrition
Affects ages from 40 to over 60	Affects ages from 40 to over 60	Peaks in seventh decade of life; affects men primarily

[a]"Pain" associated with vascular claudication may also be described as an "aching," "cramping," or "tired" feeling.
Modified from Goodman CC, Snyder TE: *Differential diagnosis in physical therapy*, ed 2, Philadelphia, 1995, W.B. Saunders Co., p 539.

TABLE **1.40**

Differential Diagnosis of Contractile Tissue (Muscle) and Inert Tissue (Ligament) Pathology

	Muscle	Ligament
Mechanism of Injury	Overstretching (overload) Crushing (pinching)	Overstretching (overload)
Contributing Factors	Muscle fatigue Poor reciprocal muscle strength Inflexibility Inadequate warm-up	Muscle fatigue Hypermobility
Active Movement	Pain on contraction (1°, 2°) Pain on stretch (1°, 2°) No pain on contraction (3°) Weakness on contraction (1°, 2°, 3°)	Pain on stretch or compression (1°, 2°) No pain on stretch (3°) ROM decreased

Continued

TABLE **1.40**

Differential Diagnosis of Contractile Tissue (Muscle) and Inert Tissue (Ligament) Pathology—cont'd

	Muscle	Ligament
Passive Movement	Pain on stretch Pain on compression	Pain on stretch (1°, 2°) No pain on stretch (3°) ROM decreased
Resisted Isometric Movement	Pain on contraction (1°, 2°) No pain on contraction (3°) Weakness on contraction (1°, 2°, 3°)	No pain (1°, 2°, 3°)
Special Tests	If test isolates muscle, weakness and pain on contraction (1°, 2°) or weakness and no pain on contraction (3°)	If test isolates ligament, ROM and pain affected
Reflexes	Normal unless 3°	Normal
Cutaneous Distribution	Normal	Normal
Joint Play Movement (in Resting Position)	Normal	Increased ROM, unless restricted by swelling
Palpation	Point tenderness at site of injury Gap if palpated early Swelling (blood ecchymosis late) Spasm	Point tenderness at site of injury Gap if palpated early Swelling (blood/synovial fluid)
Diagnostic Imaging	MRI, arthrogram, and CT scan show lesion	MRI, arthrogram, and CT scan show lesion Stress x-ray shows increased ROM

CT, Computed tomography; *MRI*, magnetic resonance imaging; *ROM*, range of motion.

Conclusion

Having completed all parts of the assessment, the examiner can look at the pertinent objective and subjective facts, note the significant signs and symptoms to determine what is causing the patient's problems, and design a proper treatment regimen based on the findings. This is the normal and correct reasoning process.[258,259] If the assessment is not followed through completely, the treatment regimen may not be implemented properly, and this may lead to unwarranted extended care of the patient and increased health care costs.

Occasionally, patients present with a mixture of signs and symptoms that indicates two or more possible problem areas. Only by adding the positive findings and subtracting the negative findings can the examiner determine the probable cause of the problem. In many cases, the decision may be an "educated guess," because few problems are "textbook perfect." Only the examiner's knowledge, clinical experience, and his or her clinical decision-making skills leading to a patient diagnosis, followed by trial treatment, can conclusively delineate the problem.[260]

Finally, when the assessment has been completed, the clinician should warn the patient about a possible exacerbation of symptoms and should not hesitate to refer the patient to another health care professional if the patient has presented with unusual signs and symptoms or if the condition appears to be beyond the scope of the examiner's practice.

References

1. Cyriax J. Textbook of orthopaedic medicine. In: *Diagnosis of Soft Tissue Lesions.* 8th ed. Vol 1. London: Balliere Tindall; 1982.
2. Weed L. Medical records that guide and teach: part I. *N Engl J Med.* 1968;278:593–600.
3. Thompson J. A practical guide to clinical medicine – history of present illness. http://medicine.ucsd.edu/clinicalmed/thinking.htm, 2007.
4. Dutton M. *Orthopedic Examination, Evaluation and Intervention.* New York: McGraw-Hill; 2004.
5. Gandhi JS, Osler W. A life in medicine. *BMJ.* 2000;321:1087.
6. Holmes F. If you listen, the patient will tell you the diagnosis. *Int J Listening.* 2007;21(2):156–161.
7. Stith JS, Sahrmann SA, Dixon KK, et al. Curriculum to prepare diagnosticians in physical therapy. *J Phys Ther Educ.* 1995;9:46–53.
8. Adams ST, Leveson SH. Clinical prediction rules. *BMJ.* 2012;344:8312–8322.
9. Moffett JK, McLean S, Roberts L. Red flags need more evaluation. *Rheumatology.* 2006;45:920–921.
10. Stewart J, Kempenaar L, Lanchlan D. Rethinking yellow flags. *Man Ther.* 2011;16:196–198.
11. Deshpande PR, Rajan S, Sudeepthi BL, Nazir A. Patient-reported outcomes: a new era in clinical research. *Perspect Clin Res.* 2011;2(4):137–144.
12. American Physical Therapy Association. Guide to physical therapist practice, second edition, American Physical Therapy Association. *Phys Ther.* 2001;81:9–746.
13. Martin RR, Mohtadi NG, Safran MR, et al. Differences in physician and patient ratings of items used to assess hip disorders. *Am J Sports Med.* 2009;37:1508–1512.
14. Maitland GD. *Neuro/Musculoskeletal Examination and Recording Guide.* Glen Osmond, South Australia: Lauderdale Press; 1992.
15. Vranceanu AM, Barsky A, Ring D. Psychosocial aspects of disabling musculoskeletal pain. *J Bone Joint Surg Am.* 2009;91:2014–2018.
16. Melzack R, Katz J. Pain. *WIREs Cognitive Science.* 2013;4:1–15.

17. Petty NJ, Moore AP. *Neuromusculoskeletal Examination and Assessment: A Handbook for Therapists*. London: Churchill-Livingstone; 1998.

18. McGuire DB. The multiple dimensions of cancer pain: a framework for assessment and management. In: McGuire DB, Yarbo CH, Ferrell BR, eds. *Cancer Pain Management*. 2nd ed. Boston: Jones & Bartlett; 1995.

19. Wiener SL. *Differential Diagnosis of Acute Pain by Body Region*. New York: McGraw-Hill; 1993.

20. Nijs J, Van Houdenove B, Oostendorp RA. Recognition of central sensitization in patients with musculoskeletal pain: application of pain neurophysiology in manual therapy practice. *Man Ther*. 2010;15:135–141.

21. Smart KM, Blake C, Staines A, et al. Clinical indicators of nociceptive, peripheral neuropathic and central mechanisms of musculoskeletal pain: a Delphi survey of clinical experts. *Man Ther*. 2010;15:80–87.

22. Travell JG, Simons DG. *Myofascial Pain and Dysfunction: The Trigger Point Manual*. Baltimore: Williams & Wilkins; 1983.

23. McKenzie RA. *The Lumbar Spine: Mechanical Diagnosis and Therapy*. Waikane, New Zealand: Spinal Publications; 1982.

24. Meadows JT. *Orthopedic Differential Diagnosis in Physical Therapy: A Case Study Approach*. New York: McGraw Hill; 1999.

25. Arendt-Nielsen L, Fernandez-de-las-Penas C, Graven-Nielson T. Basic aspects of musculoskeletal pain: from acute to chronic pain. *J Man Manip Ther*. 2011;19(4):186–193.

26. Jensen MP, Karoly P, Braver S. The measurement of clinical pain intensity: a comparison of six methods. *Pain*. 1956;27:117–126.

27. Strong J. Assessment of pain perception in clinical practice. *Manual Ther*. 1999;4:216–220.

28. Farrar JT, Young JP, LaMoreaux L, et al. Clinical importance of changes in chronic pain intensity measured on an 11-point numerical pain rating scale. *Pain*. 2001;94:149–158.

29. Hawker GA, Mian S, Kendzerska T, French M. Measures of adult pain. *Arthritis Care Res*. 2001;63(S11):S240–S252.

30. Haefeli M, Elfering A. Pain assessment. *Eur Spine J*. 2006;15:S17–S24.

31. Rowbotham MC. What is a "clinically meaningful" reduction in pain? *Pain*. 2001;94:131–132.

32. Melzack R. The McGill pain questionnaire: major properties and scoring methods. *Pain*. 1975;1:277–299.

33. Melzack R, Torgerson WS. On the language of pain. *Anesthesiology*. 1971;34:50–59.

34. Melzack R. The short-form McGill pain questionnaire. *Pain*. 1987;30:191–197.

35. Brodie DJ, Burnett JV, Walker JM, et al. Evaluation of low back pain by patient questionnaires and therapist assessment. *J Orthop Sports Phys Ther*. 1990;11:519–529.

36. Scott J, Huskisson EC. Vertical or horizontal visual analogue scales. *Ann Rheum Dis*. 1979;38:560.

37. Langley GB, Sheppeard H. The visual analogue scale: its use in pain management. *Rheumatol Int*. 1985;5:145–148.

38. Carlsson AM. Assessment of chronic pain: aspects of the reliability and validity of the visual analogue scale. *Pain*. 1983;16:87–101.

39. Huskisson EC. Measurement of pain. *Lancet*. 1974;2(7889):1127–1131.

40. Lacey RJ, Lewis M, Jordan K, et al. Interrater reliability of scoring of pain drawings in a self-report health survey. *Spine*. 2005;30:E455–E458.

41. Bennett M. The LANSS Pain Scale: the Leeds assessment of neuropathic symptoms and signs. *Pain*. 2001;92:147–157.

42. Halle JS. Neuromusculoskeletal scan examination with selected related topics. In: Flynn TW, ed. *The Thoracic Spine and Rib Cage: Musculoskeletal Evaluation and Treatment*. Boston: Butterworth-Heinemann; 1996.

43. Gleim GW, McHugh MP. Flexibility and its effect on sports injury performance. *Sports Med*. 1997;24:289–299.

44. Lee M. Biomechanics of joint movements. In: Refshauge K, Gass E, eds. *Musculoskeletal Physiotherapy*. Oxford, England: Butterworth-Heinemann; 1995.

45. Bowen MK, Warren RF. Ligamentous control of shoulder stability based on selective cutting and static translation experiments. *Clin Sports Med*. 1991;10:757–782.

46. Terry GC, Hammon D, France P, et al. The stabilizing function of passive shoulder restraints. *Am J Sports Med*. 1991;19:26–34.

47. Waddell G, Main CJ. Illness behavior. In: Waddell G, ed. *The Back Pain Revolution*. Edinburgh: Churchill Livingstone; 1998.

48. Main CJ, Waddell G. Psychologic stress. In: Waddell G, ed. *The Back Pain Revolution*. Edinburgh: Churchill Livingstone; 1998.

49. Barsky AJ, Goodson JD, Lane RS, et al. The amplification of somatic symptoms. *Psychosomatic Med*. 1988;50:510–519.

50. Chaturvedi SK. Prevalence of chronic pain in psychiatric patients. *Pain*. 1987;24:231–237.

51. Main CJ, George SZ. Psychosocial influences on low back pain: why should you care? *Phys Ther*. 2011;91:609–613.

52. Linton SJ, Shaw WS. Impact of psychological factors in the experience of pain. *Phys Ther*. 2011;91:700–711.

53. Hill JC, Fritz JM. Psychosocial influences on low back pain, disability and response to treatment. *Phys Ther*. 2011;91:712–721.

54. Nicholas MK, Linton SJ, Watson PJ, et al. Early identification and management of psychological risk factors ("yellow flags") in patients with low back pain: a reappraisal. *Phys Ther*. 2011;91:737–753.

55. Waddell G, Newton M, Henderson I, et al. A fear-avoidance beliefs questionnaire (FABQ) and the role of fear-avoidance beliefs in chronic low back pain and disability. *Pain*. 1993;52:157–168.

56. Vlaeyen J, Kole-Snijders A, Boeren R, et al. Fear of movement/(re)injury in chronic low back pain and its relation to behavioral performance. *Pain*. 1995;62:363–372.

57. Miller RP, Kori SH, Todd DD. *The Tampa Scale*. Tampa, FL: Unpublished report; 1991.

58. Murphy DR, Hurwitz EL. The usefulness of clinical measures of psychologic factors in patients with spinal pain. *J Manip Physiol Ther*. 2011;34:609–613.

59. Hapidou EG, O'Brien MA, Pierrynowski MR, et al. Fear and avoidance of movement in people with chronic pain: psychometric properties of the 11 item Tampa Scale for Kinesiophobia (TSK-11). *Physiother Can*. 2012;64:235–241.

60. Swinkels-Meewisse EJ, Swinkels RA, Verbeek AL, et al. Psychometric properties of the Tampa Scale for Kinesiophobia and the Fear-Avoidance Beliefs Questionnaire in acute low back pain. *Man Ther*. 2003;8(1):29–36.

61. Vlaeyen JW, Kole Snijders AM, Rotteveel AM, et al. The role of fear of movement/(re)injury in pain disability. *J Occup Rehabil*. 1995;5(4):235–252.

62. McCracken LM, Gross RT, Aikens J, Carnrike CL. The assessment of anxiety and fear in persons with chronic pain: a comparison of instruments. *Behav Res Ther*. 1996;34(11/12):927–933.

63. Asmundson GJ, Norton PJ, Norton GR. Beyond pain: the role of fear and avoidance in chronicity. *Clin Psychol Rev*. 1999;19(1):97–119.

64. Fritz JM, George SZ, Delitto A. The role of fear-avoidance beliefs in acute low back pain: relationships with current and future disability and work status. *Pain*. 2001;94:7–15.

65. George SZ, Stryker SE. Fear-avoidance beliefs and clinical outcomes for patients seeking outpatient physical therapy for musculoskeletal pain conditions. *J Orthop Sports Ther*. 2011;41:249–259.

66. Gray H, Adefolarin AT, Howe TE. A systematic review of instruments for the assessment of work-related psychosocial factors (blue flags) individuals with non-specific low back pain. *Man Ther*. 2011;16:531–543.

67. LoPiccolo CJ, Goodkin K, Baldewicz TT. Current issues in the diagnosis and management of malingering. *Ann Med*. 1989;31:166–174.

68. Mallinson S. Listening to respondents: a qualitative assessment of the short-form 36 Health Status Questionnaire. *Social Sci Med*. 2002;54:11–21.

69. Ware JE, Sherbourne CD. The MOS 36-item short form health survey (SF-36). *Med Care*. 1992;30(6):473–483.

70. Terwee CB, Bot SD, de Boer MR, et al. Quality criteria were proposed for measurement properties of health status questionnaires. *J Clin Epidemiol*. 2007;60:34–42.

71. Goodman CC, Snyder TE. *Differential Diagnosis in Physical Therapy*. Philadelphia: WB Saunders; 1995.

72. Keefe FJ, Block AR. Development of an observation method for assessing pain behavior in chronic low back pain patients. *Behav Ther*. 1982;13:363–375.

73. Refshauge KM, Latimer J. The physical examination. In: Refshauge KM, Gass E, eds. *Musculoskeletal Physiotherapy*. Oxford, England: Butterworth-Heinemann; 1995.

74. Delany C. Should I warn the patient first? *Aust J Physiother*. 1996;42:249–255.

75. Ross MD, Boissonnault WG. Red flags: to screen or not to screen. *J Orthop Sports Phys Ther*. 2010;40:682–684.

76. Macedo LG, Magee DJ. Differences in range of motion between dominant and nondominant sides of upper and lower extremities. *J Manip Physiol Ther*. 2008;31:577–582.

77. Thompson J. A practical guide to clinical medicine – vital signs. http://medicine.ucsd.edu/clinicalmed/thinking.htm, 2007.

78. Kaplan NM, Deveraux RB, Miller HS. Systemic hyperextension. *Med Sci Sports Exerc*. 1994;26:S268–S270.

79. Zabetakis PM. Profiling the hypertensive patient in sports. *Clin Sports Med*. 1984;3:137–152.

80. Sanders B, Nemeth WC. Preparticipation physical examination. *J Orthop Sports Phys Ther*. 1996;23:144–163.

81. Hayes KW, Petersen C, Falconer J. An examination of Cyriax's passive motion tests with patients having osteoarthritis of the knee. *Phys Ther*. 1994;74:697–708.

82. Peterson CM, Hayes KW. Construct validity of Cyriax's selective tension examination: association of end feels with pain in the knee and shoulder. *J Orthop Sports Phys Ther*. 2000;30:512–527.

83. Franklin ME, Conner-Kerr T, Chamness M, et al. Assessment of exercise-induced minor muscle lesions: the accuracy of Cyriax's diagnosis by selective tissue paradigm. *J Orthop Sports Phys Ther*. 1996;24:122–129.

84. Williams P, Warwick R, eds. *Gray's Anatomy*. 36 ed. Edinburgh: Churchill Livingstone; 1980.

85. Kandel ER, Schwartz JH, Jessell TM. *Principles of Neural Science*. New York: McGraw Hill; 2000.

86. Nitta H, Tajima T, Sugiyama H, et al. Study on dermatomes by means of selective lumbar spinal nerve block. *Spine*. 1993;18:1782–1786.

87. Downs MB, Laport E. Conflicting dermatome maps: educational and clinical implications. *J Orthop Sports Phys Ther*. 2011;41:427–434.

88. Keegan JJ, Garrett ED. The segmental distribution of the cutaneous nerves in the limbs of man. *Anat Rec*. 1948;101:409–437.

89. Grieve GP. Referred pain and other clinical features. In: Boyling JD, Palastanga N, eds. *Grieve's Modern Manual Therapy: The Vertebral Column*. 2nd ed. Edinburgh: Churchill Livingstone; 1994.

90. Smyth MJ, Wright V. Sciatica and the intervertebral disc: an experimental study. *J Bone Joint Surg Am*. 1958;40:1401–1418.

91. Seddon HJ. Three types of nerve injury. *Brain*. 1943;66:17–28.

92. Sunderland S. *Nerve and Nerve Injuries*. Edinburgh: Churchill Livingstone; 1978.

93. Wilgis EF. Techniques for diagnosis of peripheral nerve loss. *Clin Orthop*. 1982;163:8–14.

94. Tardif GS. Nerve injuries: testing and treatment tactics. *Phys Sports Med*. 1995;23:61–72.

95. Omer GE. Physical diagnosis of peripheral nerve injuries. *Orthop Clin North Am*. 1981;12:207–228.

96. Harrelson GL. Evaluation of brachial plexus injuries. *Sports Med Update*. 1989;4:3–8.

97. Wilbourn AJ. Electrodiagnostic testing of neurologic injuries in athletes. *Clin Sports Med*. 1990;9:229–245.

98. Leffert R. Clinical diagnosis, testing, and electromyographic study in brachial plexus traction injuries. *Clin Orthop*. 1988;237:24–31.

99. Upton AR, McComas AJ. The double crush in nerve-entrapment syndromes. *Lancet*. 1973;2:359–362.

100. Mackinnon SE. Double and multiple "crush" syndromes. *Hand Clin*. 1992;8:369–390.

101. Lee Dellon A, Mackinnon SE. Chronic nerve compression model for the double crush hypothesis. *Ann Plast Surg*. 1991;26:259–264.

102. Nemoto K, Matsumoto N, Tazaki K, et al. An experimental study on the "double crush" hypothesis. *J Hand Surg Am*. 1987;12:552–559.

103. Schmid AB, Coppieters MW. The double crush syndrome revisited—a Delphi study to reveal current expert views on mechanisms underlying dual nerve disorders. *Man Ther*. 2011;16:557–562.

104. Butler D. *Mobilisation of the Nervous System*. Melbourne: Churchill Livingstone; 1991.

105. Elvey RL. Treatment of arm pain associated with abnormal brachial plexus tension. *Aust J Physiother*. 1986;32:225–230.

106. Shacklock M. Neurodynamics. *Physiotherapy*. 1995;81:9–16.

107. Shacklock M, Butler D, Slater H. The dynamic central nervous system: structure and clinical neurobiomechanics. In: Boyling JD, Palastanga N, eds. *Grieve's Modern Manual Therapy: The Vertebral Column*. 2nd ed. Edinburgh: Churchill Livingstone; 1994.

108. Sahrmann SA. *Diagnosis and Treatment of Movement Impairment Syndromes*. St. Louis: Mosby; 2002.

109. Shumway-Cook A, Woollacott M. *Motor Control: Theory and Practical Applications*. Baltimore: Williams & Wilkins; 1995.

110. Schmidt RA, Lee TD. *Motor Control and Learning: A Behavioral Emphasis*. Champaign, IL: Human Kinetics; 1999.

111. Kaltenborn FM. *Manual Mobilization of the Extremity Joints*. Oslo, Norway: Olaf Norlis Bokhandel; 1980.

112. Ombregt L, Bisschop P, ter Veer HJ, et al. *A System of Orthopedic Medicine*. London: WB Saunders; 1995.

113. Jull GA. Examination of the articular system. In: Boyling JD, Palastanga N, eds. *Grieve's Modern Manual Therapy: The Vertebral Column*. 2nd ed. Edinburgh: Churchill Livingstone; 1994.

114. Myers A, Canty K, Nelson T. Are the Ottawa ankle rules helpful in ruling out the need for x-ray examination in children? *Arch Dis Child*. 2005;90:1309–1311.

115. Lea RD, Gerhardt JJ. Range-of-motion measurements. *J Bone Joint Surg Am*. 1995;77:784–798.

116. Williams JG, Callaghan M. Comparison of visual estimation and goniometry in determination of a shoulder joint angle. *Physiotherapy*. 1990;76:655–657.

117. Bovens AM, van Baak MA, Vrencken JG, et al. Variability and reliability of joint measurements. *Am J Sports Med*. 1990;18:58–63.

118. Boone DC, Azen SP, Lin CM, et al. Reliability of goniometric measurements. *Phys Ther*. 1978;58(11):1355–1360.

119. Mayerson NH, Milano RA. Goniometric measurement reliability in physical medicine. *Arch Phys Med Rehabil*. 1984;65:92–94.

120. Riddle DL, Rothstein JM, Lamb RL. Goniometric reliability in a clinical setting: shoulder measurements. *Phys Ther*. 1987;67:668–673.

121. Remvig L, Jensen DV, Ward RC. Epidemiology of general joint hypermobility and basis for the proposed criteria for benign joint hypermobility syndrome: review of the literature. *J Rheumatol*. 2007;34(4):804–809.

122. Remvig L, Jensen DV, Ward RC. Are diagnostic criteria for general joint hypermobility and benign joint hypermobility syndrome based on reproducible and valid tests? A review of the literature. *J Rheumatol*. 2007;34(4):798–803.

123. Juul-Kristensen B, Rogind H, Jensen DV, et al. Inter-examiner reproducibility of tests and criteria for generalized joint hypermobility and benign joint hypermobility syndrome. *Rheumatology*. 2007;46:1835–1841.

124. Wolf JM, Cameron KL, Owens BD. Impact of joint laxity and hypermobility on the musculoskeletal system. *J Am Acad Orthop Surg*. 2011;19(8):463–471.

125. Aslan UB, Çelik E, Cavlak U, et al. Evaluation of inter-rater and intrarater reliability of Beighton and Horan joint mobility index. *Fizyoterapi Rehabilitasyon*. 2006;17(3):113–119.

126. Hirsch C, Hirsch M, John MT, et al. Reliability of the Beighton Hypermobility Index to determine the general joint laxity performed by dentists. *J Orofacial Ortho*. 2007;68:342–352.

127. Beighton P, Grahame R, Borde H. *Hypermobility of Joints*. Berlin: Springer-Verlag; 1983.

128. Wynne-Davies R. Hypermobility. *Proc R Soc Med*. 1971;64:689–693.

129. Carter C, Wilkinson J. Persistent joint laxity and congenital dislocation of the hip. *J Bone Joint Surg Br*. 1969;46:40–45.

130. Nicholas JS, Grossman RB, Hershman EB. The importance of a simplified classification of motion in sports in relation to performance. *Orthop Clin North Am*. 1977;8:499–532.

131. Paris SV, Patla C. *E1 Course Notes: Extremity Dysfunction and Manipulation*. Atlanta: Patris; 1988.

132. Riddle DL. Measurement of accessory motion: critical issues and related concepts. *Phys Ther*. 1992;72:865–874.

133. Petersen CM, Hayes KW. Construct validity of Cyriax's selective tissue examination: association of end-feels with pain at the knee and shoulder. *J Orthop Sports Phys Ther*. 2000;30:512–521.

134. Ivanhoe CB, Reistetter TA. Spasticity: the misunderstood part of the upper motor neuron syndrome. *Am J Phys Med Rehabil*. 2004;83(suppl):S3–S9.

135. Pandyan AD, Johnson GR, Price CI, et al. A review of the properties and limitations of the Ashworth and modified Ashworth scales as measures of spasticity. *Clin Rehab*. 1999;13:373–383.

136. Haas BM, Bergstrom E, Jamous A, et al. The inter rater reliability of the original and of the modified Ashworth scale for the assessment of spasticity in patients with spinal cord injury. *Spinal Cord*. 1996;34:560–564.

137. Ward AB. Assessment of tone. *Age Aging*. 2000;29:385–386.

138. Haugh AB, Pandyan AD, Johnson GR. A systemic review of the Tardieu Scale for the measurement of spasticity. *Disability Rehabil*. 2006;28(15):899–907.

139. Glisky J. Tardieu Scale. *J Physiother*. 2016;62:229.

140. Maitland GD. Palpation examination of the posterior cervical spine: the ideal, average and abnormal. *Aust J Physiother*. 1982;28:3–11.

141. Clarkson HM, Gilewich GB. *Musculoskeletal Assessment: Joint Range of Motion and Manual Muscle Strength*. Baltimore: Williams & Wilkins; 1989.

142. Evans P. Ligaments, joint surfaces, conjunct rotation and close pack. *Physiotherapy*. 1988;74:105–114.

143. Pope MH, Frymoyer JW, Krag MH. Diagnosing instability. *Clin Orthop*. 1992;279:60–67.

144. Sapega AA. Muscle performance evaluation in orthopedic practice. *J Bone Joint Surg Am*. 1990;72:1562–1574.

145. Hislop HJ, Montgomery J. *Daniels and Worthingham's Muscle Testing: Techniques of Manual Examination*. Philadelphia: WB Saunders; 1995.

146. Bohannon RW. Manual muscle testing: does it meet the standards of an adequate screening test? *Clin Rehabil*. 2005;19:662–667.

147. Kendall HO, Kendall FP, Boynton DA. *Posture and Pain*. Huntington, NY: Robert E. Krieger; 1970.

148. American Academy of Orthopedic Surgeon. *Athletic Training and Sports Medicine*. 2nd ed. Park Ridge, IL: American Academy of Orthopedic Surgeons; 1991.

149. Khan KM, Cook JL, Bonar F, et al. Histopathology of common tendinopathies: update and implications for clinical management. *Sports Med*. 1999;27:393–408.

150. Janda V. On the concept of postural muscles and posture in man. *Aust J Physiother*. 1983;29:83–85.

151. Schlink MB. Muscle imbalance patterns associated with low back syndromes. In: Watkins RG, ed. *The Spine in Sports*. St. Louis: Mosby; 1996.

152. Jull GA, Janda V. Muscles and motor control in low back pain: assessment and management. In: Twomey LT, Taylor JR, eds. *Physical Therapy of the Low Back*. New York: Churchill Livingstone; 1987.

153. Janda V. Muscles and motor control in cervicogenic disorders: assessment and management. In: Grant R, ed. *Physical Therapy of the Cervical and Thoracic Spine*. New York: Churchill-Livingstone; 1994.

154. Watson CJ, Schenkman M. Physical therapy management of isolated serratus anterior muscle paralysis. *Phys Ther*. 1995;75:194–202.

155. Laupacis A, Sekar N, Stiell IG. Clinical prediction rules—a review and suggested modifications of methodological standards. *JAMA*. 1997;277:488–494.

156. Reiman MP, Manske RC. The assessment of function: how is it measured? A clinical perspective. *J Man Manip Ther*. 2011;19:91–99.

157. Paxton EW, Fithian DC, Stone ML, et al. The reliability and validity of knee-specific and general health instruments in assessing acute patellar dislocation outcomes. *Am J Sports Med*. 2003;31:487–492.

158. Epstein AM. The outcomes movement: will it get us where we want to go? *N Engl J Med*. 1990;323:266–270.

159. Goldstein TS. *Functional Rehabilitation in Orthopedics*. Gaithersburg, MD: Aspen; 1995.

160. Swiontkowski MF, Engelberg R, Martin DP, et al. Short musculoskeletal function assessment questionnaire: validity, reliability, and responsiveness. *J Bone Joint Surg Am*. 1999;81:1245–1260.

161. Research Foundation, State University of New York. *Guide for Use of the Uniform Data Set for Medical Rehabilitation Including the Functional*

Independence Measure (FIM). Buffalo, NY: Research Foundation, State University of; 1990.

162. Reuben DB, Siu AL. An objective measure of physical function of elderly outpatients: the physical performance test. *J Am Geriatr Soc.* 1990;38:1105–1112.

163. Jette AM. Functional status index: reliability of a chronic disease evaluation instrument. *Arch Phys Med Rehabil.* 1980;61:395–401.

164. Meenan R, Mason JH, Anderson JJ, et al. AIMS 2: the content and properties of a revised and expanded arthritis impact measurement scales health status questionnaire. *Arthritis Rheum.* 1990;25:1–10.

165. Brimer MA, Shuneman G, Allen BR. Guidelines for developing a functional assessment for an acute facility. *Phys Ther Forum.* 1993;12:22–25.

166. Gatchel RJ, Polatin PB, Mayer TG, et al. Use of the SF-36 health status survey with a chronically disabled back pain population: strength and limitations. *J Occup Rehab.* 1998;8:237–245.

167. Gatchel RJ, Mayer T, Dersh J, et al. The association of the SF-36 health status survey with 1-year socioeconomic outcomes in a chronically disabled spinal disorder population. *Spine.* 1999;24:2162–2170.

168. Bergner M, Bobbitt RA, Pollard WE, et al. The sickness impact profile: validation of a health status measure. *Medical Care.* 1976;14:57–67.

169. Swiontkowski MF, Engelberg R, Martin DP, et al. Short musculoskeletal function assessment questionnaire: validity, reliability and responsiveness. *J Bone Joint Surg Am.* 1999;81:1245–1260.

170. Strand LI, Wie SL. The sock test for evaluating activity limitation in patients with musculoskeletal pain. *Phys Ther.* 1999;79:136–145.

171. Ellexson MT. Analyzing an industry: job analysis for treatment, prevention, and placement. *Orthop Phys Ther Clin.* 1992;1;15–21.

172. McGinn TG, Guyatt GH, Wyer PC, et al. Users' guides to medical literature: XXII: how to use articles about clinical decision rules. *JAMA.* 2000;284(7):79–84.

173. Backstrom KM, Whitman JM, Flynn TW. Lumbar spinal stenosis—diagnosis and management of the aging spine. *Man Ther.* 2011;16:308–317.

174. Haskins R, Rivett DA, Osmotherly PG. Clinical prediction rules in the physiotherapy management of low back pain: a systemic review. *Man Ther.* 2012;17:9–21.

175. Flynn T, Fritz J, Whitman J, et al. A clinical prediction rule for classifying patients with low back pain who demonstrate short-term improvements with spinal manipulation. *Spine.* 2002;27:2835–2843.

176. Glynn PE, Weisbach PC. *Clinical Prediction Rules—A Physical Therapy Reference Manual.* Sudbury, MA: Jones and Bartlett Publishers; 2011.

177. Reilly BM, Evans AT. Translating clinical research into clinical practice: impact of using prediction rules to make decisions. *Ann Intern Med.* 2006;144:201–209.

178. Wasson JH, Sox HC, Neff RK, et al. Clinical prediction rules—applications and methodological standards. *N Eng J Med.* 1985;313:793–799.

179. Toll DB, Janssen KJ, Vergouwe, Moons KG. Validation, updating and impact of clinical prediction rules: a review. *J Clin Epidemiol.* 2008;61:1085–1094.

180. Beatie P, Nelson R. Clinical prediction rules: what are they and what do they tell us? *Austr J Physiother.* 2006;52:157–163.

181. Brehant JC, Stiell IG, Visentin L, et al. Clinical decision rules "in the real world": how a widely disseminated rule is used in everyday practice. *Acad Emerg Med.* 2005;12:948–957.

182. Bruce SL, Wilkerson GB. Clinical prediction rules, Part 1: Conceptual overview; Part 2: Data analysis procedures and clinical application of results. *Athletic Ther Today.* 2010;15(2):4–13.

183. Ebell M. AHRQ White Paper: use of clinical decision rules for point-of-care decision support. *Med Decision Making.* 2010;30(6):712–721.

184. Rowe CR. *The Shoulder.* Edinburgh: Churchill Livingstone; 1988.

185. Lippitt SB, Harryman DT, Matsen FA. A practical tool for evaluating function: the simple shoulder test. In: Matsen FA, Fu FH, Hawkins RJ, eds. *The Shoulder: A Balance of Mobility and Stability.* Rosemont, IL: American Academy of Orthopedic Surgeons; 1993.

186. Gerber C. Integrated scoring systems for the functional assessment of the shoulder. In: Matsen FA, Fu FH, Hawkins RJ, eds. *The Shoulder: A Balance of Mobility and Stability.* Rosemont, IL: American Academy of Orthopedic Surgeons; 1993.

187. Carroll HD. A quantitative test of upper extremity function. *J Chron Dis.* 1965;18:479–491.

188. Potvin AR, Tourtellotte WW, Dailey JS, et al. Simulated activities of daily living examination. *Arch Phys Med Rehabil.* 1972;53:476–486.

189. Cook C. The lost art of the clinical examination: an overemphasis on clinical special tests. *J Man Manip Ther.* 2010;18:3–4.

190. Hegedus EJ. Studies of quality and impact in clinical diagnosis and decision making. *J Man Manip Ther.* 2010;18:5–6.

191. Hegedus EJ, Wright AA, Cook C. Orthopedic special tests and diagnostic accuracy studies: house wine served in very cheap containers. *Br J Sports Med.* 2017;51(22):1578–1579.

192. Ransohoff DF, Feinstein AR. Problems of spectrum and bias in evaluating the efficacy of diagnostic tests. *N Engl J Med.* 1978;299:926–930.

193. Bossuyt PM, Reitsma JB, Bruns DE, et al. Towards complete and accurate reporting of studies of diagnostic accuracy: the STARD initiative. *BMJ.* 2003;326:41–42.

194. Cipriani D, Noftz J. The utility of orthopedic clinical tests for diagnosis. In: Magee DJ, Zachazewski JF, Quillen SW, eds. *Scientific Foundations and Principles of Practice in Musculoskeletal Rehabilitation.* Philadelphia: Elsevier; 2007.

195. Greenhalgh T. How to read a paper: papers that report diagnostic or screening tests. *Br Med J.* 1997;315:540–543.

196. Fritz JM, Wainner RS. Examining diagnostic tests: an evidence-based perspective. *Phys Ther.* 2001;81:1546–1564.

197. Cook CE, Hegedus EJ. *Orthopedic Physical Examination Tests—An Evidence Based Approach.* Upper Saddle River, NJ: Prentice Hall Pearson; 2008.

198. Cleland J, Koppenhaver S. *Orthopedic Clinical Examination: An Evidence-Based Approach for Physical Therapists.* 2nd ed. Philadelphia: Saunders Elsevier; 2011.

199. Portney LG, Walkins MP. *Foundations of Clinical Research: Applications to Practice.* Upper Saddle River, NJ: Prentice Hall; 2000.

200. Schwartz JS. Evaluating diagnostic tests: what is done—what needs to be done. *J Gen Int Med.* 1986;1:266–267.

201. Guyatt GH, Deyo RA, Charlson M, et al. Responsiveness and validity in health status measurement: a clarification. *J Clin Epidemiol.* 1989;42:403–408.

202. Jaeschke R, Singer J, Guyatt GH. Measurement of health status: ascertaining the minimally clinical important difference. *Control Clin Trials.* 1989;10:407–415.

203. Boyko EJ. Ruling out or ruling in disease with the most sensitive or specific diagnostic test: short cut or wrong turn? *Med Decision Making.* 1994;14:175–179.

204. Hagen MD. Test characteristics: how good is that test? *Med Decision Making.* 1995;22:213–233.

205. Jaeschke R, Guyatt GH, Sackett DL. Users' guides to the medical literature. III. How to use an article about a diagnostic test. B. What are the results and will they help me in caring for my patients? The Evidence-Based Medicine Working Group. *JAMA.* 1994;271:703–707.

206. Anderson MA, Forman TL. Return to competition: functional rehabilitation. In: Zachazewski JE, Magee DJ, Quillen WS, eds. *Athletic Injuries and Rehabilitation.* Philadelphia: WB Saunders; 1996.

207. Lijmer JG, Mol BW, Heisterkamp S, et al. Empirical evidence of design-related bias in studies of diagnostic tests. *JAMA.* 1999;282:1061–1066.

208. Schulzer M. Diagnostic tests: a statistical review. *Muscle Nerve.* 1994;17:815–819.

209. Cook C. Challenges with diagnosis: sketchy reference standards. *J Man Manip Ther.* 2012;20:111–112.

210. Sackett DL. A primer on the precision and accuracy of the clinical examination. *JAMA.* 1992;267:2638–2644.

211. Wright A, Hannon J, Hegedus EJ, et al. Clinimetrics corner: a closer look at the minimal clinically important difference (MCID). *J Man Manip Ther.* 2012;20:160–166.

212. Davidson M, Keating J. Patient-reported outcome measures (PROMS): how should I interpret reports of measurement properties? A practical guide for clinicians and researchers who are no biostatisticians. *Br J Sports Med.* 2014;48:792–796.

213. McGregor AH, Doré CJ, McCarthy ID, et al. Are subjective clinical findings and objective clinical tests related to the motion characteristics of low back pain subjects? *J Orthop Sports Phys Ther.* 1998;28:370–377.

214. Kuroda R, Hoshino Y, Kubo S, et al. Similarities and differences of diagnostic manual tests for anterior cruciate ligament insufficiency—a global survey and kinematics assessment. *Am J Sports Med.* 2012;40:91–99.

215. Jonsson T, Althoff B, Peterson L, et al. Clinical diagnosis of ruptures of the anterior cruciate ligament: a comparative study of the Lachman test and the anterior drawer sign. *Am J Sports Med.* 1982;10:100–102.

216. Rosenberg TD, Rasmussen GL. The function of the anterior cruciate ligament during anterior drawer and Lachman's testing. *Am J Sports Med.* 1984;12:318–322.

217. Cervical Spine Research Society. *The Cervical Spine.* Philadelphia: JB Lippincott; 1989.

218. Hagbarth KE, Wallen G, Burke D, et al. Effects of the Jendrassik maneuver on muscle spindle activity in man. *J Neurol Neurosurg Psych.* 1975;38:1143–1153.

219. Bland JH. *Disorders of the Cervical Spine.* Philadelphia: WB Saunders; 1987.

220. Poynton AR, O'Farrell DA, Shannon F, et al. Sparing of sensation to pin prick predicts recovery of a motor segment after injury to the spinal cord. *J Bone Joint Surg Br.* 1997;79:952–954.

221. Hockaday JM, Whitty CWM. Patterns of referred pain in the normal subject. *Brain.* 1967;90:481–495.

222. Mennell JM. *Joint Pain.* Boston: Little Brown & Co; 1972.

223. Kaltenborn FM. *Mobilization of the Extremity Joints: Examination and Basic Treatment Techniques.* Oslo, Norway: Olaf Norlis Bokhandel; 1980.

224. Lewit K, Liebenson C. Palpation: Problems and implications. *J Manip Physiol Ther.* 1993;16:586–590.

225. Gerwin RD, Shannon S, Hong CZ, et al. Interrater reliability in myofascial trigger point examination. *Pain.* 1997;17:591–595.

226. Njoo KH, Van der Does E. The occurrence and interrater reliability of myofascial trigger points in the quadratus lumborum and gluteus maximus: a prospective study in non-specific low back patients and controls in general practice. *Pain.* 1994;58:317–321.

227. Snider KT, Snider EJ, Degenhardt BF, et al. Palpatory accuracy of lumbar spinous processes using multiple bony landmarks. *J Manip Physiol Ther.* 2011;34:306–313.

228. Deyle GD. Musculoskeletal imaging in physical therapy practice. *J Orthop Sports Phys Ther.* 2005;35:708–721.

229. Deyle GD. The role of MRI in musculoskeletal practice: a clinical perspective. *J Man Manip Ther.* 2011;19(3):152–161.

230. Khan KM, Tress BW, Hare WS, et al. Treat the patient, not the x-ray: advances in diagnostic imaging do not replace the need for clinical interpretation. *Clin J Sports Med.* 1998;8:1–4.

231. Johnson TR, Steinbach LS. *Essentials of Musculoskeletal Imaging.* Rosemont, IL: American Academy of Orthopedic Surgeons; 2003.

232. Resnick D, Kransdorf MJ. *Bone and Joint Imaging.* Philadelphia: Elsevier; 2005.

233. McKinnis LN. *Fundamentals of Musculoskeletal Imaging.* Philadelphia: FA Davis; 2005.

234. Coris EE, Zwygart K, Fletcher M, et al. Imaging in sports medicine: an overview. *Sports Med Arthrosc Rev.* 2009;17:2–12.

235. Bigg-Wither G, Kelly P. Diagnostic imaging in musculoskeletal physiotherapy. In: Refshauge K, Gass E, eds. *Musculoskeletal Physiotherapy.* Oxford, England: Butterworth-Heinemann; 1995.

236. Jones MD. *Basic Diagnostic Radiology.* St. Louis: Mosby; 1969.

237. Miller WT. *Introduction to Clinical Radiology.* New York: MacMillan; 1982.

238. Gross GW. Imaging. In: Stanitski CL, DeLee JC, Drez D, eds. *Pediatric and Adolescent Sports Medicine.* Philadelphia: WB Saunders; 1994.

239. Fischbach F. *A Manual of Laboratory Diagnostic Tests.* 3nd ed. Philadelphia: JB Lippincott.; 1988.

240. Ghanem I, El Hage S, Rachkidi R, et al. Pediatric cervical spine instability. *J Child Orthop.* 2008;2:71–84.

241. Gruelich WW, Pyle SU. *Radiographic Atlas of Skeletal Development of the Wrist and Hand.* Stanford, CA: Stanford University Press; 1959.

242. Sanders JO, Khoury JG, Kishan S, et al. Predicting scoliosis progression from skeletal maturity: a simplified classification during adolescence. *J Bone Joint Surg Am.* 2008;90(3):540–543.

243. Grainger RG. The spinal canal. In: Whitehouse GH, Worthington BS, eds. *Techniques in Diagnostic Radiology.* Oxford, England: Blackwell Scientific; 1983.

244. Buckwalter KA. Computerized tomography in sports medicine. *Sports Med Arthrosc Rev.* 2009;17:13–20.

245. Evans RC. *Illustrated Essentials in Orthopedic Physical Assessment.* St. Louis: Mosby Year Book; 1994.

246. Hsu W, Hearty TM. Radionuclide imaging in the diagnosis and management of orthopedic disease. *J Am Acad Orthop Surg.* 2012;20(3):151–159.

247. Leffers D, Collins L. An overview of the use of bone scintigraphy in sports medicine. *Sports Med Arthrosc Rev.* 2009;17:21–24.

248. Black BR, Chong LR, Potter HG. Cartilage imaging in sports medicine. *Sports Med Arthrosc Rev.* 2008;17:68–80.

249. Silvis ML, Mosher TJ, Smetana BS, et al. High prevalence of pelvis and hip magnetic resonance imaging findings in asymptomatic collegiate and professional hockey players. *Am J Sports Med.* 2011;39:715–721.

250. Hurd WJ, Eby S, Kaufman KR, et al. Magnetic resonance imaging of the throwing elbow in the uninjured high school-aged baseball pitcher. *Am J Sports Med.* 2011;39:722–728.

251. Murray PJ, Shaffer BS. MR imaging of the shoulder. *Sports Med Arthrosc Rev.* 2008;17:40–48.

252. Klauser AS, Taglifico A, Allen GM, et al. Clinical indications for musculoskeletal ultrasound: a Delphi-based consensus paper of the European Society of Musculoskeletal Radiology. *Eur Radiol.* 2012;22:1140–1148.

253. Alves TI, Girish G, Brigido MK, Jacobson JA. US of the knee: Scanning techniques, pitfalls, and pathologic conditions. *Radio Graphics.* 2016;36:1759–1775.

254. Jacobson JA. Musculoskeletal Ultrasound: Focused impact on MRI. *Am J Radiol.* 2009;193:619–627.

255. Starr HM, Sedgley MD, Means KR, Murphy MS. Ultrasonography for hand and wrist conditions. *J Am Acad Orthop Surg.* 2016;24:544–554.

256. Vanderhave KL, Brighton B, Casey V, et al. Applications of musculoskeletal ultrasonography in pediatric patients. *J Am Acad Orthop Surg.* 2014;22(11):691–698.

257. Weissman BNW, Sledge CB. *Orthopedic Radiology.* Philadelphia: WB Saunders; 1986.

258. Jones MA. Clinical reasoning in manual therapy. *Phys Ther.* 1992;72:875–884.

259. Jones MA, Rivett DA. *Clinical Reasoning for Manual Therapists.* Edinburgh: Butterworth Heinemann; 2004.

260. Thompson J. A practical guide to clinical medicine – clinician decision making. http://medicine.ucsd.edu/clinicalmed/thinking.htm, 2007.

CHAPTER 2

Head and Face

Casualty officers and clinicians working in emergency care settings are often the ones who assess the head and face. In these settings, the assessment involves the bony aspects of the head and face as well as the soft tissues. The soft-tissue assessment involves primarily the sensory organs, such as the skin, eyes, nose, ears, and brain whereas the muscles are tested only as they relate to injury to these structures. Joints and their integrity are not the main objects of the assessment. Because the temporomandibular joints and cervical spine are discussed in Chapters 3 and 4, this chapter deals with only the head, the face, and their associated structures.

Applied Anatomy

The head and face are made up of the cranial vault and facial bones. The **cranial vault,** or skull, is composed of several bones: one frontal, two sphenoid, two parietal, two temporal, and one occipital (Fig. 2.1). Of these, the strongest is the occipital bone, and the weakest are the temporal bones. The frontal bone forms the forehead, and the temporal and sphenoid bones form the antero-lateral walls of the skull, or the temples of the head. The parietal bones form the top and posterolateral portions of the skull, and the occipital bones form the posterior portion of the skull. The cranial vault reaches 90% of its ultimate size by age 5.

In addition to the cranial vault bones, there are 14 **facial bones.** These bones develop more slowly than the cranial bones, reaching only 60% of their ultimate size by age 6. The facial skeleton is composed of the mandible, which forms the lower jaw; the maxilla, which forms the upper jaw on each side; the nasal bones, which form the bridge of the nose; and the palatine, lacrimal, zygomatic, and ethmoid bones, which form the remainder of the face. It is the zygomatic bone that gives the cheek its prominence. The sphenoid bones also form part of the orbital cavity. The facial skull has several cavities for the eyes (orbital), nose (nasal), and mouth (oral), as well as spaces for nerves and blood vessels to penetrate the bony structure. Weight is saved in the skull area by the addition of sinus cavities (Fig. 2.2).

The muscles of the head and face are controlled primarily by the 12 **cranial nerves.** The cranial nerves and their chief functions are shown in Table 2.1. The cranial nerves generally contain both sensory and motor fibers. However, some cranial nerves are strictly sensory (i.e., olfactory and optic), whereas others are strictly motor (i.e., oculomotor, trochlear, and hypoglossal).

The **external eye** is composed of the eyelids (upper and lower), conjunctiva (a transparent membrane covering the cornea, iris, pupil, lens, and sclera), lacrimal gland, eye muscles, and bony skull orbit (Fig. 2.3). Muscles of the eye, their actions, and their nerve supply are shown in Table 2.2. The muscles and movements of the eye are shown in Fig. 2.4. To produce some of the actions, the various muscles of the eye must work together. The **eyelids** protect the eye from foreign bodies, distribute tears over the surface of the eye, and limit the amount of light entering the eye. The **conjunctiva** is a thin membrane covering the majority of the anterior surface of the eye. It helps to protect the eye from foreign bodies and desiccation (i.e., drying up). The lacrimal gland provides tears, which keep the eye moist (Fig. 2.5). The eye itself is made up of the sclera, cornea, and iris, as well as the lens and retina (Fig. 2.6). The **sclera** is the dense white portion of the eye that physically supports the internal structures. The **cornea** is very sensitive to pain (e.g., the extreme pain that accompanies corneal abrasion) and separates the watery fluid of the anterior chamber of the eye from the external environment. It permits transmission of light through the lens to the retina. The **iris** is a circular, contractile muscular disc that controls the amount of light entering the eye and contains pigmented cells that give color to the eye. The **lens** is a crystalline structure located immediately behind the iris that permits images from varied distances to be focused on the retina. It is primarily the lens and its supporting ligaments that separate the eye into chambers: the anterior chamber (**aqueous humor**) and the posterior chamber (**vitreous humor**). Finally, the **retina** is the primary sensory structure of the eye that transforms light impulses into electrical impulses that are then transmitted by the optic nerve to the brain, which interprets the impulses as the objects seen.

The **external ear** consists of cartilage covered with skin. Its primary purpose is to direct sound and to protect the **external auditory meatus**, through which sound is transmitted to the eardrum. The external ear, which is sometimes called the *pinna, auricle,* or *trumpet,* consists of the helix and lobule around the outside and the

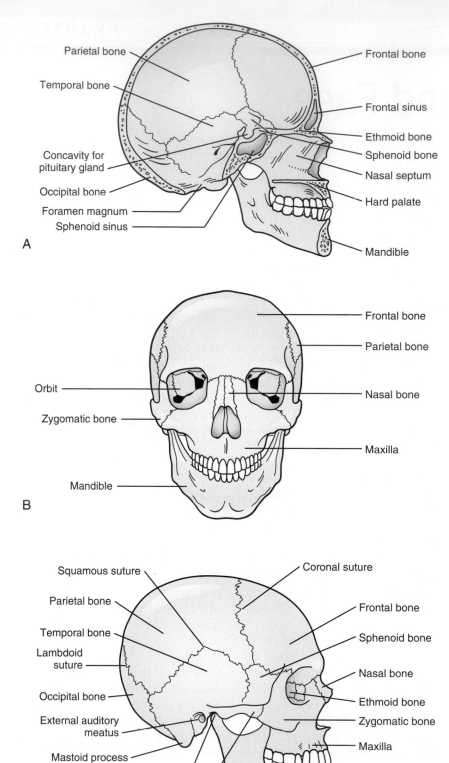

Fig. 2.1 Bones of the head and face. (A) Interior view. (B) Anterior view. (C) Lateral view. (Redrawn from Jenkins DB: *Hollinshead's functional anatomy of the limbs and back*, Philadelphia, 1991, WB Saunders, pp 332–333.)

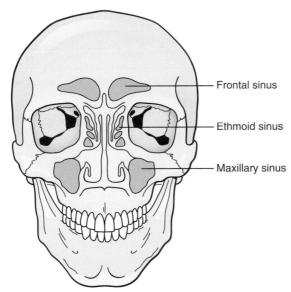

Frontal sinus

Ethmoid sinus

Maxillary sinus

Fig. 2.2 The nasal sinuses. (Modified from Swartz HM: *Textbook of physical diagnosis*, Philadelphia, 1989, WB Saunders, p 166.)

triangular fossa, antihelix, concha, tragus (a cartilaginous projection anterior to external auditory meatus), and antitragus on the inside (Fig. 2.7). The **middle ear** structures consist of the tympanic membrane, or eardrum, which vibrates when sound hits it and sends vibrations through the ossicles—called the *malleus* (hammer), *incus* (anvil), and *stapes* (stirrup)—to the cochlea. The cochlea, which is part of the inner ear, transmits the sound waves to the vestibulocochlear nerve (cranial nerve VIII), which transmits electrical impulses to the brain for interpretation. The **semicircular canals,** the other part of the inner ear, play a significant role in maintaining balance.

The **external nose,** like the external ear, consists primarily of cartilage covered with skin. Its proximal portion contains bone covered with skin. Fig. 2.8 shows the bone and cartilage makeup of the nose. The floor of the nose consists of the hard and soft palates and forms the roof of the mouth (Fig. 2.9). Cartilage and the nasal, frontal, ethmoid, and sphenoid bones form the roof of the nose. The frontal and maxillary bones form the nasal bridge. Three bony structures called *turbinates* (superior, middle, and inferior) form the lateral aspects of the nose, which increase the surface area of the nose and thereby warm, humidify, and filter more of the inspired air. The nose is divided into two chambers (vestibules) by a septum. These chambers are lined with a mucous membrane containing hairs that collect debris and other foreign substances from the inspired air. The cribriform plate of the ethmoid bone contains the sensory fibers of the olfactory nerve (cranial nerve I) for smell.

Patient History

In addition to the questions listed under "Patient History" in Chapter 1, the examiner should obtain the following

information from the patient who has sustained an injury to the head or the face:

1. *What happened?* This question determines the mechanism of injury and, potentially, the area of the brain or face injured (Table 2.3). A pathological classification for acute traumatic brain injuries is shown in the box below.[1] A forceful blow to a resting, movable head usually produces maximum brain injury beneath the point of impact (Fig. 2.10). This type of injury, called a **coup injury,** is usually caused by linear or translational acceleration.[2] It often causes focal ischemic lesions, especially in the cerebellum, leading to alterations in smooth, coordinated movements, equilibrium, and posture. If the head is moving and strikes an unyielding object, such as the ground, maximum brain injury is usually sustained in an area opposite the site of impact.

Pathological Classification of Acute Traumatic Brain Injury

- Diffuse brain injury
  - Cerebral concussion
  - Diffuse axonal injury
- Focal brain injury
  - Epidural hematoma
  - Subdural hematoma
  - Cerebral contusion
  - Intracerebral hemorrhage
  - Subarachnoid hemorrhage
  - Intraventricular hemorrhage
- Skull fracture
- Penetrating brain injury

Modified from Jordan BD: Brain injury in boxing, *Clin Sports Med* 28:561–578, 2009.

This **contrecoup injury** is the result of impact deceleration. The injury occurs on the side of the head opposite to that receiving the blow, because the head is accelerating before impact, which squeezes the cerebrospinal fluid away from the trailing edge (i.e., the side away from the impact). The fluid moves toward the impact side, thereby thickening the cerebrospinal fluid and offering a cushioning effect at the point of impact. Because of the lack of cushioning on the trailing edge, greater injury is likely to occur to the brain on the side opposite the impact. The brain may also experience a "shaking" caused by repeated reverberation within the brain after the head has been struck. **Concussion severity** can be determined only after signs and symptoms have disappeared and any neurological and cognitive testing is normal.[3] If the cervical spine is taken beyond its normal range of motion (ROM), especially into rotation or side flexion, there may be a twisting of the cerebral hemisphere, brain stem, carotid artery, or carotid sinus that can result in injury to these structures or ischemia to the brain. These areas of the brain that are most susceptible to

TABLE **2.1**

Cranial Nerves and Methods of Testing

Nerve	Afferent (Sensory)	Efferent (Motor)	Test
I. Olfactory	Smell: Nose	—	Identify familiar odors (e.g., chocolate, coffee)
II. Optic	Sight: Eye	—	Test visual fields
III. Oculomotor	—	Voluntary motor: Levator of eyelid; superior, medial, and inferior recti; inferior oblique muscle of eyeball Autonomic: Smooth muscle of eyeball	Upward, downward, and medial gaze Reaction to light
IV. Trochlear	—	Voluntary motor: superior oblique muscle of eyeball	Downward and lateral gaze
V. Trigeminal	Touch, pain: Skin of face, mucous membranes of nose, sinuses, mouth, anterior tongue	Voluntary motor: muscles of mastication	Corneal reflex Face sensation Clench teeth; push down on chin to separate jaws
VI. Abducens	—	Voluntary motor: Lateral rectus muscle of eyeball	Lateral gaze
VII. Facial	Taste: Anterior tongue	Voluntary motor: Facial muscles Autonomic: Lacrimal, submandibular, and sublingual glands	Close eyes tight Smile and show teeth Whistle and puff cheeks Identify familiar tastes (e.g., sweet, sour)
VIII. Vestibulocochlear (acoustic nerve)	Hearing: Ear Balance: Ear	—	Hear watch ticking Hearing tests Balance and coordination test
IX. Glossopharyngeal	Touch, pain: Posterior tongue, pharynx Taste: Posterior tongue	Voluntary motor: Unimportant muscle of pharynx Autonomic: Parotid gland	Gag reflex Ability to swallow
X. Vagus	Touch, pain: Pharynx, larynx, bronchi Taste: Tongue, epiglottis	Voluntary motor: Muscles of palate, pharynx, and larynx Autonomic: Thoracic and abdominal viscera	Gag reflex Ability to swallow Say "Ah"
XI. Accessory	—	Voluntary motor: Sternocleidomastoid and trapezius muscle	Resisted shoulder shrug
XII. Hypoglossal	—	Voluntary motor: Muscles of tongue	Tongue protrusion (if injured, tongue deviates toward injured side)

Adapted from Hollinshead WH, Jenkins DB: *Functional anatomy of the limbs and back*, Philadelphia, 1981, WB Saunders, p 358; Reid DC: *Sports injury assessment and rehabilitation*, New York, 1992, Churchill Livingstone, p 860.

damage include the temporal lobes, anterior frontal lobe, posterior occipital lobe, and upper portion of the midbrain.[4]

2. *Did the patient lose consciousness? If so, how long was the patient unconscious? Has the patient suffered a concussion before?* These questions are often difficult for the patient to answer or the examiner to know, because the patient may have been momentarily stunned and the time may have been so short that the patient believed there was no loss of consciousness. In other words, loss of consciousness may have been only momentary or, more traditionally, it may have lasted seconds to minutes. If the examiner is working with a sports team, accurate records are essential to record the severity and the number of concussions suffered by the athlete and to ensure that proper care is instituted so that the athlete is not allowed to return to competition too soon. If

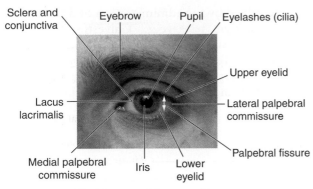

Fig. 2.3 External features of the eye.

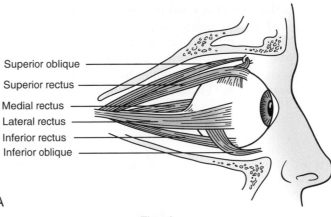

A

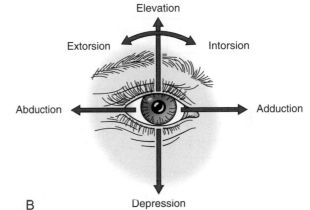

B

Fig. 2.4 Muscles (A) and movements (B) of the eye. (Modified from Swartz HM: *Textbook of physical diagnosis*, Philadelphia, 1989, WB Saunders, pp 125–126.)

TABLE **2.2**

Muscles of the Eye: Their Actions and Nerve Supply

Action	Muscles Acting	Nerve Supply
Moves pupil upward	Superior rectus	Oculomotor (CN III)
Moves pupil downward	Inferior rectus	Oculomotor (CN III)
Moves pupil medially	Medial rectus	Oculomotor (CN III)
Moves pupil laterally	Lateral rectus	Abducens (CN VI)
Moves pupil downward and laterally	Superior oblique	Trochlear (CN IV)
Moves pupil upward and laterally	Inferior oblique	Oculomotor (CN III)
Elevates upper eyelid	Levator palpebrae superioris	Oculomotor (CN III)

CN, Cranial nerve.

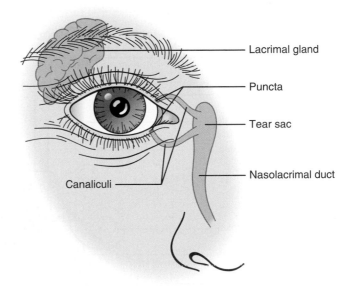

Fig. 2.5 The lacrimal apparatus. (Modified from Swartz HM: *Textbook of physical diagnosis*, Philadelphia, 1989, WB Saunders, p 126.)

unconsciousness occurs, as he or she recovers, the level of consciousness may vary. The patient may be comatose, stuporous, obtunded, lethargic, confused, or finally fully alert. The patient goes through the following stages of recovery: unconsciousness (also called **paralytic coma**), stupor, obtundity, lethargy, confusion (with or without delirium), near lucidity with automatism, and finally full alertness. **Stupor** implies that the patient is only partially conscious and has reduced responsiveness. **Obtundity** implies the patient has reduced sensitivity to painful or unpleasant stimuli. **Lethargy** implies a state of sluggishness, dullness, or serious drowsiness. **Confusion** implies that the patient is disoriented in terms of time, place, or person. **Delirium** means that the patient may experience illusions, hallucinations, restlessness, or incoherence. **Lucidity with automatism** implies that the patient appears to be alert and fully recovered but acts only mechanically and is not really aware of what he or she is doing. Both retrograde and posttraumatic amnesia are evident, and the patient demonstrates mental confusion and complains of tinnitus (i.e., ringing in the ears) and dizziness. The patient also has residual headaches and is unsteady for 5 to 10 minutes after regaining consciousness. The literature has reported that loss of consciousness, by itself, is not a good predictor of the degree of neurophysiologic loss or damage with a head injury.[5] The severity of the head injury is best determined by the administration of different neurophysiologic tests (e.g., Galveston Orientation and Amnesia Test [GOAT],[6] Hopkins Verbal Learning Test,[7] Trail Making Test, Wisconsin Card Sorting Test, Digit Symbol Substitution Test [DSST],[8] and measures of decision time[8]), as well

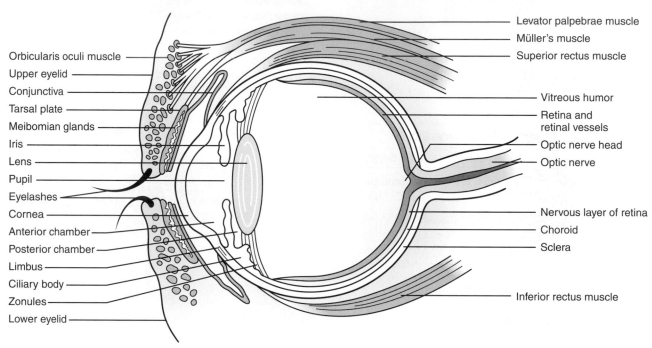

Fig. 2.6 Cross section of the eye. (Modified from Swartz HM: *Textbook of physical diagnosis,* Philadelphia, 1989, WB Saunders, p 132.)

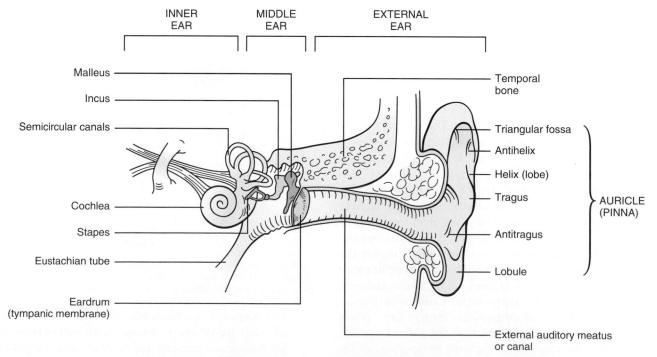

Fig. 2.7 A cross-sectional view through the ear.

as considering all signs and symptoms the patient demonstrates.[9-15] However, to ensure adequate data, these tests must also have been administered before the injury (e.g., in a preparticipation evaluation for sports).[9,16]

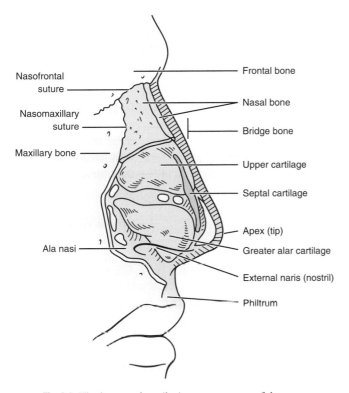

Fig. 2.8 The bony and cartilaginous structures of the nose.

Levels of Consciousness

• **Alertness**	Is readily aroused, oriented, and fully aware of surroundings
• **Confusion**	Memory is impaired
	Is confused and disoriented
• **Lethargy**	Sleeps when not stimulated
	Is drowsy and inattentive
	Responds to name
	Loses train of thought
	Shows decreased spontaneous movement
	Has slow and fuzzy thinking
• **Obtundity**	Responds to loud voice or shaking
	Responds to painful stimulus (withdrawal)
	Is confused when aroused
	Talks in monosyllables
	Mumbles and is incoherent
	Needs constant stimulation to cooperate
• **Stupor (semicoma)**	Responds to painful stimuli (withdrawal), shaking
	Groans, mumbles
	Exhibits reflex activity
• **Coma**	Does not respond to painful or any other stimuli

A **concussion** (a subset of mild traumatic brain injury [mTBI]) is a pathophysiologic process that affects the brain and is caused by direct/indirect, acceleration/deceleration biomechanical forces transmitted to the head following a blast, fall, direct impact, motor vehicle accident, or sports injury leading to primarily transient functional rather than structural changes (NOTE: structural changes may occur with greater injury severity or with

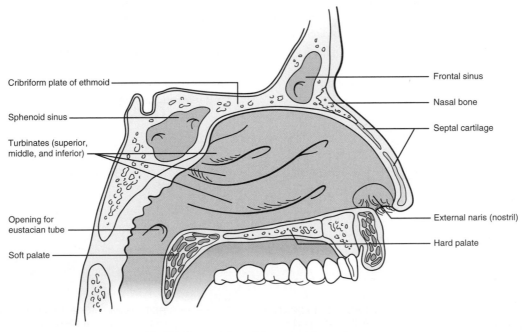

Fig. 2.9 Cross section of the nose and nasopharynx.

multiple concussions) in neurological tissue.[9,17–39] Concussions can result from a blow to the head or jaw, or a fall on the buttocks from a height. The result of a concussion commonly is posttraumatic headache, dizziness, inability to process information, and other cognitive, somatic, affective changes and sleep disturbances (Table 2.4). It may or may not involve loss of consciousness.[49] An mTBI typically includes a **Glasgow Coma Scale** rating of 13 to 15 (tested 6 hours postinjury; Table 2.5), possible loss of consciousness for up to 30 minutes (occurs in 10% of cases or less), and possible amnesia (i.e., retrograde or posttraumatic [also called anterograde]) for up to 24 hours after the injury.[22,27,29,33,50,51]

Concussion Guidelines Available on the Internet

- Ontario Neurotrauma Foundation: Guidelines for concussion/mild traumatic brain injury and persistent symptoms, ed 3, 2018.
- Ontario Neurotrauma Foundation: Guidelines for diagnosing and managing pediatric concussion, 2014.
- Physiotherapy Alberta—College and Association: Concussion management—a toolkit for physiotherapists, 2017.
- Parachute Canada: Statement on concussion baseline testing in Canada, 2017.
- Fowler/Kennedy/St. Joseph's Health Care: Postconcussion syndrome management guidelines, 2013.
- Ontario Psychological Association: Guidelines for best practice in the assessment of concussions and related symptoms, 2016.

TABLE 2.3

Areas of the Brain and Their Function

Area of the Brain	Function
Cerebrum	Cognitive aspects of motor control Memory Sensory awareness (e.g., pain, touch) Speech Special senses (e.g., taste, vision)
Cerebellum	Coordinate and integrate motor behavior Balance Motor learning Motor control (muscle contraction and force production)
Diencephalon (thalamus)	Regulation of body temperature and water balance Control of emotions Information processing to cerebrum
Brain stem	Control of respiratory and heart rates Peripheral blood flow control

Head Injury Severity Based on Score Maintained on Glasgow Coma Scale (After 6 or More Hours)

8 or less:	Severe head injury
9–11:	Moderate head injury
12 or more:	Mild head injury

Because the changes have been thought to be most commonly functional rather than structural and because normal diagnostic imaging (i.e., computed tomography [CT] scans and magnetic resonance imaging [MRI]) shows no changes with functional concussions, diagnostic imaging has not been recommended as part of the early assessment (i.e., first 24 to 48 hours) unless there is severe prolonged level of unconsciousness or disorientation, posttraumatic amnesia and/or neurological deficit, a bleed/intracranial hemorrhage in the brain (i.e., subdural, epidural, intracerebral or subarachnoid hemorrhage), skull fracture, or other major injury that would be evident by the progressive deterioration of the patient.[31,37,42,52–55] Signs and symptoms of intracranial hemorrhage include deteriorating consciousness, confusion, severe or increased

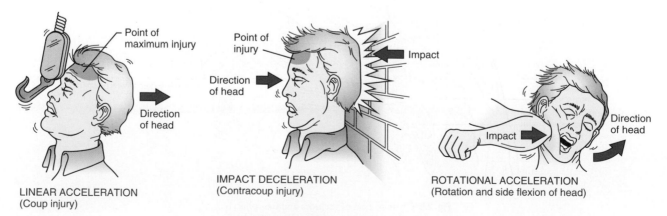

LINEAR ACCELERATION (Coup injury) — Point of maximum injury — Direction of head

IMPACT DECELERATION (Contracoup injury) — Point of injury — Direction of head — Impact

ROTATIONAL ACCELERATION (Rotation and side flexion of head) — Impact — Direction of head

Fig. 2.10 Mechanisms of injury to the brain.

TABLE **2.4**

Signs and Symptoms of a Concussion[9,32,36,40-48]

Somatic (Physical)	Cognitive	Emotional (Affective)	Sleep
• Headache • Nausea • Vomiting • Balance problems/incoordination • Dizziness/vertigo • Visual problems (e.g., blurred or double vision, saccades) • Fatigue • Sensitivity to light (photophobia) • Sensitivity to noise (phonophobia) • Numbness/tingling • Dazed • Tinnitus • Seizure	• Feeling mentally "foggy" • Feeling slowed down • Difficulty concentrating • Difficulty remembering (amnesia—retrograde and/or posttraumatic) • Forgetful of recent information and conversations (memory dysfunction) • Confused about recent events/dazed/groggy • Answers questions slowly (slurred speech) • Repeats questions • Disoriented • Light-headed • Vacant stare • Loss of consciousness (occurs in <10%)	• Irritable/low frustration tolerance • Sadness • More emotional (moody) • Nervousness • Depression • Anxiety • Personality changes	• Drowsiness/lethargy • Sleeping more than usual • Sleeping less than usual • Difficulty falling asleep

TABLE **2.5**

☑ Glasgow Coma Scale[a]

				Time 1 ( )	Time 2 ( )
Eyes	Open	Spontaneously	4		
		To verbal command	3		
		To pain	2		
		No response	1	_____	_____
Best motor response	To verbal command To painful stimulus[b]	Obeys	6		
		Localizes pain	5		
		Flexion—withdrawal	4		
		Flexion—abnormal (decorticate rigidity)	3		
		Extension (decerebrate rigidity)	2		
		No response	1	_____	_____
Best verbal response[c]		Oriented and converses	5		
		Disoriented and converses	4		
		Inappropriate words	3		
		Incomprehensible sounds	2		
		No response	1	_____	_____
Total			3–15	_____	_____

[a]The Glasgow Coma Scale, which is based on eye opening and verbal and motor responses, is a practical means of monitoring changes in level of consciousness. If responses on the scale are given numeric grades, the overall responsiveness of the patient can be expressed in a score that is the summation of the grades. The lowest score is 3, and the highest is 15.
[b]Apply knuckles to sternum; observe arms.
[c]Arouse patient with painful stimulus if necessary.

headache, repeated vomiting, seizures, and blurred or double vision. Neurological signs and symptoms of a cervical spine injury include weakness, tingling or burning in the limbs, severe neck pain, and increased persistent difficulty in walking or poor balance.[51]

Signs and Symptoms That Indicate an Individual With a Head Injury Should be Referred to an Emergency Facility[33,41,51,56,57]

- Worsening or severe headache
- Very drowsy or cannot be easily awakened
- Cannot recognize people or places
- Develops significant nausea or vomiting (i.e., emesis)
- Behaves unusually, more confused or irritable
- Develops seizures
- Weakness or numbness in the arms or legs
- Slurred speech
- Unsteadiness of gait or balance
- Nuchal (i.e., back of neck) rigidity
- Decreased level of consciousness
- Battle signs (mastoid ecchymosis; i.e., bruising over mastoid process)
- Developing blurred, double, or loss of vision
- Becomes drowsy, lethargic, or obtunded
- Develops or exhibits worsening mental/cognitive abilities (i.e., inability to answer simple questions, worsening amnesia)
- Unequal or fixed and dilated pupil(s)
- Urinary or bowel incontinence
- Numbness or burning in legs and/or arms

The need for neuroimaging should be determined by using the **Canadian CT Head Rule** or **New Orleans Criteria**.[23] However, it should be noted that new neuroimaging techniques such as diffusion tensor imaging, functional magnetic resonance imaging (fMRI), serum bile markers, positron emission tomography (PET) scan, and magnetic resonance spectroscopy have shown that there may be some structural changes with a concussion such as diffuse axonal injury which may result in headache, irritability, balance problems, nausea and vomiting, memory dysfunction, impaired functional eye movement, confusion, amnesia, fatigue/drowsiness, slurred speech, fatigue, photophobia (i.e., sensitivity to light) and phonophobia (i.e., sensitivity to sound), blurred vision, difficulty concentrating, and sleep disturbances. These diagnostic imaging techniques may be used if there are a large number of risk factors or modifiers (Table 2.6) present that may result in more severe or prolonged impairment or if the individual is not showing improvement in the signs and symptoms during the first few days.[13,19,21,22,26,29,31,40,52,54,61–66]

Canadian Computed Tomography Head Rule[a,58–60]

Computed tomography (CT) is required only for patients with minor head injury with any one of the following findings: Patients with minor head injury who present with a Glasgow Coma Scale score of 13–15 after having been witnessed to have loss of consciousness, amnesia, or confusion.

- High risk for neurosurgical intervention
  1. Glasgow Coma Scale score lower than 15 at 2 hours after injury
  2. Suspected open or depressed skull fracture
  3. Any sign of basal skull fracture[b]
  4. Two or more episodes of vomiting
  5. 65 years or older
- Medium risk for brain injury detection by CT imaging
  6. Amnesia before impact of 30 or more minutes
  7. Dangerous mechanism[c]

[a]The rule is not applicable if the patient did not experience a trauma, has a Glasgow Coma Scale score lower than 13, is younger than 16 years, is taking warfarin or has a bleeding disorder, or has an obvious open skull fracture.
[b]Signs of basal skull fracture include hemotympanum (i.e., blood behind eardrum), racoon eyes, cerebrospinal fluid otorrhea (i.e., discharge from the ear) or rhinorrhea (i.e., discharge from the nose), Battle sign.
[c]Dangerous mechanism is a pedestrian struck by a motor vehicle, an occupant ejected from a motor vehicle, or a fall from an elevation of 3 or more feet or 5 stairs.
From Stiell IG, Clement CM, Rowe BH, et al: Comparison of the Canadian CT Head Rule and the New Orleans Criteria in patients with minor head injury, *JAMA* 294(12):1512, 2005.

New Orleans Criteria[58,60]

Computed tomography (CT) is required for patients with minor head injury with any one of the following findings. The criteria apply only to patients who also have a Glasgow Coma Scale score of 15.

- Headache
- Vomiting
- Older than 60 years
- Drug or alcohol intoxication
- Persistent anterograde amnesia (deficits in short-term memory)
- Visible trauma above the clavicle
- Seizure

From Stiell IG, Clement CM, Rowe BH, et al: Comparison of the Canadian CT Head Rule and the New Orleans Criteria in patients with minor head injury, *JAMA* 294(12):1512, 2005.

Sports-related concussions generally are caused by less severe traumatic forces when compared with other injury mechanisms such as falls from a height or down stairs, or motor vehicle accidents which can have much lower Glasgow Coma Scale values. They are primarily associated with less disability and more rapid recovery from the concussion because of the athlete's higher levels of fitness and strength, the presence of less comorbidities, and the athlete's motivation to return to the game.[19] Despite these better short-term outcomes, athletes may be more vulnerable to long-term effects of mTBI because they are commonly subjected to repeated head trauma in contact and collision sports.[19] A concussion has been characterized as a clinical syndrome

TABLE **2.6**

Risk Factors That May Prolong or Complicate Recovery from Concussion

Factors	Modifier
Symptoms	Number of concussions Duration of symptoms (>10 days) Severity (intensity and duration) Fogginess or dizziness
Signs	Prolonged loss of consciousness (>1 min), amnesia (posttraumatic [anterograde] and/or retrograde)
Sequelae	Concussive convulsions
Temporal	Frequency—repeated concussions over time Timing—injuries close together in time "Recency"—recent concussion or traumatic brain injury
Threshold	Repeated concussions occurring with progressively less impact force or slower recovery after each successive concussion
Age/Gender	Child and adolescent (<18 years old) may recover slower Females may recover slower
Comorbidities and premorbidities	History of migraine Depression or other mental health disorders Attention-deficit/hyperactivity disorder (ADHD) Posttraumatic stress disorder (PTSD) Learning disabilities Sleep disorders Specific genotype Vestibular dysfunction (e.g., motion sickness) Oculomotor dysfunction (e.g., nystagmus) Anxiety Stress
Medication	Psychoactive drugs Anticoagulants
Behavior	Dangerous style of play
Sport	High-risk activity Contact and collision sport High level sport Position played Equipment used

Modified from McCrory P, Meeuwisse W, Johnston K, et al: Consensus statement on concussion in sport—The 3rd International Conference on Concussion in Sport held in Zurich, November 2008. *Clin J Sport Med* 19(3):189, 2009.

Clinical Note

At present, there is no known force threshold that can result in a concussion nor does the magnitude of the impact correlate to the clinical injury.[9,10,22,26,29,57,59,67]

---

that commonly demonstrates immediate and transient posttraumatic impairment of neural function such as altered cognitive function (i.e., information processing, decision-making, mood changes, decreased judgement, decreased reaction time, and memory loss), posttraumatic migraine headache (i.e., headache with nausea and photo- and/or phonosensitivity), possible altered level of consciousness, vision/hearing disturbance, and equilibrium problems (e.g., coordination, balance or gait problems) due to possible involvement of the brain stem, cerebrum, cerebellum, cranial nerves, and/or the vestibulo-ocular system and presents with a myriad of cognitive, physical, emotional, somatic, and sleep-related symptoms and impairment that requires a multifaceted individualized approach for assessment and management.[20,21,40,62,68–70]

It is currently widely recognized that a **neurometabolic impairment** is the foundation of a concussive injury, which involves a cascade of neurochemical, hemodynamic, structural, electrical, metabolic, and physiological changes.[34,65,71–79] Normally, cerebral blood flow is coupled with cerebral metabolism so that an increase in neuronal activity and metabolism results in increased regional and global cerebral blood flow.[20,28,50,65,71,72] When a concussion occurs, there is a mismatch between energy demand of the brain and energy supply to the brain, and this energy deficit leads to a **period of vulnerability** (i.e., the first 7 to 10 days) during which the brain is at risk for additional injury.[40] This may explain why the symptoms are exacerbated by excessive cognitive and physical exertion early after the concussion.[77,79] Disruption of the normal function of the brain results in baseline metabolic demands not being met, resulting in a **neurometabolic cascade crisis** with the brain unable to restore ionic hemostasis rapidly enough across cellular membranes.[80,81] This energy deficit accounts for the somatic, cognitive, sleep, and mood symptoms that follow a concussion.[28,65,82] Central nervous system changes result in widespread systemic effects including altered function of the autonomic nervous system, altered cardiovascular response to exercise, reduced carbon dioxide reactivity, and altered function of the renal hepatic systems.[83] The symptoms of the concussions are believed to arise as a result of the transient neurochemical and neurometabolic changes initiated by the injury,[19] resulting in the neurometabolic energy crisis in the brain.[40]

Because of the neurometabolic cascade and because it takes time for the changes to return to normal, there is an increased risk of repeated concussion for the first 7 to 10 days after the initial concussion.[54] In extremely rare cases, diffuse brain swelling, especially in children and adolescents, herniation and death may occur from a relatively minor head injury if a second injury has occurred when the brain has not fully recovered from a concussion.[28,84] This **second impact syndrome** (also called **malignant cerebral edema**) has been characterized by rapid clinical deterioration resulting from cerebral hyperemia and an increase in intracranial pressure with a high rate of mortality following a second impact to the brain which is still symptomatic and recovering from the initial head injury.[42,85–87] The 7- to 10-day window of increased susceptibility to sustaining another concussion and more severe injury is a reason for increased caution following an initial concussion, especially in children and adolescents whose brains are still developing.[29,85]

In the last few years, there has been a great deal of controversy concerning repeated head trauma in sports that may lead to the development of **chronic traumatic encephalopathy (CTE),** which is a progressive neurodegenerative disorder triggered by repetitive head trauma and characterized by brain atrophy and tau pathology occurring later in life, most commonly after the athlete has retired from sports in susceptible individuals.[19,64,88–92] There is a concern that individuals with a lifetime exposure to collision and contact sports may develop, in midlife, increased rates of depression and dementia, possibly leading to CTE (Table 2.7).[76,93] There are at least 20 different neural pathological conditions associated with abnormal tau protein aggregation in the brain, including Alzheimer disease, frontotemporal dementia, Lewy Body Disease, and other neural pathological conditions.[94] In addition, tau protein may be found in individuals undergoing the normal aging process independent of head trauma.[88–92,94] CTE is not the accumulation of symptoms from earlier injuries, but the concussions can contribute to or result in a progressive decline in neuron function in susceptible individuals and presently can be diagnosed only at autopsy.[88–92] There is no question that repeat concussions can have long-lasting harmful effects.[19,94] Because of this uncertainty of outcome, concussions must be dealt with using extra caution (e.g., "when in doubt, keep them out") and every individual suspected of having a concussion must be dealt with individually to ensure the individual has recovered fully before return to sport.

Clinical Note

If a child or adolescent receives a concussion, he or she should abstain from sport and vigorous exercise for at least 7–10 days, or until all signs and symptoms have disappeared to decrease the chance of a more severe head injury or complications.

TABLE **2.7**

Early and Late Signs and Symptoms of Chronic Traumatic Encephalopathy

Early	Late
• Short-term memory problems • Executive dysfunction (e.g., planning, organization, multitasking) • Depression and/or apathy • Emotional instability • Impulse control problems (e.g., disinhibition, having a "short fuse") • Suicidal behavior	• Worsening memory impairment • Worsening executive dysfunction • Language difficulties • Aggressive and irritable behavior • Apathy • Motor disturbance, including Parkinsonism • Dementia (i.e., memory and cognitive impairment severe enough to impair social and/or occupational functioning)

From Stern RA, Riley DO, Daneshvar DH, et al: Long-term consequences of repetitive brain trauma: chronic traumatic encephalopathy, *Phys Med Rehabil* 3:S460–S467, 2011.

It must be remembered that concussion symptoms are not specific to concussions and may resemble other comorbidities or conditions.[22,27,42,95,96] Thus a careful and thorough differential diagnosis is required. Women appear to be more susceptible to concussions than men,[97] and mTBI is different in children and adolescents compared with adults.[11,61,86] The effects of concussion are cumulative, and the risk of having another concussion following an initial concussion is 4 to 6 times greater than someone who has not had a concussion.[73,98,99] Although most concussions resolve within 2 to 4 weeks, a small percentage of concussions can lead to continued and severe problems (e.g., postconcussion syndrome, second impact syndrome).[71,98–103]

Comorbidities With Similar Signs and Symptoms to Concussion[9,23,27,44,63,66,73,104–107]

- Chronic migraines
- Depression
- Anxiety disorders
- Dehydration
- Chronic pain
- Attention-deficit/hyperactivity disorder (ADHD)
- Learning difficulties
- Developmental delays
- Sleep dysfunction
- Posttraumatic stress disorder (PTSD)
- Posttraumatic headaches
- Whiplash-associated disorders
- Anemia
- Neuroendocrine disorders
- Anorexia nervosa
- Lack of sleep
- Substance abuse

Athletes, especially those at high risk for potential concussion injury or those with a significant concussion history or other relevant comorbidities as mentioned previously, should be considered for **neuropsychological testing** on an individual basis as part of the **preparticipation examination** to provide baseline measurements that can be compared with postinjury values in the event of the suspected concussion.[15,19,20,26,29,42,108–114]

Normally, neuropsychological testing can be done every 2 years for adults (every 4 months to a year depending on maturation for children) if there have been no previous concussions.[25,115,116] If preinjury values for neuropsychological testing are not available, normative data can be used, but it is not ideal.[13,36,117] In most individuals who have suffered a concussion, the test values return to normal levels within 7 to 10 days.[9,118–120] The most common neuropsychological tests used in sport are the ImPACT (i.e., Immediate Post-Concussion

Assessment and Cognitive Testing), Computerized Cognitive Assessment Tool (CogSport), Automated Neuropsychological Assessment Metrics (ANAM), and Concussion Resolution Index.[13,16,22,26,31,35,37,40,120–134] Other neurophysiological tests are shown in Table 2.8.

Preparticipation "concussion" examinations should include a clinical history of any concussions along with somatic and cognitive symptom assessment, cranial nerve assessment, physical and neurobehavioral examination, and assessments

---

TABLE **2.8**

Examples of Neurophysiologic Tests

Test	Ability Evaluated
Continuous Performance Test	Sustained attention, reaction time
Controlled Oral Word Association Test	Word fluency, word retrieval
Delayed Recall (from Hopkins Verbal Learning Test)	Delayed learning from previously learned word list
Digit Span (from Wechsler Memory Scale—revised)	Attention span
Grooved-Pegboard Test	Motor speed and coordination
Hopkins Verbal Learning Test	Verbal memory (memory for words)
Immediate Post Concussion Assessment and Cognitive Testing (ImPACT)	Attention span, sustained and selective attention, reaction time, memory
Number/Symbol Matching	Processing speed, visual motor speed
Orientation Questionnaire	Orientation, posttraumatic amnesia
Sequential Digit Tracking	Sustained attention, reaction time
Stroop Test	Mental flexibility, attention
Symbol Digit Modalities	Visual scanning, attention
Symbol Memory	Immediate visual memory
Trail Making Test	Visual scanning, mental flexibility
Verbal Working Memory	Word memory, working memory
Visual Span	Visual attention, immediate memory
Visual Symbol Search	Visual scanning, reaction time
Word/Color Tracking	Focused attention, response inhibition

Data from Maroon JC, Lovell MR, Norwig J, et al: Cerebral concussion in athletes: evaluation and neurophysiological testing, *Neurosurg* 47:659–672, 2000.

of motor control and balance.[3,20,98,110,120,135–139] Table 2.9 outlines suggested domains of the clinical history and examination for concussions for the preseason "concussion" examination. In the preparticipation examination, the Sport Concussion Assessment Tool 5 (SCAT5; see Fig. 2.49) and the Child SCAT5 (see Fig. 2.50) can be used as part of the assessment process as the same tools are used following a concussion. Likewise, the Standardized Assessment of Concussion (SAC) Form (see eTool 2.13) can be used and is actually part of the SCAT5.

The severity stages of concussion are shown in Table 2.10.[100] Acute and late (or delayed) signs and symptoms of concussions are shown in Table 2.11.[9,29,98,109,140–142] Dizziness, fogginess, memory impairment, anxiety, and photophobia and phonophobia are considered the primary risk factors indicating the possibility of development of persistent postconcussion symptoms.[73]

There have been several different grading systems developed in the past (see past editions of *Orthopedic Physical Assessment*) that provided a severity grade for a concussion, but the use of these grading systems has been discouraged because they were not developed based on scientific knowledge regarding the process of recovery from concussion and there is no evidence that amnesia (retrograde or posttraumatic) or loss of consciousness should be weighed heavier than other markers in making decisions regarding concussions.[18,20,42,95,143,144] The Fifth International Conference on Concussion and Sport in Berlin[66] has recommended that grade scales be abandoned because concussion severity can be determined only retrospectively after all signs and symptoms have disappeared, the neurological examination is normal, and cognitive function has returned to normal.[66] For ease of description, concussions can be grouped as simple, complex, or postconcussion[110,132] based on the duration of symptoms, which means these injuries often

TABLE **2.9**

Suggested Domains of the Clinical History and Examination for "Concussion" Preseason/Preparticipation Examination

Domain	Features or Examples	How to Assess?[a]
Previous concussions	Date(s) and circumstances; presence and duration of loss of consciousness, amnesia, and symptoms with each injury	History
Concussion-related personal history	Mood disorder, learning disability, attention-deficit/hyperactivity disorder, epilepsy or seizures, sleep apnea, skull fracture, migraine headaches, potential risk factors	History
Family history	Mood disorder, learning disability, attention-deficit/hyperactivity disorder, dementia (e.g., Alzheimer disease), migraine headaches, complications from concussions	History
Symptoms	Current and recurrent	Symptom checklist or scale (SCAT5)
Mental status	Level of consciousness, attention and concentration, orientation, memory	Standardized Assessment of Concussion (SAC) SCAT5
Eye examination	Eye movements with smooth pursuit (cranial nerves [CN] III, IV, VI), nystagmus (CN VIII), pupillary reflex (CN II, III)	Clinical examination of all cranial nerves
Muscle strength	Strength evaluation of deltoids, biceps, triceps, wrist and finger flexors and extensors[b]; pronator drift; peripheral nerves; adjacent joints	Clinical examination
Motor control	Balance assessment	Balance Error Scoring System (BESS)
Cognitive function	Reaction time, working memory, delayed recall	Neurocognitive testing
Coordination	Finger to nose, dual task	Clinical examination
Gait	Look for deviations, heel-toe, dual task	Clinical examination
Oculovestibular system	Visual acuity, nystagmus, smooth pursuits, accommodation convergence, saccades, vestibulo-ocular reflex (VOR), dynamic vision acuity	Clinical examination
Reaction time	Drop ruler test	Clinical examination

[a]Assessment tools are indicated where available.
[b]Notable deficits may be associated with nerve root injury or concussion.
Modified from Broglio SP, Cantu RC, Gioia GA, et al: National Athletic Trainers Association Position Statement: management of sport concussion, *J Athletic Train* 49(2):245–265, 2014.

TABLE **2.10**

Severity Stages of Concussive Injury

Acute Concussion (7–10 Days)	Postconcussion Syndrome (Chronic Concussion)	Prolonged Postconcussion Syndrome	Chronic Traumatic Encephalopathy
• *Physical (somatic) symptoms:* Headache, dizziness, hearing loss, balance difficulty, sleep disturbances, nausea/vomiting, sensitivity to light or noise, diminished athletic performance • *Cognitive deficits:* Loss of short-term memory (anterograde and/or retrograde), difficulty with focus or concentration, confusion, loss of consciousness, disorientation, inability to focus, delayed verbal and/or motor responses, excessive drowsiness, decreased attention, diminished work or school performance • *Emotional (affective) disturbances:* Irritability, anger, fear, mood swings, decreased libido	• Persistent concussion symptoms • Usually lasting 1–6 weeks after mTBI • Self-limiting	• Symptoms lasting over 6 months • Lowered concussion threshold • Diminished athletic performance • Diminished work or school performance	• Latency period (usually 6–10 years) • Personality disturbances • Emotional lability • Marriage/personal relationship failures • Depression • Alcohol/substance abuse • Suicide attempt/completion

mTBI, Mild traumatic brain injury.
Modified from Sedney CL, Orphanos J, Bailes JE: When to consider retiring an athlete after sports-related concussion, *Clin Sports Med* 30(1):189–200, 2011.

TABLE **2.11**

Acute and Late (Delayed) Signs and Symptoms of Concussions

Acute (First 24–48 Hours)[a,b]	Late (Delayed)
• Light-headedness • Delayed motor and/or verbal responses • Memory or cognitive dysfunction • Disorientation • Amnesia (retrograde and/or posttraumatic) • Headache • Balance problems/incoordination • Vertigo/dizziness • Concentration difficulties • Loss of consciousness • Visual disturbance (e.g., blurred vision, saccades) • Vacant stare (befuddled facial expression) • Photophobia • Tinnitus • Nausea • Vomiting • Increased emotionality • Numbness • Slurred or incoherent speech	• Persistent low-grade headache • Easy fatiguability • Sleep irregularities • Inability to perform daily activities • Depression/anxiety • Lethargy • Memory dysfunction • Light-headedness • Personality changes • Low frustration tolerance/irritability • Intolerance to bright lights, loud sounds (photophobia and phonophobia) • Irritability

[a]Acute signs and symptoms may get progressively worse over 24 to 48 hours.
[b]Some signs and symptoms may take time postconcussion to be evident.

can be classified only retrospectively and not at the time of injury.[62] First, almost all individuals, whether they are suffering from a simple or complex concussion, will exhibit the most severe signs and symptoms of cognitive dysfunction and balance problems during the acute phase (first 24 to 48 hours) because it may take time for the signs and symptoms to become evident.[29,66,75] These dysfunctions and problems will then decrease at different rates depending on the individual over a period of time. A **simple concussion** implies that the injury, cognitive function, and other signs and symptoms resolve spontaneously over 7 to 10 days without complications, no neurocognitive testing or intervention is required, other than observation (i.e., linear mental status screening/testing should be performed at regular intervals over the 10 to 14 days to ensure signs and symptoms are abating).[21,22,51,62,86,110,145] Simple concussions make up 80% to 90% of concussions.[40,110,146] In contrast, **complex concussions** last longer than 10 days and/or have persistent symptoms and specific sequelae occur (e.g., convulsions, loss of consciousness for up to 1 minute, prolonged cognitive impairment) and most commonly, the condition clinically resolves within 30 days of injury.[3,95,110,132] Approximately 15% to 30% of individuals will experience symptoms that persist beyond the normal 1 (for adults) to 4 (for children and adolescents) weeks of a simple concussion. Individuals who have suffered more than one concussion, those with posttraumatic amnesia, retrograde amnesia, or disorientation lasting longer than 5 minutes fall within this group.[147] Complex concussions require a multidisciplinary approach to management.[148] In the case of complex concussions, neuropsychological testing and diagnostic imaging can play a role.[67,141,149–151] Table 2.12 shows return-to-play guidelines for simple and complex concussions.

If the symptoms persist or are protracted for 3 months or longer (approximately 1 month in children), then a **postconcussion syndrome** is present, which often has long-term consequences that severely interfere with the individual's quality of life.[19,23,26,36,39,42,43,45,48,55,104,120,152–155] It should be noted that the actual time for determining how long the persistent symptoms must be present varies between authors. The strongest and most consistent predictor of slower recovery from concussion is the severity of a person's initial symptoms on the first day or the initial few days (24 to 48 hours) after the injury. The risk of developing postconcussion syndrome is higher in those who had delayed symptom onset of greater than 3 hours postinjury, with a personal and family history of mood disorders, other psychiatric illnesses, and migraines.[44] Having a low level of symptoms in the first day after injury is a favorable prognostic indicator. A postconcussion syndrome refers to cognitive and memory deficits and at least three or more of the following symptoms: headache, nausea, dizziness, fatigue, impaired balance, sleep disturbance, irritability, atrophy, impaired blurred vision, confusion, memory impairment, fatigue, and personality change in various combinations.[73,104] The fundamental cause of postconcussion syndrome can be persistent physiological dysfunction including altered autonomic function and impaired autoregulation of cerebral blood flow.[155] Other causes of postconcussion syndrome include migraine, vestibular dysfunction, and emotional disturbance.[79,155,156] Between 10% and 15% of patients diagnosed with mTBI will continue to experience persistent and delayed return to school, work, or sports.[22,23,26,27,36,71,81,112,146,154] The presence of prolonged loss of consciousness of greater than 30 seconds to 1 minute, history of more than three concussions, amnesia, prolonged confusion, and persistent symptoms are associated with more severe and persistent injury.[154,157] Patients with affective symptoms tend to show extensive overlap between mood disorders and symptoms of postconcussion syndrome. Symptoms of major depression include depressed mood, loss of interest, fatigue, sleep disturbance, and difficulty concentrating. The **Beck Depression Inventory**[158] and the **Patient Health Questionnaire (PHQ-9)**[131] (eTool 2.1) are examples of questionnaires used to measure the level of depression.[159] Symptoms of anxiety disorders such as general anxiety disorder, PTSD, and acute stress disorder include feeling "keyed up" or "on edge," fatigability, irritability, difficulty concentrating, and difficulty falling asleep or staying asleep.[45,46,71]

The **Post Concussion Symptom Scale (PCSS)** is a 22-item checklist that can be used to help diagnose a concussion and to monitor recovery over time assessing the frequency, intensity, and duration of the postconcussion symptoms (eTool 2.2).[13,37,66,81,126,133,152,159–162] The **Rivermead Post-Concussion Symptoms Questionnaire (RPSQ)** (eTool 2.3) is a 16-item questionnaire

TABLE **2.12**

Return-to-Play Guidelines Following Simple and Complex Concussions

Grade of Concussion	On-the-Field Treatment	First Concussion	Second Concussion	Third Concussion
Simple	Remove athlete from the competition	Athlete may return to play if asymptomatic for 1 week	Obtain CT scan; athlete may return in 2 weeks if asymptomatic for 1 week	Athlete sidelined a minimum of 1 month; may return then if asymptomatic for 1 week
Complex	Remove athlete from the competition; transport athlete to a hospital for emergency evaluation of the player by a neurosurgeon and to obtain diagnostic neuroimaging	Obtain CT scan, remove from play for a minimum of 1 month or until all signs and symptoms have disappeared; athlete may then return to play if asymptomatic for 1 week	Obtain CT scan; consider terminating for season	Terminate athlete for season; athlete may return next season if asymptomatic, but permanent retirement from contact sports should be considered

CT, Computed tomography.

Modified from Warren WL, Bailes JE, Cantu RC: Guidelines for safe return to play after athletic head and neck injuries. In Cantu RC, editor: *Neurologic athletic head and spine injuries*, Philadelphia, 2000, WB Saunders.

that measures symptom severity comparing symptoms experienced in the past 24 hours with the individual's experience with the same injuries prior to injury and was devised to gauge the severity of postconcussion syndrome.[115,116,133,159,163,164] There is also the **Rivermead Head Injury Service Follow-Up Questionnaire (RHFUQ)**[116] that can be used for follow-up assessments.

Caution should be exercised when giving the diagnosis of postconcussion syndrome because there may be significant symptoms that could be the result of other atraumatic or premorbid conditions such as chronic migraines, depression, anxiety, attention problems, sleep dysfunction, and PTSD, as well as pain related to posttraumatic headaches and whiplash-associated disorders (WADs), and it is difficult to distinguish each of these conditions.[9,23,27,44,63,66,73,104–107] The presence of a psychiatric illness such as anxiety, depression, and compulsive histrionic personality disorders or those with a family history of mood disorders have been found to have a higher incidence of postconcussion syndrome.[73] Table 2.6 outlines the risk factors that may prolong or complicate recovery from concussions.[104] People with postconcussion disorders have significant exercise intolerance, whereas those with signs and symptoms coming from the cervical spine or vestibular system or having a visual dysfunction or combination of these typically do not have early significant exercise intolerance. The **Buffalo Concussion Treadmill Test** (BCTT; see eTool 2.21) is a test that uses a graded exercise program with exercise levels that do not precipitate concussion signs and symptoms.[77,104]

Regardless of the classification used for concussions, it is important to understand that each concussion should be managed individually because there is no "one size fits all" in concussion management.[21] If a concussion is suspected, the SCAT5 or Child SCAT5 should be used for the assessment. It is the most common sideline tool used and was updated in 2017 at the International Conference on Concussion and Sport in Berlin as an update of the SCAT3 and Child SCAT3.

3. If the patient has had an injury to the head, are there any associated symptoms in the neck or problems with breathing, altered vision, discharge from the nose or ears, or urinary or fecal incontinence? These symptoms indicate severe brain or spinal cord injury, and the patient must be handled with extreme care.

4. What are the sites and boundaries of pain? This question helps the examiner to determine what structures have been injured. It is important to keep in mind that the patient may be experiencing a referral of pain.

> ### Chronic Head Signs and Symptoms Requiring Specialist Care
>
> - Presence of amnesia
> - Prolonged residual symptoms
> - Loss of consciousness
> - Prolonged headache
> - Postconcussion syndrome
> - Personality changes
> - More than one concussion
> - Prolonged disorientation, unsteadiness, or confusion (more than 2–3 min)
> - Blurred vision
> - Dizziness (more than 5 min)
> - Tinnitus (more than 5 min)

5. What type of pain is the patient experiencing? The type of pain indicates the type of structure injured (see Table 1.3).

6. Is there any paresthesia, abnormal sensation, or lack of sensation? Are smell (cranial nerve I), vision (cranial nerve II), taste (cranial nerve VII), and hearing (cranial nerve VIII) normal? These questions give the examiner some idea of whether neurological structures (especially the cranial nerves) have been injured and, if so, which ones.

7. What is the age and sex of the patient? Children who suffer a concussion tend to take longer to recover than adults.[165] Children who experience a sports-related concussion usually recover, from a clinical perspective, within 1 month. However, approximately 30% of children and adolescents report persistent symptoms after 4 weeks.[166,167] The brain in children, because of continual brain, cognitive, physical, and emotional development, is more vulnerable to additional injury during the acute recovery period, which tends to be longer, and therefore caution is advised when considering returning the child to activity prior to complete recovery. Early return may result in additional deficits or problems.[13,26,86,147,152,168–170] For example, the primary concern for premature return of a child or adolescent athlete to activity is diffuse cerebral swelling which can result in delayed catastrophic deterioration commonly referred to a **Second Impact Syndrome or Malignant Cerebral Edema**.[26,32,70,171] Because there is no method for predicting which children will experience prolonged symptoms following a concussion, it is recommended that conservative management include both cognitive and physical rest followed by a stepwise return to school (Table 2.13) and sport activities (Table 2.14) for all children.[43,172] Light aerobic controlled physical activities are safe as long as they do not exacerbate the symptoms while promoting recovery by enhancing physical, psychological, and academic outcomes.[173] Accommodation in terms of returning to school and returning to activity should be individualized, depending on the symptoms or difficulties that

TABLE **2.13**

RETURN TO SCHOOL GUIDELINES

STAGES 1-3 of the Return to Activity (**RTA**) and Return to School (**RTS**) guidelines should progress together, however youth should return full-time to school activities before progressing to STAGE 4, and 5 of the RTA guidelines

STAGE 1	Short Phase of Physical and Cognitive Rest with Symptom Guided Activity 24-48 hours	**GOAL:** NO SCHOOL for at least 24 hours. Home and leisure activities as tolerated, without an increase in the number or severity of symptoms. Notify school of concussive injury. NO physical activities of any intensity for longer than 5 minutes, as long as these activities do not increase symptoms. **REST/LIGHT ACTIVITIES:** Regular daily activities that do not provoke symptoms such as self-care and easy tasks (e.g., making your bed, quiet socialization with a friend, talk on phone). LIMIT screen time (e.g. TV, video games, texting) and reading. **WHEN TO MOVE TO STAGE TWO?** → When symptoms are not exacerbated by regular daily activities or have disappeared. If symptoms persist past 1 week, then progress to STAGE 2 cautiously.
STAGE 2	Getting Ready to Go Back to School	**GOAL:** Begin simple cognitive activity at home for a maximum of 30 minutes, without worsening symptoms. If symptoms worsen, reduce activity. **ACTIVITIES:** Walking, 15 minutes of screen time/school work twice daily; socialize with 1-2 friends for no longer than 30 minutes. **WHEN TO MOVE TO STAGE THREE?** → When symptoms have disappeared, decreased, or if symptoms persist past 2 weeks then move to STAGE 3 with support from school and medical professionals.
STAGE 3	Back to School with Environmental Accommodations and Modified Academics	**GOAL:** Build up your back-to-school routines by increasing cognitive activity in a school environment with accommodations. This stage may last days or months depending on the rate of recovery. **ACADEMIC MODIFICATIONS are decided on an individual basis and guided by symptoms** **TIMETABLE/ATTENDANCE:** Start by going for one hour, half days, or every other day. Try to reduce class time, later start time, or a shortened day. **CURRICULUM:** Attend less stressful classes, allow more time to complete work, no tests, homework in 15-minute blocks for up to a maximum of 45 minutes daily. **ENVIRONMENT:** Preferential seating, avoid computer, music, and gym classes, avoid noisy/crowded environments such as the cafeteria. Use headphones or sunglasses if sound or light sensitive. Provide a quiet work space or rest breaks during class. **ACTIVITIES:** Limit screen/TV time into 15-minute blocks for up to 1 hour daily. General school activities: No school bus, lunch room, recess, and carrying heavy books. **WHEN TO MOVE TO STAGE FOUR?** → When activities are tolerated without increasing symptoms.
STAGE 4	Normal Routines, with Some Restrictions	**GOAL:** Back to full days of school, but can do less than 5 days a week if needed due to fatigue or other continued symptoms. **ACTIVITIES:** Complete as much homework as tolerated without causing or worsening symptoms. Only 1 test per week, may require shorter test or more time to complete. The student should NOT be required to catch up on missed work or exams in addition to new learning and curriculum. **WHEN TO MOVE TO STAGE FIVE?** → When symptom free.
STAGE 5	Fully Back to School	**GOAL:** Gradual return to normal routines including regular attendance, homework, tests, and extracurricular activities. **STOP** If symptoms increase or return at any STAGE, reduce activity by returning to the previous stage for 24 hours.

IMPORTANT NOTES

ANXIETY can be high after a brain injury. Many youth worry about school failure and need reassurance that accommodations will be temporary.

DEPRESSION is common during recovery from brain injury, especially when the child is unable to be active. Depression may make symptoms worse or prolong recovery.

Note: Different people recover at different rates depending on many factors, including severity of injury and previous health history. These timelines are meant to help set expectations and to be used as a guide. If you are worried about the pace of your recovery, contact a physician or brain injury specialist.

©CanChild, McMaster University 2018

From DeMatteo C, Randall S, Falla K, et al: Concussion management has changed: new pediatric protocols using the latest evidence, *Clin Pediatr (Phila)* 59:5-20, 2020.

TABLE **2.14**

Graduated Return-to-Play Protocol for Returning an Individual to Sport

Rehabilitation Stage	Functional Exercise at Each Stage of Rehabilitation	Objective of Each Stage
1. No activity (cognitive or brain rest)	Symptom limited physical and cognitive rest	Recovery
2. Light aerobic exercise	Walking, swimming, or stationary cycling, keeping intensity less than 70% maximum permitted heart rate; no resistance training	Increase heart rate
3. Sport-specific exercise	Skating drills in ice hockey, running drills in soccer; no head impact activities	Add movement
4. Noncontact training drills	Progression to more complex training drills (e.g., passing drills in football and ice hockey); may start progressive resistance training	Exercise, coordination, and cognitive load
5. Full-contact practice	Following medical clearance participate in normal training activities	Restore confidence and assess functional skills by coaching staff
6. Return to play	Normal game play, normal activity	

Note: An initial period of 24 to 48 hours of both relative physical rest and cognitive rest is recommended before beginning the return to sport progression. There should be at least 24 hours (or longer) for each step of the progression. If any symptoms worsen during exercise, the athlete should go back to the previous step. Resistance training should be added only in the later stages (stage 3 or 4 at the earliest). If symptoms are persistent (e.g., more than 10 to 14 days in adults or more than 1 month in children), the athlete should be referred to a health care professional who is an expert in the management of concussion.

Modified from McCrory P, Meeuwisse WH, Aubry M, et al: Consensus statement on concussion in sport: the 4th International Conference on Concussion in Sport held in Zurich, November 2012, *Br J Sports Med* 47(5):250–258, 2013; Halstead ME, Walter KD: Clinical report-sport related concussion in children and adolescents, *Pediatrics* 126(3):597–611, 2010.

the child is experiencing.[86] The expected duration of symptoms in children (age 5 to 12 years) is up to 4 weeks. Children should not return to sports until they have successfully returned to school.[174] Children with a history of a previous concussion, particularly recent concussion, are at a higher risk of prolonged symptoms following the concussion.[175] Routine use of baseline computerized neuropsychological testing is often not recommended for children and adolescents because of problems with reliability over time and insufficient evidence of diagnostic or prognostic value.[166]

Adolescence (age 13 to 18 years) is also a critical period for brain development, and brain injury during this stage of life may result in a greater degree of injury than that seen in an adult.[70] In addition to developmental differences, anatomic and physiological differences are possible factors that may explain the adolescents' vulnerability to concussion-related symptoms.[144] Adolescents who have greater than or equal to four concussion symptoms have double the risk of a prolonged recovery.[157]

Female athletes have been found to be at greater risk of concussion, reporting increased symptoms and demonstrating differences on baseline neuropsychological testing than males.[13,42,81,86,176–178] Females demonstrate significantly lower visual memory composite scores and complex reaction time and processing speed compared with male athletes.[177] Concussed female athletes report more drowsiness and increased sensitivity to noise (phonophobia), whereas concussed male athletes report more amnesia and confusion/disorientation.[177] It has been reported that female concussed athletes exhibited greater total concussion symptoms and poorer concentration, increased fatigue, and light-headedness compared with male concussed athletes.[179] Interestingly, although there are differences in symptoms between males and females, their recovery rate is reported to be the same.[177] Postconcussion symptoms in women also tend to be greater in number than those seen in males.[176]

8. *What activities aggravate the particular problem?* With a concussion, early activity tends to aggravate any symptoms, so any activity should be delayed until symptoms disappear or the activity can be performed at a level in which the symptoms are not evident (i.e., sub–symptom level activity).

9. *What activities ease the particular problem?* With a concussion, a **"cognitive rest period"** is recommended following a concussion. This period is usually limited to no activity for 2 to 3 days followed by sub–symptom level activity. If the athlete wants to maintain a level of fitness, the **Buffalo Concussion Treadmill Test** can be used to systematically test exercise tolerance and to provide sub-symptom activity.[77,104,142]

10. *Does the patient have a **headache**, and, if so, where* (Tables 2.15 and 2.16)? Is the headache tolerable? What type of headache is it? Is it a throbbing,

TABLE 2.15

Type of Headache Pain and Usual Causes

Type of Pain	Usual Causes
Acute	Trauma, acute infection, impending cerebrovascular accident, subarachnoid hemorrhage
Chronic, recurrent	Migraine (definite pattern or irregular interval); eyestrain; noise; excessive eating, drinking, or smoking; inadequate ventilation
Continuous, recurrent	Trauma
Severe, intense	Meningitis, aneurysm (ruptured), migraine, brain tumor
Intense, transient, shocklike	Neuralgia
Throbbing, pulsating (vascular)	Migraine, fever, hypertension, aortic insufficiency, neuralgia
Constant, tight (bandlike), bilateral	Muscle contraction

TABLE 2.16

Location of Headache and Usual Causes

Location	Usual Causes
Forehead	Sinusitis, eye or nose disorder, muscle spasm of occipital or suboccipital region
Side of head	Migraine, eye or ear disorder, auriculotemporal neuralgia
Occipital	Myofascial problems, herniated disc, eyestrain, hypertension, occipital neuralgia
Parietal	Hysteria (viselike), meningitis, constipation, tumor
Face	Maxillary sinusitis, trigeminal neuralgia, dental problems, tumor

pounding, boring, shocklike, dull, nagging, or constant-pressure type of headache? Is the pain of the headache aggravated by movement or by rest? What is the exact location of the headache? Is the headache affected by position or time of day (Table 2.17)? Does it cover the entire head, the sinus region, or behind the eyes? Does it present a "hat band" distribution, or does it affect the neck or the occiput area? It is important for the examiner to record the location, character, duration, and frequency of the headache, as well as any factors that appear to either aggravate or relieve the pain so that a diagnosis can be made and any changes can be noted (Table 2.18). eTool 2.4 shows a headache disability questionnaire that may be used to determine the severity of headache and its effect on everyday activity.[179]

TABLE **2.17**

Effect of Position or Time of Day on Headache

Position or Time of Day When Headache Is Worst	Usual Causes
Morning	Sinusitis, migraine, hypertension, alcoholism, sleeping position
Afternoon	Eyestrain, muscle tension
Night	Intracranial disease, osteomyelitis, nephritis
Bending	Sinusitis
Lying horizontal	Migraine

A headache is the most commonly reported symptom following a concussion. These posttraumatic headaches are not all alike. In fact, they may include but are not limited to mixed headaches, tension-type headaches, cluster-like headaches, and migraine-like headaches.[73,181,182] Headaches that are not associated with migraine-type symptoms are not significantly associated with protracted recovery time.[63] **Postconcussive migraine headache** symptoms include an episodic, unilateral, pounding headache, nausea, vomiting, photophobia, phonophobia, and aggravation with activity and are related to prolonged symptom recovery following a concussion.[118,182,183] These migraine-like headaches are more likely to be reported by females than males.[181]

11. *Is the patient dizzy, unsteady, or having problems with balance?* The examiner should also note whether the dizziness occurs when the patient suddenly stands up, turns, or bends, or whether it occurs without movement. Remember that "dizziness" is a word that patients sometimes use to indicate unsteadiness in walking. Dizziness is usually associated with problems of the middle ear, vestibular system, vertebrobasilar insufficiency, or problems in the upper cervical spine.[69,184] Table 2.19 outlines some common types of dizziness symptoms. Vertigo implies a rotary component; the patient's environment seems to whirl around the patient, or the patient's body seems to rotate in relation to the environment. If the patient complains of dizziness or vertigo, the time of onset and duration of these attacks should be noted. A description of the type of motion that occurs and any other associated symptoms should be included. The **Dizziness Handicapped Inventory** may be used to test dizziness following a concussion to determine if there is a problem with the vestibular and/or oculomotor system.[69,160,184] Dizziness is reported by approximately 50% of concussed athletes

and is associated with greater risk of protracted (>21 days) recovery.[69] Balance may be affected by problems within the brain or the semicircular canals in the inner ear. The examiner should also note whether the patient is talking about unsteadiness, loss of balance, or actual falling.

12. *Is the patient unduly irritated or having trouble concentrating?* The patient's state indicates the severity of the injury and possibility of concussion.

13. *Does the patient know where he or she is, who he or she is, the day, and the time of day?* Does the patient have some idea of what was happening when the injury occurred? These types of questions reveal the severity of the head injury.

14. *Does the patient have any memory of past events or what occurred before or after the injury?* This type of question tests for retrograde amnesia, posttraumatic amnesia, and injury severity, which can be determined by asking the patient straightforward questions about events in the patient's own past, such as birth date or year of graduation from high school or university. **Posttraumatic (anterograde) amnesia** is the loss of memory for events occurring immediately after wakening or from the moment of injury. Posttraumatic amnesia is considered to be the length of time from injury until conscious memory returns. In the acute state, it may take time for posttraumatic amnesia to become obvious. Sometimes, the patient will remember what happened immediately after the injury, but as time goes on (up to 1 to 2 hours after the injury), posttraumatic amnesia becomes evident. This is one of the reasons it is advisable to reassess acute head injuries every 15 to 30 minutes. Manzi and Weaver reported that a patient who had sustained a period of posttraumatic amnesia of less than 60 minutes was considered to have sustained a mild head injury.[185] **Retrograde amnesia** is loss of memory of events that occurred before the injury. It may take 5 to 10 minutes for retrograde amnesia to develop after the concussion, and amnesia may involve only a few minutes before the injury. For this reason, the patient should be questioned frequently about what happened before the injury occurred and how it occurred, to see if there is any change in the patient's memory pattern. There is always some degree of permanent retrograde amnesia with these patients.

Head Injury Severity Based on Length of Posttraumatic Amnesia

Less than 60 minutes:	Mild
1–24 hours:	Moderate
More than 1 week:	Serious (full return of neurological function unlikely)

TABLE **2.18**

Headaches: A Differential Diagnosis

Disorder	Sex/Age Predominance	Nature of Pain	Frequency	Location	Duration	Prodromal Events	Precipitating Factors	Cause	Familial Predisposition	Other Possible Symptoms
Migraine	Female/20–40 years	Builds to throbbing and intense	Usually not more than twice a week; may be nocturnal	Usually unilateral	Several hours to days	Visual disturbances can occur contralateral to pain site	Unknown, may be physical, emotional, hormonal, dietary	Vasomotor	Yes	Nausea, vomiting, pallor, photophobia, mood disturbances, fluid retention
Cluster (histamine) headache	Male/40–60 years	Excruciating, stabbing, burning, pulsating	1–4 episodes per 24 h; nocturnal manifestation	Unilateral eye, temple, forehead	Minutes to hours	Sleep disturbances or personality changes can occur	Unknown, may be serotonin, histamine, hormonal blood flow	Vasomotor	Minor	Ipsilateral sweating of face, nasal lacrimation, congestion or discharge
Hypertension headache	None	Dull, throbbing, nonlocalized	Variable	Entire cranium, especially occipital region	Variable	None	Activity that increases blood pressure	High blood pressure; diastolic >120 mm Hg	Only as related to hypertension	
Trigeminal neuralgia (tic douloureux)	Female/40–60 years	Excruciating, spontaneous, lancinating, lightning	Can occur many (12 or more) times per day	Unilateral along trigeminal nerve area	30 seconds to 1 minute	Disagreeable tingling	Touch (cold) to affected area	Neurological	None	Reddened conjunctiva, lacrimation
Glossopharyngeal neuralgia	Male/40–60 years	Excruciating, spontaneous, lancinating, lightning	Can occur many (12 or more) times per day	Unilateral retrolingual area to ear	30 seconds to 1 minute	None	Movement or contact of the pharynx	Neurological	None	
Cervical neuralgia	None	Dull pain or pressure in head		Bilateral, occipital, frontal, or facial	Variable	None	Posture or head movement	Neurological, pressure on roots of spinal nerves	None	Dizziness, auditory disturbances
Eye disorders	None	Generalized discomfort in or around the eyes	Intensifies with sustained visual effort	Entire cranium	During and after visual effort	None	Impairment of eye function	Cornea, iris, or intraocular pain	Possible	Diminished vision, sensitivity to light
Sinus, ear, and nasal disorders	None	Dull, persistent	Variable	Frontal, temporal, ear, nose, occipital	Variable	None	Infection, allergy, chemical, bending, straining	Blockage, inflammation, infection	None	

Modified from Esposto CJ, Grim GA, Binkley TK: Headaches: a differential diagnosis, *J Craniomand Pract* 4:320–321, 1986.

TABLE **2.19**

Common Types of Dizziness Symptoms

Descriptions	Common Causes
Vertigo (e.g., visualized spinning, tilting, dropping of the environment)	Imbalance in tonic vestibular signals due to unilateral peripheral or central lesion
Light-headed/woozy	Blood pressure, metabolic, drugs, vestibular, psychophysiological
Near-faint	Decreased cerebral blood flow (diffuse)
Out of body, floating, spinning inside (e.g., no visualized movement of the environment)	Psychophysiological
Motion sickness or intolerance	Sensory conflict
Gait unsteadiness	Loss of vestibular, proprioceptive, cerebellar, or motor function

From Kerber KA, Baloh RW: The evaluation of a patient with dizziness, *Neurol Clin Pract* 1(1):24–32, 2011.

The examiner may also ask questions about the injury, preceding events, memory (**Maddocks questions**), and posttraumatic events. Questions such as "What day is it?" "Who is the opposition?" "Who is winning?" and "What is your telephone number and address?" test the patient's static memory ability. The examiner must ensure that he or she or someone present at the time of the examination knows the answer to these questions. Although it is common to ask these orientation questions (e.g., time, place), it has been shown that these questions can be unreliable in sporting situations when compared with memory assessment.[186,187] The examiner can assess **recent memory** by asking the patient to remember the names for two to five persons or common objects, such as the color "red," the number "five," the name "Mr. Smith," and the word "pride," and then asking the patient to name them 5 or 10 minutes later. The patient may be asked to repeat the words two or three times when the examiner initially says them to test immediate recall or to ensure that the patient can say and recall the words. **Immediate recall,** another form of memory, is best tested by asking the patient to repeat a series of single digits. Normally, a person can repeat at least six digits, and many people can repeat eight or nine. The examiner may also ask the patient to repeat the months of the year backward in a similar type of test. Memory is generally thought to be formed and stored in certain regions of the temporal lobes. The parietal lobe of the brain is thought to enable one to appreciate the environment, to interpret visual stimuli, and to communicate.

Common Head Injury Tests

- Static memory (What day is it? Who's winning?)
- Immediate recall (repeat series of single digits)
- Recent memory (recall three common objects or names after 15 min)
- Short-term memory (What is the game plan?)
- Processing and concentration ability (minus-7 test, months backwards, multiplying)
- Abstract relationships
- Coordination (finger to nose, heel to knee, dual task)
- Balance (BESS)
- Gait (normal, heel toe, dual task)
- Myotomes
- Eye coordination (e.g., acuity, smooth pursuits, accommodation, convergence, saccades, pupil size)
- Visual disturbance tests
- Reaction time
- Vestibulo-ocular reflex (VOR)

15. *Can the patient solve simple problems?* Because concussions reduce one's ability to process information, it is important to determine the patient's **reasoning and processing ability.** For example, does the patient know his or her home telephone number? Is the patient able to do the "minus 7" or "serial 7" test (i.e., count backward from 100 by sevens)? This test gives the examiner some idea of the patient's calculating ability and concentration skills. Mathematic ability (i.e., the ability to add, subtract, multiply, and divide) can also be evaluated to test processing ability. In addition, the examiner can ask the patient to name several important people from the present in reverse chronologic order (e.g., the past three presidents of the United States) or to give the names of some familiar capital cities. Finally, the patient should be tested on his or her ability to comprehend abstract relations. For example, the examiner may quote a common proverb, such as "A bird in the hand is worth two in the bush," and then ask the patient to explain what the expression means. Patients with organic mental impairment and certain patients with schizophrenia may give a concrete answer, failing to recognize the abstract principle involved.[185] The ability to conceptualize, abstract, plan ahead, and formulate rational judgments of problems or events is largely a function of the frontal lobes.

16. *Can the patient talk normally?* Patients with lesions of the parietal lobe have difficulty communicating and understanding what is occurring around them. **Dysarthria** indicates defects in articulation, enunciation, or rhythm of speech. It usually results from extraneural problems, such as poor-fitting dentures, malformation of the oral structures, or impairment of the musculature of the tongue, palate, pharynx, or lips because of incoordination, weakness, or abnormal innervation. It is characterized by slurring, slowness of

speech, indistinct speech, and breaks in normal speech rhythm. **Dysphonia** is a disorder of vocalization characterized by the abnormal production of sounds from the larynx. Dysphonia is usually caused by various abnormalities of the larynx itself or of its innervation. The principal complaint of dysphonia is hoarseness, ranging from mild roughness of the voice to an inability to produce sound. **Dysphasia** denotes the inability to use and understand written and spoken words as a result of disorders involving cortical centers of speech or their interconnections in the dominant cerebral hemisphere. With all of these conditions, the peripheral mechanisms for speech remain intact.

17. *Does the patient have any allergies, or is the patient receiving any medication?* Allergies may affect the eyes and nose, as may medications. Medications themselves may mask some symptoms.

18. *Is the patient having any problems with the eyes and visual acuity?* Monocular **diplopia** (i.e., blurred vision when looking with one eye) may result from hyphema, a detached lens, or other trauma to the globe of the eye.[188] Binocular diplopia (i.e., blurred vision when looking through both eyes) occurs in 10% to 40% of patients with a zygoma fracture. It may be caused by soft-tissue entrapment, neuromuscular injury (intraorbital or intramuscular), hemorrhage, or edema. It disappears when one eye is closed. Double vision, which occurs when the good eye is closed, indicates that some structure of the eye is injured. If it occurs with both eyes open, something is affecting the free movement of the eyes (Tables 2.20 and 2.21). Both blurred and/or double vision may occur with a head injury. Note whether there is any nystagmus (i.e., rapid involuntary eye movements), abnormal accommodation (i.e., looking at near and far objects), convergence (i.e., inward movement of eyes), saccades (i.e., quick jerky movement of eyes), and smooth pursuits (i.e., how eyes follow an object).

19. *Does the patient wear glasses or contact lenses?* If the patient wears glasses, are the lenses treated (hardened) or made of polycarbonate? If they are hardened, how long ago were they treated? If the patient wears contact lenses, are they hard, soft, or extended-wear lenses? Did the patient wear eye protectors? If so, what type were they? Are the patient's eyes watering? Is there any pain in the eyes? Small perforating injuries may be painless. If the patient complains of flashes of bright light, "a curtain falling in front of the eye," or floating black specks, these findings may indicate retinal detachment. These questions tell the examiner whether the eyewear or eyes need to be examined in greater detail.

20. *Is the patient having any problem with hearing?* Does the patient complain of an earache? If so, when was the onset, and what is the duration of the earache? Does the patient complain of pain or a discharge from the ear? Is the earache associated with an upper respiratory tract infection, swimming, or trauma? The patient should also be questioned on his or her method of cleaning the ear. If there appears to be a hearing loss, the patient should be asked whether the hearing loss came on quickly or slowly, whether the patient hears best on the telephone (amplified sound) or in a quiet or noisy environment, and whether speech is heard soft or loud. Does the patient use a hearing aid?

21. *Is the patient having any problems with the nose?* Has the patient used nose drops or spray? If so, how much, how often, and for how long? Does the patient have any nasal discharge, and if so, is its character watery, mucoid, purulent, crusty, or bloody? Does the discharge have any odor (indicative of infection), and is it unilateral or bilateral? Does the patient exhibit any associated nasal symptoms, such as sneezing, nasal congestion, itching, or mouth breathing? Does the patient complain of a nosebleed, and has the patient had many nosebleeds? If so, how frequent are the nosebleeds, what is the amount of the bleeding, and what appears to be causing the bleeding? Positive responses to any of these questions indicate that the nose must be examined in greater detail.

TABLE **2.20**

Common Visual Eye Symptoms and Disease States

Visual Symptom	Associated Causes
Loss of vision	Optic neuritis Detached retina Retinal hemorrhage Central retinal vascular occlusion
Spots	No pathological significance[a]
Flashes	Migraine Retinal detachment Posterior vitreous detachment
Loss of visual field or presence of shadows or curtains	Retinal detachment Retinal hemorrhage
Glare, photophobia	Iritis (inflammation of the iris) Meningitis (inflammation of the meninges)
Distortion of vision	Retinal detachment Macular edema
Difficulty seeing in dim light	Myopia Vitamin A deficiency Retinal degeneration
Colored haloes around lights	Acute narrow-angle glaucoma Opacities in lens or cornea
Colored vision changes	Cataracts Drugs (digitalis increases yellow vision)
Double vision	Extraocular muscle paresis or paralysis

[a]May precede a retinal detachment or be associated with fertility drugs.
From Swartz MH: *Textbook of physical diagnosis*, Philadelphia, 1989, WB Saunders, p 132.

TABLE **2.21**

Common Nonvisual Eye Symptoms and Disease States

Nonvisual Symptom	Associated Causes
Itching	Dry eyes Eye fatigue Allergies
Tearing	Emotional states Hypersecretion of tears Blockage of drainage
Dryness	Sjögren syndrome Decreased secretion as a result of aging
Sandiness, grittiness	Conjunctivitis
Fullness of eyes	Proptosis (bulging of the eyeball) Aging changes in the lids
Twitching	Fibrillation of orbicularis oculi
Eyelid heaviness	Fatigue Lid edema
Dizziness	Refractive error Cerebellar disease
Blinking	Local irritation Facial tic
Lids sticking together	Inflammatory disease of lids or conjunctivae
Foreign body sensation	Foreign body Corneal abrasion
Burning	Uncorrected refractive error Conjunctivitis Sjögren syndrome
Throbbing, aching	Acute iritis (inflammation of the iris) Sinusitis (inflammation of the sinuses)
Tenderness	Lid inflammations Conjunctivitis Iritis
Headache	Refractive errors Migraine Sinusitis
Drawing sensation	Uncorrected refractive errors

From Swartz MH: *Textbook of physical diagnosis*, Philadelphia, 1989, WB Saunders, p 133.

22. If the examiner is concerned about the mouth and teeth or the temporomandibular joints, questions related to these areas can be found in Chapter 4. However, it is important to ensure that the patient's dental occlusion and biting alignment have not been altered. Are all the teeth present, and are they symmetric? Is there any swelling or bleeding around the teeth? Are the teeth mobile, or is part of a tooth missing? Is the pulp exposed? Each of these questions helps to determine whether the teeth have been injured. Teeth that have been avulsed, if intact, should be reimplanted as quickly as possible. If reimplanted after cleansing (rinsed in saline solution or water) within less than 30 minutes, the tooth has a 90% chance of being retained. If it is not possible to reimplant the tooth, it should be kept moist in saline, or the patient should keep it between the gum and cheek while dental care is sought.

23. Questions concerning the neck and cervical spine can be found in Chapter 3.

Observation

For proper observation[186–192] of the head and face, any hat, helmet, mouth guard, or face guard should be removed. If a neck injury is suspected or if the patient presents an emergency situation, the examiner may take the time to remove only those items that are interfering with immediate emergency care. If a neck injury is suspected, extreme caution should be observed when removing the item. When assessing the head and face, the examiner must also observe and assess the posture of the cervical spine and the temporomandibular joints; see Chapters 3 and 4 for detailed descriptions of observation of these areas.

When observing the head and face, it is essential that the examiner look at the face to note the position and shape of the eyes, nose, mouth, teeth, and ears and look for deformity, asymmetry, facial imbalance, swelling, lacerations, foreign bodies, or bleeding during rest, with movement, or with different facial expressions.[193] One should also note, as much as possible, the individual's normal facial expression. A patient's facial expression often reflects the patient's general feeling and well-being. A dazed or vacant look often indicates problems. While talking to the patient, the examiner should watch for any asymmetry of facial motion or change in facial expression when the patient answers; slight facial asymmetry is common. In addition, small degrees of paralysis may not be obvious unless one attempts an exaggerated expression. If some facial paralysis is suspected, the examiner should ask the patient to make exaggerated facial expressions that will demonstrate the paralysis. If facial asymmetry is present, one should note whether all of the features on one side of the face are affected or only a portion of the face is affected. For example, with facial nerve (cranial nerve VII) paralysis, the entire side of the face is affected, although the most noticeable differences will occur around one eye and one side of the mouth. If only one side of the mouth is involved, then a problem with the trigeminal nerve (cranial nerve V) should be suspected. Any changes in the shape of the face or unusual features (e.g., masses, edema, puffiness, coarseness, prominent eyes, amount of facial hair, excessive perspiration, or skin color) should be noted. Eye puffiness is often one of the earliest signs of edema in the face. Skin color may include cyanosis, pallor, jaundice, or pigmentation, and each may be indicative of different systemic problems.

The examiner should view the patient from the front, side, behind, and above, noting the area behind the ears, at the hairline, and around the crown of the head as well as on the face (Fig. 2.11). An examiner who suspects a skull

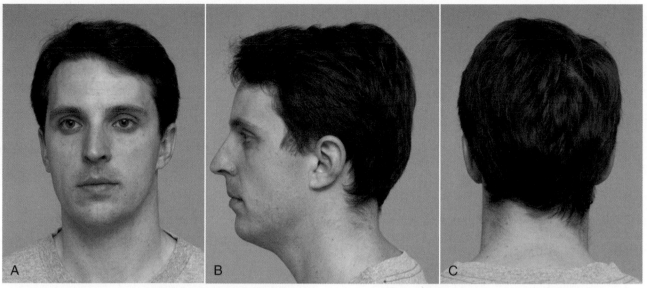

Fig. 2.11 Views of the head and face. (A) Anterior. (B) Side. (C) Posterior.

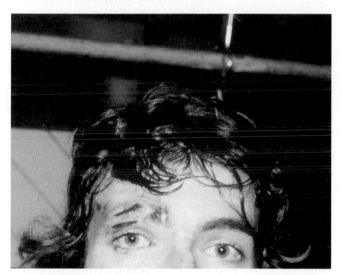

Fig. 2.12 Lacerations to the upper eyelid and eyebrow.

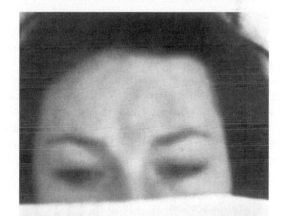

Fig. 2.13 Contusion to the forehead caused by a racquetball ball.

(cranial vault) injury should look behind the ears (**Battle sign** [see Fig. 2.17]), at the hairline, and around the crown of the head for any deformity, bruising, or laceration.

Viewing from the front, the examiner should observe the patient's hairline, noting any abnormalities. The soft tissues (e.g., the eyelids, eyebrows, cheeks, lips, nose, and chin) should be inspected for lacerations, bruising, or hematoma (Figs. 2.12 and 2.13). The eyes should be level. For example, a zygoma fracture causes the eye on the affected side to drop (Fig. 2.14). The two eyes should be compared for prominence or retraction (Fig. 2.15). If there appears to be any bulging, especially unilaterally, the examiner should tilt the patient's head forward or back and, looking from above, compare each cornea with the lid below, noting whether one or both corneas bulge beyond the lid margins. If one or both eyes appear to bulge, the

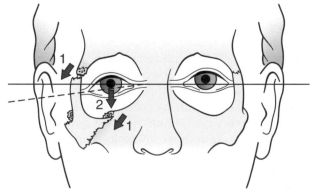

Fig. 2.14 Inferior displacement of the zygoma *(1)* results in depression of the lateral canthus and pupil *(2)* because of depression of the suspensory ligaments that attach to the lateral orbital, Whitnall tubercle. (Modified from Ellis E: Fractures of the zygomatic complex and arch. In Fonseca RJ, Walker RV, editors: *Oral and maxillofacial trauma*, Philadelphia, 1991, WB Saunders, p 446.)

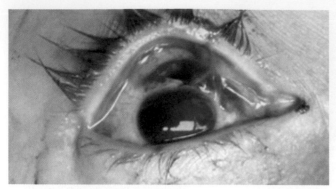

Fig. 2.15 Ruptured globe of the right eye from trauma. There is a visible puncture wound superior to the pupil, an irregularly shaped pupil, and endophthalmos (posterior displacement of the eyeball). (From Gragossian A, Vearrier D: Ruptured globe in a 35-year-old male, *Visual J Emerg Med* 13:50–51, 2018.)

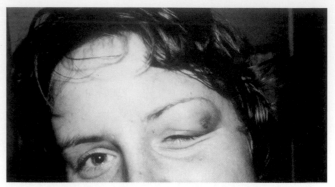

Fig. 2.16 Black eye (periorbital ecchymosis).

Eye Signs and Symptoms Requiring Specialist Care

- Foreign body that is not easily removed
- Eye does not move properly
- Altered pupil action
- Abnormal pupil size or shape[a]
- Double vision
- Blurred vision
- Decreased or partial vision
- Loss of part or all of visual field
- Laceration of eye or eyelid
- Blood between cornea and iris (i.e., hyphema)
- Impaired eyelid function
- Penetration of eye or eyelid
- Eye pain
- Sharp or throbbing eye pain
- Protrusion or retraction of eye

[a]In some individuals, this is normal and should be picked up in preseason evaluation.

examiner can use a pocket ruler to approximately measure the distance from the angle of the eye to the corneal apex.

Immediate referral for further examination by a specialist is required for an embedded corneal foreign body; haze or blood in the anterior chamber (i.e., hyphema); decreased or partial vision; irregular, asymmetric, or poor pupil action; diplopia or double vision; laceration of the eyelid or impaired lid function; perforation or laceration of the globe; broken contact lens or shattered eyeglass in the eye; unexplained eye pain that is stabbing or deep and throbbing; blurred vision that does not clear with blinking; loss of all or part of the visual field; protrusion of one eye relative to the other; an injured eye that does not move as fully as the uninjured eye; or abnormal pupil size or shape. A teardrop pupil usually indicates iris entrapment in a corneal or scleral laceration. In addition, the eyes should be observed from the lateral aspect. The normal distance from the cornea to the angle of the eye is 16 mm or less. The distances between the upper and lower lids should be the same for both eyes. When the eyes open, the superior eyelid should cover a portion of the iris but not the pupil itself. If it covers more of the iris than the other upper eyelid does or if it extends over the iris or pupil, ptosis or drooping of that eyelid should be suspected. If the eyelid does not cover part of the iris, retraction of the eyelid should be suspected. Are the eyelids everted or inverted? Normally, they are neither. The examiner should also note whether the patient can close both eyes completely. If an eye injury is suspected, this action should be done carefully, because closing the eyes can increase intraocular pressure. The lids should be pressed together only enough to bring the eyelashes together. Any inflammation or masses, especially on the lid margin, should be noted. If present, a "black eye," or periorbital contusion, should also be noted (Fig. 2.16). The lashes should be viewed to see if there is even distribution along the lid margins. "Racoon eyes," (Fig. 2.17) which are purple discolorations of the eyelids and orbital regions, may indicate orbital fractures, basilar skull fractures, or a fracture of the base of the anterior cranial fossa.[189] This sign takes several hours to develop.

The conjunctiva should be inspected for hemorrhage, laceration, and foreign bodies.[193] If the patient complains of "something in the eye," eversion of the upper eyelid usually reveals a foreign body that can often be easily brushed away. Displaced contact lenses are often found in this upper area of the eye. The conjunctival covering of the lower lid may be examined by having the patient look upward while the examiner draws the lower lid downward. The conjunctiva should be examined as being a continuous sheet of epithelium from the globe to the lids. The color of the sclera should also be noted. Posttraumatic conjunctival hemorrhage (Fig. 2.18) and possible scleral lacerations (Fig. 2.19) should be noted, if present. In dark-skinned patients, pigmented areas may show up as small dark spots or patches near the limbus. The shape and color of the cornea should be inspected. The anterior chambers of the eye should be inspected and compared for clarity and depth.[194] If present, hyphema in the form of haze or actual blood pooling (Fig. 2.20) in the anterior eye chamber should be noted.[188] If there is any potential for or evidence of bleeding in the anterior chamber of the eye, the patient's activity should be curtailed, because increased activity increases the chances of secondary hemorrhage during the first week after injury. Examination

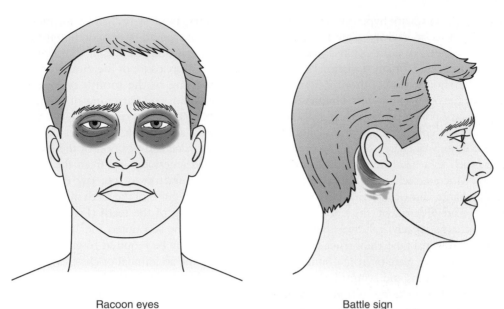

Racoon eyes   Battle sign

Fig. 2.17 Battle sign and racoon (panda) eyes for basilar skull fracture.

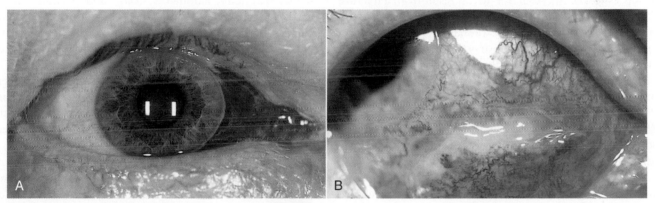

Fig. 2.18 Conjunctival hemorrhage and laceration. (A) Trauma resulted in a large hemorrhage in the nasal conjunctiva. (B) Conjunctival laceration present in another patient. (From Yanoff M, Sassani J: *Ocular pathology*, ed 7, Philadelphia, 2015, Saunders/Elsevier.)

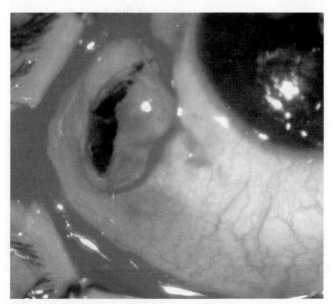

Fig. 2.19 Penetrating scleral wounds. Radial anterior scleral laceration with ciliary and vitreous prolapse. (From Eagling EM, Roper-Hall MJ: *Eye injuries: an illustrated guide*, London, 1986, Butterworth-Heinemann.)

of the cornea with a penlight shone obliquely on the eye should be carried out to look for foreign bodies, abrasions, or lacerations. Corneal injuries can lead to lacrimation (tearing), photophobia (intolerance to light), or blepharospasm (spasm of the eyelid orbicular muscle), as well as extreme pain from exposure of sensory nerve endings. A fluorescein strip dipped into tears that are exposed as the lower lid is pulled downward will readily outline abrasions.

The **pupillary size** (diameter range, 2 to 6 mm; mean, 3.5 mm), shape (round), and symmetry should be compared with those of the other eye. Elliptical pupils often indicate a corneal laceration. The color of the irises of the eyes should be compared. When looking at the pupils, the examiner should note whether the pupils are equal. Are the pupils smaller or larger than normal? Are they round or irregularly shaped? The pupils are normally slightly unequal in 5% of the population, but inequality of pupil size should initially be viewed with suspicion. For example, some medications can affect pupil dilation, or unilateral dilation could be the result of a sympathetic nerve response following a blow to the face.[4] Pupils tend to be smaller in infants, the elderly, and persons with hyperopia (farsightedness), whereas they tend to be slightly dilated in persons with myopia (nearsightedness) or light-colored irises.

The nose should be inspected for any deviations in shape, size, or color.[193] The skin should be smooth without swelling and should conform to the color of the face. The airways are usually oval and symmetrically proportioned. If a discharge is present, its character (i.e., color, smell, texture) should be noted and described. Bloody discharge occurs as a result of epistaxis or trauma, such as a nasal fracture, zygoma fracture, or skull fracture. Mucoid discharge is typical of rhinitis. Bilateral purulent discharge can occur with upper respiratory tract infection. Unilateral purulent, thick, greenish, and often malodorous discharge usually indicates the presence of a foreign body. Cerebrospinal fluid rhinorrhea may occur with a fracture of the cribriform plate or frontal sinus due to a tear in the dura.[195] Other signs and symptoms associated with cerebral spinal fluid leak include positional headaches (better when lying down), nausea, vomiting, neck pain and stiffness, imbalance, ringing in ears, and photophobia.

Depression of the nasal bridge can result from a fracture of the nasal bone. Nasal flaring is associated with respiratory distress, whereas narrowing of the airways on inspiration may indicate chronic nasal obstruction and be associated with mouth breathing. The nasal mucosa should be deep pink and glistening. A film of clear discharge is often apparent on the nasal septum. The nasal septum should be close to midline and fairly straight, appearing thicker anteriorly than posteriorly. If present, a hematoma in the septal area should be noted. Asymmetric posterior nasal cavities may indicate a deviation of the nasal septum.

With the patient's mouth closed, the lips should be observed for symmetry, color, edema, and surface abnormalities. Lipstick should be removed before the assessment. The lips should be pink and have vertical and horizontal symmetry, both at rest and with movement. Dry, cracked lips may be caused by dehydration from wind or low humidity, whereas deep fissures at the corners of the mouth may indicate overclosure of the mouth or riboflavin deficiency.

Drooping of the mouth on one side, sagging of the lower eyelid, and flattening of the nasolabial fold suggest possible facial nerve (cranial nerve VII) involvement. The patient is also unable to pucker the lips to whistle.

The shape and position of the jaw and teeth should also be noted anteriorly and from the side.[193] Asymmetry may indicate a fracture of the jaw Fig. 2.21, whereas bleeding around the gums of the teeth may indicate fracture, avulsion, or loosening of the teeth (Fig. 2.22). If teeth are missing, they must be accounted for. If they are not accounted for, an x-ray may be required to ensure that the teeth have not entered the abdominal or chest cavity. Pain on percussion of the teeth often indicates damage to the periodontal ligament.

From the side, the examiner should look for any asymmetry or depression, which may indicate pathology. The examiner should inspect the auricles of the ears for size, shape, symmetry, landmarks, color, and position on the head. To determine the position of the auricle, the examiner can draw an imaginary line between the outer canthus of the eye and occipital protuberance (Fig. 2.23). The top of the auricle should touch or be above this line.[12] The examiner can then draw another imaginary line perpendicular to the previous line and just anterior to the auricle. The auricle's position should be almost vertical. If the angle is more than 10° posterior or anterior, it is considered

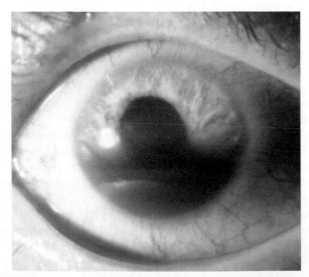

Fig. 2.20 Traumatic hyphema. Note the visible blood in the anterior chamber. (From Bowling B: *Kanski's clinical ophthalmology: a systematic approach*, ed 8, China, 2016, Elsevier.)

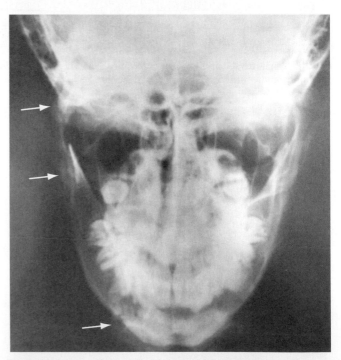

Fig. 2.21 Fracture of the neck of the condyle on the right *(upper arrows)* with fracture through the mandible on the same side *(lower arrow)*. When one fracture is shown in the mandible, search carefully for the second. (From O'Donoghue DH: *Treatment of injuries to athletes*, Philadelphia, 1984, WB Saunders, p 115.)

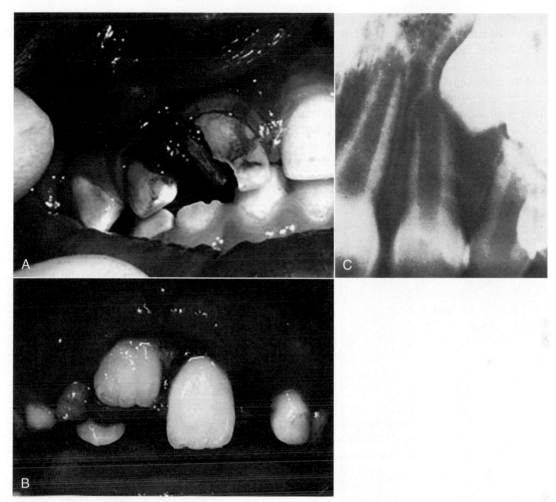

Fig. 2.22 (A) A small hard object trauma, in this case a stone, caused a severe localized dental injury. (B) A larger soft object injury caused widespread dental injuries involving displacement of soft tissues, intrusion, luxation, and avulsion of teeth and bone fractures. (C) Radiograph of root canal with wide-open apex. (A and B, From Moule AJ, Moule CA: Minor traumatic injuries to the permanent dentition, *Dent Clin North Am* 53(4):639–659, 2009. Courtesy Richard Widmer, BDSc, MDSc, Sydney, NSW, Australia. C, From Torg JS: *Athletic injuries to the head, neck and face*, Philadelphia, 1982, Lea & Febiger, p 247.)

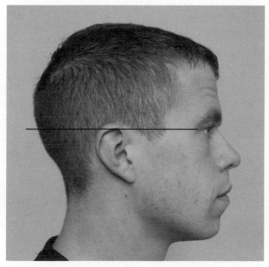

Fig. 2.23 Auricle alignment. Normal position shown.

abnormal. An auricle that is set low or is at an unusual angle may indicate chromosomal aberrations or renal disorders. In addition, the lateral and medial surfaces and surrounding tissues should be examined, noting any deformities, lesions, or nodules. The auricles should be the same color as the facial skin without moles, cysts, or other lesions or deformities. Athletes, especially wrestlers, may exhibit a **cauliflower ear** (hematoma auris), which is a keloid scar forming in the auricle because of friction to or twisting of the ear (Fig. 2.24). Blueness may indicate some degree of cyanosis. Pallor or excessive redness may be the result of vasomotor instability or increased temperature. Frostbite can cause extreme pallor or blistering (Fig. 2.25).

The examiner should look posteriorly for any asymmetry or depression. The positions of the ears (height, protrusion) can be compared by observing them from behind. A low hairline may indicate conditions such as

Klippel-Feil syndrome. The examiner should also look for the presence of **Battle sign** and **racoon (or panda) eyes** (see Fig. 2.17), which may take as long as 24 hours to appear, are demonstrated by purple and blue discoloration of the skin in the mastoid area and the eyes, and may indicate a temporal bone or basilar skull fracture.

The examiner then views the patient from overhead (superior view) to note any asymmetry from above (Fig. 2.26). This method is especially useful when looking for a possible fracture of the zygoma (Fig. 2.27). The deformity is easier to detect if the examiner carefully places the index fingers below the infraorbital margins along the zygomatic bodies and then gently pushes into the edema to reduce the effect of the edema (Fig. 2.28).

▼ **Signs and Symptoms of Maxillary and Zygomatic Fractures**

- Facial asymmetry
- Loss of cheek prominence
- Palpable steps
  - Infraorbital rim (zygomaticomaxillary suture)
  - Lateral orbital rim (frontozygomatic suture)
  - Root of zygoma intraorally
  - Zygomatic arch between the ear and the eye (zygomaticotemporal suture)
- Hypoesthesia/anesthesia
  - Cheek, side of nose, upper lip, and teeth on the injured side
  - Compression of the infraorbital nerve as it courses along the floor of the orbit to exit into the face via the foramen beneath the orbital rim

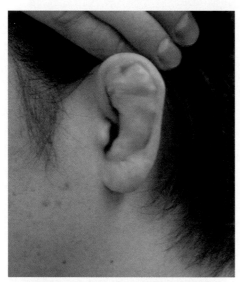

Fig. 2.24 Cauliflower ear (hematoma auris).

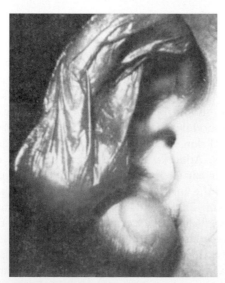

Fig. 2.25 Auricular frostbite with development of massive vesicles that are beginning to resolve spontaneously. (From Schuller DE, Bruce RA: Ear, nose, throat and eye. In Strauss RH, editor: *Sports medicine*, ed 2, Philadelphia, 1991, WB Saunders, p 191.)

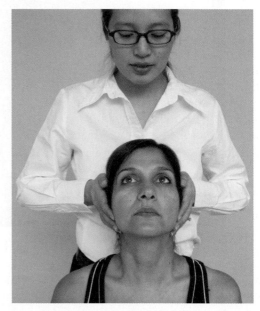

Fig. 2.26 View of the patient from above to look for bilateral symmetry of the face.

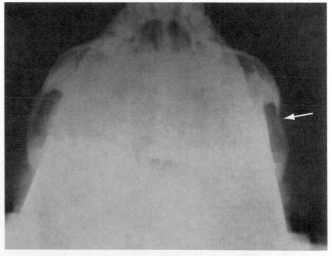

Fig. 2.27 Typical fracture of zygomatic arch on the right *(arrow)*. Note normal arch on the left. (From O'Donoghue DH: *Treatment of injuries to athletes*, Philadelphia, 1984, WB Saunders, p 114.)

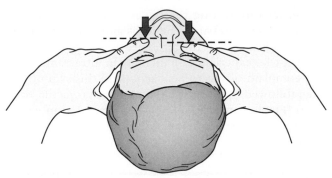

Fig. 2.28 Method of assessing posterior displacement of the zygomatic complex from behind the patient. The examiner should firmly but carefully depress the fingers into the edematous soft tissues while palpating along the infraorbital areas. (Modified from Ellis E: Fractures of the zygomatic complex and arch. In Fonseca RJ, Walker RV, editors: *Oral and maxillofacial trauma*, Philadelphia, 1991, WB Saunders, p 443.)

Examination

The examination of the head and face differs from the orthopedic assessment of other areas of the body because the assessment does not involve joints. The only joints that could be included in the assessment are the temporomandibular joints, and these joints are discussed in Chapter 4.

Examination of the Head

Many problems in the head and face may be problems referred from the cervical spine, temporomandibular joint, or teeth. However, if one suspects a head injury, it is necessary to keep a close watch on the patient, noting any changes and when these changes occur. The examiner should implement a **Neural Watch** so that any changes that occur over time can be determined easily (Table 2.22). The testing should occur at 15- or 30-minute intervals, depending on the severity of the injury and the changes recorded.

Head Examination

- Concussion
- Headache
- Memory tests
- Neural Watch and Glasgow Coma Scale
- Expanding intracranial lesion
- Proprioception
- Coordination
- Head injury card

Presently, it is recommended that an athlete not return to competition or practice if he or she has suffered a concussion. In fact, activity should be limited until all symptoms have disappeared. Research has shown that the

TABLE **2.22**

Neural Watch Chart

Unit		Time 1 ( )	Time 2 ( )	Time 3 ( )
I Vital signs	Blood pressure			
	Pulse			
	Respiration			
	Temperature			
II Conscious and	Oriented			
	Disoriented			
	Restless			
	Combative			
III Speech	Clear			
	Rambling			
	Garbled			
	None			
IV Will awaken to	Name			
	Shaking			
	Light pain			
	Strong pain			
V Nonverbal reaction to pain	Appropriate			
	Inappropriate			
	"Decerebrate"			
	None			
VI Pupils	Size on right			
	Size on left			
	Reacts on right			
	Reacts on left			
VII Ability to move	Right arm			
	Left arm			
	Right leg			
	Left leg			
VIII Sensation	Right side (normal/ abnormal)			
	Left side (normal/ abnormal)			
	Dermatome affected (specify)			
	Peripheral nerve affected (specify)			

Modified from American Academy of Orthopedic Surgeons: *Athletic training and sports medicine*, Park Ridge, IL, 1984, AAOS, p 399.

brain is vulnerable to reinjury for 3 to 5 days following concussions because of altered blood flow and metabolic dysfunction.[140] If the examiner is contemplating allowing the patient to return to activity because all symptoms have disappeared, return-to-school (see Table 2.13) and return-to-play protocols (see Table 2.14) should be followed when considering allowing the individual to return to school or activity. Provocative stress tests are commonly related to the sport but may include jumping jacks, sit-ups, push-ups, deep knee bends, and lying supine for 1 minute with feet elevated or similar activities that may be related to what the patient will return to functionally (e.g., rapid head movements, straining or holding breath). These activities should be viewed as actions that increase intracranial pressure and can cause a different physiological response in concussed athletes,[196] which may lead to symptoms.[4,197] Although the guidelines outlined in Tables 2.13 and 2.14 may appear excessively precautionary, they are designed to prevent **second impact syndrome,** especially in children, which is potentially catastrophic injury with a mortality rate close to 50% or permanent brain injury.[101,198–203]

Red Flags[a] for Concussions in Acute Phase[33]

- Worsening headache
- Nuchal rigidity
- Battle sign and/or racoon eyes (late sign)
- Developing blurred, double or loss of vision
- Becoming drowsy or lethargic
- Worsening mental/cognitive ability
- Unusual behavior
- Slurred speech
- Inability to recognize people
- Worsening memory
- Inability to answer simple questions
- Seizures
- Urinary or bowel incontinence

[a]Implies patient should be seen by a physician or emergency department.

The examiner should always be looking for the possibility of an **expanding intracranial lesion** resulting from a leaking or torn blood vessel. Normally, the brain has a fixed volume that is enclosed in a nonexpansile structure, namely, the skull and dura mater. These lesions may be caused by epidural hemorrhage (usually tearing of one of the meningeal arteries as a result of high-speed impact), subarachnoid hemorrhage (usually as a result of an aneurysm), or subdural hemorrhage (usually as a result of tearing of bridging veins between the brain and cavernous sinus).[198] These injuries are emergency conditions that must be looked after immediately because of their high mortality rate (as much as 50%). An expanding intracranial lesion is indicated by an altered lucid state (i.e., state of consciousness), development of inequality of the pupils, unusual slowing of the heart rate that primarily occurs after a lucid interval, irregular eye movements, and eyes that no longer track properly. There is also a tendency for the patient to demonstrate increased body temperature and irregular respirations. Normal intracranial pressure measures from 4 to 15 mm Hg, and an intracranial pressure of more than 20 mm Hg is considered abnormal. Intracranial pressure of 40 mm Hg causes neurological dysfunction and impairment. Although in the

emergency care setting there is no way of determining the intracranial pressure, the signs and symptoms mentioned indicate that the pressure is increasing. Most patients who experience an increase in intracranial pressure complain of severe headache, and this symptom is often followed by vomiting (sometimes projectile vomiting). Finally, an expanding intracranial lesion causes increased weakness on the side of the body opposite that on which the lesion has occurred.

Signs and Symptoms of an Expanding Intracranial Lesion

- Altered state of consciousness
- Nystagmus
- Pupil inequality
- Irregular eye movements
- Abnormal slowing of heart
- Irregular respiration
- Severe headache
- Intractable vomiting
- Positive expanding intracranial lesion tests (lateralizing)
- Positive coordination tests
- Decreasing muscle strength
- Seizure

Signs and symptoms that indicate a good possibility of recovery from a head injury, especially after the patient experiences unconsciousness, include response to noxious stimuli, eye opening, pupil activity, spontaneous eye movement, intact oculovestibular reflexes, and appropriate motor function responses. Neurological signs that indicate a poor prognosis after a head injury include nonreactive pupils, absence of oculovestibular reflexes, severe extension patterns or no motor function response at all, and increased intracranial pressure.[185]

It is important when examining the unconscious or conscious patient for a possible head injury to determine the individual's level of consciousness, which may be determined using the **Glasgow Coma Scale** ✓ (see Table 2.5 and Special Tests section for description).

The **Rancho Los Amigos Scale of Cognitive Function** may also be used to assess the patient's cognitive abilities. This scale is an eight-level progression from level I, in which the patient is nonresponsive, to level VIII, in which the patient's behavior is purposeful and appropriate (Table 2.23). The Rancho Los Amigos Scale provides an assessment of cognitive function and behavior only, not of physical functioning.[185]

If a person receives a head injury, such as a mild concussion, and is not referred to the hospital, the examiner should ensure that someone accompanies the person home and that someone at home knows what has happened so he or she can monitor the patient in case the patient's condition worsens. Appropriate written instructions should be

TABLE **2.23**

Rancho Los Amigos Scale of Cognitive Function

Level I	No response
Level II	Generalized response
Level III	Localized response
Level IV	Confused, agitated
Level V	Confused, inappropriate
Level VI	Confused, appropriate
Level VII	Automatic, appropriate
Level VIII	Purposeful, appropriate

From Hagen C, Malkmus D, Durham P: Levels of cognitive functioning. In *Rehabilitation of the brain injured adult–comprehensive management*, Downey, CA, 1980, Professional Staff Association of Rancho Los Amigos.

sent home concerning the individual. The **Home Head Injury Card** is an example (Fig. 2.29).

Levin and colleagues reported the use of the **Galveston Orientation and Amnesia Test (GOAT)**,[6] which they believe measures orientation to person, place, and time and the memory of events preceding and following head trauma (eTool 2.5). As the patient improves, the total GOAT score should increase.

As part of the head examination, the **cranial nerves** should be tested (see Table 2.1). The most commonly affected cranial nerve is the olfactory nerve (cranial nerve I), followed by the facial nerve (cranial nerve VII). If multiple cranial nerves are affected, the most frequent associations are reported to be cranial nerves II, III, IV, and VI; cranial nerves VI and VII; and cranial nerve VII and cranial nerves VII and VIII.[195,204,205]

The examiner may also wish to determine whether the patient has suffered an **upper motor neuron lesion**. Testing the deep tendon reflexes (see Table 1.30) or the pathological reflexes (see Table 1.32) or having the patient perform various balance and coordination tests may help to determine whether this type of lesion has occurred. However, the pathological reflexes may not be elicited owing to shock. Deep tendon reflexes are accentuated on the side of the body opposite that on which the brain injury has occurred.

Balance can play an important role in the assessment of a head-injured patient. Balance control is a complex activity and involves activities such as an ability to maintain a body position, an ability to provide postural responses to external perturbations, an ability to provide gait stability, and an ability to allow anticipatory postural adjustments and sensory integration.[206–208] For correct balance, information from the somatosensory, visual, and vestibular systems and an intact central nervous system to maintain an upright stance are required.[82] Balance involves the integration of several inputs (e.g., from the visual, proprioceptive, and vestibular systems) that are analyzed by the

---

Home Health Care Guidelines: Head Injury Care

The person you have been asked to watch has suffered a head injury, which at this time does *not* appear to be severe. However, to ensure proper care, please ensure that the following guidelines are followed for the next 24 hours.

1. Limited physical activity for at least 24 hours **(rest quietly, do not drive a vehicle).**

2. Liquid diet only for the next 8 to 24 hours **(no alcohol).**

3. Apply ice to the head for approximately 15 minutes every hour to relieve discomfort and swelling.

4. Tylenol may be given as needed but NO aspirin. No other medication for 24 hours without doctor's approval.

5. Awaken the patient every 2 hours during the next ____ hours and be aware of any symptoms in #6.

6. Appearance of any of the following signs and symptoms means that you should consult a doctor or go to an emergency room at a hospital **immediately:**

   - Nausea and/or vomiting
   - Weakness or numbness in arm, leg, or any other body part
   - Any visual difficulties or dizziness
   - Ringing in the ears
   - Mental confusion or disorientation, irritability, restlessness, forgetfulness
   - Loss of coordination
   - Unusual sleepiness or difficulty in awakening
   - Progressively worsening headache
   - Persistent intense headache after 48 hours
   - Unequal pupil size; slow or no pupil reaction to light
   - Difficulty breathing
   - Irregular heartbeat
   - Convulsions or tremors

7. Call to arrange an appointment with your doctor or the team physician/therapist* for a follow-up visit. If unable to contact your doctor, go to an emergency room as soon as possible for an evaluation.

   *Consult: _____ at _____
   phone number

   or: _____ at _____
   phone number

SPECIAL INSTRUCTIONS, APPOINTMENTS:

Fig. 2.29 Example of home health care guidelines for patients with head injuries. (Modified from Allman FL, Crow RW: On-field evaluation of sports injuries. In Griffin LY, editor: *Orthopedic knowledge update: sports medicine*, Rosemont, IL, 1994, American Academy of Orthopaedic Surgeons, p 14.)

brain to allow a proper action. For example, in standing, the body is inherently unstable, and only the integration of input from various sources enables the patient to stand and to make appropriate corrections to maintain proper standing posture. Balance and coordination can be tested in several ways. The examiner can ask the patient to stand

and walk a straight line with the eyes open and then with the eyes closed while the examiner is noting any difference. The **Balance Error Scoring System (BESS)** (see Special Tests—Balance for description) has been developed as an objective test for balance, which is the balance test most commonly used and is part of the SCAT5 tool.[137,154,209–214] Other balance tests that may be considered include the **4-Stage Balance Test** (see eTool 2.14), the **BESTest** (i.e., Balance Evaluation-Systems Test; see Table 2.26), the **Mini BESTest** (see eTool 2.17), and **Star Excursion Balance Test** (SEBT; sec Fig. 2.53).[206,207,215]

Coordination can be tested by the Finger-to-Nose test or Heel-to-Knee test (see Special Test section).

Gait may be tested by asking the individual to walk a certain distance or by completing gait tests such as the **Dynamic Gait Index (DGI)** (eTool 2.6),[216,217] **Functional Gait Assessment** (eTool 2.7), the **Modified Gait Abnormality Rating Scale (GARS-M)** (eTool 2.8), and **Timed Up and Go (TUG) Test** (see eTool 2.16).[49,216,218–220] When assessing gait, the examiner is watching for excessive side to side motion to counter imbalance, excessive hip movement, upper extremity movement, or the inability to coordinate the foot movement in the tandem stance.[33]

Balance and gait can be made more difficult by doing them as a **dual task activity.** This means the patient is asked to do a second activity while balancing or walking (e.g., "walking and talking").[144,221–225] Dual task balance assessments, in particular, have been reported to provide a more sensitive detection of neurological deficits that persist, so it may help to identify compromise processes that may require more healing following a concussion.[144]

Clinical **reaction time** is another component that may be considered as part of the multifaceted concussion assessment battery. A prolonged reaction time is common following concussion and is one of the more sensitive indices of neurocognitive change following injury. Testing for clinical reaction time is a physical motor test in which the individual is asked to catch a falling ruler by closing a hand around the ruler after its release by the examiner. It has been reported that a 13% total prolongation of clinical reaction time and athletes tested within 72 hours of concussion as compared with baseline.[226] (Also see Special Tests section.)

Because dizziness and potential balance problems are related and because the vestibular system is a complex sensory network that provides a subjective sense of self motion, the integrity and function of the vestibulo-ocular system needs to be assessed as 40% to 50% of athletes who have suffered a concussion report balance dysfunction and dizziness, respectively, which could reflect underlying impairments of the vestibular system (i.e., the vestibulo-ocular and vestibulospinal systems).[148] The **Vestibular/Ocular Motor Screening (VOMS)** (see eTool 2.20) involves using several tests to evaluate for vestibular and oculomotor symptoms (e.g., migraine-like headache, dizziness, nausea, floppiness)

following a concussion. The VOMS includes testing smooth pursuit, saccades, the vestibulo-ocular reflex (VOR), vision motion sensitivity (VMS), and near point of convergence (NPC) distance (see Special Tests section).[69,148] More than 60% of patients with a concussion experience symptom provocation on greater than or equal to one VOMS item.[148] Posttraumatic vision or oculomotor problems have been reported in 30% to 65% of patients with mTBI and in nearly 30% of patients with concussion. Vision impairment after concussion may include diplopia (i.e., double vision), blurred vision, eye fatigue, difficulty tracking a moving target or words appearing to be moving on page when reading, loss of visual field integrity, binocular vision (i.e., lack of convergence), difficulty with accommodation (i.e., focusing), saccadic disorders (i.e., abnormal eye movements), headaches, and, to a lesser extent, dizziness and nausea symptoms, and impairment may result in visual discomfort and vision-mediated functional difficulties such as slow reading and tearing during academic or occupational activities.[161,227,228]

Muscle tone and strength may also play a role in assessing the patient for head injury. Increased unilateral muscle tone usually implies contralateral cerebral peduncle compression. Flaccid muscle tone implies brain stem infarction, spinal cord transaction, or spinal shock. Unilateral effects, such as hemiparesis, may be seen with a stroke.

Examination of the Face[190–194,229]

Once a head injury has been ruled out or if no head injury is suspected, the examiner can inspect the face for injury. Major trauma and subsequent injury to the face should be assessed first. If major trauma has not occurred, only those areas of the face that have been affected by the trauma (e.g., eyes, nose, ears) need be assessed. The patient may initially be tested for fractures with the use of a tongue depressor if the patient can open her or his mouth. The patient is asked to bite down as hard as possible on the tongue depressor while the examiner twists the tongue depressor and tries to break it (Fig. 2.30A). The examiner should note whether the patient is able to bite down strongly and hold the contraction and where any pain is elicited.

Facial Examination

- Bone and soft-tissue contours
- Fractures
- Mandible
- Maxilla
- Zygoma
- Skull
- Cranial nerves
- Facial muscles

To test for a maxillary fracture, the examiner grasps the anterior aspect of the maxilla with the fingers of one hand and places the fingers of the other hand over the bridge of the patient's nose or forehead. The examiner then gently pulls the maxilla forward (Fig. 2.31). If the fingers of the other hand at the nose feel movement or the examiner feels the test hand moving forward, a Le Fort II or III fracture may be present (Fig. 2.32). If the maxilla moves without movement at the nose, either the maxilla is horizontally fractured or a Le Fort I fracture is present. With a Le Fort I fracture, the palate is separated from the superior portion of the maxilla, and the upper tooth-bearing segment of the face moves alone. The nasal bones, midportion of the face, and maxilla move if a Le Fort II fracture is present. With a Le Fort III fracture, the middle third of the face separates from the upper third of the face; this is often called a *craniofacial separation*. The patient may complain of lip or cheek anesthesia and double vision (diplopia) with any of these fractures.

The examiner then asks the patient to open his or her mouth slightly. The examiner carefully applies pressure bilaterally at the angles of the mandible (Fig. 2.30B). Localized pain, lower lip anesthesia, and intraoral laceration may indicate a fracture of the mandible. Malocclusion of the teeth is often seen with fractures of the mandible or maxilla (Fig. 2.33). Alterations in smell (cranial nerve I) are often seen with frontobasal and nasoethmoidal fractures. Skull fractures are often associated with clear nasal discharge (i.e., spinal fluid rhinorrhea), clear ear discharge (i.e., otorrhea), or a salty taste. If blood accompanies the fluid, the examiner can use a gauze pad to collect the fluid. If cerebrospinal fluid is mixed with the blood, the examiner may observe a "halo" effect as the fluid collects on the gauze pad (Fig. 2.34). If the eardrum has not been perforated, blood may be visible behind it. Skull fractures may also result in blurred or double vision, loss of smell (i.e., anosmia), dizziness, tinnitus, and nausea and vomiting, as well as signs and symptoms of concussion. Orbital floor fractures or dislocations are often accompanied by anesthesia of the skin in the midface or anesthesia of the cheek, lip, maxillary teeth, and gingiva.[230] Zygoma fractures are detected by observation

(see Fig. 2.28). They may also cause unilateral epistaxis, double vision, and anesthesia and be associated with eye injuries. Mouth opening may also be affected.

After major trauma has been ruled out, the examiner may test the muscles of the face (Table 2.24), especially if injury to these structures is suspected. Excluding the temporomandibular joint, the muscles of the face are different from most muscles in that they move the skin and soft tissues rather than joints. For example, the frontalis muscle may be weak if the eyebrows do not raise symmetrically. The corrugator muscle draws the eyebrows medially and downward (frowning). The orbicularis oris muscle approximates and

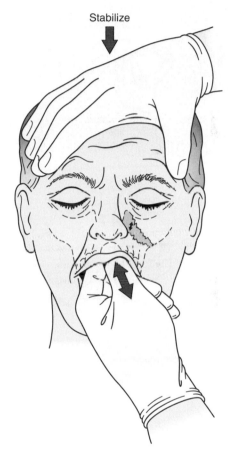

Stabilize

Fig. 2.31 Testing for maxillary fracture.

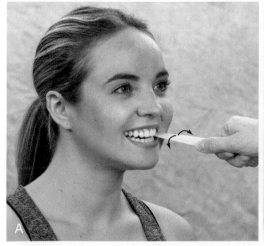

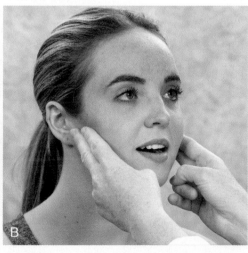

Fig. 2.30 Testing for mandibular fracture. (A) Patient bites down on tongue depressor while examiner tries to twist the tongue depressor and break it (tongue blade test). (B) Pressure at the angles of the mandible.

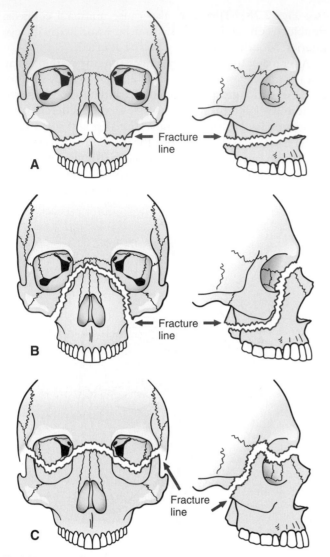

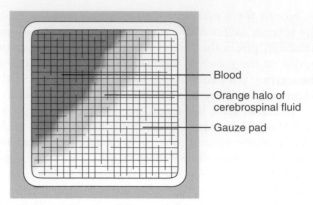

Fig. 2.34 An orange halo will form around the blood on a gauze pad if cerebrospinal fluid is present because of the different densities of blood and cerebrospinal fluid.

Fig. 2.32 Le Fort fractures. (A) Le Fort I. (B) Le Fort II. (C) Le Fort III.

compresses the lips, whereas the zygomaticus muscles raise the lateral angle of the mouth (smiling).

Examination of the Eye[190–193]

If the eyelids are swollen shut, the examiner should initially assume that the globe has been ruptured. A penetrating wound of the eyelid should be assessed carefully, because it may be associated with an injury to the globe of the eye. The examiner should not force the eyelid open, because intraocular pressure can force extrusion of the ocular contents if the globe has been ruptured. The patient should also be instructed not to squeeze the eyelids tight, because this action can increase the intraocular pressure from a normal value of 15 mm Hg up to approximately 70 mm Hg.

To examine the **normal functioning of the eye muscles** and several of the cranial nerves (II, III, IV, and VI), the examiner asks the patient to move through the **six cardinal positions of gaze** (up to the left, up to the right, down to the left, down to the right, laterally, and medially; Fig. 2.35). The examiner holds the patient's chin steady with one hand and asks the patient to follow the examiner's other hand while the examiner traces a large "H" in the air. The examiner should hold the index finger or pencil approximately 25 cm (10 inches) from the patient's nose. From the midline, the finger or pencil is moved approximately 30 cm (12 inches) to the patient's right and held. It is then moved up approximately 20 cm (8 inches) and held, moved down 40 cm (16 inches; 20 cm relative to midline) and held, and moved slowly back to midline. The same movement is repeated on the other side. The examiner should observe movement of both eyes, noting whether the eyes follow the finger or pencil smoothly. The examiner should also observe any parallel movement of the eyes in all directions. If the eyes do not move in unison or if only one eye moves, something is affecting the action of the muscles. One of the most common causes of one eye's not moving after trauma to the eye is a blowout fracture of the orbital floor (Fig. 2.36). Because the inferior muscles become "caught" in

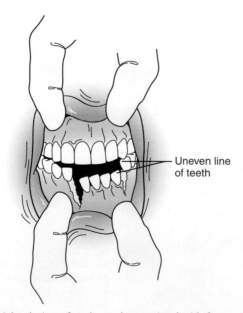

Fig. 2.33 Malocclusion of teeth may be associated with fracture of mandible or maxilla.

TABLE **2.24**

Muscles of the Face

	Action	Cranial Nerve
Muscles of the Mouth		
Orbicularis oris	Compresses lips against anterior teeth, closes mouth, protrudes lips	VII (Zygomatic, buccal, and mandibular branches)
Depressor anguli oris	Depresses angle of mouth	VII (Buccal and mandibular branches)
Levator anguli oris	Elevates angle of mouth	VII (Zygomatic and buccal branches)
Zygomaticus major	Draws angle of mouth upward and back	VII (Zygomatic and buccal branches)
Risorius	Draws angle of mouth laterally	VII (Zygomatic and buccal branches)
Muscle of the Lips		
Levator labii superioris	Elevates upper lip, flares nostril	VII (Zygomatic and buccal branches)
Muscle of the Cheek		
Buccinator	Compresses cheeks against molar teeth; sucking and blowing	VII (Buccal branches)
Muscle of the Chin		
Mentalis	Puckers skin of chin, protrudes lower lip	VII (Mandibular branches)
Muscle of the Nose		
Nasalis	Compresses nostrils	VII (Zygomatic and buccal branches)
	Dilates or flares nostrils	
Muscle of the Eye		
Orbicularis oculi	Closes eye forcefully	VII (Temporal and zygomatic branches)
	Closes eye gently	
	Squeezes lubricating tears against eyeball	
Muscles of the Forehead		
Procerus	Transverse wrinkling of bridge of nose	VII (Temporal and zygomatic branches)
Corrugator	Vertical wrinkling of bridge of nose	VII (Temporal branches)
Frontalis	Pulls scalp upward and back	VII (Temporal branches)

Adapted from Liebgott B: *The anatomical basis of dentistry*, St Louis, 1986, Mosby, pp 242–243.

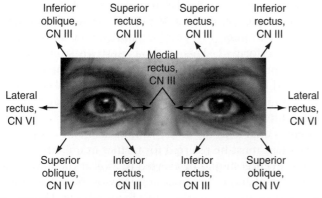

Fig. 2.35 The six cardinal fields of gaze, showing eye muscles and cranial nerves involved in the movement.

> ### Eye Examination
>
> - Six cardinal gaze positions
> - Pupils (size, equality, reactivity)
> - Nystagmus
> - Visual field (peripheral vision)
> - Visual acuity (eye chart)
> - Symmetry of gaze
> - Foreign objects/corneal abrasion
> - Surrounding bone and soft tissue
> - Hyphema
> - Saccades (horizontal and vertical)
> - Accommodation
> - Near point of convergence
> - Smooth pursuits
> - Vestibulo-ocular reflex (VOR)
> - Tracking

the fracture site, the affected eye demonstrates limited movement (Fig. 2.37), especially upward. The patient with this type of fracture may also demonstrate depression of the eye globe, blurred vision, double vision, and conjunctival hemorrhage.

Occasionally, when looking to the extreme side, the eyes will develop a rhythmic motion called *end-point nystagmus*.

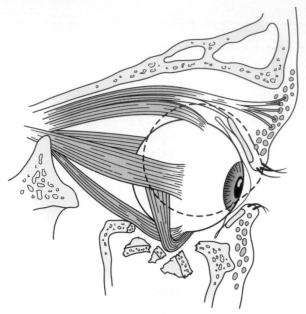

Fig. 2.36 Blowout fracture of the orbital floor. The *dashed line* indicates normal position of the globe. The inferior oblique and inferior rectus muscles are "caught" in the fracture site, preventing the eye from returning to its normal position. (Modified from Paton D, Goldberg MF: *Management of ocular injuries*, Philadelphia, 1976, WB Saunders, p 63.)

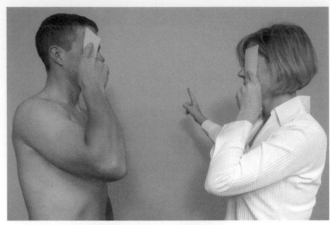

Fig. 2.38 Confrontation eye test.

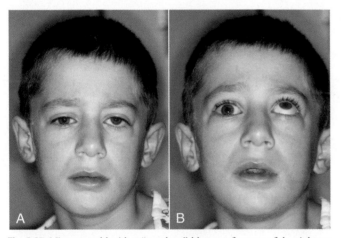

Fig. 2.37 Nine-year-old with a "trapdoor" blowout fracture of the right orbital floor and entrapment of the inferior rectus muscle. This injury represents a surgical emergency; the orbit must be explored and the muscle released expeditiously. (A) Frontal gaze. (B) Upward gaze. Note how the right eye does not elevate when the patient is asked to look up. (From Bell RB, Al-Bustani SS: Orbital fractures. In Bagheri S, Bell RB, Khan HA, editors: *Current therapy in oral and maxillofacial surgery*, Philadelphia, 2012, Saunders.)

Nystagmus is a rhythmic movement of the eyes with an abnormal slow drifting away from fixation and rapid return. With end-point nystagmus, there is a quick motion in the direction of the gaze followed by a slow return. This test differentiates end-point nystagmus from pathological nystagmus, in which there is a quick movement of the eyes in the same direction regardless of gaze. Pathological nystagmus exists in the region of full binocular vision, not just at the periphery. Cerebellar nystagmus is greater when the eyes are deviated toward the side of the lesion.

While testing the cardinal positions, the examiner should also watch for **lid lag**. Normally, the upper lid covers the top of the iris, rising when the patient looks up and quickly lowering as the eye lowers. With lid lag, the upper lid delays lowering as the eye lowers.

Peripheral vision, or **the visual field** (peripheral limits of vision), can be tested with the **confrontation test** (Fig. 2.38). The patient is asked to cover the right eye while the examiner covers his or her own left eye so that the open eyes of the examiner and of the patient are directly opposite each other. While the examiner and the patient look into each other's eye, the examiner fully extends his or her right arm to the side, midway between the patient and the examiner, and then moves it toward them with the fingers waving. The patient tells the examiner when he or she first sees the moving fingers. The examiner then compares the patient's response with the time or distance at which the examiner first noted the fingers. The test is then repeated to the other side.

The nasal, temporal, superior, and inferior fields should all be tested in a similar fashion. The visual field should describe angles of 60° nasally, 90° temporally, 50° superiorly, and 70° inferiorly. Double simultaneous testing may also be performed. This method uses two stimuli (e.g., moving fingers) that are simultaneously presented in the right and left visual fields, and the patient is asked which finger is moving. Normally, the patient should say "both," without hesitation. With any loss of vision field (i.e., if the patient is unable to see in the same visual fields as before), the patient must be referred for further examination.

The **eyelids** should be everted to look at the underside of the eyelid and to give a clearer view of the globe, especially if the patient complains of a foreign body. The upper eyelid may be everted with the use of a special lid retractor or a cotton swab (Fig. 2.39). The patient is asked to look down and to the right and then down and to the left while the superior aspect of the eye is examined. The examiner can check the inferior aspect of the eye and its conjunctival lining by carefully pulling the lower eyelid downward and gently holding it against the bony orbit. Next, the patient is asked to look up and to the right and then up

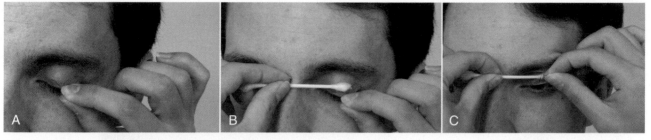

Fig. 2.39 Eversion of the eyelid. (A) Grasping eyelash. (B) Putting moistened cotton-tipped applicator over eyelid. (C) Everting eyelid over the cotton-tipped applicator.

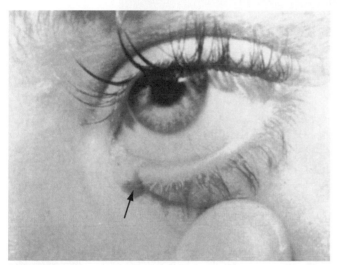

Fig. 2.40 A lower lid laceration *(arrow).* (From Pashby TJ, Pashby RC: Treatment of sports eye injuries. In Schneider RC, et al, editors: *Sports injuries: mechanisms, prevention and treatment,* Baltimore, 1985, Lippincott Williams & Wilkins, p 576.)

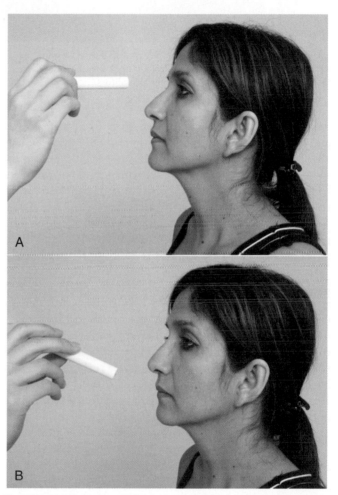

Fig. 2.41 Testing the pupils for reaction to light. (A) Light shining in eye. (B) Light shining away from eye.

and to the left while the inferior aspect of the eye is examined. These two techniques may also be used to look for a contact lens that has migrated away from the cornea.

Both eyelids should be checked for laceration. Lacerations in the area of the lacrimal gland are especially important to detect because, if they are not looked after properly, the tearing function of the lacrimal gland may be lost (Fig. 2.40).

The **reaction of the pupils** to light should then be tested. First, the light in the room is dimmed. The pupils dilate in a dark environment or with a long focal distance and constrict in a light environment or with a short focal distance. The examiner shines a penlight directly into one of the patient's eyes for approximately 5 seconds (Fig. 2.41). Normally, constriction of the pupil occurs, followed by slight dilation. The pupillary reaction is classified as brisk (normal), sluggish, nonreactive, or fixed. An oval or slightly oval pupil or one that is fixed and dilated indicates increased intracranial pressure. The fixation and dilation of both pupils is a terminal sign of anoxia and ischemia to the brain. If the dilation is significant, an injury to the optic nerve may be suspected. If both pupils are midsize, midposition, and nonreactive, midbrain damage is usually indicated. In a fully conscious, alert patient

who has sustained a blow near the eye, a dilated, fixed pupil usually implies injury to the ciliary nerves of the eye rather than brain injury. The other eye is tested similarly, and the results are compared.

Normally, both pupils constrict when a light is shined in one eye. The reaction of the eye being tested is called the **direct light reflex;** the reaction of the other pupil is called the **consensual light reflex.** This reaction is brisker in the young and people with blue eyes.[194] If the optic nerve is damaged, the affected pupil constricts in response to light in the opposite eye (consensual) and dilates in response to light shined into it (direct). If the oculomotor

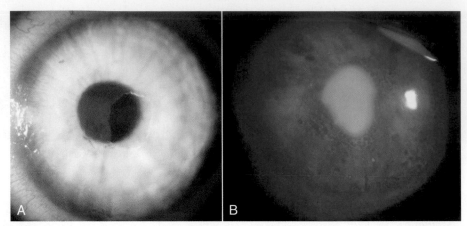

Fig. 2.42 Corneal epithelial abrasion. (A) Epithelial defect without fluorescein highlighting the defect. An irregularity in the otherwise smooth corneal surface is the key to identifying the defect if no fluorescein is available. (B) Classic fluorescein staining of an epithelial defect. (From Broocker G., et al: Ocular trauma. In Palay DA, Krachmer JH, editors: *Primary care ophthalmology*, ed 2, Philadelphia, 2005, Mosby.)

nerve is affected, the affected pupil is fixed and dilated and does not respond to light, either directly or consensually. If the pupils do not react, it is an indication of injury to the oculomotor nerve and its connections or of injury to the head. The eye also appears laterally displaced owing to paresis of the medial rectus muscle.

The pupil is then tested for accommodation. The patient is asked to look at a distant object and then at a test object—a pencil or the examiner's finger held 10 cm (4 inches) from the bridge of the nose. The pupils dilate when the patient looks at a far object and constrict when the patient focuses on the near object (i.e., accommodation). The eyes also adduct (i.e., go "cross-eyed") when the patient looks at the close object (i.e., convergence). These actions are called the **accommodation-convergence reflex.**[194] When looking at distant objects, the eyes should be parallel. Deviation or lack of parallelism is called **strabismus** and indicates weakness of one of the extraocular muscles or lack of neural coordination.[231]

When inspected under normal overhead light, the **lens** of the eye should be transparent. Shining a light on the lens may cause it to appear gray or yellow. The cornea should be smooth and clear. If the patient has extreme pain in the corneal area, a corneal abrasion should be suspected (Fig. 2.42). An appropriate specialist may test for corneal abrasion by using a fluorescein strip and a slit lamp. The cornea should be crystal clear when it is viewed, and the iris details should match those of the other eye.

To check for depth of the **anterior chamber of the eye** or a narrow corneal angle, the examiner shines a light obliquely across each eye. Normally, it illuminates the entire iris. If the corneal angle is narrow because of a shallow anterior chamber, the examiner will be able to see a crescent-shaped shadow on the side of the iris away from the light (Fig. 2.43). This finding indicates an anatomical predisposition to narrow-angled glaucoma.

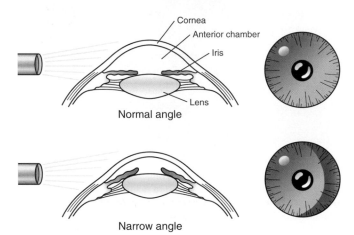

Fig. 2.43 Normal and narrow corneal angle (depth of anterior chamber). (Modified from Swartz HM: *Textbook of physical diagnosis*, Philadelphia, 1989, WB Saunders, p 144.)

To test for **symmetry of gaze,** the examiner aims a light source approximately 60 cm (24 inches) from the patient while standing directly in front of the patient and holding the light distant enough to prevent convergence of the patient's gaze. The patient is asked to stare at the light. The dots of reflected light on the two pupils should be in the same relative location (Fig. 2.44). When one eye does not look directly at the light, the reflected dot of light moves to the side opposite the deviation. For example, if the eye deviates medially, the reflection appears more laterally placed than in the other eye. The examiner can approximate the angle of deviation by noting the position of the reflection. Each millimeter of displacement in the reflection represents approximately 7° of ocular deviation. To bring out a mild deviation, the examiner may use a **cover-uncover test** (Fig. 2.45). The patient looks at a specific point, such as the bridge of the examiner's nose. One of the patient's eyes is then covered with a card. Normally, the uncovered eye will not move. If it moves, it was not straight before the other eye was covered. The other eye is then tested in a similar fashion.

Visual acuity is tested using a vision chart. **Visual acuity** is the ability of the eye to perceive fine detail, for example, when reading. If a standard eye wall chart is not available, a pocket visual acuity card may be used. This pocket card is usually viewed at a distance of 35 to 36 cm (14 inches). As with the wall chart, the patient is asked to examine the smallest line possible. If neither eye chart is available, any printed material may be used. A patient who wears glasses or contact lenses should be tested both without and with the corrective lenses. The test is done quickly so that the patient cannot memorize the chart. Visual acuity is recorded as a fraction in which the numerator indicates the distance of the patient from the chart (e.g., 20 feet) and the denominator indicates the distance at which the normal eye can read the line. Thus 20/100 means the patient can read at 20 feet what the average person can read at 100 feet—the smaller the fraction, the worse the myopia (i.e., nearsightedness). Patients with corrected vision of less than 20/40 should be referred to the appropriate specialist.[194] Intraocular examination with an ophthalmoscope, if available, may reveal lens, vitreous, or retinal damage.

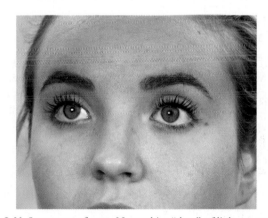

Fig. 2.44 Symmetry of gaze. Note white "dots" of light on pupils.

Examination of the Nose[190–194,198,232]

Patency of the nasal passages can be determined by occluding one of the patient's nostrils by pushing a finger against the side of the nostril. The box below outlines the items to be considered when assessing the nose. The patient is then asked to breathe in and out of the opposite nostril with the mouth closed. The process is repeated on the other side. Normally, no sound is heard, and the patient can breathe easily through the open nostril.

Nasal Examination

- Patency
- Nasal cavities
- Sinuses
- Fracture
- Nasal discharge (bloody, straw colored, clear)

If available, a nasal speculum and light may be used to inspect the nasal cavity. The nasal mucosa and turbinates can be inspected for color, foreign bodies, and abnormal masses (e.g., polyp). The **nasal septum** should be in midline and straight and is normally thicker anteriorly than posteriorly. If the nasal cavities are asymmetric, it may indicate a deviated septum. If the patient demonstrates a septal hematoma, it must be treated fairly quickly, because the hematoma may cause excessive pressure on the septum, making it avascular. This avascularity can result in a "saddle nose" deformity owing to necrosis and absorption of the underlying cartilage (Fig. 2.46).

Illumination of the **frontal and maxillary sinuses** may be performed if sinus tenderness is present or infection is suspected. The examination must be performed in a completely darkened room. To illuminate the maxillary sinuses, the examiner places the light source lateral to the patient's nose just beneath the medial aspect of the eye. The examiner then looks through the patient's open mouth for

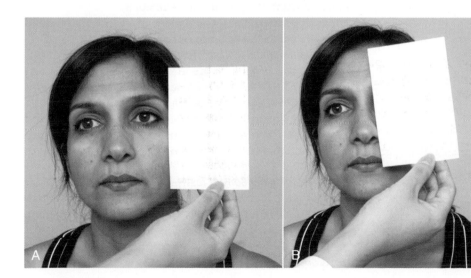

Fig. 2.45 Cover-uncover test for mild ocular deviation. As patient gazes at a specific point (A), examiner covers one eye and looks for movement in uncovered eye (B).

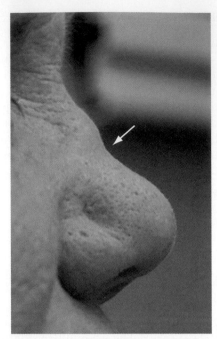

Fig. 2.46 "Saddle nose" deformity *(arrow)* following recurrent nasal cartilage inflammation and as a result, there is loss of septal cartilage. (From Mathew SD, Battafarano DF, Morris MJ: Relapsing polychondritis in the department of defense population and review of the literature, *Sem Arthr Rheum* 42[1]:70–83, 2012.)

illumination of the hard palate. To illuminate the frontal sinuses, the examiner places the light source against the medial aspect of each supraorbital rim. The examiner looks for a dim red glow as light is transmitted just below the eyebrow. The sinuses usually show differing degrees of illumination. The absence of a glow indicates either that the sinus is filled with secretions or that it has never developed.

Examination of the Teeth[190–194,198,232]

The examiner should observe the teeth to see if they are in normal position and whether any teeth are missing, chipped, or depressed (see Fig. 2.22). Using the gloved index finger and thumb, the examiner applies mild pressure to each tooth, pressing inward toward the tongue and outward toward the lips. Normally, a small amount of movement is observed. If a tooth is loose, excessive movement or increased pain or numbness relative to other teeth indicates a positive test. A tooth that has been avulsed may be cleansed with warm water and reinserted into the socket. The patient is then referred to the appropriate specialist for stabilization and root canal work.

Tooth Examination

- Number of teeth
- Position of teeth
- Movement of teeth
- Condition of teeth
- Condition of gums

Examination of the Ear[189–193]

Examination of the ear deals primarily with whether the patient is able to hear. Several tests may be used to examine hearing (see Special Tests section).

Ear Examination

- Tenderness (exterior and interior)
- Ear discharge (bloody, straw colored, clear)
- Hearing
- Balance

Conductive hearing loss implies that the patient experiences a reduction of all sounds rather than difficulty in interpreting sounds. **Sensorineural or perceptual hearing loss** indicates that the patient has difficulty interpreting the sounds.

To examine the internal structure of the ear, the examiner may use an otoscope if one is available. In this case, the examiner would observe the canal and the eardrum (tympanic membrane), noting any blockage, excessive wax, swelling, redness, transparency (usually pearly gray), bulging, retraction, or perforation of the eardrum.

Special Tests

Examiners perform only those special tests that they think will have value in helping to confirm a diagnosis. For example, the tests for expanding intracranial lesions would not be performed with a facial injury unless an associated injury to the brain or other neurological tissues is suspected.

For the reader who would like to review them, the reliability, validity, specificity, sensitivity, and odds ratios of some of the special tests used for the head and face are available in eAppendix 2.1.

Tests for Expanding Intracranial Lesions

For each of these tests, the patient must be able to stand normally when the eyes are open.

❓ *Neurological Control Test—Upper Limb.* The examiner asks the patient to stand with his or her arms forward flexed 90° and eyes closed. The patient holds this position for approximately 30 seconds. If the examiner notes that one arm tends to move or drift outward and downward, the test is considered positive for an expanding intracranial lesion on the side opposite the side with the drift.

❓ *Neurological Control Test—Lower Limb.* The examiner asks the patient to sit on the edge of a table or in a chair with his or her legs extended in front and not touching the ground. The patient closes his or her eyes for approximately 20 to 30 seconds. If the examiner notes that one leg tends to move or drift, the test is considered positive for an expanding intracranial lesion on the side opposite that with the drift.

⚠️ *Walk or Stand in Tandem Test.* Patients with expanding intracranial lesions demonstrate increasing difficulty in walking in tandem ("walking a line") or standing in tandem (i.e., one foot in front of other). Standing in tandem is more difficult to perform than walking in tandem.

Tests for Concussion

☑️ *Acute Concussion Evaluation.* There are different forms making up the Acute Concussion Evaluation (ACE)—one for the physician/clinician office (eTool 2.9), one for the emergency department, and one for a care plan. The ACE consists of questions related to concussion characteristics such as loss of consciousness, amnesia, concussion symptoms, and risk factors that may predict recovery. It may be used serially to track recovery or changes over time to help make clinical management decisions.[133,233]

☑️ *Brief Symptom Inventory (BSI–18).* The BSI-18[234] may be helpful in identifying the influence of depression, anxiety, and somatic isolation both preinjury and postinjury and protracted recovery from concussion.[142] It is a short reliable instrument used to determine psychological distress.[235]

☑️ *Concussion Symptom Inventory.* The Concussion Symptom Inventory (CSI) (eTool 2.10) is a 12-item scale that was developed to test for concussion symptoms within the first 24 hours of a concussion. It measures cognitive processing speed, working memory, attention, concentration, learning, memory, and executive functioning.[109,162] It is not designed to be used in isolation but as part of a number of tests that will help to confirm a concussion and its severity.[109] It may also be used to track recovery.[133]

☑️ *Glasgow Coma Scale.* The Glasgow Coma Scale (see Table 2.5) is a scoring scale of eye opening and motor and verbal responses that can be administered to individuals to objectively measure the level of consciousness and severity of the head injury. The responses are scored between 1 and 5 with a combined total score of 3 to 15, with 15 being normal. An initial score of less than 5 is associated with an 80% chance of being in a lasting vegetative state or death. An initial score of greater than 11 is associated with 90% chance of recovery. Concussions are usually rated between 13 and 15. Its primary use in evaluating individuals for concussion is to rule out more severe brain injury and to help determine which individuals need immediate emergent medical attention.[133]

The first test relates to eye opening. Eye opening may occur spontaneously, in response to speech or pain, or there may be no response at all. Each of these responses is given a numeric value: spontaneous eye opening—*4;* response to speech—*3;* response to pain—*2;* and no response—*1.* Spontaneous opening of the eyes indicates functioning of the ascending reticular activating system.

This finding does not necessarily mean that the patient is aware of the surroundings or of what is happening, but it does imply that the patient is in a state of arousal. A patient who opens his or her eyes in response to the examiner's voice is probably responding to the stimulus of sound, not necessarily to the command to open the eyes. If unsure, the examiner may use different sound-making objects (e.g., bell, horn) to elicit an appropriate response.

The second test involves motor response; the patient is given a grade of 6 if there is a response to a verbal command. Otherwise, the patient is graded on a 5-point scale depending on the motor response to a painful stimulus (see Table 2.5). When scoring motor responses, it is the ease with which the motor responses are elicited that constitutes the criterion for the best response. Commands given to the patient should be simple, such as, "Move your arm." The patient should not be asked to squeeze the examiner's hand, nor should the examiner place something in the patient's hand and then ask the patient to grasp it. This action may cause a **grasp reflex**, not a response to a command.[185]

If the patient does not give a motor response to a verbal command, then the examiner should attempt to elicit a motor response to a painful stimulus. It is the type and quality of the patient's reaction to the painful stimulus that constitute the scoring criteria. The stimulus should not be applied to the face, because painful stimulus in the facial area may cause the eyes to close tightly as a protective reaction. The painful stimulus may consist of applying a knuckle to the sternum, squeezing the trapezius muscle, or squeezing the soft tissue between the thumb and index finger (Fig. 2.47). If the patient moves a limb when the painful stimulus is applied to more than one point or tries to remove the examiner's hand that is applying the painful stimulus, the patient is localizing and a value of 5 is given. If the patient withdraws from the painful stimulus rapidly, a normal **withdrawal reflex** is being shown and a value of 4 is given.

However, if application of a painful stimulus creates a decorticate or decerebrate posture (Fig. 2.48), an abnormal response is being demonstrated and a value of 3 is given for the decorticate posture (i.e., injury above red nucleus) or a value of 2 is given for decerebrate posture (i.e., brain stem or midbrain injury). **Decorticate posturing** results from lesions of the diencephalon area, whereas decerebrate posturing results from lesions of the midbrain. With decorticate posturing, the arms, wrists, and fingers are flexed, the upper limbs are adducted, and the legs are extended, medially rotated, and plantar flexed. **Decerebrate posturing,** which has a poorer prognosis, involves extension, adduction, and hyperpronation of the arms, whereas the lower limbs are the same as for decorticate posturing.[236] Decerebrate rigidity is usually bilateral. If the patient exhibits no reaction to the painful stimulus, a value of 1 is given. **Note**: It is important to be sure the "no" response is caused by a head injury and not a spinal cord injury leading to lack of feeling or sensation. Any

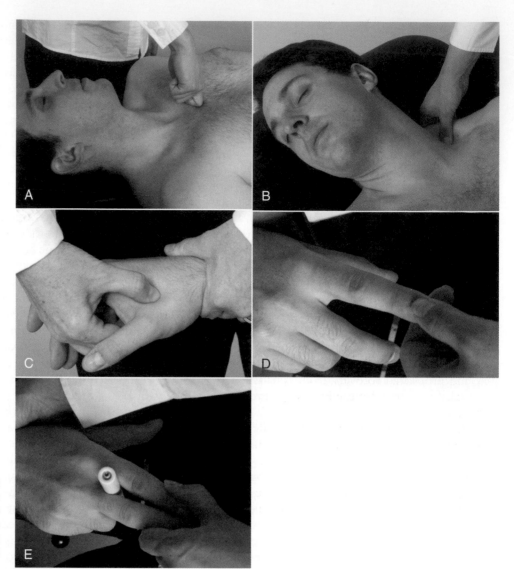

Fig. 2.47 Examples of painful stimuli applied by the examiner. (A) Knuckle to sternum. (B) Squeezing trapezius muscle. (C) Squeezing tissue between the thumb and index finger. (D) Squeezing a fingertip. (E) Squeezing an object between two fingers.

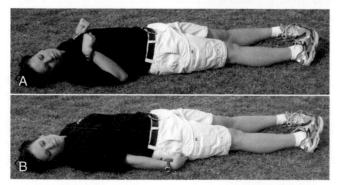

Fig. 2.48 (A) Decorticate rigidity. (B) Decerebrate rigidity.

difference in reaction between limbs should be carefully noted; this finding may indicate a specific focal injury.[185]

In the third test, verbal response is graded on a 5-point scale to measure the patient's speech in response to simple questions, such as "Where are you?" or "Are you winning the game?" For verbal responses, the patient who converses appropriately and shows proper orientation, being aware of oneself and the environment, is given a grade of 5. The patient who is confused is disoriented and unable to completely interact with the environment; this patient is able to converse using the appropriate words and is given a grade of 4. The patient exhibiting inappropriate speech is unable to sustain a conversation with the examiner; this person would be given a grade of 3. A vocalizing patient only groans or makes incomprehensible sounds; this finding leads to a grade of 2. Again, the examiner should note any possible mechanical reason for the inability to verbalize. If the patient makes no sounds and thus has no verbal response, a grade of 1 is assigned.

It is vital that the initial score on the Glasgow Coma Scale be obtained as soon as possible after the onset of the injury. The scale can then be repeated at 15- or 30-minute intervals, especially in the early stages, if changes are noted. If the score is between 3 and 8, emergency care is required. With the Glasgow Coma Scale, the initial score is used as a basis for determining the severity of the patient's head injury. Patients who maintain a score of 8 or lower on the Glasgow Coma Scale for 6 hours or longer are considered to have a serious head injury. A patient who scores between 9 and 11 is considered to have a moderate head injury, and one who scores 12 or higher is considered to have a mild head injury.[185]

☑ *Head Injury Scale.* This 16-item scale (eTool 2.11) is completed by the injured individual to determine the severity of the head injury.[237] The presence of a headache, nausea, and balancing difficulties are related to the neuropsychological symptoms, whereas fatigue, having trouble falling asleep, and drowsiness are related to the neurophysiologic group. Feeling slowed down, feeling "in a fog," and having difficulty concentrating are related to the cognitive symptoms.[237]

☑ *Maddocks Questions/Score.* The Maddocks Questions/ Score (see SCAT5; Fig. 2.49) are questions asked of a patient and are designed to specifically measure orientation following a suspected concussion in an athletic event.[33,42,57,186]

☑ *Scandinavian Guidelines for Head Injury.* The Scandinavian Guidelines for Head Injury (eTool 2.12) is a management algorithm that may be used in the treatment of minimal, mild, and moderate head injuries in adults.[238,239]

☑ *Sport Concussion Assessment Tool 5.* The SCAT (Fig. 2.49) is one of the more common concussion assessment tools used currently. It has been developed through four iterations (there is no SCAT4 or Child SCAT4).[240,241] The SCAT5 is used for youths and adults (13 years of age plus), and the Child SCAT5 is used for children (5 to 12 years of age; Fig. 2.50).[133,241] It may be used to establish preseason baseline values and following a concussion. Individuals with comorbid conditions (e.g., headaches, learning disability/dyslexia, attention-deficit/hyperactivity disorder [ADHD], depression, anxiety, or other psychological history) all report higher symptoms in severity score at baseline.[242,243] The tool includes the Glasgow Coma Scale, the SAC, modified Maddocks questions, a brief assessment of orientation, memory and concentration, an evaluation of the cervical spine, and an assessment of balance (BESS testing), as well as information on the mechanism of injury and background information on comorbidities (e.g., history of concussions, headaches, migraines, depression, and/or anxiety).[66,133,162,243,244] The tool was originally developed to help with return to play decisions but currently is used to identify concussions and to provide initial management ideas for a suspected concussion.[240] The tool should not be used in isolation, nor should it be used solely to make a diagnosis of concussion. During the acute phase, the tool is repeated to see if symptoms are increasing or decreasing and is often combined with neuropsychological testing a few days after the concussion.[33,110] After the SCAT5 and any other testing has been completed, the clinician must still make a clinical judgment as to whether the individual has suffered a concussion and when he or she should be allowed to return to school, work, practice, and/or play.[33]

☑ *Standardized Assessment of Concussion.* The SAC (eTool 2.13) is a neurocognitive test that may be used alone or as part of the SCAT5.[129,245] It should take no more than 10 minutes to complete, and it should be administered in the resting state.[54,110,133,154,228,240] The test is used to evaluate cognitive function and includes standard questions of orientation (i.e., place, time, months, year), working memory (i.e., immediate recall of selected words), concentration (i.e., recalling a list of numbers backward), and remote memory (i.e., delayed recall—e.g., remembering some words that were previously memorized). The SAC is sensitive to the immediate effects of concussion and is most effective in the first 48 hours following a concussion.[15,54,57,110] The SAC score drops an average of 2.9 points immediately after concussion and returns to baseline within 5 to 7 days.[41,54] Like the SCAT5, it is not used in isolation but is supported by neurocognitive testing, postural stability testing, and other tests following a concussion.[110,246,247] Likewise, it is used as one of the tests for preseason baseline testing.[248,249] It is used for orientation, immediate and delayed memory, and concentration.[133,248] Differences in baseline values have been found in females and young athletes between the ages of 9 and 14 years of age.[133]

Tests for Balance

If one is contemplating doing a balance test, there are several considerations that must be taken into account. First, the individual must be rested for at least 20 minutes after vigorous activity so that fatigue does not interfere with the test. Secondly, the test could be different from any baseline testing if the shoes the individual is wearing are different, tape is being used on the ankle or foot, a brace is being worn, or there is another lower limb injury.[9,32,214,250] The sensitivity of balance testing is highest immediately after injury, and the sensitivity decreases from days 1 to 10.[41,57,75,82,110,154,251]

Balance problems are present approximately 30% of the time following a concussive injury. Only headache, dizziness, confusion, disorientation, and blurred vision occur more frequently with a concussion.[213] Commonly, the results of balance testing return to normal within 3 to 5 days following a concussion.[75] Balance disturbances may be an indicator of concussion but, as with the other tests, cannot be used in isolation as other conditions can lead to balance disturbances.

☑ *4-Stage Balance Test.* The 4-Stage Balance Test (eTool 2.14) is used to test balance but is more likely to be used in older people. With this group, it may be combined with the **30-Second Chair Stand Test** (eTool 2.15) and the **Timed Up and Go (TUG) Test** (eTool 2.16) to determine the risk of an individual falling. For the balance test, the patient is asked to stand in four positions as outlined in eTool 2.14 for 10 seconds in each position, holding the arms out or moving the body if desired to maintain balance but the feet must not move. The patient is asked to hold each position until he or she is told to stop (i.e., at 10 seconds).

☑ *Balance Error Scoring System.* The BESS is a clinical balance assessment tool developed to evaluate static postural stability following a concussion.[9,82,154,213,214,252] The

Text continued on page 134.

SCAT5©   SPORT CONCUSSION ASSESSMENT TOOL — 5TH EDITION

DEVELOPED BY THE CONCUSSION IN SPORT GROUP
FOR USE BY MEDICAL PROFESSIONALS ONLY

supported by

Patient details

Name: _____

DOB: _____

Address: _____

ID number: _____

Examiner: _____

Date of Injury: _____   Time: _____

WHAT IS THE SCAT5?

The SCAT5 is a standardized tool for evaluating concussions designed for use by physicians and licensed healthcare professionals[1]. The SCAT5 cannot be performed correctly in less than 10 minutes.

If you are not a physician or licensed healthcare professional, please use the Concussion Recognition Tool 5 (CRT5). The SCAT5 is to be used for evaluating athletes aged 13 years and older. For children aged 12 years or younger, please use the Child SCAT5.

Preseason SCAT5 baseline testing can be useful for interpreting post-injury test scores, but is not required for that purpose. Detailed instructions for use of the SCAT5 are provided on page 7. Please read through these instructions carefully before testing the athlete. Brief verbal instructions for each test are given in italics. The only equipment required for the tester is a watch or timer.

This tool may be freely copied in its current form for distribution to individuals, teams, groups and organizations. It should not be altered in any way, re-branded or sold for commercial gain. Any revision, translation or reproduction in a digital form requires specific approval by the Concussion in Sport Group.

Recognise and Remove

A head impact by either a direct blow or indirect transmission of force can be associated with a serious and potentially fatal brain injury. If there are significant concerns, including any of the red flags listed in Box 1, then activation of emergency procedures and urgent transport to the nearest hospital should be arranged.

Key points

- Any athlete with suspected concussion should be REMOVED FROM PLAY, medically assessed and monitored for deterioration. No athlete diagnosed with concussion should be returned to play on the day of injury.

- If an athlete is suspected of having a concussion and medical personnel are not immediately available, the athlete should be referred to a medical facility for urgent assessment.

- Athletes with suspected concussion should not drink alcohol, use recreational drugs and should not drive a motor vehicle until cleared to do so by a medical professional.

- Concussion signs and symptoms evolve over time and it is important to consider repeat evaluation in the assessment of concussion.

- The diagnosis of a concussion is a clinical judgment, made by a medical professional. The SCAT5 should NOT be used by itself to make, or exclude, the diagnosis of concussion. An athlete may have a concussion even if their SCAT5 is "normal".

Remember:

- The basic principles of first aid (danger, response, airway, breathing, circulation) should be followed.

- Do not attempt to move the athlete (other than that required for airway management) unless trained to do so.

- Assessment for a spinal cord injury is a critical part of the initial on-field assessment.

- Do not remove a helmet or any other equipment unless trained to do so safely.

Echemendia RJ, *et al. Br J Sports Med* 2017;**51**:851–858. doi:10.1136/bjsports-2017-097506SCAT5

Fig. 2.49 Sports Concussion Assessment Tool—5th Edition (SCAT5). (Copyright Concussion in Sport Group 2017. From Echemendia RJ, Meeuwisse W, McCrory P, et al: The Sport Concussion Assessment Tool 5th Edition (SCAT5): Background and rationale, *Br J Sports Med* 51[11]:851–858, 2017.)

Br J Sports Med: first published as 10.1136/bjsports-2017-097506SCAT5 on 26 April 2017. Downloaded from http://bjsm.bmj.com/ on 29 October 2018 by guest. Protected by copyright.

1

IMMEDIATE OR ON-FIELD ASSESSMENT

The following elements should be assessed for all athletes who are suspected of having a concussion prior to proceeding to the neurocognitive assessment and ideally should be done on-field after the first first aid / emergency care priorities are completed.

If any of the "Red Flags" or observable signs are noted after a direct or indirect blow to the head, the athlete should be immediately and safely removed from participation and evaluated by a physician or licensed healthcare professional.

Consideration of transportation to a medical facility should be at the discretion of the physician or licensed healthcare professional.

The GCS is important as a standard measure for all patients and can be done serially if necessary in the event of deterioration in conscious state. The Maddocks questions and cervical spine exam are critical steps of the immediate assessment; however, these do not need to be done serially.

STEP 1: RED FLAGS

RED FLAGS:

- Neck pain or tenderness
- Double vision
- Weakness or tingling/ burning in arms or legs
- Severe or increasing headache
- Seizure or convulsion
- Loss of consciousness
- Deteriorating conscious state
- Vomiting
- Increasingly restless, agitated or combative

STEP 2: OBSERVABLE SIGNS

Witnessed ☐   Observed on Video ☐

Lying motionless on the playing surface	Y	N
Balance / gait difficulties / motor incoordination: stumbling, slow / laboured movements	Y	N
Disorientation or confusion, or an inability to respond appropriately to questions	Y	N
Blank or vacant look	Y	N
Facial injury after head trauma	Y	N

STEP 3: MEMORY ASSESSMENT MADDOCKS QUESTIONS[2]

"I am going to ask you a few questions, please listen carefully and give your best effort. First, tell me what happened?"

_____

_____

Mark Y for correct answer / N for incorrect

What venue are we at today?	Y	N
Which half is it now?	Y	N
Who scored last in this match?	Y	N
What team did you play last week / game?	Y	N
Did your team win the last game?	Y	N

Note: Appropriate sport-specific questions may be substituted.

Name:	_____
DOB:	_____
Address:	_____
ID number:	_____
Examiner:	_____
Date:	_____

STEP 4: EXAMINATION
GLASGOW COMA SCALE (GCS)[3]

Time of assessment			
Date of assessment			
Best eye response (E)			
No eye opening	1	1	1
Eye opening in response to pain	2	2	2
Eye opening to speech	3	3	3
Eyes opening spontaneously	4	4	4
Best verbal response (V)			
No verbal response	1	1	1
Incomprehensible sounds	2	2	2
Inappropriate words	3	3	3
Confused	4	4	4
Oriented	5	5	5
Best motor response (M)			
No motor response	1	1	1
Extension to pain	2	2	2
Abnormal flexion to pain	3	3	3
Flexion / Withdrawal to pain	4	4	4
Localizes to pain	5	5	5
Obeys commands	6	6	6
Glasgow Coma score (E + V + M)			

CERVICAL SPINE ASSESSMENT

Does the athlete report that their neck is pain free at rest?	Y	N
If there is NO neck pain at rest, does the athlete have a full range of ACTIVE pain free movement?	Y	N
Is the limb strength and sensation normal?	Y	N

In a patient who is not lucid or fully conscious, a cervical spine injury should be assumed until proven otherwise.

Echemendia RJ, *et al. Br J Sports Med* 2017;**51**:851–858. doi:10.1136/bjsports-2017-097506SCAT5

Fig. 2.49, cont'd

OFFICE OR OFF-FIELD ASSESSMENT

Please note that the neurocognitive assessment should be done in a distraction-free environment with the athlete in a resting state.

STEP 1: ATHLETE BACKGROUND

Sport / team / school: _____

Date / time of injury: _____

Years of education completed: _____

Age: _____

Gender: M / F / Other

Dominant hand: left / neither / right

How many diagnosed concussions has the
athlete had in the past?: _____

When was the most recent concussion?: _____

How long was the recovery (time to being cleared to play)
from the most recent concussion?: _____ (days)

Has the athlete ever been:

Hospitalized for a head injury?	Yes	No
Diagnosed / treated for headache disorder or migraines?	Yes	No
Diagnosed with a learning disability / dyslexia?	Yes	No
Diagnosed with ADD / ADHD?	Yes	No
Diagnosed with depression, anxiety or other psychiatric disorder?	Yes	No

Current medications? If yes, please list:

_____

_____

_____

_____

_____

Name: _____

DOB: _____

Address: _____

ID number: _____

Examiner: _____

Date: _____

2

STEP 2: SYMPTOM EVALUATION

The athlete should be given the symptom form and asked to read this instruction paragraph out loud then complete the symptom scale. For the baseline assessment, the athlete should rate his/her symptoms based on how he/she typically feels and for the post injury assessment the athlete should rate their symptoms at this point in time.

Please Check: ☐ Baseline ☐ Post-Injury

Please hand the form to the athlete

	none	mild		moderate		severe	
Headache	0	1	2	3	4	5	6
"Pressure in head"	0	1	2	3	4	5	6
Neck Pain	0	1	2	3	4	5	6
Nausea or vomiting	0	1	2	3	4	5	6
Dizziness	0	1	2	3	4	5	6
Blurred vision	0	1	2	3	4	5	6
Balance problems	0	1	2	3	4	5	6
Sensitivity to light	0	1	2	3	4	5	6
Sensitivity to noise	0	1	2	3	4	5	6
Feeling slowed down	0	1	2	3	4	5	6
Feeling like "in a fog"	0	1	2	3	4	5	6
"Don't feel right"	0	1	2	3	4	5	6
Difficulty concentrating	0	1	2	3	4	5	6
Difficulty remembering	0	1	2	3	4	5	6
Fatigue or low energy	0	1	2	3	4	5	6
Confusion	0	1	2	3	4	5	6
Drowsiness	0	1	2	3	4	5	6
More emotional	0	1	2	3	4	5	6
Irritability	0	1	2	3	4	5	6
Sadness	0	1	2	3	4	5	6
Nervous or Anxious	0	1	2	3	4	5	6
Trouble falling asleep (if applicable)	0	1	2	3	4	5	6

Total number of symptoms:	of 22
Symptom severity score:	of 132
Do your symptoms get worse with physical activity?	Y N
Do your symptoms get worse with mental activity?	Y N
If 100% is feeling perfectly normal, what percent of normal do you feel?	

If not 100%, why?

_____

_____

_____

Please hand form back to examiner

© Concussion in Sport Group 2017

Echemendia RJ, *et al. Br J Sports Med* 2017;**51**:851–858. doi:10.1136/bjsports-2017-097506SCAT5

Fig. 2.49, cont'd

3

STEP 3: COGNITIVE SCREENING
Standardised Assessment of Concussion (SAC)[4]

ORIENTATION

What month is it?	0	1
What is the date today?	0	1
What is the day of the week?	0	1
What year is it?	0	1
What time is it right now? (within 1 hour)	0	1
Orientation score		of 5

Name:	
DOB:	
Address:	
ID number:	
Examiner:	
Date:	

IMMEDIATE MEMORY

The Immediate Memory component can be completed using the traditional 5-word per trial list or optionally using 10-words per trial to minimise any ceiling effect. All 3 trials must be administered irrespective of the number correct on the first trial. Administer at the rate of one word per second.

Please choose EITHER the 5 or 10 word list groups and circle the specific word list chosen for this test.

I am going to test your memory. I will read you a list of words and when I am done, repeat back as many words as you can remember, in any order. For Trials 2 & 3: I am going to repeat the same list again. Repeat back as many words as you can remember in any order, even if you said the word before.

List		Alternate 5 word lists				Score (of 5) Trial 1 Trial 2 Trial 3
A	Finger	Penny	Blanket	Lemon	Insect	
B	Candle	Paper	Sugar	Sandwich	Wagon	
C	Baby	Monkey	Perfume	Sunset	Iron	
D	Elbow	Apple	Carpet	Saddle	Bubble	
E	Jacket	Arrow	Pepper	Cotton	Movie	
F	Dollar	Honey	Mirror	Saddle	Anchor	
				Immediate Memory Score		of 15
				Time that last trial was completed		

List		Alternate 10 word lists				Score (of 10) Trial 1 Trial 2 Trial 3
G	Finger	Penny	Blanket	Lemon	Insect	
	Candle	Paper	Sugar	Sandwich	Wagon	
H	Baby	Monkey	Perfume	Sunset	Iron	
	Elbow	Apple	Carpet	Saddle	Bubble	
I	Jacket	Arrow	Pepper	Cotton	Movie	
	Dollar	Honey	Mirror	Saddle	Anchor	
				Immediate Memory Score		of 30
				Time that last trial was completed		

CONCENTRATION

DIGITS BACKWARDS

Please circle the Digit list chosen (A, B, C, D, E, F). Administer at the rate of one digit per second reading DOWN the selected column.

I am going to read a string of numbers and when I am done, you repeat them back to me in reverse order of how I read them to you. For example, if I say 7-1-9, you would say 9-1-7.

Concentration Number Lists (circle one)

List A	List B	List C			
4-9-3	5-2-6	1-4-2	Y	N	0
6-2-9	4-1-5	6-5-8	Y	N	1
3-8-1-4	1-7-9-5	6-8-3-1	Y	N	0
3-2-7-9	4-9-6-8	3-4-8-1	Y	N	1
6-2-9-7-1	4-8-5-2-7	4-9-1-5-3	Y	N	0
1-5-2-8-6	6-1-8-4-3	6-8-2-5-1	Y	N	1
7-1-8-4-6-2	8-3-1-9-6-4	3-7-6-5-1-9	Y	N	0
5-3-9-1-4-8	7-2-4-8-5-6	9-2-6-5-1-4	Y	N	1

List D	List E	List F			
7-8-2	3-8-2	2-7-1	Y	N	0
9-2-6	5-1-8	4-7-9	Y	N	1
4-1-8-3	2-7-9-3	1-6-8-3	Y	N	0
9-7-2-3	2-1-6-9	3-9-2-4	Y	N	1
1-7-9-2-6	4-1-8-6-9	2-4-7-5-8	Y	N	0
4-1-7-5-2	9-4-1-7-5	8-3-9-6-4	Y	N	1
2-6-4-8-1-7	6-9-7-3-8-2	5-8-6-2-4-9	Y	N	0
8-4-1-9-3-5	4-2-7-9-3-8	3-1-7-8-2-6	Y	N	1
		Digits Score:			of 4

MONTHS IN REVERSE ORDER

Now tell me the months of the year in reverse order. Start with the last month and go backward. So you'll say December, November. Go ahead.

Dec - Nov - Oct - Sept - Aug - Jul - Jun - May - Apr - Mar - Feb - Jan	0 1
Months Score	of 1
Concentration Total Score (Digits + Months)	of 5

Echemendia RJ, *et al. Br J Sports Med* 2017;**51**:851–858. doi:10.1136/bjsports-2017-097506SCAT5

Fig. 2.49, cont'd

4

STEP 4: NEUROLOGICAL SCREEN

See the instruction sheet (page 7) for details of test administration and scoring of the tests.

	Y	N
Can the patient read aloud (e.g. symptom check-list) and follow instructions without difficulty?	Y	N
Does the patient have a full range of pain-free PASSIVE cervical spine movement?	Y	N
Without moving their head or neck, can the patient look side-to-side and up-and-down without double vision?	Y	N
Can the patient perform the finger nose coordination test normally?	Y	N
Can the patient perform tandem gait normally?	Y	N

BALANCE EXAMINATION

Modified Balance Error Scoring System (mBESS) testing[5]

Which foot was tested (i.e. which is the non-dominant foot) ☐ Left ☐ Right

Testing surface (hard floor, field, etc.) _____

Footwear (shoes, barefoot, braces, tape, etc.) _____

Condition	Errors
Double leg stance	of 10
Single leg stance (non-dominant foot)	of 10
Tandem stance (non-dominant foot at the back)	of 10
Total Errors	of 30

Name: _____
DOB: _____
Address: _____
ID number: _____
Examiner: _____
Date: _____

5

STEP 5: DELAYED RECALL:

The delayed recall should be performed after 5 minutes have elapsed since the end of the Immediate Recall section. Score 1 pt. for each correct response.

Do you remember that list of words I read a few times earlier? Tell me as many words from the list as you can remember in any order.

Time Started ▢

Please record each word correctly recalled. Total score equals number of words recalled.

_____
_____
_____

Total number of words recalled accurately: of 5 or of 10

6

STEP 6: DECISION

Domain	Date & time of assessment:		
Symptom number (of 22)			
Symptom severity score (of 132)			
Orientation (of 5)			
Immediate memory	of 15 / of 30	of 15 / of 30	of 15 / of 30
Concentration (of 5)			
Neuro exam	Normal Abnormal	Normal Abnormal	Normal Abnormal
Balance errors (of 30)			
Delayed Recall	of 5 / of 10	of 5 / of 10	of 5 / of 10

Date and time of injury: _____

If the athlete is known to you prior to their injury, are they different from their usual self?
☐ Yes ☐ No ☐ Unsure ☐ Not Applicable
(If different, describe why in the clinical notes section)

Concussion Diagnosed?
☐ Yes ☐ No ☐ Unsure ☐ Not Applicable

If re-testing, has the athlete improved?
☐ Yes ☐ No ☐ Unsure ☐ Not Applicable

I am a physician or licensed healthcare professional and I have personally administered or supervised the administration of this SCAT5.

Signature: _____
Name: _____
Title: _____
Registration number (if applicable): _____
Date: _____

SCORING ON THE SCAT5 SHOULD NOT BE USED AS A STAND-ALONE METHOD TO DIAGNOSE CONCUSSION, MEASURE RECOVERY OR MAKE DECISIONS ABOUT AN ATHLETE'S READINESS TO RETURN TO COMPETITION AFTER CONCUSSION.

Echemendia RJ, et al. Br J Sports Med 2017;**51**:851–858. doi:10.1136/bjsports-2017-097506SCAT5

Fig. 2.49, cont'd

CLINICAL NOTES:

_____

_____

_____

_____

Name: _____

DOB: _____

Address: _____

ID number: _____

Examiner: _____

Date: _____

_____

_____

_____

_____

_____

_____

_____

_____

_____

✂ ·

CONCUSSION INJURY ADVICE

(To be given to the person monitoring the concussed athlete)

This patient has received an injury to the head. A careful medical examination has been carried out and no sign of any serious complications has been found. Recovery time is variable across individuals and the patient will need monitoring for a further period by a responsible adult. Your treating physician will provide guidance as to this timeframe.

If you notice any change in behaviour, vomiting, worsening headache, double vision or excessive drowsiness, please telephone your doctor or the nearest hospital emergency department immediately.

Other important points:

Initial rest: Limit physical activity to routine daily activities (avoid exercise, training, sports) and limit activities such as school, work, and screen time to a level that does not worsen symptoms.

1) Avoid alcohol

2) Avoid prescription or non-prescription drugs without medical supervision. Specifically:

  a) Avoid sleeping tablets

  b) Do not use aspirin, anti-inflammatory medication or stronger pain medications such as narcotics

3) Do not drive until cleared by a healthcare professional.

4) Return to play/sport requires clearance by a healthcare professional.

Clinic phone number: _____

Patient's name: _____

Date / time of injury: _____

Date / time of medical review: _____

Healthcare Provider: _____

© Concussion in Sport Group 2017

Contact details or stamp

Echemendia RJ, *et al. Br J Sports Med* 2017;**51**:851–858. doi:10.1136/bjsports-2017-097506SCAT5

Fig. 2.49, cont'd

INSTRUCTIONS

Words in *Italics* throughout the SCAT5 are the instructions given to the athlete by the clinician

Symptom Scale

The time frame for symptoms should be based on the type of test being administered. At baseline it is advantageous to assess how an athlete "typically" feels whereas during the acute/post-acute stage it is best to ask how the athlete feels at the time of testing.

The symptom scale should be completed by the athlete, not by the examiner. In situations where the symptom scale is being completed after exercise, it should be done in a resting state, generally by approximating his/her resting heart rate.

For total number of symptoms, maximum possible is 22 except immediately post injury, if sleep item is omitted, which then creates a maximum of 21.

For Symptom severity score, add all scores in table, maximum possible is 22 x 6 = 132, except immediately post injury if sleep item is omitted, which then creates a maximum of 21x6=126.

Immediate Memory

The Immediate Memory component can be completed using the traditional 5-word per trial list or, optionally, using 10-words per trial. The literature suggests that the Immediate Memory has a notable ceiling effect when a 5-word list is used. In settings where this ceiling is prominent, the examiner may wish to make the task more difficult by incorporating two 5–word groups for a total of 10 words per trial. In this case, the maximum score per trial is 10 with a total trial maximum of 30.

Choose one of the word lists (either 5 or 10). Then perform 3 trials of immediate memory using this list.

Complete all 3 trials regardless of score on previous trials.

"I am going to test your memory. I will read you a list of words and when I am done, repeat back as many words as you can remember, in any order." The words must be read at a rate of one word per second.

Trials 2 & 3 MUST be completed regardless of score on trial 1 & 2.

Trials 2 & 3:

"I am going to repeat the same list again. Repeat back as many words as you can remember in any order, even if you said the word before."

Score 1 pt. for each correct response. Total score equals sum across all 3 trials. Do NOT inform the athlete that delayed recall will be tested.

Concentration

Digits backward

Choose one column of digits from lists A, B, C, D, E or F and administer those digits as follows:

Say: *"I am going to read a string of numbers and when I am done, you repeat them back to me in reverse order of how I read them to you. For example, if I say 7-1-9, you would say 9-1-7."*

Begin with first 3 digit string.

If correct, circle "Y" for correct and go to next string length. If incorrect, circle "N" for the first string length and read trial 2 in the same string length. One point possible for each string length. Stop after incorrect on both trials (2 N's) in a string length. The digits should be read at the rate of one per second.

Months in reverse order

"Now tell me the months of the year in reverse order. Start with the last month and go backward. So you'll say December, November ... Go ahead"

1 pt. for entire sequence correct

Delayed Recall

The delayed recall should be performed after 5 minutes have elapsed since the end of the Immediate Recall section.

"Do you remember that list of words I read a few times earlier? Tell me as many words from the list as you can remember in any order."

Score 1 pt. for each correct response

Modified Balance Error Scoring System (mBESS)[5] testing

This balance testing is based on a modified version of the Balance Error Scoring System (BESS)[5]. A timing device is required for this testing.

Each of 20-second trial/stance is scored by counting the number of errors. The examiner will begin counting errors only after the athlete has assumed the proper start position. The modified BESS is calculated by adding one error point for each error during the three 20-second tests. The maximum number of errors for any single condition is 10. If the athlete commits multiple errors simultaneously, only

one error is recorded but the athlete should quickly return to the testing position, and counting should resume once the athlete is set. Athletes that are unable to maintain the testing procedure for a minimum of five seconds at the start are assigned the highest possible score, ten, for that testing condition.

OPTION: For further assessment, the same 3 stances can be performed on a surface of medium density foam (e.g., approximately 50cm x 40cm x 6cm).

Balance testing – types of errors

1. Hands lifted off iliac crest
2. Opening eyes
3. Step, stumble, or fall
4. Moving hip into > 30 degrees abduction
5. Lifting forefoot or heel
6. Remaining out of test position > 5 sec

"I am now going to test your balance. Please take your shoes off (if applicable), roll up your pant legs above ankle (if applicable), and remove any ankle taping (if applicable). This test will consist of three twenty second tests with different stances."

(a) Double leg stance:

"The first stance is standing with your feet together with your hands on your hips and with your eyes closed. You should try to maintain stability in that position for 20 seconds. I will be counting the number of times you move out of this position. I will start timing when you are set and have closed your eyes."

(b) Single leg stance:

"If you were to kick a ball, which foot would you use? [This will be the dominant foot] *Now stand on your non-dominant foot. The dominant leg should be held in approximately 30 degrees of hip flexion and 45 degrees of knee flexion. Again, you should try to maintain stability for 20 seconds with your hands on your hips and your eyes closed. I will be counting the number of times you move out of this position. If you stumble out of this position, open your eyes and return to the start position and continue balancing. I will start timing when you are set and have closed your eyes."*

(c) Tandem stance:

"Now stand heel-to-toe with your non-dominant foot in back. Your weight should be evenly distributed across both feet. Again, you should try to maintain stability for 20 seconds with your hands on your hips and your eyes closed. I will be counting the number of times you move out of this position. If you stumble out of this position, open your eyes and return to the start position and continue balancing. I will start timing when you are set and have closed your eyes."

Tandem Gait

Participants are instructed to stand with their feet together behind a starting line (the test is best done with footwear removed). Then, they walk in a forward direction as quickly and as accurately as possible along a 38mm wide (sports tape), 3 metre line with an alternate foot heel-to-toe gait ensuring that they approximate their heel and toe on each step. Once they cross the end of the 3m line, they turn 180 degrees and return to the starting point using the same gait. Athletes fail the test if they step off the line, have a separation between their heel and toe, or if they touch or grab the examiner or an object.

Finger to Nose

"I am going to test your coordination now. Please sit comfortably on the chair with your eyes open and your arm (either right or left) outstretched (shoulder flexed to 90 degrees and elbow and fingers extended), pointing in front of you. When I give a start signal, I would like you to perform five successive finger to nose repetitions using your index finger to touch the tip of the nose, and then return to the starting position, as quickly and as accurately as possible."

References

1. McCrory et al. Consensus Statement On Concussion In Sport – The 5th International Conference On Concussion In Sport Held In Berlin, October 2016. British Journal of Sports Medicine 2017 (available at www.bjsm.bmj.com)

2. Maddocks, DL; Dicker, GD; Saling, MM. The assessment of orientation following concussion in athletes. Clinical Journal of Sport Medicine 1995; 5: 32-33

3. Jennett, B., Bond, M. Assessment of outcome after severe brain damage: a practical scale. Lancet 1975; i: 480-484

4. McCrea M. Standardized mental status testing of acute concussion. Clinical Journal of Sport Medicine. 2001; 11: 176-181

5. Guskiewicz KM. Assessment of postural stability following sport-related concussion. Current Sports Medicine Reports. 2003; 2: 24-30

Echemendia RJ, *et al. Br J Sports Med* 2017;**51**:851–858. doi:10.1136/bjsports-2017-097506SCAT5

Fig. 2.49, cont'd

CONCUSSION INFORMATION

Any athlete suspected of having a concussion should be removed from play and seek medical evaluation.

Signs to watch for

Problems could arise over the first 24-48 hours. The athlete should not be left alone and must go to a hospital at once if they experience:

- Worsening headache
- Drowsiness or inability to be awakened
- Inability to recognize people or places

- Repeated vomiting
- Unusual behaviour or confusion or irritable
- Seizures (arms and legs jerk uncontrollably)

- Weakness or numbness in arms or legs
- Unsteadiness on their feet.
- Slurred speech

Consult your physician or licensed healthcare professional after a suspected concussion. **Remember, it is better to be safe.**

Rest & Rehabilitation

After a concussion, the athlete should have physical rest and relative cognitive rest for a few days to allow their symptoms to improve. In most cases, after no more than a few days of rest, the athlete should gradually increase their daily activity level as long as their symptoms do not worsen. Once the athlete is able to complete their usual daily activities without concussion-related symptoms, the second step of the return to play/sport progression can be started. The athlete should not return to play/sport until their concussion-related symptoms have resolved and the athlete has successfully returned to full school/learning activities.

When returning to play/sport, the athlete should follow a stepwise, **medically managed exercise progression, with increasing amounts of exercise.** For example:

Graduated Return to Sport Strategy

Exercise step	Functional exercise at each step	Goal of each step
1. Symptom-limited activity	Daily activities that do not provoke symptoms.	Gradual reintroduction of work/school activities.
2. Light aerobic exercise	Walking or stationary cycling at slow to medium pace. No resistance training.	Increase heart rate.
3. Sport-specific exercise	Running or skating drills. No head impact activities.	Add movement.
4. Non-contact training drills	Harder training drills, e.g., passing drills. May start progressive resistance training.	Exercise, coordination, and increased thinking.
5. Full contact practice	Following medical clearance, participate in normal training activities.	Restore confidence and assess functional skills by coaching staff.
6. Return to play/sport	Normal game play.	

In this example, it would be typical to have 24 hours (or longer) for each step of the progression. If any symptoms worsen while exercising, the athlete should go back to the previous step. Resistance training should be added only in the later stages (Stage 3 or 4 at the earliest).

Written clearance should be provided by a healthcare professional before return to play/sport as directed by local laws and regulations.

Graduated Return to School Strategy

Concussion may affect the ability to learn at school. The athlete may need to miss a few days of school after a concussion. When going back to school, some athletes may need to go back gradually and may need to have some changes made to their schedule so that concussion symptoms do not get worse. If a particular activity makes symptoms worse, then the athlete should stop that activity and rest until symptoms get better. To make sure that the athlete can get back to school without problems, it is important that the healthcare provider, parents, caregivers and teachers talk to each other so that everyone knows what the plan is for the athlete to go back to school.

Note: If mental activity does not cause any symptoms, the athlete may be able to skip step 2 and return to school part-time before doing school activities at home first.

Mental Activity	Activity at each step	Goal of each step
1. Daily activities that do not give the athlete symptoms	Typical activities that the athlete does during the day as long as they do not increase symptoms (e.g. reading, texting, screen time). Start with 5-15 minutes at a time and gradually build up.	Gradual return to typical activities.
2. School activities	Homework, reading or other cognitive activities outside of the classroom.	Increase tolerance to cognitive work.
3. Return to school part-time	Gradual introduction of schoolwork. May need to start with a partial school day or with increased breaks during the day.	Increase academic activities.
4. Return to school full-time	Gradually progress school activities until a full day can be tolerated.	Return to full academic activities and catch up on missed work.

If the athlete continues to have symptoms with mental activity, some other accomodations that can help with return to school may include:

- Starting school later, only going for half days, or going only to certain classes
- More time to finish assignments/tests
- Quiet room to finish assignments/tests
- Not going to noisy areas like the cafeteria, assembly halls, sporting events, music class, shop class, etc.

- Taking lots of breaks during class, homework, tests
- No more than one exam/day
- Shorter assignments
- Repetition/memory cues
- Use of a student helper/tutor
- Reassurance from teachers that the child will be supported while getting better

The athlete should not go back to sports until they are back to school/learning, without symptoms getting significantly worse and no longer needing any changes to their schedule.

© Concussion in Sport Group 2017

Echemendia RJ, et al. Br J Sports Med 2017;**51**:851–858. doi:10.1136/bjsports-2017-097506SCAT5

Fig. 2.49, cont'd

Child SCAT5©

SPORT CONCUSSION ASSESSMENT TOOL
FOR CHILDREN AGES 5 TO 12 YEARS
FOR USE BY MEDICAL PROFESSIONALS ONLY

supported by

Patient details

Name: _____

DOB: _____

Address: _____

ID number: _____

Examiner: _____

Date of Injury: _____ Time: _____

WHAT IS THE CHILD SCAT5?

The Child SCAT5 is a standardized tool for evaluating concussions designed for use by physicians and licensed healthcare professionals[1].

If you are not a physician or licensed healthcare professional, please use the Concussion Recognition Tool 5 (CRT5). The Child SCAT5 is to be used for evaluating Children aged 5 to 12 years. For athletes aged 13 years and older, please use the SCAT5.

Preseason Child SCAT5 baseline testing can be useful for interpreting post-injury test scores, but not required for that purpose. Detailed instructions for use of the Child SCAT5 are provided on page 7. Please read through these instructions carefully before testing the athlete. Brief verbal instructions for each test are given in italics. The only equipment required for the tester is a watch or timer.

This tool may be freely copied in its current form for distribution to individuals, teams, groups and organizations. It should not be altered in any way, re-branded or sold for commercial gain. Any revision, translation or reproduction in a digital form requires specific approval by the Concussion in Sport Group.

Recognise and Remove

A head impact by either a direct blow or indirect transmission of force can be associated with a serious and potentially fatal brain injury. If there are significant concerns, including any of the red flags listed in Box 1, then activation of emergency procedures and urgent transport to the nearest hospital should be arranged.

Key points

- Any athlete with suspected concussion should be REMOVED FROM PLAY, medically assessed and monitored for deterioration. No athlete diagnosed with concussion should be returned to play on the day of injury.

- If the child is suspected of having a concussion and medical personnel are not immediately available, the child should be referred to a medical facility for urgent assessment.

- Concussion signs and symptoms evolve over time and it is important to consider repeat evaluation in the assessment of concussion.

- The diagnosis of a concussion is a clinical judgment, made by a medical professional. The Child SCAT5 should NOT be used by itself to make, or exclude, the diagnosis of concussion. An athlete may have a a concussion even if their Child SCAT5 is "normal".

Remember:

- The basic principles of first aid (danger, response, airway, breathing, circulation) should be followed.

- Do not attempt to move the athlete (other than that required for airway management) unless trained to do so.

- Assessment for a spinal cord injury is a critical part of the initial on-field assessment.

- Do not remove a helmet or any other equipment unless trained to do so safely.

© Concussion in Sport Group 2017

Fig. 2.50 Sports Concussion Assessment Tool for children ages 5 to 12 years (Child SCAT5) (Copyright Concussion in Sport Group 2017. Taken from McCrory P, Meeuwisse W, Dvořák J, et al: Consensus statement on concussion in sport. *Br J Sports Med* 51:838-847, 2017.)

1

IMMEDIATE OR ON-FIELD ASSESSMENT

The following elements should be assessed for all athletes who are suspected of having a concussion prior to proceeding to the neurocognitive assessment and ideally should be done on-field after the first first aid / emergency care priorities are completed.

If any of the "Red Flags" or observable signs are noted after a direct or indirect blow to the head, the athlete should be immediately and safely removed from participation and evaluated by a physician or licensed healthcare professional.

Consideration of transportation to a medical facility should be at the discretion of the physician or licensed healthcare professional.

The GCS is important as a standard measure for all patients and can be done serially if necessary in the event of deterioration in conscious state. The cervical spine exam is a critical step of the immediate assessment, however, it does not need to be done serially.

STEP 1: RED FLAGS

RED FLAGS:

- Neck pain or tenderness
- Double vision
- Weakness or tingling/burning in arms or legs
- Severe or increasing headache
- Seizure or convulsion
- Loss of consciousness
- Deteriorating conscious state
- Vomiting
- Increasingly restless, agitated or combative

STEP 2: OBSERVABLE SIGNS

Witnessed ☐   Observed on Video ☐

Lying motionless on the playing surface	Y	N
Balance / gait difficulties / motor incoordination: stumbling, slow / laboured movements	Y	N
Disorientation or confusion, or an inability to respond appropriately to questions	Y	N
Blank or vacant look	Y	N
Facial injury after head trauma	Y	N

STEP 3: EXAMINATION
GLASGOW COMA SCALE (GCS)[2]

Time of assessment			
Date of assessment			

Best eye response (E)

No eye opening	1	1	1
Eye opening in response to pain	2	2	2
Eye opening to speech	3	3	3
Eyes opening spontaneously	4	4	4

Best verbal response (V)

No verbal response	1	1	1
Incomprehensible sounds	2	2	2
Inappropriate words	3	3	3
Confused	4	4	4
Oriented	5	5	5

Best motor response (M)

No motor response	1	1	1
Extension to pain	2	2	2
Abnormal flexion to pain	3	3	3
Flexion / Withdrawal to pain	4	4	4
Localizes to pain	5	5	5
Obeys commands	6	6	6
Glasgow Coma score (E + V + M)			

Name: _____

DOB: _____

Address: _____

ID number: _____

Examiner: _____

Date: _____

CERVICAL SPINE ASSESSMENT

Does the athlete report that their neck is pain free at rest?	Y	N
If there is NO neck pain at rest, does the athlete have a full range of ACTIVE pain free movement?	Y	N
Is the limb strength and sensation normal?	Y	N

In a patient who is not lucid or fully conscious, a cervical spine injury should be assumed until proven otherwise.

OFFICE OR OFF-FIELD ASSESSMENT
STEP 1: ATHLETE BACKGROUND

Please note that the neurocognitive assessment should be done in a distraction-free environment with the athlete in a resting state.

Sport / team / school: _____

Date / time of injury: _____

Years of education completed: _____

Age: _____

Gender: M / F / Other

Dominant hand: left / neither / right

How many diagnosed concussions has the athlete had in the past?: _____

When was the most recent concussion?: _____

How long was the recovery (time to being cleared to play) from the most recent concussion?: _____ (days)

Has the athlete ever been:

Hospitalized for a head injury?	Yes	No
Diagnosed / treated for headache disorder or migraines?	Yes	No
Diagnosed with a learning disability / dyslexia?	Yes	No
Diagnosed with ADD / ADHD?	Yes	No
Diagnosed with depression, anxiety or other psychiatric disorder?	Yes	No

Current medications? If yes, please list: _____

© Concussion in Sport Group 2017

Fig. 2.50, cont'd

STEP 2: SYMPTOM EVALUATION

The athlete should be given the symptom form and asked to read this instruction paragraph out loud then complete the symptom scale. For the baseline assessment, the athlete should rate his/her symptoms based on how he/she typically feels and for the post injury assessment the athlete should rate their symptoms at this point in time.

To be done in a resting state

Please Check: ☐ **Baseline** ☐ **Post-Injury**

Name: _____

DOB: _____

Address: _____

ID number: _____

Examiner: _____

Date: _____

Child Report[3]

	Not at all/ Never	A little/ Rarely	Somewhat/ Sometimes	A lot/ Often
I have headaches	0	1	2	3
I feel dizzy	0	1	2	3
I feel like the room is spinning	0	1	2	3
I feel like I'm going to faint	0	1	2	3
Things are blurry when I look at them	0	1	2	3
I see double	0	1	2	3
I feel sick to my stomach	0	1	2	3
My neck hurts	0	1	2	3
I get tired a lot	0	1	2	3
I get tired easily	0	1	2	3
I have trouble paying attention	0	1	2	3
I get distracted easily	0	1	2	3
I have a hard time concentrating	0	1	2	3
I have problems remembering what people tell me	0	1	2	3
I have problems following directions	0	1	2	3
I daydream too much	0	1	2	3
I get confused	0	1	2	3
I forget things	0	1	2	3
I have problems finishing things	0	1	2	3
I have trouble figuring things out	0	1	2	3
It's hard for me to learn new things	0	1	2	3
Total number of symptoms:				of 21
Symptom severity score:				of 63
Do the symptoms get worse with physical activity?			Y	N
Do the symptoms get worse with trying to think?			Y	N

Overall rating for child to answer:

	Very bad			Very good
On a scale of 0 to 10 (where 10 is normal), how do you feel now?		0 1 2 3 4 5 6 7 8 9 10		

If not 10, in what way do you feel different?:

_____

Parent Report

The child:

	Not at all/ Never	A little/ Rarely	Somewhat/ Sometimes	A lot/ Often
has headaches	0	1	2	3
feels dizzy	0	1	2	3
has a feeling that the room is spinning	0	1	2	3
feels faint	0	1	2	3
has blurred vision	0	1	2	3
has double vision	0	1	2	3
experiences nausea	0	1	2	3
has a sore neck	0	1	2	3
gets tired a lot	0	1	2	3
gets tired easily	0	1	2	3
has trouble sustaining attention	0	1	2	3
is easily distracted	0	1	2	3
has difficulty concentrating	0	1	2	3
has problems remembering what he/she is told	0	1	2	3
has difficulty following directions	0	1	2	3
tends to daydream	0	1	2	3
gets confused	0	1	2	3
is forgetful	0	1	2	3
has difficulty completing tasks	0	1	2	3
has poor problem solving skills	0	1	2	3
has problems learning	0	1	2	3
Total number of symptoms:				of 21
Symptom severity score:				of 63
Do the symptoms get worse with physical activity?			Y	N
Do the symptoms get worse with mental activity?			Y	N

Overall rating for parent/teacher/coach/carer to answer

On a scale of 0 to 100% (where 100% is normal), how would you rate the child now?

_____

If not 100%, in what way does the child seem different?

_____

Fig. 2.50, cont'd

3

STEP 3: COGNITIVE SCREENING
Standardized Assessment of Concussion - Child Version (SAC-C)[4]

IMMEDIATE MEMORY

The Immediate Memory component can be completed using the traditional 5-word per trial list or optionally using 10-words per trial to minimise any ceiling effect. All 3 trials must be administered irrespective of the number correct on the first trial. Administer at the rate of one word per second.

Please choose EITHER the 5 or 10 word list groups and circle the specific word list chosen for this test.

I am going to test your memory. I will read you a list of words and when I am done, repeat back as many words as you can remember, in any order. For Trials 2 & 3: I am going to repeat the same list again. Repeat back as many words as you can remember in any order, even if you said the word before.

List	Alternate 5 word lists					Score (of 5)		
						Trial 1	Trial 2	Trial 3
A	Finger	Penny	Blanket	Lemon	Insect			
B	Candle	Paper	Sugar	Sandwich	Wagon			
C	Baby	Monkey	Perfume	Sunset	Iron			
D	Elbow	Apple	Carpet	Saddle	Bubble			
E	Jacket	Arrow	Pepper	Cotton	Movie			
F	Dollar	Honey	Mirror	Saddle	Anchor			
					Immediate Memory Score			of 15
					Time that last trial was completed			

List	Alternate 10 word lists					Score (of 10)		
						Trial 1	Trial 2	Trial 3
G	Finger	Penny	Blanket	Lemon	Insect			
	Candle	Paper	Sugar	Sandwich	Wagon			
H	Baby	Monkey	Perfume	Sunset	Iron			
	Elbow	Apple	Carpet	Saddle	Bubble			
I	Jacket	Arrow	Pepper	Cotton	Movie			
	Dollar	Honey	Mirror	Saddle	Anchor			
					Immediate Memory Score			of 30
					Time that last trial was completed			

Name: _____

DOB: _____

Address: _____

ID number: _____

Examiner: _____

Date: _____

CONCENTRATION

DIGITS BACKWARDS

Please circle the Digit list chosen (A, B, C, D, E, F). Administer at the rate of one digit per second reading DOWN the selected column.

I am going to read a string of numbers and when I am done, you repeat them back to me in reverse order of how I read them to you. For example, if I say 7-1-9, you would say 9-1-7.

List A	List B	List C			
5-2	4-1	4-9	Y	N	0
4-1	9-4	6-2	Y	N	1
4-9-3	5-2-6	1-4-2	Y	N	0
6-2-9	4-1-5	6-5-8	Y	N	1
3-8-1-4	1-7-9-5	6-8-3-1	Y	N	0
3-2-7-9	4-9-6-8	3-4-8-1	Y	N	1
6-2-9-7-1	4-8-5-2-7	4-9-1-5-3	Y	N	0
1-5-2-8-6	6-1-8-4-3	6-8-2-5-1	Y	N	1
7-1-8-4-6-2	8-3-1-9-6-4	3-7-6-5-1-9	Y	N	0
5-3-9-1-4-8	7-2-4-8-5-6	9-2-6-5-1-4	Y	N	1

List D	List E	List F			
2-7	9-2	7-8	Y	N	0
5-9	6-1	5-1	Y	N	1
7-8-2	3-8-2	2-7-1	Y	N	0
9-2-6	5-1-8	4-7-9	Y	N	1
4-1-8-3	2-7-9-3	1-6-8-3	Y	N	0
9-7-2-3	2-1-6-9	3-9-2-4	Y	N	1
1-7-9-2-6	4-1-8-6-9	2-4-7-5-8	Y	N	0
4-1-7-5-2	9-4-1-7-5	8-3-9-6-4	Y	N	1
2-6-4-8-1-7	6-9-7-3-8-2	5-8-6-2-4-9	Y	N	0
8-4-1-9-3-5	4-2-7-3-9-8	3-1-7-8-2-6	Y	N	1
		Digits Score:			of 5

DAYS IN REVERSE ORDER

Now tell me the days of the week in reverse order. Start with the last day and go backward. So you'll say Sunday, Saturday. Go ahead.

Sunday - Saturday - Friday - Thursday - Wednesday - Tuesday - Monday	0 1
Days Score	of 1
Concentration Total Score (Digits + Days)	of 6

Fig. 2.50, cont'd

4

STEP 4: NEUROLOGICAL SCREEN

See the instruction sheet (page 7) for details of test administration and scoring of the tests.

Can the patient read aloud (e.g. symptom check-list) and follow instructions without difficulty?	Y	N
Does the patient have a full range of pain-free PASSIVE cervical spine movement?	Y	N
Without moving their head or neck, can the patient look side-to-side and up-and-down without double vision?	Y	N
Can the patient perform the finger nose coordination test normally?	Y	N
Can the patient perform tandem gait normally?	Y	N

BALANCE EXAMINATION

Modified Balance Error Scoring System (BESS) testing[5]

Which foot was tested (i.e. which is the non-dominant foot)	☐ Left ☐ Right

Testing surface (hard floor, field, etc.) _____

Footwear (shoes, barefoot, braces, tape, etc.) _____

Condition	Errors			
Double leg stance		of 10		
Single leg stance (non-dominant foot, 10-12 y/o only)		of 10		
Tandem stance (non-dominant foot at back)		of 10		
Total Errors	5-9 y/o	of 20	10-12 y/o	of 30

Name: _____

DOB: _____

Address: _____

ID number: _____

Examiner: _____

Date: _____

5

STEP 5: DELAYED RECALL:

The delayed recall should be performed after 5 minutes have elapsed since the end of the Immediate Recall section. Score 1 pt. for each correct response.

Do you remember that list of words I read a few times earlier? Tell me as many words from the list as you can remember in any order.

Time Started [   ]

Please record each word correctly recalled. Total score equals number of words recalled.

_____
_____
_____

Total number of words recalled accurately:	of 5	or	of 10

6

STEP 6: DECISION

Domain	Date & time of assessment:		
Symptom number Child report (of 21) Parent report (of 21)			
Symptom severity score Child report (of 63) Parent report (of 63)			
Immediate memory	of 15 of 30	of 15 of 30	of 15 of 30
Concentration (of 6)			
Neuro exam	Normal Abnormal	Normal Abnormal	Normal Abnormal
Balance errors (5-9 y/o of 20) (10-12 y/o of 30)			
Delayed Recall	of 5 of 10	of 5 of 10	of 5 of 10

Date and time of injury: _____

If the athlete is known to you prior to their injury, are they different from their usual self?

☐ Yes ☐ No ☐ Unsure ☐ Not Applicable

(If different, describe why in the clinical notes section)

Concussion Diagnosed?

☐ Yes ☐ No ☐ Unsure ☐ Not Applicable

If re-testing, has the athlete improved?

☐ Yes ☐ No ☐ Unsure ☐ Not Applicable

I am a physician or licensed healthcare professional and I have personally administered or supervised the administration of this Child SCAT5.

Signature: _____

Name: _____

Title: _____

Registration number (if applicable): _____

Date: _____

SCORING ON THE CHILD SCAT5 SHOULD NOT BE USED AS A STAND-ALONE METHOD TO DIAGNOSE CONCUSSION, MEASURE RECOVERY OR MAKE DECISIONS ABOUT AN ATHLETE'S READINESS TO RETURN TO COMPETITION AFTER CONCUSSION.

Fig. 2.50, cont'd

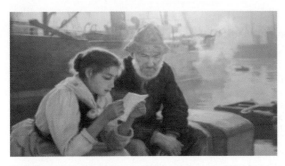

Name: _____

DOB: _____

Address: _____

ID number: _____

Examiner: _____

Date: _____

For the Neurological Screen (page 5), if the child cannot read, ask him/her to describe what they see in this picture.

CLINICAL NOTES:

_____

_____

_____

_____

_____

_____

✂ ·

Concussion Injury advice for the child and parents/carergivers

(To be given to the person monitoring the concussed child)

This child has had an injury to the head and needs to be carefully watched for the next 24 hours by a responsible adult.

If you notice any change in behavior, vomiting, dizziness, worsening headache, double vision or excessive drowsiness, please call an ambulance to take the child to hospital immediately.

Other important points:

Following concussion, the child should rest for at least 24 hours.

· The child should not use a computer, internet or play video games if these activities make symptoms worse.

· The child should not be given any medications, including pain killers, unless prescribed by a medical doctor.

· The child should not go back to school until symptoms are improving.

· The child should not go back to sport or play until a doctor gives permission.

Clinic phone number: _____

Patient's name: _____

Date / time of injury: _____

Date / time of medical review: _____

Healthcare Provider: _____

© Concussion in Sport Group 2017

Contact details or stamp

Fig. 2.50, cont'd

INSTRUCTIONS

Words in *Italics* throughout the Child SCAT5 are the instructions given to the athlete by the clinician

Symptom Scale

In situations where the symptom scale is being completed after exercise, it should still be done in a resting state, at least 10 minutes post exercise.

At Baseline	On the day of injury	On all subsequent days
• The child is to complete the Child Report, according to how he/she feels today, and	• The child is to complete the Child Report, according to how he/she feels now.	• The child is to complete the Child Report, according to how he/she feels today, and
• The parent/carer is to complete the Parent Report according to how the child has been over the previous week.	• If the parent is present, and has had time to assess the child on the day of injury, the parent completes the Parent Report according to how the child appears now.	• The parent/carer is to complete the Parent Report according to how the child has been over the previous 24 hours.

For Total number of symptoms, maximum possible is 21

For Symptom severity score, add all scores in table, maximum possible is 21 x 3 = 63

Standardized Assessment of Concussion Child Version (SAC-C)

Immediate Memory

Choose one of the 5-word lists. Then perform 3 trials of immediate memory using this list.

Complete all 3 trials regardless of score on previous trials.

"I am going to test your memory. I will read you a list of words and when I am done, repeat back as many words as you can remember, in any order." The words must be read at a rate of one word per second.

OPTION: The literature suggests that the Immediate Memory has a notable ceiling effect when a 5-word list is used. (In younger children, use the 5-word list). In settings where this ceiling is prominent the examiner may wish to make the task more difficult by incorporating two 5–word groups for a total of 10 words per trial. In this case the maximum score per trial is 10 with a total trial maximum of 30.

Trials 2 & 3 MUST be completed regardless of score on trial 1 & 2.

Trials 2 & 3: *"I am going to repeat the same list again. Repeat back as many words as you can remember in any order, even if you said the word before."*

Score 1 pt. for each correct response. Total score equals sum across all 3 trials. Do NOT inform the athlete that delayed recall will be tested.

Concentration

Digits backward

Choose one column only, from List A, B, C, D, E or F, and administer those digits as follows:

"I am going to read you some numbers and when I am done, you say them back to me backwards, in reverse order of how I read them to you. For example, if I say 7-1, you would say 1-7."

If correct, circle "Y" for correct and go to next string length. If incorrect, circle "N" for the first string length and read trial 2 in the same string length. One point possible for each string length. Stop after incorrect on both trials (2 N's) in a string length. The digits should be read at the rate of one per second.

Days of the week in reverse order

"Now tell me the days of the week in reverse order. Start with Sunday and go backward. So you'll say Sunday, Saturday ... Go ahead"

1 pt. for entire sequence correct

Delayed Recall

The delayed recall should be performed after at least 5 minutes have elapsed since the end of the Immediate Recall section.

"Do you remember that list of words I read a few times earlier? Tell me as many words from the list as you can remember in any order."

Circle each word correctly recalled. Total score equals number of words recalled.

Neurological Screen

Reading

The child is asked to read a paragraph of text from the instructions in the Child SCAT5. For children who can not read, they are asked to describe what they see in a photograph or picture, such as that on page 6 of the Child SCAT5.

Modified Balance Error Scoring System (mBESS)[5] testing

These instructions are to be read by the person administering the Child SCAT5, and each balance task should be demonstrated to the child. The child should then be asked to copy what the examiner demonstrated.

Each of 20-second trial/stance is scored by counting the number of errors. The This balance testing is based on a modified version of the Balance Error Scoring System (BESS)[5].

A stopwatch or watch with a second hand is required for this testing.

"I am now going to test your balance. Please take your shoes off, roll up your pants above your ankle (if applicable), and remove any ankle taping (if applicable). This test will consist of two different parts."

OPTION: For further assessment, the same 3 stances can be performed on a surface of medium density foam (e.g., approximately 50cm x 40cm x 6cm).

(a) Double leg stance:

The first stance is standing with the feet together with hands on hips and with eyes closed. The child should try to maintain stability in that position for 20 seconds. You should inform the child that you will be counting the number of times the child moves out of this position. You should start timing when the child is set and the eyes are closed.

(b) Tandem stance:

Instruct or show the child how to stand heel-to-toe with the non-dominant foot in the back. Weight should be evenly distributed across both feet. Again, the child should try to maintain stability for 20 seconds with hands on hips and eyes closed. You should inform the child that you will be counting the number of times the child moves out of this position. If the child stumbles out of this position, instruct him/her to open the eyes and return to the start position and continue balancing. You should start timing when the child is set and the eyes are closed.

(c) Single leg stance (10-12 year olds only):

"If you were to kick a ball, which foot would you use? [This will be the dominant foot] Now stand on your other foot. You should bend your other leg and hold it up (show the child). Again, try to stay in that position for 20 seconds with your hands on your hips and your eyes closed. I will be counting the number of times you move out of this position. If you move out of this position, open your eyes and return to the start position and keep balancing. I will start timing when you are set and have closed your eyes."

Balance testing – types of errors

1. Hands lifted off iliac crest	3. Step, stumble, or fall	5. Lifting forefoot or heel
2. Opening eyes	4. Moving hip into > 30 degrees abduction	6. Remaining out of test position > 5 sec

Each of the 20-second trials is scored by counting the errors, or deviations from the proper stance, accumulated by the child. The examiner will begin counting errors only after the child has assumed the proper start position. The modified BESS is calculated by adding one error point for each error during the 20-second tests. The maximum total number of errors for any single condition is 10. If a child commits multiple errors simultaneously, only one error is recorded but the child should quickly return to the testing position, and counting should resume once subject is set. Children who are unable to maintain the testing procedure for a minimum of five seconds at the start are assigned the highest possible score, ten, for that testing condition.

Tandem Gait

Instruction for the examiner - Demonstrate the following to the child:

The child is instructed to stand with their feet together behind a starting line (the test is best done with footwear removed). Then, they walk in a forward direction as quickly and as accurately as possible along a 38mm wide (sports tape), 3 metre line with an alternate foot heel-to-toe gait ensuring that they approximate their heel and toe on each step. Once they cross the end of the 3m line, they turn 180 degrees and return to the starting point using the same gait. Children fail the test if they step off the line, have a separation between their heel and toe, or if they touch or grab the examiner or an object.

Finger to Nose

The tester should demonstrate it to the child.

"I am going to test your coordination now. Please sit comfortably on the chair with your eyes open and your arm (either right or left) outstretched (shoulder flexed to 90 degrees and elbow and fingers extended). When I give a start signal, I would like you to perform five successive finger to nose repetitions using your index finger to touch the tip of the nose as quickly and as accurately as possible."

Scoring: 5 correct repetitions in < 4 seconds = 1

Note for testers: Children fail the test if they do not touch their nose, do not fully extend their elbow or do not perform five repetitions.

References

1. McCrory et al. Consensus Statement On Concussion In Sport – The 5th International Conference On Concussion In Sport Held In Berlin, October 2016. British Journal of Sports Medicine 2017 (available at www.bjsm.bmj.com)

2. Jennett, B., Bond, M. Assessment of outcome after severe brain damage: a practical scale. Lancet 1975; i: 480-484

3. Ayr, L.K., Yeates, K.O., Taylor, H.G., Brown, M. Dimensions of postconcussive symptoms in children with mild traumatic brain injuries. Journal of the International Neuropsychological Society. 2009; 15:19–30

4. McCrea M. Standardized mental status testing of acute concussion. Clinical Journal of Sports Medicine. 2001; 11: 176-181

5. Guskiewicz KM. Assessment of postural stability following sport-related concussion. Current Sports Medicine Reports. 2003; 2: 24-30

Fig. 2.50, cont'd

CONCUSSION INFORMATION

If you think you or a teammate has a concussion, tell your coach/trainer/ parent right away so that you can be taken out of the game. You or your teammate should be seen by a doctor as soon as possible. YOU OR YOUR TEAMMATE SHOULD NOT GO BACK TO PLAY/SPORT THAT DAY.

Signs to watch for

Problems can happen over the first 24-48 hours. You or your teammate should not be left alone and must go to a hospital right away if any of the following happens:

- New headache, or headache gets worse
- Neck pain that gets worse
- Becomes sleepy/ drowsy or can't be woken up
- Cannot recognise people or places

- Feeling sick to your stomach or vomiting
- Acting weird/strange, seems/feels confused, or is irritable
- Has any seizures (arms and/or legs jerk uncontrollably)

- Has weakness, numbness or tingling (arms, legs or face)
- Is unsteady walking or standing
- Talking is slurred
- Cannot understand what someone is saying or directions

Consult your physician or licensed healthcare professional after a suspected concussion. Remember, it is better to be safe.

Graduated Return to Sport Strategy

After a concussion, the child should rest physically and mentally for a few days to allow symptoms to get better. In most cases, after a few days of rest, they can gradually increase their daily activity level as long as symptoms don't get worse. Once they are able to do their usual daily activities without symptoms, the child should gradually increase exercise in steps, guided by the healthcare professional (see below).

The athlete should not return to play/sport the day of injury.

NOTE: An initial period of a few days of both cognitive ("thinking") and physical rest is recommended before beginning the Return to Sport progression.

Exercise step	Functional exercise at each step	Goal of each step
1. Symptom-limited activity	Daily activities that do not provoke symptoms.	Gradual reintroduction of work/school activities.
2. Light aerobic exercise	Walking or stationary cycling at slow to medium pace. No resistance training.	Increase heart rate.
3. Sport-specific exercise	Running or skating drills. No head impact activities.	Add movement.
4. Non-contact training drills	Harder training drills, e.g., passing drills. May start progressive resistance training.	Exercise, coordination, and increased thinking.
5. Full contact practice	Following medical clearance, participate in normal training activities.	Restore confidence and assess functional skills by coaching staff.
6. Return to play/sport	Normal game play.	

There should be at least 24 hours (or longer) for each step of the progression. If any symptoms worsen while exercising, the athlete should go back to the previous step. Resistance training should be added only in the later stages (Stage 3 or 4 at the earliest). The athlete should not return to sport until the concussion symptoms have gone, they have successfully returned to full school/learning activities, and the healthcare professional has given the child written permission to return to sport.

If the child has symptoms for more than a month, they should ask to be referred to a healthcare professional who is an expert in the management of concussion.

Graduated Return to School Strategy

Concussion may affect the ability to learn at school. The child may need to miss a few days of school after a concussion, but the child's doctor should help them get back to school after a few days. When going back to school, some children may need to go back gradually and may need to have some changes made to their schedule so that concussion symptoms don't get a lot worse. If a particular activity makes symptoms a lot worse, then the child should stop that activity and rest until symptoms get better. To make sure that the child can get back to school without problems, it is important that the health care provider, parents/caregivers and teachers talk to each other so that everyone knows what the plan is for the child to go back to school.

Note: If mental activity does not cause any symptoms, the child may be able to return to school part-time without doing school activities at home first.

Mental Activity	Activity at each step	Goal of each step
1. Daily activities that do not give the child symptoms	Typical activities that the child does during the day as long as they do not increase symptoms (e.g. reading, texting, screen time). Start with 5-15 minutes at a time and gradually build up.	Gradual return to typical activities.
2. School activities	Homework, reading or other cognitive activities outside of the classroom.	Increase tolerance to cognitive work.
3. Return to school part-time	Gradual introduction of schoolwork. May need to start with a partial school day or with increased breaks during the day	Increase academic activities.
4. Return to school full-time	Gradually progress school activities until a full day can be tolerated.	Return to full academic activities and catch up on missed work.

If the child continues to have symptoms with mental activity, some other things that can be done to help with return to school may include:

- Starting school later, only going for half days, or going only to certain classes
- More time to finish assignments/tests
- Quiet room to finish assignments/tests
- Not going to noisy areas like the cafeteria, assembly halls, sporting events, music class, shop class, etc.

- Taking lots of breaks during class, homework, tests
- No more than one exam/day
- Shorter assignments
- Repetition/memory cues
- Use of a student helper/tutor
- Reassurance from teachers that the child will be supported while getting better

The child should not go back to sports until they are back to school/ learning, without symptoms getting significantly worse and no longer needing any changes to their schedule.

Fig. 2.50, cont'd

test has become commonly used when assessing concussions because concussions have an adverse effect on balance, especially in the first 24 hours.[81,253] As such, the BESS has become part of the SCAT5 assessment tool.[211] Any balance deficits in the case of a concussion are attributed to the inability of the patient to integrate sensory information from the vestibular and visual components of the balance mechanism in the brain.[26] The test has six parts—three on a solid floor and three on a foam surface (Fig. 2.51).[206,247] On each surface, three progressive stances are attempted: double leg stance, single leg stance, and heel-to-toe tandem stance. Each of the six stances is evaluated for 20 seconds with the patient closing the eyes and with hands on the iliac crests. The examiner counts a number of errors for each test (Table 2.25). Provided one has a baseline score,

TABLE **2.25**

Balance Error Scoring System (BESS) Countable Errors

Errors

- Hands lifted off the iliac crests
- Opening eyes
- Step, stumble, or fall
- Moving a hip into more than 30° of flexion or extension
- Lifting the forefoot or heel
- Remaining out of the testing position for more than 5 seconds

From Guskiewicz KM, Ross SE, Marshall SW: Postural stability and neuropsychological deficits after concussion in collegiate athletes, *J Athl Train* 36(3):265, 2001.

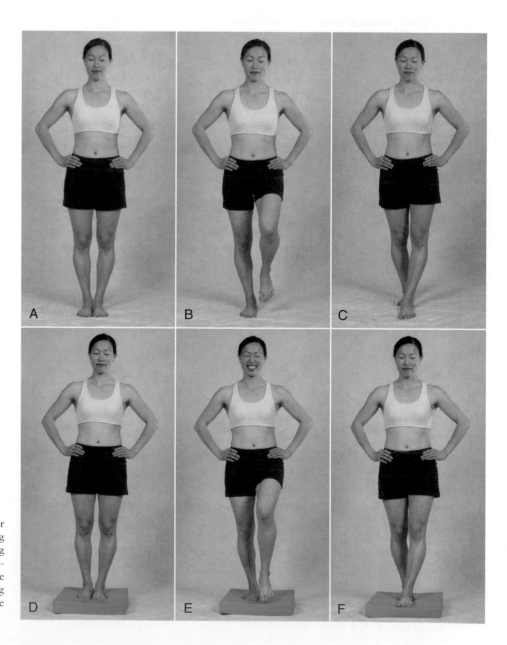

Fig. 2.51 Stances for the Balance Error Scoring System (BESS). (A) Double leg stance on a solid floor. (B) Single leg stance on a solid floor. (C) Heal to toe tandem stance on a solid floor. (D) Double leg stance on a foam surface. (E) Single leg stance on a foam surface. (F) Heel to toe tandem stance on a foam surface.

a score of 3 or more errors from baseline indicates a balance impairment[35,54,129,137,154,207,209–214,254] and may be an indicator of a concussion.[110] High school level of competition, ADHD, and learning disabilities have been associated with a poor BESS baseline performance.[41,248] When evaluating children 12 years of age or younger, it has been suggested that the child be tested only on a solid surface (called a **mini-BESS**) and using only the double leg and tandem stances as children, when tested preconcussion, have significantly worse performance on balance tests than older age groups.[249] The BESS is a static test which tests only the vestibulospinal aspect of the vestibular system. It does not address the dynamic aspects of the system or the vestibulo-ocular control.

✓ *Balance Evaluation Systems Test (BESTest) and mini-BESTest.*[206,207] The BESTest is a multitest dynamic balance assessment developed to identify specific postural control problems such as biomechanical constraints, stability limits, postural responses, anticipatory postural adjustments, sensory orientation, dynamic balance during gait, and cognitive effects (Table 2.26).[206,207] It is designed to distinguish the underlying systems and for treating balance problems in patients. It involves more than the BESS and takes approximately 30 to 45 minutes to complete.[207,215,255]

A shorter version (**14-item mini-BESTest**) (eTool 2.17) has been developed and is useful for predicting falls.[206] It tests some skill transition/anticipatory postural control, reaction postural control, sensory orientation and stability, and gait and takes approximately 10 to 15 minutes to complete.[215,255]

⚠ *Dual Task Gait Stability Test.*[54] Following a concussion, there may be deficits in sensory integration used to maintain optimal balance or locomotion.[256] Dual test balance assessment has been reported to provide a sense of persistent neurological deficits and may help to identify compromised processes that may require more healing time following a concussion as the assessment involves more than doing just one task (e.g., balancing) which makes the test more difficult for the patient.[144,223] This is called a **dual test paradigm**.[49,221] The patient is being asked to do a second task while

TABLE **2.26**

Summary of Balance Evaluation Systems Test (BESTest) Items Under Each System Category[206,207]

I. Biomechanical Constraints	II. Stability Limits/Verticality	III. Anticipatory Postural Adjustments	IV. Postural Responses	V. Sensory Orientation	VI. Stability in Gait
1. Base of support	6. Sitting vertically (left and right) and lateral lean (left and right)	9. Sit to stand	14. In-place response, forward	19. Sensory integration for balance (modified CTSIB) Stance on firm surface, EO Stance on firm surface, EC Stance on foam, EO Stance on foam, EC	21. Gait, level surface
2. CoM alignment	7. Functional reach forward	10. Rise to toes	15. In-place response, backward		22. Change in gait speed
3. Ankle strength and ROM	8. Functional reach lateral (left and right)	11. Stand on one leg (left and right)	16. Compensatory stepping correction, forward		23. Walk with head turns, horizontal
4. Hip/trunk lateral strength		12. Alternate stair touching	17. Compensatory stepping correction, backward	20. Incline, EC	24. Walk with pivot turns
5. Sit on floor and stand up		13. Standing arm raise	18. Compensatory stepping correction, lateral (left and right)		25. Step over obstacles
					26. Timed "Get Up and Go" Test
					27. Timed "Get Up and Go" Test with dual task

CoM, Center of mass; *CTSIB,* Clinical Test of Sensory Integration for Balance; *EC,* eyes closed; *EO,* eyes open; *ROM,* range of motion.
From Horak FB, Wrisley DM, Frank J: The balance evaluation systems test (BESTest) to differentiate balance deficits, *Phys Ther* 89(5):487, 2009.

walking or balancing. If the demands of executing the two tasks simultaneously exceeds cognitive capacity, the performance on one or both tasks may be diminished leading to postural instability.[223] The diminished performance in a dual test condition is called a **dual task cost**. Most activities of daily living involve simultaneous performance of cognition and motor tasks,[221] so the test is attempting to duplicate a more functional activity that includes balance.

The subject is asked to balance or to walk barefoot at a self-selected speed along the walkway while completing a second task. The patient should try not to focus his or her attention on either task.[257] The second task involves a mental task (e.g., adding, subtracting, multiplying, reciting months of the year backwards) or some physical task (e.g., stepping over obstacles).[144,221,223,258] The demands of balance control and gait are very dependent on the complexity of the task and the type of secondary test to be performed.[259] Concussed athletes will have significantly slower walking velocity while performing a secondary cognitive task, greater time in double leg stance support, less time in single leg stance support (i.e., shorter steps), and wider step width throughout the gait cycle.[258,260] This is called a **Conservative Gait Strategy**. Conservative gait strategy is defined as reduced gait velocity and increased time in double support, with identified altered postural control dynamics.[144,221,222,261] Children and adolescents who have suffered a concussion exhibit slower tandem gait walking and more time in double support than controls.[221]

⚠ *Obstructive Stroop Dual Task.* This is a dual task event that is conducted along a 7-m-long walkway and requires the patient, using a tandem gait (i.e., heel-toe), to step over a stationary obstacle that is normalized to 30% of the patient's lower leg length defined as a distance from the tibial plateau to the ground.[225]

⚠ *Romberg Test.* This is a static test and involves relaxed standing with the eyes closed. The examiner asks the patient to stand with feet together and arms by the sides with the eyes open. The examiner notes whether the patient has any problem with balance. The patient then closes his or her eyes for at least 20 seconds, and the examiner notes any differences. A positive Romberg test is elicited if the patient sways excessively or falls to one side when the eyes are closed. This reaction indicates an expanding intracranial lesion, possible disease of the spinal cord posterior columns, or proprioceptive problems. Several authors feel this test is too subjective.[110,214,252]

☑ *Sensory Organization Test.* The Sensory Organization Test (SOT) is a "balance device" in which the patient stands on a force plate surrounded by a visual image (Fig. 2.52) which objectively measures postural sway and center of pressure under three different visual conditions (i.e., eyes open, eyes closed, and sway referenced) on two

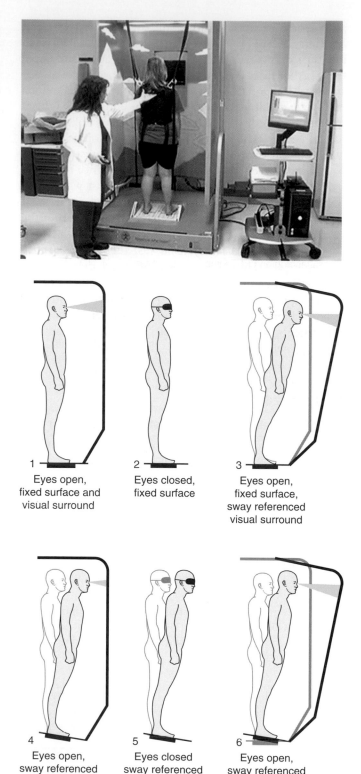

Fig. 2.52 Sensory Organization Test (SOT). (From Graham V, Napier-Dovorany K: Multifactoral measures of fall risk in the visually impaired population: a pilot study, *J Body Mov Ther* 20[1]:104–109, 2015; Lew HL, Tanaka C, Hirohata E, Goodrich GL: Auditory, vestibular, and visual impairments. In Cifu DX, Kaelin DL, Kowalske KJ, et al., editors: *Braddom's physical medicine and rehabilitation*, ed 5, Philadelphia, 2016, Elsevier [line drawings courtesy of Natus Medical Incorporated].)

different surface conditions (fixed and sway referenced [i.e., surface moves]).[54,252] The term "sway referenced" involves the tilting (i.e., moving up and down) of the support surface and/or visual surround area to directly affect the patient's center of gravity sway. It is measuring the patient's ability to maintain equilibrium.[54] The test protocol consists of three trials under three different visual conditions (i.e., eyes open, eyes closed, sway referenced) on two different surface conditions (i.e., fixed and sway referenced) for a total of 18 tests. The patient is asked to stand as motionless as possible for each test in a normal stance with his or her feet shoulder-width apart.[213] The test is used to show whether that patient has decreased sensory interaction and/or decreased postural stability.[214]

⚠ *Star Excursion Balance Test (SEBT).* This dynamic test measures the ability of an individual to maintain a single leg stance while the contralateral leg reaches as far as possible in eight different directions (i.e., anterior, anteromedial, medial, posteromedial, posterior, posterolateral, lateral, and anterolateral). To begin with, the examiner places four strips of tape with a length of 6 to 8 feet in a star pattern as shown in Fig. 2.53A. All the lines are separated from each other by a 45° angle. The patient stands in the center of the star balancing on one leg while extending the other leg out in different directions of the star (Fig. 2.53B). The examiner measures how far the patient is able to reach in each direction along the star using a measuring tape. The test begins with balancing on the dominant or good leg and concludes with the other leg, and the values are compared. If the examiner has preconcussion values, they can be used to compare with postconcussion values which should show decreases bilaterally with the concussion.[262,263] If the values decrease unilaterally, it is probably due to a leg injury. The most important directions are anterior, posteromedial, and posterolateral.[262,264] The **Y-Balance Test** is a modification or refinement of this test doing only the anterior, posteromedial, and posterolateral movement using a specific Y-shaped device in which boxes are pushed along a metal line while the patient balances on one foot on the center box (Fig. 2.54).

Standing on LEFT Limb   Standing on RIGHT Limb

1. Anterior	5. Posterior
2. Anteromedial	6. Posterolateral
3. Medial	7. Lateral
4. Posteromedial	8. Anterolateral

A

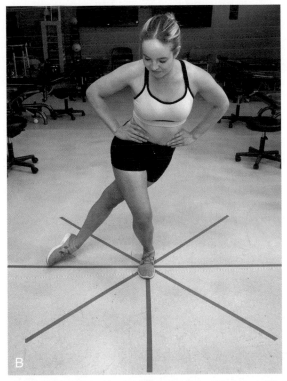

Fig. 2.53 Star Excursion Balance Test (SEBT). (A) Setup. (B) Patient testing balance on right leg in lateral direction.

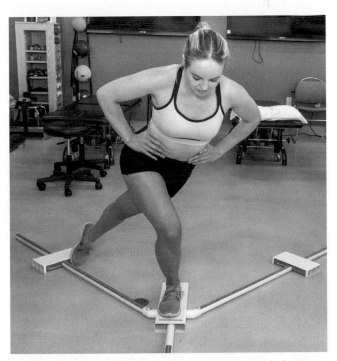

Fig. 2.54 Y-Balance Test showing patient balancing on right leg in posterolateral position. Note how white boxes have been pushed as far as possible.

Tests for Coordination

⚠ *Finger Drumming Test.* The patient drums the index and middle finger of one hand up and down as quickly as possible on the back of the other hand. The test is repeated with the opposite hand. The examiner compares the two sides for coordination and speed. Both sides should be equal. A positive test would be slower movement on the affected side.

❓ *Finger-Thumb Test.* The patient touches each finger with the thumb of the same hand. The normal or uninjured side is tested first, followed by the injured side. The examiner compares the two sides for coordination and timing. Both sides should be equal. A positive test would be slower movement on the affected side.

⚠ *Finger-to-Nose Test.* The patient stands or sits with the eyes open and brings the index finger to the nose (Fig. 2.55A). The test is repeated with the eyes closed. Both arms are tested several times with increasing speed. Normally, the tests should be accomplished easily, smoothly, and quickly with the eyes open and closed.[33]

❓ *Hand "Flip" Test.* The patient touches the back of the opposite, stationary hand with the anterior aspect of the fingers, flips the test hand over, and touches the opposite hand with the posterior aspect of the fingers. The movement is repeated several times with both sides being tested. The examiner compares the two sides for coordination and speed.

❓ *Hand-Thigh Test.* The patient pats his or her thigh with the hand as quickly as possible. The uninjured side is tested first. The patient may be asked to supinate and pronate the hand between each hand-thigh contact to make the test more complex. The examiner watches for speed and coordination and compares the two sides.

❓ *Heel-to-Knee Test.* The patient, who is lying supine with the eyes open, takes the heel of one foot and touches the opposite knee with the heel and then slides the heel down the shin (Fig. 2.55B). The test is repeated with the eyes closed, and both legs are tested. The test can be repeated several times with increasing speed. The examiner notes any differences in coordination or the presence of tremor. Normally, the test should be accomplished easily, smoothly, and quickly with the eyes open or closed.

❓ *Past Pointing Test.* The patient and examiner face each other. The examiner holds up both index fingers approximately 15 cm (6 inches) apart. The patient is asked to lift his or her arms over the head and then bring the arms down to touch the patient's index fingers to the examiner's index fingers (Fig. 2.56). The test is repeated with the patient's eyes closed. Normally, the test can be performed without difficulty. Patients with vestibular disease have problems with past pointing. The test may also be used to test proprioception.

Tests for Cognitive Function

Cognitive assessment involves orientation, immediate memory, concentration, delayed recall, and a total score. eTool 2.18 shows an example of a cognitive assessment following a concussion.[204]

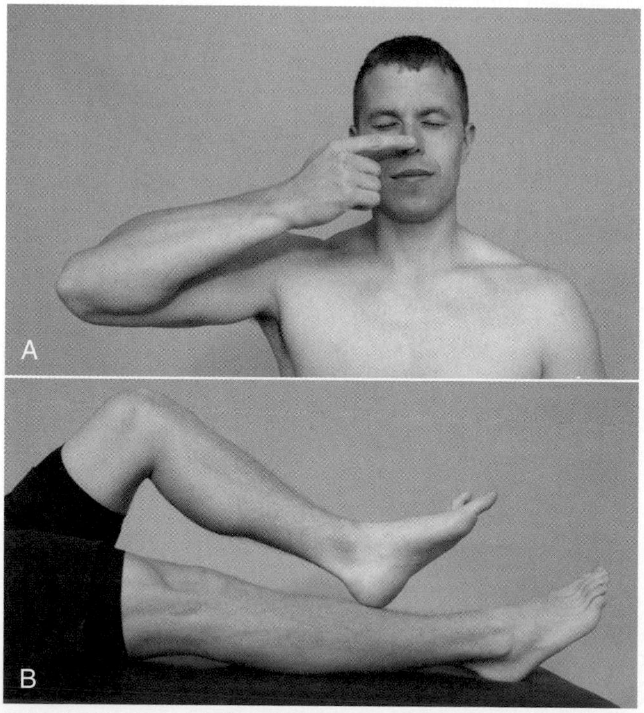

Fig. 2.55 Performing coordination testing. (A) Touching nose with index finger with eyes closed. (B) Touching knee with opposite heel with eyes closed.

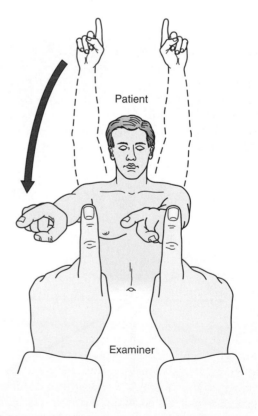

Fig. 2.56 Past pointing. (Redrawn from Reilly BM: *Practical strategies in outpatient medicine*, Philadelphia, 1991, WB Saunders, p 195.)

⚠️ *Trail Making Test.* The Trail Making Test is a neuro-psychological test in which the patient is asked to sequentially trace with a pen or pencil a list of 25 numbers on a piece of paper as fast as possible while still maintaining accuracy. The time taken to complete the task is recorded along with the number of errors. This task measures orientation, concentration, visual spatial capacity, and problem-solving abilities.[252,265,266]

⚠️ *Visual Stroop Test.* The Visual Stroop Test is designed to assess cognitive flexibility and attention span by examining a patient's ability to separate word and color naming stimuli through the use of three separate subtests. Each subtest contains 100 items presented in 5 columns of 20 items. Patients have 45 seconds to complete each subtest, with a total score calculated from the sum of each of the subtests. During the first subtest, the patient is asked to read aloud the color names such as red, green, or blue written in black ink. The reader's time to complete the task and any errors are recorded. For the second subtest, the patient is asked to repeat the test with a new list of words reading aloud color names such as red, green, or blue, but this time the named colors are written in a different color than the word (e.g., the word "blue" is written in red). Again, the time to complete the task and number of errors is recorded. In the third subtest, the patient is asked to repeat the second subtest but should say the colors that the words are printed in (e.g., when red is printed in green, the patient should say green). Again, the time to complete the task and the number of errors is recorded.[224,252,268] The error rate and not the speed is the index of inhibitory cognitive control.[224,225]

⚠️ *Wechsler Digit Span Test.* The Wechsler Digit Span Test involves two parts and is used to examine a child's concentration and immediate memory recall. It is designed for children from age 5 to 15.[267] In both parts of the test, the subject is presented with a series of numbers, words, or letters and asked to repeat the numbers, words, or letters either in the same order (i.e., digits forward) for the first part or in reverse order (i.e., digits backward) for the second part. The number of successful trials for each part is recorded as a total score (i.e., digits total).[252]

Tests of the Vestibular System

The vestibular system is made up of a complex network that includes small sensory organs in the inner ear (i.e., utricle, saccule, and semicircular canals) along with connections to the brain stem, cerebellum, cerebral cortex, ocular system, and postural muscles.[69] The system provides information related to head movements and maintaining balance control.[69] It is organized into two distinct functional units: the **vestibulo-ocular system** for visual stability when the head moves, and the vestibulospinal system for postural control.[69] Symptoms of dizziness and vision problems are related to the vestibulo-ocular system and problems with balance are related to the **vestibulo-spinal system**.[69]

Dizziness is defined as a subjective sensation of spinning around and potentially losing one's balance. It is a very subjective symptom which can have several causes (see Table 2.19). When looking for causes of dizziness, the examiner should focus first on the cardiovascular system, including cardiac rhythm and orthostatic blood pressure measurements. Secondly, the neurological exam should focus on oculomotor function and balance.[269] The key characteristics when assessing for dizziness include the date of onset, whether the dizziness is constant or episodic, its duration, what triggers the dizziness, any aggravating or alleviating factors, and/or any other patterns associated with the symptoms.[269] The **Dizziness Handicap Inventory**[184] or **Modified Dizziness Handicap Inventory** (eTool 2.19) may be used to determine how much the dizziness affects the patient.

Clinical examination of a patient suspected of having a vestibular disorder should begin with examination of the eyes. The patient is asked to move the eyes in six different **cardinal gaze** positions (see Fig. 2.35).[27,270] The examiner should watch for nystagmus, **abnormal visual tracking** (e.g., saccadic eye motion with symptoms during smooth pursuit testing), or abnormal **near point convergence (NPC)** (normal is 6 to 10 cm from the nose).

There are several oculomotor conditions that can indicate disturbance in the vestibular system. **Saccades** are jerky quick simultaneous movement of both eyes that occur as a patient tries to fixate on two widely spaced targets with both eyes as the eyes move back and forth between the targets.[245,271] **Smooth pursuits** are predictable smooth visual tracking movements (i.e., the eyes move smoothly instead of "in jumps" [i.e., saccades]) when a person looks between two objects. Smooth pursuits can be used to assess cognitive function because the motion requires attention, anticipation, and working memory as well as smooth and, at times, saccadic eye movements to maintain gaze on a fixed target.[76] **Pursuits** are tested by having the patient fixate and follow slowly moving objects. To test smooth pursuits, the patient is asked to visually track an object moving slowly in horizontal and vertical directions at approximately 10°/sec to 20°/sec while keeping the head stationary. **Spontaneous nystagmus** is movement of the eyes without some stimulus. Nystagmus indicates an imbalance within the central or peripheral vestibular system.[269] Unidirectional horizontal spontaneous nystagmus is a characteristic of acute peripheral vestibular imbalance. Nystagmus is secondary to a direction specific imbalance of the VOR which activates brain stem neuronal activity. **Accommodation** is a process by which the eye changes the shape of the lens to maintain focus on an object.[76] **Convergence** is a simultaneous adduction of the eyes to maintain binocular fusion (i.e., both eyes fixate on the same object at the same time).[76] **NPC** is a measurement of how close the patient can bring a target to the nose while maintaining normal fusion. Normally it is less than 6 cm (2.4 inches) from the nose to the target. The patient is asked to focus on the target which is slowly brought toward the tip of the patient's nose while the patient is focusing on the target with both eyes. The patient is instructed to stop moving the target when the patient sees two distinct images or when the examiner observes that there was deviation of one eye. The NPC is measured as a mean of three separate measurement trials consecutively measured without rest. The mean NPC measurements of less than or equal to 5 cm are considered normal and the NPC measurements greater than 5 cm are considered abnormal.[227] **Convergence insufficiency** is a condition in which the patient's eyes are unable to work together when looking at a nearby object. It is a common binocular vision disorder characterized by **exophoria** (i.e., a tendency of one eye to deviate outward from the midline).[227]

Vestibular problems can be caused by both peripheral and central vestibular deficits and are difficult to assess because they are subjective and are a result of a variety of sensations reported by the patient.[270] There are two mechanisms for vestibular dysfunction following cerebral concussion. First, the peripheral receptors may be damaged, which alters accurate senses of motion. Secondly, there may be impairment of the central integration of vestibular, visual, and somatosensory information in the brain. There may also be various combinations of peripheral and central deficits that lead to symptoms.[26,213] Approximately three-quarters of the vestibular disorders are peripheral involving the ear or vestibular nerve. The most common peripheral vestibular disorder is **benign paroxysmal positional vertigo (BPPV)** which results in dizziness, oscillopsia (i.e., objects appear to oscillate), nystagmus, nausea, and postural imbalance.[270] This type of vertigo occurs when one rapidly stands up from a relaxed supine or seated position and does not necessarily indicate the presence of pathology. It is the result of lack of blood flow to the brain caused by a quick change in position. It may also be due to an inner ear problem.[270] **Semicircular canal dysfunction** signs and symptoms typically include rotational vertigo and deviation of perceived straight ahead (i.e., deviation of what the patient thinks is straight ahead when asked to look straight ahead), spontaneous vestibular nystagmus with oscillopsia, postural imbalance, altered past pointing, nausea, and vomiting.[270] The most common pathological central causes of dizziness and vertigo are cerebrovascular disorders, cerebral disease, migraine, multiple sclerosis, tumors in the posterior fossa, neurodegenerative disorders, and psychiatric disorders.[105] Dysfunction of the oculomotor system is one of the most commonly reported visual problems in individuals suffering from mild to moderate brain injury (mTBI).[64,245,272]

✓ *Dix-Hallpike Maneuver or Test.*[270,273,274] This test is used to identify **BPPV**, a condition in which patients experience episodes of dizziness, or vertigo, especially if the head and neck are moved to different positions. The test is performed by having the patient long-sit on a plinth with the head rotated approximately 30° to 45° (Fig. 2.57A). The examiner stands behind the patient with one hand supporting the head/neck and the other hand supporting the trunk. The patient is then assisted into a supine position with the patient's head slightly below the horizontal plane, and the position is maintained for 30 to 60 seconds (Fig. 2.57B). The test is performed with the head rotated to both sides starting with the unaffected side. Signs of dizziness and nystagmus (involuntary eye movement) are considered a positive test. The affected ear is the ear closest to the examiner (i.e., lower ear). The **Epley Maneuver** and **Semont Maneuver** are exercises that may be prescribed to relieve the dizziness caused by BPPV.

⚠ *Head Heave Test.* The Head Heave Test (HHT) (Fig. 2.58) is also used to test decreased vestibular function in one ear or the other. The examiner stands facing the patient. The

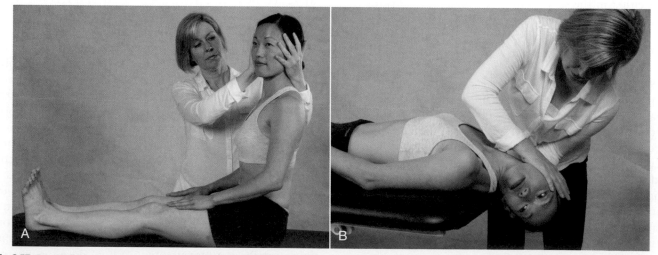

Fig. 2.57 Dix-Hallpike maneuver or test. (A) This test is performed by having the patient long-sit on a plinth with the head rotated approximately 30° to 45° to the unaffected side first. (B) The patient is assisted into a supine position with the patient's head slightly below the horizontal plane while maintaining the rotation. The position is maintained for 30 to 60 seconds. Rotation both ways is tested.

patient sits on the examining table and is asked to fixate on the examiner's nose. The examiner holds the patient's head to enable the patient's neck muscles to relax and abruptly accelerates and decelerates the head laterally (i.e., a side glide) at high speed. As the movement is completed, the examiner watches the patient's eyes to see whether or not a fixation saccade is needed to bring the patient's eyes back to the examiner's nose. If the test is positive, it is probably an inner ear problem.[270,275] Like the Head Impulse Test (HIT), the test depends on subjective judgment of the examiner.

⚠ *Head Impulse Test.* The HIT, also called the **Vestibular Head Impulse Test (VHIT)** or the **Halmagyi—Curthoys Head Impulse Test** (Fig. 2.59), is used to diagnose decreased vestibular function in one ear or the other.[270] The examiner stands facing the patient. The patient sits on an examining table and is told to fixate on the examiner's nose. The examiner holds the patient's head to enable the patient to relax the neck muscles and abruptly accelerates and then

decelerates the head moving rapidly approximately 20° to the right or left. After stopping the movement, the examiner watches the patient's eyes to see whether or not a refixation saccade occurs to get the patient's eyes onto the examiner's nose. If the test is positive, it is probably an inner ear problem.

⚠ *Head Shake Test.* The Head Shake Test is a test for nystagmus. The patient is seated facing the examiner. The examiner flexes the patient's head 20° to 30°. In this position, the examiner asks the patient to rotate the head from side to side 20 times with the eyes closed and then stop. The patient then looks straight ahead while the examiner observes the eyes for nystagmus (Fig. 2.60).

⚠ *Head Thrust Test.* This test is used to test the VOR (Fig. 2.61). The examiner stands facing the patient. The patient sits on the examining table and fixates on the examiner's nose. The examiner holds the patient's head to enable the patient's neck muscles to relax and rotates the head to the right or left and while doing so, abruptly accelerates the motion and then returns to the same slower speed of motion to approximately 20°. As the examiner moves the patient's head, the examiner watches the patient's eyes to see whether or not a fixation saccade is needed to bring the patient's eyes back to the examiner's nose. The test is very similar to the HIT test. The only difference is the quick thrust during the movement of rotation.[269,270]

✔ *King-Devick Test.* The King-Devick Test (Fig. 2.62) is an oculomotor test of visual tracking and is used to detect subtle cognitive visual scanning impairments such as saccadic rhythm, language, and other correlates of suboptimal brain function following acute concussions and other neurological disorders.[31,33,271,276,277] The test was originally developed in the 1970s as a screening tool to identify learning disabilities in young people.[271,278] The test is a quick 2- to 3-minute visual scanning test in which the patient is asked to read, as quickly as possible, a sequence of numbers on three different cards from left to right with varying degrees of visual difficulty (e.g.,

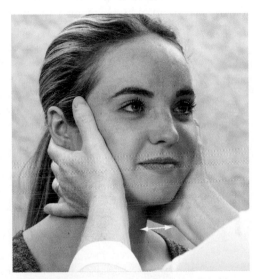

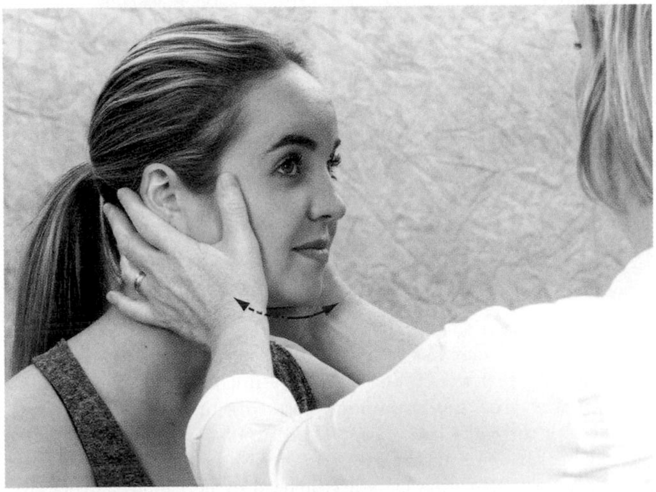

Fig. 2.58 Head heave test. Head is quickly side glided by examiner.

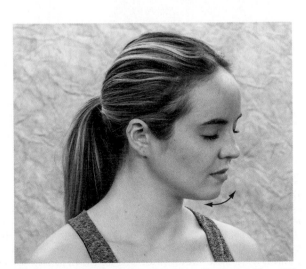

Fig. 2.59 Head impulse test. The examiner quickly rotates the head left or right while the patient continues to watch the examiner's nose.

Fig. 2.60 Head shake test. The patient flexes the neck 20° to 30° and then rotates the head from side to side 20 times with eyes closed.

different spacing of the numbers).[133,277] The patient is shown a demonstration card first to show how the test is done. This is followed by the three test cards (see Fig. 2.62). The test cards have rows of single-digit numbers that are read from left to right as quickly as possible without making any errors.[64,133,245,277,279] The examiner times how long it takes the patient to complete each of the three test cards and sums a total time it takes the patient to read all three test cards. The number of errors made reading each test card is also recorded.[133,277] Normally, the patient would have received a baseline score during his or her preseason evaluation. This baseline assessment allows the examiner to determine if there has been any increase in the time required to complete three tests. Concussed athletes tend to take 5 to 7 seconds longer than normal to complete the test.[33,277] It must be remembered that there is a learning effect with this test so it is not good for serial assessments.[245,271] The test does not evaluate pursuit, convergence, or accommodation[69] which also should be tested if a concussion is suspected as deficits related to oculomotor dysfunction and mTBI include anticipatory saccades during smooth pursuits, antisaccades (i.e., voluntary eye movements away from the side to which the stimulus was presented), nystagmus, and an altered VOR.[57,64,76,276,280]

⚠ *Vestibular Oculomotor Screening for Concussion.* In general, isolated posttraumatic vestibular injuries present with symptoms of true positional vertigo (i.e., a sensation of motion and nausea precipitated by head motion and typically without other associated postconcussion symptoms). Vestibular symptoms caused primarily by concussion, although they may be temporarily exacerbated by head position, typically do not demonstrate nystagmus; the Dix-Hallpike maneuver is almost always present at rest with or without head motion and is associated with multiple other postconcussion symptom complaints such as light-headedness and cognitive problems.[79]

The **VOR**, located in the brain stem, is the most important structure of the vestibular system. It has three main planes of action: horizontal head rotation about a vertical

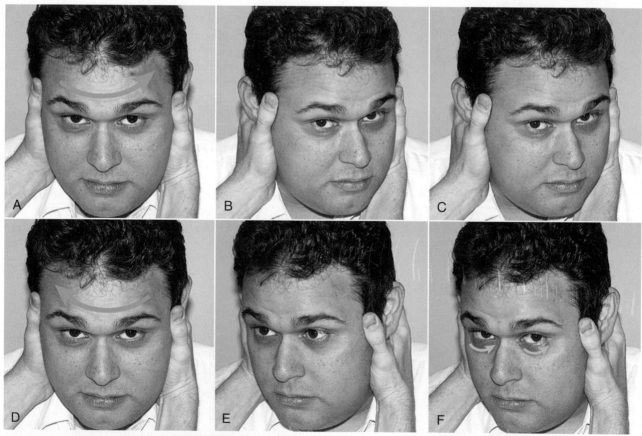

Fig. 2.61 Head thrust test. The examiner asks the subject to fix the gaze on the examiner's nose. The examiner rapidly turns the subject's head but only by approximately 10° to 15°; larger angles of rotation are unnecessary and may risk injury to the neck. The acceleration must be ≥3000 degrees/s², and the peak velocity must be 150 to 300 degrees/s, meaning that the rotation must be finished in 150 ms. (A–C) Show a head thrust to the left, exciting the left horizontal canal (HC). The eyes stay on the examiner's nose throughout the maneuver, indicating normal left HC function. (D–F) show a head thrust to the right, exciting the right HC. The eyes do not stay on target but move with the head during the head thrust (D and E). A refixation saccade brings the eyes back on target after completion of the head movement (F). This is a "positive" head-thrust sign for the right HC, which indicates hypofunction of that canal. (From Carey JP, Della Santina CC: Principles of applied vestibular physiology. In Flint PW, Haughey BH, Lund V, et al., eds. *Cummings otolaryngology*, ed 6, Philadelphia, 2015, Saunders.)

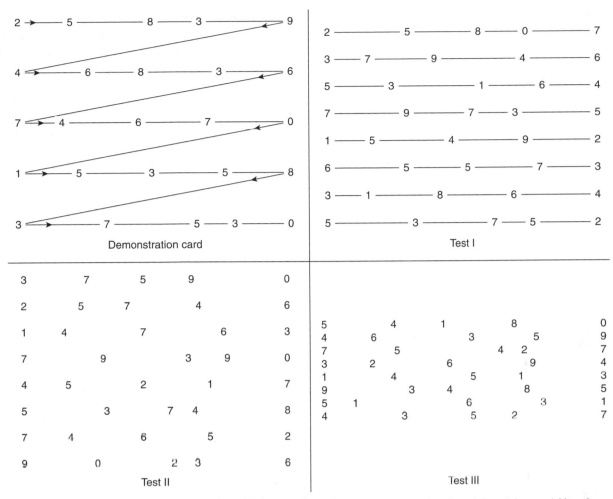

Fig. 2.62 King-Devick (K-D) Test. To perform the K-D test, the participant is asked to read the numbers from left to right as quickly as he or she can without making any errors. The tester should start the stopwatch when the subject reads the first number and stop the watch when the last number has been read. Time required to complete each card is recorded in seconds using a stopwatch, and the K-D time score is based on the cumulative time taken to read all three test cards. The number of errors made in reading the test cards is also recorded; misspeaks on numbers are recorded as errors if the subject does not immediately correct the mistake before continuing on to the next number. (From Leong DF, Balcer LJ, Galetta SL, et al: The King-Devick Test for sideline concussion screening in collegiate football, *J Optometry* 8:131–139, 2015.)

axis (yaw), head extension or flexion about the horizontal axis (pitch), and lateral head tilt about the horizontal x-axis (roll).[270] Yaw plane signs include horizontal nystagmus, altered past-pointing, and horizontal deviation from looking straight ahead (i.e., patient thinks he or she is looking straight ahead). Roll plane signs include torsional nystagmus, skewed deviation, ocular torsion, tilt of the head or body, and an ocular tilt reaction. Pitch plane signs are upbeat or downbeat nystagmus, forward or backward tilts and falls, and vertical deviation of the procedure from looking straight ahead.[270] Bilateral or peripheral loss of vestibular function is shown via oscillopsia during head movements, and instability of gait and posture which increases in the darkness or on uneven ground. Unilateral acute or subacute failure of the vestibular system is shown via a rotary vertigo or apparent body tilt, nystagmus, oscillopsia, nausea, and a tendency to fall.[270]

The **Vestibular/Ocular Motor Screening (VOMS)** (eTool 2.20) is an extensive screen of control of eye movements that indicate vestibular oculomotor causes of vertigo or dizziness. The screen includes tests for smooth pursuits, horizontal saccades, vertical saccades, convergence, the horizontal VOR test, the vertical VOR test, a test for visual motion sensitivity (VMS), accommodation, ocular motor palsies, and visual tracking (i.e., saccadic eye motion with symptoms during smooth pursuit testing or abnormal NPC).[69] To properly diagnose vestibular symptoms resulting in vertigo or dizziness, it is important to determine the type of vertigo and its duration, what triggers or exacerbates the vertigo, and whether the vertigo is associated with auditory dysfunction, headache or nonvestibular neurological signs and symptoms.[270] Table 2.27 describes the ocular changes that may be seen during the VOMS test.[160]

TABLE **2.27**

Vestibulo-Ocular Motor Screening Description

Ocular Test	Targeted Functional Ability
Smooth pursuits	Ability to follow a slowly moving target
Saccades-horizontal, saccades-vertical	Ability of the eyes to move between targets without head movement in each directional plane
Vestibulo-ocular reflex, horizontal; vestibulo-ocular reflex, vertical	Ability to stabilize vision during head movement in each directional plane
Visual motion sensitivity test	Ability to inhibit vestibular-induced eye movements using vision and motion sensitivity

Before beginning the screening test, participants rate headache, dizziness, nausea, and mental fogginess on a 6-point Likert scale in a similar fashion to the Postconcussion Symptoms Scale or 10-point visual analog scale. After each component, participants provide a rating for each of the four symptoms. The targeted function is described in the above table for each component of the screening.

Modified from Henry LC, Elbin RJ, Collins MW, et al: Examining recovery trajectories after sport related concussion with a multimodal clinical assessment approach, *Neurosurgery* 78(2):232–241, 2016.

Tests for Clinical Reaction Time

A prolonged reaction time is common following concussion and is one of the most sensitive indices of neurocognitive change following injury. A greater than 10% increase in reaction time in athletes tested within 72 hours of concussion has been reported as compared with baseline.[226]

⚠ *Drop Ruler Test.* The Drop Ruler Test is a simple reaction time test that can be used in the clinical setting.[281] To do this test, the examiner holds a long ruler or measuring stick vertically. The patient sits with the dominant arm resting on the table with a hand positioned over the edge of the table. The examiner holds a ruler vertically such that the ruler is in line with the top of the patient's open hand (Fig. 2.63A). The patient's hand is open or surrounding the ruler without touching the ruler. It is important that the distance between the patient's thumb and index finger at the start of the test remain constant during all trials. When the patient is ready, and using random intervals ranging from 2 to 5 seconds, the examiner releases the ruler and the patient catches it as quickly as possible by closing the thumb and index finger around the ruler (Fig 2.63B). The distance the ruler has fallen before the patient grasps the ruler is measured at the superior aspect of the ruler. The patient is given two practice trials and then completes three recorded trials. The mean

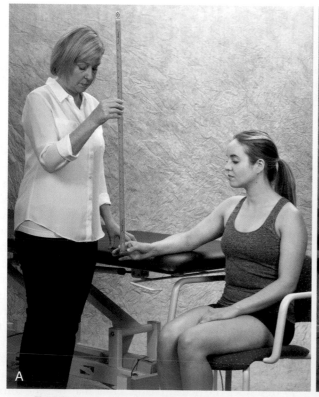
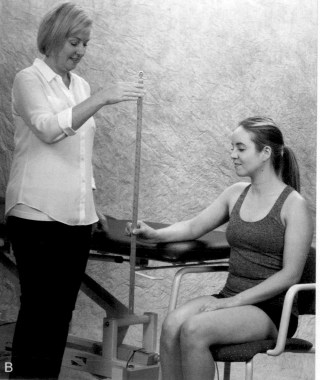

Fig. 2.63 Drop ruler test. (A) Starting position. (B) Examiner releases the ruler and the patient catches it as quickly as possible.

clinical reaction time is calculated using the formula for a body under the influence of gravity (distance × ½ gravity × time falling squared [G. = −9.8 m/s²]).[133,226,281–283]

Tests for Proprioception

❓ *Past Pointing Test.* The test is performed as described under Tests for Coordination.

⚠️ *Proprioceptive Finger-Nose Test.* The patient keeps the eyes closed. The examiner lightly touches one of the patient's fingers and asks the patient to touch the patient's nose with that finger. The examiner then touches another finger on the other hand, and the patient again touches the nose. Patients with proprioceptive loss have difficulty doing the test without visual input.

❓ *Proprioceptive Movement Test.* With the patient's eyes closed, the examiner moves the patient's finger or toe slowly up or down by grasping it on the sides to lessen clues given by pressure. The patient then tells the examiner which way the digit moved.

❓ *Proprioceptive Space Test.* With the patient's eyes closed, the examiner places one of the patient's hands or feet in a selected position in space. The patient then imitates that position with the other limb or finds the hand or foot with the other limb. True proprioceptive loss causes the patient to be unable to properly position or to find the normal limb with the limb that has proprioceptive loss.

Tests for Hearing

⚠️ *Rinne Test.* The Rinne test is performed by placing the base of the vibrating tuning fork against the patient's mastoid bone and starts a stopwatch. The patient tells the examiner when he or she no longer hears the sound, and the examiner notes the seconds on the stopwatch. The examiner then quickly positions a still-vibrating tine 1 to 2 cm (0.5 to 0.8 inch) from the auditory canal and asks patient to indicate when he or she no longer hears the sound. The examiner then compares the number of seconds the sound was heard by bone conduction (first time in seconds) and by air conduction (second time in seconds). The counting or timing of the interval between the two sounds determines the length of time that sound is heard by air conduction (Fig. 2.64). Air-conducted sound should be heard twice as long as bone-conducted sound. For example, if bone conduction is heard for 15 seconds, the air conduction should be heard for 30 seconds.[189–191]

❓ *Schwabach Test.* This test compares the patient's and examiner's hearing by bone conduction. The examiner alternately places the vibrating tuning fork against the patient's mastoid process and against the examiner's mastoid bone until one of them no longer hears a sound. The examiner and patient should hear the sound for equal amounts of time.[189,190]

❓ *Ticking Watch Test.* The ticking watch test uses a non-electric ticking watch to test high-frequency hearing. The examiner positions the watch approximately 15 cm (6 inches) from the ear to be tested, slowly moving it toward the ear.

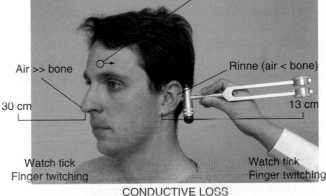

Fig. 2.64 Bedside hearing tests and results with sensorineural or conductive loss in left ear and with normal hearing.

The patient then indicates when he or she hears the ticking sound. The distance can be measured and will give some idea of the patient's ability to hear high-frequency sound.[189,190]

❓ *Weber Test.* The examiner places the base of a vibrating tuning fork on the midline vertex of the patient's head. The patient should hear the sound equally well in both ears (Fig. 2.65). If the patient hears better in one ear (i.e., the sound is lateralized), the patient is asked to identify which ear hears the sound better. To test the reliability of the patient's response,

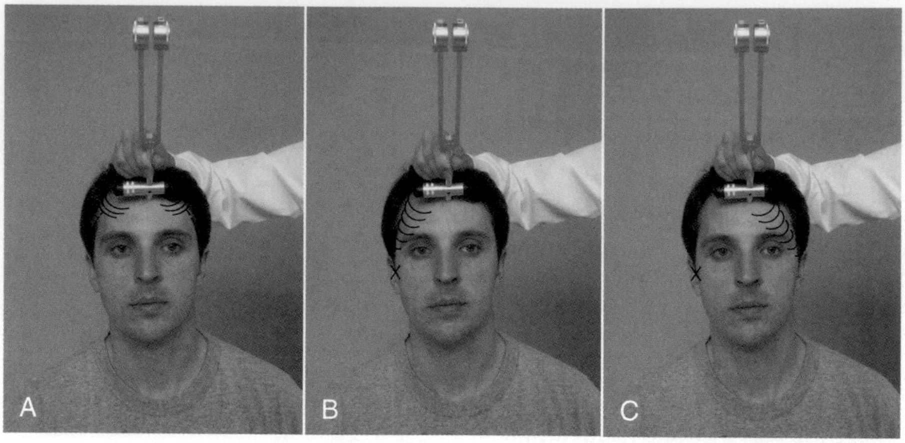

Fig. 2.65 The Weber test. (A) When a vibrating tuning fork is placed on the center of the forehead, the sound is heard in the center without lateralization to either side (normal response). (B) In the presence of a conductive hearing loss, the sound is heard on the side of the conductive loss. (C) In the presence of sensorineural loss, the sound is better heard on the opposite (unaffected) side.

the examiner repeats the procedure while occluding one ear with a finger and asks the patient which ear hears the sound better. It should be heard better in the occluded ear.[189,190]

❓ *Whispered Voice Test.* The patient's response to the examiner's whispered voice can be used to determine hearing ability. The examiner masks the hearing in one of the patient's ears by placing a finger gently in the patient's ear canal. Standing approximately 30 to 60 cm (12 to 24 inches) away from the patient, the examiner whispers one- or two-syllable words and asks the patient to repeat them. If the patient has difficulty, the examiner gradually increases his or her volume until the patient responds appropriately. The procedure is repeated in the other ear. The patient should be able to hear whispered words in each ear at a distance of 30 to 60 cm (12 to 24 inches) and respond correctly at least 50% of the time.[189,190]

Graded Exercise After Concussion

Normally, especially in children and adolescents, a period of 2 to 3 days of **cognitive rest** should be observed following a concussion. Prolonged rest beyond the first couple of days may hinder rather than aid recovery because the patient may not respond well to prolonged removal from the social and physical environment which may lead to the prolonged rest adversely affecting the physiology of the concussion.[77,284,285] Symptom limited activity is safe as long as one uses a predetermined stopping criteria **prior to symptom exacerbation** and can be used to help the patient maintain aerobic capacity.[77] Aerobic exercise may help concussion-related physiological dysfunction because exercise increases parasympathetic activity, reduces sympathetic activation, and improves cerebral blood flow.[31,77,156] Aerobic exercise is also useful in treating depression.[156]

☑️ *Buffalo Concussion Treadmill Test.* This test (eTool 2.21) was developed to systematically evaluate exercise tolerance in individuals with prolonged concussion symptoms (i.e., more than 3 to 6 weeks). The test is based on the **Balke Cardiac Treadmill Test,**[286,287] (eTool 2.22) which requires a gradual increase in workload while walking and has been shown to be safe and reliable in

patients with cardiac problems.[79] Before the BCTT can begin, the patient must be asymptomatic of any concussion symptoms at rest. By determining **subthreshold exercise heart rate**, the test helps to determine when the individual can start doing exercises to regain or restore physical fitness and the level that the individual can work at while not causing symptoms.[156] The data from the test allow the examiner to develop an individualized exercise treatment program to restore the physiology to normal enhancing recovery.[77,104,142] If symptoms were provoked during vestibular oculomotor testing, then cycling may be chosen as the exercise device to minimize head movement compared with the treadmill. Regardless of the modality used, patients are instructed to inform the examiner whether there is any worsening of symptoms.[47] If needed, the Buffalo Concussion Physical Examination (eTool 2.23) can be completed before the treadmill test. Exercise testing should be considered only for patients without orthopedic or vestibular problems that increase the risk of falling off the treadmill, bike, or elliptical machine and only if the patient does not suffer from cardiac disease (Tables 2.28 and 2.29).[77]

The test is performed on a treadmill and begins at a speed of 3.2 to 3.6 mph, depending on the patient's age and height, and 0° incline. This is a warm-up speed, and the speed and time can be altered as necessary. After the warm-up, the test then begins. During the first minute of the test, the speed and incline remain the same (i.e., 3.2 to 3.6 mph at 0°). The incline is then increased by 1° each minute while maintaining the same walking speed until symptoms become evident (usually well short of normal age-predicted maximum exercise capacity) or the maximum incline is reached, and the patient is instructed to stop.[77] The examiner should be cautious because neurological symptoms have also been reported in healthy individuals after intense exercise and cervical symptoms, and migraine headaches can occasionally be exacerbated during the final stages of the test.[77] During the test, the heart rate (using a chest strap) and blood pressure are measured every 2 minutes. At the start of the third

TABLE **2.28**

Absolute and Relative Contraindications to the Buffalo Concussion Treadmill Test[77,79]

Absolute Contraindications

History	Unwilling to exercise Increased risk for cardiopulmonary disease[a]
Physical examination	Focal neurologic deficit (i.e., a problem with brain, spinal cord, or nerve function) Significant balance/vestibular deficit, visual deficit, or orthopedic injury/motor dysfunction that does represent a significant risk for walking/running on a treadmill Score higher than 7 out of 10 on symptom severity scale

Relative Contraindications

History	β-Blocker use Major depression (may not comply with directions or prescription) Does not understand English
Physical examination	Minor balance deficit, visual deficit, or orthopedic injury that increases risk for walking/running on a treadmill Resting systolic BP >140 mm Hg or diastolic BP > 90 mm Hg Obesity: body mass index >30 kg/m^2

BP, Blood pressure.

[a]Individuals with known cardiovascular, pulmonary, or metabolic disease; signs and symptoms suggestive of cardiovascular or pulmonary disease; or individuals greater than 45 years who have more than one risk factor, including (1) family history of myocardial infarction, coronary revascularization, or sudden death before age 55 years; (2) cigarette smoking; (3) hypertension; (4) hypercholesterolemia; (5) impaired fasting glucose level; or (6) obesity (body mass index >30 kg/m^2).
Modified from Leddy JJ, Willer B: Use of graded exercise testing in concussion and return-to-activity management, *Curr Sports Med Rep* 12(6):372, 2013.

minute and each minute thereafter, the grade is increased by 1° while the heart rate and rate of perceived exertion (Fig. 2.66) and any symptom occurrence are noted. The test is stopped if there are any significant exacerbation of symptoms (defined as greater than or equal to three points from that day's pre–treadmill test overall symptom score of rest on a visual analog scale [see eTool 2.21] or at exhaustion). (Note: If a cycle ergometer is used, the protocol cadence is maintained at 60 rpm and the resistance is initially set at level 1 being increased by one level every minute). If the patient reaches maximum incline and can still continue, the speed is increased by 0.04 mph for each subsequent minute until stopping criteria are fulfilled.[48,79] The safety protocol dictates that exercise be stopped according to a predetermined stopping criterion.[104] Once the diagnosis of a physiological concussion has been established (i.e., the symptoms are due to a concussion) by treadmill testing and the patient symptoms threshold target heart rate is established, the patient is prescribed exercise at 80% to 90% of the *symptom threshold* **heart rate** which becomes his or her individual target heart rate. The patient is then asked to exercise for 20 minutes per day at 80% to 90% of the symptom threshold heart rate with a 5-minute warm-up and 5-minute cooldown for a total exercise duration of 30 minutes per day for 6 or 7 days per week. The use of a heart rate monitor is important to prevent athletes from overexerting, which will precipitate symptoms. The patient is advised to stop exercise if symptoms are exacerbated or after 20 minutes of exercise (i.e., 30 minutes total time) has been reached, whichever comes first. The patient may be advised to do the exercise program on the bicycle ergometer or elliptical machine to minimize any provocation of vestibular problems and then progress to treadmill running. The symptoms threshold heart rate is increased by 5 to 10 beats/min every 1 to 2 weeks, depending on how fast the patient responds to the exercise and the absence of any symptoms. Once the patient is able to do exercise at a greater than or equal to 85% of the symptoms threshold heart rate for 20 minutes, the patient should be evaluated to see if he or she can return to school, work, practice, or games. Advice on return to play is based not only on the test but also on history (e.g., depending on a number of prior concussions and the presence of other signs and symptoms [e.g., ocular or vestibular dysfunction] that need to be resolved) before full return to practice, work, or school is advised.[77,104] It is advisable to have someone present during the exercise training for safety monitoring and who should terminate exercise at the first sign of symptom exacerbation. The test can be repeated every 2 to 3 weeks to establish new symptom threshold heart rate until symptoms are no longer exacerbated on the bike, elliptical, or treadmill, or one can establish the symptoms threshold heart rate on the initial test and increase exercise heart rate by 5 to 10 beats/min every 2 weeks, provided the patient responds favorably.[79] Physiological resolution of postconcussion symptoms is defined as the ability to exercise to volunteer exhaustion at 85% to 90% of **age-predicted maximum heart rate** for 20 minutes without exacerbation of symptoms.[79] If no postconcussion symptoms are occurring at this level, the patient can be cleared to return to practice, work, or games and follow the return to practice/game protocols.[32,79,288]

Stopping Criteria for the Buffalo Concussion Treadmill Test

- Exacerbation of symptoms
- Feeling faint or light-headed
- Borg scale rating of 6 or more
- Nausea
- Symptom severity scale >1

TABLE **2.29**

Summary of Pathophysiology, Predominant Symptoms, Pertinent Physical Examination Findings, Graded Treadmill Test Results, and Treatment Options in Patients with Postconcussion Disorders[71,79]

	Physiological PCD	Vestibulo-ocular PCD	Cerviogenic PCD
Pathophysiology	• Persistent alterations in neuronal depolarization, cell membrane permeability, mitochondrial function, cellular metabolism, and cerebral blood flow	• Dysfunction of the vestibular and oculomotor symptoms	• Muscle trauma and inflammation • Dysfunction of cervical spine proprioception
Predominant symptoms	• Headache exacerbated by physical and cognitive activity • Nausea, intermittent vomiting, photophobia, phonophobia, dizziness, fatigue, difficulty concentrating, slowed speech, light-headedness, pressure in head	• Dizziness, vertigo, nausea, light-headedness, gait instability and postural instability at rest • Blurred or double vision, difficulty tracking objects and focusing, motion sensitivity, photophobia, eye strain or brow-ache, and headache exacerbated by activities that worsen vestibulo-ocular symptoms (e.g., when reading)	• Neck pain, stiffness, and decreased range of motion • Occipital headaches exacerbated by head movements and not physical or cognitive activity • Light-headedness and postural imbalance
Physical exam findings	• No focal neurological findings • Elevated resting HR	• Impairments on standardized balance and gait testing • Impaired VOR, fixation, convergence, horizontal and vertical saccades	• Decreased cervical lordosis and range of motion • Paraspinal and suboccipital muscle tenderness/spasm • Impaired head-neck position sense (i.e., proprioception)
Graded treadmill test	• Graded treadmill tests are often terminated early due to symptom onset or exacerbation	• Patients typically reach maximal exertion without exacerbation of vestibulo-ocular symptoms on graded treadmill tests	• Patients typically reach maximal exertion without exacerbation of cervicogenic symptoms on graded treadmill tests
Management options	• Physical and cognitive rest • School accommodations • Sub–symptom threshold aerobic exercise programs should be considered for adolescent and adult athletes	• Vestibular rehabilitation program • Vision therapy program • School accommodations • Sub–symptom threshold aerobic exercise programs should be considered for adolescent athletes	• Cervical spine manual therapy • Head-neck proprioception retraining • Balance and gaze stabilization exercises • Sub–symptom threshold aerobic exercise programs should be considered for adolescent and adult athletes

HR, Heart rate; *PCD,* postconcussion disorders; *VOR,* vestibulo-ocular reflex.
Modified from Ellis MJ, Leddy JJ, Willer B: Physiological, vestibulo-ocular and cervicogenic postconcussion disorders: An evident space classification system with directions for treatment, *Brain Inj* 29(2):241, 2015.

If, during the test, the patient can exercise to exhaustion without reproduction of or exacerbation of the headache or other concussion symptoms, and he or she demonstrates a normal physiological response to exercise, then it can be concluded that the symptoms the patient is having are not due to a physiological concussion but to other problems such as a cervical injury, vestibular/ocular dysfunction, or a posttraumatic headache syndrome such as migraine.[79]

Reflexes and Cutaneous Distribution

With a head injury patient, deep tendon reflexes (see Table 1.30) should be tested. Accentuation of one or more of the reflexes may indicate trauma to the brain on the opposite side. Pathological reflexes (see Table 1.32) may also be altered with a head injury.

The **corneal reflex** (trigeminal nerve, cranial nerve V) is used to test for damage or dysfunction to the pons. In some cases, the patient may look to one side to avoid involuntary blinking. The examiner touches the cornea (not the eyelashes or conjunctiva) with a small, fine point of cotton (Fig. 2.67). The normal response is a bilateral blink because the reflex arc connects both facial nerve nuclei. If the reflex is absent, the test is considered positive.

The **gag reflex** may be tested using a tongue depressor that is inserted into the posterior pharynx and depressed

Borg RPE Scale®

Use this scale to tell how strenuous and tiring the work feels to you. RPE stand for Ratings ® of Perceived (P) Exertion (E). The exertion is mainly felt as fatigue in your muscles and as breathlessness or possibly aches. When the exercise is hard it also becomes difficult to talk. It is your own feeling of exertion that is important. Don't underestimate it, but don't overestimate it either. For common exercise, such as cycling, running or walking, 11-15 is a good level. For strength and high-intensity interval training (HIIT), 15-19 is good. If you are sick follow your doctor's advice. Look at the scale and the descriptions and then assign a number. Use whatever numbers you want, even numbers between the descriptions.

6	No exertion at all	No muscle fatigue, breathlessness or difficulty in breathing.
7	Extremely light	Very, very light.
8		
9	Very light	Like walking slowly for a short while. Very easy to talk.
10		
11	Light	Like a light exercise at your own pace.
12	Moderate	
13	Somewhat hard	Fairly strenuous and breathless. Not so easy to talk.
14		
15	Hard	Heavy and strenuous. An upper limit for fitness training, as when running or walking fast.
16		
17	Very hard	Very strenuous and tiring. Very difficult to talk.
18		
19	Extremely hard	The most strenuous effort you have ever experienced.
20	Maximal exertion	Maximal heaviness.

Borg RPE Scale®
© Gunnar Borg, 1970, 1998, 2017
English

Fig. 2.66 Borg scale of perceived exertion. (Copyright Gunnar Borg, 1970, 1985, 1994, 1998. From Borg G: *Borg's perceived exertion and pain scales.* Champaign, IL, 1998, Human Kinetics.)

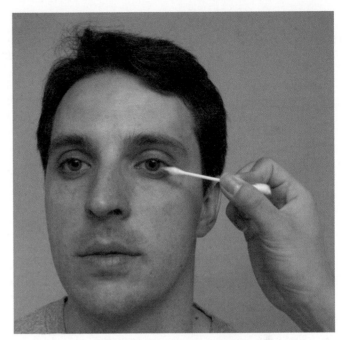

Fig. 2.67 Test of corneal reflex.

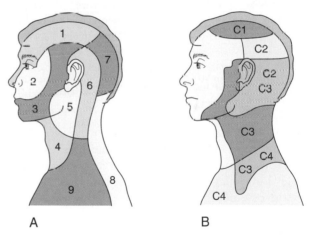

Fig. 2.68 (A) Sensory nerve distribution of the head, neck and face. *1*, Ophthalmic nerve; *2*, maxillary nerve; *3*, mandibular nerve; *4*, transverse cutaneous nerve of neck (C2–C3); *5*, greater auricular nerve (C2–C3); *6*, lesser auricular nerve (C2); *7*, greater occipital nerve (C2–C3); *8*, cervical dorsal rami (C3–C5); *9*, suprascapular nerve (C5–C6). (B) Dermatome pattern of the head, neck, and face. Note the overlap of C3.

toward the hypopharynx. The reflex tests cranial nerves IX and X, and its absence in a trauma setting may indicate caudal brain stem dysfunction.

Consensual light reflex may be tested by shining a light into one eye. This action causes the lighted pupil to constrict. If there is normal communication between the two oculomotor nerves, the nonlighted pupil also constricts.

The **jaw reflex** is usually tested only if the temporomandibular joint or cervical spine is being examined.

The examiner should check the sensation of the head and face, keeping in mind the differences in dermatome and sensory nerve distributions (Fig. 2.68). Lip anesthesia or paresthesia is often seen in patients with mandibular fracture.

Nerve Injuries of the Head and Face

Bell's palsy involves paralysis of the facial nerve (cranial nerve VII) and usually occurs where the nerve emerges from the stylomastoid foramen. Pressure in the foramen caused by inflammation or trauma affects the nerve and therefore the muscles of the face (i.e., occipitofrontalis, corrugator, orbicularis oculi, and the nose and mouth muscles) on one side. The inflammation may result from a middle ear infection, viral infection, chilling of the face, or tumor. The observable result is smoothing of the face on the affected side owing to loss of muscle action, the eye on the affected side remaining open, and the lower eyelid sagging. The patient is unable to wink, whistle, purse the lips, or wrinkle the forehead. Speech sounds, especially those requiring pursing of the lips, are affected, resulting in slurred speech. The mouth droops, and it and the nose may deviate to the opposite side, especially in longstanding cases, of which there are remarkably few (90% of patients recover completely

TABLE **2.30**

House-Brackmann Facial Nerve Grading System

Parameter	Grade I	Grade II	Grade III	Grade IV	Grade V	Grade VI
Overall appearance	Normal	Slight weakness on close inspection	Obvious but not disfiguring difference between both sides	Obvious weakness and/or disfiguring asymmetry	Only barely perceptible motion	No movement
At rest	Normal symmetry	Normal symmetry	Normal symmetry	Normal symmetry	Asymmetry	Asymmetry
Forehead movement	Normal with excellent function	Moderate to good function	Slight to moderate function	None	None	None
Eyelid closure	Normal closure	Complete with minimum effort	Complete with maximal effort	Incomplete closure with maximal effort	Incomplete closure with maximal effort	No movement
Mouth	Normal and symmetric	Slight asymmetry	Slight asymmetry with maximum effort	Asymmetry with maximum effort	Slight movement	No movement
Synkinesis[a] contracture and/or hemifacial spasm	None	May have very slight synkinesis; no contracture or hemifacial spasm	Obvious but not disfiguring synkinesis contracture and/or hemifacial spasm	Synkinesis contracture and/or asymmetrical facial spasm leading to disfiguring severe enough to interfere with function	Synkinesis contracture and/or hemifacial spasm usually absent	No movement

[a]*Synkinesis*: an abnormal voluntary muscle movement causing simultaneous contraction of other muscles.
Modified from Dutton M: *Orthopedic examination, evaluation, and intervention*, New York, 2004, McGraw Hill, p 1130. Adapted from Houie JW, Brackmann HE: Facial nerve grading system, *Otolaryngol Head Neck Surg* 93:146–147, 1985.

within 2 to 8 weeks). Facial sensation on the affected side is lost, and taste sensation is sometimes lost as well. The House-Brackmann Facial Nerve Grading System (Table 2.30) may be used to grade the level of facial nerve involvement.[289]

Joint Play Movements

Because no articular joints are involved in the assessment of the head and face, there are no joint play movements to test.

Palpation

During palpation of the head and face, the examiner should note any tenderness, deformity, crepitus, or other signs and symptoms that may indicate the source of pathology. The examiner should note the texture of the skin and surrounding bony and soft tissues. Normally, the patient is palpated in the sitting or supine position, beginning with the skull and moving from anterior to posterior, to the face, and finally to the lateral and posterior structures of the head.

The skull is palpated by a gentle rotary movement of the fingers, progressing systematically from front to back. Normally, the skin of the skull moves freely and has no tenderness, swelling, or depressions.

The temporal area and temporalis muscle should be laterally palpated for tenderness and deformity. The external ear or auricle and the periauricular area should also be palpated for tenderness or lacerations.

The occiput should be palpated posteriorly for tenderness. The presence of **Battle sign** (see Fig. 2.17) should be noted, if observed, because this signals a possible basilar skull fracture. The sign may take 2 or 3 days to become visible.

The face is palpated beginning superiorly and working inferiorly in a systematic manner. Like the skull, the forehead is palpated by gentle rotary movements of the fingers, feeling the movement of the skin and the occipitofrontalis muscle underneath. Normally, the skin of the forehead moves freely and is smooth and even with no tender areas. The examiner then palpates around the eye socket or orbital rim, moving over the eyebrow and supraorbital rims, around the lateral side of the eye, and along the zygomatic arch to the infraorbital rims, looking for deformity, crepitus, tenderness, and lacerations/scarring from previous lacerations (Fig. 2.69A and B). The orbicularis oculi muscles surround the orbit, and the medial side of the orbital rim and nose are then palpated for tenderness, deformity, and fracture. The nasal bones, including the lateral and alar cartilage, are palpated for any crepitus or deviation (Fig. 2.69C). The septum should be inspected to see if it has widened, possibly indicating a septal hematoma, which often occurs with a fracture. It should also be determined whether the patient can breathe through the nose or smell.

The frontal and maxillary sinuses should be inspected for swelling. To palpate the frontal sinuses, the examiner uses the thumbs to press up under the bony brow on each side of the nose (Fig. 2.70A). The examiner then presses under the zygomatic processes using either the thumbs or index and middle fingers to palpate the maxillary sinuses (Fig. 2.70B). No tenderness or swelling over the soft tissue should be present. The sinus areas may also be percussed to detect tenderness. A light tap directly over each sinus with the index finger can be used to detect tenderness.

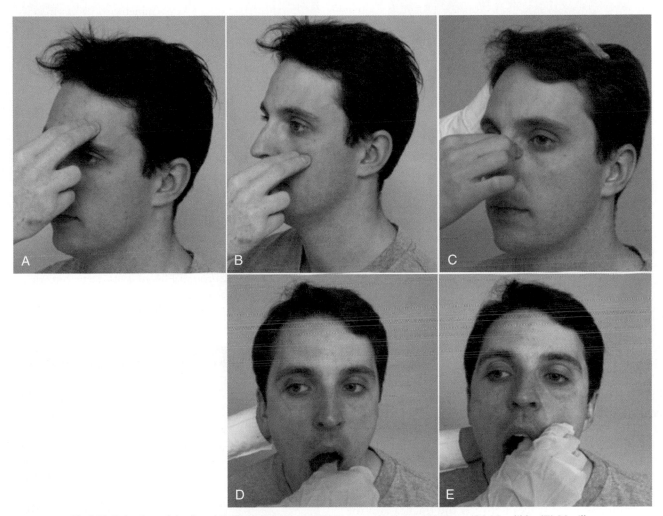

Fig. 2.69 Palpation of the face. (A) Upper orbital rim. (B) Lower orbital rim. (C) Nose. (D) Mandible. (E) Maxilla.

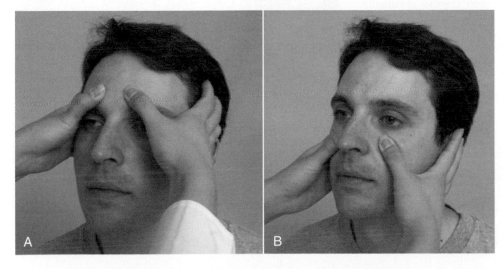

Fig. 2.70 (A) Palpation of frontal sinuses. (B) Palpation of maxillary sinuses.

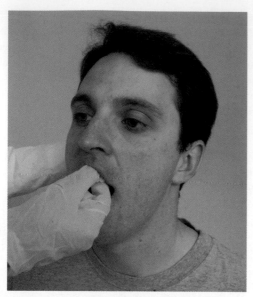

Fig. 2.71 Palpation of maxillary fracture with anteroposterior rocking motion.

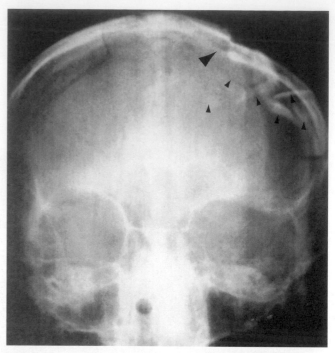

Fig. 2.72 Normal anteroposterior view of the head and face showing a depressed parietal skull fracture *(large arrowhead)* with multiple bony fragments into the brain *(small arrowheads)*. (From Albright JP, et al: Head and neck injuries in sports. In Scott WN, et al, editors: *Principles of sports medicine*, Baltimore, 1984, Lippincott Williams & Wilkins, p 53.)

The examiner then moves inferiorly to palpate the jaw. The examiner palpates the mandible along its entire length, noting any tenderness, crepitus, or deformity. The examiner, wearing a rubber glove, may also palpate along the mandible interiorly, noting any tenderness or pain (Fig. 2.69D). The outside hand may be used to stabilize the jaw during this procedure. The mandible may also be tapped with a finger along its length to see if signs of tenderness are elicited. The muscles of the cheek (buccinator) and mouth (orbicularis oris) should be palpated at the same time.

The maxilla may be palpated in a similar fashion, both internally and externally, noting position of the teeth, tenderness, and any deformity (Fig. 2.69E). The examiner may grasp the teeth anteriorly to see if the teeth and mandible or maxilla move in relation to the rest of the face, which may indicate a Le Fort fracture (Fig. 2.71).

The trachea should be palpated for midline position. The examiner places a thumb along each side of the trachea, comparing the spaces between the trachea and the sternocleidomastoid muscle, which should be symmetric. The hyoid bone and the thyroid and cricoid cartilages should be identified. Normally, they are smooth and nontender and move when the patient swallows.

Diagnostic Imaging

Plain Film Radiography

Common x-rays taken involving the head and face are outlined in the following box.

Common X-Ray Views of the Head and Face Depending on Pathology

- Anteroposterior view (Fig. 2.72)
- Lateral view (Fig. 2.73)

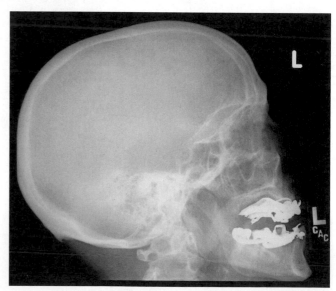

Fig. 2.73 Normal lateral view of the head and face.

Anteroposterior View. The examiner should note the normal bone contours, looking for fractures of the various bones (Figs. 2.74 and 2.75; see Fig. 2.72).

Lateral View. The examiner should again note bony contours, looking for the possibility of fractures (Fig. 2.76).

Computed Tomography

CT scans help to differentiate between bone and soft tissue and give a more precise view of fractures (Figs. 2.77 and 2.78). The **Canadian Computed Tomography Head Rule** or **New Orleans Criteria** have been developed to help the clinician decide when to use CT scans in minor head injury patients.[59] The authors of the rule have defined minor head injury as witnessed loss of consciousness, definite amnesia, or witnessed disorientation in patients with a Glasgow Coma Scale score of 13 to 15. CT scans are not usually recommended in concussion cases unless there is a suspected skull fracture, intracranial hemorrhage, neurological deficit, prolonged level of unconsciousness, or progressive deterioration of the patient.[31,37,42,52–55]

Magnetic Resonance Imaging

MRI is especially useful for demonstrating lesions of the soft tissues of the head and face and for differentiating between bone and soft tissue (Figs. 2.79 and 2.80). As with CT scans, MRI is not usually recommended in concussion cases except with the same suspicions.[31,37,42,52–55]

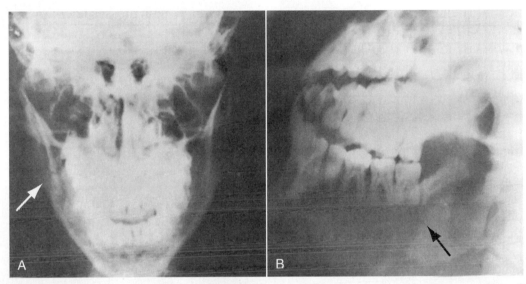

Fig. 2.74 Incomplete fracture of angle of mandible on the left side *(arrows)*. (A) Anteroposterior view. (B) Lateral view. (From O'Donoghue DH: *Treatment of injuries to athletes*, Philadelphia, 1984, WB Saunders, p 114.)

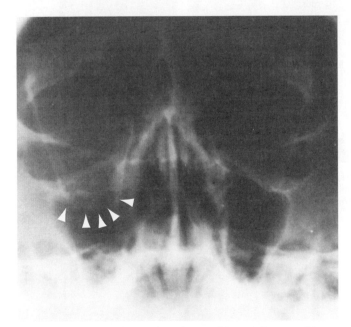

Fig. 2.75 Plain posteroanterior view showing blowout fracture of the orbit *(arrowheads)*. (From Paton D, Goldberg MF: *Management of ocular injuries*, Philadelphia, 1976, WB Saunders, p 70.)

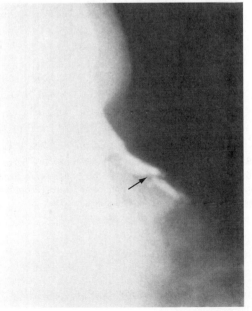

Fig. 2.76 Lateral radiograph of the nasal bones demonstrating a nasal fracture *(arrow)*. (From Torg JS: *Athletic injuries to the head, neck and face*, Philadelphia, 1982, Lea & Febiger, p 229.)

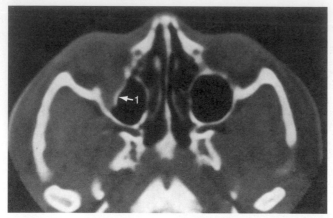

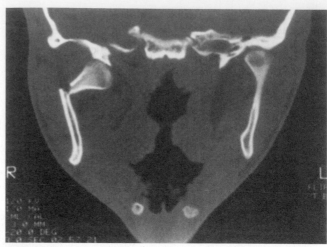

Fig. 2.77 Axial computed tomogram of orbital blowout fracture showing fracture of the orbit *(1)* with orbital contents herniated into the maxillary sinus. (From Sinn DP, Karas ND: Radiographic evaluation of facial injuries. In Fonseca RJ, Walker RV, editors: *Oral and maxillofacial trauma*, Philadelphia, 1991, WB Saunders.)

Fig. 2.78 The computed tomographic scan is ideal for condylar fractures as seen in the right condyle. (From Bruce R, Fonseca RJ: Mandibular fractures. In Fonseca RJ, Walker RV, editors: *Oral and maxillofacial trauma*, Philadelphia, 1991, WB Saunders, p 389.)

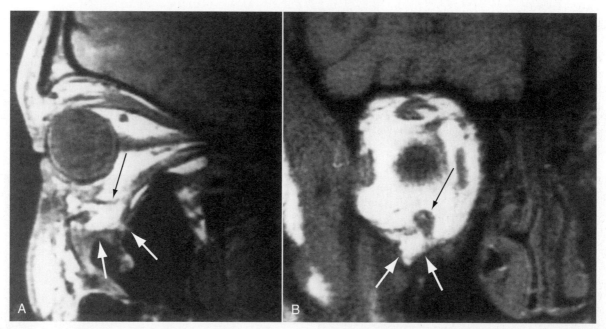

Fig. 2.79 Magnetic resonance images showing blowout fracture. Sagittal (A) and coronal (B) T1-weighted scans demonstrate a blowout fracture of the right orbit with depression of the orbital floor *(white arrows)* into the superior maxillary sinus. The inferior rectus muscle *(long arrow)* is clearly identified and is not entrapped by the floor fracture. (From Harms SE: The orbit. In Edelman RR, Hesselink JR, editors: *Clinical magnetic resonance imaging*, Philadelphia, 1990, WB Saunders, p 619.)

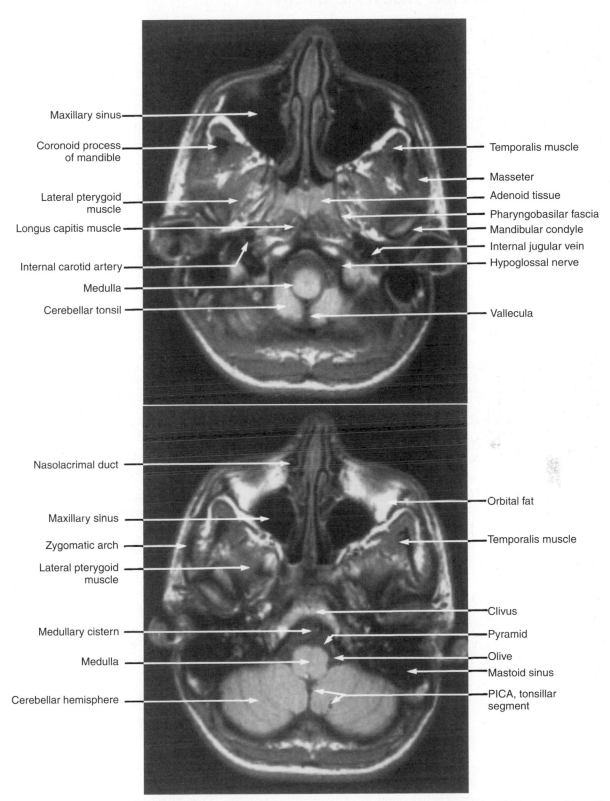

Fig. 2.80 T1-weighted axial magnetic resonance images of the head and brain at two levels. *PICA,* Posterior inferior cerebellar artery. (From Greenberg JJ, et al: Brain: indications, techniques, and atlas. In Edelman RR, Hesselink JR, editors: *Clinical magnetic resonance imaging,* Philadelphia, 1990, WB Saunders, p 384.)

PRÉCIS OF THE HEAD AND FACE ASSESSMENT[a]

NOTE: Suspected pathology will determine which *Special Tests* are to be performed.

History (sitting)
Observation (sitting)
Examination[a] (sitting)
  Head injury
    Neural Watch
    Glasgow Coma Scale
    Concussion
    Memory tests
    Headache
    Expanding intracranial lesion
    Proprioception
    Coordination
    Head injury card
  Facial injury
    Bone and soft-tissue contours
    Fractures
    Cranial nerves
    Facial muscles
  Eye injury
    Six cardinal gaze positions
    Pupils (size, equality, reactivity)
    Visual field (peripheral vision)
    Visual acuity
    Symmetry of gaze
    Hyphema
    Foreign objects, corneal abrasion
    Nystagmus
    Surrounding bone and soft tissue
    Saccades (horizontal and vertical)
    Accommodation
    Near point of convergence
    Smooth pursuits

    Vestibulo-ocular reflex (VOR)
    Tracking
  Nasal injury
    Patency
    Nasal cavities
    Sinuses
    Fracture
    Nose discharge (bloody, straw colored, clear)
  Tooth injury
    Number of teeth
    Position of teeth
    Movement of teeth
    Condition of teeth
    Condition of gums
  Ear injury
    Tenderness or pain
    Ear discharge (bloody, straw colored, clear)
    Hearing tests
    Balance
  Special tests
    Tests for expanding intracranial lesions
    Tests for concussion
    Tests for balance
    Tests for coordination
    Tests for cognitive function
    Tests of the vestibular system
    Tests for clinical reaction time
    Tests for proprioception
    Tests for hearing
    Graded exercise after concussion
  Reflexes and cutaneous distribution
  Palpation
  Diagnostic imaging

[a]When examining the head and face, if only one area has been injured (e.g., the nose), then only that area needs to be examined, provided the examiner is certain that adjacent structures have not also been injured. After any examination, the patient should be warned of the possibility of exacerbation of symptoms as a result of the assessment.

CASE STUDIES

When doing these case studies, the examiner should list the appropriate questions to be asked and why they are being asked, identify what to look for and why, and specify what things should be tested and why. Depending on the patient's answers (and the examiner should consider different responses), several possible causes of the patient's problem may become evident (examples are given in parentheses). A differential diagnosis chart should be made up (see Table 2.31 as an example). The examiner can then decide how different diagnoses may affect the treatment plan.

1. You are providing medical coverage of a local mixed martial arts (MMA) event. A 30-year-old grappler takes a beating and loses in the third round from a technical knockout. Although he did not actually lose consciousness, he continues to be dizzy and has headache even 30 minutes after the fight. He has tinnitus and some retrograde amnesia. Does this athlete have a concussion or an intracranial lesion? What other findings would you expect to see with the diagnosis that you made? What would be your immediate plan of care for this athlete?

2. You are providing coverage for a little league baseball tournament. A 10-year-old male baseball player, while sliding into home plate, is hit in the maxillary central incisor on the right with a baseball. There is severe bleeding from the right incisor. His right central incisor is loose but remains held in place by surrounding soft tissues and gums. Are there any other tests that need

CASE STUDIES—cont'd

to be done to determine the overall extent of maxillary or tooth damage? How is the extent of damage determined? As you are doing these other procedures, the tooth falls out into your hand. What would now be your plan of care for this athlete?

3. A 27-year-old man was playing football. He received a "knee to the head," rendering him unconscious for approximately 3 minutes. How would you differentiate between a first-time, fourth-degree concussion and an expanding intracranial lesion?

4. A 13-year-old boy received an elbow in the nose and cheek while play-wrestling. The nose is crooked and painful and bled after the injury, and the cheek is sore. Describe your assessment plan for this patient (nasal fracture vs. zygoma fracture).

5. A 23-year-old woman was in an automobile accident. She was a passenger in the front seat and was not wearing a seat belt. The car in which she was riding hit another car that had run a red light. The woman's face hit the dashboard, and she received a severe facial injury. Describe your assessment plan for this patient (Le Fort fracture vs. mandibular fracture).

6. An 83-year-old man tripped in the bathroom and hit his chin against the bathtub, knocking himself unconscious. Describe your assessment plan for this patient (cervical spine lesion vs. mandibular fracture).

7. An 18-year-old woman was playing squash. She was not wearing eye protectors and was hit in the eye with the ball. Describe your assessment plan for this patient (ruptured globe vs. blowout fracture).

8. A 15-year-old boy was playing field hockey. He was not wearing a mouth guard and was hit in the mouth and jaw by the ball. There was a large amount of blood. Describe your assessment plan for this patient (tooth fracture vs. mandible fracture).

9. A 16-year-old male wrestler comes to you complaining of ear pain. He has just finished a match, which he lost. Describe your assessment plan for this patient (cauliflower car vs. external otitis).

10. A 17-year-old female basketball player comes to you complaining of eye pain. She says she received a "finger in the eye" when she went up to get the ball. Describe your assessment plan for this patient (hyphema vs. corneal abrasion).

TABLE **2.31**

Differential Diagnosis of Concussion[a] and Intracranial Lesion

Sign or Symptom	Concussion[a]	Intracranial Lesion
Confusion	Yes, but should improve with time	Will have increased confusion with time
Amnesia	Posttraumatic, retrograde	Not usually
Loss of consciousness	Yes, but recovers	Lucid interval varies
Tinnitus	Severe	Not a factor
Dizziness	Severe, but improves	May get worse
Headache	Often	Severe
Nystagmus or irregular eye movements	Not usually	Possible
Pupil inequality	Not usually	Possible early; present later
Irregular respiration	No	Possible early; present later
Slowing of heart	No	Possible early; present later
Intractable vomiting	Not usually	Possible
Lateralization	No	Yes
Coordination affected	Yes, but improves	Yes, and gets worse
Seizure	Not usually	Possible early; probable late
Personality change	Possible	Possible

[a]Presence of particular signs and symptoms may depend on severity of concussion.

References

1. Jordan BD. Brain injury in boxing. *Clin Sports Med.* 2009;28:561–578.
2. McAlindon RJ. On field evaluation and management of head and neck injured athletes. *Clin Sports Med.* 2002;21:1–14.
3. McCrory P, Johnston K, Meeuwisse W, et al. Summary and agreement statement of the 2nd International Conference on concussion in sport, Prague 2004. *Clin J Sports Med.* 2005;15:48–55.
4. Albright JP, Van Gilder J, El Khoury G, et al. Head and neck injuries in sports. In: Scott WN, Nisonson B, Nicholas JA, eds. *Principles of Sports Medicine.* Baltimore: Williams & Wilkins; 1984.
5. Lovell MR, Iverson GL, Collins MW, et al. Does the level of consciousness predict neurophysiological decrements after concussion? *Clin J Sports Med.* 1999;9:193–198.
6. Levin HS, O'Donnell VM, Grossman RG. The Galveston orientation and amnesia test: a practical scale to assess cognition after head injury. *J Nerv Ment Dis.* 1979;167:675–684.
7. Brandt J. The Hopkins verbal learning test: development of a new memory test with six equivalent forms. *Clin Neuropsychologist.* 1991;5:125–142.
8. Maddocks D, Saling M. Neurophysiological deficits following concussion. *Brain Inj.* 1996;10:99–103.
9. Harmon KG, Drezner JA, Gammons M, et al. American Medical Society for Sports Medicine position statement: concussion in sport. *Br J Sports Med.* 2013;47:15–26.
10. McCrory P, Meeuwisse WH, Aubry M, et al. Consensus statement on concussion in sport: the 4th International Conference on concussion in sport held in Zurich, November 2012. *Br J Sports Med.* 2013;47:250–258.
11. Meehan WP, Taylor AM, Proctor M. The pediatric athlete: younger athletes with sport-related concussion. *Clin Sports Med.* 2011;30:133–144.
12. Putukian M, Echemendia RJ. Managing successive minor head injuries: which tests guide return to play? *Phys Sportsmed.* 1996;24(11):25–38.
13. Johnson EW, Kegel NE, Collins MW. Neurophysiological assessment of sports-related concussion. *Clin Sports Med.* 2011;30:73–88.
14. Solomon GS, Dott S, Lovell MR. Long-term neurocognitive dysfunction in sports: what is the evidence? *Clin Sports Med.* 2011;30:165–177.
15. Echemendia RJ, Iverson GL, McCrea M, et al. Advances in neurophysiological assessment of sport-related concussion. *Br J Sports Med.* 2013;47:294–298.
16. Lovell MR, Collins MW. Neurophysiological assessment of the college football players. *J Head Trauma Rehabil.* 1998;13(2):9–26.
17. Kerr ZY, Mihalik JP, Guskiewicz KM, et al. Agreement between athlete-recalled and clinically documented concussion histories in former collegiate athletes. *Am J Sports Med.* 2015;43(3):606–613.
18. Pfaller AY, Nelson LD, Apps JN, et al. Frequency and outcomes of a symptom-free waiting after sport-related concussion. *Am J Sports Med.* 2016;44(11):2941–2946.
19. Rabinowitz AR, Li X, Levin HS. Sport and nonsport etiologies of mild traumatic brain injury: similarities and differences. *Annu Rev Psychol.* 2014;65:301–331.
20. Maroon JC, Lovell MR, Norwig J, et al. Cerebral concussion in athletes: evaluation and neurophysiological testing. *Neurosurg.* 2000;47:659–672.
21. Echemendia RJ, Giza CC, Kutcher JS. Developing guidelines for return to play: consensus and evidence-based approaches. *Brain Inj.* 2015;29(2):85–194.
22. Putukian M. The acute symptoms of sport-related concussion: diagnosis and on-field management. *Clin Sports Med.* 2011;30:49–61.
23. Ontario Neurotrauma Foundation. *Guidelines for Concussion/mild Traumatic Brain Injury and Persistent Symptoms.* 2nd ed. 2013.
24. Ontario Ministry of Tourism, Culture and Sport: *Concussion guidelines.* Available at: http://www.health.gov.on.ca/en/public/programs/concussions/.
25. Kerr ZY, Mihalik JP, Guskiewicz KM, et al. Agreement between athlete-recalled and clinically documented concussion histories in former collegiate athletes. *Am J Sports Med.* 2015;43(3):606–613.
26. Broglio SP, Cantu RC, Gioia GA, et al. National Athletic Trainers' Association Position Statement: management of sport concussion. *J Athl Train.* 2014;49(2):245–265.
27. Marshall S, Bayley M, McCullagh S, et al. Updated clinical practice guidelines for concussion/mild traumatic brain injury and persistent symptoms. *Brain Inj.* 2015;29(6):688–700.
28. Kanani AN, Hartshorn S. Fifteen minute consultation: a structured approach to the recognition and management of concussion in children and adolescents. *Arch Dis Child Educ Pract Ed.* 2016;101(2):71–76.
29. McCrory P, Meeuwisse WH, Echemendia EJ, et al. What is the lowest threshold for making a diagnosis of concussion? *Br J Sports Med.* 2013;47:268–271.
30. Emery CA, Black AM, Kolstad A, et al. What strategies can be used to effectively reduce the risk of concussion in sport? A systematic review. *Br J Sports Med.* 2017;51(12):970–984.
31. Register-Mihalik JK, Kay MC. The current state of sports concussion. *Neurol Clin.* 2017;35:387–402.
32. Harmon KG, Drezner J, Gammons M, et al. American Medical Society for Sport Medicine position statement: concussion in sport. *Clin J Sports Med.* 2013;23(1):1–18.
33. Podell K, Presley C, Derman H. Sideline sports concussion assessment. *Neurol Clin.* 2017;35(3):435–450.
34. Steenerson K, Starling AJ. Pathophysiology of sports-related concussion. *Neurol Clin.* 2017;35(3):403–405.
35. Sufrinko A, McAllister-Deitrick J, Womble M, Kontos A. Do sideline concussion assessments predict subsequent neurocognitive impairment after sport-related concussion? *J Athl Train.* 2017;52(7):676–681.
36. Grindel SH, Lovell MR, Collins MW. The assessment of sport-related concussion: the evidence behind neuropsychological testing and management. *Clin J Sports Med.* 2001;11:134–143.
37. Lovell MR, Iverson GL, Collins MH, et al. Measurement of symptoms following sports-related concussion: reliability and normative data for the post-concussion scale. *Appl Neuropsychol.* 2006;13:166–174.
38. Carl RL, Kinsella SB. Pediatricians' knowledge of current sport concussion legislation and guidelines and comfort with sports concussion management: a cross sectional study. *Clin Pediatr.* 2014;53(7):689–697.
39. Azouvi P, Arnould A, Dromer E, Vallat-Azouvi C. Neuropsychology of traumatic brain injury: an expert overview. *Rev Neurol (Paris).* 2017;173:461–472.
40. Collins MW, Kontos AP, Reynolds E, et al. A comprehensive, targeted approach to the clinical care of athletes following sport-related concussion. *Knee Surg Sports Traumatol Arthrosc.* 2014;22:235–246.
41. Putukian M. Clinical evaluation of the concussed athlete: a view from the sideline. *J Athl Train.* 2017;52(3):236–244.
42. Halstead ME, Walter KD, McCambridge TM, et al. Clinical report – sport-related concussion in children and adolescents. *Pediatrics.* 2010;126(3):597–615.
43. Zemek RL, Farion KJ, Sampson M, McGahern C. Prognosticators of persistent symptoms following pediatric concussion: a systematic review. *JAMA Pediatr.* 2013;167(3):259–265.
44. Morgan CD, Zuckerman SL, Lee YM, et al. Predictors of postconcussion syndrome after sports-related concussion in young athletes: a matched case-control study. *J Neurosurg Pediatr.* 2015;15:589–598.
45. Lau BC, Collins MW, Lovell MR. Cut off scores in neurocognitive testing and symptom clusters that predict protracted recovery from concussions in high school athletes. *Neurosurgery.* 2012;70(2):371–379.
46. Potter S, Leigh E, Wade D, Fleminger S. The Rivermead Post Concussion Symptoms Questionnaire: a confirmatory factor analysis. *J Neurol.* 2006;253(12):1603–1614.
47. Grabowski P, Wilson J, Walker A, et al. Multimodal impairment-based physical therapy for the treatment of patients with post-concussion syndrome: a retrospective analysis on safety and feasibility. *Phys Ther Sport.* 2017;23:22–30.
48. Kozlowski KF, Graham J, Leddy JJ, et al. Exercise intolerance in individuals with postconcussion syndrome. *J Athl Train.* 2013;48(5):627–635.
49. Alsalaheen BA, Mucha A, Morris LO, et al. Vestibular rehabilitation for dizziness and balance disorders after concussion. *J Neurol Phys Ther.* 2010;34(2):87–93.
50. Kozlowski K. Exercise in concussion, part 1: local and systemic alterations and normal function. *Int J Athl Ther Train.* 2014;19(2):23–27.
51. Brooks J, Kemp S, Newth A, Sylvester R. Managing recovery from concussion. *BMJ.* 2016;355:5629–5630.
52. Johnson KM, Ptito A, Chankowsky J, Chen JK. New frontiers in diagnostic imaging in concussive head injury. *Clin J Sports Med.* 2001;11(3):166–175.
53. May KH, Marshall DL, Burns TG, et al. Pediatric sports specific return to play guidelines following concussion. *Int J Sports Phys Ther.* 2014;9(2):242–255.
54. Giza CC, Kutcher JS, Ashwal S, et al. Summary of evidence-based guideline update: evaluation and management of concussion in sports: report of the Guideline Development Subcommittee of the American Academy of Neurology. *Neurology.* 2013;80(24):2250–2257.
55. Johnston KM, McCrory P, Mohtadi NG, Meeuwisse W. Evidence-based review of sport-related concussion: clinical science. *Clin J Sports Med.* 2001;11(3):150–159.
56. Hides JA, Franettovich MM, Mendis MD, et al. Self-reported concussion history and sensorimotor tests predict head/neck injuries. *Med Sci Sports Exerc.* 2017;49(12):2385–2393.
57. Putukian M, Raftery M, Guskiewicz K, et al. Onfield assessment of concussion in the adult athlete. *Br J Sports Med.* 2013;47(5):285–288.
58. Stiell IG, Clement CM, Rowe BH, et al. Comparison of the Canadian CT Head Rule and the New Orleans Criteria in patients with minor head injury. *J Am Med Assoc.* 2005;294(12):1511–1518.
59. Stiell IG, Wells GA, Vandemkeen K, et al. The Canadian CT Head Rule for patients with minor head injury. *Lancet.* 2001;357:1391–1396.
60. Mata-Mbemba D, Mugikura S, Nakagawa A, et al. Canadian CT Head Rule and New Orleans Criteria in mild traumatic brain injury: comparison at a

tertiary referral Hospital in Japan. *SpringerPlus.* 2016;5:176–182.

61. McCrory P, Meeuwisse W, Johnston K, et al. Consensus statement on concussion in sport—3rd International Conference on concussion in sport, held in Zurich, November 2008. *Clin J Sports Med.* 2009;19:185–195.

62. Makdissi M. Is the simple versus complex classification of concussion a valid and useful differentiation? *Br J Sports Med.* 2009;43(suppl 1):i23–i27.

63. Brooks BL, Mannix R, Maxwell B, et al. Multiple past concussions in high school football players: are there differences in cognitive functioning and symptom reporting? *Am J Sports Med.* 2016;44(12):3243–3251.

64. Leong DF, Balcer LJ, Galetta SL, et al. The King-Devick test for sideline concussion screening in collegiate football. *J Optom.* 2015;8:131–139.

65. Wells EM, Goodkin HP, Griesbach GS. Challenges in determining the role of rest and exercise in the management of mild traumatic brain injury. *J Child Neurol.* 2015;31(1):86–92.

66. McCrory P, Meeuwisse W, Dvorak J, et al. Consensus statement on concussion in sport – the 5th International Conference on concussion in sport held in Berlin, October 2016. *Br J Sports Med.* 2017;51(11):838–847.

67. Hinton-Bayre AD, Geffen G. Severity of sports-related concussion and neurophysiological test performance. *Neurology.* 2002;59:1068–1070.

68. Sawyer AR, Hamdallah M, White D, et al. A high school coaches' assessments, intentions to use, and use of a concussion prevention toolkit: Centers for Disease Control and Prevention's heads up: concussion in high school Sports. *Health Promot Pract.* 2010;11(1):33–43.

69. Mucha A, Collins MW, Elbin RJ, et al. A brief vestibular/ocular motor screening (VOMS) assessment to evaluate concussions: preliminary findings. *Am J Sports Med.* 2014;42(10):2479–2486.

70. Purcell L. What are the most appropriate return-to-play guidelines for concussed child athletes? *Br J Sports Med.* 2009;43(suppl 1):i51–i55.

71. Ellis MJ, Leddy JJ, Willer B. Physiological, vestibulo-ocular and cervicogenic post-concussion disorders: an evidence-based classification system with directions for treatment. *Brain Inj.* 2015;29(2):238–248.

72. Giza CC, Hovda DA. The new neural metabolic cascade of concussion. *Neurosurgery.* 2014;75:S24–S33.

73. Phillips MM, Reddy CC. Managing patients with prolonged recovery following concussion. *Phys Med Rehabil Clin North Am.* 2016;27:455–474.

74. Cancelliere C, Hincapie CA, Keighley M, et al. Systematic review of prognosis and returned to play after sport concussion: results of the International Collaboration on Mild Traumatic Brain Injury Prognosis. *Arch Phys Med Rehabil.* 2014;95(suppl 3):S210–S229.

75. McCrea M, Guskiewicz KM, Marshall SW, et al. Acute effects and recovery time following concussion in collegiate football players: the NCAA Concussion Study. *J Am Med Assoc.* 2003;290(19):2556–2563.

76. Ventura RE, Balcer LJ, Galetta SL. The neuro-ophthalmology of head trauma. *Lancet Neurol.* 2014;13(10):1006–1016.

77. Leddy J, Hinds A, Sirica D, Willer B. The role of controlled exercise in concussion management. *Phys Med Rehabil.* 2016;8(suppl 3):S91–S100.

78. Buckley TA, Oldham JR, Caccese JB. Postural control deficits identify lingering post-concussion neurological deficits. *J Sports Health Sci.* 2016;5(1):61–69.

79. Leddy JJ, Willer B. Use of graded exercise testing in concussion and return-to-activity management. *Curr Sports Med Rep.* 2013;12(6):370–376.

80. Collins MW, Lovell MR, Iverson GL, et al. Cumulative effects of concussion in high school athletes. *Neurosurgery.* 2002;51(5):1175–1181.

81. Kontos AP, Elbin RJ, Schatz P, et al. A revised factor structure for the post-concussion symptoms scale: baseline and post-concussion factors. *Am J Sports Med.* 2012;40(10):2375–2384.

82. Susco TM, McLeod TC, Gansneder BM, Shultz SJ. Balance recovers within 20 minutes after exertion as measured by the balance error scoring system. *J Athl Train.* 2004;39(3):241–246.

83. Schneider K. Concussion in sport – where have we been and where do we need to go? *Physiother Pract.* 2018;8(1):10–13.

84. Guha A. Management of traumatic brain injury: some current evidence and applications. *Postgrad Med J.* 2004;80(949):650–653.

85. Pellman EJ, Viano DC, Casson IR, et al. Concussion in professional football: repeat injuries—part 4. *Neurosurgery.* 2004;55(4):860–876.

86. Makdissi M, Davis G, Jordan B, et al. Revisiting the modifiers: how should the evaluation and management of acute concussions differ in specific groups. *Br J Sports Med.* 2013;47:314–320.

87. McCrory P. Does second impact syndrome exist? *Clin J Sports Med.* 2001;11(3):144–149.

88. Gavett BE, Stern RA, McKee AC. Chronic traumatic encephalopathy: a potential late effect of sport-related concussive and subconcussive head trauma. *Clin Sports Med.* 2011;30(1):179–188.

89. McKee AC, Stein TD, Nowinski CJ, et al. The spectrum of disease in chronic traumatic encephalopathy. *Brain.* 2013;136(Pt 1):43–64.

90. McKee AC, Cairns NJ, Dickson DW, et al. The first NINDS/NIBIB consensus meeting to define neuropathological criteria for the diagnosis of chronic traumatic encephalopathy. *Acta Neuropathol.* 2016;131:75–86.

91. Stern RA, Riley DO, Daneshvar DH, et al. Long-term consequences of repetitive brain trauma: chronic traumatic encephalopathy. *Phys Med Rehabil.* 2011;3:S460–S467.

92. Mez J, Solomon TM, Daneshvar DH, et al. Pathologically confirmed chronic traumatic encephalopathy in a 25-year-old former college football player. *JAMA Neurol.* 2016;73(3):353–355.

93. Martini DN, Eckner JT, Meehan SK, Broglio SP. Long-term effects of adolescent sport concussion across the age spectrum. *Am J Sports Med.* 2017;45(6):1420–1428.

94. Love S, Solomon GS. Talking with parents of high school football players about chronic traumatic encephalopathy: a concise summary. *Am J Sports Med.* 2015;43(5):1260–1264.

95. Meehan WP, Bachur RG. Sport-related concussion. *Pediatrics.* 2009;123(1):114–123.

96. Kerr ZY, Register-Mihalik JK, Marshall SW, et al. Disclosure and non-disclosure of concussion and concussion symptoms in athletes: review and application of the socio-ecological framework. *Brain Inj.* 2014;28(8):1009–1021.

97. Covassin T, Elbin RJ. The female athlete: the role of gender in the assessment and management of sport related concussion. *Clin Sports Med.* 2011;30:125–131.

98. Kelly JP, Rosenberg JH. Diagnosis and management of concussion in sports. *Neurology.* 1997;48:575–580.

99. Gronwell D, Wrightson P. Cumulative effect of concussion. *Lancet.* 1975;2:995–997.

100. Sedney CL, Orphanos J, Bailes JE. When to consider retiring an athlete after sports-related concussion. *Clin Sports Med.* 2011;30:189–200.

101. McCrory PR, Berkovic SF. Second impact syndrome. *Neurology.* 1998;50:677–683.

102. Evans RW. The post concussion syndrome: 130 years of controversy. *Semin Neurol.* 1994;14:32–39.

103. d'Hemecourt P. Subacute symptoms of sports-related concussion: outpatient management and return to play. *Clin Sports Med.* 2011;30:63–72.

104. Leddy J, Baker JG, Haider MN, et al. A physiological approach to prolonged recovery from sport-related concussion. *J Athl Train.* 2017;52(3):299–308.

105. Buckley TA, Munkasy BA, Clouse BP. Acute cognitive and physical rest may not improve concussion recovery time. *J Head Trauma Rehabil.* 2016;31(4):233–241.

106. Bernard CO, Ponsford JL, McKinlay A, et al. Do concussive symptoms really resolve in young children? *J Head Trauma Rehabil.* 2017;32(6):413–424.

107. Makdissi M, Cantu RC, Johnston KM, et al. The difficult concussion patient: what is the best approach to investigation and management of persistent (>10 days) postconcussive symptoms? *Br J Sports Med.* 2013;47(5):308–313.

108. Nakayama Y, Covassin T, Schatz P, et al. Examination of the test-retest reliability of a computerized neurocognitive test battery. *Am J Sports Med.* 2014;42(8):2000–2005.

109. Randolph C, Millis S, Barr WB, et al. Concussion symptom inventory: an empirically derived scale for monitoring resolution of symptoms following sport-related concussion. *Arch Clin Neuropsychol.* 2009;24(3):219–229.

110. Broglio JP, Guskiewicz KM, Norwig J. If you're not measuring, you're guessing: the advent of objective concussion assessments. *J Athl Train.* 2017;52(3):160–166.

111. Creighton DW, Shrier I, Shultz R, et al. Return-to-play in sport: a decision-based model. *Clin J Sports Med.* 2010;20(5):379–385.

112. Barlow KM. Postconcussion syndrome: a review. *J Child Neurol.* 2016;31(1):57–67.

113. Cottle JE, Hall EE, Patel K, et al. Concussion baseline testing: preexisting factors, symptoms, and neurocognitive performance. *J Athl Train.* 2017;52(2):77–81.

114. Parachute Canada. *Statement on Concussion Baseline Testing in Canada;* 2017.

115. King NS, Crawford S, Wenden FJ, et al. The Rivermead Post Concussion Symptoms Questionnaire: a measure of symptoms commonly experienced after head injury and its reliability. *J Neurol.* 1995;242(9):587–592.

116. Crawford S, Wenden FJ, Wade DT. The Rivermead Head Injury Follow Up Questionnaire: a study of a new rating scale and other measures to evaluate outcome after head injury. *J Neurol Neurosurg Psychiatry.* 1996;60(5):510–514.

117. Schmidt JD, Register-Mihalik JK, Mihalik JP, et al. Identifying impairments after concussion: normative data vs individualized baselines. *Med Sci Sports Exerc.* 2012;44:1621–1628.

118. Pellman EJ, Viano DC, Casson IR, et al. Concussion in professional football: injuries involving 7 or more days out—part 5. *Neurosurgery.* 2004;55(5):1100–1119.

119. Pellman EJ, Lovell ML, Viano DC, et al. Concussion in professional football: neuropsychological testing—part 6. *Neurosurgery.* 2004;55(6):1290–1305.

120. Lovell MR, Collins MW. Neuropsychological assessment of the college football player. *J Head Trauma Rehabil.* 1998;13:9–26.

121. Schatz P, Putz BO. Cross-validation of measures used for computer-based assessment of concussion. *Appl Neuropsychol.* 2006;13(3):151–159.

122. Elbin RJ, Schatz P, Covassin T. One year test-retest reliability of the online version of ImPACT in high school athletes. *Am J Sports Med.* 2011;39:2319–2324.

123. Schatz P, Sandel N. Sensitivity and specificity of the online version of ImPACT in high school and collegiate athletes. *Am J Sports Med.* 2013;11:321–326.

124. Echemendia RJ, Herring S, Bailes J. Who should conduct and interpret the neuropsychological assessment in sports related concussion? *Br J Sports Med.* 2009;43(suppl 1):i32–i35.

125. Schatz P, Pardini JE, Lovell MR, et al. Sensitivity and specificity of the ImPACT test battery for concussion in athletes. *Arch Clin Neuropsychol.* 2006;21(1):91–99.

126. Pellman EJ, Lovell MR, Vianao DC, Casson IR. Concussion in professional football: recovery of NFL and high school athletes assessed by computerized neuropsychological testing–part 12. *Neurosurgery.* 2006;58(2):263–274.

127. Schatz P, Zillmer ER. Computer-based assessment of sports-related concussion. *Appl Neuropsychol.* 2003;10(1):42–47.

128. Erlanger D, Feldman D, Kutner K, et al. Development and validation of a web-based neuropsychological test protocol for sports-related return-to-play decision-making. *Arch Clin Neuropsychol.* 2003;18:293–316.

129. Barr WB, Prishep LS, Chabot R, et al. Measuring brain electrical activity to track recovery from sport-related concussion. *Brain Inj.* 2012;26(1):58–66.

130. Lichenstein JD, Moser RS, Schatz P. Age and test setting affect the prevalence of invalid baseline scores on neurocognitive tests. *Am J Sports Med.* 2013;42(2):479–484.

131. Nelson LD, Pfaller AY, Rein LE, McCrea MA. Rates and predictors of invalid baseline test performance in high school and collegiate athletes for 3 computerized neurocognitive tests: ANAM, Axon Sports and ImPACT. *Am J Sports Med.* 2015;43(9):2018–2026.

132. Iverson G. Predicting slow recovery from sport-related concussion: the new simple-complex distinction. *Clin J Sports Med.* 2007;17(1):31–37.

133. Graham R, Rivara FP, Ford MA, et al. *Sports-related Concussions in Youth: Improving the Science, Changing the Culture. Appendix C: Clinical Evaluation Tools-Concussion Assessment Tools.* Committee on Sports-Related Concussions in Youth; Board on Children, Youth and Families; Institute of Medicine; National Research Council. Washington: National Academies Press (US); 2014.

134. Farnsworth JL, Dargo L, Ragan BG, Kang M. Reliability of computerized neurocognitive tests for concussion assessment: a meta-analysis. *J Athl Train.* 2017;52(9):826–833.

135. LaBotz M, Martin MR, Kimura IF, et al. A comparison of a preparticipation evaluation history form and a symptom-based concussion survey in the identification of previous head injury in collegiate athletes. *Clin J Sports Med.* 2005;15:73–78.

136. Piland SG, Motl RW, Guskiewicz KM, et al. Structural validity of a self-report concussion-related symptoms scale. *Med Sci Sports Exerc.* 2006;38:27–32.

137. Broglio SP, Guskiewicz KM. Concussion in sports: the sideline assessment. *Sports Health.* 2009;1(6):361–369.

138. Makdissi M, Darby D, Maruff P, et al. Natural history of concussion in sport-markers of severity and implications for management. *Am J Sports Med.* 2010;38:464–471.

139. Baugh CM, Kroshus E, Stamm JM, et al. Clinical practices in collegiate concussion management. *Am J Sports Med.* 2016;44(6):1391–1399.

140. Wojtys EM, Hovda D, Landry G, et al. Concussion in sports. *Am J Sports Med.* 1999;27:676–686.

141. Kelly JP, Rosenberg JH. Practice parameter: the management of concussions in sports: report of the quality standards subcommittee. *Neurology.* 1997;48:581–585.

142. Makdissi M, Schneider KJ, Feddermann-Demont N, et al. Approach to investigation and treatment of persistent symptoms following sport-related concussion: a systematic review. *Br J Sports Med.* 2017;51(12):958–968.

143. Sullivan SJ, Schneiders AG, McCrory P, Gray A. Physiotherapists' use of information identifying a concussion: an extended Delphi approach. *Br J Sports Med.* 2008;42(3):175–177.

144. Howell DR, Osternig LR, Chou LS. Adolescents demonstrate greater gait balance control deficits after concussion than young adults. *Am J Sports Med.* 2014;43(3):625–632.

145. Tsao JW, Perry BN, Kennedy CH, Beresford R. Predicting prolonged recovery after concussion. *Neurology.* 2014;83(24):2196–2197.

146. Yengo-Kahn AM, Johnson DJ, Zuckerman SL, Solomon GS. Concussions in the National Football League: a current concepts review. *Am J Sports Med.* 2015;44(3):801–811.

147. Lovell MR, Collins MW, Iverson GL, et al. Recovery from mild concussion in high school athletes. *J Neurosurg.* 2003;98(2):96–301.

148. Kontos AP, Sufrinko A, Elbin RJ, et al. Reliability and associated risk factors for performance on the vestibular/ocular motor screening (VOMS) tool in healthy collegiate athlete. *Am J Sports Med.* 2016;44(6):1400–1406.

149. Mrazik M, Ferrara MS, Peterson CL, et al. Injury severity and neurophysiological and balance outcomes of four college athletes. *Brain Inj.* 2000;14:921–931.

150. Collins MW, Grindell SH, Lovell MR, et al. Relationship between concussion and neurophysiological performance in college football players. *J Am Med Assoc.* 1999;282:964–970.

151. Bleiberg J, Cernich A, Cameron K, et al. Duration of cognitive impairment after sports concussion. *Neurosurgery.* 2004;54:1073–1080.

152. Zemek R, Barrowman N, Freedman SB, et al. Clinical risk score for persistent postconcussion symptoms among children with acute concussion in the ED. *J Am Med Assoc.* 2016;315(10):1014–1025.

153. Guskiewicz KM, McCrea M, Marshall SW, et al. Cumulative effects associated with recurrent concussion in collegiate football players: the NCAA concussion study. *J Am Med Assoc.* 2003;290(19):2549–2555.

154. Ellenberg D, Henry LC, Macciocchi SN, et al. Advances in sport concussion assessment: from behavioral to brain imaging measures. *J Neurotrauma.* 2009;26(12):2365–2382.

155. Baker JG, Freitas MS, Leddy JJ, et al. Return to full functioning after graded exercise assessment and progressive exercise treatment of postconcussion syndrome. *Rehabil Res Pract.* 2012:705309. Epub 2012 Jan 16.

156. Leddy JJ, Kozlowski K, Donnelly JP, et al. A preliminary study of subsymptom threshold exercise training for refractory post-concussion syndrome. *Clin J Sports Med.* 2010;20(1):21–27.

157. Covassin T, Moran R, Wilhelm K. Concussion symptoms and neurocognitive performance of high school and college athletes who incur multiple concussions. *Am J Sports Med.* 2013;41(12):2885–2889.

158. Beck AT, Ward CH, Mendelson M, et al. An inventory for measuring depression. *Arch Gen Psychiatry.* 1961;4(6):561–571.

159. Sullivan K, Garden N. A comparison of the psychometric properties of 4 postconcussion syndrome measures in a nonclinical sample. *J Head Trauma Rehabil.* 2011;26(2):170–176.

160. Henry LC, Elbin RJ, Collins MW, et al. Examining recovery trajectories after sport-related concussion with a multimodal clinical assessment approach. *Neurosurgery.* 2016;78(2):232–241.

161. Master CL, Scheiman M, Gallaway M, et al. Vision diagnoses are common after concussion in adolescents. *Clin Pediatr.* 2016;55(3):260–267.

162. McCrea M, Iverson GL, Echemendia RJ, et al. Date of injury assessment of sport-related concussion. *Br J Sports Med.* 2013;47(5):272–284.

163. Eyres S, Carey A, Gilworth G, et al. Construct validity and reliability of the Rivermead Postconcussion Symptoms Questionnaire. *Clin Rehab.* 2005;19(8):878–887.

164. Rush AJ, Trivedi MH, Ibrahim HM, et al. The 16-item Quick Inventory of Depressive Symptomatology (QIDS), clinician rating (QIDS-C) and self-report (QIDS-SR): a psychometrics evaluation in patients with chronic major depression. *Biol Psychiatry.* 2003;54(5):573–583.

165. DeMatteo C, Stazyk K, Singh SK, et al. Development of a conservative protocol to return children and youth to activity following concussive injury. *Clin Pediatr (Phila).* 2015;54(2):152–163.

166. Davis GA, Anderson V, Babl FE, et al. What is the difference in concussion management in children as compared with adults? A systematic review. *Br J Sports Med.* 2017;51(12):949–957.

167. Iverson GL, Gardner AJ, Terry DP, et al. Predictors of clinical recovery from concussion: a systematic review. *Br J Sports Med.* 2017;51(12):941–948.

168. McCrea M, Guskiewicz K, Randolph C, et al. Effects of a symptom-free waiting period on clinical outcome and risk of reinjury after sport-related concussion. *Neurosurgery.* 2009;65(5):876–882.

169. Yeates KO, Beauchamp M, Craig W, et al. Advancing Concussion Assessment in Pediatrics (A-CAP): a prospective, concurrent cohort, longitudinal study of mild traumatic brain injury in children: protocol study. *Br Med J Open.* 2017;7(7):e17012.

170. Zemek KJ, Farion M, Sampson M, McGahern C. Prognosticators of persistent symptoms following pediatric concussion: a systematic review. *JAMA Pediatrics.* 2013;167(3):259–265.

171. Meehan WP, Mannix RC, Stracciolini A, et al. Symptom severity predicts prolonged recovery after sport-related concussion, but age and amnesia do not. *J Pediatr.* 2013;163:721–725.

172. Field M, Collins MW, Lovell MR, Maroon J. Does age play a role in recovery from sports-related concussion? A comparison of high school and collegiate athletes. *J Pediatr.* 2003;142:546–553.

173. Grool AM, Aglipay M, Momoli F, et al. Association between early participation in physical activity following acute concussion and persistent postconcussive symptoms in children and adolescents. *J Am Med Assoc.* 2016;316(23):2504–2514.

174. Collie A, Makdissi M, Maruff P, et al. Cognition in the days following concussion: comparison of symptomatic versus asymptomatic athletes. *J Neurol Neurosurg Psychiatry.* 2006;77(2):241–245.

175. Eisenberg MA, Andrea J, Meehan W, Mannix R. Time interval between concussions and symptom duration. *Pediatrics.* 2013;132(1):8–17.

176. Covassin T, Schatz P, Swanik CB. Sex differences in neuropsychological function and post-concussion symptoms of concussed collegiate athletes. *Neurosurgery.* 2007;61(2):345–351.

177. Ono KE, Burns TG, Bearden DJ, et al. Sex-based differences as a predictor of recovery trajectories in young athletes after a sports-related concussion. *Am J Sports Med.* 2016;44(3):748–752.

178. Covassin T, Swanik CB, Sachs M, et al. Sex differences in baseline neuropsychological function and

concussion symptoms in collegiate athletes. *Br J Sports Med.* 2006;40(11):923–927.

179. Covassin T, Elbin RJ, Bleecker A, et al. Are there differences in neurocognitive function and symptoms between male and female soccer players after concussions? *Am J Sports Med.* 2013;41(12):2890–2895.

180. Niere K, Quin A. Development of a headache-specific disability questionnaire for patients attending physiotherapy. *Man Ther.* 2009;14:45–51.

181. Mihalik JP, Register-Mihalik J, Kerr ZY, et al. Recovery of posttraumatic migraine characteristics in patients after mild traumatic brain injury. *Am J Sports Med.* 2013;41(7):1490–1496.

182. Kontos AP, Elbin RJ, Lau B, et al. Posttraumatic migraine as a predictor of recovery and cognitive impairment after sport-related concussion. *Am J Sports Med.* 2013;41(7):1497–1504.

183. Seifert T. Headache and sports. *Curr Pain Headache Rep.* 2014;18(9):448–455.

184. Jacobson GP, Newman CW. The development of the dizziness headache inventory. *Arch Otolatyngol Head Neck Surg.* 1990;116(4):424–427.

185. Manzi DB, Weaver PA. *Head Injury: The Acute Care Phase.* Thorafare, NJ: Slack; 1987.

186. Maddocks DL, Dicker GD, Saling MM. The assessment of orientation following concussion in athletes. *Clin J Sports Med.* 1995;5:32–35.

187. McCrea M, Kelly JP, Kluge J, et al. Standardized assessment of concussion in football players. *Neurology.* 1997;48:586–588.

188. Stilger VG, Alt JM, Robinson TW. Traumatic hyphema in an intercollegiate baseball player: a case report. *J Athl Train.* 1999;34:25–28.

189. Seidel HM, Ball JW, Dains JE, et al. *Mosby's Guide to Physical Examination.* St Louis: Mosby; 1987.

190. Swartz MH. *Textbook of Physical Diagnosis.* Philadelphia: WB Saunders; 1989.

191. Reilly BM. *Practical Strategies in Outpatient Medicine.* Philadelphia: WB Saunders; 1984.

192. Novey DW. *Rapid Access Guide to the Physical Examination.* Chicago: Year Book Medical; 1988.

193. Kelly JP. Maxillofacial injuries. In: Zachazewski JE, Magee DJ, Quillen WS, eds. *Athletic Injuries and Rehabilitation.* Philadelphia: WB Saunders; 1996.

194. Pashby TJ, Pashby RC. Treatment of sports eye injuries. In: Fu FH, Stone DA, eds. *Sports Injuries: Mechanisms, Prevention, and Treatment.* Baltimore: Williams & Wilkins; 1994.

195. Coello AF, Canals AG, Gonzalez JM, Martin JJ. Cranial nerve injury after minor head trauma. *J Neurosurg.* 2010;113(3):547–555.

196. Gall B, Parkhouse W, Goodman D. Heart rate variability of recently concussed athletes at rest and exercise. *Med Sci Sports Exerc.* 2004;36:1269–1274.

197. Kelly JP, Nichols JS, Filley CM, et al. Concussion in sports: guidelines for the prevention of catastrophic outcome. *J Am Med Assoc.* 1991;266:2867–2869.

198. Durand P, Adamson GJ. On-the-field management of athletic head injuries. *J Am Acad Orthop Surg.* 2004;12. 191-145.

199. Macciocchi SN, Barth JT, Littlefield LM. Outcome after mild head injury. *Clin Sports Med.* 1998;17(1):27–36.

200. Polin RS, Alves WM, Jane JA. Sports and head injuries. In: Evans RW, ed. *Neurology and Trauma.* Philadelphia: WB Saunders; 1996.

201. Cantu RC. Return to play guidelines after a head injury. *Clin Sports Med.* 1998;17(1):45–60.

202. Fick DS. Management of concussion in collision sports: guidelines for the sidelines. *Postgrad Med.* 1995;97:53–60.

203. Cantu RC. Second-impact syndrome. *Clin Sports Med.* 1998;17:37–44.

204. Matuszak JM, McVige J, McPherson J, et al. A practical concussion physical examination toolbox. *Sports Health.* 2016;8(3):260–269.

205. Patel P, Kalyanaraman S, Reginald J, et al. Posttraumatic cranial nerve injury. *Indian J Neurotrauma.* 2005;2(1):27–32.

206. Tsang CS, Liao L-R, Chung RC, Pang MY. Psychometrics properties of the Mini-Balance Evaluation Systems Test (Mini-BESTest) in community-dwelling individuals with chronic stroke. *Phys Ther.* 2013;93(8):1102–1115.

207. Horak FB, Wrisley DM, Frank J. The Balance Evaluation Systems Test (BESTest) to differentiate balance deficits. *Phys Ther.* 2009;89(5):485–498.

208. Shumway-Cook A, Woollacott M. Attention demands and postural control: the effect of sensory context. *J Gerontol Biol Med Sci.* 2000;55(1):M10–M16.

209. Riemann BL, Guskiewicz KM, Shields EW. Relationship between clinical and forceplate measures of postural stability. *J Sports Rehab.* 1999;8:71–82.

210. Valovich-McLeod TC, Barr WB, McCrea M, et al. Psychometric and measurement properties of concussion assessment tools in youth sports. *J Athl Train.* 2006;41:399–408.

211. McCrea M, Barr WB, Guskiewicz K, et al. Standard regression-based methods for measuring recovery from sport-related concussion. *J Int Neuropsychol Soc.* 2005;11:58–69.

212. Guskiewicz KM, Ross SE, Marshall SW. Postural stability and neuropsychological deficits after concussion in collegiate athletes. *J Athl Train.* 2001;36:263–273.

213. Guskiewicz KM. Balance assessment in the management of sport-related concussion. *Clin Sports Med.* 2011;30(1):89–102.

214. Guskiewicz KM. Postural stability assessment following concussion: one piece of the puzzle. *Clin J Sports Med.* 2001;11(3):182–189.

215. Franchignoni F, Horak F, Godi M, et al. Using psychometric techniques to improve The Balance Evaluation Systems Test: The Mini-Bestest. *J Rehabil Med.* 2010;42(4):323–331.

216. Whitney S, Wrisley D, Furman J. Concurrent validity of the Berg Balance scale and the Dynamic Gait Index in people with vestibular dysfunction. *Physiother Res Int.* 2003;8(4):178–186.

217. Jonsdottir J, Cattaneo D. Reliability and validity of the dynamic gait index in persons with chronic stroke. *Arch Phys Med Rehabil.* 2007;88:1410–1415.

218. Perell KL, Nelson A, Goldman RL, et al. Fall risk assessment measures: an analytical review. *J Gerontol A Biol Sci Med Sci.* 2001;56(12):M761–M766.

219. VanSwearingen JM, Paschal KA, Bonino P, Yang JF. The Modified Gait Abnormality Rating Scale for recognizing the risk of recurrent falls in community-dwelling elderly adults. *Phys Ther.* 1996;76:994–1002.

220. Herman T, Inbar-Borovsky N, Brozgol M, et al. The dynamic gait index in healthy older adults: the role of stair climbing, fear of falling and gender. *Gait Posture.* 2009;29(2):237–241.

221. Kleiner M, Wong L, Dubé A, et al. Dual-task assessment protocols in concussion assessment: a systematic literature review. *J Orthop Sports Phys Ther.* 2018;48(2):87–103.

222. Cossette I, Gagné ME, Ouellet MC, et al. Executive dysfunction following a mild traumatic brain injury revealed in early adolescence with locomotor-cognitive dual-tasks. *Brain Inj.* 2016;30(13–14):1648–1655.

223. Howell DR, Osternig LR, Chou LS. Single-task and dual-task tandem gait test performance after concussion. *J Sci Med Sport.* 2017;20(7):622–626.

224. Morgan AL, Brandt JF. An auditory Stroop effect for pitch, loudness and time. *Brain Lang.* 1989;36(4):592–603.

225. Worden TA, Mendes M, Singh P, Vallis LA. Measuring the effects of a visual or auditory Stroop task on dual-task cost during obstacle crossing. *Gait Posture.* 2016;50:159–163.

226. Eckner JT, Kutcher JS, Broglio SP, Richardson JK. Effect of sport-related concussion on clinically measured simple reaction time. *Br J Sports Med.* 2014;48(2):112–118.

227. Pearce KL, Sufrinko A, Lau BC, et al. Near point of convergence after a sport-related concussion: measurement reliability and relationship to neurocognitive impairment and symptoms. *Am J Sports Med.* 2015;43(12):3055–3061.

228. Alla S, Sullivan SJ, Hale L, McCrory P. Self-report scales/checklists for the measurement of concussion symptoms: a systematic review. *Br J Sports Med.* 2009;43(suppl 1):i3–i12.

229. Fonseca RJ, Walker RV. *Oral and Maxillofacial Trauma.* Philadelphia: WB Saunders; 1991.

230. Pollock RA, Dingman RO. Management and reconstruction of athletic injuries of the face, anterior neck, and upper respiratory tract. In: Schneider RC, Kennedy JC, Plant ML, eds. *Sports Injuries: Mechanisms, Treatment and Prevention.* Baltimore: Williams & Wilkins; 1985.

231. Simpson JF, Magee KR. *Clinical Evaluation of the Nervous System.* Boston: Little, Brown; 1973.

232. Cantu RC. Guidelines for return to contact sports after cerebral concussion. *Phys Sportsmed.* 1986;14:75–83.

233. Gioia G, Collins M, Isquith PK. Improving identification and diagnosis of mild hematocrit injury with evidence: psychometric support for the acute concussion evaluation. *J Head Trauma Rehabil.* 2008;23(4):230–242.

234. Derogatis LR. *BSI Brief Symptom Inventory. Administration, Scoring, and Procedures Manual.* 4th ed. Minneapolis: National Computer Systems; 1993.

235. Franke GH, Jarger S, Glaesmer H, et al. Psychometric analysis of the brief symptom inventory 18 (BSI-18) in a representative German sample. *BMC Med Res Methodol.* 2017;17(1):14–21.

236. Topel JL. Examination of the comatose patient. In: Weiner WJ, Goetz CG, eds. *Neurology for the Non-neurologist.* Philadelphia: JB Lippincott; 1989.

237. Piland SG, Motl RW, Ferrara MS, Peterson CL. Evidence for the factorial and construct validity of a self-report concussion symptoms scale. *J Athl Train.* 2003;38(2):104–112.

238. Undén J, Ingebrigtsen T, Romner B. The Scandinavian Neurotrauma Committee: Scandinavian guidelines for initial management of minimal, mild, and moderate head injuries in adults: an evidence and consensus-based update. *BMC Med.* 2013;11:50–63.

239. Ingebrigtsen T, Romner B, Kock-Jensen C. Scandinavian guidelines for initial management of minimal, mild, and moderate head injuries. The Scandinavian Neurotrauma Committee. *J Trauma.* 2000;48(4):760–766.

240. Echemendia RJ, Meeuwisse W, McCrory P, et al. The Sport Concussion Assessment Tool Fifth edition (SCAT5). *Br J Sports Med.* 2017;51(11):848–850.

241. Davis GA, Purcell L, Schneider KJ, et al. The child Sport Concussion Assessment Tool Fifth edition (child SCAT5): background and rationale. *Br J Sports Med.* 2017;5111:859–861.

242. Snedden TR, Brooks MA, Hetzel S, McGuine T. Normative values of the Sport Concussion Assessment Tool 3 (SCAT3) in high school athletes. *Clin J Sports Med.* 2017;27(5):462–467.

243. Chin EY, Nelson LD, Barr WB, et al. Reliability and validity of the Sport Concussion Assessment Tool-3 (SCAT3) in high school and collegiate athletes. *Am J Sports Med.* 2016;44(9):2276–2285.

244. Davis GA, Makdissi M. Concussion tests: clarifying potential confusion regarding sideline assessment and cognitive testing. *Br J Sports Med.* 2012;46(14):959–960.

245. Ventura RE, Jancuska JM, Balcer LJ, Galetta SL. Diagnostic tests for concussion: is vision part of the puzzle. *J Neuro Ophthalmol.* 2015;35(1):73–81.

246. Valovich TC, Perron DH, Gansneder BM. Repeat administration elicits a practice effect with a Balance Error Scoring System but not with the Standardized Assessment of Concussion in high school athletes. *J Athl Train.* 2003;38(1):51–56.

247. McCrea M. Standardized mental status testing on the sideline after sport-related concussion. *J Athl Train.* 2001;36(3):274–279.

248. McCrea M. Standardized mental status assessment of sport concussion. *Clin J Sports Med.* 2001;11(3):176–181.

249. Breen EO, Howell DR, Stracciolini A, et al. Examination of age-related differences on clinical tests of postural stability. *Sports Health.* 2016;8(3):244–249.

250. Wilkins JC, Valovich McLeod TC, Perrin DH, Gansneder BM. Performance on the balance error scoring system decreases after fatigue. *J Athl Train.* 2004;39(2):156–161.

251. DeMatteo C, Stazyk K, Giglia L, et al. A balanced protocol for return to school for children and youth following concussive injury. *Clin Pediatr (Phila).* 2015;54(8):783–792.

252. Guskiewicz KM, Rieman BL, Perrin DH, Nashner LM. Alternative approaches to the assessment of mild head injury in athletes. *Med Sci Sports Exerc.* 1997;29(suppl 7):S213–S221.

253. Iverson GL, Koehle MS. Normative data for the modified balance error scoring system in adults. *Brain Inj.* 2013;27(5):596–599.

254. Kosinski M, Bayless MS, Bjoner JB, et al. A six-item short-form survey for measuring headache impact: the HIT-6. *Qual Life Res.* 2003;12(8):963–974.

255. Potter K, Brandfuss K. The Mini-Balance Evaluation Systems Test (Mini-BESTest). *J Physiother.* 2015;61(4):225.

256. Broglio SP, Macciocchi SN, Ferrar MS. Sensitivity of the concussion assessment battery. *Neurosurgery.* 2007;60(6):1050–1057.

257. Howell DR, Osternig LR, Christie AD, Chou LS. Return to physical activity timing and dual-task gait stability are associated 2 months following concussion. *J Head Trauma Rehabil.* 2016;31(4):262–268.

258. Martini DN, Sabin MJ, DePesa SA, et al. A chronic effects of concussion on gait. *Arch Phys Med Rehabil.* 2011;92(4):585–589.

259. Woollacott M, Shumway-Cook A. Attention and the control of posture and gait: a review of an emerging area of research. *Gait Posture.* 2002;16(1):1–14.

260. Buckley TA, Vallabhajosula S, Oldham JR, et al. Evidence of a conservative gait strategy in athletes with a history of concussions. *J Sport Health Sci.* 2016;5(4):417–423.

261. Martini DN, Goulet GC, Gates DH, Broglio SP. Long-term effects of adolescent concussion history on gait, across age. *Gait Posture.* 2016;49:264–270.

262. Shaffer SW, Teyhen DS, Lorenson CL, et al. Y-balance test: a reliability study involving multiple raters. *Mil Med.* 2013;178(11):1264–1270.

263. Gribble PA, Hertel J. Considerations for normalizing measures of the star excursion balance test. *Measurement Phys Educ Exerc Sci.* 2003;7(2):89–100.

264. Hertel J, Braham RA, Hale SA, Olmstead-Kramer LC. Simplify the star excursion balance test: analysis of subjects with and without chronic ankle instability. *J Orthop Sports Phys Ther.* 2006;36(3):131–137.

265. Reitan RM. Validity of the trail making test as an indicator of organic brain damage. *Percept Mot Skills.* 1958;8(3):271–276.

266. Tombaugh TN. Trail making test A and B: normative data stratified by age and education. *Arch Clin Neuropsychol.* 2004;19(2):203–214.

267. Wechsler D. A standardized memory scale for clinical use. *J Psychol.* 1945;19(1):87–95.

268. Scarpina F, Tagini S. The Stroop color and word test. *Front Psychol.* 2017;8:557.

269. Kerber KA, Baloh RW. The evaluation of a patient with dizziness. *Neurol Clin Pract.* 2011;1(1):24–33.

270. Brandt T, Strupp M: General vestibular testing. *Clin Neurophysiol* 116(2):406-426, 205.

271. Oberlander TJ, Olson BL, Weidauer L. Test-retest reliability of the King-Devick test in an adolescent population. *J Athl Train.* 2017;52(5):439–445.

272. Kontos AP, Sufrinko A, Elbin RJ, et al. Reliability and associated risk factors for performance on the vestibular/ocular motor screening (VOMS) tool in healthy collegiate athletes. *Am J Sports Med.* 2016;44(6):1400–1406.

273. Herdman SJ. *Vestibular Rehabilitation.* 3rd ed. Philadelphia: FA Davis; 2007.

274. Johnson EG, Landel R, Kusunose RS, et al. Positive patient outcome after manual cervical spine management despite a positive vertebral artery test. *Man Ther.* 2008;13:367–371.

275. Kessler P, Tomlinson D, Blakeman A, et al. The high-frequency/acceleration head heave test in detecting otolith diseases. *Otol Neurotol.* 2007;28(7):896–904.

276. Galetta KM, Barrett J, Allen M, et al. The King-Devick test as a determinant of head trauma and concussion in boxers and MMA fighters. *Neurology.* 2011;76(17):1456–1462.

277. Galetta KM, Brandes LE, Maki K, et al. The King-Devick test and sports-related concussion: study of a rapid visual screening tool in a collegiate cohort. *J Neurol Sci.* 2011;309(1–2):34–39.

278. King D, Brughelli M, Hume P, Gissane C. Concussions in amateur rugby union identified with the use of a rapid visual screening tool. *J Neurol Sci.* 2013;326(1–2):59–63.

279. Oride MK, Marutani JK, Rouse MW, DeLand PN. Reliability study of the Pierce and King-Devick saccade tests. *Am J Optometry Physiol Opt.* 1986;63(6):419–424.

280. Molloy JH, Murphy I, Gissane C. The King-Devick (K-D) test and concussion diagnosis in semi-professional rugby union players. *J Sci Med Sport.* 2017;20(8):708–711.

281. Del Rossi G. Evaluating the recovery curve for clinically assessed reaction time after concussion. *J Athl Train.* 2017;52(8):766–770.

282. MacDonald J, Wilson J, Young J, et al. Evaluation of a simple test of reaction time for baseline concussion testing in the population of high school athletes. *Clin J Sports Med.* 2015;25(1):43–48.

283. Eckner JT, Kutcher JS, Richardson JK. Effect of concussion on clinically measured reaction time in 9 NCAA division I collegiate athletes: a preliminary study. *Phys Med Rehabil.* 2010;3(3):212–218.

284. Silverberg ND, Iverson GL. Is rest after concussion "the best medicine"?: Recommendations for activity resumption following concussion and athletes, civilians, and military service members. *J Head Trauma Rehabil.* 2013;28(4):250–259.

285. Griesbach GS, Tio DL, Vincelli J, et al. Differential effects of voluntary and forced exercise on stress responses after traumatic brain injury. *J Neurotrauma.* 2012;29(7):1426–1433.

286. Balke B, Ware RW. An experimental study of physical fitness in Air Force personnel. *U S Armed Forces Med J.* 1959;10(6):675–688.

287. Froelicher VF, Thompson AJ, Davis G, et al. Prediction of maximum oxygen consumption: comparison of the Bruce and Balke Treadmill Protocols. *Chest.* 1975;68(3):331–336.

288. Leddy JJ, Baker JG, Kozlowski K, et al. Ability of a graded exercise test for assessing recovery from concussion. *Clin J Sports Med.* 2011;21(2):89–94.

289. House JW, Brackmann DE. Facial nerve grading system: otolaryngol. *Head Neck Surg.* 1985;93:146–147.

290. Caccese JB, Kaminski TW. Comparing computer-derived and human-observed scores for the balance error scoring system. *J Sport Rehabil.* 2016;25(2):133–136.

291. Sheehan DP, Lafave MR, Katz L. Intra-rater and inter-rater reliability of the Balance Error Scoring System in pre-adolescent school children. *Meas Educ Exerc Sci.* 2011;15(3):234–243.

292. Broglio SP, Zhu W, Sopiarz K, Park Y. Generalizability theory analysis of Balance Error Scoring System reliability in healthy young adults. *J Athletic Train.* 2009;44(5):497–502.

293. Ozinga SJ, Linder SM, Koop MM, et al. Normative performance on the Balance Error Scoring System by youth, high school, and collegiate athletes. *J Athl Train.* 2018;53(7):636–645.

294. Iverson GL, Koehle MS. Normative data for the balance error scoring system in adults. *Rehabil Res Pract.* 2013;2013:846418.

295. Leddy AL, Crowner BE, Earhart GM. Functional gait assessment and balance evaluation system test: reliability, validity, sensitivity, and specificity for identifying individuals with Parkinson disease who fall. *Phys Ther.* 2011;91(1):102–113.

296. Mital S, Ramalingam T, Dibyendunarayan B, et al. Intra and inter-rater reliability of brief balance evaluation system test in patients with total knee arthroplasty. *Indian J Physiother Occup Ther.* 2018;12(1):144–150.

297. Duncan RP, Leddy AL, Cavanaugh JT, et al. Comparative utility of the BESTest, Mini-BESTest, and Brief-BESTest for predicting falls in individuals with Parkinson disease: a cohort study. *Phys Ther.* 2013;93(4):542–550.

298. Jacobson CP, Means ED. Efficacy of a monothermal warm water caloric screening test. *Ann Otol Rhinol Laryngol.* 1985;94:377–381.

299. Shupak A, Kaminer M, Gilbey P, Tal D. Monothermal caloric testing in the screening of vestibular function. *Aviat Space Env Med.* 2010;81(4):369–374.

300. Shumway-Cook A, Taylor CS, Matsuda, PN et al. Expanding the scoring system for the dynamic gait index. *Phys Ther.* 93(11):1493–1506.

301. Arceneaux JM. Validity and reliability of rapidly alternating movement's tests. *Int J Neurosci.* 1997;89:281–286.

302. Swaine BR, Sullivan SJ. Reliability of the cores for the finger to nose tests in adults with traumatic brain injury. *Phys Ther.* 1993;73(2):71–78.

303. Feys PG, Davies-Smith A, Jones R, et al. Intention tremor rated according to different finger-to-nose test protocols: a survey. *Arch Phys Med Rehabil.* 2003;84:79–82.

304. Schneiders AG, Sullivan SJ, Gray AR, et al. Normative values for three clinical measures of

motor performance used in the neurological assessment of sports concussion. *J Sci Med Sport.* 2010;13:196–201.

305. Nilsagård Y, Kollén L, Axelsson H, et al. Functional gait assessment: reliability and validity in people with peripheral vestibular disorders. *Int J Ther Rehabil.* 2014;21(8):367–373.

306. Yang Y, Wang Y, Zhou Y, et al. Validity of the Functional Gait Assessment in patients with Parkinson disease: construct, concurrent, and predictive validity. *Phys Ther.* 2014;94(3):392–400.

307. Juarez VJ, Lyons M. Interrater reliability of the Glasgow coma scale. *J Neurosci Nurs.* 1995;27(5):283–286.

308. Pettigrew LEL, Wilson JTL, Teasdale GM. Reliability of rating on the Glasgow Outcome Scales from in-person and telephone structured interviews. *J Head Trauma Rehabil.* 2003;18(3):252–258.

309. Rowley G, Fielding K. Reliability and accuracy of the Glasgow Coma Scale with experienced and inexperienced users. *Lancet.* 1991;337:535–538.

310. Fielding K, Rowley G. Reliability of assessments by skilled observers using the Glasgow Coma Scale. *Aust J Adv Nurs.* 1990;7(4):13–17.

311. Gill MR, Reiley DG, Green SM. Interrater reliability of Glasgow Coma Scale scores in the emergency department. *Ann Emerg Med.* 2004;43(2):215–223.

312. Awadie A, Holdstein Y, Kaminer M, Shupak A. The head impulse test as a predictor of video nystagmography caloric test lateralization according to the level of examiner experience: a prospective open-label study. *Ent Ear Nose Throat J.* 2018;97(1/2):16–23.

313. Singh N, Govindaswamy R, Jagadish N. Efficacy of vestibulo-ocular reflex gain and reflxation saccades of video head impulse test in identifying vestibular pathologies. *Ind J Otol.* 2017;23(4):247–251.

314. Heick JD, Bay C, Dompier TP, Valovich McLeod TC. The psychometric properties of the King-Devick Test and the influence of age and sex in healthy individuals aged 14 to 24 years. *Athletic Train Sports Health Care.* 2016;8(5):222–229.

315. Alsalaheen B, Haines J, Yorke A, Diebold J. King-Devick Test reference values and associations with balance measures in high school American football players. *Scand J Med Sci Sports.* 2016;26(2):235–239.

316. Vartiainen MV, Holm A, Peltonen K, et al. King-Devick test normative reference values for professional male ice hockey players. *Scand J Med Sci Sports.* 2015;25(3):e327–e330.

317. Hecimovich M, King D, Dempsey A, Murphy M. The King-Devick test is a valid and reliable tool for assessing sport-related concussion in Australian football: a prospective cohort study. *J Sci Med Sport.* 2018;21(10):1004–1007.

318. Hale L, McIlraith L, Miller C, et al. The interrater reliability of the modified Gait Abnormality Rating Scale for use with people with intellectual disability. *J Intellect Dev Disabil.* 2010;5(2):77–81.

319. Brach JS, VanSwearingen JM. Physical impairment and disability: relationship to performance of activities of daily living in community-dwelling older men. *Phys Ther.* 2002;82(8):752–761.

320. Franchignoni F, Tesio L, Martino MT, et al. Reliability of four simple, quantitative tests of balance and mobility in health elderly females. *Aging Clin Exp Res.* 1998;10(1):26–31.

321. Johnston DF. A new modification of the Rinne test. *Clin Otolaryngol.* 1992;17:322–326.

322. Thyssen HH, Brynskov J, Jansen EC, et al. Normal ranges and reproducibility for the quantitative Romberg's test. *Acta Neurol Scand.* 1982;66:100–104

323. Geer F, Letz R, Green RC. Relationships between quantitative measures and neurologist's clinical rating of tremor and standing steadiness in two epidemiological studies. *Neurotoxicology.* 2000;21(5):753–760.

324. Jacobson GP, McCaslin DL, Piker EG, et al. Insensitivity of the "Romberg test of standing balance on firm and compliant support surfaces" to the results of caloric and VEMP tests. *Ear Hear.* 2011;32(6):e1–e5.

325. Undén L, Calcagnile O, Undén J, et al. Validation of the Scandinavian guidelines for initial management of minimal, mild and moderate traumatic brain injury in adults. *BMC Med.* 2015;13:1–9.

326. Undén J, Dalziel SR, Borland ML, et al. External validation of the Scandinavian guidelines for management of minimal, mild and moderate head injuries in children. *BMC Med.* 2018;16(1):176.

327. Shaikh AA, Walunjkar RN. Reliability of the Star Excursion Balance test (SEBT) in healthy children of 12-16 years. *Indian Physiother Occup Ther.* 2014;8(2):29–32.

328. Hyong IH, Kim JH. Test of intrarater and interrater reliability for the star excursion balance test. *J Phys Ther Sci.* 2014;26(8):1139–1141.

329. van Lieshout R, Reijneveld EA, van den Berg SM, et al. Reproducibility of the modified star excursion balance test composite and specific reach direction scores. *Int J Sports Phys Ther.* 2016;11(3):356–365.

330. Gribble PA, Kelly SE, Refshauge KM, Hiller CE. Interrater reliability of the star excursion balance test. *J Athletic Train.* 2013;48(5):621–626.

331. Munro AG, Herrington LC. Between-session reliability of the star excursion balance test. *Phys Ther Sport.* 2010;11(4):128–132.

CHAPTER 3

Cervical Spine

Examination of the cervical spine involves determining whether the injury or pathology occurs in the cervical spine or in a portion of the upper limb. Cyriax[1] called this assessment the **scanning examination.** In the initial assessment of a patient who complains of pain in the neck and/or upper limb, this procedure is always carried out unless the examiner is absolutely sure of the location of the lesion. If the injury is in the neck, the scanning examination is definitely called for to rule out neurological involvement. After the lesion site has been determined, a more detailed assessment of the affected area is performed if it is outside the cervical spine.

Because many conditions affecting the cervical spine can be manifested in other parts of the body, the cervical spine is a complicated area to assess properly, and adequate time must be allowed to ensure that as many causes or problems are examined as possible.

Applied Anatomy

The cervical spine consists of several pairs of joints. It is an area in which stability has been sacrificed for mobility, making the cervical spine particularly vulnerable to injury because it sits between a heavy, mobile head and a stable thoracic spine and ribs. The cervical spine is divided into two areas—the **cervicoencephalic** for the upper cervical spine and the **cervicobrachial** for the lower cervical spine. The cervicoencephalic or cervicocranial region (C0 to C2) shows the relationship between the cervical spine and the occiput, and injuries in this region have the potential of involving the brain, brain stem, and spinal cord (Fig. 3.1).[2,3] Injuries in this area lead to symptoms of headache, fatigue, vertigo, poor concentration, hypertonia of the sympathetic nervous system, and irritability. In addition, there may be a cognitive dysfunction and a cranial nerve dysfunction.[2,3]

The **atlanto-occipital joints** (C0 to C1) are the two uppermost joints. The principal motion of these two joints is flexion-extension (15° to 20°), or nodding of the head. Side flexion is approximately 10°, whereas rotation is negligible. The **atlas** (C1) has no vertebral body as such. During development, the vertebral body of C1 evolves into the **odontoid process,** which is part of C2. The atlanto-occipital joints are ellipsoid and act in unison. Along with the atlanto-axial joints, these joints are the most complex articulations of the axial skeleton.

There are several ligaments that stabilize the atlanto-occipital joints. Anteriorly and posteriorly are the atlanto-occipital membranes. The anterior membrane is strengthened by the anterior longitudinal ligament. The posterior membrane replaces the ligamentum flavum between the atlas and occiput. The tectorial membrane, which is a broad band covering the dens and its ligaments, is found within the vertebral canal and is a continuation of the posterior longitudinal ligament. The alar ligaments are two strong rounded cords found on each side of the upper dens passing upward and laterally to attach on the medial sides of the occipital condyles. The alar ligaments limit flexion and rotation and play a major role in stabilizing C1 and C2, especially in rotation.[4]

The **atlanto-axial joints** (C1–C2) constitute the most mobile articulations of the spine. Flexion-extension is approximately 10°, and side flexion is approximately 5°. Rotation, which is approximately 50°, is the primary movement of these joints. With rotation, there is a decrease in height of the cervical spine at this level as the vertebrae approximate because of the shape of the facet joints. The odontoid process of C2 acts as a pivot point for the rotation. This middle, or median, joint is classified as a **pivot (trochoidal) joint.** The lateral atlanto-axial, or facet, joints are classified as **plane joints.** Generally, if a person can talk and chew, there is probably some motion occurring at C1–C2. At the atlanto-axial joints, the main supporting ligament is the **transverse ligament of the atlas,** which holds the dens of the axis against the anterior arch of the atlas. It is this ligament that weakens or ruptures in rheumatoid arthritis. As the ligament crosses the dens, there are two projections off the ligament, one going superiorly to the occiput and one inferiorly to the axis. The ligament and the projections form a cross, and the three parts taken together are called the **cruciform ligament of the atlas** (Fig. 3.2).

The vertebral artery—part of the vertebrobasilar system that passes through the transverse processes of the cervical vertebrae usually starting at C6 but entering as high as C4—supplies 20% of the blood supply to the brain (primarily the hindbrain) along with the internal carotid artery (80%) (Fig. 3.3).[5,6] In its path, the vertebral artery lies close to the facet joints and vertebral body where it

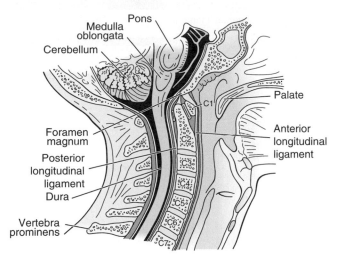

Fig. 3.1 This sagittal view of the cervical spine shows the relations among the brain stem, the medulla oblongata, the foramen magnum, the spinal canal, and the cervical spine. The lower portion of the medulla is outside and below the foramen; therefore, with subluxation of the atlas on the axis, compression of the brain stem can occur through pressure of the odontoid against the upper spinal cord and the lower medulla. Note that the anterior arch of the atlas is only millimeters from the pharynx. (Redrawn from Bland JH: *Disorders of the cervical spine*, Philadelphia, 1994, W.B. Saunders, p 47.)

may be compressed by osteophyte formation or injury to the facet joint. In addition, in older individuals, atherosclerotic changes and other vascular risk factors (e.g., hypertension, high fat or cholesterol levels, diabetes, smoking) may contribute to altered blood flow in the arteries.[7] The vertebral and internal carotid arteries are stressed primarily by rotation, extension, and traction movements, but other movements may also stretch the artery.[8–10] Rotation and extension of as little as 20° have been shown to significantly decrease vertebral artery blood flow.[11,12] The greatest stresses are placed on the vertebral arteries in four places: where it enters the transverse process of C6, within the bony canals of the vertebral transverse processes, between C1 and C2, and between C1 and the entry of the arteries into the skull.[13,14] These latter two areas have the greatest potential for problems (e.g., thrombosis, dissection, stroke) related to treatment and their concomitant stress on the vertebral arteries.[15] Dutton[13] reports that the most common mechanism for nonpenetrating injury to the vertebral artery is neck extension, with or without side flexion or rotation.[16,17] Given the type of injury possible, symptoms may be delayed.[18,19] Symptoms related to the vertebral artery include vertigo, balance deficits, arm paresthesia, nausea, tinnitus, "drop attacks" (i.e., falling without fainting), visual disturbances, or, in rare cases, stroke or death.[20]

The lower cervical spine (C3 to C7) is called the **cervicobrachial area**, since pain in this area is commonly referred into the upper extremity.[2,3] Pathology in this region leads to neck pain alone, arm pain alone, or both neck and arm pain. Thus, symptoms include neck and/or arm pain, headaches, restricted range of motion

(ROM), paresthesia, altered myotomes and dermatomes, and radicular signs. Cognitive dysfunction and cranial nerve dysfunction are not commonly symptoms of injuries in this area although sympathetic dysfunction may be. Injury to both areas, if severe enough, may result in psychosocial issues.

There are 14 **facet (apophyseal) joints** in the cervical spine (C1 to C7). The upper four facet joints in the two upper thoracic vertebrae (T1 to T2) are often included in the examination of the cervical spine. The superior facets of the cervical spine face upward, backward, and medially; the inferior facets face downward, forward, and laterally (Fig. 3.4). This plane facilitates flexion and extension, but it prevents simple rotation or side flexion without both occurring to some degree together. This is called a **coupled movement** with rotation and side flexion both occurring with either movement.[21] Ishii et al.[22,23] reported that between C0 and C2, as well as C7 and T1, the two movements occur in opposite directions while between C2 and C7, they occur in the same direction. These joints move primarily by gliding and are classified as **synovial (diarthrodial) joints**. The capsules are lax to allow sufficient movement. At the same time, they provide support and a check-rein type of restriction at end range. The greatest flexion-extension of the facet joints occurs between C5 and C6; however, there is almost as much movement at C4 to C5 and C6 to C7. Because of this mobility, degeneration is more likely to be seen at these levels. The neutral or resting position of the cervical spine is slightly extended. The close packed position of the facet joints is complete extension.

Cervical Spine	
Resting position:	Midway between flexion and extension
Close packed position:	Full extension
Capsular pattern:	Side flexion and rotation equally limited extension

The **recurrent meningeal,** or **sinuvertebral, nerve** innervates the anterior dura sac, the posterior annulus fibrosus, and the posterior longitudinal ligament. The facet joints are innervated by the medial branch of the dorsal primary rami.[24] For C3 to C7, the main ligaments are the anterior longitudinal ligament, the posterior longitudinal ligament, the ligamentum flavum, and the supraspinal and interspinal ligaments (Fig. 3.5). There are also ligaments between the transverse processes (intertransverse ligaments), but in the cervical spine, they are rudimentary.

Some anatomists[25–28] refer to the costal or uncovertebral processes as **uncinate joints** or **joints of Luschka** (Fig. 3.6). These structures were described by von Luschka in 1858. The uncus gives a "saddle"

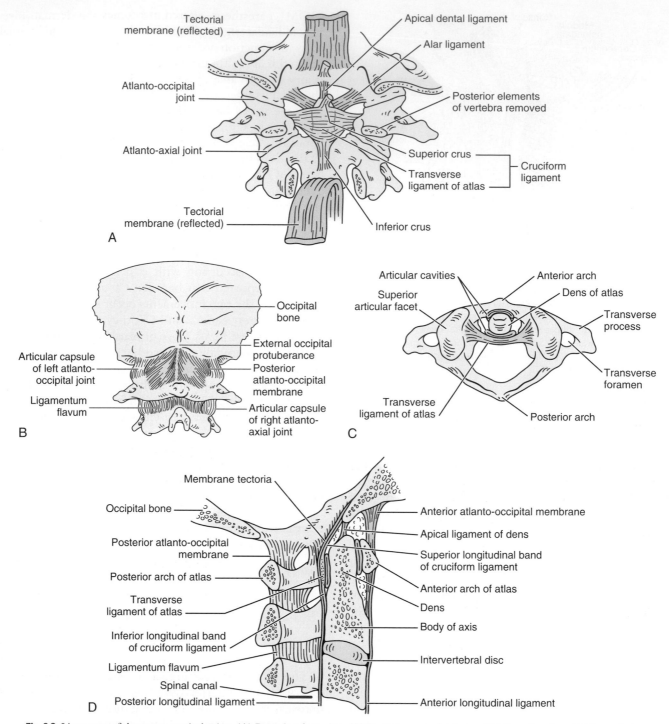

Fig. 3.2 Ligaments of the upper cervical spine. (A) Posterior deep view. (B) Posterior superficial view. (C) Superior view. (D) Lateral view.

form to the upper aspect of the cervical vertebra, which is more pronounced posterolaterally; it has the effect of limiting side flexion. Extending from the uncus is a "joint" that appears to form because of a weakness in the annulus fibrosus. The portion of the vertebra above, which "articulates" or conforms to the uncus, is called the *échancrure,* or notch. Notches are found from C3 to T1, but according to most authors,[25–28] they are not seen until age 6 to 9 years and are not fully developed

until 18 years of age. There is some controversy as to whether they should be classified as real joints because some authors believe they are the result of degeneration of the intervertebral disc.

The **intervertebral discs** make up approximately 25% of the height of the cervical spine. No disc is found between the atlas and the occiput (C0–C1) or between the atlas and the axis (C1–C2). It is the discs rather than the vertebrae that give the cervical spine its lordotic shape

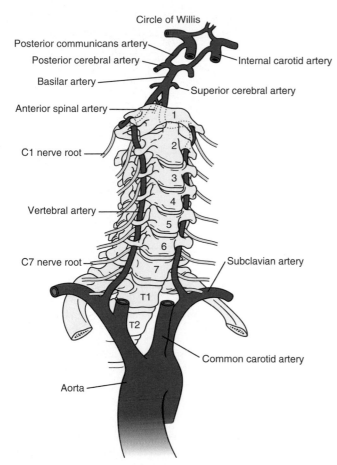

Fig. 3.3 Anterolateral drawing of the course of the vertebral artery from C6 to C1 through the bony rings of the foramina transversaria. Note the double U-turn the artery makes from C2 to C1 and the posterior course around the lateral mass of the atlas. (Modified from Bland JH, Nakano KK: Neck pain. In Kelley WN, et al., eds: *Textbook of rheumatology*, ed 1, Philadelphia, 1981, W.B. Saunders.)

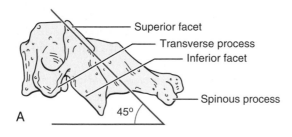

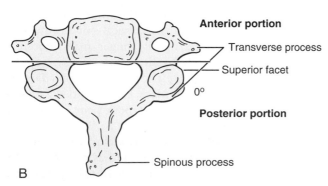

Fig. 3.4 Cervical spine-plane of facet joints. (A) Lateral view. (B) Superior view.

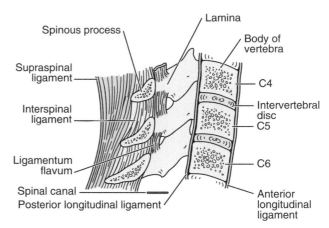

Fig. 3.5 Median section of C4 to C6 vertebrae to illustrate the intervertebral disc and the ligaments of the cervical spine.

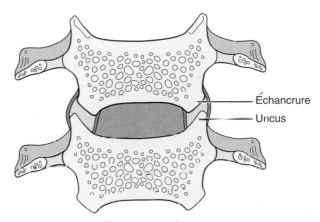

Fig. 3.6 Joints of Luschka.

(Fig. 3.7). The **nucleus pulposus** functions as a buffer to axial compression in distributing compressive forces, whereas the **annulus fibrosus** acts to withstand tension within the disc. The intervertebral disc has some innervation on the periphery of the annulus fibrosus.[29,30]

There are seven vertebrae in the cervical spine with the body of each vertebra (except C1) supporting the weight of those above it. The facet joints may bear some of the weight of the vertebrae above, but this weight is minimal if the normal lordotic posture is maintained. However, even this slight amount of weight bearing can lead to spondylitic changes in these joints. The outer ring of the vertebral body is made of cortical bone, and the inner part is made of cancellous bone covered with the cartilaginous end plate. The vertebral arch protects the spinal cord, while the spinous processes, most of which are bifid in the cervical spine, provide for attachment of muscles. The transverse processes have basically the same function. In the cervical spine, the transverse processes are made up of two parts: the anterior portion that provides the foramen for the vertebral body, and the posterior portion containing the two articular facets (see Fig. 3.4B). In the cervical spine, the

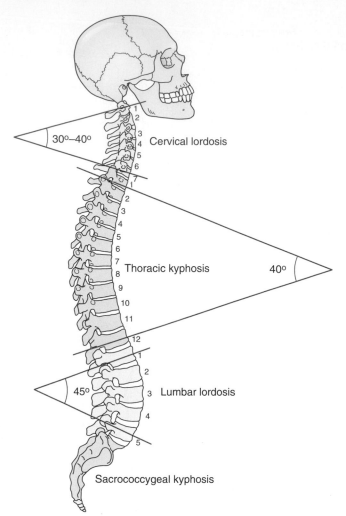

Fig. 3.7 The normal sagittal plane curvatures across the regions of the vertebral column. The curvatures represent the normal resting postures of the region. (Modified from Neumann DA: Kinesiology of the musculoskeletal system—foundations for physical rehabilitation, St Louis, 2002, Mosby, p 276.)

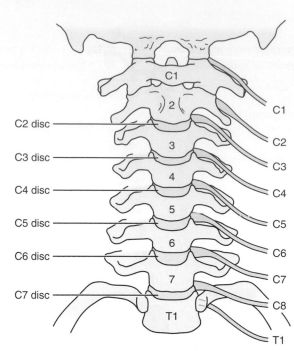

Fig. 3.8 Anterior view of cervical spine showing nerve roots. Note how each cervical nerve root is numbered for the vertebra below it.

Patient History

In addition to the questions listed under Patient History in Chapter 1, the examiner should obtain the following information from the patient:

1. *What is the patient's age?* Spondylosis (also called *spondylosis deformans*) is often seen in persons 25 years of age or older, and it is present in 60% of those older than 45 years and 85% of those older than 65 years of age.[31,32] It is a generalized disease of aging initiated by intervertebral disc degeneration. Symptoms of osteoarthritis do not usually appear until a person is 60 years of age or older (Table 3.1).

2. *What are the signs and symptoms, and which are most severe?* Table 3.2 outlines many of the signs and symptoms that may arise from cervical spine pathology.[33] Where are the symptoms most severe—in the neck, the shoulder, above or below the elbow, in the hands, and/or fingers?[34] Location of the symptoms may help determine what level of the cervical spine is involved (e.g., tingling in the middle finger may indicate a problem at C6 to C7). Are the symptoms constant, intermittent, or variable?[34] The Bone and Joint Decade 2000–10 Task Force on Neck Pain and its Associated Disorders recommended that neck pain sufferers be divided into four groups (Table 3.3).[35]

Watkins[36] provided a severity scale for neurological injury in football that can be used as a guideline for injury severity involving the cervical spine, especially if one is contemplating allowing the patient to return to activity (Fig. 3.9). A combined score (A + B) of

spinous processes are at the level of the facet joints of the same vertebra. Generally, the spinous process is considered to be absent or at least rudimentary on C1. This is why the first palpable vertebra descending from the external occiput protuberance is the spinous process of C2.

Although there are seven cervical vertebrae, there are eight **cervical nerve roots.** This difference occurs because there is a nerve root exiting between the occiput and C1 that is designated the C1 nerve root. In the cervical spine, each nerve root is named for the vertebra below it. As an example, C5 nerve root exists between the C4 and C5 vertebrae (Fig. 3.8). In the rest of the spine, each nerve root is named for the vertebra above; the L4 nerve root, for example, exists between the L4 and L5 vertebrae. The switch in naming of the nerve roots from the one below to the one above is made between the C7 and T1 vertebrae. The nerve root between these two vertebrae is called C8, accounting for the fact that there are eight cervical nerve roots and only seven cervical vertebrae.

TABLE **3.1**

Differential Diagnosis of Cervical Spondylosis, Spinal Stenosis, and Disc Herniation

	Cervical Spondylosis	Cervical Spinal Stenosis	Cervical Disc Herniation[a]
Pain	Unilateral	May be unilateral or bilateral	May be unilateral (most common) or bilateral
Distribution of pain	Into affected dermatomes	Usually several dermatomes affected	Into affected dermatomes
Pain on extension	Increases	Increases	May increase (most common)
Pain on flexion	Decreases	Decreases	May increase or decrease[b] (most common)
Pain relieved by rest	No	Yes	No
Age group affected	60% of those older than 45 years	11–70 years	17–60 years
	85% of those older than 65 years	Most common: 30–60 years	
Instability	Possible	No	No
Levels commonly affected	C5–C6, C6–C7	Varies	C5–C6
Onset	Slow	Slow (may be combined with spondylosis or disc herniation)	Sudden
Diagnostic imaging	Diagnostic	Diagnostic	Diagnostic (be sure clinical signs support)

[a]Posterolateral protrusion.
[b]Depends on the direction of the herniation.

TABLE **3.2**

Signs and Symptoms Arising From Cervical Spine Pathology

Signs	Symptoms
• Anesthesia (lack of sensation)	• Arm and leg pain and ache
• Asymmetry	• Auditory disturbance
• Ataxia	• Cough
• Atrophy	• Depressed mood
• Drop attack	• Diarrhea
• Dysesthesia (abnormal sensation)	• Diplopia
• Falling	• Dizziness
• Fasciculation	• Fatigue
• Hyperesthesia (increased sensitivity)	• Gait disturbance
• Nystagmus	• Headache
• Pathologic gait	• Insomnia
• Reflex changes	• Muscle twitch
• Spastic gait	• Nausea
• Sweating or lack of sweating	• Pain
• Tender bones	• Paresthesia
• Tender muscles	• Poor balance
• Tender scalp	• Restless arms and legs
• Transient loss of hearing, consciousness, sight	• Sneeze
• Upper extremity weakness	• Speech disturbance
	• Stiff neck
	• Threatened faint
	• Tinnitus
	• Torticollis
	• Vertigo
	• Visual disturbance

Modified from Bland JH: *Disorders of the Cervical Spine*, Philadelphia, 1994, W.B. Saunders Co, p 161.

TABLE **3.3**

Grading of Patients Suffering From Neck Pain

Grade	Clinical Presentation
1	No signs of major pathology
	Little or no interference with ADL
2	No signs of major pathology
	Interference with ADL
3	Pain with neurological signs of nerve compression (radiculopathy)
4	Signs of major pathology (e.g., instability, infection)

ADL, Activities of daily living.
Adapted from Guzman J, Haldeman S, Carroll LJ, et al: Clinical practice implications of the Bone and Joint Decade 2000–2010 Task Force on Neck Pain and Its Associated Disorders: from concepts and findings to recommendations, *J Manipulative Physiol Ther* 32(2 Suppl):235, 2009.

4 is considered a mild episode, 4 to 7 is a moderate episode, and 8 to 10 is a severe episode. This scale can be combined with radiologic information on canal size (score C) to give a general determination of the possibility of symptoms returning if the patient returns to activity. In this case, a score of 6 (A + B + C) indicates minimum risk, 6 to 10 is moderate risk, and 10 to 15 is severe risk. Watkins[36] also points out that extenuating factors (such as age of patient, level of activity, and risk versus benefit) also play a role and, although not included in the score, must be considered. Table 3.4

Watkins' Severity Scale for Neurological Deficit

Grade	Neurological Deficit
1	Unilateral arm numbness or dysesthesia; loss of strength
2	Bilateral upper extremity loss of motor and sensory function
3	Ipsilateral arm, leg, and trunk loss of motor and sensory function
4	Transient quadriparesis (temporary sensory loss in all 4 limbs)
5	Transient quadriplegia (temporary motor loss in all 4 limbs)
Score:_____ (A)	

Grade	Time Symptoms Present
1	Less than 5 min
2	Less than 1 h
3	Less than 24 h
4	Less than 1 week
5	Greater than 1 week
Score:_____ (B)	

Severity Score: A + B = _____
(≤4: mild episode; 4–7: moderate episode; 8–10: severe episode)

Grade	Central Canal Diameter
1	>12 mm
2	Between 10 and 12
3	10 mm
4	8–10 mm
5	<8 mm
Score:_____ (C)	

Return to Activity Score: A + B + C = _____
(≤6: minimum risk; 6–10: moderate risk; 10–15: severe risk)

Fig. 3.9 Watkins Severity Scale for Neurologic Deficit. (Data from Watkins RG: Neck injuries in football. In Watkins RG, editor: *The spine in sports,* St. Louis, 1996, Mosby-Year Book, p 327.)

outlines some of the factors that increase the chances of recovery from neck pain. **Chronic post-whiplash syndrome** can lead to anxiety, pain catastrophizing (negative or heightened orientation toward pain), and other adverse psychosocial factors over time, and it can play a major role in the symptoms felt by the patient.[37] Table 3.5 outlines yellow flags related to fear-avoidance beliefs and possible long-term disability.

3. *What was the mechanism of injury?* Was trauma, stretching, or overuse involved? Was the patient moving when the injury occurred? Table 3.6 outlines warning signs and symptoms (red flags) of serious cervical spine disorders.[38] These questions help determine the type and severity of injury. For example, trauma may cause a whiplash-type (acceleration) injury or **whiplash-associated disorder (WAD)** (Table 3.7),[39] stretching may lead to "burners," overuse or sustained postures may result in thoracic outlet symptoms, and

a report of an insidious onset in someone older than 55 years of age may indicate cervical spondylosis. Was the patient hit from the side, front, or behind? Did the patient see the accident coming?[40] "Burners" or "stingers" typically occur from a blow to part of the brachial plexus or from stretching or compression of the brachial plexus (Table 3.8; Fig. 3.10). **Backpack palsy (BPP)**[41] is sometimes reported from carrying a heavy backpack especially without waist support and the symptoms, commonly bilateral, are related to the brachial plexus (i.e., paresis, numbness, paresthesia, and painless motor weakness in the shoulder girdle and elbow flexor muscles). The answers to these questions help the examiner determine how the injury occurred, the tissues injured, and the severity of the injuries.

4. *Has the patient had neck pain before?* Table 3.9 outlines factors that decrease chances of a new

TABLE **3.4**

Factors That Increase Chances of Recovery From an Episode of Neck Pain

Scenario and Grade of Neck Pain	Likely Increase	Might Increase	No Effect	Not Enough Evidence to Make Determination
General population	Younger age, no previous neck pain, good physical and psychological health, good coping, good social support	Being employed	—	Gender, general exercise or fitness prior to pain episode, cervical disc changes
At work	Exercise and sports, no prior pain or prior sick leave	Changing jobs (for certain job types), white collar job, greater influence over work	Age, ergonomics/physical job demands, work-related psychosocial factors (but many such factors not studied)	Gender, compensation, litigation, obesity, smoking, cervical disc changes
After a traffic collision	No prior pain or sick leave, fewer initial symptoms, less symptom severity, Grade I WAD, good psychological health (e.g., not coping passively, no fear of movement, no post-injury anxiety), no early "overtreatment"	No prior pain problems, good prior health, non-tort insurance, no lawyer involvement, lower collision speed	Collision-specific factors (such as head position when struck, position in vehicle, direction of collision)	Age, gender, culture, prior physical fitness, cervical disc changes

WAD, Whiplash-associated disorder.

From Guzman J, Haldeman S, Carroll LJ, et al: Clinical practice implications of the Bone and Joint Decade 2000–2010 Task Force on Neck Pain and its Associated Disorders: from concepts and findings to recommendations, *J Manipulative Physiol Ther* 32(2 Suppl):234, 2009.

episode of neck pain.[35] In chronic cases of pain or headache, a **pain diary** may be useful to help determine pain patterns or factors that trigger the pain or headaches.

5. *What is the patient's usual activity or pastime?* Do any particular activities or postures bother the patient? What type of work does the patient do? Are there any positions that the patient holds for long periods (e.g., when sewing, typing, or working at a desk)? Does the patient wear glasses? If so, are they bifocals or trifocals? Upper cervical symptoms may result from excessive nodding as the patient tries to focus through the correct part of the glasses. Cervicothoracic (lower cervical/upper thoracic spine) joint problems are often painful when activities that require push-and-pull motion (such as lawn mowing, sawing, and cleaning windows) are performed. What movements bother the patient? For example, extension can aggravate symptoms in patients with radicular signs and symptoms.[42]

6. *Did the head strike anything, or did the patient lose consciousness?* If the injury was caused by a motor vehicle accident, it is important to know whether the patient was wearing a seat belt, the type of seat belt (lap or shoulder), and whether the patient saw the accident coming. These questions give some idea of the severity and mechanisms of injury. If the patient was unconscious or unsteady, the character of each episode of altered consciousness should be noted (see Chapter 2).

7. *Did the symptoms come on right away?* Bone pain usually occurs immediately, but muscle or ligamentous pain can either come on immediately (e.g., a tear) or occur several hours or days later (e.g., stretching caused by a motor vehicle accident). Seventy percent of whiplash patients reported immediate symptom occurrence while the rest reported delayed symptoms.[33,43–47] How long have the symptoms been present? Myofascial pain syndromes demonstrate generalized aching and at least three trigger points, which have lasted for at least 3 months with no history of trauma.[48]

8. *What are the sites and boundaries of the pain?* Have the patient point to the location or locations of the pain. Symptoms do not go down the arm for a C4 nerve root injury or for nerve roots above that level. For example, C2 and C3 nerve roots go to the lateral neck while C4 and C5 nerve roots go to the lateral neck and shoulders. **Cervical radiculopathy,** or injury to the nerve roots in the cervical spine, presents primarily with unilateral motor and sensory symptoms into the upper limb, with muscle weakness (myotome), sensory alteration (dermatome), reflex hypoactivity, and sometimes focal activity being the primary signs.[49–52] Acute

TABLE 3.5

Clinical Yellow Flags Indicating Heightened Fear-Avoidance Beliefs and Risk of Patient Developing Long-Term Disability

Attitudes and Beliefs	Behaviors
• Belief that pain is harmful or disabling, resulting in guarding and fear of movement • Belief that all pain must be abolished before returning to activity • Expectation of increased pain with activity or work, lack of ability to predict capabilities • Catastrophizing, expecting the worst • Belief that pain is uncontrollable • Passive attitude to rehabilitation	• Use of extended rest • Reduced activity level with significant withdrawal from daily activities • Avoidance of normal activity and progressive substitution of lifestyle away from productive activity • Reports of extremely high pain intensity • Excessive reliance on aids (braces, crutches, and so on) • Sleep quality reduced following the onset of back pain • High intake of alcohol or other substances with an increase since the onset of back pain • Smoking

From Childs JD, Fritz JM, Piva SR, et al: Proposal of a classification system for patients with neck pain, *J Orthop Sports Phys Ther* 34:686–700, 2004. Data from Kendall, et al: *Guide to assessing psychosocial yellow flags in acute low back pain: risk factors for long-term disability and work loss*, Wellington, New Zealand, 2002, Accident Rehabilitation and Compensation Insurance Corporation of New Zealand and the National Health Committee.

radiculopathies are commonly associated with disc herniations, whereas chronic types are more related to spondylosis.[50] Disc herniations in the cervical spine commonly cause severe neck pain that may radiate into the shoulder, scapula, and/or arm; limit ROM; and cause an increase in pain on coughing, sneezing, jarring, or straining.[47] Using discography, it has been demonstrated that disc injury in the cervical spine can refer pain to the thoracic spine, especially along the medial scapular border.[53] C3–C4 disc referral of pain is to the cervicothoracic junction and ipsilateral upper trapezius, C4–C5 is to the superomedial border of the scapula, C5–C6 to mid-scapular area, and C6–C7 to lower scapular area and along the medial scapular border. **Cervical myelopathy,** or injury to the spinal cord itself, is more likely to present with spastic weakness, paresthesia, and possible incoordination in one or both lower limbs, as well as proprioceptive and/or sphincter dysfunction (Tables 3.10 and 3.11).[54] With cervical myelopathy, hand symptoms may be evident early. This **myelopathic hand** results in weakness then loss of adduction and extension of the ulnar two or three fingers (**finger escape sign** or **Wartenberg sign**—difficulty with little finger adduction) and the patient has an inability to grip and release (**grip and release test**) these fingers rapidly.[55] To do the test, the patient is asked to

TABLE 3.6

Warning Signs and Symptoms of Serious Cervical Spine Disorders (Red Flags), Some of Which Will Necessitate Immediate Imaging Studies

Potential Cause	Clinical Characteristics
Fracture	Clinically relevant trauma in adolescent or adult Minor trauma in elderly patient Ankylosing spondylitis Follow Canadian C-Spine Rules
Neoplasm (cancer)	Pain worse at night Unexplained weight loss History of neoplasm Age of more than 50 or less than 20 years Previous history of cancer Constant pain, no relief with bed rest
Infection	Fever, chills, night sweats Unexplained weight loss History of recent systemic infection Recent invasive procedure Immunosuppression Intravenous drug use
Neurologic injury	Progressive neurologic deficit Upper- and lower-extremity symptoms Bowel or bladder dysfunction
Cervical myelopathy	Muscle wasting of hand intrinsic muscles Sensory disturbance in the hands Unsteady gait Hoffman's reflex present Hyperreflexia Bowel and bladder disturbances Multisegmental weakness and/or sensory changes Clonus (a series of involuntary, rhythmic muscle contractions) Inverted supinator sign
Upper cervical ligamentous instability	Occipital headache and numbness Severe limitation during neck active ROM in all directions Signs of cervical myelopathy Post trauma Rheumatoid arthritis Down syndrome
Vertebral artery insufficiency	Drop attacks Dizziness or light-headedness related to neck movement Dysphasia (difficulty swallowing) Dysarthria (difficulty speaking) Diplopia (double vision) Positive cranial nerve signs Ataxia (lack of muscle coordination) Nausea
Inflammatory or systemic disease	Temperature more than 37°C (98.6°F) Blood pressure more than 160/95 mm Hg Resting pulse more than 100 bpm Resting respiration more than 25 bpm Fatigue

ROM, Range of motion.
Modified from Rao RD, Currier BL, Albert TJ, et al: Degenerative cervical spondylosis: clinical syndromes, pathogenesis, and management, *J Bone Joint Surg Am* 89(6):1360–1378, 2007; Childs JD, Fritz JM, Piva SR, et al: Proposal of a classification system for patients with neck pain, *J Orthop Sports Phys Ther* 34:688, 2004.

TABLE **3.7**

The Quebec Severity Classification of Whiplash-Associated Disorders

Grade	Clinical Presentation
0	No neck symptoms, no physical sign(s)
1	No physical sign(s); neck pain; stiffness or tenderness only; neck complaints predominate; normal ROM; normal reflexes, dermatomes, and myotomes
2	Neck symptoms (pain, stiffness) and musculoskeletal sign(s), such as decreased ROM and point tenderness; soft-tissue complaints (pain, stiffness) into shoulders and back; normal reflexes, dermatomes, and myotomes
3	Neck symptoms (pain, stiffness, restricted ROM) and neurological sign(s), such as decreased or absence of deep tendon reflexes, weakness (positive myotomes), and sensory (positive dermatome) deficits; x-ray shows no fracture; CT/MRI may show nerve involvement; possible disc lesion
4	Neck symptoms (pain, stiffness, restricted ROM) with fracture or dislocation and objective neurological signs, possible spinal cord signs

CT, Computed tomography; *MRI,* magnetic resonance imaging; *ROM,* range of motion.
Modified from Spitzer WO, Skovron ML, Salmi LR, et al: Scientific monograph of the Quebec Task Force on Whiplash-Associated Disorders: redefining "whiplash" and its management, *Spine* 20(8 Suppl):8S–58S, 1995.

grip and release for 10 seconds. Normally, 20 or more repetitions are possible.

9. *Is there any radiation of pain?* It is helpful to correlate this answer with dermatome and sensory peripheral nerve findings when performing sensation testing and palpation later in the examination. Is the pain deep, superficial, shooting, burning, or aching? For example, when an athlete experiences a "burner," the sensation is a lightning-like, burning pain into the shoulder and arm, followed by a period of heaviness or loss of function in the arm. Fig. 3.11 shows the radiation of pain with facet (apophyseal) joint pathology.[56,57]

10. *Is the pain affected by laughing, coughing, sneezing, or straining?* If so, an increase in intrathoracic or intra-abdominal pressure may be contributing to the problem.

11. *Does the patient have any headaches? If so, where? How frequently do they occur?* Cervicogenic headaches occur as a symptom of musculoskeletal dysfunction in the cervical spine, especially C1, C2, and C3.[58–61] Table 3.12 outlines the clinical criteria for a cervicogenic headache.[58] If the patient complains of a headache, the examiner should record the headache history, its temporal pattern, symptoms behavior, and medication intake to ensure the headache is benign and can be classified.[62] For example, do they occur every day, two times per day, two days per week, or one day per month?[63] How intense are they? How long do they last? Are they affected by medication and, if so, by how much medication, and

TABLE **3.8**

Differential Diagnosis of Cervical Nerve Root and Brachial Plexus Lesion

	Cervical Nerve Root Lesion	Brachial Plexus Lesion
Cause	Disc herniation Stenosis Osteophytes Swelling with trauma Spondylosis	Stretching of cervical spine Compression of cervical spine Depression of shoulder
Contributing factors	Congenital defects	Thoracic outlet syndrome
Pain	Sharp, burning in affected dermatomes	Sharp, burning in all or most of arm dermatomes, pain in trapezius
Paresthesia	Numbness, pins and needles in affected dermatomes	Numbness, pins and needles in all or most arm dermatomes (more ambiguous distribution)
Tenderness	Over affected area of posterior cervical spine	Over affected area of brachial plexus or lateral to cervical spine
Range of motion	Decreased	Decreased but usually returns rather quickly
Weakness	Transient paralysis usually Myotome may be affected	Transient muscle weakness Myotomes affected
Deep tendon reflexes	Affected nerve root may be depressed	May be depressed
Provocative test	Side flexion, rotation, and extension with compression increase symptoms Cervical traction decreases symptoms Upper limb tension tests positive	Side flexion with compression (same side) or stretch (opposite side) may increase symptoms Upper limb tension tests may be positive

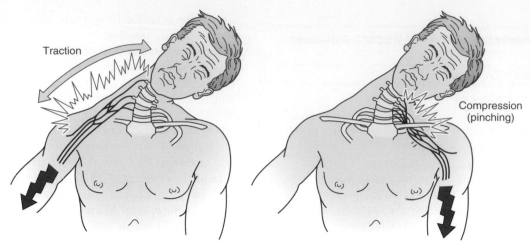

Fig. 3.10 Mechanism of injury for brachial plexus (burner or stinger) pathology.

TABLE **3.9**

Factors That Decrease Chances of Getting a New Episode of Neck Pain

Scenario and Grade of Neck Pain	Likely Decrease	Might Decrease	No Effect	Not Enough Evidence to Make Determination
General population	No previous neck pain, no other musculoskeletal problems, good psychological health	Younger age, male gender, non-smoking, changing rules in sports (like in ice hockey)	Obesity	Weight of school bags, cervical disc changes (on imaging)
At work	Younger age (peak risk in fourth and fifth decades), male gender, no previous pain in the neck, back or upper limbs, little psychological job strain, good coworker support, active work (nonsedentary), less repetitive or precision work	Not being an immigrant or a visible minority, higher strength or endurance of the neck, not working with the neck bent for prolonged periods, non-smoking, no previous headaches, good physical health, "non-type A" personality, not working in awkward positions, light physical work, adequate keyboard position, no awkward head, elbow and shoulder posture, no screen glare	Physical or sports activity during leisure, sleep quality, time spent on domestic activities, time spent on hobbies	Marital status, education, occupational class duration of employment, obesity, self-assessed health status, mental stress, job satisfaction, working with hands above the shoulder level, height of computer screen, cervical disc changes
After a traffic collision	—	Male gender, no previous neck pain, riding in back seat, side collision, no compensation for pain and suffering, specially engineered car seats and headrests	Tow bars in the car, age, type of child seat restraint	Awareness of collision, head position at time of collision, severity of collision impact, cervical disc changes (on imaging)

From Guzman J, Haldeman S, Carroll LJ, et al: Clinical practice implications of the Bone and Joint Decade 2000–2010 Task Force on Neck Pain and Its Associated Disorders: from concepts and finding to recommendations, *J Manipulative Physiol Ther* 32(2 Suppl):233, 2009.

what kind? Are there any precipitating factors (e.g., food, stress, posture)? See Tables 2.15–2.17, which indicate the influence of time of day, body position, headache location, and type of pain on diagnosis of the type of headache that the patient may have. Table 2.18 outlines the salient features of some of the more common headaches. Craniovertebral joint dysfunction commonly is accompanied by headaches. For example, C1 headaches occur at the base and top of the head, whereas C2 headaches are referred to the temporal area. **Cervical arterial dissection**, although rare, may result in neck pain and

TABLE **3.10**

Signs and Symptoms in Cervical Myelopathy

Motor Changes	Sensory Changes
Initial Symptoms (Predominantly Lower Limbs)	• Headache and head pain
• Spastic paraparesis	• Neck, eye, ear, throat, or sinus pain
• Stiffness and heaviness, scuffing of the toe, difficulty climbing stairs	• Sensory symptoms in the pharynx and larynx
• Weakness, spasms, cramps, easy fatigability	• Paroxysmal hoarseness and aphonia
• Decreased power, especially of flexors (dorsiflexors of ankles and toes; flexors of hips)	• Rotary vertigo
• Hyperreflexia of knee and ankle jerks, with clonus	• Tinnitus synchronous with pulse or continuous whistling noises
• Positive Babinski sign, extensor hypertonia	• Deafness
• Decreased or absent superficial abdominal and cremasteric reflexes	• Oculovisual changes (e.g., blurring, photophobia, scintillating scotomata, diplopia, homonymous hemianopsia, and nystagmus)
• Drop foot, crural monoplegia	• Autonomic disturbance (e.g., sweating, flushing, rhinorrhea, salivation, lacrimation, nausea, and vomiting)
Later Symptoms (In Order of Occurrence)	• Weakness in one or both legs, drop attacks with or without loss of consciousness
• Various combinations of upper and lower limb involvement	• Numbness on one or both sides of the body
• Mixed picture of upper and lower motoneuron dysfunction	• Dysphagia or dysarthria
• Atrophy, weakness, hypotonia, hyperreflexia to hyporeflexia, and absent deep tendon reflexes	• Myoclonic jerks
	• Hiccups
	• Respiratory changes (e.g., Cheyne-Stokes respiration, Biot respiration, or ataxic respiration)

Modified from Bland JH: *Disorders of the cervical spine*, Philadelphia, 1994, W.B. Saunders, pp 215–216.

a migraine-like headache.[20] Dissection of a cervical artery (i.e., vertebral or internal carotid artery [Fig. 3.12]) usually results in "unusual" acute moderate to severe neck pain that is different from anything previously experienced. This may be followed by a **transient ischemic attack (TIA)** or stroke.[20] Vertebral artery dissection signs and symptoms include balance disturbances, ataxia (i.e., slurred speech, stumbling, falling [like being drunk]), syncope (i.e., fainting), drop attacks, dysphagia (i.e., difficulty swallowing), dysarthria (i.e., difficulty speaking), and visual defects (i.e., blurred vision) (Table 3.13).[20,64] Many of these patients have transient neurological signs and symptoms days or weeks prior to dissection.[20] Internal carotid artery dissection presents with unilateral frontal or retro-orbital pain as well as constriction of the pupil (i.e., miosis) or facial palsy.[20]

If the headache is a major complaint especially following trauma, then the examiner should take a blood pressure measurement, assess the mental state of the patient as is done with a concussion (see Chapter 2 SCAT5), and assess the cranial nerves (see Table 2.1).[65]

12. *Does a position change alter the headache or pain?* If so, which positions increase or decrease the pain? The patient may state that the pain and referred symptoms are decreased or relieved by placing the hand or arm of the affected side on top of the head. This is called **Bakody sign,** and it is usually indicative of problems in the C4 or C5 area.[66,67]

13. *Is paresthesia (a "pins and needles" feeling) present?* This sensation occurs if pressure is applied to the nerve root. It may become evident if pressure is relieved from a nerve trunk. Numbness and/or paresthesia in the hands or legs and deteriorating hand function all may relate to cervical myelopathy (see Table 3.10).

14. *Does the patient experience any tingling in the extremities?* Are the symptoms bilateral? Bilateral symptoms usually indicate either systemic disorders (e.g., diabetes, alcohol abuse) that are causing neuropathies or central space–occupying lesions.

15. *Are there any risk factors present?* For example, hypertension can be a risk factor for carotid and vertebral artery disease.[68] Instability due to problems with the craniovertebral ligaments could compromise neurological and vascular tissues in the upper cervical spine.[68] Other risk factors related to vertebrobasilar insufficiency include cardiovascular disease, TIA, blood clotting disorders, anticoagulant therapy, oral contraceptives, smoking, long-term use of steroids, and past history of trauma to the neck.

16. *Are there any lower-limb symptoms?* This finding may indicate a severe problem affecting the spinal cord (myelopathy; see Table 3.10). These symptoms may include numbness, paresthesia, stumbling, difficulty walking, and lack of balance or agility. All of these symptoms could indicate cervical myelopathy. Likewise, signs of sphincter (bowel or bladder) or sexual dysfunction may be related to cervical myelopathy.

TABLE **3.11**

Differential Diagnosis of Neurological Disorders of the Cervical Spine and Upper Limb

Cervical Radiculopathy (Nerve Root Lesion)	Cervical Myelopathy	Brachial Plexus Lesion (Plexopathy)	Burner (Transient Brachial Plexus Lesion)	Peripheral Nerve (Upper Limb)
Arm pain in dermatome distribution	Hand numbness, head pain, hoarseness, vertigo, tinnitus, deafness	Pain more localized to shoulder and neck (sometimes face)	Temporary pain in dermatome	No pain
Pain increased by extension and rotation or side flexion	Extension, rotation, and side flexion may all cause pain	Pain on compression of brachial plexus	Pain on compression or stretch of brachial plexus	No pain early; if contracture occurs (late), pain on stretching
Pain may be relieved by putting hand on head (C5, C6)	Arm positions have no effect on pain	Arm positions have no effect on pain[a]	Arm positions have no effect on pain[a]	Arm positions have no effect on pain[a]
Sensation (dermatome) affected	Sensation affected, abnormal pattern	Sensation (dermatome) affected	Sensation (dermatome) affected	Peripheral nerve sensation affected
Gait not affected	Wide-based gait, drop attacks, ataxia; proprioception affected	Gait not affected	Gait not affected	Gait not affected
Altered hand function	Loss of hand function	Loss of arm function	Loss of function temporary	Loss of function of muscles supplied by nerve
Bowel and bladder not affected	Possible loss of bowel and bladder control	Bowel and bladder not affected	Bowel and bladder not affected	Bowel and bladder not affected
Weakness in myotome but no spasticity	Spastic paresis (especially in lower limb early, upper limb affected later)	Weakness in myotome	Temporary weakness in myotome	Weakness of muscles supplied by nerve
DTR hypoactive	Lower limb DTR hyperactive Upper limb DTR hyperactive	DTR hypoactive	DTR not affected	DTR may be decreased
Negative pathological reflex	Positive pathological reflex	Negative pathological reflex	Negative pathological reflex	Negative pathological reflex
Negative superficial reflex	Decreased superficial reflex	Negative superficial reflex	Negative superficial reflex	Negative superficial reflex
Atrophy (late sign), hard to detect early	Atrophy	Atrophy	Atrophy possible	Atrophy (not usually with neuropraxia)

[a]Except in neurotension test positions.
DTR, Deep tendon reflexes.

17. *Does the patient have any difficulty walking? Does the patient have problems with balance?* Does the patient stumble when walking, have trouble walking in the dark, or walk with feet wide apart? Positive responses may indicate a cervical myelopathy. Abnormality of the cranial nerves combined with gait alterations may indicate systemic neurological dysfunction.[69]

18. *Does the patient experience dizziness, faintness, or seizures?* What is the degree, frequency, and duration of the dizziness? Is it associated with certain head positions or body positions? Semicircular canal problems or vertebral artery problems (Table 3.14) can lead to dizziness. Dizziness from a vertebral artery problem is commonly associated with other symptoms. Falling with no provocation while remaining conscious is sometimes called a **drop attack.**[70] Has the patient experienced any visual disturbances? Disturbances such as diplopia (double vision), nystagmus ("dancing eyes"), scotomas (depressed visual field), and loss of acuity may indicate severity of injury, neurological injury, and sometimes increased intracranial pressure (see Chapter 2).[66]

19. *Does the patient exhibit or complain of any sympathetic symptoms?* There may be injury to the cranial nerves or the sympathetic nervous system, which lies in the soft tissues of the neck anterior and lateral to the

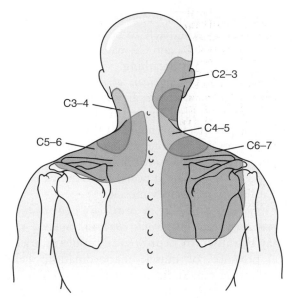

Fig. 3.11 Referred pain patterns suggested with pathology of the apophyseal (facet) joints. (Redrawn from Porterfield JA, DeRosa C: *Mechanical neck pain—perspective in functional anatomy*, Philadelphia, 1995, W.B. Saunders, p 104. Adapted from Dwyer A, April C, Bogduk N: Cervical zygapophyseal joint pain patterns, *Spine* 15:453–457, 1990.)

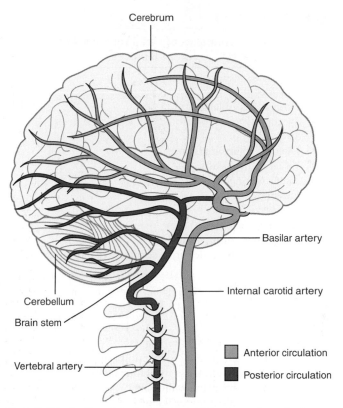

Fig. 3.12 Distribution of the internal carotid, basilar, and vertebral artery via the Circle of Willis. (Redrawn from Haneline M: The etiology of cervical artery dissection, *J Chiro Med* 6:111, 2007.)

TABLE **3.12**

Clinical Criteria for the Diagnosis of Cervicogenic Headache

- Unilateral headache without side-shift with an occipital or suboccipital component
- Symptoms and signs of neck involvement: pain triggered by neck movement or sustained awkward posture and/or external pressure in the posterior neck or occipital region; ipsilateral neck, shoulder, and arm pain; reduced range of motion; abnormal mobility at C0–C1
- Pain episodes of varying duration or fluctuating continuous pain
- Moderate, nonexcruciating pain, usually of a nonthrobbing nature
- Pain starting in the neck, spreading to oculo-fronto-temporal areas; suboccipital or nuchal tenderness
- Anesthetic blockades abolish the pain transiently provided complete anesthesia is obtained, or occurrence of sustained neck trauma shortly before onset
- Various attack-related events and sensory abnormalities: autonomic symptoms and signs, nausea, vomiting, ipsilateral edema and flushing in the peri-ocular area, dizziness, photophobia, phonophobia, or blurred vision in the ipsilateral eye

Satisfying the first five criteria above qualifies for a diagnosis of possible cervicogenic headache

Satisfying an additional three criteria above advances the diagnosis to probably cervicogenic headache

Modified from Bogduk N, Govind J: Cervicogenic headache: an assessment of the evidence on clinical diagnosis, invasive tests and treatment, *Lancet Neurol* 8(10):959–968, 2009. Adapted from Antonaci F, Ghirmai S, Bono S, et al: Cervicogenic headache: evaluation of the original diagnostic criteria, *Cephalalgia* 21:573–583, 2001.

TABLE **3.13**

Differentiation Between Features of Cervical Artery Dissection and Vertebrobasilar Insufficiency

Cervical Artery Dissection	Vertebrobasilar Insufficiency
Acute onset of neck pain or headache	Longstanding neck pain or headache
Young-middle age (30–50 years)	Older person (>65 years of age)
History of recent trauma or infection	No report of recent trauma or infection
No clear link of signs and symptoms with head movement	Link of symptoms with head position or neck movement
Headache, neck pain	Neck pain
Moderate/severe pain	Mild-moderate pain
5 Ds (i.e., dizziness, diplopia, dysarthria, dysphagia, drop attacks), other symptoms (e.g., limb paresthesia or weakness, Horner syndrome)	5 Ds (i.e., dizziness, diplopia, dysarthria, dysphagia, drop attacks), presyncope

From Thomas LC: Cervical arterial dissection: an overview and implications for manipulative therapy practice, *Man Ther* 21:2–9, 2016.

TABLE 3.14

Signs and Symptoms of Vertebrobasilar Artery Insufficiency[a]

- Dizziness, vertigo
- Giddiness
- Drop attacks, blackouts
- Syncope (loss of consciousness)
- Stroke
- Diplopia, blurred vision
- Visual hallucination
- Tinnitus (ringing in the ears)
- Flushing
- Sweating
- Lacrimation (tearing)
- Rhinorrhea (runny nose)
- Scotomata (visual defect in defined area of eye[s])
- Hiccups
- Myotonic jerks
- Tremor and rigidity
- Disorientation
- Vertigo
- Photophobia (sensitivity to light)
- Numbness and tingling (around lips or face)
- Quadriparesis (weakness in all four limbs)
- Dysphagia (difficulty swallowing)
- Dysarthria (difficulty speaking)
- Photopsia (sensation of flashing lights)
- Visual anosognosia (unawareness of visual defect)
- Nystagmus
- Ataxia (lack of voluntary muscle coordination/ unsteady gait)
- Nausea/vomiting
- Headache

[a]These paraspinal symptoms result mainly from rotation and extension of the neck, although they sometimes occur during flexion. The spectrum of neurologic symptoms and signs is as broad as that of the structures potentially involved. In a complex, bizarre, and poorly explained neurologic syndrome, vertebrobasilar artery insufficiency should be suspected.
Modified from Bland JH: *Disorders of the cervical spine*, Philadelphia, 1994, W.B. Saunders Co., p 217.

cervical vertebrae. The cranial nerves and their functions are shown in Table 2.1. Severe injuries (e.g., acceleration/whiplash type) can lead to hypertonia of the sympathetic nervous system.[2] Some of the sympathetic signs and symptoms the examiner may elicit are "ringing" in the ears (tinnitus), dizziness, blurred vision, photophobia, rhinorrhea, sweating, lacrimation, and loss of strength.

20. *Is the condition improving, worsening, or staying the same?* The answers to these questions give the examiner some indication of the condition's progress.

21. *Which activities aggravate the problem? Which activities ease the problem?* Are there any head or neck positions that the patient finds particularly bothersome? These positions should be noted. For example, does reading (flexed cervical spine) bother the patient?

If symptoms are not varied by a change in position, the problem is not likely to be mechanical in origin. Lesions of C3, C4, and C5 may affect the diaphragm and thereby affect breathing.

22. *Does the patient complain of any restrictions when performing movements?* If so, which movements are restricted? It is important that the patient not demonstrate the movements at this stage; the actual movements will be done during the examination.

23. *Is the patient a mouth breather?* Mouth breathing encourages forward head posture and increases activity of accessory respiratory muscles.

24. *Is there any difficulty in swallowing (dysphagia), or have there been any voice changes?* Such a change may be caused by neurological problems, mechanical pressure, or muscle incoordination. Pain on swallowing may indicate soft-tissue swelling in the throat, vertebral subluxation, osteophyte projection, or disc protrusion into the esophagus or pharynx. In addition, swallowing becomes more difficult and the voice becomes weaker as the neck is extended.

25. *What can be learned about the patient's sleeping position and nighttime symptoms?* Is there any problem sleeping? How many pillows does the patient use, and what type are they (e.g., feather, foam, buckwheat)? Foam pillows tend to retain their shape and have more "bounce"; they do not offer as much support as a good feather or buckwheat pillow. What type of mattress does the patient use (e.g., hard, soft)? Does the patient "hug" the pillow or abduct the arms when sleeping? These positions can increase the stress on the lower cervical nerve roots.

26. *Does the patient display any cognitive dysfunction?* If a possible head injury is suspected, the clinician should also consider testing for mental status (see Chapter 2).

27. *Are there any behavioral or psychological problems present that may be contributing to the problem?* These problems may be related to issues such as economic issues, coping skills, fear avoidance, pain catastrophizing, litigation, occupational issues, stress, and/ or quality of life.[71–73] These concepts were developed from work by Waddell et al. on the lumbar spine.[74] Table 3.15 outlines the tests that can be performed to determine if there is a psychological component to the patient's problems.[71,75,76] Issues such as depression can be screened using the **Beck Depression Inventory**, the **Depression Anxiety Stress Scales (DASS-21)**,[77] and the **Impact of Event Scale–Revised**.[78,79]

28. *Does the patient have any problems with the temporomandibular joints (TMJs)?* The TMJ can refer pain to the cervical spine (see Chapter 4) and the cervical spine can refer pain to the TMJ.[80,81]

TABLE **3.15**

Reliable Behavioral (Nonorganic) Signs in the Cervical Spine and the Criteria for a Positive Test[a]

Sign	Test Site	Criteria for a Positive Test
Palpation		
• Superficial tenderness	Palpation of cervical spine region and upper thoracic region	Patient complains of pain with light touch or light pinching of the skin
• Nonanatomic tenderness	Deep palpation of the cervical, thoracic, lumbar, and brachial region	Patient complains of widespread tenderness that is outside of the cervical and upper thoracic region
Simulation		
• Rotation of head/shoulders/trunk/pelvis while standing	Examiner rotates patient's head, shoulders, trunk, and pelvis	Patient complains of neck pain with rotation
Cervical Range of Motion	Patient rotates head as far as possible to the right and then left	Rotation is less than 50% of normal in each direction
Regional Disturbance		
• Sensory loss	Light touch or pinprick	Patient reports diminished sensation in a pattern that does not correspond to a specific dermatome of a nerve root(s) or peripheral nerve(s)
• Motor loss	Formal manual muscle testing, observation	Weakness detected in a nonanatomic pattern, the hallmark being "giveway weakness" Also positive if patient is observed to have normal muscle strength but on formal test exhibits weakness
Overreaction	Examiner's observation	Examiner feels the patient is "overreacting" during the examination. Reliable behaviors include: • Moderate to extremely stiff, rigid, or slow movements • Rubbing the affected area for more than 3 seconds • Clutching, grasping, or squeezing the area for more than 3 seconds • Grimacing due to pain • Sighing

[a]Waddell considered three positive tests out of five as a cutoff for significant nonorganic problems affecting the patient.
From Sobel JB, Sollenberger P, Robinson R, et al: Cervical nonorganic signs: a new clinical tool to assess abnormal illness behavior in neck pain patients: a pilot study, *Arch Phys Med Rehabil* 81(2):172, 2000.

Observation

For a proper observation, the patient must be suitably undressed. However, the examiner should also watch the patient as he or she enters the examination room, and before or while he or she undresses. The spontaneous movements of these activities can be very helpful in determining the patient's problems. For example, can the patient easily move the head when undressing? A male patient should remove clothing above the waist, and a female patient should wear a bra for this part of the assessment. In some cases, the bra may have to be removed to determine whether there are any problems, such as thoracic outlet syndrome, thoracic symptoms being referred to the cervical spine or to the sensory distribution of a thoracic nerve that radiates anteriorly along the ribs, or functional restriction of movement of the ribs. The examiner should note the willingness of the patient to move and the patterns of movement demonstrated. Facial expression of the patient can often give the examiner an indication of the amount of pain the patient is experiencing. If the patient is supporting the head and neck during the history and

observation and is afraid to move the head (i.e., **Rust's sign**), it may be an indication of cervical instability and the examiner should proceed with caution as this action by the patient may indicate a fracture or ligamentous injury leading to instability in the upper cervical spine.

The patient may be seated or standing. Usually, a standing posture is best because the posture of the whole body can be observed (see Chapter 15). Abnormalities in one area frequently affect another area. For example, excessive lumbar lordosis may cause a "poking" chin (cervical spine is in extension) to compensate for the lumbar deformity and to maintain the body's center of gravity centered beneath the base of support. In the cervical spine region, the examiner should note the following:

Head and Neck Posture (Standing). Is the head in the midline, and does the patient have a normal lordotic curvature (30° to 40°) (see Figs. 3.7 and 3.13)? This curvature along with the other spinal curvatures in the lower spine provides a shock absorption mechanism for the spine and helps the body maintain its center of gravity.[82] From the front, the chin should be in line with the sternum (manubrium) and from the side, the ears should be in line with the shoulder

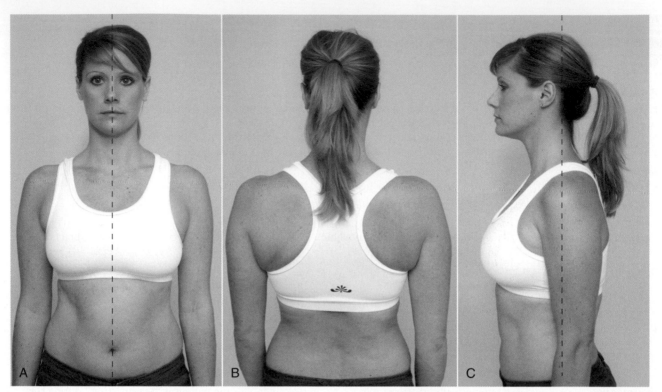

Fig. 3.13 Observation views of head and neck. (A) Anterior view. (B) Posterior view. (C) Lateral or side view. With normal posture, the ear should be in line with the shoulder and the forehead vertical. Note that this model is a "chin poker" with the head sitting anteriorly, which leads to a decrease in the lordotic curve.

and the forehead vertical. Is there evidence of torticollis (congenital or acquired) (Fig. 3.14), Klippel-Feil syndrome (congenital fusion of some cervical vertebra, usually C3 to C5) (Fig. 3.15), or other neck deformity? With acute torticollis due to a disc problem, the head is side flexed away from the painful side. Does the patient exhibit a poking chin or a "military posture?" A habitual poking chin can result in adaptive shortening of the occipital muscles. It also causes the cervical spine to change alignment resulting in increased comprehensive stress of the facet joints and posterior discs and other posterior elements (Fig. 3.16). The position may also lead to weaknesses of the deep neck flexors.[83] Janda[84] described a cervical **"upper crossed syndrome"** to show the effect of a "poking chin" posture on the muscles. With this syndrome, the deep neck flexors are weak, as are the rhomboids, serratus anterior, and often the lower trapezius. Opposite these weak muscles are tight pectoralis major and minor, along with upper trapezius and levator scapulae (Fig. 3.17). Does the head sit in the middle of the shoulders? Is the head tilted or rotated to one side or the other, indicating possible torticollis? Does this posture appear to be habitual (in other words, does the patient always go back to this posture)? Habitual posture may result from postural compensation, weak muscles, hearing loss, temporomandibular joint problems, or wearing of bifocals or trifocals. The trapezius neck line should be equal on both sides. Head and neck posture should be checked with the patient sitting and then standing, and any differences should be noted.

Shoulder Levels. Usually the shoulder on the dominant side will be slightly lower than that on the nondominant

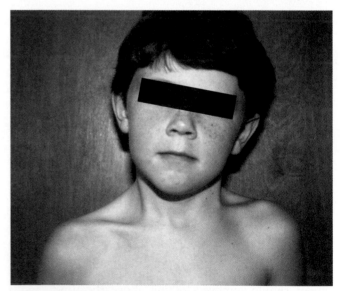

Fig. 3.14 Seven-year-old boy with left congenital muscular torticollis. (From Mauck BM: Congenital anomalies of the trunk and upper extremity. In Azar FM, Beaty JH, Canale ST, editors: *Campbell's operative orthopedics*, ed 13, Philadelphia, 2017, Elsevier.)

side. This is known as part of **handedness**. With injury, the injured side may be elevated to provide protection (e.g., upper trapezius and/or levator scapulae) or because of muscle spasm. Rounded shoulders may be the result of or the cause of a poking chin. Rounding also causes the scapulae to protract, the humerus to medially rotate, and the anterior structures of the shoulder to tighten and posterior structures to be lengthened.

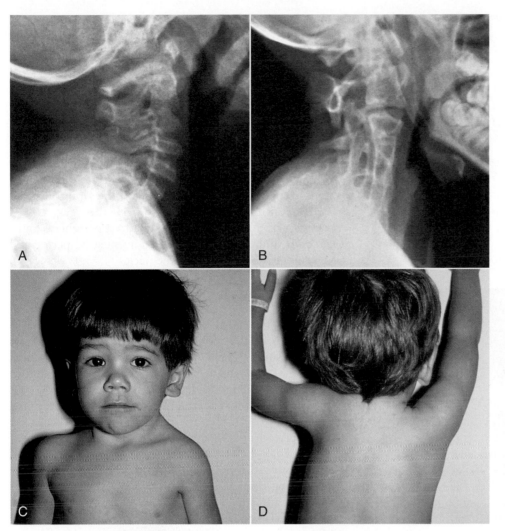

Fig. 3.15 Klippel-Feil syndrome. (A) This radiograph shows mild osseous involvement with fusion of the upper cervical segments. (B) In this radiograph, a different patient has severe osseous involvement in which C3 to C7 are fused and hypoplastic (i.e., underdeveloped). (C) Clinically the neck appears short and broad in the anterior view of this young child. (D) In this posterior view, the hairline is low and an associated Sprengel Deformity is present, the left scapula being hypoplastic and high riding. As a result, the patient is unable to fully raise his left arm. Typical webbing of the neck is not appreciable in this child. (From Deeney VF, Arnold J: Orthopedics. In Zitelli BJ, McIntire SC, Nowalk AJ, editors: *Zitelli and Davis' atlas of pediatric physical diagnosis*, ed 7, Philadelphia, 2018, Elsevier.)

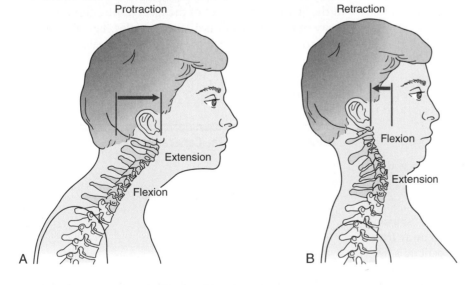

Fig. 3.16 Protraction and retraction of the cranium. (A) During protraction of the cranium, the lower-to-mid cervical spine flexes as the upper craniocervical region extends. (B) During retraction of the cranium, in contrast, the lower-to-mid cervical spine extends as the upper craniocervical region flexes. Note the change in distance between the C1–C2 spinous processes during the two movements. (Modified from Neumann DA: Kinesiology of the musculoskeletal system—foundations for physical rehabilitation, St Louis, 2002, Mosby, p 284.)

Muscle Spasm or Any Asymmetry. Is there any atrophy of the deltoid muscle (axillary nerve palsy) or torticollis (muscle spasm, tightness, or prominence of the sternocleidomastoid muscle) (see Fig. 3.14)? Another example is trapezius atrophy due to spinal accessory nerve palsy.

Facial Expression. The examiner should observe the patient's facial expression as the patient moves from position to position, makes different movements, and explains the problem. Such observation should give the examiner an idea of how much the patient is subjectively suffering.

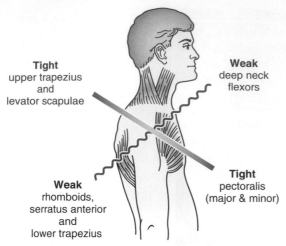

Tight
upper trapezius
and
levator scapulae

Weak
deep neck
flexors

Weak
rhomboids,
serratus anterior
and
lower trapezius

Tight
pectoralis
(major & minor)

Fig. 3.17 Upper crossed syndrome.

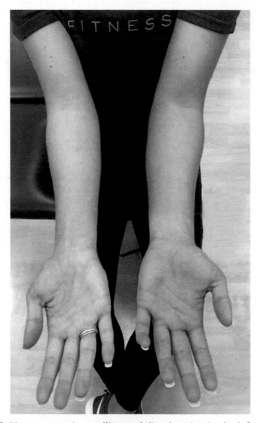

Fig. 3.18 Upper extremity swelling and discoloration in the left arm due to venous thoracic outlet syndrome.

Bony and Soft-Tissue Contours. If the cervical spine is injured, the head tends to be tilted and rotated away from the pain, and the face is tilted upward. If the patient is hysterical, the head tends to be tilted and rotated toward the pain, and the face is tilted down.

Evidence of Ischemia in Either Upper Limb. The examiner should note any altered coloration of the skin, ulcers, or vein distention as evidence of upper limb ischemia (Fig. 3.18).

Normal Sitting Posture. The nose should be in line with the manubrium and xiphoid process of the sternum. From the side, the earlobe should be in line with the acromion process and the high point on the iliac crest for proper postural alignment. The normal curve of the cervical spine is a lordotic type of curve. Referred pain from conditions, such as spondylosis, tends to occur in the shoulder and arm rather than the neck.

Examination

A complete examination of the cervical spine must be performed, including the neck, upper thoracic spine, upper ribs, and both upper limbs.[85] Many of the symptoms that occur in an upper limb originate from the neck. Unless there is a history of definite trauma to a peripheral joint, an upper limb scanning examination must be performed to rule out problems within the neck.

Active Movements

The first movements that are carried out are the active movements of the cervical spine with the patient in the sitting position. The examiner is looking for differences in range of movement, the pattern of movement, and in the patient's willingness to do the movement.[86] If the pattern of movement is aberrant or uncontrolled, it is called **cervical movement control dysfunction**.[87] The ROM taking place in this phase is the summation of all movements of the entire cervical spine, not just at one level. This combined movement allows for greater mobility in the cervical spine while still providing a firm support for the trunk and appendages. The ROM available in the cervical spine is the result of many factors, such as the flexibility of the intervertebral discs, the shape and inclination of the articular processes of the facet joints, and the slight laxity of the ligaments and joint capsules. Female patients tend to have a greater active ROM than males, except in flexion, but the differences are not great. The range available decreases with age, except rotation at C1–C2, which may increase.[88,89]

Active Movements of the Cervical Spine

- Flexion
- Extension
- Side flexion left and right
- Rotation left and right
- Combined movements (if necessary)
- Repetitive movements (if necessary)
- Sustained positions (if necessary)

The movements should be done in a particular order so that the most painful movements are done last, and no residual pain is carried over from the previous movement.[1] If the patient has complained of pain on specific movements in the history, these movements are done last. In the very acute cervical spine, only some movements—those that give the most information—are performed to avoid undue symptom exacerbation.

If, when doing the active and passive movements, the symptoms are relieved when the patient returns to neutral, the condition is nonirritable. If the symptoms are not relieved, then the condition is irritable and movements may be restricted depending on the intensity of the symptoms.

While the patient performs the active movements, the examiner looks for limitation of movement and possible reasons for pain, spasm, stiffness, or blocking. As the patient reaches the full active ROM, passive **overpressure** may be applied very carefully, but only if the movement appears to be full and not too painful (see passive movement in a later discussion). If, when doing active as well as passive movements, the patient is able to hold the end range position, the symptoms would not be considered severe. If the patient cannot hold the end range position, any symptoms would be considered more severe and overpressure should not be applied. The overpressure helps the examiner to test the end feel of the movement as well as differentiating between physiological (active) end range and anatomical (passive) end range. The examiner must be careful when applying overpressure to rotation or any combination of rotation, side flexion, and extension.[8] In these positions, the vertebral artery is often compressed, which can lead to a decrease in blood supply to the brain. Should this occur, the patient may complain of dizziness or feel faint. If the patient exhibits these symptoms, the examiner must use extreme care during these movements, the rest of the assessment, and treatment.

The examiner can differentiate between movement in the upper and lower cervical spine. During flexion, **nodding** occurs in the upper cervical spine, whereas **flexion** occurs in the lower cervical spine. If the nodding movement does not occur, it indicates restriction of movement in the upper cervical spine; if flexion does not occur, it indicates restriction of motion in the lower cervical spine. Movement can occur between C1 and C2 without affecting the other vertebrae, but this is not true with other cervical vertebrae. In other words, for C2 to C7, if one vertebra moves, the ones adjacent to it will also move. Thus, the active movements in the cervical spine can be divided into two parts: those testing the upper cervical spine (C0 to C2) and those involving the rest of the cervical spine (C2 to C7) (Fig. 3.19). Table 3.16 gives the approximate ROMs in the different parts of the cervical spine.[90]

Flexion

To test flexion movement in the upper cervical spine, the patient is asked to nod or place the chin on the Adam's apple. Normally this movement is pain free. Positive symptoms (e.g., tingling in feet, electric shock sensation down the neck [**Lhermitte sign**], severe pain, nausea, cord signs) all indicate severe pathology (e.g., meningitis, tumor, dens fracture) as the dura in the cervical and thoracic spine is also being stretched.[13] While the patient is flexing (nodding) the head, the examiner can palpate the relative movement between the mastoid and transverse process of C1 on each side comparing both sides for hypomobility or hypermobility between C0 and C1.[13] Likewise, the examiner can palpate the posterior arch of C1 and the lamina of C2 during the nodding movement to compare the relative movement.[13] For flexion, or forward bending, of the lower cervical spine, the maximum ROM is 80° to 90°. The extreme of ROM is normally found when the chin is able to reach the chest with the mouth closed; however, up to two finger-widths between chin and chest is considered normal. If the deep neck flexors are weak, the sternocleidomastoid muscles will initiate the flexion movement, causing the jaw to lead the movement, not the nose, since the sternocleidomastoid muscles will cause the chin to initially elevate before flexion occurs.[63,91,92] In flexion, the intervertebral disc widens posteriorly and narrows anteriorly. The intervertebral foramen is 20% to 30% larger on flexion than on extension. The vertebrae shift forward in flexion and backward in extension (Figs. 3.20 and 3.21). Also, the mastoid process moves away from the C1 transverse process on flexion and extension. As the patient forward flexes, the examiner should look for a posterior bulging of the spinous process of the axis (C2). This bulging may result from forward subluxation of the atlas, which allows the spinous process of the axis to become more prominent. If this sign appears, the examiner should exercise extreme caution during the remainder of the cervical assessment. To verify the subluxation, the Sharp-Purser test (see under Special Tests) may be performed, but only with extreme care.

Extension

To test extension in the upper cervical spine, the patient is asked to lift the chin up without moving the neck. The examiner can lift the occiput at the same time. If serious symptoms arise (e.g., tingling in the feet, loss of balance, drop attack), it is suggestive of spinal cord compression or vertebrobasilar dysfunction.[13] Extension, or backward bending of the cervical spine, is normally limited to 70°. Because there is no anatomic block to stop movement going past this position, problems often result from whiplash or cervical strain. Normally, there is sufficient extension to allow the plane of the nose and forehead to be nearly horizontal. When the head is held in extension, the atlas tilts upward, resulting in posterior compression between the atlas and occiput.

Side Flexion

Side, or lateral, flexion is approximately 20° to 45° to the right and left (Fig. 3.22). As the patient does the movement, the examiner can palpate adjacent transverse processes on the convex side to determine relative movement at each level. When the patient does the movement, the

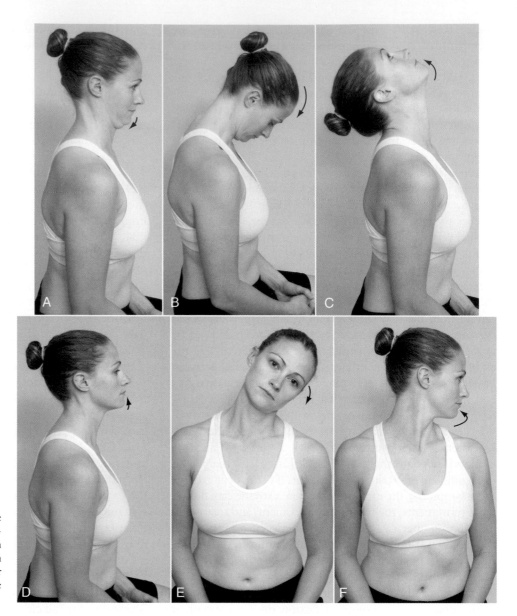

Fig. 3.19 Active movements of the cervical spine. (A) Anterior nodding (upper cervical spine). (B) Flexion (lower cervical spine). (C) Extension (lower cervical spine). (D) Posterior nodding (upper cervical spine). (E) Side flexion. (F) Rotation.

TABLE **3.16**

Approximate Range of Motion for the Three Planes of Movement for the Joints of the Craniocervical Region[a]

Joint or Region	Flexion and Extension (Sagittal Plane, Degrees)	Axial Rotation (Horizontal Plane, Degrees)	Lateral Flexion (Frontal Plane, Degrees)
Atlanto-occipital joint	Flexion: 5 Extension: 10 *Total: 15*	Negligible	About 5
Atlanto-axial joint complex	Flexion: 5 Extension: 10 *Total: 15*	40–45	Negligible
Intracervical region (C2–C7)	Flexion: 35 Extension: 70 *Total: 105*	45	35
Total across craniocervical region	Flexion: 45–50 Extension: 85 *Total: 130–135*	90	About 40

[a]The horizontal and frontal plane motions are to one side only. Data are compiled from multiple sources and subject to large intersubject variations. From Neumann DA: Kinesiology of the musculoskeletal system—foundations for physical rehabilitation, St Louis, 2002, Mosby, p 278.

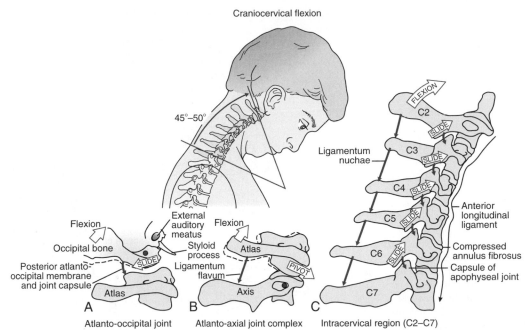

Fig. 3.20 Kinematics of craniocervical flexion. (A) Atlanto-occipital joint. (B) Atlanto-axial joint complex. (C) Intracervical region (C2 to C7). Note in **C** that flexion slackens the anterior longitudinal ligament and increases the space between the adjacent laminae and spinous processes. Elongated and taut tissues are indicated by *thin arrows;* slackened tissue is indicated by *a wavy arrow.* (Modified from Neumann DA: Kinesiology of the musculoskeletal system—foundations for physical rehabilitation, St. Louis, 2002, Mosby, p 281.)

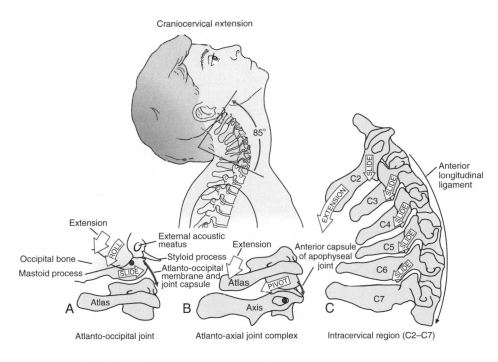

Fig. 3.21 Kinematics of craniocervical extension. (A) Atlanto-occipital joint. (B) Atlanto-axial joint complex. (C) Intracervical region (C2 to C7). Elongated and taut tissues are indicated by *thin arrows.* (Modified from Neumann DA: *Kinesiology of the musculoskeletal system—foundations for physical rehabilitation*, St. Louis, 2002, Mosby, p 280.)

examiner should ensure that the ear moves toward the shoulder and not the shoulder toward the ear.

Rotation

Normally, rotation is 70° to 90° right and left, and the chin does not quite reach the plane of the shoulder (Fig. 3.23). Rotation and side flexion always occur together (coupled movement) but not necessarily in the same direction.[21,22] This combined movement, which may or may not be visible in a given patient, occurs because of the shape of the articular surfaces of the facet joints; this shape is coronally oblique. Most of the rotation occurs between C1 and C2. If the patient can rotate 40° to 50°, then it is unlikely that the C1/C2 articulation is at fault.[13] If, however, side flexion occurs early to allow full motion, C1–C2 is probably involved.[13]

If, in the history, the patient has complained that **repetitive movements** or **sustained postures** have

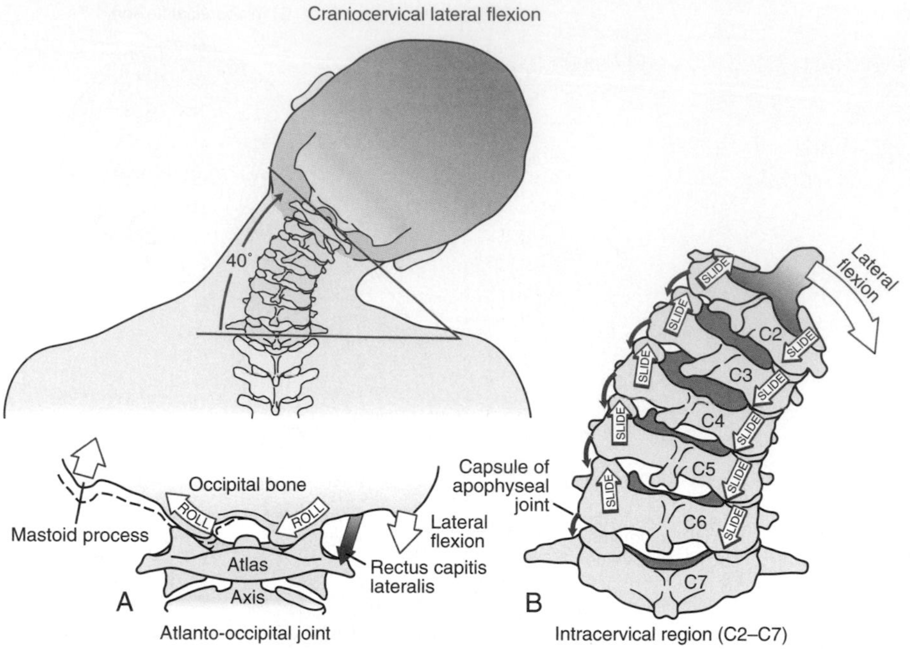

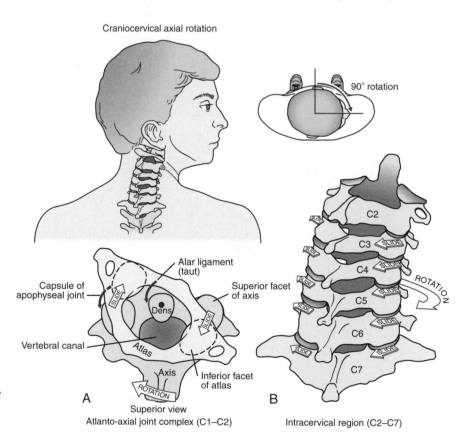

Craniocervical lateral flexion

Fig. 3.22 Kinematics of craniocervical lateral flexion. (A) Atlanto-occipital joint. The primary function of the rectus capitis lateralis is to laterally flex this joint. Note the slight compression and distraction of the joint surfaces. (B) Intracervical region (C2 to C7). Note the ipsilateral coupling pattern between axial rotation and lateral flexion. Elongated and taut tissue is indicated by *thin arrows.* (Modified *from Neumann DA: Kinesiology of the musculoskeletal system—foundations for physical rehabilitation,* St. Louis, 2002, Mosby, p 286.)

Craniocervical axial rotation

Fig. 3.23 Kinematics of craniocervical axial rotation. (A) Atlanto-axial joint complex. (B) Intracervical region (C2 to C7). (Modified from Neumann DA: *Kinesiology of the musculoskeletal system—foundations for physical rehabilitation,* St. Louis, 2002, Mosby, p 285.)

caused problems, not only should the specific movements be performed, but they should be either repeated several times or sustained to see if the symptoms are exacerbated. If a patient has complained in the history that a movement in other than a cardinal plane or a **combined movement** (e.g., side flexion, rotation, and extension combined) exacerbates the symptoms, then these movements should be performed as well. For example, the **cervical flexion-rotation test** ☑ in which the patient flexes the cervical spine to the point of pain or discomfort and then, while holding the position, rotates the head, is considered positive for pain and dysfunction arising from the C1–C2 segment in cervicogenic headaches if pain occurs with the rotation as well.[93–95] Table 3.17 outlines examples of movement restrictions and possible causes.

TABLE **3.17**

Movement Restriction and Possible Causes

Movement Restriction	Possible Causes
Extension and right side bending	Right extension hypomobility Left flexor muscle tightness Anterior capsular adhesions Right subluxation Right small disc protrusion
Flexion and right side bending	Left flexion hypomobility Left extensor muscle tightness
Extension and right side bending restriction greater than extension and left side bending	Left posterior capsular adhesions Left subluxation Left capsular pattern (arthritis, arthrosis)
Flexion and right side bending restriction equal to extension and left side flexion	Left arthrofibrosis (very hard capsular end feel)
Side bending in neutral, flexion, and extension	Uncovertebral hypomobility or anomaly

From Dutton M: *Orthopedic examination, evaluation and intervention*, New York, 2004, McGraw Hill, p 1050.

Passive Movements

If the patient does not have full active ROM or the examiner has not applied overpressure to determine the end feel of the movement, the patient should be asked to lie in a supine position. The examiner then passively tests flexion, extension, side flexion, and rotation, as in the active movements. The passive ROM with the patient supine is normally greater than the active and passive ROM with the patient sitting. For example, in sitting, active side flexion is about 45°, whereas in supine lying, passive side flexion is 75° to 80° with the examiner often able to take the ear to the shoulder. This increased range in the supine position results from relaxation of the muscles that, in sitting, are trying to hold the head up against gravity. For the cervical spine, therefore, passive movements with overpressure should be performed along with active movements. Active movements with overpressure at end of range do not give a true impression of end feel for the cervical spine. When doing passive flexion with overpressure, if pain is felt in the lower extremities, it may indicate a lower-extremity radiculopathy of one of the lower limb peripheral nerves as the movement stretches the dura (**Lindner test**).[96] If the examiner's second hand is placed over the sternum to prevent thoracic flexion, the test is called the **Soto-Hall test**.

Passive Movements of the Cervical Spine and Normal End Feel

- Flexion (tissue stretch)
- Extension (tissue stretch)
- Side flexion right and left (tissue stretch)
- Rotation right and left (tissue stretch)

During passive movements, the examiner can palpate between adjacent vertebra to feel the relative amount of movement on each side. For flexion, the examiner palpates between the mastoid process and the transverse process for movement between C0 and C1 (Fig. 3.24A) and between the arch of C1 and spinous process of C2 for movement between C1 and C2 (Fig. 3.24B). For the rest of the cervical spine and upper thoracic spine, the examiner can palpate between the spinous processes at each level while passively and progressively flexing

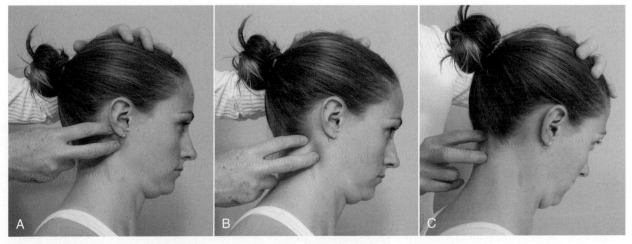

Fig. 3.24 Testing passive movement in the cervical spine. (A) Position testing for atlanto-occipital joint. (B) Position testing for atlanto-axial joint. (C) Flexion testing of C2 to T1.

the spine. To feel the movement, the examiner will find that as one works down the spine from C2 to C7, more flexion is required to feel the movement (Fig. 3.24C). Movement at each segment during side flexion and rotation may be felt by palpating the adjacent transverse processes on each side while doing the movement (Fig. 3.25). To test rotation between the occiput and C1, the examiner holds the patient's head in position and palpates the transverse processes of C1 (Fig. 3.26). The examiner must first find the mastoid process on each side and then move the fingers inferiorly and anteriorly until a hard bump (i.e., the transverse process of C1) is palpated on each side (usually below the earlobe and just behind the jaw). Palpation in the area of the C1 transverse process is generally painful, so care must be taken and the patient warned that the palpation may be painful. The examiner then rotates the patient's head while palpating the transverse processes; the transverse process on the side to which the head is rotated will seem to disappear (bottom one) while the other side (top one) seems to be accentuated in the normal case. If this disappearance/accentuation does not occur, there is restriction of movement between C0 and C1 on that side. To test rotation at C1 to C2, the examiner stands beside the seated patient and side bends the head and neck, followed by rotation to the opposite side. As the rotation is performed, the examiner palpates the relative position of the C1 and C2 transverse processes as the head is rotated. To limit side flexion to a specific segment, as the examiner side flexes the head, the examiner applies an opposing translation force in the opposite direction to the passive movement to limit movement below that being tested.[13] With all of these movements, the end feel should be a solid tissue stretch.

If the passive movements with overpressure are normal and pain free, the examiner may, with great care, test other positions. For the flexion-rotation test, the patient lies supine while the examiner flexes the neck fully and, while holding this position, passively rotates the head as far as possible within the patient's comfort limits.[97] Hall and Robinson[97] report significant restriction in rotation in patients complaining of cervicogenic headache indicating C1 to C2 segmental dysfunction. The quadrant position is end-range extension, side flexion, and rotation, a position that increases the vulnerability of anterior, posterior, and lateral tissues of the neck, including the vertebral artery.[98] If overpressure is applied in the quadrant position and symptoms result, it is highly suggestive of nerve root pathology (radicular signs), apophyseal joint involvement (localized pain), or vertebral artery involvement (dizziness, nausea).[63]

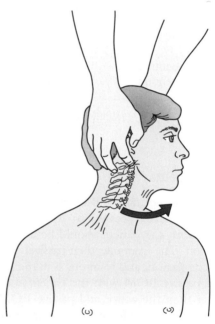

Fig. 3.26 Left rotation of the occiput on C1. Note the index finger palpating the right transverse process of C1.

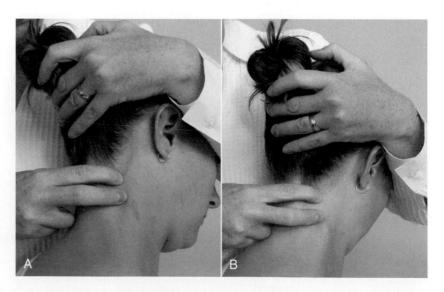

Fig. 3.25 Testing passive movement in the cervical spine. (A) Side flexion. (B) Rotation.

In addition to the passive movements of the whole cervical spine, physiological movements between each pair of vertebrae may be performed. These are called **passive physiological intervertebral movements (PPIVMs).** By stabilizing or blocking the movement of one vertebra (usually the distal one) and then passively moving the head through the different physiological movements (e.g., flexion, extension, side flexion, rotation), each segment can be tested. Needless to say, the amount of movement of each segment will be considerably less than the whole.[99]

Passive movements are performed to determine the end feel of each movement. This may give the examiner an idea of the pathology involved. The normal **end feels** of the cervical spine motions are tissue stretch for all four movements. As with active movements, the most painful movements are done last. The examiner should also note whether a **capsular pattern** (i.e., side flexion and rotation equally limited; extension less limited) is present. Overpressure may be used to test the entire spine (Fig. 3.27A) by testing it at the end of the ROM, or proper positioning may be used to test different parts of the cervical spine.[100] For example, end feel for movement of the lower cervical spine into extension is tested with minimal extension and the head pushed directly posterior (Fig. 3.27C), whereas the upper cervical spine is tested by "nodding" the head into extension and pushing posteriorly at an approximate 45° angle (Fig. 3.27B).[101]

Resisted Isometric Movements

The same movements that were done actively (flexion, extension, side flexion, and rotation) are then tested isometrically to determine relative muscle strength of each movement and to compare opposite movements.[102] It is better for the examiner to place the patient in the resting position and then say, "Don't let me move you," rather than to tell the patient, "Contract the muscle as hard as possible." In this way, the examiner ensures that the movement is as isometric as possible and that a minimal amount of movement occurs (Fig. 3.28). The examiner should ensure that these movements are done with the cervical spine in the neutral position and that painful movements are done last. Neck flexion tests cranial nerve XI and the C1 and C2 myotomes as well as muscle strength or state. By using Table 3.18 and looking at the various combinations of muscles that cause the movement (Fig. 3.29), the examiner is often able to decide which muscle is at fault (Fig. 3.30). If, in the history, the patient has complained that certain loaded or combined movements (those movements giving resistance other than gravity) are painful, the examiner should not hesitate to carefully test these movements isometrically to better ascertain the problem. If a neurological injury is suspected, the examiner must carefully assess for muscle weakness to determine the structures injured. If a severe neuropraxia or axonotmesis has occurred, there may be residual weakness even though muscle atrophy may not be evident.

Resisted Isometric Movements of the Cervical Spine

- Flexion
- Extension
- Side flexion right and left
- Rotation right and left

Scanning Examination

Peripheral Joint Scan

After the resisted isometric movements to the cervical spine have been completed, a peripheral joint scanning examination is performed to rule out obvious pathology in the extremities and to note areas that may need more detailed assessment.[1] The following joints are scanned bilaterally:

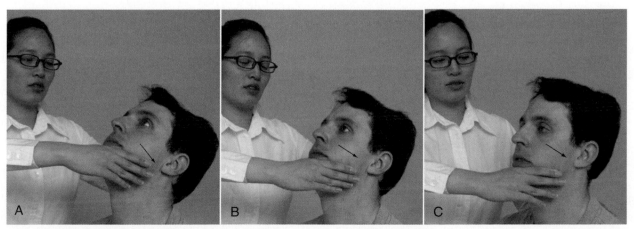

Fig. 3.27 (A) Overpressure to the whole cervical spine. (B) Overpressure to the upper cervical spine. (C) Overpressure to the low cervical spine. Clinician must differentiate between temporomandibular joint symptoms and cervical symptoms.

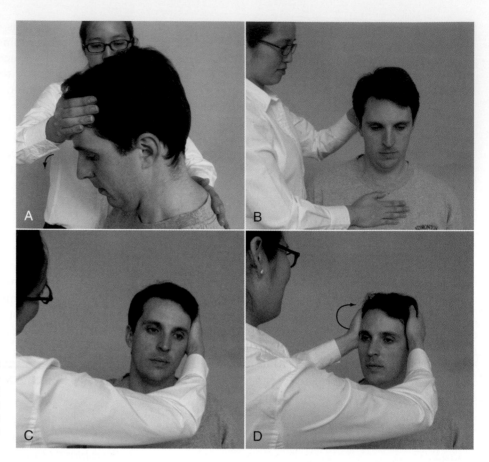

Fig. 3.28 Positioning for resisted isometric movement. (A) Flexion. Note slight flexion of neck before giving resistance. (B) Extension. Note slight flexion of neck before giving resistance. (C) Side flexion (left-side flexion shown). (D) Rotation (left rotation shown).

Peripheral Joint Scanning Examination

Temporomandibular joints	Open mouth
	Closed mouth
Shoulder joints	Elevation through abduction
	Elevation through forward flexion
	Elevation through plane of scapula (SCAPTION)
	Apley's scratch test (right and left)
	Rotation in 90° abduction
Elbow joints	Flexion
	Extension
	Supination
	Pronation
Wrist and hand joints	Flexion
	Extension
	Radial deviation
	Ulnar deviation
	Abduction of the fingers/thumb
	Adduction of the fingers/thumb
	Opposition of thumb and little finger

Temporomandibular Joints. The examiner checks the movement of the joints by placing the index or little fingers in the patient's ears (Fig. 3.31). The pulp aspect of the finger is placed facing forward to feel for equality of movement of the condyles of the TMJs and for clicking or grinding as well as to ensure that the ears are clear. Pain or tenderness, especially on closing the mandible, usually indicates posterior capsulitis. As the patient opens the mouth, the condyle normally moves forward. To open the mouth fully, the condyle must rotate and translate equally bilaterally. If this does not occur, mouth opening will be limited and/or deviation of the mandible will occur (see Chapter 4). The examiner should observe the patient as he or she opens and closes the mouth and should watch for any deviation during the movement.

Shoulder Girdle. The examiner quickly scans this complex of joints (glenohumeral, acromioclavicular, sternoclavicular, and "scapulothoracic" joint) by asking the patient to first actively elevate the shoulders ("lift your shoulders to your ears," "shrug your shoulders") and then to actively elevate each arm through abduction, followed by active elevation through forward flexion and elevation through the plane of the scapula (SCAPTION). These movements check the mobility of the scapula on the thorax and movement of the upper ribs. In addition, the examiner quickly tests medial and lateral rotation of each shoulder with the arm at the side and with the arm abducted to 90°. Any pattern of restriction should be noted. If the patient is able to reach full abduction without difficulty or pain, the examiner

TABLE **3.18**

Muscles of the Cervical Spine: Their Actions and Nerve Supply

Action	Muscles Acting	Nerve Supply
Forward flexion of head	1. Rectus capitis anterior	C1, C2
	2. Rectus capitis lateralis	C1, C2
	3. Longus capitis	C1–C3
	4. Hyoid muscles	Inferior alveolar, facial, hypoglossal, ansa cervicalis
	5. Obliquus capitis superior	C1
	6. Sternocleidomastoid (if head in neutral or flexion)	Accessory, C2
Extension of head	1. Splenius capitis	C4–C6
	2. Semispinalis capitis	C1–C8
	3. Longissimus capitis	C6–C8
	4. Spinalis capitis	C6–C8
	5. Trapezius	Accessory, C3, C4
	6. Rectus capitis posterior minor	C1
	7. Rectus capitis posterior major	C1
	8. Obliquus capitis superior	C1
	9. Obliquus capitis inferior	C1
	10. Sternocleidomastoid (if head in some extension)	Accessory, C2
Rotation of head (muscles on one side contract)	1. Trapezius (face moves to opposite side)	Accessory, C3, C4
	2. Splenius capitis (face moves to the same side)	C4–C6
	3. Longissimus capitis (face moves to same side)	C6–C8
	4. Semispinalis capitis (face moves to same side)	C1–C8
	5. Obliquus capitis inferior (face moves to same side)	CI
	6. Sternocleidomastoid (face moves to opposite side)	Accessory, C2
Side flexion of head	1. Trapezius	Accessory, C3, C4
	2. Splenius capitis	C4–C6
	3. Longissimus capitis	C6–C8
	4. Semispinalis capitis	C1–C8
	5. Obliquus capitis inferior	C1
	6. Rectus capitis lateralis	C1, C2
	7. Longus capitis	C1–C3
	8. Sternocleidomastoid	Accessory, C2
Flexion of neck	1. Longus colli	C2–C6
	2. Scalenus anterior	C4–C6
	3. Scalenus medius	C3–C8
	4. Scalenus posterior	C6–C8
	5. Infrahyoid muscles	Ansa cervicalis, hypoglossal
	6. Suprahyoid muscles	Inferior alveolar, facial, C1
Extension of neck	1. Splenius cervicis	C6–C8
	2. Semispinalis cervicis	C1–C8
	3. Longissimus cervicis	C6–C8
	4. Levator scapulae	C3, C4, Dorsal scapular
	5. Iliocostalis cervicis	C6–C8
	6. Spinalis cervicis	C6–C8
	7. Multifidus	C1–C8
	8. Interspinalis cervicis	C1–C8
	9. Trapezius	Accessory
	10. Rectus capitis posterior major	C3, C4
	11. Rotatores brevis	C1
	12. Rotatores longi	C1–C8
Side flexion of neck	1. Levator scapulae	C3, C4, Dorsal scapular
	2. Splenius cervicis	C4–C6
	3. Iliocostalis cervicis	C6–C8
	4. Longissimus cervicis	C6–C8
	5. Semispinalis cervicis	C1–C8
	6. Multifidus	C1–C8
	7. Intertransversarii	C1–C8

TABLE **3.18**

Muscles of the Cervical Spine: Their Actions and Nerve Supply—cont'd

Action	Muscles Acting	Nerve Supply
	8. Scaleni	C3–C8
	9. Sternocleidomastoid	Accessory, C2
	10. Obliquus capitis inferior	C1
	11. Rotatores breves	C1–C8
	12. Rotatores longi	C1–C8
	13. Longus colli	C2–C6
Rotation[a] of neck (muscles on one side contract)	1. Levator scapulae (face moves to same side)	C3, C4, Dorsal scapular
	2. Splenius cervicis (face moves to same side)	C4–C6
	3. Iliocostalis cervicis (face moves to same side)	C6–C8
	4. Longissimus cervicis (face moves to same side)	C6–C8
	5. Semispinalis cervicis (face moves to same side)	C1–C8
	6. Multifidus (face moves to opposite side)	C1–C8
	7. Intertransversarii (face moves to same side)	C1–C8
	8. Scaleni (face moves to opposite side)	C3–C8
	9. Sternocleidomastoid (face moves to opposite side)	Accessory, C2
	10. Obliquus capitis inferior (face moves to same side)	C1
	11. Rotatores brevis (face moves to same side)	C1–C8
	12. Rotatores longi (face moves to same side)	C1–C8

[a]Occurs in conjunction with side flexion owing to direction of facet joints.

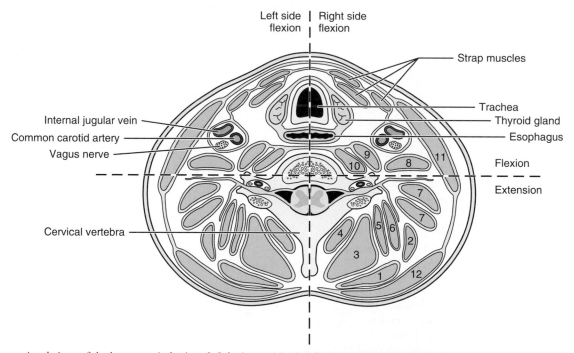

Fig. 3.29 Anatomic relations of the lower cervical spine. *1*, Splenius capitis. *2*, Splenius cervicis. *3*, Semispinalis cervicis and capitis. *4*, Multifidus and rotatores. *5*, Longissimus capitis. *6*, Longissimus cervicis. *7*, Levator scapulae. *8*, Scalenus posterior. *9*, Scalenus medius. *10*, Scalenus anterior. *11*, Sternocleidomastoid. *12*, Trapezius.

may decide that there is no problem with the shoulder complex (see Chapter 5).

Elbow Joints. The elbow joints are actively moved through flexion, extension, supination, and pronation. Any restriction of movement or abnormal signs and symptoms should be noted, because they may be indicative of pathology (see Chapter 6).

Wrist and Hand. The patient actively performs flexion, extension, and radial and ulnar deviation of the wrist. Active movements (flexion, extension, abduction, adduction, and opposition) are performed for the fingers and thumb. These actions can be accomplished by having the patient make a fist and then spread the fingers and thumb wide. Again, any alteration in signs

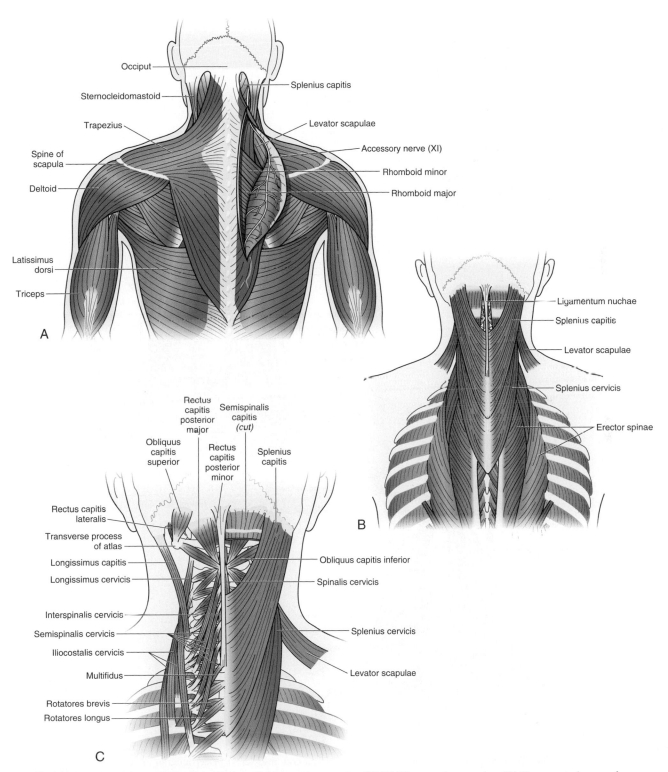

Fig. 3.30 Muscles of the cervical spine. (A) Superficial posterior muscles. (B) Middle posterior muscles. (C) Deep posterior muscles.

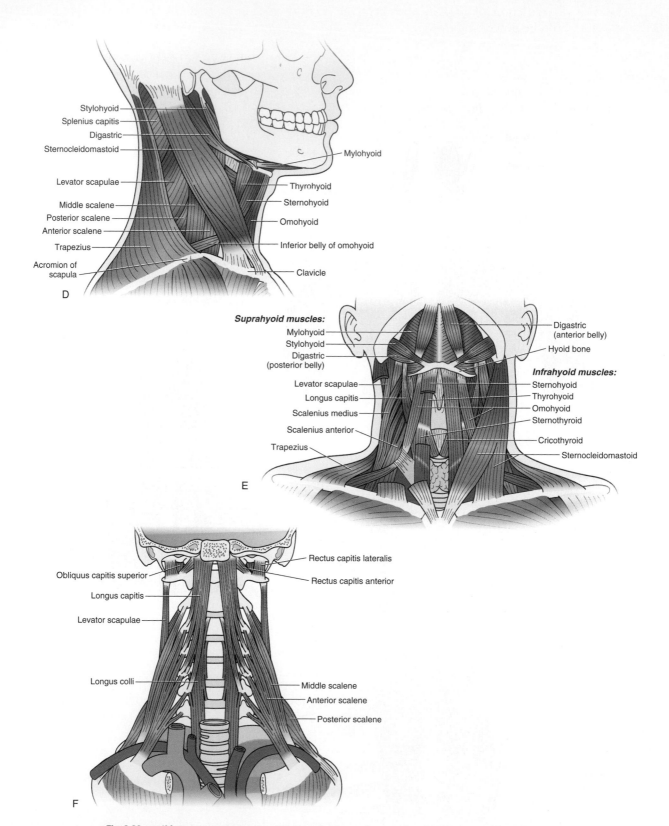

Fig. 3.30, cont'd (D) Lateral muscles. (E) Superficial anterior muscles. (F) Deep anterior muscles.

and symptoms or restriction of motion or differences between sides should be noted (see Chapter 7).

Myotomes

Having completed the peripheral joint scanning examination, the examiner should then determine muscle power and possible neurological weakness originating from the nerve roots in the cervical spine by testing the myotomes (Table 3.19; Fig. 3.32). Myotomes are tested by resisted isometric contractions with the joint at or near the resting position. As with the resisted isometric movements previously mentioned, the examiner should position the seated patient and say, "Don't let me move you," so that an isometric contraction is obtained.

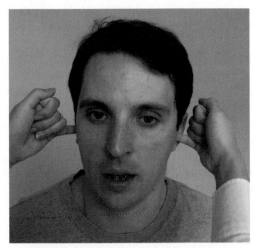

Fig. 3.31 Testing temporomandibular joints.

Cervical Myotomes

- Neck flexion: C1–C2
- Neck side flexion: C3 and cranial nerve XI
- Shoulder elevation: C4 and cranial nerve XI
- Shoulder abduction/shoulder lateral rotation: C5
- Elbow flexion and/or wrist extension: C6
- Elbow extension and/or wrist flexion: C7
- Thumb extension and/or ulnar deviation: C8
- Abduction and/or adduction of hand intrinsics: T1

The contraction should be held for *at least 5 seconds* so that weakness, if any, can be noted. Where applicable, both sides are tested at the same time to provide a comparison.

TABLE 3.19

Myotomes of the Upper Limb

Nerve Root	Test Action	Muscles[a]
C1–C2	Neck flexion	Rectus lateralis, rectus capitis anterior, longus capitis, longus coli, longus cervicis, sternocleidomastoid
C3	Neck side flexion	Longus capitis, longus cervicis, trapezius, scalenus medius
C4	Shoulder elevation	Diaphragm, trapezius, levator scapulae, scalenus anterior, scalenus medius
C5	Shoulder abduction	Rhomboid major and minor, deltoid, supraspinatus, infraspinatus, teres minor, biceps, scalenus anterior and medius
C6	Elbow flexion and wrist extension	Serratus anterior, latissimus dorsi, subscapularis, teres major, pectoralis major (clavicular head), biceps, coracobrachialis, brachialis, brachioradialis, supinator, extensor carpi radialis longus, scalenus anterior, medius and posterior
C7	Elbow extension and wrist flexion	Serratus anterior, latissimus dorsi, pectoralis major (sternal head), pectoralis minor, triceps, pronator teres, flexor carpi radialis, flexor digitorum superficialis, extensor carpi radialis longus, extensor carpi radialis brevis, extensor digitorum, extensor digiti minimi, scalenus medius and posterior
C8	Thumb extension and ulnar deviation	Pectoralis major (sternal head), pectoralis minor, triceps, flexor digitorum superficialis, flexor digitorum profundus, flexor pollicis longus, pronator quadratus, flexor carpi ulnaris, abductor pollicis longus, extensor pollicis longus, extensor pollicis brevis, extensor indicis, abductor pollicis brevis, flexor pollicis brevis, opponens pollicis, scalenus medius and posterior
T1	Hand intrinsics	Flexor digitorum profundus, intrinsic muscles of the hand (except extensor pollicis brevis), flexor pollicis brevis, opponens pollicis

[a]Muscles listed may be supplied by additional nerve roots; only primary nerve root sources are listed.

If possible, the examiner must not apply pressure over the joints, because this action may mask symptoms if the joints are tender.

To test neck flexion (C1–C2 myotome), the patient's head should be slightly flexed. The examiner applies pressure to the forehead while stabilizing the trunk with a hand between the scapulae (see Fig. 3.32A). The examiner should ensure the neck does not extend when applying pressure to the forehead. To test neck side flexion (C3 myotome and cranial nerve XI), the examiner places one hand above the patient's ear and applies a side flexion force while stabilizing the trunk with the other hand on the opposite shoulder (see Fig. 3.32B). Both right and left side flexion must be tested.

The examiner then asks the patient to elevate the shoulders (C4 myotome and cranial nerve XI) to about half of full elevation. The examiner applies a downward force on both of the patient's shoulders while the patient attempts to hold them in position (see Fig. 3.32C). The examiner should ensure that the patient is not "bracing" the arms against the thighs if testing is done while sitting.

To test shoulder abduction (C5 myotome), the examiner asks the patient to elevate the arms to about 75° to 80° in the scapular plane with the elbows flexed to 90° and the forearms pronated or in neutral (see Fig. 3.32D). The examiner applies a downward force on the humerus while the patient attempts to hold the arms in position. To prevent rotation, the examiner places his or her forearms over the patient's forearms while applying pressure to the humerus.

To test elbow flexion and extension, the examiner asks the patient to put the arms by the sides with the elbows flexed to 90° and forearms in neutral. The examiner applies a downward isometric force (see Fig. 3.32E) to the forearms to test the elbow flexors (C6 myotome) and an upward isometric force (see Fig. 3.32G) to test the elbow

extensors (C7 myotome). For testing of wrist movements (extension, flexion, ulnar deviation) the patient's arms are by the side; elbows at 90°; forearms pronated; and wrists, hands, and fingers in neutral. The examiner applies a downward force (see Fig. 3.32F) to the hands to test wrist extension (C6 myotome), and an upward force (see Fig. 3.32H) to test wrist flexion (C7 myotome). To apply a lateral force (radial deviation) to test ulnar deviation (C8 myotome), the clinician stabilizes the patient's forearm with one hand and applies a radial deviation force to the side of the hand.

In the test for thumb extension (C8 myotome), the patient extends the thumb just short of full ROM (see Fig. 3.32I). The examiner applies an isometric force to bring the thumbs into flexion. To test hand intrinsics (T1 myotome), the patient squeezes a piece of paper between the fingers while the examiner tries to pull it away; the patient may squeeze the examiner's fingers, or the patient may abduct the fingers slightly with the examiner isometrically adducting them (see Fig. 3.32J).

Sensory Scanning Examination

The examiner then tests sensation by doing a **sensory scanning examination.** This "sensory scan" is accomplished by running relaxed hands over the patient's head (sides and back); down over the shoulders, upper chest, and back; and down the arms, being sure to cover all aspects of the arm. If any difference is noted between the sides in this "sensation scan," the examiner may then use a pinwheel, pin, cotton batting, or brush (or a combination of these) to map out the exact area of sensory difference and to determine if any sensory difference is due to a nerve root (see later section on reflexes and cutaneous distribution), peripheral nerve, or some other neurological deficit. The sensory scanning examination may also include the testing of

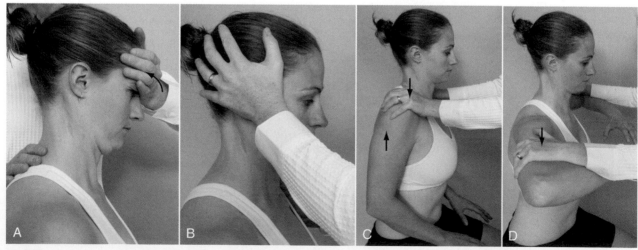

Fig. 3.32 Positioning to test myotomes. (A) Neck flexion (C1, C2). (B) Neck side flexion to the right (C3). (C) Shoulder elevation (C4). (D) Shoulder abduction (C5).

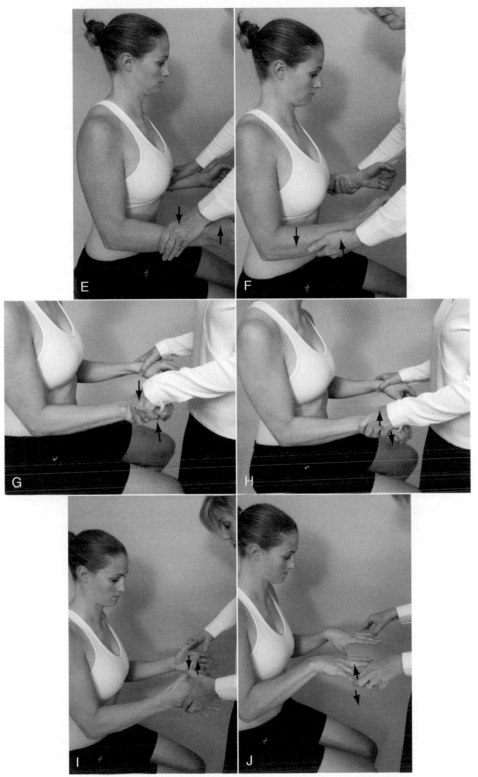

Fig. 3.32, cont'd (E) Elbow flexion (C6). (F) Elbow extension (C7). (G) Wrist extension (C6). (H) Wrist flexion (C7). (I) Thumb extension (C8). (J) Finger abduction (T1).

reflexes, especially the deep tendon reflexes, to test for upper and lower neuron pathology and pathological reflexes for upper motor neuron pathology, and the performance of selected neurodynamic tests (e.g., upper limb tension test, slump test) if peripheral nerve irritability is suspected.

Functional Assessment

If, in the history, the patient has complained of functional difficulties or the examiner suspects some functional impairment, a series of functional tests or movements may be performed to determine the patient's functional

---

Functional Assessment of the Cervical Spine

- Activities of daily living (ADLs)
- Numerical scoring table (if desired)

---

capacity, keeping in mind the patient's age and health. These tests may include activities of daily living (ADLs) such as the following:

Breathing. Normal, unlabored breathing should be seen with the mouth closed. There should be no gulping or gasping.

Swallowing. This is a complex movement involving muscles of the lips, tongue, jaw, soft palate, pharynx, and larynx as well as the suprahyoid and infrahyoid muscles.

Looking Up at the Ceiling. At least 40° to 50° of neck extension is usually necessary for everyday activities. If this range is not available, the patient will bend the back or the knees, or both, to obtain the desired range.

Looking Down at Belt Buckle or Shoe Laces. At least 60° to 70° of neck flexion is necessary. If this range is not available, the patient will flex the back to complete the task.

Shoulder Check. At least 60° to 70° of cervical rotation is necessary. If this range is not available, the patient will rotate the trunk to accomplish this task.

Tuck Chin In. This action produces upper cervical flexion with lower cervical extension.[101]

Poke Chin Out. This action produces upper cervical extension with lower cervical flexion.[101]

Neck Strength. In athletes, neck strength should be approximately equivalent to 30% of body weight to decrease chance of injury.[103]

Paresthesia. Paresthesia, especially referred to the hands, may make cooking and handling utensils or power tools particularly difficult or even dangerous.

Table 3.20 lists functional strength tests that can give the examiner some indication of the patient's functional strength capacity. For flexion, if the jaw juts forward at the beginning of the movement, it indicates an imbalance pattern of strong sternocleidomastoid and weak deep neck flexors.[13]

Pinfold and others[104,105] developed the **Whiplash Disability Questionnaire (WDQ)** (eTool 3.1) to assess the impact of WADs including social and emotional problems.[106,107] Vernon and Mior[108] have developed a numerical scoring functional test called the **Neck Disability Index (NDI)**[109,110] (eTool 3.2), which is a modification of the Oswestry low back pain index.[111] This index and similar tests (e.g., **Bournemouth Questionnaire** [eTool 3.3],[112] the **Copenhagen Neck Functional Disability Scale** [eTool 3.4],[113] and the **Northwick Park Neck Pain Questionnaire** [eTool 3.5][114,115]) can be used to detect change in patients over time.[116,117] The **Whiplash Activity and Participation List (WAL)** has been developed to determine the activity limitation and participation restrictions in patients with WAD.[118,119]

Special Tests

There are several special tests that may be performed if the examiner believes they are relevant and to help confirm a diagnosis. The tests should never be used in isolation and are sometimes combined to give better results.[120–122] Some of these tests should always be performed (e.g., instability tests, vertebral artery tests), especially if treatment is to be given to the upper cervical spine, while others should be performed only if the

---

TABLE **3.20**

Functional Strength Testing of the Cervical Spine

Starting Position	Action	Functional Test[a]
Supine lying	Lift head keeping chin tucked in (neck flexion)	6–8 repetitions: Functional 3–5 repetitions: Functionally fair 1–2 repetitions: Functionally poor 0 repetitions: Nonfunctional
Prone lying	Lift head backward (neck extension)	Hold 20–25 seconds: Functional Hold 10–19 seconds: Functionally fair Hold 1–9 seconds: Functionally poor Hold 0 seconds: Nonfunctional
Side lying (pillows under head so head is not side flexed)	Lift head sideways away from pillow (neck side flexion) (must be repeated for other side)	Hold 20–25 seconds: Functional Hold 10–19 seconds: Functionally fair Hold 1–9 seconds: Functionally poor Hold 0 seconds: Nonfunctional
Supine lying	Lift head off bed and rotate to one side keeping head off bed or pillow (neck rotation) (must be repeated both ways)	Hold 20–25 seconds: Functional Hold 10–19 seconds: Functionally fair Hold 1–9 seconds: Functionally poor Hold 0 seconds: Nonfunctional

[a]Younger patients should be able to do the most repetitions and for the longest time; with age, time and repetitions decrease.
Adapted from Palmer ML, Epler M: *Clinical assessment procedures in physical therapy,* Philadelphia, 1990, J.B. Lippincott, pp 181–182.

examiner wants to use them as confirming tests. Some tests are provocative and should only be used if the examiner wants to cause symptoms. Other tests relieve symptoms and are used when the symptoms are present. The reliability of many of these tests commonly depends on the experience and skill of the examiner and whether the patient is sufficiently relaxed to allow the test to be performed.[123,124]

Key Tests Performed on the Cervical Spine Depending on Suspected Pathology[a]

- **For cervical muscle (deep neck flexors) strength:**
  - ☑ Craniocervical flexion test
  - ⚠ Deep neck flexor endurance test
- **For neurologic symptoms:**
  - ☑ Brachial plexus tension test
  - ☑ Brachial plexus provocation test
  - ⚠ Doorbell sign
  - ☑ Distraction test (if symptoms are severe)
  - ☑ Foraminal compression test (three stages) (if symptoms are absent or mild)
  - ☑ Upper limb neurodynamic (tension) tests (specific to particular nerve/nerve root symptoms)
- **For myelopathy:**
  - ☑ Romberg test
- **For vascular signs[b]:**
  - ❓ Hold planned mobilization/manipulation position for at least 30 seconds watching for vertebral-basilar artery signs
- **For cervical instability[c]:**
  - ❓ Anterior shear stress test
  - ❓ Lateral flexion alar ligament stress test
  - ⚠ Lateral shear test
  - ⚠ Posterior atlanto-occipital membrane test
  - ❓ Rotational alar ligament stress test
  - ⚠ Transverse ligament stress test
- **For cervical spine mobility:**
  - ☑ Cervical flexion rotation test
- **For first rib mobility:**
  - ☑ First rib mobility

[a]The authors recommend these key tests be learned by the clinician to facilitate a diagnosis. See Chapter 1, Key for Classifying Special Tests.
[b]These tests should be performed if the examiner anticipates doing end-range mobilization or manipulation techniques to the cervical spine, especially the upper cervical spine. If instability of vascular signs are present, mobilization and/or manipulation should **not** be performed.
[c]Before these tests are performed, the C-spine rule for radiographs should be administered, and the results should indicate that no radiographs are required.

For the reader who would like to review them, the reliability, validity, specificity, sensitivity, and odds ratios of some of the special tests used in the cervical spine are available in eAppendix 3.1.

Tests for Cervical Muscle Strength

☑ *Craniocervical Flexion Test.*[32,125–128] The craniocervical flexion (CCF) test is a test of the deep cervical flexor muscle function.[125] A pneumatic pressure device is needed for this test. The patient lies in supine with knees bent (crook lying)

with head and neck in midrange, and an inflatable pressure sensor is placed under the cervical spine (Fig. 3.33). Towels may be used to keep the head and neck in midrange neutral (two parallel lines: one from forehead to chin and one from tragus of ear to the line of the longitudinal neck). The pressure device is inflated to 20 mm Hg to "fill in" the lordotic curve of the cervical spine. While keeping the head/occiput stationary (no pushing down or lifting up), the patient flexes the cervical spine by nodding the head to five graded segments of increasing pressure (22, 24, 26, 28, and 30 mm Hg) and holds each for 10 seconds with 10 seconds rest between each segment. Superficial cervical muscles (e.g., sternocleidomastoid, platysma, hyoid) must remain relaxed during the test.[129] Normally, young and middle-aged patients should be able to increase pressure to between 26 and 30 mm Hg and hold for 10 seconds without utilizing the superficial muscles. Elderly people are more likely to make greater use of the sternocleidomastoid muscle during the test.[130] A positive test is considered if the patient cannot increase pressure to at least 26 mm Hg, is unable to hold a contraction for 10 seconds, uses the superficial neck muscles, or extends the head. The performance index is calculated as the increase in pressure times the number of repetitions, while the activation score is the maximum pressure achieved and held for 10 seconds. Signs of reduced endurance include an inability to hold the pressure steady or it decreases over time, the superficial flexors are or become active, and the pressure is held but with a jerky action.[125]

⚠ *Deep Neck Flexor Endurance Test.*[32,131] The patient lies supine in crook lying. The chin is maximally retracted by the patient and maintained while the patient lifts the head and neck until the head is approximately 2 to 5 cm (1 inch) above the examining table. The examiner places a hand on the table under the patient's head (occiput). The examiner watches the skin folds resulting from the chin tuck and neck flexion. As soon as the skin folds separate (due to loss of chin tuck) or the patient's head touches the examiner's hand, the test is terminated. Normal people

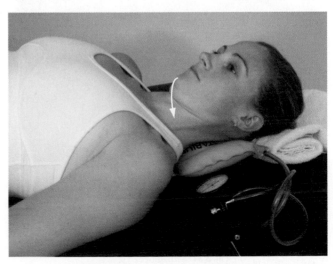

Fig. 3.33 Craniocervical flexion test.

should be able to hold for 39 ± 26 seconds while those with neck pain average 24 seconds.[131]

Tests for Neurological Symptoms

These tests are designed to provoke neurological symptoms in most cases (distraction test is the exception) to determine the effect of applying pressure or stretching to the nervous tissue. They are specific to neurological tissue (i.e., they produce neurological symptoms), but they do not necessarily tell where the pathology is originating. The pathology may be the result of trauma, degeneration, or anatomical anomalies that may occur anywhere along the path of the affected nerve or nerve root.[132,133]

Tests for neurological symptoms that involve movement of the nerve are called **neurodynamic tests,** because they assess the sensitivity of nerve roots and peripheral nerves to movement and tension caused by the movement. This sensitivity has also been called *neurologic mechanosensitivity*.[134]

Neurodynamic Tests[134]

During neurodynamic testing, a positive test is considered present only when one or more of the following occur:
- There is a reproduction of the patient's symptoms.
- There is asymmetric sensation between right and left limbs.
- There is significant deviation from normal sensation.
- Symptoms change with sensitizing movements.

❓ *Arm Squeeze Test*.[135] This test is used to differentiate cervical nerve root compression from shoulder lesions. The patient is seated and the examiner firmly squeezes the upper arm including the biceps and triceps on the side of shoulder pain (Fig. 3.34). A positive test is indicated by intense local pain in the arm and indicates a nerve root lesion (one or more nerve roots from C5 to T1). If pain results in the shoulder, it is a shoulder problem.

☑ *Brachial Plexus Compression Test*.[136] The examiner applies firm compression to the brachial plexus by squeezing the plexus under the thumb or fingers at the neck-shoulder interface (Fig. 3.35). Pain at the site is not diagnostic; the test is positive only if pain radiates into the shoulder or upper extremity. It is positive for mechanical cervical lesions having a mechanical component.

☑ *Brachial Plexus Provocation Test*.[137] The patient lies supine. Starting with the unaffected side or side with less symptoms, the examiner abducts the patient's shoulder to about 90° with the elbow flexed and wrist extended while preventing shoulder elevation either with one hand (Fig. 3.36A) or using the elbow (Fig. 3.36B). The examiner then extends the patient's elbow. Loss of ≥30° of elbow extension and moderate pain are considered positive for brachial plexus involvement. With whiplash, the test may be positive bilaterally. The test will not work if the shoulder is not kept depressed.

☑ *Distraction Test*. The distraction test is used for patients who have complained of radicular symptoms in the history and show radicular signs during the examination. It is used to alleviate symptoms. To perform the distraction test, the examiner places one hand under the patient's chin and the other hand around the occiput, then slowly lifts the patient's head (Fig. 3.37)—in effect, applying traction to the cervical spine. The test is classified as positive if the pain is relieved or decreased when the head is lifted or distracted, indicating pressure on nerve roots that has been relieved. This test may also be used to check radicular signs referred to the shoulder complex anteriorly or posteriorly. If the patient abducts the arms while traction is applied, the symptoms are often further relieved or lessened in the shoulder, especially if C4 or C5 nerve roots are involved. In this case, the test would still be indicative of nerve root pressure in the cervical

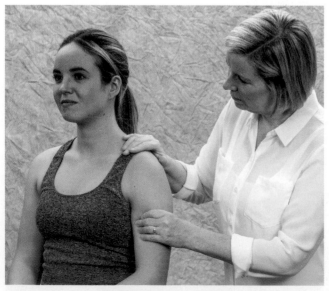
Fig. 3.34 Arm squeeze test.

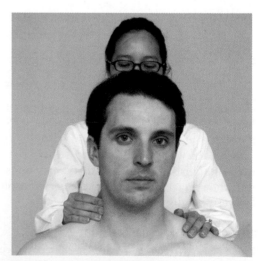
Fig. 3.35 Maneuver to compress and squeeze the brachial plexus at the neck-shoulder interface. Right side is demonstrated.

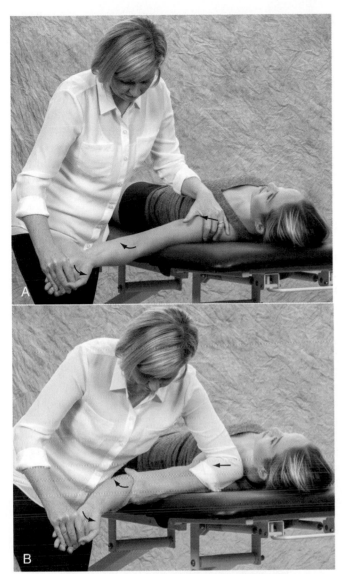

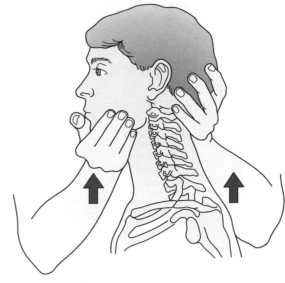

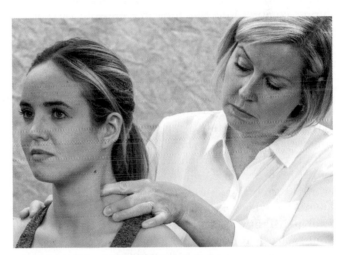

Fig. 3.37 Distraction test.

Fig. 3.38 Doorbell sign.

Fig. 3.36 Brachial plexus provocation test. (A) Method one—the examiner keeps the patient's shoulder depressed with the left hand while the patient's elbow is extended and wrist and fingers extended. (B) Method two—the examiner keeps the patient's shoulder depressed using the examiner's left elbow while the patient's elbow is extended and wrist and fingers extended.

spine, not shoulder pathology. Increased pain on distraction may be the result of muscle spasm, ligament sprain, muscle strain, dural irritability, or disc herniation.[13]

⚠ *Doorbell Sign.*[138] This doorbell sign is also called the **anterior cervical door push button sign**. The patient is seated and the examiner stands behind the patient carefully moving the sternocleidomastoid muscle laterally out of the way and then with the index finger of the same hand, palpates the nerve roots in the vertebral gutter of each vertebra where they exit the gutter. The examiner applies a moderate pressure for 2 to 3 seconds to the nerve root (Fig. 3.38). The process is repeated with each nerve root. The examiner must be careful not to apply pressure to the carotid artery. A positive test would be symptoms of the particular nerve root into the arm or mid-thoracic

area (i.e., somatic referral pattern). Reproduction of arm symptoms suggests a radicular (i.e., nerve root) problem.

✓ *Foraminal Compression (Spurling) Test.*[139] This test is performed if, in the history, the patient has complained of nerve root symptoms, which at the time of examination are diminished or absent. This test is designed to provoke symptoms. The patient bends or side flexes the head to the unaffected side first, followed by the affected side (Fig. 3.39). The examiner carefully presses straight down on the head. Bradley and colleagues[69] advocate doing this test in three stages, each of which is increasingly provocative; if symptoms are produced, one does not proceed to the next stage. The first stage involves compression with the head in neutral. The second stage involves compression with the head in extension, and the final stage is with the head in extension and rotation to the unaffected side, then to the side of complaint with compression. The third part of the test more closely follows the test as described

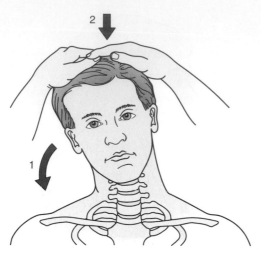

Fig. 3.39 Foraminal compression test. Patient flexes head to one side *(1)*, and examiner presses straight down on head *(2)*.

by Spurling.[139] A test result is classified as positive if pain radiates into the arm toward which the head is side flexed during compression; this indicates pressure on a nerve root (cervical radiculitis). **Radiculitis** implies pain in the dermatomal distribution of the nerve root affected.[69] Neck pain with no radiation into the shoulder or arm does not constitute a positive test. The dermatome distribution of the pain and altered sensation can give some indication as to which nerve root is involved. The test positions narrow the intervertebral foramen so that the following conditions may lead to symptoms: stenosis; cervical spondylosis; osteophytes; trophic, arthritic, or inflamed facet joints; herniated disc, which also narrows the foramen; or even vertebral fractures. If the pain is felt in the opposite side to which the head is taken, it is called a **reverse Spurling sign** and is indicative of muscle spasm in conditions such as tension myalgia and WADs.[140]

A very similar test is called the **maximum cervical compression test** ✓. With this test, the patient side flexes the head and then rotates it to the same side. The test is repeated to the other side. A positive test is indicated if pain radiates into the arm.[30] If the head is taken into extension (as well as side flexion and rotation) and compression is applied, the intervertebral foramina close maximally to the side of movement and symptoms are accentuated. Pain on the concave side indicates nerve root or facet joint pathology, whereas pain on the convex side indicates muscle strain (Fig. 3.40).[141] This second position may also compress the vertebral artery. If one is testing the vertebral artery, the position should be held for 20 to 30 seconds to elicit symptoms (e.g., dizziness, nystagmus, feeling faint, nausea) that would indicate compression of the vertebral artery.

✓ *Jackson Compression Test.* This test is also a modification of the foraminal compression test. The patient rotates the head to one side. The examiner then carefully presses straight down on the head (Fig. 3.41). The test is repeated with the head rotated to the other side. The test

is positive if pain radiates into the arm, indicating pressure on a nerve root. The pain distribution (dermatome) can give some indication of which nerve root is affected.[66]

❓ *Scalene Cramp Test.*[48] The patient sits and rotates the head to the affected side and pulls the chin down into the hollow above the clavicle by flexing the cervical spine. If pain increases, it is usually in the trigger points of the scalenes toward which the head rotates. Radicular signs may indicate plexopathy or thoracic outlet symptoms.

⚠ *Shoulder Abduction (Relief) Test.* This test is used to test for radicular symptoms, especially those involving the C4

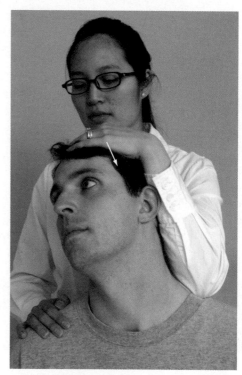

Fig. 3.40 Maximum cervical compression test.

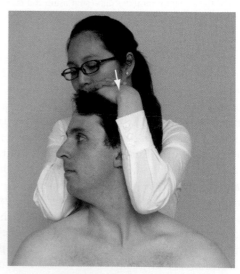

Fig. 3.41 Jackson compression test.

or C5 nerve roots. The patient is sitting or lying down, and the examiner passively or the patient actively elevates the arm through abduction so that the hand or forearm rests on top of the head (Fig. 3.42).[66,142] A decrease in or relief of symptoms indicates a cervical extradural compression problem, such as a herniated disc, epidural vein compression, or nerve root compression, usually in the C4–C5 or C5–C6 area. Differentiation is by the dermatome (and possible myotome) distribution of the symptoms. This finding is also called **Bakody's sign**.[67] Abduction of the arm decreases the length of the neurological pathway and decreases the pressure on the lower nerve roots.[142,143] If the pain increases with the positioning of the arm, it implies that pressure is increasing in the interscalene triangle.[67]

Shoulder Depression Test. This test may be used to evaluate for brachial plexus lesions (see Table 3.11), since the test position is the mechanism of injury for these lesions, plexopathies, and radiculopathies. With brachial plexus lesions, more than one nerve root is commonly affected. The examiner side flexes the patient's head to one side (e.g., the left) while applying a downward pressure on the opposite shoulder (e.g., the right) (Fig. 3.43). If the pain is increased, it indicates irritation or compression of the nerve roots or foraminal encroachments, such as osteophytes in the area on the side being compressed, or adhesions around the dural sleeves of the nerve and adjacent joint capsule or a hypomobile joint capsule on the side being stretched. Differentiation is by the dermatome (and possibly myotome) distribution of symptoms.

Tinel Sign for Brachial Plexus Lesions.[144] The patient sits with the neck slightly side flexed. The examiner taps the area of the brachial plexus (Fig. 3.44) with a finger along the nerve trunks in such a way that the different nerve roots are tested. Pure local pain implies that there is an underlying cervical plexus lesion. A positive Tinel sign (tingling sensation in the distribution of a nerve) means the lesion is anatomically intact and some recovery is occurring. If pain is elicited in the distribution of a peripheral nerve, the sign is positive for a neuroma and indicates a disruption of the continuity of the nerve.

☑ **Upper Limb Neurodynamic (Tension) Tests (Brachial Plexus Tension or Elvey Test).** The upper limb neurodynamic tests (ULNT) are equivalent to the straight leg raising (SLR) test in the lumbar spine. They are tension tests designed to put stress on the neurological structures of the upper limb by stretching them, although, in truth, stress is put on all the tissues of the upper limb. The neurological tissue is differentiated by what is defined as sensitizing tests (e.g., neck flexion with the SLR test). This test, first described by Elvey,[100] has since been divided

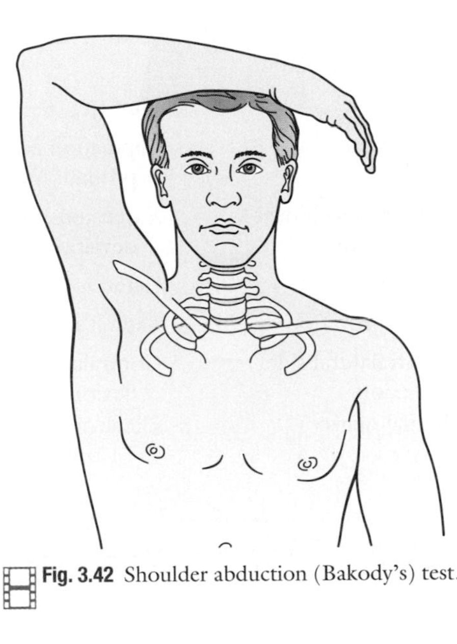

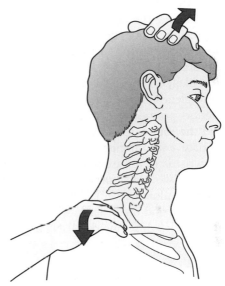

Fig. 3.43 Shoulder depression test.

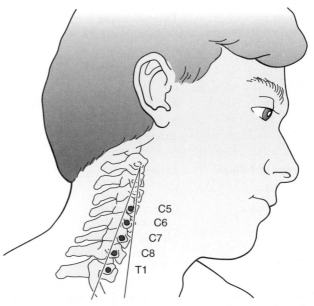

Fig. 3.44 Tinel sign for brachial plexus lesions. *Dots* indicate percussion points.

Fig. 3.42 Shoulder abduction (Bakody's) test.

into four tests (Table 3.21). Modification of the position of the shoulder, elbow, forearm, wrist, and fingers places greater stress on specific nerves (nerve bias).[146]

Each test begins by testing the good side first and positioning the shoulder, followed by the forearm, wrist, fingers, and last, because of its large ROM, the elbow. Davis et al.[147] felt the tests should be considered positive only if neurological symptoms were manifested before 60° of elbow extension when elbow extension was the last movement performed. Each phase is added until symptoms are produced. To further "sensitize" the test, side flexion of the cervical spine may be performed.[100,141] Symptoms are more easily aggravated into the upper limb than the lower limb when doing tension tests,[146,148] and if the neurological signs are worsening or in the acute phase, or if a cauda equina or spinal cord lesion is present, these stress tests are contraindicated.[146]

When positioning the shoulder, it is essential that a constant depression force be applied to the shoulder girdle so that, even with abduction, the shoulder girdle remains depressed. If the shoulder is not held depressed, the test is less likely to work. While the shoulder girdle is depressed, the glenohumeral joint is taken to the appropriate abduction position (110° or 10°, depending on the test), and the forearm, wrist, and fingers are taken to their appropriate end-of-range position; for example, in ULNT2 the wrist is in full extension (Fig. 3.45). Elbow extension stresses the radial and median nerves, whereas flexion stresses the ulnar nerve. Wrist and finger extension stresses the median and ulnar nerve while releasing stress on the radial nerve.[146] If required (ULNT2, 3, and 4), the

glenohumeral joint is appropriately rotated and held. The elbow position is often not performed until last because the large elbow ROM is easiest to measure when recording available range to show improvement over time. As the elbow is taken toward its extreme (end-of-range) position, symptoms are usually felt.[148] Some of these symptoms are normal (Table 3.22), and some are pathological. If symptoms are minimal or no symptoms appear, the head and cervical spine are taken into contralateral side flexion. This final movement is sometimes referred to as a **sensitizing test.** This sensitizing test may be within or near the test limb (e.g., neck side flexion in ULNT), or it may be in another quadrant (e.g., right ULNT and right SLR).

The tests are designed to stress tissues. Although they stress the neurological tissues, they also stress some contractile and inert tissues. Differentiation among the types of tissues depends on the signs and symptoms presented (Table 3.23).

Finally, although specific ULNTs are described, if the patient describes neurological symptoms when doing functional movements (e.g., getting wallet out of back pocket) these movements should also be tested by positioning the limb and taking the joints toward their end range.

Evans[67] described a modification of the ULNT that he called the **brachial plexus tension test** ✓. The sitting patient abducts the arms with the elbows extended, stopping just short of the onset of symptoms. The patient laterally rotates the shoulder just short of symptoms, and the examiner then holds this position. Finally, the patient flexes the elbows so that the hands lie behind the head

TABLE **3.21**

Upper Limb Neurodynamic (Tension) Tests Showing Order of Joint Positioning[a] and Nerve Bias

	ULNT1[133]	ULNT2	ULNT3[145]	ULNT4
Shoulder	Depression and abduction (110°)	Depression and abduction (10°)	Depression, shoulder medial rotation, abduction (40°), and extension (25°)	Depression and abduction (10° to 90°), hand to ear
Elbow	Extension	Extension	Extension	Flexion
Forearm	Supination	Supination	Pronation	Supination or pronation
Wrist	Extension	Extension	Flexion and ulnar deviation	Extension and radial deviation
Fingers and thumb	Extension	Extension	Flexion	Extension
Shoulder	—	Lateral rotation	Medial rotation	Lateral rotation
Cervical spine	Contralateral side flexion	Contralateral side flexion	Contralateral side flexion	Contralateral side flexion
Nerve bias	Median nerve, anterior interosseous nerve, C5, C6, C7	Median nerve, musculocutaneous nerve, axillary nerve	Radial nerve	Ulnar nerve, C8 and T1 nerve roots

[a]The elbow motion is often done last as the elbow ROM increase or decrease can be used to determine whether the patient is improving or regressing over time.

ULNT, Upper limb neurodynamic tests.

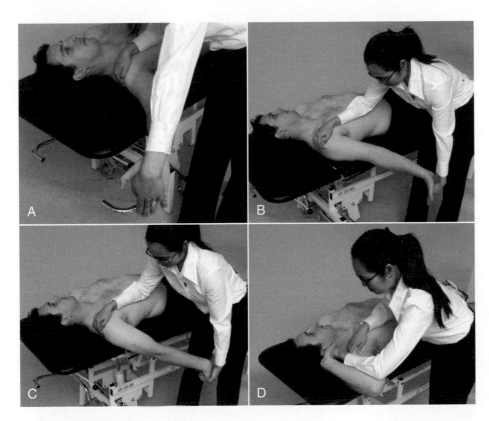

Fig. 3.45 Upper limb neurodynamic (tension) tests (Elvey tests). (A) Upper limb neurodynamic test (ULNT)1. (B) ULNT2. (C) ULNT3. (D) ULNT4.

TABLE **3.22**

Upper Limb Neurodynamic (Tension) Test: Normal and Pathological Signs and Symptoms

Normal (Negative)	Pathological (Positive)
• Deep ache or stretch in cubital fossa (99%) • Deep ache or stretch into anterior and radial aspect of forearm and radial aspect of hand (80%) • Tingling to the fingers supplied by appropriate nerve (nerve bias) • Stretch in anterior shoulder area • Above responses increased with contralateral cervical side flexion (90%) • Above responses decreased with ipsilateral cervical side flexion (70%)	• Production of patient's symptoms (most important feature) • A sensitizing test in the ipsilateral quadrant alters the symptoms • Different symptoms between right and left (contralateral quadrant)

Adapted from Butler DS: *Mobilisation of the nervous system*, Melbourne, 1991, Churchill Livingstone.

(Fig. 3.46). Reproduction of radicular symptoms with elbow flexion is considered a positive test. This test is similar to ULNT4 and stresses primarily the ulnar nerve and the C8 and T1 nerve roots.

Evans[67] outlined a second similar test. The seated patient abducts the arm to 90° with the elbow fully flexed. The arm is extended at the shoulder and then the elbow is extended (Fig. 3.47). If radicular pain results, the test is positive **(Bikele's sign)**. This test in reality is a modification of the ULNT4 done actively.

☑ **Valsalva Test.** This test is used to determine the effect of increased pressure on the spinal cord. The examiner asks the patient to take a deep breath and hold it while bearing down, as if moving the bowels. A positive test is indicated by increased pain, which may be caused by increased intrathecal pressure. This increased pressure within the spinal cord usually results from a space-occupying lesion, such as a herniated disc, a tumor, stenosis, or osteophytes. Test results are very subjective. The test should be performed with care and caution because the patient may become dizzy and pass out during the test or shortly afterward if the procedure blocks the blood supply to the brain.

Tests for Upper Motor Neuron Lesions (Cervical Myelopathy)

In addition to the tests below, positive pathological reflexes (e.g., Babinski, Hoffman), hyperreflexia of the deep tendon reflexes, and clonus may indicate a cervical myelopathy.[149]

❓ *Grip and Release Test (10-Second Test).*[55,150] Normally, patients can perform rapid grip and release from full finger flexion to full finger extension 20 times in 10 seconds. If the movement becomes slower over the 10 seconds (i.e., cannot do 20 times) or if exaggerated wrist extension occurs with finger extension or exaggerated wrist flexion occurs with finger flexion, the test is considered positive for a cervical myelopathy.

❓ *Lhermitte Sign.* This is a test for the spinal cord itself and a possible upper motor neuron lesion. The patient is in the long leg sitting position on the examining table.

TABLE **3.23**

Differential Diagnosis of Contractile, Inert, and Nervous Tissue Based on Stretch or Tension

	Contractile Tissue	Inert Tissue (Ligament)	Neurogenic Tissue
Pain	Cramping, dull, ache	Dull → sharp	Burning, bright, lightning-like
Tingling	No	No	Yes
Constancy	Intermittent	Intermittent	Longer symptom duration
Dermatome pattern	No	No	Yes (if nerve root pathological)
Peripheral nerve sensory distribution	No	No	Yes (if peripheral nerve or nerve root is affected)
Resistance to stretch	Muscle spasm	Boggy, hard capsular	Soft tissue stretch

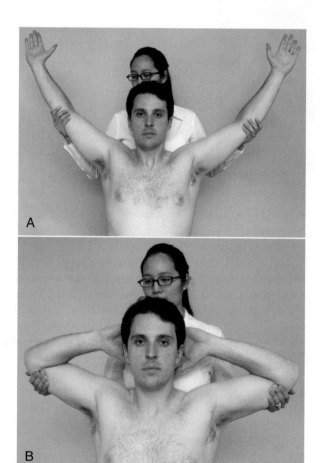

Fig. 3.46 Brachial plexus tension test. (A) The patient abducts and then laterally rotates the arms until symptoms are felt; the patient then lowers the arms until symptoms disappear, and the examiner holds the patient's arms in the position. (B) While the shoulders are held in position, the patient flexes the elbows and places the hands behind the head. A positive test is indicated by return of symptoms.

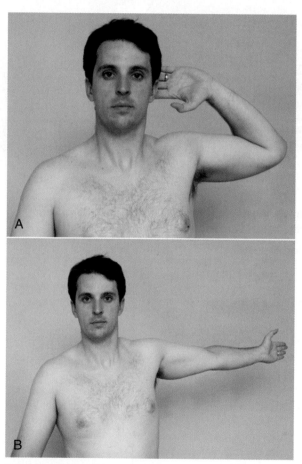

Fig. 3.47 Bikele's sign. (A) The arm is abducted to 90° with the elbow fully flexed. (B) The arm and then the elbow are extended.

The examiner passively flexes the patient's head and one hip simultaneously with the leg kept straight (Fig. 3.48). A positive test occurs if there is a sharp, electric shock-like pain down the spine and into the upper or lower limbs; it indicates dural or meningeal irritation in the spine or possible cervical myelopathy.[67] Coughing or sneezing may produce similar results. The test is similar to a combination of the Brudzinski test and the SLR test (see Chapter 9).

If the patient actively flexes the head to the chest while in the supine lying position, the test is called the **Soto-Hall test.** If the hips are flexed to 135°, greater traction is placed on the spinal cord.[66]

✓ ***Romberg Test.*** For the Romberg test, the patient is standing and is asked to close the eyes. The position is held for 20 to 30 seconds. If the body begins to sway excessively or the patient loses balance, the test is considered positive for an upper motor neuron lesion.

△ ***Ten-Second Step Test.***[151] The patient, while standing, is asked to step "in place" by lifting the thigh of one leg

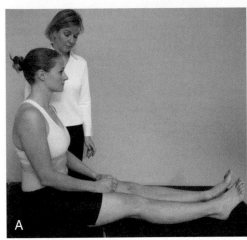
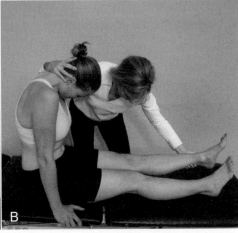

Fig. 3.48 Lhermitte sign. (A) Patient in long sitting position. (B) Examiner flexes patient's head and hip simultaneously.

parallel to the floor (i.e., hip and knees at 90°) and then lifting the other leg in a similar manner as though walking at maximum speed while not holding on to any object. The number of steps in 10 seconds is counted (Table 3.24).

Tests for Vascular Signs (Vascular "Clearing" Tests)

Vertebral and internal carotid artery testing is an important component of the cervical spine assessment in cases where end range mobilization and manipulation treatment techniques are contemplated, especially if the techniques involve a rotary component (>45°) and the upper cervical spine (C0 to C3).[152–154] The vertebral artery is especially vulnerable to injury as it transitions from its protective area in the foramen transversarium within the cervical spine transverse processes, then looping before it enters the cranial vault behind the first vertebra. Vertebrobasilar insufficiency leads to ischemic symptoms from the pons, medulla, and cerebellum (see Fig. 3.1).[155] Several authors[152,155–159] have reported that the vertebral artery tests have not been conclusively proven to be effective in indicating stretching and occlusion of the vertebral artery or internal carotid artery but do say that the tests should be performed to decrease the risk of potentially catastrophic complications when doing end-range mobilization or manipulation, especially of the upper cervical spine. Thus, risk factors must be considered when doing the examination.[68] In any case, it appears that although circulation may be slowed in one vessel, there is "enough slack in the system" that other vessels are able to compensate by increasing flow provided there is not significant disease processes present in the vessels.[160] Table 3.25 outlines vertebral and internal carotid artery signs and symptoms associated with pathology.[161] Although the following text discusses many vertebral artery tests, not all of them have to be performed. However, it is imperative that the patient be tested in the position in which the treatment will be given and held in that position for at least 10 to 30 seconds ✓, especially if the technique is an end-range technique or involves the upper cervical

TABLE 3.24

Normal Values (Number of Steps) of Ten-Second Step Test in Each Gender and Age Group

Age	Male	Female
20–29	21.9 ± 2.6	20.6 ± 3.5
30–39	21.4 ± 3.7	20.9 ± 4.4
40–49	20.9 ± 3.5	19.9 ± 2.2
50–59	19.9 ± 3.1	19.0 ± 2.7
60–69	18.3 ± 2.8	18.2 + 2.2
70–79	17.5 ± 3.1	16.9 ± 2.3
Average	20.0 ± 3.5	19.2 ± 3.3

Modified from Yukawa Y, Kato F, Ito K, et al: "Ten second step test" as a new quantifiable parameter of cervical myelopathy, *Spine* 34(1):82–86, 2009.

spine.[6,162–164] This is called **provocative positional testing**.[68] Any of the signs and symptoms that indicate vertebral-basilar artery problems would indicate the treatment should not be given (Table 3.26). When doing more than one test, 10 seconds should elapse between each test to ensure there are no latent symptoms from the previous test. It is recommended that if mobilization or manipulation of the cervical spine is contemplated, the clinician should follow the Australian Physiotherapy Association's protocol for pre-manipulative testing of the cervical spine.[165] If, when performing the vertebral artery tests, or if in the history, the patient complains of signs and symptoms that may be related to the vertebral artery, care should be taken when mobilizing the upper cervical spine.[153,166–168]

Carotid and Vertebral Artery Risk Factors[68]

- Hypertension
- Hypermobility of craniovertebral ligaments (transverse and alar ligaments, tectorial membrane)
- Cardiovascular disease

Signs and Symptoms That May Indicate Possible Vertebral-Basilar Artery Problems[152,155]

- Dizziness/vertigo
- Dysphagia (difficulty swallowing)
- Drop attacks
- Malaise and nausea
- Vomiting
- Unsteadiness when walking, incoordination
- Visual disturbances
- Severe headaches
- Weakness in extremities
- Sensory changes in face or body
- Dysarthria (difficulty with speech)
- Unconsciousness, disorientation, light-headedness
- Hearing difficulties
- Facial paralysis

Note: Similar symptoms may be seen with other conditions (e.g., benign paroxysmal positional vertigo, head injury, epilepsy, ear disease).

These tests are often more effective if performed with the patient sitting because the blood must flow against gravity and there is a restriction caused by the passive movement. However, the supine position allows greater passive range of movement.[169] Movements to the right tend to have more effect on the left vertebral artery, and movements to the left tend to have more effect on the right artery.[168]

❓ *Barré Test.*[170] The patient stands with the shoulders forward flexed to 90°, elbows straight and forearms supinated, palms up and eyes closed, holding the position for 10 to 20 seconds. The test is considered positive if one arm slowly falls with simultaneous forearm pronation. The cause is thought to be diminished blood flow to the brain stem. This test is identical to the first part of Hautant's test.

❓ *Hautant's Test.*[67,171] This test has two parts and is used to differentiate dizziness or vertigo caused by articular problems from that caused by vascular problems.

TABLE **3.25**

Vascular Pathology Signs and Symptoms Related to the Vertebral and Internal Carotid Arteries

Factors to Consider When Assessing Cervical Vascular Problems	***Vascular Risk Factors***
• Risk factors	• Hypertension
• Position testing (especially rotation and extension)	• Hypercholesterolemia (high cholesterol)
• Cranial nerve examination	• Hyperlipidemia (high fat)
• Eye examination	• Hyperhomocysteinemia (hardening of the arteries)
• Cognitive function	• Diabetes mellitus
• Blood pressure examination	• General clotting disorders
• "Headache like no other"	• Infection
	• Smoking
Vertebral Artery Nonischemic (Local) Signs and Symptoms	• Direct vessel trauma
• Ipsilateral posterior neck pain	• Iatrogenic causes (surgery, medical interventions)
• Occipital headache	
• C5–C6 cervical root impairment (rare)	***Internal Carotid Nonischemic (Local) Signs and Symptoms***
	• Head/neck pain
Vertebral Artery Ischemic Signs and Symptoms	• Horner syndrome: a rare condition caused by injury to the sympathetic nerves of the face; involves a collection of symptoms including sinking of the eyeball into the face (enophthalmia), small (constricted) pupils (miosis), ptosis (drooping eyelid), anhidrosis (facial dryness)
• "Headache like no other"	• Pulsatile tinnitus
• Ipsilateral posterior upper cervical pain	• Cranial nerve palsies (most commonly cranial nerve IX–XII)
• Occipital headache	• Ipsilateral carotid bruit (less common)
• Hindbrain transient ischemic attack: dizziness, diplopia, dysarthria, dysphagia, drop attacks, nausea, nystagmus, facial numbness, ataxia, vomiting, hoarseness, loss of short-term memory, weakness, hypotonia/limb weakness (arm or leg), anhidrosis (lack of facial sweating), hearing disturbances, malaise, perioral dysesthesia, photophobia, papillary changes, clumsiness, and agitation	• Scalp tenderness (less common)
	• Neck swelling (less common)
	• Cranial nerve VI palsy (less common)
	• Orbital pain (less common)
	Internal Carotid Artery Ischemic Signs and Symptoms
• Hindbrain stroke: Wallenberg syndrome (a neurological condition caused by a stroke in the vertebral or posterior inferior cerebral artery of the brain stem), symptoms include difficulty in swallowing, hoarseness, dizziness, nausea and vomiting, rapid involuntary movements of the eyes (nystagmus), and problems with balance and gait coordination	• Ipsilateral frontal temporal headache (clusterlike, thunderclap, migraine without aura, or simply "different from previous headaches")
	• Upper/middle and anterolateral cervical pain, facial pain and sensitivity (carotidynia)
	• Transient ischemic attack
	• Ischemic stroke
	• Retinal infarction
	• Amaurosis fugax (transient episodic blindness caused by decreased blood flow to the retina)

Data from Kerry R, Taylor AJ: Cervical artery dysfunction assessment and manual therapy, *Man Ther* 11:243–253, 2006.

The patient sits and forward flexes both arms to 90° (Fig. 3.49). The eyes are then closed. The examiner watches for any loss of arm position. If the arms move, the cause is nonvascular. The patient is then asked to rotate, or extend and rotate, the neck; this position is held while the eyes are again closed. If wavering of the arms occurs, the dysfunction is caused by vascular impairment to the brain. Each position should be held for 10 to 30 seconds.

❓ *Naffziger Test.*[67,172] The patient is seated, and the examiner stands behind the patient with his or her fingers over the patient's jugular veins (Fig. 3.50). The examiner compresses the veins for 30 seconds (Naffziger recommended 10 minutes!) and then asks the patient to cough. Pain may indicate a nerve root problem or space-occupying lesion (e.g., tumor). If light-headedness or similar symptoms occur with compression of the jugular veins, the test should be terminated.

❓ *Static Vertebral Artery Tests.* The examiner may test the following passive movements with the patient supine or sitting, as advocated by Grant,[173] watching for eye nystagmus and complaints by the patient of dizziness, lightheadedness, or visual disturbances. Each of these tests is increasingly provocative; if symptoms occur with the first test, there is no need to progress to the next test.

TABLE **3.26**

Differential Diagnosis of Internal Carotid Artery Disease, Vertebrobasilar Artery Disease, and Upper Cervical Instability

	Internal Carotid Artery Disease	Vertebrobasilar Artery Disease	Upper Cervical Instability
Early presentation	Mid-upper cervical pain, pain around ear and jaw (carotidynia), head pain (fronto-temporo-parietal) Ptosis Lower cranial nerve dysfunction (VIII–XII) Acute onset of pain described as "unlike any other"	Mid-upper cervical pain, occipital headache Acute onset of pain described as "unlike any other"	Neck and head pain Feeling of instability Cervical muscle hyperactivity Constant support needed for head Worsening symptoms
Late presentation	Transient retinal dysfunction (scintillating scotoma, amaurosis fugax) Transient ischemic attack Cerebrovascular accident	Hindbrain transient ischemic attack (dizziness, diplopia, dysarthria, dysphagia, drop attacks, nausea, nystagmus, facial numbness, ataxia, vomiting, hoarseness, loss of short-term memory, vagueness, hypotonia/limb weakness [arm or leg], anhidrosis [lack of facial sweating], hearing disturbances, malaise, perioral dysesthesia, photophobia, papillary changes, clumsiness, and agitation) Cranial nerve dysfunction Hindbrain stroke (e.g., Wallenberg syndrome, locked-in syndrome)	Bilateral foot and hand dysesthesias Feeling of lump in throat Metallic taste in mouth (VII) Arm and leg weakness Lack of coordination bilaterally

From Rushton A, Rivett D, Carlesso L, et al: International framework for examination of the cervical region for potential of cervical arterial dysfunction prior to orthopedic manual therapy intervention, *Man Ther* 19(3):222–228, 2014.

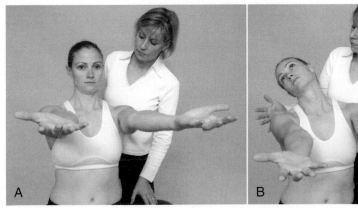
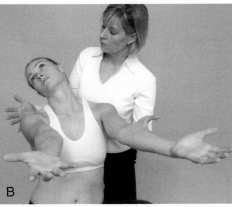

Fig. 3.49 Positioning for Hautant test. (A) Forward flexion of both arms to 90°. (B) Rotation and extension of neck with arms forward flexed to 90°.

In the sitting position:
1. Sustained full neck and head extension
2. Sustained full neck and head rotation, right and left (if this movement causes symptoms, it is sometimes called a positive **Barré-Lieou sign**)[67]
3. Sustained full neck and head rotation with extension right and left **(DeKleyn test)**[67]
4. Provocative movement position (implies movement into the position that provokes symptoms)
5. Quick head movement into provocative position
6. Quick repeated head movement into provocative position
7. Head still, sustained trunk movement left and right (10 to 30 seconds)
8. Head still, repeated trunk movement left and right

In supine position:
1. Sustained full neck and head extension
2. Sustained full neck and head rotation left and right

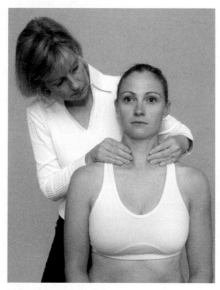

Fig. 3.50 Naffziger test (compression of jugular veins).

3. Sustained full neck and head rotation with extension left and right (if combined with side flexion, it is called the **Hallpike maneuver**[67]). Extension combined with rotation has been found to be the position most likely to occlude the vertebral artery.[152]
4. Unilateral posteroanterior oscillation (Maitland grade IV) of C1 to C2 facet joints (prone lying) with head rotated left and right
5. Simulated mobilization and manipulation position

Each position should be held for at least 10 to 30 seconds unless symptoms are evoked. Extension in isolation is more likely to test the patency of the intervertebral foramen, whereas rotation and side flexion or, especially, rotation and extension are more likely to test the vertebral artery (Table 3.27).[10] If symptoms are evoked, care should be taken concerning any treatment to follow.

Aspinall[174] advocated the use of a progressive series of clinical tests to evaluate the vertebral artery. With these tests, the examiner progressively moves from the lower cervical spine and lower vertebral artery to the upper cervical spine and upper vertebral artery where it is more vulnerable to pathology. Table 3.28 demonstrates Aspinall progressive clinical tests for the vertebral arteries.

❓ *Underburg's Test.*[67] The patient stands with the shoulders forward flexed to 90°, elbows straight, and forearms supinated. The patient then closes the eyes and marches in place while holding the extended and rotated head to one side. The test is repeated with head movement to the opposite side. The test is considered positive if there is dropping of the arms, loss of balance, or pronation of the hands; a positive result indicates decreased blood supply to the brain.

❓ *Vertebral Artery (Cervical Quadrant) Test.* With the patient supine, the examiner passively takes the patient's head and neck into extension and side flexion (Fig. 3.51).[175] After this movement is achieved, the examiner rotates the patient's neck to the same side and holds it for approximately 30 seconds. A positive test provokes referring symptoms if the

TABLE 3.27

Relationship of Head Position to Blood Flow to Head and Neurological Function

Head Position	Blood Flow	Neurological Space
Neutral	Normal	Normal
Flexion	Normal	Normal
Extension	Usually normal	Decreased
Side flexion	Slight decrease in ipsilateral artery; normal in contralateral artery	Decrease on ipsilateral side; increase on contralateral side
Rotation	Slight decrease in ipsilateral artery; significant decrease in contralateral artery	Decrease on ipsilateral side; increase on contralateral side
Extension and rotation	Bilateral decrease, greater in contralateral artery	Bilateral decrease, greater on ipsilateral side
Flexion and rotation	Bilateral decrease	Decrease on ipsilateral side; increase on contralateral side

TABLE **3.28**

Aspinall's Progressive Clinical Tests for Vertebral Artery Pathology

Vertebral Artery Area	Sitting	Lying	Test
Area 1 (lower cervical spine)	X		Active cervical rotation
Area 2 (middle cervical spine)	X		Active cervical rotation
	X	X	Passive cervical rotation
	X		Active cervical extension
	X	X	Passive cervical extension
	X	X	Passive cervical extension with rotation
	X		Passive segmental extension with rotation
	X	X	Passive cervical flexion
	X	X	Cervical flexion with traction
		X	Accessory oscillatory anterior/posterior movement—transverse processes C2–C7 in combined extension and rotation
		X	Sustained manipulation position
Area 3 (upper cervical spine)	X		Active cervical rotation
	X	X	Passive cervical rotation
	X		Active cervical extension
	X	X	Passive cervical extension
	X	X	Passive cervical rotation with extension
	X	X	Cervical rotation with extension and traction
	X		Cervical rotation with flexion
		X	Accessory oscillatory anterior/posterior movement—transverse processes C1–C2 in combined rotation and extension
		X	Sustained manipulation position

From Aspinall W: Clinical testing for the craniovertebral hypermobility syndrome, *J Orthop Sports Phys Ther* 12:180–181, 1989.

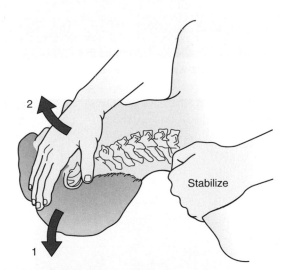

Fig. 3.51 Vertebral artery (cervical quadrant) test. Examiner passively moves patient's head and neck into extension and side flexion *(1)*, then rotation *(2)*, holding for 30 seconds.

opposite artery is affected. This test must be done with care. If dizziness or nystagmus occurs, it is an indication that the vertebral arteries are being compressed. The **DeKleyn-Nieuwenhuyse test**[69,170] ❓ performs a similar function but involves extension and rotation instead of extension and side flexion. Both tests may also be used to assess nerve root

compression in the lower cervical spine. To test the upper cervical spine, the examiner "pokes" the patient's chin and follows with extension, side flexion, and rotation.

Tests for Vertigo and Dizziness

❓ *Dizziness Test.* The patient sits, and the examiner grasps the patient's head. The examiner actively rotates the patient's head as far as possible to the right and then to the left, holding the head at the extreme of motion for a short time (10 to 30 seconds) while the shoulders remain stationary. The patient's head is then returned to neutral. Next, the patient's shoulders are actively rotated as far to the right as possible, held for 10 to 30 seconds, and then to the left as far as possible, and held for 10 to 30 seconds while keeping the head facing straight ahead. If the patient experiences dizziness in both cases, the problem lies in the vertebral arteries, because in both cases the vertebral artery may be "kinked," decreasing the blood flow. If the patient experiences dizziness only when the head is rotated, the problem lies within the semicircular canals of the inner ear.

Fitz-Ritson[176] advocates a modification of this test. For the first part of the test, he advocates that the examiner hold the shoulders still while the patient rapidly rotates the head left and right with eyes closed. If vertigo results, the problem is in the vestibular nuclei or muscles and joints of the cervical spine. In addition, patients may lose their balance, veer to one side, or possibly vomit. The second stage is the same as previously mentioned, except that the eyes are closed. If vertigo is experienced this time, Fitz-Ritson believes that the problem is in the cervical spine because the vestibular apparatus is not being moved.

✓ **Hallpike-Dix Maneuver or Test.**[177,178] See Chapter 2 for description.

❓ **Temperature (Caloric) Test.**[179] The examiner alternately applies hot and cold test tubes several times just behind the patient's ears on the side of the head; each side is done in turn. A positive test is associated with the inducement of vertigo, which indicates inner ear problems.

Tests for Cervical Instability (Instability "Clearing" Tests)

Instability in the cervical spine is most commonly the result of ligament damage (e.g., transverse ligament, alar ligaments), bone or joint damage (e.g., fracture or dislocation), or weak muscles (e.g., deep flexors or extensors). The instability may be the result of chronic arthritic conditions (e.g., rheumatoid arthritis), trauma, long-term corticosteroid use, congenital malformations, Down syndrome, and osteoporosis.[13] One commonly should have a high level of suspicion of instability if in the history the patient complains of instability, a lump in the throat, lip paresthesia, severe headache (especially with movement), muscle spasm, nausea, or vomiting.[13] If the examiner anticipates doing mobilization (especially end-range techniques) or manipulation techniques to the cervical spine, especially the upper cervical spine, a selection of appropriate "clearing" tests should be performed to rule out instability. If instability is present, mobilization and/or manipulation should **not** be performed.

> ### Signs and Symptoms of Cervical Instability
> - Severe muscle spasm
> - Patient does not want to move head (especially into flexion)
> - Lump in throat
> - Lip or facial paresthesia
> - Severe headache
> - Dizziness
> - Nausea
> - Vomiting
> - Soft-end feel
> - Nystagmus
> - Pupil changes

❓ **Anterior Shear or Sagittal Stress Test.**[70,180,181] This test is designed to test the integrity of the supporting ligamentous and capsular tissues of the cervical spine. It is similar to the **posteroanterior central vertebral pressure (PACVP)** testing in the joint play section. The patient lies supine with the head in neutral resting on the bed. The examiner applies an anteriorly directed force through the posterior arch of C1 or the spinous processes of C2 to T1

or bilaterally through the lamina of each vertebral body. In each case, the normal end feel is tissue stretch with an abrupt stop (Fig. 3.52). Positive signs, especially when the upper cervical spine is tested, include nystagmus, pupil changes, dizziness, soft end feel, nausea, facial or lip paresthesia, and a lump sensation in the throat.[69]

❓ **Lateral Flexion Alar Ligament Stress Test.**[124,171,180,182] The patient lies supine with the head in the physiological neutral position while the examiner stabilizes the axis with a wide pinch grip around the spinous process and lamina (Fig. 3.53). The examiner then attempts to side flex the head and axis. Normally, if the ligament is intact, minimal side flexion occurs with a strong capsular end feel and a solid stop.

⚠ **Lateral (Transverse) Shear Test.**[171,180] This test is used to determine instability of the atlanto-axial articulation caused by odontoid dysplasia. The patient lies supine with

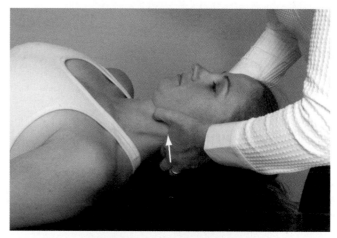

Fig. 3.52 Anterior sagittal stress test.

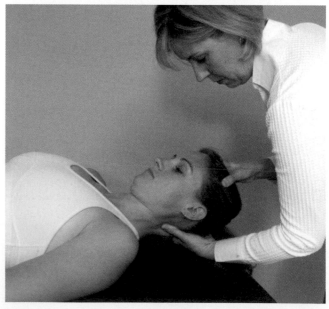

Fig. 3.53 Lateral flexion alar ligament stress test. Examiner attempts to side flex the patient's head while stabilizing the axis.

the head supported. The examiner places the radial side of the second metacarpophalangeal (MCP) joint of one hand against the transverse process of the atlas and the MCP joint of the other hand against the opposite transverse process of the axis. The examiner's hands are then carefully pushed together, causing a shear of one bone on the other (Fig. 3.54). Normally, minimal motion and no symptoms (spinal cord or vascular) are produced. Because this test is normally painful because of the compression of soft tissues against the bone, the patient should be warned beforehand that pain is a normal sensation to be expected. The test can also be used to test other levels of the cervical spine (i.e., C2 to C7).

⚠ *Posterior Atlanto-Occipital Membrane Test.*[183] This test assesses the stability between the occiput and atlas in the posterior part of the neck. The patient is seated and the patient's head is cradled against the examiner's chest. The fingers of the examiner's upper hand grip the occiput while the lower hand stabilizes C1 by applying a downward pressure with fingers placed on the lateral mass of the atlas (Fig. 3.55). The test is performed by the examiner pulling with the left hand in the opposite direction to the downward pressure of the other hand. The pulling is repeated through different angles of neck flexion and on both sides starting with the uninjured or side with no symptoms. A positive test is indicated by abnormal motion relative to the other (uninjured) side and possible pain.

❓ *Rotational Alar Ligament Stress Test.*[180,182] The patient is in sitting position. The examiner grips the lamina and spinous process of C2 between the finger and thumb. While stabilizing C2, the examiner passively rotates the patient's head left or right moving to the "no symptom" side first. If more than 20° to 30° rotation is possible without C2 moving, it is indicative of injury to the contralateral alar ligament especially if the lateral flexion alar stress test is positive in the same direction. If the excessive motion is in the opposite direction for both tests, the instability is due to an increase in the neutral zone in the joint (Fig. 3.56).

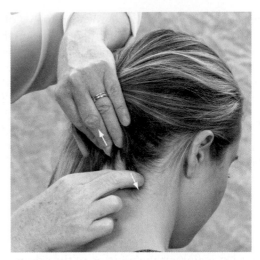

Fig. 3.55 Posterior atlanto-occipital membrane test.

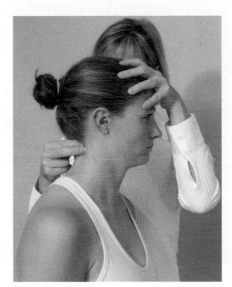

Fig. 3.56 Rotational alar ligament stress test. While the examiner grips the lamina of C2, the patient's head is rotated left and right with the other hand.

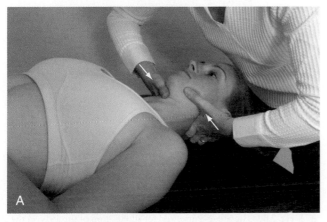

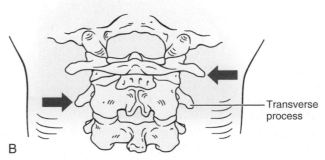

Transverse process

Fig. 3.54 (A) Atlanto-axial lateral shear test. (B) Metacarpophalangeal joints against transverse processes.

Kaale et al.[183] advocated doing the test ❓ in a different fashion. They advocate placing the patient in sitting position. The examiner supports the patient's head against his or her body and places both hands on the same side of the patient's occipitocervical junction. The lower hand (Fig. 3.57) stabilizes C2 by pressing the second and third fingers against the lateral aspect of C2 pulling it backwards. The other hand is placed above with the third finger under the lateral mass of the atlas and the second finger under the mastoid process pulling upward into rotation (see Fig. 3.57). The test is performed in different angles of rotation to locate the position of maximum movement between C1 and C2.

⚠ *Sharp-Purser Test.* This test should be performed *with extreme caution.* It is a test to determine subluxation of the atlas on the axis (Fig. 3.58). If the transverse ligament that maintains the position of the odontoid process relative to C1 (Fig. 3.59) is torn, C1 will translate forward (sublux) on C2 on flexion. Thus, the examiner may find the patient reticent to do forward flexion if the transverse ligament has been damaged. The examiner places one hand over the patient's forehead while the thumb of the other hand is placed over the spinous process of the axis to stabilize it (Fig. 3.60). The patient is asked to slowly flex the head; while this is occurring, the examiner presses backward with the palm. A positive test is indicated if the examiner feels the head slide backward during the movement. The slide backward indicates that the subluxation of the atlas has been reduced, and the slide may be accompanied by a "clunk."

Aspinall[184] advocates use of an additional test if the Sharp-Purser test is negative (**Aspinall transverse ligament test**). The patient is placed in supine. The examiner stabilizes the occiput on the atlas in flexion and holds the occiput in this flexed position. The examiner then applies an anteriorly directed force to the posterior aspect of the atlas (Fig. 3.61). Normally, no movement or symptoms are perceived by the patient. For the test to be positive, the patient should feel a lump in the throat as the atlas

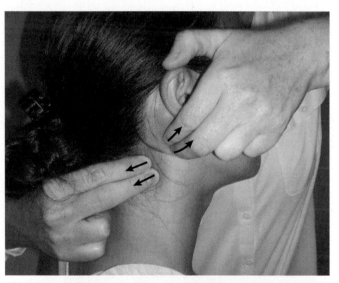

Fig. 3.57 Rotational alar ligament stress test. Kaale's alternate method.

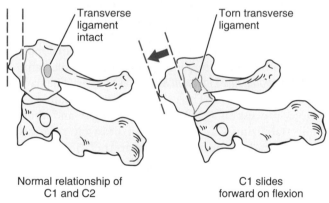

Normal relationship of C1 and C2

C1 slides forward on flexion

Fig. 3.59 Forward translation of C1 on C2 during flexion as a result of torn transverse ligament.

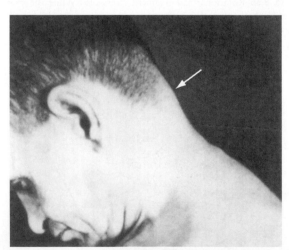

Fig. 3.58 Subluxation of the atlas on neck flexion. Note the bulge in the posterior neck caused by the forward subluxation of the atlas, bringing the spinous process of the axis into prominence beneath the skin *(arrow).* (Courtesy Harold S. Robinson, MD, Vancouver, BC.)

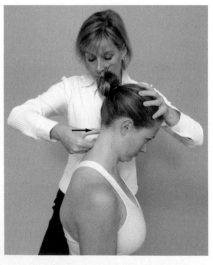

Fig. 3.60 The Sharp-Purser test for subluxation of the atlas on the axis.

moves toward the esophagus; this is indicative of hypermobility at the atlanto-axial articulation.

Rey-Eiriz et al.[185] advocated doing a similar test to test for hypomobility in the middle cervical spine (**posterior-anterior middle cervical spine gliding test ❓**). The head and cervical

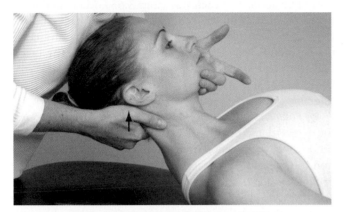

🎞 **Fig. 3.61** Aspinall transverse ligament test.

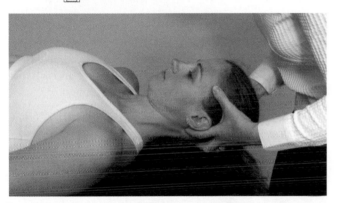

Fig. 3.62 Testing the transverse ligament of C1. Examiner's hands support head and C1.

spine are held in neutral and the examiner pushes anteriorly on the lamina of C3, C4, or C5. Hypomobility for the test was defined as abnormal resistance to movement, abnormal end feel, and/or reproduction of local or referred pain.

⚠ *Transverse Ligament Stress Test.*[171,180] The patient lies supine with the examiner supporting the occiput with the palms and the third, fourth, and fifth fingers. The examiner places the index fingers in the space between the patient's occiput and C2 spinous process so that the fingertips are overlying the neural arch of C1. The head and C1 are then carefully lifted anteriorly together, allowing no flexion or extension (Fig. 3.62). This anterior shear is normally resisted by the transverse ligament (Fig. 3.63). The position is held for 10 to 20 seconds to see whether symptoms occur, indicating a positive test. Positive symptoms include soft end feel; muscle spasm; dizziness; nausea; paresthesia of the lip, face, or limb; nystagmus; or a lump sensation in the throat. The test indicates hypermobility at the atlanto-axial articulation.

Kaale et al.[183] advocated doing the test ❓ by stabilizing C2 from the front of the neck with the fingers pressed against the anterior aspect of the side of the transverse process on one side and the thumb in the same position on the opposite side of C2 (Fig. 3.64). *Do not choke the patient!* The examiner's other hand is similarly placed on the posterior aspect of the transverse processes of C1 and against the inferior part of the occiput. C1 is pressed forward while C2 is pressed backward testing the translation of the dens of the atlas.

Tests for Upper Cervical Spine Mobility

✅ *Cervical Flexion Rotation Test.*[61,97,186,187] The test is used to determine the mobility of the upper cervical spine (C1–C2) and to determine if the upper cervical spine is the

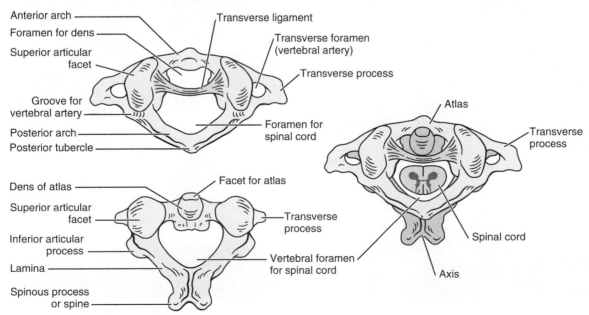

Fig. 3.63 Relationship of C1 to C2 and the position of the transverse ligament.

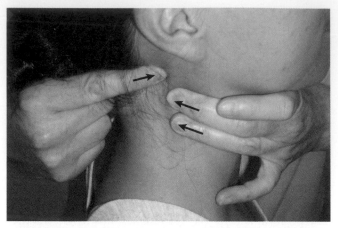

Fig. 3.64 Transverse ligament stress test. Kaale's alternate method.

cause of a cervicogenic headache.[61,188–190] The patient is in supine lying position. The examiner sits or stands at the head of the patient and flexes the cervical spine fully. While holding the flexed position, the examiner then rotates the head left and right. Normal rotation in the flexed position should be about 45° each way (Fig. 3.65). Maintaining the flexed position is more likely to isolate the rotation to the C1–C2 area so that C1–C2 dysfunction may be evident if the rotation is less (hypomobility) or more (hypermobility) than normal. If the patient also has a headache, the restricted ROM to one side is likely to be cervicogenic in nature, not a migraine or other type of headache.[190]

? *Pettman's Distraction Test.*[180,181] This test is used to test the tectorial membrane. The patient lies supine with the head in neutral position. The examiner applies gentle traction to the head. Provided no symptoms are produced, the patient's head is lifted forward, flexing the spine, and traction is reapplied. If the patient complains of symptoms, such as pain, or paresthesia in the second position, then the test is considered positive for a lax tectorial membrane (Fig. 3.66).

Tests for Movement Control Dysfunction

Tests for movement control are designed to test the ability of the patient to do an active movement correctly. Table 3.29 outlines how these tests are performed and what to look for to ensure proper controlled movement.[87]

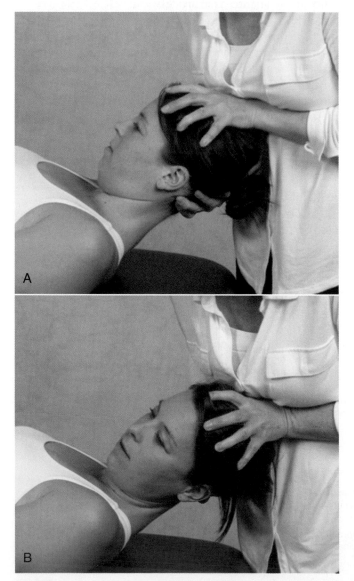

Fig. 3.65 Cervical flexion rotation test. (A) Flexion. (B) Rotation in flexion.

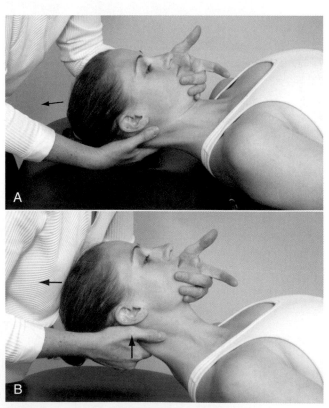

Fig. 3.66 Pettman's distraction test. (A) First position. (B) Second (flexed) position.

TABLE **3.29**

Operational Definitions for the Movement Control Tests of the Cervical Spine

Movement Control Tests	Muscles/Direction of Movement Control	Correct Performance	Impaired Performance
1. Active cervical extension in 4-point kneeling Instruction: *Imagine you have a book between your hands. Look down to flex the head and neck together as far as you can and then curl your head back up as far as you can (lower and mid cervical spine), but maintain your eyes on the book.* The patient is to perform cervical extension, while keeping the craniocervical region in neutral.	Bias toward semispinalis cervicis/multifidus which act only on the cervical spine and against superficial extensors, which also extend the head	Patient is able to dissociate mid-lower from upper cervical extension: head remains in a neutral position while performing mid-lower cervical extension to about 20°.	Patient is unable to dissociate mid-lower from upper cervical extension. Different impairments can be observed: 1. The patient cannot reach 20° of cervical extension while keeping the craniocervical region in neutral. 2. The patient adopts a poor coordination strategy and uses superficial cervical muscles excessively, indicated by craniocervical extension (poked chin) and excessive use of the semispinalis capitis muscles indicated by their marked prominence on the back of the neck.
2. Active upper cervical rotation in 4-point kneeling Instruction: *Rotate the head while keeping the cervical region still, as if saying 'No.'* Examiner gently stabilizes the C2 vertebra (only for the practice sessions) to assist patient in locating the movement to the upper cervical region. Patient is instructed to perform small ranges of craniocervical rotation to both sides (no greater than 40°), while maintaining cervical spine in a neutral position.	Bias toward the suboccipital rotators (obliquus capitis superior and inferior)	Patient is able to dissociate upper cervical rotation movement from movement at the mid-lower cervical region: no motion of the mid-lower cervical spine occurs.	Patient is unable to dissociate upper cervical rotation movement from movement at the typical cervical region: excessive motion of the typical cervical region occurs.
3. Active cervical flexion in 4-point kneeling Instruction: *Look down to flex the head and neck together as far as you can.*	Extensor muscles	The flexion movement is predominantly anterior sagittal plane rotation of the head and cervical spine.	Movement: The head and the cervical spine translate anteriorly with diminished anterior sagittal plane rotation during the flexion movement. Lower cervical flexion greater than upper thoracic flexion.
4. Active cervical extension in sitting Instruction: *Look toward the ceiling and follow the ceiling back with the eyes as far as possible.*	Flexor muscles (eccentric control)	Head extends behind the frontal plane to 15°–20°. A pattern of smooth and even neck extension of upper, mid, and lower cervical regions should be observed.	Dominant upper cervical spine extension with minimal, if any, movement of the head posteriorly. The head moves backward but then reaches a point of extension where it appears to drop or translate backward.

TABLE **3.29**

Operational Definitions for the Movement Control Tests of the Cervical Spine—cont'd

Movement Control Tests	Muscles/Direction of Movement Control	Correct Performance	Impaired Performance
5. Return to neutral from the cervical extension position in sitting Instruction: *Return to neutral from the cervical extension position.*	Flexor muscles (concentric control)	Return to neutral position starts with craniocervical flexion followed by lower cervical flexion.	Initiation of returning to neutral position with sternocleidomastoid and anterior scalene muscles resulting in lower cervical flexion but not upper craniocervical flexion. Craniocervical flexion is the last rather than first component of the pattern of movement.
6. Active bilateral arm flexion in standing Instruction: *Raise and lower your arms (palms facing in) as far as you can while keeping your head steady.*	Flexor, extensor muscle co-contraction	Cervical spine remains still during 180° of bilateral arm flexion.	Compensatory/excessive forward head movement or extension of the cervical spine observed during 180° of bilateral arm flexion.
7. Rocking backward in 4-point kneeling Instruction: *Rock backward slowly as far as you can.*	Flexor, extensor muscle co-contraction	Cervical spine remains in a neutral position during the movement.	Compensatory motion or excessive cervical extension is observed during the quadruped rocking back.
8. Active unilateral arm flexion in standing Instruction: *Raise and lower each arm separately (palms facing in) as far as you while keeping the head in a neutral position.*	Flexor, extensor muscle co-contraction	Cervical spine remains stable via observation during single-arm flexion to 180° to both sides	Compensatory motion of cervical rotation/lateroflexion is noted during arm flexion to 180° in either side.
9. Active cervical rotation in sitting Instruction: *Rotate your head and neck as far as you can to each side while maintaining the plane of the face vertical and eyes horizontal.* Note: bilateral cervical rotation is assessed with the scapula in a neutral position (hands on thighs).	Rotation movement control	A pattern of smooth and even head rotation around a vertical axis should be observed to each side (70°–80° rotation to each side). The plane of the face should stay vertical with the eyes horizontal and with concurrent upper and lower cervical movement. No other components of motion (i.e., lateroflexion, extension, or flexion) should be observed.	Rotation to either side occurs with concurrent/simultaneous lateral flexion, extension, or flexion and/or forward translation of the head and neck.

From Segarra V, Dueñas L, Torres R, et al: Inter- and intra-tester reliability of a battery of cervical movement control dysfunction tests, *Man Ther* 20(4):572, 2015.

Tests for First Rib Mobility

Although the first rib would normally be included with assessment of the thoracic spine, the examiner should always test for mobility of the first rib when examining the cervical spine, especially if side flexion is limited and there is pain or tenderness in the area of the first rib or T1.

For the first test ✅, the patient lies supine while fully supported. The examiner palpates the first rib bilaterally lateral to T1 and places his or her fingers along the path of the patient's ribs just posterior to the clavicles (Fig. 3.67A). While palpating the ribs, the examiner notes the movement of both first ribs as the patient takes a deep breath in and out, and any asymmetry is noted. The examiner then palpates one first rib and side flexes the head to the opposite side until the rib is felt to move up. The range of neck side flexion is noted. The side flexion is then repeated to the opposite side, and results from the two sides are compared. Asymmetry may be caused by hypomobility of the first rib or tightness of the scalene muscles on the same side.

For the second test, the patient lies prone, and the examiner again palpates the first rib (Fig. 3.67B). Using the thumb, reinforced by the other thumb, the examiner pushes the rib caudally, noting the amount of movement, end feel, and presence of pain. The other first rib is tested in a similar fashion, and the two sides are compared. Normally, a firm

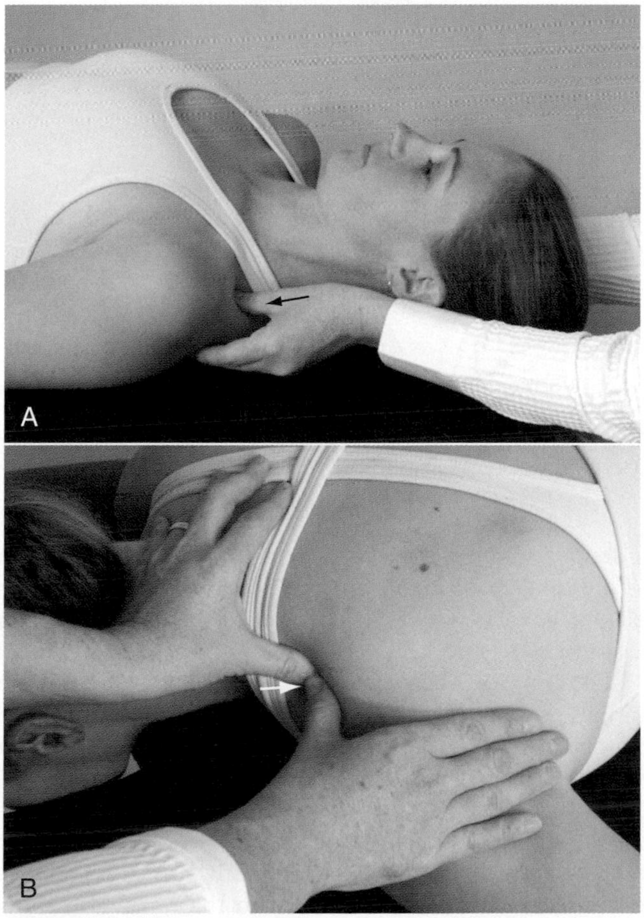

Fig. 3.67 Testing mobility of the first rib. (A) In supine. (B) In prone.

tissue stretch is felt with no pain, except possibly where the examiner's thumbs are compressing soft tissue against the rib.

Tests for Thoracic Outlet Syndrome

See Special Tests in Chapter 5.

Reflexes and Cutaneous Distribution

If the examiner suspects neurological involvement during the assessment, reflex testing and cutaneous sensation should be tested. For the cervical spine, the following reflexes should be checked for differences between the two sides, as shown in Fig. 3.68: biceps (C5–C6), the brachioradialis (C5–C6), the triceps (C7–C8), and the jaw jerk (cranial nerve V). Bland[33] felt the jaw jerk was a useful diagnostic test. A normal (negative) jaw jerk combined with positive (exaggerated) tendon reflexes in the upper limb suggested the lesion was below the foramen magnum. If both reflexes were abnormal, then the lesion is above the pons.

The reflexes are tested with a reflex hammer. The examiner tests the biceps and jaw jerk reflexes by placing his or her thumb over the patient's biceps tendon or at midpoint of the chin and then tapping the thumbnail with the reflex hammer to elicit the reflex. The jaw reflex may also be tested with a tongue depressor (see Fig. 3.68B). The examiner holds the tongue depressor firmly against the lower teeth while the patient relaxes the jaw and then strikes the tongue depressor with the reflex hammer. The brachioradialis and triceps reflexes are tested by directly tapping the tendon or muscle.

Common Reflexes Checked in Cervical Spine Assessment

- Biceps (C5, C6)
- Triceps (C7, C8)
- Hoffmann sign (if upper motor neuron lesion suspected)
- Inverted supinator sign (if upper motor neuron lesion suspected)

If the examiner suspects involvement of the cranial nerves, then each of the cranial nerves should be tested (see Table 2.1). These nerves are more likely to be affected by a head injury but head and neck injuries can occur in unison so the examiner should test any cranial nerves that may be involved especially if the patient has complained about any signs or symptoms affecting the cranial nerves while the history is being taken.

If an upper motor neuron lesion is suspected, the pathological reflexes (e.g., **Babinski reflex**) should be checked (see Table 1.32) and the deep tendon reflexes (see Table 1.30) may show hyperreflexia. **Hoffmann sign** is the upper limb equivalent of the Babinski test although its efficacy has been questioned.[191] To test for Hoffmann sign, the examiner holds the patient's middle finger and briskly flicks the distal phalanx. A positive sign is noted if the interphalangeal joint of the thumb of the same hand flexes/adducts (Fig. 3.69). The fingers may also flex. Denno and Meadows[192] advocated a dynamic

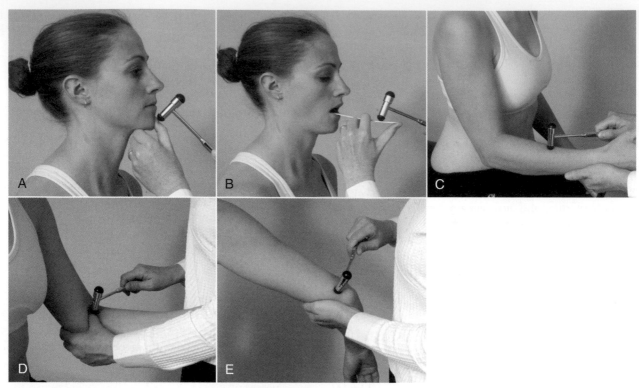

Fig. 3.68 Testing of upper limb reflexes. (A) Jaw. (B) Jaw (tongue depressor method). (C) Brachioradialis. (D) Biceps. (E) Triceps.

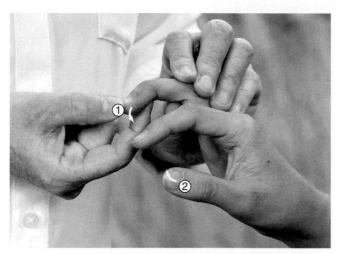

Fig. 3.69 Hoffmann sign. The examiner flicks the distal phalanx of the patient's middle finger (third digit) (*1*). In a positive test, such action causes the patient's thumb to flex and/or adduct (*2*).

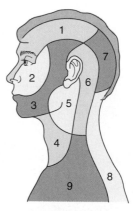

Fig. 3.70 Sensory nerve distribution of the head, neck, and face. *1,* Ophthalmic nerve. *2,* Maxillary nerve. *3,* Mandibular nerve. *4,* Transverse cutaneous nerve of neck (C2–C3). *5,* Greater auricular nerve (C2–C3). *6,* Lesser auricular nerve (C2). *7,* Greater occipital nerve (C2–C3). *8,* Cervical dorsal rami (C3–C5). *9,* Suprascapular nerve (C5–C6).

Hoffmann sign. The patient is asked to repeatedly flex and extend the head, and then the test is performed as described previously. Denno and Meadows believed that the dynamic test showed positive results earlier than the static or normal Hoffmann sign. The **inverted supinator sign** (also called the **inverted brachioradialis jerk**) is a pathological reflex. Using a reflex hammer, the examiner rapidly taps near the styloid process at the wrist. A positive test results in finger flexion and slight elbow extension.[193,194] Because an upper motor neuron lesion affects both the upper and lower limb, initially unilaterally and at later stages bilaterally, the Babinski test may be performed

if desired. Clonus, most easily seen by sudden dorsiflexion of the ankle resulting in three to five reflex twitches of the plantar flexors, is also a sign of an upper motor neuron lesion.[195,196]

The examiner then checks the dermatome pattern of the various nerve roots as well as the sensory distribution of the peripheral nerves (Figs. 3.70 and 3.71) using a sensation scan (see previous discussion). Dermatomes vary from person to person and overlap a great deal, and the diagrams shown are estimations only. For example, C5 dermatome may stop distally on the radial side of the arm at the elbow, forearm, or wrist. Cervical radiculopathies may also show modified patterns. Levine et al.[50] point out that about 45%

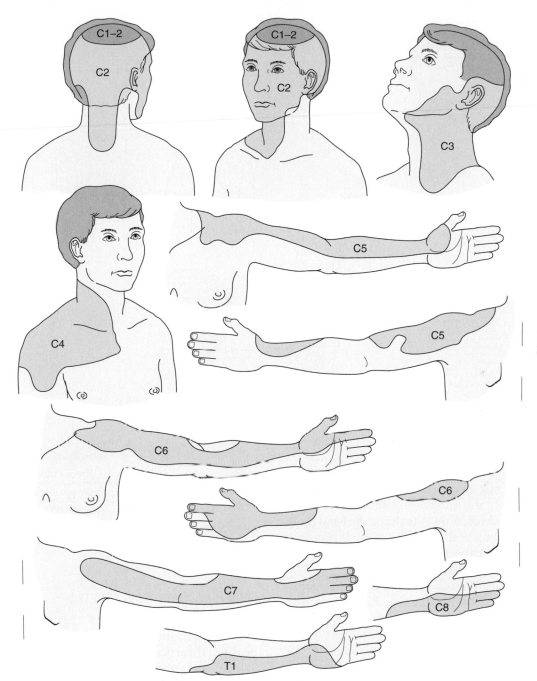

Fig. 3.71 Dermatomes of the cervical spine.

of patients have modified patterns and do not follow strict dermatome patterns. Classically, these patients also have referred pain into the trapezius and periscapular area posteriorly, and some will have pain into the breast area anteriorly.

Because of the spinal cord and associated nerve roots and their relation to the other bony and soft tissues in the cervical spine, referred pain is a relatively common experience in lesions of the cervical spine. Within the cervical spine, the intervertebral discs, facet joints, and other bony and soft tissues may refer pain to other segments of the neck (dermatomes) or to the head, the shoulder, the scapular area, and the whole of the upper limb (Figs. 3.72

and 3.73).[48,88] Table 3.30 shows the muscles of the cervical spine and their referral of pain.

Brachial Plexus Injuries of the Cervical Spine[197,198]

Brachial plexus injuries often result in paresthesia in one or both hands and all digits. If the injury is due to external pressure, the pins and needles may only be felt after the compression is removed. This is called a **release phenomenon** and can occur when the pressure is relieved on any peripheral nerve.

Erb-Duchenne Paralysis. This paralysis is an upper brachial plexus injury involving injury to the upper nerve

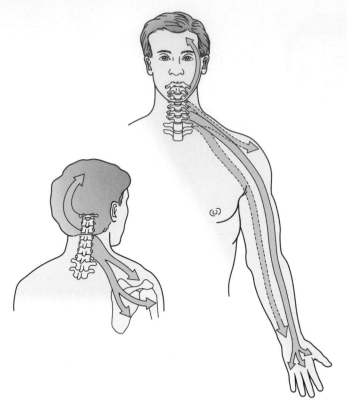

Fig. 3.72 Referral of symptoms from the cervical spine to areas of the spine, head, shoulder girdle, and upper limb.

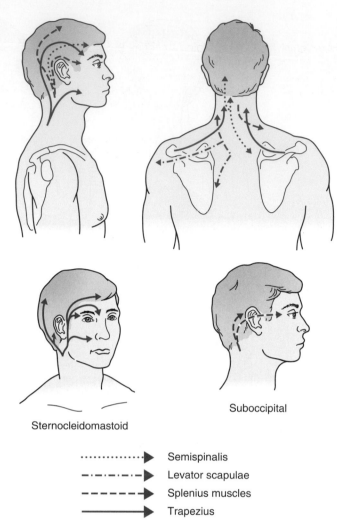

Sternocleidomastoid

Suboccipital

·············▶ Semispinalis
─·─·─·─▶ Levator scapulae
─ ─ ─ ─▶ Splenius muscles
━━━━▶ Trapezius

Fig. 3.73 Muscles and their referred pain patterns. Diagram shows primarily one side.

roots (C5, C6) as a result of compression or stretching. The injury frequently occurs at Erb's point. With this injury, it is primarily the muscles of the shoulder region and elbow that are affected; the muscles of the hand (especially the intrinsic muscles) are not involved. However, sensation over the radial surfaces of the forearm and hand and the deltoid area are affected.

Klumpke (Dejerine-Klumpke) Paralysis. This injury involves the lower brachial plexus and results from compression or stretching of the lower nerve roots (C8, T1). Atrophy and weakness are evident in the muscles of the forearm and hand as well as in the triceps. The obvious changes are in the distal aspects of the upper limb. The resultant injury is a functionless hand. Sensory loss occurs primarily on the ulnar side of the forearm and hand.

Brachial Plexus Birth Palsy.[199] These injuries to the brachial plexus occur in 0.1% to 0.4% of births with the majority showing full recovery within 2 months. Those infants who have not recovered within 3 months are at considerable risk of decreased strength and ROM in the upper limb.

Burners and Stingers.[200,201] These are transient injuries to the brachial plexus, which may be the result of trauma (see Fig. 3.10) combined with factors such as stenosis or a degenerative disc (spondylosis). Recurrent burners are not associated with more severe neck injury, but their effect on the nerve may be cumulative.[200]

Joint Play Movements

The joint play movements that are carried out in the cervical spine may be general movements (called **passive intervertebral movements [PIVMs]**) that involve the entire cervical spine (first four below) or specific movements isolated to one segment. As the joint play movements are performed, the examiner should note any decreased ROM, pain, or difference in end feel.

Joint Play Movements of the Cervical Spine

- Side glide of the cervical spine (general)
- Anterior glide of the cervical spine (general)
- Posterior glide of the cervical spine (general)
- Traction glide of the cervical spine (general)
- Rotation of the occiput on C1 (specific)
- Posteroanterior central vertebral pressure (specific)
- Posteroanterior unilateral vertebral pressure (specific)
- Transverse vertebral pressure (specific)

TABLE **3.30**

Muscles of the Cervical Spine and Their Referral of Pain

Muscle	Referral Pattern
Trapezius	Right and left occiput, lateral aspect of head above ear to behind eye, tip of jaw
	Spinous processes to medial border of scapula and along spine of scapula; may also refer to lateral aspect of upper arm
Sternocleidomastoid	Back and top of head, front of ear over forehead to medial aspect of eye; cheek
	Behind ear, ear to forehead
Splenius capitis	Top of head
Splenius cervicis	Posterior neck and shoulder angle, side of head to eye
Semispinalis cervicis	Back of head
Semispinalis capitis	Band around head at level of forehead
Multifidus	Occiput to posterior neck and shoulder angle to base of spine of scapula
Suboccipital	Lateral aspect of head to eye
Scalenes	Medial border of scapula and anterior chest down posterolateral aspect of arm to anterolateral and posterolateral aspect of hand

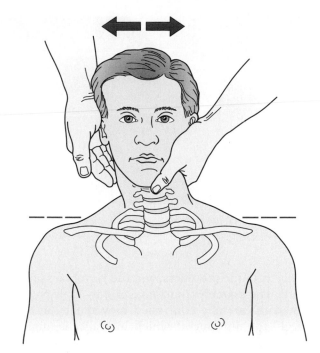

Fig. 3.74 Side glide of the cervical spine. Glide to the right is illustrated.

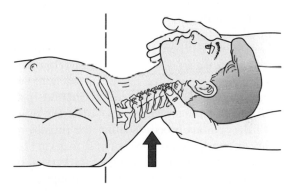

Fig. 3.75 Anterior glide of the cervical spine.

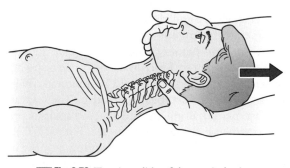

Fig. 3.76 Traction glide of the cervical spine.

Side Glide. The examiner holds the patient's head and moves it from side to side, keeping the head parallel to the shoulders (Fig. 3.74).[202]

Anterior and Posterior Glide. The examiner holds the patient's head with one hand around the occiput and one hand around the chin, taking care to ensure that the patient is not choked.[101] The examiner then draws the head forward in the same plane as the shoulders for anterior glide (Fig. 3.75) and posteriorly for posterior glide. While doing these movements, the examiner must prevent flexion and extension of the head.

Traction Glide. The examiner places one hand around the patient's chin and the other hand on the occiput.[103] Traction is then applied in a straight longitudinal direction with the majority of the pull being through the occiput (Fig. 3.76).

Vertebral Pressures. For the last three joint play movements (Fig. 3.77), the patient lies prone with the forehead resting on the back of the hands.[175] These techniques are specific to each vertebra and are applied to each vertebra in turn, or at least to the ones that the examination has indicated may be affected by pathology. They are sometimes called **passive accessory intervertebral movements (PAIVMs)**.[99] The

examiner palpates the spinous processes of the cervical spine, starting at the C2 spinous process and working downward to the T2 spinous process. The positions of the examiner's hands, fingers, and thumbs in performing PACVPs are shown in Fig. 3.77A. Pressure is then applied through the examiner's thumbs pushing

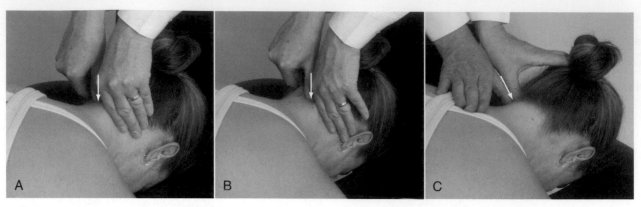

Fig. 3.77 Vertebral pressures to the cervical spine. (A) Posteroanterior central vertebral pressure on tip of spinous process. (B) Posteroanterior unilateral vertebral pressure on posterior aspect of transverse process. (C) Transverse vertebral pressure on side of spinous process.

carefully from the shoulders, and the vertebra is pushed forward. The examiner must take care to apply pressure slowly, with carefully controlled movements, in order to "feel" the movement, which in reality is minimal. This "springing test" may be repeated several times to determine the quality of the movement and the end feel. Hypomobility would be indicated by abnormal resistance to movement, abnormal end feel, or reproduction of local or referred pain.[185] End range can be determined by feeling the adjacent spinous process (above or below). When the adjacent spinous process begins to move, the end range of the vertebra to which the PACVP is being applied has been reached.

For **posteroanterior unilateral vertebral pressure (PAUVP),** the examiner's fingers move laterally away from the tip of the spinous process so that the thumbs rest on the lamina or transverse process, about 2 to 3 cm (1 to 1.5 inches) lateral to the spinous process of the cervical or thoracic vertebra (see Fig. 3.77B). Anterior springing pressure is applied as in the central pressure technique. This pressure causes a minimal rotation of the vertebral body. If one was to palpate the spinous process while doing the technique, the spinous process would be felt to move to the side the pressure is applied. Similarly, end range can be determined by feeling the adjacent spinous process (above or below). When the adjacent spinous process begins to rotate, the end range of the vertebra to which the PAUVP is being applied has been reached. Both sides should be done and compared.

For **transverse vertebral pressure,** the examiner's thumbs are placed along the side of the spinous process of the cervical or thoracic spine (see Fig. 3.77C). The examiner then applies a transverse springing pressure to the side of the spinous process, feeling for the quality of movement. This pressure also causes rotation of the vertebral body, and end range can be determined by feeling for rotation of the adjacent spinous process.

Palpation

If, after completing the examination of the cervical spine, the examiner decides the problem is in another joint,

palpation should be delayed until that joint is completely examined. However, during palpation of the cervical spine, the examiner should note any tenderness, trigger points, muscle spasm, or other signs and symptoms that may indicate the source of the pathology. Pain provocation and landmark location has been found to have the greatest intrarater reliability with palpation.[203] As with any palpation, the examiner should note the texture of the skin and surrounding bony and soft tissues on the posterior, lateral, and anterior aspects of the neck. Usually, palpation is performed with the patient supine so that maximum relaxation of the neck muscles is possible. However, the examiner may palpate with the patient sitting (patient resting the head on forearms that are resting on something at shoulder height) or lying prone (on a table with a face hole) if it is more comfortable for the patient.

To palpate the posterior structures, the examiner stands at the patient's head behind the patient. With the patient lying supine, the patient's head is "cupped" in the examiner's hand while the examiner palpates with the fingers of both hands. For the lateral and anterior structures, the examiner stands at the patient's side. If the examiner suspects that the problem is in the cervical spine, palpation is done on the following structures (Fig. 3.78).

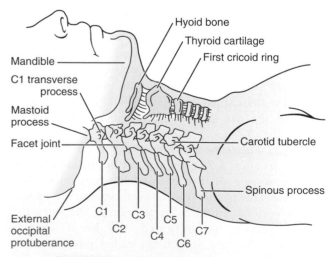

Fig. 3.78 Palpation landmarks of the cervical spine.

Posterior Aspect

External Occipital Protuberance. The protuberance may be found in the posterior midline. The examiner palpates the posterior skull in midline and moves caudally until coming to a point where the fingers "dip" inward. The part of the bone just before the dip is the external occipital protuberance. The inion, or "bump of knowledge," is the most obvious point on the external occipital protuberance and lies in the midline of the occiput.

Spinous Processes and Facet Joints of Cervical Vertebrae. The spinous processes of C2, C6, and C7 are the most obvious. If the examiner palpates the occiput of the skull and descends in the midline, the C2 spinous process will be palpated as the first bump. The next spinous processes that are most obvious are C6 and C7, although C3, C4, and C5 can be differentiated with careful palpation and by flexing the spine. The examiner can differentiate between C6 and C7 by passively flexing and extending the patient's neck. With this movement, the C6 spinous process moves in and out, and the C7 spinous process remains stationary. The movements between the spinous processes of C2 through C7 or T1 may be palpated by feeling between each set of spinous processes. While palpating between the spinous processes, the examiner can use the opposite hand or his/her chest to push the head into nodding flexion and releasing, causing the cervical spine to flex and extend; the palpating finger will feel the movement between the two spinous processes and tension (when flexing) in the interspinous and supraspinous ligaments. Relative movement between the cervical vertebrae can then be determined (i.e., hypomobility, normal movement, or hypermobility).[101] The facet joint may be palpated 1.3 to 2.5 cm (0.5 to 1 inch) lateral to the spinous process. Usually the facet joints are not felt as distinct structures but rather as a hard bony mass under the fingers. The muscles in the adjacent area may be palpated for tenderness, swelling, and other signs of pathology. Careful palpation should also include the suboccipital structures.

Mastoid Processes (Below and Behind Earlobe). If the examiner palpates the skull following the posterior aspect of the ear, there will be a point on the skull at which the finger again dips inward. The point just before the dip is the mastoid process.

Lateral Aspect

Transverse Processes of Cervical Vertebrae. The C1 transverse process is the easiest to palpate. The examiner first palpates the mastoid process and then moves inferiorly and slightly anteriorly until a hard bump is felt. If the examiner applies slight pressure to the bump, the patient should say it feels uncomfortable. These bumps are the transverse processes of C1. If the examiner rotates the patient's head while palpating the transverse processes of C1, the uppermost transverse process will protrude farther, and the lower one will seem to disappear. If this does not occur, the segment is hypomobile. The other transverse processes may be palpated if the musculature is sufficiently relaxed. After the C1 transverse process has been located, the examiner moves caudally, feeling for similar bumps. Normally, the bumps are not directly inferior but rather follow the lordotic path of the cervical vertebrae under the sternocleidomastoid muscle. These structures are situated more anteriorly than one might suspect (see Fig. 3.78). During flexion, the space between the mastoid and the transverse processes increases. On extension, it decreases. On side flexion, the mastoid and transverse processes approach one another on the side to which the head is side flexed and separate on the other side.[101]

Lymph Nodes and Carotid Arteries. The lymph nodes are palpable only if they are swollen. The nodes lie along the line of the sternocleidomastoid muscle. The carotid pulse may be palpated in the midportion of the neck, between the sternocleidomastoid muscle and the trachea. The examiner should determine whether the pulse is normal and equal on both sides.

Temporomandibular Joints, Mandible, and Parotid Glands. The TMJ may be palpated anterior to the external ear. The examiner may either palpate directly over the joint or place the little or index finger (pulp forward) in the external ear to feel for movement in the joint. The examiner can then move the fingers along the length of the mandible, feeling for any abnormalities. The angle of the mandible is at the level of the C2 vertebra. Normally, the parotid gland is not palpable, because it lies over the angle of the mandible. If it is swollen, however, it is palpable as a soft, boggy structure.

Anterior Aspect

Hyoid Bone, Thyroid Cartilage, and First Cricoid Ring. The hyoid bone may be palpated as part of the superior part of the trachea above the thyroid cartilage anterior to the C2–C3 vertebrae. The thyroid cartilage lies anterior to the C4–C5 vertebrae. With the neck in a neutral position, the thyroid cartilage can be moved easily. In extension, it is tight and crepitations may be felt. Adjacent to the cartilage is the thyroid gland, which the examiner should palpate. If the gland is abnormal, it will be tender and enlarged. The cricoid ring is the first part of the trachea and lies above the site for an emergency tracheostomy. The ring moves when the patient swallows. Rough palpation of the ring may cause the patient to gag. While palpating the hyoid bone, the examiner should ask the patient to swallow; normally, the bone should move and cause no pain. The cricoid ring and thyroid cartilage also move when palpated as the patient swallows.

Paranasal Sinuses. Returning to the face, the examiner should palpate the paranasal sinuses (frontal and maxillary) for signs of tenderness and swelling (Fig. 3.79).

First Three Ribs. The examiner palpates the manubrium sternum and, moving the fingers laterally, follows the path of the first three ribs posteriorly, feeling whether one rib

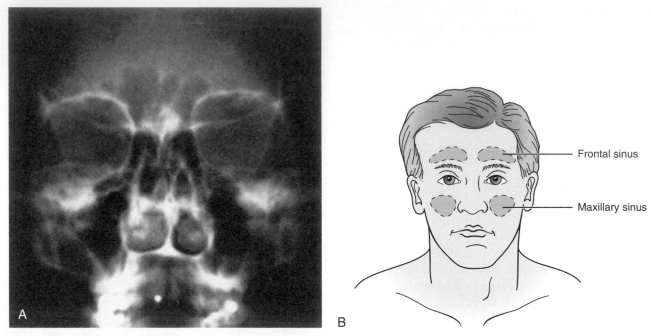

Fig. 3.79 Paranasal sinuses. Radiograph (A) and illustration (B) of frontal and maxillary sinuses.

is protruded more than the others. The examiner should palpate the ribs individually and with care, because it is difficult to palpate the ribs as they pass under the clavicle. The patient should be asked to breathe in and out deeply a few times so that the examiner can compare the movements of the ribs during breathing. Normally, there is equal mobility on both sides. The first rib is more prone to pathology than the second and third ribs and can refer pain to the neck and/or shoulder.

Supraclavicular Fossa. The examiner can palpate the supraclavicular fossa, which is superior to the clavicle. Normally, the fossa is a smooth indentation. The examiner should palpate for swelling after trauma (possible fractured clavicle), abnormal soft tissue (possible swollen glands), and abnormal bony tissue (possible cervical rib). In addition, the examiner should palpate the sternocleidomastoid muscle along its length for signs of pathology, especially in cases of torticollis.

Diagnostic Imaging

Imaging techniques should primarily be performed as an adjunct to the clinical examination. The appearance of many degenerative changes or anatomical or congenital variations is relatively high in the cervical spine, and many of the changes have no relationship with the patient's complaints.[204]

Plain Film Radiography

Normally, a standard set of x-rays for the cervical spine is made up of an anteroposterior (AP) view, a lateral view, and an open or odontoid ("through-the-mouth") view. Other views that may be included are the oblique view, flexion stress view (lateral view in flexion), and

extension stress view (lateral view in extension). For osteoarthritis, the x-rays commonly taken are AP (C3 to C7), lateral, and oblique. In cases of trauma and an alert and stable patient, the Canadian C-Spine Rule[205–207] may be used to determine if diagnostic imaging is required (Fig. 3.80). **The National Emergency X-Radiography Utilization Study (NEXUS)** low-risk criteria is another clinical decision rule related to the use of x-rays.[208,209]

Common X-Ray Views of the Cervical Spine

- Anteroposterior view (see Figs. 3.81 and 3.82)
- Lateral view (see Fig. 3.83A)
- Open mouth of odontoid view (following trauma) (see Fig. 3.90)
- Oblique view (see Fig. 3.92)
- Flexion stress view (lateral view in flexion) (see Fig. 3.83B)
- Extension stress view (lateral view in extension (see Fig. 3.83C)
- Swimmer's view (following trauma) (see Chapter 5, Fig. 5.219B)

 NEXUS Low-Risk Criteria for Cervical Radiographs[208,209]

Cervical spine radiographs are indicated for patients with trauma unless they meet all of the following criteria:
- No posterior or midline cervical spine tenderness
- Normal levels of alertness
- No motor or sensory neurological deficit
- No clinically apparent painful injury that may distract patient from cervical injury
- No evidence of intoxication

NEXUS, National Emergency X-Radiography Utilization Study.

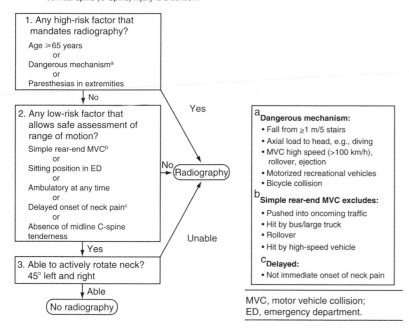

For alert (Glasgow Coma Scale Score = 15) and stable trauma patients where cervical spine (C-Spine) injury is a concern

1. Any high-risk factor that mandates radiography?

Age ≥65 years
or
Dangerous mechanism[a]
or
Paresthesias in extremities

→ No

2. Any low-risk factor that allows safe assessment of range of motion?

Simple rear-end MVC[b]
or
Sitting position in ED
or
Ambulatory at any time
or
Delayed onset of neck pain[c]
or
Absence of midline C-spine tenderness

Yes →

No → Radiography

Unable →

→ Yes

3. Able to actively rotate neck? 45° left and right

→ Able

No radiography

[a]**Dangerous mechanism:**
• Fall from ≥1 m/5 stairs
• Axial load to head, e.g., diving
• MVC high speed (>100 km/h), rollover, ejection
• Motorized recreational vehicles
• Bicycle collision

[b]**Simple rear-end MVC excludes:**
• Pushed into oncoming traffic
• Hit by bus/large truck
• Rollover
• Hit by high-speed vehicle

[c]**Delayed:**
• Not immediate onset of neck pain

MVC, motor vehicle collision; ED, emergency department.

Fig. 3.80 ✓ The Canadian C-spine rule. (From Stiell IG, Wells GA, Vandemheen KL, et al: The Canadian C-spine rule for radiography in alert and stable trauma patients, *JAMA* 286[15]:1846, 2001.)

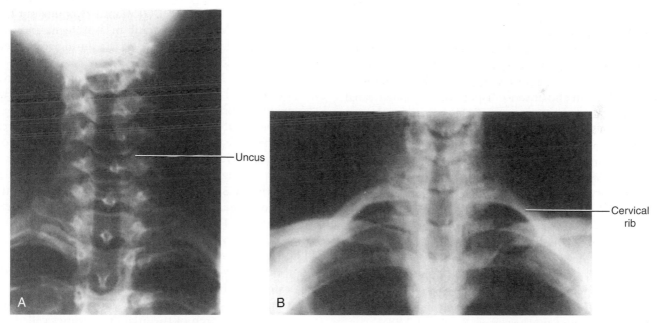

Uncus

Cervical rib

Fig. 3.81 Anteroposterior films of the cervical spine. (A) Normal spine. (B) Cervical rib.

Anteroposterior View. The examiner should look for or note the following (Figs. 3.81 and 3.82): the shape of the vertebrae, the presence of any lateral wedging or osteophytes, the disc space, and the presence of a cervical rib. Frontal alignment should also be ascertained.

Lateral View. Lateral views of the cervical spine give the greatest amount of radiological information. The examiner should look for or note the following (Figs. 3.83–3.86):

1. *Normal or abnormal curvature.* The curvature may be highly variable, because 20% to 40% of normal spines have a straight or slightly kyphotic curve in neutral position.[210] McAviney et al.[211] reported the normal lordosis in the cervical spine as 30° to 40° (see Fig. 3.7) when measuring the lines intersecting the posterior aspects of the vertebral bodies of C2 and C7. They felt patients with a cervical lordosis of less than 20° were more likely to experience

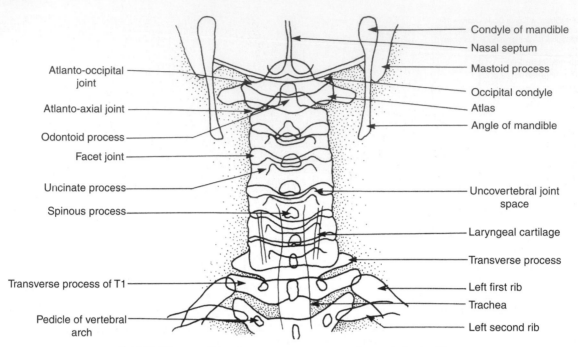

Fig. 3.82 Diagram of structures seen on anteroposterior cervical spine film.

cervicogenic symptoms. Are the "lines" of the vertebrae normal? The line joining the anterior portion of the vertebral bodies (anterior vertebral line) should form a smooth, unbroken arc from C2 to C7 (see Fig. 3.84). Similar lines should be seen for the posterior vertebral bodies (posterior vertebral line), which form the anterior aspect of the spinal canal, and the posterior aspect of the spinal canal (posterior canal line). Disruption of any of these lines would be an indication of instability possibly caused by ligamentous injury.

2. *"Kinking" of the cervical spine.* Kinking may be indicative of a subluxation or dislocation in the cervical spine.

3. *General shape of the vertebrae.* Is there any fusion, collapse, or wedging? The examiner should count the vertebrae, because x-ray films do not always show C7 or T1, and it is essential that they be visualized for a proper radiological examination.

4. *Displacement.* Do the vertebrae sit in normal alignment with one another (Figs. 3.87 and 3.88)?

5. *Disc space.* Is it normal? Narrow? Narrowing may indicate cervical spondylosis (also called spondylosis deformans).

6. *Lipping at the vertebral edges.* Lipping indicates degeneration (see Figs. 3.83A and 3.84).

7. *Osteophytes.* Osteophytes indicate degeneration or abnormal movement (instability) (see Figs. 3.83A and 3.84).

8. *Ratio of the spinal canal diameter.* Normally, the ratio of the spinal canal diameter to the vertebral body diameter (Torg ratio) in the cervical spine is 1. If this ratio is less than 0.8, it is an indication of possible cervical stenosis.[54,212–215] This comparison is shown in Fig. 3.85 (ratio AB:BC). Cantu[213] points out that this measurement is a static measurement and may not apply to stenosis that occurs during movement of the cervical spine.

9. *Prevertebral soft-tissue width.* Measured at the level of the anteroinferior border of the C3 vertebra, this width is normally 7 mm.[216] Edema or hemorrhage is suspected if the space is wider than 7 mm. The retropharyngeal space, lying between the anterior border of the vertebral body and the posterior border of the pharyngeal air shadow, should be 2 to 5 mm in width at C3. From C4 to C7, the space is called the **retrotracheal space** and should be 18 to 22 mm in width (see Fig. 3.85).

10. *Subluxation of the facets.*

11. *Abnormal soft-tissue shadows.*

12. *Forward shifting of C1 on C2.* This finding indicates instability between C1 and C2. Normally, the joint space between the odontoid process and the anterior arch of the atlas (sometimes called the **atlas-dens index** or **atlantodens interval [ADI]**) does not exceed 2.5 to 3 mm in the adult (4.5 to 5 mm in children). Instability is present when there is 3.5 mm ADI difference in flexion views. An ADI of more than 5 mm in adults commonly indicates a rupture of the transverse ligament. A 7-mm difference may imply disruption of alar ligaments. The **space available for cord (SAC)** is measured between the posterior dens and the anterior cortex of the posterior ring of the atlas. In adults and teenagers, the SAC should be greater than 13 mm (Fig. 3.89).[217]

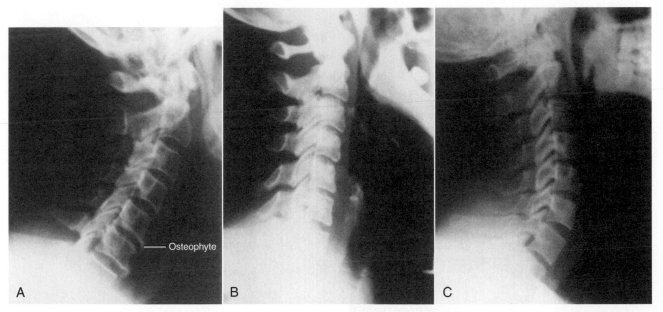

Fig. 3.83 Lateral radiograph of the cervical spine. (A) Normal curve showing osteophytic lipping. (B) Cervical spine in flexion. (C) Cervical spine in extension.

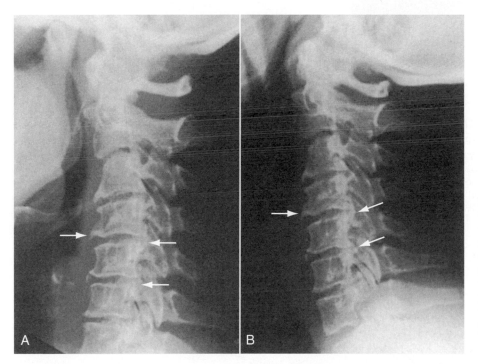

Fig. 3.84 X-ray films of a 68-year-old man with multiple radiologic signs of cervical osteoarthritis *(arrows)*. (A) The cervical spine in flexion, which is very limited. Note that the atlas tips up, as compared with that in B. All intervertebral disc spaces below C2 to C3 are very narrow. Anterior and posterior osteophytes are apparent *(arrows)*. The spine extends very little in (B) and is quite straight in (A) (i.e., no significant flexion). (From Bland JH: *Disorders of the cervical spine*, Philadelphia, 1994, W.B. Saunders, p 213.)

13. *Instability.* Instability is present when more than 3.5 mm of horizontal displacement of one vertebra occurs in relation to the adjacent vertebra (see Fig. 3.87).

Open or Odontoid ("Through-the-Mouth") View. This AP view enables the examiner to determine the state of the odontoid process of C2 and its relation with C1 (Fig. 3.90; see Fig. 3.88). It may also show the atlanto-occipital and atlanto-axial joints.

Oblique View. This view provides information on the neural foramen and posterior elements of the cervical spine. The examiner should look for or note the following (Figs. 3.91 and 3.92):

1. Lipping of the joints of Luschka (osteophytes)
2. Overriding of the facet joints (subluxation, spondylosis)
3. Facet joints and intervertebral foramen (see Fig. 3.92)

Pillar View. This special view is used to evaluate the lateral masses of the cervical spine and especially the facet joints (Fig. 3.93). It is usually reserved for patients with suspected facet fractures.[218]

Computed Tomography

Computed tomography (CT) helps to delineate the bone and soft-tissue anatomy of the cervical spine in cross section and can show, for example, a disc prolapse. It also

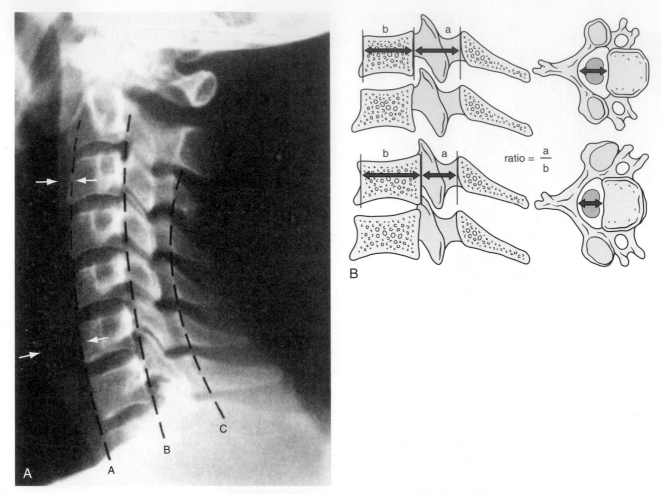

Fig. 3.85 (A) Normal cervical spine. Lateral projection. Note the alignment and appearance of the facet joints: *A*, anterior vertebral line; *B*, posterior vertebral line; *C*, posterior canal line. Retropharyngeal space *(between top arrows)* should not exceed 5 mm. Retrotracheal space *(between bottom arrows)* should not exceed 22 mm. (B) The Torg ratio is calculated by dividing the shortest distance between the posterior vertebral body and the spinolaminar line *(a)* by the vertebral body width *(b)*. (A, Modified from Forrester DM, Brown JC: *The radiology of joint disease*, Philadelphia, 1987, W.B. Saunders, p 408. B, Redrawn from McAlindon RJ: On field evaluation and management of head and neck injured athletes, *Clin Sports Med* 21:10, 2002. Adapted from Torg JS, Pavlov H: Cervical spinal stenosis with cord neurapraxia and transient quadriplegia, *Clin Sports Med* 6:115–133, 1987; with permission.)

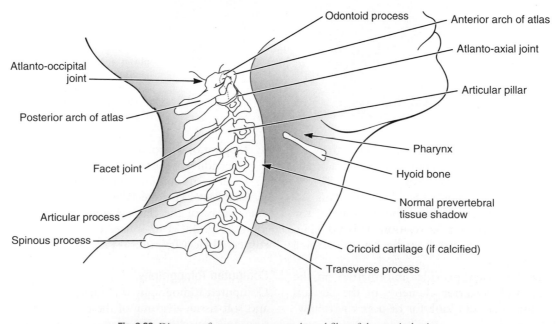

Fig. 3.86 Diagram of structures seen on lateral film of the cervical spine.

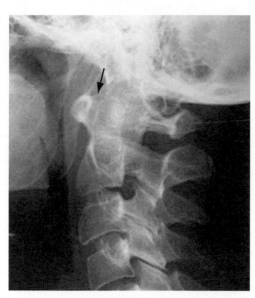

Fig. 3.87 Atlanto-axial subluxation. Flexion view shows abnormal widening of the atlanto-axial space *(arrow)*, which measures 4 mm. (From Resnick D, Kransdorf MJ: *Bone and joint imaging*, Philadelphia, 2005, Saunders, p 883.)

shows the true size and extent of osteophytes better than do plain x-rays (Fig. 3.94). CT scans are especially useful for showing bone fragments in the spinal canal after a fracture and bony defects in the vertebral bodies and neural arches. CT scans may be combined with myelography to outline the spinal cord and nerve roots inside the thecal sac (Fig. 3.95). CT scans are used only after conventional radiographs have been taken and a need for them is shown.

Diagnostic Ultrasound Imaging

Diagnostic ultrasound is used rarely in the cervical spine. It may be used intermittently to examine the brachial plexus. Several specific areas should be addressed when examining the brachial plexus and include the extraforaminal area of the lower five nerve roots (i.e., C5, C6, C7, C8, T1), the intrascalene area including five nerve roots and three nerve trunks, the supraclavicular area with the six subdivisions, the infraclavicular area and the three nerve cords, and the axillary area and the five terminal nerve branches (i.e., musculocutaneous, axillary, radial, median and ulnar nerves) (see Fig. 1.8).[219] Placing the transverse transducer at the anterolateral lower neck will

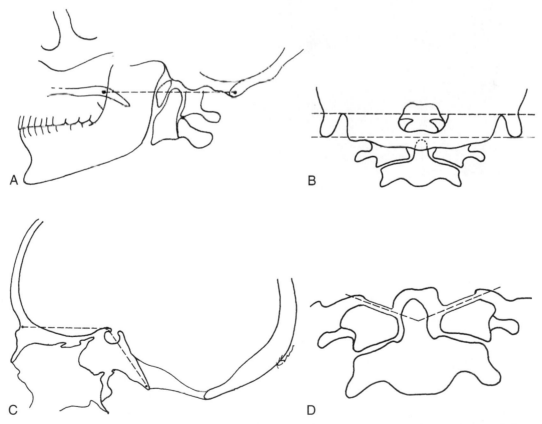

Fig. 3.88 Cervicobasilar junction: Normal osseous relationships. (A) Chamberlain line is drawn from the posterior margin of the hard palate to the posterior border of the foramen magnum. The odontoid process normally does not extend more than 5 mm above this line. (B) The bimastoid line *(lower line)*, connecting the tips of the mastoids, is normally within 2 mm of the odontoid tip. The digastric line *(upper line)*, connecting the digastric muscle fossae, is normally located above the odontoid process. (C) The basilar angle, which normally exceeds 140°, is formed by the angle of intersection of two lines—one drawn from the nasion to the tuberculum sellae, and the second drawn from the tuberculum sellae to the anterior edge of the foramen magnum. (D) The atlanto-occipital joint angle, constructed on frontal tomograms by the intersection of two lines drawn along the axes of these articulations, is normally not greater than 150°. (From Resnick D, Kransdorf MJ: *Bone and joint imaging*, Philadelphia, 2005, Saunders, p 37.)

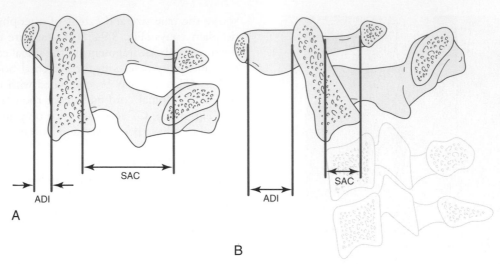

Fig. 3.89 The atlantodens interval *(ADI)* and the space available for cord *(SAC)* are used in determining atlanto-axial instability. The ADI increases as the SAC decreases. A SAC less than 13 mm is significant. (A) Normal. (B) Subluxation. (Redrawn from Ghanem I, El Hage S, Rachkidi R, et al: Pediatric cervical spine instability, *J Child Orthop* 2[2]:71–84, 2008.)

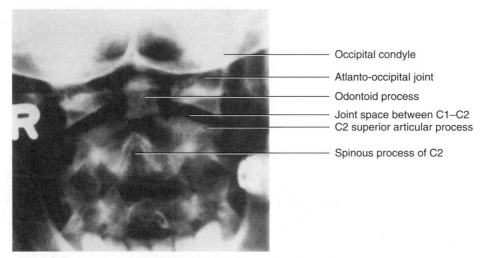

— Occipital condyle

— Atlanto-occipital joint

— Odontoid process

— Joint space between C1–C2
— C2 superior articular process

— Spinous process of C2

Fig. 3.90 Through-the-mouth radiograph.

demonstrate the hypoechoic nerve roots of the brachial plexus exiting the neural foramina (Fig. 3.96). Moving down the neck to the interscalene area demonstrates the five hypoechoic nerve roots of the brachial plexus (Fig. 3.97). Fig. 3.98 demonstrates the supraclavicular area which appears as a "cluster of grapes" dorsally and cranially to the subclavian artery and first rib.

Myelography
Myelograms are the modality of choice with brachial plexus avulsions, either Erb-Duchenne paralysis (C5 and C6) or Klumpke paralysis (C7, C8, and T1). They may also be used to demonstrate narrowing in the intervertebral foramen and cervical spinal stenosis. They may be used to outline the contour of the thecal sac, nerve roots, and spinal cord (Fig. 3.99).

Magnetic Resonance Imaging
This noninvasive technique can differentiate between various soft tissues and bone (Figs. 3.100 and 3.101). Because it shows differences based on water content,

magnetic resonance imaging (MRI) can differentiate between the nucleus pulposus and the annulus fibrosus. MRI may be used to reveal disc protrusions, but it has been reported that patients showing these lesions are often asymptomatic, highlighting the fact that diagnostic imaging abnormalities should be considered only in relation to the history and clinical examination.[220] An MRI allows visualization of the nerve roots, spinal cord, and thecal sac as well as the bone and bone marrow. It is also used to identify postoperative scarring and disc herniation.[221] **Magnetic resonance angiography (MRA)** is an MRI examination of the blood vessels in which a dye is introduced into the bloodstream in a vein in the hand or forearm to see the vessels more clearly in the neck when the MRI is taken. It is also useful for determining the patency and status of the vertebral artery.[222–224]

Xeroradiography
Xeroradiography helps to delineate bone and soft tissue by enhancing the interfaces between tissues (Fig. 3.102).

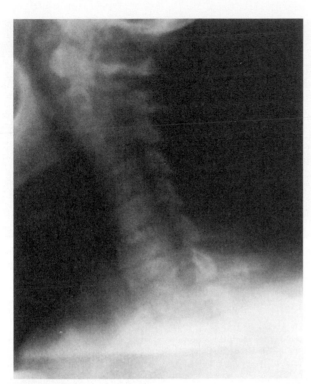

Fig. 3.91 Abnormal x-ray findings on oblique view. Note loss of normal curve; narrowing at C4, C5, and C6; osteophytes and lipping of C4, C5, and C6; and encroachment on intervertebral foramen at C4–C5, C5–C6, and C6–C7.

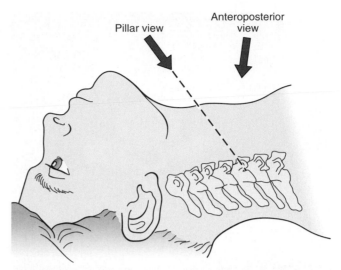

Fig. 3.93 Diagram of pillar view showing orientation of facet joints.

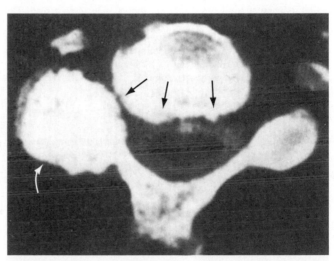

Fig. 3.94 Foraminal stenosis caused by hypertrophic facet arthropathy and by spondylosis. Metrizamide-enhanced computed tomography scan through C5 foramina details the markedly overgrown facet *(white arrow)* and the bony "bar," or spondylotic spurring *(black arrows)*. The right foramen is almost occluded by abnormal bone. (From Dorwart RH, LaMasters DL: Application of computed tomographic scanning of the cervical spine, *Orthop Clin North Am* 16:386, 1985.)

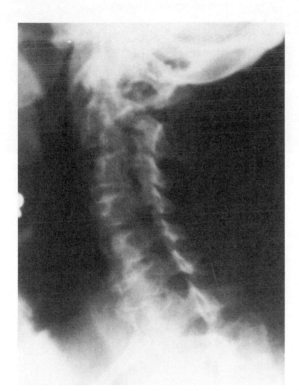

Fig. 3.92 Oblique radiograph of the cervical spine showing intervertebral foramen and facet joints. Severe lipping in lower cervical spine and spondylosis are also evident.

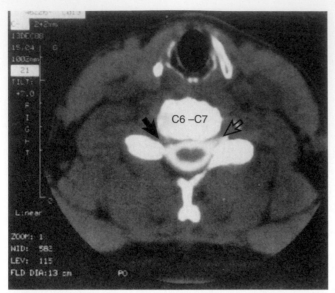

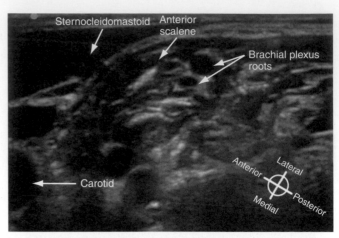

Fig. 3.95 Postcontrast computed tomogram showing normally patent neural foramen at the C6–C7 level on the left side *(open arrow)*. The nerve root sleeve fills with contrast medium and enters the neural foramen. On the right side *(closed arrow)*, there is no evidence of filling of the nerve root sleeve within the neural foramen as a result of lateral C6 disc herniation. (From Bell GR, Ross JS: Diagnosis of nerve root compression: myelography, computed tomography, and MRI, *Orthop Clin North Am* 23:410, 1992.)

Fig. 3.97 Transverse entry into the intrascalene area showing hypoechoic roots of the brachial plexus. (From Weller RS: Ultrasound of the brachial plexus. In Walker FO, Cartwright MS, editors: *Neuromuscular ultrasound*, Philadelphia, 2011, Saunders/Elsevier)

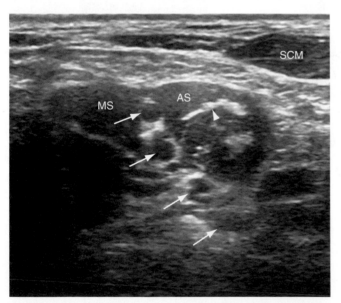

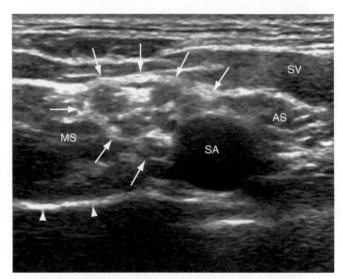

Fig. 3.96 Transverse ultrasound image of anterolateral lower neck shows hypoechoic roots of brachial plexus as they exit the neural foramina and move to the intrascalene area. Circular hypoechoic C5–C8 nerve roots *(upper arrow to lower arrow, respectively)* traversing the space between the hyperechoic fascicular pattern of the anterior scalene *(AS)* and middle scalene *(MS)* muscle. The anterior scalene *(arrowhead)* and the sternocleidomastoid *(SCM)* are visualized. (From Haun DW, Cho JC, Clark TB, Kettner NW: Normative cross-sectional area of the brachial plexus and subclavian artery using ultrasonography, *J Manip Physiol Ther* 32[7]:566, 2009.)

Fig. 3.98 Transverse ultrasound at supraclavicular area shows hypoechoic divisions of the brachial plexus located dorsocranial to the subclavian artery *(SA)* akin to a "cluster of grapes." Also seen are the shadow of first rib *(arrowheads)*, the anterior scalene *(AS)*, the middle scalene *(MS)*, and the subclavian vein *(SV)* which lies superficial to the AS. (From Haun DW, Cho JC, Clark TB, Kettner NW: Normative cross-sectional area of the brachial plexus and subclavian artery using ultrasonography, *J Manip Physiol Ther* 32[7]:566, 2009)

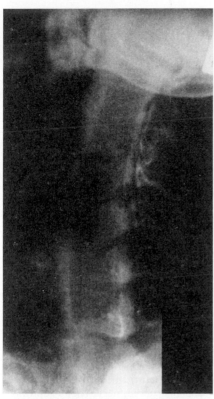

Fig. 3.99 Myelogram of cervical spine.

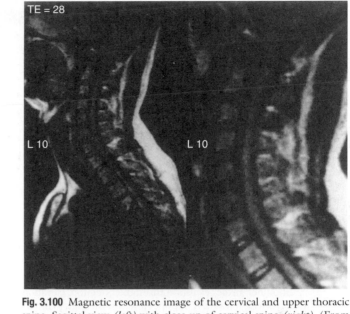

Fig. 3.100 Magnetic resonance image of the cervical and upper thoracic spine. Sagittal view *(left)* with close-up of cervical spine *(right)*. (From Foreman SM, Croft AC: *Whiplash injuries: the cervical acceleration/deceleration syndrome*, Baltimore, 1988, Williams & Wilkins, p 126.)

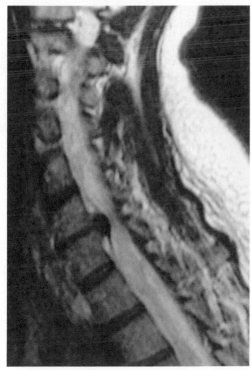

Fig. 3.101 Posterior disc displacement: magnetic resonance (MR) imaging findings. Sagittal T2-weighted (TR/TE, 2608/96) fast spin echo MR image reveals an extruded paracentral disc of low signal intensity at the C6–C7 spinal level. (From Resnick D, Kransdorf MJ: *Bone and joint imaging*, Philadelphia, 2005, Saunders, p 415. Courtesy D. Goodwin, MD, Hanover, NH.)

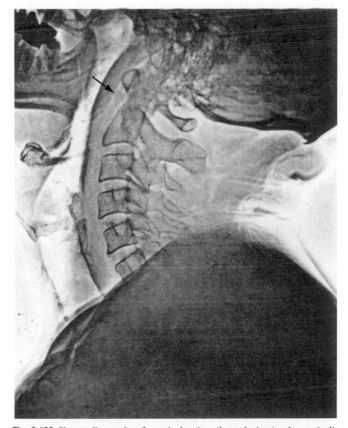

Fig. 3.102 Xeroradiograph of cervical spine (lateral view). *Arrow* indicates calcified mass. (From Forrester DM, Brown JC: *The radiology of joint disease*, Philadelphia, 1987, W.B. Saunders, p 420.)

PRÉCIS OF THE CERVICAL SPINE ASSESSMENT[a]

NOTE: Suspected pathology will determine which *Special Tests* are to be performed.

History
Observation (standing or sitting)
Examination (sitting)
Active movements
    Flexion
    Extension
    Side flexion (right and left)
    Rotation (right and left)
    Combined movements (if necessary)
    Repetitive movements (if necessary)
    Sustained positions (if necessary)
Resisted isometric movements (as in active movements)
Scanning examination
    Peripheral joint:
        Temporomandibular joints (open mouth and closed mouth)
        Shoulder girdle (elevation through abduction, elevation through forward flexion, elevation through plane of scapula, medial and lateral rotation with arm at side; medial and lateral rotation at 90° abduction)
        Elbow (flexion, extension, supination, pronation)
        Wrist (flexion, extension, radial, and ulnar deviation)
        Fingers and thumb (flexion, extension, abduction, adduction)
    Myotomes:
        Neck flexion (C1, C2)
        Neck side flexion (C3)
        Shoulder elevation (C4)
        Shoulder abduction (C5)
        Elbow flexion (C6) and/or extension (C7)
        Wrist flexion (C7) and/or extension (C6)
        Thumb extension (C8) and/or ulnar deviation (C8)
        Hand intrinsics (abduction or adduction) (T1)
    Sensory scanning examination
Functional assessment
Special tests[b] (sitting)
    For neurological symptoms:
        Brachial plexus tension test
        Distraction test (if symptoms severe)
        Doorbell sign
        Foraminal compression test (three stages) (if symptoms absent or mild)
    For myelopathy:
        Romberg test
    For cervical instability:
        Posterior atlanto-occipital membrane test
    For movement control dysfunction:
        Active cervical extension
        Active cervical rotation
        Return to neutral from the cervical extension position
Reflexes and cutaneous distribution
    Biceps (C5, C6)
    Triceps (C7, C8)
    Hoffmann sign (or Babinski test)
    Sensory scan

Examination (standing)
Special tests (standing)
    For movement control dysfunction:
        Active bilateral arm flexion
        Active unilateral arm flexion
Examination (4-point kneeling)
Special tests (4-point kneeling)
    For movement control dysfunction:
        Active cervical extension
        Active cervical flexion
        Active upper cervical rotation
        Rocking backwards
Examination (supine)
Passive movements
    Flexion
    Extension
    Side flexion
    Rotation
Special tests[b] (lying)
    For cervical muscle (deep neck flexors) strength:
        Craniocervical flexion test
        Deep neck flexor endurance test
    For neurological symptoms:
        Brachial plexus provocation test
        Upper limb neurodynamic (tension) tests (specific to particular nerve/nerve root symptoms)
    For vascular signs[c]:
        Hold planned mobilization/manipulation position for at least 30 seconds watching for vertebral-basilar artery signs
    For cervical instability[c]:
        Anterior shear stress test
        Lateral shear test
        Lateral flexion alar ligament stress test
        Rotational alar ligament stress test
        Transverse ligament stress test
    For cervical spine mobility:
        Cervical flexion rotation test
    For first rib mobility:
        First rib mobility
Joint play movements
    Side glide of cervical spine
    Anterior glide of cervical spine
    Posterior glide of cervical spine
    Traction glide of cervical spine
    Rotation of occiput on C1
    Palpation
Examination, prone
Joint play movements
    Posteroanterior central vertebral pressure (PACVP)
    Posteroanterior unilateral vertebral pressure (PAUVP)
    Transverse vertebral pressure (TVP)
Palpation
Diagnostic imaging
After any examination, the patient should be warned of the possibility of exacerbation of symptoms as a result of the assessment.

[a]The précis is shown in an order that limits the amount of moving that the patient has to do but ensures that all necessary structures are tested.
[b]The authors recommend these key tests be learned by the clinician to facilitate a diagnosis.
[c]These tests should be performed if the examiner anticipates doing end-range mobilization or manipulation techniques to the cervical spine, especially the upper cervical spine. If instability of vascular signs are present, mobilization and/or manipulation should not be performed.

CASE STUDIES

When doing these case studies, the examiner should list the appropriate questions to be asked and why they are being asked, what to look for and why, and what things should be tested and why. Depending on the answers of the patient (and the examiner should consider different responses), several possible causes of the patient's problems may become evident (examples are given in parentheses). A differential diagnosis chart should be made up (see Table 3.31 as an example). The examiner can then decide how different diagnoses may affect the treatment plan.

1. A 59-year-old male, who works as a supervisor on a factory floor, comes to see you with a complaint of headaches and neck stiffness. He denies numbness or tingling into his extremities. He does have limited cervical active and passive ROM mostly right-side rotation and side bending. He also has intermittent headaches at the base of the skull. Describe your assessment plan (migraine versus tension headache vs. facet syndrome).

2. A 61-year-old female comes to you with complaints of neck pain and right radicular pain that radiates distally to her hand and fingers. Her pain is intermittent and seems to be worse after sleeping and after any strenuous lifting using her upper extremities. There is intermittent numbness and tingling into radial and medial nerve distribution. Reflexes are normal and symmetrical, and there is no loss of upper extremity strength. Cervical ROM is limited into right side bending and right rotation. Flexion and extension cervical ROM appear normal. Describe your assessment plan (cervical spondylosis vs. cervical disc lesion).

3. A 2-month-old baby is brought to you by a concerned parent. The child does not move the head properly, and the sternocleidomastoid muscle on the left side is prominent. Describe your assessment plan before beginning treatment (congenital torticollis vs. Klippel-Feil syndrome).

4. A 54-year-old man comes to you complaining of neck stiffness, especially on rising; sometimes he has numbness into his left arm. Describe your assessment plan (cervical spondylosis vs. subacromial bursitis).

5. An 18-year-old male football player comes to you complaining of a "dead arm" after a tackle he made 2 days ago. Although he can now move the left arm, it still does not feel right. Describe your assessment plan (brachial plexus lesion vs. acromioclavicular sprain).

6. A 23-year-old woman comes to you after a motor vehicle accident. Her car was hit from behind while stopped for a red light. She could tell the accident was going to occur because she could see in the rearview mirror that the car behind her was not going to be able to stop. The car that hit her was going 50 kph (30 mph), and skid marks were visible for only 5 m from the location of her car.

Describe your assessment plan (cervical sprain vs. cervical facet syndrome).

7. A 35-year-old woman comes to you complaining of persistent headaches that last for days at a time. She has recently lost her job. She complains that she sometimes sees flashing lights and cannot stand having anyone around her when the pain is very bad. Describe your assessment plan for this patient (migraine vs. tension headache).

8. A 26-year-old man comes to you complaining of pain in his neck. The pain was evident yesterday when he got up and has not decreased significantly since then. He thinks that he may have "slept wrong." There is no previous history of trauma. Describe your assessment plan for this patient (acquired torticollis vs. cervical disc lesion).

9. A 75-year-old woman comes to you complaining primarily of neck pain but also of stiffness. She exhibits a dowager's hump. There is no history of trauma. Describe your assessment plan for this patient (osteoporosis vs. cervical spondylosis).

10. A 47-year-old man comes to you complaining of elbow and neck pain. There is no recent history of trauma, but he remembers being in a motor vehicle accident 19 years ago. He now works at a desk all day. Describe your assessment for this patient (cervical spondylosis vs. tennis elbow vs. double crush injury).

11. A 16-year-old boy comes to you with a complaint of having hurt his neck. While "fooling" with some friends at the lake, he ran away from them and dove into the water to get away. The top of his head hit the bottom, and he felt a burning pain. The pain decreased as he came out of the water, but he still has a residual ache. Describe your plan for this patient (cervical fracture vs. cervical sprain).

12. A 14-year-old girl comes to you complaining of neck pain. She has long hair. She states that when she "whipped" her hair out of her eyes, which she has done many times before, she felt a sudden pain in her neck. Although the pain intensity has decreased, it is still there, and she cannot fully move her neck. Describe your assessment plan for this patient (cervical sprain vs. acquired torticollis).

TABLE **3.31**

Differential Diagnosis of Cervical Facet Syndrome, Cervical Nerve Root Lesion, and Thoracic Outlet Syndrome

Signs and Symptoms	Facet Syndrome	Cervical Nerve Root	Thoracic Outlet Syndrome
Pain referral	Possible	Yes	Possible
Pain on hyperextension and rotation	Yes (often without increased referral of symptoms)	Yes with increased symptoms	No
Spine stiffness	Yes	Possible	Possible
Paresthesia	No	Yes	Possible
Reflexes	Not affected	May be affected	May be affected
Muscle spasm	Yes	Yes	Yes
Tension tests	May or may not be positive	Positive	May be positive
Pallor and coolness	No	No	Possible
Muscle weakness	No	Possible	Not early (later small hand muscles)
Muscle fatigue and cramps	No	No	Possible

References

1. Cyriax J. *Textbook of Orthopaedic Medicine: Diagnosis of Soft Tissue Lesions.* Vol. 1. London: Bailliere Tindall; 1982.
2. Porterfield JA, DeRosa C. *Mechanical Neck Pain—Perspective in Functional Anatomy.* Philadelphia: WB Saunders; 1995.
3. Radanov BP, Dvorak J, Valach L. Cognitive deficits in patients after soft tissue injury of the cervical spine. *Spine.* 1992;17:127–131.
4. Panjabi M, Dvorak J, Crisco J, et al. Flexion, extension, and lateral bending of the upper cervical spine in response to alar ligament transactions. *J Spinal Disord.* 1991;4(2):157–167.
5. Rieger P, Huber G. Fenestration and duplicate origin of the left vertebral artery in angiography: report of three cases. *Neuroradiology.* 1983;25(1):45–50.
6. Taylor AJ, Kerry R. Neck pain and headache as a result of internal carotid artery dissection: implications for manual therapists. *Man Ther.* 2005;10:73–77.
7. Castaigne P, Lhermitte F, Gautier JC, et al. Arterial occlusions in the vertebro-basilar system: a study of 44 patients with post-mortem data. *Brain.* 1973;96(1):133–154.
8. Toole J, Tucker SH. Influence of head position upon cerebral circulation. *Arch Neurol.* 1960;2:616–623.
9. Brown BS, Tissington-Tatlow WF. Radiographic studies of the vertebral arteries in cadavers. *Radiology.* 1963;81:80–88.
10. Haynes MJ. Doppler studies comparing the effects of cervical rotation and lateral flexion on vertebral artery blood flow. *J Manip Physiol Ther.* 1996;19:378–384.
11. Endo K, Ichimaru K, Shimura H, et al. Cervical vertigo after hair shampoo treatment at a hair dressing salon: a case report. *Spine.* 2000;25:632.
12. Nagler W. Vertebral artery obstruction by hyperextension of the neck: report of three cases. *Arch Phys Med Rehabil.* 1973;54:237–240.
13. Dutton M. *Orthopedic Examination, Evaluation and Intervention.* New York: McGraw Hill; 2004.
14. Miyachi S, Okamura K, Watanabe M, et al. Cerebellar stroke due to vertebral artery occlusion after cervical spine trauma: two case reports. *Spine.* 1994;19:83–89.
15. Hart RG, Easton JD. Dissections. *Stroke.* 1985;16:925–927.
16. Hayes P, Gerlock AJ, Cobb CA. Cervical spine trauma: a cause of vertebral artery injury. *J Trauma.* 1980;20:904–905.
17. Schwarz N, Buchinger W, Gaudernak T, et al. Injuries of the cervical spine causing vertebral artery trauma: case reports. *J Trauma.* 1991;31:127–133.
18. Auer RN, Krcek J, Butt JC. Delayed symptoms and death after minor head trauma with occult vertebral artery injury. *J Neurol Neurosurg Psychiatry.* 1994;57:500–502.
19. Bose B, Northrup BE, Osteoholm JL. Delayed vertebrobasilar insufficiency following cervical spine injury. *Spine.* 1985;10:108–110.
20. Thomas LC. Cervical arterial dissection: an overview and implications for manipulative therapy practice. *Man Ther.* 2016;21:2–9.
21. Kapandji IA. *The Physiology of Joints: The Trunk and the Vertebral Column.* Vol. 3. New York: Churchill Livingstone; 1974.
22. Ishii T, Mukai Y, Hosono N, et al. Kinematics of the cervical spine in lateral bending in vivo three-dimensional analysis. *Spine.* 2006;31:155–160.
23. Ishii T, Mukai Y, Hosono N, et al. Kinematics of the subaxial cervical spine in rotation in vivo three-dimensional analysis. *Spine.* 2004;29:2826–2931.
24. Bogduk N. The innervation of the lumbar spine. *Spine.* 1983;8:286–293.
25. Boreadis AG, Gershon-Cohen J. Luschka joints of the cervical spine. *Radiology.* 1956;66:181–187.
26. Hall MC. *Luschka's Joint.* Springfield, IL: Charles C Thomas; 1965.
27. Silberstein CE. The evolution of degenerative changes in the cervical spine and an investigation into the "joint of Luschka. *Clin Orthop.* 1965;40:184–204.
28. Willis TA. Luschka's joints. *Clin Orthop.* 1966;46:121–125.
29. Ferlic D. The nerve supply of the cervical intervertebral disc in man. *Johns Hopkins Hosp Bull.* 1963;113:347.
30. Mendel T, Wink CS, Zimny ML. Neural elements in human cervical intervertebral discs. *Spine.* 1992;17:132–135.
31. Rao RD, Currier BL, Albert TJ, et al. Degenerative cervical spondylosis: cervical syndromes, pathogenesis and management. *J Bone Joint Surg Am.* 2007;89:1360–1378.
32. Childs JD, Cleland JA, Elliott JM, et al. Neck pain: clinical guidelines linked to the international classification of functioning, disability and health. *J Orthop Sports Phys Ther.* 2008;38:A1–A34.
33. Bland JH. *Disorders of the Cervical Spine.* Philadelphia: WB Saunders; 1994.
34. Cleland J. *Orthopedic Clinical Examination—An Evidence Based Approach for Physical Therapists.* Carlstadt, NJ: Icon Learning Systems; 2005.
35. Guzman J, Haldeman S, Carroll L, et al. Clinical practice implications of the Bone and Joint Decade 2000–2010 Task Force on Neck Pain and Its Associated Disorders: from concepts and findings to recommendations. *J Manip Physiol Ther.* 2009;32(suppl 2):227–243.
36. Watkins RG. Neck injuries in football. In: Watkins RG, ed. *The Spine in Sports.* St Louis: Mosby-Year Book; 1996.
37. Buitenhuis J, de Jong PJ, Jaspers JP, et al. Catastrophizing and causal beliefs in whiplash. *Spine.* 2008;33:2427–2433.
38. Greenhalgh S, Selfe J. A qualitative investigation of red flags for serious spinal pathology. *Physiotherapy.* 2009;95(3):223–226.
39. Spitzer WO, Skovron ML, Salmi LR, et al. Scientific monograph of the Quebec Task Force on Whiplash-Associated Disorders: redefining "whiplash" and its management. *Spine.* 1995;20(suppl 8):S1–S73.
40. Siegmund GP, Davis MB, Quinn KP, et al. Head-turned postures increase the risk of cervical facet capsule injury during whiplash. *Spine.* 2008;33:1643–1649.
41. Nyland T, Mattila VM, Salmi T, et al. Recovery of brachial plexus lesions resulting from heavy backpack use: a follow-up case series. *BMC Musculoskel Dis.* 2011;12(1):62–68.
42. Kitigawa T, Fujiwara A, Kobayashi N, et al. Morphologic changes in the cervical neural foramen due to flexion and extension–in vivo imaging study. *Spine.* 2004;29:2821–2825.
43. Benoist M. Natural evolution and resolution of the cervical whiplash syndrome. In: Gunzburg R, Szpalski M, eds. *Current concepts with prevention, diagnosis and treatment of cervical whiplash syndrome.* Philadelphia: Lippincott-Raven; 1998.
44. Suissa S, Harder S, Veilleux M. The Quebec whiplash-associated disorders cohort study. *Spine.* 1995;20:S12–S20.
45. Evans RW. Some observations on whiplash injuries. *Neurol Sci.* 1992;10:975–997.
46. Deans GT, Magalliard JN, Kerr M, et al. Neck sprain—a major disability following car events. *Injury.* 1987;18:10–12.
47. Wiener SL. *Differential Diagnosis of Acute Pain by Body Region.* New York: McGraw Hill; 1993.

48. Travell TG, Simons DG. *Myofascial Pain and Dysfunction: The Trigger Point Manual.* Vol. 1. Baltimore: Williams & Wilkins; 1983.

49. Malanga GA. The diagnosis and treatment of cervical radiculopathy. *Med Sci Sports Exer.* 1997;29:S236–S245.

50. Levine MJ, Albert TJ, Smith MD. Cervical radiculopathy diagnosis and nonoperative management. *J Am Acad Orthop Surg.* 1996;4:305–316.

51. Ellenberg MR, Honet JC, Treanor WJ. Cervical radiculopathy. *Arch Phys Med Rehabil.* 1994;75:342–352.

52. Carette S, Fehlings MG. Cervical radiculopathy. *N Engl J Med.* 2005;353:392–399.

53. Cloward RB, diskography Cervical. A contribution to etiology and mechanism of neck, shoulder and arm pain. *Ann Surg.* 1959;150(6):1052–1064.

54. Tsairis P, Jordan B. Neurological evaluation of cervical spinal disorders. In: Camins MB, O'Leary PF, eds. *Disorders of the Cervical Spine.* Baltimore: Williams & Wilkins; 1992.

55. Ono K, Ebara S, Fuji T, et al. Myelopathy hand. New clinical signs of cervical cord damage. *J Bone Joint Surg Br.* 1987;69(2):215–219.

56. Dywer A, April C, Bogduk N. Cervical zygapophyseal joint pain patterns. *Spine.* 1990;15:453–457.

57. Fukui S, Ohseto K, Shiotani M, et al. Referred pain distribution of the cervical zygapophyseal joints and cervical dorsal rami. *Pain.* 1996;68(1):79–83.

58. Bogduk N, Govind. Cervicogenic headache: an assessment of the evidence on clinical diagnosis, invasive tests, and treatment. *Lancet Neurol.* 2009;8(10):959–968.

59. Hall T, Briffa K, Hopper D, Robinson K. Reliability of manual examination and frequency of symptomatic cervical motion segment dysfunction in cervicogenic headache. *Man Ther.* 2010;15(6):542–546.

60. Fernández-de-las-Peñas C, Cuadrado ML. Cervicogenic headache. In: Aminoff MJ, Daroff RB, eds. *Encyclopedia of the Neurological Sciences.* 2nd ed. London: Academic Press/Elsevier; 2014.

61. Rubio-Ochoa J, Benitez-Martinez J, Lluch E, et al. Physical examination tests for screening and diagnosis of cervicogenic headache: a systematic review. *Man Ther.* 2016;21:35–40.

62. Luedtke K, Boissonnault W, Caspersen N, et al. International consensus on the most useful physical examination tests used by physiotherapists for patients with headache: a Delphi study. *Man Ther.* 2016;23:17–24.

63. Petty NJ, Moore AP. *Neuromusculoskeletal Examination and Assessment—A Handbook for Therapists.* London: Churchill Livingstone; 1998.

64. Thomas LC, Rivett DA, Attia JR, Levi C. Risk factors and clinical presentation of cervical arterial dissection: preliminary results of the prospective case-control study. *J Orthop Sports Phys Ther.* 2015;45(7):503–511.

65. Donohoe CD. The role of the physical examination in the evaluation of headache. *Med Clin North Am.* 2013;97(2):197–216.

66. Foreman SM, Croft AC. *Whiplash Injuries: The Cervical Acceleration/Deceleration Syndrome.* Baltimore: Williams & Wilkins; 1988.

67. Evans RC. *Illustrated Essentials in Orthopedic Physical Assessment.* St Louis: Mosby-Year Book; 1994.

68. Rushton A, Rivett D, Carlesso L, et al. International framework for examination of the cervical region for potential of cervical arterial dysfunction prior to orthopedic manual therapy intervention. *Man Ther.* 2014;19(3):222–228.

69. Bradley JP, Tibone JE, Watkins RG. History, physical examination, and diagnostic tests for neck and upper extremity problems. In: Watkins RG, ed. *The Spine in Sports.* St Louis: Mosby-Year Book; 1996.

70. Meadows JT. *Orthopedic Differential Diagnosis in Physical Therapy—A Case Study Approach.* New York: McGraw-Hill; 1999.

71. Sobel JB, Sollenberger P, Robinson R, et al. Cervical nonorganic signs: a new clinical tool to assess abnormal illness behavior in neck pain patients: a pilot study. *Arch Phys Med Rehabil.* 2000;81(2):170–175.

72. Sullivan MJ, Adams H, Rhodenizer T, Stanish WD. A psychosocial risk factor–targeted intervention for the prevention of chronic pain and disability following whiplash injury. *Phys Ther.* 2006;86(1):8–18.

73. Adams H, Ellis T, Stanish WD, Sullivan MJ. Psychosocial factors related to return to work following rehabilitation of whiplash injuries. *J Occup Rehabil.* 2007;17(2):305–315.

74. Waddell G, Main CJ, Morris EW, et al. Chronic low-back pain, psychologic distress, and illness behavior. *Spine.* 1984;9(2):209–213.

75. Jorritsma W, Dijkstra PU, De Vries GE, et al. Physical dysfunction and nonorganic signs in patients with chronic neck pain: exploratory study into interobserver reliability and construct validity. *J Orthop Sports Phys Ther.* 2014;44(5):366–376.

76. Novy DM, Collins HS, Nelson DV, et al. Waddell signs: distributional properties and correlates. *Arch Phys Med Rehabil.* 1998;79(7):820–822.

77. Antony MM, Bieling PJ, Cox BJ, et al. Psychometric properties of the 42-item and 21-item versions of the depression anxiety stress scales in clinical groups and a community sample. *Psychol Assessment.* 1998;10(2):176–181.

78. Horowitz M, Wilner N, Alvarez W. Impact of event scale: a measure of subjective stress. *Psychosom Med.* 1979;41(3):209–218.

79. Motlagh H. Impact of event scale–revised. *J Physiother.* 2010;56(3):203.

80. Armijo-Olivo S, Bravo J, Magee DJ, et al. The association between head and cervical posture and temporomandibular disorders: a systematic review. *J Orofac Pain.* 2005;20(1):9–23.

81. Armijo-Olivo S, Magee DJ. Cervical musculoskeletal impairments and temporomandibular disorders. *J Oral Maxillofac Res.* 2012;3(4):1–18.

82. Levangie PK, Norkin CC. *Joint Structure and Function: A Comprehensive Analysis.* Philadelphia: FA Davis; 2005.

83. Watson D, Trott P. Cervical headache: an investigation of natural head posture and upper cervical flexor muscle performance. *Cephalalgia.* 1993;13:272–284.

84. Janda V. Muscles and motor control in cervicogenic disorders: assessment and management. In: Grant R, ed. *Physical Therapy of the Cervical and Thoracic Spine.* New York: Churchill Livingstone; 1994.

85. Tsang SM, Szeto GP, Lee RY. Normal kinematics of the neck: the interplay between the cervical and thoracic spine. *Man Ther.* 2013;18(5):431–437.

86. Prushansky T, Dvir Z. Cervical motion testing: methodology and clinical implications. *J Manip Physiol Ther.* 2008;31:518–524.

87. Segarra V, Dueñas L, Torres R, et al. Inter- and intra-tester reliability of a battery of cervical movement control dysfunction tests. *Man Ther.* 2015;20(4):570–579.

88. Youdas JW, Garrett TR, Suman VJ, et al. Normal range of motion of the cervical spine: an initial goniometric study. *Phys Ther.* 1992;72:770–780.

89. Dvorak J, Antinnes JA, Panjabi M, et al. Age and gender related normal motion of the cervical spine. *Spine.* 1992;17:S393–S398.

90. Neumann DA. *Kinesiology of the Musculoskeletal System—Foundations for Physical Rehabilitation.* St Louis: CV Mosby; 2002.

91. Reese NB. *Muscle and Sensory Testing.* Philadelphia: WB Saunders; 1999.

92. Janda V. Muscles and cervicogenic pain syndrome. In: Grant R, ed. *Physical Therapy of the Cervical And Thoracic Spine.* New York: Churchill Livingstone; 1988.

93. Smith K, Hall T, Robinson K. The influence of age, gender, lifestyle factors and sub-clinical neck pain on the cervical flexion rotation test and cervical range of motion. *Man Ther.* 2008;13:552–559.

94. Takasaki H, Hall T, Oshiro S, et al. Normal kinematics of the upper cervical spine during the flexion-rotation test—in vivo measurements using magnetic resonance imaging. *Man Ther.* 2011;16:167–171.

95. Hall T, Briffa K, Hopper D, et al. Long-term stability and minimal detectable change of the cervical flexion-rotation test. *J Orthop Sports Phys Ther.* 2010;40:225–229.

96. Miller KJ. Physical assessment of lower extremity radiculopathy and sciatica. *J Chiropr Med.* 2007;6(2):75–82.

97. Hall T, Robinson K. The flexion-rotation test and active cervical mobility—a comparative measurement study in cervicogenic headache. *Man Ther.* 2004;9:147–202.

98. Yi-Kai L, Yun-Kun Z, Cai-Mo L, et al. Changes and implications of blood flow velocity of the vertebral artery during rotation and extension of the head. *J Manip Physiol Ther.* 1999;22:91–95.

99. Magarey ME. Examination of the cervical and thoracic spine. In: Grant R, ed. *Physical Therapy of the Cervical and Thoracic Spine.* New York: Churchill Livingstone; 1988.

100. Elvey RL. The investigation of arm pain. In: Boyling JD, Palastanga N, eds. *Grieve's Modern Manual Therapy: the Vertebral Column.* 2nd ed. Edinburgh: Churchill Livingstone; 1994.

101. Magarey ME. Examination of the cervical spine. In: Grieve GP, ed. *Modern Manual Therapy of the Vertebral Column.* Edinburgh: Churchill Livingstone; 1986.

102. Dvir Z, Pruchansky T. Cervical muscle strength testing: methods and clinical implications. *J Manip Physiol Ther.* 2008;31:518–524.

103. Schneider R, Gosch H, Norrell H, et al. Vascular insufficiency and differential distortion of brain and cord caused by cervicomedullary football injuries. *J Neurosurg.* 1970;33:363–375.

104. Pinfold M, Niere KR, O'Leary EF, et al. Validity and internal consistency of a whiplash-specific disability measure. *Spine.* 2004;29(3):263–268.

105. Willis C, Niere R, Hoving JL, et al. Reproducibility and responsiveness of the whiplash disability questionnaire. *Pain.* 2004;110(3):681–688.

106. Stupar M, Côté P, Beaton DE, et al. A test-retest reliability study of the whiplash disability questionnaire in patients with acute whiplash-associated disorders. *J Manipulative Physiol Ther.* 2015;38(9):629–636.

107. Stupar M, Cote P, Beaton DE, et al. Structural and construct validity of the whiplash disability questionnaire in adults with acute whiplash-associated disorders. *Spine J.* 2015;15(11):2369–2377.

108. Vernon H, Mior S. The neck disability index: a study of reliability and validity. *J Manip Physiol Ther.* 1991;14:409–415.

109. Vernon H. The neck disability index: state-of-the-art, 1991–2008. *J Manip Physiol Ther.* 2008;31:491–502.

110. Macdermid JC, Walton DM, Avery S, et al. Measurement properties of the neck disability index: a systemic review. *J Orthop Sports Phys Ther.* 2009;39:400–417.

111. Stratford PW, Riddle DL, Binkley JM, et al. Using the neck disability index to make decisions concerning individual patients. *Physiother Can.* 1999;51:107–112.

112. Bolton JE, Humphreys BK. The Bournemouth Questionnaire: a short-form comprehensive outcome measure. II. Psychometric properties in neck pain patients. *J Manipulative Physiol Ther.* 2002;25(3):141–148.

113. Manniche JA, Mosdal C, Hindsberger C. The Copenhagen Functional Disability Scale: a study of reliability and validity. *J Manip Physiol Ther.* 1998;21:520–527.

114. Leak AM, Cooper J, Dyer S, et al. The Northwick Park Neck Pain Questionnaire, devised to measure neck pain and disability. *Br J Rheumatol.* 1994;33:469–474.

115. Hoving JL, O'Leary EF, Niere KR, et al. Validity of the neck disability index, Northwick Park neck pain questionnaire, and problem elicitation technique for measuring disability associated with whiplash associated disorders. *Pain.* 2003;102(3):273–281.

116. Bolton JE. Sensitivity and specificity of outcome measures in patients with neck pain: detecting clinically significant improvement. *Spine.* 2004;29:2410–2417.

117. Bolton JE, Humphreys BK. The Bournemouth Questionnaire: a short-form comprehensive outcome measure. II Psychometric properties in neck pain patients. *J Manip Physiol Ther.* 2002;25:141–148.

118. Stenneberg MS, Schmitt MA, van Trijffel E, et al. Validation of a new questionnaire to assess the impact of whiplash associated disorders: the whiplash activity and participation list (WAL). *Man Ther.* 2015;20(1):84–89.

119. Schmitt MA, Stenneberg MS, Schrama PP, et al. Measurement of clinically relevant functional health perceptions in patients with whiplash-associated disorders: the development of the whiplash specific activity and participation list (WAL). *Eur Spine J.* 2013;22(9):2097–2104.

120. Cook C, Hegedus E. Diagnostic utility of clinical tests for spinal dysfunction. *Man Ther.* 2011;16(1):21–25.

121. Schneider GM, Jull G, Thomas K, Salo P. Screening of patients suitable for diagnostic cervical facet joints blocks – a role for physiotherapists. *Man Ther.* 2012;17(2):180–183.

122. Schneider GM, Jull G, Thomas K, et al. Derivation of a clinical decision guide in the diagnosis of cervical facet joint pain. *Arch Phys Med Rehabil.* 2014;95(9):1695–1701.

123. Cattrysse E, Swinkels RA, Oostendorp RA, et al. Upper cervical instability: are clinical tests reliable? *Man Ther.* 1997;2:91–97.

124. Olson KA, Paris SV, Spohr C, et al. Radiographic assessment and reliability study of the craniovertebral sidebending test. *J Man Manip Ther.* 1998;6:87–96.

125. Jull GA, O'Leary SP, Falla DL. Clinical assessment of the deep cervical flexor muscles: the craniocervical flexion test. *J Manip Physiol Ther.* 2008;31:525–533.

126. Falla DL, Jull GA, Hodges PW. Patients with neck pain demonstrate reduced electromyographic activity of the deep cervical flexor muscles during performance of the craniocervical flexion tests. *Spine.* 2004;29:2108–2114.

127. Jull GA. Physiotherapy management of neck pain of mechanical origin. In: Giles LG, Singer KP, eds. *Clinical Anatomy and Management of Cervical Spine Pain.* London: Butterworth-Heinemann; 1998.

128. Jull G, Barrett C, Magee R, et al. Further clinical clarification of the muscle dysfunction in cervical headache. *Cephalalgia.* 1999;19:179–185.

129. Jull G, Falla D. Does increased superficial neck flexor activity in the craniocervical flexion test reflect reduced deep flexor activity in people with neck pain? *Man Ther.* 2016;25:43–47.

130. Uthaikhup S, Jull G. Performance in the cranio-cervical flexion test is altered in elderly subjects. *Man Ther.* 2009;14:475–479.

131. Harris KD, Heer DM, Roy TC, et al. Reliability of a measurement of neck flexor muscle endurance. *Phys Ther.* 2005;85:1349–1355.

132. Van Hoof T, Vangestel C, Forward M, et al. The impact of muscular variation on the neurodynamic test for the median nerve in a healthy population with Langer's axillary arch. *J Manip Physiol Ther.* 2008;31:414–483.

133. Vanti C, Conteddu L, Guccione A, et al. The upper limb neurodynamic test 1: intra- and inter-tester reliability and the effect of several repetitions on pain and resistance. *J Manip Physiol Ther.* 2010;33:292–299.

134. Boyd BS, Wanek L, Gray AT, et al. Mechanosensitivity of the lower extremity nervous system during straight leg raise neurodynamic testing in healthy individuals. *J Orthop Sports Phys Ther.* 2009;39:780–790.

135. Gumina S, Carbone S, Albino P, et al. Firm squeeze test: a new clinical test to distinguish neck from shoulder pain. *Eur Spine J.* 2013;22:1558–1563.

136. Uchihara T, Furukawa T, Tsukagoshi H. Compression of brachial plexus as a diagnostic test of a cervical cord lesion. *Spine.* 1994;19:2170–2173.

137. Sterling M, Kenardy J. Physical and psychological aspects of whiplash: important considerations for primary care assessment. *Man Ther.* 2008;13(2):93–102.

138. Maigne R, Nieves WL, Jommer HM. *Diagnosis and Treatment of Pain of Vertebral Origin, A Manual Medicine Approach.* Baltimore: Williams & Wilkins; 1996.

139. Spurling RG, Scoville WB. Lateral rupture of the cervical intervertebral disc. *Surg Gynec Obstet.* 1944;78:350–358.

140. Kelly JJ. Neurological problems in the athlete's shoulder. In: Pettrone FA, ed. *Athletic Injuries of the Shoulder.* New York: McGraw-Hill; 1995.

141. Wells P. Cervical dysfunction and shoulder problems. *Physiotherapy.* 1982;68:66–73.

142. Davidson RI, Dunn EJ, Metzmaker JN. The shoulder abduction test in the diagnosis of radicular pain in cervical extradural compressive monoradiculopathies. *Spine.* 1981;6:441–446.

143. Farmer JC, Wisneski RJ. Cervical spine nerve root compression: an analysis of neuroforaminal pressure with varying head and arm positions. *Spine.* 1994;19:1850–1855.

144. Landi A, Copeland S. Value of the Tinel sign in brachial plexus lesions. *Ann R Coll Surg Engl.* 1979;61:470–471.

145. Manvell JJ, Manvell N, Snodgrass SL, Reid SA. Improving the radial nerve neurodynamic test: an observation of tension of the radial, median and ulnar nerves during upper limb positioning. *Man Ther.* 2015;20(6):790–796.

146. Butler DS. *Mobilisation of the Nervous System.* Melbourne: Churchill Livingstone; 1991.

147. Davis DS, Anderson IB, Carson MG, et al. Upper limb neural tension and seated slump tests: the false positive rate among healthy young adults without cervical or lumbar symptoms. *J Man Manip Ther.* 2008;16:136–141.

148. Slater H, Butler DS, Shacklock MO. The dynamic central nervous system: examination and assessment using tension tests. In: Boyling JD, Palastanga N, eds. *Grieve's Modern Manual Therapy: The Vertebral Column.* 2nd ed. Edinburgh: Churchill Livingstone; 1994.

149. Cook CE, Wilhelm M, Cook AE, et al. Clinical tests for screening and diagnosis of cervical spine myelopathy: a systemic review. *J Manip Physiol Ther.* 2011;34:539–546.

150. Yukawa Y, Nakashima H, Ito K, et al. Quantifiable tests for cervical myelopathy; 10-sec grip and release test and 10-s step test: standard values and aging variation from 1230 healthy volunteers. *J Orthop Sci.* 2013;18(4):509–513.

151. Yukawa Y, Kato F, Ito K, et al. "Ten second step test" as a new quantifiable parameter of cervical myelopathy. *Spine.* 2009;34:82–86.

152. Grant R. Vertebral artery testing—the Australian Physiotherapy Association Protocol after 6 years. *Man Ther.* 1996;1:149–153.

153. Kunnasmaa KT, Thiel HW. Vertebral artery syndrome: a review of the literature. *J Orthop Med.* 1994;16:17–20.

154. Bolton PS, Stick PE, Lord RS. Failure of clinical tests to predict cerebral ischemia before neck manipulation. *J Manip Physiol Ther.* 1989;12:304–307.

155. Magarey ME, Rebbeck T, Coughlan B, et al. Premanipulative testing of the cervical spine review, revision and new clinical guidelines. *Man Ther.* 2004;9:95–108.

156. Rivett DA, Sharples KJ, Milburn PD. Effects of premanipulative test on vertebral artery and internal carotid artery blood flow: a pilot study. *J Manip Physiol Ther.* 1999;22(6):368–375.

157. Thiel H, Rix G. Is it time to stop functional pre-manipulation testing of the cervical spine? *Man Ther.* 2005;10:154–158.

158. Kerry R, Taylor AJ, Mitchell J, et al. Cervical arterial dysfunction and manual therapy: a critical literature review to inform professional practice. *Man Ther.* 2008;13:278–288.

159. Bowler N, Shamley D, Davies R. The effect of a simulated manipulation position on internal carotid and vertebral artery blood flow in healthy individuals. *Man Ther.* 2011;16:87–93.

160. Thomas LC, McLeod LR, Osmotherly PG, Rivett DA. The effect of end-range cervical rotation on vertebral and internal carotid arterial blood flow and cerebral inflow: a sub analysis of an MRI study. *Man Ther.* 2015;20(3):475–480.

161. Willett GM, Wachholtz NA. A patient with internal carotid artery dissection. *Phys Ther.* 2011;91(8):1266–1274.

162. Arnold C, Bourassa R, Langer T, et al. Doppler studies evaluating the effect of a physical therapy screening protocol on vertebral artery blood flow. *Man Ther.* 2004;9:13–21.

163. Fast A, Zinicola DF, Marin EL. Vertebral artery damage complicating cervical manipulation. *Spine.* 1987;12:840–842.

164. Golueke P, Sclafani S, Phillips T, et al. Vertebral artery injury—diagnosis and management. *J Trauma.* 1987;27:856–865.

165. Australian Physiotherapy Association. Protocol for pre-manipulative testing of the cervical spine. *Aust J Physiother.* 1988;34:97–100.

166. Rivett DA. The premanipulative vertebral artery testing protocol. *N Z J Physiother.* 1995;23:9–12.

167. Barker S, Kesson M, Ashmore J, et al. Guidance for pre-manipulative testing of the cervical spine. *Man Ther.* 2000;5:37–40.

168. Mitchell J. Vertebral artery blood flow velocity changes associated with cervical spine rotation: a meta-analysis of the evidence with implications for professional practice. *J Man Manip Ther.* 2009;17:46–56.

169. Wadsworth CT. *Manual Examination and Treatment of the Spine and Extremities.* Baltimore: Williams & Wilkins; 1988.

170. Ombregt L, Bisschop P, ter Veer HJ, et al. *A System of Orthopedic Medicine.* London: WB Saunders; 1995.

171. Meadows JJ, Magee DJ. An overview of dizziness and vertigo for the orthopedic manual therapist. In: Boyling JD, Palastanga N, eds. *Grieve's Modern Manual Therapy: The Vertebral Column.* 2nd ed. Edinburgh: Churchill Livingstone; 1994.

172. Gird RB, Naffziger HC. Prolonged jugular compression: a new diagnostic test of neurological value. *Trans Am Neurol Assoc.* 1940;66:45–49.

173. Grant R. Vertebral artery insufficiency: a clinical protocol for pre-manipulative testing of the cervical spine. In: Boyling JD, Palastanga N, eds. *Grieve's Modern Manual Therapy: The Vertebral Column*. 2nd ed. Edinburgh: Churchill Livingstone; 1994.

174. Aspinall W. Clinical testing for cervical mechanical disorders which produce ischemic vertigo. *J Orthop Sports Phys Ther*. 1989;11:176–182.

175. Maitland GD. *Vertebral Manipulation*. London: Butterworths; 1973.

176. Fitz-Ritson D. Assessment of cervicogenic vertigo. *J Manip Physiol Ther*. 1991;14:193–198.

177. Herdman SJ. *Vestibular Rehabilitation*. 3rd ed. Philadelphia: FA Davis; 2007.

178. Johnson EG, Landel R, Kusunose RS, et al. Positive patient outcome after manual cervical spine management despite a positive vertebral artery test. *Man Ther*. 2008;13:367–371.

179. Goncalves DU, Felipe L, Lima TM. Interpretation and use of caloric testing. *Braz J Otorhinolaryngol*. 2008;74(3):440–446.

180. Pettman E. Stress tests of the craniovertebral joints. In: Boyling JD, Palastanga N, eds. *Grieve's Modern Manual Therapy: The Vertebral Column*. 2nd ed. Edinburgh: Churchill Livingstone; 1994.

181. Osmotherly PG, Rivett DA, Rowe LJ. The anterior shear and distraction tests for craniocervical instability: an evaluation using magnetic resonance imaging. *Man Ther*. 2012;17:416–421.

182. Osmotherly PG, Rivett DA, Rowe LJ. Construct validity of clinical tests for alar ligament integrity: an evaluation using magnetic resonance imaging. *Phys Ther*. 2012;92:718–725.

183. Kaale BR, Krakenes J, Albrektsen G, Wester K. Clinical assessment techniques for detecting ligament and membrane injuries in the upper cervical spine region—a comparison with MRI results. *Man Ther*. 2008;13:397–403.

184. Aspinall W. Clinical testing for the craniovertebral hypermobility syndrome. *J Orthop Sports Phys Ther*. 1990;12:47–54.

185. Rey-Eiriz G, Alburque-Sendin F, Barrera-Mellado I, et al. Validity of the posterior-anterior middle cervical spine gliding test for the examination of the intervertebral joint hypomobility in mechanical neck pain. *J Manip Phyiol Ther*. 2010;33:279–285.

186. Hall TM, Robinson KW, Fujinawa O, et al. Intertester reliability and diagnostic validity of the cervical flexion-rotation test. *J Manip Physiol Ther*. 2008;31(4):293–300.

187. Ogince M, Hall T, Robinson K. The diagnostic validity of the cervical flexion-rotation test in C1/2 related cervicogenic headache. *Man Ther*. 2007;12:256–262.

188. Hall T, Briffa K, Hopper D. The influence of lower cervical joint pain on range of motion and interpretation of the flexion-rotation test. *J Man Manip Ther*. 2010;18(3):126–131.

189. Greenbaum T, Dvir Z, Reiter S, Winocur E. Cervical flexion-rotation test and physiological range of motion – a comparative study of patients with myogenic temporomandibular disorder versus healthy subjects. *Musculoskelet Sci Pract*. 2017;27:7–13.

190. Hall TM, Briffa K, Hopper D, Robinson K. Comparative analysis and diagnostic accuracy of the cervical flexion-rotation test. *J Headache Pain*. 2010;11(5):391–397.

191. Glaser JA, Cure JK, Bailey KL, Morrow DL. Cervical spinal cord compression and the Hoffman sign. *Iowa Orthop J*. 2001;21:49–52.

192. Denno JJ, Meadows GR. Early diagnosis of cervical spondylotic myelopathy: a useful clinical sign. *Spine*. 1991;16:1353–1355.

193. Estañol BV, Marin OS. Mechanism of the inverted supinator reflex. A clinical and neurophysiological study. *J Neurol Neurosurg Psychiatry*. 1976;39:905–908.

194. Kiely P, Baker JF, O'hEireamhoin S, et al. The evaluation of the inverted supinator reflex in asymptomatic patients. *Spine*. 2010;35(9):955–957.

195. Refshauge K, Gass E. The neurological examination. In: Refshauge K, Gass E, eds. *Musculoskeletal Physiotherapy*. Oxford: Butterworth-Heinemann; 1995.

196. Cook C, Roman M, Stewart KM, et al. Reliability and diagnostic accuracy of clinical special tests for myelopathy in patients seen for cervical dysfunction. *J Orthop Sports Phys Ther*. 2009;39:172–178.

197. Coene LN. Mechanisms of brachial plexus lesions. *Clin Neuro Neurosurg*. 1993;95S:S24–S29.

198. Benjamin K. Injuries to the brachial plexus: mechanisms of injury and identification of risk factors. *Adv Neonatal Care*. 2005;5:181–189.

199. Waters PM. Obstetric brachial plexus injuries: evaluation and management. *J Am Acad Orthop Surg*. 1997;5:205–214.

200. Cantu RC. Stingers, transient quadriplegia, and cervical spinal stenosis: return to play criteria. *Med Sci Sports Exer*. 1997;29:S233–S235.

201. Weinstein SM. Assessment and rehabilitation of the athlete with a "stinger." A model for the management of noncatastrophic athletic cervical spine injury. *Clin Sports Med*. 1998;17:127–135.

202. Mennell JM. *Joint Pain*. Boston: Little, Brown; 1964.

203. Seffinger MA, Najm WI, Mishra SI, et al. Reliability of spinal palpation for diagnosis of back and neck pain. *Spine*. 2004;19:E413–E425.

204. Johnson MJ, Lucas GL. Value of cervical spine radiographs as a screening tool. *Clin Orthop Relat Res*. 1997;340(–108):102.

205. Stiell IG, Wells GA, Vandemheen KL, et al. The Canadian C-spine rule for radiography in alert and stable trauma patients. *JAMA*. 2001;286(15):1841–1848.

206. Dreahut JC, Stiell IG, Graham ID. Will a new clinical decision rule be widely used? The case of the Canadian C-spine rule. *Acad Emerg Med*. 2006;13:413–420.

207. Stiell IG, Wells GA, Vandemhaven K, et al. The Canadian CT Head Rule for patients with minor head injury. *Lancet*. 2001;357(9266):1391–1396.

208. Stiell IG, Clement CM, McKnight RD, et al. The Canadian C-spine rule versus the NEXUS low risk criteria in patients with trauma. *N Eng J Med*. 2003;349:2510–2518.

209. Cook CE, Hegedus EJ. *Orthopedic Physical Examination Tests—An Evidence Based Approach*. Upper Saddle River, NJ: Pearson/Prentice Hall; 2008.

210. Helliwell PS, Evans PF, Wright V. The straight cervical spine: does it indicate muscle spasm? *J Bone Joint Surg Br*. 1994;76:103–106.

211. McAviney J, Schulz D, Bock R, et al. Determining the relationship between cervical lordosis and neck complaints. *J Manip Physiol Ther*. 2005;28:187–193.

212. Pavlov H, Torg JS, Robie B, et al. Cervical spine stenosis: determination with vertebral body method. *Radiology*. 1987;164:771–775.

213. Cantu RC. Functional cervical spinal stenosis: a contraindication to participation in contact sports. *Med Sci Sports Exerc*. 1993;25:316–317.

214. Castro FP, Ricciardi J, Brunet ME, et al. Stingers, the Torg ratio, and the cervical spine. *Am J Sports Med*. 1997;25:603–608.

215. Torg JS, Pavlov H, Genuario SE, et al. Neurapraxia of the cervical spinal cord with transient quadriplegia. *J Bone Joint Surg Am*. 1986;68(9):1354–1370.

216. Templeton PA, Young JW, Mirvis SE, et al. The value of retropharyngeal soft tissue measurements in trauma of the adult cervical spine. *Skeletal Radiol*. 1987;18:98–104.

217. Ghanem I, El Hage S, Rachkidi R, et al. Pediatric cervical spine instability. *J Child Orthop*. 2008;2(2):71–84.

218. Harris JH. Radiographic evaluation of spinal trauma. *Orthop Clin North Am*. 1986;17:75–86.

219. Griffith JF. *Diagnostic Ultrasound Musculoskeletal*. Philadelphia: Elsevier; 2015.

220. Reid DC. *Sports Injury Assessment and Rehabilitation*. New York: Churchill Livingstone; 1992.

221. Bigg-Wither G, Kelly P. Diagnostic imaging in musculoskeletal physiotherapy. In: Refshauge K, Gass E, eds. *Musculoskeletal Physiotherapy*. Oxford: Butterworth-Heinemann; 1995.

222. Vaccaro AR, Klein GR, Flanders AE, et al. Long-term evaluation of vertebral artery injuries following cervical spine trauma using magnetic resonance angiography. *Spine*. 1998;23:789–795.

223. Furumoto T, Nagase J, Takahashi K, et al. Cervical myelopathy caused by the anomalies vertebral artery—a case report. *Spine*. 1996;21:2280–2283.

224. Combs SB, Triano JJ. Symptoms of neck artery compromise: case presentations of risk estimate for treatment. *J Manip Physiol Ther*. 1997;20:274–278.

225. Wainner RS, Fritz JM, Irrgang JJ, et al. Reliability and diagnostic accuracy of the clinical examination and patient self-report measures for cervical radiculopathy. *Spine*. 2003;28(1):52–62.

226. Lauder TD, Dillingham TR, Andary M, et al. Predicting electrodiagnostic outcome in patients with upper limb symptoms: are the history and physical exam helpful? *Arch Phys Med Rehabil*. 2000;81:436–441.

227. Selvaratnam PJ, Matyas TA, Glasgow EF. Noninvasive discrimination of brachial plexus involvement in upper limb pain. *Spine*. 1994;19(1):26–33.

228. Viikari-Juntura E, Porras M, Laasonen EM. Validity of clinical tests in the diagnosis of root compression in cervical disc disease. *Spine*. 1989;14(3):253–257.

229. Viikari-Juntura E. Interexaminer reliability of observations in physical examinations of the neck. *Phys Ther*. 1987;67:1526–1532.

230. Quintner JL. A study of upper limb pain and paraesthesia following neck injury in motor vehicle accidents: Assessment of the brachial plexus tension test of Elvey. *Br J Rheumatol*. 1989;28:528–533.

231. Nordin M, Carragee EJ, Hogg-Johnson S, et al. Assessment of neck pain and its associated disorders: results of the Bone and Joint Decade 2000–2010 Task Force on Neck Pain and Its Associated Disorders. *J Manip Physiol Ther*. 2009;32(suppl 2):S117–S140.

232. Lindgren KA, Leino E, Manninen H. Cervical rotation lateral flexion test in brachialgia. *Arch Phys Med Rehabil*. 1992;73:735–737.

233. Cote P, Kreitz BG, Cassidy JD, et al. The validity of the extension-rotation test as a clinical screening procedure before neck manipulation: a secondary analysis. *J Manip Physiol Ther*. 1996;19(3):159–164.

234. Sakagnchi M, Kitagawa K, Hougakti H, et al. Mechanical compression of the extracranial vertebral artery during neck rotation. *Neurology*. 2003;61:845–847.

235. Sandmark H, Nisell R. Validity of five common manual neck pain provoking tests. *Scand J Rehab Med*. 1995;27:131–136.

236. Tong HC, Haig AJ, Yamakawa K. The Spurling test and cervical radiculopathy. *Spine*. 2002;27:156–159.

237. Shabat S, Leitner Y, David R, Folman Y. The correlation between Spurling test and imaging studies in detecting cervical radiculopathy. *J Neuroimaging*. 2012;22(4):375–378.

238. Shah KC, Rajshekhar V. Reliability of diagnosis of soft cervical disc prolapse using Spurling's test. *Br J Neurosurg*. 2004;18(5):480–483.

239. Jull G, Bogduk N, Marsland A. The accuracy of manual diagnosis for cervical zygapophyseal joint pain syndromes. *Med J Austr*. 1988;148:233–236.

240. Viikari-Juntura E, Takala E-S, Riijimaki H, et al. Predictability of symptoms and signs in the neck and shoulders. *J Clin Epidemiol*. 2000;53:800–808.

241. Cleland JA, Fritz JM, Whitman JM, et al. The reliability and construct validity of the neck disability index and patient specific scale in patients with cervical radiculopathy. *Spine*. 2006;31(5):598–602.

242. Young IA, Cleland JA, Michener LA, Brown C. Reliability, construct validity, and responsiveness of the neck disability index, patient-specific functional scale, and numeric pain rating scale in patients with cervical radiculopathy. *Am J Phys Med Rehabil*. 2010;89:831–839.

243. Carreon LY, Glassman SD, Campbell MJ, et al. Neck Disability Index, short form-36 physical component summary and pain scales for neck and arm pain: the minimum clinically important difference and substantial clinical benefit after cervical spine fusion. *Spine J*. 2010;10:469–474.

244. Cleland JA, Childs JD, Whitman JM. Psychometric properties of the Neck Disability Index and Numeric Pain Rating Scale in patients with mechanical neck pain. *Arch Phys Med Rehabil*. 2008;89(1):69–74.

245. Humphreys BK, Delahaye M, Pederson CK. An investigation into the validity of cervical spine motion palpation using subjects with congenital vertebrae as a "gold standard. *BMC Musculoskelet Disord*. 2004;5:19.

246. Westaway MD, Stratford PW, Binkley JM. The patient-specific functional scale: validation of its use in persons with neck dysfunction. *J Orthop Sports Phys Ther*. 1998;27(5):331–338.

247. Singh A, Gnanalignham K, Casey A, et al. Quality of life assessment using the Short Form-12 (SF-12) questionnaire in patients with cervical spondylotic myelopathy: comparison with SF-36. *Spine*. 2006;31(6):639–643.

248. Brazier JE, Harper R, Jones NM, et al. Validating the SF-36 health survey questionnaire: new outcome measure for primary care. *BMJ*. 1992;305(6846):160–164.

249. Mathews JA. Atlanto-axial subluxation in rheumatoid arthritis. *Ann Rheum Dis*. 1969;28:260–266.

250. Stevens JC, Cartlidge NE, Saunders M, et al. Atlanto-axial subluxation and cervical myelopathy in rheumatoid arthritis. *Quart J Med*. 1971;40:391–408.

251. Uitvlugt G, Indenbaum S. Clinical assessment of atlantoaxial instability using the Sharp-Purser test. *Arthr Rheum*. 1988;31(7):918–922.

252. Bertilson BC, Grunnesjo M, Strender L-S. Reliability of clinical tests in the assessment of patients with neck/shoulder problems—impact of history. *Spine*. 2003;28:2222–2231.

253. Petersen SM, Covill LG. Reliability of the radial and ulnar nerve biased upper extremity neural tissue provocation tests. *Physiother Theory Pract*. 2010;26(7):476–482.

254. Heide BVD, Zusman AM. Pain and muscular responses to a neural tissue provocation test in the upper limb. *Man Ther*. 2001;6(3):154–162.

255. Coppieters M, Stappaerts K, Janssens K, et al. Reliability of detecting "onset of pain" and "submaximal pain" during neural provocation testing of the upper quadrant. *Physiother Res Int*. 2002;7(3):146–156.

256. Kleinrensink GJ, Stoeckart R, Mulder PG, et al. Upper limb tension tests as tools in the diagnosis of nerve and plexus lesions: anatomical and biomechanical aspects. *Clin Biomech*. 2000;15(1):9–14.

257. Refshauge KM. Rotation: a valid premanipulative dizziness test? Does it predict safe manipulation. *J Manip Physiol Ther*. 1994;17(1):15–19.

CHAPTER 4

Temporomandibular Joint

The temporomandibular joints (TMJs) are two of the most frequently used joints in the body, but they probably receive the least attention. It has been shown that temporomandibular disorders (TMDs) affect 10% to 15% of adults.[1] Without these joints, one would be severely hindered when talking, eating, yawning, kissing, or sucking. The TMJs should be included in any examination of the head and neck. TMDs consist of several complex multifactorial ailments involving many interrelating factors, including psychosocial issues.[2–4] Oral lesions (e.g., herpes zoster, herpex simplex, oral ulcers), muscle overuse (e.g., clenching, bruxism), trauma, systemic lupus erythematosus, rheumatoid arthritis, headaches, and cancer pain can mimic TMDs.[5–7] Three cardinal features of TMDs are orofacial pain, restricted jaw motion, and joint noise.[2] Much of the work in this chapter has been developed from the teachings of Rocabado.[8]

Applied Anatomy

The TMJs are located just anterior to the external auditory meatus (the ear).[9] The TMJ is a synovial, condylar, modified ovoid, and hinge-type joint with fibrocartilaginous surfaces rather than hyaline cartilage[10,11] and an articular disc; this disc completely divides each joint into two cavities (Fig. 4.1). Both joints, one on each side of the jaw, must be considered together in any examination. Along with the teeth, these joints are considered to be a "trijoint complex."

Gliding, translation, or **sliding movement** occurs in the upper cavity of the temporomandibular joint, whereas **rotation** or **hinge movement** occurs in the lower cavity (Fig. 4.2). Rotation occurs from the beginning to the midrange of movement. The upper head of the lateral pterygoid muscle draws the disc, or **meniscus,** anteriorly and prepares for condylar rotation during movement. The rotation occurs through the two condylar heads between the articular disc and the condyle. In addition, the disc provides congruent contours and lubrication for the joint. Gliding, which occurs as a second movement, is a translatory movement of the condyle and disc along the slope of the articular eminence. Both gliding and rotation are essential for full opening

and closing of the mouth (Fig. 4.3). The capsule of the TMJs is thin and loose. In the resting position, the mouth is slightly open, the lips are together, and the teeth are not in contact but slightly apart. In the close packed position, the teeth are tightly clenched, and the heads of the condyles are in the posterior aspect of the joint. **Centric occlusion** is the relation of the jaw and teeth when there is maximum contact of the teeth, and it is the position assumed by the jaw in swallowing. The position in which the teeth are fully interdigitated is called the **median occlusal position.**[12]

Temporomandibular Joints	
Resting position:	Mouth slightly open, lips together, teeth not in contact
Close packed position:	Teeth tightly clenched
Capsular pattern:	Limitation of mouth opening

The TMJs actively displace only anteriorly and slightly laterally. When the mouth is opening, the condyles of the joint rest on the disc in the articular eminences, and any sudden movement, such as a yawn, may displace one or both condyles forward. As the mandible moves forward on opening, the disc moves medially and posteriorly until the collateral ligaments and lateral pterygoid stop its movement. The disc is then "seated" on the head of the mandible, and both disc and mandible move forward to full opening. If this "seating" of the disc does not occur, full range of motion (ROM) at the TMJ is limited. In the first phase, mainly rotation occurs, primarily in the inferior joint space. In the second phase, in which the mandible and disc move together, mainly translation occurs in the superior joint space.[13]

The hyoid bone, found in the anterior throat region, is sometimes referred to as the skeleton of the tongue.[12] It serves as an attachment for the extrinsic tongue muscles and infrahyoid muscles and, by so doing, provides reciprocal stabilization during swallowing; through its muscle attachments, it can affect cervical and even shoulder function. Fig. 4.4 outlines the effect of a forward head posture and the relation to the hyoid bone and related muscles.

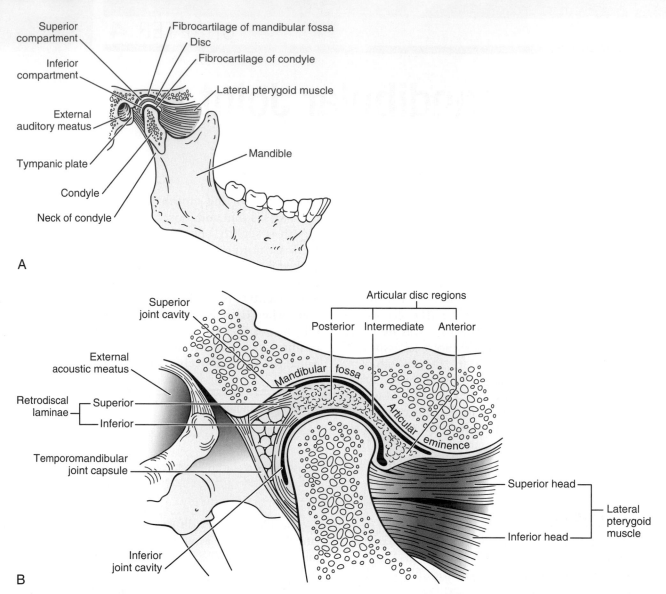

Fig. 4.1 (A) The temporomandibular joint. (B) Close-up of temporomandibular joint. (B, Redrawn from Neumann DA: *Kinesiology of the musculoskeletal system—foundations for physical rehabilitation*, St Louis, 2002, CV Mosby, p. 357.)

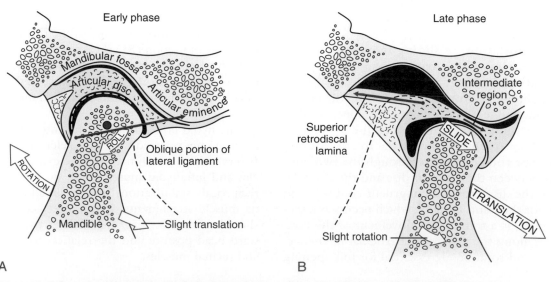

Fig. 4.2 Arthrokinematics of opening the mouth: (A) Early phase. (B) Late phase. (Modified from Neumann DA: *Kinesiology of the musculoskeletal system—foundations for physical rehabilitation*, St Louis, 2002, CV Mosby, p. 360.)

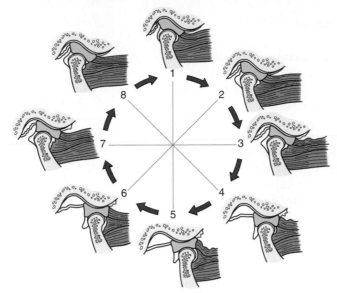

Fig. 4.3 Normal functional movement of the condyle and disc during the full range of opening and closing. Note that the disc is rotated posteriorly on the condyle as the condyle is translated out of the fossa. The closing movement is the exact opposite of the opening movement.

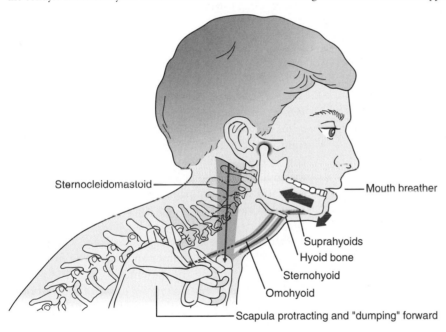

Sternocleidomastoid

Mouth breather

Suprahyoids
Hyoid bone
Sternohyoid
Omohyoid
Scapula protracting and "dumping" forward

Fig. 4.4 A forward head posture shows one mechanism by which passive tension in selected suprahyoid and infrahyoid muscles alter the resting posture of the mandible. The mandible is pulled inferiorly and posteriorly, changing the position of the condyle within the temporomandibular joint. Note the interrelationship to the cervical spine and shoulder. (Modified from Neumann DA: *Kinesiology of the musculoskeletal system—foundations for physical rehabilitation*, St Louis, 2002, CV Mosby, p. 366.)

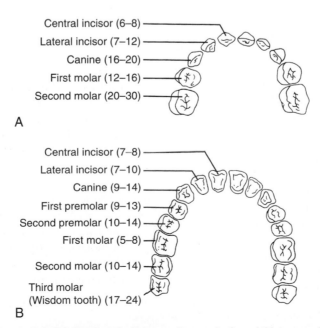

Central incisor (6–8)
Lateral incisor (7–12)
Canine (16–20)
First molar (12–16)
Second molar (20–30)

A

Central incisor (7–8)
Lateral incisor (7–10)
Canine (9–14)
First premolar (9–13)
Second premolar (10–14)
First molar (5–8)
Second molar (10–14)
Third molar
(Wisdom tooth) (17–24)

B

Fig. 4.5 Teeth in a child (A) and in an adult (B). Numbers indicate age (in months for a child, in years for an adult) at which teeth erupt.

The TMJs are innervated by branches of the auriculo-temporal nerve and masseteric branches of the mandibular nerve. The disc is innervated along its periphery but is aneural and avascular in its intermediate (force-bearing) zone.

The **temporomandibular,** or **lateral, ligament** restrains movement of the lower jaw and prevents compression of the tissues behind the condyle. In reality, this collateral ligament is a thickening in the joint capsule. The **sphenomandibular** and **stylomandibular ligaments** act as "guiding" restraints to keep the condyle, disc, and temporal bone firmly opposed. The stylomandibular ligament is a specialized band of deep cerebral fascia with thickening of the parotid fascia.

In the human, there are 20 deciduous, or temporary ("baby"), teeth and 32 permanent teeth (Fig. 4.5). The temporary teeth are shed between the ages of 6 and 13 years. In the adult, the incisors are the front teeth (four maxillary and four mandibular), with the maxillary incisors being larger than the mandibular incisors. The incisors are designed to cut food. The canine teeth (two maxillary and two mandibular) are the longest permanent teeth and are designed to cut and tear food. The premolars crush and break down the food for digestion; they usually have two cusps. There are eight premolars in all, two on each side, top and bottom. The final set of teeth is the molars, which crush and grind food for digestion. They have 4 or 5 cusps, and there are 2 or 3 on each side, top and bottom (total 8 to 12). The third molars are called **wisdom teeth.** Missing teeth, abnormal tooth eruption, malocclusion, or dental caries (decay) may lead to problems of the TMJ. By convention, the teeth are divided into four quadrants—upper left, upper right, lower left, and lower right (Fig. 4.6).

Patient History

In 1992, the Clinical Diagnostic Criteria for Temporomandibular Disorders (CDC/TMD) were published to provide a standardized definition of diagnostic subgroups of patients with orofacial pain and TMDs, including masticatory muscle disorders, TMJ internal derangements, and TMJ degenerative joint disease.[14,15] The criteria were revised in 2010.[9,16,17] Some have found the criteria too limiting relative to the diversity of TMJ patients, as the criteria do not take into account involvement of the cervical spine, nor do they deal with pain in a scientific manner.[9] The latest criteria are now called Diagnostic Criteria for Temporomandibular Disorders (DC/TMD) and are appropriate for clinical and research purposes.[18] Table 4.1 outlines some conditions that can mimic TMDs[5] and Table 4.2 provides a classification and lists the clinical patterns of TMDs.[9]

In addition to the questions listed under "Patient History" in Chapter 1, the examiner should obtain the following information from the patient[19,20]:

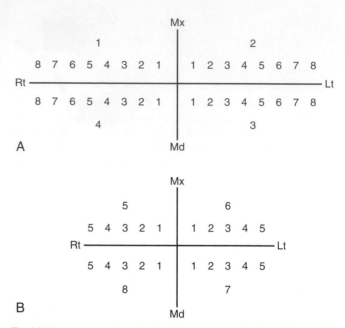

Fig. 4.6 Numeric symbols for dentition in an adult (A) and in a child (B). (From Liebgott B: *The anatomical basis of dentistry,* St Louis, 1986, CV Mosby.)

1. *Where is the pain? Is it in the face, jaw, temple, front of the ear?* When did the pain begin? Is the pain constant, recurrent, or a one-time problem? How would you rate your pain (see Fig. 1.2)?[9] These questions will give the examiner some idea of the patient's pain level and where the pain is felt.

2. *Does the patient have any difficulty chewing, eating soft or hard food, smiling or laughing, cleaning teeth or face, yawning, swallowing or talking?* These questions will give the examiner an idea of the functional limitations affecting the patient.

3. *Is there pain or restriction on opening or closing of the mouth?* Pain and other symptoms of TMJ dysfunction are usually associated with jaw movement.[5] Signs and symptoms of TMJ dysfunction include facial pain, ear discomfort, headache, and jaw discomfort.[5] Pain in the fully opened position (e.g., pain associated with opening to bite an apple, yawning) is probably caused by an extra-articular problem, whereas pain associated with biting firm objects (e.g., nuts, raw fruit and vegetables) (i.e., dynamic loading) is probably caused by an intra-articular problem.[21] Limited opening may be due to displacement of the disc anteriorly, inert tissue tightness, or muscle spasm. Restriction can lead to anxiety in patients because of its effect on everyday activities (e.g., eating, talking).[4]

4. *Is there pain on eating or dynamic loading? Does the patient chew on the right? Left? Both sides equally?* Loss of molars or worn dentures can lead to loss of vertical dimension, which can make chewing painful. **Vertical dimension** is the distance between any two arbitrary

points on the face, one of these points being above and the other below the mouth, usually in midline. Often, chewing on one side is the result of malocclusion.[21]

5. *What movements of the jaw cause pain? Do the symptoms change over a 24-hour period?* The examiner should watch the patient's jaw movement while the patient is talking. A history of stiffness on waking with pain on function that disappears as the day goes on suggests osteoarthritis.[22]

6. *Do any of these actions cause pain or discomfort: yawning, biting, chewing, swallowing, speaking, or shouting? If so, where?* All of these actions cause movement, compression, and/or stretching of the soft tissues of the TMJs.

7. *Does the patient breathe through the nose or the mouth?* Normal breathing is through the nose with the lips closed and no "air gulping." If the patient is a "mouth breather," the tongue does not sit in the proper position against the palate. In the young, if the tongue does not push against the palate, developmental abnormalities may occur, because the tongue normally provides internal pressure to shape the mouth. The buccinator and orbicularis oris muscle complex provides external pressure to counterbalance the internal pressure of the tongue. Loss of normal neck balance often results in the individual becoming a mouth breather and an upper respiratory breather, making greater use of the accessory muscles of respiration. Conditions (such as adenoids, tonsillitis, and upper respiratory tract infections) may cause the same problem.

8. *Has the patient complained of any **crepitus or clicking**?* Normally, the condyles of the TMJ slide out of the concavity and onto the rim of the disc. Clicking is the result of abnormal motion of the disc and man-

TABLE 4.1

Conditions That May Mimic Temporomandibular Disorders

Condition	Location	Pain Characteristics	Aggravating Factors	Typical Findings
Dental conditions				
Caries/abscess	Affected tooth	Intermittent to continuous dull pain	Hot or cold stimuli	Visible decay
Cracked tooth	Affected tooth	Intermittent dull or sharp pain	Biting, eating	Often difficult to visualize crack
Dry socket	Affected tooth	Continuous, deep, sharp pain	Hot or cold stimuli	Loss of clot, exposed bone
Giant cell arteritis	Temporal region	Sudden onset of continuous dull pain	Visual disturbance, loss of vision	Scalp tenderness, absence of temporal artery pulse
Migraine headache	Temporal region, behind the eye, cutaneous allodynia	Acute throbbing, occasionally with aura	Activity, nausea, phonophobia, photophobia	Often normal, aversion during ophthalmoscopic examination, normal cranial nerve findings
Neuropathic conditions				
Glossopharyngeal neuralgia	Most often ear, occasionally neck or tongue	Paroxysmal attacks of electrical or sharp pain	Coughing, swallowing, touching the ear	Pain with light touch
Postherpetic neuralgia	Site of dermatomal nerve and its distribution	Continuous, burning, sharp pain	Eating, light touch	Hyperalgesia
Trigeminal neuralgia	Unilateral trigeminal nerve	Paroxysmal attacks of sharp pain	Cold or hot stimuli, eating, light touch, washing	Pain with light touch
Salivary stone	Submandibular or parotid region	Intermittent dull pain	Eating	Tenderness at gland, palpable stone, no salivary flow
Sinusitis	Maxillary sinus, intraoral upper quadrant	Continuous dull ache	Headache, nasal discharge, recent upper respiratory infection	Tenderness over maxillary sinus or upper posterior teeth

From Gauer RL, Semidey MJ: Diagnosis and treatment of temporomandibular disorders. *Am Fam Physician* 91(6):380, 2015.

TABLE **4.2**

Classification and Clinical Patterns of Primary Recurrent Temporomandibular Disorder

Myogenic	Arthrogenic	Disc Displacement with Reduction	Disc Displacement without Reduction	Cervical Spine Involvement
• Associated with stress, anxiety, clenching, bruxism; secondary component to all other forms of TMD • Palpable tenderness of musculature (temporalis, masseter, pterygoids) • Palpable MTrPs of TMJ musculature • Provocation with activity (mastication, bruxing, etc.) • Often bilateral when the primary disorder • Confirmed through muscular management techniques and patient education to reduce contributing factors	• Associated with joint line pain, arthritis or arthrosis, arthralgia, hypermobility and joint pain with movement • Palpable joint line tenderness • Crepitus (palpable or audible to the patient and/or clinician) • Positive joint compression test • Accessory motion irregularities • Confirmed through joint techniques including joint mobilization when applicable patient education for hypermobile joints	• Associated with joint noises (popping/clicking) and blocked opening, may resolve spontaneously • Opening and/or reciprocal noise • Generally not associated with severe locking of the joint • Positive joint compression test • Generally unilateral • Confirmed through response to joint intervention, poor clinical differentiation of different disc displacements	• Associated with blocked opening and possibly a history of displacement with reduction • May have a history of opening and/or reciprocal noise • Locking that does not permit functional range • Positive joint compression test • Generally unilateral • Confirmed through response to joint intervention, poor clinical differentiation of different disc displacements	• Generally present across all patients with TMD • Upper cervical spine and/or head pain • Accessory movement restrictions • Multiple levels may be involved • Unilateral or bilateral • Confirmed through manual therapy and symptom reduction (high error rate with diagnostic imaging)

MTrPs, Myofascial trigger points; *TMD,* temporomandibular disorder; *TMJ,* temporomandibular joint.
From Shaffer SM, Brismée JM, Sizer PS, Courtney CA: Temporal mandibular disorders. Part one: Anatomy and examination/diagnosis, *J Man Manip Ther* 22(1):5, 2014.

dible. Early clicking implies a developing dysfunction, whereas late clicking is more likely to mean a chronic problem. Clicking may occur when the condyle slides back off the rim into the center (Fig. 4.7).[23] If the disc sticks or is bunched slightly, opening causes the condyle to move abruptly over the disc and into its normal position, resulting in a single click on opening (see Fig. 4.7).[24] There may be a partial anterior displacement (subluxation) or dislocation of the disc, which the condyle must override to reach its normal position when the mouth is fully open (Fig. 4.8). This override may also cause a click. Similarly, a click may occur if the disc is displaced anteriorly and/or medially, causing the condyle to override the posterior rim of the disc later than normal during mouth opening. It may also occur with closing, which is referred to as **disc displacement with reduction.** If clicking occurs in both directions, it is called **reciprocal clicking** (Fig. 4.9). The opening click occurs at some point during the opening or protrusive path, indicating that the condyle is slipping over the thicker posterior border of the disc to its position in the thinner middle or intermediate zone. The closing (reciprocal) click occurs near the end of the closing or retrusive path as the pull of the superior lateral pterygoid muscle causes the disc to slip more anteriorly and the condyle to move over its posterior border.

Clicks may also be caused by adhesions (Fig. 4.10), especially in people who clench their teeth **(bruxism).** These "adhesive" clicks occur in isolation, after the period of clenching.[25] If adhesions occur in the superior or inferior joint space, translation or rotation will be limited. This presents as a temporary closed lock, which then opens with a click.

If the articular eminence is abnormally developed (i.e., short, steep posterior slope or long, flat anterior slope), the maximum anterior movement of the disc may be reached before maximum translation of the condyle has occurred. As the condyle overrides the disc, a loud crack is heard, and the condyle-disc leaps or jogs (subluxes) forward.[25]

The "soft" or "popping" clicks that are sometimes heard in normal joints are caused by ligament movement, articular surface separation, or sucking of loose tissue behind the condyle as it moves forward. These clicks usually result from muscle incoordination. "Hard" or "cracking" clicks are more likely to indicate joint pathology or joint surface defects. Soft crepitus (like rubbing knuckles together) is a sound that sometimes occurs in symptomless joints and is not necessarily an indication of pathology.[26] Hard crepitus (like a footstep on gravel) is indicative of

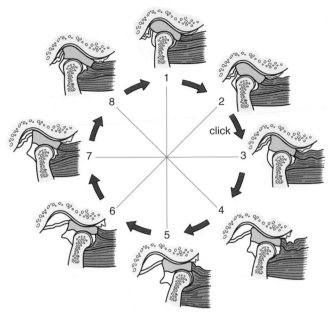

Fig. 4.7 Single click. Between positions *2* and *3*, a click is felt as the condyle moves across the posterior border into the intermediate zone of the disc. Normal condyle-disc function occurs during the remaining opening and closing movement. In the closed joint position *(1)*, the disc is again displaced forward (and medially) by activity of the superior lateral pterygoid muscle.

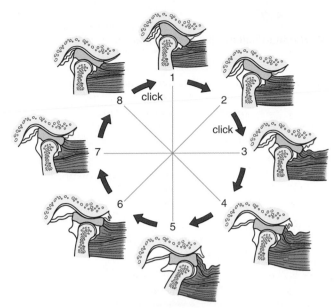

Fig. 4.9 Reciprocal click. Between positions *2* and *3*, a click is felt as the condyle moves across the posterior border of the disc. Normal condyle-disc function occurs during the remaining opening and closing movement until the closed joint position is approached. A second click is heard as the condyle once again moves from the intermediate zone to the posterior border of the disc between positions *8* and *1*.

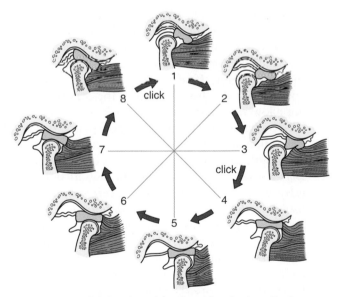

Fig. 4.8 Functional dislocation of the disc with reduction. During opening, the condyle passes over the posterior border of the disc into the intermediate area of the disc, thus reducing the dislocated disc.

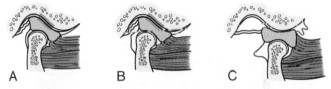

Fig. 4.10 (A) Adhesion in the superior joint space. (B) The presence of the adhesion limits the joint to rotation only. (C) If the adhesion is freed, normal translation can occur.

arthritic changes in the joints. The clicking may be caused by uncoordinated muscle action of the lateral pterygoid muscles, a tear or perforation in the disc, osteoarthrosis, or occlusal imbalance. Normally the upper head of the lateral pterygoid muscle pulls the disc forward. If the disc does not move first, the condyle clicks over the disc as it is pulled forward by the lower head of the lateral pterygoid muscle.

Iglarsh and Snyder-Mackler[13] have divided disc displacement into four stages (Table 4.3).

9. *Has the mouth or jaw ever locked?* Locking may imply that the mouth does not fully open (i.e., closed lock) or it does not fully close (i.e., open lock) and is often related to problems of the disc or joint degeneration. Locking is usually preceded by reciprocal clicking. If the jaw has locked in the closed position, the locking is probably caused by a disc with the condyle being posterior or anteromedial to the disc. Even if translation is blocked (e.g., "locked" disc), the mandible can still open 30 mm by rotation. If there is functional dislocation of the disc with reduction (see Fig. 4.8), the disc is usually positioned anteromedially and opening is limited. The patient complains that the jaw "catches" sometimes, so the locking occurs only occasionally; at those times opening is limited. If there is functional anterior dislocation of the disc without reduction, a **closed lock** occurs. Closed lock implies there has been anterior and/or medial displacement of the disc so that the disc does not return to its normal position during

TABLE **4.3**

Temporomandibular Disc Dysfunction

Stage	Characteristics
Stage 1	Disc slightly anterior and medial on mandibular condyle Inconsistent click (may or may not be present) Mild or no pain
Stage 2	Disc anterior and medial Reciprocal click present (early on opening, late on closing) Severe consistent pain
Stage 3	Reciprocal consistent click present (later on opening, earlier on closing) Most painful stage
Stage 4	Click rare (disc no longer relocates) No pain

Data from Iglarsh ZA, Snyder-Mackler L: Temporomandibular joint and the cervical spine. In Richardson JK, Iglarsh ZA (editors): *Clinical orthopedic physical therapy*, Philadelphia, 1994, WB Saunders.

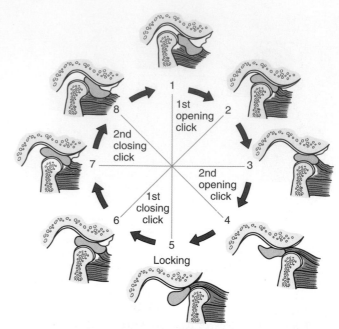

Fig. 4.12 Open lock (disc incoordination). *1,* The disc always stays in anterior position with the jaw closed. *1-4,* Disc is displaced posterior to the condyle with one or two opening clicks. *5-6,* The disc disturbs jaw closing after maximum opening. *6-1,* The disc is again displaced to anterior position from the posterior with one or two clicks.

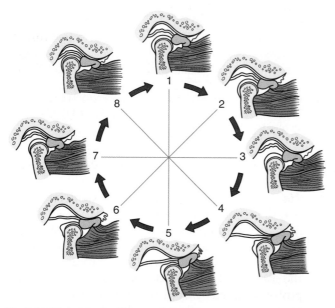

Fig. 4.11 Closed lock. The condyle never assumes a normal relation to the disc but instead causes the disc to move forward ahead of it. This condition limits the distance the condyle can translate forward.

the entire movement of the condyle. In this case opening is limited to about 25 mm, the mandible deviates to the affected side (Fig. 4.11), and lateral movement to the uninvolved side is reduced.[25] If locking occurs in the open position, it is probably caused by subluxation of the joint or possibly by posterior disc displace-

ment (see Fig. 4.11). With an **open lock,** there are two clicks on opening, when the condyle moves over the posterior rim of the disc and then when it moves over the anterior rim of the disc; then there are two clicks on closing. If, after the second click occurs on opening, the disc lies posterior to the condyle, it may not allow the condyle to slide back (Fig. 4.12).[27] If the condyle dislocates outside the fossa, it is a true dislocation with open lock; the patient cannot close the mouth, and the dislocation must be reduced.[27]

10. *Does the patient have any habits, such as smoking a pipe, using a cigarette holder, leaning on the chin, chewing gum, biting the nails, chewing hair, pursing and chewing lips, continually moving the mouth, or any other nervous habits?* All these activities place additional stress on the TMJs.

11. *Does the patient grind the teeth or hold them tightly?* **Bruxism** is the forced clenching and grinding of the teeth, especially during sleep. This may lead to facial, jaw, or tooth pain or headaches in the morning along with muscle hypertrophy. If the front teeth are in contact and the back ones are not, facial and temporomandibular pain may develop as a result of malocclusion. Normally the upper teeth cover the upper third to half of the bottom teeth (Fig. 4.13).

12. *Does there appear to be any related psychosocial problems or stress-related issues?* Temporomandibular dysfunction is often accompanied by related psychosocial issues.[2,28] Table 4.4 outlines psychosocial factors that may affect the TMJ.

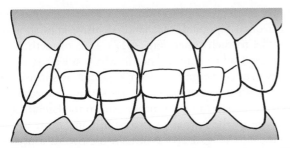

Fig. 4.13 Normally the maxillary anterior teeth overlap the mandibular anterior teeth almost half the length of the mandibular crowns. (From Okeson JP: *Management of temporomandibular disorders and occlusion*, St Louis, 1998, CV Mosby, p. 84.)

TABLE **4.4**

Checklist of Psychological and Behavioral Factors

1. Clinically significant anxiety or depression
2. Evidence of drug abuse
3. Repeated failures with conventional therapies
4. Evidence of secondary gain
5. Major life events; for example, new job, marriage or divorce, death
6. Pain duration greater than 6 months
7. History of possible stress-related disorders
8. Inconsistency in response to drugs
9. Inconsistent, inappropriate, and vague reports of pain, or both
10. Overdramatization of symptoms
11. Symptoms that vary with life events

Note: The first two factors are the most significant and warrant further evaluation by a mental health professional; factors 3 through 6 need at least one more factor for consideration of referral; and factors 7 through 11 require three or more factors for consideration of referral to a mental health professional.
From McNeili C, Mohl ND, Rugh JD, et al: Temporomandibular disorders: diagnosis, management, education and research, *J Am Dent Assoc* 120:259, 1990.

13. *Are any teeth missing? If so, which ones, and how many?* Loss of one or more teeth is called **partial edentulism.** The presence or absence of teeth and their relation to one another must be noted on a table similar to the one shown in Fig. 4.6. Their presence or absence can have an effect on the TMJs and their muscles. If some teeth are missing, others may deviate to fill in the space, altering the occlusion.
14. *Are any teeth painful or sensitive?* This finding may be indicative of dental caries or abscess. Tooth pain may lead to incorrect biting when chewing, which puts abnormal stresses on the TMJs.
15. *Does the patient have any difficulty swallowing? Does the patient swallow normally or gulp? What happens to the tongue when the patient swallows? Does it move normally, anteriorly, or laterally? Is there any evidence of tongue thrust or thumbsuck-*

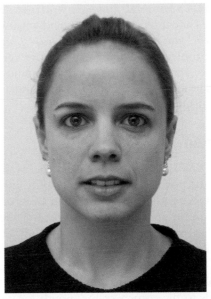

Fig. 4.14 Normal resting position of the tongue. Tongue position cannot be seen because of teeth but upper and lower teeth are not in contact.

ing? For example, the facial nerve (CN VII) and the trigeminal nerve (CN V), which control facial expression and mastication and contribute to speech, also control anterior lip seal. If lip seal is weakened, the teeth may move anteriorly, an action that would be accentuated in "tongue thrusters." The normal **resting position of the tongue** is against the anterior palate (Fig. 4.14). It is the position in which one would place the tongue to make a "clicking" sound.
16. *Are there any ear problems, such as hearing loss, ringing in the ears, blocking of the ears, earache, or dizziness?* Symptoms such as these may be caused by inner ear, cervical spine, vestibular dysfunction, or TMJ problems.
17. *Does the patient have any habitual head postures?* For example, holding the telephone between the ear and the shoulder compacts the TMJ on that side. Reading or listening to someone while leaning one hand against the jaw has the same effect.
18. *Has the patient noticed any voice changes?* Changes may be caused by muscle spasm.
19. *Does the patient have headaches? If so, where?* TMJ problems can refer pain to the head. Is there any history of infection or swollen glands?
20. *Does the patient ever feel dizzy or faint?*
21. *Has the patient ever worn a dental splint or other dental appliance? If so, when? For how long?*
22. *Has the patient ever been seen by a dentist, such as a periodontist (a dentist who specializes in the study of tissues around the teeth and diseases of these tissues), an orthodontist (a dentist who specializes in correction and prevention of irregularities of the teeth), or an endodontist (a dentist who specializes in the treatment of diseases of the*

tooth pulp, root canal, and periapical areas)? If so, why did the patient see the specialist, and what was done?

23. *Does the patient have any cervical spine problems?* TMJ problems can refer pain to the cervical spine and vice versa. If there are cervical spine symptoms, the examiner should include an examination of the cervical spine (see Chapter 3).

Observation

When the TMJs are being assessed, the examiner must also assess the posture of the cervical spine and head. For example, it is necessary that the head be "balanced" on the cervical spine and be in proper postural alignment.

1. Is the face symmetrical horizontally and vertically, and are facial proportions normal (Fig. 4.15)? The examiner should check the eyebrows, eyes, nose, ears, length of mandible from center line, and distance from the nasolabial folds to the corners of the mouth for symmetry on both horizontal and vertical planes. Horizontally, the face of an adult is divided into thirds (Fig. 4.16); this demonstrates normal vertical dimension. Usually the upper and lower teeth are used to measure vertical dimension. The horizontal bipupital, otic, and occlusive lines should be parallel to each other (Fig. 4.17). Loss of teeth on one side can lead to convergence in which at least two of the lines may converge because the jawline is short on one side relative to the other. A quick way to measure the vertical dimension is to measure from the lateral edge of the eye to the corner of the mouth and from the nose to the chin (Fig. 4.18). Normally the two measurements are equal, as are the lateral edges of the eye to the corner of the mouth bilaterally. If the second measurement is smaller than the first by 1 mm or more, there has been a loss of vertical dimension, which may have resulted from loss of teeth, overbite, or TMJ dysfunction. In children, elderly persons, and those with massive tooth loss, the lower third of the face is not well developed (lack of teeth) or has recessed (Fig. 4.19). As the teeth grow, the lower third develops into its normal proportion. The examiner should notice whether there is any paralysis, which could be indicated by ptosis (drooping of an eyelid) or by drooping of the mouth on one side (Bell's palsy).

2. The examiner should note whether the teeth are normally aligned or there is any crossbite, underbite, or overbite (Fig. 4.20). With **crossbite,** the teeth of the mandible

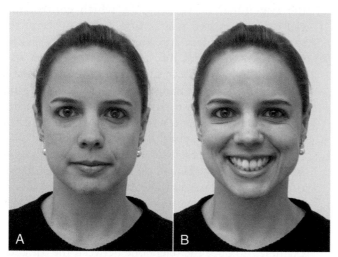

Fig. 4.15 Facial symmetry. Look for asymmetry both vertically and horizontally. Asymmetric changes may be seen with no smile (A) or with smile (B). These asymmetrical differences may or may not be related to pathology.

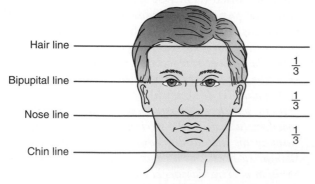

Fig. 4.16 Divisions of the face (vertical dimension).

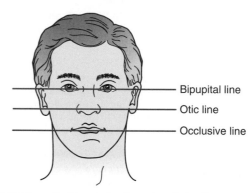

Fig. 4.17 Normally, bipupital, otic, and occlusive lines are parallel.

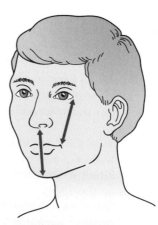

Fig. 4.18 A quick measurement of vertical dimension. Normally, the bilateral distance from the lateral edge of the eye to the corner of the mouth should be equal and each one should equal the distance from nose to point of chin.

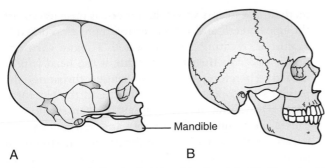

Fig. 4.19 Human skull at birth (A) and in the adult (B). Note the difference brought about by development of the teeth and lower jaw in the adult.

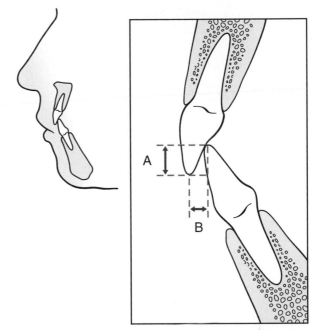

Fig. 4.21 Overlap of maxillary anterior teeth. (A) Vertical overlap (overbite). (B) Horizontal overlap (overjet). (Redrawn from Friedman MH, Weisberg J: The temporomandibular joint. In Gould JA, editor: *Orthopedics and sports physical therapy*, St Louis, 1990, CV Mosby, p. 578.)

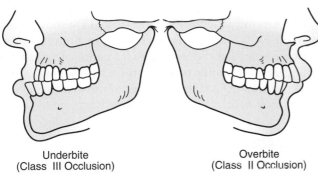

Underbite
(Class III Occlusion)

Overbite
(Class II Occlusion)

Fig. 4.20 Underbite and overbite.

are lateral to the upper (maxillary) teeth on one side and medial on the opposite side. There is abnormal interdigitation of the teeth. With anterior crossbite, the lower incisors are ahead of the upper incisors. With posterior crossbite, there is a transverse abnormal relation of the teeth. In **underbite,** the mandibular teeth are unilaterally, bilaterally, or in pairs in **buccoversion** (i.e., they lie anterior to the maxillary teeth). In **overbite,** the anterior maxillary incisors extend below the anterior mandibular incisors when the jaw is in centric occlusion. A small amount of overbite (1 to 2 mm) (i.e., the upper teeth lie slightly ahead of lower teeth) anteriorly is the most common position of the teeth (i.e., **normal dental occlusion**).[5] This is because the maxillary arch is slightly longer than the mandibular arch. **Overjet** (Fig. 4.21) is the distance that the maxillary incisors close over the mandibular incisors when the mouth is closed. This distance is normally 2 to 3 mm. **Occlusal interference** refers to premature contact of the teeth, which tends to deflect the jaw laterally and/or anteriorly.[29] Any orthodontic appliances or false teeth present should also be evaluated for fit and possible sore spots.

3. The examiner should note whether there is any **malocclusion** that could result in a faulty bite. Malocclusion may be a major factor in the development of disc problems of the TMJs. Occlusion occurs when the teeth are in contact and the mouth is closed. Malocclusion is defined as any deviation from normal occlusion.

Class I occlusion refers to the normal anteroposterior relation of the maxillary teeth to mandibular teeth. A slight modification with only the incisors affected and overjet slightly larger is sometimes classified as a Class I malocclusion. Class II malocclusion (i.e., **overbite**) occurs when the mandibular teeth are positioned posterior to their normal position relative to the maxillary teeth. This malocclusion deformity involves all the teeth, including the molars. The designation class II division 1 malocclusion (also called **large overjet** or **horizontal overlap**) indicates that the maxillary incisors demonstrate significant overjet. Class II division 2 malocclusion (also called **deep overlap** or **vertical overlap**) implies that overjet is not significant but that there is overbite and lateral flaring of the lateral maxillary incisors.[30] Class III malocclusion (i.e., **underbite**) occurs when the mandibular teeth are positioned anterior to their normal position relative to the maxillary teeth. If maxillary and mandibular teeth are on the same vertical plane, a class III malocclusion would be present.

4. What is the facial profile? The orthognathic profile is the normal, "straight-jawed" form. With this facial profile, a vertical line dropped perpendicular to the bipupital line would touch the upper and lower lips and the tip of the chin. In a person with a retrognathic profile, the chin would lie behind the vertical line and the person would be said to have a "receding chin." With the prognathic profile, the chin would be in front of the vertical line and the person would have a protruded or "strong" chin (Fig. 4.22).[30]

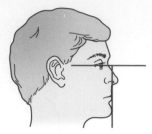

Orthognathic

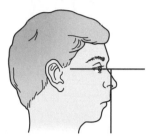

Retrognathic

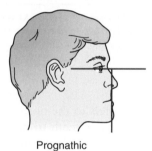

Prognathic

Fig. 4.22 Facial profiles.

5. The examiner should note whether the patient demonstrates normal bony and soft tissue contours. When the patient bites down, do the masseter muscles bulge as they normally should? Hypertrophy caused by overuse may lead to abnormal wear of the teeth. In looking at the soft tissues, it is important to note symmetry. The upper lip should normally cover two-thirds of the maxillary teeth at rest. If it does not, the lip is said to be short.[13] If the lip can be drawn over the upper teeth, however, the upper lip is said to be functional and no treatment is necessary. The lower lip normally covers the mandibular teeth and, when the mouth is closed, part of the maxillary teeth.

6. Is the patient able to move the tongue properly? Can the patient move the tongue up to and against the palate? Restriction may be caused by the small fold of mucous membrane (i.e., the **lingual frenulum**) extending from the floor of the mouth to the midline of the underside of the tongue. Can the tongue be protruded or rolled? Is the patient able to "click" the tongue? **Tongue thrusting** refers to forward movement of the tongue, usually to push against the lower teeth; it also occurs when the tongue is pushed against the upper teeth and the lower teeth are closed firmly against it, creating an oral seal.[31] Tongue thrusters find it easier to thrust the tongue if the head is protruded. Therefore, to test for tongue thrusting, the patient's head posture is corrected and the patient is asked to swallow. In the tongue thruster, swallowing causes the tongue to move forward resulting in protrusion of the head. Tongue thrusting may be due to hyperactivity of the masticatory muscles. When one swallows, the hyoid bone should move up and down quickly. If it moves only upward and slowly, and the suboccipital muscles posteriorly contract, it is suggestive of a tongue thrust.[32]

7. Where does the tongue rest? Is the tongue bitten frequently? Does the tongue have any scalloping or ridges? Does the patient swallow normally? Do the lips part when swallowing? What is the tongue position when swallowing? Do the facial muscles tighten on swallowing? All of these factors give the examiner some idea of the mobility of the structures of the mouth and jaw and their neurological mechanisms.

Examination

The examiner must remember that many problems of the TMJs may be the result of or related to problems in the cervical spine or teeth. Therefore, the cervical spine is at least partially included in any temporomandibular assessment.

Active Movements

With the patient in the sitting position, the examiner watches the active movements, noting whether they deviate from what would be considered normal ROM and whether the patient is willing to do the movement. The patient is first asked to carry out active movements of the cervical spine. As the active cervical movements are carried out by the patient, the examiner watches not only the movement in the cervical spine but also notes any changes in position of the mandible, as its position can have an effect on cervical ROM (especially in the upper cervical spine).[33] The most painful movements, if any, should be done last.

Active Movements of the Cervical Spine

- Flexion
- Extension
- Side flexion, left and right
- Rotation, left and right
- Combined movements (if necessary)
- Repetitive movements (if necessary)
- Sustained positions (if necessary)

During flexion of the neck, the mandible moves up and forward and the posterior structures of the neck become tight. During extension, the mandible moves down and back and the anterior structures of the neck become tight. The examiner should note whether the patient can flex and extend the neck while keeping the mouth closed or whether the patient must open the mouth to do these movements. The patient should be asked to place a fist under the chin and then to open the mouth while keeping the fist in place and the lower jaw against it. If the mouth opens in this way, movement of the neck into extension is occurring because the head is rotating backward on the temporomandibular condyles. This test movement would be especially important if the patient subjectively felt that there was a loss of neck extension. With side flexion of the neck to the right, maximal occlusion occurs on the right. Side flexion and rotation of the neck occur to the same side; therefore, if these movements are carried out to the right, maximal occlusion also occurs to the right.

Having observed the neck movements, the examiner goes on to note the active movements of the TMJs. The movements of the mandible can be measured with a millimeter ruler, depth gauge, or Vernier calipers. When the examiner is using the ruler, he or she should pick a midline point from which to measure opening and lateral deviation.[34] This same ruler can be used to measure protrusion and retrusion. Table 4.5 gives the active range of movement for the TMJ.

Active Movements of the Temporomandibular Joints

- Opening of the mouth
- Closing of the mouth
- Protrusion of the mandible
- Lateral deviation of the mandible, right and left

Opening and Closing of the Mouth

With opening (i.e., mandibular depression) and closing of the mouth (i.e., mandibular elevation), the normal arc of movement of the jaw is smooth and unbroken; that is, both TMJs are working in unison with no asymmetry or sideward movement, and both joints are bilaterally rotating and translating equally. Normally the mandible should open more than 30 to 35 mm[5] and chewing typically requires an opening of about 18 mm. Any alteration may cause or indicate potential problems in the TMJs. To observe any asymmetries, opening and closing of the mouth must be done slowly. The first phase of opening is rotation, which can be tested by having the patient open the mouth as widely as possible while maintaining the tongue against the roof (hard palate) of the mouth. Usually this movement causes minimal pain and occurs even in the presence of acute TMJ dysfunction. The second phase of opening is translation and rotation as the condyles move along the slope of the eminence. This phase begins when the tongue loses contact with the roof of the mouth.[3] Most of the clicking sensations occur during this phase. While the patient does the active movements, the examiner can palpate both joints simultaneously to compare the movement qualities occurring in both joints.[9]

The lateral pterygoid muscle is the primary opener of the mouth and is the strongest contributor to protrusion and medial and lateral deviation of the jaw.[9] The temporalis, masseter, and medial pterygoids are the primary closers (Table 4.6).[9]

Normally the mandible should open and close in a straight line (Figs. 4.23 and 4.24) provided that the bilateral action of the muscles is equal and the inert tissues have normal pliability. Each movement is done at least three times to determine whether any deviation is present with each repetition and to enable the examiner to find out whether the deviation is due to muscular, neuromuscular, or mechanical dysfunction.[35] This linear tracking

---

TABLE **4.5**

Active Range-of-Motion Measurements by Age and Sex for the Temporomandibular Joints

Active Motion	AGE			
	6 Years	12–14 Years	18–25 Years (Women)	18–25 Years (Men)
Mean opening (mm) (±SD)	44.8 (±4.3) Range 33–60	53.9 (±5.9) Range 41–73	51.0 (±5.7) Range 39–75	55.5 (±7.1) Range 42–77
Mean lateral deviation (mm) (±SD)	8.2 (±1.3) Range 5–13	10.0 (±1.7) Range 6–15	9.7 (±1.1) Range 5–15	10.0 (±2.1) Range 6–16
Mean protrusion (mm) (±SD)	0.6	1.4	2.3–10	3.0–10
Retrusion (mm)			1–3	1–3

SD, Standard deviation.
Modified from Shaffer SM, Brismée JM, Sizer PS, Courtney CA: Temporal mandibular disorders. Part one: Anatomy and examination/diagnosis, *J Man Manip Ther* 22(1):7, 2014.

TABLE **4.6**

Muscles of the Temporomandibular Joint: Their Actions and Nerve Supply

Action	Muscles Acting	Nerve Supply
Opening of mouth (depression of mandible)	1. Lateral (external) pterygoid 2. Mylohyoid[a] 3. Geniohyoid[a] 4. Digastric[a]	Mandibular (CN V) Inferior alveolar (CN V) Hypoglossal (CN XII) Inferior alveolar (CN V) Facial (CN VII)
Closing of mouth (elevation of mandible or occlusion)	1. Masseter 2. Temporalis 3. Medial (internal) pterygoid	Mandibular (CN V) Mandibular (CN V) Mandibular (CN V)
Protrusion of mandible	1. Lateral (external) pterygoid 2. Medial (internal) pterygoid 3. Masseter[a] 4. Mylohyoid[a] 5. Geniohyoid[a] 6. Digastric[a] 7. Stylohyoid[a] 8. Temporalis (anterior fibers) [a]	Mandibular (CN V) Mandibular (CN V) Mandibular (CN V) Inferior alveolar (CN V) Hypoglossal (CN XII) Inferior alveolar (CN V) Facial (CN VII) Facial (CN VII) Mandibular (CN V)
Retraction of mandible	1. Temporalis (posterior fibers) 2. Masseter[a] 3. Digastric[a] 4. Stylohyoid[a] 5. Mylohyoid[a] 6. Geniohyoid[a]	Mandibular (CN V) Mandibular (CN V) Inferior alveolar (CN V) Facial (CN VII) Inferior alveolar (CN V) Inferior alveolar (CN V) Hypoglossal (CN XII)
Lateral deviation of mandible	1. Lateral (external) pterygoid (ipsilateral muscle) 2. Medial (internal) pterygoid (contralateral muscle) 3. Temporalis[a] 4. Masseter[a]	Mandibular (CN V) Mandibular (CN V) Mandibular (CN V) Mandibular (CN V)

[a]Act only when assistance is required.
CN, Cranial nerve.

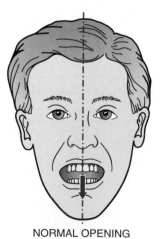
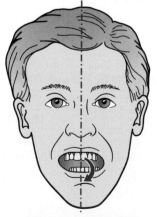
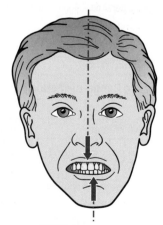

Fig. 4.23 Mandibular motion.

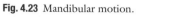 NORMAL OPENING   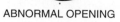 ABNORMAL OPENING   ABNORMAL CLOSED

is sometimes called **mandibular gait.**[35] If deviation or deflection occurs to the left on opening (see Fig. 4.23; a C-type curve) or to the right (a reverse C-type curve), hypomobility is evident toward the side of the deviation caused either by a displaced disc without reduction or unilateral muscle hypomobility;[20] if the deviation is an S-type or reverse S-type curve, the problem is probably muscular imbalance or medial displacement as the condyle "walks

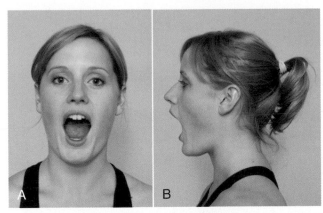

Fig. 4.24 Active opening of mouth. (A) Anteroposterior view. (B) Side view.

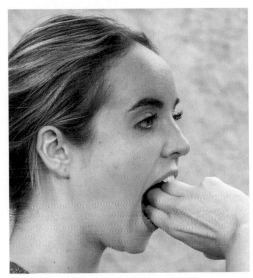

Fig. 4.25 Functional opening "knuckle" test.

around" the disc on the affected side.[20] The chin deviates toward the affected side, usually because of spasm of the pterygoid or masseter muscles or an obstruction in the joint. Both of these curves return to midline. If there is deviation to one side that does not return to midline, it is due to muscle spasm or adhesions. Early deviation on opening is usually caused by muscle spasm, whereas late deviation on opening is usually a result of capsulitis or a tight capsule. Pain or tenderness, especially on closing, indicates posterior capsulitis.

The examiner should then determine whether the patient's mouth can functionally be opened. The **functional** or **full active opening** is determined by having the patient try to place two or three flexed proximal interphalangeal joints within the mouth opening (Fig. 4.25).[36] This opening should be approximately 35 to 55 mm.[4] Normally only about 25 to 35 mm of opening is needed for everyday activity. If the patient has pain on opening, the examiner should also measure the amount

of opening to the point of pain and compare this distance with functional opening.[19] If the space is less than this, the TMJs are said to be hypomobile. Kropmans et al.[37] have pointed out that for treatment, at least 6 mm of change must be seen to be a detectable difference when more than one measurement is being made or to determine the effect of treatment.

As the mouth opens, the examiner should palpate the external auditory meatus with the index or little finger (fleshy part anterior). The patient is then asked to close the mouth. When the examiner first feels the condyle touch the finger, the TMJs are in the resting position. This resting position of the TMJs is called the **freeway space,** or **interocclusal space.** The freeway space is the potential space or vertical distance found between the teeth when the mandible is in the resting position. To determine the freeway space, the examiner marks a point on the chin and a point vertically above on the upper lip below the nose. The patient closes the mouth into centric occlusion, and the distance between the two points is measured. Then the patient is asked to say three simple words (e.g., "boy, boy, boy") and then maintain this position of the jaw without moving. The distance between the two points is measured again. The difference between the two measurements is the freeway space.[29] Normally, the space between the front teeth at this point is 2 to 4 mm.

If rotation does not occur at the TMJ, the mouth cannot open fully. There may be gliding at the TMJ, but rotation has not occurred. If translation (gliding) does not occur, the mandible may still open up to 30 mm as a result of rotation. Normally, when the mouth opens, the disc moves forward approximately 7 mm, and the condyle moves forward approximately 14 mm.[38]

If clicking (see question 8 in the earlier "History" section) occurs on opening, the examiner should ask the patient to open the mouth with the jaw protruded and retruded. If the clicking is eliminated with protrusion and accentuated with retrusion, the problem is probably an anterior disc displacement with reduction.[39] Anterior disc displacement without reduction cannot be determined as confidently.[40]

Protrusion of the Mandible

The examiner asks the patient to protrude or jut the lower jaw out past the upper teeth (Fig. 4.26A). The patient should be able to do this without difficulty. The normal movement is more than 7 mm, measured from the resting position to the protruded position.[4] The normal values vary depending on the degree of overbite (greater movement) or underbite (less movement).

Retrusion of the Mandible

The examiner asks the patient to retrude or pull the lower jaw in or back as far as possible (Fig. 4.26B). In full retention or centric relation, the TMJ is in a close packed position. The normal movement is 3 to 4 mm.[21]

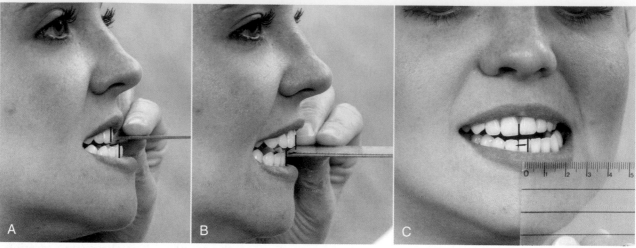

Fig. 4.26 Other active movements of the temporomandibular joint. (A) Protrusion. (B) Retrusion. (C) Lateral deviation left and right. Note position of lower teeth relative to upper teeth.

Lateral Deviation or Excursion of the Mandible

For lateral deviation, the teeth are slightly disoccluded and the patient moves the mandible laterally, first to one side and then to the other (Fig. 4.26C). With the joints in the resting position, two points are picked on the upper and lower teeth that are at the same level. When the mandible is laterally deviated, the two points, which have moved apart, are measured, giving the amount of lateral deviation. The normal lateral deviation is 10 to 15 mm.[4] During lateral deviation, the opposite condyle moves forward, down, and toward the motion side. The condyle on the motion side (e.g., left condyle on left lateral deviation) remains relatively stationary and becomes more prominent.[21] Any lateral deviation from the normal opening position or abnormal protrusion to one side indicates that the lateral pterygoid, masseter, or temporalis muscle, the disc, or the lateral ligament on the opposite side is affected.

When any changes are being charted, the examiner should note the type of opening deviation as well as the functional opening and any lateral deviation (Fig. 4.27).

Mandibular Measurement

Next, the examiner should measure the mandible from the posterior aspect of the TMJ to the notch of the chin (Fig. 4.28). Both sides are measured and compared for equality (the normal distance is 10 to 12 cm). Any difference indicates a developmental problem or structural change leading to left or right convergence; the patient may not be able to obtain balancing in the midline.

Swallowing and Tongue Position

The patient is asked to relax, then swallow, and leave the tongue in the position it assumed when swallowing occurred (normally close to the roof of the mouth). The examiner, wearing rubber gloves, then separates the lips and notes the position of the tongue (e.g., between the teeth or at upper anterior palate?).[29] During the swallowing, the examiner can also watch the action of the suprahyoid muscles.

Cranial Nerve Testing

If injury to the cranial nerves is suspected, these nerves should be tested.

Cranial Nerve Testing

CN I	Smell coffee or some similar substance with eyes closed.
CN II (optic nerve)	Read something with one eye closed.
CN III, IV, VI	Eye movements; note any ptosis.
CN V (trigeminal nerve)	Contract muscles of mastication (masseter and temporalis).
CN VII (facial nerve)	Move eyebrows up and down, purse lips, show teeth. This cranial nerve is the most commonly injured one. If the patient is unable to whistle or wink or close an eye on one side, the symptoms may be indicative of Bell's palsy (paralysis of the facial nerve).
CN VIII (auditory nerve)	Eyes closed; talk to patient and have him or her repeat what was said.
CN IX	Have patient swallow.
CN X (vagus nerve)	Have patient swallow.
CN XI (spinal accessory)	Have patient contract sternomastoid.
CN XII	Have patient stick out tongue, move it to the right and left.

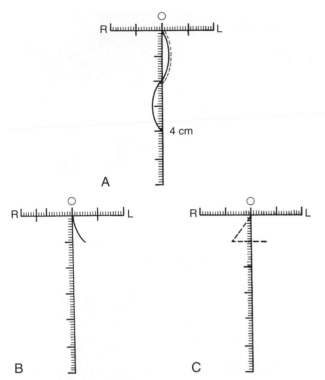

Fig. 4.27 Charting temporomandibular motion. (A) Deviation to both right *(R)* and left *(L)* on opening; maximum opening, 4 cm; lateral deviation equal (1 cm each direction); protrusion on functional opening *(dashed lines)*. (B) Capsule-ligamentous pattern; opening limited to 1 cm; lateral deviation greater to right than left; deviation to left on opening. (C) Protrusion is 1 cm; lateral deviation to right on protrusion (indicates weak lateral pterygoid on opposite side).

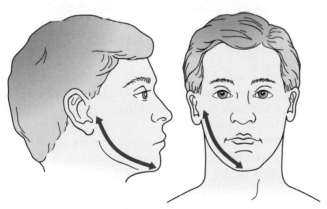

Fig. 4.28 Measurement of the mandible.

Passive Movements

Very seldom are passive movements carried out for the TMJs except when the examiner is attempting to determine the end feel of the joints. The amount of passive opening (full passive stretch) may also be measured and compared with the functional opening amount.[19] The normal end feel of these joints is tissue stretch on opening and teeth contact ("bone to bone") on closing. When the teeth are in maximal contact, the horizontal overjet is sometimes measured. The **overjet**

is the horizontal distance from the edge of the upper central incisors to the lower central incisors (see Fig. 4.21). If the lower teeth extend over the upper teeth, this malocclusion condition is called an **underbite**. **Overbite** is the vertical overlap of the teeth.

Normal End Feel at the Temporomandibular Joints

- Opening: Tissue stretch
- Closing: Bone to bone

Resisted Isometric Movements

Resisted isometric movements of the TMJs are relatively difficult to test. The jaw should be in the resting position. The examiner applies firm but gentle resistance to the joints and asks the patient to hold the position, saying "Don't let me move you." It is also important to test the muscles of the cervical spine (see Chapter 3) because there is a close correlation between muscles of the neck and those of the TMJs.[1]

Resisted Isometric Movements of the Temporomandibular Joints

- Depression (opening)
- Occlusion (closing)
- Lateral deviation left and right

Opening of the Mouth (Depression). This movement may be tested by applying resistance at the chin or, using a rubber glove, over the teeth with one hand while the other hand rests behind the head or neck or over the forehead to stabilize the head (Fig. 4.29A; see Table 4.6).

Closing of the Mouth (Elevation or Occlusion). One hand is placed over the back of the head or neck to stabilize the head while the other hand is placed under the chin of the patient's slightly open mouth to resist the movement (Fig. 4.29B). In a second method, the examiner uses a rubber glove and places two fingers over the patient's lower teeth (mandible) to resist the movement (Fig. 4.29C).

Lateral Deviation of the Jaw. One of the examiner's hands is placed over the side of the head above the TMJ to stabilize the head. The other hand is placed along the jaw of the patient's slightly open mouth and the patient pushes out against it (Fig. 4.29D). Each side is tested individually.

Functional Assessment

After the basic movements of the TMJs have been tested, the examiner should test functional activities or activities of daily living involving the use of the TMJs. These activities include chewing, swallowing, coughing, talking, and blowing. If the patient complains of pain while eating, the examiner can ask the patient to bite down on a tongue

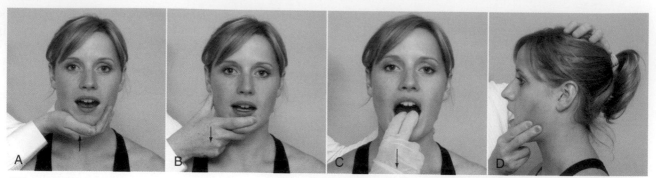

Fig. 4.29 Resisted isometric movements for the muscles controlling the temporomandibular joint. (A) Opening of the mouth (depression). (B) Closing of the mouth (elevation or occlusion). (C) Closing of the mouth (alternative method). (D) Lateral deviation of the jaw.

depressor held between the teeth in different positions to see if the compressive movement is painful in the teeth or the TMJ. Biting down on one side stresses the TMJ on the opposite side.[12]

In addition, there are a number of function questionnaires that may be used as part of the functional assessment: the Research Diagnostic Criteria for Temporomandibular Disorders (RDC/TMD),[16,17,41–44] the Limitations of Daily Function Questionnaire (TMJ; eTool 4.1),[45] the Jaw Functional Limitation Scale (there are 8- and 20-item scales; eTool 4.2),[46] the Mandibular Function Impairment Questionnaire (MFIQ) (eTool 4.3),[47–49] the History Questionnaire for Jaw Pain, and the TMJ Scale (eTool 4.4).

Special Tests

There are no routine special tests for the TMJs.

❷ *Chvostek Test.* This test may be used to determine whether there is pathology involving the seventh cranial (facial) nerve (Fig. 4.30). The examiner taps the parotid gland overlying the masseter muscle. If the facial muscles twitch, the test is considered positive.

If the patient is suffering from a facial nerve injury (Bell's palsy), the examiner may use the facial nerve grading system (see Table 2.30) developed by the American Academy of Otolaryngology.[19]

⚠ *Flexion/Extension Test.*[35] The patient is in sitting position and, before doing any movement, is asked to keep the mouth closed and the tongue in contact with the roof of the mouth and front teeth in contact. While holding this position, the patient is asked to flex and extend the cervical spine. If, when doing these two movements, the patient loses contact with the roof of the mouth, it may indicate hyoid hypertonicity or a tight lingual frenulum.

❷ *Joint Compression Test.*[9] The patient is in side-lying position with the head supported. The examiner pushes the mandible in a posterior and cranial direction with one hand to compress the condyle against the temporal bone while the other hand provides a counterforce on the

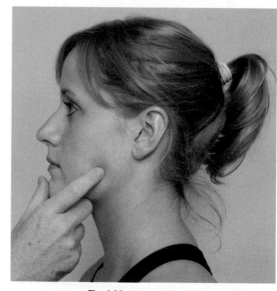

Fig. 4.30 Chvostek test.

cranium (Fig. 4.31A). The test may also be done with the patient in supine position and pushing both condyles in and up at the same time (**cranial loading;** Fig. 4.31B). A positive test results in pain.

❷ *Pressure Test.*[35] The examiner applies about 1 kg (2.2 lb) pressure over the temporalis (see Fig. 4.39A). If the muscle is tender, it indicates a pain generator and can help separate muscle pain from joint pain.

⚠ *Reload Test.*[35] This test is used if clicking or popping is heard during the examination. The patient is seated and asked to open the mouth to the point where the clicking occurred. The examiner inserts a tongue depressor vertically between the molars on the clicking side (Fig. 4.32). With the tongue depressor inserted, the patient is asked again to open and close the mouth. If the click is eliminated with the tongue depressor in place, the splint is helping to reduce posterior loading of the joint and allows the disc to reposition.

⚠ *Separation Clench Test.*[35] The patient is in sitting position and, starting with the unaffected side, is asked

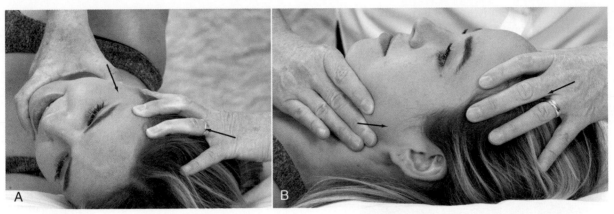

Fig. 4.31 Joint compression test. (A) In side lying. (B) In supine lying. Both condyles are compressed at the same time.

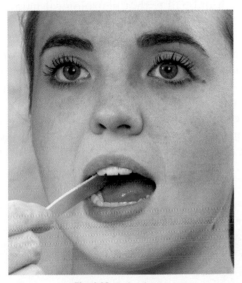

Fig. 4.32 Reload test.

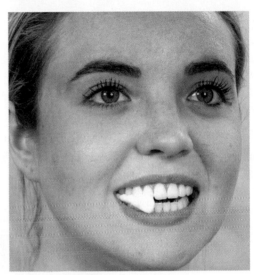

Fig. 4.33 Separation clench test.

to bite down on a cotton roll or similar object placed between the mandibles (Fig. 4.33). The test is repeated on the other side. The placing of the cotton roll distracts the ipsilateral TMJ and compresses the contralateral joint. If the pain is in the muscle that closes the mouth, the affected muscle could be on either side. If the pain is in the joint on the distraction side, it suggests a capsular problem. If the pain is on the contralateral side, it indicates inflammation in the joint.

⚠ *Tongue Blade Test.*[9,50–53] This test is used to rule out mandibular fractures. The uninvolved side is tested first. The patient is asked to bite down on a tongue depressor as it lies over the molars on one side. The examiner then attempts to twist and break the tongue depressor (see Fig. 2.30A). If the examiner is able to do so, the test is negative. If the patient cannot stabilize the tongue depressor because of pain, the test is positive and indicates the need for diagnostic imaging.

The examiner can listen to (auscultate) the TMJs during movement (Fig. 4.34). The movements "listened to" include opening and closing of the mouth, lateral deviation of the mandible to the right and left, and mandibular protrusion. Normally, a sound would be heard only on occlusion. This is a single solid sound, not a "slipping" sound. A slipping sound could occur if the teeth were not hitting simultaneously. The most common joint noise is reciprocal clicking (see Fig. 4.9), which occurs when the mouth opens and when it closes. The clicking ☑ is clinical evidence that the condyle is slipping over the disc and then self-reducing. The opening click results when the condyle slips under the posterior aspect of the disc (reduces) or slips anterior to the disc (subluxes) on opening. The second click, which is quieter, occurs when the condyle slips posterior to the disc (subluxes) or into its proper position and reduces. A single click may occur if the condyle gets caught behind the disc on opening (see Fig. 4.7) or if the condyle slips behind the disc on closing. On opening, the later the click occurs, the more anterior lies the disc. The later the opening click, the more the disc is displaced anteriorly and the more likely it is to lock. A closing click is usually caused by loosening of the structures attaching the disc to the condyle. Clicking is more likely to occur in hypermobile joints.[54,55]

Grating noise (crepitus) is usually indicative of degenerative joint disease or a perforation in the disc. Painful crepitus usually means that the disc has eroded, the condyle bone and temporal bone are rubbing together, and much of the fibrocartilage has been lost. While the examiner is listening, each movement should be done four or five times to ensure a correct diagnosis.

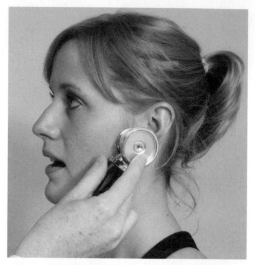

Fig. 4.34 Auscultation of the left temporomandibular joint.

For the reader who would like to review them, the reliability, validity, specificity, sensitivity, and odds ratios of some of the special tests used in the TMJ are available in eAppendix 4.1.

Reflexes and Cutaneous Distribution

The reflex of the TMJs is called the **jaw reflex.** The examiner's thumb or finger is placed on the chin of the patient with the patient's mouth relaxed and open in the resting position. The patient is asked to close the eyes. If this is not done, the patient commonly tenses as he or she sees the reflex hammer being swung toward the examiner's thumb/finger or the tongue depressor, and the test does not work. The examiner then taps the thumbnail with a neurological hammer (Fig. 4.35A). The jaw reflex may also be tested by using a tongue depressor (Fig. 4.35B). The examiner holds the tongue depressor firmly against the bottom teeth; while the patient relaxes the jaw muscles, the examiner taps the tongue depressor with the reflex hammer. The reflex closes the mouth and is a test of CN V.

The examiner must be aware of the dermatome patterns for the head and neck (Fig. 4.36) as well as the sensory nerve distribution of the peripheral nerves (see

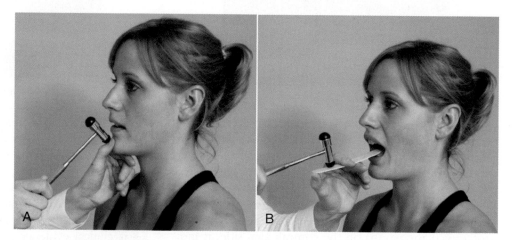

Fig. 4.35 Testing of the jaw reflex. (A) Hitting examiner's thumb. (B) Hitting tongue depressor.

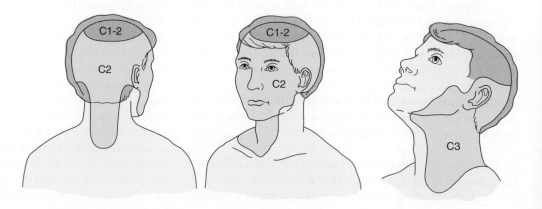

Fig. 4.36 Dermatomes of the head.

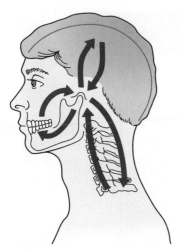

Fig. 4.37 Referred pain patterns to and from the temporomandibular joint in the teeth, head, and neck.

TABLE 4.7

Temporomandibular Muscles and Referral of Pain

Muscle	Referral Pattern
Masseter	Cheek, mandible to forehead or ear
Temporalis	Maxilla to forehead and side of head above ear
Medial pterygoid	Posterior mandible to temporomandibular joint
Lateral pterygoid	Cheek to temporomandibular joint
Digastric	Lateral cervical spine to posterolateral skull
Occipitofrontal	Above eye, over eyelid, and up over lateral aspect of skull

Fig. 3.70). Pain may be referred from the TMJ to the teeth, neck, or head, and vice versa (Fig. 4.37). Table 4.7 shows the muscles of the TMJ and their referral of pain.

Joint Play Movements

The joint play movements of the TMJs are then tested. Pain on performing these tests may indicate articular problems or pathology to the retrodiscal tissues.[56]

Longitudinal Cephalad (Distraction) and Anterior Glide. Wearing rubber gloves, the examiner places the thumb on the patient's lower teeth inside the mouth with the index finger on the mandible outside the mouth. The mandible is then distracted by pushing down with the thumb and pulling down and forward with the index finger while the other fingers push against the chin, acting as a pivot point. The examiner should feel the tissue stretch of the joint. Each joint is done individually while the other hand and arm stabilize the head (Fig. 4.38A).

Lateral Glide of the Mandible. The patient lies supine with the mouth slightly open and the mandible relaxed. The examiner places the thumb inside the mouth along the medial side of the mandible and teeth. By pushing the thumb laterally, the mandible glides laterally.[32] Each joint is done individually (Fig. 4.38B).

Medial Glide of the Mandible. The patient is in side-lying position with the mandible relaxed. The examiner places the thumb (or overlapping thumbs) over the lateral aspect of the mandibular condyle outside the mouth and applies a medial pressure to the condyle, gliding the condyle medially.[32] Each joint is done individually (Fig. 4.38C).

Posterior Glide of the Mandible. The patient is in side-lying position with the mandible relaxed. The examiner places the thumb (or overlapping thumbs) over the anterior aspect of the mandibular condyle outside the mouth and applies a posterior pressure to the condyle, gliding the condyle posteriorly.[32] Each joint is done individually (Fig. 4.38D).

Caudal-Anterior-Medial (CAM) Glide. The patient is placed in the same position as for medial glide. The mobilizing hand is placed over the proximal (upper) mandibular ramus and pushes the ramus caudally, anteriorly, and medially, causing a CAM glide. The test can be performed in various amounts of mouth opening and tests the temporomandibular ligament.[9]

Palpation

Palpation should be carried out carefully because of the sensitivity of the tissues around the TMJ. To palpate the TMJs, the examiner places the fingers (padded part anteriorly) in the patient's external auditory canals and asks the patient to actively open and close the mouth. As this is being done, the examiner determines whether both sides are moving simultaneously and whether the movement is smooth. If the patient feels pain on closing, the posterior capsule is usually involved. While palpating, the examiner looks to see if there is any tenderness and whether the joint is irritable or nonirritable. If the joint or structure being palpated (applying about 2 to 3 lb [approximately 1 kg] of force) is **irritable,** the patient's symptoms increase with minimal pressure and it takes a relatively longer time for the sensation to return to baseline. If the joint or structure is **nonirritable,** the patient's symptoms become evident only with more pressure and the time of the sensation to return to baseline is relatively short.[9] The examiner can also apply pressure to the facial muscles (Fig. 4.39) to see if they are pain generators by comparing degrees of tenderness.[35]

The examiner then places the index fingers over the mandibular condyles and feels for elicited pain or tenderness on opening and closing of the mouth. The examiner may also palpate the medial pterygoid, the medial and lower border of the inferior head of the lateral pterygoid, the temporalis and its tendon, and the masseter muscles

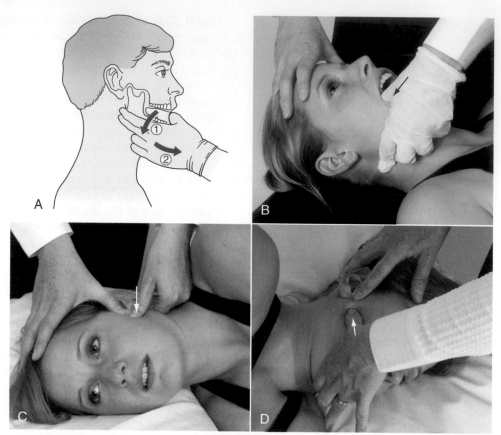

Fig. 4.38 Joint play of the temporomandibular joints when each side is tested individually. (A) Longitudinal cephalad and anterior glide. (B) Lateral glide of the mandible. Examiner pushes mandible laterally. (C) Medial glide of the mandible. Examiner pushes mandible medially while palpating temporomandibular joint with the other thumb. This causes the other temporomandibular joint to move laterally. (D) Posterior glide of the mandible. Examiner pushes mandible posteriorly while palpating temporomandibular joint with the other thumb.

and any other soft tissues for tenderness or indications of pathology (see Fig. 4.39). This procedure is followed by palpation of the following structures.

Mandible. The examiner palpates the mandible along its entire length, feeling for any differences between the left and right sides. As the examiner moves along the superior aspect of the angle of the mandible, the fingers pass over the parotid gland. Normally the gland is not palpable, but with pathology (e.g., mumps), the site feels "boggy" rather than having the normal hard and bony feel.

Teeth. The examiner should note the position, absence, or tenderness of the teeth. The examiner wears a rubber glove and palpates inside the patient's mouth. At the same time, the interior cheek region and gums may be palpated for pathology.

Hyoid Bone (Anterior to C2, C3 Vertebrae). While palpating the hyoid bone (Fig. 4.40), the examiner asks the patient to swallow. Normally the bone moves and causes no pain. The hyoid bone is part of the superior trachea.

Thyroid Cartilage (Anterior to C4, C5 Vertebrae). When the patient's neck is in neutral position, the thyroid cartilage can easily be moved; when the neck is in extension, it is tight and the examiner may feel crepitations. The thyroid

gland, which is adjacent to the cartilage, may be palpated at the same time. If it is abnormal or inflamed, it will be tender and enlarged.

Mastoid Processes. The examiner should palpate the skull, following the posterior aspect of the ear. The examiner will come to a point on the skull where the finger dips inward. The point just before the dip is the mastoid process (see Fig. 3.78).

Cervical Spine. Beginning on the posterior aspect at the occiput, the examiner systematically palpates the posterior structures of the neck (spinous processes, facet joints, and muscles of the suboccipital region), working from the head toward the shoulders. On the lateral aspect, the transverse processes of the vertebrae, the lymph nodes (palpable only if swollen), and the muscles should be palpated for tenderness. A more detailed description of the palpation of these structures is given in Chapter 3.

Diagnostic Imaging

Diagnostic imaging should be used only when it will generate information that will influence treatment decisions.[57,58]

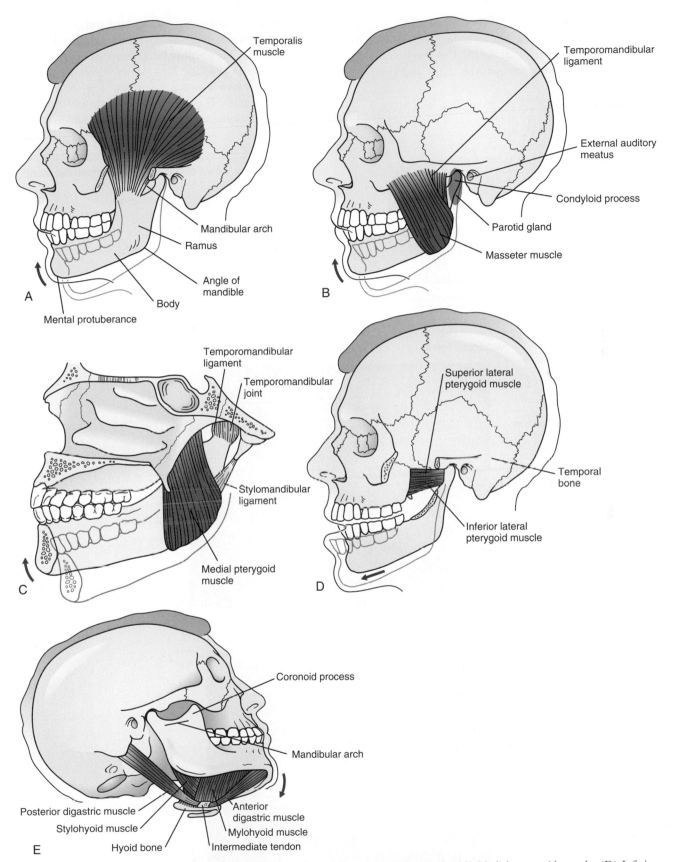

Fig. 4.39 Muscles of the temporomandibular joint. (A) Temporalis muscle. (B) Masseter muscle. (C) Medial pterygoid muscle. (D) Inferior and superior lateral pterygoid muscles. (E) Digastric muscle. (Modified from Okeson JP: *Management of temporomandibular disorders and occlusion*, St Louis, 1998, CV Mosby, pp. 18–20, 22.)

Plain Film Radiography

On the anteroposterior view, the examiner should look for condylar shape and normal contours. On the lateral view, the examiner should look for condylar shape and contours, position of condylar heads in the opened and closed positions (Fig. 4.41), amount of condylar movement (closed vs. open), and relation of TMJ to other bony structures of the skull and cervical spine (Fig. 4.42). X-ray views commonly taken for the TMJ are shown in the following box. A dental panoramic radiograph (Fig. 4.43) may sometimes be taken by a dentist to allow comparison of teeth on both sides of the jaw.

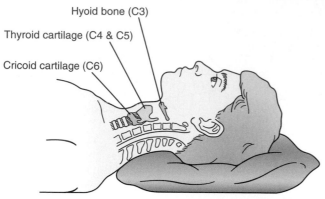

Fig. 4.40 Position of the hyoid bone, thyroid cartilage, and cricoid cartilage.

Common X-Ray Views of the Temporomandibular Joints

- Anteroposterior view (mouth closed) (Fig. 4.44)
- Lateral view (open and closed mouth) of TMJ (Fig. 4.45)
- Lateral view (closed mouth) (Fig. 4.46)
- Lateral view (TMJ and cervical spine) (see Fig. 4.42)
- Transcranial (lateral oblique) view (Fig. 4.47)
- Submentovertex view (Fig. 4.48)
- Dental panoramic view (see Fig. 4.43)

TMJ, Temporomandibular joint.

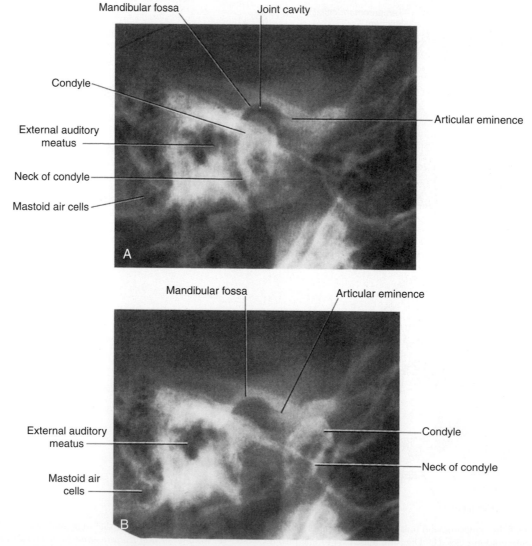

Fig. 4.41 Radiographs of the right temporomandibular joint. (A) Mouth closed. (B) Mouth open. (From Liebgott B: *The anatomical basis of dentistry,* St Louis, 1986, CV Mosby, p. 295; Courtesy Dr. Friedman.)

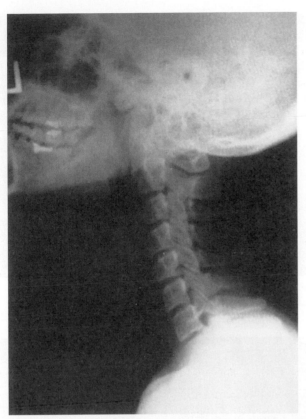

Fig. 4.42 Lateral radiographs of the skull, left temporomandibular joint, and cervical spine.

Diagnostic Ultrasound Imaging

Diagnostic ultrasound imaging (DUSI) is beginning to be used in assessment of the TMJ. Its advantage is that it can project dynamic opening and closing of the joint.[59–61] To be used for imaging the TMJ, high-resolution devices (≥12 MHz) should be used.[57,62] Similar to magnetic resonance imaging (MRI), DUSI can be used to detect the normal condyle-disc relationship, anterior disc displacement with and without reduction, joint effusion, and bone pathologies (Fig. 4.49).[57,62,63] As with all DUSI techniques, the quality will depend on the operator's experience and training.[57,64]

Magnetic Resonance Imaging

MRI is considered by dentists to be the gold standard imaging technique for testing the reliability of clinical findings in the TMJ.[14,59,60,62,64] This technique is used to differentiate the soft tissue of the joint, mainly the disc, from the bony structures. It has the advantage of using nonionizing radiation (Figs. 4.50 and 4.51). MRIs are contraindicated in patients with pacemakers, intracranial vascular clips, and metal particles in the eye or other vital structures.[57]

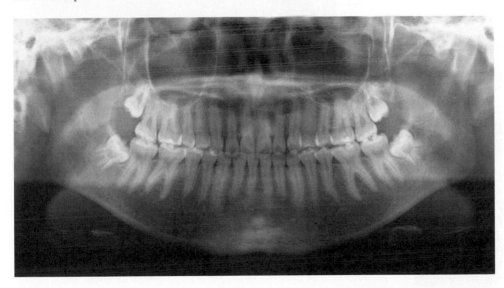

Fig. 4.43 Dental panoramic radiograph. (From Kaneda T, Weber AL, Scrivani SJ, et al: Cysts, tumors, and nontumorous lesions of the jaw. In Som PM, Curtin HD, editors: *Head and neck imaging*, ed 5, St. Louis, 2011, Mosby, Inc.)

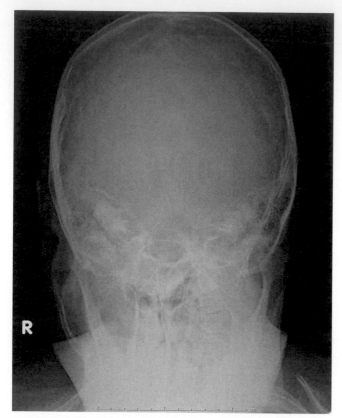

Fig. 4.44 Anteroposterior view of the temporomandibular joints (closed mouth).

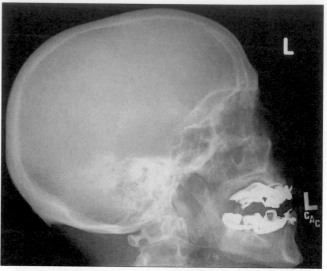

Fig. 4.46 Lateral view of the skull (closed mouth).

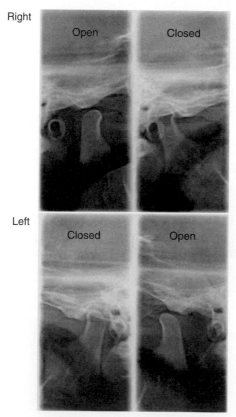

Fig. 4.45 Lateral view of the temporomandibular joints (open and closed mouth).

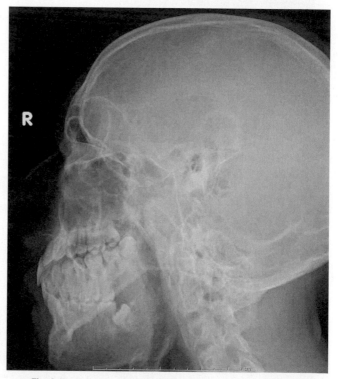

Fig. 4.47 Transcranial (lateral oblique) view (closed mouth).

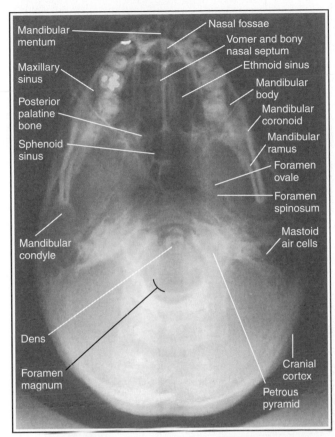

Mandibular mentum
Maxillary sinus
Posterior palatine bone
Sphenoid sinus
Mandibular condyle
Dens
Foramen magnum

Nasal fossae
Vomer and bony nasal septum
Ethmoid sinus
Mandibular body
Mandibular coronoid
Mandibular ramus
Foramen ovale
Foramen spinosum
Mastoid air cells
Cranial cortex
Petrous pyramid

Fig. 4.48 Submentovertex (Schueller) cranial image with accurate positioning. (From McQuillen Martensen K: *Radiographic image analysis*, ed 3, St Louis, 2011, WB Saunders Company, p. 525.)

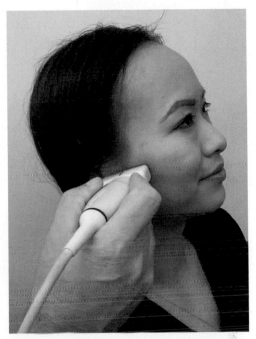

Fig. 4.49 Ultrasound examination of the temporomandibular joint.

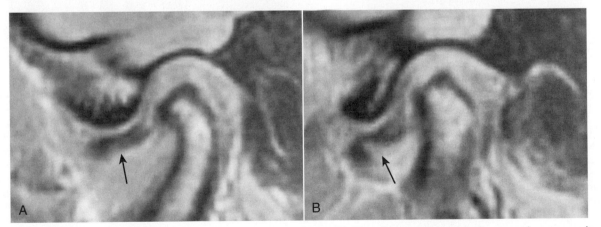

A   B

Fig. 4.50 Acute temporomandibular joint lock from a nonreducing displaced disc. (A) T1-weighted sagittal spin-echo magnetic resonance image with the mouth closed shows the dislocated disc *(arrow)* anterior to the condyle. (B) With attempted mouth opening, no appreciable anterior translation of the condyle occurs, but the disc folds on itself in the thin intermediate zone because of increased pressure from the condyle. The normal biconcave configuration of the disc and the normal intradiscal signal intensity are maintained *(arrow)*. (From Resnick D, Kransdorf MJ: *Bone and joint imaging*, Philadelphia, 2005, WB Saunders, p. 516.)

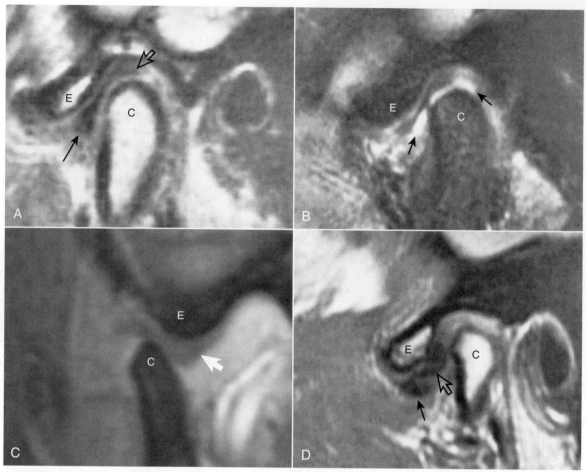

Fig. 4.51 Magnetic resonance (MR) imaging of the temporomandibular joint (TMJ). (A) T1-weighted sagittal spin-echo MR image of a normal TMJ. View with the mouth closed shows high signal intensity from the condylar marrow *(C)* and articular eminence *(E)*. Surrounding cortical bone is devoid of signal. The disc, of low signal intensity, is interposed between the condyle and the fossa; the intermediate zone articulates with the condyle and eminence where they are most closely apposed. The *solid arrow* points to the anterior band and the *open arrow* to the posterior band of the disc. (B) Sagittal gradient echo MR image used for fast (pseudodynamic) scanning shows a normal position of the disc with the mouth closed. Marrow becomes low in signal intensity with this sequence, and fluid in the inferior joint space becomes bright *(arrows);* the disc remains low in signal intensity. (C) Sagittal gradient image of a normal TMJ with the mouth open. The intermediate zone of the disc maintains its position between the condyle *(C)* and the eminence *(E)*, whereas the posterior band slides posterior to the condyle *(arrow)*. (D) T1-weighted sagittal spin-echo MR image in a patient with clicking and pain demonstrates internal derangement with both the anterior *(solid arrow)* and posterior *(open arrow)* bands of the disc displaced anteriorly relative to the condyle *(C)*. *C,* Condyle; *E,* eminence. (From Resnick D, Kransdorf MJ: *Bone and joint imaging*, Philadelphia, 2005, WB Saunders, p. 509.)

PRÉCIS OF TEMPOROMANDIBULAR JOINT ASSESSMENT[a]

NOTE: Suspected pathology will determine which *Special Tests* are to be performed.

History
Observation
Examination

Active movements
Neck flexion
Neck extension
Neck side flexion, left and right
Neck rotation, left and right
Extend neck by opening mouth
Assess functional opening
Assess freeway space
Open mouth
Closed mouth (occlusion)
Measure protrusion of mandible
Measure retrusion of mandible
Measure lateral deviation of mandible, left and right
Measure mandibular length
Swallowing and tongue position
Cranial nerve testing, if necessary

Passive movements (as in active movements), if necessary
Resisted isometric movements
Open mouth
Closed mouth (occlusion)
Lateral deviation of jaw
Functional assessment
Special tests
Reflexes and cutaneous distribution
Joint play movements
Palpation
Diagnostic imaging

[a]The entire assessment is usually done with the patient sitting. After any examination, the patient should be warned of the possibility of exacerbation of symptoms as a result of the assessment.

CASE STUDIES

When doing these case studies, the examiner should list the appropriate questions to be asked and why they are being asked, what to look for and why, and what things should be tested and why. Depending on the answers of the patient (and the examiner should consider different responses), several possible causes of the patient's problem may become evident (examples are given in parentheses). A differential diagnosis chart should be made up (see Table 4.8 as an example). The examiner can then decide how different diagnoses may affect the treatment plan.

1. A 52-year-old housewife is being seen for painful clicking in her right jaw. She reports recent onset of jaw pain following a visit to the dentist for a standard tooth filling. The pain is unilateral and is increased with eating. She has pain near her TMJ on that side but also reports that she thinks she is still having tooth pain as she did prior to the dental procedure, including sharp pain with drinking hot or cold drinks. Describe how you would determine whether her problem is arising from TMJ, the dental procedure, or both?

2. You are treating a 28-year-old male who competes in competitive Taekwondo. During a recent event, he was kicked in the mouth. Although he was wearing a mouth guard, the kick was hard enough that it caused damage to several of his teeth; and, he is also having left jaw pain. He has pain to opening and closing of his mouth on the left side only. This is even painful at times to open mouth enough to speak. Because of bruising present over his lateral face, you anticipate some of his problem may be soft tissue in origin. What muscles that affect TMJ function would be important to palpate for this patient? Additionally, what muscles would be important to manual muscle test and how would you test each of those muscles?

3. A 49-year-old woman comes to you complaining of neck and left temporomandibular joint pain. The pain is worse when she eats, especially if she chews on the left. Describe your assessment plan for this patient (cervical spondylosis versus temporomandibular dysfunction; see Table 4.8).

4. A 33-year-old woman comes to you complaining of pain and clicking when opening her mouth, especially when the mouth is open wide. She states that there is a small click on closing but minimal pain. Describe your assessment plan for this patient (temporomandibular joint arthritis vs. temporomandibular disc dysfunction).

5. An 18-year-old male hockey player comes to you stating that he was hit in the jaw while playing. He is in severe pain and has difficulty speaking. Describe your assessment plan for this patient (cervical sprain vs. temporomandibular joint dysfunction).

6. A 35-year-old man comes to you with his jaw locked open. Describe your assessment plan for this patient (temporomandibular disc dysfunction vs. temporomandibular arthritis).

7. A 42-year-old woman comes to you complaining of jaw pain and headaches. She slipped on some wet stairs 3 days ago and fell, hitting her chin on the stairs. Describe your assessment plan for this patient (temporomandibular joint dysfunction vs. head injury).

8. A 27-year-old nervous woman comes to you complaining of jaw pain. She has recently had a new dental plate installed. Describe your assessment plan for this patient (cervical sprain vs. temporomandibular joint dysfunction).

TABLE **4.8**

Differential Diagnosis of Cervical Spondylosis and Temporomandibular Joint Dysfunction

	Cervical Spondylosis	Temporomandibular Joint Dysfunction
History	Insidious onset May complain of referred pain into shoulder, arm, or head Stiff neck	Insidious onset May be related to biting something hard Pain may be referred to neck or head
Observation	Muscle guarding of neck muscles	Minimal or no muscle guarding
Active movements	Cervical spine movements limited TMJ movements normal	Cervical movements may be limited if they compress or stress TMJ TMJ movements may or may not be painful but range of motion is altered
Passive movements	Restricted May have altered end feel: muscle spasm or bone-to-bone	Restricted
Resisted isometric movements	Relatively normal Myotomes may be affected	Normal
Special tests	Spurling's test may be positive Distraction test may be positive	None
Reflexes and cutaneous distribution	Deep tendon reflexes may be hyporeflexic See history for referred pain	No effect See history for referred pain

TMJ, Temporomandibular joint.

References

1. Armijo-Olivo S, Fuentes J, Major PW, et al. The association between neck disability and jaw disability. *J Oral Rehab.* 2010;37(9):670–679.
2. Dimitroulis G. Temporomandibular disorders: a clinical update. *BMJ.* 1998;317:190–194.
3. Clark GT, Seligman DA, Solberg WK, et al. Guidelines for the examination and diagnosis of temporomandibular disorders. *J Craniomand Disord.* 1989;3:7–14.
4. Dimitroulis G, Dolwick MF, Gremillion HA. Temporomandibular disorders: clinical evaluation. *Aust Dent J.* 1995;40:301–305.
5. Gauer RL, Semidey MJ. Diagnosis and treatment of temporomandibular disorders. *Am Fam Physician.* 2015;91(6):378–386.
6. Okeson JP, de Leeuw R. Differential diagnosis of temporomandibular disorders and other orofacial pain disorders. *Dent Clin North Am.* 2011;55(1):105–120.
7. Zakrzewska JM. Differential diagnosis of facial pain and guidelines for management. *Br J Anesth.* 2013;111(1):95–104.
8. Rocabado M. *Course Notes: Course on Temporomandibular Joints.* Edmonton: Canada; 1979.
9. Shaffer SM, Brismée JM, Sizer PS, Courtney CA. Temporal mandibular disorders. Part one: anatomy and examination/diagnosis. *J Man Manip Ther.* 2014;22(1):2–12.
10. Rees LA. The structure and function of the mandibular joint. *Br Dent J.* 1954;96:125–133.
11. Kuroda S, Tanimoto K, Izawa T, et al. Biomechanical and biochemical characteristics of the mandibular condylar cartilage. *Osteoarthritis Cartilage.* 2009;17(11):1408–1415.
12. Dutton M. *Orthopedic Examination, Evaluation and Intervention.* New York: McGraw Hill; 2004.
13. Iglarsh ZA, Snyder-Mackler L. Temporomandibular joint and the cervical spine. In: Richardson JK, Iglarsh

ZA, eds. *Clinical Orthopedic Physical Therapy.* Philadelphia: W.B. Saunders; 1994.
14. Emshoff R, Brandlmaier I, Bosch R, et al. Validation of the clinical diagnostic criteria for temporomandibular disorders for the diagnostic subgroup—disc derangement with reduction. *J Oral Rehab.* 2002;29:1139–1145.
15. Emshoff R, Brandlmaier I, Bertram S, Rudisch A. Comparing methods for diagnosing temporomandibular joint disk displacement without reduction. *J Am Dent Assoc.* 2002;133(4):442–451.
16. List T, Greene CS. Moving forward with the RDC/TMD. *J Oral Rehab.* 2010;37:731–733.
17. Schiffman EL, Truelove EL, Ohrbach R, et al. The research diagnostic criteria for temporomandibular disorders I: overview and methodology for assessment of validity. *J Orofacial Pain.* 2010;24:7–24.
18. Schiffman E, Ohrbach R, Truelove E, et al. Diagnostic criteria for temporomandibular disorders (DC/TMD) for clinical and research applications: recommendations of the International RDC/TMD Consortium Network and Orofacial pain special interest Group. *J Oral Facial Pain Headache.* 2014;28(1):6–27.
19. House JW, Brackmann DE. Facial nerve grading system. *Otolaryngol Head Neck Surg.* 1985;93:146–147.
20. Okeson JP. *Management of Temporomandibular Disorders and Occlusion.* St Louis: CV Mosby; 1998.
21. Trott PH. Examination of the temporomandibular joint. In: Grieve G, ed. *Modern Manual Therapy of the Vertebral Column.* Edinburgh: Churchill Livingstone; 1986.
22. Day LD. History taking. In: Morgan DH, House LR, Hall WP, et al., eds. *Diseases of the Temporomandibular Apparatus.* St Louis: C.V. Mosby; 1982.
23. Isberg-Holm AM, Westesson PL. Movement of the disc and condyle in temporomandibular joints with clicking. *Acta Odontol Scand.* 1982;40:151–164.

24. Bush FM, Butler JH, Abbott DM. The relationship of TMJ clicking to palpable facial pain. *J Craniomand Pract.* 1983;1:44–48.
25. Bourbon B. Craniomandibular examination and treatment. In: Myers R, ed. *Saunders Manual of Physical Therapy Practice.* Philadelphia: W.B. Saunders; 1995.
26. Kaplan AS. Examination and diagnosis. In: Kaplan AS, Assael LA, eds. *Temporomandibular Disorders—Diagnosis and Treatment.* Philadelphia: W.B. Saunders; 1991.
27. Hondo T, Shimoda T, Moses JJ, et al. Traumatically induced posterior disc displacement without reduction of the TMJ. *J Craniomand Pract.* 1994;12:128–132.
28. McNeill C, Mohl ND, Rugh JD, et al. Temporomandibular disorders: diagnosis, management, education and research. *J Am Dent Assoc.* 1990;120:253–260.
29. Curnette DC. The role of occlusion in diagnoses and treatment planning. In: Morgan DH, House LR, Hall WP, et al., eds. *Diseases of the Temporomandibular Apparatus.* St Louis: C.V. Mosby; 1982.
30. Enlow DH. *Handbook of Facial Growth.* Philadelphia: W.B. Saunders; 1975.
31. Mew J. Tongue posture. *Br J Orthod.* 1981;8:203–211.
32. Petty NJ, Moore AP. *Neuromusculoskeletal Examination and Assessment—A Handbook for Therapists.* London: Churchill Livingstone; 1998.
33. Grondin F, Hall T, von Piekartz H. Does altered mandibular position and dental occlusion influence upper cervical movement: a cross sectional study of asymptomatic people. *Musculoskel Sci Pract.* 2017;27:85–90.
34. Walker N, Bohanen RW, Cameron D. Discriminant validity of temporomandibular joint range of motion measurements obtained with a ruler. *J Orthop Sports Phys Ther.* 2000;30:484–492.
35. Mitchel B, Cummins C, LeFebvre R. *Temporal Mandibular Joint Disorders (TMD): A Clinical Assessment.* University of Western States College of Chiropractic; 2015.

36. Friedman M, Weisberg J. Screening procedures for temporomandibular joint dysfunction. *Am Fam Physician.* 1982;25:157–160.

37. Kropmans T, Dijkstra P, Stegenga B, et al. Smallest detectable difference of maximal mouth opening in patients with painful restricted temporomandibular joint function. *Eur J Oral Sci.* 2000;108:9–13.

38. Friedman MH, Weisberg J. The temporomandibular joint. In: Gould JA, ed. *Orthopedic and Sports Physical Therapy.* St Louis: C.V. Mosby; 1990.

39. Yatani H, Sonoyama W, Kuboki T, et al. The validity of clinical examination for diagnosing anterior disc displacement with reduction. *Oral Surg Oral Med Oral Pathol Oral Radiol Endod.* 1998;85:647–653.

40. Yatani H, Suzuki K, Kuboki T, et al. The validity of clinical examination for diagnosing anterior disc displacement without reduction. *Oral Surg Oral Med Oral Pathol Oral Radiol Endod.* 1998;85:654–660.

41. Look JO, John MT, Tai F, et al. The research diagnostic criteria for temporomandibular disorders II: reliability of axis I diagnoses and selected clinical measures. *J Orofacial Pain.* 2010;24:25–34.

42. Ohrbach R, Turner JA, Sherman JJ, et al. The research diagnostic criteria for temporomandibular disorders IV: evaluation of psychometric properties of the axis II measures. *J Orofacial Pain.* 2010;24:48–62.

43. Schiffman EL, Ohrbach R, Truelove EL, et al. The research diagnostic criteria for temporomandibular disorders V: methods used to establish and validate revised axis I diagnostic algorithms. *J Orofacial Pain.* 2010;24:63–78.

44. Anderson GC, Gonzalez YM, Ohrbach R, et al. The research diagnostic criteria for temporomandibular disorders VI: future directions. *J Orofacial Pain.* 2010;24:79–88.

45. Sugisaki M, Kino K, Yoshida N, et al. Development of a new questionnaire to assess pain-related limitations of daily functions in Japanese patients with temporomandibular disorders. *Community Dent Oral Epidemiol.* 2005;33:384–395.

46. Ohrbach R, Larsson P, List T. The jaw functional limitation scale: development, reliability and validity of 8-item and 20-item versions. *J Orofacial Pain.* 2008;22:219–230.

47. Stegenga B, de Bont LG, de Lecuw R, et al. Assessment of mandibular function impairment associated with temporomandibular joint osteoarthrosis and internal derangement. *J Orofacial Pain.* 1993;7:183–195.

48. Kropmans TJ, Dijkstra PU, van Veen A, et al. The smallest detectable difference of mandibular function impairment in patients with a painfully restricted temporomandibular joint. *J Dent Res.* 1999;78:1445–1449.

49. Sudheesh KM, Desai R, Bharani S, Katta N. Assessment of mandibular function using mandibular function impairment questionnaire after closed treatment of unilateral mandibular condyle fractures. *Int J Oral Health Med Res.* 2016;3(1):28–30.

50. Caputo ND, Raja A, Shields C, Menke N. Re-evaluating the diagnostic accuracy of the tongue blade test: still useful as a screening tool for mandibular fractures? *J Emerg Med.* 2013;45(1):8–12.

51. Alonso LL, Purcell TB. Accuracy of the tongue blade test and patients with suspected mandibular fracture. *J Emerg Med.* 1995;13(3):297–304.

52. Schwab RA, Genners K, Robinson WA. Clinical predictors of mandibular fractures. *Am J Emerg Med.* 1998;16(3):304–305.

53. Malhotra R, Dunning J. The utility of the tongue blade test for the diagnosis of mandibular fracture. *Emerg Med J.* 2003;20(6):552–553.

54. Friedman MH, Weisberg J. Application of orthopedic principles in evaluation of the temporomandibular joint. *Phys Ther.* 1982;62:597–603.

55. Rocabado M. Arthrokinematics of the temporomandibular joint. *Dent Clin North Am.* 1983;27:573–594.

56. Langendoen J, Muller J, Jull GA. Retrodiscal tissue of the temporomandibular joint: clinical anatomy and its role in diagnosis and treatment of arthropathies. *Man Ther.* 1997;2:191–198.

57. Bas B, Yilmaz N, Gökce E, Akan H. Diagnostic value of ultrasonography and temporomandibular disorders. *J Oral Maxillofac Surg.* 2011;69(5):1304–1310.

58. Emshoff R, Innerhofer K, Rudisch A, Bertram S. Clinical versus magnetic resonance imaging findings with internal derangement of the temporomandibular joint: an evaluation of anterior disc displacement without reduction. *J Oral Maxillofacial Surg.* 2002;60(1):36–41.

59. Emshoff R, Bertram S, Rudisch A, Gassner R. The diagnostic value of ultrasonography to determine the temporomandibular joint disk position. *Oral Surg Oral Med Oral Pathol Oral Radiol Endod.* 1997;84(6):688–696.

60. Hechler BL, Phero JA, Van Mater H, Matthews NS. Ultrasound versus magnetic resonance imaging of the temporomandibular joint and juvenile idiopathic arthritis: a systematic review. *Int J Oral Maxillofac Surg.* 2018;47(1):83–89.

61. Klatkiewicz T, Gawriolek K, Radzikowska MP, Czajka-Jakubowska A. Ultrasonography in the diagnosis of temporomandibular joints: a meta-analysis. *Med Sci Monit.* 2018;24:812–817.

62. Kaya K, Dulgeroglu D, Unsal-Delialioglu S, et al. Diagnostic value of ultrasonography evaluation of temporomandibular joint anterior disc displacement. *J Cranio-Maxillo-Fac Surg.* 2010;38(5):391–395.

63. Kundu H, Basavaraj P, Kote S, et al. Assessment of TMJ disorders using ultrasonography as a diagnostic tool: a review. *J Clin Diagn Res.* 2013;7(12):3116–3120.

64. Manfredini D, Guarda-Nardini L. Ultrasonography of the temporomandibular joint: a literature review. *Int J Oral Maxillofac Surg.* 2009;38(12):1229–1236.

65. Neiner J, Free R, Caldito G, et al. Tongue blade bite test predicts mandibular fractures. *Craniomaxillofac Trauma Reconstr.* 2016;9(2):121–124.

CHAPTER 5

Shoulder

The prerequisite to any treatment of a patient with pain in the shoulder region is a precise and comprehensive picture of the signs and symptoms as they present during the assessment and as they existed before that time. This knowledge ensures that the techniques used will suit the condition and that the degree of success will be estimated against this background. Shoulder pain can be caused by intrinsic disease of the shoulder joints, more than one structure in the shoulder or pathology in the periarticular structures, or it may originate from the cervical spine, chest, or visceral structures. To compound the issue, there is no one pain pattern that is distinct for one particular tissue in the shoulder. Most pain tissues in the shoulder show a similar pain pattern.[1] For example, tendon injuries, rotator cuff syndrome, superior labrum anteroposterior (SLAP) lesions, osteoarthritis, and shoulder instability show similar symptoms.[1] Pathology is commonly related to the level of activity, and age can play a significant role. The shoulder complex is difficult to assess because of its many structures (most of which are located in a small area), its many movements, and the many lesions that can occur either inside or outside the joints. Influences such as referred pain from the cervical spine and the possibility of more than one lesion being present simultaneously, as well as the difficulty in deciding what weight to give to each response, make the examination even more difficult to understand. Assessment of the shoulder region often necessitates an evaluation of the cervical spine (see Chapter 3) and thoracic spine (see Chapter 8), especially the ribs, to rule out referred symptoms. The examiner must be prepared to include the cervical spine and its scanning examination in any shoulder assessment in order to clear any issues involving peripheral nerves and nerve roots.

Applied Anatomy

The **glenohumeral joint** is a multiaxial ball-and-socket synovial joint that depends primarily on the muscles and ligaments rather than bones for its support, stability, and integrity.[2] Thus assessment of the muscles and ligaments/capsule can play a major role in assessment of the shoulder. The **labrum,** which is the ring of fibrocartilage, surrounds and deepens the glenoid concavity of the scapula by about 30% to 50% (Fig. 5.1).[3,4] The labrum functions as a "chock block," increases the depth of the glenoid, resists translation, enables **concavity compression** (i.e.,

when the head of the humerus is compressed into the glenoid by the rotator cuff), centralizes the humeral head in the glenoid, and helps to maintain a negative intra-articular pressure within the joint, all of which help to stabilize the glenohumeral joint.[4] Only part of the humeral head is in contact with the glenoid at any one time. This joint has three axes and three degrees of freedom. The resting position of the glenohumeral joint is 55° of abduction and 30° of horizontal adduction. The close packed position of the joint is full abduction and lateral rotation. When it is relaxed, the humerus sits centered in the glenoid cavity; with contraction of the rotator cuff muscles, it is compressed and pushed or translated anteriorly, posteriorly, inferiorly, superiorly, or in any combination of these movements. This movement is small, but full movement is impossible if it does not occur. The glenoid in the resting position has 5° of superior tilt or inclination and 7° of retroversion (slight medial rotation). **Humeral torsion** is the relative position of the humeral head and the axis of the elbow at the distal humerus (Fig. 5.2).[5] The amount of torsion is determined by genetic as well as activity-related factors, with greater retrotorsion commonly found in the dominant limb. It is greatest at birth, decreases up to early adolescence, and normally stabilizes in teenagers.[6–9] The amount of torsion present affects medial and lateral rotation of the shoulder and normally ranges from –5° to +50°, with a smaller angle in children.[10,11] The larger the angle of torsion (i.e., less retroversion), the greater the amount of lateral rotation the patient can accomplish.[10,12] The angle between the humeral neck and shaft is about 130°, and the humeral head is retroverted 25° to 30° in adults (from about 75° in babies) relative to the line joining the epicondyles (Fig. 5.3).[4,13,14] The retroversion may be larger in overhead-throwing athletes (i.e., the retrotorsion is restricted by repetitive throwing) such as pitchers and tennis players, who try to maintain maximum lateral rotation in the shoulder.[5,6,14–21] This can

Glenohumeral Joint

Resting position:	40°–55° abduction, 30° horizontal adduction (scapular plane)
Close packed position:	Full abduction, lateral rotation
Capsular pattern:	Lateral rotation, abduction, medial rotation

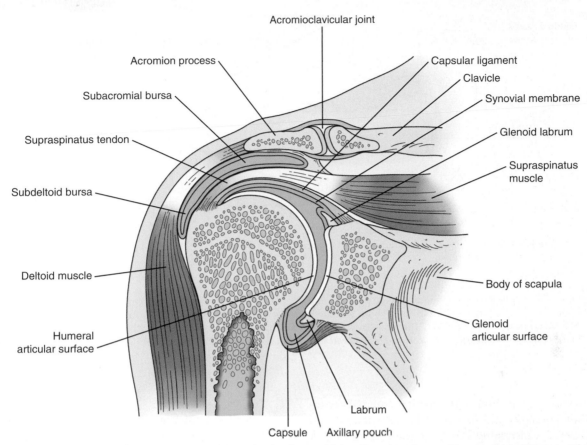

Fig. 5.1 Anterior view of a frontal plane cross section of the right glenohumeral joint. Note the subacromial and subdeltoid bursa within the sub-acromial space. Bursa and synovial lining are depicted in *blue*. The deltoid and supraspinatus muscles are also shown. (Redrawn from Neuman DA: *Kinesiology of the musculoskeletal system: foundations for rehabilitation*, ed 2, St Louis, 2010, Mosby/Elsevier, p 143.)

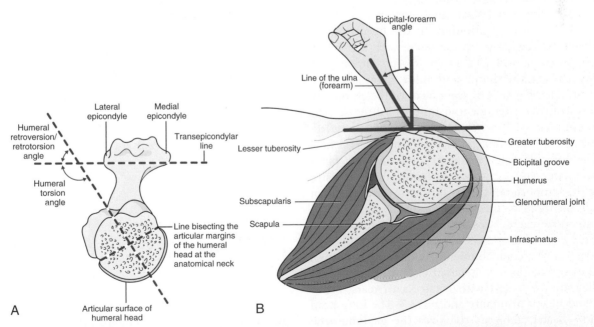

Fig. 5.2 (A) The humeral head retroversion angle is the angle between a line bisecting the humeral articular margins and a line joining the epicondyles at the elbow. (B) The bicipital-forearm angle (BFA): the angle between the epicondylar axis (distal humerus) and a line connecting the two tuberosities (proximal humerus) represents the torsion of the humerus. Because the ulna is perpendicular to the epicondylar axis, the angle between the ulna and vertical is a measure of **humeral retroversion**. (A, Modified from Van Hoof T, Vangestel C, Shacklock M, et al: Asymmetry of the ULNT1 elbow extension range-of-motion in a healthy population: consequences for clinical practice and research. *Phys Ther Sport* 13:141-149, 2011. B, Redrawn from Dashottar A, Borstad JD: Validity of measuring humeral torsion using palpation of bicipital tuberosities, *Physiother Theory Pract* 29(1):67-74, 2013.)

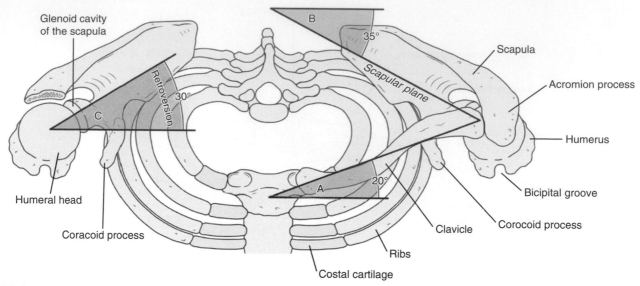

Fig. 5.3 Superior view of both shoulders in the anatomical position. *Angle A:* The clavicle is deviated about 20° posterior to the frontal plane. *Angle B:* The scapula (scapular plane or "scaption") is deviated about 35° anterior to the frontal plane. *Angle C:* Retroversion of the humeral head about 30° posterior to the mediolateral axis at the elbow. The right clavicle and acromion have been removed to expose the top of the right glenohumeral joint. (Redrawn from Neuman DA: *Kinesiology of the musculoskeletal system: foundations for rehabilitation,* ed 2, St Louis, 2010, Mosby/Elsevier, p 123.)

lead to increased **glenohumeral internal (medial) rotation deficit (GIRD)** and increased lateral rotation and possible posterior instability.[22–25] Swimmers, on the other hand, show almost equal retroversion in both dominant and nondominant shoulders because swimming is a bilateral sport in which both shoulders commonly perform the same action (i.e., in freestyle swimming).[26]

The rotator cuff muscles play an integral role in shoulder movement. Their positioning on the humerus may be visualized by "cupping" the shoulder with the thumb anteriorly, as shown in Fig. 5.4. The biceps tendon (Fig. 5.5) runs between the thumb and index finger just anterior to the index finger. The long head of biceps tendon originates from the supraglenoid tubercle of the scapula and is about 9 cm (3.5 inches) long.[27] The **biceps reflection pulley** consists of the superior glenohumeral ligament, the coracohumeral ligament, and the deep fibers of supraspinatus and subscapularis tendons and helps to stabilize the long head of biceps as it passes over the joint line. It is anchored to the superior labrum and makes a 30° to 40° turn where it is stabilized by the structures of the rotator interval as it exits the joint.[28–30] The tendon travels deep to the coracohumeral ligament and through the rotator interval before it exits the joint.[30] Injuries to the pulley are associated with rotator cuff tears, SLAP lesions, and biceps instability and tears.[28] The long head (and short head) of biceps stabilizes the glenohumeral joint anteriorly and acts as a dynamic depressor of the humeral head.[30,31] The pulley has the greatest chance of injury by shear loading on forward flexion in neutral or medial rotation.[27,30] The rotator cuff controls osteokinematic and arthrokinematic motion of the humeral head

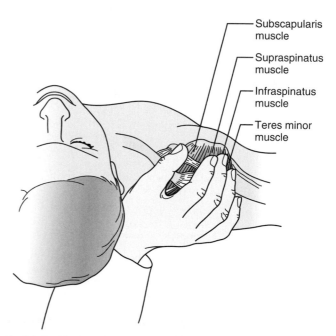

Fig. 5.4 Positioning of the rotator cuff with thumb over subscapularis, index finger over supraspinatus, middle finger over infraspinatus, and ring finger over teres minor.

in the glenoid and, along with the biceps, depresses the humeral head during movements into elevation.

The primary ligaments of the glenohumeral joint—the superior, middle, and inferior glenohumeral ligaments and the coracohumeral ligament—play an important role in stabilizing the shoulder (Fig. 5.6).[32,33] The superior glenohumeral ligament's primary role is limiting inferior

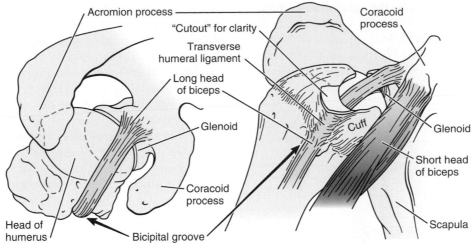

Fig. 5.5 The biceps apparatus.

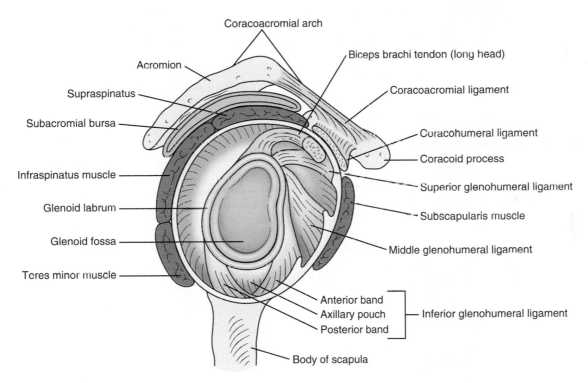

Fig. 5.6 Lateral aspect of the internal surface of the right glenohumeral joint. The humerus has been removed to expose the capsular ligaments and the glenoid fossa. Note the prominent coracoacromial arch and underlying subacromial bursa *(blue)*. The four rotator cuff muscles are shown in *red*. (Redrawn from Neuman DA: *Kinesiology of the musculoskeletal system: foundations for rehabilitation*, ed 2, St Louis, 2010, Mosby/Elsevier, p 139.)

translation in adduction. It also restrains anterior translation and lateral rotation up to 45° of abduction. The middle glenohumeral ligament, which is absent in 30% of the population, limits lateral rotation between 45° and 90° of abduction. The inferior glenohumeral ligament is the most important of the three ligaments. It has an anterior and posterior band with a thin "axillary pouch" in between, so it acts much like a hammock or sling. It supports the humeral head above 90° abduction, limiting inferior translation while the anterior band tightens on lateral rotation and the posterior band tightens on

medial rotation.[34] Excessive lateral rotation, as seen in throwing, may lead to stretching of the anterior portion of the ligament (and capsule), thereby increasing glenohumeral laxity.[35] The coracohumeral ligament primarily limits inferior translation and helps to limit lateral rotation below 60° of abduction. It also helps to stabilize the long head of biceps.[29] This ligament is found in the rotator interval between the anterior border of the supraspinatus tendon and the superior border of the subscapularis tendon; thus, the ligament unites the two tendons anteriorly (Fig. 5.7).[36–38] The **rotator interval** is the anatomic space bound by the subscapularis, supraspinatus, and the coracoid.[39] It consists of fibers of the coracohumeral ligament, middle and superior glenohumeral ligament, long head of biceps tendon and biceps tendon pulley, glenohumeral joint capsule, and part of the tendons of supraspinatus and subscapularis.[38,40] Its

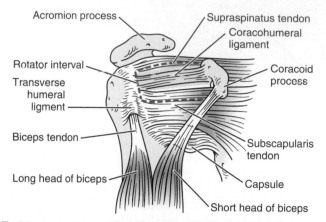

Fig. 5.7 Rotator interval *(between dashed lines)* showing the relationship between the supraspinatus tendon, subscapularis tendon, and the coracohumeral ligament.

role is as a passive stabilizer of the glenohumeral joint and to act as a "check rein" against excessive movement and posteroinferior glenohumeral translation.[39,40] Injury to these structures can lead to contractures (e.g., frozen shoulder), biceps tendon instability, and anterior glenohumeral instability.[38] See Table 5.1 for structures limiting movement in different degrees of abduction.[34,41] The coracoacromial ligament forms an arch over the humeral head, acting as a block to superior translation.[42] The transverse humeral ligament forms a roof over the bicipital groove to hold the long head of biceps tendon within the groove. The capsular pattern of the glenohumeral joint is most limited in lateral rotation, followed by abduction and medial rotation. Branches of the posterior cord of the brachial plexus and the suprascapular, axillary, and lateral pectoral nerves innervate the joint.

The **acromioclavicular joint** is a plane synovial joint that augments the range of motion (ROM) of the humerus in the glenoid (Fig. 5.8). The bones making up this joint are the acromion process of the scapula and the lateral end of the clavicle. The acromion may have different undersurface shapes or types: type I, flat (17%); type II, curved (43%); type III, hooked (39%); and type IV,

TABLE **5.1**

Structures Limiting Movement in Different Degrees of Abduction

Angle of Abduction	Lateral Rotation	Neutral	Medial Rotation
0°	Superior GH ligament Anterior capsule	Coracohumeral ligament Superior GH ligament Capsule (anterior and posterior) Supraspinatus	Posterior capsule
0°–45° (note: 30°–45° of abduction in the scapular plane [resting position]—maximal looseness of shoulder)	Coracohumeral ligament Superior GH ligament Anterior capsule	Middle GH ligament Posterior capsule Subscapularis Infraspinatus Teres minor	Posterior capsule
45°–60°	Middle GH ligament Coracohumeral ligament Inferior GH ligament (anterior band) Anterior capsule	Middle GH ligament Inferior GH ligament (especially anterior band) Subscapularis Infraspinatus Teres minor	Inferior GH ligament (posterior band) Posterior capsule
60°–90°	Inferior GH ligament (anterior band) Anterior capsule	Inferior GH ligament (especially posterior band) Middle GH ligament	Inferior GH ligament (posterior band) Posterior capsule
90°–120°	Inferior GH ligament (anterior band) Anterior capsule	Inferior GH ligament	Inferior GH ligament (posterior band) Posterior capsule
120°–180°	Inferior GH ligament (anterior band) Anterior capsule	Inferior GH ligament	Inferior GH ligament (posterior band) Posterior capsule

GH, Glenohumeral.
Data from Curl LA, Warren RF: Glenohumeral joint stability—selective cutting studies on the static capsular restraints, *Clin Orthop Relat Res* 330:54–65, 1996; and Peat M, Culham E: Functional anatomy of the shoulder complex, In Andrews JR, Wilks KE, editors: *The athlete's shoulder,* New York, 1994, Churchill Livingstone.

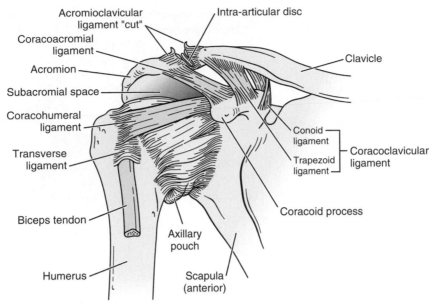

Fig. 5.8 Anterior view of the right glenohumeral and acromioclavicular joints. Note the subacromial space or supraspinatus outlet located between the top of the humeral head and the underside of the acromion. (Modified from Neumann DA: *Kinesiology of the musculoskeletal system: foundations for rehabilitation*, St Louis, 2002, Mosby, p 107.)

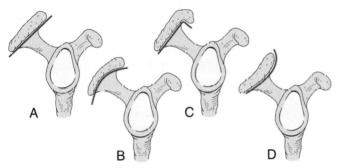

Fig. 5.9 Acromion morphology. (A) Flat. (B) Curved. (C) Hooked. (D) Convex (upturn).

convex (upturned) (1%) (Fig. 5.9).[43] About 70% of rotator cuff tears are associated with a hooked acromion.[43] Some believe that the hooked acromion is not an anatomical variant but rather the result of ossification of the coracoacromial ligament at its attachment to the acromion.[44] The joint has three degrees of freedom. The capsule, which is fibrous, surrounds the joint. An articular disc may be found within the joint. Rarely, the disc separates the acromion and clavicular articular surfaces. This joint depends on ligaments for its strength. The acromioclavicular ligaments surround the joint and control horizontal motion of the clavicle.[45] These are commonly the first ligaments injured when the joint is stressed. The coracoclavicular ligament is the primary support of the acromioclavicular joint. It has two portions: the conoid (medial) and trapezoid (lateral) parts; they control the vertical motion of the clavicle.[45,46] If a step deformity is found, this ligament has been torn. In the resting position of the joint, the arm rests by the side in the normal, standing position. In the

close packed position of the acromioclavicular joint, the arm is abducted to 90°. The indication of a capsular pattern in the joint is pain at the extreme ROM, especially in horizontal adduction (cross flexion) and full elevation. This joint is innervated by branches of the suprascapular and lateral pectoral nerve.

Acromioclavicular Joint

Resting position:	Arm resting by side in normal physiological position
Close packed position:	90° abduction
Capsular pattern:	Pain at extremes of range of motion, especially horizontal adduction and full elevation

The **sternoclavicular joint,** along with the acromioclavicular joint, enables the humerus in the glenoid to move through a full 180° of abduction (Fig. 5.10). It is a saddle-shaped synovial joint with three degrees of freedom and is made up of the medial end of the clavicle, the manubrium of the sternum, and the cartilage of the first rib. It is the joint that joins the appendicular skeleton to the axial skeleton.[47] A substantial disc lies between the two bony joint surfaces, and the capsule is thicker anteriorly than posteriorly. The disc separates the articular surfaces of the clavicle and sternum and adds significant strength to the joint because of its attachments, thereby preventing medial displacement of the clavicle. As in the case of the acromioclavicular joint, this joint depends on ligaments for its strength. The ligaments of the sternoclavicular joint include the anterior

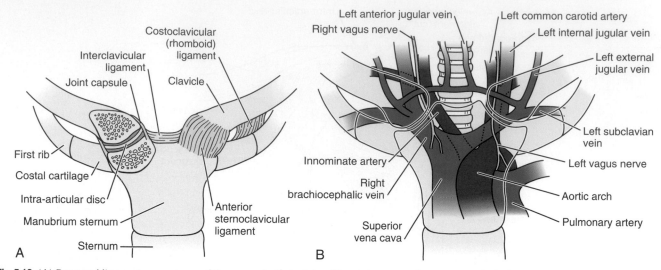

Fig. 5.10 (A) Bony and ligamentous anatomy of the sternoclavicular joint. The major supporting structures include the anterior capsule, the posterior capsule, the interclavicular ligament, the costoclavicular (rhomboid) ligament, and the intra-articular disc and ligament. (B) Retrosternal anatomy. Note the proximity of the sternoclavicular joint to the trachea, aortic arch, and brachiocephalic vein. (Redrawn from Higginbotham TO, Kuhn JE: Atraumatic disorders of the sternoclavicular joint, *J Am Acad Ortho Surg* 13:139, 2005.)

and posterior sternoclavicular ligaments, which support the joint anteriorly and posteriorly; the interclavicular ligament; and the costoclavicular ligament running from the clavicle to the first rib and its costal cartilage. This is the main ligament maintaining the integrity of the sternoclavicular joint. The movements possible at this joint and at the acromioclavicular joint are elevation, depression, protraction, retraction, and rotation. The close packed position of the sternoclavicular joint involves full or maximum rotation of the clavicle, which occurs when the upper arm is in full elevation. The resting position and capsular pattern are the same as with the acromioclavicular joint. The joint is innervated by branches of the anterior supraclavicular nerve and the nerve to the subclavius muscle. Major vessels and the trachea lie close behind the sternum and the sternoclavicular joint (see Fig. 5.10B).[47]

Sternoclavicular Joint

Resting position:	Arm resting by side in normal physiological position
Close packed position:	Full elevation and protraction
Capsular pattern:	Pain at extremes of range of motion, especially horizontal adduction and full elevation

---

Although the **scapulothoracic joint** is not a true joint, it functions as an integral part of the shoulder complex and must be considered in any assessment because a stable scapula enables the rest of the shoulder to function correctly. Some texts call this structure the scapulocostal joint. This "joint" consists of the body of

the scapula and the muscles covering the posterior chest wall. The muscles acting on the scapula help to control its movements. The medial border of the scapula is not parallel with the spinous processes but is angled about 3° away (top to bottom), and the scapula lies 20° to 30° forward relative to the sagittal plane.[32] Because it is not a true joint, it does not have a capsular pattern nor a close packed position. The resting position of this joint is the same as for the acromioclavicular joint. The scapula extends from the level of T2 spinous process to T7 or T9 spinous process, depending on its size. The scapula acts as a stable base for the rotator cuff muscles; the muscles controlling its movements must be strong and balanced because the joint funnels the forces of the trunk and legs into the arm.[48]

When the shoulder is being assessed, especially in athletes and people who work overhead, it is important to look not only at the shoulder but also the whole kinetic chain (Table 5.2).[49] **Kinetic chain** refers to the linkage of multiple segments of the body that allow the transfer of forces and motion starting at the feet, lower extremities, core, and trunk, which provide a base of support and generate energy or power that can be transferred to the shoulder, arm, and hand.[50–53] Changes, deficits, or breaks in any of these segments can cause performance to decrease and injuries to occur.[18,50] When assessing active individuals, it is often important to consider looking at the whole kinetic chain to determine which part or parts of the chain is/are contributing to the problem. Table 5.3 provides an example of a whole-body kinetic chain involved in throwing and issues that can arise when there are deficits in a throwing kinetic chain.[50]

TABLE 5.2

Proximal to Distal Kinetic Chain Evaluation

Examination Emphasis	Normal	Abnormal	Result	Evaluation
One-leg stability: stance	Negative Trendelenburg	Positive Trendelenburg	Decreased force to shoulder	Gluteus medius strength
One-leg stability: squat	Control of knee varus/valgus during descent	Knee valgus or corkscrewing during descent	Altered arm position during task	Dynamic postural control
Hip rotation	Bilateral symmetry within known normal limits	Side-to-side asymmetry and/or not within normal limits	Decreased trunk flexibility and rotation	Medial and lateral rotation of hip
Plank	Ability to maintain body position for at least 30 seconds	Inability to maintain body position	Decreased core stability and strength	Dynamic postural control in suspended horizontal position
Scapular dyskinesis	Bilateral symmetry with no inferior angle or medial border prominence	Side-to-side asymmetry or bilateral prominence of inferior angle and/or medial border	Decreased rotator cuff function and increased risk of internal and/or external impingement	Scapular muscle control of scapular position ("yes/no" clinical evaluation, manual corrective maneuvers)
Shoulder rotation	Side-to-side asymmetry or medial and lateral rotation values <15° or <5°	Side-to-side asymmetry of 15° or more in medial and/or lateral rotation or 5° or more of total ROM	Altered kinematics and increased load on the glenoid labrum	Medial and lateral rotation of glenohumeral joint
Shoulder muscle flexibility	Normal mobility of pectoralis minor and latissimus dorsi	Tight pectoralis minor and/or latissimus dorsi	Scapular protraction	Palpation of pectoralis minor and latissimus dorsi
Shoulder strength	Normal resistance to testing in anterior and posterior muscles	Weakness and/or imbalance of anterior and posterior muscles	Scapular protraction; decreased arm elevation, strength, and concavity compression	Muscle strength from a stabilized scapula
Joint internal derangement	All provocative and stress testing negative	Pop, click, slide, pain, stiffness, possible "dead arm"	Loss of concavity compression and functional stability	Labral injury, rotator cuff injury or weakness, glenohumeral instability, biceps tendinopathy

ROM, Range of motion.
From Kibler WB, Wilkes T, Sciascia A: Mechanics and pathomechanics in the overhead athlete, *Clin Sports Med* 32:637–651, 2013.

TABLE 5.3

Phases of Throwing and the Kinetic Chain

Phase	Required Motions/ Normal Mechanics	Function	Deficits/Pathomechanics	Evaluation
Phase 1: Windup	*Stance leg:* Hip abduction, extension Knee flexion (isometric knee extensor contraction)	Provides a stable base for the kinetic chain	Weakness in hip abductors, extensors and knee Unstable base "Catch-up" phenomenon Potential injury in distal kinetic chain Overload of lower extremity muscles to stabilize unstable balance Premature forward motion, poor balance Increase forces on distal kinetic chain	*Stance leg:* Single leg balance (standing, partial squat) Hip abduction strength (side-lying, single-leg stance) Hip extensor strength (standing, prone) Quadriceps strength

Continued

TABLE **5.3**

Phases of Throwing and the Kinetic Chain—cont'd

Phase	Required Motions/ Normal Mechanics	Function	Deficits/Pathomechanics	Evaluation
Phase 2: Stride	*Stance leg:* Hip abduction, extension Knee extension Hip medial rotation *Stride leg:* Hip lateral rotation Foot positioned toward target *Shoulder:* Shoulder lateral rotation, abduction Scapular protraction, forward tilt, lateral rotation	Provides a stable base for kinetic chain Prepares the throwing arm for the next phases of throwing	Hip and knee weakness: unstable base Hip medial rotation deficits Premature opening up or forward pelvic rotation Increased demand on distal kinetic chain Hip external range deficits → Altered foot positioning Foot positions that close the body increase load on obliques, hip Foot positions that open the body increase load on abdominals, shoulder, medial elbow	*Stance leg:* Single leg balance and hip/knee strength Hip medial rotation ROM *Stride leg:* Hip lateral rotation ROM Foot positioning of stride leg *Shoulder:* Glenohumeral ROM Scapular dyskinesis evaluation
Phase 3: Arm cocking	*Stride leg:* Knee extension	Decelerates flexed knee (eccentric) Stabilizes stride leg (isometric) Provides stable base	Weakness or tightness of knee extensors: Decreased stability Impaired kinetic chain energy transfer distally Loss of velocity and accuracy Overuse injuries (shoulder, elbow)	Quadriceps strength
	Trunk: Pelvis rotation toward target Lumbar spine hyperextension Upper torso rotation	Eccentric control of abdominal obliques to prevent hyperextension	Early trunk rotation Increase valgus strain on elbow Hyperextension of lumbar spine	Timing of trunk rotation Trunk flexibility
	Throwing arm: Elbow flexion Shoulder lateral rotation Shoulder abduction to 90° Scapular retraction, lateral rotation, posterior tilt Hand on top of ball	Elbow and hand lag behind shoulder Rotator cuff activation provides stability to glenohumeral joint Maintains subacromial space Avoids impingement	GIRD >18°–20° Risk of shoulder, elbow injury Increased glenohumeral lateral rotation Risk of SLAP tears, impingement, rotator cuff tears Increased valgus elbow strain Scapular dyskinesis → external impingement, internal impingement, decreased rotator cuff strength, anterior capsular strain Decreased elbow flexion → increased valgus elbow strain Hand is under or on the side of the ball → increased valgus elbow strain	Glenohumeral ROM Elbow ROM Scapular dyskinesis Hand positioning
Phase 4: Acceleration	*Throwing arm:* Elbow extension Shoulder medial rotation Shoulder abduction to 90° Scapular protraction *Trunk:* Forward flexion *Stride leg:* Hip flexion, knee extension	Lag between elbow extension and shoulder medial rotation to decrease rotational resistance along longitudinal axis Stable base of support	If throwing elbow is dropped below 90° of abduction Increased valgus load on the elbow Hyperlordosis or back extension Increased load on the abdominals Creates a "slow arm" Increased compression loads at the shoulder	Positioning of elbow Scapular dyskinesis Eccentric and concentric control of lumbar motion in standing position

TABLE **5.3**

Phases of Throwing and the Kinetic Chain—cont'd

Phase	Required Motions/ Normal Mechanics	Function	Deficits/Pathomechanics	Evaluation
Phase 5: **Deceleration**	*Arm/shoulder:* Arm deceleration Shoulder medial rotation deceleration Elbow extension deceleration Scapula returns to anterior tilted position	Decelerates throwing arm Counterbalance large medial rotation torque Rotator cuff contraction, posterior capsule limits excessive anterior humeral translation	Most overuse injuries of the posterior arm or trunk occur in this phase or at follow-through Energy must be safely dissipated	Rotator cuff strength Scapular dyskinesis
Phase 6: **Follow-through**	*Trunk deceleration* *Shoulder deceleration* *Scapular deceleration* *Elbow deceleration*	Stride leg stabilizes and absorbs forces eccentrically	Most overuse injuries of the posterior arm or trunk occur in this phase or the late deceleration phase Energy must be safely dissipated	Lumbar flexion Scapular dyskinesis Shoulder horizontal adduction ROM

GIRD, Glenohumeral internal rotation deficit; *ROM,* range of motion; *SLAP,* superior labrum anterior to posterior.
Modified from Chu SK, Jayabalan P, Kibler WB, Press J: The kinetic chain revisited: new concepts on throwing mechanics in injury, *Phys Med Rehabil* 8(3 Suppl):S72, 2016. Adapted from Kibler WB, Wilkes T, Sciascia A: Mechanics and pathomechanics in the overhead athlete, *Clin Sports Med* 32:637–651, 2013.

Patient History

In addition to the questions listed under "Patient History" in Chapter 1, the examiner should obtain the following information from the patient.[54] Most commonly the patient complains of pain, especially on movement; restricted motion; or shoulder instability.

1. *What is the patient's age?* Many problems of the shoulder can be age-related. For example, rotator cuff degeneration usually occurs in patients who are between 40 and 60 years of age. Rotator cuff tears, which can occur at any age, are more likely to be seen in individuals over 65 years of age (especially full-thickness tears).[55] Litaker et al.[56] suggested that external rotation weakness, night pain, and age over 65 are indicative of rotator cuff tears. Murrell and Watson reported that there was a 98% chance of having a full-thickness rotator cuff tear if the patient's age was greater than 60 years, there was weakness in abduction, and the patient had a positive impingement sign.[57] Park and colleagues reported that having a positive painful arc sign, a positive drop-arm sign, and weakness in shoulder lateral rotation equated with a greater than 90% chance of having a full-thickness rotator cuff tear.[58] Primary impingement due to degeneration and weakness is usually seen in patients above 35 years of age, whereas secondary impingement due to instability caused by weakness in the scapular or humeral control muscles is more common in people in their late teens or their twenties, especially those involved in vigorous overhead activities such as swimming or pitching in baseball.[59] Calcium deposits may occur between the ages of 20 and 40 years.[60] Chondrosarcomas may be seen in those above 30 years of age, whereas frozen shoulder resulting from causes other than trauma is seen in persons between the ages of 45 and 60 years (Tables 5.4 and 5.5). Frozen shoulder due to trauma can occur at any age but is more common with increased age. Overuse damage to the proximal humeral physis (i.e., Little Leaguer's shoulder or apophysitis) may be seen in young, skeletally immature baseball pitchers and tennis players due to chronic repetitive, microtraumatic shear, torque, or traction forces to the physis when the arm is used.[61]

2. *Does the patient support the upper limb in a protected position* (Fig. 5.11) *or hesitate to move it?* This action could mean that one of the joints of the shoulder complex is unstable or that there is an acute problem in the shoulder. In some cases, patients with lax shoulders ask, "What happens when I do this?" In effect, the patient is subluxing the shoulder (Fig. 5.12). This may or may not be pathological, but it is a sign of voluntary instability in which the patient uses his or her muscles to sublux the humerus in the glenoid, stressing the labrum and inert tissues.

3. *If there was an injury, what exactly was the mechanism of injury?* Did the patient injure himself or herself

TABLE **5.4**

Differential Diagnosis of Rotator Cuff Degeneration, Frozen Shoulder, Atraumatic Instability, and Cervical Spondylosis

	Rotator Cuff Lesions	Frozen Shoulder	Atraumatic Instability	Cervical Spondylosis
History	Age 30–50 years Pain and weakness after eccentric load	Age 45+ (insidious type) Insidious onset or after trauma or surgery Functional restriction of lateral rotation, abduction, and medial rotation	Age 10–35 years Pain and instability with activity No history of trauma	Age 50+ years Acute or chronic
Observation	Normal bone and soft-tissue outlines Protective shoulder hike may be seen	Normal bone and soft-tissue outlines	Normal bone and soft-tissue outlines	Minimal or no cervical spine movement Torticollis may be present
Active movement	Weakness of abduction or rotation, or both Crepitus may be present	Restricted ROM Shoulder hiking	Full or excessive ROM	Limited ROM with pain
Passive movement	Pain if impingement occurs	Limited ROM, especially in lateral rotation, abduction, and medial rotation (capsular pattern)	Normal or excessive ROM	Limited ROM (symptoms may be exacerbated)
Resisted isometric movement	Pain and weakness on abduction and lateral rotation	Normal when arm by side	Normal	Normal except if nerve root compressed Myotome may be affected
Special tests	Drop-arm test positive Empty: can test positive	None	Load and shift test positive Apprehension test positive Relocation test positive Augmentation tests positive	Spurling's test positive Distraction test positive ULNT positive Shoulder abduction test positive
Sensory function and reflexes	Not affected	Not affected		Dermatomes affected Reflexes affected
Palpation	Tender over rotator cuff	Aching, not painful unless capsule is stretched	Anterior or posterior pain	Tender over appropriate vertebra or facet
Diagnostic imaging	Radiography: Upward displacement of humeral head; acromial spurring MRI diagnostic	Radiography: Negative Arthrography: Decreased capsular size	Negative	Radiography: Narrowing osteophytes

MRI, Magnetic resonance imaging; *ROM,* range of motion; ULNT, upper limb neurodynamic (tension) test.

with a fall on outstretched hand (FOOSH), which could indicate a fracture or dislocation of the glenohumeral joint? Did the patient fall on or receive a blow to the tip of the shoulder, or did the patient land on the elbow, driving the humerus up against the acromion? This finding may indicate an acromioclavicular dislocation or subluxation.[62,63] A blow to the posterolateral shoulder can cause the lateral clavicle to be pushed anteriorly while the medial clavicle is pushed posteriorly, which may lead to complications

TABLE **5.5**

Differential Diagnosis of Shoulder Pathology

Pathology	Symptoms
External primary impingement (stage I)	Intermittent mild pain with overhead activities Over age 35
External primary impingement (stage II)	Mild to moderate pain with overhead activities or strenuous activities
External primary impingement (stage III)	Pain at rest or with activities Night pain may occur Scapular or rotator cuff weakness is noted
Rotator cuff tears (full thickness)	Classic night pain Weakness noted predominantly in abduction and lateral rotators Loss of motion
Adhesive capsulitis (idiopathic frozen shoulder)	Inability to perform ADLs owing to loss of motion Loss of motion may be perceived as weakness
Anterior instability (with or without external secondary impingement)	Apprehension to mechanical shifting limits activities Slipping, popping, or sliding may present as instability Apprehension usually associated with horizontal abduction and lateral rotation Anterior or posterior pain may be present Weak scapular stabilizers
Posterior instability	Slipping or popping of the humerus out the back This may be associated with forward flexion and medial rotation while the shoulder is under a compressive load
Multidirectional instability	Looseness of shoulder in all directions This may be most pronounced while the patient is carrying luggage or turning over while asleep Pain may or may not be present

ADLs, Activities of daily living.
Modified from Maughon TS, Andrews JR: The subjective evaluation of the shoulder in the athlete, In Andrews JR, Wilk KE, editors: *The athlete's shoulder*, New York, 1994, Churchill Livingstone, p 36.

because of the close association of the neurovascular structures behind the medial end of the clavicle (see Fig. 5.10B).[64] Does the shoulder feel unstable or feel as if it were "coming out" during movement? Does the arm "go dead" when engaged in an activity? "Going dead" implies that the patient cannot use

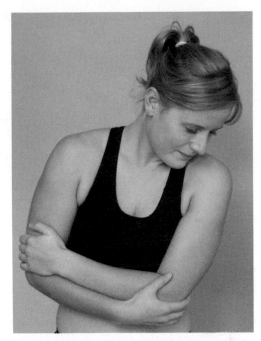

Fig. 5.11 Patient supporting the left upper arm in protected position.

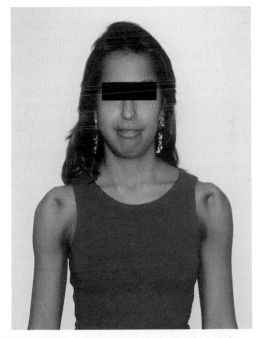

Fig. 5.12 Voluntary instability. Note how the patient uses her muscles to sublux the humerus posteriorly in the glenoid, resulting in an anterior sulcus in each shoulder.

the arm functionally because of pain and a subjective feeling of unease when the arm is used.[65] Patients with instability may appear normal on clinical examination, especially if the shoulder muscles are not fatigued. Many overuse injuries are more evident immediately after the patient does an activity repeatedly.[66] This may indicate gross or anatomical instability, as in recurrent shoulder dislocation, subluxation, or

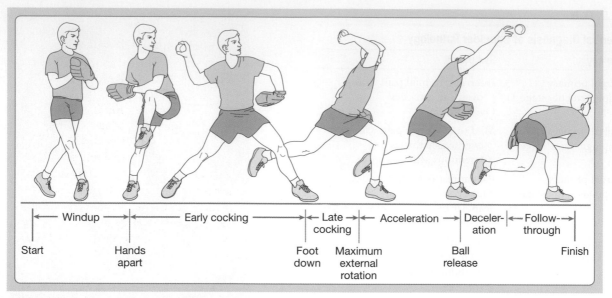

Fig. 5.13 Phases of overhead throwing and key events. Similar patterns are seen when equipment is used (e.g., in tennis or football). Note how the whole kinetic chain is involved in the activity. (From Harrast MA, Laker SR, Maslowski E, De Luigi AJ: Sports medicine and adaptive sports. In Cifu DX, Kaelin DL, Kowalske KJ et al., editors: *Braddom's physical medicine and rehabilitation*, ed 5, Philadelphia, 2016, Elsevier.)

subtle translational instability. The spectrum of instability varies from gross or anatomical instability—the TUBS type (**T**raumatic onset, **U**nidirectional anterior with a **B**ankart lesion responding to **S**urgery) to a more subtle translational instability—the AMBRI type (**A**traumatic cause, **M**ultidirectional with **B**ilateral shoulder findings with **R**ehabilitation as appropriate treatment and, rarely, **I**nferior capsular shift surgery).

4. *Are there any movements or positions that cause the patient pain or symptoms?* If so, which ones? The examiner must keep in mind that cervical spine movements may cause pain in the shoulder. Persons who have had recurrent dislocations/instability of the shoulder may find that any movement involving lateral rotation bothers them, because this movement is involved in anterior dislocations of the shoulder. With subacromial impingement, the pectoralis minor tends to be overactive during elevation activities.[67] Questions related to instability should include the following[68]:
   a. How many episodes have there been in the last year?
   b. Was there an injury that precipitated this?
   c. In which direction does the shoulder "go out" most times?
   d. Have you ever needed help getting the shoulder back into proper position within the joint (i.e., reduced dislocation)?

   If the patient complains of pain with overhead activity, especially if the patient is an athlete, the examiner will want to know what phase of the movement causes pain (Fig. 5.13) and how it affects the kinetic chain.[69,70] With an unstable and painful shoulder, the patient may complain of pain when his or her hand is placed behind the head with the elbow backward (i.e., the **siesta sign**) (Fig. 5.14A) or when the patient is carrying a heavy weight with the arm extended along the body (i.e., the **suitcase sign**) (Fig. 5.14B).

Recurrent dislocators may sometimes show pain at extreme medial rotation when the humeral head is "tightened" against the anterior glenoid. Pathology of the long head of biceps causes pain that moves medially and laterally with medial and lateral rotation of the shoulder.[71] Excessive abduction and lateral rotation may lead to the dead-arm syndrome, in which the patient feels a sudden paralyzing pain and weakness in the shoulder.[65] This finding often indicates altered shoulder mechanics, commonly involving a tight posterior capsule, altered arthrokinematics of the glenohumeral joint, and **scapular dyskinesia.**[65,72,73] In throwers, the condition may be referred to as a **"SICK" scapula** (malposition of **S**capula, prominence of **I**nferior medial border of scapula, **C**oracoid pain and malposition, and scapular dys**K**inesia).[74] If the patient complains of pain during specific phases of pitching (for example, during the late cocking and acceleration phases), anterior instability should be considered even in the presence of minimal clinical signs.[75] Commonly, instability and secondary impingement occur together. Secondary impingement implies that although impingement signs are present, they result from a primary problem somewhere else, commonly in the scapular or humeral

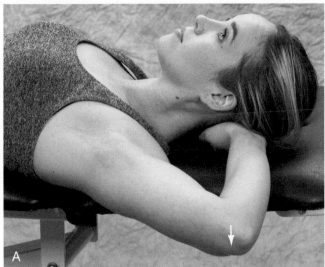

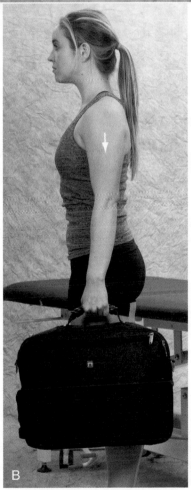

Fig. 5.14 (A) Siesta sign. (B) Suitcase sign.

control or stabilizer muscles. Primary impingement implies that impingement or pinching is the primary cause of the pain.

Stability of the shoulder depends on both dynamic stabilizers (the muscles) and static stabilizers (e.g., the capsule and the labrum).[34] Night pain and resting

pain are often related to rotator cuff tears and on occasion to tumors; activity-related pain usually signifies paratenonitis. Arthritis pain commonly arises, at least initially, at the extremes of motion. Acromioclavicular pain is especially evident at greater than 90° of abduction and tends to be localized to the joint. Similarly, sternoclavicular pain is localized to the joint and increases on horizontal adduction and sometimes can be referred to the lateral neck area and can overlap pain from the acromioclavicular joint and the subacromial space.[76] In addition, the injured joint will be painful on shoulder protraction and retraction.[76]

5. *What is the extent and behavior of the patient's pain?* For example, deep, boring, toothache-like pain in the neck, shoulder region, or both may indicate **thoracic outlet syndrome** (Fig. 5.15)[77] or acute brachial plexus neuropathy. Strains of the rotator cuff usually cause dull, toothache-like pain that is worse at night, whereas acute calcific tendinitis usually causes a hot, burning type of pain. Sprain of the first or second rib from direct trauma or sudden contraction of the scaleni may mimic an acute impingement or rotator cuff injury.[78]

6. *Are there any activities that cause or increase the pain?* For example, bicipital paratenonitis or tendinosis[79] are often seen in skiers and may result from holding on to a ski tow; in cross-country skiing, it may result from poling (using the pole for propulsion). Paratenonitis is inflammation of the paratenon of the tendon. The paratenon is the outer covering of the tendon, whether or not it is lined with synovium. Tendinosis is actual degeneration of the tendon itself. With chronic overuse, tendinosis is more likely than paratenonitis (Table 5.6; see Table 1.20).[79,80] Elite swimmers may train for more than 15,000 m daily, which can lead to stress overload (repetitive microtrauma) of the structures of the shoulder. Does throwing or reaching alter the pain? If so, what positions cause pain or discomfort? These questions may indicate which structures are injured.

7. *Do any positions relieve the pain?* Patients with nerve root pain may find that elevating the arm over the head relieves symptoms. For a patient with instability or inflammatory conditions, lifting the arm over the head usually exacerbates shoulder problems.

8. *What is the patient unable to do functionally?* Is the patient able to talk or swallow? Is the patient hoarse? These signs could indicate an injury to the sternoclavicular joint (if there is swelling) or a posterior dislocation of the joint because pressure is being applied to the trachea. In addition, determining whether the shoulder has been overstressed or overused is important.[81] For example, in swimmers and baseball pitchers, it is important to determine the following[82]:

   a. The age when the patient first began the activity
   b. The total years of throwing/swimming

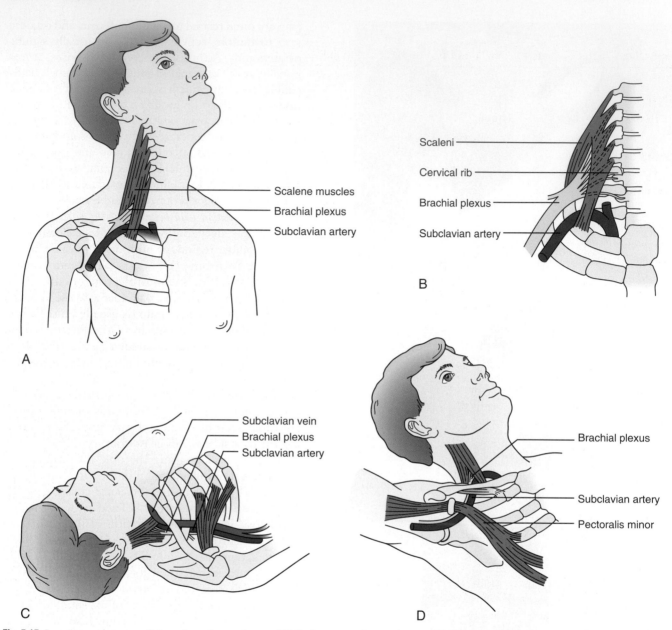

Fig. 5.15 Location and causes of thoracic outlet syndrome. (A) Scalenus anterior syndrome. (B) Cervical rib syndrome. (C) Costoclavicular space syndrome. (D) Hyperabduction syndrome (abduction, extension, and lateral rotation).

c. The number of pitches thrown per outing
d. The number of games/innings pitched per year
e. The distances swam per week
f. The strokes used/types of pitches thrown
g. The amount of rest between outings
h. Whether there was any complete rest from activity during the year
i. Whether there was any previous injury related to the activity
j. The phase of activity that produces the symptoms

9. *How long has the problem bothered the patient?* For example, an idiopathic frozen shoulder goes through three stages: the condition becomes progressively worse, eventually plateaus, and then progressively improves, with each stage lasting 3 to 5 months.[83,84]

10. *Is there any indication of muscle spasm, deformity, bruising, wasting, paresthesia, or numbness?*[85] These findings can help the examiner to determine the acuteness of the condition and potentially the structures injured.

11. *Does the patient complain of weakness and heaviness in the limb after activity?* Does the limb tire easily? These findings may indicate vascular involvement. Are there any venous symptoms, such as swelling or stiffness, that may extend all the way to the fingers? Are there any arterial symptoms, such as coolness or

TABLE **5.6**

Implications of the Diagnosis of Tendinosis Compared With Tendinitis

Trait	Overuse Tendinosis	Overuse Tendinitis
Prevalence	Common	Rare
Time for recovery, early presentation	6–10 weeks	Several days to 2 weeks
Time for full recovery, chronic presentation	3–6 months	4–6 weeks
Likelihood of full recovery to sport from chronic symptoms	Approximately 80%	99%
Focus of conservative therapy	Encouragement of collagen-synthesis, maturation and strength	Anti-inflammatory modalities and drugs
Role of surgery	Excise abnormal tissue	Not known
Prognosis for surgery	70%–85%	95%
Time for recovery from surgery	4–6 months	3–4 weeks

From Khan KM, Cook JL, Taunton JE, et al: Overuse tendinosis, not tendonitis. Part 1: a new paradigm for a difficult clinical problem, *Phys Sportsmed* 28:43, 2000. Reproduced with permission of McGraw Hill.

pallor in the upper limb? These complaints may result from pressure on an artery, a vein, or both. An example is thoracic outlet syndrome (see Fig. 5.15), in which pressure may be applied to the vascular or neurological structures as they enter the upper limb in three locations: at the scalene triangle, at the costoclavicular space, and under the pectoralis minor and the coracoid process.[86,87] Excessive repetitive demands placed on the shoulder (such as, those seen in pitching) may lead to thoracic outlet syndrome, axillary artery occlusion, effort thrombosis, or pressure in the quadrilateral space. (The quadrilateral space has as its boundaries the medial border of the humerus laterally, the lateral border of the long head of triceps medially, the inferior border of the teres minor, and the superior border of the teres major.)[88]

12. *Is there any indication of nerve injury?* The examiner should evaluate the nerves and the muscles supplied by the nerves to determine possible nerve injury. Any history of weakness, numbness, or paresthesia may indicate nerve injury (Table 5.7). For example, the suprascapular nerve may be injured as it passes through the suprascapular notch under the transverse scapular ligament, leading to atrophy and paralysis of the supra- and infraspinatus muscles. The examiner should listen to the patient's account carefully, because this condition can mimic a third-degree (rupture) strain of the supraspinatus tendon. Another potential nerve injury is one to the axillary (circumflex) nerve (Fig. 5.16) or musculocutaneous nerve (Fig. 5.17)

after dislocation of the glenohumeral joint. With an axillary nerve injury, the deltoid and teres minor muscles are atrophied and weak or paralyzed. The radial nerve (see Fig. 5.16) is sometimes injured as it winds around the posterior aspect of the shaft of the humerus. The injury frequently occurs when the humeral shaft is fractured. If the nerve is damaged in this location, the extensors of the elbow, wrist, and fingers are affected, and an altered sensation occurs in the radial nerve's sensory distribution.

13. *Which hand is dominant?* Often the dominant shoulder is lower than the nondominant shoulder and the ROM may not be the same for both. The dominant shoulder usually shows greater muscularity and can show a different ROM from that of the nondominant shoulder.[89]

Causes of Primary and Secondary Shoulder Impingement Syndrome

- Abnormal glenohumeral arthrokinematics (secondary)
- Abnormal scapulothoracic arthrokinematics (secondary)
- "Slouched" (chin poking) posture (secondary)
- Muscle weakness or fatigue (secondary)
- Muscle hypomobility (secondary)
- Capsule tightness, especially posterior (secondary)
- Inflammation in the subacromial space (primary)
- Degeneration of the rotator cuff tendon (primary)
- Adhesions, especially inferiorly (secondary)
- Osteophytes under the acromioclavicular joint (primary)
- Hooked acromion (primary)
- Hypermobility of the glenohumeral joint (primary)

TABLE **5.7**

Peripheral Nerve Injuries (Neuropathy) About the Shoulder

Affected Nerve (Root)	Muscle Weakness	Sensory Alteration	Reflexes Affected	Mechanism of Injury
Suprascapular nerve (C5, C6)	Supraspinatus, infraspinatus (arm lateral rotation)	Top of shoulder from clavicle to spine of scapula Pain in posterior shoulder radiating into arm	None	Compression in suprascapular notch Stretch into scapular protraction plus horizontal adduction Compression in spinoglenoid notch Direct blow Space-occupying lesion (e.g., ganglion)
Axillary (circumflex) nerve (posterior cord; C5, C6)	Deltoid, teres minor (arm abduction)	Deltoid area Anterior shoulder pain	None	Anterior glenohumeral dislocation or fracture of surgical neck of humerus Forced abduction Surgery for instability
Radial nerve (C5–C8, T1)	Triceps, wrist extensors, finger extensors (shoulder, wrist, and hand extension)	Dorsum of hand	Triceps	Fracture humeral shaft Pressure (e.g., crutch palsy)
Long thoracic nerve (C5, C6, [C7])	Serratus anterior (scapular control)	None	None	Direct blow Traction Compression against internal chest wall (backpack injury) Heavy effort above shoulder height Repetitive strain
Musculocutaneous nerve (C5–C7)	Coracobrachialis, biceps, brachialis (elbow flexion)	Lateral aspect of forearm	Biceps	Compression Muscle hypertrophy Direct blow Fracture (clavicle or humerus) Dislocation (anterior) Surgery (Putti-Platt, Bankart)
Spinal accessory nerve (cranial nerve XI; C3, C4)	Trapezius (shoulder elevation)	Brachial plexus symptoms possible because of drooping of shoulder Shoulder aching	None	Direct blow Traction (shoulder depression and neck rotation to opposite side) Biopsy
Subscapular nerve (posterior cord; C5, C6)	Subscapularis, teres major (arm medial rotation)	None	None	Direct blow Traction
Dorsal scapular nerve (C5)	Levator scapulae, rhomboid major, rhomboid minor (scapular retraction and elevation)	None	None	Direct blow Compression
Lateral pectoral nerve (C5, C6)	Pectoralis major, pectoralis minor	None	None	Direct blow
Thoracodorsal nerve (C6, C7, [C8])	Latissimus dorsi	None	None	Direct blow Compression
Supraclavicular nerve	None	Mild clavicular pain Sensory loss over anterior shoulder	None	Compression

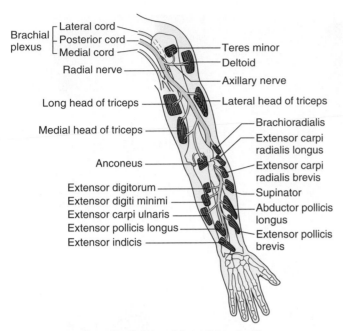

Fig. 5.16 Motor distribution of the radial and axillary nerves.

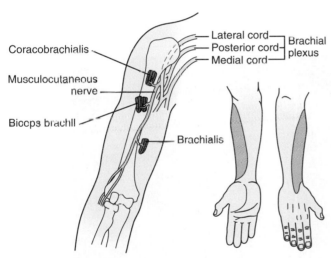

Fig. 5.17 Motor and sensory distribution of musculocutaneous nerve.

Observation

The patient must be suitably undressed so that the examiner can observe the bony and soft-tissue contours of both shoulders and determine whether they are normal and symmetric. While observing the shoulder, the examiner looks at the head, the cervical spine, the thorax (especially the posterior aspect), and the entire upper limb. The hand, for example, may show vasomotor changes that result from problems in the shoulder, including shiny skin, hair loss, swelling, and muscle atrophy.

It is important to observe the patient as he or she removes clothes from the upper body and later replaces them. For example, does the patient undress the affected arm last or dress it first? This pattern indicates that the patient is limiting the movement of the arm as much as possible, signifying

possible pathology. The patient's actions give some indication of functional restriction, pain, or weakness in the upper limb.

As part of the observation, noting whether the patient can assume a "neutral pelvis" position is important, because an abnormal pelvic position can lead to an abnormal scapulothoracic, glenohumeral, and cervical spine position and abnormal kinematics in these joints (i.e., alteration in the kinetic chain). In addition, kinematics plays a role in how much force that contributes to an activity can be generated by the lower quadrant. For example, about 50% of the force of throwing is normally generated by the lower quadrant or kinetic chain. Three questions must be asked by the examiner related to the "neutral pelvic" position:

1. Can the patient get into the "neutral pelvis" position?
2. Can the patient hold the static neutral pelvis position while making distal dynamic movements (e.g., shoulder movements)?
3. Can the patient control a dynamic neutral pelvis while making dynamic shoulder movements?

If the answer to any of the questions is negative, the examiner must consider including the pelvis and any restricted parts of the lower quadrant or kinetic chain in the treatment plan for the shoulder.

Anterior View

When the examiner is looking at the patient from the anterior view (Fig. 5.18A), he or she should begin by ensuring that the head and neck are in the midline of the body and observing their relation to the shoulders. A forward head posture is often associated with rounded shoulders, a medially rotated humerus, and a protracted scapula. This will result in the humeral head translating anteriorly; a tight posterior capsule; tightness of the pectoral, upper trapezius, and levator scapulae muscles; and weakness of the lower scapular stabilizers and deep neck flexors.[90] While observing the shoulder, the examiner should look for the possibility of a **step deformity** (Fig. 5.19A). Such a deformity may be caused by an acromioclavicular dislocation with the distal end of the clavicle lying superior to the acromion process. Seen at rest, a step deformity indicates both the acromioclavicular and coracoclavicular ligaments have been torn. The deformity may be accentuated by asking the patient to horizontally adduct the arm or to medially rotate the shoulder and bring the hand up the back as high as possible. Occasionally swelling is evident anterior to the acromioclavicular joint. This is called the **fountain sign** and indicates that degeneration has caused communication between the acromioclavicular joint and swollen subacromial bursa underneath.[91] If a **sulcus deformity** appears when traction is applied to the arm, it may be caused by multidirectional instability or loss of muscle control due to nerve injury or a stroke, leading to inferior subluxation of the glenohumeral joint (Fig. 5.19B). This deformity is lateral to the acromion and should not be confused with

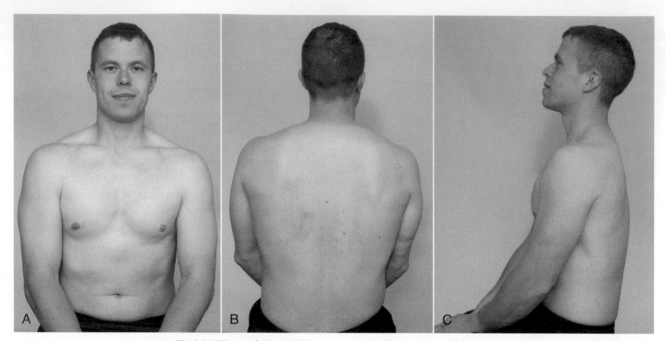

Fig. 5.18 Views of the shoulder. (A) Anterior. (B) Posterior. (C) Side.

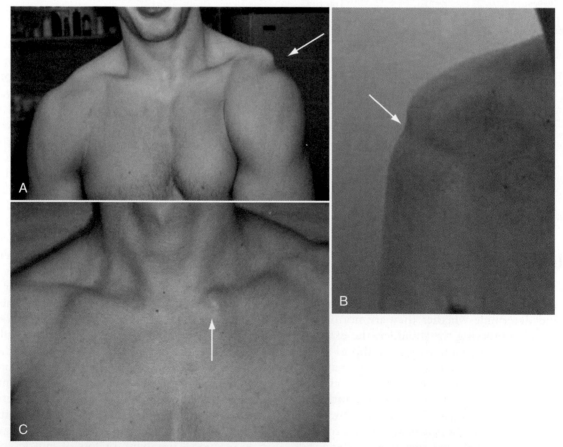

Fig. 5.19 (A) Step deformity resulting from acromioclavicular dislocation *(arrow)*. (B) Subluxation of glenohumeral joint following a stroke (paralysis of deltoid muscle). (C) Anterior dislocation at the sternoclavicular joint *(arrow)*.

a step deformity. This is also referred to as a **sulcus sign** because of the appearance of a sulcus or groove below the acromion process. Subluxation or dislocation at the sternoclavicular joint may be seen (Fig. 5.19C), although swelling may hide a subluxation. With a posterior dislocation, the examiner must be aware of vascular tissues behind the joint, which may be injured (see Fig. 5.10). Flattening of the normally round deltoid muscle area may indicate an anterior dislocation of the glenohumeral joint or paralysis of the deltoid muscle (Fig. 5.20). With an anterior dislocation, note also how the arm is held abducted because of the location of the humeral head below the glenoid. If the examiner palpated in the axilla, he or she would feel the head of the humerus. The examiner should note any abnormal bumps or malalignment in the bones that may indicate past injury, such as a healed fracture of the clavicle.

In most people, the dominant side is lower than the nondominant side. This difference may be caused by extra use of the dominant side, which stretches the ligaments, joint

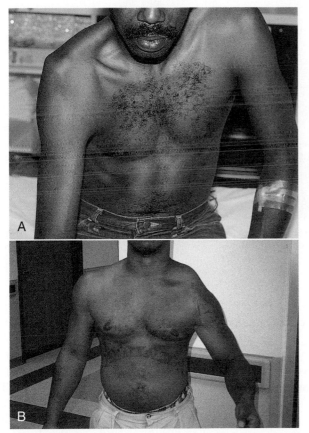

Fig. 5.20 (A) Typical manifestation of an anterior right shoulder dislocation. The shoulder is very painful; thus the patient resists movement. The outer round contour of the shoulder is flattened, and the displaced humeral head can be appreciated in the subcoracoid area or axilla. Frequently, the patient abducts the arm slightly, bends the torso toward the injured side, and supports the flexed elbow on the injured side with the other hand. (B) Obvious left shoulder dislocation—a chronic dislocation that frequently occurs with minimal trauma. In this case the patient was able to dislocate it at will and feign a new injury, thus being able to obtain narcotics from multiple emergency departments. (From Naples RM, Ufberg JW: Management of common dislocations. In Roberts JR, Custalow CB, Thomsen TW, editors: *Roberts and Hedges' clinical procedures in emergency medicine and acute care,* ed 7, Philadelphia, 2019, Elsevier.)

capsules, and muscles, allowing the arm to sag slightly. Tennis players[92] and others who stretch their upper limbs in a reaching action show even greater differences, along with gross hypertrophy of the muscles on the dominant side (Fig. 5.21). If the patient is protective of the shoulder, however, it may appear that the injured shoulder, whether dominant or nondominant, is higher than the normal side (see Fig. 5.11).

The examiner notes whether the patient is able to assume the normal functional position for the shoulder, which is in the scapular plane with 60° of abduction and the arm in neutral or no rotation. In this position or with the arm abducted to 90°, rupture or congenital absence of the pectoralis major may be evident (Figs. 5.22 and 5.23) or the presence of the **axillopectoral muscle (i.e., Langer Axillary Arch)** may be present, which is the most common anomalous muscle in the axillary fossa (Fig. 5.24) and should not be confused with congenital absence of the sternal head of pectoralis major.[93–96] Rupture of the pectoralis major is often accompanied by a tearing sensation and pop, along with weakness, painful limitation of movement, and ecchymosis.[93] If the patient's arm is medially rotated from this position to bring the hand into midline, the biceps tendon is forced against the lesser tuberosity of the medial wall of the bicipital (intertubercular) groove. If this position is maintained for long periods, there may be increased wear on the biceps tendon, which can lead to bicipital tendinitis or paratenonitis. If the arm is horizontally adducted while it is medially rotated, anterior pain indicates impingement symptoms (Hawkins-Kennedy test—see "Special Tests," later). The width and depth of the bicipital groove may vary (Fig. 5.25), possibly leading to problems if the shoulder is overused. Especially wide or deep grooves lead to the greatest problems. The wide grooves tend to allow the tendon too much lateral movement, leading to inflammation of the paratenon (paratenonitis)[79]; the deep grooves tend to be too narrow, thus compressing the tendon, especially if it becomes inflamed.[97]

Posterior View

When the patient is viewed from behind (Fig. 5.18B), the examiner again notes bony and soft-tissue contours and body alignment, especially scapular malpositioning.[98] The scapula plays a major role in the shoulder.[99] First, it provides an origin for the rotator cuff muscles as well as the biceps and triceps muscles; therefore it provides a stable dynamic base from which these muscles act. Second, it maintains the glenohumeral alignment within physiological limits that facilitates congruency and concavity compression capability at the glenohumeral joint through the full ROM. Third, the attachment of the acromion to the clavicle leads to scapular upward rotation and posterior tilt to allow maximum arm elevation. Finally, the scapula facilitates force transfer from the shoulder to the core (and vice versa), acting like a funnel for efficient energy transfer. This transfer of forces can involve the whole kinetic chain. By using this "chain" correctly, the patient can decrease the stresses on the shoulder itself.

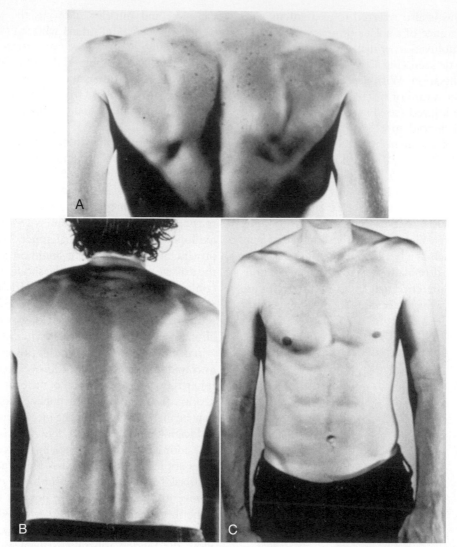

Fig. 5.21 Depressed right shoulder in a right-dominant individual—in this case, a tennis player. (A) Hypertrophy of playing shoulder muscles. (B) With muscles relaxed, the distance between spinous processes and the medial border of the scapula is widened on the right. (C) Depressed shoulder. (From Priest JD, Nagel DA: Tennis shoulder, *Am J Sports Med* 4:33, 1976.)

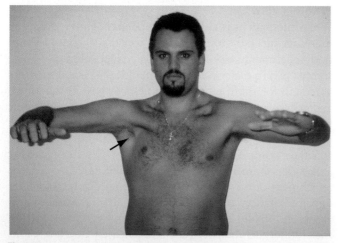

Fig. 5.22 Congenital absence of the sternal head of the pectoralis major. Note the axillopectoral muscle *(arrow)*.

Atrophy of the upper trapezius may indicate spinal accessory nerve palsy, whereas atrophy of supraspinatus or infraspinatus may indicate supraspinous nerve palsy.[100] The spines of the scapulae, which begin medially at the level of the third thoracic (T3) vertebra, should be at the same angle. The scapula itself should extend from the T2 or T3 spinous process to the T7 or T9 spinous process of the thoracic vertebrae with the medial border parallel to the thoracic midline.[101] The scapula on the dominant side will sit lower and further away from the spine than on the nondominant side. Sobush and associates developed a method for measuring the scapular position called the **Lennie test.**[102] In this test, they measured from the spinous processes horizontally to three scapular positions: the medial aspect of the most superior point (superior angle), the root of the spine of the scapula, and the inferior angle (Fig. 5.26).[102] If the scapula is sitting lower than normal

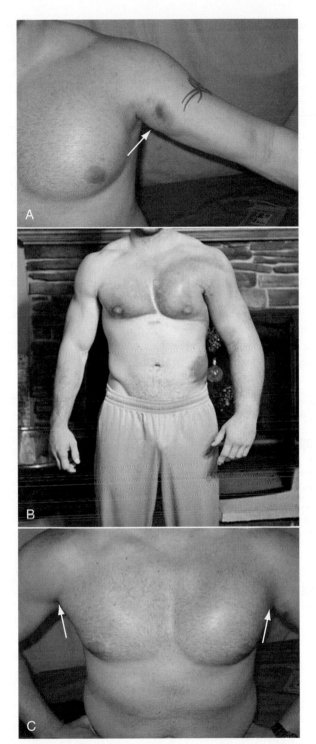

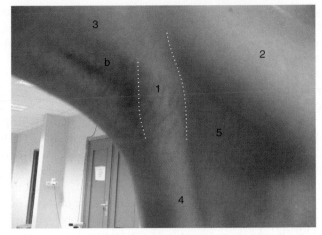

Fig. 5.24 Langer axillary arch *(1, outlined in dashed lines)*; pectoralis major *(2)*; biceps brachii *(3)*; insertion tendon of latissimus dorsi *(4)*; subscapularis *(5)*; and neurovascular bundle *(b)*. (From Van Hoof T, Vangestel C, Shacklock M, et al: Asymmetry of the ULNT1 elbow extension range-of-motion in a healthy population: Consequences for clinical practice and research. *Phys Ther Sport* 13(3):141–149, 2011.)

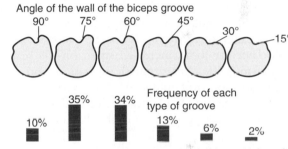

Fig. 5.25 Different shapes of the bicipital groove. (Adapted from Hitchcock HH, Bechtol CO: Painful shoulder: observation on the role of the tendon of the long head of the biceps brachii in its causation, *J Bone Joint Surg Am* 30:267, 1948.)

Fig. 5.23 Rupture of the pectoralis major. (A) Ecchymosis and swelling, with *arrow* illustrating the sternal head rupture of pectoralis major. (B) Massive swelling and bruising after rupture of the pectoralis major. (C) Loss of axillary fold on the left side due to a pectoralis major tear creates an asymmetry compared with the normal right side. (From Provencher MT, Handfield K, Boniquit NT, et al: Injuries to the pectoralis major muscle—diagnosis and management, *Am J Sports Med* 38:1693–1705, 2010.)

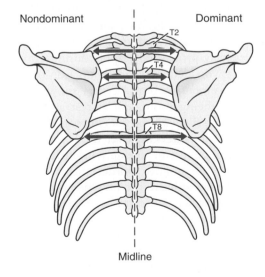

Fig. 5.26 Lennie test. Measurements are taken at three positions on the scapula, and the dominant and nondominant sides are compared.

against the chest wall, the superior medial border of the scapula may "washboard" over the ribs, causing a snapping or clunking sound (snapping scapula) during abduction and adduction.[103–107] Other causes of snapping may be spinal kyphosis, rounded shoulders, forward tipped scapula, and a chin poking posture.[108] The inferior angles of the scapulae should be equidistant from the spine.

In some patients, morphological **"subacromial dimples"** are found over the posteromedial deltoid of both shoulders about 1 cm (0.4 inch) below and medial to the posterior angle of the acromion. They are present at all times whether the shoulder is at rest, moving, or stressed. It has been postulated that these dimples are associated with recurrent posterior positional instability.[109] In odd cases where both atrophy and weakness are present bilaterally, the examiner should consider inherited myogenic disorders such as **limb girdle muscular dystrophy (LGMD)** or **facioscapulohumeral dystrophy (FSHD)**.[110]

Scapular dyskinesia, or **scapular dysfunction**, although not an injury itself, can lead to altered glenohumeral joint angulation, abnormal stress on shoulder ligaments, altered subacromial space, overload of the acromioclavicular joint, increased strain on the scapular stabilizing muscles, altered muscle activation, and modified arm position and motion.[99] For example, a tight pectoralis minor muscle can lead to secondary impingement caused by the anterior tilt of the scapula and medial rotation of its inferior angle.[111] Abnormal positions of the scapula are defined as tilting, winging, or **dysrhythmia** (i.e., abnormality [premature, excessive or stuttering] in movement rhythm) (Fig. 5.27).[72,101,112] The sequencing of muscle activation patterns and muscle performance and length that help stabilize the scapula along with inhibition due to pain are altered with dyskinesia.[112–114] These alterations are commonly the result of an excessively protracted scapula during arm motion. Kibler et al.[115] divided scapular dysfunction or dyskinesia into four movement patterns. Type I shows the inferior medial border being prominent at rest and the inferior angle tilting dorsally with movement (scapular tilt), while the acromion tilts anteriorly over the top of the thorax. It may be seen at rest or during concentric or eccentric movement. If the inferior border tilts away from the chest wall, it may indicate the presence of weak muscles (e.g., lower trapezius, latissimus dorsi, serratus anterior) or a tight pectoralis minor or major pulling, or tilting, the scapula forward from above.[74] Type II is the classic winging of the scapula with the whole medial border of the scapula being prominent and lifting away from the posterior chest wall both statically and dynamically (Fig. 5.28). It too may be seen at rest or during eccentric or concentric movements. This deformity may indicate the presence of a SLAP lesion to the biceps; weakness of the serratus anterior; rhomboids; lower, middle, and upper trapezius; a long thoracic nerve problem; or tight humeral

rotators.[74] Type III is illustrated by the superior border of the scapula being elevated at rest and during movement; a shoulder shrug initiates the movement, and there is minimal winging. This deformity is seen with active movement and may result from overactivity of the levator scapula and upper trapezius along with imbalance of the upper and lower trapezius force couple (Fig. 5.29). It is associated with impingement and rotator cuff lesions.[74] In the type IV pattern, which is normal, both scapulae are symmetrical at rest and during motion; they rotate symmetrically upward with the inferior angles rotating laterally away from midline (rotary winging). It is seen during movement and may indicate that the scapular control muscles are stabilizing the scapula. Huang et al.[116,117] added further to Kibler's classification by including mixed scapular dyskinesia patterns (Table 5.8), noting that the patterns may be different during the elevation (through forward flexion and abduction) and lowering phases with the lowering phases showing more dramatic loss of control. To increase the loss of scapular control and increase the deformity, the examiner can have the patient hold a weight in the hand during the movement.[118,119]

Causes of Scapular Dyskinesia[99]

BONY
- Thoracic kyphosis
- Clavicular fracture nonunion
- Clavicular fracture malunion

JOINT
- Acromioclavicular instability
- Acromioclavicular arthrosis
- Glenohumeral internal derangement

NEUROLOGICAL
- Cervical radiculopathy
- Long thoracic nerve palsy
- Spinal accessory nerve palsy

SOFT TISSUE
- Intrinsic muscle pathology (1°, 2°, or 3° strain)
- Hypomobility (e.g., short head of biceps, pectoralis minor)
- Glenohumeral internal rotation deficit (GIRD)
- Altered muscle activation patterns
- Altered muscle force-couple action

MYOGENIC DISORDERS
- Limb girdle muscular dystrophy (LGMD)
- Facioscapulohumeral dystrophy (FSHD)

Kibler et al.[99] advocated a **dynamic scapular motion test** ✓ to test for scapular dyskinesia. The patient, while holding a 3-lb to 5-lb (1.4-kg to 2.3-kg) weight in the hand, is asked to fully elevate and lower the arms three to five times into forward flexion or scaption. The examiner

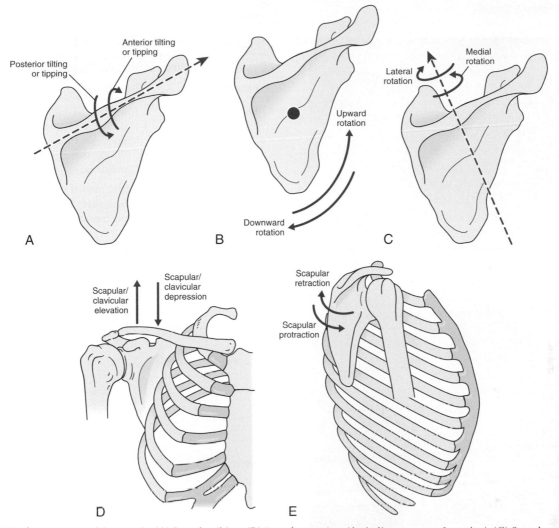

Fig. 5.27 Individual movements of the scapula. (A) Scapular tilting. (B) Scapular rotation (*dot indicates center of rotation*). (C) Scapular rotation winging. (D) Scapular/clavicular elevation. (E) Scapular protraction and retraction along the chest wall. (Modified from McClure PW, Bialker J, Neff N, et al: Shoulder function and 3-dimensional kinematics in people with shoulder impingement syndrome before and after a 6-week exercise program, *Phys Ther* 84[9]:832–848, 2004.)

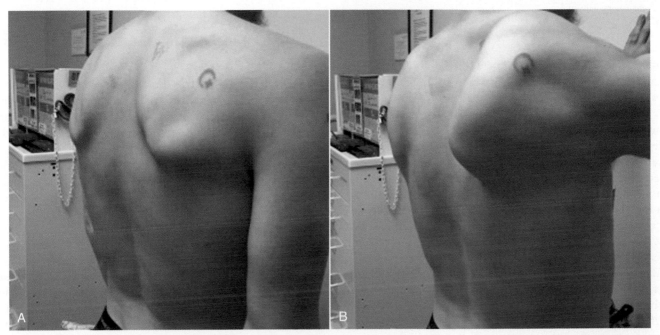

Fig. 5.28 Winging of the medial border of the scapula. (A) At rest, the patient has subtle prominence of the medial border of the right scapula. (B) When the patient flexes his arm forward and pushes against a wall, the medial border of the right scapula protrudes from the posterior chest wall ("winged scapula"). (From Chiu EF, Miller TA, Canders CP: Winged scapula, *Visual J Emerg Med* 13:135–136, 2018.)

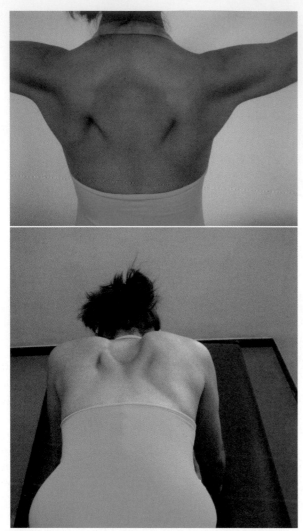

Fig. 5.29 Imbalance pattern of the upper and lower trapezius. Note over-development of the upper trapezius and the lower trapezius working to prevent rotary winging.

TABLE **5.8**

Detailed Descriptions of Scapular Dyskinesis Patterns

Pattern	Descriptions
Pattern I	Inferomedial angle of the scapula is displaced posteriorly from the posterior thorax and is prominent during dynamic observation and palpation
Pattern II	Entire medial border of the scapula is displaced posteriorly from the posterior thorax and is prominent during dynamic observation and palpation
Pattern III	Early scapular elevation or excessive/insufficient scapular upward rotation (dysrythmia) during dynamic observation and palpation compared with asymptomatic side
Pattern IV (normal)	1. No evidence of posterior displacement in medial border/inferior angle of the scapula and excessive/insufficient scapular movement 2. Minimal motion during the initial 30°–60° of scapulohumeral elevation, then smoothly and continuously rotating upward and downward during humeral elevation and lowering, respectively
Mixed patterns	Mixed condition of abnormal patterns: (1) patterns I + II; (2) patterns II + III; (3) pattern I + III; (4) pattern I + II + III

From Huang TS, Huang HY, Wang TG, et al: Comprehensive classification test of scapular dyskinesis: a reliability study, *Man Ther* 20(3):429, 2015.

watches for prominence of the medial border of the scapula (i.e., classic winging), which indicates a positive test.[120]

Primary scapular winging implies that the winging is the result of muscle weakness of one of the scapular muscle stabilizers. This, in turn, disrupts the normal muscle force couple balance of the scapulothoracic complex.[121] **Secondary scapular winging** implies that the normal movement of the scapula is altered because of pathology in the glenohumeral joint.[121] **Dynamic scapular winging** (i.e., winging with movement) may be caused by a lesion of the long thoracic nerve affecting serratus anterior, trapezius palsy (spinal accessory nerve), rhomboid weakness, multidirectional instability, voluntary action, or a painful shoulder resulting in splinting of the glenohumeral joint, which in turn causes reverse scapulohumeral rhythm.[122] This splinting of the glenohumeral joint leads to reverse origin-insertion of the rotator cuff muscles so that instead

of moving the humerus as they normally would, they work in reverse fashion and move the scapula. Commonly, with pathology, the scapular control muscles are weak and cannot counteract this action, resulting in protraction of the scapula and dynamic winging. The two other common causes of dynamic winging—long thoracic nerve palsy and spinal accessory nerve palsy—cause different scapular positioning and different winging patterns. Spinal accessory nerve palsy causes the scapula to depress and move laterally with the inferior angle rotated laterally. If the trapezius is weak or paralyzed, the winging of the scapula occurs before 90° abduction, and there is little winging on forward flexion.[123] Long thoracic nerve palsy causes the scapula to elevate and move medially with the inferior angle rotating medially (Fig. 5.30).[124,125] If the serratus anterior is weak or paralyzed, the winging of the scapula occurs on abduction and forward flexion (especially with a "punch out" forward against resistance) (see Fig. 5.28B).[123,126] Radiculopathies at C3, C4 (trapezius), C5 (rhomboids), and C7 (serratus anterior, rhomboids) can also cause winging.[127,128]

Static winging (i.e., winging occurring at rest) is usually caused by a structural deformity of the scapula, clavicle, spine, or ribs.[129]

Sprengel's deformity, which is a developmental condition leading to a high or undescended scapula (Fig. 5.31), is rare, but it is the most common congenital deformity of the shoulder complex.[130–133] With this deformity, the scapular muscles are poorly developed or are replaced by a fibrous band. The condition may be unilateral or bilateral, and the range of the shoulder abduction decreases, leading to decreased shoulder

function. Usually, the scapula is smaller than normal and is medially rotated. It may be associated with other anomalies (e.g., scoliosis, Klippel-Feil syndrome, rib anomalies).[133]

The shoulder muscles may be accentuated by having the patient place the hands on the hips and contract the muscles. The examiner should check closely for wasting in the supraspinatus and infraspinatus muscles (suprascapular nerve palsy), the serratus anterior muscle (long thoracic nerve palsy), and the trapezius muscle (spinal accessory nerve palsy), all of which can lead to winging of the scapula.

Examination

Because assessment of the shoulder may include an assessment of the cervical spine, the examination can be an extensive one. If the examiner has any doubt as to the location of the lesion, a cervical spine assessment (see Chapter 3) should be performed. In addition, the examiner must remember that the arm, of which the shoulder is an integral part, may act as an open kinetic chain when the hand is free to move or as a closed kinetic chain when the hand is fixed to some relatively immovable object. For example, scapular instability may be evident with a closed kinetic chain when the arm is fixed and the rotator cuff muscles work in reverse order (reverse origin-insertion; for example, the insertion of the muscles into the humerus becomes the stable part because the arm is fixed, whereas the scapula becomes the mobile part and is more likely to move) (Fig. 5.32). It may also

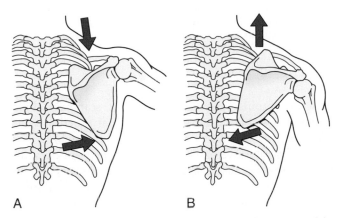

Fig. 5.30 Scapular movement resulting in scapular winging caused by trapezius palsy (A) and serratus anterior palsy (B).

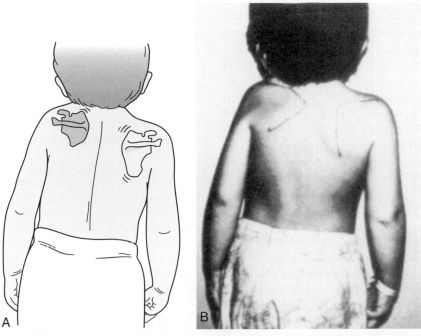

Fig. 5.31 Sprengel's deformity. Diagram (A) and photograph (B) of child with Sprengel's deformity. Note elevated shoulder and poorly developed scapula on the left. (A, Modified from Gartland JJ: *Fundamentals of orthopaedics*, Philadelphia, 1979, WB Saunders, p 73. B, Courtesy Dr. Roshen Irani.)

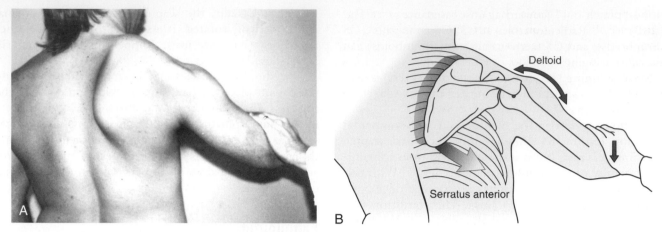

Fig. 5.32 The pathomechanics of "classic winging" of the scapula. (A) Winging of the right scapula caused by marked weakness of the right serratus anterior. The winging of the medial border of the scapula is exaggerated when resistance is applied against a shoulder abduction effort. Note how the stabilization occurs where the examiner's hand is offering resistance. Instead of the arm moving, the scapula moves because its stabilizing muscles are weak. (B) Kinesiologic analysis of the winging scapula. Without an adequate upward rotation force from the serratus anterior *(fading arrow)*, the scapula becomes unstable and cannot resist the pull of the deltoid. Subsequently, the force of the deltoid *(bidirectional arrow)* causes the scapula to rotate downward and the glenohumeral joint to partially abduct (reverse origin-insertion). (From Neumann DA: *Kinesiology of the musculoskeletal system: foundations for physical rehabilitation*, St Louis, 2002, Mosby, p 107.)

be evident with an open kinetic chain, especially during high-speed movements when the scapula must be stabilized (e.g., when hitting a ball) or when the scapular muscles should be working eccentrically to slow or stop a movement (i.e., they are unable to do so because of weakness). With an open kinetic chain, the scapula acts as the base or origin of the muscles, whereas the insertion into the humerus is more mobile. Knowledge of muscle balance and muscle force couples becomes imperative in determining a diagnosis. For example, the legs, pelvis, and trunk act as force generators, whereas the shoulder acts as a funnel and force regulator with the arm acting as the force delivery system.[74] These **kinetic chains** and the intricate and complex interplay of the components of the kinetic chain have different effects on the shoulder. Eating, reaching, and dressing are considered open-kinetic-chain activities, whereas crutch walking and pushing up from a chair are considered closed-kinetic-chain movements.

As with any assessment, the examiner is comparing one side of the body with the other. This comparison is necessary because of individual differences among normal people.

Active Movements

The first movements to be examined are the active movements. These are usually done in such a way that the painful movements are performed last, so that pain does not carry over to the next movement. It is important to remember that shoulder movements are a combination of not only glenohumeral, scapulothoracic, acromioclavicular, and sternoclavicular movements but also of maximum end-range movement, which can involve the thoracic spine and ribs.[134] Thus, being able to differentiate

between scapular movement and the scapula's ability to act as a stable base for glenohumeral function while allowing itself to move is essential, as is watching how glenohumeral movements are accomplished during active movements, because scapular movement often compensates for restricted glenohumeral movement, leading to weak and often lengthened scapular control muscles. This, in turn, leads to rotator cuff overuse as the body attempts to control upper kinetic chain movement.[135] If scapular dyskinesis is present without pain, individuals who use their shoulder excessively, especially with overhead movement, will have a high risk of developing shoulder pain.[136] In effect, they have a "time bomb" shoulder, which, if overused or overstressed, will start to develop problems, including weak muscles (e.g., scapular control muscles, rotator cuff), tight muscles (e.g., pectoralis minor), and an unstable glenohumeral joint.

Active Movements of the Shoulder Complex

- Elevation through abduction (170°–180°)
- Elevation through forward flexion (160°–180°)
- Elevation through the plane of the scapula (170°–180°)
- Lateral (external) rotation (80°–90°)
- Medial (internal) rotation (60°–100°)
- Extension (50°–60°)
- Adduction (50°–75°)
- Horizontal adduction/abduction (cross flexion/cross extension; 130°)
- Circumduction (200°)
- Scapular protraction
- Scapular retraction
- Combined movements (if necessary)
- Repetitive movements (if necessary)
- Sustained positions (if necessary)

Scapular dysrhythmia is demonstrated by premature excessive elevation or protraction of the scapula, unsmooth or stuttering motion on elevation or especially on lowering, or rapid downward rotation during arm lowering.[101] In addition, posture can affect the ROM at the shoulder. A slouched (i.e., rounded shoulder) posture with forward-head posture causes the scapula to have more superior translation between 0° and 90° of elevation, along with more anterior tilt and less upward rotation (i.e., more medial rotation) between 90° and maximum abduction, and slightly more medial rotation during abduction with less serratus anterior activity during forward flexion.[51,137,138] In forward flexion, there is more scapular medial rotation.[139] Thus active shoulder movement should be observed in the patient's normal posture and in a corrected position (i.e., if the patient can hold the corrected position) to see if signs and symptoms and/or ROM changes or whether other parts of the kinetic chain need correction to restore normal kinetic chain movement.

An understanding of the **force couples** acting on the shoulder complex and the necessity of balancing the muscle strength and endurance of these muscles is especially important when the shoulder is being assessed.[140] Force couples are groups of counteracting muscles that show obvious action when a movement is loaded or done quickly.[141] With a particular movement, one group of muscles (the agonists) acts concentrically or as "movers," whereas the other group (the antagonists) acts eccentrically and as dynamic stabilizers in a controlled, harmonized fashion to produce smooth movement. Thus these muscles may work by co-contraction or co-activation to provide a stabilizing effect and joint control. If these functions are altered or lost, then movement is altered, often leading to stress overload and pain.[142] Table 5.9 gives examples of some of the force couples acting about the shoulder.

Active elevation through abduction is normally 170° to 180°. The extreme of the ROM occurs when the arm is abducted and lies against the ear on the same side of the head (Fig. 5.33). The examiner must watch that the

TABLE **5.9**

Force Couples About the Shoulder

Movement	Agonist/Stabilizer	Antagonist/Stabilizer
Protraction (scapula)	Serratus anterior[a] Pectoralis major[b] and minor[b]	Trapezius Rhomboids
Retraction (scapula)	Trapezius Rhomboids	Serratus anterior[a] Pectoralis major[b] and minor[b]
Elevation (scapula)	Upper trapezius[b] Levator scapulae[b]	Serratus anterior[a] Lower trapezius[a]
Depression (scapula)	Serratus anterior[a] Lower trapezius[a]	Upper trapezius[b] Levator scapulae[b]
Lateral rotation (upward rotation of inferior angle of scapula)	Trapezius (upper[b] and lower[a] fibers) Serratus anterior[a]	Levator scapulae[b] Rhomboids Pectoralis minor[b]
Medial rotation (downward rotation of inferior angle of scapula)	Levator scapulae[b] Rhomboids Pectoralis minor[b]	Trapezius (upper[b] and lower[a] fibers) Serratus anterior[a]
Scapular stabilization	Upper trapezius[b] Lower trapezius[a] Rhomboids	Serratus anterior[a]
Abduction (humerus)	Deltoid	Supraspinatus
Medial rotation (humerus)	Subscapularis[b] Pectoralis major[b] Latissimus dorsi Anterior deltoid Teres major	Infraspinatus[a] Teres minor Posterior deltoid
Lateral rotation (humerus)	Infraspinatus Teres minor Posterior deltoid	Subscapularis[b] Pectoralis major[b] Latissimus dorsi Anterior deltoid

[a]Muscles prone to weakness.
[b]Muscles prone to tightness.

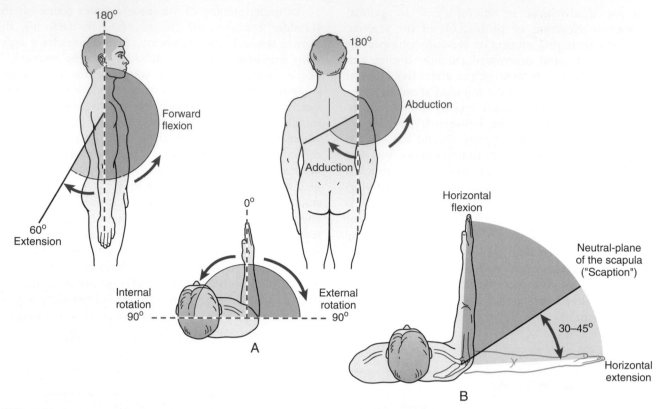

Fig. 5.33 Movement in the shoulder complex. (A) Range of motion of the shoulder. (B) Axes of arm elevation. (Adapted from Perry J: Anatomy and biomechanics of the shoulder in throwing, swimming, gymnastics, and tennis, *Clin Sports Med* 2:255, 1983.)

patient does not shrug (i.e., elevate the scapula) the shoulders when the movement is being done. This **"shrug sign"** indicates an inability to lift the arm to 90° without elevating the scapula. The shrug sign is commonly associated with adhesive capsulitis, large rotator cuff tears, and glenohumeral arthritis.[98,142,143] As the patient elevates the upper extremity by abducting the shoulder, the examiner should note whether a **painful arc** ⚠ is present (Fig. 5.34).[144] A painful arc may be caused by subacromial bursitis, calcium deposits, a peritenonitis or tendinosis[79,80] of the rotator cuff muscles, or most commonly by an unstable scapula. The pain results from the pinching of inflamed or tender structures under the acromion process and the coracoacromial ligament. Initially, the structures are not pinched under the acromion process, so the patient is able to abduct the arm 45° to 60° with little difficulty. As the patient abducts further (60° to 120°), the structures (e.g., subacromial bursa, rotator cuff tendon insertions, especially supraspinatus) become pinched, and the patient is often unable to abduct fully because of pain. If full abduction is possible, however, the pain diminishes after approximately 120° because the pinched soft tissues have passed under the acromion process and are no longer being pinched. Often, the pain is greater going up (against gravity) than coming down, and there is more pain on active abduction than on passive abduction. If the movement is very painful, the patient often elevates the arm through forward flexion or hikes the shoulder, using the upper

trapezius and levator scapulae in an attempt to decrease the pain. In some cases, retracting the scapula and holding it retracted slightly enlarges the space under the coracoacromial space, which may decrease the pain. It has been reported that the painful arc sign, a positive drop-arm test, and a positive infraspinatus test are strong indicators of a full-thickness rotator cuff tear.[58] A second painful arc in the shoulder may be seen during the same abduction movement. This painful arc (see Fig. 5.34) occurs toward the end of abduction, in the last 10° to 20° of elevation, and is caused by pathology in the acromioclavicular joint or by a positive impingement test. In the case of the acromioclavicular joint lesion, the pain tends to be localized to the joint. With the impingement syndrome, the pain is usually found in the anterior shoulder region. Table 5.10 presents the signs and symptoms of three types of painful arc in the shoulder with the superior type being the most common. The arc of pain may also be present during elevation through forward flexion and scaption, although the pain is usually less severe on these movements. The interconnection of the subacromial, subcoracoid, and subscapularis bursae with each other and with the glenohumeral joint capsule often produces a broad area of signs and symptoms, which may result in a painful arc.

When examining the movement of elevation through abduction, the examiner must take time to observe **scapulohumeral rhythm** of the shoulder complex (Fig. 5.35), both anteriorly and posteriorly.[145-147]

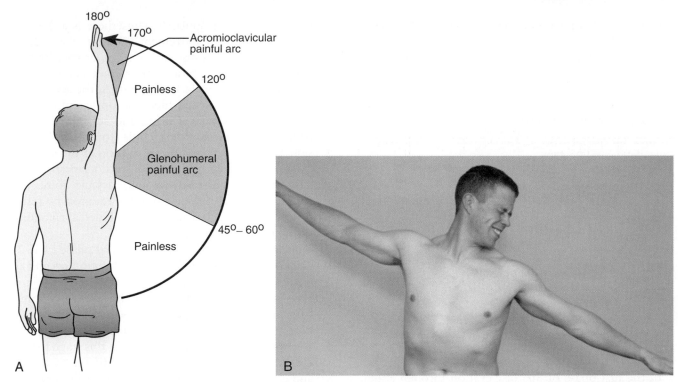

Fig. 5.34 Painful arc in the shoulder. (A) Painful arc of the glenohumeral joint. In the case of acromioclavicular joint problems only, the range of 170° to 180° would elicit pain. (B) Note impingement, which is causing pain on the left at approximately 85°. (A, Modified from Hawkins RJ, Hobeika PE: Impingement syndrome in the athletic shoulder, *Clin Sports Med* 2:391–405, 1983.)

TABLE 5.10

Classification of Glenohumeral Painful Arcs

	Anterior	Posterior	Superior
Night pain	Yes	Yes	Maybe
Age	50+	50+	40+
Sex ratio	F > M	F > M	M > F
Aggravated by	Lateral rotation and abduction	Medial rotation and abduction	Abduction
Tenderness	Lesser tuberosity	Posterior aspect of greater tuberosity	Greater tuberosity
Acromioclavicular joint involvement	No	No	Often
Calcification (if present)	Supraspinatus, infraspinatus, and/or subscapularis	Supraspinatus and/or infraspinatus	Supraspinatus and/or subscapularis
Third-degree strain biceps brachii (long head)	No	No	Occasional
Prognosis	Good	Very good	Poor (without surgery)

From Kessel L, Watson M: The painful arc syndrome, *J Bone Joint Surg Br* 59:166, 1977.

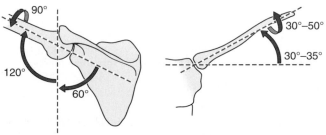

Fig. 5.35 Movement of the scapula, humerus, and clavicle during scapulohumeral rhythm.

That is, during 180° of abduction, there is roughly a 2:1 ratio of movement of the humerus to the scapula with 120° of movement occurring at the glenohumeral joint and 60° at the scapulothoracic joint; one should be aware, however, that there is a great deal of variability among individuals and may depend on the speed of movement,[148] and authors do not totally agree on the exact amounts of each movement.[146,147,149] Although all authors concede that there is more movement in the glenohumeral joint than in the scapulothoracic joint, Davies and Dickoff-Hoffman believe the ratio is greater, at least to 120° of abduction,[150] whereas Poppen and Walker[151] and others[36,152] believe the ratio is less (5:4 or 3:2) after 30° of abduction. During this total simultaneous movement at the four joints, there are three phases; the reader should understand that others will give values of the amount of each movement that vary from those noted here.

Scapulohumeral Rhythm

Phase 1:	Humerus	30° abduction
	Scapula	Minimal movement (setting phase)
	Clavicle	0°–5° elevation
Phase 2:	Humerus	40° abduction
	Scapula	20° rotation, minimal protraction or elevation, and possibly posteriorly tilt
	Clavicle	15° elevation and posterior rotation at sternoclavicular joint
Phase 3:	Humerus	60° abduction, 90° lateral rotation
	Scapula	30° rotation
	Clavicle	30°–50° posterior rotation, up to 15° elevation

---

1. In the first phase of 30° of elevation through abduction, the scapula is said to be "setting." This setting phase means that the scapula may rotate slightly in, rotate slightly out, or not move at all.[126] Thus, there is no 2:1 ratio of movement during this phase. The angle between the scapular spine and the clavicle may also increase up to 5° by elevating at the sternoclavicular and acromioclavicular joints,[145] but this depends on whether the scapula moves during this phase. The clavicle rotates upward minimally during this stage.

2. During the next 60° of elevation (second phase), the scapula rotates upward (inferior angle moves out) about 20° and begins to posteriorly tilt,[153] and the humerus elevates 40° with minimal protraction or elevation of the scapula.[145] Thus there is a 2:1 ratio of scapulohumeral movement. During phase 2, the clavicle elevates because of the scapular rotation[36,145] and begins to rotate posteriorly, retract, and minimally elevate at the sternoclavicular joint. At the acromioclavicular joint, the clavicle tilts posteriorly and upwardly and rotates medially. During the second and third phases, the rotation of the scapula (total of 60°) is possible because there are 20° of motion at the acromioclavicular joint and 40° at the sternoclavicular joint. The sternoclavicular and acromioclavicular joints contribute to scapulothoracic upward rotation by retraction at the sternoclavicular joint and medial rotation at the acromioclavicular joint.[153]

3. During the final 90° of motion (third phase), the 2:1 ratio of scapulohumeral movement continues and the angle between the scapular spine and the clavicle increases an additional 10°. Thus the scapula continues to rotate and now begins to elevate. The amount of protraction continues to be minimal when the abduction movement is performed. It is in this stage that the clavicle rotates posteriorly 30° to 50° on a long axis and elevates up to a further 15°.[36] In reality, the clavicle rotates only 5° to 8° relative to the acromion because of scapular rotation.[154,155] Also during this final stage, the humerus finishes its lateral rotation to 90°, so that the greater tuberosity of the humerus avoids the acromion process. Tables 5.11 and 5.12 outline the shoulder kinematics in healthy and pathological states.[156]

In the unstable shoulder, scapulohumeral rhythm is commonly altered because of incorrect dynamic functioning of the scapular or humeral stabilizers or both.[157] This may be related to incorrect arthrokinematics at the glenohumeral joint; therefore the examiner must be sure to check for normal joint play and the presence of

---

TABLE **5.11**

Summary of Scapular Kinematics During Arm Elevation in Healthy and Pathologic States

Group	Healthy (Normal)	Impingement or Rotator Cuff Disease	Glenohumeral Joint Instability	Adhesive Capsulitis
Primary scapular motion	Upward rotation	Lesser upward rotation	Lesser upward rotation	Greater upward rotation
Secondary scapular motion	Posterior tilting	Lesser posterior tilting	No consistent evidence for alteration	No consistent evidence for alteration
Accessory scapular motion	Variable medial/lateral rotation	Greater medial rotation	Greater medial rotation	No consistent evidence for alteration
Presumed implications	Maximize shoulder ROM and available subacromial space	Presumed contributory to subacromial or internal impingement	Presumed contributory to lesser inferior and anterior joint stability	Presumed compensatory to minimize functional shoulder ROM loss

ROM, Range of motion.
Adapted with permission from Ludewig PM, Reynolds JF: The association of scapular kinematics and glenohumeral joint pathologies, *J Orthop Sports Phys Ther* 39:95, 2009.

TABLE **5.12**

Mechanisms of Scapular Dyskinesia

Mechanism	Associated Effects
Inadequate serratus anterior activation	Lesser scapular upward rotation and posterior tilt
Excess upper trapezius activation	Greater clavicular elevation
Pectoralis minor tightness	Greater scapular medial rotation and anterior tilt
Posterior glenohumeral joint soft-tissue tightness	Greater scapular anterior tilt
Thoracic kyphosis or flexed posture	Greater scapular medial rotation and anterior tilt, lesser scapular upward rotation

Modified from Ludewig PM, Reynolds JF: The association of scapular kinematics and glenohumeral joint pathologies, *J Orthop Sports Phys Ther* 39:97, 2009.

hypomobile structures that could lead to these abnormal motions.[157] Kon et al. advocated using a 3-kg (6.6-lb) weight when checking scapulohumeral rhythm during the active movements, especially elevation, as the extra weight when these movements are being done requires greater muscle stabilization.[158]

Kibler pointed out that it is important to watch the movement, especially of the scapula, in both the ascending and descending phases of abduction.[159] Commonly weakness of the scapular control muscles is more evident during descent, and an instability jog, hitch, or jump may occur when the patient loses control of the scapula.

The speed of abduction may also have an effect on the ratio.[160] Therefore it is more important to look for asymmetry between the injured and the good sides than to be concerned with the actual degrees of movement occurring at each joint. That being said, if the clavicle does not rotate and elevate, elevation through abduction at the glenohumeral joint is limited to 120°.[145] If the glenohumeral joint does not move, elevation through abduction is limited to 60°, which occurs totally in the scapulothoracic joint. If there is no lateral rotation of the humerus during abduction, the total movement available is 120°, 60° of which occurs at the glenohumeral joint and 60° of which occurs at the scapulothoracic articulation.[36] The normal end of ROM is reached when there is contact of a surgical neck of humerus with the acromion process. **Reverse scapulohumeral rhythm** (Fig. 5.36) means that the scapula moves more than the humerus. This occurs in conditions like the frozen shoulder. The patient appears to "hike" the entire shoulder complex (the **shrug sign**) rather than produce a smooth coordinated abduction movement.

Active elevation through forward flexion is normally 160° to 180°, and at the extreme of the ROM, the arm

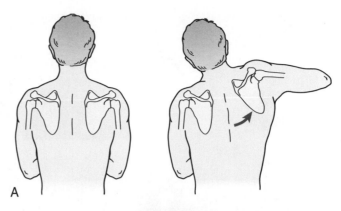

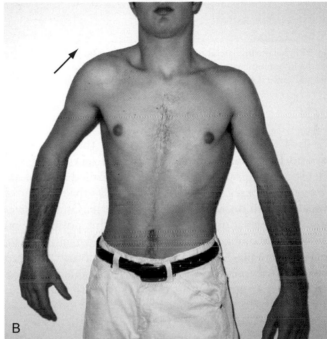

Fig. 5.36 Reverse scapulohumeral rhythm (notice shoulder hiking) and excessive scapular movement. Examples include frozen shoulder (A) or tear of rotator cuff (B). In (B), the patient with a complete rotator cuff tear of the right arm is unable to hold the arm in the abducted position, and it falls to the patient's side. The patient often shrugs or hitches the shoulder forward so as to use the intact muscles of the rotator cuff and the deltoid to keep the arm in the abducted position. (B, From Waldman SD: *Physical diagnosis of pain: an atlas of signs and symptoms*, Philadelphia, 2006, Saunders.)

is in the same position as for active elevation through abduction. As the movement is attempted, the examiner watches the movement of the scapula (i.e., is the movement the same on both sides?), the humerus and the clavicle. As well, the examiner may palpate the C7 to T4 spinal segments to feel for movement. Normally, in the last 30° of forward flexion elevation, the spinous processes will rotate to the same (i.e., ipsilateral) side. If they do not move, then either the facet joints or ribs are restricting the movement. These spinal and rib movements may have to be assessed to ensure normal movement of the kinetic chain.[161] Active elevation (170° to 180°) through the plane of the scapula (30° to 45° of

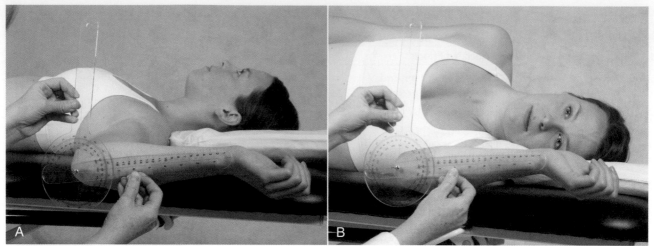

Fig. 5.37 Measuring lateral rotation. (A) Supine. The patient's arm is rotated until the scapula is felt to move and until an endpoint is reached. A handheld goniometer is used to measure medial and lateral rotation. (B) Side lying. The examiner rotates the arm until the scapula is seen to move and resistance is felt. The amount of lateral and medial rotation can be examined in this manner with a handheld goniometer.

forward flexion), termed **scaption,** is the most natural and functional motion of elevation (see Fig. 5.33). Elevation in this position is sometimes called *neutral elevation.* The exact angle is determined by the contour of the chest wall on which the scapula rests. Often, movement into elevation is less painful in this position than elevation through abduction in which the glenohumeral joint is actually in extension, or elevation in forward flexion. Movement in the plane of the scapula puts less stress on the capsule and surrounding musculature and is the position in which most of the functions of daily activity are commonly performed. Strength testing in this plane also gives higher values. It has been reported that elevation performed within a 30° arc of the scapular plane results in no change in shoulder muscle activation patterns.[162] Patients with weakness spontaneously choose this plane when elevating the arm.[163,164] During scaption elevation, scapulohumeral rhythm is similar to that of abduction, although there is greater individual variability. The three phases are similar, but there are differences. For example, in scaption elevation, there is little or no lateral rotation of the head of the humerus in the third phase.[152] Also, the total elevation in scaption is about 170° with scapular rotation being about 65° and humeral abduction about 105°; although there is slightly more scapular rotation in scaption, this difference again may result from individual variation.[152] More scapular protraction is likely to occur in scaption elevation, especially in elevation through forward flexion.

Active lateral rotation is normally 80° to 90°, but it may be greater in some athletes, such as gymnasts and baseball pitchers. Care must be taken when applying overpressure with this movement, because it could lead to anterior dislocation of the glenohumeral joint, especially in those with recurrent dislocation problems. If glenohumeral lateral rotation is limited, the patient will compensate by retracting the scapula. To minimize scapular movement, lateral rotation may be measured with the patient in the supine or side-lying position with the arm abducted to 90° and the elbow at 90° (Fig. 5.37). Wilk et al.[165] have recommended that rotation be tested in supine with the arm abducted to 90°, the elbow at 90°, and the scapula stabilized to increase reliability.

Active medial rotation is normally 60° to 100°. This is usually assessed by measuring the height of the "hitchhiking" thumb (i.e., thumb in extension) reaching up the patient's back (Fig. 5.38A and B). Common reference points include the greater trochanter, buttock, waist, and spinous processes with T5 to T10 representing the normal degree of medial rotation.[166] Van den Dolder et al.[167] recommended drawing a line to join the two posterior superior iliac spines and then measuring up to the tip of the thumb (Fig. 5.39) and comparing both sides. When the test is done in this fashion, the examiner must be aware that, in reality, the range measured is not that of the glenohumeral joint alone. In fact, much of the range is gained by winging the scapula. In the presence of tight medial glenohumeral motion, greater winging and protraction of the scapula occurs. Awan et al.[168] advised testing medial rotation in supine with the shoulder abducted to 90° and the elbow flexed to 90°. The examiner passively or the patient actively rotates the arm medially, and as soon as the scapula begins to lift, the movement is stopped and the amount of medial rotation is measured. This method eliminates the scapular movement that commonly contributes to the medial rotation and gives the true medial rotation occurring at the glenohumeral joint as body weight stabilizes or prevents the scapula from moving. The examiner may have to stabilize the scapula manually as medial rotation is attempted

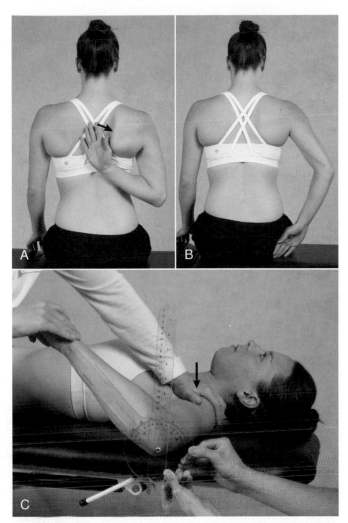

Fig. 5.38 Measuring medial rotation. (A) Reaching up the patient's back. Note winging of scapula *(arrow)* so that the result is made up of glenohumeral and scapular movement. (B) Position of hand when scapula begins to wing indicates end of true medial rotation at the glenohumeral joint. (C) Supine. Glenohumeral medial rotation passive range-of-motion measurement using stabilization of the scapula by holding the coracoid process and the scapula down *(arrow)*.

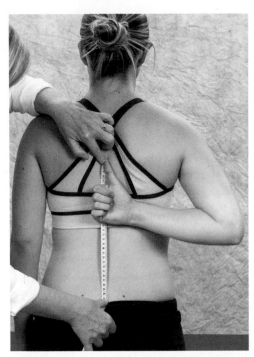

Fig. 5.39 Assessing active medial rotation. The examiner is measuring from the patient's thumb to an imaginary line joining the two posterior superior iliac spines *(dots)*.

and tested (Fig. 5.38C). Lateral rotation may be tested in the same position, but in this case the examiner palpates for the first movement of the scapula, stops the movement, and measures the true lateral rotation at the glenohumeral joint.

Doing the rotation testing in 90° abduction (if the patient can achieve this position) will give a clearer indication of the glenohumeral joint's true medial and lateral rotation, measured when the scapula starts to move (see Fig. 5.38C). If rotation is tested in 90° of abduction and crepitus is present on rotation, it indicates abrasion of torn tendon margins against the coracoacromial arch and is called the **abrasion sign.**[103]

It is important to compare medial and lateral rotation, especially in active people who use their dominant arm at extremes of motion and under high-load situations.

Most of this change in medial rotation gain is due to soft-tissue changes in the capsule and muscles, but some of it may be due to humeral retrotorsion changes from high-load stress in overhead activities.[169] Normally, any gain in lateral rotation is accompanied by a comparable loss in medial rotation. Thus it is important to note any **GIRD** (Fig. 5.40),[65] which is the difference in medial rotation between the patient's two shoulders. Small changes in GIRD can lead to biomechanical changes in passive glenohumeral motion.[170] For example, the loss of medial rotation may be due to thickness, contracture, or elasticity of the posteroinferior capsule, which in turn can lead to a SLAP lesion.[81,171] Normally, the difference should be within 20°, or 10% of total rotation of the opposite arm.[65,172,173] This may also be compared with the **glenohumeral external (lateral) rotation gain (GERG)** (see Fig. 5.40). If the GIRD/GERG ratio is greater than 1, the patient will probably develop shoulder problems.[74,174]

Wilk et al.[174,175] advocate adding medial and lateral rotation bilaterally at 90° of abduction (giving *total rotational motion*) for both limbs and said that in throwing athletes, the dominant (throwing) arm should be within 5° of the nondominant limb if injuries were to be prevented. (This does not imply that the amounts of medial and lateral rotation are the same as in the dominant limb.) There may be a gain in lateral rotation and a deficit in medial rotation or vice versa. This change may be due to humeral retroversion (HR), which can vary depending on the age of the individual and his or her overhead activities.[10–12,24,176] Normally,

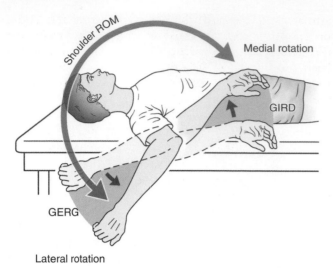

Lateral rotation

Fig. 5.40 Range of shoulder motion showing glenohumeral internal (medial) rotation deficit *(GIRD)* and glenohumeral external (lateral) rotation gain *(GERG)*. *ROM,* Range of motion.

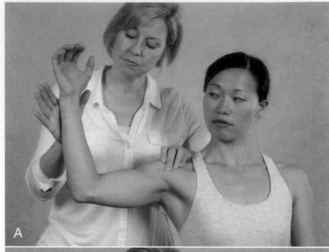

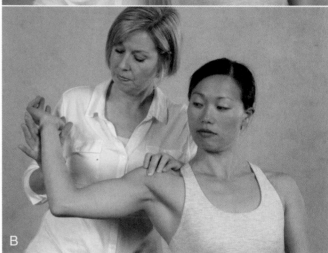

Fig. 5.41 Dynamic rotary instability test demonstrating two different positions in which humeral head control can be evaluated. The examiner's left hand is placed over the humeral head in order to detect any translation that may occur during contraction of the rotators. Isometric lateral rotation is resisted in midrange (A) and end range (B) in a position functionally relevant for a thrower.

humeral retrotorsion decreases with age; however, with high-stress overload activities (e.g., pitching in baseball, playing tennis) into lateral rotation, the amount of retrotorsion decrease is slowed down and, when measured, gives the appearance of being greater than on the unaffected side.[176] Excessive lateral rotation may lead to posterior internal impingement.[177]

In the unstable shoulder, it has been advocated that the examiner do the **dynamic rotary stability test (DRST),** ⚠ which assesses the rotator cuff's ability to maintain the humeral head in the glenoid through the arc of rotation (i.e., the ability of the rotator cuff to maintain arthrokinematic control).[178–180] The patient is positioned in sitting or lying with the arm abducted to about 90° and the elbow flexed to about 90°. The examiner controls the patient's arm position with one hand while the other hand palpates the position of the humerus in the glenoid (it is best to palpate the joint line) (Fig. 5.41). The examiner places the patient's glenohumeral joint in different positions of flexion and abduction close to the position where the patient has symptoms. The patient is asked to do an isometric contraction against light to moderate resistance and then isotonically (concentrically or eccentrically [eccentric break] depending on what movements caused the patient's symptoms). While the patient does the contraction, the examiner palpates the joint line to see if and when arthrokinematic control is lost (i.e., does the humeral head slip or translate?).[179] During the test, the scapula should be stable and should not translate. If the scapula protracts during the test, it indicates lack of scapular control.

Magarey and Jones[179] also advocated doing the **dynamic relocation test (DRT),** ⚠ which tests the ability of the rotator cuff to stabilize the humeral head through cocontraction of the rotator cuff muscles. The

patient is seated with the arm supported in 60° to 80° abduction in the scapular plane (scaption) (Fig. 5.42). With the middle finger of one hand palpating the subscapularis and the thumb along the outer edge of the acromion, the examiner uses the other hand to apply traction (longitudinal distraction) to the arm while asking the patient to pull the arm up into the socket. As the patient pulls the arm in and up, the examiner should feel for contraction of the rotator cuff, especially the subscapularis. If the pectoral muscles are overactive, the examiner may palpate the rotator cuff posteriorly.[178] During the test, the scapula should not move. If the scapula protracts, it indicates an unstable scapula.

Active extension is normally 50° to 60°. The examiner must ensure that the movement is in the shoulder and not in the spine because some patients may flex the spine or bend forward, giving the appearance of increased shoulder extension. Similarly, retraction of the scapula increases the appearance of glenohumeral extension. Weakness of full extension commonly implies weakness of the posterior deltoid in one arm and is sometimes called the **swallow-tail sign** because both arms do not extend the same amount either due to injury to the muscle itself or to the axillary nerve.[181]

Adduction is normally 50° to 75° if the arm is brought in front of the body. Horizontal adduction, or cross flexion, is normally 130°. To accomplish this movement, the patient first abducts the arm to 90° and then moves the

arm across the front of the body. Horizontal abduction, or cross extension, is approximately 45°. After abducting the arm to 90°, the patient moves the straight arm in a backward direction. In both cases, the examiner should watch the relative amount of scapular movement between the normal and pathological sides. If movement is limited in the glenohumeral joint, greater scapular movement occurs. Circumduction is normally approximately 200° and involves taking the arm in a circle in the vertical plane.

In addition to the aforementioned movements, several of which involve movement of the humerus and scapula, the patient should actively perform two distinct movements of the scapulae: scapular retraction and scapular protraction (Fig. 5.43). For scapular retraction, the examiner asks the patient to squeeze the shoulder blades (scapula) together. Normally, the medial borders of the scapula remain parallel to the spine but move toward the spine with the soft tissue bunching up between the scapula (see Fig. 5.43B). Ideally, the patient should be able to do this movement without excessive contraction of the upper trapezius muscles. For scapular protraction, the patient tries to bring the shoulders together anteriorly so that the scapula moves away from midline with the inferior angle of the scapula commonly moving laterally more than the superior angle so that some lateral rotation of the inferior angle occurs (see Fig. 5.43C). Pain in the sternoclavicular joint during protraction may indicate a problem with the sternoclavicular joint.[70] This protraction/retraction cycle may cause a clicking or snapping near the inferior angle or supramedial corner, which is sometimes called a **snapping scapula,** caused by the scapula rubbing over the underlying ribs at the scapulothoracic "articulation."[106] The condition may be due to incongruence between the concave scapula and the

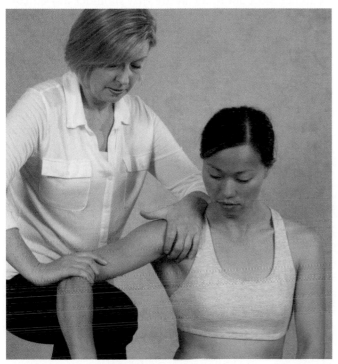

Fig. 5.42 Dynamic relocation test.

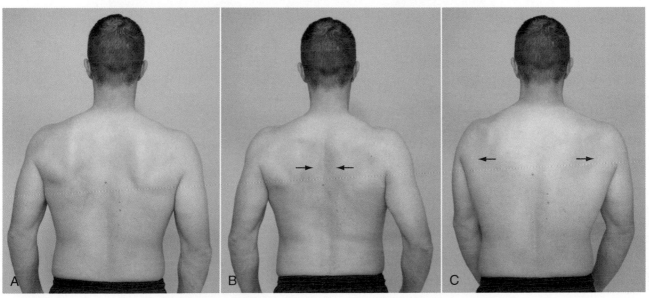

Fig. 5.43 (A) Resting position. (B) Scapular retraction. (C) Scapular protraction.

convex thoracic wall, muscle imbalance or tightness, posture especially a kyphotic posture, or an inflamed bursa, resulting in pain and/or crepitus.[182]

Injury to the individual muscles can affect several movements. For example, if the serratus anterior muscle is weak or paralyzed, the scapula "wings" away from the thorax on its medial border. It also assists upper rotation of the scapula during abduction. Injury to the muscle or its nerve may therefore limit abduction. In fact, loss or weakness of serratus anterior affects all shoulder movements because scapular stabilization is lost.[141] Similarly, weakness of the lower trapezius muscle can alter scapular mechanics resulting in anterior secondary impingement. Many of the tests for these muscles are described in the section titled "Special Tests," later.

When these movements are being observed, the examiner may ask the patient to perform them in combination, especially if the patient history has indicated that combined movements are bothersome. For example, the **Apley's scratch test** combines medial rotation with adduction and lateral rotation with abduction (Fig. 5.44). This method may decrease the time required to do the assessment. In addition, by having the patient do the combined movements, the examiner gains some idea of the patient's functional capacity. For example, abduction combined with flexion and lateral rotation or adduction combined with extension and medial rotation is needed to comb the hair, to zip a back zipper, or to reach for a wallet in a back pocket. However, the examiner must take care to notice which movements are restricted and which are not, because several movements are performed at the same time. Some examiners prefer doing the same motion in both arms at the same time: neck reach (abduction, flexion, and lateral rotation at the glenohumeral joint) and back reach (adduction, extension, and medial rotation at the glenohumeral joint). Some believe this method makes comparison easier (Fig. 5.45).[91] Often, the dominant shoulder shows greater restriction than the nondominant shoulder, even in normal people. An exception would be patients who continually use their arms at the extremes of motion (e.g., baseball pitchers). Because of the extra ROM developed over time doing the activity, the dominant arm may show greater ROM. However, the examiner must always be aware that shoulder movements include movements of the scapula and clavicle as well as the glenohumeral joint and that many of the perceived glenohumeral joint problems are in reality scapular muscle control problems. These may secondarily lead to glenohumeral joint problems, especially in people under 40 years of age. If, in the history, the patient has complained that shoulder movements in certain postures are painful or that sustained or repetitive movements increase symptoms, the examiner should consider having the patient hold a sustained arm position (10 to 60 seconds) or do the movements repetitively (10 to 20 repetitions). Ideally, these repeated movements should be performed at the speed and with the load that the patient was using when the symptoms were elicited. Thus the volleyball player should do the spiking motion in which he or she jumps up to hit the imaginary ball.

Capsular tightness, although commonly tested during passive movement, can affect active movement by limiting some or all movements in the glenohumeral joint with compensating excessive movement of the scapula. Just as

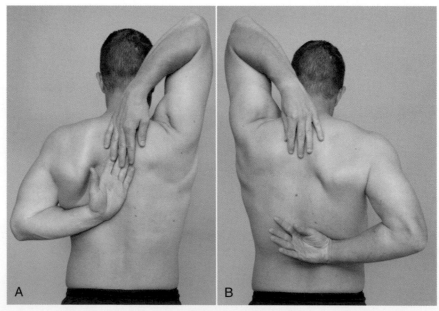

Fig. 5.44 Apley's scratch test. (A) The right arm is in lateral rotation, flexion, and abduction and the left arm is in medial rotation, extension, and adduction. (B) The left arm is in lateral rotation, flexion, and abduction and the right arm is in medial rotation, extension, and adduction. Note the difference in medial rotation and scapular winging in the right arm compared with the left arm in (A).

The biceps tendon does not move in the bicipital groove during movement; rather, the humerus moves over the fixed tendon. From adduction to full elevation of abduction, a given point in the groove moves along the tendon at least 4 cm. If the examiner wants to keep excursion of the bicipital groove along the biceps tendon to a minimum, the arm should be elevated with the humerus in medial rotation; elevating the arm with the humerus laterally rotated causes maximum excursion of the bicipital groove along the biceps tendon. Patients who have deltoid or supraspinatus pathology sometimes use this laterally rotated position because lateral rotation allows the biceps tendon to be used as a shoulder abductor in a "cheating" movement.

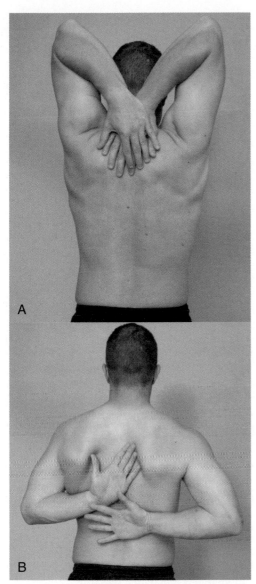

Fig. 5.45 (A) Neck reach. (B) Back reach. Note the difference in medial rotation on both sides and greater winging of left scapula.

Humeral Movement Faults

Superior humeral translation:	Scapular downward rotators are predominating
Anterior humeral translation:	Weak subscapularis and teres major; tight infraspinatus, teres minor
Inferior humeral translation:	Weak upward scapular rotators; poor glenohumeral rotation timing
Decreased lateral rotation:	Short pectoralis major and/or latissimus dorsi
Excessive scapular retraction during lateral rotation:	Tight anterior capsule; tight medial rotators; poor scapulothoracic muscle control

As the patient does the various movements, the examiner watches to see whether the components of the shoulder complex move in normal, coordinated sequence and whether the patient exhibits any apprehension when doing a movement. With **anterior instability** of the shoulder, the shoulder girdle often droops, and excessive scapulothoracic movement may occur on abduction. With **posterior instability,** horizontal adduction (cross flexion) may cause excessive scapulothoracic movement. Any apprehension on movement suggests the possibility of instability. The examiner should also watch for **winging of the scapula** on active movements. Winging of the medial border of the scapula indicates injury to the serratus anterior muscle or the long thoracic nerve; rotary winging of the scapula or scapular tilt indicates upper trapezius pathology or injury to the spinal accessory nerve (cranial nerve XI; Table 5.14).[100,166,183] Scapular tilt (the inferior angle of scapula moves away from the rib cage) may also be caused by a weak lower trapezius or a tight pectoralis minor. In some cases, it may be necessary to load the appropriate muscle isometrically (holding the contraction for 10 to 15 seconds) to demonstrate abnormal scapular stability. It has been reported that application of a resistance to adduction at 30° and at 60° of shoulder abduction is the best way to show scapular winging.[166] Eccentric loading of the shoulder in different positions,

a frozen shoulder can affect all movements, selected tightness due to particular pathologies may affect only part of the capsule. For example, with anterior shoulder instability, posterior capsular tightness is a common finding combined with weak lower trapezius and serratus anterior muscles. Table 5.13 shows common selected capsular tightness and states their effect on movement.

Likewise, muscle tightness can affect both active and passive movement. For example, with anterior shoulder instability, the following muscles may be found to be tight: subscapularis, pectoralis minor and major, latissimus dorsi, upper trapezius, levator scapulae, sternocleidomastoid, scalenes, and rectus capitus. Weak muscles include serratus anterior, middle and lower trapezius, infraspinatus, teres minor, posterior deltoid, rhomboids, longus colli, and longus capitus.[106]

TABLE **5.13**

Capsular Tightness: Its Effect and Resulting Humeral Head Translation

Where	Effect (Signs and Symptoms)	Resulting Translation
Posterior	Cross flexion decreased Medial rotation decreased Flexion (end range) decreased Decreased posterior glide Impingement signs in medial rotation Weak external rotators Weak scapular stabilizers	Anterior (with medial rotation)
Posteroinferior	Elevation anteriorly Medial rotation of elevated arm decreased Horizontal adduction decreased	Superior Anterosuperior Anterosuperior
Posterosuperior	Medial rotation limited	Anterosuperior
Anterosuperior	Flexion (end range) decreased Extension (end range) decreased Lateral rotation decreased Horizontal extension decreased Abduction (end range) decreased Decreased posteroinferior glide Impingement in medial rotation and cross flexion Increased night pain Weak rotator cuff May have positive ULNT Biceps tests may be positive	Posterior (with lateral rotation)
Anteroinferior	Abduction decreased Extension decreased Lateral rotation decreased Horizontal extension decreased Increased posterior glide	Posterior (with lateral rotation of elevated arm)

ULNT, Upper limb neurodynamic test.
Data from Matsen FA, et al: *Practice evaluation and management of the shoulder*, Philadelphia, 1994, WB Saunders.

TABLE **5.14**

Winging of the Scapula: Dynamic Causes and Effects

Cause	Effect (Signs and Symptoms)
Trapezius or spinal accessory nerve lesion	Inability to shrug shoulder
Serratus anterior or long thoracic nerve lesion	Difficulty elevating arm above 120°
Strain of rhomboids	Difficulty pushing elbow back against resistance (with hand on hip)
Muscle imbalance or contractures	Winging of upper margin of scapula on adduction and lateral rotation

Causes of Scapular Imbalance Patterns

Increased protraction:	Tight pectoralis minor Weak/lengthened lower trapezius Weak/lengthened serratus anterior
Increased depression:	Weak upper trapezius
Loss of scapular stabilization:	Early/excessive protraction Early/excessive lateral rotation of scapula Early/excessive elevation of scapula Tight lateral rotators Secondary impingement

Indications of Loss of Scapular Control

- Scapula protracting along chest wall, especially under load
- Early contraction of upper trapezius on abduction, especially under load
- Increased work of rotator cuff and biceps, especially with closed chain activity (reverse origin-insertion)
- Altered scapulohumeral rhythm

especially into horizontal adduction, may also demonstrate winging or loss of scapular control. Weakness of the scapular control muscles often leads to overactivity of the rotator cuff and biceps muscle, leading to overuse pathology in those structures.

Scapular Winging Faults

On concentric elevation:	Long/weak serratus anterior
On eccentric forward flexion:	Overactive rotator cuff; underactive scapular control muscles
Tilting of inferior angle:	Tight pectoralis minor; weak lower trapezius

If the scapula appears to wing, the examiner should ask the patient to forward flex the shoulder to 90°. The examiner then pushes the straight arm toward the patient's body while the patient resists. If there is weakness of the upper or lower trapezius muscle, the serratus anterior muscle, or the nerves supplying these muscles, their inability to contract will cause the scapula to wing. Another way to test winging of the scapula is to have the patient stand and lean against a wall. The examiner then asks the patient to do a push-up away from the wall while the examiner watches for winging (see Figs. 5.28B and 5.46A). Similarly, asking the patient

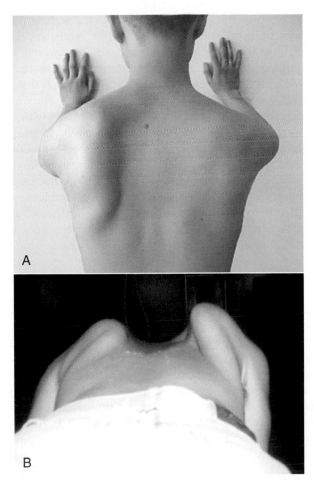

A

B

Fig. 5.46 Scapular winging is demonstrated by having the patient push against a wall (unilateral weakness demonstrated on left) (A) or the floor (bilateral weakness) (B) with both arms forward flexed to 90°. (A, From Li T, Yang ZZ, Deng Y, et al: Indirect transfer of the sternal head of the pectoralis major with autogenous semitendinosus augmentation to treat scapular winging secondary to long thoracic nerve palsy, *J Shoulder Elbow Surg* 26[11]:1970–1977, 2017.)

to do a floor push-up may demonstrate this winging (Fig. 5.46B). The patient should be tested in a relaxed starting position and be asked to do the push-up. Sometimes the winging is visible at rest only (static winging), sometimes during rest and activity, and sometimes only with the activity (dynamic winging).

Injury to other nerves in the shoulder region must not be overlooked (Table 5.15). As previously mentioned, damage to the suprascapular nerve may affect both the supraspinatus and infraspinatus muscles, or it may affect only the infraspinatus, depending on where the pathology lies (see Fig. 5.188), whereas injury to the musculocutaneous nerve can lead to paralysis of the coracobrachialis, biceps, and brachialis muscles. These changes affect elbow flexion and supination and forward flexion of the shoulder. There is also a loss of the biceps reflex. Injury to the axillary (circumflex) nerve leads to paralysis of the deltoid and teres minor muscles, affecting abduction and lateral rotation of the shoulder. A sensory loss over the deltoid insertion area also occurs. Damage to the radial nerve affects all of the extensor muscles of the upper limb, including the triceps. Triceps paralysis may be overlooked when examining the shoulder unless arm extension is attempted along with elbow extension against gravity. Both of these movements are affected in high radial nerve palsy, although some triceps function may remain (e.g., in radial nerve palsy after a humeral shaft fracture).

Passive Movements

If the ROM is not full during the active movements and the examiner is unable to test the end feel, the examiner should perform all passive movements of the shoulder to determine the end feel, and any restriction should be

TABLE **5.15**

Signs and Symptoms of Possible Peripheral Nerve Involvement

Spinal accessory nerve	Inability to abduct arm beyond 90° Pain in shoulder on abduction
Long thoracic nerve	Pain on flexing fully extended arm Inability to flex fully extended arm Winging starts at 90° forward flexion
Suprascapular nerve	Increased pain on forward shoulder flexion Shoulder weakness (partial loss of humeral control) Pain increases with scapular abduction Pain increases with cervical rotation to opposite side
Axillary (circumflex) nerve	Inability to abduct arm with neutral rotation
Musculocutaneous nerve	Weak elbow flexion with forearm supinated

noted. This passive examination should include not only the mobility of the four shoulder joints but also the ribs and spine as limitations in rib and spinal movement can restrict shoulder movement.

Passive Movements of the Shoulder Complex and Normal End Feel

- Elevation through forward flexion of the arm (tissue stretch)
- Elevation through abduction of the arm (bone-to-bone or tissue stretch)
- Elevation through abduction of the glenohumeral joint only (bone-to-bone or tissue stretch)
- Lateral rotation of the arm (tissue stretch)
- Medial rotation of the arm (tissue stretch)
- Extension of the arm (tissue stretch)
- Adduction of the arm (tissue approximation)
- Horizontal adduction (tissue stretch or approximation) and abduction of the arm (tissue stretch)
- Quadrant test

When the ROM in the shoulder is being considered and both sides are compared, the total ROM for the dominant side should be no greater than 8°, side-to-side GIRD should be 20° or less, and glenohumeral lateral rotation should be 5° or less between sides. Any values above these values would indicate that treatment intervention should be considered.[52,184–186] **Anterior hyperlaxity** is defined as lateral rotation greater than 85° with the arm at the side; **inferior hyperlaxity** is a positive hyperabduction test in which a side-to-side difference greater than 20° is positive.[187]

The end feel of capsular tightness is different from the tissue stretch end feel of muscle tightness.[188] Capsular tightness has a harder, more elastic feel to it and usually occurs earlier in the ROM. If one is unsure of the end feel, the patient can be asked to contract the muscles acting in the opposite direction, 10% to 20% of maximum voluntary contraction (MVC), and then to relax. The examiner then attempts to move the limb further into range. If the range increases, the problem is muscular and not capsular.

If the problem is capsular, capsular tightness should be measured. For example, a tight posterior capsule can cause increased scapular protraction and depression, leading to anterior tilting and insufficient scapular elevation, which in turn can lead to impingement.[81] In addition, it can limit horizontal adduction, and posteroinferior tightness can increase the risk of injury to the rotator cuff.[189] A **frozen shoulder** (i.e., **adhesive capsulitis**) can limit movements in all directions but primarily limits movements into lateral rotation, abduction, and medial rotation (i.e., a capsular pattern) and results in a reverse scapulohumeral rhythm (i.e., the scapula has greater ROM than the humerus, and on elevation movements, the patient exhibits the **shrug sign**).[190] Frozen shoulder can be divided into primary, which is associated with an idiopathic onset and lasts about 12 months before "unthawing," and secondary, which

is the result of forced inactivity following trauma.[190] To measure posterior capsular tightness, the patient, suitably undressed (no shirt for males; bra for females), is placed in supine lying with the arm forward flexed to 90° and the elbow flexed to 90°. The examiner stands beside the patient and palpates the lateral edge of the scapula. The examiner then passively retracts the scapula and holds the retracted position with one hand. With the other hand, the examiner holds the distal humerus in 90° abduction and 0° rotation. The examiner then horizontally adducts the patient's arm. As soon as the examiner feels the scapula begin to move or the humerus begin to rotate, the horizontal adduction is stopped and the angle relative to the vertical position is measured.[191] Both sides, starting with the normal side, are measured (Fig. 5.47A).[192] The test may also be done in side lying, but it is then harder to stabilize the scapula (Fig. 5.47B).[193,194] The angle from the vertical to the arm indicates the passive ROM available and should be compared with the opposite side.[191] If the pathological side has less ROM and the end feel is capsular, capsular tightness is present. This capsular tightness should correlate well with decreased medial rotation provided the scapula is not allowed to move in compensation.[193,194] Similarly, passive medial rotation at the glenohumeral joint is measured with the subject in supine and the humerus in 90° of abduction (a towel may be placed under the humerus so that the humerus is horizontal to the examining table). The examiner then passively rotates the humerus medially with one hand while the other hand palpates the scapula. As soon as the scapula starts to move, the medial humeral rotation is stopped and the angle is measured and compared.[191]

Particular attention must be paid to passive medial and lateral rotation if the examiner suspects a problem with the glenohumeral joint capsule (see previous discussion of GIRD). Lunden et al.[195] recommend that rotation, especially medial rotation, should be measured in side lying for greater reliability (Fig. 5.48). Ropars et al.[143] recommend that lateral rotation should be measured using the "elbow on the table" (EOT) method as, according to them, it showed better reproducibility than other methods. The patient is in supine with the arm by the side and the elbow flexed to 90°. The examiner passively rotates the shoulder laterally. Ropars et al.[143] considered a patient to be hyperlax if lateral rotation was more than 90° (Fig. 5.49). Excessive scapular movement may be seen as compensation for a tight glenohumeral joint. **Subcoracoid bursitis** may limit full lateral rotation, and **subacromial bursitis** may limit full abduction because of compression or pinching of these structures. If lateral rotation of the shoulder is limited, the examiner should check forearm supination with the arm forward flexed to 90°. Patients who have a posterior dislocation at the glenohumeral joint exhibit restricted lateral rotation of the shoulder and limited supination in forward flexion (**Rowe sign ❓**).[196] Lateral rotation is the movement most commonly affected with a frozen shoulder and often a capsular pattern of lateral

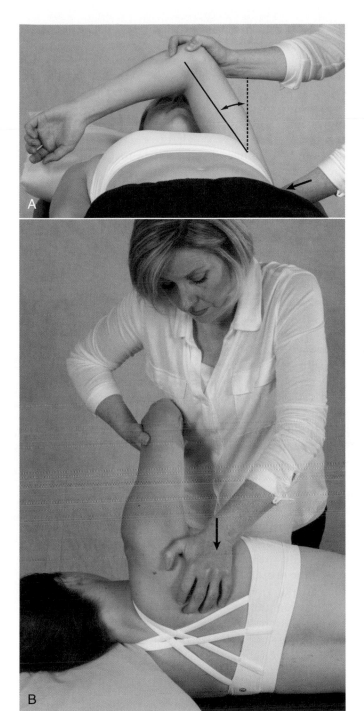

Fig. 5.47 Testing for posterior capsular tightness. (A) Supine lying. Angle created by the end position of the humerus with respect to the starting position to determine glenohumeral horizontal adduction range of motion. Note stabilization of the scapula *(arrow)*. (B) Starting position for the posterior shoulder flexibility measurement with the patient positioned in side lying. Note the scapular stabilization *(arrow)* with the torso perpendicular to the examining table. As soon as the scapula begins to move, the examiner stops.

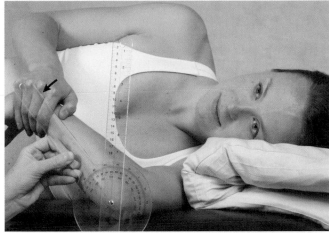

Fig. 5.48 Measuring medial rotation in the sleeper stretch position.

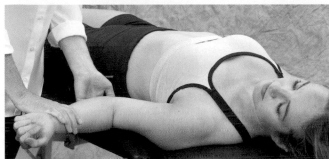

Fig. 5.49 "Elbow on the table" (EOT) method to measure lateral rotation of shoulder.

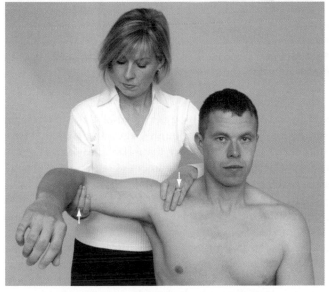

Fig. 5.50 Passive abduction of the glenohumeral joint.

rotation, abduction, and medial rotation (in that order) may be found.[197] Even if overpressure has been applied on active movement, it is still necessary for the examiner to perform elevation through abduction of the glenohumeral joint only (Fig. 5.50) and the quadrant test.

The examiner performs passive elevation through abduction or scaption of the glenohumeral joint with the clavicle and scapula fixed to determine the amount of abduction in the glenohumeral joint alone (see Fig. 5.50). This can give an indication of capsular tightness or

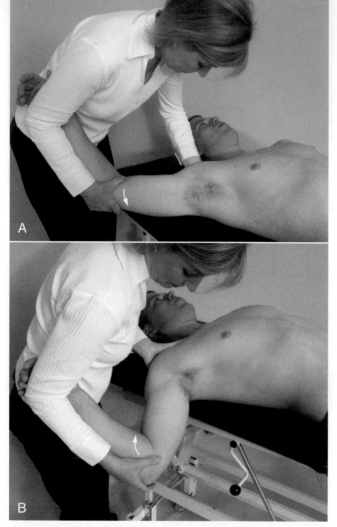

Fig. 5.51 Quadrant position. (A) Adduction test. (B) Abduction test (locked quadrant).

the unconscious rotation occurring at the glenohumeral joint. Thus the quadrant test is designed to demonstrate whether the automatic or subconscious rotation is occurring during movement. The examiner should not only feel the movement but also determine the quality of the movement and the amount of anterior humeral movement. This test and the following locked quadrant test assess one area or quadrant of the 200° of circumduction. The humerus must rotate in the quadrant of the circumduction movement to allow full pain-free movement. Although both of these tests should normally be pain free, the examiner should be aware that they place a high level of stress on the soft tissues of the glenohumeral joint, and discomfort should not be misinterpreted as pathological pain. If movement is painful and restricted, the tests indicate early stages of shoulder pathology.[201]

To test the **quadrant position,**[202,203] the examiner stabilizes the scapula and clavicle by placing the forearm under the patient's scapula on the side to be tested and extending the hand over the shoulder to hold the trapezius muscle and prevent shoulder shrugging (Fig. 5.51). To test the position, the upper limb is elevated to rest alongside the patient's head with the shoulder rotated laterally. The patient's shoulder is then adducted. Because adduction occurs on the coronal plane, a point (the quadrant position) is reached at which the arm moves forward slightly from the coronal plane. At approximately 60° of adduction (from the arm beside the head), this position of maximum forward movement occurs (i.e., at about 120° of abduction) even if a backward pressure is applied. As the shoulder is further adducted, the arm falls back to the previous coronal plane. The quadrant position indicates the position at which the arm has medially rotated during its descent to the patient's side.

The quadrant position also may be found by abducting the medially rotated shoulder while maintaining extension. In this case, the quadrant position is reached (at about 120° of abduction) when the shoulder no longer abducts, because it is prevented from laterally rotating by the catching of the greater tuberosity in the subacromial space. This position is referred to as the **locked quadrant position.**[204] If the arm is allowed to move forward, lateral rotation occurs and full abduction can be achieved. Both the quadrant and locked quadrant simply indicate where the rotation normally occurs during shoulder abduction/adduction.

The capsular pattern of the shoulder is lateral rotation showing the greatest restriction, followed by abduction and medial rotation. Each of these movements normally has a tissue-stretch end feel. Other movements may be limited, but not in the same order and not with as much restriction. Early capsular patterns may exhibit only limitations of lateral rotation or possibly lateral rotation and

subacromial space pathology.[91] Normally, this movement should be up to 120°, although Gagey and Gagey[198] have stated that anything greater than 105° indicates laxity in the inferior glenohumeral ligament (**Gagey hyperabduction test** ⚠️).[199]

The rotation of the humerus in the quadrant position demonstrates the Codman "pivotal paradox"[164,200] and MacConaill[201] conjunct rotation (rotation that automatically or subconsciously occurs with movement) in diadochal movement (a succession of two or more distinct movements). For example, if the arm, with the elbow flexed, is laterally rotated when the arm is at the side and then abducted in the coronal plane to 180°, the shoulder will be in 90° of medial rotation even though no apparent rotation has occurred. The path traced by the humerus during the quadrant test, in which the humerus moves forward at approximately 120° of abduction, is abduction. Finding of limitation, but not in the order described, indicates a noncapsular pattern.

Resisted Isometric Movements

Having completed the active and passive movements, which are done while the patient is standing, sitting, or lying supine (in the case of quadrant test), the patient lies supine to do the resisted isometric movements (Fig. 5.52). The disadvantage of this position is that the examiner cannot observe the stabilization of the scapula during the testing. Normally, the scapula should not move during isometric testing. Scapular protraction, winging, or tilting during isometric testing indicates weakness of the scapular control muscles. Although all the muscles around the shoulder can be tested in supine lying, it has been advocated that the muscles should be tested in more than one position (e.g., different amounts of abduction or forward flexion) to determine the mechanical effect of the contraction in different situations. If, in the history, the patient complained of pain in one or more positions, these positions should be tested as well. If the initial position causes pain, other positions (e.g., position of injury, position of mechanical advantage) may be tried to further differentiate the specific contractile tissue that has been injured. During the active movements, the examiner should have noted which movements caused discomfort or pain so that this information can be correlated with that obtained from resisted isometric movements. By carefully noting which movements cause pain on isometric testing, the examiner should be able to determine which muscle or muscles are at fault (Fig. 5.53; Table 5.16). The rotator cuff (especially supraspinatus and subscapularis in overhead athletes), biceps, and triceps should receive particular attention along with the scapular control muscles (i.e., trapezius, serratus anterior, levator scapulae, and pectoralis minor).[205] For example, if the patient experiences pain primarily on medial rotation but also on

abduction and adduction, the examiner would suspect a problem in the subscapularis muscle, because the other muscles involved in these actions were found to be pain free in other movements. To do the initial resisted isometric tests, the examiner positions the patient's arm at the side with the elbow flexed to 90°. The muscles of the shoulder are then tested isometrically with the examiner positioning the patient and saying, "Don't let me move you."

Resisted Isometric Movements of the Shoulder Complex

- Forward flexion of the shoulder
- Extension of the shoulder
- Adduction of the shoulder
- Abduction of the shoulder
- Medial rotation of the shoulder
- Lateral rotation of the shoulder
- Flexion of the elbow
- Extension of the elbow

Resisted isometric elbow flexion and extension must be performed, because some of the muscles (e.g., biceps, triceps) act over the elbow as well as the shoulder. In addition, the region of hypovascularity of the long head of biceps is 1.2 to 3 cm (0.5 to 1.2 inches) from its origin at the coracoid process, where it may rupture.[27,206] The examiner should watch for the possibility of a third-degree strain (rupture) of the long head of biceps tendon (at the shoulder) ("Popeye muscle" or **Popeye sign**) as the muscle will bulge distally (i.e., toward the elbow) while a distal rupture (at the elbow) will cause the bulge to be more proximal when testing isometric elbow flexion (Fig. 5.54).[27] It has been reported that 96% of all biceps ruptures occur to the long head.[27]

During testing, the examiner will find differences in the relative strengths of the various muscle groups around the shoulder. The relative percentages for isometric testing will be altered for tests at faster speeds and tests in different planes. If, in the history, the patient complained that concentric, eccentric, or econcentric (biceps and triceps) movements were painful or caused symptoms, these movements should also be tested, with loading or no loading as required.

Relative Isometric Muscle Strengths

- Abduction should be 50%–70% of adduction
- Forward flexion should be 50%–60% of adduction
- Medial rotation should be 45%–50% of adduction
- Lateral rotation should be 65%–70% of medial rotation
- Forward flexion should be 50%–60% of extension
- Horizontal adduction should be 70%–80% of horizontal abduction

---

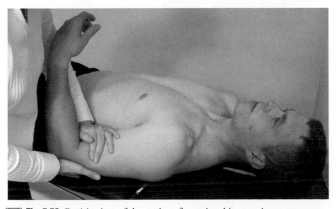

Fig. 5.52 Positioning of the patient for resisted isometric movements.

Superficial   **Deep**

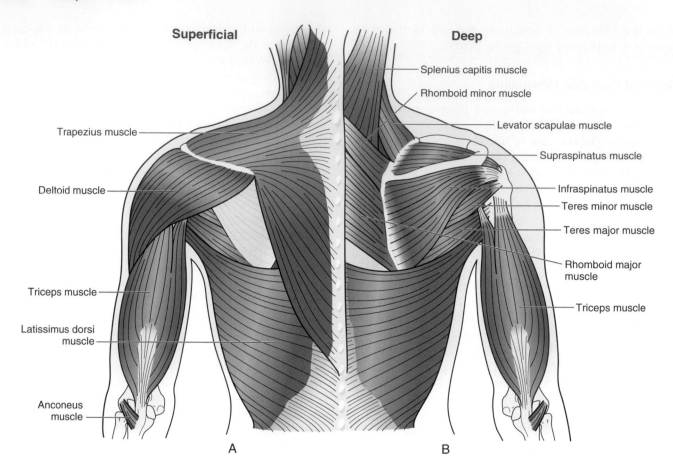

Splenius capitis muscle

Rhomboid minor muscle

Levator scapulae muscle

Supraspinatus muscle

Infraspinatus muscle

Teres minor muscle

Teres major muscle

Rhomboid major muscle

Triceps muscle

Trapezius muscle

Deltoid muscle

Triceps muscle

Latissimus dorsi muscle

Anconeus muscle

A   B

Superficial   **Deep**

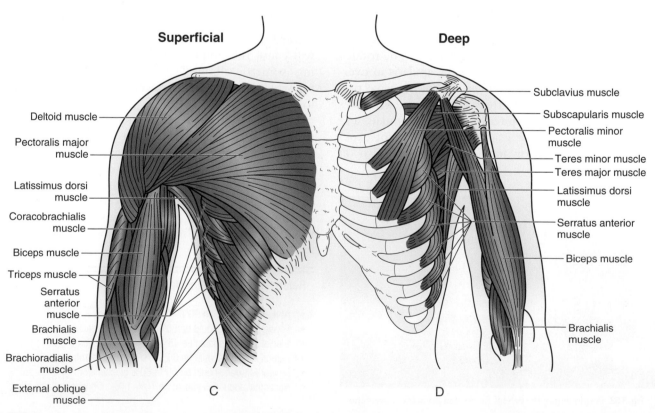

Subclavius muscle

Subscapularis muscle

Pectoralis minor muscle

Teres minor muscle

Teres major muscle

Latissimus dorsi muscle

Serratus anterior muscle

Biceps muscle

Brachialis muscle

Deltoid muscle

Pectoralis major muscle

Latissimus dorsi muscle

Coracobrachialis muscle

Biceps muscle

Triceps muscle

Serratus anterior muscle

Brachialis muscle

Brachioradialis muscle

External oblique muscle

C   D

Fig. 5.53 Muscles about the shoulder. Posterior view of superficial (A) and deep (B) muscles. Anterior view of superficial (C) and deep (D) muscles.

TABLE **5.16**

Muscles About the Shoulder: Their Actions, Nerve Supply, and Nerve Root Derivation

Action	Acting Muscles	Nerve Supply	Nerve Root Derivation Retraction
Forward flexion	1. Deltoid (anterior fibers) 2. Pectoralis major (clavicular fibers) 3. Coracobrachialis 4. Biceps (when strong contraction required)	Axillary (circumflex) Lateral pectoral Musculocutaneous Musculocutaneous	C5, C6 (posterior cord) C5, C6 (lateral cord) C5–C7 (lateral cord) C5–C7 (lateral cord)
Extension	1. Deltoid (posterior fibers) 2. Teres major 3. Teres minor 4. Latissimus dorsi 5. Pectoralis major (sternocostal fibers) 6. Triceps (long head)	Axillary (circumflex) Subscapular Axillary (circumflex) Thoracodorsal Lateral pectoral Medial pectoral Radial	C5, C6 (posterior cord) CS, C6 (posterior cord) C5, C6 (posterior cord) C6–C8 (posterior cord) C5, C6 (lateral cord) C8, T1 (medial cord) C5–C8, T1 (posterior cord)
Horizontal adduction	1. Pectoralis major 2. Deltoid (anterior fibers)	Lateral pectoral Axillary (circumflex)	C5, C6 (lateral cord) C5, C6 (posterior cord)
Horizontal abduction	1. Deltoid (posterior fibers) 2. Teres major 3. Teres minor 4. Infraspinatus	Axillary (circumflex) Subscapular Axillary (circumflex) Suprascapular	C5, C6 (posterior cord) C5, C6 (posterior cord) C5, C6 (brachial plexus trunk) C5, C6 (brachial plexus trunk)
Abduction	1. Deltoid 2. Supraspinatus 3. Infraspinatus 4. Subscapularis 5. Teres minor 6. Long head of biceps (if arm laterally rotated first, trick movement)	Axillary (circumflex) Suprascapular Suprascapular Subscapular Axillary (circumflex) Musculocutaneous	C5, C6 (posterior cord) C5, C6 (brachial plexus trunk) C5, C6 (brachial plexus trunk) C5, C6 (posterior cord) C5, C6 (posterior cord) C5–C7 (lateral cord)
Adduction	1. Pectoralis major 2. Latissimus dorsi 3. Teres major 4. Subscapularis 5. Coracobrachialis	Lateral pectoral Thoracodorsal Subscapular Subscapular Musculocutaneous	C5, C6 (lateral cord) C6–C8 (posterior cord) C5, C6 (posterior cord) C5, C6 (posterior cord) C5–C7 (lateral cord)
Medial rotation	1. Pectoralis major 2. Deltoid (anterior fibers) 3. Latissimus dorsi 4. Teres major 5. Subscapularis (when arm is by side)	Lateral pectoral Axillary (circumflex) Thoracodorsal Subscapular Subscapular	C5, C6 (lateral cord) C5, C6 (posterior cord) C6–C8 (posterior cord) C5, C6 (posterior cord) CS, C6 (posterior cord)
Lateral rotation	1. Infraspinatus 2. Deltoid (posterior fibers) 3. Teres minor	Suprascapular Axillary (circumflex) Axillary (circumflex)	C5, C6 (brachial plexus trunk) C5, C6 (posterior cord) C5, C6 (posterior cord)
Elevation of scapula	1. Trapezius (upper fibers) 2. Levator scapulae 3. Rhomboid major 4. Rhomboid minor	Accessory C3, C4 nerve roots C3, C4 nerve roots Dorsal scapular Dorsal scapular Dorsal scapular	CN XI C3, C4 C3, C4 C5 (C4), C5 (C4), C5
Depression of scapula	1. Serratus anterior 2. Pectoralis major 3. Pectoralis minor 4. Lattissimus dorsi 5. Trapezius (lower fibers)	Long thoracic Lateral pectoral Medial pectoral Thoracodorsal Accessory C3, C4 nerve roots	C5, C6 (C7) C5, C6 (lateral cord) C8, T1 (medial cord) C6–C8 (posterior cord) CN XI C3, C4

Continued

TABLE **5.16**

Muscles About the Shoulder: Their Actions, Nerve Supply, and Nerve Root Derivation—cont'd

Action	Acting Muscles	Nerve Supply	Nerve Root Derivation Retraction
Protraction (forward movement) of scapula	1. Serratus anterior 2. Pectoralis major 3. Pectoralis minor 4. Latissimus dorsi	Long thoracic Lateral pectoral Medial pectoral Thoracodorsal	C5, C6 (C7) C5, C6 (lateral cord) C8, T1 (medial cord) C6–C8 (posterior cord)
Retraction (backward movement) of scapula	1. Trapezius 2. Rhomboid major 3. Rhomboid minor	Accessory Dorsal scapular Dorsal scapular	CN XI (C4), C5 (C4), C5
Lateral (upward) rotation of inferior angle of scapula	1. Trapezius (upper and lower fibers) 2. Serratus anterior	Accessory Long thoracic	CN XI C3, C4 C5, C6 (C7)
Medial (downward) rotation of inferior angle of scapula	1. Levator scapulae 2. Rhomboid major 3. Rhomboid minor 4. Pectoralis minor	C3, C4 nerve roots Dorsal scapular Dorsal scapular Dorsal scapular Medial pectoral	C3, C4 C5 (C4), C5 (C4), C5 C8, T1 (medial cord)
Flexion of elbow	1. Brachialis 2. Biceps brachii 3. Brachioradialis 4. Pronator teres 5. Flexor carpi ulnaris	Musculocutaneous Musculocutaneous Radial Median Ulnar	C5, C6 (C7) CS, C6 C5, C6 (C7) C6, C 7 C7, C8
Extension of elbow	1. Triceps 2. Anconeus	Radial Radial	C6–C8 C7, C8, (T1)

CN, Cranial nerve.

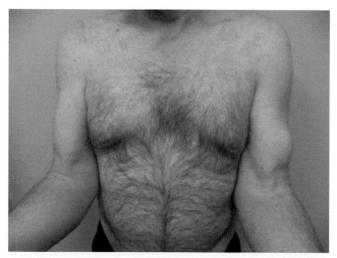

Fig. 5.54 In most patients with an acute full-thickness tear of the long head of biceps tendon at the shoulder, the "Popeye" deformity on the left arm is readily apparent on observation. (From McFarland EG, Borade A: Examination of the biceps tendon, *Clin Sport Med* 35[1]:32, 2016.)

Functional Assessment

The shoulder complex plays an integral role in the activities of daily living (ADLs), sometimes acting as part of an open kinetic chain and sometimes acting as part of a closed kinetic chain. Assessment of function plays an important part of the shoulder evaluation.[207] Limitation of function can greatly affect the patient. For example, placing the hand behind

TABLE **5.17**

Range of Motion Necessary at the Shoulder to Do Certain Activities of Daily Living

Activity	Range of Motion
Eating	70°–100° horizontal adduction[a] 45°–60° abduction
Combing hair	30°–70° horizontal adduction[a] 105°–120° abduction 90° lateral rotation
Reach perineum	75°–90° horizontal abduction 30°–45° abduction 90°+ medial rotation
Tuck in shirt	50°–60° horizontal abduction 55°–65° abduction 90° medial rotation
Place hand behind head	10°–15° horizontal adduction[a] 110°–125° forward flexion 90° lateral rotation
Put something on a shelf	70°–80° horizontal adduction 70°–80° forward flexion 45° lateral rotation
Wash opposite shoulder	60°–90° forward flexion 60°–120° horizontal adduction[a]

[a]Horizontal adduction is from 0° to 90° of abduction.
Adapted from Matsen FA, et al: *Practical evaluation and management of the shoulder*, Philadelphia, 1994, WB Saunders, p 20, 24.

TABLE **5.18**

Scoring for Functional Shoulder Movements of the Arm

Hand-To-Back of Neck (Test 1)

0	The fingers reach the posterior median line of the neck with the shoulder in full abduction and lateral rotation. The wrist is not dorsally extended.
1	The fingers reach the median line of the neck but do not have full abduction and/or lateral rotation.
2	The fingers reach the median line of the neck, but with compensation by adduction (over 20° in the horizontal plane) or by shoulder elevation.
3	The fingers touch the neck.
4	The fingers do not reach the neck.

Hand-To-Scapula (From Behind) (Test 2)

0	The hand reaches behind the trunk to the opposite scapula or 5 cm beneath it in full medial rotation. The wrist is not laterally deviated.
1	The hand reaches the opposite scapula 6–15 cm beneath it.
2	The hand reaches the opposite iliac crest.
3	The hand reaches the buttock.
4	The hand cannot be moved behind the trunk.

Hand-To-Opposite Scapula (From In Front) (Test 3)

0	The hand reaches the spine of the opposite scapula in full adduction without wrist flexion.
1	The hand reaches the spine of the opposite scapula in full adduction.
2	The hand passes the midline of the trunk.
3	The hand cannot pass the midline of the trunk.

Modified from Mannerkorpi K, Svantesson U, Carlsson J, et al: Tests of functional limitations in fibromyalgia syndrome: a reliability study, *Arthr Care Res* 12(3):195, 1999; and Dutton M: *Dutton's orthopedic examination, evaluation and intervention*, ed 3, New York, 2012, McGraw-Hill, p 511.

the head (e.g., to comb the hair) requires almost full lateral rotation, whereas placing the hand in the small of the back (e.g., to get a wallet out of a back pocket or undo a bra) requires almost full medial rotation. Matsen et al.[103] have listed the functional ROM necessary to do some of the functional ADLs (Table 5.17), and Mannerkorpi et al.[208] and Dutton[209] have outlined functional movements of the arm (Table 5.18). The tables point out that although full ROM is desirable, most functional tasks can be performed with less than full ROM.[210] Test 1 in Table 5.18 measures the ability to do activities such as arm reach, pulling or hanging an object overhead, combing one's hair, or drinking from a cup. Test 2 measures the ability to do activities such as getting something out of a back pocket, scratching one's back, or hooking a bra. Test 3 measures the ability to do such tasks as fastening a seatbelt or turning a steering wheel.[208,209]

The functional assessment may be based on a particular joint, structure (e.g., **Nottingham Clavicle Score**) (eTool 5.1),[211] ADLs, work, or recreation and outcomes measures,[212,213] because these activities are of most concern to the patient (eTool 5.2),[214–220] or it may be based on numerical scoring charts (eTools 5.3 to 5.5 are examples), which are derived from clinical measures as well as functional measures. Some numerical evaluation scales

are designed for specific populations, such as athletes (see eTool 5.3), level of disability[221–224] (see eTool 5.5), or specific injuries, such as instability.[225–228] Other shoulder rating scales are also available.[229–241] When numerical scoring charts are being used, the examiner should not place total reliance on the scores, because most of these charts are based primarily on the examiner's clinical measures and not the patient's subjective functional hoped-for outcome, which is the patient's primary concern, and there has been concern whether the most appropriate data (based on the patient's desired outcome) are being recorded.[242–244] Probably the most functional numerical shoulder tests from a patient's perspective are the **simple shoulder test** (eTool 5.6) developed by Lippitt, Matsen, and associates[103,216,227,245–248]; the **Disabilities of the Arm, Shoulder, and Hand (DASH) test** from Hudak et al. (eTool 5.7)[216,249–251] and its modification—the **Quick DASH**[227,251–254]; the **Western Ontario Shoulder Instability Index (WOSI)** (eTool 5.8)[238]; the **Instability Severity Index Score (ISIS)** to select patients for stabilization surgery[255,256]; the **Shoulder Pain and Disability Index (SPADI)** (see eTool 5.4)[222,223,227,257,258]; the **Penn Shoulder Score** (eTool 5.9) by Leggin et al.[259,260]; the **American Shoulder and Elbow Surgeons (ASES) Shoulder Score** (eTool 5.10)[235,247,257,261]; the **Oxford**

TABLE **5.19**

Functional Testing of the Shoulder

Starting Position	Action	Function Test[a]
Sitting	Forward flexing of arm to 90°	Lift 4-lb to 5-lb weight: functional Lift 1-lb to 3-lb weight: functionally fair Lift arm weight: functionally poor Cannot lift arm: nonfunctional
Sitting	Shoulder extension	Lift 4-lb to 5-lb weight: functional Lift 1-lb to 3-lb weight: functionally fair Lift arm weight: functionally poor Cannot lift arm: nonfunctional
Side lying (may be done in sitting with pulley)	Shoulder medial rotation	Lift 4-lb to 5-lb weight: functional Lift 1-lb to 3-lb weight: functionally fair Lift arm weight: functionally poor Cannot lift arm: nonfunctional
Side lying (may be done in sitting with pulley)	Shoulder lateral rotation	Lift 4-lb to 5-lb weight: functional Lift 1-lb to 3-lb weight: functionally fair Lift arm weight: functionally poor Cannot lift arm: nonfunctional
Sitting	Shoulder abduction	Lift 4-lb to 5-lb weight: functional Lift 1-lb to 3-lb weight: functionally fair Lift arm weight: functionally poor Cannot lift arm: nonfunctional
Sitting	Shoulder adduction (using wall pulley)	Lift 4-lb to 5-lb weight: functional Lift 1-lb to 3-lb weight: functionally fair Lift arm weight: functionally poor Cannot lift arm: nonfunctional
Sitting	Shoulder elevation (shoulder shrug)	5–6 repetitions: functional 3–4 repetitions: functionally fair 1–2 repetitions: functionally poor 0 repetitions: nonfunctional
Sitting	Sitting push-up (shoulder dysfunction)	5–6 repetitions: functional 3–4 repetitions: functionally fair 1–2 repetitions: functionally poor 0 repetitions: nonfunctional

[a]Younger, more fit patients should easily be able to do more than the values given for these tests. A comparison between the good side and the injured side gives the examiner some idea about the patient's functional strength capacity.
Data from Palmer ML, Epler M: *Clinical assessment procedures in physical therapy*, Philadelphia, 1990, JB Lippincott, pp 68–73.

Shoulder Instability Score[227,262]; and the **Constant-Murley Shoulder Score**.[233,263–266] However, some authors[264,265] have questioned the last score and what it measures. Table 5.19 provides the examiner with a method of determining the patient's functional shoulder strength and endurance. This table is based on the general population and would not indicate a true functional reading of athletes or persons who do heavy work involving the shoulders. Ahmad et al.[267] have developed a **Youth Throwing Score (YTS)** (eTool 5.11) for the injury assessment of young (i.e., 10 to 19 years of age) baseball players, and the Kerlan-Jobe Clinic has developed the **Kerlan-Jobe Orthopedic Clinic Shoulder and Elbow Score** (eTool 5.12) for adult overhead athletes.[249,268,269] There is also the **Degree of Shoulder Involvement in Sports (DOSIS) Scale,** which can be used to determine how much the shoulder is used. It is similar to the **Teglar Activity Scale** for the knee.[270] For athletes or those applying significant

load to their shoulders while forward flexed, the **one-arm hop test** has been developed (Fig. 5.55). To do this test, the patient assumes the push-up position, balancing on one arm. The patient then hops up onto a 10-cm (4-inch) step and then back to the floor. The hop is repeated five times and the time is noted. The patient starts with the good arm and then uses the injured arm, and the two times are compared. Provided that the patient is trained, completing this action in less than 10 seconds is considered normal.[271]

Burkhart et al. felt it was important to test core stability (i.e., testing kinetic chain function) and flexibility when the shoulder was being assessed so as to ensure the proper transfer of forces from the legs to the trunk and the shoulder as part of the kinetic chain.[74] They advocated testing one-legged stance (not Trendelenburg), one-legged squat (stable pelvis), one-legged step up and step down (stable pelvis), normal hip medial rotation bilaterally, and strength of hip abductors, trunk flexors, and abdominal muscles.

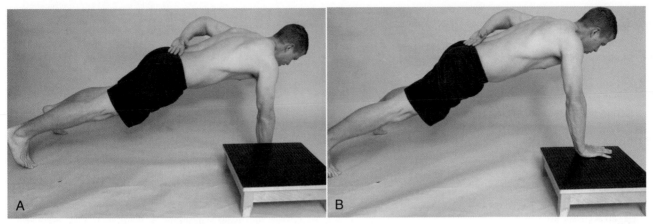

Fig. 5.55 One-arm hop test. (A) Start position. (B) End position.

Special Tests

Special tests are often used in shoulder examinations to confirm findings or to make a tentative diagnosis. Many of the tests, especially those involving the labrum, have not shown high sensitivity or specificity; therefore a combination of tests (i.e., test clusters, **clinical prediction rules**) may often be more helpful,[272-279] although even in these cases, the tests are not necessarily definitive or discriminatory.[1,280] The problem is that too many pain-generating structures in the shoulder cause the same painful symptoms (e.g., tendinitis, rotator cuff tears, SLAP lesions, instability, impingement). Thus the tests are rarely diagnostic but do raise the clinician's level of suspicion as to whether the injury is treatable conservatively or should be referred to a surgeon.[1,281]

The examiner must be proficient in those tests that he or she decides to use. Proficiency increases the reliability of the findings, although the reliability of some of the tests has been questioned.[273,282,283] Depending on the patient history, some tests are compulsory and others may be used as confirming or excluding tests. As with all passive tests, results are more likely to be positive in the presence of pathology when the muscles are relaxed, the patient is supported, and there is minimal or no muscle spasm.

Key Tests Performed at the Shoulder Depending on Suspected Pathology[a]

- *For anterior shoulder (glenohumeral) instability:*
  - ✓ Apprehension (crank) release ("surprise") test and Jobe relocation tests and modifications
  - ⚠ Anterior drawer test of the shoulder
  - ⚠ Bony apprehension test
  - ⚠ Load and shift test
  - ❓ Andrews anterior instability test
  - ❓ Anterior instability (Leffert's) test
  - ❓ Dugas test
  - ❓ Fulcrum test
  - ❓ Protzman test
  - ❓ Rockwood test
  - ❓ Rowe test
  - ❓ Supine apprehension test
- *For posterior shoulder (glenohumeral) instability:*
  - ✓ Jerk (Jahnke) test
  - ⚠ Load and shift test
  - ⚠ Norwood test
  - ❓ Circumduction test
  - ❓ Miniaci test
  - ❓ Posterior apprehension or stress test
  - ❓ Posterior drawer test
  - ❓ Posterior subluxation test
  - ❓ Push-pull test

- *For inferior and multidirectional shoulder (glenohumeral) instability:*
  - ✓ Sulcus sign
  - ⚠ Feagin test (abduction inferior stability test)
  - ⚠ Hyperabduction test (Gagey hyperabduction test)
  - ⚠ Hyperextension–internal (medial) rotation (HERI) test
  - ⚠ Knee–shoulder test
  - ❓ Rowe test
- *For anterior impingement:*
  - ✓ Coracoid impingement sign
  - ✓ Hawkins-Kennedy test
  - ✓ Neer test and modification
  - ✓ Supine impingement test
  - ✓ Yokum test
  - ✓ Zaslav test (internal rotation resistance strength test [IRRST])
  - ❓ Impingement sign
  - ❓ Reverse impingement (impingement relief) test
- *For posterior impingement:*
  - ❓ Posterior internal impingement test
- *For labral lesions[b]:*
  - ✓ Active compression test of O'Brien
  - ✓ Kim test I (biceps load test II)
  - ✓ Porcellini test
  - ⚠ Anterior slide test
  - ⚠ Biceps load test (Kim test II)

Continued

Key Tests Performed at the Shoulder Depending on Suspected Pathology—cont'd[a]

- *For labral lesions (cont'd):*
  - ⚠ Biceps tension test
  - ⚠ Clunk test
  - ⚠ Compression rotation test
  - ⚠ Forced shoulder abduction and elbow flexion test
  - ⚠ Mayo shear test
  - ⚠ Pain provocation (Mimori) test
  - ⚠ Passive distraction test
  - ⚠ Resisted supination external rotation test (RSERT)
  - ⚠ Supine flexion resistance test
  - ⚠ Throwing test
  - ❓ Labral crank test
  - ❓ Labral tension test
  - ❓ O'Driscoll SLAP (dynamic labral shear) test
  - ❓ Passive compression test
  - ❓ SLAP prehension test
- *For scapular dyskinesia:*
  - ✅ Scapular dyskinesia test
  - ✅ Scapular load test
  - ⚠ Lateral scapular slide test
  - ⚠ Scapular retraction test (SRT)
  - ⚠ Wall/floor push-up
  - ❓ Kinetic medial rotation test
  - ❓ Scapular assistance test
  - ❓ Scapular isometric pinch or squeeze test
- *For acromioclavicular joint pathology:*
  - ✅ Horizontal adduction (cross-body adduction) test
  - ✅ Paxinos sign
  - ⚠ Acromioclavicular shear test
  - ❓ Ellman's compression rotation test
- *For ligament and capsule pathology:*
  - ✅ Crank test
  - ⚠ Low flexion test
  - ❓ Coracoclavicular ligament test
  - ❓ Posterior inferior glenohumeral ligament test
- *For muscle pathology[b]:*
  - Biceps
    - ⚠ Biceps tightness test
    - ⚠ Speed's test
    - ⚠ Yergason's test
    - ❓ Gilchrest's test
    - ❓ Heuter's sign
    - ❓ Lippman's test
    - ❓ Ludington's test
    - ❓ Upper-cut test
  - Deltoid
    - ⚠ Deltoid extension lag (swallow-tail) sign
  - Rotator cuff stability
    - ⚠ Dynamic relocation test (DRT)
    - ⚠ Dynamic rotary stability test (DRST)
    - ⚠ Lateral Jobe test
    - ❓ Abrasion test
  - Rotator cuff (general)
    - ✅ Rent test
    - ✅ Whipple test
    - ⚠ Drop-arm (Codman's) test
  - Supraspinatus
    - ✅ Champagne toast position
    - ✅ "Empty can" test (Jobe or supraspinatus test)
    - ⚠ Drop-arm test
  - Subscapularis
    - ✅ External rotation lag sign (ERLS)
    - ✅ Lift-off sign (Gerber's test)
    - ✅ Medial rotation lag or "spring back" test
    - ⚠ Belly-off sign
    - ⚠ Belly press test (abdominal compression or Napoleon test)
    - ❓ Bear-hug test
  - Infraspinatus
    - ✅ Infraspinatus test
    - ✅ Lateral rotation lag sign
    - ⚠ Dropping sign
    - ⚠ Infraspinatus scapula retraction test (ISRT)
  - Teres minor
    - ✅ Hornblower's sign (Patte's test)
    - ✅ Lateral rotation lag sign
    - ❓ Teres minor test
  - Trapezius, rhomboids
    - ✅ Trapezius test (three positions)
    - ⚠ Rhomboid weakness
  - Latissimus dorsi, pectoralis major, pectoralis minor
    - ⚠ Latissimus dorsi weakness
    - ⚠ Pectoralis major contracture test
    - ⚠ Pectoralis minor tightness
    - ⚠ Scapula backward tipping test (pectoralis minor)
    - ⚠ Tightness of latissimus dorsi, pectoralis major, pectoralis minor
  - Serratus anterior
    - ⚠ Punch out test
    - ⚠ Triangle sign
- *For neurological function:*
  - ✅ Upper limb neurodynamic (tension) test (ULNT)
    - Median nerve (ULNT I)
    - Median nerve (ULNT II)
    - Radial nerve (ULNT III)
    - Ulnar nerve (ULNT IV)
  - ⚠ Scratch collapse test (axillary nerve, long thoracic nerve)
  - ❓ Active elevation lag
  - ❓ Tinel's sign
- *For thoracic outlet syndrome:*
  - ⚠ Roos test
  - ❓ Adson maneuver
  - ❓ Costoclavicular (military thrust) syndrome
  - ❓ Halstead maneuver
  - ❓ Provocative elevation test
  - ❓ Shoulder girdle passive elevation
  - ❓ Wright test
- *Other:*
  - ⚠ Olecranon-manubrium percussion sign

[a]See Chapter 1, Key for Classifying Special Tests.
[b]Research has shown that no single test or even a group of tests can accurately diagnose a superior labrum anteroposterior (SLAP) or rotator cuff lesion.[98,275,284–289]

For the reader who would like to review them, the reliability, validity, specificity, sensitivity, and odds ratios of some of the special tests used in the shoulder are available in eAppendix 5.1.

Instability and Pseudolaxity Impingement

Anterior shoulder pain is commonly seen in patients young and old complaining of shoulder pain and dysfunction. Instability at the shoulder manifests itself as symptomatic abnormal motion within the shoulder complex, including the scapula. This abnormal motion may be the result of several intrinsic and extrinsic factors such as abnormal scapular or glenohumeral muscle patterning, hypo- or hypermobility of the capsule (most commonly a tight posterior capsule) or ribs, a labral tear (a Bankart or SLAP lesion), a rotator cuff or biceps injury, altered surface area of contact between the glenoid and humeral head, and/or a problem with the central or peripheral nervous system.[178,290] Kuhn et al.[68,291] advocated using the **FEDS System** (i.e., frequency, etiology, direction, and severity) for diagnosing glenohumeral instability. Lewis et al.[292–294] suggested using the **Shoulder Symptom Modification Procedure (SSMP)** as part of the shoulder examination to demonstrate to the patient that rotator cuff symptoms are modifiable, which may increase individual confidence to move and to adhere to any treatment plans. However, the usefulness of the SSMP has been questioned.[295]

In the older patient (40 years old or older), mechanical impingement occurs because of degenerative changes to the rotator cuff, the acromion process, the coracoid process, and the anterior tissues from stress overload. In this case, impingement is the primary problem (thus the term **primary impingement**). It may be intrinsic because of rotator cuff degeneration or extrinsic because of the shape of the acromion and degeneration of the coracoacromial ligament.[296]

In the young patient (15 to 35 years old), anterior shoulder pain is primarily caused by problems with muscle dynamics, with an upset in the normal force couple action leading to muscle imbalance and abnormal movement patterns at both the glenohumeral joint and the scapulothoracic articulation. These altered muscle dynamics lead to symptoms of anterior impingement (thus the term **secondary impingement**). The impingement signs are a secondary result of altered muscle dynamics in the scapula or glenohumeral joint.[296]

As secondary impingement is primarily a problem with muscle dynamics, it commonly presents in conjunction with instability, either of the scapula or at the glenohumeral joint. A hypermobile or lax joint does not imply instability.[297] Laxity implies that there is a certain amount of nonpathological "looseness" in a joint, so that ROM is greater in one or more directions and the shoulder complex functions normally. It is usually found bilaterally.

Instability implies that the patient is unable to control or stabilize a joint during motion or in a static position either because static restraints have been injured (as would be noted in an anterior dislocation with tearing of the capsule and labrum, also called **gross** or **anatomical instability**), or because the muscles controlling the joint are weak or the force couples are unbalanced (also called **translational instability**).[298]

Both primary and second impingements occur anteriorly (thus, the terms *anterior primary impingement* or *anterior secondary impingement*). Because the areas of impingement are in the supraspinatus outlet area, they are also called **outlet impingement syndromes.**[90]

Jobe and colleagues believed that impingement and instability often occur together in throwing athletes and, based on that assumption, developed the following classification[75,299]:
- Grade I: Pure impingement with no instability (often seen in older patients)
- Grade II: Secondary impingement and instability caused by chronic capsular and labral microtrauma
- Grade III: Secondary impingement and instability caused by generalized hypermobility or laxity
- Grade IV: Primary instability with no impingement

In this classification, secondary impingement implies that the impingement occurs secondarily and that the main problem is instability.

A third type of impingement is termed **internal impingement** or nonoutlet impingement. This type of impingement is found posteriorly rather than anteriorly, mostly in overhead athletes. It involves contact of the undersurface of the rotator cuff (primarily supraspinatus and infraspinatus) with the posterosuperior glenoid labrum when the arm is abducted to 90° and laterally rotated fully.[271,300–305]

If the patient history indicates instability, then at least one test each for anterior, posterior, and multidirectional instability should be performed. Because of the interrelation of impingement and instability, tests for both should be applied if the patient history indicates that either condition may be present.[305] Traumatic first-time subluxations and dislocations may result in a torn labrum (Bankart or SLAP lesion), Hill-Sach lesion, osteochondral lesion, and/or capsular damage; therefore the examiner should consider the possibility of these problems existing during the assessment.[306]

When one is looking at shoulder instability, it is important to realize that instability includes a spectrum of conditions from gross or anatomical instability (as seen with the TUBS lesion) to translational instability (muscle weakness) (as seen with AMBRI lesions) (Table 5.20).[103] Burkhart et al.[65] also included **pseudolaxity,** which includes altered glenohumeral arthrokinematics because of the presence of a SLAP lesion, a tight posteroinferior capsule, and often

TABLE **5.20**

Differential Diagnosis of Shoulder Instability (AMBRI Lesion) versus Traumatic Anterior Dislocation (TUBS Lesion)

	Shoulder Instability	Traumatic Anterior Dislocation
History	Feeling of shoulder slippage with pain Feeling of insecurity when doing specific activities No history of injury	Arm elevated and laterally rotated relative to body Feeling of insecurity when in specific position (of dislocation) Recurrent episodes of apprehension
Observation	Normal	Normal (if reduced; if not, loss of rounding of deltoid caused by anterior dislocation)
Active movement	Normal ROM May be abnormal or painful at activity speed	Apprehension and decreased ROM in abduction and lateral rotation
Passive movement	Normal ROM Pain at extreme of ROM possible	Muscle guarding and decreased ROM in apprehension position
Resisted isometric movement	Normal in test position May be weak in provocative position	Pain into abduction and lateral rotation
Special tests	Load and shift test positive	Apprehension positive Augmentation positive Relocation positive
Reflexes and cutaneous distribution	Normal reflexes and sensation	Reflexes normal Sensation normal, unless axillary or musculocutaneous nerve is injured
Palpation	Normal	Anterior shoulder is tender
Diagnostic imaging	Normal	Normal, unless still dislocated; defect possible

AMBRI, Atraumatic cause, Multidirectional with Bilateral shoulder findings with Rehabilitation as appropriate treatment and, rarely, Inferior capsular shift surgery; *ROM,* range of motion; *TUBS,* Traumatic onset, Unidirectional anterior with a Bankart lesion responding to Surgery.

scapular dyskinesia. They felt that the apparent increased anterior laxity resulted from the decreased cam effect in the glenohumeral joint combined with functional lengthening of the anteroinferior capsule and glenohumeral ligament.[65] A posterosuperior SLAP lesion permits laxity on the opposite side (the circle concept of instability).[65] With the instability tests, the examiner is trying to duplicate the patient's symptoms as well as to feel for abnormal movement. Therefore, a response of "that's what my shoulder feels like when it bothers me" is much more significant than the degree of laxity or translation found.[103]

Tests for Anterior Shoulder Instability

❓ *Andrews' Anterior Instability Test.*[307] The patient lies supine with the shoulder abducted 130° and laterally rotated 90°. The examiner stabilizes the elbow and distal humerus with one hand and uses the other hand to grasp the humeral head and lift it forward (Fig. 5.56). A reproduction of the patient's symptoms gives a positive test for anterior instability. If the examiner hears a clunk, an anterior labral tear may be present. This test is a modification of the load and shift test.

⚠ *Anterior Drawer Test of the Shoulder.*[308] The patient lies supine. The examiner places the hand of the affected shoulder in the examiner's axilla, holding the patient's hand with the arm so that the patient remains relaxed. The shoulder to be tested is abducted between 80° and

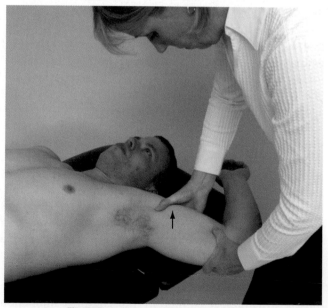

Fig. 5.56 Andrews' anterior instability test.

120°, forward flexed up to 20°, and laterally rotated up to 30°. The examiner then stabilizes the patient's scapula with the opposite hand, pushing the spine of the scapula forward with the index and middle fingers. The examiner's thumb exerts counterpressure on the patient's coracoid process. Using the arm that is holding the patient's hand, the examiner places his or her hand around the patient's relaxed upper arm and draws the humerus forward. The movement may be accompanied by a click, by patient apprehension, or both. The amount of movement available is compared with that of the normal side. A positive test indicates anterior instability (Fig. 5.57), depending on the amount of anterior translation. The click may indicate a labral tear or slippage of the humeral head over the glenoid rim. This test is a modification of the load and shift test.

? *Anterior Instability Test (Leffert's Test).*[309] The examiner stands behind the shoulder being examined while the patient sits. The examiner places his or her near hand over the shoulder so that the index finger is over the head of the humerus anteriorly and the middle finger is over the coracoid process. The thumb is placed over the posterior humeral head. The examiner's other hand grasps the patient's wrist and carefully abducts and laterally rotates the arm (Fig. 5.58). If, on movement of the arm, the finger palpating the anterior humeral head moves forward, the test is said to be positive for anterior instability. Normally, the two fingers remain in the same plane. With a positive test, when the arm is returned to the starting position, the index finger returns to the starting position as the humeral head glides backward.

✓ *Apprehension (Crank) Test for Anterior Shoulder Dislocation.*[273] This test is primarily designed to check for traumatic instability problems causing gross or anatomical

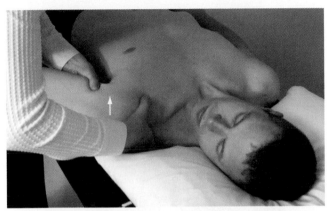

Fig. 5.57 Anterior drawer test of the shoulder.

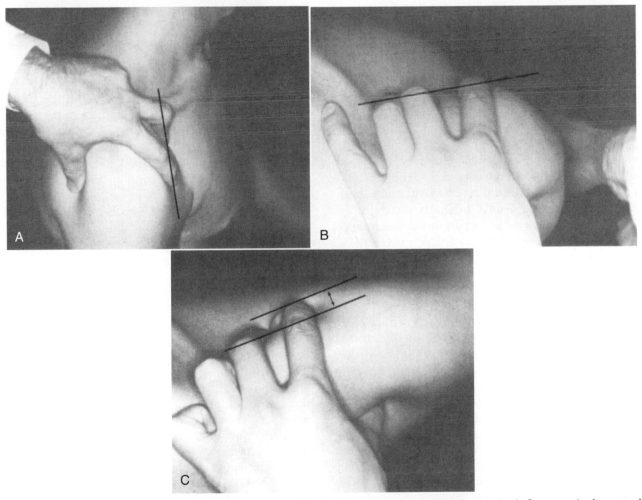

Fig. 5.58 Anterior instability test. (A) Side view. (B) Superior view. With the patient's arm by the side, the examiner's fingers are in the same plane. (C) With a positive test, on abduction and lateral rotation, the index and middle fingers are no longer in the same plane. (Adapted from Leffert RD, Gumbery G: The relationship between dead arm syndrome and thoracic outlet syndrome, *Clin Orthop Relat Res* 223:22–23, 1987.)

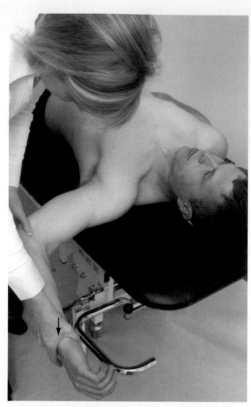

Fig. 5.59 Anterior apprehension (crank) test.

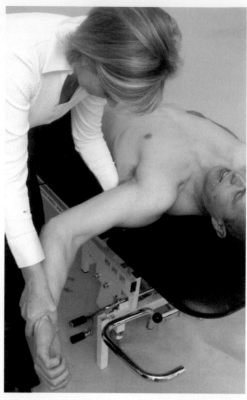

Fig. 5.60 Fulcrum test with the left fist pushing the head of the humerus anteriorly.

instability of the shoulder, although the relocation portion of the test is sometimes used to differentiate between instability and impingement. The examiner abducts the arm to 90° and laterally rotates the patient's shoulder slowly (Fig. 5.59). By placing a hand under the glenohumeral joint to act as a fulcrum (Fig. 5.60), the apprehension test becomes the **fulcrum test.**[310] Kvitne and Jobe[75] recommended applying a mild anteriorly directed force to the posterior humeral head when in the test position to see if the patient's apprehension or pain increases (Fig. 5.61). If posterior pain increases, this indicates posterior internal impingement.[304] Hamner et al.[311] suggested that if posterior superior internal impingement is suspected, the relocation test should be done in 110° and 120° of abduction. Translation of the humeral head in the glenoid is less than with other tests, provided the joint is normal, because the test is taking the joint into the close packed position.[312] A positive test is indicated when the patient looks or feels apprehensive or alarmed and resists further motion. Thus the patient's apprehension is greater than the complaint of pain (i.e., apprehension predominates). The patient may also state that the feeling resembles what it felt like when the shoulder was dislocated. This test *must* be done slowly. If the test is done too quickly, the humerus may dislocate. Hawkins and Bokor noted that the examiner should observe the amount of lateral rotation that exists when the patient becomes apprehensive and compare the range with the uninjured side.[313]

Castagna et al.[314] recommended doing the **Castagna test** ⚠, which is similar to the apprehension test but is done with the arm at 45° abduction instead of 90° and the elbow at 90° and then laterally rotated (Fig. 5.62A). Posterosuperior pain indicates a loose anterior capsule and injury to the middle glenohumeral ligament. If the pain is relieved with relocation (see Jobe relocation test later) (Fig. 5.62B), the test is positive. Similarly, Bak[315] recommended doing the apprehension test in swimmers at 135° abduction, as this is the position of the arm at the initiation of the pull-through phase.

If the examiner then applies a posterior translation stress to the head of the humerus or the arm **(relocation test),** the patient commonly loses the apprehension, any pain that is present commonly decreases, and further lateral rotation is possible before the apprehension or pain returns (see Figs. 5.61A and 5.61C). This relocation is sometimes referred to as the **Fowler sign or test** ✓ or the **Jobe relocation test** ✓. The test is considered positive if pain decreases during the maneuver even if there was no apprehension.[316,317] If the patient's symptoms decrease or are eliminated during the relocation test, the diagnosis is glenohumeral instability, subluxation, dislocation, or impingement. If apprehension predominated during the crank test and disappears with the relocation test, the diagnosis is glenohumeral instability, subluxation, or dislocation. If pain predominated during the crank test and disappears

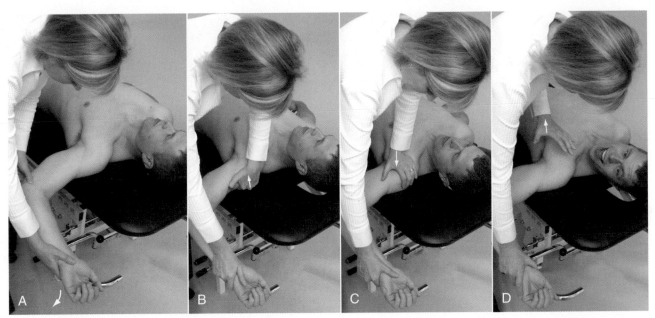

Fig. 5.61 Crank and relocation test. (A) Abduction and lateral rotation (crank test). (B) Abduction and lateral rotation combined with anterior translation of the humerus, which may cause anterior subluxation or posterior joint pain. (C) Abduction and lateral rotation combined with posterior translation of the humerus (relocation test). (D) "Surprise" test.

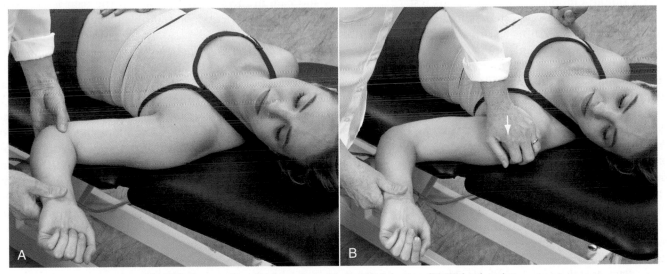

Fig. 5.62 Castagna test. (A) Lateral rotation in 45° abduction. (B) With relocation.

with the relocation test, the diagnosis is pseudolaxity or anterior instability either at the glenohumeral joint or scapulothoracic joint with secondary impingement or a posterior SLAP lesion.[318] The relocation test does not alter the pain for patients with primary impingement.[75,307,319] If, when the relocation test is done posteriorly, posterior pain decreases, it is a positive test for posterior internal impingement.[304,320] If the arm is released (**anterior release** or **"surprise" test** ✓ [see Fig. 5.61D]) in the newly acquired range, pain and forward translation of the head are noted in positive tests.[305,317,321] The resulting pain from this release procedure may be caused by anterior shoulder instability, a labral lesion (Bankart lesion or SLAP lesion—superior labrum, anterior posterior), or bicipital peritenonitis or tendinosus. Most commonly it is related to anterior instability because the pain is temporarily produced by the anterior translation.[321] It has also been reported to cause pain in older patients with rotator cuff pathology and no instability.[322] This release maneuver should be done with care because it often causes apprehension and distrust on the part of the patient, and it could cause a dislocation, especially in patients who have had recurrent dislocations. For most patients, therefore, when the relocation test is done, lateral rotation should be released before the posterior stress is released.

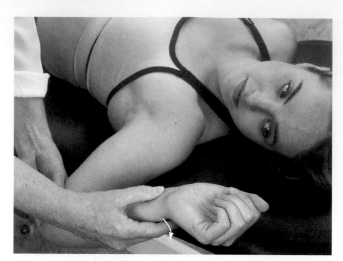

Fig. 5.63 Supine apprehension test.

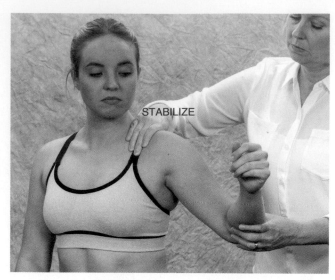

STABILIZE

Fig. 5.64 Bony apprehension test.

The crank test may be modified to test lateral rotation at different degrees of abduction (see bony apprehension test, further on), depending on the patient history and mechanism of injury.[323] The Rockwood test described later is simply a modification of the crank test.

Milgrom et al.[324] suggested that the **supine apprehension test** ❓ would be useful to determine the risk of recurrent instability in patients who had been rehabilitated following an anterior dislocation. The patient is lying supine with the affected arm in 90° of abduction with the elbow in 90° of flexion (Fig. 5.63). The examiner uses one hand to support the patient's elbow and grasps the patient's distal forearm with the other hand, then quickly rotates the arm laterally to about 90° of lateral rotation. If the patient shows apprehension or resists the movement, the test is considered positive and the patient is not allowed to return to full activity because further rehabilitation should occur before returning to activity. Milgrom et al. felt that the test could be performed at any time after 3 to 6 weeks following reduction of the dislocation.

⚠️ *Bony Apprehension Test.*[325–327] This test is designed to look for bony defects (e.g., a Hill-Sach or Bankart lesion) in the patient with an anterior instability. The patient is tested in standing or sitting first with the arm abducted to 90° and the elbow flexed 90°. Then the examiner, while holding the patient's elbow and hand, laterally rotates the arm, watching for apprehension (this part of the test is similar to the apprehension test). The examiner then repeats the test in 45° of abduction and 45° of lateral rotation (Fig. 5.64). If the patient shows apprehension with or without pain in both of these positions, the test is positive for a bony defect contributing to the anterior instability and confirmatory diagnostic imaging is required.

❓ *Dugas' Test.*[328] This test is used if an unreduced anterior shoulder dislocation is suspected. The patient

is asked to place the hand of the test arm on the opposite shoulder and then attempt to lower the elbow to the chest. With an anterior dislocation, this is not possible, and pain in the shoulder results. If the pain is only over the acromioclavicular joint, problems in that joint should be suspected.

⚠️ *Load and Shift Test.*[166,316] This test is designed to check primarily atraumatic instability problems of the glenohumeral joint. The patient sits with no back support and with the hand of the test arm resting on the thigh. Ideally, the patient should be sitting in a properly aligned posture (i.e., earlobe, tip of acromion, and high point of iliac crest in a straight line). If the patient slouches forward, the scapula protracts, causing the humeral head to translate anteriorly in the glenoid and narrowing the subacromial space.[329] For best results, the muscles about the shoulder should be as relaxed as possible. The examiner stands or sits slightly behind the patient and stabilizes the shoulder with one hand over the patient's clavicle and scapula (Fig. 5.65A). With the other hand, the examiner grasps the head of the humerus with the thumb over the posterior humeral head and the fingers over the anterior humeral head (Fig. 5.65B). The examiner runs his or her fingers along the anterior humerus and the thumb along the posterior humerus to feel where the humerus is seated relative to the glenoid (Fig. 5.66). If the fingers "dip in" anteriorly as they move medially but the thumb does not, it indicates that the humeral head is sitting anteriorly. Normally the humeral head feels a bit more anterior (i.e., the "dip" is slightly greater anteriorly) when it is properly "seated" in the glenoid. Protraction of the scapula causes the glenoid head to shift anteriorly in the glenoid. The examiner must be careful with the finger and thumb placement. In the presence of anterior or posterior pathology, finger and thumb placement may cause pain. If necessary, the humerus is then gently pushed anteriorly

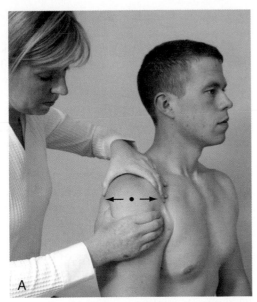
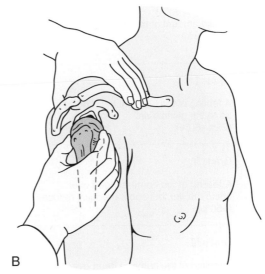

Fig. 5.65 (A) Load and shift test in sitting starting position. Note that the humerus is loaded or "centered" in the glenoid to begin. The examiner then shifts the humerus anteriorly or posteriorly. (B) Line drawing showing the position of the examiner's hands in relation to the bones of the patient's shoulder. Notice that the examiner's left thumb holds the spine of the scapula for stability.

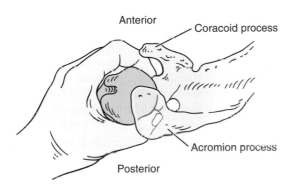

Fig. 5.66 Superior view of the shoulder showing palpation of the anterior and posterior glenohumeral joint to ensure that the humeral head is centered in the glenoid.

or posteriorly (most common) in the glenoid to seat it properly in the glenoid fossa.[305] The seating places the head of the humerus in its normal position relative to the glenoid.[91] This is the "load" portion of the test. If the load is not applied (as in the anterior drawer test), there is no "normal" or standard starting position for the test. The examiner then pushes the humeral head anteriorly (anterior instability) or posteriorly (posterior instability), noting the amount of translation and end feel. This is the "shift" portion of the test.

With anterior translation, if the head is not centered, posterior translation will be greater than anterior translation, giving a false-negative test. If the head is properly centered first, however, with anterior instability present, anterior translation is possible, but posterior translation is virtually absent because of the tight posterior capsule that accompanies a positive anterior instability. Differences between affected and normal sides should be compared in terms of the amount of translation and the ease with which it occurs. This comparison, along with reproduction of the patient's symptoms, is often considered more important than the amount of movement obtained. If the patient has multidirectional instability, both anterior and posterior translation may be excessive on the affected side compared with the normal side. The test may also be done with the patient in lying supine.

Translation of 25% or less of the humeral head diameter anteriorly is considered normal, although results vary.[313,330] Generally, anterior translation is less than posterior translation, although some authors disagree with this and say that anterior and posterior translation are virtually equal.[331,332] Sauers et al.[332] and Ellenbecker et al.[333] stated that hand dominance does not affect the amount of translation, but Lintner et al.[334] disagreed, saying that the nondominant shoulder shows more translation. Hawkins and Mohtadi,[316] Silliman and Hawkins,[305] and Altchek et al.[335] advocated a three-grade system for anterior translation (Fig. 5.67). These authors feel that the head normally translates 0% to 25% of the diameter of the humeral head. Up to 50% of humeral head translation, with the head riding up to the glenoid rim and spontaneous reduction, is considered grade I. For grade II, the humeral head has more than 50% translation; the head feels as though it were riding over the glenoid rim but reduces spontaneously. Normal hypermobile shoulders may show grade II translation in any direction.[334] Grade III implies that the humeral head rides over the glenoid rim and does not spontaneously reduce. For posterior translation, translation of 50% of the diameter of the humeral head is considered normal, although results vary.[305] Thus one would normally expect greater posterior translation than anterior translation when this test is done. However, all authors do not support this view.

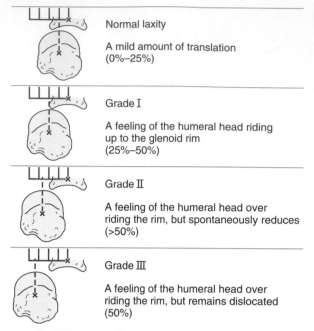

Normal laxity

A mild amount of translation
(0%–25%)

Grade I

A feeling of the humeral head riding
up to the glenoid rim
(25%–50%)

Grade II

A feeling of the humeral head over
riding the rim, but spontaneously reduces
(>50%)

Grade III

A feeling of the humeral head over
riding the rim, but remains dislocated
(50%)

Fig. 5.67 Grades of anterior glenohumeral translation.

The load and shift test may also be done with the patient lying supine.[323] To test anterior translation, the patient's arm is taken to 45° to 60° scaption (abduction in the plane of the scapula) and in neutral rotation by the examiner, who is holding the forearm near the wrist (Fig. 5.68). The examiner then places the other hand around the patient's upper arm near the deltoid insertion with the thumb anterior and the fingers posterior, feeling the movement of the humeral head in the glenoid while applying an anterior or anteroinferior translation force (with the fingers) or a posterior translation force (with the thumb). Ideally, the humerus should be "loaded" in the glenoid before starting the test. With the hand holding the forearm, the examiner controls the arm position and applies an axial load to the humerus. During the translation movements with the thumb or fingers, the scapula should not move. As the anterior or anteroinferior translation force is applied, the examiner, using the other hand (the one holding the forearm), rotates the humerus laterally and incrementally (see Fig. 5.68B). This causes greater involvement of the anterior band of the inferior glenohumeral ligament, which, if intact, will limit movement so that the amount of anterior translation decreases as lateral rotation increases. To test posterior translation (posterior instability), the arm is placed in scaption with 45° to 60° of lateral rotation (Fig. 5.69). In this case, the thumb pushes the humerus posteriorly.[323,336] Incrementally, while applying the posterior translation, the examiner rotates the arm medially. Medial rotation causes the posterior band of the inferior glenohumeral ligament and the posteroinferior capsule to

become increasingly tight, so that posterior translation decreases as medial rotation increases.

❓ *Prone Anterior Instability Test.*[307] The patient lies prone. The examiner abducts the patient's arm to 90° and laterally rotates it 90°. While holding this position with one hand at the elbow, the examiner places the other hand over the humeral head and pushes it forward (Fig. 5.70). A reproduction of the patient's symptoms indicates a positive test for anterior instability. This test is a modification of the load and shift test.

❓ *Protzman Test for Anterior Instability.*[337] The patient is sitting. The examiner abducts the patient's arm to 90° and supports the arm against the examiner's hip so that the patient's shoulder muscles are relaxed. The examiner palpates the anterior aspect of the head of the humerus with the fingers of one hand deep in the patient's axilla while the fingers of the other hand are placed over the posterior aspect of the humeral head. The examiner then pushes the humeral head anteriorly and inferiorly (Fig. 5.71). If this movement causes pain and if palpation indicates abnormal anteroinferior movement, the test is positive for anterior instability. Anterior translation should normally be no more than 25% of the diameter of the humeral head.[338] A click may sometimes be palpated as the humeral head slides over the glenoid rim. The test can also be done with the patient in the supine-lying position with the elbow supported on a pillow.

❓ *Rockwood Test for Anterior Instability.*[339] The examiner stands behind the seated patient. With the patient's arm at the patient's side, the examiner rotates the shoulder laterally. The arm is then abducted to 45° and passive lateral rotation is repeated. The same procedure is repeated at 90° and 120° (Fig. 5.72). These different positions are performed because the stabilizers of the shoulder vary as the angle of abduction changes (see Table 5.1). For the test to be positive, the patient must show marked apprehension with primarily posterior pain when the arm is tested at 90°. At 45° and 120°, the patient shows some uneasiness and some pain; at 0°, there is rarely apprehension.

Similarly, the Rowe and fulcrum tests stress the anterior shoulder structures. They are more likely to bring on apprehension sooner, because they stress the anterior structures sooner (i.e., the examiner pushes the head of the humerus forward). In effect, they are the opposite of the relocation test; they are therefore called **augmentation tests.**

❓ *Rowe Test for Anterior Instability.*[340] The patient lies supine and places the hand of the affected side behind his or her head. The examiner places one hand (clenched fist) against the posterior humeral head and pushes up while extending the arm slightly (Fig. 5.73). This part is similar to the fulcrum test. If the patient appears to be apprehensive or in pain, a positive test for anterior instability is

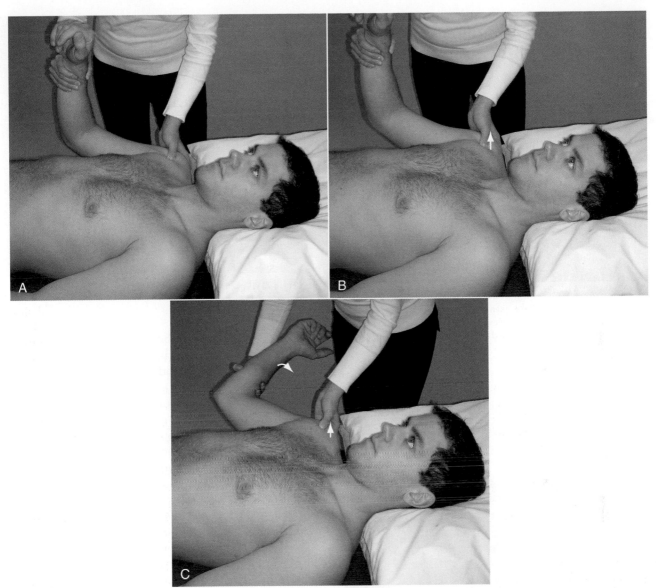

Fig. 5.68 (A) Initial position for load and shift test for anterior instability testing of the shoulder in the supine-lying position. The examiner's hand grasps the patient's upper arm with the fingers posterior. The examiner's arm positions the patient's arm and controls its rotation. The arm is placed in the plane of the scapula, abducted 45° to 60°, and maintained in 0° of rotation. The examiner's arm places an axial load on the patient's arm through the humerus. The examiner's fingers then shift the humeral head anteriorly and anteroinferiorly over the glenoid rim. (B) The second position for the load and shift test for anterior stability is as described in (A) for the initial position except that the arm is progressively laterally rotated in 10° to 20° increments while the anterior dislocation force is alternatively applied and released. (C) The examiner quantifies the degree of lateral rotation required to reduce the translation from grade 3 or 2 to grade 1. The examiner compares the normal and abnormal shoulders for this difference in translation with the humeral rotation. The degree of rotation required to reduce the translation is an indicator of the functional laxity of the antero-inferior capsular ligaments.

indicated. A clunk or grinding sound may indicate a torn anterior labrum (see clunk test under "Tests for Labral Tears").

Tests for Posterior Shoulder Instability[341]
Posterior instability is not as common as anterior instability in the shoulder, but the examiner should take care to also assess for posterior instability, especially in the presence of anterior instability and labral disruption.[342]

Without careful assessment, posterior dislocations have been missed even when the humeral head is posteriorly dislocated. A **posterior humeral avulsion of the glenohumeral ligament (HAGL) lesion** can lead to persistent posterior shoulder instability.[264] These lesions are best assessed by doing a posterior load and shift test with the arm abducted to 90° and in neutral rotation coupled with a posteriorly directed axial load.[342–345] With posterior instability, glenoid retroversion is

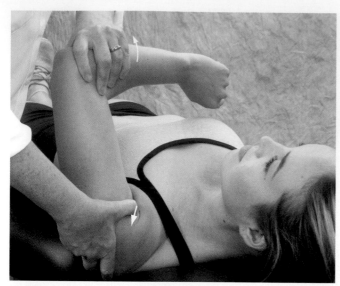

Fig. 5.69 Load-and-shift test for posterior instability testing of the shoulder. The patient is supine on the examining table. The arm is brought into approximately 90° of forward elevation in the plane of the scapula. A posteriorly directed force is applied to the humerus with the arm in varying degrees of lateral rotation.

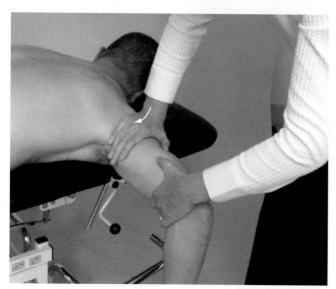

Fig. 5.70 Prone anterior instability test. The examiner stabilizes the arm in 90° of abduction and lateral rotation and then pushes anteriorly on the humerus.

increased, there is deep posterior pain, and a positive finding in the other relevant tests (i.e., jerk test, Kim test, posterior load and shift test, and posterior stress test) are positive.[346]

❓ *Circumduction Test.*[347] The patient is in the standing position. Standing behind the patient, the examiner grasps the patient's forearm with his or her hand. The examiner begins circumduction by extending the patient's arm

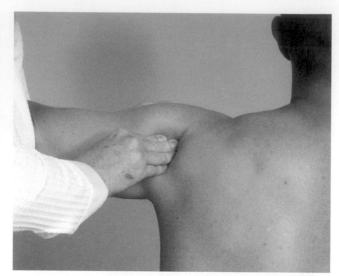

Fig. 5.71 Protzman test for anterior instability (posterior view).

while maintaining slight abduction. As the circumduction continues into elevation, the arm is brought over the top and into the flexed and adducted position. As the arm moves into forward flexion and adduction from above, it is vulnerable to posterior subluxation if the patient is unstable posteriorly. If the examiner palpates the posterior aspect of the patient's shoulder as the arm moves downward in forward flexion and adduction, the humeral head will be felt to sublux posteriorly in a positive test, and the patient will say, "That's what it feels like when it bothers me" (Fig. 5.74).

✓ *Jerk Test (Jahnke Test).*[310,348,349] The patient sits with the arm medially rotated and forward flexed to 90°. The examiner grasps the patient's elbow and axially loads the humerus in a proximal direction. While maintaining the axial loading, the examiner moves the arm horizontally (cross flexion/horizontal adduction) across the body (Fig. 5.75). A positive test for recurrent posterior instability is the production of a sudden jerk or clunk as the humeral head slides off (subluxes) the back of the glenoid (Fig. 5.76). When the arm is returned to the original 90° of abduction, a second jerk may be felt as the head reduces. Kim et al.[349] reported that the positive signs also indicate a positive test for a posteroinferior labral tear.

⚠ *Load and Shift Test.* This test is described under "Tests for Anterior Shoulder Instability."

❓ *Miniaci Test for Posterior Subluxation.*[350] The patient lies supine with the shoulder off the edge of the examining table. The examiner uses one hand to flex (70° to 90°), adduct, and medially rotate the arm while pushing the humerus posteriorly. The patient may become apprehensive during this maneuver, because these motions cause the humerus to sublux posteriorly. With the other hand, the examiner palpates the anterior

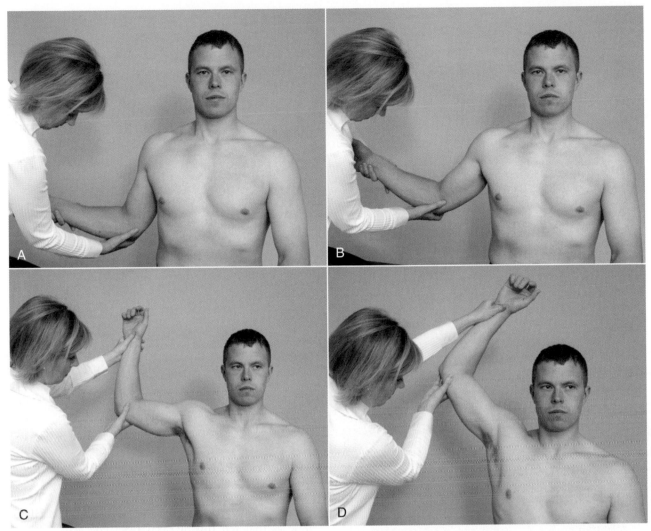

Fig. 5.72 Rockwood test for anterior instability. (A) Arm at side. (B) Arm at 45°. (C) Arm at 90°. (D) Arm at 120°.

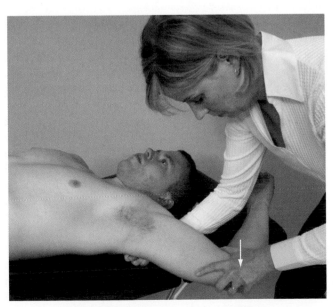

Fig. 5.73 Rowe test for anterior instability.

and posterior shoulder. The examiner then abducts and laterally rotates the arm, a clunk is heard, and the humerus reduces (relocates), indicating a positive test (Fig. 5.77).

Norwood Stress Test for Posterior Instability.[351] The patient lies supine with the shoulder abducted 60° to 100° and laterally rotated 90° and with the elbow flexed to 90°, so that the arm is horizontal. The examiner stabilizes the scapula with one hand, palpating the posterior humeral head with the fingers, and stabilizes the upper limb by holding the forearm and elbow at the elbow or wrist. The examiner then brings the patient's arm into horizontal adduction to the forward flexed position. At the same time, the examiner feels the humeral head slide posteriorly with his or her fingers (Fig. 5.78). Cofield and Irving recommend medially rotating the forearm approximately 20° after the forward flexion then pushing the elbow posteriorly to enhance the effect of the test.[352] Similarly, the thumb may push the humeral head posteriorly as horizontal adduction in forward flexion is

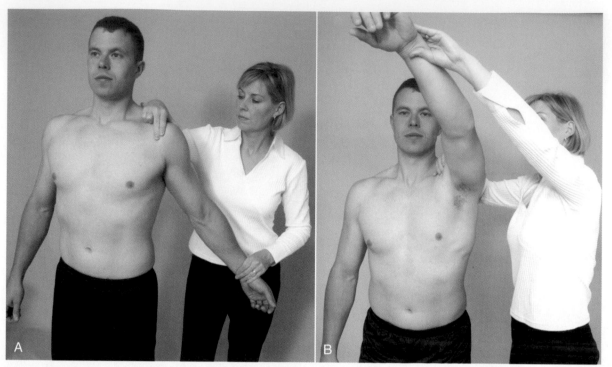

Fig. 5.74 Circumduction test. (A) Starting position. (B) The flexed adducted position where the shoulder is vulnerable to posterior subluxation.

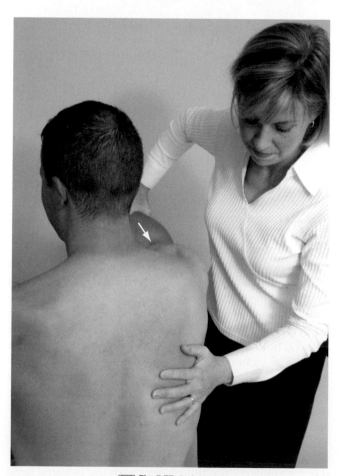

Fig. 5.75 Jerk test.

carried out to enhance the effect making the test similar to the posterior apprehension test. A positive test is indicated if the humeral head slips posteriorly relative to the glenoid. Care must be taken because the test does not always cause apprehension before subluxation or dislocation. The patient confirms that the sensation felt is the same as that felt during activities. The arm is returned to the starting position, and the humeral head is felt to reduce. A clicking caused by the passage of the head over the glenoid rim may accompany either subluxation or reduction.

❓ *Posterior Apprehension or Stress Test.*[336,353] The patient is in a supine or sitting position. The examiner elevates the patient's shoulder in the plane of the scapula to 90° while stabilizing the scapula with the other hand (Fig. 5.79). The examiner then applies a posterior force on the patient's elbow. While applying the axial load, the examiner horizontally adducts and medially rotates the arm. A positive result is indicated by a look of apprehension or alarm on the patient's face and the patient's resistance to further motion or the reproduction of the patient's symptoms. Pagnani and Warren reported that pain production is more likely than apprehension in a positive test.[354] They reported that with atraumatic multidirectional (inferior) instability, the test is negative. If the test is done with the patient in the sitting position, the scapula must be stabilized. A positive test indicates a posterior instability or dislocation of the humerus. The test should also be performed with the arm in 90° of abduction. The examiner palpates the head of

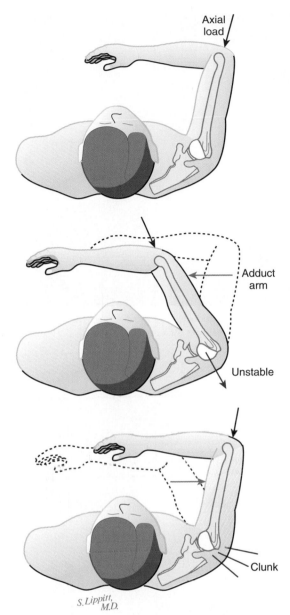

Axial load

Adduct arm

Unstable

Clunk

S. Lippitt, M.D.

Fig. 5.76 Positive jerk test. The humeral head of the axially loaded arm slides out the back of the shoulder when the arm is adducted across the body and clunks back in when the arm position is aligned with the scapula. (From Matsen FA III, Lippitt SB: *Shoulder surgery: principles and procedures*, Philadelphia, 2004, WB Saunders.)

the humerus with one hand while the other hand pushes the head of the humerus posteriorly. Translation of 50% of the humeral head diameter or less is considered normal, although results vary.[312] If the humeral head moves posteriorly more than 50% of its diameter (Fig. 5.80), posterior instability is evident.[338] The movement may be accompanied by a clunk as the humeral head passes over the glenoid rim.

❓ *Posterior Drawer Test of the Shoulder.*[308,355] The patient lies supine. The examiner stands at the level of

the shoulder and grasps the patient's proximal forearm with one hand, flexing the patient's elbow to 120° and the shoulder to between 80° and 120° of abduction and between 20° and 30° of forward flexion. With the other hand, the examiner stabilizes the scapula by placing the index and middle fingers on the spine of the scapula and the thumb on the coracoid process. (The examining table partially stabilizes the scapula as well.) The examiner then rotates the upper arm medially and forward flexes the shoulder to between 60° and 80° while taking the thumb of the other hand off the coracoid process and pushing the head of the humerus posteriorly. The head of the humerus can be felt by the index finger of the same hand (Fig. 5.81). The test is usually not painful, but the patient may exhibit apprehension. A positive test indicates posterior instability and demonstrates significant posterior translation (more than 50% humeral head diameter). This test is similar to the Norwood test without the horizontal adduction.

❓ *Posterior Subluxation Test.*[356] The patient is in sitting or standing. Starting with the unaffected shoulder, the examiner places the test arm into adduction, medial rotation, and 70° to 90° forward flexion. The examiner then applies a posteriorly directed force at the patient's elbow while slowly moving the shoulder into horizontal abduction and lateral rotation (Fig. 5.82). The affected shoulder is then tested. If a clunk is heard, the test is positive, indicating that the humeral head has reduced into the glenoid during the movement.

❓ *Push-Pull Test.*[310] The patient lies supine. The examiner holds the patient's arm at the wrist, abducts the arm 90°, and forward flexes it 30°. The examiner places the other hand over the humerus close to the humeral head. The examiner then pulls up on the arm at the wrist while pushing down on the humerus with the other hand (Fig. 5.83). Normally, 50% posterior translation can be accomplished. If more than 50% posterior translation occurs or if the patient becomes apprehensive or pain results, the examiner should suspect posterior instability.[339]

Tests for Inferior and Multidirectional Shoulder Instability
It is believed that if a patient demonstrates inferior instability, multidirectional instability is also present. Therefore, the patient with inferior instability also demonstrates anterior or posterior instability. The primary complaint of these patients is pain rather than instability with symptoms most commonly in midrange. Transient neurological symptoms may also be present.[357]

⚠ *Feagin Test (Abduction Inferior Stability [ABIS] Test).*[339] The Feagin test is a modification of the sulcus sign test with the arm abducted to 90° instead of being at the patient's side (Fig. 5.84). Some authors consider it to be

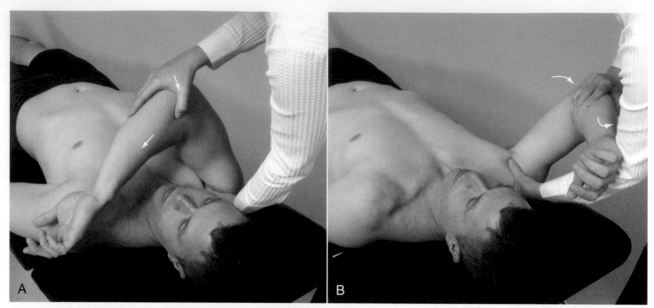

Fig. 5.77 Miniaci test for posterior subluxation. (A) To start, the examiner uses one hand to flex, adduct, and medially rotate the arm while pushing the humerus posteriorly. (B) The arm is then abducted and laterally rotated while the examiner palpates for a clunk.

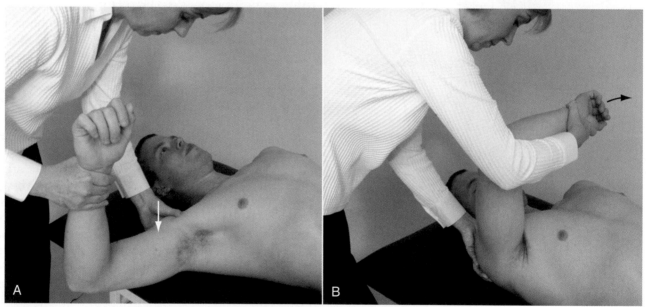

Fig. 5.78 Norwood stress test for posterior shoulder instability. (A) The arm is abducted 90°. (B) The arm is horizontally adducted to the forward flexed position.

the second part of the sulcus test.[358] The patient stands with the arm abducted to 90° and the elbow extended and resting on the top of the examiner's shoulder. The examiner's hands are clasped together over the patient's humerus, between the upper and middle thirds. The examiner pushes the humerus down and forward (see Fig. 5.84A). The test can also be done with the patient in a sitting position. In this case, the examiner holds the patient's arm at the elbow (elbow straight) abducted to 90° with one hand and arm holding the arm against the examiner's body. The other hand is placed just lateral to the acromion over the humeral head. Ensuring the shoulder musculature is relaxed, the examiner pushes the head of the humerus down and forward (see Fig. 5.84B). Doing the test this way often gives the examiner greater control when doing the test. A sulcus may also

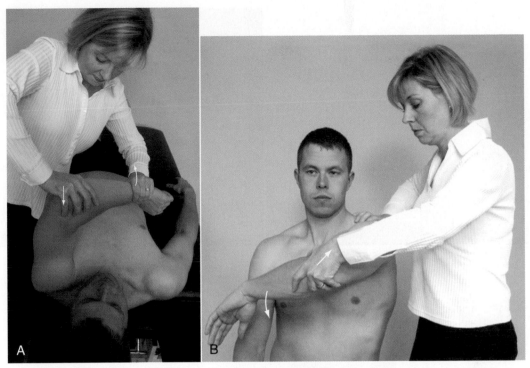

Fig. 5.79 Posterior apprehension test. (A) Supine. (B) Sitting, arm medially rotated and adducted.

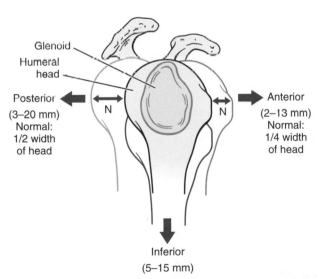

Fig. 5.80 Normal translation movement of humeral head in glenoid. (Redrawn from Harryman DT II, Slides JA, Harris SL, et al: Laxity of the normal glenohumeral joint: a quantitative in vivo assessment, *J Shoulder Elbow Surg* 1:73, 1992.)

be seen above the coracoid process (Fig. 5.85). A look of apprehension on the patient's face indicates a positive test and the presence of inferior capsular laxity.[359] If both the sulcus sign and Feagin test are positive, it is a greater indication of multidirectional instability rather than just laxity, but it should only be considered positive

if the patient is symptomatic (e.g., pain/ache on activity, shoulder does not "feel right" with activity).[359] This test position also places more stress on the inferior glenohumeral ligament.

▲ *Hyperabduction Test (Gagey Hyperabduction Test).*[199] This test is designed to test the inferior glenohumeral ligament. The patient is in sitting or standing and the examiner stands behind the patient. The examiner grasps the patient's elbow (elbow is at 90°) and passively abducts the arm with one hand while stabilizing the scapula and clavicle with the other hand (Fig. 5.86). The examiner passively abducts the arm until the scapula and clavicle start to elevate. If the glenohumeral joint elevation is greater than 105°, the test is considered positive for laxity in the inferior glenohumeral ligament and a possible inferior labral tear. It should be noted however that, subjectively, normal passive scapulohumeral rhythm can show up to 120° of abduction at the glenohumeral joint.

▲ *Hyperextension–Internal Rotation (HERI) Test.*[360] This test is designed to assess the inferior glenohumeral ligament and inferior capsule with decreased risk of dislocation. The examiner stands behind the patient. Starting with the normal shoulder, the examiner carefully elevates the patient's non-test limb to maximum elevation to prevent movement of the thoracic spine and scapulothoracic joint while at the same time medially rotating the test arm and extending it maximally (Fig. 5.87). This must

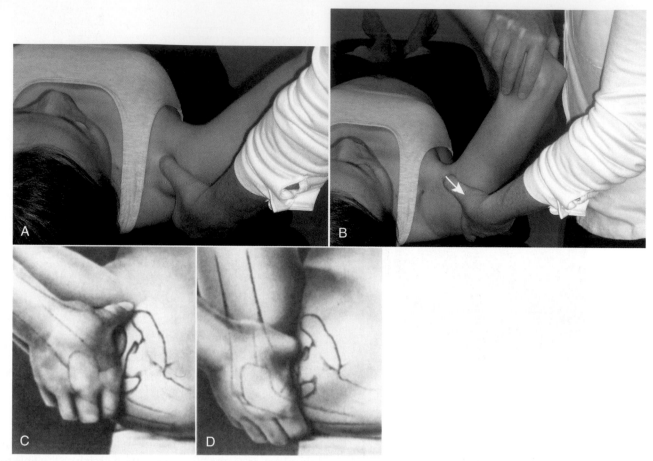

Fig. 5.81 Posterior drawer test of the shoulder. (A) The examiner first palpates the coracoid process and then slides the thumb laterally over onto the head of the humerus. (B) The arm is positioned and the examiner then pushes the humeral head posteriorly. (C and D) Superimposed view of bones involved in the test.

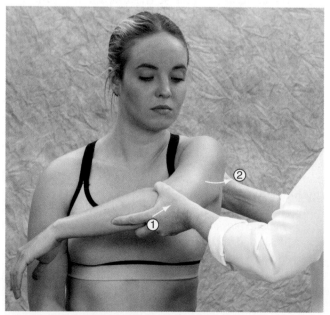

Fig. 5.82 Posterior subluxation test. The arm is pushed posteriorly *(1)* while the patient's arm is abducted horizontally and rotated laterally *(2)*.

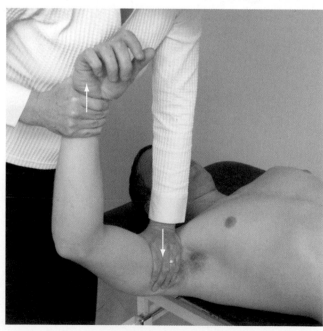

Fig. 5.83 Push-pull test.

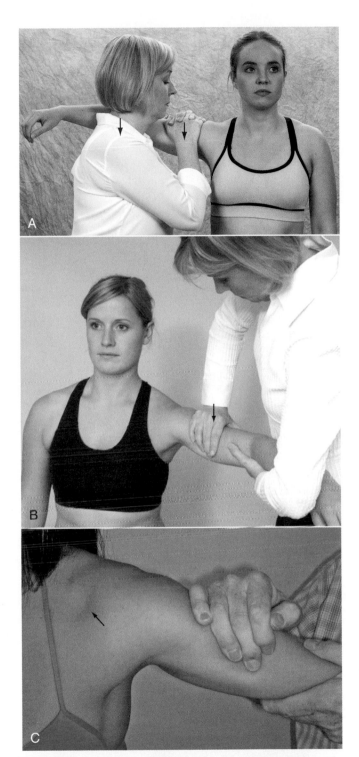

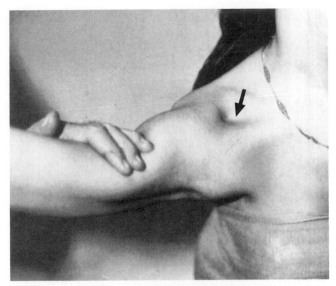

Fig. 5.85 A 21-year-old female whose shoulder could be dislocated inferiorly and anteriorly and subluxated posteriorly. Note sulcus *(arrow)* anteriorly when the Feagin test is performed. She was unable to carry books, reach overhead, or use the arm for activities such as tennis or swimming. Associated episodes of numbness and weakness of the entire upper extremity sometimes lasted for 1 or 2 days. (From Neer CS, Foster CR: Inferior capsular shift for involuntary inferior and multidirectional instability of the shoulder, *J Bone Joint Surg Am* 62:900, 1980.)

Fig. 5.84 Feagin test. (A) In standing. (B) In sitting. (C) Positive Feagin—note sulcus *(arrow)*.

be done carefully as the patient may become apprehensive when the injured arm is elevated. Then the problem shoulder is tested. For a positive test, the extension of the affected arm must be greater than 10° relative to the normal arm.

⚠ *Knee-Shoulder Test.*[361] The patient is seated and is asked to grasp one knee with both hands (Fig. 5.88). If pain results in the shoulder, it is considered a positive test. The patient will also feel the shoulder sliding out of the socket or an anteroinferior drawer will be visible. This is a test for anterior and multidirectional instability.

❓ *Rowe Test for Multidirectional Instability.*[340] The patient stands forward flexed at the waist to 45° with the arms relaxed and pointing to the floor. The examiner places one hand over the patient's shoulder so that the examiner's index and middle fingers sit over the anterior aspect of the humeral head and the thumb sits over the posterior aspect of the humeral head. The examiner then pulls the arm down slightly (Fig. 5.89). To test for anterior instability, the humeral head is pushed anteriorly with the thumb while the arm is extended 20° to 30° from the vertical position. To test for posterior instability, the humeral head is pushed posteriorly with the examiner's index and middle fingers while the patient's arm is flexed 20° to 30° from the vertical position. For inferior instability, more traction is applied to the arm and the sulcus sign becomes evident.

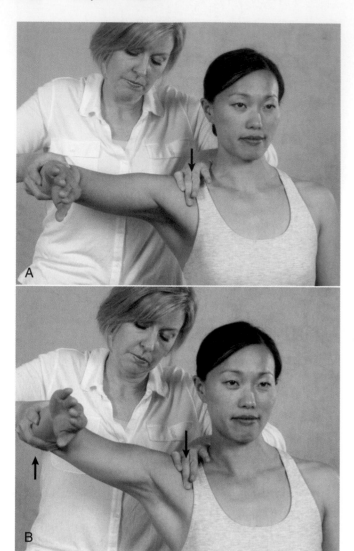

Fig. 5.86 Hyperabduction test (Gagey hyperabduction test). (A) Start position. (B) End position.

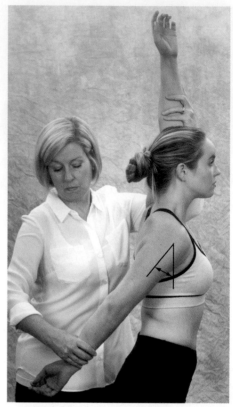

Fig. 5.87 Hyperextension–internal (medial) rotation (HERI) test.

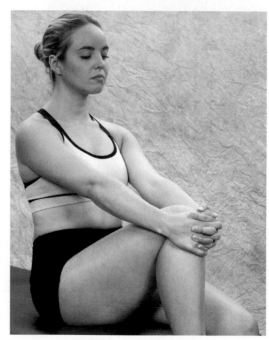

Fig. 5.88 Knee–shoulder test.

✓ *Test for Inferior Shoulder Instability (Sulcus Sign).*[308,310] The patient stands with the arm by the side and shoulder muscles relaxed. The examiner grasps the patient's forearm below the elbow and pulls the arm distally (Fig. 5.90A). The presence of a **sulcus sign** (Fig. 5.90B) may indicate inferior instability or glenohumeral laxity[362] but should only be considered positive for instability if the patient is symptomatic (e.g., pain/ache on activity, shoulder does not "feel right" with activity).[359] A bilateral sulcus sign is not as clinically significant as unilateral laxity on the affected side.[358] The sulcus sign with a feeling of subluxation is also clinically significant.[358] The sulcus sign may be graded by measuring from the inferior margin of the acromion to the humeral head. A +1 sulcus implies a distance of less than 1 cm; +2 sulcus, 1 to 2 cm (some authors say a +1 grade is <1.5 cm and a +2 grade is 1.5 to 2.0 cm[98,305]); and +3 sulcus, more than 2 cm. Humeral head displacement of more than 2 cm from the acromion has been reported to be indicative of a high degree of glenohumeral laxity.[359] Note: a sulcus sign is seen further laterally than a step deformity, which is seen with a 3° acromioclavicular sprain.

The best position to test for inferior instability is at 20° to 50° of abduction with neutral rotation. Also, rotation causes the capsule to tighten anteriorly (lateral rotation) or posteriorly

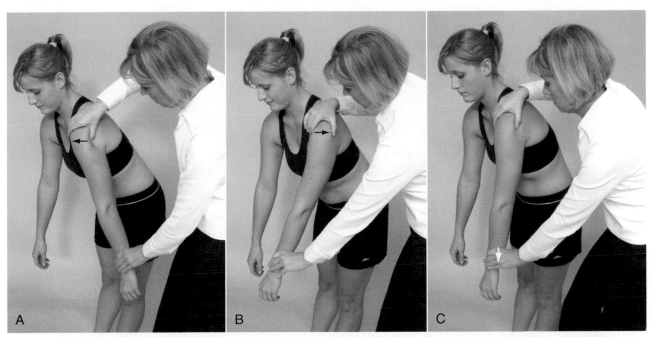

Fig. 5.89 Rowe test for multidirectional instability. (A) Testing for anterior instability. (B) Testing for posterior instability. (C) Testing for inferior instability.

(medial rotation), and the sulcus distance decreases.[323] Thus more than one position should be tested.[124,354,363] Depending on the patient history, the examiner should test the patient in the position in which the sensation of instability is reported. Ren and Bicknell[361] advocated also doing the sulcus test in 30° of lateral rotation (Fig. 5.90C). If the amount of inferior translation does not decrease when the test is done in 30° of lateral rotation, it suggests that the superior glenohumeral ligament and the structures in the **rotator interval** are lax and not holding the humeral head up in the glenoid the way they should.[39,40]

Tests for Impingement

Anterior shoulder impingement, regardless of its cause (i.e., rotator cuff pathology, bicipital paratenonitis/tendinosis, scapular or humeral instability, labral pathology), results from structures being compressed in the anterior aspect of the humerus between the head of the humerus and the coracoid process under the acromion process (Fig. 5.91).[364–369] Park et al.[58] found that better results were achieved by combining the tests. They found that the Hawkins-Kennedy test, the painful arc sign, and a positive infraspinatus test gave the best probability of anterior impingement, whereas the painful arc sign, drop-arm test, and the infraspinatus test were best for full-thickness rotator cuff tears. Abduction and lateral rotation (i.e., the cocking position in throwing) may cause the posterosuperior labrum to contact the rotator cuff, resulting in a posterosuperior impingement.[370,371]

✓ *Hawkins-Kennedy Impingement Test.*[82,273,372] The patient stands while the examiner forward flexes the arm to 90° and then forcibly rotates the shoulder medially (see Fig. 5.96B). This movement pushes the supraspinatus tendon against the anterior surface[373] of the coracoacromial ligament and coracoid process.[374–376] The test can also be performed in different degrees of forward flexion (vertically "circling the shoulder") or horizontal adduction (horizontally "circling the shoulder"). Pain indicates a positive test for supraspinatus paratenonitis/tendinosis or secondary impingement.[79] It has also been advocated that the examiner place an arm under the patient's arm and hold the opposite shoulder (Fig. 5.92).[356] This will allow the patient to relax the arm on the examiner's arm. A positive test would indicate pinching of structures rather than strain of a muscle. McFarland et al.[377] described the **coracoid impingement sign** ✓, which is the same as the Hawkins-Kennedy test but involves horizontally adducting the arm across the body 10° to 20° before doing the medial rotation (Fig. 5.93). This is more likely to approximate the lesser tuberosity of the humerus and the coracoid process. The **Yocum test** ✓ is a modification of this test in which the patient's hand is placed on his or her opposite shoulder and the examiner elevates the elbow.[92,378] Pain indicates a positive test.

⊘ *Impingement Test.*[379] The patient is seated. The examiner takes the arm to 90° of abduction and full lateral rotation. This is the same position as that for the apprehension test. However, if there is no history of possible traumatic subluxation or dislocation, the movement can also can cause anterior translation of the humerus, resulting in secondary impingement of the rotator cuff. Therefore, a positive test indicates a grade II or III shoulder lesion based on the Jobe classification (see the previous discussion).[299] A positive test depends on production

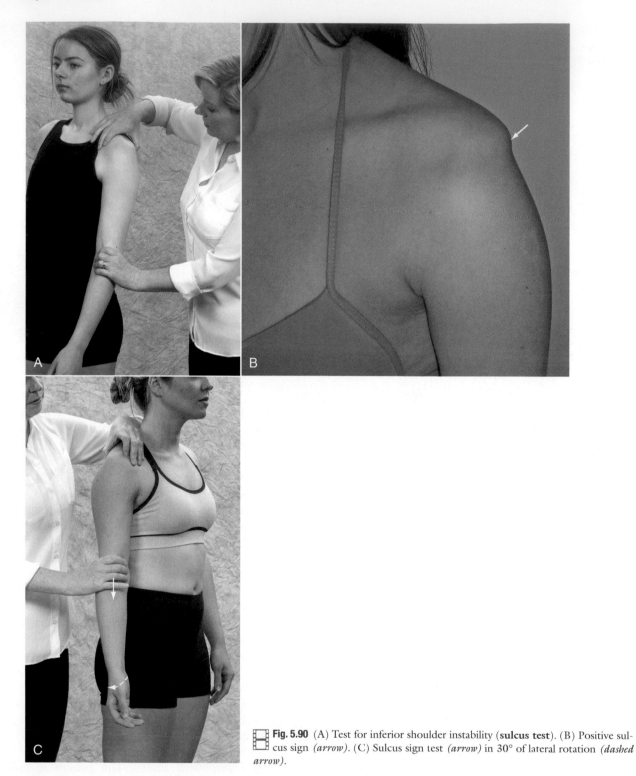

Fig. 5.90 (A) Test for inferior shoulder instability (**sulcus test**). (B) Positive sulcus sign *(arrow)*. (C) Sulcus sign test *(arrow)* in 30° of lateral rotation *(dashed arrow)*.

of the patient's symptoms, anterior or posterior shoulder pain, or both.

Branch et al.[380] advocated testing the anterior capsule in a position of 30° to 40° abduction and 0° to 10° flexion. Lateral rotation is then passively applied to stress the anterior capsule. To test the posterior capsule, they advocated placing the humerus in 60° to 70° of abduction and 20° to 30° of flexion followed by passive medial rotation to stress the posterior capsule. By testing below 70° of abduction, they felt impingement signs would be less.

☑ *Internal (Medial) Rotation Resistance Strength Test (IRRST) (Zaslav Test).*[381] This test is a follow-up to a Neer test. The patient stands with the arm abducted to 90° and laterally rotated 80° to 85°. The examiner then applies an isometric resistance into lateral rotation followed by isometric resistance into medial rotation (Fig. 5.94).

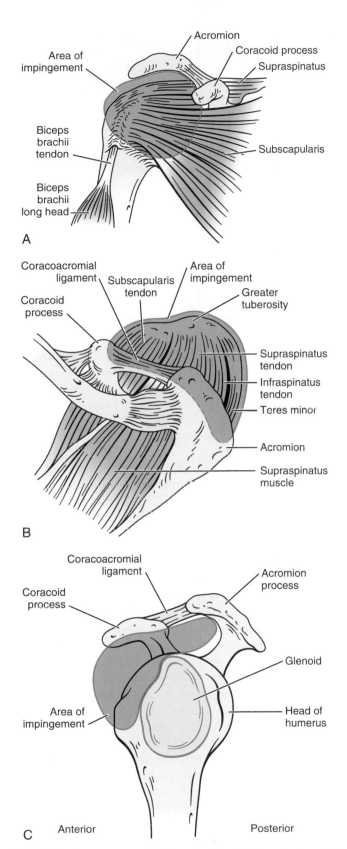

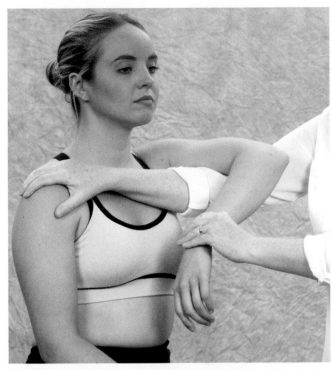

Fig. 5.92 Modified Hawkins-Kennedy impingement test. Note the position of the examiner's right arm.

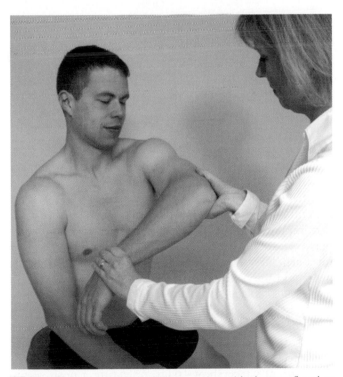

Fig. 5.93 The coracoid impingement sign with the arm flexed to 90°, adducted to 10°, and rotated internally. The test is positive if it produces pain in the area of the coracoid.

Fig. 5.91 Impingement zone. (A) Anterior view. (B) Superior view. (C) Lateral view.

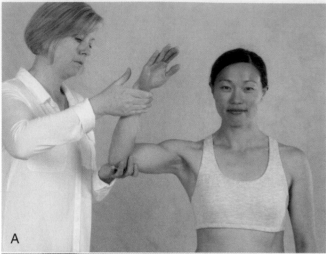

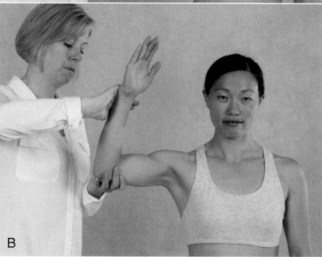

Fig. 5.94 Medial rotation resistance strength test. The patient is asked to maximally resist medial rotation (A) followed by lateral rotation (B).

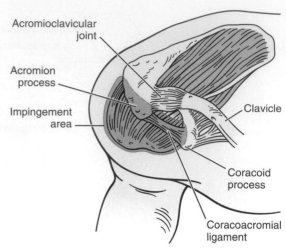

Fig. 5.95 The functional arc of elevation of the proximal humerus is forward, as proposed by Neer. The greater tuberosity impinges against the anterior one-third of the acromial surface. This critical area comprises the supraspinatus and bicipital tendons and the subacromial bursa.

The test is considered positive in a patient who has a positive impingement test if the patient has good strength in lateral rotation but not medial rotation; it indicates an internal impingement. If the patient exhibits more weakness on lateral rotation, it indicates a classic external anterior impingement. This test may be used to differentiate between an outlet (subacromial) impingement and an intra-articular (nonoutlet) problem when the examiner has found the Neer test to be positive.

☑ *Neer Impingement Test.*[82,273,382] The patient's arm is passively and forcibly fully elevated in the scapular plane with the arm medially rotated by the examiner. This passive stress causes the greater tuberosity to jam against the anteroinferior border of the acromion (Fig. 5.95).[374] The patient's face shows pain, reflecting a positive test result (Fig. 5.96A). The test indicates an overuse injury to the supraspinatus and sometimes to the biceps tendon. If the test is positive when done with the arm laterally rotated, the examiner should check the acromioclavicular joint (**acromioclavicular differentiation test**).[383]

Guosheng et al.[384] recommend doing the Neer test in two positions, calling the test the **Modified Neer Test** ☑. The first part of the test (Fig. 5.97A) is done similar to the Neer test with the patient seated and the examiner stabilizes the clavicle and scapula with one hand while abducting the test arm, in which the elbow is flexed to 90° and the palm faces the floor, as far as possible. The examiner then laterally rotates the abducted arm (Fig. 5.97B). A disappearance of pain with the second part of the test is considered a positive sign for impingement. If the pain did not disappear in the second part of the test or if the patient is unable to abduct the arm, the test is negative for impingement.

❓ *Posterior Internal Impingement Test.*[104,320,371,385–387] This type of impingement is found primarily in overhead athletes, although it may be found in others who hold their arm in the vulnerable position. The impingement occurs when the rotator cuff impinges against the posterosuperior edge of the glenoid when the arm is abducted, extended beyond the coronal plane, and laterally rotated (Fig. 5.98).[300,371,388,389] The result is that of a "kissing" labral lesion posteriorly. The resulting impingement is between the rotator cuff and greater tuberosity on the one hand and the posterior glenoid and labrum on the other. It often accompanies anterior instability or pseudolaxity, and the deltoid activity increases to compensate for weakened rotator cuff muscles. The patient complains of pain posteriorly in late cocking and early acceleration phase of throwing. To perform the test, the patient is placed in the supine position. The examiner passively abducts the shoulder to 90° to 110°, with 15° to 20° extension and maximum lateral rotation (Fig. 5.99). The test is considered positive if it elicits localized pain in the posterior shoulder.[104]

❓ *Reverse Impingement Sign (Impingement Relief Test).*[322] This test is used if the patient has a positive painful arc or pain on lateral rotation. The patient lies supine.

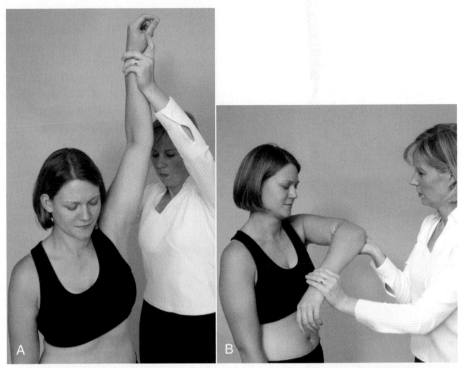

Fig. 5.96 Impingement sign. (A) A positive Neer impingement sign is present if pain and its resulting facial expression are produced when the examiner forcibly flexes the arm forward, jamming the greater tuberosity against the anteroinferior surface of the acromion. (B) An alternative method (Hawkins-Kennedy impingement test) demonstrates the impingement sign by forcibly medially rotating the proximal humerus when the arm is flexed forward to 90°.

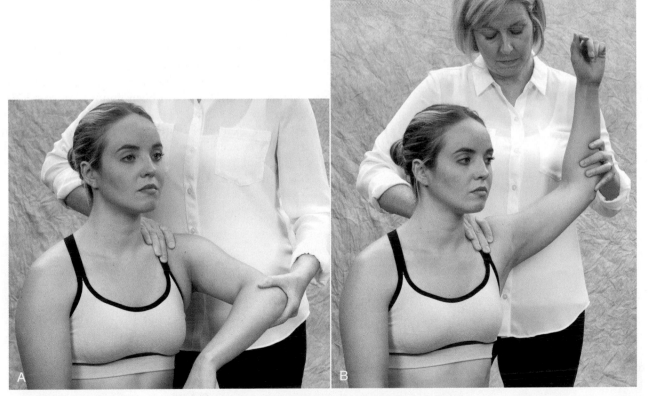

Fig. 5.97 Modified Neer test. (A) Start position. (B) End position.

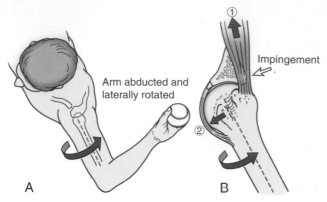

Fig. 5.98 Internal impingement of the undersurface of the rotator cuff against the posterior aspect of the labrum in maximum lateral rotation and abduction. (A) Lateral rotation. (B) Area of impingement *(open arrow)* when rotator cuff contracts *(1)* and humeral head is pushed anteriorly *(2)*.

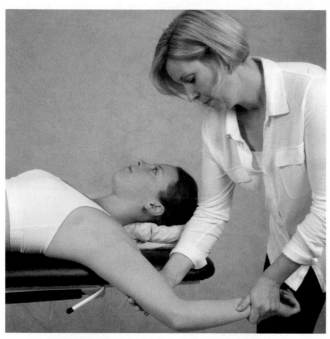

Fig. 5.99 Posterior internal impingement test.

The examiner pushes the head of the humerus inferiorly as the arm is abducted or laterally rotated. Corso advocated doing the test in the standing position.[390] He also advocated an inferior glide of the humerus during abduction but suggested using a posteroinferior glide of the humeral head during forward flexion. He advocated applying the glide just before the ROM where pain occurred on active movement. If the pain decreases or disappears when repeating the movements with the humeral head depressed, it is considered a positive test for mechanical impingement under the acromion (Fig. 5.100).

☑ *Supine Impingement Test.*[56,280] The patient is supine with the examiner at the side by the shoulder to be tested (Fig. 5.101). The examiner holds the patient's wrist and humerus (near the elbow) and elevates the patient's arm to end range (approximately 170° to 180°). The examiner then laterally rotates the arm and adducts it into further elevation with the supinated arm against the patient's ear. The examiner then medially rotates the patient's arm. If the medial rotation causes a significant increase in pain, the test is considered positive for an impingement and rotator cuff pathology (nonspecific) because of narrowing and compression in the subacromial space.

Tests for Labral Tears

Injuries to the labrum are relatively common, especially in throwing athletes where the labrum plays a key role in glenohumeral stability but are hard to diagnose using only special tests.[74] A detailed history is also required.[391] In the young, the tensile strength of the labrum is less than that of the capsule, so it is more prone to injury when anterior stress (e.g., anterior dislocation) is applied to the glenohumeral joint.[392] The tear may be a **Bankart lesion,** in which the anteroinferior labrum is torn, or the superior labrum may have been injured, causing a **SLAP lesion** (to the biceps) (Fig. 5.102).[393–395] These injuries are classic examples of the **circle concept of instability.** This concept suggests that injury in one direction of the joint results in injury to structures on the other side of the joint. A Bankart lesion occurs most commonly

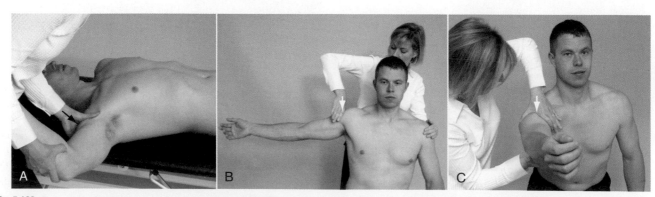

Fig. 5.100 Reverse impingement sign (impingement relief test). (A) In supine. (B) In standing, doing the test in abduction. (C) In standing, doing the test in forward flexion.

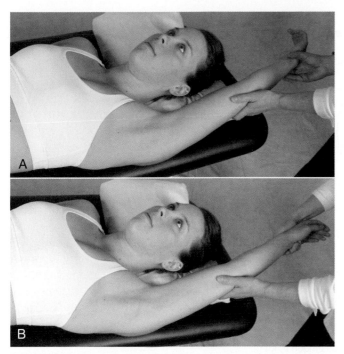

Fig. 5.101 Supine impingement test. (A) Arm in lateral rotation. (B) Arm in medial rotation.

with a traumatic anterior dislocation leading to anterior instability. In the right shoulder, for example, this injury results in the labrum being detached anywhere from the 3 o'clock to the 7 o'clock position, resulting in both anterior and posterior structural injury (see Fig. 5.102A). Not only is the labrum torn, but the stability of the inferior glenohumeral ligament is lost.[396] A **reverse Bankart** occurs with a posterior glenohumeral dislocation and results in the labrum being detached from the 6 o'clock to the 9 o'clock position on the glenoid fossa (see Fig. 5.102B). The SLAP lesion has the labrum detaching (pulled or peeled, depending on the mechanism) from the 10 o'clock to the 2 o'clock position (see Fig. 5.102B). The injury often results from a FOOSH injury, occurs during deceleration when throwing, or arises when sudden traction is applied to the biceps.[397,398] If the biceps tendon also detaches, the shoulder becomes unstable and the support of the superior glenohumeral ligament is lost. Snyder and colleagues[399] have divided these SLAP lesions into four types:

- Type I: Superior labrum markedly frayed but attachments intact
- Type II: Small tear in the superior labrum; instability of the labral-biceps complex (most common)
- Type III: Bucket-handle tear of labrum that may displace into the joint; labral biceps attachment intact
- Type IV: Bucket-handle tear of labrum that extends to the biceps tendon, allowing the tendon to sublux into the joint

Burkhart et al.[65,400] described a **"peel back" mechanism** that resulted in a posterior type II SLAP lesion

in overhead athletes; they demonstrate increased lateral rotation, decreased medial rotation, and a tight posterior capsule that results in posterosuperior migration of the head during maximum lateral rotation, causing a tear of the posterosuperior labrum.[401–403] Fig. 5.103 shows three possible mechanisms of SLAP injuries.

Research has shown that no single test can accurately diagnose a SLAP lesion. In most cases, there are no definitive tests. Testing most often leads only to a higher level of suspicion of a labral lesion.[99,275,284–287,391,404,405] There are several tests for labral lesions. Labral lesion tests, especially those for SLAP lesions, show sensitivity but lack specificity. Part of the reason for this is that SLAP lesions commonly occur along with other shoulder injuries (e.g., instability, muscle tears, and tendon ruptures) and there is no specific pain pattern associated with SLAP lesions leading to a cascade of mechanical problems in the shoulder, and patients are often unable to accurately describe the location of the pain, give a precise history, or point to a mechanism of injury.[391,406] At present, there is no convincing evidence for accurate tests to detect a SLAP lesion.[275,288,289]

✓ *Active Compression Test of O'Brien.*[82,104,286,318,407–410] This test is designed to detect SLAP (type II) or superior labral lesions. The patient is placed in the standing position with the arm forward flexed to 90° and the elbow fully extended. The arm is then horizontally adducted 10° to 15° (starting position) and medially rotated so the thumb faces downward. The examiner stands behind the patient and applies a downward eccentric force to the arm (Fig. 5.104). The arm is returned to the starting position and the palm is supinated so that the shoulder is rotated laterally; then the downward eccentric load is repeated. If pain on the joint line or deep painful clicking is produced inside the shoulder (not over the acromioclavicular joint) in the first part of the test and eliminated or decreased in the second part, the test is considered positive for labral abnormalities. The test also "locks and loads" the acromioclavicular joint in medial rotation, so that the examiner must take care to differentiate between labral and acromioclavicular (pain over acromioclavicular joint) pathology.[63]

It has been suggested that the test should be modified in the following way to give clearer results. The patient is asked to forward flex both arms to 90° so that the backs of the hands are close to each other and the thumbs face the floor (shoulder is in medial rotation). The examiner stands in front of the patient and applies a uniform downward force to both arms at the same time noting any differences (Fig. 5.105A). The patient is then asked to laterally rotate the shoulders so the hands are close together with the palms up. The examiner then applies a downward force to both arms noting any differences (Fig. 5.105B). The outcomes would be the same as for the original test, but doing the test in this way enables better standardization.[411]

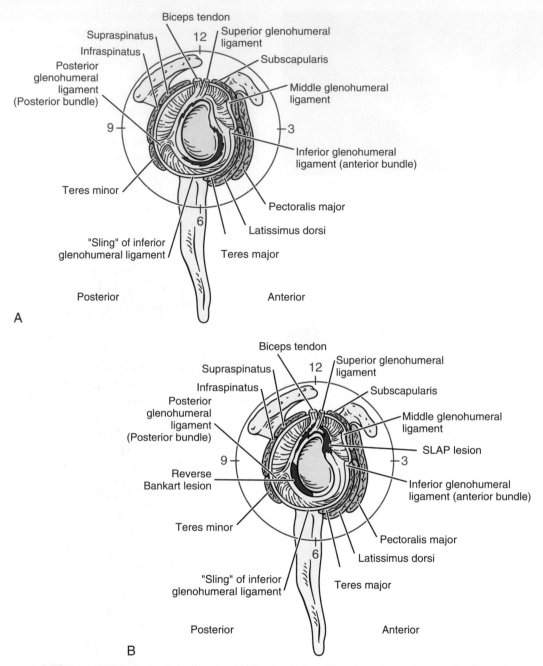

Fig. 5.102 Labral lesions to the right shoulder. (A) Bankart lesion. (B) SLAP lesion and reverse Bankart lesion.

⚠ ***Anterior Slide Test.***[82,289,408,412,413] The patient is sitting with the hands on the waist, thumbs posterior. The examiner stands behind the patient and stabilizes the scapula and clavicle with one hand. With the other hand, the examiner applies an anterosuperior force at the elbow (Fig. 5.106A). If the labrum is torn (SLAP lesion), the humeral head slides over the labrum with a pop or crack with pain on the joint line, and the patient complains of anterosuperior pain. McFarland et al.[82] have described the test as the examiner applying an axial upward load to the glenohumeral joint that the patient resists (Fig. 5.106B). The test is positive if a pain or click is produced deep in the shoulder.

⚠ ***Biceps Load Test (Kim Test II).***[285,414] This test is designed to check the integrity of the superior labrum. The patient is in the supine or seated position with the shoulder abducted to 120° and laterally rotated with the elbow flexed to 90° and the forearm supinated, as it is for the apprehension or crank test. The examiner performs an apprehension test on the patient by taking the arm into full lateral rotation. If apprehension appears, the examiner stops lateral rotation and holds the position. The patient is then asked to flex the elbow against the examiner's resistance at the wrist. If apprehension decreases or the patient feels more comfortable, the test is negative for a SLAP lesion. If the apprehension remains the same or the shoulder becomes more painful, the test is considered positive for a SLAP lesion in the presence of recurrent dislocations (Fig. 5.107). Wilk et al.[415] also advocate doing the test with the forearm pronated (**pronated biceps load test ❓**). If the pain is located deep in the superior glenohumeral joint, the test is considered positive.

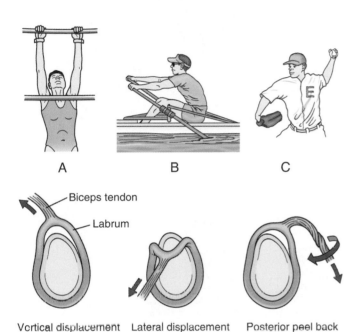

Fig. 5.103 Mechanisms of injury for SLAP lesions. (A) Vertical displacement. (B) Lateral displacement. (C) Posterior peel back.

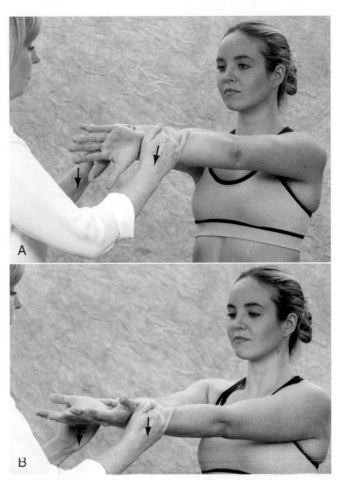

Fig. 5.105 Modified O'Brien test. (A) In medial rotation with backs of hands together. (B) In lateral rotation with palms up.

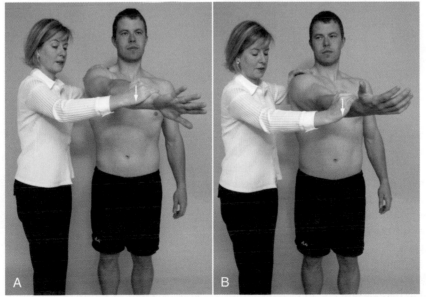

Fig. 5.104 Active compression test of O'Brien. (A) Position 1: The patient forward flexes the arm to 90° with the elbow extended and adducted 15° medial to the midline of the body and with the thumb pointed down. The examiner applies a downward force to the arm that the patient resists. (B) Position 2: The test is performed with the arm in the same position but the patient fully supinates the arm with the palm facing the ceiling. The same maneuver is repeated. The test is positive for a superior labral injury if pain is elicited in the first step and reduced or eliminated in the second step of this maneuver.

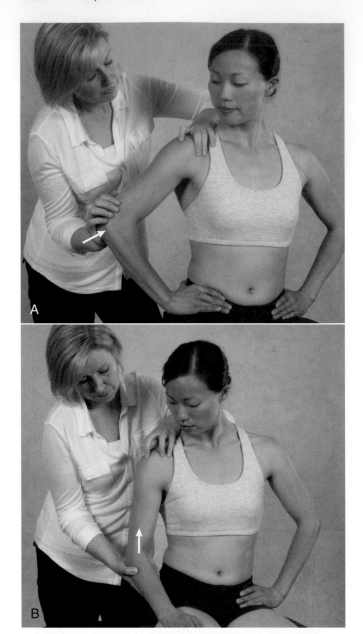

Fig. 5.106 (A) Anterior slide testing. Note the position of the examiner's hands and the patient's arms. (B) McFarland's anterior slide test.

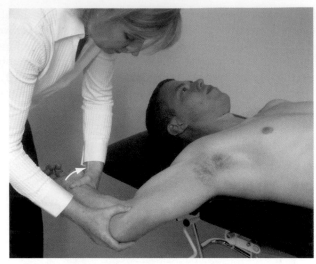

Fig. 5.107 Biceps load test (Kim test II).

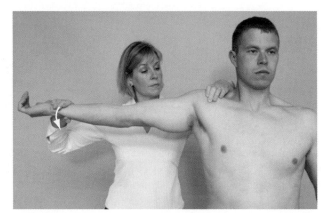

Fig. 5.108 Biceps tension test. The patient's arm is abducted to 90° and laterally rotated. The examiner then applies an eccentric adduction force.

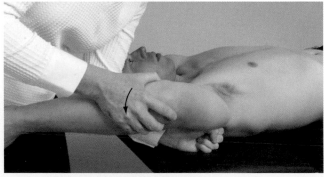

Fig. 5.109 Clunk test.

⚠ *Biceps Tension Test.*[273] This test determines whether a SLAP lesion is present. The patient, in standing, abducts and laterally rotates the arm to 90° with the elbow extended and forearm supinated. The examiner then applies an eccentric adduction force to the arm. A reproduction of the patient's symptoms is a positive test (Fig. 5.108). The examiner should also do a Speed test (discussed later) to rule out biceps pathology.

⚠ *Clunk Test.* The patient lies supine. The examiner places one hand on the posterior aspect of the shoulder over the humeral head. The examiner's other hand holds the humerus above the elbow. The examiner fully abducts the arm over the patient's head. The examiner then pushes anteriorly with the hand over the humeral head (a fist may be used to apply more anterior pressure) while the other hand rotates the humerus into lateral rotation (Fig. 5.109). A clunk or grinding sound indicates both a positive test and a tear of the labrum.[416] The test may also cause apprehension if anterior instability is present. Walsh indicated that if the examiner follows these maneuvers with horizontal adduction that relocates the humerus, he

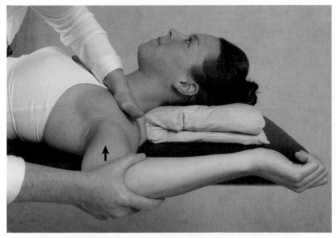

Fig. 5.110 Compression rotation test.

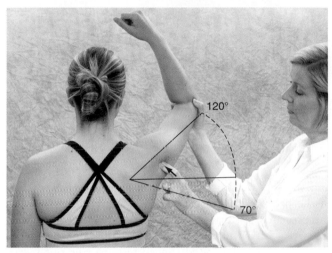

Fig. 5.111 Dynamic labral shear test (O'Driscoll SLAP test). Arm in 120° in the plane of the scapula. Examiner's fingers apply an anterior shearing force *(arrow)*.

or she may also hear a clunk or a click, indicating a tear of the labrum.[417]

The examiner may also position the arm in different amounts of abduction (vertically "circling the shoulder") and perform the test. This will stress different parts of the labrum.

Compression Rotation Test.[276,289,418] The patient is supine with the examiner standing beside the test shoulder. The examiner passively abducts the shoulder to between 20° and 90° with the patient's elbow at 90°. The examiner applies an axial compression force through the long axis of the humerus (pushing up through the elbow) while passively rotating the humerus back and forth (small and large circles) to try to trap the labrum within the joint (Fig. 5.110). If pain, clicking, or a catching sensation is elicited, the test is considered positive for a torn labrum.

Dynamic Labral Shear Test (O'Driscoll's SLAP Test).[419] The patient is in sitting, standing (most common), or supine with the arm at the side and the elbow

flexed to 90°. If the patient is supine, the arm should not rest on the table. The examiner laterally rotates the arm to tightness and takes the arm into 70° abduction in the scapular plane (Fig. 5.111). Maintaining the flexed elbow, the examiner then abducts the arm from 70° to 120° while applying a shear load to the joint moving back and forth from 70° to 120° to 70°. A positive test is indicated by pain and possibly a click between 90° and 120° of abduction. Kibler et al.[408] modified the test by taking the arm above 120° before placing the arm in maximum horizontal abduction. The examiner then lowers the arm to 60° of abduction.[420]

Forced Shoulder Abduction and Elbow Flexion Test.[421] The patient is seated with the examiner standing behind on the test side. The examiner passively abducts the patient's shoulder fully with the patient's elbow in full extension noting whether there is any pain in the posterosuperior aspect of the shoulder (Fig. 5.112A). The examiner then passively flexes the patient's elbow and notes whether the pain is decreased (Fig. 5.112B). If the pain is greater when the elbow is extended than when it is flexed, the test is considered positive for a superior labral tear.

Kim Test (Biceps Load Test I).[285,348,410] The patient sits with the back supported. The arm is abducted to 90° with the elbow supported in 90° flexion. The examiner's hand, while supporting the elbow and forearm, applies an axial compression force to the glenoid through the humerus. While maintaining the axial compression force, the examiner elevates the arm diagonally upward using the same hand while the other hand applies a downward and backward force to the proximal arm (Fig. 5.113). A sudden onset of posterior shoulder pain and click indicates a positive test for a posteroinferior labral lesion.

Labral Crank Test.[422] The patient is in the supine lying or sitting position. The examiner elevates the arm to 160° in the scapular plane. With the patient in this position, the examiner applies an axial load to the humerus with one hand while the other hand rotates the humerus medially and laterally. A positive test is indicated by pain on rotation, especially lateral rotation, with or without a click or reproduction of the patient's symptoms (Fig. 5.114).

Labral Tension Test.[275] The patient lies supine. The examiner first places the patient's arm in 120° of abduction with the forearm in neutral and then into full lateral rotation (Fig. 5.115). In this position, the examiner holds the patient's hand and asks the patient to supinate the forearm against resistance from the neutral forearm position. If the patient has increased pain on supination of the forearm, it is considered a positive test for a SLAP lesion.

Mayo Shear Test.[409] The patient stands with the examiner standing behind. The examiner elevates the patient's arm to about 70° and then laterally rotates the arm. Once laterally rotated, the patient's arm is taken into full elevation. The examiner then brings the arm down while maintaining lateral rotation and applying an anterior directed

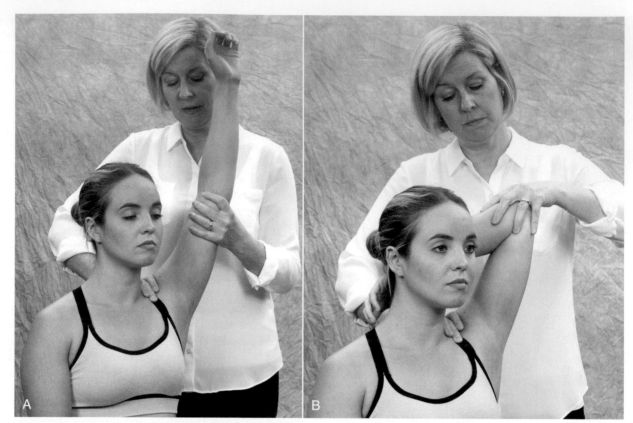

Fig. 5.112 Forced shoulder abduction (A) and elbow flexion (B) test.

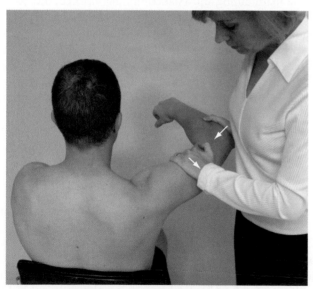

Fig. 5.113 Kim test (biceps load test I).

force with the hand on the posterior shoulder (Fig. 5.116). The test is considered positive if the patient reports pain or a click in the posterior or posterosuperior shoulder and indicates a superior labral (SLAP) tear.

⚠ *Pain Provocation (Mimori) Test.*[423] With the patient seated and the arm abducted to between 90° and 100°, the examiner laterally rotates the arm by holding the wrist (Fig. 5.117). The forearm is taken into maximum supination

and then maximum pronation. If pain is provoked only in the pronated position or if the pain is more severe in the pronated position, the test is considered positive for a superior (SLAP) tear. As with other superior labral tests, the biceps must be tested (Speed test) to rule out biceps pathology causing the pain.

❓ *Passive Compression Test.*[325,424] The patient is in side lying with the test arm uppermost and the examiner behind the patient. The examiner stabilizes the shoulder with one hand over the scapula and clavicle while the other hand holds the arm in 30° abduction at the elbow. The patient's shoulder is laterally rotated and the patient's arm is pushed proximally and extended by the examiner's hand on the elbow. This movement causes compression of the superior labrum on the glenoid. A positive test for superior labral (SLAP) tears is indicated by a click or pain in the glenohumeral joint.

⚠ *Passive Distraction Test (PDT).*[325,425] The patient lies supine with the test arm abducted to 150° with the elbow extended and the forearm supinated (Fig. 5.118A). The examiner stabilizes the upper arm (humerus) to prevent rotation. While maintaining the humerus in the same position, the forearm is pronated (Fig. 5.118B). Pain felt deep in the shoulder (anteriorly or posteriorly) is considered a positive test for a SLAP lesion. This test mimics the position of the arm and glenohumeral joint when a backstroke swimmer's hand enters the water.

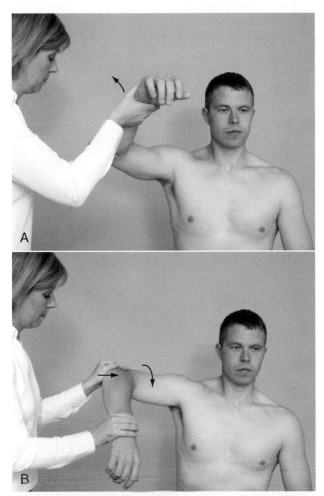

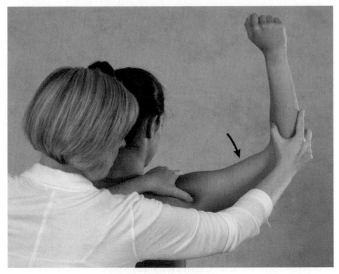

Fig. 5.116 Mayo shear test.

Fig. 5.114 Labral crank test. (A) Crank test in sitting with lateral humeral rotation. (B) Crank test in sitting with medial humeral rotation.

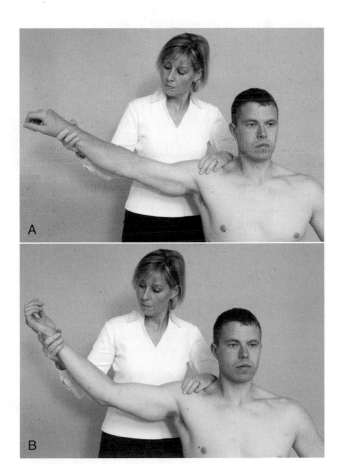

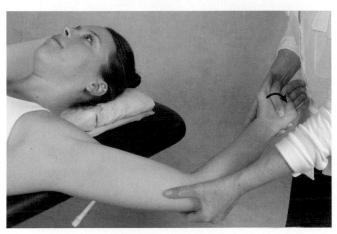

Fig. 5.115 Labral tension test.

Fig. 5.117 Pain provocation test. (A) Test with the forearm pronated. (B) Test with the forearm supinated.

☑ *Porcellini Test.*[426] This test is used to test for posterior instability and posterior labral tears. The patient is standing and the examiner stands behind the patient. The patient's arm is forward flexed to 90°, abducted 10° to 15° and maximally medially rotated (similar to part of the O'Brien test). The examiner stabilizes the scapula with

one hand while the patient is asked to elevate the arm while the examiner's other hand pushes the patient's arm down (Fig. 5.119A). Pain and level of strength are noted. Then, with the patient in the same position, the examiner places the thumb of the hand stabilizing the scapula just lateral to the glenohumeral posterior joint line to stabilize the posterior head of humerus and maintains an anterior force with the thumb to prevent the humeral head from subluxating posteriorly (Fig. 5.119B). If the pain is reduced with or without a change in strength with the second part of the test, the test is considered positive.

⚠ *Resisted Supination External Rotation Test (RSERT)*.[285,397] This test is designed to check for SLAP lesions and is thought to re-create the peel-back mechanism of the superior labrum. The patient is placed in the supine position with the scapula near the edge of the bed. The examiner stands beside the patient, holding the arm to be examined at the elbow and hand. The patient's arm is placed with the shoulder abducted to 90°, the elbow flexed to 65° to 70°, and the forearm is neutral or slight pronation. The patient is then asked to maximally supinate the hand while the examiner resists. While the patient continues to supinate against the examiner's resistance, the examiner rotates the shoulder laterally to end range (Fig. 5.120).

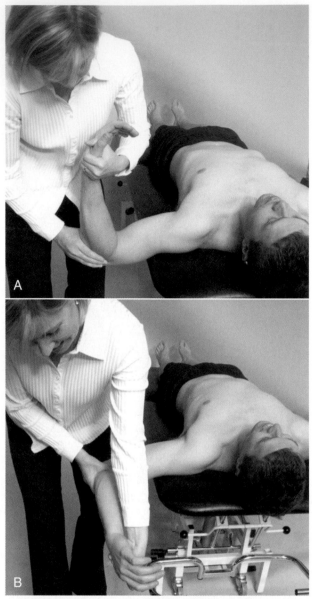

Fig. 5.120 Resisted supination external rotation test (RSERT). (A) The examiner supports the limb in the starting position. The patient attempts to supinate his hand as the examiner resists. (B) The shoulder is then gently externally rotated to the maximal point.

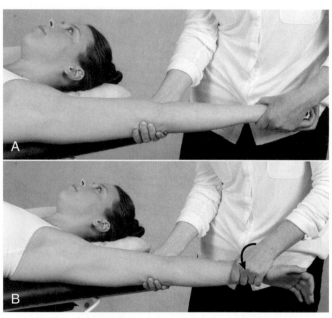

Fig. 5.118 Passive distraction test. (A) Arm abducted to 150°, elbow extended and forearm supinated. (B) Forearm pronated.

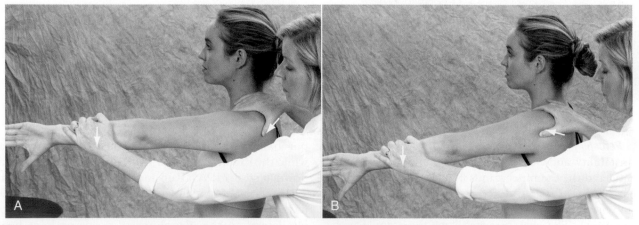

Fig. 5.119 Porcellini test. (A) Examiner stabilizing the scapula. (B) Examiner stabilizing the posterior head of the humerus using the right thumb.

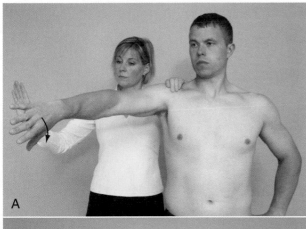

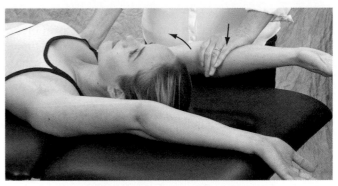

Fig. 5.122 Supine flexion resistance test.

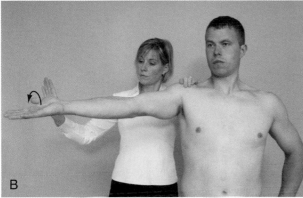

Fig. 5.121 SLAP prehension test. (A) Start position 1: Arm abducted to 90° with the elbow extended and forearm pronated. The patient then horizontally adducts the arm. (B) Start position 2: Same as position 1, but the forearm is supinated. The patient again adducts the arm horizontally. If position 1 is painful and position 2 is not, the test is considered positive.

The test is considered positive if the patient has anterior or deep shoulder pain, there is clicking or catching in the shoulder, or the symptoms are reproduced. The test is considered negative if there is posterior shoulder pain, no pain, or apprehension.

❷ SLAP Prehension Test.[427] The patient is in the sitting or standing position. The arm is abducted to 90° with the elbow extended and the forearm pronated (thumb down and shoulder medially rotated). The patient is then asked to adduct the arm horizontally. The movement is repeated with the forearm supinated (thumb up and shoulder laterally rotated). If the patient feels pain in the bicipital groove in the first case (pronation) but the pain lessens or is absent in the second case (supination), the test is considered positive for a SLAP lesion (Fig. 5.121).

⚠ Supine Flexion Resistance Test.[360] The patient is lying supine with both arms fully elevated over the head with the palms facing the ceiling (Fig. 5.122). The examiner stands beside the patient's head on the side to be tested, testing the good arm first, and grasps the arm just distal to the elbow. The patient is then asked to perform a forward flexion movement of the arm as if simulating a throwing motion while the examiner resists the movement. The test

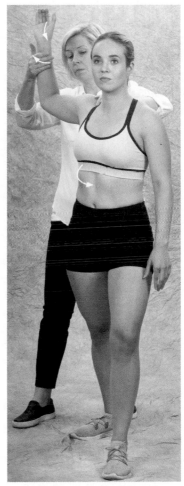

Fig. 5.123 Throwing test.

is considered positive for a SLAP lesion if pain is elicited deep inside the shoulder or at the dorsal aspect along the joint line.

⚠ Throwing Test.[428] The patient is standing with the test arm in 90° abduction, the elbow flexed to 90°, and the shoulder in maximum lateral rotation, mimicking the late cocking phase of pitching (Fig. 5.123). The patient then steps forward with the contralateral leg, moving into the early phase of acceleration (see Fig. 5.13). As the patient moves forward, the examiner provides isometric resistance to the shoulder. A positive test would indicate pain in the long head of biceps tendon or a torn labrum. If the "three-pack examination" of O'Brien testing, the throwing test, and the bicipital tunnel palpation are negative, it is unlikely that the biceps is involved in any pathology.[428]

Tests for Scapular Stability (Scapular Dyskinesia)

For the muscles of the glenohumeral joint to work in a normal coordinated fashion, the scapula must be stabilized by its muscles to act as a firm base for the glenohumeral muscles. Thus, when doing these tests, the examiner is watching for movement patterns of the scapula as well as scapular dyskinesia and the ability of the scapula to dynamically stabilize during movement. It has been reported that no physical examination test of the scapula has been found useful in differentially diagnosing shoulder pathologies.[429]

Signs and Symptoms of "SICK" Scapula [74]

- Insidious onset
- Prominence of inferomedial border of scapula
- Protraction of scapula
- Acromion less prominent
- Coracoid very tender to palpation
- Tight pectoralis minor
- Lack of full forward flexion
- Tight short head of biceps

? *Kinetic Medial Rotation Test.*[101,430] This test is designed to test dynamic control of the scapula during medial rotation of the glenohumeral joint. The patient is in supine lying with the test arm abducted to 90° in scaption and elbow flexed to 90° so the hand faces the ceiling. The patient is asked to perform 60° of medial rotation at the glenohumeral joint while keeping the scapula still (Fig. 5.124). The test is considered positive if the scapula tilts forward, rotates downward, or elevates.

▲ *Lateral Scapular Slide Test.*[107,151,431–433] This test determines the stability of the scapula during glenohumeral movements. The patient sits or stands with the arm resting at his or her side. The examiner measures the distance from the base of the spine of the scapula to the spinous process of T2 or T3 (most common), from the inferior angle of the scapula to the spinous process of T7 to T9, or from T2 to the superior angle of the scapula. The patient is then tested holding two (Fig. 5.125)[431] or four[150] other positions: 45° abduction (hands on waist, thumbs posteriorly),[150,431] 90° abduction with medial rotation,[150,431] 120° abduction,[150] and 150° abduction.[150] Davies and Dickoff-Hoffman[150] and Kibler[431] stated that in each position, the distance measured should not vary more than 1 to 1.5 cm (0.5 to 0.75 inch) from the original measure. However, there may be increased distances above 90° as the scapula rotates during scapulohumeral rhythm. Minimal protraction of

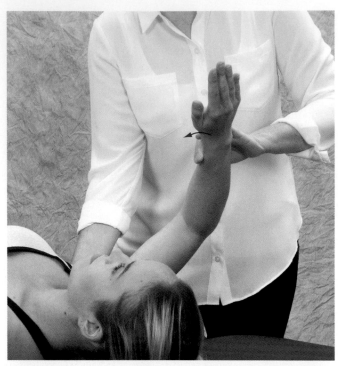

Fig. 5.124 Kinetic medial rotation test. Note how the examiner palpates the scapula to ensure no movement while the patient does the test.

the scapula should occur, however, during full elevation through abduction. Looking for asymmetry of movement between left and right sides is important, as well as noticing the amount of movement when determining scapular stability.

The test may also be performed by loading the arm (providing resistance) at 45° and greater abduction (**scapular load test ✓**) to see how the scapula stabilizes under dynamic load.[433] This load may be applied anteriorly, posteriorly, inferiorly, or superiorly to the arm and can be from 1 kg (2.2 lb) to 3 kg (6.6 lb) (Fig. 5.126). Again, the scapula should not move more than 1.5 cm (0.75 inch). Odom and associates[434] have stated that the test has poor reliability for differentiating normal and pathological shoulders. However, loading the scapula, either by the weight of the arm or by applying a load to the arm, indicates the stabilizing ability of the scapular control muscles and whether abnormal winging or abnormal movement patterns occur.

In the different positions, the examiner may test for scapular and humeral stability by performing an eccentric movement at the shoulder by pushing the arm forward (**eccentric hold test**). One arm is tested at a time. As the arm is pushed forward eccentrically, the examiner should watch the relative movement at the scapulothoracic joint (protraction) and the glenohumeral joint (horizontal adduction). Normally, slightly more movement (relatively) occurs at the glenohumeral joint. If instability due to muscle weakness exists at either joint, excessive movement is evident at that joint relative to the other joint. In addition, the examiner should watch for winging of the scapula, which indicates scapular instability.

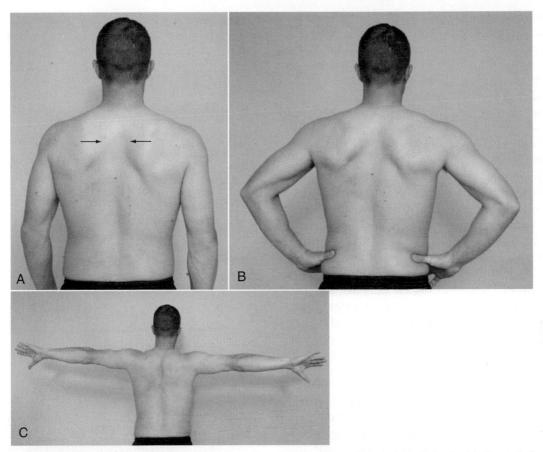

Fig. 5.125 Lateral scapular slide test. The examiner measures from the spinous process to the scapula at the level of the base of spine of the scapula (*arrows* in A). (A) Arms at side. (B) Arms abducted, hands on waist, thumbs back. (C) Arms abducted to 90°, thumbs down.

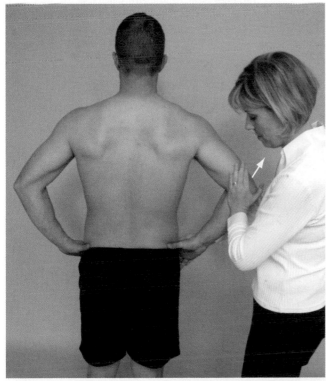

Fig. 5.126 Scapular load test in 45° of abduction. Examiner is pushing anteriorly.

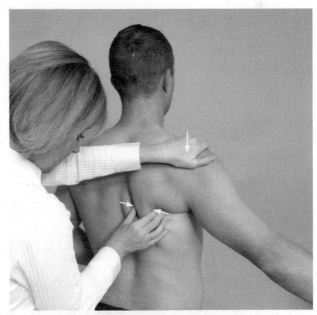

Fig. 5.127 Scapular assistance test (SAT).

? *Scapular Assistance Test (SAT).* [99,107,159,435,436] This test (Fig. 5.127) evaluates scapular and acromial involvement in patients with impingement symptoms. The patient is in a standing position, and the examiner stands behind the patient. The examiner places the fingers of one hand over the clavicle with the heel of the hand over the spine of the scapula. This stabilizes the clavicle and scapula and holds the scapula retracted. The examiner's other hand holds the inferior angle of the scapula. As the patient actively abducts or forward flexes the arm, the examiner stabilizes and pushes the inferior medial border of the scapula up and laterally while keeping the scapula retracted. Decreased pain would be a positive test and would indicate that the scapular control muscles are weak as the assistance by the examiner simulates the activity of serratus anterior and lower trapezius during elevation (see Fig. 5.127). During treatment, the test may be used as a method to increase the subacromial space or acromiohumeral distance.[437] The test may be done with or without weights.[438]

✓ *Scapular Dyskinesia Test.*[118,119,439,440] The patient is in standing with the back exposed so the examiner who is standing behind the patient can watch the scapula move while the patient does elevation through abduction and elevation through forward flexion. The patient is asked to hold a weight of 1.4 kg (3 lb) if the patient weighs less than 68 kg (150 lb) and 2.3 kg (5 lb) if the patient weighs more than 68 kg (150 lb). The patient is asked to simultaneously abduct both arms to full elevation with the thumbs up to a 3-second count and then lower to a 3-second count, and the movement is repeated three times (Fig. 5.128A). The patient then forward flexes to full elevation and then lowers in a similar fashion (Fig. 5.128B). While the patient does the movements, the examiner watches for any abnormal movement in the scapula. If scapular dyskinesia is present, it is more likely to be seen during the lowering movement.

❷ *Scapular Isometric Pinch or Squeeze Test.*[159] The patient is in a standing position and is asked to actively "pinch" or retract the scapulae together as hard as possible and to hold the position for as long as possible (Fig. 5.129). Normally, an individual can hold the contractions for 15 to 20 seconds

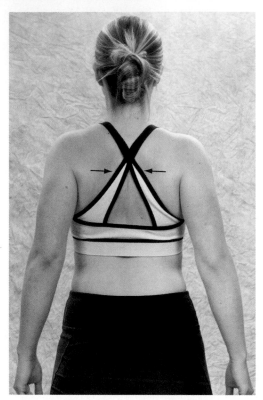

Fig. 5.129 Scapular isometric pinch test.

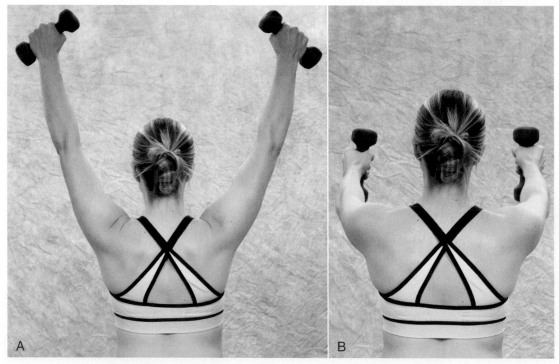

Fig. 5.128 Scapular dyskinesia test. (A) In abduction. (B) In forward flexion.

with no burning pain or obvious muscle weakness. If burning pain occurs in less than 15 seconds, the scapular retractors are weak. When doing the test, the examiner must watch the patient carefully. Subconsciously, many patients will relax the contraction a slight amount, which is barely noticeable but allows the patient to hold the contraction in a comfort zone for longer periods with no burning.

⚠ *Scapular Retraction Test (SRT).*[99,107,159,435,436] The patient is in the standing position. The examiner, standing behind the patient, places the fingers of one hand over the clavicle with the heel of the hand over the spine of the scapula to stabilize the clavicle and scapula and to hold the scapula retracted. The examiner's other hand compresses the scapula against the chest wall (Fig. 5.130). Holding the scapula in this position provides a firm stable base for the rotator cuff muscles, and often rotator cuff strength (if tested by a second examiner) improves. The test may also be positive in patients with a positive relocation test. If scapular retraction decreases the pain, when the relocation test is performed, it indicates that the weak scapular stabilizers must be addressed in the treatment.[436] This test may also be done in supine. In patients with a SICK scapula, if the scapula is repositioned, forward flexion improves.[74]

⚠ *Wall Push-up Test.*[159,435] The patient stands arms' length from a wall. The patient is then asked to do a "wall push-up" 15 to 20 times (Fig. 5.131). Any weakness of the scapular muscles or winging usually shows up with 5 to 10 push-ups. For stronger or younger people, a normal push-up on the floor shows similar scapular changes, usually with fewer repetitions. Goldbeck and Davies have taken this test further in what they describe as a **closed kinetic chain upper extremity stability test.**[441–443] In this test, two markers (e.g., tape) are placed 91 cm (36 inches) apart. Patients assume the push-up position with one hand on each marker. When the examiner says "go," the subject moves one hand to touch the other, returns it to the original position, and then does the same with the other hand, repeating the motions for 15 seconds. Females use a modified push-up position (on knees instead of feet). The examiner counts the number of touches or crossovers made in the allotted time. The test is repeated three times, and the average is the test score. This test is designed primarily for young, active patients.

Other Shoulder Joint Tests

Scheibel et al.[444] have developed an acromioclavicular joint instability (ACJI) scoring system to determine disability associated with injury to the acromioclavicular joint.

☑ *Acromioclavicular Crossover, Cross-Body, or Horizontal Adduction Test.* The patient stands and reaches the hand across to the opposite shoulder. The examiner may also passively perform the test. With the patient in a sitting position, the examiner passively forward flexes the arm to 90° and then horizontally adducts the arm as far as possible (Fig. 5.132).[91,415] If the patient feels localized pain over the acromioclavicular joint, the test is positive.[445–447] Localized pain in the sternoclavicular joint indicates that joint is at fault.

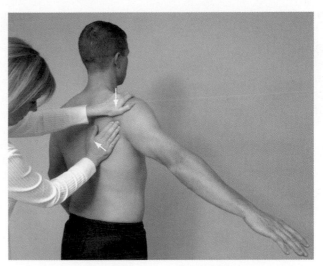

Fig. 5.130 Scapular retraction test. Examiner's hands stabilize the clavicle and scapula.

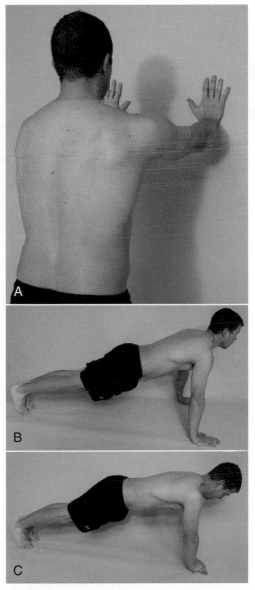

Fig. 5.131 Wall (A) and floor (B) push-up tests. (C) Closed kinetic chain stability test of the upper extremity touching the opposite hand.

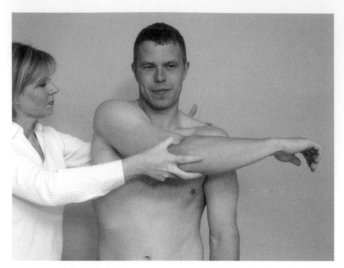

Fig. 5.132 Acromioclavicular crossover, cross-body, or horizontal adduction test.

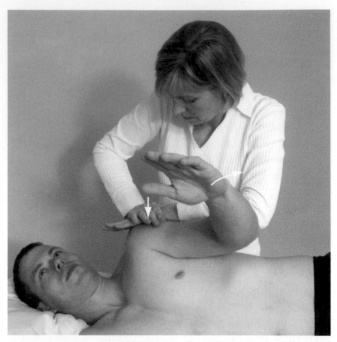

Fig. 5.134 Ellman's compression-rotation test for glenohumeral arthritis.

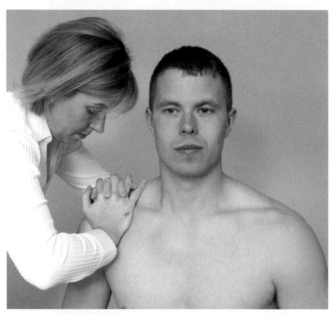

Fig. 5.133 Acromioclavicular shear test.

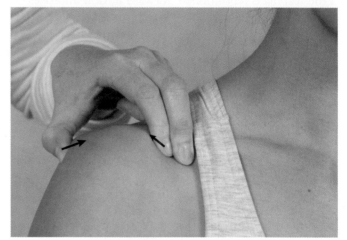

Fig. 5.135 Paxinos sign.

Acromioclavicular Shear Test.[338] With the patient in the sitting position, the examiner cups his or her hands over the deltoid muscle with one hand on the clavicle and one hand on the spine of the scapula. The examiner then squeezes the heels of the hands together (Fig. 5.133). Abnormal movement and pain at the acromioclavicular joint indicate a positive test as well as acromioclavicular joint pathology.

Ellman's Compression Rotation Test.[448,449] The patient lies on the unaffected side. The examiner compresses the humeral head into the glenoid while the patient rotates the shoulder medially and laterally. If the patient's symptoms are reproduced, glenohumeral arthritis is suspected (Fig. 5.134).

Paxinos Sign.[450] The patient is seated with the test arm relaxed at the side. The examiner stands beside the test arm and places one hand over the shoulder so that the thumb is under the posterolateral aspect of the acromion and the index and long fingers of the same hand (the fingers of the opposite hand may also be used instead) over the middle part of the clavicle on the same side (Fig. 5.135). The examiner then applies pressure to the acromion with the thumb anterosuperiorly while applying an inferior directed counterforce to the clavicle with the fingers. The test is considered positive if pain in the area of acromioclavicular joint is increased.

Tests for Ligament and Capsule Pathology

Coracoclavicular Ligament Test. The integrity of the conoid portion of the coracoclavicular ligament may be

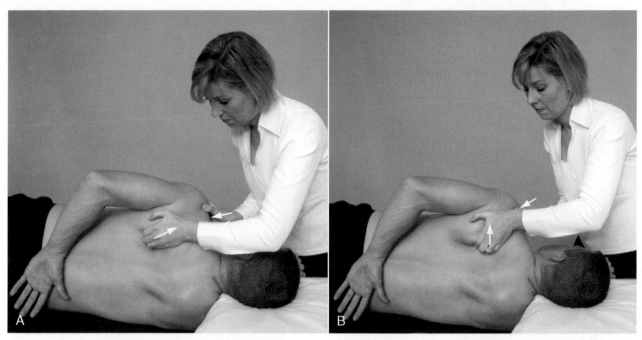

Fig. 5.136 Coracoclavicular ligament test. (A) Conoid portion. (B) Trapezoid portion.

tested by placing the patient in a side-lying position on the unaffected side with the hand resting against the lower back. The examiner stabilizes the clavicle while pulling the inferior angle of the scapula away from the chest wall. The trapezoid portion of the ligament may be tested from the same position. The examiner stabilizes the clavicle and pulls the medial border of the scapula away from the chest wall (Fig. 5.136). Pain in either case in the area of the ligament (anteriorly under the clavicle between the outer one-third and inner two-thirds) constitutes a positive test.

☑ *Crank Test.* The crank test (see also under "Tests for Anterior Shoulder Instability") may also be used to evaluate the different glenohumeral ligaments (Fig. 5.137). For example, when the crank test is done with the arm by the side, primarily the superior glenohumeral ligament and capsule are being tested. At 45° to 60° abduction, the middle glenohumeral ligament, the coracohumeral ligament, the inferior glenohumeral ligament (anterior band), and anterior capsule are being tested. Over 90° abduction, the inferior glenohumeral ligament and anterior capsule are being tested (see Table 5.1).[451,452]

⚠ *Low Flexion Test.*[453,454] The patient is seated. The examiner forward flexes the test arm to 40° (or 60°) and then medially rotates the arm (Fig. 5.138). These two positions provide maximum strain to the posterior glenohumeral joint capsule. Both sides are compared. The test may be done in supine to stabilize the scapula. The angle formed between the horizontal and the forearm may be used to quantify the amount of medial rotation and capsular restriction.

❓ *Posteroinferior Glenohumeral Ligament Test.*[412] Just as the crank test may be used to test the superior

glenohumeral ligament, middle glenohumeral ligament, and the anterior portion of the inferior glenohumeral ligament, the posterior inferior glenohumeral test may be used to test the posterior portion of the inferior glenohumeral ligament. The patient sits while the examiner forward flexes the arm to between 80° and 90° and then horizontally adducts the arm 40° with medial rotation (Fig. 5.139). While doing the movement, the examiner palpates the posteroinferior region of the glenoid. If the humerus protrudes or pain is felt in the area, the test is considered positive and indicates a lesion of the posterior portion of the inferior glenohumeral ligament. If movement (i.e., horizontal adduction) is restricted, it may also indicate a tight posterior capsule.

Tests for Muscle or Tendon Pathology

Ideally, an examiner would like to be able to isolate the problem muscle or tendon when examining for rotator cuff tears and subacromial tissues. In fact, no test or series of tests have been shown to be able to do this reliably and with reproducibility and validity.[292] Thus, the tests for shoulder muscles should be tested in the patient's normal posture, and if the body is not aligned, the posture should be altered to as close to the correct posture as possible and the test repeated with the scapula stabilized. Lewis's **SSMP** may be used.[293] It is also important to remember that when the muscles are tested, one is testing not only the muscle and its tendon but also the peripheral nerve that supplies that muscle (also see "Resisted Isometric Movements" earlier). Whether the injury is to the muscle or nerve may depend on the mechanism of injury and the signs and symptoms presented.

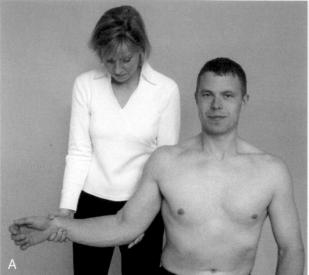

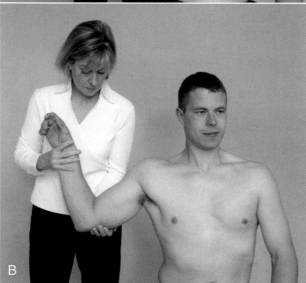

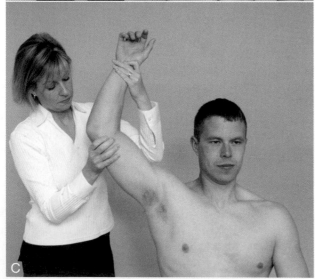

Fig. 5.137 Crank test used to test the glenohumeral ligaments. (A) With arm by the side, superior glenohumeral ligament tested. (B) With 45° to 60° abduction, middle glenohumeral ligament tested. (C) Over 90° abduction, inferior glenohumeral ligament tested.

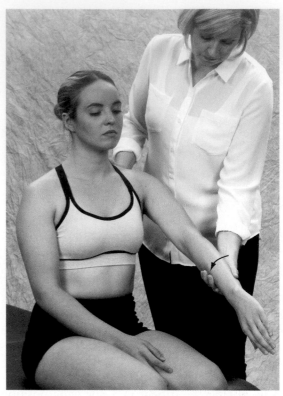

Fig. 5.138 Low flexion test to stress the posterior glenohumeral joint capsule.

⚠ *Abdominal Compression Test (Belly-Press or Napoleon Test).*[273,408,410,455–459] This test checks the subscapularis muscle, especially if the patient cannot medially rotate the shoulder enough to take it behind the back. The patient is in a standing position. The examiner places a hand on the abdomen below the xiphoid process so that the examiner can feel how much pressure the patient is applying to the abdomen. The patient places his or her hand of the shoulder being tested on the examiner's hand and pushes the hand as hard as he or she can into the stomach (medial shoulder rotation). While pushing the hand into the abdomen, the patient attempts to bring the elbow forward to the scapular plane, causing greater medial shoulder rotation. If the patient is unable to maintain the pressure on the examiner's hand while moving the elbow forward, or posteriorly flexes the wrist or extends the shoulder, the test is positive for a tear of the subscapularis muscle (Fig. 5.140). It has also been suggested that when the patient brings the elbow forward and straightens the wrist, the examiner measures the final belly press angle of the wrist with a goniometer (i.e., **modified belly-press test**). A difference of 10° or more indicates a positive test for subscapularis.[325,460]

❓ *Abrasion Sign.*[103] The patient sits and abducts the arm to 90° with the elbow flexed to 90°. The patient then medially and laterally rotates the arm at the shoulder.

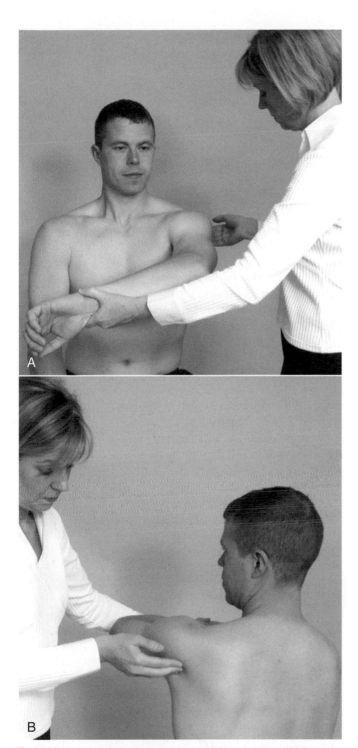

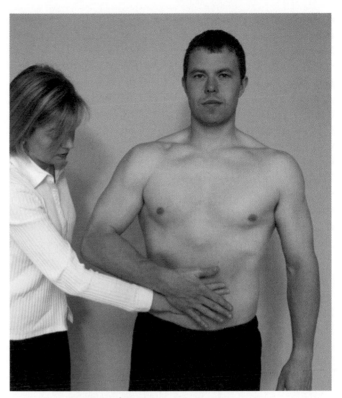

Fig. 5.140 Abdominal compression test.

Fig. 5.139 Posteroinferior ligament test. (A) Anterior view. (B) Posterior view.

Normally there are no signs and symptoms. If crepitus occurs, it is a sign that the rotator cuff tendons are frayed and are abrading against the undersurfaces of the acromion process and the coracoacromial ligament.

❓ *Active Elevation Lag Test.* [461] The patient is in standing. Prior to the test, the examiner ensures there is full passive ROM especially elevation through forward flexion. The examiner then places one hand over the patient's lumbar spine. Starting with the unaffected

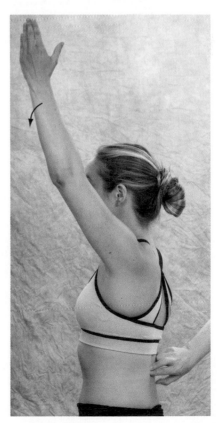

Fig. 5.141 Active elevation lag test. The examiner is palpating when the patient's lumbar spine moves.

side, the patient is then asked to forward flex the arm into as full elevation as possible. As the patient forward flexes the arm, the examiner feels when the lumbar spine starts to extend but allows the patient to continue to as full elevation as possible. When the greatest elevation is reached, the patient is asked to bring the arm back down to where the lumbar lordosis corrects to normal (Fig. 5.141). With a trapezius palsy (i.e., spinal accessory nerve problem), the increase in lumbar lordosis occurs earlier in the elevation through forward flexion. The difference in forward flexion between the two sides with the lumbar spine in normal lordosis is called the **active elevation lag** and is the result of injury to the trapezius muscle itself or its nerve supply (i.e., the spinal accessory nerve).

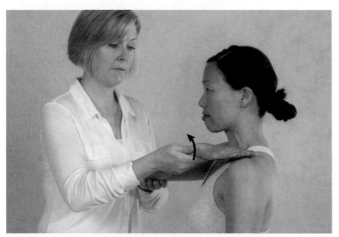

Fig. 5.142 Bear-hug test.

❓ *Bear-Hug Test.*[273,408,459,462] The patient stands with the hand of the test shoulder on top of the other shoulder (Fig. 5.142) with the fingers extended and the elbow in front of the body. The examiner stands in front of the patient and tries to lift the hand away from the shoulder applying a perpendicular lateral rotation force while the patient resists the movement. The examiner's other hand stabilizes the patient's elbow. If the patient cannot hold the hand on top of the shoulder because of weakness, it is considered a positive test for subscapularis strain.

⚠ *Belly-Off Sign.*[325,460,463] The patient is seated or standing. The examiner stands in front of the patient and passively moves the test limb into flexion and maximum medial rotation with the elbow flexed to 90°. The examiner supports the patient's elbow while the examiner's other hand brings the arm into maximum medial rotation, placing the patient's hand on the abdomen (Fig. 5.143A). The patient is then asked to keep the wrist straight and actively maintain the medial rotation while the examiner releases the wrist (Fig. 5.143B). If the patient is not able to maintain the position, the wrist flexes or a lag (i.e., hand moves away from abdomen) occurs, the test is positive for an injured subscapularis muscle.

⚠ *Biceps Entrapment Test.*[1,408] This test may be found to be positive during active movement testing. The biceps entrapment is caused by bulbous swelling (i.e., **"hourglass" biceps**) just outside the glenohumeral joint in the bicipital groove.[29,30,40,464] The swelling acts like a trigger finger, so that full active or passive elevation of the shoulder is not possible without pain (patients lack 10° to 20°). The diagnosis can be made only at surgery.

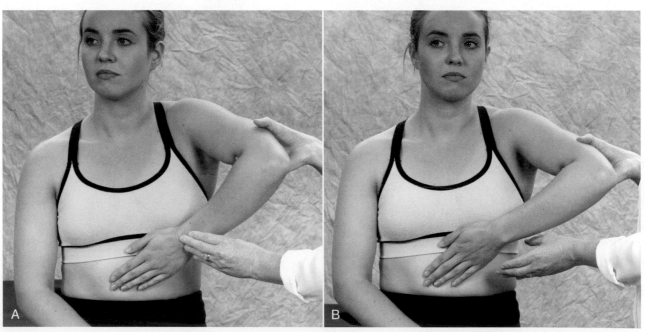

Fig. 5.143 Belly-off sign. (A) Start position. The examiner is keeping the elbow forward while placing the patient's hand on her stomach. (B) End position.

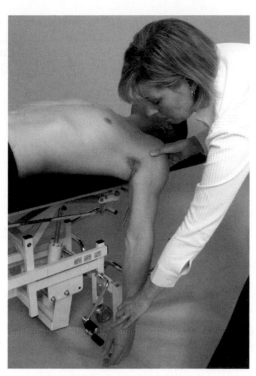

Fig. 5.144 Testing for biceps tightness.

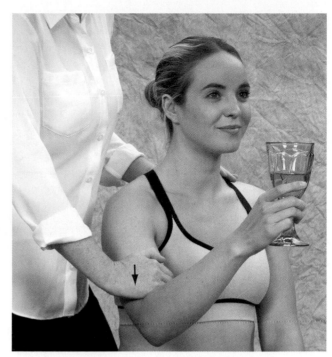

Fig. 5.145 Champagne toast test for supraspinatus.

🔺 *Biceps Tightness.* The patient lies supine with the shoulder in extension over the edge of the examining table with the elbow flexed and the forearm supinated. The examiner then extends the elbow, which would normally have a bone-to-bone end feel if the biceps flexibility is normal. If the biceps is tight, full elbow extension does not occur, and the end feel is a muscular tissue stretch (Fig. 5.144).[465]

✅ *Champagne Toast Position.*[466] The patient is seated and positions the arm in 30° abduction, slight lateral rotation and 30° forward flexion, and elbow in 90° flexion (Fig. 5.145) which replicates the position when one is giving a "toast." The examiner applies downward isometric resistance at the elbow. A positive test of pain and/or weakness indicates an injury to the supraspinatus muscle.

🔺 *Deltoid Extension Lag Sign (Swallow-Tail Sign).*[181,467] The patient is standing or sitting. Starting with the uninjured side, the examiner extends the arm fully ensuring no forward flexion of the trunk on the part of the patient (Fig. 5.146A). The patient is asked to maintain the position for 5 to 10 seconds if possible (Fig. 5.146B). The test is repeated on the injured side. If the extension does not equal the uninjured side, then there has been an injury to the posterior deltoid muscle or its innervation, the axillary nerve, which most commonly occurs after an anterior glenohumeral dislocation. The test may also be done bilaterally in order to compare sides (Fig. 5.146C).

🔺 *Drop-Arm (Codman's) Test.* The examiner abducts the patient's shoulder to 90° and then asks the patient to slowly lower the arm to the side in the same arc of movement (Fig. 5.147). A positive test is indicated if the patient is unable to return the arm to the side slowly or has severe pain when attempting to do so. A positive result indicates a tear in the rotator cuff complex.[468] A complete tear (3° strain) of the rotator cuff is more common in older patients (50 years old or older). In younger people, a partial tear (1° or 2° strain) is more likely to occur when the patient is abducting the arm and a strong downward, eccentric load is applied to the arm.

🔺 *Dropping Sign.*[469] The patient stands with the test arm by the side. The examiner stands by the test side and passively places the patient's elbow in 90° flexion (Fig. 5.148A) with the arm in 45° of lateral rotation. The patient is then asked to isometrically laterally rotate the arm against resistance and then relax. If the patient is not able to maintain the laterally rotated position and the arm drops back to the neutral position (Fig. 5.148B), the test is considered positive for an infraspinatus tear.

❓ *Gilchrest's Sign.*[338,470] While standing, the patient lifts a 2-kg to 3-kg (5-lb to 7-lb) weight overhead. The arm is laterally rotated fully and lowered to the side in the coronal plane. A positive test is indicated by discomfort or pain in the bicipital groove. A positive test indicates bicipital paratenonitis or tendinosis.[79] In some cases, an audible snap or pain may be felt at between 90° and 100° abduction.

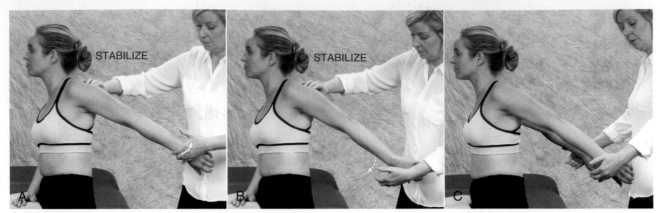

Fig. 5.146 Deltoid extension lag sign. (A) The examiner extends the patient's arm fully. (B) The patient attempts to actively maintain the position (*arrow* indicates lag when examiner releases patient's arm). (C) The test may be done bilaterally to compare both sides.

❓ *Heuter's Sign.*[470] Normally, if elbow flexion is resisted when the arm is pronated, some supination occurs as the biceps attempts to help the brachialis muscle flex the elbow. This supination movement is called *Heuter's sign.* If it is absent, the distal biceps tendon has been disrupted.

✓ *Hornblower's Sign (Signe de Clairon).*[298,469,471,472] This test, also called the **Patte test**, is designed to test the strength of teres minor. The patient is in a standing position (Fig. 5.149A). The examiner elevates the patient's arm to 90° in the scapular plane (scaption). The examiner then flexes the elbow to 90°, and the patient is asked to laterally rotate the shoulder against resistance. A positive test is indicated when the patient is unable to laterally rotate the arm and indicates a tear of teres minor.[473]

McClusky offered a second way to do the test.[298] The patient is standing with the arms by the side and then is asked to bring the hands to the mouth. With a massive posterior rotator cuff tear, the patient is unable to do this without abducting the arm first (Fig. 5.149B). This abduction with hands to the mouth is called the **hornblower's sign.**

✓ *Infraspinatus Test.* The patient stands with the arm at the side with the elbow at 90° and the humerus medially rotated to 45°. The examiner then applies a medial rotation force that the patient resists. Pain or the inability to resist medial rotation indicates a positive test for an infraspinatus strain (Fig. 5.150).

It has been advocated that the examiner should ensure the scapula is retracted and supported by the examiner before the patient does the resisted lateral rotation.[474] This has been called the **infraspinatus scapular retraction test (ISRT)** ⚠ (Fig. 5.151). The reason for the scapular retraction is to stabilize the scapula before doing the test.

⚠ *Lateral Jobe Test.*[325,475] The patient is in standing with the test arm abducted to 90° with the elbow flexed to 90°, the shoulder is medially rotated so that the fingers point to the ground and the thumb towards the body (Fig. 5.152). The examiner then applies an inferior (i.e., downward) force to the arm at the elbow. A positive test is indicated by pain, weakness, or inability to hold the position. It indicates rotator cuff pathology.

✓ *Lateral Rotation Lag Sign (Infraspinatus and Teres Minor "Spring-Back" Test).*[298,472,476] The patient is seated or in standing position with the arm by the side and the elbow flexed to 90°. The examiner passively abducts the arm to 90° in the scapular plane, laterally rotates the shoulder to end range (some authors say 45°)[469] and asks the patient to hold it (Fig. 5.153A). For a positive test, the patient cannot hold the position and the hand springs back anteriorly toward midline, indicating infraspinatus and teres minor cannot hold the position due to weakness or pain (Fig. 5.153B).[477,478] The examiner will also find passive medial rotation will have increased on the affected side.

If the test is performed with the arm in 20° abduction or by the side in the scapular plane with the elbow at 90° and the shoulder laterally rotated, the examiner then takes the arm into maximum lateral rotation and asks the patient to hold the position (Fig. 5.154A). If the supraspinatus and infraspinatus are torn, the arm will medially rotate and spring back anteriorly, indicating a positive test (Fig. 5.154B). If it rotates more than 40°, there is a problem with the teres minor. This test has also been called the **external rotation lag sign (ERLS) test** ✓. Hertel et al.[476] described a **drop sign** ✓, in which the patient is standing and abducts the arm to 90° with the elbow flexed to 90°. The examiner

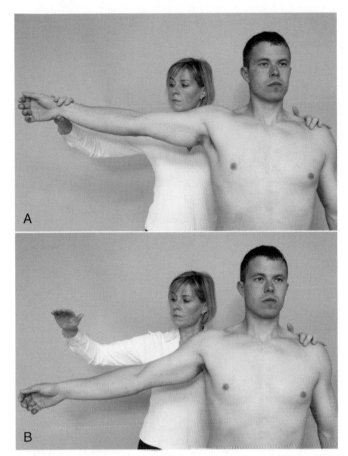

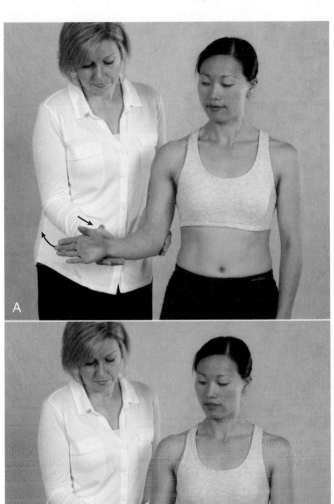

Fig. 5.147 Drop-arm test. (A) The patient abducts his arm to 90°. (B) The patient tries to lower the arm slowly and is unable to do so; instead, the arm drops to his side. The examiner's hand illustrates the start position.

Fig. 5.148 Dropping sign. (A) Start position with the examiner resisting the patient's lateral rotation at 45° of lateral rotation. (B) Arm dropping back to neutral position *(arrow)* because of infraspinatus weakness.

rotates the arm laterally and maximally, and the patient is asked to hold the position. If the arm falls or drops into medial rotation, the test is considered positive for tears to the infraspinatus and supraspinatus and perhaps subscapularis (Fig. 5.155).[280,377,469,476] If the patient is able to hold the position, the strength of the infraspinatus can be graded as three or greater, depending on the resistance to the examiner's medially rotated force.[469]

⚠ *Latissimus Dorsi Weakness.*[341] The patient is in a standing position with the arms elevated in the plane of the scapula to 160°. Against resistance of the examiner, the patient is asked to medially rotate and extend the arm downward as if climbing a ladder (Fig. 5.156).

☑ *Lift-Off Sign (Gerber's Test).*[273,455,456,459,477,479,480] The patient stands and places the dorsum of the hand on his or her back pocket or against the midlumbar spine. Great subscapularis activity is shown with the second position (Fig. 5.157).[481] The patient then lifts the hand away from the back. An inability to do so indicates a lesion of the subscapularis muscle.

Abnormal motion in the scapula during the test may indicate scapular instability. If the patient is able to take the hand away from the back, the examiner should apply a load pushing the hand toward the back to test the strength of the subscapularis and to test how the scapula acts under dynamic loading. With a torn subscapularis tendon, passive (and active) lateral rotation increases.[480]

If the patient's hand is passively rotated medially as far as possible and the patient is asked to hold the position, it will be found that the hand moves toward

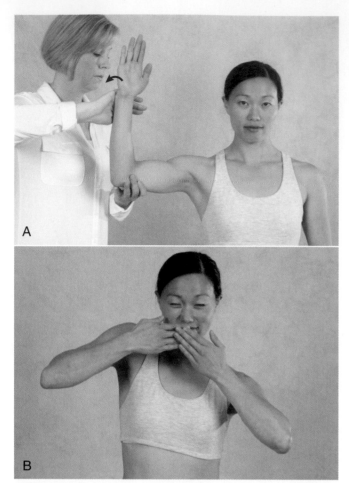

Fig. 5.149 Hornblower's sign (*signe du clairon*). (A) The patient is in a standing position. The examiner elevates the patient's arm to 90° in the scapular plane (scaption). The examiner then flexes the elbow to 90° and the patient is asked to laterally rotate the shoulder against resistance. (B) McClusky modification: patient is asked to abduct the arms to bring the hands to the mouth. A positive test is shown.

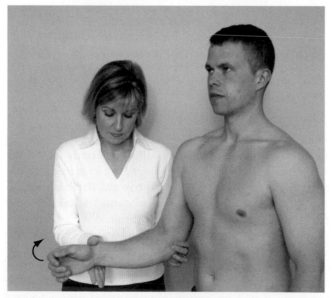

Fig. 5.150 Infraspinatus test.

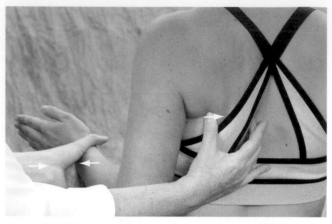

Fig. 5.151 Infraspinatus scapular retraction test (ISRT).

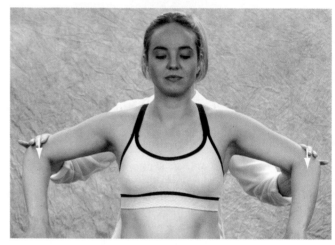

Fig. 5.152 Lateral Jobe test done bilaterally.

the back (**subscapularis** or **medial rotation, "spring-back," or lag test ✓**) because subscapularis cannot hold the position due to weakness or pain (Fig. 5.158).[310,476] This test is also called the **modified lift-off test.**[471,480] A small lag between maximum passive medial rotation and active medial rotation implies a partial tear (1°, 2°) of subscapularis.[455] This modified test is reported to be more accurate in diagnosing a rotator cuff tear.[476] The test may also be used to test the rhomboids. Medial border winging of the scapula during the test may indicate that the rhomboids are affected. Stefko et al. reported that maximum isolation of the subscapularis was achieved by placing the hand against the postero-inferior border of the scapula (**maximum medial rotation test ❓**) and then attempting the lift-off.[482] In the other positions for lift-off, teres major, latissimus dorsi, posterior deltoid, or rhomboids may compensate for a weak subscapularis.

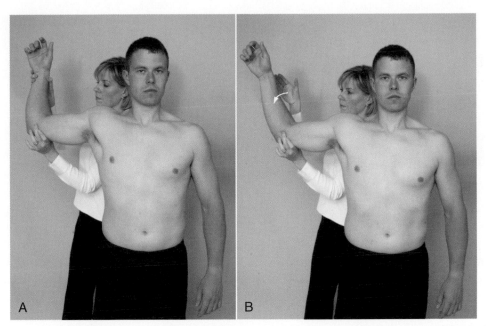

Fig. 5.153 Lateral rotation lag test to test the teres minor and infraspinatus. (A) Arm is abducted 90°. (B) Note how the hand springs forward when it is released by the examiner *(arrow)*.

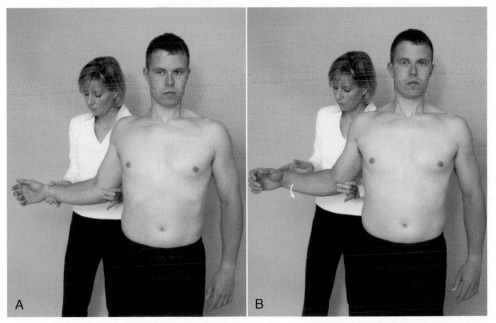

Fig. 5.154 External rotation lag sign (ERLS) or drop test. (A) Start position. (B) Position in positive test.

❓ *Lippman's Test.*[483] The patient sits or stands while the examiner holds the arm flexed to 90° with one hand. With the other hand, the examiner palpates the biceps tendon 7 to 8 cm (2.5 to 3 inches) below the glenohumeral joint and moves the biceps tendon from side to side in the bicipital groove. A sharp pain is a positive test, indicating bicipital paratenonitis or tendinosis.[79]

❓ *Ludington's Test.*[484] The patient clasps both hands on top of or behind the head, allowing the interlocking fingers to support the weight of the upper limbs

(Fig. 5.159A). This action allows maximum relaxation of the biceps tendon in its resting position. The patient then alternately contracts and relaxes the biceps muscles. While the patient does the contractions and relaxations, the examiner palpates the biceps tendon, which will be felt on the uninvolved side but not on the affected side if the test result is positive. A positive result indicates that the long head of biceps tendon has ruptured. The test can also be used to compare the symmetry of the biceps muscle bilaterally (Fig. 5.159B).

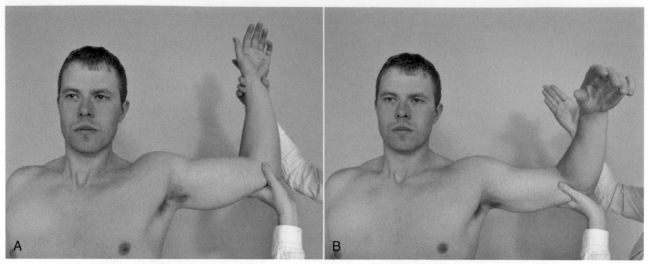

Fig. 5.155 The drop sign. (A) The examiner places the arm in 90° of abduction and maximal external rotation and then asks the patient to hold the position. (B) If the patient cannot hold this position and the arm falls into internal rotation, the test is positive.

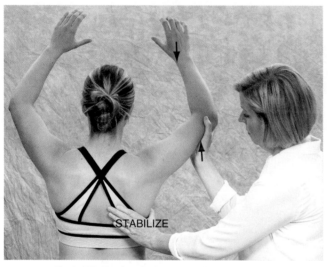

STABILIZE

Fig. 5.156 Testing for latissimus dorsi weakness.

⚠ *Pectoralis Major Contracture Test.* The patient lies supine and clasps the hands together behind the head. The arms are then lowered until the elbows touch the examining table (Fig. 5.160A). A positive test occurs if the elbows do not reach the table and indicates a tight pectoralis major muscle.

⚠ *Pectoralis Minor Tightness.* Pectoralis minor functions along with the rhomboids and levator scapulae to stabilize the scapula during arm extension. Tightness of the pectoralis minor can lead to increased scapular protraction and tilting of the inferior angle of the scapula posteriorly. Tightness of the pectoralis minor can be tested by having the patient in a supine-lying position with arm forward flexed 30°.[485] The examiner places the heel of the hand over the coracoid process and pushes it toward the examining table retracting the scapula (Fig. 5.160B). Normally, the posterior movement occurs with no discomfort to the patient, and the scapula lies flat against the table. However, if there is tightness (muscle tissue stretch) over the pectoralis minor muscle during the posterior movement, the test is considered positive. One can also measure the distance between the examination table and the posterior border of the acromion while the patient is in a relaxed supine position with the arms by the side and the elbows flexed so that the hands rest on the body. If the pectoralis minor is of proper length, the distance should not exceed 2.54 cm (1 inch).[486,487]

☑ *Rent Test.*[488] The patient is seated with his or her arm by the side and the examiner standing behind (Fig. 5.161). The examiner palpates the anterior margin of the patient's acromion with one hand while holding the patient's elbow at 90° with the other hand. The examiner then passively extends the patient's arm and slowly medially and laterally rotates the patient's humerus while palpating the greater tuberosity and rotator cuff tendons. The presence of a depression ("rent" or defect) of about one finger-width or a more prominent greater tuberosity (relative to the other side) indicates a positive test for a rotator cuff tear.

⚠ *Rhomboid Weakness.*[297,489] The patient is in a prone-lying position or sitting with the test arm behind the body so that the hand is on the opposite side (opposite back pocket). The examiner places the index finger along and under the medial border of the scapula while asking the patient to push the shoulder forward slightly against resistance to relax the trapezius (Fig. 5.162A). The patient then is asked to raise the forearm and hand away from the body. If the rhomboids are normal, the fingers are pushed away from under the scapula (Fig. 5.162B).

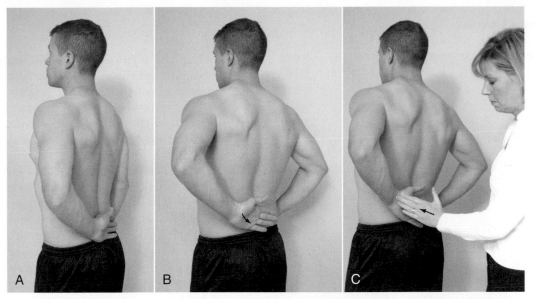

Fig. 5.157 Lift-off sign. (A) Start position. (B) Lift-off position. (C) Resistance to lift off is provided by the examiner. The examiner tests the strength of the subscapularis and watches the positioning of scapula.

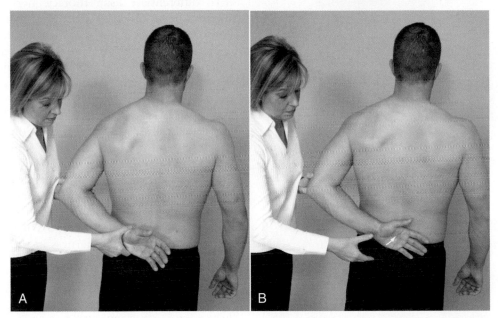

Fig. 5.158 Subscapularis spring-back or lag test. (A) Start position. (B) The patient is unable to hold the start position and the hand springs forward toward the lower back.

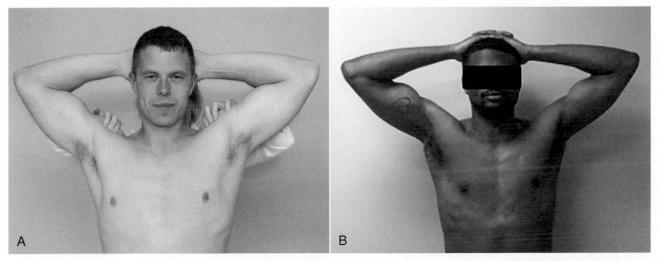

Fig. 5.159 (A) Ludington's test. (B) The test is helpful for evaluating the asymmetry of the biceps muscles, especially after biceps tenodesis. Note the small size of the left biceps. (B, From McFarland EG, Borade A: Examination of the biceps tendon, *Clin Sport Med* 35[1]:33, 2016.)

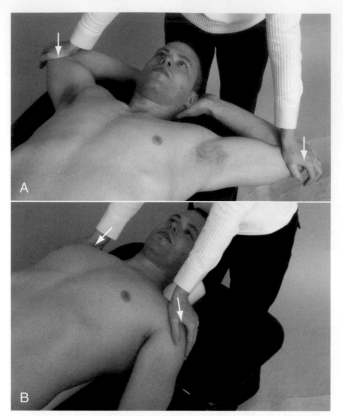

Fig. 5.160 Testing for tightness of (A) the pectoralis major and (B) the pectoralis minor. The examiner is testing end feel. Note the position of the examiner's hand on (A) the humerus and (B) the coracoid process.

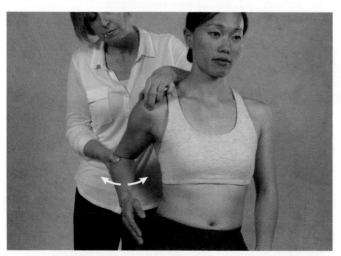

Fig. 5.161 Rent test for rotator cuff tear.

Rhomboid and levator scapulae strength may also be tested by having the patient place hands on hips while the examiner pushes the elbows anteriorly.[121]

⚠ Scapula Backward Tipping Test.[490] The patient lies prone with the head in neutral and the arms by the side with the palms facing downward. The examiner places one hand on the inferior angle of the scapula to stabilize the scapula and the fingers of the other hand hook the undersurface of the coracoid process, initiating an upward force while sensing for tightness and observing the movement of the acromion to the tragus of the ear (Fig. 5.163). If tightness occurs, it means that the pectoralis minor muscle is tight.

⚠ Serratus Anterior Weakness (Punch-Out Test).[489] The patient is in a standing position and forward flexes the arm to 90°. The examiner applies a backward force to the arm (Fig. 5.164). If serratus anterior is weak or paralyzed, the medial border of the scapula wings (classic winging). The patient also has difficulty abducting or forward flexing the arm above 90° with a weak serratus anterior, but it still may be possible with lower trapezius compensation.[123] A similar finding may be accomplished by doing a wall or floor push-up.

To differentiate long thoracic nerve palsy (serratus anterior) from posterior instability that causes serratus anterior dysfunction, the examiner should ask the patient to laterally rotate the arm and then forward flex the arm. In this case, if scapular winging is eliminated, then the problem is posterior instability due to serratus anterior weakness.[121]

⚠ Speed's Test (Biceps or Straight-Arm Test). The examiner resists shoulder forward flexion by the patient while the patient's forearm is first supinated, then pronated, and the elbow is completely extended. The test can also be performed by forward flexing the patient's arm to 90° and then asking the patient to resist an eccentric movement into extension first with the arm supinated, then pronated (Fig. 5.165).[408,491] A positive test elicits increased tenderness in the bicipital groove especially with the arm supinated and is indicative of bicipital paratenonitis or tendinosis.[79] The Speed's test is more effective than the Yergason's test because the bone moves over more of the tendon during the Speed test. It has been reported that this test may cause pain; therefore it is positive if a SLAP (type II) lesion is present.[362] If profound weakness is found on resisted supination, a severe second- or third-degree (rupture) strain of the distal biceps should be suspected.[492] It has been reported that it is hard to get consistent results with this test.[493]

✓ Supraspinatus ("Empty Can" or Jobe) Test.[273,494] The patient's arm is abducted to 90° with neutral (no) rotation, and the examiner provides resistance to abduction. The shoulder is then medially rotated and angled forward 30° ("empty can" position) so that the patient's thumbs point toward the floor (Fig. 5.166) in the plane of the scapula. Others have said that testing the arm with the thumb up ("full can") is best for maximum contraction of supraspinatus.[479] Resistance to abduction is again given while the examiner looks for weakness or pain, reflecting a positive test result. A positive test result indicates a tear of

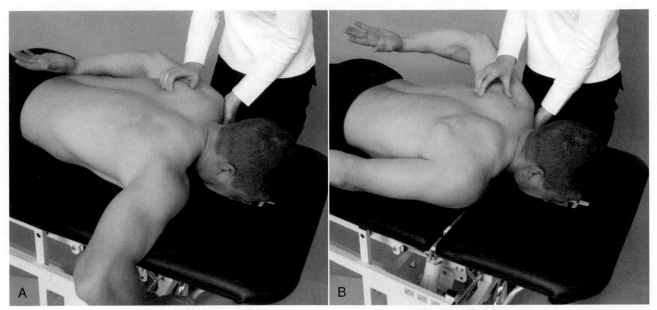

Fig. 5.162 Testing for rhomboid weakness. (A) Start position. (B) Test position.

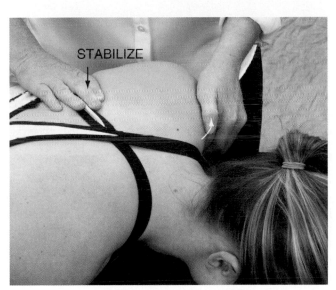

Fig. 5.163 Scapula backward tipping test.

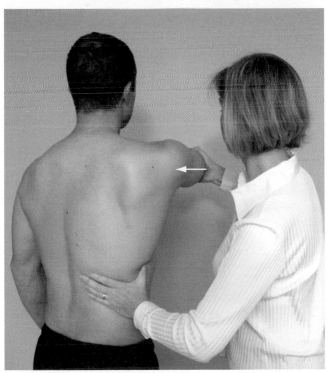

Fig. 5.164 Testing for serratus anterior weakness. Punch-out test: The examiner applies a backward force.

the supraspinatus tendon or muscle, or neuropathy of the suprascapular nerve.

Teres Minor Test. The patient lies prone and places the hand on the opposite posterior iliac crest. The patient is then asked to extend and adduct the medially rotated arm against resistance. Pain or weakness indicates a positive test for teres minor strain (Fig. 5.167).

Tightness of Latissimus Dorsi, Pectoralis Major, and Pectoralis Minor. The patient is placed in the supine position and is asked to fully elevate the arms through forward flexion. If the three muscles have normal length, the arms will extend to rest against the examining table. If the

scapula does not lie flat against the table, it indicates that the pectoralis minor, pectoralis major, or latissimus dorsi is tight (the scapula remains protracted) (Fig. 5.168).[495]

Trapezius Weakness.[489] The patient sits down and places the hands together over the head. The examiner

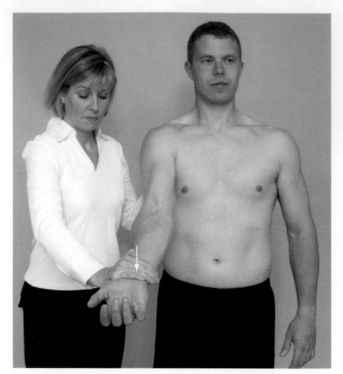

Fig. 5.165 Speed's test (biceps or straight-arm test).

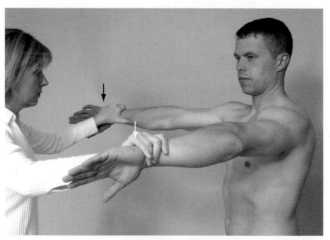

Fig. 5.166 Supraspinatus "empty can" test.

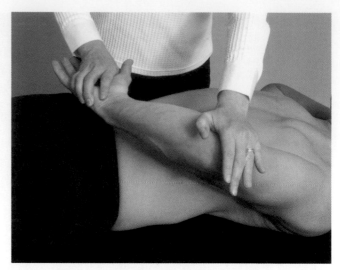

Fig. 5.167 Teres minor test.

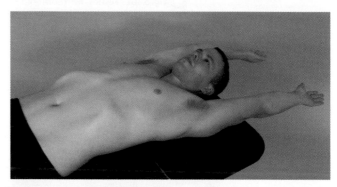

Fig. 5.168 Testing for tightness of the latissimus dorsi, pectoralis major, and pectoralis minor as a group.

stands behind the patient and pushes the elbows forward. Normally the three parts of the trapezius contract to stabilize the scapula (Fig. 5.169A). The upper trapezius can be tested separately by elevating the shoulder with the arm slightly abducted or to resisted shoulder abduction and head side flexion (Fig. 5.169B).[495,496] If the shoulder is elevated with the arm by the side, levator scapulae and rhomboids are more likely to be involved as well. The middle trapezius can be tested with the patient in a prone position with the arm abducted to 90° and laterally rotated. The test involves the examiner resisting horizontal extension of the arm watching for retraction of the scapula, which should normally occur (Fig. 5.169C).[495,496] If scapular protraction occurs, the middle fibers of trapezius are weak. To test the lower trapezius, the patient is in prone lying with arm abducted to 120° and the shoulder laterally rotated. The examiner applies resistance to diagonal extension and watches for scapular retraction that should normally occur (Fig. 5.169D). If scapular protraction occurs, the lower trapezius is weak.[495] Paralysis of the trapezius muscle causes the scapula to translate inferiorly, and the inferior angle of the scapula is rotated laterally.[121] If the scapula is elevated more than normal, it may indicate a tight trapezius or the presence of cervical torticollis.

⚠ *Triangle Sign.*[461]   The patient is in prone with both arms elevated about 120°. The patient is then asked to elevate both arms maximally. In the prone position, the patient will be unable to elevate the arms further in the presence of muscle problem or nerve injury. If the patient tries to elevate further, the lumbar spine will extend to provide more apparent elevation.

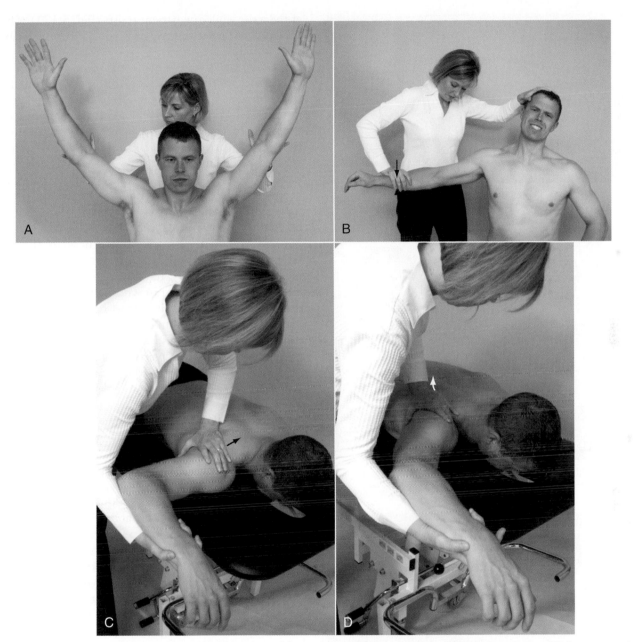

Fig. 5.169 Testing for trapezius weakness. (A) All portions of the trapezius. (B) Upper trapezius. (C) Middle trapezius. (D) Lower trapezius.

Normally, the patient should be able to elevate the arm fully without extending the spine. With pathology, the arm, trunk, and table form a triangle (Fig. 5.170) as the patient extends the lumbar spine to gain more elevation. The angle between the trunk and arm gives an indication of the injury severity to the trapezius muscle or its nerve supply, the spinal accessory nerve. Typically the angle on the injured side is approximately 90°; thus the starting position is obtained only with the help of the examiner; any additional movement would be the result of spinal extension. A patient with serratus anterior weakness will also show medial scapular winging.

Triceps Tightness. The patient is in a sitting position. The arm is fully elevated through forward flexion and lateral rotation. While stabilizing the humerus, the examiner flexes the elbow (see Fig. 6.16C).[465] Normally, the end feel would be soft-tissue approximation. If the triceps is tight, elbow flexion is limited and the end feel is muscular tissue stretch.

"Upper-Cut" Test.[408] The patient stands with the shoulder in neutral by the side and the elbow flexed to 90°. The forearm is supinated and the hand is in a fist (Fig. 5.171). The examiner puts a hand over the fist to resist the patient's movement. The patient then actively

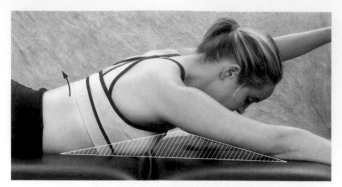

Fig. 5.170 Triangle sign.

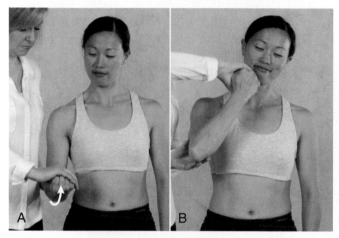

Fig. 5.171 "Upper-cut" test. (A) Start position. (B) End position.

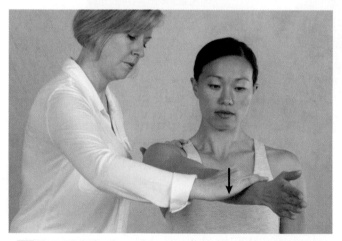

Fig. 5.172 Whipple test for rotator cuff and superior labral tears.

and quickly brings the hand up and toward the chin doing a "boxing upper-cut punch." A positive test is indicated by pain or a painful pop over the anterior shoulder and is an indication of a biceps injury.

✓ *Whipple Test.*[74] The patient stands with the arm forward flexed to 90° and adducted until the hand is opposite the other shoulder. The examiner pushes downward

at the wrist while the patient resists (Fig. 5.172). The test is considered positive for partial rotator cuff tears and/or superior labrum tears.

⚠ *Yergason's Test.* This test is primarily designed to check the ability of the coracohumeral ligament and the transverse humeral ligament to hold the biceps tendon in the bicipital groove.[31] With the patient's elbow flexed to 90° and stabilized against the thorax and with the forearm pronated, the examiner resists supination while the patient also laterally rotates the arm against resistance (Fig. 5.173).[497] If the examiner palpates the biceps tendon in the bicipital groove during the supination and lateral rotation movement, the tendon will be felt to "pop out" of the groove if the transverse humeral ligament is torn. Tenderness in the bicipital groove alone without the dislocation may indicate bicipital paratenonitis/tendinosis.[79] This test is not as effective as the Speed's test when testing the biceps tendon, because the bicipital groove moves only slightly over the tendon affecting only a small part of the tendon during the test and biceps tendon pain tends to occur with motion or palpation rather than with tension. It has been reported that it is hard to get consistent results with the test.[493]

Tests for Neurological Function

⚠ *Scratch Collapse Test for Axillary Nerve.*[498] The patient is seated facing the examiner. The patient elevates the arms in scaption to 90° with the elbows and wrists extended and the hands in a "fist" position. The examiner then isometrically horizontally adducts the arms while the patient resists by isometrically and horizontally abducting the arms (Fig. 5.174A). The examiner then scratches over the pathway of the axillary nerve (posterior aspect of the deltoid) (Fig. 5.174B) and then quickly repeats the test. If the patient has allodynia (i.e., increased pain response) due to compression neuropathy of the axillary nerve, a brief loss of horizontal adduction (i.e., loss of posterior deltoid strength) will occur. The axillary nerve may be compressed by fibrous bands, scarring after injury, compression in the quadrangular space (see Fig. 5.187), or muscle hypertrophy.

⚠ *Scratch Collapse Test for Long Thoracic Nerve.*[499] The patient is in standing with the elbows flexed to 90° and the wrists in neutral so that the examiner can resist shoulder medial rotation by doing resisted isometric lateral rotation. The examiner tests the patient's isometric lateral rotation bilaterally (Fig. 5.175A). The examiner then scratches the patient's skin over the pathway of the long thoracic nerve (i.e., along the midaxillary line just anterior to the latissimus dorsi muscle) on the lateral sides of the trunk (Fig. 5.175B) and then quickly has the patient again resist isometric medial rotation by providing a laterally rotating force (Fig. 5.175C). If the patient has allodynia due to a compression neuropathy, a

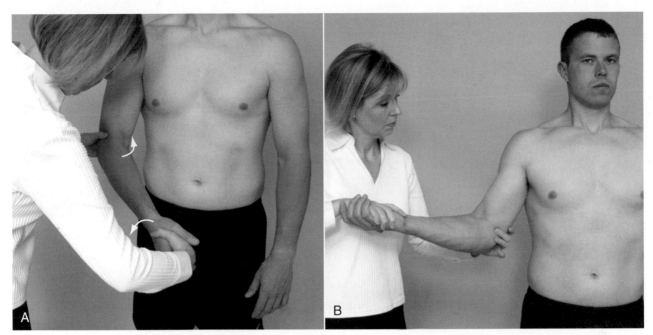

Fig. 5.173 Yergason's test. (A) Start position. (B) End position.

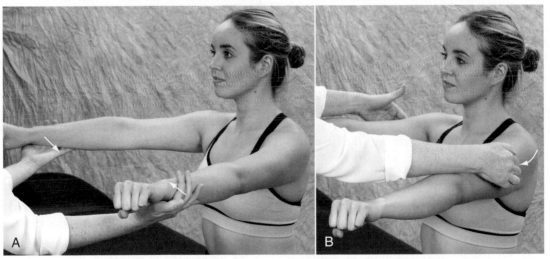

Fig. 5.174 Scratch collapse test for axillary nerve. (A) The test: the examiner isometrically and horizontally adducts the patient's arms. (B) The examiner scratches over the posterior deltoid and then (A) is repeated.

brief loss of lateral rotation will occur. Potential areas of compression include the scalenus medius muscle, a fascial band from the brachial plexus, angulation over the second rib, and compression by traversing vessels overlying the thorax.[499]

Tinel Sign (at the Shoulder). The area of the brachial plexus above the clavicle in the area of the scalene triangle is tapped. A positive sign is indicated by a tingling sensation in one or more of the nerve roots.

Upper Limb Neurodynamic (Tension) Test (ULNT) (Brachial Plexus Tension Test).[500] This test is the upper limb equivalent of the straight leg raising test of the lower limb. It is used when the patient has presented with upper limb radicular signs or peripheral nerve symptoms. The patient is positioned to stress the neurological tissue entering the arm. The patient lies supine. The test may be performed by placing the joints of the upper limb in different positions to stress each of the neurological tissues differently.[501] There are, in effect, four upper limb tension tests (ULNT 1 to 4) (see Table 3.21 and Fig. 3.45).[502] The key to performing the tests correctly is to ensure that the shoulder is held in depression. If it is allowed to elevate, tension is taken off the neurological structures. Depending on the patient

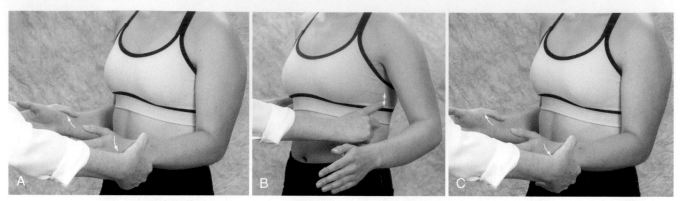

Fig. 5.175 Scratch collapse test for long thoracic nerve. (A) The patient does isometric lateral rotation. (B) The examiner scratches skin over the nerve's pathway. (C) The patient repeats isometric lateral rotation.

history, the examiner picks the ULNT that stresses the appropriate neurological tissue. Pain in the form of tingling or a stretch or ache in the cubital fossa indicates stretching of the dura mater in the cervical spine. The available range of passive movement at the elbow as compared with the normal side can indicate the restriction. Lateral or side flexion of the cervical spine to the opposite side can enhance the effect. If full ROM is not available in the shoulder, the test can still be performed by taking the shoulder to the point just short of pain in abduction and lateral rotation and performing the other maneuvers of the arm or by passively side flexing the cervical spine. The upper limb tension tests put tension on the upper limb neurological tissues even in normal individuals. Therefore reproduction of the patient's symptoms, rather than stretching, constitutes a positive sign. This finding indicates the neurological tissue is being stressed, but it does not tell the examiner where or why it is being stressed.

Tests for Thoracic Outlet Syndrome

Thoracic outlet syndromes may combine neurological and vascular signs; the signs and symptoms of neurological deficit, restriction of arterial flow, or restriction of venous flow may be seen individually.[503] The patient may complain of fatigue in the shoulder, vague shoulder pain, achiness, and sense of heaviness in the shoulder, all of which can affect speed and control while doing activity (e.g., throwing, swimming), especially with the arm in abduction and lateral rotation (Table 5.21).[81] For this reason a diagnosis of thoracic outlet syndrome is usually one of exclusion, in which all other causes have been eliminated.[504–507] In fact, neurogenic signs are rare in thoracic outlet syndrome, and there is poor correlation between the vascular signs of the condition and neurological involvement. *Thoracic outlet tests must not only*

decrease the pulse but also reproduce the patient's symptoms to be considered positive.[508] The tests do not show high reliability.

With thoracic outlet tests that involve taking the pulse, the examiner must find the pulse before positioning the patient's arm or cervical spine. Because the pulse may be diminished even in a "normal" individual, looking for the reproduction of symptoms is more important than looking for diminution of the pulse. Unless stated, the duration of these provocative tests should be no more than 1 to 2 minutes.[505]

? ***Adson Maneuver.***[77,509] This test is probably one of the most common methods of testing for thoracic outlet syndrome reported in the literature. The examiner locates the radial pulse. The patient's head is rotated to face the test shoulder (Fig. 5.176). The patient then extends the head while the examiner laterally rotates and extends the patient's shoulder. The patient is instructed to take a deep breath and hold it. A disappearance of the pulse and reproduction of symptoms indicates a positive test.

? ***Costoclavicular Syndrome (Military Brace) Test.***[77] The examiner palpates the radial pulse and then draws the

TABLE **5.21**

Thoracic Outlet Signs and Symptoms[506]

| Neurological | VASCULAR | |
	Arterial	Venous
• Numbness • Tingling • Weak grip • Loss of manual dexterity (intrinsics)	• Cool, pale extremity	• Swelling • Mottled discoloration

patient's shoulder down and back (Fig. 5.177). A positive test is indicated by an absence of the pulse and reproduction of symptoms, and implies possible thoracic outlet syndrome (costoclavicular syndrome). This test is particularly effective in patients who complain of symptoms while wearing a backpack or heavy coat.

❓ Halstead Maneuver. The examiner finds the radial pulse and applies a downward traction on the test extremity while the patient's neck is hyperextended and the head is rotated to the opposite side (Fig. 5.178). Absence or disappearance of a pulse and reproduction of symptoms indicates a positive test for thoracic outlet syndrome.

❓ Provocative Elevation Test.[310] The patient elevates both arms above the horizontal and is asked to rapidly open and close the hands 15 times. If fatigue, cramping, tingling or reproduction of symptoms occurs during the test, the test is positive for vascular insufficiency and thoracic outlet syndrome. This test is a modification of the Roos test.

⚠ Roos Test (Elevated Arm Stress Test [EAST]).[77,510] The patient stands and abducts the arms to 90°, laterally rotates the shoulder, and flexes the elbows to 90° so that the elbows are slightly behind the frontal plane. The patient then opens and closes the hands slowly for 3 minutes (Fig. 5.179). If the patient is unable to keep the arms in the starting position for 3 minutes or suffers ischemic pain, heaviness or profound weakness of the arm, or numbness and tingling of the hand during the 3 minutes, the test is considered positive for thoracic outlet syndrome on the affected side. Minor fatigue and distress are considered negative tests. The test is sometimes called the **positive abduction and external rotation (AER) position test,** the **"hands up" test,** or the **elevated arm stress test (EAST)** ⚠.[510–513]

❓ Shoulder Girdle Passive Elevation.[322] This test is used on patients who already present with symptoms. The patient sits and the examiner grasps the patient's arms from behind and passively elevates the shoulder girdle up and forward into full elevation (a passive bilateral shoulder shrug); the position is held for 30 or more seconds (Fig. 5.180). Arterial relief is evidenced by stronger pulse, skin color change (more pink), and increased hand temperature. Venous relief is shown by decreased cyanosis and venous engorgement. Neurological signs go from numbness to pins and needles or tingling, as well as some pain, as the ischemia to the nerve is released. This is referred to as a *release phenomenon.*

❓ Wright Test or Maneuver.[77] Wright advocated "hyperabducting" the arm so that the hand is brought over the head with the elbow and arm in the coronal plane with the shoulder laterally rotated (Fig. 5.181A).[514] He advocated doing the test in the sitting and then the supine

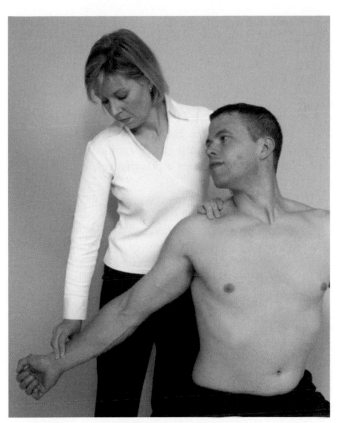

Fig. 5.176 Adson maneuver.

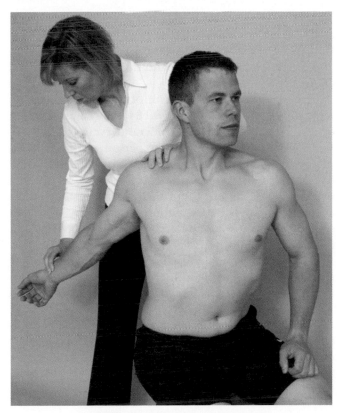

Fig. 5.177 Costoclavicular syndrome test.

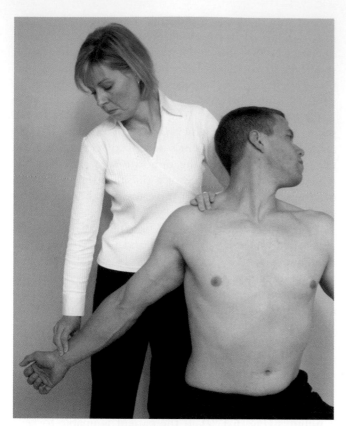

Fig. 5.178 Halstead maneuver.

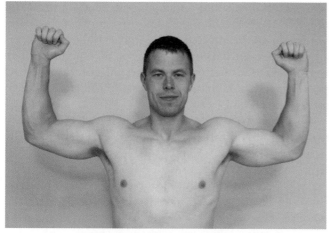

Fig. 5.179 Roos test position.

positions. Having the patient take a breath or rotating or extending the head and neck may have an additional effect of reproducing symptoms. The pulse is palpated for differences. This test is used to detect compression in the costoclavicular space and is similar to the costoclavicular syndrome test.

Examiners have modified this test over time so that it has come to be described as follows. The examiner flexes the patient's elbow to 90° while the shoulder is extended horizontally and rotated laterally (Fig. 5.181B). The patient then rotates the head away from the test side. The examiner palpates the radial pulse, which becomes absent (disappears) when the head is rotated away from the test side. The test done in this fashion has also been called the **Allen maneuver.** The pulse disappearance and reproduction of symptoms indicates a positive test result for thoracic outlet syndrome.

Other Tests of the Shoulder

⚠ *Olecranon Manubrium Percussion Sign.*[515] This test is designed to test the integrity of the bony structures of the upper limb from the humerus to the sternum. The patient is in sitting with the elbows bent to 90°. The examiner places the bell of the stethoscope over the patient's manubrium sternum (Fig. 5.182). Starting with the uninjured side, the olecranon process of the ulna is percussed while the examiner listens to the sound and compares both sides for pitch and loudness. Normally, the sounds are the same bilaterally. If there has been any bony disruption (e.g., fracture), then the sound will be duller.

Reflexes and Cutaneous Distribution

The reflexes in the shoulder region that are often assessed include the pectoralis major, clavicular portion (C5 to C6), sternocostal portion (C7 to C8 and T1), the biceps (C5 to C6), and the triceps (C7 to C8) (Fig. 5.183).

The examiner must be aware of the dermatome patterns of the nerve roots (Fig. 5.184) as well as the cutaneous distribution of the peripheral nerves (Fig. 5.185). Dermatomes vary from person to person, so the diagrams offer estimates only. A scanning test for altered sensation is performed by running the relaxed hands and fingers over the neck, shoulders, and anterior and posterior chest area. Any difference in sensation between the two sides should be noted. These differences can be mapped more exactly using a pinwheel, a pin, a brush, or cotton batting. In this way, the examiner can use sensation to help differentiate between a peripheral nerve lesion and a nerve root lesion referred from the cervical spine.

True shoulder pain rarely extends below the elbow. Pain in the acromioclavicular or sternoclavicular joint tends to be localized to the affected joint and usually does not spread or radiate. Pain can be referred to the shoulder and surrounding tissues from many structures,[516,517] including the cervical spine, elbow, lungs,

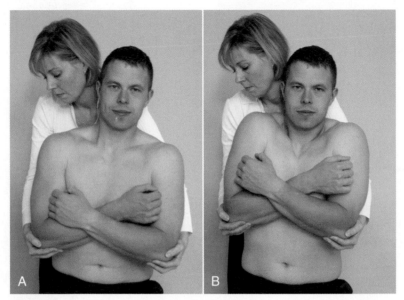

Fig. 5.180 Shoulder girdle passive elevation. (A) Start position. (B) Relief position.

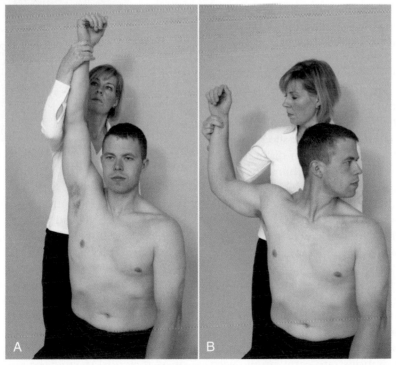

Fig. 5.181 (A) Wright test. (B) Modified Wright test or maneuver (Allen maneuver).

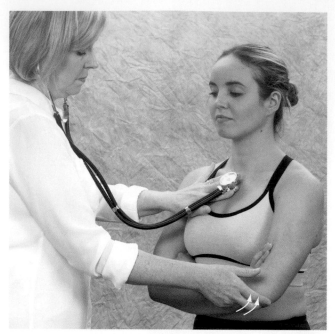

Fig. 5.182 Olecranon manubrium percussion sign.

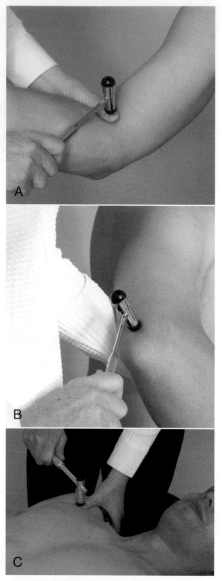

Fig. 5.183 Positioning to test the reflexes around the shoulder. (A) Biceps (C5–C6). (B) Triceps (C7–C8). (C) Pectoralis major (C5–C6).

heart, diaphragm, gallbladder, and spleen (Fig. 5.186; Table 5.22).

Peripheral Nerve Injuries About the Shoulder

Individual nerves can be injured about the shoulder, as shown further on. The examiner should not forget, however, that these nerves can be injured before they branch off the brachial plexus as individual nerves. Thus the thoracic outlet syndrome must be considered, especially in the throwing athlete, if symptoms arise with abduction and lateral rotation of the arm.[81]

Axillary (Circumflex) Nerve (C5 to C6). The axillary nerve is the most commonly injured nerve in the shoulder. The most common cause of its injury is anterior dislocation of the shoulder or fracture of the neck of the humerus.[518,519] The nerve injury may occur during the dislocation itself or during the reduction. Other traumatic events (e.g., fracture or bullet/stab wounds) or brachial plexus injuries, compression (e.g., crutches), quadrilateral space entrapment (Fig. 5.187), or shoulder surgery may also affect the axillary nerve.[520]

Motor loss (see Tables 5.7 and 5.15) includes an inability to abduct the arm (deltoid), although the patient may attempt to rotate the arm laterally and use the long head of biceps to abduct the arm (trick movement). In some cases, the patient is asymptomatic, although he or she may demonstrate early fatigue with strenuous activities.[520] There is weakness of lateral rotation owing to loss of the teres minor.[520] The patient may attempt to use scapular movement (i.e., trapezius or serratus anterior) to compensate for the muscle loss (trick movement). Atrophy of the deltoid leads to loss of the lateral roundness (flattening) of the shoulder. Sensory loss is over the deltoid with the main loss being a small, 2- to 3-cm (1-inch) circular area at the deltoid insertion (see Fig. 5.185).

Suprascapular Nerve (C5 to C6). The suprascapular nerve may be injured by a fall on the posterior shoulder, stretching, repeated microtrauma, or fracture of the scapula.[514,520,521] Commonly the nerve is injured as it passes through the suprascapular notch under the transverse scapular (suprascapular) ligament or as it winds around the spine of the scapula under the spinoglenoid ligament (Fig. 5.188).[122,520,522–528] It is often hard to distinguish from rotator cuff syndrome; therefore the patient history and mechanism of injury become important for differential diagnosis. Most commonly, the condition is seen in people who

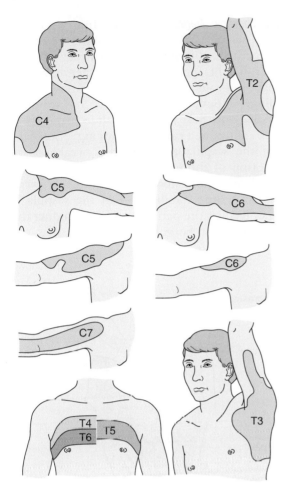

Fig. **5.184** Dermatome pattern of the shoulder. Dermatomes on one side only are illustrated.

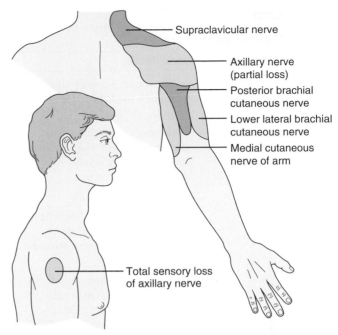

Fig. **5.185** Cutaneous distribution of the peripheral nerves around the shoulder.

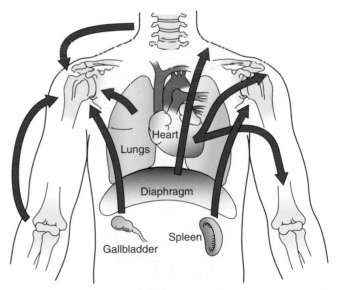

Fig. **5.186** Structures referring pain to the shoulder.

work with their arms overhead or in activities involving cocking and following through (e.g., volleyball spiking, pitching).[104,523,529,530]

Signs and symptoms include persistent rear shoulder pain and paralysis of the supraspinatus (suprascapular notch) and infraspinatus (suprascapular notch and spine of scapula), leading to decreased strength of abduction (supraspinatus) and lateral rotation (infraspinatus) of the shoulder. Wasting may also be evident in the muscles over the scapula.

Musculocutaneous Nerve (C5 to C6). This nerve is not commonly injured, although it may be injured by trauma (e.g., humeral dislocation or fracture) or in conjunction with injury to the brachial plexus or adjacent axillary artery. Injury to this nerve (see Tables 5.7 and 5.15) results primarily in loss of elbow flexion (biceps and brachialis), shoulder forward flexion (biceps and coracobrachialis), and decreased supination strength (biceps). In addition, injury to its sensory branch, the antebrachial cutaneous nerve, leads to altered sensation in the anterolateral aspect of the

forearm (see Fig. 5.17). This sensory branch is sometimes compressed as it passes under the distal biceps tendon, resulting in **musculocutaneous nerve tunnel syndrome.** The injury results in sensory loss in the forearm; it is usually the result of forced elbow hyperextension or repeated pronation (e.g., excessive screwdriving, backhand tennis strokes) and may be misdiagnosed as tennis elbow.

TABLE 5.22

Shoulder Muscles and Referral of Pain

Muscle	Referral Pattern
Levator scapulae	Over muscle to posterior shoulder and along medial border of scapula
Latissimus dorsi	Interior angle of scapula up to posterior and anterior shoulder into posterior arm; may refer to area above iliac crest
Rhomboids	Medial border of scapula
Supraspinatus	Over shoulder cap and above spine of scapula; sometimes down lateral aspect of arm to proximal forearm
Infraspinatus	Anterolateral shoulder and medial border of scapula; may refer down lateral aspect of arm
Teres minor	Near deltoid insertion, up to shoulder cap, and down lateral arm to elbow
Subscapularis	Posterior shoulder to scapula and down posteromedial and anteromedial aspects of arm to elbow
Teres major	Shoulder cap down lateral aspect of arm to elbow
Deltoid	Over muscle and posterior glenoid area of shoulder
Coracobrachialis	Anterior shoulder and down posterior arm

Long Thoracic Nerve (C5 to C8). Injury to the long thoracic nerve, although not common, may occur from repetitive microtrauma with heavy effort above shoulder height, pressure on the nerve from backpacking, vigorous upper limb activities[507,531] (e.g., shoveling, chopping, stretching), or wounds (see Tables 5.7 and 5.15). The result is paralysis of the serratus anterior, causing winging (medial border) of the scapula and pain and weakness on forward flexion of the extended arm.[104,123,126,141,518,519,524,532,533] Abduction above 90° is difficult because of scapular winging. Stabilization of the scapula by the examiner enables the patient to further abduct the arm. Recovery time can be as long as 2 years.

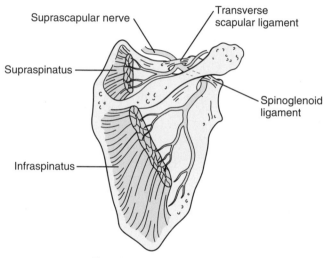

Fig. 5.188 Suprascapular nerve.

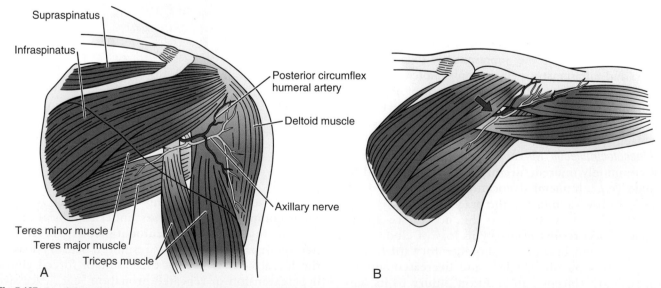

Fig. 5.187 Quadrilateral space entrapment, posterior view of the shoulder. (A) With the arm in adduction or at the side, there is no compression of the axillary nerve and posterior circumflex humeral artery. (B) A mechanism of intermittent compression of the axillary nerve and posterior circumflex humeral artery as a result of shearing and closing down of the space by the teres major and teres minor. (Redrawn from Safran MR: Nerve injury about the shoulder in athletes. Part 1: suprascapular nerve and axillary nerve, *Am J Sports Med* 32:814, 2004.)

Spinal Accessory Nerve (C3 to C4). The spinal accessory nerve is vulnerable to traumatic injury as it passes the posterior triangle of the neck; injury spares the sternocleidomastoid muscles but affects the trapezius muscle.[531] A common example would be abnormal pressure from a poorly fitting backpack (see Tables 5.7 and 5.15). Shoulder drooping (scapula is translated laterally and rotates downward) and scapular winging (medial superior portion) with medial rotation of the inferior angle, especially on abduction, may be evident, along with deepening of the supraclavicular fossa (asymmetric neck line) as a result of trapezius atrophy (Fig. 5.189).[104,534,535] The patient has difficulty abducting the arm above 90°.[518] Interestingly, Safran reported that spinal accessory palsy results in scapular winging on abduction but not on forward flexion.[507]

Joint Play Movements

Joint play movements are usually performed with the patient lying supine.[126,536] The examiner compares the amount of available movement and end feel on the affected side with the movement on the unaffected side and notes whether the movements affect the patient's symptoms.

To perform the backward joint play movement of the humerus, the examiner grasps the patient's upper limb, placing one hand over the anterior humeral head. The other hand is placed around the humerus above and near the elbow while the patient's hand is held against the examiner's thorax by the examiner's arm (Fig. 5.190A). The examiner then applies a backward force (similar to a posterior shift), keeping the patient's arm parallel to the patient's body so that no rotation or torsion occurs at the glenohumeral joint.

Joint Play Movements of the Shoulder Complex

- Backward glide of the humerus
- Forward glide of the humerus
- Lateral distraction of the humerus
- Caudal glide of the humerus (long arm traction)
- Backward glide of the humerus in abduction
- Lateral distraction of the humerus in abduction
- Anteroposterior and cephalocaudal movements of the clavicle at the acromioclavicular joint
- Anteroposterior and cephalocaudal movements of the clavicle at the sternoclavicular joint
- General movement of the scapula to determine mobility
- Ribs - anteroposterior glide, springing
- Thoracic spine - posteroanterior central vertebral pressure (PACVP), posteroanterior unilateral vertebral pressure (PAUVP), transverse vertebral pressure (TVP)

Forward joint play movement of the humerus is carried out in a similar fashion with the examiner's hands placed as shown in Fig. 5.190B. The examiner applies an anterior force (anterior drawer), keeping the patient's arm parallel to the body so that no rotation or torsion occurs at the glenohumeral joint.

To apply a lateral distraction joint play movement to the humerus, the examiner's hands are placed as shown in Fig. 5.190C. A lateral distraction force is applied to the glenohumeral joint with the patient's arm kept parallel to the body so that no rotation or torsion occurs at

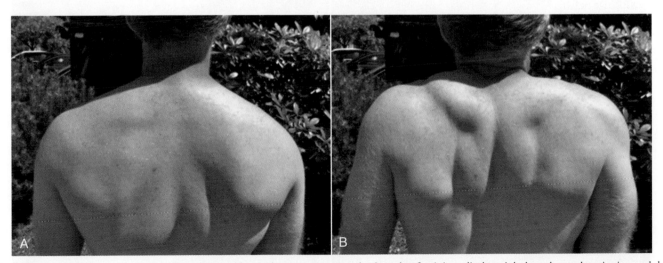

Fig. 5.189 Spinal accessory nerve palsy. The patient with spinal accessory nerve palsy 2 weeks after injury displays right lateral scapular winging and decreased tone in the trapezius (A) and decreased elevation as a result of dysfunction of the right trapezius (B). (From Coulter JM, Warme WJ: Complete spinal accessory nerve palsy from carrying climbing gear, *Wilderness Environ Med* 26[3]:384–386, 2015.)

the glenohumeral joint. The examiner must be careful to apply the lateral distraction force with the flat of the hand, because one sometimes has a tendency, in applying a force, to turn the hand so that the distraction is applied through the side of the index finger. This is uncomfortable for the patient.

A caudal glide (long arm traction) joint play movement is performed with the patient in the same supine position. The examiner grasps the arm above the patient's wrist with one hand and palpates with the other hand below the distal spine of the scapula posteriorly and below the distal clavicle anteriorly over the glenohumeral joint line (Fig. 5.190D). The examiner then applies a traction force to the shoulder while palpating to see whether the head of the humerus drops down (moves distally) in the glenoid cavity, as it normally should. If the patient complains of pain in the elbow, the test may be done with the hands positioned as in Fig. 5.190E.

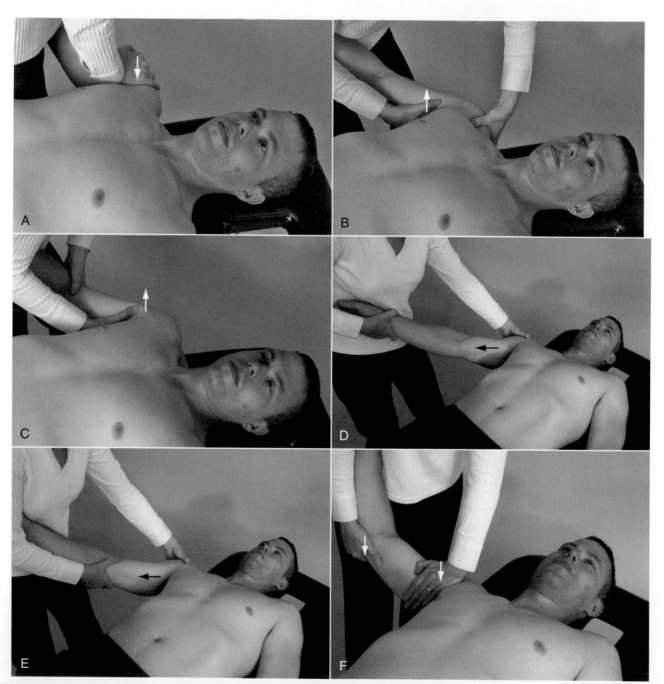

Fig. 5.190 Joint play movements of the shoulder complex. (A) Backward glide of the humerus. (B) Forward glide of the humerus. (C) Lateral distraction of the humerus. (D) Long arm traction applied below the elbow. (E) Long arm traction applied above the elbow. (F) Backward glide of the humerus in abduction. Note that the examiner allows the elbow to drop the same amount as the movement at the shoulder to minimize torque at the shoulder.

Continued

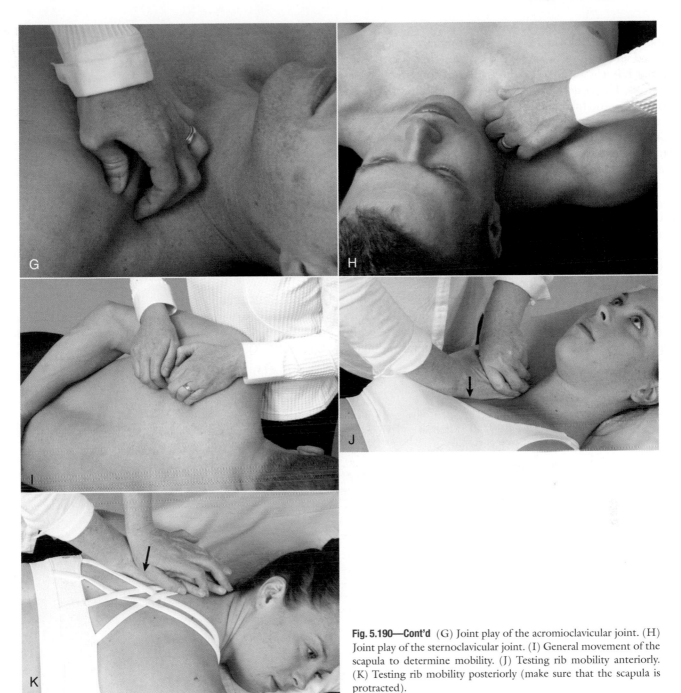

Fig. 5.190—Cont'd (G) Joint play of the acromioclavicular joint. (H) Joint play of the sternoclavicular joint. (I) General movement of the scapula to determine mobility. (J) Testing rib mobility anteriorly. (K) Testing rib mobility posteriorly (make sure that the scapula is protracted).

The examiner then abducts the patient's arm to 90°, grasping the arm above the patient's wrist with one hand while stabilizing the thorax with the other hand. The examiner applies a long arm traction force to determine joint play in this position.

With the patient's arm abducted to 90°, the examiner places one hand over the anterior humerus while stabilizing the patient's arm with the other hand and stabilizing the patient's hand against the thorax with the same arm. A backward force is then applied, keeping the patient's arm parallel to the body. This is a backward joint play movement of the humerus in abduction (Fig. 5.190F).

To assess the acromioclavicular and sternoclavicular joints (Fig. 5.190G and H, respectively), the examiner gently grasps the clavicle as close to the joint to be tested as possible and moves it in and out or up and down while palpating the joint with the other hand. Because the bone lies just under the skin, these techniques are uncomfortable for the patient where the examiner grasps the clavicle. The examiner should warn the patient before attempting this technique. A comparison of the amount of movement available is made between the two sides. Care should be taken not to squeeze the clavicle, because this too may cause pain.

For a determination of mobility of the scapula, the patient lies on one side to fixate the thorax with the arm relaxed and resting behind the low back (hand by opposite back pocket). The uppermost scapula is tested in this position. The examiner faces the patient, placing the lower hand along the medial border of the patient's scapula. The hand of the examiner's other arm holds the upper (cranial) dorsal surface of the patient's scapula. To relax the scapula further, the patient is asked to relax against the examiner and the examiner uses his or her body to push the patient's test shoulder posteriorly, retracting it to obtain a better hold on the scapula. By holding the scapula in this way, the examiner is able to move it medially, laterally, caudally, cranially, and away from the thorax (Fig. 5.190I).

With any shoulder examination, the ribs and spine should be checked for normal mobility, as restrictions in these areas can restrict shoulder movement. To test the mobility of the ribs generally, the examiner can apply anterior rib springing using the side of the thenar eminence of the hand (Fig. 5.190J). By pressing down several times, the examiner can compare the bilateral mobility of the ribs. If this is done posteriorly (Fig. 5.190K), the examiner must ensure the scapula is protracted out of the way. Mobility of the thoracic spine is shown in Fig. 8.55.

Palpation

When palpating the shoulder complex, the examiner should note any muscle spasm, tenderness, abnormal bumps, or other signs and symptoms that may indicate the source of pathology. The examiner should perform palpation in a systematic manner, beginning with the anterior structures and working around to the posterior structures. Findings on the injured side should be compared with those on the unaffected side. Any differences between the two sides should be noted, because they may indicate the cause of the patient's problems.

Anterior Structures

The anterior structures of the shoulder may be palpated with the patient in the supine lying or sitting position (Fig. 5.191A).

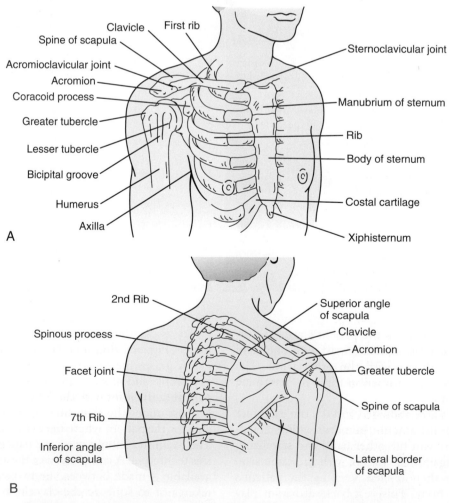

Fig. 5.191 Bony landmarks of the shoulder region. (A) Anterior view. (B) Posterior view.

Clavicle. The clavicle should be palpated along its full length to look for tenderness or abnormal bumps, such as callus formation after a fracture, and to ensure that it is in its resting position relative to the uninjured side. That is, it may be rotated anteriorly or posteriorly more than the unaffected side, or one end may be higher than that of the uninjured side, indicating a possible subluxation or dislocation at the sternoclavicular or acromioclavicular joint.

Sternoclavicular Joint. The sternoclavicular joint should be palpated for normal positioning in relation to the sternum and first rib. Palpation should also include the supporting ligaments and sternocleidomastoid muscle. Adjacent to the joint, the suprasternal notch may be palpated. From the notch, the examiner moves the fingers laterally and posteriorly to palpate the first rib. The examiner should apply slight caudal pressure to the first rib on both sides and note any difference. Spasm of the scalene muscles or pathology in the area may elevate the first rib on the affected side.

Acromioclavicular Joint. Like the sternoclavicular joint, the acromioclavicular joint should be palpated for normal positioning and tenderness. Likewise, supporting ligaments (acromioclavicular and coracoclavicular) and the trapezius, subclavius, and deltoid (anterior, middle, and posterior fibers) muscles should be palpated for tenderness and spasm.

Coracoid Process. The coracoid process may be palpated approximately 2.5 cm (1 inch) below the junction of the lateral one-third and medial two-thirds of the clavicle. The short head of biceps and coracobrachialis muscles originate from this process and the pectoralis minor inserts into it. With a SICK scapula syndrome, the coracoid is often very tender.[74]

Sternum. In the midline of the chest, the examiner should palpate the three portions of the sternum (manubrium, body, and xiphoid process), noting any abnormality or tenderness.

Ribs and Costal Cartilage. Adjacent to the sternum, the examiner should palpate the sternocostal and costochondral articulations, noting any swelling, tenderness, or other abnormality. These "articulations" are sometimes sprained or subluxed, or a costochondritis (Tietze syndrome) may be evident. The examiner should palpate the ribs as they extend around the chest wall, seeking any potential pathology and noting whether they are aligned with each other or one protrudes more than the adjacent ones as sometimes occurs with anterior shoulder pathology.

Humerus and Rotator Cuff Muscles. Moving laterally from the chest and caudally from the acromion process, the examiner should palpate the humerus and its surrounding structures for potential pathology. The examiner first palpates the lateral tip of the acromion process and then moves inferiorly to the greater tuberosity of the humerus. The examiner should then laterally rotate the humerus. During palpation, the long head of biceps in the bicipital groove will slip under the fingers, followed by the lesser tuberosity of the humerus (Fig. 5.192). As with all palpation, the testing should be done gently and carefully to prevent causing the patient undue pain. By rotating the humerus alternately laterally and medially, the smooth progression over the three structures is normally noted **(de Anquin test),** and the lesser tuberosity is felt at the level of the coracoid process. Dashottar and Borstad[10] advocated that one should palpate the two borders of the bicipital groove (i.e., the greater and lesser tuberosities) to determine the **bicipital-forearm angle (BFA)** (see Fig. 5.2B). To do this, the patient sits with the elbow flexed to 90° while the examiner palpates both tuberosities. Because the ulna is virtually perpendicular to the line joining the two epicondyles at the elbow, the angle between the ulna and the vertical can be used to quantify **humeral retroversion (HR).** The BFA and HR are inversely related so that as the BFA gets smaller, the HR gets bigger.[10,11] If the examiner then palpates along the lesser tuberosity and the lip of the bicipital groove, the fingers will rest on the tendon of the subscapularis muscle. The subscapularis may also be palpated in the triangle made up of the superior border of pectoralis major, the clavicle, and the medial border of the deltoid.[537] If the examiner places the thumb over the lesser tuberosity and "grips" the shoulder between the second, third, and fourth fingers (as shown in Fig. 5.4), the fingers will be over the insertion of the other three rotator cuff muscles: supraspinatus, infraspinatus, and teres minor. Moving laterally over the bicipital groove to its other lip, the examiner may palpate the insertion of the pectoralis major muscle. The patient is then asked to further medially rotate the humerus so that the forearm rests behind the back, and the examiner palpates 2 cm inferior to the anterior aspect of the acromion process for the supraspinatus tendon. Any tenderness of the tendon should be noted. The examiner then passively abducts the patient's shoulder to between 80° and 90° and palpates the notch formed by the acromion and spine of the scapula with the clavicle. In the notch, the examiner is palpating the musculotendinous junction of the supraspinatus muscle. With the arm in 10° medial rotation at the side and the elbow flexed, the examiner can palpate the long head of biceps under the pectoralis major tendon by having the patient laterally rotate the humerus 30° while flexing and extending the elbow to identify the long head of biceps under the tendon of pectoralis major in the axilla (see Fig. 5.192C). Both sides should be compared.[1,94] If the examiner then elevates the patient's arm into full abduction and lateral rotation, followed by bringing the arm down by the side (adducting the arm) while progressively medially rotating the shoulder and a click or pop occurs, it indicates the tendon is sliding in and out of the bicipital grooves indicating dynamic instability of the long head of biceps.[1,40]

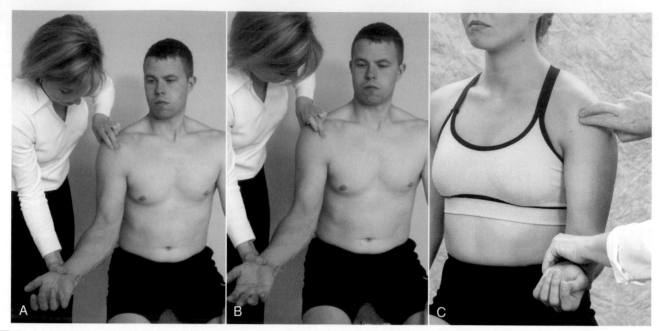

Fig. 5.192 Palpation around the shoulder. (A) The greater tuberosity. (B) The lesser tuberosity. The bicipital groove lies between these two landmarks. (C) Palpation of the biceps tendon.

The examiner should then palpate the head of the humerus and its relationship to the glenoid cavity. By placing the fingers over the anterior humeral head and the thumb over the posterior humeral head, the examiner then slides the fingers and thumbs medially (see Fig. 5.66). As the humeral head is larger than the glenoid with only about 25% to 30% of the head in contact with the glenoid at any one time, the examiner's fingers and thumb will "dip in" as they approach the glenohumeral joint. This "dipping in" should be slightly greater anteriorly. If there is no dipping anteriorly or posteriorly, it means the humeral head is sitting further posteriorly or anteriorly than it should. Once the examiner has found the glenohumeral joint (at the point of hardness after dipping in), he or she can palpate along the joint line superiorly and inferiorly on the anterior and posterior surfaces, feeling for any pain or the presence of pathology (torn labrum, ligament, or capsule). The examiner can determine the joint line by medially and laterally rotating the humerus while palpating. The examiner should be able to differentiate the glenoid (does not move) from the humerus (rotates). As the technique is uncomfortable to the patient, the patient should be warned about possible discomfort, and the results should be compared with those from the normal side. With care, the examiner can palpate all of the glenoid edge except superiorly, where the proximity of the acromion to the humerus will not allow it. The examiner can palpate most of the anterior joint line (see Fig. 5.66). If the painful shoulder demonstrates more pain than the uninjured shoulder, it may indicate a problem with structures (i.e., labrum, capsule) along the joint line.[361]

Axilla. With the shoulder slightly abducted (20° to 30°), the examiner palpates the structures of the axilla, latissimus dorsi muscle (posterior wall), pectoralis major muscle (anterior wall), serratus anterior muscle (medial wall), lymph nodes (palpable only if swollen), and brachial artery. The inferior glenohumeral joint and glenoid edge may also be palpated in the axilla. The patient is then asked to lie prone on the elbows (sphinx position) with the shoulders slightly laterally rotated and the elbow slightly adducted in relation to the shoulder. The examiner then palpates just inferior to the most lateral aspect of the scapula for the insertion of the infraspinatus muscle. Just distal to this insertion, the examiner may be able to palpate the insertion of the teres minor.

Posterior Structures

To complete the palpation, the patient may be either sitting or lying prone with the upper limb by the trunk (Fig. 5.191B).

Spine of Scapula. From the acromion process the examiner moves his or her hands along the spine of the scapula, noting any tenderness or abnormality.

Scapula. The examiner follows the spine of the scapula to the medial border of the scapula and then follows the outline of the scapula, which normally extends from the spinous process of T2 to the spinous process of T9, depending on the size of the scapula. The superior angle lies at the level of the T2 spinous process. The base or root of the spine of the scapula lies between T3 and T4, and the inferior angle lies between T7 and T9. Along the medial border and spine of the scapula, the examiner can palpate the trapezius muscle (upper, middle, and lower parts) and the rhomboids. At the inferior angle, the latissimus dorsi may be palpated. The examiner then moves around the inferior angle of the scapula and along its lateral border. Against the lateral border and along the ribs, the serratus anterior can be palpated. Near the glenoid, long head of triceps and teres minor may be palpated. After the borders of the scapula have been palpated, the posterior surface (supraspinatus and infraspinatus muscles) may be palpated for tenderness, atrophy, or spasm. By positioning the arm in forward flexion (60°), adduction and lateral rotation, infraspinatus and teres minor may be palpated just under and slightly inferior to the posterior aspect of the acromion.[537]

Spinous Processes of the Lower Cervical and Thoracic Spine. In the midline, the examiner may palpate the cervical and thoracic spinous processes for any abnormality or tenderness. This is followed by palpation of the trapezius muscle.

Diagnostic Imaging

Diagnostic imaging is used in conjunction with a physical examination to determine a diagnosis. It should never be used in isolation, but any findings should be related to clinical signs to rule out false-positive indications or age-related changes.[538–510]

Plain Film Radiography[541–543]

Anteroposterior View. This may be a true anteroposterior view or a tilt view (Figs. 5.193 and 5.194). It may be used

---

Common X-Ray Views of the Shoulder

- Anteroposterior view (see Figs. 5.193 and 5.194)
- Anteroposterior lateral rotation view (glenohumeral joint) (see Fig. 5.196A)
- Anteroposterior medial rotation view (glenohumeral joint) (see Fig. 5.196B)
- Transscapular (Y) lateral view (fracture or dislocation suspected) (see Fig. 5.196D and E)
- Stress x-ray of acromioclavicular joint (see Fig. 5.202)
- Anteroposterior view (true) (glenohumeral joint) (also called the Rockwood view) (Figs. 5.203 and 5.204; see Fig. 5.193)
- Anteroposterior view of sternoclavicular joint (Fig. 5.205)
- Anteroposterior view of acromioclavicular joint (Fig. 5.206)
- Lateral view of shoulder (Fig. 5.207)
- Axillary lateral view (fracture or dislocation suspected) (see Fig. 5.208)
- Stryker notch view (instability, Hill-Sach lesion) (see Fig. 5.213)
- West point view (instability, anterior glenoid rim) (see Fig. 5.215)
- Zanca view (10°–15° cephalad anteroposterior) (see Fig. 5.217)
- Swimmer's view (Figs. 5.218 and 5.219)
- Serendipity for sternoclavicular joint (beam 40° off vertical caudal, centered on sternum, patient supine)

---

to assess the acromioclavicular joint's width, spurring of the acromioclavicular undersurface, lateral tilt of the acromion, and the distance between the humeral head and anterior acromion (Fig. 5.195).[544] A great deal of information can be obtained from either view (Fig. 5.196).

1. The relation of the humerus to the glenoid cavity should be examined. The "empty glenoid" sign may recognize posterior dislocations. Normally the radiograph shows overlapping shadows of the humerus and glenoid. With a posterior dislocation, this shadow is reduced or absent (Fig. 5.197).[546]
2. The relation of the clavicle to the acromion process and the humerus to the glenoid should also be observed.
3. The examiner should determine whether the epiphyseal plate of the humeral head is present and if so, whether it is normal.
4. The examiner should note whether there are any calcifications in any of the tendons (Fig. 5.198), especially those of the supraspinatus or infraspinatus muscles, or fractures.[547,548]
5. The examiner should note the configuration of the undersurface of the acromion (see Figs. 5.9 and 5.196D)[549,550] and the presence of any subacromial spurs (Fig. 5.199).
6. Medial rotation of the humerus with this view may show a defect on the lateral aspect of the humeral head from recurrent dislocations. This defect, in reality a compression fracture of the posterosuperolateral humeral head, is called a **Hill-Sachs lesion** (Fig. 5.200) (i.e., a pathological depressed fracture) and may be classed as engaged or nonengaged.[551–553] *Engaged* implies that the area of the lesion articulates with the glenoid when the arm is in abduction and lateral rotation. Any defect and its size will increase glenohumeral instability[554] and may affect the stability of the joint.[555] Posterior dislocations may sometimes result in an anteromedial humeral head impression fracture (also called **reverse Hill-Sachs lesion [RHSL]**, **Malgaigne lesion**, or **McLaughlin lesion**).[556] The lesion can be seen on x-ray, computed tomography (CT) scan, or magnetic resonance imaging (MRI) and occurs in 30% to 90% of posterior dislocations.[109,556–558]
7. The examiner should look at the acromiohumeral interval (the space between the acromion and the humerus) and see whether it is normal.[559] The normal interval is 7 to 14 mm (Fig. 5.201). If this distance decreases, it may indicate a rotator cuff tear.[560] Likewise, if the arm is medially rotated and the view shows the coracohumeral distance of less than 11 mm, its indicates impingement and rotator cuff pathology.[561] If the arm is x-rayed in 90° of abduction, the acromiohumeral distance will be much less (see Fig. 5.195D).[544]
8. The normal coracoclavicular interspace (distance between the coracoid process and the clavicle) is 1.1 to 1.3 cm.[562]

Routine A-P shoulder

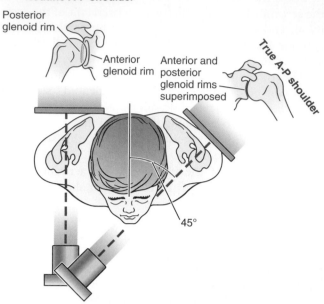

Fig. 5.193 Positioning for the anteroposterior radiographic view.

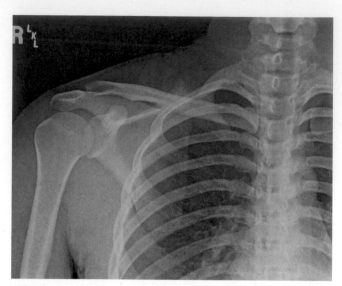

Fig. 5.194 Anteroposterior view (routine) of the shoulder. Note the glenoid sitting partially behind the humerus.

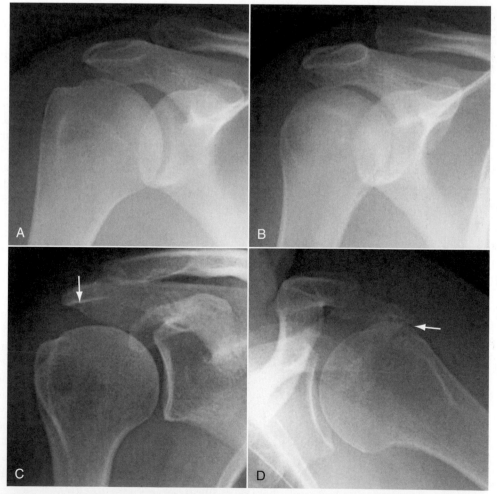

Fig. 5.195 (A) Anteroposterior lateral rotation. Note the greater tubercle in profile, the humeral-acromial distance, and the coracoclavicular interspace. (B) Anteroposterior medial rotation. Note the smooth rounded contour of the humeral head. (C) Grashey projection. The glenohumeral joint appears more "open." Note the **sourcil sign** *(arrow)*, a white line on the bottom of the acromion that is purported to be a sign of sclerosis.[545] (D) Active abduction view. Note the narrowing of the acromiohumeral distance *(arrow)* in this patient with a rotator cuff tear (normal, more than 2 mm). (From Anderson MW, Brennan C, Mittal A: Imaging evaluation of the rotator cuff, *Clin Sports Med* 31[4]:613, 2012.)

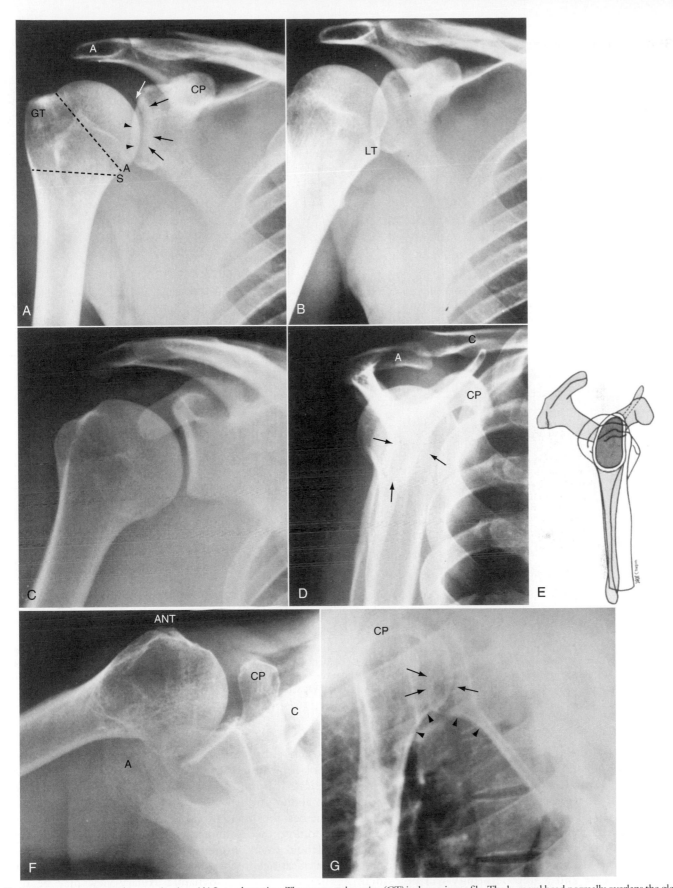

Fig. 5.196 Normal radiographic examination. (A) Lateral rotation. The greater tuberosity *(GT)* is shown in profile. The humeral head normally overlaps the glenoid on this view. The anterior *(black arrows)* and posterior *(arrowheads)* glenoid margins are well shown and do not overlap because of the anterior tilt of the glenoid. The anatomical *(black A)* and surgical *(S)* necks of the humerus are indicated. A vacuum phenomenon *(white arrow)* is present. (B) Medial rotation. The overlap of the greater tuberosity and humeral head produces a rounded appearance of the proximal humerus. A small exostosis is noted projecting from the humeral metaphysis. (C) Posterior oblique view. The glenohumeral cartilage space is shown in profile with no overlap of the humerus and glenoid. (D) Normal scapular Y view. This true lateral view of the scapula (anterior oblique view of the shoulder) shows the humeral head centered over the glenoid *(arrows).* (E) Diagram of the normal scapular Y view. (F) Axillary view. (G) Normal transthoracic view. The smooth arch formed by the inferior border of the scapula and the posterior aspect of the humerus is indicated *(arrowheads).* A faint view of the coracoid process *(CP)* shown. The margins of the glenoid are indicated *(arrows).* This view is slightly oblique, allowing the glenoid to be shown more en face than usual. *A,* Acromion; *A (white),* acromion process: *ANT,* anterior; *C,* clavicle; *CP,* coracoid process; *LT,* lesser tuberosity. (From Weissman BNW, Sledge CB: *Orthopedic radiology,* Philadelphia, 1986, WB Saunders, p 219.)

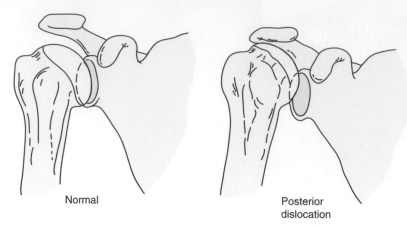

Normal

Posterior dislocation

Fig. 5.197 "Empty glenoid" sign of posterior dislocation on an anteroposterior radiograph. The head of the humerus fills the glenoid in the normal radiograph *(left)*. With a posterior dislocation, the glenoid is "empty," especially in its anterior portion *(right)*. (From Magee DJ, Reid DC: Shoulder injuries, In Zachazewski JE et al., editors: *Athletic injuries and rehabilitation*, Philadelphia, 1996, WB Saunders, p 523.)

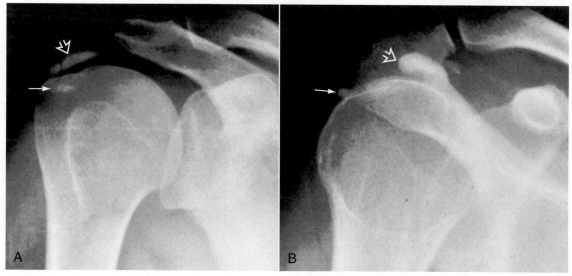

Fig. 5.198 Calcific tendinitis—supraspinatus and infraspinatus. (A) Lateral rotation view shows calcification projected over the base of the greater tuberosity *(white arrow)* and above the greater tuberosity *(open arrow)*. (B) Medial rotation view projects the infraspinatus calcification *(white arrow)* in profile and documents its posterior location. The supraspinatus calcification *(open arrow)* is rotated medially and maintains its superior location. (From Weissman BNW, Sledge CB: *Orthopedic radiology*, Philadelphia, 1986, WB Saunders, p 227.)

9. A stress anteroposterior radiograph may be used to gap the injured acromioclavicular joint to see whether there has been a third-degree sprain or to show an inferior laxity at the glenohumeral joint (Fig. 5.202). Equal weights of 9 kg (20 lb) are tied to each of the patient's hands to apply traction to the arms. If a third-degree acromioclavicular sprain has occurred, the coracoclavicular distance will increase and a step deformity will be evident. However, these radiographs are not routinely done.[63]

Axillary Lateral View. This view shows the relation of the humeral head to the glenoid and the coracohumeral distance (Fig. 5.208).[544] It is used to diagnose anterior and posterior dislocations at the glenohumeral joint and to look for avulsion fractures of the glenoid or a Hill-Sachs lesion. It does, however, require the patient to be able to abduct the arm 70° to 90° (Fig. 5.209). This view is the best for observation of the acromioclavicular joint. In addition, the examiner should note the relations of the glenoid cavity, humerus, scapula, and clavicle and any calcifications in the subscapularis, infraspinatus, or teres minor muscles. A dynamic axillary view may be used to show horizontal instability of the acromioclavicular joint.[563]

Transscapular (Y) Lateral (Outlet) View. This view (Fig. 5.210) shows the position of the humerus relative to the glenoid and the shape of the acromion and coracoid

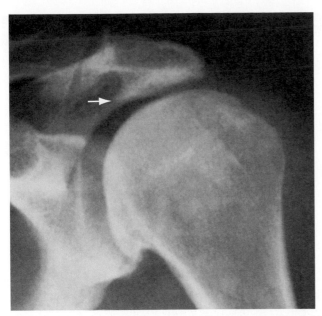

Fig. 5.199 External subacromial impingement syndrome-radiographic abnormalities. A frontal radiograph of the shoulder shows a large enthesophyte *(arrow)* extending from the anteroinferior portion of the acromion; it is associated with osteophytes at the acromioclavicular joint and in the inferior portion of the humeral head. (From Resnick D, Kransdorf MJ: *Bone and joint imaging*, Philadelphia, 2005, WB Saunders, p 922.)

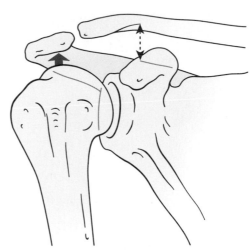

Fig. 5.201 Acromiohumeral interval *(solid arrow)* and coracoclavicular interspace *(dashed arrows)*.

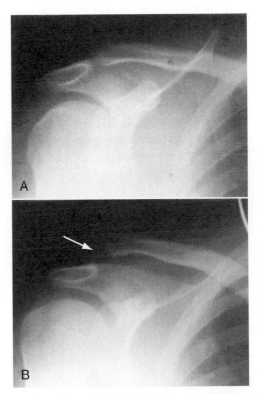

Fig. 5.202 Stress radiograph for third-degree acromioclavicular sprain. (A) No stress. (B) Stress. Note the increase (step) in the distance between the acromion process and the clavicle *(arrow)*.

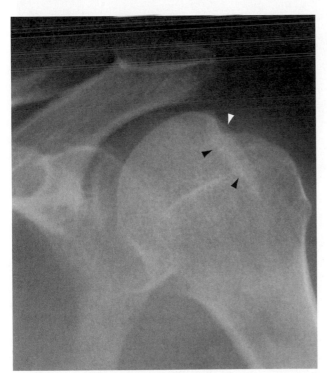

Fig. 5.200 Glenohumeral joint: **Hill-Sachs lesion**. In a patient with a previous anterior dislocation, an internal rotation view reveals the extent of the Hill-Sachs lesion *(arrowheads)*. (From Resnick D, Kransdorf MJ: *Bone and joint imaging*, Philadelphia, 2005, WB Saunders, p 833.)

processes. This view is the true lateral view of the scapula (see Fig. 5.196D and E). This view may be used to determine the coracoacromial outlet shape and its role in impingement (Fig. 5.211).[564–566]

Stryker Notch View. For this view, the patient lies supine with the arm forward flexed and the hand on top of the head (Fig. 5.212). The radiograph centers on the coracoid

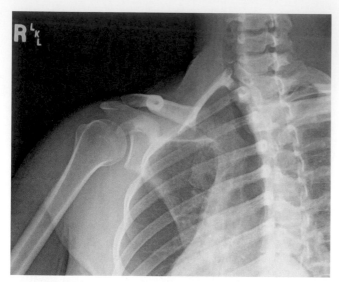

Fig. 5.203 Anteroposterior view (true) of the glenohumeral joint (Rockwood view).

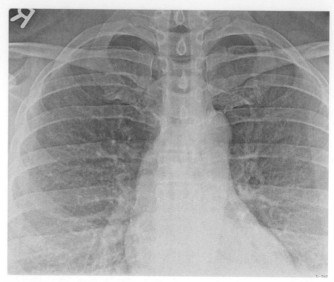

Fig. 5.205 Anteroposterior view of the sternoclavicular joint.

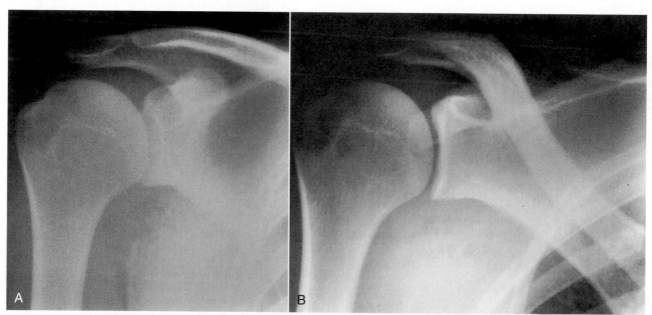

Fig. 5.204 (A) A radiograph of the shoulder in the plane of the thorax. (B) A radiograph of the shoulder taken in the plane of the scapula. (Modified from Rockwood CA, Green DP, editors: *Fractures*, 3 vols, ed 2, Philadelphia, 1984, JB Lippincott.)

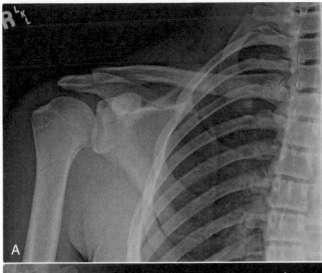

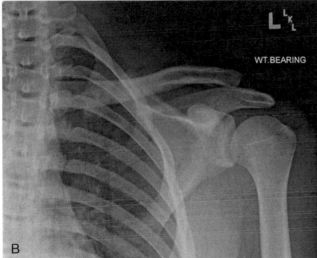

Fig. 5.206 (A) Anteroposterior view of the acromioclavicular joint. Note that the clavicle is in line with the acromion. (B) If there is a 3° sprain of the acromioclavicular joint and the arm is loaded, the clavicle will be seen to be above the acromion.

process. This view is used to assess fractures of the coracoid, a Hill-Sachs lesion (Fig. 5.213), or a Bankart lesion.[63,544,567]

West Point View. The patient is positioned prone (Fig. 5.214). This projection gives a good view of the glenoid (Fig. 5.215) to delineate glenoid fractures and bony abnormalities of the anterior glenoid rim.[568]

Arch View. This lateral view is used to determine the width and height of the subacromial arch. It helps the examiner determine the type of acromial arch (Fig. 5.216).

Zanca View. The Zanca view may be used to detect posterior dislocations of the acromioclavicular joint by

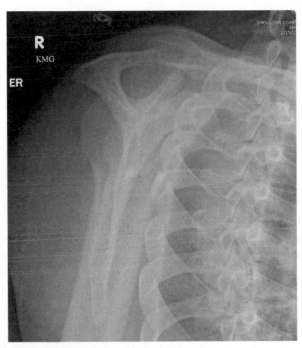

Fig. 5.207 Lateral view of the shoulder.

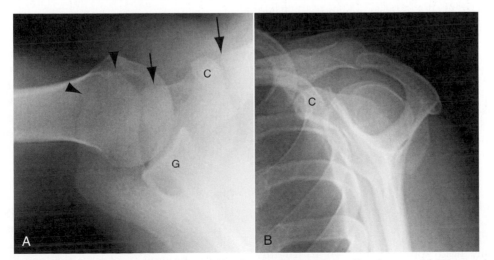

Fig. 5.208 (A) An axillary view reveals the relationship of the humeral head to the glenoid *(G)* as well as the coracoid *(C)*, acromion *(arrowheads)*, and distal clavicle *(arrows)*. (B) An outlet view shows the the humeral head centered on the glenoid, the coracoid process *(C)* anteriorly, and the acromioclavicular joint in profile. (From Anderson MW, Brennan C, Mittal A: Imaging evaluation of the rotator cuff, *Clin Sports Med* 31[4]:614, 2012.)

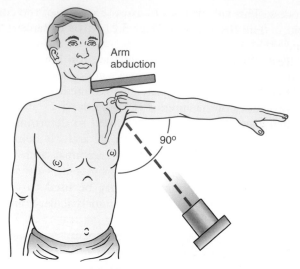

Fig. **5.209** Axillary lateral view.

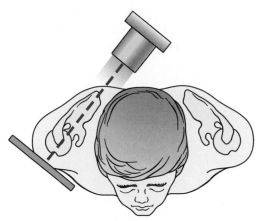

Fig. **5.210** Positioning for transscapular (Y) lateral view.

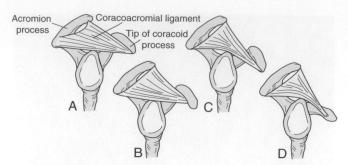

Fig. **5.211** Illustrations demonstrating variations in the shape of the **coracoacromial outlet** as described by Kragh et al.[564] The variations are based on the position of the coracoid relative to the glenoid. (A) Rhomboid outlet. This is a normal variant with a large outlet. (B) Triangular outlet, which is a normal variant. (C) Mild circumflex outlet, in which the coracoid tip is slightly inferior to the supraglenoid tubercle. Outlet capacity is adequate. (D) Chevron-shaped outlet in which the coracoid tip is near the equator of the glenoid or the humeral head. Anterior capacity is limited. (Adapted with permission from Kragh JF Jr, Doukas WC, Basamania CJ: Primary coracoid impingement syndrome. *Am J Orthop [Belle Mead NJ]* 33:229-232, 2004. Adapted from Kragh JF Jr, Doukas WC, Basamania CJ: Primary coracoid impingement syndrome, *Am J Orthop [Belle Mead NJ]* 33[5]:229–232, 2004.)

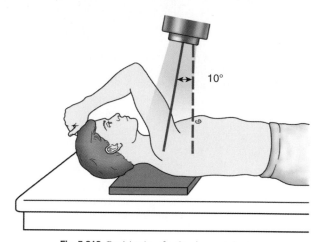

Fig. **5.212** Positioning for Stryker notch view.

measuring the distance between the end of the acromion and the end of the clavicle and this space is called the **AC width index (ACI)** (Fig. 5.217), which is calculated using the following formula:

$$ACI = \frac{(\text{Width of injured side - width of normal side})}{\text{width of normal (uninjured) side}} \times 100\%$$

If the index is ≥60%, the patient has suffered a posterior acromioclavicular dislocation.[569] The view may also show degenerative changes in the acromioclavicular joint.

Arthrography

An arthrogram of the shoulder is useful for delineating many of the soft tissues and recesses around the glenohumeral joint (Figs. 5.220 and 5.221).[350,570–572] The joint can normally hold approximately 16 to 20 mL of solution. With adhesive capsulitis (idiopathic frozen shoulder), the amount the joint can hold may decrease to 5 to 10 mL. The arthrogram shows a decrease in the capacity of the joint and obliteration of the axillary fold. Also, there is an almost complete lack of filling of the subscapular bursa with adhesive capsulitis (Fig. 5.222). Tearing of any structures, such as the supraspinatus tendon and rotator cuff, may result in extravasation of the radiopaque dye.[573]

Diagnostic Ultrasound

Diagnostic ultrasound imaging (DUSI) is becoming a more frequently used device for assessment of the shoulder by physical therapists. Ultrasound (US) imaging can be used to observe the long head of biceps, the

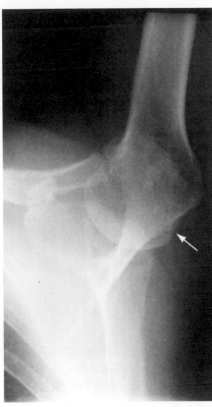

Fig. 5.213 Stryker notch view demonstrates a notch in the posterolateral aspect of the humeral head, representing a large Hill-Sachs lesion *(arrow)* on the humerus.

acromiohumeral distance, the subacromial/subdeltoid bursa, the amount of joint laxity, and the rotator cuff anatomy including subscapularis, supraspinatus, infraspinatus and teres minor, for both normal appearances and pathological changes.

Anterior View. The US position for examining the long head of biceps starts with the patient's arm in supination with the palm up and the arm resting on the patient's own leg. The transducer is placed in the transverse plane along the long head of biceps to visualize the tendon (Fig. 5.223). This position allows visualization of the tendon in the short axis. When the transducer is in the correct perpendicular position, a hyperechoic and well-defined humeral cortex is seen underneath the biceps tendon (Fig. 5.224, *arrows*). The tendon is examined from proximal to distal and viewed as a fibrillary (i.e., thread-like) structure presenting as a high-intensity, hyperechoic round, tubular shaped structure. The biceps tendon is normally fibrillar in appearance. Additionally, care should be taken to observe the tendon's placement between the greater and lesser tuberosities in the bicipital groove, which create a thin hyperechoic rim just deep to the tendon (see Fig. 5.224).[574] Recent effusion around the long head of biceps has been shown to have a moderate to high degree of correlation with ROM, and

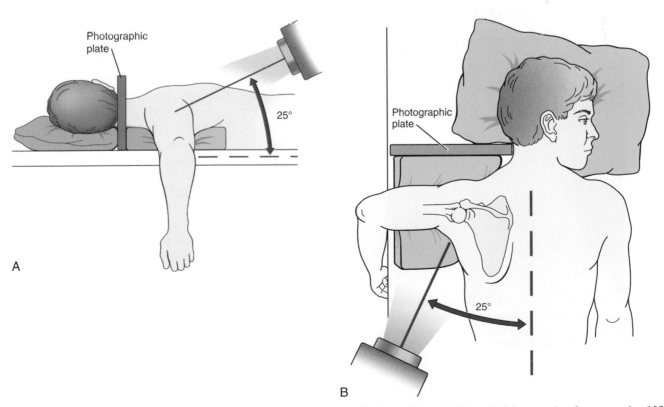

Fig. 5.214 Positioning of patient for West Point axillary view. (A) Side view. (B) The beam *(bottom left)* is angled downward to form an angle of 25° from the horizontal plane.

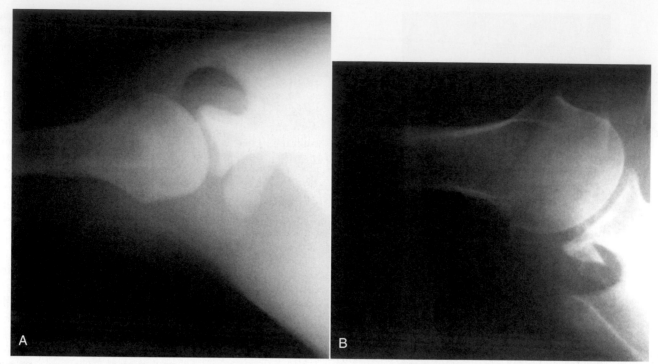

Fig. 5.215 (A) The result of a West Point view of the glenohumeral joint. Note the acromion superior to the glenoid and the coracoid process, which is inferior to the glenoid in this view. (B) Plain film x-ray in an axillary or West Point view of a fracture of the glenoid, a **Bankart fracture**. (From Swain J, Bush KW: *Diagnostic imaging for physical therapists*, St. Louis, 2009, Saunders/Elsevier, pp 196, 208.)

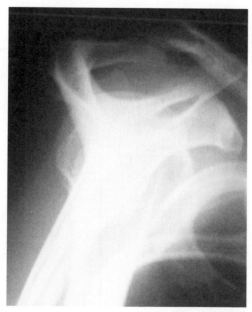

Fig. 5.216 Arch view of the acromioclavicular joint. Notice the separation of the clavicle and acromion. This view also shows the relation of the humerus to the glenoid (Y view).

a low degree with functional scores and visual analogue scale for pain in shoulder disease.[575]

The DUSI transducer can then be rotated 90° to visualize the long axis of the tendon. The tendon can be viewed from proximal at the humeral head to distal near the pectoralis major tendon (Fig. 5.225). The tendon should be viewed as described previously. However, due to anisotropy, the transducer may need to be toggled or rocked back and forth along the width of the tendon to obtain a good visualization of the tendon in the longitudinal view (Fig. 5.226).

The acromioclavicular joint is assessed initially by placing the transducer superiorly in the transverse plane or the short axis, over the distal acromioclavicular joint (Fig. 5.227). A hypoechoic joint space or a hyperechoic joint disc may be seen. The cortical outline of the acromion and the clavicle may also be seen. By visualizing the acromion and the clavicle, the **acromioclavicular space** can be measured and the hyperechoic interposed fibrocartilage disc, if present (Fig. 5.228). Joint widening can occur in those with acromioclavicular joint

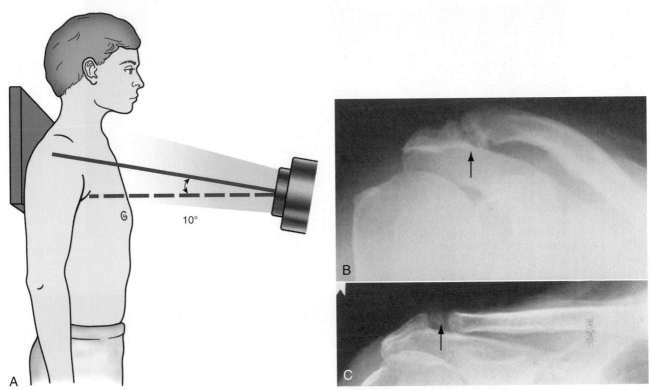

Fig. 5.217 (A) Positioning of patient for a Zanca view of the acromioclavicular joint. (B) A Zanca view of the joint reveals significant degenerative changes *(arrow)*. (C) With the Zanca view, a loose body is clearly noted within the joint *(arrow)*. The space between the end of the acromion and the end of the clavicle is called the **acromioclavicular width index**. (B and C, From Rockwood CA: *The shoulder*, ed 4, Philadelphia, 2009, WB Saunders.)

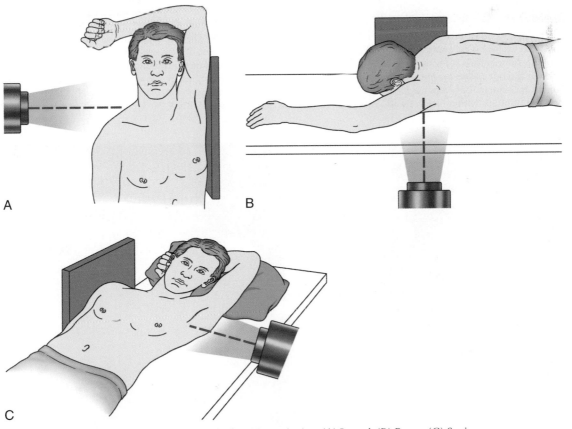

Fig. 5.218 Patient positioning for swimmer's view. (A) Lateral. (B) Prone. (C) Supine.

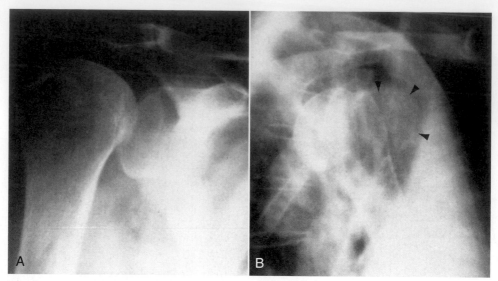

Fig. 5.219 (A) Posterior dislocation of the humerus. (B) Swimmer's view. (From Sutton D, Young JWR: *A concise textbook of clinical imaging*, ed 2, St Louis, 1995, Mosby.)

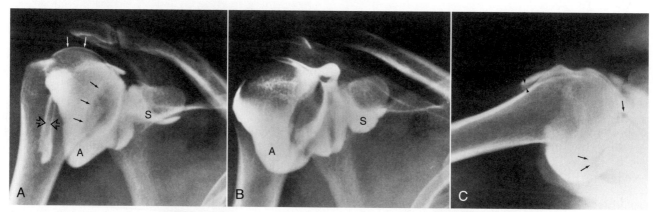

Fig. 5.220 Normal single-contrast arthrogram. (A) Lateral rotation. (B) Medial rotation. The humeral articular cartilage is coated with contrast medium *(white arrows)*. There is no contrast agent in the subacromial-subdeltoid bursa. The defect created by the glenoid labrum *(black arrows)* is shown. Filling of the subscapularis recess is often poor on lateral rotation views because of bursal compression by the subscapularis muscle. (C) In the axillary view, the anterior *(single arrow)* and posterior *(double arrows)* glenoid labral margins are shown. The biceps tendon *(arrowheads)* is surrounded by contrast medium in the biceps tendon sheath. No contrast agent overlies the surgical neck of the humerus. *A*, Axillary recess; *open arrows*, tendon of long head of biceps within biceps sheath; *S*, subscapularis recess (From Weissman BNW, Sledge CB: *Orthopedic radiology*, Philadelphia, 1986, WB Saunders, p 222.)

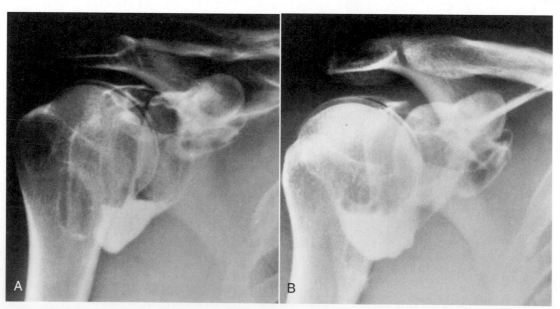

Fig. 5.221 Normal double-contrast arthrogram. Upright views of the patient with a sandbag suspended from the wrist and the humerus in lateral rotation (A) and medial rotation (B) show the structures noted on single-contrast examination and allow better appreciation of the articular cartilages. (From Weissman BNW, Sledge CB: *Orthopedic radiology*, Philadelphia, 1986, WB Saunders, p 222.)

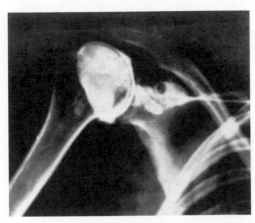

Fig. 5.222 Typical arthrographic picture in adhesive capsulitis. Note the absence of a dependent axillary fold and poor filling of the biceps. (From Neviaser JS: Arthrography of the shoulder joint: study of the findings of adhesive capsulitis of the shoulder, *J Bone Joint Surg Am* 44:1328, 1962.)

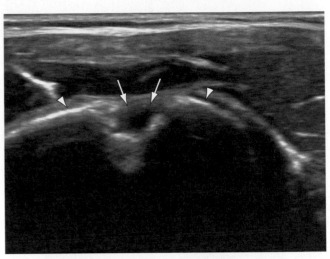

Fig. 5.224 DUSI transverse image of the biceps tendon *(between arrows)* pointing out the greater (on the right) and lesser tuberosities (on the left) *(at the arrowheads).*

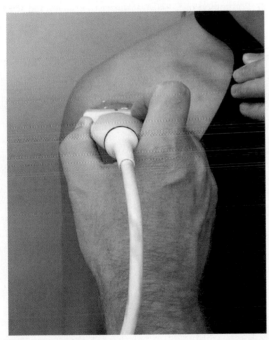

Fig. 5.223 Positioning of DUSI transducer to view the long head of biceps brachii tendon in the short axis.

separation (i.e., 3° sprain). When a disruption exists, the distal end of the clavicle will be elevated with movement. This will be seen if the patient actively moves the arm from "hand on knee" position to "hand on opposite shoulder."

Acromiohumeral interval distance (see Fig. 5.201) is measured between the inferior surface (most lateral edge) of the acromion and the superior surface of the humeral head.[576,577] The importance of this measurement is that poor surgical outcomes, large rotator cuff tears, and superior humeral migration have been shown when the acromiohumeral interval distance is decreased.[229,578,579] The transducer is then moved in a coronal oblique plane vertically along the most lateral aspect of the acromion. In this position, one can see the acromion and the greater tuberosity of the humerus.[580]

Using the same position, the examiner can view the subacromial/subdeltoid bursa. After viewing the acromioclavicular joint, the transducer is moved laterally. The bursa is directly above the supraspinatus muscle. The bursa will appear as a small anechoic rim, which is indicative of the collapsed subacromial bursa.[581–583] When the patient actively moves the shoulder into abduction, pooling of the subacromial fluid may be seen as an enlarged bursa.

Standard DUSI examination positions for the rotator cuff muscles can be seen in (Fig. 5.229). The subscapularis tendon is examined with the shoulder laterally rotated. Initially, the transducer is placed in a long axis parallel to the tendon (Fig. 5.230). The tendon should appear hyperechoic and can be traced laterally to the lessor tubercle of the humerus (Fig. 5.231). The tendon is viewed in its entirety from superior to inferior with emphasis being placed on its superior insertion, as this is the location that is most commonly injured in supraspinatus rotator cuff tears.[584] Rotation of the transducer 90° will allow visualization of the subscapularis tendon along its short axis (Fig. 5.232). Just above the outline of the humeral head, one can see a transverse cut of the subscapularis (Fig. 5.233). It is common to see areas of hypoechoic striations of muscle or interfaces between the several tendon bundles.

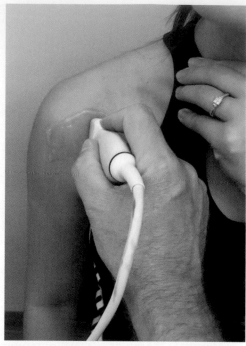

Fig. 5.225 Positioning of the DUSI transducer to view the long head of biceps brachii tendon in the long axis.

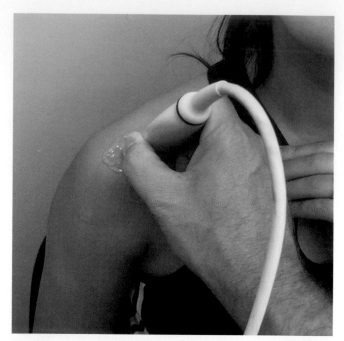

Fig. 5.227 Positioning of DUSI transducer to examine the acromioclavicular joint.

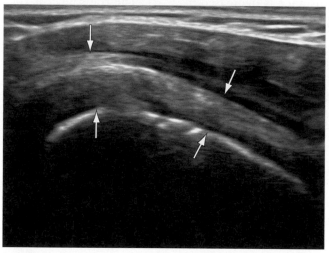

Fig. 5.226 DUSI sagittal image showing the long head of biceps tendon *(between arrows)*.

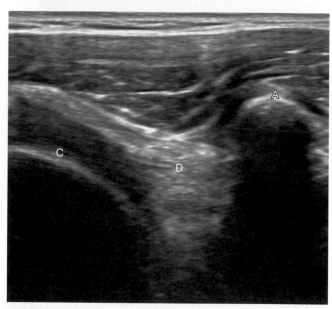

Fig. 5.228 DUSI image of the acromioclavicular joint. *A*, Acromion; *C*, clavicle; *D*, joint disc.

The supraspinatus is the most common rotator cuff tendon torn; therefore, it is critical to visualize this muscle during any shoulder DUSI examination.[574] To begin examination of the supraspinatus, the patient is asked to place the hand of the affected shoulder on the ipsilateral hip, known as the "modified Crass" position (Fig. 5.234). By extending the humerus, the greater tuberosity and the supraspinatus tendon are moved from underneath the acromion to allow them to be exposed anteriorly. To view the supraspinatus longitudinally, the transducer is placed parallel to the supraspinatus fibers in line with the ipsilateral humerus. The transducer can be moved both anteromedially and posterolaterally to view the tendon in its entirety

from anterior to posterior. The healthy tendon will appear hyperechoic and fibrillary. By rotating the transducer 90°, the tendon is seen in its short axis as a transverse cut. This position will place the transducer perpendicular to the long axis of the ipsilateral humerus. A hyperechoic rim of the humerus will lie below the hypoechoic articular cartilage (Fig. 5.235). The supraspinatus will lie just superior to the hypoechoic articular cartilage. The anterior border of the supraspinatus can be seen just lateral to the long head of biceps tendon.

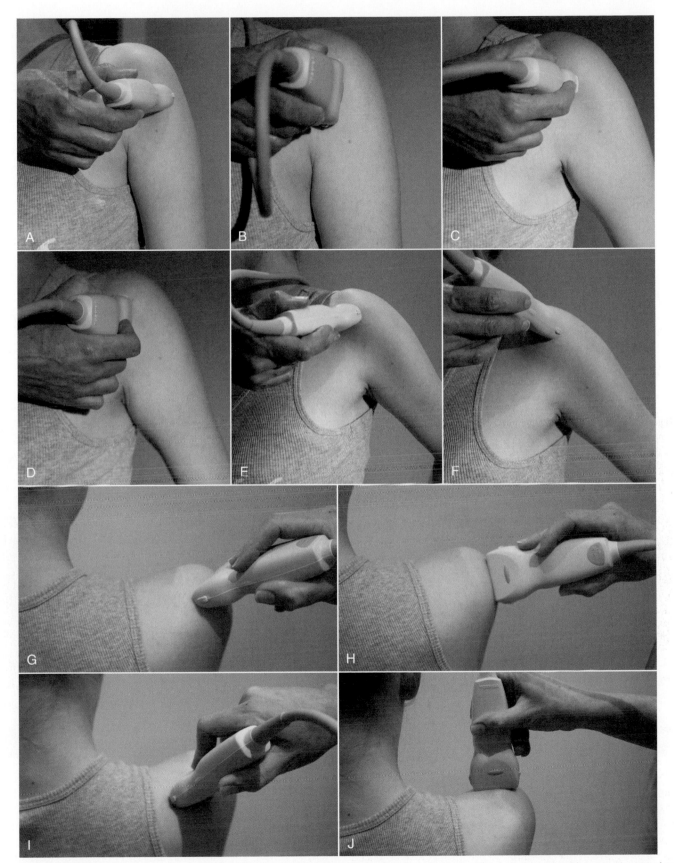

Fig. 5.229 Standard DUSI examination positions. (A and B) Dorsum of hand on patient's knee (same side) with some shoulder extension: used to visualize the biceps tendon in short and long axes. (C and D) Shoulder extended, hand-by-side position for subscapularis (lateral rotation can also be used). (E and F) Patient's hand on back pocket; used for supraspinatus short and long axes. (G–J) Arm across anterior chest for teres. (From McNally E: *Practical musculoskeletal ultrasound*, ed 2, China, 2014, Elsevier.)

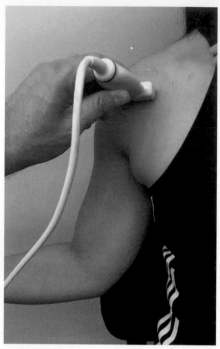

Fig. 5.230 Positioning of DUSI transducer to view the subscapularis tendon in long axis.

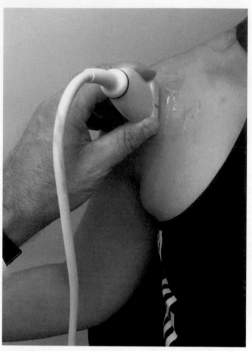

Fig. 5.232 Positioning of DUSI transducer to view subscapularis tendon in short axis.

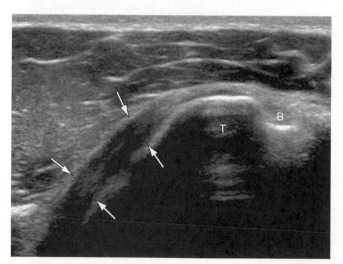

Fig. 5.231 DUSI evaluation of subscapularis tendon: long-axis image shows tendon (*between arrows*). *B,* Biceps tendon; *T,* lesser tuberosity. (From Jacobson JA: *Fundamentals of musculoskeletal ultrasound,* ed 3, Philadelphia, 2018, Elsevier.)

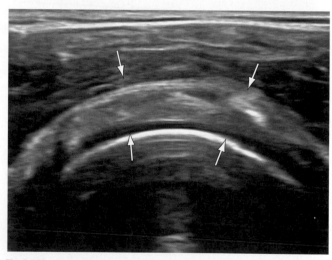

Fig. 5.233 DUSI image of subscapularis tendon showing hyperechoic appearance *(between arrows).*

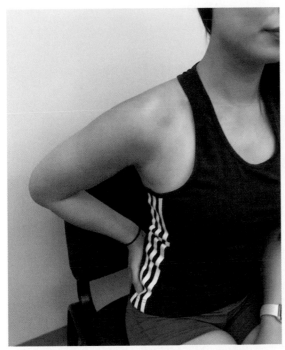

Fig. 5.234 The modified Crass position for DUSI examination of the shoulder.

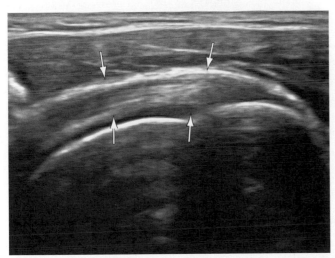

Fig. 5.235 DUSI image of a normal supraspinatus tendon viewed in the long axis *(between arrows).*

Posterior View. If the US transducer is moved posteriorly, the infraspinatus can be visualized. The infraspinatus is best viewed with the patient seated with the shoulder in medial rotation and the ipsilateral hand and forearm resting on the patient's medial thigh. The transducer is placed longitudinally parallel with the tendon fibers just below the scapular spine. The tendon fibers will appear hyperechoic while lying above the humeral head and under the deltoid muscle fibers. The fibers are followed laterally to the attachment

on the greater tuberosity. The transverse plane view of the infraspinatus can be seen by rotating the transducer 90° so that the transducer runs parallel to the posterior humerus.

Lastly, humeral torsion can be determined by use of DUSI. Humeral torsion is the relative difference in osseous rotation between the proximal and distal articular surfaces of the humerus and significantly influences shoulder ROM.[585-587] Ultrasonography can be used to determine humeral torsion by aligning the apices of the greater and lesser tuberosities and measuring the corresponding forearm angle.

Computed Tomography (CT)

CT, especially when combined with radiopaque dye **(computed tomoarthrogram [CTA]),** is effective in diagnosing bone and soft-tissue anomalies and injuries around the shoulder, including tears of the labrum (Figs. 5.236 through 5.238) and the rotator cuff.[560,588] This technique helps delineate capsular redundancy, glenoid rim abnormalities, and loose bodies.[550,589-591]

Magnetic Resonance Imaging (MRI)

MRI is proving to be useful in diagnosing soft-tissue injuries to the shoulder and has, in fact, become the method of choice for demonstrating soft-tissue abnormalities of the shoulder, such as labral and rotator cuff pathology along with MR arthrography.[28,40,543,592-598] However, it is important that these abnormalities be correlated with clinical findings.[593,597] It is possible to differentiate bursitis, peritenonitis/tendinosis, muscle strains, especially with injuries to the rotator cuff.[599] It is also useful for differentially diagnosing causes of impingement and instability syndromes. Labral tears, Hill-Sachs lesions, glenoid irregularities, and the state of bone marrow can also be diagnosed in the shoulder with the use of MRI (Figs. 5.239 through 5.245).[349,543,548,600-605] A **Buford complex** which is a congenital glenoid labral variant in which the anterosuperior labrum is absent in the 1 to 3 o'clock position and the middle glenohumeral ligament is a thick cord-like structure that originates from the superior labrum, may be seen on MRI and may mimic a torn labrum (Fig. 5.246).[606,607] Magnetic resonance arthrography has been found to increase the sensitivity to detecting partial-thickness tears.[599,608]

Angiography

Angiography is examination of the blood or lymph vessels using the introduction of a radiopaque substance followed by an x-ray. In the case of thoracic outlet syndromes and other syndromes involving arterial impingement, angiograms are sometimes used to demonstrate blockage of the subclavian artery during certain movements (Fig. 5.247).

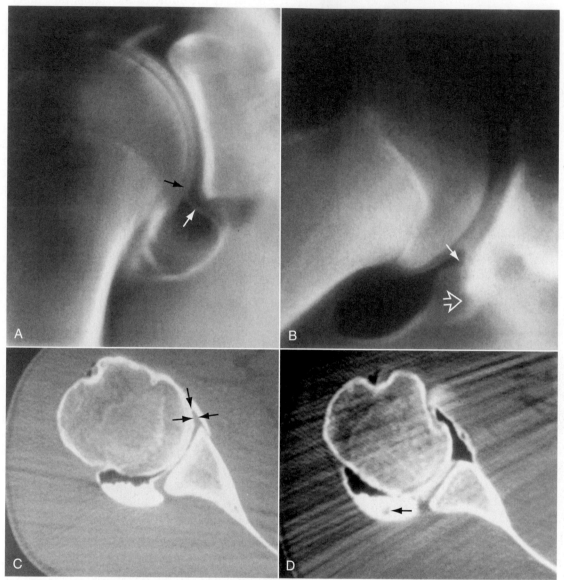

Fig. 5.236 Tomogram and computed tomography scan of the glenoid labrum. (A) Normal glenoid labrum on posterior oblique double-contrast arthrotomography. Tomographic section through the anterior margin of the glenoid in the posterior oblique position shows smooth articular cartilage on the humeral head *(black arrow)* and glenoid and a smooth contour to the glenoid labrum *(white arrow)*. (B) Abnormal glenoid labrum. Tomographic section shows a triangular defect in the labrum *(white arrow)*. The bony margin of the glenoid is also irregular *(open arrow)*. The patient had suffered a single anterior dislocation. (C) Normal glenoid labrum on computed tomography after double-contrast arthrography. The sharply pointed anterior *(arrows)* and slightly rounder posterior margins of the labrum are visible. (D) Computed tomoarthrogram shows absence of the anterior labrum and a loose body *(arrow)* posteriorly. (B, Courtesy Dr. Ethan Braunstein, Brigham and Women's Hospital, Boston, MA; C and D, Courtesy Dr. Arthur Newberg, Boston, MA. From Weissman BNW, Sledge CB: *Orthopedic radiology*, Philadelphia, 1986, WB Saunders, p 257.)

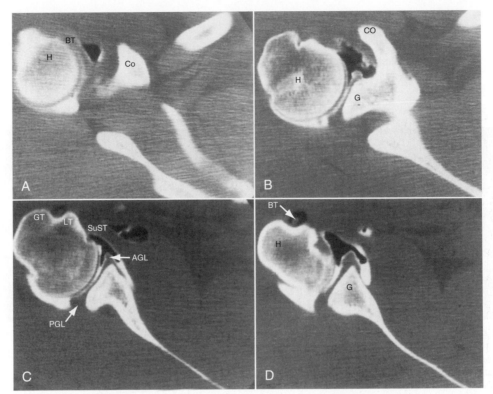

Fig. 5.237 Normal shoulder, computed arthrotomography. Normal anatomy is demonstrated by computed arthrotomographic sections at the level of the bicipital tendon origin (A), the coracoid process (B), the subscapularis tendon, (C) and the inferior joint level (D). *AGL,* Anterior glenoid labrum; *BT,* bicipital tendon; *Co,* coracoid process; *G,* glenoid process; *GT,* greater tuberosity; *H,* humeral head; *LT,* lesser tuberosity; *PGL,* posterior glenoid labrum; *SuST,* subscapularis tendon. (From De Lee JC, Drez D, editors: *Orthopedic sports medicine: principles and practice,* Philadelphia, 1994, WB Saunders, p 721.)

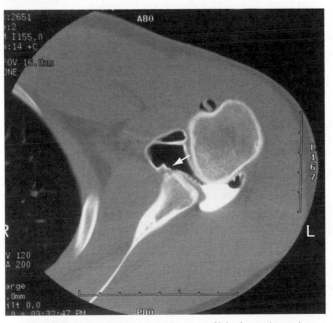

Fig. 5.238 Computed tomography scan of labral tear *(arrow).*

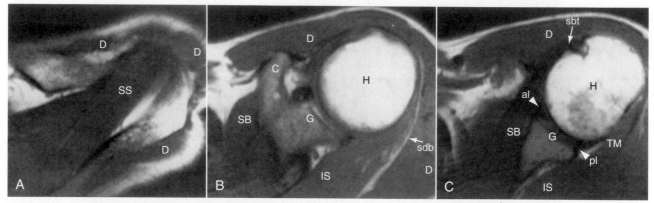

Fig. 5.239 T1-weighted axial magnetic resonance images from cranial (A) to caudal (C). *al,* Anterior labrum; *C,* coracoid; *D,* deltoid muscle; *G,* glenoid of scapula; *H,* humerus; *IS,* infraspinatus muscle; *pl,* posterior labrum; *SB,* subscapularis muscle; *sbt,* subscapularis tendon; *sdb,* subdeltoid-subacromial bursa; *SS,* supraspinatus muscle; *TM,* teres minor muscle. (From Meyer SJF, Dalinka MK: Magnetic resonance imaging of the shoulder, *Orthop Clin North Am* 21:499, 1990.)

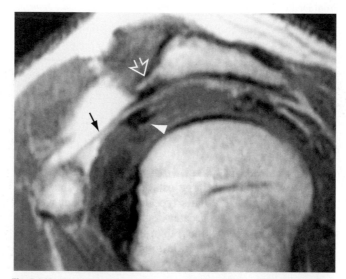

Fig. 5.240 Shoulder impingement syndrome: subacromial enthesophyte. Sagittal oblique T1-weighted (TR/TE, 800/20) spin-echo magnetic resonance image shows the enthesophyte *(open arrow)*, which is intimate with the coracoacromial ligament *(solid arrow)* and supraspinatus tendon *(arrowhead)*. (From Resnick D, Kransdorf MJ: *Bone and joint imaging*, Philadelphia, 2005, WB Saunders, p 375.)

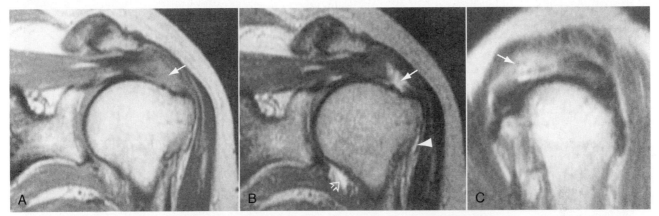

Fig. 5.241 Full-thickness rotator cuff tear: magnetic resonance (MR) imaging. In the coronal oblique plane, intermediate-weighted (TR/TE, 2000/20) (A) and T2-weighted (TR/TE, 2000/80) (B) spin-echo MR images show fluid in a gap *(solid arrow)* in the supraspinatus tendon; the fluid is of increased signal intensity in (B). Also in (B), note the increased signal intensity related to fluid in the glenohumeral joint *(open arrow)* and subdeltoid bursa *(arrowhead)*. Osteoarthritis of the acromioclavicular joint is evident. (C) In the same patient, sagittal oblique T2-weighted (TR/TE, 2000/60) spin-echo MR images show the site *(arrow)* of disruption of the supraspinatus tendon, which is of high signal intensity. (From Resnick D, Kransdorf MJ: *Bone and joint imaging*, Philadelphia, 2005, WB Saunders, p 925.)

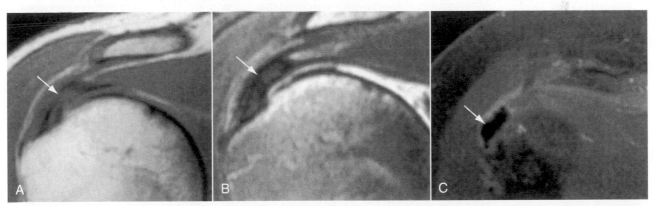

Fig. 5.242 (A) T1-weighted coronal image demonstrating mild thickening of the supraspinatus tendon with intermediate signal *(arrow)* present within the substance of the tendon. (B) A T2-weighted coronal image at the same level also demonstrates thickening of the tendon with intermediate signal *(arrow)* within the tendon. The presence of intermediate signal within the tendon is diagnostic of tendinopathy, whereas bright (fluid) signal within the tendon is diagnostic of a tear. (C) A globular area of low signal abnormality *(arrow)* in the infraspinatus tendon and mild surrounding edema is consistent with calcific bursitis. (From Sanders TG, Miller MD: A systematic approach to magnetic resonance imaging interpretation of sports medicine injuries of the shoulder, *Am J Sports Med* 33:1094, 2005.)

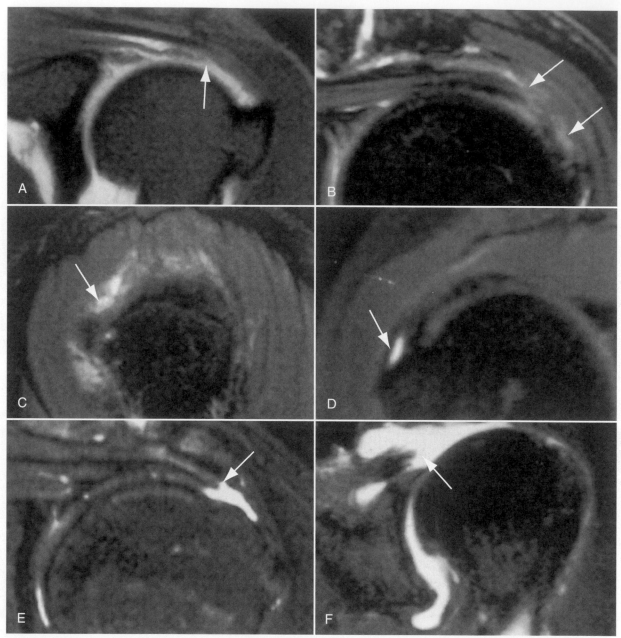

Fig. 5.243 Rotator cuff tear. Criteria for diagnosing a rotator cuff tear on magnetic resonance (MR) imaging include the presence of fluid in the expected location of the tendon or retraction of the tendon. (A) MR arthrogram of a partial-thickness articular surface tear of the supraspinatus tendon as contrast *(arrow)* extends into the substance of the tendon but not completely through the thickness of the tendon. (B) Conventional T2-weighted coronal image. (C) Sagittal image. Both (B) and (C) demonstrate fluid signal intensity *(arrows)* extending partially through the thickness of the tendon involving the bursal surface. (D) An interstitial tear *(arrow)* of the supraspinatus tendon. Fluid signal intensity *(arrow)* is present within the substance of the tendon but does not extend to either its articular or bursal surface. (E) A full-thickness tear with bright fluid signal *(arrow)* extending all the way through the thickness of the tendon from top to bottom. (F) A complete tear of the supraspinatus tendon extending from front to back, with approximately 3 cm of retraction of the musculotendinous junction *(arrow)*. (From Sanders TG, Miller MD: A systematic approach to magnetic resonance imaging interpretation of sports medicine injuries of the shoulder, *Am J Sports Med* 33:1094, 2005.)

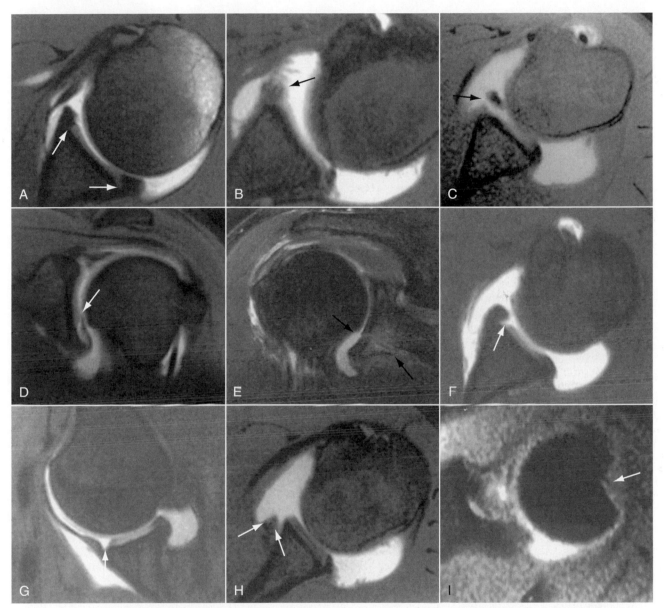

Fig. 5.244 Bankart lesions. (A) Cartilage undermining *(arrows)* the anterior and posterior labrum. The articular cartilage is intermediate in signal intensity; it is smooth and tapering because it undermines the fibrocartilage of the glenoid labrum. This image should not be confused with that of a tear, which would be irregular in appearance and usually extend completely beneath the labrum. (B) Marked irregularity and fraying *(arrow)* of the anteroinferior labrum. (C) A displaced Bankart lesion *(arrow)*. (D) A T2-weighted coronal image through the level of the anterior labrum demonstrates an irregular fluid collection *(arrow)* located within a tear of the anterior labrum, between the labrum and the glenoid. This irregularity is referred to as the "double axillary pouch" sign and is very common for an anterior labral tear. (E) A minimally displaced Bankart fracture *(arrows)* through the inferior glenoid. (F) Axial image with intra-articular contrast. (G) Abduction external rotation image with intra-articular contrast. Both F and G demonstrate a small collection of contrast *(arrows)* extending partially beneath the anterior labrum, representing a nondisplaced Bankart (Perthes) lesion. (H) A medialized Bankart lesion *(arrows)*. (I) This T2-weighted axial image through the superior aspect of the humeral head demonstrates a concavity *(arrow)* of the posterosuperior humeral head, representing a Hill-Sachs deformity. The humeral head should be round on the top three images, with no flattening or concavity. (From Sanders TG, Miller MD: A systematic approach to magnetic resonance imaging interpretation of sports medicine injuries of the shoulder, *Am J Sports Med* 33:1097, 2005.)

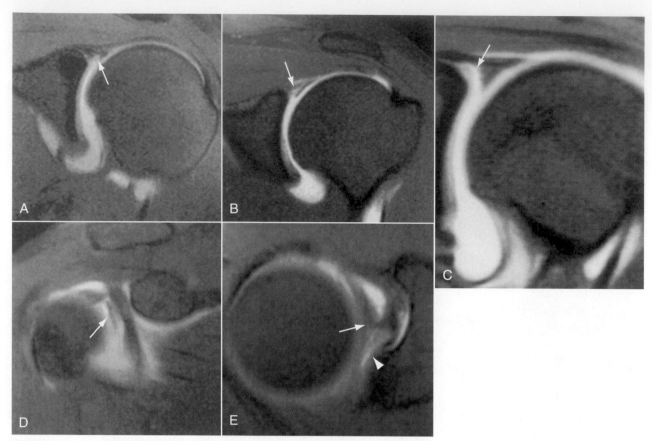

Fig. 5.245 Superior labral anteroposterior (SLAP) tear. (A) Fraying and irregularity *(arrow)* of the undersurface of the superior labrum, consistent with a SLAP tear. (B) A linear area of high signal *(arrow)* extending into the substance of the superior labrum. The presence of any high signal within the substance of the superior labrum is diagnostic of a SLAP tear. (C) Displacement *(arrow)* of the superior labrum away from the glenoid. This image represents a type II SLAP tear. (D) A bucket-handle tear (type III SLAP tear) of the superior labrum with the bucket-handle fragment *(arrow)* dangling in the superior joint. (E) Axial image demonstrating an irregular collection of contrast extending into the biceps anchor; this is consistent with a type IV SLAP tear with involvement of the biceps anchor. (From Sanders TG, Miller MD: A systematic approach to magnetic resonance imaging interpretation of sports medicine injuries of the shoulder, *Am J Sports Med* 33:1096, 2005.)

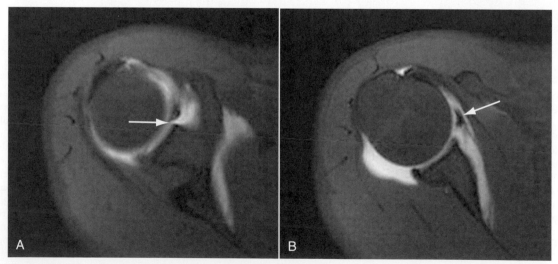

Fig. 5.246 (A) An axial FSE T2-weighted image with fat suppression through the upper part of the joint shows the anterior labrum separated from the bony glenoid *(arrow)*. (B) Lower in the joint the anterior labrum is firmly attached to the glenoid, but a thick, cordlike middle glenohumeral ligament is present *(arrow)*. This is a **Buford complex**. In (A), the anterior labrum is absent and a thick middle glenohumeral ligament is simulating the anterior labrum. (From Helms CA: *Fundamentals of skeletal radiology*, ed 4, Philadelphia, 2014, Elsevier.)

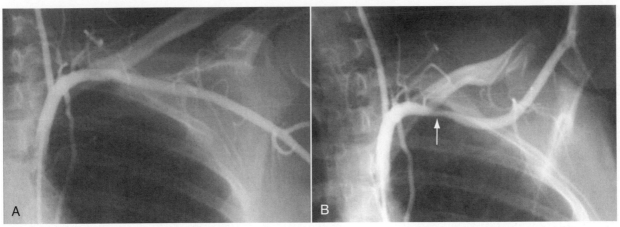

Fig. 5.247 Left subclavian angiogram shows normal-appearing artery at neutral position (A). Note compression of the artery between the clavicle and the first rib when the arm is abducted and externally rotated (B), consistent with thoracic outlet syndrome. (From Kalva SP, Hedgire S, Waltman AC: Upper extremity arteries. In Abbara S, Kalva SP, eds: *Problem solving in cardiovascular imaging,* Philadelphia, 2013, Saunders, pp 758–771.)

PRÉCIS OF THE SHOULDER ASSESSMENT[a]

NOTE: Suspected pathology will determine which *special tests* are to be performed.

Patient history (sitting)

Observation (sitting or standing)

Examination

  Active movements (sitting or standing)
    Elevation through forward flexion of the arm
    Elevation through abduction of the arm
    Elevation through the plane of the scapula (i.e., scaption)
    Medial rotation of the arm
    Lateral rotation of the arm
    Adduction of the arm
    Horizontal adduction and abduction of the arm
    Circumduction of the arm

  Passive movements (sitting)
    Elevation through abduction of the arm
    Elevation through forward flexion of the arm
    Elevation through abduction at the glenohumeral joint only
    Lateral rotation of the arm
    Medial rotation of the arm
    Extension of the arm
    Adduction of the arm
    Horizontal adduction and abduction of the arm

  Functional assessment

  Special tests (sitting or standing)
    For anterior shoulder instability:
      Bony apprehension test
      Load and shift test
    For posterior shoulder instability:
      Jerk test (Jahnke test)
      Load and shift test

For inferior and multidirectional shoulder instability:
  Feagin test (abduction inferior stability [ABIS] test)
  Hyperabduction test (Gagey hyperabduction test)
  Hyperextension–internal rotation (HERI) test
  Knee–shoulder test
  Sulcus sign

For anterior impingement:
  Coracoid impingement sign
  Hawkins-Kennedy test
  Neer test and modification
  Yokum test
  Zaslav test (internal rotation resistance strength test [IRRST])

For labral lesions:[b]
  Active compression test of O'Brien
  Anterior slide test
  Biceps load test (Kim test II)
  Biceps tension test
  Dynamic labral shear test
  Forced shoulder abduction and elbow flexion test
  Jerk test
  Kim test I (biceps load test II)
  Mayo shear test
  Pain provocation (Minori) test
  Porcellini test
  Throwing test

For scapular dyskinesia:
  Lateral scapular slide test
  Scapular dyskinesia test
  Scapular load test
  Scapular retraction test
  Wall/floor push-up

PRÉCIS OF THE SHOULDER ASSESSMENT[a]—CONT'D

For acromioclavicular joint pathology:
    Acromioclavicular shear test
    Horizontal adduction test (cross body adduction)
    Paxinos sign
For ligament and capsule pathology:
    Low flexion test
For muscle pathology:[b]
    Biceps tightness
    Upper-cut test (biceps)
    Yergason's test (biceps)
    Deltoid extension lag (swallow-tail) sign (deltoid)
    Dynamic relocation test (DRT) (rotator cuff stability)
    Dynamic rotary stability test (DRST) (rotator cuff stability)
    Lateral Jobe test (rotator cuff stability)
    Drop arm (Codman's test) (rotator cuff—general)
    Rent test (rotator cuff—general)
    Whipple test (rotator cuff—general)
    Champaign toast position (supraspinatus)
    Drop arm test (supraspinatus)
    "Empty can" test (Jobe or supraspinatus test) (supraspinatus)
    Abdominal compression (belly press or Napoleon) test (subscapularis)
    Belly-off sign (subscapularis)
    Belly press test (abdominal compression or Napoleon test) (subscapularis)
    External rotation lag sign (subscapularis)
    Lift-off sign (Gerber's test) (subscapularis)
    Medial rotation lag or "spring back" test (subscapularis)
    Dropping sign (infraspinatus)
    Infraspinatus scapula retraction test (ISRT) (infraspinatus)
    Infraspinatus test (infraspinatus)
    Lateral rotation lag sign (infraspinatus)
    Hornblower's sign (teres minor)
    Lateral rotation lag sign (teres minor)
    Trapezius test (three positions)
    Latissimus dorsi weakness
    Punch-out test (serratus anterior)
For neurological function:
    Scratch collapse test (axillary nerve, long thoracic nerve)
For thoracic outlet syndrome:
    Roos test
Other:
    Olecranon-manubrium percussion sign
Reflexes and cutaneous distribution (sitting)
Reflexes
Sensory scan
Peripheral nerves
    Axillary nerve
    Suprascapular nerve
    Musculocutaneous nerve
    Long thoracic nerve
    Spinal accessory nerve
Palpation (sitting)
Resisted isometric movements (supine lying)
    Forward flexion of the shoulder
    Extension of the shoulder
    Abduction of the shoulder
    Adduction of the shoulder
    Medial rotation of the shoulder
    Lateral rotation of the shoulder
    Flexion of the elbow
    Extension of the elbow
Special tests (supine lying)
    For anterior shoulder instability:
        Apprehension (crank) release ("surprise") test and Jobe relocation test and modifications
    For posterior shoulder instability:
        Norwood test
    For anterior impingement:
        Supine impingement test
    For labral lesions:[b]
        Clunk test
        Compression rotation test
        Passive distraction test
        Resisted supination external rotation test (RSERT)
        Supine flexion resistance test
    For ligament pathology:
        Crank test
    For muscle pathology:[b]
        Pectoralis major contracture test
        Pectoralis minor test
        Rhomboid weakness (prone lying)
        Scapula backward tipping test (pectoralis minor) (prone lying)
        Trapezius test (three positions) (prone lying)
        Triangle sign (trapezius) (prone lying)
    For neurological function:
        Upper limb neurodynamic (tension) test (ULNT)
            Median nerve (ULNT I)
            Median nerve (ULNT II)
            Radial nerve (ULNT III)
            Ulnar nerve (ULNT IV)
Joint play movements (supine lying)
Backward glide of the humerus
Forward glide of the humerus
Lateral distraction of the humerus
Long arm traction
Backward glide of the humerus in abduction
Anteroposterior and cephalocaudal movements of the clavicle at the acromioclavicular joint
Anteroposterior and cephalocaudal movements of the clavicle at the sternoclavicular joint
General movement of the scapula to determine mobility
Diagnostic imaging

[a]The précis is shown in an order that limits the amount of movement that the patient has to do but ensures that all necessary structures are tested. After any examination, the patient should be warned of the possibility that symptoms may be exacerbated as a result of the assessment.
[b]Research has shown that no single test or even group of tests can accurately diagnose a superior labrum anteroposterior or rotator cuff lesion.[98,394–399]

CASE STUDIES

When these case studies are being completed, the examiner should list the appropriate questions to ask the patient and should specify why they are being asked, what to look for and why, as well as what things should be tested and why. Depending on the patient's answers (and the examiner should consider numerous responses), several possible causes of the patient's problem may become evident (examples are given in parentheses). The examiner should therefore prepare a differential diagnosis chart. He or she can then decide how different diagnoses may affect the treatment plan. For example, a 23-year-old man comes to the clinic complaining of shoulder pain. He says that 2 days earlier he was playing touch football. When his friend threw the ball, he reached for it, lost his balance, and fell on the tip of his shoulder but managed to hang on to the ball. How would you differentiate between acromioclavicular sprain and supraspinatus tendinitis? Table 5.23 demonstrates a differential diagnosis chart for the two conditions.

1. A 49-year-old female comes to see you owing to a 1-week history of pain in her dominant shoulder, which began following a long day spent in taking down holiday decorations. She is unable to lift her arm past 30° of elevation. She is having extensive nighttime pain. She does not complain of numbness or tingling. Her strength is acceptable at 4/5 throughout most shoulder movements. Attempting to lift anything overhead causes her worst symptoms. She has seen her primary care physician who performed radiographs, which were negative for any pathological findings. She has a prescription for therapy to treat a "frozen shoulder." Describe your assessment plan and your differential diagnosis.

2. A 17-year-old male right-hand-dominant baseball player comes to see you following a lengthy bout of shoulder pain that progressively worsened over the previous 12 months. He noticed some generalized shoulder pain a year earlier, which has gradually become worse. He initially had pain only while throwing, but now he has pain at rest in between throwing sessions. He reports that over the preceding 3 months he was unable to get his shoulder loose. He feels that he has lost command of his pitches, and his velocity has decreased. He has noticed an occasional clicking in his shoulder, which is not painful. Describe your assessment plan and your differential diagnosis.

3. A 47-year-old male comes to you complaining of pain in his left shoulder. There is no history of overuse. The pain that occurs when he elevates his shoulder is referred to his neck and sometimes down the arm to his wrist. Describe your assessment plan for this patient (cervical spondylosis vs. subacromial bursitis).

4. An 18-year-old female comes to your office. She reports that she recently had a Putti-Platt procedure for a recurring dislocation of the left shoulder. When you see her, her arm is still in a sling, but the surgeon wants you to begin treatment. Describe your assessment of this patient.

5. A 68-year-old female comes to you complaining of pain and restricted ROM in her right shoulder. She tells you that 3 months earlier she slipped on a rug on a tile floor and landed on her elbow. Both her elbow and shoulder hurt at that time. Describe your assessment plan for this patient (olecranon bursitis vs. adhesive capsulitis).

6. A 5-year-old male is brought in by his parents. They state that he was running around the recreation room chasing a friend when he tripped over a stool and landed on his shoulder. He refuses to move his arm and is still crying, as the accident occurred only 2 hours earlier. Describe your assessment plan for this patient (clavicular fracture vs. humeral epiphyseal injury).

7. A 35-year-old female master swimmer comes to you complaining of shoulder pain. She states that she has been swimming approximately 2000 m/day in two training sessions, and she recently increased her swimming from 1500 m/day to get ready for a competition in 3 weeks. Describe your assessment plan for this patient (subacromial bursitis vs. biceps tendinitis).

8. A 20-year-old male tennis player comes to you complaining that when he serves the ball, his arm "goes dead." He has had this problem for 3 weeks but never before. He had increased his training during the past month. Describe your assessment plan for this patient (thoracic outlet syndrome vs. brachial plexus lesion).

9. A 15-year-old female competitive swimmer comes to you complaining of diffuse shoulder pain. She notices the problem most when she does the backstroke. She complains that her shoulder sometimes feels unstable when she is doing this stroke. Describe your assessment plan for this patient (anterior instability vs. supraspinatus tendinitis).

10. A 48-year-old male comes to you complaining of neck and shoulder pain. He states that he has difficulty abducting his right arm. There is no history of trauma, but he remembers being in a car accident 10 years earlier. Describe your assessment plan for this patient (cervical spondylosis vs. adhesive capsulitis).

TABLE **5.23**

Differential Diagnosis of Acromioclavicular Joint Sprain and Supraspinatus Paratenonitis

	Acromioclavicular Joint Sprain	Supraspinatus Paratenonitis
Observation	Step deformity (third degree)	Normal
Active movement	Pain, especially at extreme of motion (horizontal adduction and full elevation especially painful)	Pain on active movement, especially of abduction
Passive movement	Pain on horizontal adduction and elevation Muscle spasm end feel at end of ROM possible	No pain except if impingement occurs
Resisted isometric movement	May have some pain if test causes stress on joint (e.g., abduction)	Pain on abduction May have some pain on stabilizing for other movements
Functional tests	Pain on extremes of movement	Pain on any abduction movement
Special tests	Acromioclavicular shear test painful	"Empty can" test positive Impingement tests positive
Reflexes and cutaneous distribution	Negative	Negative
Joint play	Acromioclavicular joint play movements painful	Negative
Palpation	Acromioclavicular joint painful	Supraspinous tendon and insertion tender or painful

ROM, Range of motion.

References

1. McFarland EG, Borade A. Examination of the biceps tendon. *Clin Sport Med*. 2016;35(1):29–45.
2. Hess SA. Functional stability of the glenohumeral joint. *Manual Therapy*. 2000;5:63–71.
3. Tillman B, Petersen W. Clinical anatomy. In: Wulker N, Mansat M, Fu F, eds. *Shoulder Surgery: An Illustrated Textbook*. London: Martin Dunitz; 2001.
4. Smith C, Funk L. The glenoid labrum. *Shoulder and Elbow*. 2010;2:87–93.
5. Greenberg EM, Fernandez-Fernandez A, Lawrence JT, McClure PW. The development of humeral retrotorsion and its relationship to throwing sports. *Sports Health*. 2015;7(6):489–496.
6. Kurokawa D, Yamamoto N, Ishikawa H, et al. Differences in humeral retroversion in dominant and nondominant sides of young baseball players. *J Shoulder Elbow Surg*. 2017;26(6):1083–1087.
7. Whiteley RJ, Adams RD, Nicholson LL, Ginn KA. Reduced humeral torsion predicts throwing-related injury in adolescent baseballers. *J Sci Med Sport*. 2010;13(4):392–396.
8. Oyama S, Hibberd EE, Myers JB. Preseason screening of shoulder range of motion and humeral retrotorsion does not predict injury in high school baseball players. *J Shoulder Elbow Surg*. 2017;26(7):1182–1189.
9. Oyama S, Hibberd EE, Myers JB. Changes in humeral torsion and shoulder rotation range of motion in high school baseball players over a 1-year period. *Clin Biomech*. 2013;28(3):268–272.
10. Dashottar A, Borstad JD. Validity of measuring humeral torsion using palpation of bicipital tuberosities. *Physiother Theory Pract*. 2013;29(1):67–74.
11. Ito N, Eto M, Maeda K, et al. Ultrasonographic measurements of humeral torsion. *J Shoulder Elbow Surg*. 1995;4(3):157–161.
12. Roach NT, Lieberman DE, Gill TJ, et al. The effect of humeral torsion on rotational range of motion in the shoulder and throwing performance. *J Anat*. 2010;220(3):293–301.
13. Edelson G. Variations in the retroversion of the humeral head. *J Shoulder Elbow Surg*. 1999;8(2):142–145.

14. Itami Y, Mihata T, Shibano K, et al. Site and severity of the increased humeral retroversion in symptomatic baseball players: a three-dimensional computed tomographic analysis. *Am J Sports Med*. 2016;44(7):1825–1831.
15. Reuther KE, Sheridan S, Thomas SJ. Differentiation of bony and soft-tissue adaptations of the shoulder in professional baseball pitchers. *J Shoulder Elbow Surg*. 2018;27(8):1491–1496.
16. Chant CB, Litchfield R, Griffin S, Thain LM. Humeral head retroversion in competitive baseball players and its relationship to glenohumeral rotation range of motion. *J Orthop Sports Phys Ther*. 2007;37(9):514–520.
17. Polster JM, Bullen J, Obuchowski NA, et al. Relationship between humeral torsion and injury in professional baseball pitchers. *Am J Sports Med*. 2013;41(9):2015–2021.
18. Miyashita K, Urabe Y, Kobayashi H, et al. The role of shoulder maximum external rotation during throwing for elbow injury prevention in baseball players. *J Sports Sci Med*. 2008;7(2):223–228.
19. Yamamoto N, Itoi E, Minagawa H, et al. Why is the humeral retroversion of throwing athletes greater in dominant shoulders than in nondominant shoulders? *J Shoulder Elbow Surg*. 2006;15(5):571–575.
20. Noonan TJ, Shanley E, Bailey LB, et al. Professional pitchers with glenohumeral internal rotation deficit (GIRD) display greater humeral retrotorsion than pitchers without GIRD. *Am J Sports Med*. 2015;43(6):1448–1454.
21. Noonan TJ, Thigpen CA, Bailey LB, et al. Humeral torsion as a risk factor for shoulder and elbow injury in professional baseball players. *Am J Sports Med*. 2016;44(9):2214–2219.
22. Lee BJ, Garrison JC, Conway JE, et al. The relationship between humeral retrotorsion and shoulder range of motion in baseball players with an ulnar collateral ligament tear. *Am J Sports Med*. 2016;4(10):1–6.
23. Hall K, Borstad JD. Posterior shoulder tightness: to treat or not to treat? 2018;48(3):133–136.

24. Tokish JM, Curtin MS, Kim YK, et al. Glenohumeral internal rotation deficit in the asymptomatic professional pitcher and its relation to humeral retroversion. *J Sports Sci Med*. 2008;7(1):78–83.
25. Owens BD, Campbell SE, Cameron KL. Risk factors for posterior shoulder instability in young athletes. *Am J Sports Med*. 2013;41(11):2645–2649.
26. Holt K, Boettcher C, Halaki M, Ginn KA. Humeral torsion and shoulder rotation range of motion parameters in elite swimmers. *J Sci Med Sport*. 2017;20(5):469–474.
27. Elser F, Braun S, Dewing CB, et al. Anatomy, function, injuries and treatment of the long head of biceps brachii tendon. *Arthroscopy*. 2011;27(4):581–592.
28. Martetschlager F, Tauber M, Habermeyer P. Injuries to the biceps pulley. *Clin Sports Med*. 2016;35(1):19–27.
29. Taylor SA, O'Brien SJ. Clinically relevant anatomy and biomechanics of the proximal biceps. *Clin Sports Med*. 2016;35:1–18.
30. Khazzam M, George MS, Churchill RS, Kuhn JE. Disorders of the long head of biceps tendon. *J Shoulder Elbow Surg*. 2012;21(1):136–145.
31. Beall DP, Williamson EE, Ly JQ, et al. Association of biceps tendon tears with rotator cuff abnormalities: degree of correlation with tears of the anterior and superior portions of the rotator cuff. *Am J Roentgenol*. 2003;180(3):633–639.
32. Warner JJ. The gross anatomy of the joint surfaces, ligaments, labrum and capsule. In: Matsen FA, Fu FH, Hawkins RJ, eds. *The Shoulder: A Balance of Mobility and Stability*. Rosemont, IL: American Academy of Orthopedic Surgeons; 1993.
33. LU Bigliani, Kelkar R, Flatow EL, et al. Glenohumeral stability: biomechanical properties of passive and active stabilizers. *Clin Orthop Relat Res*. 1996;330:13–30.
34. Curl LA, Warren RF. Glenohumeral joint stability: selective cutting studies on the static capsular restraints. *Clin Orthop Relat Res*. 1996;330:54–65.
35. Mihata T, McGarry MH, Abe M, et al. Excessive humeral external rotation results in increased shoulder laxity. *Am J Sports Med*. 2004;32:1278–1285.

36. Lucas DB. Biomechanics of the shoulder joint. *Arch Surg*. 1973;107:425–432.
37. Peat M. Functional anatomy of the shoulder complex. *Phys Ther*. 1986;66:1855–1865.
38. Hunt SA, Kwon YW, Zuckerman JD. The rotator interval—anatomy, pathology and strategies for treatment. *J Am Acad Orthop Surg*. 2007;15:218–227.
39. Gaskill TR, Braun S, Millett PJ. The rotator interval: pathology and management. *Arthroscopy*. 2011;27(4):556–567.
40. Morag Y, Bedi A, Jamadar DA. The rotator interval and long head of biceps tendon: anatomy, function, pathology, and magnetic resonance imaging. *Magn Reson Imaging Clin N Am*. 2012;20(2):229–259.
41. Peat M, Culham E. Functional anatomy of the shoulder complex. In: Andrews JR, Wilk KE, eds. *The Athlete's Shoulder*. New York: Churchill-Livingstone; 1994.
42. Soslowsky LJ, An CH, DeBano CM, et al. Coracoacromial ligament: in situ load and viscoelastic properties in rotator cuff disease. *Clin Orthop Relat Res*. 1996;330:40–44.
43. Bigliani LH, Morrison DS, April EW. The morphology of the acromion and its relation to rotator cuff tears. *Orthop Trans*. 1986;10:228
44. Edelson JG. The "hooked" acromion revisited. *J Bone Joint Surg Br*. 1995;77:284–287.
45. Fukuda K, Craig EV, An KN, et al. Biomechanical study of the ligamentous system of the acromioclavicular joint. *J Bone Joint Surg*. 1986;68:434–440.
46. Izadpanah K, Weitzel E, Honal M, et al. In vivo analysis of coracoclavicular ligament kinematics during shoulder abduction. *Am J Sports Med*. 2012;40:185–192.
47. Higginbotham TO, Kuhn JE. Atraumatic disorders of the sternoclavicular joint. *J Am Acad Ortho Surg*. 2005;13:138–145.
48. Kibler WB. The role of the scapula in athletic shoulder function. *Am J Sports Med*. 1998;26:325–337.
49. Kibler WB, Wilkes T, Sciascia A. Mechanics and pathomechanics in the overhead athlete. *Clin Sports Med*. 2013;32(4):637–651.
50. Chu SK, Jayabalan P, Kibler WB, Press J. The kinetic chain revisited: new concepts on throwing mechanics in injury. *Phys Med Rehabil*. 2016;8(suppl 3):S69–S77.
51. Lewis JS, Green A, Wright C. Subacromial impingement syndrome: the role of posture and muscle imbalance. *J Shoulder Elbow Surg*. 2005;14(4):385–392.
52. Kibler WB, Sciascia A. The shoulder at risk: scapular dyskinesis and altered glenohumeral rotation. *Oper Tech Sports Med*. 2016;24(3):162–169.
53. Solomito MJ, Garibay EJ, Woods JR, et al. Lateral trunk lean in pitchers affects both ball velocity and upper extremity joint moments. *Am J Sports Med*. 2015;43(5):1235–1240.
54. Maughon TS, Andrews JR. The subjective evaluation of the shoulder in the athlete. In: Andrews JR, Wilk KE, eds. *The Athlete's Shoulder*. New York: Churchill-Livingstone; 1994.
55. Tarkin IS, Morganti CM, Zillmer DA, et al. Rotator cuff tears in adolescent athletes. *Am J Sports Med*. 2005;33:596–601.
56. Litaker D, Pioro M, El Bilbeisi H, et al. Returning to the bedside: using the history and physical examination to identify rotator cuff tears. *J Am Geriatr Soc*. 2000;48(12):1633–1637.
57. Murrell GA, Watson JR. Diagnosis of rotator cuff tears. *Lancet*. 2001;357:769–770.
58. Park HB, Yokota A, Gill HS, et al. Diagnostic accuracy of clinical tests for the different degrees of subacromial impingement syndrome. *J Bone Joint Surg Am*. 2005;87:1446–1455.
59. Kauffman J, Jobe FW. Anterior capsulolabral reconstruction for recurrent anterior instability. *Sports Med Arthro Rev*. 2000;8:272–279.

60. Wolf WB. Calcific tendinitis of the shoulder: diagnosis and simple effective treatment. *Phys Sportsmed*. 1999;27:27–33.
61. Heyworth BE, Kramer DE, Martin DJ, et al. Trends in the presentation, management, and outcomes of little league shoulder. *Am J Sports Med*. 2016;44(6):1431–1438.
62. Hutchinson MR, Ahuja CO. Diagnosing and treating clavicle injuries. *Phys Sportsmed*. 1996;24:26–36.
63. Simovitch R, Sanders B, Ozbzydar M, et al. Acromioclavicular joint injuries: diagnosis and management. *J Am Acad Orthop Surg*. 2009;17:207–219.
64. Tepolt F, Carry PM, Heyn PC, Miller NH: Posterior sternoclavicular joint injuries in the adolescent population: a meta-analysis. *Am J Sports Med*. 42(10):2517–2524.
65. Burkhart SS, Morgan CD, Kibler WB. The disabled throwing shoulder: spectrum of pathology, part one: pathoanatomy and biomechanics. *Arthroscopy*. 2003;19:404–420.
66. Su KA, Johnson MP, Gracely EJ, et al. Scapular rotation in swimmers with and without impingement syndrome: practice effects. *Med Sci Sports Exerc*. 2004;31:1117–1123.
67. Castelein B, Cagnie B, Parlevliet T, Cools A. Scapulothoracic muscle activity during elevation exercises measured with surface and fine wire EMG: a comparative study between patients with subacromial impingement syndrome and healthy controls. *Man Ther*. 2016;23:33–39.
68. Kuhn JE. A new classification system for shoulder instability. *Br J Sports Med*. 2010;44:341–346.
69. Oyama S. Baseball pitching kinematics, joint loads, and injury prevention. *J Sports Health Sci*. 2012;1(2):80–91.
70. Rubin BD. Evaluation of the overhead athlete: examination and ancillary testing. *Arthroscopy*. 2003;19(10)(suppl 1):42–40.
71. Krupp RJ, Kevern MA, Gaines MD, et al. Long head of biceps tendon pain: differential diagnosis and treatment. *J Orthop Sports Phys Ther*. 2009;39:55–70.
72. Kibler WB, Sciascia A. Current concepts: scapular dyskinesis. *Br J Sports Med*. 2010;44:300–305.
73. Borsa PA, Laudner KG, Sauers EL. Mobility and stability adaptations in the shoulder of the overhead athlete—a theoretical and evidence-based perspective. *Sports Med*. 2008;38:17–36.
74. Burkhart SS, Morgan CD, Kibler WB. The disabled throwing shoulder: spectrum of pathology, part three: the SICK scapula, scapular dyskinesia, the kinetic chain, and rehabilitation. *Arthroscopy*. 2003;19:641–661.
75. Kvitne RS, Jobe FW. The diagnosis and treatment of anterior instability in the throwing athlete. *Clin Orthop*. 1993;291:107–123.
76. Van Tongel A, Karelse A, Berghs B, et al. Diagnostic value of active protraction and retraction for sternoclavicular joint pain. *BMC Musculoskelet Disord*. 2014;15:421–427.
77. Watson LA, Pizzari T, Balster S. Thoracic outlet syndrome. Part 1: clinical manifestations, differentiation and treatment pathways. *Manual Therapy*. 2009;14:586–595.
78. Boyle JJ. Is the pain and dysfunction of shoulder impingement lesion really second rib syndrome in disguise? Two case reports. *Manual Therapy*. 1999;4:44–48.
79. Khan KM, Cook JL, Taunton JE, et al. Overuse tendinosis, not tendinitis. Part 1: a new paradigm for a difficult clinical problem. *Phys Sportsmed*. 2000;28:38–48.
80. Khan KM, Cook JL, Bonar F, et al. Histopathology of common tendinopathies: update and implications for clinical management. *Sports Med*. 1999;27:393–408.

81. Seroyer ST, Nho SJ, Bach BR, et al. Shoulder pain in the overhead throwing athlete. *Sports Health*. 2009;1:108–120.
82. McFarland EG, Tanaka MJ, Papp DF. Examination of the shoulder in the overhead and throwing athlete. *Clin Sports Med*. 2008;27:553–578.
83. Cyriax J. Textbook of orthopaedic medicine. In: *Diagnosis of Soft Tissue Lesions*. vol 1. London: Bailliere Tindall; 1982.
84. Griggs SM, Ahn A, Green A. Idiopathic adhesive capsulitis: a prospective functional outcome study of non-operative treatment. *J Bone Joint Surg Am*. 2000;82:1398–1407.
85. Butcher JD, Siekanowicz A, Pettrone F. Pectoralis major rupture: ensuring accurate diagnosis and effective rehabilitation. *Phys Sportsmed*. 1996;24:37–44.
86. Nichols HM. Anatomic structures of the thoracic outlet syndrome. *Clin Orthop*. 1967;51:17–25.
87. Riddell DH. Thoracic outlet syndrome: thoracic and vascular aspects. *Clin Orthop*. 1967;51:53–64.
88. Baker CL, Liu SH. Neurovascular injuries to the shoulder. *J Orthop Sports Phys Ther*. 1993;18:360–364.
89. Conte AL, Marques AP, Cararotto RA, Amado-Joâo SM. Handedness influences passive shoulder range of motion in non athlete adult women. *J Manip Physiol Ther*. 2009;32:149–153.
90. Dutton M. *Orthopedic Examination, Evaluation and Intervention*. New York: McGraw-Hill; 2004.
91. Rudert M, Wulker M. Clinical evaluation. In: Wulker N, Mansat M, Fu F, eds. *Shoulder Surgery: An Illustrated Textbook*. London: Martin Dunitz; 2001.
92. Priest JD, Nagel DA. Tennis shoulder. *Am J Sports Med*. 1976;4:28–42.
93. Petilon J, Carr DR, Sekiya JK, et al. Pectoralis major muscle injuries: evaluation and management. *J Am Acad Ortho Surg*. 2005;13:59–68.
94. Mazzocca AD, Cote MP, Arciero CL, et al. Clinical outcomes after subpectoral biceps tendonosis with an interference screw. *Am J Sports Med*. 2008;36:1922–1929.
95. Provencher MT, Handfield K, Boniquit NT, et al. Injuries to the pectoralis major muscle—diagnosis and management. *Am J Sports Med*. 2010;38:1693–1705.
96. Herbst KA, Miller LS. Symptomatic axillopectoral muscle in a swimmer: a case report. *Am J Sports Med*. 2013;41(6):1400–1403.
97. Hitchcock HH, Bechtol CO. Painful shoulder: observation on the role of the tendon of the long head of the biceps brachii in its causation. *J Bone Joint Surg Am*. 1948;30:263–273.
98. McFarland EG, Garzon-Muvdi J, Jia X, et al. Clinical and diagnostic tests for shoulder disorders: a critical review. *Br J Sports Med*. 2010;44:328–332.
99. Kibler WB, Sciascia A, Wilkes T. Scapular dyskinesia and its relation to shoulder injury. *J Am Acad Orthop Surg*. 2012;20:364–372.
100. Silliman JF, Dean MT. Neurovascular injuries to the shoulder complex. *J Orthop Sports Phys Ther*. 1993;18:442–448.
101. Struyf F, Nijs J, Mottram S, et al. Clinical assessment of the scapula: a review of the literature. *Br J Sports Med*. 2014;48(11):883–890.
102. Sobush DC, Simoneau GG, Dietz KE, et al. The Lennie test for measuring scapular position in healthy young adult females: a reliability and validity study. *J Orthop Sports Phys Ther*. 1996;23:39–50.
103. Matsen FA, Lippitt SB, Sidles JA, et al. *Practical Evaluation and Management of the Shoulder*. Philadelphia: WB Saunders; 1994.
104. Meister K. Injuries to the shoulder in the throwing athlete. Part II: evaluation/treatment. *Am J Sports Med*. 2000;28:587–601.
105. Milch H. Snapping scapula. *Clin Orthop Relat Res*. 1961;20:139–150.

106. Manske RC, Reiman MP, Stovak ML. Nonoperative and operative management of snapping scapula. *Am J Sports Med.* 2004;32:1554–1565.

107. Kibler WB. Scapular dyskinesis and its relation to shoulder pain. *J Am Acad Ortho Surg.* 2003;11:142–151.

108. Lazar MA, Kwon YW, Rokuti AS. Snapping scapula syndrome. *J Bone Joint Surg Am.* 2009;91:2251–2262.

109. Von Raebrox A, Campbell B, Ramesh R, Bunker T. The association of subacromial dimples with recurrent posterior dislocation of the shoulder. *J Shoulder Elbow Surg.* 2006;15(5):591–593.

110. Dori Z, Sarig Bahat H. Unusual scapular winging – a case report. *Man Ther.* 2016;24:75–80.

111. Provencher MT, Kirby H, McDonald LS, et al. Surgical release of the pectoralis minor tendon for scapular dyskinesia and shoulder pain. *Am J Sports Med.* 2016;45(1):173–178.

112. Kibler WB, Ludewig PM, McClure PW, et al. Clinical implications of scapular dyskinesis in shoulder injury: the 2013 consensus statements from the 'Scapular Summit'. *Br J Sports Med.* 2013;47:877–885.

113. Reijneveld EA, Noten S, Michener LA, et al. Clinical outcomes of a scapular-focused treatment in patients with subacromial pain syndrome: a systematic review. *Br J Sports Med.* 2017;51(5):436–441.

114. Huang TS, Huang CY, Ou HL, Lin JJ. Scapular dyskinesis: patterns, functional disability and associated factors in people with shoulder disorders. *Man Ther.* 2016;26:165–171.

115. Kibler WB, Uhl TL, Maddux JW, et al. Qualitative clinical evaluation of scapular dysfunction: a reliability study. *J Shoulder Elbow Surg.* 2002;11:550–556.

116. Huang TS, Huang HY, Wang TG, et al. Comprehensive classification test of scapular dyskinesis: a reliability study. *Man Ther.* 2015;20(3):427–432.

117. Huang TS, Ou HL, Huang CY, Lin JJ. Specific kinematics and associated muscle activation in individuals with scapular dyskinesia. *J Shoulder Elbow Surg.* 2015;24(8):1227–1234.

118. McClure P, Tate AR, Kareha S, et al. A clinical method for identifying scapular dyskinesis, part 1: reliability. *J Athl Train.* 2009;44(2):160–164.

119. Tate AR, McClure P, Kareha S, et al. A clinical method for identifying scapular dyskinesis, part 2: validity. *J Athl Train.* 2009;44(2):165–173.

120. Uhl TL, Kibler WB, Gecewich B, et al. Evaluation of clinical assessment methods for scapular dyskinesia. *Arthroscopy.* 2009;25:1240–1248.

121. Meininger AK, Figuerres BF, Goldberg BA. Scapular winging: an update. *J Am Acad Orthop Surg.* 2011;19:453–462.

122. Butters KP. Nerve lesions of the shoulder. In: De Lee JC, Drez D, eds. *Orthopedic Sports Medicine: Principles and Practice.* Philadelphia: WB Saunders; 1994.

123. Schultz JS, Leonard JA. Long thoracic neuropathy from athletic activity. *Arch Phys Med Rehabil.* 1992;73:87–90.

124. Bowen M, Warren R. Ligamentous control of shoulder stability based on selective cutting and static translation. *Clin Sports Med.* 1991;10:757–782.

125. Duralde X. Surgical management of neurologic and vascular lesions in the athlete's shoulder. *Sports Med Arthro Rev.* 2000;8:289–304.

126. Foo CL, Swann M. Isolated paralysis of the serratus anterior: a report of 20 cases. *J Bone Joint Surg Br.* 1983;65:552–556.

127. Makin GJ, Brown WF, Webers GC. C7 radiculopathy: importance of scapular winging in clinical diagnosis. *J Neurol Neurosurg Psych.* 1986;49:640–644.

128. Saeed MA, Gatens PF, Singh S. Winging of the scapula. *Am Fam Physician.* 1981;24:139–143.

129. Fiddian NJ, King RJ. The winged scapula. *Clin Orthop.* 1984;185:228–236.

130. Carson WC, Lovell WW, Whitesides TE. Congenital elevation of the scapula. *J Bone Joint Surg Am.* 1981;63:1199–1207.

131. Cavendish ME. Congenital elevation of the scapula. *J Bone Joint Surg Br.* 1972;54:395–408.

132. McMurtry I, Bennet GC, Bradish C. Osteotomy for congenital elevation of the scapula (Sprengel's deformity). *J Bone Joint Surg Br.* 2005;87:986–989.

133. Harvey EJ, Bernstein M, Desy NM, et al. Sprengel deformity: pathogenesis and management. *J Am Acad Orthop Surg.* 2012;20(3):177–186.

134. Miyashita K, Kobayashi H, Koshida S, et al. Glenohumeral, scapular and thoracic angles at maximum shoulder external rotation in throwing. *Am J Sports Med.* 2010;38:363–368.

135. McClure PW, Michener LA, Sennett BJ, Karduna AR. Direct 3-dimensional measurement of scapular kinematics during dynamic movements in vivo. *J Shoulder Elbow Surg.* 2001;10(3):269–277.

136. Hickey D, Solvig V, Cavalheri V, et al. Scapular dyskinesis increases the risk of future shoulder pain by 43% in asymptomatic athletes: a systematic review and meta-analysis. *Br J Sports Med.* 2017;51:1–10.

137. Kebaetse M, McClure P, Pratt NA. Thoracic position effect on shoulder range of motion, strength, and three-dimensional scapular kinematics. *Arch Phys Med Rehabil.* 1999;80:945–950.

138. Cole AK, McGrath ML, Harrington SE, et al. Scapular bracing and alteration of posture and muscle activity in overhead athletes with poor posture. *J Athl Train.* 2013;48(1):12–24.

139. Thigpen CA, Padua DA, Michener LA, et al. Head and shoulder posture affect scapular mechanics and muscle activity in overhead tasks. *J Electromyogr Kinesiol.* 2010;20(4):701–709.

140. Payne LZ, Deng XH, Craig EV, et al. The combined dynamic and static contributions to subacromial impingement: a biomechanical analysis. *Am J Sports Med.* 1997;25:801–808.

141. Watson CJ, Schenkman M. Physical therapy management of isolated serratus anterior muscle paralysis. *Phys Ther.* 1995;75:194–202.

142. Jia X, Ji JH, Petersen SA, et al. Clinical evaluation of the shoulder shrug sign. *Clin Orthop Relat Res.* 2008;466(11):2813–2819.

143. Ropars M, Fournier A, Campillo B, et al. Clinical assessment of external rotation for diagnosis of anterior shoulder hyperlaxity. *Orthop Traumatol Surg Res.* 2010;96(suppl 8):S84–S87.

144. Kessel L, Watson M. The painful arc syndrome. *J Bone Joint Surg Br.* 1977;59:166–172.

145. Inman VT, Saunders M, Abbott LC. Observations on the function of the shoulder joint. *J Bone Joint Surg Br.* 1944;26:1–30.

146. Reid DC. The shoulder girdle: its function as a unit in abduction. *Physiotherapy.* 1969;55:57–59.

147. Saha SK. Mechanism of shoulder movements and a plea for the recognition of "zero position" of glenohumeral joint. *Clin Orthop.* 1983;173:3–10.

148. Sugamoto K, Harada T, Machida A, et al. Scapulohumeral rhythm: relationship between motion velocity and rhythm. *Clin Orthop Relat Res.* 2002;401:119–124.

149. Boody SG, Freedman L, Waterland JC. Shoulder movements during abduction in the scapular plane. *Arch Phys Med Rehabil.* 1970;51:595–604.

150. Davies GJ, Dickoff-Hoffman S. Neuromuscular testing and rehabilitation of the shoulder complex. *J Orthop Sports Phys Ther.* 1993;18:449–458.

151. Poppen NK, Walker PS. Normal and abnormal motion of the shoulder. *J Bone Joint Surg Am.* 1976;58:195–201.

152. Freedman L, Munro RR. Abduction of the arm in the scapular plane: scapular and glenohumeral movements. *J Bone Joint Surg Am.* 1966;48:1503–1510.

153. Kibler WB, Ludewig PA, McClure P, et al. Scapular Summit 2009: introduction and the consensus statements. *J Orthop Sports Phys Ther.* 2009;39(11):A1–A13.

154. Flatow EL. The biomechanics of the acromioclavicular, sternoclavicular and scapulothoracic joints. *Instr Course Lect.* 1993;42:237–245.

155. Stanley E, Rauh MJ, Michener LA, et al. Shoulder range of motion measures as risk factors for shoulder and elbow injuries in high school softball and baseball players. *Am J Sports Med.* 2011;39:1997–2006.

156. Ludewig PM, Reynolds JF. The association of scapular kinematics and glenohumeral joint pathologies. *J Orthop Sports Phys Ther.* 2009;39:90–104.

157. van Eisenhart-Rothe R, Matsen FA, Eckstein F, et al. Pathomechanics in atraumatic shoulder instability. *Clin Orthop Relat Res.* 2005;433:82–89.

158. Kon Y, Nishinaka N, Gamada K, et al. The influence of handheld weight on the scapulohumeral rhythm. *J Shoulder Elbow Surg.* 2008;17(6):943–946.

159. Kibler WB. Evaluation and diagnosis of scapulothoracic problems in the athlete. *Sports Med Arthro Rev.* 2000;8:192–202.

160. Michiels I, Grevenstein J. Kinematics of shoulder abduction in the scapular plane: on the influence of abduction velocity and external load. *Clin Biomech.* 1995;10:137–143.

161. Baertschi E, Swanenburg J, Brunner F, Kool J. Interrater reliability of clinical tests to evaluate scapulothoracic motion. *BMC Musculoskelet Disord.* 2013;14:315–323.

162. Reed D, Cathers I, Halaki M, Ginn KA. Does changing the plane of abduction influence shoulder muscle recruitment patterns in healthy individuals? *Man Ther.* 2016;21:63–68.

163. Perry J. Biomechanics of the shoulder. In: Rowe CR, ed. *The Shoulder.* Edinburgh: Churchill Livingstone; 1988.

164. Kapandji IA. The physiology of joints. In: *Upper Limb.* vol 1. New York: Churchill Livingstone; 1970.

165. Wilk KE, Reinold MM, Macrina LC, et al. Glenohumeral internal rotation measurements differ depending on stabilization techniques. *Sports Health.* 2009;1:131–136.

166. Boublik M, Silliman JF. History and physical examination. In: Hawkins RJ, Misamore GW, eds. *Shoulder Injuries in the Athlete.* New York: Churchill Livingstone; 1996.

167. Van den Dolder PA, Ferreira PH, Refshauge K. Intra- and inter-reliability of a modified measure of hand behind back range of motion. *Man Ther.* 2014;19:72–76.

168. Awan R, Smith J, Boon AJ. Measuring shoulder internal rotation range of motion: a comparison of 3 techniques. *Arch Phys Med Rehabil.* 2002;83(9):1229–1234.

169. Whitley R, Oceguera M. GIRD, TRROM, and humeral torsion-based classification of shoulder risk in throwing athletes are not in agreement and should not be used interchangeably. *J Sci Med Sport.* 2016;19(10):816–819.

170. Gates JJ, Gupta A, McGarry MH, et al. The effect of glenohumeral internal rotation deficit due to posterior capsular contracture on passive glenohumeral joint motion. *Am J Sports Med.* 2012;40:2794–2800.

171. Takenaga T, Sugimoto K, Goto H, et al. Posterior shoulder capsules are thicker and stiffer in the throwing shoulders of healthy college baseball players: a quantitative assessment using shear-wave ultrasound elastography. *Am J Sports Med.* 2015;43(12):2935–2942.

172. Lo IK, Nonweiler B, Woolfrey M, et al. An evaluation of the apprehension, relocation, and surprise tests for anterior shoulder instability. *Am J Sports Med.* 2004;32(2):301–307.

173. Naredo E, Aguado P, De Miguel E, et al. Painful shoulder: comparison physical examination and ultrasonographic findings. *Ann Rheum Dis.* 2002;61:132–136.

174. Wilk KE, Macrina LC, Fleisig GS, et al. Correlation of glenohumeral internal rotation deficit and total rotational motion to shoulder injuries in professional baseball players. *Am J Sports Med.* 2011;39:329–335.

175. Wilk KE, Macrina LC, Fleiseg GS, et al. Deficits in glenohumeral passive range of motion increase risk of shoulder injury in professional baseball players: a prospective study. *Am J Sports Med.* 2014;42(9):2075–2081.

176. Hibberd EE, Oyama S, Myers JB. Increase in humeral retrotorsion accounts for age-related increase in glenohumeral internal rotation deficit in youth and adolescent baseball players. *Am J Sports Med.* 2014;42(4):851–858.

177. McClincy JW, Arner JW, Bradley JP. Posterior shoulder instability in throwing athletes: a case-matched comparison of throwers and non-throwers. *Arthroscopy.* 2015;31(6):1041–1051.

178. Jaggi A, Lambert S. Rehabilitation of shoulder instability. *Br J Sports Med.* 2010;44:333–340.

179. Magarey ME, Jones MA. Dynamic evaluation and early management of altered motor control around the shoulder complex. *Manual Therapy.* 2003;8:195–206.

180. Howell SM, Galiant BJ, Renzi AJ, et al. Normal and abnormal mechanics of the glenohumeral joint in the horizontal plane. *J Bone Joint Surg Am.* 1988;70:227–232.

181. Nishijima N, Yamamuro T, Fujio K, et al. The swallowtail sign: a test for deltoid function. *J Bone Joint Surg Br.* 1994;77:152–153.

182. Warth RJ, Spiegl UJ, Millet PJ. Scapulothoracic bursitis and snapping scapula syndrome: a critical review of current evidence. *Am J Sports Med.* 2014;43(1):236–245.

183. Kuhn JC, Plancher KD, Hawkins RJ. Scapular winging. *J Am Acad Orthop Surg.* 1995;3:319–325.

184. Kibler WB, Kuhn JE, Wilk K, et al. The disabled throwing shoulder: spectrum of pathology – 10 year update. *Arthroscopy.* 2013;29(1):141–161.

185. McClure P, Balaicuis J, Heiland D, et al. A randomized controlled comparison of stretching procedures for posterior shoulder tightness. *J Orthop Sports Phys Ther.* 2007;37(3):108–114.

186. Wilk KE, Macrina LC, Arrigo C. Passive range of motion characteristics in the overhead baseball pitcher and their implications for rehabilitation. *Clin Orthop Relat Res.* 2012;470(6):1586–1594.

187. Balg F, Boileau P. The instability severity index score. A simple pre-operative score to select patients for arthroscopic or open shoulder stabilization. *J Bone Joint Surg Br.* 2007;89(11):1470–1477.

188. Petersen CM, Hayes KW. Construct validity of Cyriax's selective tension examination: association of end feels with pain in the knee and shoulder. *J Orthop Sports Phys Ther.* 2000;30:512–521.

189. Muraki T, Yamamoto N, Zhao KD, et al. Effect of posteroinferior capsular tightness on contact pressure and area beneath the coracoacromial arch during pitching motion. *Am J Sports Med.* 2010;38:600–607.

190. Lewis J. Frozen shoulder contracture syndrome – aetiology, diagnosis and management. *Man Ther.* 2015;20(1):2–9.

191. Land H, Gordon S, Watt K. Clinical assessment of subacromial shoulder impingement – which factors differ from the asymptomatic population? *Musculoskelet Sci Pract.* 2017;27:49–56.

192. Laudner KG, Meline MT, Meister K. The relationship between forward scapular posture and posterior shoulder tightness among baseball players. *Am J Sports Med.* 2010;38:2106–2112.

193. Tyler TF, Roy T, Nicholas SJ, et al. Reliability and validity of a new method of measuring posterior shoulder tightness. *J Orthop Sports Phys Ther.* 1999;29:262–274.

194. Tyler TF, Nicholas SJ, Roy T, et al. Quantification of posterior capsule tightness and motion loss in patients with shoulder impingement. *Am J Sports Med.* 2000;28:668–673.

195. Lunden JB, Muffenbier M, Giveans MR, et al. Reliability of shoulder internal rotation passive range of motion measurements in the supine vs sidelying position. *J Orthop Sports Phys Ther.* 2010;40:589–594.

196. Pagnani MJ, Galinat BJ, Warren RF. Glenohumeral instability. In: De Lee JC, Drez D, eds. *Orthopedic Sports Medicine: Principles and Practice.* Philadelphia: WB Saunders; 1994.

197. Sawyer EE, McDevitt AW, Louw A, et al. Use of pain neuroscience education, tactile discrimination, and graded motor imagery in an individual with frozen shoulder. *J Orthop Sports Phys Ther.* 2018;48(3):174–184.

198. Gagey OJ, Gagey N. The hyperabduction test: an assessment of the laxity of the inferior glenohumeral ligament. *J Bone Joint Surg Br.* 2000;82:69–74.

199. Cadet ER. Evaluation of glenohumeral instability. *Orthop Clin North Am.* 2010;41:287–295.

200. Rowe CR. Unusual shoulder conditions. In: Rowe CR, ed. *The Shoulder.* Edinburgh: Churchill Livingstone; 1988.

201. MacConaill MA, Basmajian JV. *Muscles and Movements: A Basis for Human Kinesiology.* Baltimore: Williams & Wilkins; 1969.

202. Corrigan B, Maitland GD. *Practical Orthopedic Medicine.* London: Butterworths; 1985.

203. Maitland GD. *Peripheral Manipulation.* London: Butterworths; 1977.

204. Mullen F, Slade S, Briggs C. Bony and capsular determinants of glenohumeral "locking" and "quadrant" positions. *Aust J Physio.* 1989;35:202–206.

205. Polster JM, Lynch TS, Bullen JA, et al. Throwing-related injuries of the subscapularis in professional baseball players. *Skeletal Radiol.* 2016;45(1):41–47.

206. Cheng NM, Pan WR, Vally F, et al. The arterial supply of the long head of biceps tendon: anatomical study with implications for tendon rupture. *Clin Anat.* 2010;23(6):683–692.

207. Richards RR. Outcomes analysis in the shoulder and elbow. In: Norris TR, ed. *Orthopedic Knowledge Update: Shoulder and Elbow.* Rosemont, IL: American Academy of Orthopedic Surgeons; 2002.

208. Mannerkorpi K, Svantesson U, Carlsson J, et al. Tests of functional limitations in fibromyalgia syndrome: a reliability study. *Arthr Care Res.* 1999;12(3):193–199.

209. Dutton M. *Dutton's Orthopedic Examination, Evaluation and Intervention.* 3rd ed. New York: McGraw-Hill; 2012.

210. Namdari S, Yagnik G, Ebaugh DD, et al. Defining functional shoulder range of motion for activities of daily living. *J Shoulder Elbow Surg.* 2012;21:1177–1183.

211. Charles ER, Kumar V, Blacknall J, et al. A validation of the Nottingham clavicle score: a clavicle, acromioclavicular joint and sternoclavicular joint-specific patient-reported outcome measure. *J Shoulder Elbow Surg.* 2017;26(10):1732–1739.

212. Wright RW, Gaumgarten KM. Shoulder outcome measures. *J Am Acad Orthop Surg.* 2010;18:436–444.

213. Roller AS, Mounts RA, DeLong JM, Hanypsiak BT. Outcome instruments for the shoulder. *Arthroscopy.* 2013;29(5):955–964.

214. Ellenbecker TS, Manske R, Davies GJ. Closed kinetic chain testing techniques of the upper extremities. *Orthop Phys Ther Clin North Am.* 2000;9:219–229.

215. Brophy RH, Beauvais RL, Jones EC, et al. Measurement of shoulder activity level. *Clin Orthop Relat Res.* 2005;439:101–108.

216. Roy JS, MacDermid JC, Woodhouse LJ. Measuring shoulder function: a systematic review of four questionnaires. *Arthritis Rheum.* 2009;61(5):623–632.

217. Brophy RH, Lin KM, Skillington A, et al. Shoulder activity level is associated with type of employment and income in the normal population without shoulder disorders. *Clin Orthop Relat Res.* 2016;474(10):2269–2276.

218. Hepper CT, Smith MV, Steger-May K, Brophy RH. Normative data of shoulder activity level by age and sex. *Am J Sports Med.* 2013;41(5):1146–1151.

219. Brophy RH, Levy B, Chu S, et al. Shoulder activity level varies by diagnosis. *Knee Surg Sports Traumatol Arthrosc.* 2009;17(12):1516–1521.

220. Brophy RH, Dunn WR, Kuhn JE, MOON Shoulder Group. Shoulder activity level is not associated with the severity of symptomatic, atraumatic rotator cuff tears in patients electing nonoperative treatment. *Am J Sports Med.* 2014;42(5):1150–1154.

221. Roach KE, Budiman-Mak E, Songsiridej N, et al. Development of a shoulder pain and disability index. *Arthritis Care Res.* 1991;4(4):143–149.

222. Breckenridge JD, McAuley JH. Shoulder pain and disability index (SPADI). *J Physiotherapy.* 2011;57(3):197.

223. Williams JW, Holleman DR, Simel DL. Measuring shoulder function with the shoulder pain and disability index. *J Rheumatol.* 1995;22(4):727–732.

224. Heald SL, Riddle DL, Lamb RL. The shoulder pain and disability index: the construct validity and responsiveness of a region-specific disability measure. *Phys Ther.* 1997;77:1079–1089.

225. Slobogean GP, Slobogean BL. Measuring shoulder injury function: common scales and checklists. *Injury.* 2011;42(3):248–252.

226. Kirkley A, Griffin S, Dainty K. Scoring systems for the functional assessment of the shoulder. *Arthroscopy.* 2003;19(10):1109–1120.

227. Angst F, Schwyzer HK, Aeschlimann A, et al. Measures of adult shoulder function: Disabilities of the Arm, Shoulder, and Hand Questionnaire (DASH) and its short version (QuickDASH), Shoulder Pain and Disability Index (SPADI), American Shoulder and Elbow Surgeons (ASES) Society standardized shoulder assessment form, Constant (Murley) Score (CS), Simple Shoulder Test (SST), Oxford Shoulder Score (OSS), Shoulder Disability Questionnaire (SDQ), and Western Ontario Shoulder Instability Index (WOSI). *Arthritis Care Res.* 2011;63(S11):S174–S188.

228. Wolke J, Herrmann DA, Krannich A, Scheibel M. Influence of bony defects on preoperative shoulder function in recurrent anteroinferior shoulder instability. *Am J Sports Med.* 2016;44(5):1131–1136.

229. Ellman H, Hanker G, Bayer M. Repair of the rotator cuff: end result study of factors influencing reconstruction. *J Bone Joint Surg Am.* 1986;68:1136–1144.

230. Patte D. Directions for the use of the index of severity for painful and/or chronically disabled shoulder. In: *Abstracts from First Open Congress.* Paris, France: European Society of Surgery of the Shoulder and Elbow; 1987:36–41.

231. Rowe CR, Patel D, Southmayd WW. Bankart procedure: a long term end result study. *J Bone Joint Surg Am.* 1978;60:1–6.

232. Macdonald DA. The shoulder and elbow. In: Pynsent PB, Fairbank JC, Carr A, eds. *Outcome Measures in Orthopedics, Appendices 8-1 Through 8-7.* Oxford: Butterworth-Heinemann; 1993.

233. Constant CR, Murley AHG. A clinical method of functional assessment of the shoulder. *Clin Orthop.* 1987;214:160–164.

234. Williams GH, Gangel TJ, Arciero RA, et al. Comparison of the single assessment numeric evaluation method and two shoulder rating scales: outcome measures after shoulder surgery. *Am J Sports Med.* 1999;27:214–221.

235. Richards RR, An KN, LU Bagliani, et al. A standardized method for the assessment of shoulder function. *J Shoulder Elbow Surg.* 1994;3:347–352.

236. L'Insalata JC, Warren RF, Cohen SB, et al. A self-administered questionnaire for assessment of symptoms and function of the shoulder. *J Bone Joint Surg Am.* 1997;79:738–748.

237. Leggin BG, Iannotti JP. Shoulder outcome measurement. In: Iannotti JP, Williams CR, eds. *Disorders of the Shoulder.* Philadelphia: Lippincott Williams & Wilkins; 1999.

238. Kirkley A, Alverez C, Griffin S. The development and evaluation of a disease-specific quality-of-life questionnaire for disorders of the rotator cuff: the Western Ontario Rotator Cuff Index. *Clin J Sports Med.* 2003;13:84–92.

239. Lopes AD, Ciconelli R, Carrera EF, et al. Validity and reliability of the Western Ontario Rotator Cuff Index (WORC) for use in Brazil. *Clin J Sports Med.* 2008;18:226–272.

240. Alberta FG, El Attrache NS, Bissell S, et al. The development and validcation of a functional assessment tool for the upper extremity in the overhead athlete. *Am J Sports Med.* 2010;38:903–911.

241. Huang H, Grant JA, Miller BS, et al. A systematic review of the psychometrics properties of patient-reported outcome instruments for use in patients with rotator cuff disease. *Am J Sports Med.* 2015;43(10):2572–2582.

242. Romeo AA, Bach BR, O'Halloran KL. Scoring systems for shoulder conditions. *Am J Sports Med.* 1996;24:472–476.

243. Placzek JD, Lukens SC, Badalanmenti S, et al. Shoulder outcome measures: a comparison of six functional tests. *Am J Sports Med.* 2004;32:1270–1277.

244. Makhni EC, Saltzman BM, Meyer MA, et al. Outcomes after shoulder and elbow injury in baseball players: are we reporting what matters? *Am J Sports Med.* 2017;45(2):495–500.

245. Lippitt SB, Harryman DT, Matsen FA. A practical tool for evaluating function: the simple shoulder test. In: Matsen FA, Fu FH, Hawkins RJ, eds. *The Shoulder: A Balance of Mobility and Stability.* Rosemont, IL: American Academy of Orthopedic Surgeons; 1993.

246. Roy JS, Macdermid JC, Faber KJ, et al. The simple shoulder test is responsive in assessing change following shoulder arthroplasty. *J Orthop Sports Phys Ther.* 2010;40:143–421.

247. Tashjian RZ, Hung M, Keener JD, et al. Determining the minimal clinically important difference for the American Shoulder and Elbow Surgeons score, simple shoulder test, and visual analogue scale (VAS) measuring pain after shoulder arthroplasty. *J Shoulder Elbow Surg.* 2017;26(1):144–148.

248. Hsu JE, Russ SM, Somerson JS, et al. Is the simple shoulder test a valid outcome instrument for shoulder arthroplasty? *J Shoulder Elbow Surg.* 2017;26(10):1693–1700.

249. Hudak PL, Amadio PC, Bombardier C. Development of an upper extremity outcome measure: the DASH (disabilities of the arm, shoulder and hand) [corrected]: The Upper Extremity Collaborative Group (UECG). *Am J Ind Med.* 1996;29(6):602–608.

250. Bot SD, Terwee CB, van der Windt DA, et al. Clinimetric evaluation of shoulder disability questionnaires: a systematic review the literature. *Ann Rheum Dis.* 2004;63(4):335–341.

251. Kobler MJ, Salamh PA, Hanney WJ, Cheng MS. Clinimetric evaluation of the disabilities of the arm, shoulder and hand (DASH) and QuickDASH questionnaires for patients with shoulder disorders. *Phys Ther Rev.* 2014;19(3):163–173.

252. Beaton DE, Wright JG, Katz JN. Upper extremity collaborative group. Development of the Quick DASH: comparison of three item reduction approaches. *J Bone Joint Surg Am.* 2005;87:1038–1046.

253. Gummesson C, Ward MM, Atroshi I. The shortened disabilities of the arm, shoulder and hand questionnaire (QuickDASH): validity and reliability based on responses within the full-length DASH. *BMC Musculoskeletal Disord.* 2006;7:44–51.

254. Kennedy CA, Beaton DE, Smith P, et al. Measurement properties of the QuickDASH (disabilities of the arm, shoulder and hand) outcome measure and cross-cultural adaptations of the QuickDASH: a systematic review. *Qual Life Res.* 2013;22(9):2509–2547.

255. Balg F, Boileau P. The instability severity index score. A simple pre-operative score to select patients for arthroscopic or open shoulder stabilization. *J Bone Joint Surg Br.* 2007;89(11):1470–1477.

256. Phadnis J, Arnold C, Elmorsy A, Flannery M. Utility of the instability index severity score in predicting failure after arthroscopic anterior stabilization of the shoulder. *Am J Sports Med.* 2015;43(8):1983–1988.

257. Goodman J, Lau BC, Krupp RJ, et al. Clinical measurements versus patient-reported outcomes: analysis of the American Shoulder and Elbow Surgeons physician assessment in patients undergoing reverse total shoulder arthroplasty. *JSES Open Access.* 2018;2(2):144–149.

258. Riley SP, Cote MP, Swanson B, et al. The shoulder pain and disability index: is it sensitive and responsive to immediate change? *Man Ther.* 2015;20(3):49–498.

259. Leggin BG, Iannotti JP. Shoulder outcome measurement. In: Iannotti JP, Williams GR, eds. *Disorders of the Shoulder: Diagnosis and Management.* Philadelphia, Lippincott: Williams & Wilkins; 1999.

260. Leggin BG, Michener LA, Shaffer MA, et al. The Penn shoulder score: reliability and validity. *J Orthop Sports Phys Ther.* 2006;36:138–151.

261. Michener LA, McClure PW, Sennet BJ. American shoulder and elbow surgeons standardized shoulder assessment form, patient self-reported selection: reliability, validity and responsiveness. *J Shoulder Elbow Surg.* 2002;11(6):587–594.

262. Dawson J, Fitzpatrick R, Carr A. The assessment of shoulder instability. The development and validation of a questionnaire. *J Bone Joint Surg Br.* 1999;81(3):420–426.

263. Yian EH, Ramappa AJ, Arneberg O, Gerber C. The Constant score in normal shoulders. *J Shoulder Elbow Surg.* 2005;14(2):128–133.

264. Roy JS, MacDermid JC, Woodhouse LJ. A systematic review of the psychometric properties of the Constant-Murley score. *J Shoulder Elbow Surg.* 2010;19(1):157–164.

265. Conboy VB, Morris RW, Kiss J, Carr AJ. An evaluation of the Constant-Murley shoulder assessment. *J Bone Joint Surg Br.* 1996;78(2):229–232.

266. Blonna D, Scelsi M, Marini E, et al. Can we improve the reliability of the Constant- Murley score? *J Shoulder Elbow Surg.* 2012;21(1):4–12.

267. Ahmad CS, Padaki AS, Noticewala MS, et al. The Youth Throwing Score: validating injury assessment in young baseball players. *Am J Sports Med.* 2016;45(2):317–324.

268. Kraeutler MJ, Ciccotti MG, Dodson CC, et al. Kerlan-Jobe Orthopaedic Clinic overhead athlete scores in asymptomatic professional baseball pitchers. *J Shoulder Elbow Surg.* 2013;22(3):329–332.

269. Fronek J, Yang J, Osbahr DC, et al. Shoulder functional performance status of the minor league professional baseball pitchers. *J Shoulder Elbow Surg.* 2015;24(1):17–23.

270. Blonna D, Bellato E, Bonasia DE, et al. Design and testing of the degree of shoulder involvement in sports (DOSIS) scale. *Am J Sports Med.* 2015;43(10):2423–2430.

271. Falsone SA, Gross MT, Guskiewicz KM, et al. One-arm hop test: reliability and effects of arm dominance. *J Orthop Sports Phys Ther.* 2002;32:98–103.

272. Abrams GD, Safran MR. Diagnosis and management of superior labrum anterior posterior lesions in overhead athletes. *Br J Sports Med.* 2010;44:311–318.

273. Hegedus EJ, Goode A, Campbell S, et al. Physical examination tests of the shoulder: a systematic review with meta-analysis of individual tests. *Br J Sports Med.* 2008;42:80–92.

274. Somerville LE, Willets K, Johnson AM, et al. Clinical assessment of physical examination maneuvers for rotator cuff lesions. *Am J Sports Med.* 2014;42(8):1911–1919.

275. Cook C, Beaty S, Kissenberth MJ, et al. Diagnostic accuracy of five orthopedic clinical tests for diagnosis of superior labrum anterior posterior (SLAP) lesions. *J Shoulder Elbow Surg.* 2012;21:13–22.

276. Oh JH, Kim JY, Kim WS, et al. The evaluation of various physical examinations for the diagnosis of type II superior labrum anterior and posterior lesions. *Am J Sports Med.* 2008;36:353–359.

277. Hegedus EJ, Goode AP, Cook CE, et al. Which physical examination tests provide clinicians with the most value when examining the shoulder? Update of a systematic review with meta-analysis of individual tests. *Br J Sports Med.* 2012;46(14):964–978.

278. Kuijpers T, van derWindt DA, Boeke AJ, et al. Clinical prediction rules for the prognosis of shoulder pain in general practice. *Pain.* 2006;120(3):276–285.

279. Lange T, Matthijs O, Jain NB, et al. Reliability of specific physical examination tests for the diagnosis of shoulder pathologies: a systematic review and meta-analysis. *Br J Sports Med.* 2017;51(6):511–518.

280. Moen MH, de Vos RJ, Ellenbecker TS, et al. Clinical tests in shoulder examination: how to perform them. *Br J Sports Med.* 2010;44:370–375.

281. Rosas S, Krill MK, Amoo-Achampong K, et al. A practical, evidence-based, comprehensive (PEC) physical examination for diagnosing pathology of the long head of biceps. *J Shoulder Elbow Surg.* 2017;26(8):1484–1492.

282. Levy AS, Lintner S, Kenter K, et al. Intra- and interobserver reproducibility of the shoulder laxity examination. *Am J Sports Med.* 1999;27:460–463.

283. Sciascia AD, Spigelman T, Kibler WB, Uhl TL. Frequency of use of clinical shoulder examination tests by experienced shoulder surgeons. *J Athl Train.* 2012;47(4):457–466.

284. Parentis MA, Glousman RE, Mohr KS, et al. An evaluation of the provocative tests for superior labral anterior posterior lesions. *Am J Sports Med.* 2006;34:265–268.

285. Dessaur WA, Magarey ME. Diagnostic accuracy of clinical tests for superior labral anterior posterior lesions: a systemic review. *J Orthop Sports Phys Ther.* 2008;38:341–352.

286. Meserve BB, Cleland JA, Boucher TR. A meta-analysis examining clinical test utility for assessing superior labral anterior posterior lesions. *Am J Sports Med.* 2009;37:2252–2258.

287. Munro W, Healy R. The validity and accuracy of clinical tests used to detect labral pathology of the shoulder—a systematic review. *Manual Therapy.* 2009;14:119–130.

288. Knesek M, Skendzel JG, Dines JS, et al. Diagnosis and management of superior labral anterior posterior tears in throwing athletes. *Am J Sports Med.* 2013;41:444–460.

289. McFarland EG, Kim TK, Savino RM. Clinical assessment of three common tests for superior labral anterior-posterior lesions. *Am J Sports Med.* 2002;30(6):810–815.

290. Braman JP, Zhao KD, Lawrence RL, et al. Shoulder impingement revisited: evolution of diagnostic understanding in orthopedic surgery and physical therapy. *Med Biol Eng Comput.* 2014;52(3):211–219.

291. Kuhn JE, Helmer TT, Dunn WR, Throckmorton TW. Development and reliability testing of the frequency, etiology, direction, and the severity (FEDS) system for classified glenohumeral instability. *J Shoulder Elbow Surg.* 2011;20(4):548–556.

292. Lewis JS, McCreesh K, Barratt E, et al. Inter-rater reliability of the Shoulder Symptom Modification Procedure in people with shoulder pain. *BMJ Open Sport Exerc Med.* 2016;2(1):e000181.

293. Lewis J. Rotator cuff tendinopathy/subacromial impingement syndrome: is it time for a new method of assessment? *Br J Sports Med.* 2009;43(4):259–264.

294. Lewis J. Rotator cuff related shoulder pain: assessment, management and uncertainties. *Man Ther.* 2016;23:57–68.

295. Meakins A, May S, Littlewood C. Reliability of the Shoulder Symptom Modification Procedure and association of within-session and between-session changes with functional outcomes. *BMJ Open Sport Exerc Med.* 2018;4(1):e000342.

296. Cleeman E, Flatow EL. Classification and diagnosis of impingement and rotator cuff lesions in athletes. *Sports Med Arthro Rev.* 2000;8:141–157.

297. Brown GA, Tan JL, Kirkley A. The lax shoulders in females. *Clin Orthop Relat Res.* 2000;372:110–122.

298. McClusky CM. Classification and diagnosis of glenohumeral instability in athletes. *Sports Med Arthro Rev.* 2000;8:158–169.

299. Jobe FW, Kvitne RS. Shoulder pain in the overhand or throwing athlete: the relationship of anterior instability and rotator cuff impingement. *Orthop Rev.* 1989;18:963–975.

300. Walch G, Boileau P, Noel E, et al. Impingement of the deep surface of the supraspinatus tendon on the posterosuperior glenoid rim: an arthroscopic study. *J Shoulder Elbow Surg.* 1992;1:238–245.

301. Jobe CM. Posterior superior glenoid impingement: expanded spectrum. *Arthroscopy J Arthro Relat Surg.* 1995;11:530–536.

302. Davidson PA, Elattrache NS, Jobe CM, et al. Rotator cuff and posterosuperior glenoid labrum injury associated with increased glenohumeral motion: a new site of impingement. *J Shoulder Elbow Surg.* 1995;4:384–390.

303. Jobe CM. Evidence for a superior glenoid impingement upon the rotator cuff. *J Shoulder Elbow Surg.* 1993;2:319.

304. Jobe CM. Superior glenoid impingement. *Orthop Clin North Am.* 1997;28:137–143.

305. Silliman JF, Hawkins RJ. Classification and physical diagnosis of instability of the shoulder. *Clin Orthop.* 1993;291:7–19.

306. Owens BD, Nelson BJ, Duffey ML, et al. Pathoanatomy of first time, traumatic anterior glenohumeral subluxation events. *J Bone Joint Surg.* 2010;92:1605–1611.

307. Andrews JA, Timmerman LA, Wilk KE. Baseball. In: Pettrone FA, ed. *Athletic Injuries of the Shoulder.* New York: McGraw-Hill; 1995.

308. Gerber C, Ganz R. Clinical assessment of instability of the shoulder. *J Bone Joint Surg Br.* 1984;66:551–556.

309. Leffert RD, Gumley G. The relationship between dead arm syndrome and thoracic outlet syndrome. *Clin Orthop.* 1987;223:20–31.

310. Matsen FA, Thomas SC, Rockwood CA. Glenohumeral instability. In: Rockwood CA, Matsen FA, eds. *The Shoulder.* Philadelphia: WB Saunders; 1990.

311. Hamner DL, Pink MM, Jobe FW. A modification of the relocation test: arthroscopic findings associated with a positive test. *J Shoulder Elbow Surg.* 2000;9:263–267.

312. Harryman DT, Sidles JA, Harris SL, et al. Laxity of the normal glenohumeral joint: a quantitative in vivo assessment. *J Shoulder Elbow Surg.* 1992;1:66–76.

313. Hawkins RJ, Bokor DJ. Clinical evaluation of shoulder problems. In: Rockwood CA, Matsen FA, eds. *The Shoulder.* Philadelphia: WB Saunders; 1990.

314. Castagna A, Nordenson U, Garofalo R, Karlsson J. Minor shoulder instability. *Arthroscopy.* 2007;23(2):211–215.

315. Bak K. The practical management of swimmer's painful shoulder: etiology, diagnosis and treatment. *Clin J Sports Med.* 2010;20(5):386–390.

316. Hawkins RJ, Mohtadi NG. Clinical evaluation of shoulder instability. *Clin J Sports Med.* 1991;1:59–64.

317. Luime JJ, Verhagen AP, Miedema HS, et al. Does this patient have instability of the shoulder or a labrum lesion? *JAMA.* 2004;292:1989–1999.

318. Burkhart SS, Morgan CD, Kibler WB. The disabled throwing shoulder: spectrum of pathology, part two: evaluation and treatment of SLAP lesions in throwers. *Arthroscopy.* 2003;19:531–539.

319. Speer KP, Hannafin JA, Altcek DW, et al. An evaluation of the shoulder relocation test. *Am J Sports Med.* 1994;22:177–183.

320. Davidson PA, Elattrache NS, Jobe CM, et al. Rotator cuff and posterior-superior glenoid labrum injury associated with increased glenohumeral motion: a new site of impingement. *J Shoulder Elbow Surg.* 1995;4:384–390.

321. Gross ML, Distefano MC. Anterior release test: a new test for occult shoulder instability. *Clin Orthop Relat Res.* 1997;339:105–108.

322. Kelley MJ. Evaluation of the shoulder. In: Kelley MJ, Clark WA, eds. *Orthopedic Therapy of the Shoulder.* Philadelphia: JB Lippincott; 1995.

323. Matthews LS, Pavlovich LJ. Anterior and anteroinferior instability: diagnosis and management. In: Iannotti JP, Williams CR, eds. *Disorders of the Shoulder.* Philadelphia: Lippincott Williams & Wilkins; 1999.

324. Milgrom C, Milgrom Y, Radeva-Petrova D, et al. The supine apprehension test helps predict the risk of recurrent instability after a first-time anterior shoulder dislocation. *J Shoulder Elbow Surg.* 2014;23:1838–1842.

325. Myer CA, Hegedus EJ, Tarara DT, Myer DM. A user's guide to performance of the best shoulder physical examination tests. *Br J Sports Med.* 2013;47(14):903–907.

326. Bushnell BD, Creighton RA, Herring MM. The bony apprehension test for instability of the shoulder: a perspective pilot analysis. *Arthroscopy.* 2008;24(9):974–982.

327. Miniaci A, Gish MW. Management of anterior glenohumeral instability associated with large Hill-Sachs defects. *Techniques Shoulder Elbow Surg.* 2004;5:170–175.

328. Evans RC. *Illustrated Essentials in Orthopedic Physical Assessment.* St Louis: Mosby Year Book; 1994.

329. Solem-Bertoft E, Thomas KA, Westerberg CE. The influence of scapular retraction and protraction on the width of the subacromial space. *Clin Orthop Relat Res.* 1993;296:99–103.

330. Borsa PA, Sauers EL, Herling DE. Patterns of glenohumeral joint laxity and stiffness in healthy men and women. *Med Sci Sports Exerc.* 2000;32:1685–1690.

331. Sauers EL, Borsa PA, Herling DE, et al. Instrumented measurement of glenohumeral joint laxity and its relationship to passive range of motion and generalized joint laxity. *Am J Sports Med.* 2001;29:143–150.

332. Sauers EL, Borsa PA, Herling DE, et al. Instrumental measurement of glenohumeral joint laxity: reliability and normative data. *Knee Surg Sports Traumatol Arthros.* 2001;9:34–41.

333. Ellenbecker TS, Mattalino AJ, Elam E, et al. Quantification of anterior translation of the humeral head in the throwing shoulder: manual assessment vs. stress radiography. *Am J Sports Med.* 2000;28:161–167.

334. Lintner SA, Levy A, Kenter K, et al. Glenohumeral translation in the asymptomatic athlete's shoulder and its relationship to other clinically measureable anthropometric variables. *Am J Sports Med.* 1996;24:716–720.

335. Altchek DA, Warren RF, Skyhar MJ, et al. T-plasty: a technique for treating multidirectional instability in the athlete. *J Bone Joint Surg Am.* 1991;73:105–112.

336. Ramsey ML, Klimkiewicz JJ. Posterior instability: diagnosis and management. In: Iannotti JP, Williams CR, eds. *Disorders of the Shoulder.* Philadelphia: Lippincott Williams & Wilkins; 1999.

337. Protzman RR. Anterior instability of the shoulder. *J Bone Joint Surg Am.* 1980;62:909–918.

338. Davies GJ, Gould JA, Larson RL. Functional examination of the shoulder girdle. *Phys Sports Med.* 1981;9:82–104.

339. Rockwood CA. Subluxations and dislocations about the shoulder. In: Rockwood CA, Green DP, eds. *Fractures in Adults.* Philadelphia: JB Lippincott; 1984.

340. Rowe CR. Dislocations of the shoulder. In: Rowe CR, ed. *The Shoulder.* Edinburgh: Churchill Livingstone; 1988.

341. Provencher MT, LeClere LE, King S, et al. Posterior instability of the shoulder—diagnosis and management. *Am J Sports Med.* 2011;39:874–886.

342. Rebolledo BJ, Nwachukwu BU, Konin GP, et al. Posterior humeral avulsion of the glenohumeral ligament and associated injuries: assessment using magnetic resonance imaging. *Am J Sports Med.* 2015;43(12):2913–2917.

343. Murrell GA, Warren RF. The surgical treatment of posterior shoulder instability. *Clin Sports Med.* 1995;14(4):903–915.

344. Boileau P, Zumstein M, Balg F, et al. The unstable painful shoulder (UPS) as a cause of pain from unrecognized anteroinferior instability in the young athlete. *J Shoulder Elbow Surg.* 2011;20(1):98–106.

345. Wolf EM, Cheng JC, Dickson K. Humeral avulsion of glenohumeral ligaments as a cause of anterior shoulder instability. *Arthroscopy.* 1995;11(5):600–607.

346. Frank RM, Romeo AA, Provencher MT. Posterior glenohumeral instability: evidence-based treatment. *J Am Acad Orthop Surg.* 2017;25(9):610–623.

347. Arcand MA, Reider B. Shoulder and upper arm. In: Reider B, ed. *The Orthopedic Physical Examination.* Philadelphia: WB Saunders; 1999.

348. Kim SH, Park JS, Jeong WK, et al. The Kim test: a novel test for posteroinferior labral lesion of the shoulder—a comparison to the jerk test. *Am J Sports Med.* 2005;33:1188–1191.

349. Kim SH, Park JC, Park JS, et al. Painful jerk test: a predictor of success in nonoperative treatment of posteroinferior instability of the shoulder. *Am J Sports Med.* 2004;32:1849–1855.

350. Miniaci A, Salonen D. Rotator cuff evaluation: imaging and diagnosis. *Orthop Clin North Am.* 1997;28:43–58.

351. Norwood LA, Terry GC. Shoulder posterior and subluxation. *Am J Sports Med.* 1984;12:25–30.

352. Cofield RH, Irving JF. Evaluation and classification of shoulder instability. *Clin Orthop.* 1987;223:32–43.

353. Pollack RG, LU Bigliani. Recurrent posterior shoulder instability: diagnosis and treatment. *Clin Orthop.* 1993;291:85–96.

354. Pagnani MJ, Warren RF. Multidirectional instability in the athlete. In: Pettrone FA, ed. *Athletic Injuries of the Shoulder.* New York: McGraw-Hill; 1995.

355. McFarland EG, Campbell C, McDowell J. Posterior shoulder laxity in asymptomatic athletes. *Am J Sports Med.* 1996;24:468–471.

356. Cools AM, Cambier D, Witvrouw EE. Screening the athlete's shoulder for impingement symptoms: a clinical reasoning algorithm for early detection of shoulder pathology. *Br J Sports Med.* 2008;42(8):628–635.

357. Schenk TJ, Brems JJ. Multidirectional instability of the shoulder: pathophysiology, diagnosis and management. *J Am Acad Orthop Surg.* 1998;6:65–72.

358. McClusky GM. Classification and diagnosis of glenohumeral instability in athletes. *Sports Med Artho Rev.* 2000;8:158–169.

359. Gaskill TR, Taylor DC, Millett PJ. Management of multidirectional instability of the shoulder. *J Am Acad Orthop Surg.* 2011;19:758–767.

360. Ebinger N, Magosch P, Lichtenberg S, Habermeyer P. A new SLAP test: the supine flexion resistance test. *Arthroscopy.* 2008;24(5):500–505.

361. Ren H, Bicknell RT. From the unstable painful shoulder to multidirectional instability in the young athlete. *Clin Sports Med.* 2013;32(4):815–823.

362. LU Bigliani, Codd TP, Conner PM, et al. Shoulder motion and laxity in the professional baseball player. *Am J Sports Med.* 1997;25:609–613.

363. Helmig P, Sojbjerg J, Kjaersgaard-Andersen P, et al. Distal humeral migration as a component of multidirectional shoulder instability. *Clin Orthop.* 1990;252:139–143.

364. Cleeman E, Flatow EL. Classification and diagnosis of impingement and rotator cuff lesions in athletes. *Sports Med Arthro Rev.* 2000;8:141–157.

365. Ferrick MR. Coracoid impingement: a case report and review of the literature. *Am J Sports Med.* 2000;28:117–119.

366. Lukasiewicz AC, McClure P, Michner L, et al. Comparison of 3-dimensional scapular position and orientation between subjects with and without shoulder impingement. *J Orthop Sports Phys Ther.* 1999;29:574–586.

367. LU Bigliani, Levine WN. Subacromial impingement syndrome. *J Bone Joint Surg Am.* 1997;79:1854–1868.

368. Harrison AK, Flatow EL. Subacromial impingement syndrome. *J Am Acad Orthop Surg.* 2011;19:701–708.

369. Ludewig PM, Braman JP. Shoulder impingement: biomechanical considerations in rehabilitation. *Manual Therapy.* 2011;16:33–39.

370. Kaplan LD, McMahon PJ, Towers J, et al. Internal impingement: findings on magnetic resonance imaging an arthroscopic evaluation. *Arthroscopy.* 2004;20(7):701–704.

371. Castagna A, Garofalo R, Cesari E, et al. Posterior superior internal impingement: an evidence-based review. *Br J Sports Med.* 2009;44:382–388.

372. Hawkins RJ, Kennedy JC. Impingement syndrome in athletics. *Am J Sports Med.* 1980;8:151–163.

373. Brossmann J, Preidler KW, Pedowitz KA, et al. Shoulder impingement syndrome: influence of shoulder position on rotator cuff impingement: an anatomic study. *Am J Roentgenol.* 1992;167:1511–1515.

374. Valadic AL, Jobe CM, Pink MM, et al. Anatomy of provocative tests for impingement syndrome of the shoulder. *J Shoulder Elbow Surg.* 2000;9:36–46.

375. Gerber C, Terrier F, Ganz R. The role of the coracoid process in the chronic impingement syndrome. *J Bone Joint Surg Br.* 1985;67:703–708.

376. Tucker S, Taylor NF, Green RA. Anatomical validity of the Hawkins-Kennedy test—a pilot study. *Manual Therapy.* 2011;16:399–402.

377. McFarland EG, Selhi HS, Keyurapan E. Clinical evaluation of impingement: what to do and what works. *J Bone Joint Surg Am.* 2006;88:432–441.

378. Leroux JL, Thomas E, Bonnel F, et al. Diagnostic value of clinical tests for shoulder impingement. *Rev Rheum.* 1995;62:423–428.

379. Miniaci A, Dowdy PA. Rotator cuff disorders. In: Hawkins RJ, Misamore GW, eds. *Shoulder Injuries in the Athlete.* New York: Churchill Livingstone; 1996.

380. Branch TP, Lawton RL, Jobst CA, et al. The role of glenohumeral capsular ligaments in internal and external rotation of the humerus. *Am J Sports Med.* 1995;23:632–637.

381. Zaslav KR. Internal rotation resistance strength tests: a new diagnostic test to differentiate intraarticular pathology from outlet (Neer) impingement syndrome in the shoulder. *J Shoulder Elbow Surg.* 2001;10:23–27.

382. Neer CS, Welsh RP. The shoulder in sports. *Orthop Clin North Am.* 1977;8:583–591.

383. Buchberger DJ. Introduction of a new physical examination procedure for the differentiation of acromioclavicular joint lesions and subacromial impingement. *J Manip Physio Ther.* 1999;22:316–321.

384. Guosheng Y, Chongxi R, Guoqing C, et al. The diagnostic value of a modified Neer test in identifying subacromial impingement syndrome. *Eur J Orthopedic Surg Traumatol.* 2017;27(8):1063–1067.

385. Jobe CM. Posterior superior glenoid impingement: expanded spectrum. *Arthroscopy.* 1995;11:530–536.

386. Jobe CM. Superior glenoid impingement. *Clin Orthop Relat Res.* 1996;330:98–107.

387. Giombini A, Rossi F, Pettrone FA, et al. Posterosuperior glenoid rim impingement as a cause of shoulder pain in top level waterpolo players. *J Sports Med Phys Fit.* 1997;37:273–278.

388. Mihata T, McGarry MH, Kinoshita M, et al. Excessive glenohumeral horizontal abduction as occurs during late cocking phase of the throwing motion can be critical for internal impingement. *Am J Sports Med.* 2010;38:369–374.

389. Heyworth BE, Williams RJ. Internal impingement of the shoulder. *Am J Sports Med.* 2009;37:1024–1037.

390. Corso G. Impingement relief test: an adjunctive procedure to traditional assessment of shoulder impingement syndrome. *J Orthop Sports Phys Ther.* 1995;22:183–192.

391. Calvert E, Chambers GK, Regan W, et al. Special physical examination tests for superior labrum anterior posterior shoulder tears are clinically limited and invalid: a diagnostic systematic review. *J Clin Epidemiol.* 2009;62(5):558–563.

392. Reeves B. Experiments on the tensile strength of the anterior capsular structures of the shoulder in man. *J Bone Joint Surg Br.* 1968;50:858–865.

393. Mileski RA, Snyder SJ. Superior labral lesions of the shoulder: pathoanatomy and surgical management. *J Am Acad Orthop Surg.* 1998;6:121–131.

394. Richards DB. Injuries to the glenoid labrum: a diagnostic and treatment challenge. *Phys Sportsmed.* 1999;22:73–85.

395. Huijbregts PA. SLAP lesions: structure, function and physical therapy diagnosis and treatment. *J Man Manip Ther.* 2001;9:71–83.

396. Pappas AM, Goss TP, Kleinman PK. Symptomatic shoulder instability due to lesions of the glenoid labrum. *Am J Sports Med.* 1983;11:279–288.

397. Myers TH, Zemanovic JR, Andrews JR. The resisted supination external rotation test: a new test for the diagnosis of superior labral anterior posterior lesions. *Am J Sports Med.* 2005;33:1315–1320.

398. Grossman MG, Tibone JE, McGarry MH, et al. A cadaveric model of the throwing shoulder: a possible etiology of superior labrum anterior-to-posterior lesions. *J Bone Joint Surg Am.* 2005;87:824–831.

399. Snyder SJ, Karzel RP, Del Pizzo W, et al. SLAP lesions of the shoulder. *Arthroscopy.* 1990;6:274–279.

400. Burkhart SS, Morgan CD. The peel-back mechanism—its role in producing and extending posterior type II SLAP lesions and its effect on SLAP repair rehabilitation. *Arthroscopy.* 1998;14:637–640.

401. Morgan CD, Burkhart SS, Palmari M, et al. Type II SLAP lesions: three subtypes and their relationships to superior instability and rotator cuff tears. *Arthroscopy.* 1998;14:553–565.

402. Braun S, Kokmeyer D, Millett PJ. Shoulder injuries in the throwing athlete. *J Bone Joint Surg Am.* 2009;91:966–978.

403. Keener JD, Brophy RH. Superior labral tears of the shoulder: pathogenesis, evaluation and treatment. *J Am Acad Orthop Surg.* 2009;17:627–637.

404. Kibler WB, Sciascia A. Current practice for the diagnosis of a SLAP lesion: systematic review and physician survey. *Arthroscopy.* 2015;31(12):2456–2469.

405. Guanche CA, Jones DC. Clinical testing for tears of the glenoid labrum. *Arthroscopy.* 2003;19(5):517–523.

406. Sodha S, Srikumaran U, Choi K, et al. Clinical assessment of the dynamic labral shear test for superior labrum anterior and posterior lesions. *Am J Sports Med.* 2017;45(4):775–781.

407. O'Brien SJ, Pagnoni MJ, Fealy S, et al. The active compression test: a new and effective test for diagnosing labral tears and acromioclavicular joint abnormality. *Am J Sports Med.* 1998;26:610–613.

408. Kibler WB, Sciascia AD, Hester P, et al. Clinical utility of traditional and new tests in the diagnosis of biceps tendon injuries and superior labrum anterior and posterior lesions in the shoulder. *Am J Sports Med.* 2009;37:1840–1847.

409. Pandya NK, Colton A, Webner D, et al. Physical examination and magnetic resonance imaging in the diagnosis of superior labrum anterior-posterior lesions of the shoulder: a sensitivity analysis. *Arthroscopy.* 2008;24:311–317.

410. Cadogan A, Laslett M, Hing W, et al. Interexaminer reliability of orthopedic special tests used in the assessment of shoulder pain. *Manual Therapy.* 2011;16:131–135.

411. Urch E, Taylor SA, Zitkovsky H, et al. A modification of the active compression test for the shoulder biceps-labrum complex. *Arthrosc Tech.* 2017;6(3):e859–e862.

412. Kibler WB. Clinical examination of the shoulder. In: Pettrone FA, ed. *Athletic Injuries of the Shoulder.* New York: McGraw-Hill; 1995.

413. Kibler WB. Specificity and sensitivity of the anterior slide test in throwing athletes with superior glenoid labral tears. *Arthroscopy.* 1995;11:296–300.

414. Kim SH, Ha KI, Han KY. Biceps load test: a clinical test for superior labrum anterior and posterior lesions in shoulder with recurrent anterior dislocations. *Am J Sports Med*. 1999;27:300–303.

415. Wilk KE, Reinold MM, Dugas JR, et al. Current concepts in the recognition and treatment of superior labral (SLAP) lesions. *J Orthop Sports Phys Ther*. 2005;35:273–291.

416. Andrews JR, Gillogly S. Physical examination of the shoulder in throwing athletes. In: Zarins B, Andrews JR, Carson WG, eds. *Injuries to the Throwing Arm*. Philadelphia: WB Saunders; 1985.

417. Walsh DA. Shoulder evaluation of the throwing athlete. *Sports Med Update*. 1989;4:24–27.

418. Guidi EJ, Suckerman JD. Glenoid labral lesions. In: Andrews JR, Wilk KE, eds. *The Athlete's Shoulder*. New York: Churchill Livingstone; 1994.

419. Cook C, Beaty S, Kissenberth MJ, et al. Diagnostic accuracy of five orthopedic clinical tests for diagnosis of superior labrum anterior posterior (SLAP) lesions. *J Shoulder Elbow Surg*. 2012;21:13–22.

420. Manske R, Prohaskab D. Superior labrum anterior and posterior (SLAP) rehabilitation in the overhead athlete. *Phys Ther Sport*. 2010;30:1–12.

421. Nakagawa S, Yoneda M, Hayashida K, et al. Forced shoulder abduction and elbow flexion test: a new simple clinical test to detect superior labral injury in the throwing shoulder. *Arthroscopy*. 2005;21:1290–1295.

422. Liu SH, Henry MH, Nuccion SL. A prospective evaluation of a new physical examination in predicting glenoid labral tears. *Am J Sports Med*. 1996;24:721–725.

423. Mimori K, Muneta T, Nakagawa T, et al. A new pain provocation test for superior labral tears of the shoulder. *Am J Sports Med*. 1999;27:137–142.

424. Kim YS, Kim JM, Ha KY, et al. The passive compression test—a new clinical test for superior labral tears of the shoulder. *Am J Sports Med*. 2007;35:1489–1494.

425. Schlechter JA, Summa S, Rubin BD. The passive distraction test: a new diagnostic aid for clinically significant superior labral pathology. *Arthroscopy*. 2009;25:1374–1379.

426. Morey VM, Singh H, Paladini P, et al. The Porcellini test: a novel test for accurate diagnosis of posterior labral tears of the shoulder: comparative analysis with established tests. *Musculoskelet Surg*. 2016;100(3):199–205.

427. Berg EE, Ciullo JV. A clinical test for superior glenoid labral or "SLAP" lesions. *Clin J Sports Med*. 1998;8:121–123.

428. Taylor SA, Newman AM, Dawson C, et al. The "3-pack" examination is critical for comprehensive evaluation of the biceps-labrum complex and the bicipital tunnel: a prospective study. *Arthroscopy*. 2017;33(1):28–38.

429. Wright AA, Wassinger CA, Frank M, et al. Diagnostic accuracy of scapular physical examination tests for shoulder disorders: a systematic review. *Br J Sports Med*. 2013;47(14):886–892.

430. Struyf F, Nijs J, De Graeve J, et al. Scapular positioning in overhead athletes with and without shoulder pain: a case control study. *Scand J Med Sci Sports*. 2011;21(6):809–818.

431. Kibler WB. Role of the scapula in the overhead throwing motion. *Contemp Orthop*. 1991;22:525–533.

432. Shadmehr A, Bagheri H, Ansari NN, Sarafraz H. The reliability measurements of lateral scapular slide test at three different degrees of shoulder joint abduction. *Br J Sports Med*. 2010;44(4):289–293.

433. Shadmehr A, Sarafraz H, Blooki MH, et al. Reliability, agreement and diagnostic accuracy of the modified lateral scapular slide test. *Man Ther*. 2016;24:18–24.

434. Odom CJ, Taylor AB, Hurd CE, et al. Measurement of scapular asymmetry and assessment of shoulder dysfunction using the lateral scapular slide test: a reliability and validity study. *Phys Ther*. 2001;81:799–809.

435. Kibler WB. The role of the scapula in athletic shoulder function. *Am J Sports Med*. 1998;26:325–337.

436. Burkhart SS, Morgan CD, Kibler WB. Shoulder injuries in overhead athletes: the "dead arm" revisited. *Clin Sports Med*. 2000;19:125–158.

437. Seitz AL, McClure PW, Lynch SS, et al. Effects of scapular dyskinesis and scapular assistance test on subacromial space during static arm elevation. *J Shoulder Elbow Surg*. 2012;21:631–640.

438. Kopkow C, Lange T, Schmitt J, Kasten P. Interrater reliability of the modified scapular assistance test with and without handheld weights. *Man Ther*. 2015;20(6):868–874.

439. Christiansen DH, Moller AD, Vestergaard JM, et al. The scapular dyskinesis test: reliability, agreement, and predicted values in patients with subacromial impingement syndrome. *J Hand Ther*. 2017;30(2):208–213.

440. Lopes AD, Timmons MK, Grover M, et al. Visual scapular dyskinesis: kinematics and muscle activity alterations in patients with subacromial impingement syndrome. *Arch Phys Med Rehabil*. 2015;96(2):298–306.

441. Goldbeck TG, Davies GJ. Test-retest reliability of the closed kinetic chain–upper extremity stability test: a clinical field test. *J Sports Rehab*. 2000;9:35–43.

442. Roush JR, Kitamura J, Waits MC. Reference values for the closed kinetic chain upper extremity stability test (CKCUEST) for a collegiate baseball players. *North Am J Sports Phys Ther*. 2007;2(3):159–163.

443. Tucci HT, Martins J, de Carvalho Sposito G, et al. Closed kinetic chain upper extremity stability test (CKCUES test): a reliability study in persons with and without shoulder impingement syndrome. *BMC Musculoskelet Disord*. 2014;15:1–9.

444. Scheibel M, Droschel S, Gerhardt C, et al. Arthroscopically assisted stabilization of acute high-grade acromioclavicular joint separations. *Am J Sports Med*. 2011;39:1507–1516.

445. Axe MJ. Acromioclavicular joint injuries in the athlete. *Sports Med Arthro Rev*. 2000;8:182–191.

446. Clark HD, McCann PD. Acromioclavicular joint injuries. *Orthop Clin North Am*. 2000;31:177–187.

447. Shaffer BS. Painful conditions of the acromioclavicular joint. *J Am Acad Orthop Surg*. 1999;7:176–188.

448. Petersen SA. Arthritis and arthroplasty. In: Hawkins RJ, Misamore GW, eds. *Shoulder Injuries in the Athlete*. New York: Churchill Livingstone; 1996.

449. Ellman H, Harris E, Kay SP. Early degenerative joint disease simulating impingement syndrome: arthroscopic findings. *Arthroscopy*. 1992;8:482–487.

450. Walton J, Mahajan S, Paxinos A, et al. Diagnostic values of tests for acromioclavicular joint pain. *J Bone Joint Surg Am*. 2004;86:807–812.

451. Blasier RB, Guldberg RE, Rothman ED. Anterior shoulder stability: contributions of rotator cuff forces and the capsular ligaments in a cadaver model. *J Shoulder Elbow Surg*. 1992;1:140–150.

452. Turkel SJ, Panio MW, Marshall JL, et al. Stabilizing mechanisms preventing anterior dislocation of the glenohumeral joint. *J Bone Joint Surg Am*. 1981;63:1208–1217.

453. Borstad JD, Dashottar A. Quantifying strain on posterior shoulder tissues during 5 simulated clinical tests: a cadaver study. *J Orthop Sports Phys Ther*. 2011;41(2):90–99.

454. Borstad JD, Dashottar A, Stoughton T. Validity and reliability of the low flexion measurement for posterior glenohumeral joint capsule tightness. *Man Ther*. 2015;20(6):875–878.

455. Gerber C, Krushell RJ. Isolated ruptures of the tendon of the subscapularis muscle. *J Bone Joint Surg Br*. 1991;73:389–394.

456. Lyons RP, Green A. Subscapularis tendon tears. *J Am Acad Ortho Surg*. 2005;13:353–363.

457. Williams GR. Complications of rotator cuff surgery. In: Iannotti JP, Williams CR, eds. *Disorders of the Shoulder*. Philadelphia: Lippincott Williams & Wilkins; 1999.

458. Tokish JM, Decker MJ, Ellis HB, et al. The belly-press test for the physical examination of the subscapularis muscle: electrodiagnostic validation and comparison to the lift-off test. *J Shoulder Elbow Surg*. 2003;12:427–430.

459. Pennock AT, Pennington WW, Torry MR, et al. The influence of arm and shoulder position on the bear-hug, belly-press and lift-off tests. *Am J Sports Med*. 2011;39:2338–2346.

460. Bartsch M, Greiner S, Haas NP, Scheibel M. Diagnostic values of clinical test for subscapularis lesions. *Knee Surg Sports Traumatol Arthrosc*. 2010;18(12):1712–1717.

461. Levy O, Relwani JG, Mullett H, et al. The active elevation lag sign and the triangle sign: new clinical signs of trapezius palsy. *J Shoulder Elbow Surg*. 2009;18:573–576.

462. Barth JR, Burkhart SS, DeBeer JF. The bear-hug test: a new and sensitive test for diagnosing a subscapularis tear. *Arthroscopy*. 2006;22:1076–1084.

463. Scheibel M, Magosch P, Pritsch M, et al. The belly-off sign: a new clinical diagnostic sign for subscapularis lesions. *Arthroscopy*. 2005;21(10):1229–1235.

464. Boileau P, Ahrens PM, Hatzidakis AM. Entrapment of the long head of biceps tendon: the hourglass biceps – a cause of pain and locking of the shoulder. *J Shoulder Elbow Surg*. 2004;13(3):249–267.

465. Clarkson HM. *Musculoskeletal Assessment: Joint Range of Motion and Manual Muscle Strength*. 3rd ed. Philadelphia: Lippincott Williams & Wilkins; 2013.

466. Chalmers PN, Cvetanovich GL, Kupfer N, et al. The champagne toast position isolates the supraspinatus better than the Jobe test: an electromyographic study of shoulder physical examination tests. *J Shoulder Elbow Surg*. 2016;25(2):322–329.

467. Hertel R, Lambert SM, Ballmer FT. The deltoid extension lag sign for diagnosis and grading of axillary nerve palsy. *J Shoulder Elbow Surg*. 1998;7:97–99.

468. Moseley HF. Disorders of the shoulder. *Clin Symp*. 1960;12:1–30.

469. Walch G, Boulahia A, Calderone S, et al. The "dropping" and "hornblower's" signs in evaluating rotator cuff tears. *J Bone Joint Surg Br*. 1998;80:624–628.

470. Post M. *Physical Examination of the Musculoskeletal System*. Chicago: Year Book Medical; 1987.

471. Arroyo JS, Flatow EL. Management of rotator cuff disease: intact and repairable cuff. In: Iannotti JP, Williams GR, eds. *Disorders of the Shoulder*. Philadelphia: Lippincott Williams & Wilkins; 1999.

472. Collin P, Treseder T, Denard PJ, et al. What is the best clinical test for assessment of teres minor in massive rotator cuff tears? *Clin Orthop Relat Res*. 2015;473(9):2959–2966.

473. Pearl MD, Wong KA. Shoulder kinematics and kinesiology. In: Norris TR, ed. *Orthopedic Knowledge Update: Shoulder and Elbow*. Rosemont, IL: American Academy of Orthopedic Surgeons; 2002.

474. Merolla G, De Santis E, Sperling JW, et al. Infraspinatus strength assessment before and after scapular muscles rehabilitation in professional volleyball players with scapular dyskinesis. *J Shoulder Elbow Surg*. 2010;19(8):1256–1264.

475. Gillooly JJ, Chidambaram R, Mok D. The lateral Jobe test: a more reliable method of diagnosing rotator cuff tears. *Int J Shoulder Surg*. 2010;4(2):41–43.

476. Hertel R, Ballmer FT, Lambert SM, et al. Lag signs in the diagnosis of rotator cuff rupture. *J Shoulder Elbow Surg*. 1996;5:307–313.

477. Greis PE, Kuhn JE, Schultheis J, et al. Validation of the lift-off sign test and analysis of subscapularis activity during maximal internal rotation. *Am J Sports Med*. 1996;24:589–593.

478. Cordasco FA, Bigliani LU. Large and massive tears: technique of open repair. *Orthop Clin North Am*. 1997;28:179–193.

479. Kelly BT, Kadrmas WR, Speer KP. The manual muscle examination for rotator cuff strength: an electromyographic investigation. *Am J Sports Med*. 1996;24:581–588.

480. Ticker JB, Warner JJ. Single-tendon tears of the rotator cuff: evaluation and treatment of subscapularis tears. *Orthop Clin North Am*. 1997;28:99–116.

481. Greis PE, Kuhn JE, Schultheis J, et al. Validation of the lift-off test and analysis of subscapularis activity during maximal internal rotation. *Am J Sports Med*. 1996;24:589–593.

482. Stefko JM, Jobe FW, Vanderwilde RS, et al. Electromyographic and nerve block analysis of the subscapularis lift off test. *J Shoulder Elbow Surg*. 1997;6:347–355.

483. Lippman RK. Frozen shoulder: periarthritis, bicipital tendinitis. *Arch Surg*. 1943;7:283–296.

484. Ludington NA. Rupture of the long head of the biceps flexor cubiti muscle. *Ann Surg*. 1923;77:358–363.

485. Muraki T, Aoki M, Izumi T, et al. Lengthening of the pectoralis minor muscle during passive shoulder motions and stretching techniques—a cadaveric biomechanical study. *Phys Ther*. 2009;89:333–341.

486. Sahrmann S. *Diagnosis and Treatment of Movement Impairment Syndromes*. St. Louis: CV Mosby; 2002.

487. Lewis JS, Valentine RE. The pectoralis minor length test: a study of the intra-rater reliability and diagnostic accuracy in subjects with and without shoulder symptoms. *BMC Musculoskelet Disord*. 2007;8:64–74.

488. Wolf EM, Agrawal V. Transdeltoid palpation (the rent test) in the diagnosis of rotator cuff tears. *J Shoulder Elbow Surg*. 2001;10:470–473.

489. Brunnstrom S. Muscle testing around the shoulder girdle: a study of the function of shoulder blade fixators in 17 cases of shoulder paralysis. *J Bone Joint Surg Am*. 1941;23:263–272.

490. Sebastian D, Chovvath R, Malladi R. The scapula backward tipping test: an inter-rater reliability study. *J Body Mov Ther*. 2017;21(1):69–73.

491. Bennett WF. Specificity of the Speed's test: arthroscopic technique for evaluating the biceps tendon at the level of the bicipital groove. *Arthroscopy*. 1998;14:789–796.

492. Bell RH, Noble JB. Biceps disorders. In: Hawkins RJ, Misamore GW, eds. *Shoulder Injuries in the Athlete*. New York: Churchill Livingstone; 1996.

493. Holtby R, Razmjou H. Accuracy of the Speed's and Yergason's tests in detecting biceps pathology and SLAP lesions: comparison with arthroscopic findings. *Arthroscopy*. 2004;20(3):231–236.

494. Jobe FW, Moynes DR. Delineation of diagnostic criteria and a rehabilitation program for rotator cuff injuries. *Am J Sports Med*. 1982;10:336–339.

495. Kendall HO, Kendall FP. *Muscles: Testing and Function*. Baltimore: Williams & Wilkins; 1999.

496. Reese MB. *Muscle and Wensory Testing*. Philadelphia: WB Saunders; 1999.

497. Yergason RM. Supination sign. *J Bone Joint Surg*. 1931;13:160.

498. Hagert E, Hagert CG. Upper extremity nerve entrapments: the axillary and radial nerves – clinical diagnosis and surgical treatment. *Plast Reconstr Surg*. 2014;134:71–79.

499. Pinder EM, Ng CV. Scratch collapse test is a useful clinical sign in assessing long thoracic nerve entrapment. *J Hand Microsurg*. 2016;8:122–124.

500. Elvey RL. The investigation of arm pain. In: Grieve GP, ed. *Modern Manual Therapy of the Vertebral Column*. Edinburgh: Churchill Livingstone; 1986.

501. Coppieters MW, Stappaerts KH, Everaert DG, et al. Addition of test components during neurodynamic testing: effect of range of motion and sensory responses. *J Orthop Sports Phys Ther*. 2001;31:226–237.

502. Butler DS. *Mobilisation of the Nervous System*. Melbourne: Churchill Livingstone; 1991.

503. Aval SM, Durand P, Shankwiler JA. Neurovascular injuries to the athlete's shoulder: part II. *J Am Acad Orthop Surg*. 2007;15:281–289.

504. Leffert RD, Perlmutter GS. Thoracic outlet syndrome: results of 282 transaxillary first rib resections. *Clin Orthop Relat Res*. 1999;368:66–79.

505. Atasoy E. Thoracic outlet compression syndrome. *Orthop Clin North Am*. 1996;27:265–303.

506. Ault J, Suutala K. Thoracic outlet syndrome. *J Man Manip Ther*. 1998;6:118–129.

507. Safran MR. Nerve injury about the shoulder in athletes. Part 2: long thoracic nerve, spinal accessory nerve, burners/stingers, thoracic outlet syndrome. *Am J Sports Med*. 2004;32:1063–1076.

508. Kozin SH. Injuries to the brachial plexus. In: Iannotti JP, Williams CR, eds. *Disorders of the Shoulder*. Philadelphia: Lippincott Williams & Wilkins; 1999.

509. Adson AW, Coffey JR. Cervical rib: a method of anterior approach for relief of symptoms by division of the scalenus anticus. *Ann Surg*. 1927;85:839–857.

510. Roos DB. Congenital anomalies associated with thoracic outlet syndrome. *J Surg*. 1976;132:771–778.

511. Liebenson CS. Thoracic outlet syndrome: diagnosis and conservative management. *J Manip Physiol Ther*. 1988;11:493–499.

512. Ribbe EB, Lindgren SH, Norgren NE. Clinical diagnosis of thoracic outlet syndrome: evaluation of patients with cervicobrachial symptoms. *Manual Med*. 1986;2:82–85.

513. Sallstrom J, Schmidt H. Cervicobrachial disorders in certain occupations with special reference to compression in the thoracic outlet. *Am J Ind Med*. 1984;6:45–52.

514. Wright IS. The neurovascular syndrome produced by hyperabduction of the arms. *Am Heart J*. 1945;29:1–19.

515. Adams SL, Yarnold PR, Mathews JJ. Clinical use of the olecranon-manubrium percussion sign in shoulder trauma. *Ann Emerg Med*. 1988;17:484–487.

516. Brown C. Compressive, invasive referred pain to the shoulder. *Clin Orthop*. 1983;173:55–62.

517. Goodman CC. Screening for medical problems in patients with upper extremity signs and symptoms. *J Hand Ther*. 2010;23(2):105–126.

518. Kelly JJ. Neurologic problems in the athlete's shoulder. In: Pettrone FA, ed. *Athletic Injuries of the Shoulder*. New York: McGraw-Hill; 1995.

519. Perlmutter GS. Axillary nerve injury. *Clin Orthop Relat Res*. 1999;368:28–36.

520. Safran MR. Nerve injury about the shoulder in athletes. Part 1: suprascapular nerve and axillary nerve. *Am J Sports Med*. 2004;32:803–819.

521. Piasecki DP, Romeo AA, Bach BR, et al. Suprascapular neuropathy. *J Am Acad Orthop Surg*. 2009;17:665–676.

522. Plancher KD, Peterson RK, Johnston JC, et al. The spinoglenoid ligament: anatomy, morphology and histological findings. *J Bone Joint Surg Am*. 2005;87:361–365.

523. Ferretti A, De Carli A, Fontana M. Injury of the suprascapular nerve at the spinoglenoid notch: the natural history of infraspinatus atrophy in volleyball players. *Am J Sports Med*. 1998;26(6):759–763.

524. Kaminsky SB, Baker CL. Neurovascular injuries in the athlete's shoulder. *Sports Med Arthro Rev*. 2000;8:170–181.

525. Cummins CA, Messer TM, Nuber GW. Suprascapular nerve entrapment. *J Bone Joint Surg Am*. 2000;82:415–424.

526. Cummins CA, Bowen M, Anderson K, et al. Suprascapular nerve entrapment at the spinoglenoid notch in a professional baseball pitcher. *Am J Sports Med*. 1999;27:810–812.

527. Moen TC, Babatunde OM, Hsu SH, et al. Suprascapular neuropathy: what does the literature show? *J Shoulder Elbow Surg*. 2012;21:835–846.

528. Fabre T, Piton C, Leclouerec G, et al. Entrapment of the suprascapular nerve. *J Bone Joint Surg Br*. 1999;81(3):414–419.

529. Pecina MM, Krmpotic-Nemanic J, Markiewitz AD. *Tunnel Syndromes*. Boca Raton, FL: CRC Press; 1991.

530. Fealy S, Altchek DW. Athletic injuries and the throwing athlete: shoulder. In: Norris TR, ed. *Orthopedic Knowledge Update: Shoulder and Elbow*. Rosemont, IL: American Academy of Orthopedic Surgeons; 2002.

531. Aval SM, Durand P, Shankwiler JA. Neurovascular injuries to the athlete's shoulder: part I. *J Am Acad Orthop Surg*. 2007;15:249–256.

532. White SM, Witten CM. Long thoracic nerve palsy in a professional ballet dancer. *Am J Sports Med*. 1993;21:626–628.

533. Bertelli JA, Ghizoni MF. Long thoracic nerve: anatomy and functional assessment. *J Bone Joint Surg Am*. 2005;87:993–998.

534. Patten C, Hillel AD. The 11th nerve syndrome: accessory nerve palsy or adhesive capsulitis. *Arch Otolaryngol Head Neck Surg*. 1993;119:215–220.

535. Wiater JM, LU Biglian. Spinal accessory nerve injury. *Clin Orthop Relat Res*. 1999;368:5–16.

536. Kaltenborn EM. *Mobilization of the Extremity Joints*. Oslo: Olaf Norlis Bokhandle; 1980.

537. Mattingly GE, Mackarey PJ. Optimal methods of shoulder tendon palpation: a cadaver study. *Phys Ther*. 1996;76:166–174.

538. Bonsell S, Pearsall AW, Heitman RJ, et al. The relationship of age, gender and degenerative changes observed on radiographs of the shoulder in asymptomatic individuals. *J Bone Joint Surg Br*. 2000;82:1135–1139.

539. Liu SH, Henry MH, Nuccion S, et al. Diagnosis of glenoid labral tears: a comparison between magnetic resonance imaging and clinical examination. *Am J Sports Med*. 1996;24:149–154.

540. DiGiovine NM. Glenohumeral instability and imaging technique. *Orthop Phys Ther Clin North Am*. 1995;4:123–142.

541. Schwartz ML. Diagnostic imaging of the shoulder complex. In: Andrews JR, Wilk KE, eds. *The Athlete's Shoulder*. New York: Churchill-Livingstone; 1994.

542. Terry GC, Patton WC. Radiographic views and imaging of the shoulder. *Sports Med Arthro Rev*. 2000;8:203–206.

543. Sanders TG, Morrison WB, Miller MD. Imaging techniques for the evaluation of glenohumeral instability. *Am J Sports Med*. 2000;28:414–434.

544. Anderson MW, Brennan C, Mittal A. Imaging evaluation of the rotator cuff. *Clin Sports Med*. 2012;31:605–631.

545. Smith C, Dattani R, Deans V, Drew S. The sourcil sign: a useful finding on plain x-ray? *Shoulder and Elbow*. 2010;2:9–12.

546. Magee DJ, Reid DC. Shoulder injuries. In: Zachazewski JE, Magee DJ, Quillen WS, eds. *Athletic Injuries and Rehabilitation*. Philadelphia: WB Saunders; 1996.

547. Uhthoff HK, Loehr JW. Calcific tendinopathy of the rotator cuff: pathogenesis, diagnosis and management. *J Am Acad Orthop Surg*. 1997;5:183–191.

548. King LJ, Healy JC. Imaging of the painful shoulder. *Manual Therapy*. 1999;4:11–18.

549. Epstein RE, Schweitzer ME, Frieman BG, et al. Hooked acromion: prevalence on MR images of painful shoulders. *Radiology*. 1993;187:479–481.

550. LU Bigliani, Tucker JB, Flatow EL, et al. The relationship of acromial architecture to rotator cuff disease. *Clin Sports Med*. 1991;10:823–838.

551. Burkhart SS. Recurrent anterior shoulder instability. In: Norris TR, ed. *Orthopedic Knowledge Update: Shoulder and Elbow*. Rosemont, IL: American Academy of Orthopedic Surgeons; 2002.

552. Provencher M, Frank RM, LeClere LE, et al. The Hill-Sach lesion: diagnosis, classification and management. *J Am Acad Orthop Surg*. 2012;20:242–252.

553. Burkhart SS, De Beer JF. Traumatic glenohumeral bone defects and their relationship to failure of arthroscopic Bankart repairs: significance of the inverted-pear glenoid and the humeral engaging Hill-Sachs lesion. *Arthroscopy*. 2000;16(7):677–694.

554. Arciero RA, Parrino A, Bernhardson AS, et al. The effect of a combined glenoid and Hill-Sachs defect on glenohumeral stability: a biomechanical cadaveric study using 3-dimensional modeling of 142 patients. *Am J Sports Med*. 2015;43(6):1422–1429.

555. Kaar SG, Fening SD, Jones MH, et al. Effect of humeral head defect size on glenohumeral stability—a cadaveric study of simulated Hill-Sachs defects. *Am J Sports Med*. 2010;38:594–599.

556. Moroder P, Tauber M, Scheibel M, et al. Defect characteristics of reverse Hill-Sachs lesions. *Am J Sports Med*. 2016;44(3):708–714.

557. Griffin JW, Brockmeier SF. Shoulder instability with concomitant bone loss in the athlete. *Clin Sports Med*. 2013;32(4):741–760.

558. Tannenbaum EP, Sekiya JK. Posterior shoulder instability in the contact athlete. *Clin Sports Med*. 2013;32(4):781–796.

559. Weiner DS, Macnab I. Superior migration of the humeral head. *J Bone Joint Surg Br*. 1970;52:524–527.

560. Nové-Josserand L, Edwards TB, O'Conner DP, et al. The acromioclavicular and coracohumeral intervals are abnormal in rotator cuff tears with muscular fatty degeneration. *Clin Orthop Relat Res*. 2005;433:90–96.

561. Bonutti PM, Norfray JF, Friedman RJ, et al. Kinematic MRI of the shoulder. *J Comput Assist Tomogr*. 1993;17:666–669.

562. Bearden JM, Hughston JC, Whatley GS. Acromioclavicular dislocation: method of treatment. *J Sports Med*. 1973;1:5–17.

563. Tauber M, Koller H, Hitzl W, et al. Dynamic radiographic evaluation of horizontal instability in acute acromioclavicular joint dislocations. *Am J Sports Med*. 2010;38:1188–1195.

564. Kragh JF, Doukas WC, Basamania CJ. Primary coracoid impingement syndrome. *Am J Orthop (Belle Mead NJ)*. 2004;33(5):229–232.

565. Okoro T, Reddy VR, Pimpelmarkar A. Coracoid impingement syndrome: a literature review. *Curr Rev Musculoskelet Med*. 2009;2(1):51–55.

566. Freehill MQ. Coracoid impingement: diagnosis and treatment. *J Am Acad Orthop Surg*. 2011;19(4):191–197.

567. Pavlov H, Warren RF, Weiss CB, et al. The roentgenographic evaluation of anterior shoulder instability. *Clin Orthop*. 1985;194:153–158.

568. Engebretsen L, Craig EV. Radiologic features of shoulder instability. *Clin Orthop*. 1993;291:29–44.

569. Vaisman A, Villalon Montenegro IE, Tuca De Diego MJ, Valderrama Ronco JV. A novel radiographic index for the diagnosis of posterior acromioclavicular joint dislocations. *Am J Sports Med*. 2014;42(1):112–116.

570. Kernwein GA, Rosenberg B, Sneed WR. Arthrographic studies of the shoulder joint. *J Bone Joint Surg Am*. 1957;39:1267–1279.

571. Neviaser JS. Arthrography of the shoulder joint: study of the findings of adhesive capsulitis of the shoulder. *J Bone Joint Surg Am*. 1962;44:1321–1330.

572. Reeves B. Arthrography of the shoulder. *J Bone Joint Surg Br*. 1966;48:424–435.

573. Nevasier TJ, Nevasier RJ, Nevasier JS. Incomplete rotator cuff tears: a technique of diagnosis and treatment. *Clin Orthop*. 1994;306:12–16.

574. Amoo-Achampong K, Nwachukwu BU, McCormick F. An orthopedist's guide to shoulder ultrasound: a systematic review of examination protocols. *Phys Sportsmed*. 2016;44(4):407–416.

575. Lee HJ, Bae SH, Lee KY, et al. Evaluation of the effusion within biceps long head tendon sheath using ultrasonography. *Clin Orthop Surg*. 2015;7(3):351–358.

576. Azzoni R, Cabitza P, Parrini M. Sonographic evaluation of subacromial space. *Ultrasonics*. 2004;42(1-9):683–687.

577. Deseules F, Minville L, Riederer B, et al. Acromiohumeral distance variation measured by ultrasonography and its association with the outcome of rehabilitation for shoulder impingement syndrome. *Clin J Sport Med*. 2004;14(4):197–205.

578. Norwood LA, Barrack R, Jacobson KE. Clinical presentation of complete tears of the rotator cuff. *J Bone Joint Surg Am*. 1989;71(4):499–505.

579. Seitz AL, Michener LA. Ultrasonographic measures of subacromial space in patients with rotator cuff disease: a systematic review. *J Clin Ultrasound*. 2011;39(3):146–154.

580. Bailey LB, Beattie PF, Shanley E, et al. Current rehabilitation applications for shoulder ultrasound imaging. *J Ortho Sports Phys Ther*. 2015;45(5):394–405.

581. Gaitini D, Dahiya N. The shoulder: rotator cuff pathology and beyond. *Ultrasound Clin*. 2012;7(4):425–438.

582. Gaitini D. Shoulder ultrasonography: performance and common findings. *J Clin Imaging Sci*. 2012;2(1):38.

583. Jacobson JA. Shoulder US: anatomy, technique, and scanning pitfalls. *Radiology*. 2011;260(1):6–16.

584. Zakurai G, Ozaki J, Tomita Y, et al. Incomplete tears of the subscapularis tendon associated with tears of the supraspinatus tendon: cadaveric and clinical studies. *J Shoulder Elbow Surg*. 1998;7(5):510–515.

585. Ellenbecker TS, Roetert EP, Bailie DS, et al. Glenohumeral joint total rotation range of motion in elite tennis players and baseball pitchers. *Med Sci Sports Exerc*. 2002;34(12):2052–2056.

586. Oshbar DC, Cannon DL, Speer KP. Retroversion of the humerus in the throwing shoulder of college baseball pitchers. *Am J Sports Med*. 2002;30(3):347–353.

587. Whiteley R, Ginn K, Nicholson L, Adams R. Indirect ultrasound measurement of humeral torsion in adolescent baseball players and non-athletic adults: reliability and significance. *J Sci Med Sport*. 2006;9:310–318.

588. Charousset C, Bellaiche L, Duranthon LD, et al. Accuracy of CT arthrography in the assessment of tears of the rotator cuff. *J Bone Joint Surg Br*. 2005;87:824–828.

589. Collaghan JJ, McNeish LM, Dehaven JP, et al. A prospective comparison study of double contrast computed tomography (CT) arthrography and arthroscopy of the shoulder. *Am J Sports Med*. 1988;16:13–20.

590. Bernageau J. Roentgenographic assessment of the rotator cuff. *Clin Orthop*. 1990;254:87–91.

591. Speer KP, Ghelman B, Warren RF. Computed tomography arthrography of the shoulder. In: Andrews JR, Wilk KE, eds. *The Athlete's Shoulder*. New York: Churchill-Livingstone; 1994.

592. Sanders TG, Miller MD. A systematic approach to magnetic resonance imaging interpretation of sports medicine injuries of the shoulder. *Am J Sports Med*. 2005;33:1088–1105.

593. Jost B, Zumstein M, Pfirrmann CW, et al. MRI findings in throwing shoulders. *Clin Orthop Relat Res*. 2005;434:130–137.

594. Chiapat L, Palmer WE. Shoulder magnetic resonance imaging. *Clin Sports Med*. 2006;25:371–386.

595. Moosikasuwan JB, Miller TT, Hines DM. Imaging of the painful shoulder in throwing athletes. *Clin Sports Med*. 2006;25:433–444.

596. Bencardino JT, Rosenberg ZS. Entrapment neuropathies of the shoulder and elbow in the athlete. *Clin Sports Med*. 2006;25:465–488.

597. Murray PJ, Shaffer BS. MR imaging of the shoulder. *Sports Med Arthrosc Rev*. 2008;17:40–48.

598. Cook TS, Stein JM, Simonson S, Kim W. Normal and variant anatomy of the shoulder on MRI. *Magn Reson Imaging Clin N Am*. 2011;19(3):581–594.

599. Toyoda H, Ito Y, Tomo H, et al. Evaluation of rotator cuff tears with magnetic resonance arthrography. *Clin Orthop Relat Res*. 2005;439:109–115.

600. Oxner KG. Magnetic resonance imaging of the musculoskeletal system: part 6 the shoulder. *Clin Orthop Relat Res*. 1997;334:354–373.

601. Connell DA, Potter HG, Wickiewicz TL, et al. Non-contrast magnetic resonance imaging of superior labral lesions: 102 cases confirmed at arthroscopic surgery. *Am J Sports Med*. 1999;27:208–213.

602. Miniaci A, Burman ML, Mascia AT. Role of magnetic resonance imaging for evaluating shoulder injuries in the athlete. *Sports Med Arthro Rev*. 2000;8:207–218.

603. Wall MS, O'Brien SJ. Arthroscopic evaluation of the unstable shoulder. *Clin Sports Med*. 1995;14:817–839.

604. Herzog RJ. Magnetic resonance imaging of the shoulder. *J Bone Joint Surg Am*. 1997;79:934–953.

605. Kneeland JB. Magnetic resonance imaging: general principles and techniques. In: Iannotti JP, Williams CR, eds. *Disorders of the Shoulder*. Philadelphia: Lippincott Williams & Wilkins; 1999.

606. Williams MM, Snyder SJ, Buford D. The Buford complex – the "cord-like" middle glenohumeral ligament and absent anterosuperior labrum complex: a normal anatomic capsulolabral variant. *Arthroscopy*. 1994;10(3):241–247.

607. Tirman PF, Feller JF, Palmer WE, et al. The Buford complex – a variation of normal shoulder anatomy: MR arthrographic imaging features. *Am J Reoentgenol*. 1966;166(4):869–873.

608. Stetson WB, Phillips T, Deutsch A. The use of magnetic resonance arthrography to detect partial-thickness rotator cuff tears. *J Bone Joint Surg Am*. 2005;87(S2):81–88.

609. Chronopoulus E, Kim TK, Park HB, et al. Diagnostic value of physical tests for isolated chronic acromioclavicular lesions. *Am J Sports Med*. 2004;32(3):655–661.

610. Burns SA, Cleland JA, Carpenter K, Mintken PE. Interrater reliability of the cervicothoracic and shoulder physical examination in patients with a primary complaint of shoulder pain. *Phys Ther Sport*. 2016;18:46–55.

611. Stetson WB, Templin K. The crank test, the O'Brien test, and routine magnetic resonance imaging scans in the diagnosis of labral tears. *Am J Sports Med*. 2002;30(6):806–809.

612. Jia X, Petersen SA, Khosravi AH, et al. Examination of the shoulder: the past, the present and the future. *J Bone Joint Surg Am.* 2009;91(suppl 6):10–18.

613. Saccomanno MF, Ieso CD, Milano G. Acromioclavicular joint instability: anatomy, biomechanics and evaluation. *Joints.* 2014;2(2):87–92.

614. Beaton D, Richards RR. Assessing the reliability and responsiveness of 5 shoulder questionnaires. *J Shoulder Elbow Surg.* 1998;7(6):565–572.

615. Kocher MS, Horan MP, Briggs KK, et al. Reliability, validity, and responsiveness of the American Shoulder and Elbow Surgeons subjective shoulder scale in patients with shoulder instability, rotator cuff disease and glenohumeral arthritis. *J Bone Joint Surg Am.* 2005;87:2006–2011.

616. Tzannes A, Paxinos A, Callanan M, et al. An assessment of the interexaminer reliability of tests for shoulder instability. *J Shoulder Elbow Surg.* 2004;13(1):18–23.

617. Michael G, Michael D. Anterior release test: a new test for occult shoulder instability. *Clin Orthop.* 1997;339:105–108.

618. Farber AJ, Castillo R, Clough M, et al. Clinical assessment of three common tests for traumatic anterior shoulder instability. *J Bone Joint Surg Am.* 2006;88(7):1467–1474.

619. Biederwolf NE. A proposed evidence-based shoulder special testing examination algorithm: clinical utility based on a systematic review of the literature. *Int J Sports Phys Ther.* 2013;8(4):427–440.

620. Kappe T, Sgroi M, Reichel H, Daexle M. Diagnostic performance of clinical tests for subscapularis tendon tears. *Knee Surg Sports Traumatol Arthrosc.* 2018;26(1):176–181.

621. Jain NB, Luz J, Higgins LD, et al. The diagnostic accuracy of special tests for rotator cuff tear. *Am J Phys Med Rehabil.* 2017;96(3):176–183.

622. Lasbleiz S, Quintero N, Ea K, et al. Diagnostic value of clinical tests for degenerative rotator cuff disease in medical practice. *Ann Phys Rehabil Med.* 2014;57:228–243.

623. Kim SH, Ha KI, Ahn JH, et al. Biceps load test II: a clinical test for SLAP lesions of the shoulder. *Arthroscopy.* 2001;17(2):160–164.

624. Hegedus EJ, Cook C, Lewis J, et al. Combining orthopedic special tests to improve diagnosis of shoulder pathology. *Phys Ther Sport.* 2015;16:87–92.

625. Calis M, Akgun K, Birtane M, et al. Diagnostic values of clinical diagnostic tests in subacromial impingement syndrome. *Ann Rheum Dis.* 2000;59(1):44–47.

626. Toprak U, Ustuner E, Ozer D, et al. Palpation tests versus impingement tests in Neer stage I and II subacromial impingement syndrome. *Knee Surg Sports Traumatol Arthrosc.* 2013;21(2):424–429.

627. Beaton DE, Katz JN, Fossel AH, et al. Measuring the whole or the parts? Validity, reliability, and responsiveness of the disabilities of the arm, shoulder and hand outcome measure in different regions of the upper extremity. *J Hand Ther.* 2001;14:128–146.

628. Getahun TY, MacDermid JC, Patterson SD. Concurrent validity of patient rating scales in assessment of outcome after rotator cuff repair. *J Musculoskelet Res.* 2000;4:119–127.

629. Maier M, Maier-Bosse T, Schulz CU, et al. Inter and intraobserver variability in DePalma's classification of shoulder calcific tendinitis. *J Rheumatol.* 2003;30(5):1029–1031.

630. Alqunaee M, Galvin R, Rahey T. Diagnostic accuracy of clinical tests for subacromial impingement syndrome: a systematic review and meta-analysis. *Arch Phys Med Rehabil.* 2012;93(2):229–236.

631. van Kampen DA, van den Berg T, van der Woude HJ, et al. The diagnostic value of the combination of patient characteristics, history, and clinical shoulder tests for the diagnosis of rotator cuff tear. *J Orth Surg Res.* 2014;9(70). https://doi.org/10.1186/s13018-014-0070-y.

632. Itoi E, Kido T, Sano A, et al. Which is more useful, the "full can test" or the "empty can test" in detecting torn supraspinatus tendon? *Am J Sports Med.* 1999;27:65–68.

633. Hayes KW, Petersen CM. Reliability of assessing end-feel and pain and resistance sequence in subjects with painful shoulders and knees. *J Orthop Sports Phys Ther.* 2001;31(8):432–445.

634. Hicks GE, Fritz JM, Delitto A, et al. Interrater reliability of clinical examination measures for identification of lumbar segmental instability. *Arch Phys Med Rehabil.* 2003;84(12):1858–1864.

635. MacDonald PB, Clark P, Sutherland K. An analysis of the diagnostic accuracy of the Hawkins and Neer subacromial impingement signs. *J Shoulder Elbow Surg.* 2000;9(4):299–301.

636. Villafane JH, Valdes K, Anselmi F, et al. The diagnostic accuracy of five tests for diagnosing partial-thickness tears of supraspinatus tendon: a cohort study. *J Hand Ther.* 2015;28:247–252.

637. Dover G, Powers ME. Reliability of joint position sense and force reproduction measures during internal and external rotation of the shoulder. *J Athl Train.* 2003;38:304–310.

638. Rajasekar S, Bangera RK, Sekaran P. Inter-rater and intra-rater reliability of a movement control test in shoulder. *J Bodyw Mov Ther.* 2017;21(3):739–742.

639. Yoon JP, Chung SW, Kim SH, Oh JH. Diagnostic value of four clinical tests for the evaluation of subscapularis integrity. *J Shoulder Elbow Surg.* 2013;22(9):1186–1192.

640. Koslow PA, Prosser LA, Strony GA, et al. Specificity of the lateral scapular slide test in asymptomatic competitive athletes. *J Orthop Sports Phys Ther.* 2003;33(6):331–336.

641. Jorgensen U, Bak K. Shoulder instability: assessment of anterior-posterior translation with a knee laxity tester. *Acta Orthop Scand.* 1995;66(5):398–400.

642. Pizzari T, Kolt GS, Remedios I. Measurement of anterior-to-posterior translation on the glenohumeral joint using the KT-1000. *J Orthop Sports Phys Ther.* 1999;29(10):602–608.

643. Jee WH, McCauley TR, Katz LD, et al. Superior labral anterior posterior (SLAP) lesions of the glenoid labrum: reliability and accuracy of MR arthrography for diagnosis. *Radiology.* 2001;218(1):127–132.

644. Smith TO, Daniell H, Geere JA, et al. The diagnostic accuracy of MRI for detection of partial- and full-thickness rotator cuff tears in adults. *Mag Reson Imag.* 2012;30:336–346.

645. Sandrey MA. Special physical examination tests for superior labrum anterior-posterior shoulder tears: an examination of clinical usefulness. *J Athl Train.* 2013;48(6):856–858.

646. Teefey SA, Rubin DA, Middleton WD, et al. Detection and quantification of rotator cuff tears: comparison of ultrasonographic, magnetic resonance imaging, and arthroscopic findings in seventy-one consecutive cases. *J Bone Joint Surg Am.* 2004;86(4):708–716.

647. Day M, McCormack RA, Nayyar S, Jazrawi L. Physician Training: ultrasound and accuracy of diagnosis in rotator cuff tears. *Bull Hosp Joint Dis.* 2016;74(3):207–211.

648. Roy JS, Braen C, Leblond J, et al. Diagnostic accuracy of ultrasonography, MRI, and MR arthrography in the characterization of rotator cuff disorders: a systematic review and meta-analysis. *Br J Sports Med.* 2015;49:1316–1328.

649. Walton J, Mahajan S, Paxinos A, et al. Diagnostic values of tests for acromioclavicular joint pain. *J Bone Joint Surg Am.* 2004;86:812–817.

650. Boyd EA, Torrance GM. Clinical measures of shoulder subluxation: their reliability. *Can J Public Health.* 1992;83(suppl 2):S24–S28.

651. Meister K, Buckley B, Batts J. The posterior impingement sign: diagnosis of rotator cuff and posterior labral tears secondary to internal impingement in overhand athletes. *Am J Orthop.* 2004;33(8):412–415.

652. Wolf EM, Agrawal V. Trans-deltoid palpation (the rent test) in the diagnosis of rotator cuff tears. *J Shoulder Elbow Surg.* 2001;10:470–473.

653. Bennett WF. Specificity of the speed's test: arthroscopic technique for evaluating the biceps tendon at the level of the bicipital groove. *Arthroscopy.* 1998;14:789–796.

654. Holtby R, Razmjou H. Validity of the supraspinatus test as a single clinical test in diagnosing patients with rotator cuff pathology. *J Orthop Sports Phys Ther.* 2004;34:194–200.

655. Reish R, Williams K. ULNT2—Median nerve bias: examiner reliability and sensory responses in asymptomatic subjects. *J Man Manip Ther.* 2005;13(1):44–55.

656. Patrik GE, Kuhn JE. Validation of the life-off test and analysis of subscapularis activity during maximal internal rotation. *Am J Sports Med.* 1996;24(5):589.

CHAPTER 6

Elbow

The elbow's primary role in the upper limb complex is to help an individual position his or her hand in the appropriate location to perform its function. Once the shoulder has positioned the hand in a gross fashion, the elbow allows for adjustments in height and length of the limb, allowing one to position the hand correctly. In addition, the forearm rotates, in part at the elbow, to place the hand in the most effective position to perform its function.

Applied Anatomy

The elbow consists of a complex set of joints that require careful assessment for proper treatment. The treatment must be geared to the pathology of the condition, because the joint responds poorly to trauma, harsh treatment, or incorrect treatment.

Because they are closely related, the joints of the elbow complex make up a compound synovial joint with injury to any one part affecting the other components as well (Fig. 6.1). In addition, the ulnar and humeral articulations "fit" together rather intimately, which does not allow much "give" as compensation when an injury occurs. Thus, this joint often does not respond well to trauma. The elbow articulations are made up of the ulnohumeral joint and the radiohumeral joint. In addition, the complexity and intricate relation of the elbow articulations are further increased by the superior radioulnar joint, which has continuity with the elbow articulations. These three joints make up the **cubital** articulations. The capsule and joint cavity are continuous for all three joints. The combination of these joints allows 2° of freedom at the elbow. The trochlear joint allows 1° of freedom (flexion-extension), and the radiohumeral and superior radioulnar joints allow the other° of freedom (rotation).

The **ulnohumeral** or **trochlear joint**, which is the major determinant of elbow stability (see Fig. 6.1), is found between the trochlea of the humerus and the trochlear notch of the ulna and is classified as a uniaxial hinge joint. The bones of this joint are shaped so that the axis of movement is not horizontal but instead passes downward and medially, going through an arc of movement. This position leads to the carrying angle at

the elbow (Fig. 6.2). The resting position of this joint is with the elbow flexed to 70° and the forearm supinated 10°. The neutral position (0°) is midway between supination and pronation in the thumb-up position (Fig. 6.3). The capsular pattern is flexion more limited than extension, and the close packed position is extension with the forearm in supination. On full extension, the medial part of the olecranon process is not in contact with the trochlea; on full flexion, the lateral part of the olecranon process is not in contact with the trochlea. This change allows the side-to-side joint play movement necessary for supination and pronation. A small amount of rotation occurs at this joint. In early flexion, 5° of medial rotation occurs; in late flexion, 5° of lateral rotation occurs.

Ulnohumeral (Trochlear) Joint

Resting position:	70° elbow flexion, 10° supination
Close packed position:	Extension with supination
Capsular pattern:	Flexion, extension

The **radiohumeral joint** is a uniaxial hinge joint between the capitulum of the humerus and the head of the radius (see Fig. 6.1). The resting position is with the elbow fully extended and the forearm fully supinated. The close packed position of the joint is with the elbow flexed to 90° and the forearm supinated 5°. As with the trochlear joint, the capsular pattern is flexion more limited than extension.

Radiohumeral Joint

Resting position:	Full extension and full supination
Close packed position:	Elbow flexed to 90°, forearm supinated to 5°
Capsular pattern:	Flexion, extension, supination, pronation

The ulnohumeral and radiohumeral joints are supported medially by the **ulnar (medial) collateral ligament** (also called the **medial ulnar collateral ligament—MUCL**),[1] a fan-shaped structure, and laterally by the **radial (lateral) collateral ligament** and the **lateral ulnar collateral ligament (LUCL)**,[1] a cord-like structure (Fig. 6.4).[2] These ligaments, along with

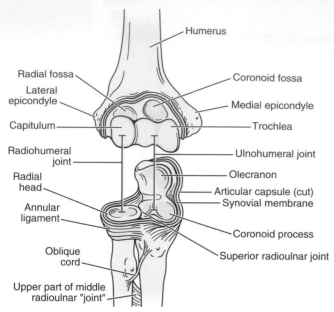

Fig. 6.1 Anterior view of the right elbow disarticulated to expose the ulnohumeral and radiohumeral joints. The margin of the proximal radioulnar joint is shown within the elbow's capsule.

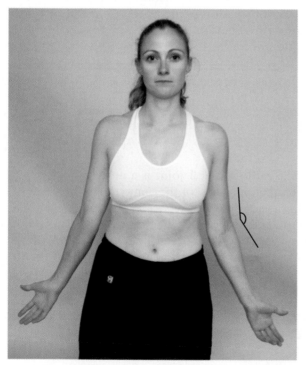

Fig. 6.2 Carrying angle of the elbow.

the ulnohumeral articulation, are the primary restraints to instability in the elbow.[3] The lateral (radial) collateral ligament is the primary restraint to posterolateral instability (most common instability), whereas the medial (ulnar) collateral ligament is the primary restraint to valgus instability.[3] In extension, the medial collateral ligament, the anterior capsule, and the ulnohumeral articulation resist valgus translation. In

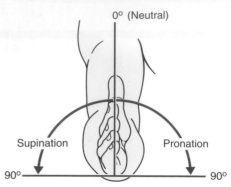

Fig. 6.3 "Thumb-up" or neutral (zero) position between supination and pronation.

90° of flexion, the anterior bundle of the medial collateral ligament provides the main restraint against valgus translation.[4]

The lateral collateral ligament complex is made up of several structures—the radial (lateral) collateral ligament, the annular ligament, the accessory lateral collateral ligament, and the LUCL.[1] It is these structures along with the extensor muscles that protect the elbow from rotary instability. The radial head plays a significant role in tensioning the lateral ligament complex.[4] Disruption of the complex results in posterolateral rotary instability.[4]

The ulnar collateral ligament has three parts, which along with the flexor carpi ulnaris muscle, form the **cubital tunnel** through which passes the ulnar nerve (see Fig. 6.4). Any injury or blow to the area or injury that increases the carrying angle puts an abnormal stress on the nerve as it passes through the tunnel. This can lead to problems such as **tardy ulnar palsy,** the symptoms of which can occur many years after the original injury and may be caused by the "double crush" phenomenon of a cubital tunnel problem combined with a cervical spine problem.

The **superior radioulnar joint** is a uniaxial pivot joint. The head of the radius is held in proper relation to the ulna and humerus by the **annular ligament** (see Figs. 6.1 and 6.4), which makes up four-fifths of the joint.[5] The resting position of this joint is supination of 35° and elbow flexion of 70°. The close packed position is supination of 5°. The capsular pattern of this joint is equal limitation of supination and pronation.

Superior Radioulnar Joint

Resting position:	35° supination, 70° elbow flexion
Close packed position:	5° supination
Capsular pattern:	Equal limitation of supination and pronation

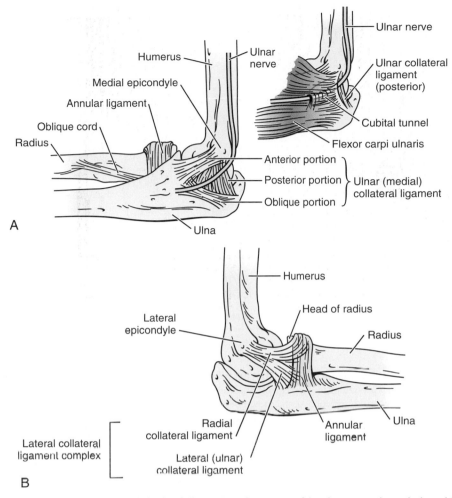

Fig. 6.4 Ligaments of the elbow. (A) Ligaments on medial side of elbow. Note the passage of the ulnar nerve through the cubital tunnel. (B) Ligaments on the lateral side of elbow.

The three elbow articulations are innervated by branches from the musculocutaneous, median, ulnar, and radial nerves. The **middle radioulnar articulation** is not a true joint but is made up of the radius and ulna and the interosseous membrane between the two bones. The **interosseous membrane** is tense only midway between supination and pronation (neutral position). Although this "joint" is not part of the elbow joint complex, it is affected by injury to the elbow joints; conversely, injury to this area can affect the mechanics of the elbow articulations. The interosseous membrane prevents proximal displacement of the radius on the ulna. The displacement is most likely to occur with pushing movements, or a fall on the outstretched hand (FOOSH). The **oblique cord** connects the radius and ulna, running from the lateral side of the **ulnar tuberosity** to the radius slightly below the **radial tuberosity**. Its fibers run at right angles to those of the interosseous membrane (see Fig. 6.1). The cord assists in preventing displacement of the radius on the ulna, especially during movements involving pulling or when a distractive force is exerted on the radius.

Patient History

In addition to the questions listed under the "Patient History" section in Chapter 1, the examiner should obtain the following information from the patient:

1. *How old is the patient? What is the patient's occupation?* Tennis elbow (lateral epicondylitis) problems usually occur in persons 35 years of age or older and in those who use a great deal of wrist flexion and extension in their occupations or activities, requiring wrist stabilization in slight extension (functional position). If the patient is a child who complains of pain in the elbow and lacks supination on examination, the examiner could suspect a dislocation of the head of the radius. This type of injury is often seen in young children. A parent may give the child a sharp "come-along" tug on the arm, or the child may trip while the parent is holding the hand, dislocating the head of the radius. Between the ages of 15 and 20, osteochondritis dissecans may be found.[6] Older individuals may show decreased range of motion (ROM) because of degenerative

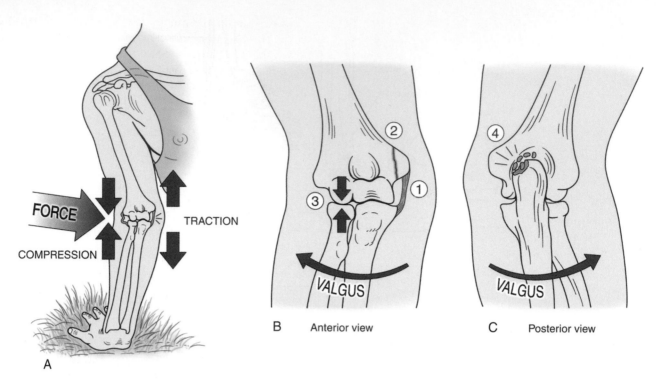

Fig. 6.5 Valgus overload to the elbow. (A) Mechanism of injury. (B) Anterior view. (C) Posterior view. Injury may lead to (1) stretching of medial collateral ligament, (2) stress on epicondylar growth plate (pitcher's or little leaguer's elbow), (3) compression at radiohumeral joint, or (4) compression of the olecranon in the fossa, which may lead to osteophyte and loose body formation.

processes or aging (e.g., osteophytes, loose bodies, osteoporosis, osteoarthritis) and disease processes such as rheumatoid arthritis may lead to swelling, pain, damaged joints, ankylosis, or deformation of the joints.

2. *What was the mechanism of injury?* Did the patient experience a FOOSH injury or a fall on the tip of the elbow? Catching oneself from falling (Fig. 6.5) or repetitive stress in sports (e.g., throwing) can create a severe valgus extension force to the elbow, causing a medial side traction injury (e.g., sprain of the medial collateral ligament) and a lateral side compression injury.[7–9] This can lead to injury at the radiohumeral joint, abnormal stress at the medial epicondyle ("little leaguer's elbow"—if from repetitive stress from throwing), and osteochondral damage either on the olecranon process or olecranon fossa. If the injury is due to overuse from throwing, then the examiner will have to consider the age of the patient, the number of pitches thrown per day, the kind of pitches thrown (e.g., fastball, curve ball), throwing motion (see Fig. 5.13), the amount of retrotorsion of the humerus (those with greater humeral retrotorsion are more likely to have elbow injuries), and posture.[10,11] Were any repetitive

activities involved? Does the patient's job involve any repetitive activities? Did the patient perform any unusual activities in the previous week? Did the patient feel a "pop" when throwing or doing other activity? If the pop was followed by pain and swelling on the medial side of the elbow, it may indicate an ulnar collateral ligament sprain.[12] A centralized pop and weakness of elbow flexion may be the result of a distal biceps rupture. Such questions help determine the structure injured and the degree of injury.

3. *How long has the patient had the problem? Does the condition come and go? What activities aggravate the problem?* Such questions indicate the seriousness of the condition and how much it bothers the patient.

4. *What are the details of the present pain and other symptoms?* What are the sites and boundaries of the pain? Is the pain radiating, does it ache, and is it worse at night? Aching pain over the lateral epicondyle that radiates may indicate a tennis-elbow problem. Depending on the patient's age and past history, the examiner may want to consider referral of pain from the cervical spine or the possibility of a double crush neurological injury. Also, multiple joint diseases (e.g., rheumatoid arthritis, osteoarthritis) must be

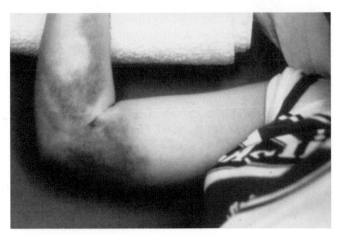

Fig. 6.6 Bruising around elbow following dislocation *(now reduced).*

considered if the patient complains of pain in several joints.

5. *Are there any activities that increase or decrease the pain? Does pulling (traction), twisting (torque), or pushing (compression) alter the pain?* For example, writing, twisting motions of the arm (e.g., turning key, opening door), ironing, gripping, carrying, and leaning on forearm all stress the elbow.[13] Such questions may indicate the tissues being stressed or the tissues injured.

6. *Are there any positions that relieve the pain?* Patients often protectively hold the elbow to the side (in the resting position) and hold the wrist for support, especially in acute conditions.

7. *Is there any indication of deformity, bruising (Fig. 6.6), wasting, muscle spasm, or instability?* Patients with posterolateral rotary instability have pain and discomfort in the elbow along with possible locking, clicking, snapping, or slipping, most likely noted at 40° of flexion as the arm goes into an extension arc of motion, especially with the forearm supinated.[4]

8. *Are any movements impaired?* Which movements make the patient feel restricted? If flexion or extension is limited, two joints may be involved, the ulnohumeral or the radiohumeral. If supination or pronation is problematic, any one of five joints could be involved: the radiohumeral, superior radioulnar at the elbow, middle radioulnar, inferior radioulnar, or ulnomeniscocarpal joints at the wrist.

9. *What is the patient unable to do functionally?* Which hand is dominant? Is the patient able to position the hand properly? Are abnormal movements of the upper limb complex necessary to position the hand? A neuropathy at the elbow may result in hand and grip problems. Specific questions related to precision hand pinch activities that are controlled by the intrinsic muscles should be asked. These would include questions such as difficulty doing up buttons, opening bottles, and difficulty typing.[14] Questions such as these help the examiner determine how functionally limiting the condition is to the patient and whether a peripheral nerve or nerve root may be involved.

10. *What is the patient's usual activity or pastime? Have any of these activities been altered or increased in the past month?*

11. *Does the patient complain of any abnormal nerve distribution pain?* The examiner should note the presence and location of any tingling or numbness for reference when checking dermatomes and peripheral nerve distribution later in the examination. Snapping on the medial side may indicate recurrent dislocation of the ulnar nerve or the medial head of the triceps dislocating over the medial epicondyle.[6]

12. *Does the patient have a history of previous overuse injury or trauma?* This question is especially important in regard to the elbow because the ulnar nerve may be affected by tardy ulnar palsy.

Observation

The patient must be suitably undressed so that both arms are exposed to allow the examiner to compare the two sides. If the history indicates an insidious onset of elbow problems, the examiner should take the time to observe full body posture, especially the neck and shoulder areas, for possible referral of symptoms.

The examiner first places the patient's arm in the anatomic position to determine whether there is a normal **carrying angle** (see Fig. 6.2).[15] It is the angle formed by the long axis of the humerus and the long axis of the ulna and is most evident when the elbow is straight (i.e., 180°) and the forearm is fully supinated (Fig. 6.7). In the adult, there is a slight valgus deviation between the humerus and the ulna when the forearm is supinated and the elbow is extended. In males, the normal carrying angle is 11° to 14°; in females, it is 13° to 16°.[16] If the carrying angle is more than 15°, it is called **cubitus valgus**; if it is less than 5° to 10°, it is called **cubitus varus** (Fig. 6.8). Because of the shape of the humeral condyles that articulate with the radius and ulna, the carrying angle changes linearly depending on the° of extension or flexion. Cubitus valgus is greatest in extension. The angle decreases as the elbow flexes, reaching varus in full flexion.[17] If there has been a fracture or epiphyseal injury to the distal humerus and a cubitus varus results, a **gunstock deformity** may occur in full extension (Fig. 6.9; see Fig. 6.8). This is

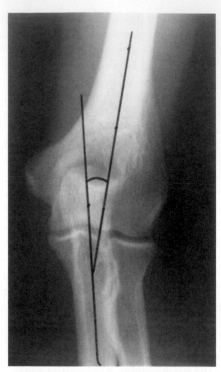

Fig. 6.7 Carrying angle. The carrying angle may be determined by noting the angle of intersection between a line connecting midpoints in the distal humerus and a line connecting midpoints in the proximal ulna.

often the result of damage to the epiphyseal (growth) plate in the presence of a supracondylar fracture in the adolescent.

If swelling exists, all three joints of the elbow complex are affected because they have a common capsule. Joint swelling is often most evident in the triangular space between the radial head, tip of olecranon, and lateral epicondyle (Fig. 6.10). Swelling resulting from olecranon bursitis (student's elbow) is more discrete, being more sharply demarcated as a "goose egg" over the olecranon process (Fig. 6.11). With swelling, the joint would be held in its resting position, with the elbow held in approximately 70° of flexion, because it is in the resting position that the joint has maximum volume.

The examiner should look for normal bony and soft-tissue contours anteriorly and posteriorly. Often, athletes (such as pitchers, tennis players, other throwers, and rodeo riders) have a much larger forearm because of muscle and bone hypertrophy on the dominant side.

The examiner should note whether the patient can assume the normal position of function of the elbow (Fig. 6.12). A normal functional position is 90° of flexion with the forearm midway between supination and pronation.[18] The forearm may also be considered to be in a

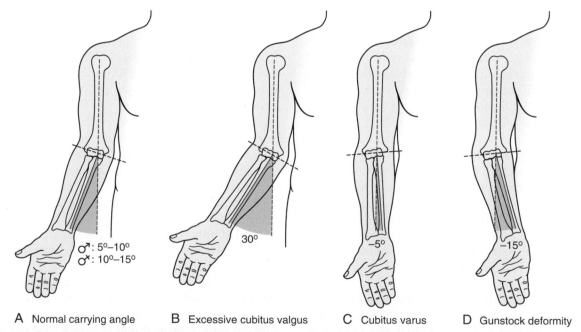

A Normal carrying angle   **B** Excessive cubitus valgus   **C** Cubitus varus   **D** Gunstock deformity

Fig. 6.8 (A) The elbow's axis of rotation extends slightly, obliquely in a medial-lateral direction through the capitulum and the trochlea. Normal carrying angle of the elbow is shown with the forearm deviated laterally from the longitudinal axis of the humerus axis between 5° and 15°. (B) Excessive cubitus valgus deformity is shown with the forearm deviated laterally 30°. (C) Cubitus varus deformity is depicted with the forearm deviated medially −5°. (D) Gunstock deformity with −15° medial deviation. (A–C, Redrawn from Neumann DA: *Kinesiology of the musculoskeletal system: foundations for physical rehabilitation*, St Louis, 2002, Mosby, p 138.)

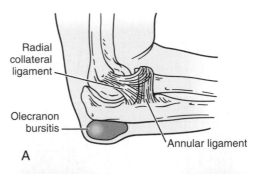

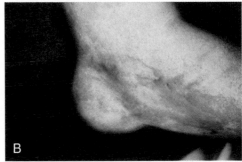

Fig. 6.11 (A) Olecranon bursitis. (B) Actual inflamed bursa. The orange color is from disinfectant applied before aspiration.

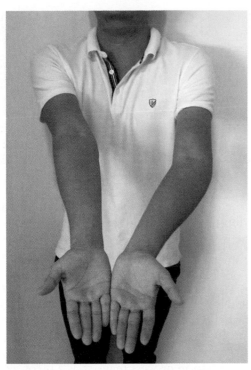

Fig. 6.9 A 29-year-old man presented with left cubitus varus ("gunstock") deformity. (From Murase T: Morphology and kinematics studies of the upper extremity and its clinical application in deformity correction, *J Orthop Sci* 23(5):722–733, 2018.)

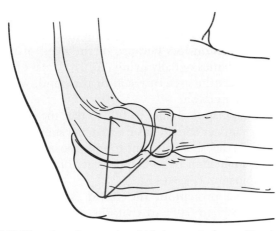

Fig. 6.10 The triangular area in which intra-articular swelling is most evident in the elbow.

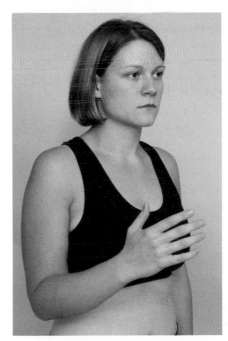

Fig. 6.12 Position of most common function of the elbow—90° flexion, midway between supination and pronation.

functional position when slightly pronated, as in writing. From this position, forward flexion of the shoulder along with slightly more elbow flexion (up to 120°) enables the person to bring food to the mouth; supination of the forearm decreases the amount of shoulder flexion necessary to accomplish this. At 90° of elbow flexion, the olecranon process of the ulna and the medial and lateral epicondyles of the humerus normally form a scalene triangle (i.e., three unequal sides).[19] (Note: Some authors believe it is an isosceles triangle—two sides of

equal length; Fig. 6.13) When the arm is fully extended, the three points normally form a straight line.[20] The triangle is sometimes called the **triangle sign.** If there is a fracture, dislocation, or degeneration leading to loss of bone or cartilage, the distance between the apex and the base decreases and the triangle no longer exists. The triangle can be measured on x-ray films.[17]

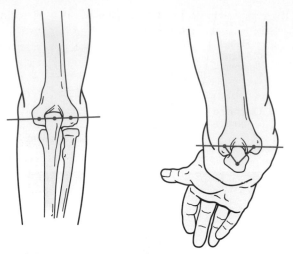

Fig. 6.13 Relation of the medial and lateral epicondyles and the olecranon at the elbow in extension *(left)* and flexion *(right)*.

Examination

If the history indicates an insidious onset of elbow symptoms, and if the patient has complained of weakness and pain, the examiner may consider performing an examination of the cervical spine, which includes the upper limb peripheral joint scanning examination and myotome testing. Because of the potential referral of symptoms from the cervical spine and the necessity of differentiating nerve root symptoms from peripheral nerve lesions, the consideration to include cervical assessment is essential.

Active Movements

The examination is performed with the patient in the sitting position. As always, active movements are done first, and it is important to remember that the most painful movements are done last. In addition, structures outside the joint may affect ROM. For example, with lateral epicondylitis, the long extensors of the forearm are often found to be tight or shortened, so the position of the wrist and fingers may affect movement.

Active Movements of the Elbow Complex

- Flexion of the elbow (140° to 150°)
- Extension of the elbow (0° to 10°)
- Supination of the forearm (90°)
- Pronation of the forearm (80° to 90°)
- Combined movements (if necessary)
- Repetitive movements (if necessary)
- Sustained positions (if necessary)

Active elbow flexion is 140° to 150°. Movement is usually stopped by contact of the forearm with the muscles of the arm.

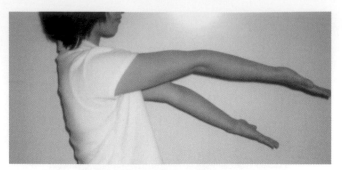

Fig. 6.14 Normal elbow hyperextension.

Active elbow extension is 0°, although up to a 10° hyperextension may be exhibited, especially in women. This hyperextension is considered normal if it is equal on both sides and there is no history of trauma. For example, collegiate and professional baseball players commonly show loss of elbow extension on the throwing arm. Normally, the movement is arrested by the locking of the olecranon process of the ulna into the olecranon fossa of the humerus. In some cases, under violent compressive loads (e.g., gymnastics, weightlifting), the olecranon process may act as a pivot, resulting in posterior dislocation of the elbow. This mechanism of injury is more likely to occur in someone with elbows that normally hyperextend (Fig. 6.14). Loss of elbow extension is a sensitive indicator of intra-articular pathology. It is the first movement lost after injury to the elbow and the first regained with healing. However, terminal flexion loss is more disabling than the same° of terminal extension loss because of the need of flexion for many activities of daily living (ADLs). Loss of either motion affects the area of reach of the hand, which in turn affects function.

Active supination should be 90° so that the palm faces up. The examiner should ensure that the shoulder is not adducted further in an attempt to give the appearance of increased supination or to compensate for a lack of sufficient supination (Fig. 6.15).[21]

For active pronation, the ROM is approximately the same (80° to 90°) so that the palm faces down. The examiner should be sure that the patient does not abduct the shoulder in an attempt to increase the amount of pronation or to compensate for a lack of sufficient pronation.[21] However, for both supination and pronation, only about 75° of movement occurs in the forearm articulations. The remaining 15° is the result of wrist action.

If, in the history, the patient has complained that combined movements, repetitive movements, or sustained positions cause pain, these specific movements should be included in the active movement assessment. If the patient has difficulty or cannot complete a movement, but it is pain-free, the examiner must consider a severe injury to the contractile tissue (rupture) or a neurological injury, and further testing is necessary.

In some cases, the examiner may want to determine whether muscles crossing the elbow are tight. If the muscles are tight, the end feel will be a muscle stretch, and ROM at one of the joints that the muscle passes over will be restricted (usually the joint that is the last to be stretched). If the muscle is normal, the end feel will be the normal joint tissue stretch end feel and the ROM will be normal. To test biceps length (Fig. 6.16A and B), the patient is placed in supine with the shoulder to be tested off the edge of the bed. The shoulder is passively extended to end range and then the elbow is extended.[22] Normally, elbow extension should be the same as that seen with active movement.

To test triceps length (Fig. 6.16C), the patient is placed in sitting position. The examiner passively forward flexes the arm to full elevation while the elbow is in extension. The elbow is then passively flexed.[18] Normally, elbow flexion should be similar to that seen with active movement.

To test the length of the long wrist extensors (as one would want to do with lateral epicondylitis), the examiner passively flexes the fingers and then flexes the wrist (Fig. 6.16D and E).[22] Normally, wrist flexion and finger flexion should be the same as found with active movement.

To test the length of the long wrist flexors, the examiner passively extends the fingers and then the wrist (Fig. 6.16F and G).[22] Normally, wrist extension and finger extension should be the same as that found with active movement.

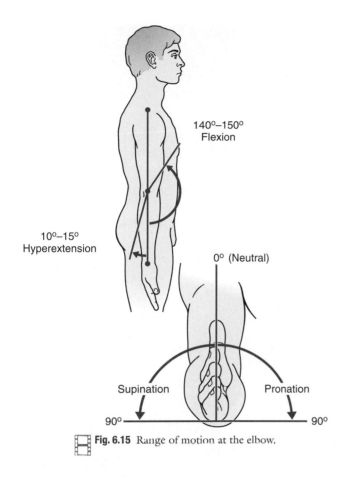

Fig. 6.15 Range of motion at the elbow.

Passive Movements

If the ROM is full on active movements, overpressure may be gently applied to test the end feel in each direction. If the movement is not full, passive movements should be carried out carefully to test the end feel and to test for a capsular pattern.

> **Passive Movements of the Elbow Complex and Normal End Feel**
>
> - Elbow flexion (tissue approximation)
> - Elbow extension (bone-to-bone)
> - Forearm supination (tissue stretch)
> - Forearm pronation (tissue stretch)

It should be pointed out that although tissue approximation is the normal end feel of elbow flexion, in thin patients the end feel may be bone to bone as a result of the coronoid process hitting in the coronoid fossa. Likewise, in thin individuals, pronation may be bone to bone.

In addition to the end feel tests during passive movements, the examiner should note whether a capsular pattern is present. The capsular pattern for the elbow complex as a whole is more limitation of flexion than extension.

Resisted Isometric Movements

For proper testing of the muscles of the elbow complex, the movement must be resisted and isometric. Muscle flexion power around the elbow is greatest in the range of 90° to 110° with the forearm supinated. At 45° and 135°, flexion power is only 75% of maximum.[18] Isometrically, research shows that men are two times stronger than women at the elbow; extension is 60% of flexion, and pronation is about 85% of supination.[23] To perform the resisted isometric tests, the patient is seated (Fig. 6.17). If the examiner finds that a particular movement or movements cause pain, Table 6.1 can be used to help differentiate the cause. Carrying out wrist extension and flexion is also necessary, because a large number of muscles (Fig. 6.18) act over the wrist as well as the elbow.

> **Resisted Isometric Movements of the Elbow Complex**
>
> - Elbow flexion
> - Elbow extension
> - Supination
> - Pronation
> - Wrist flexion
> - Wrist extension

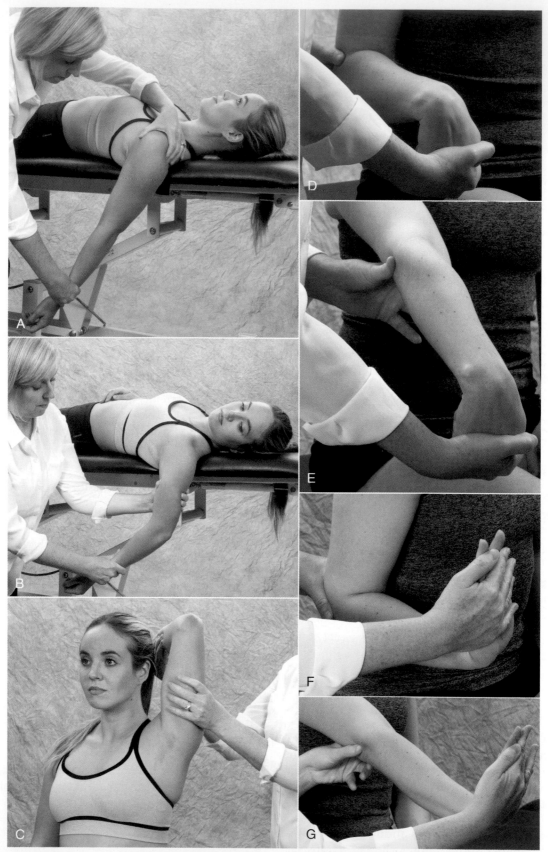

Fig. 6.16 Testing length of tight muscles. (A) Biceps—method 1: hyperextend shoulder with elbow straight. (B) Biceps—method 2: first hyperextend shoulder with elbow bent, then extend elbow to tightness and measure elbow flexion. (C) Triceps. (D) Long wrist extensors—start position. (E) Long wrist extensors—end position. (F) Long wrist flexors—start position. (G) Long wrist flexors—end position.

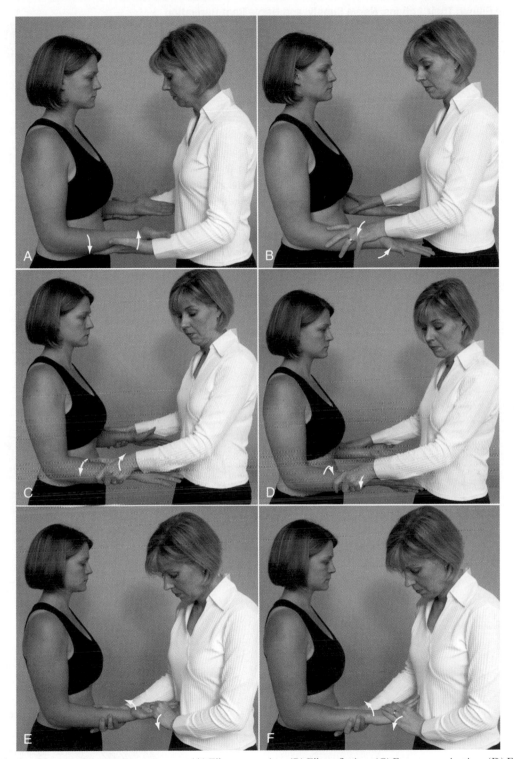

Fig. 6.17 Positioning for resisted isometric movements. (A) Elbow extension. (B) Elbow flexion. (C) Forearm supination. (D) Forearm pronation. (E) Wrist flexion. (F) Wrist extension.

If, in the history, the patient has complained that combined movements under load, repetitive movements under load, or sustained positions under load cause pain, the examiner should carefully examine these resisted isometric movements and positions as well, but only after the basic movements have been tested isometrically. For example, the biceps is a strong supinator and flexor of the elbow, but its ability to generate force depends on the position of the elbow. The biceps play a greater role in elbow flexion when the forearm is supinated than when it is pronated. At 90° of elbow flexion, biceps makes the greatest contribution

TABLE **6.1**

Muscles About the Elbow: Their Actions, Nerve Supply, and Nerve Root Derivation

Action	Muscles Acting	Nerve Supply	Nerve Root Derivation
Flexion of elbow	1. Brachialis	Musculocutaneous	C5, C6, (C7)
	2. Biceps brachii	Musculocutaneous	C5, C6
	3. Brachioradialis	Radial	C5, C6, (C7)
	4. Pronator teres	Median	C6, C7
	5. Flexor carpi ulnaris	Ulnar	C7, C8
Extension of elbow	1. Triceps	Radial	C6-C8
	2. Anconeus	Radial	C7, C8, (T1)
Supination of forearm	1. Supinator	Posterior interosseous (radial)	C5, C6
	2. Biceps brachii	Musculocutaneous	C5, C6
Pronation of forearm	1. Pronator quadratus	Anterior interosseous (median)	C8, T1
	2. Pronator teres	Median	C6, C7
	3. Flexor carpi radialis	Median	C6, C7
Flexion of wrist	1. Flexor carpi radialis	Median	C6, C7
	2. Flexor carpi ulnaris	Ulnar	C7, C8
Extension of wrist	1. Extensor carpi radialis longus	Radial	C6, C7
	2. Extensor carpi radialis brevis	Posterior interosseous (radial)	C7, C8
	3. Extensor carpi ulnaris	Posterior interosseous (radial)	C7, C8

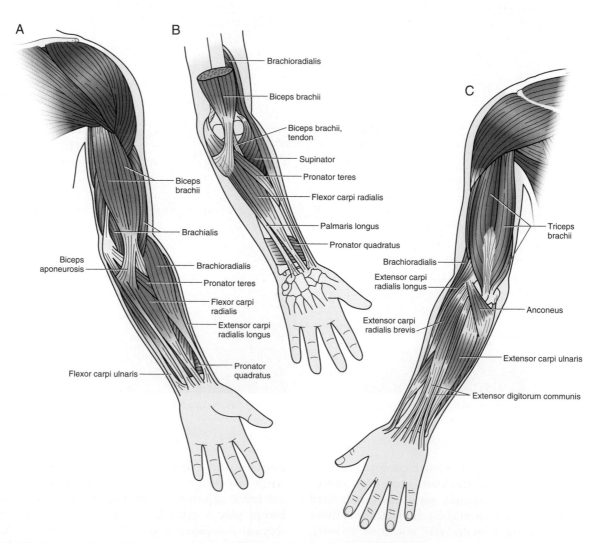

Fig. 6.18 Muscles about the elbow. (A) Anterior muscles. (B) Deep anterior muscles. (C) Posterior muscles.

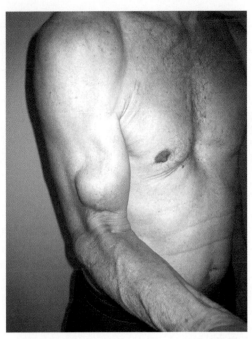

Fig. 6.19 Popeye sign. Rupture of the biceps tendon at the distal attachment at the elbow. (From Boileau P, Chuinard C: Arthroscopic biceps tenotomy: technique and results, *Oper Tech Sports Med* 15(1):35–44, 2007.)

to supination.[24] If the history indicates that concentric, eccentric, or econcentric movements have caused symptoms, these movements should also be tested with load or no load, as required.

If the resisted isometric contraction is weak and pain-free, the examiner must consider a major injury to the contractile tissue (third-degree strain) or neurological injury. For example, weakness of elbow flexion and supination may occur with a rupture of the distal biceps tendon, especially if these findings follow a sudden sharp pain in the antecubital fossa when an extension force is applied to the flexing elbow.[24] This may result in a **Popeye sign** indicating either a tear of the long head of the biceps at the shoulder or a tear of the distal end of the biceps tendon at the elbow (Fig. 6.19). If there is no history of trauma, the most likely cause is neurological, either a nerve root or peripheral nerve lesion. By selectively testing the muscles and sensory distribution (Table 6.2) and by having a knowledge of nerve compression sites (see the "Reflexes and Cutaneous Distribution" section), the examiner should be able to determine the neurological tissue injured and where the injury has occurred.

Functional Assessment

When assessing the elbow, it is important to remember that the elbow is the middle portion of an integral upper limb kinetic chain. It allows the hand to be positioned in space, helps stabilize the upper extremity for power and detailed work activities, and provides power to the arm for lifting activities.[25] Motion in the

elbow allows the hand to be positioned so that daily functions can be performed easily. Thus, functionally, the elbow is often one important part of a functional assessment that may also involve the shoulder and/or hand. This is especially true for athletes who put several joints in the kinetic chain under stress at the same time. For example, the Kerlan-Jobe Orthopaedic Clinic (KJOC) shoulder and elbow score (see eTool 5.12) is designed to look at a functional outcome score involving the shoulder and elbow in overhead athletes.[26,27]

The full range of elbow movements is not necessary to perform these activities; most ADLs are performed at between 30° and 130° of flexion and between 50° of pronation and 50° of supination (Figs. 6.20 and 6.21).[28] To reach the head, approximately 140° of flexion is needed. The activities of combing or washing the hair, reaching a back zipper, and walking with crutches require a greater ROM. Activities such as pouring fluid, drinking from a container, cutting with a knife, reading a newspaper, and using a screwdriver require an adequate range of supination and pronation. Figs. 6.22 and 6.23 show the ROM or arc of movement necessary to do certain activities or the ROM needed to touch parts of the body. Examiners must remember that elbow injuries may preclude lifting objects as light as a cup of coffee, owing to lifting mechanics. Because of the length of the lever arm of the forearm when the elbow is at 90°, loads at the hand are magnified tenfold at the elbow.[29] eTool 6.1 is a numerical scoring assessment form that can be used to assess the elbow and includes an important functional component. Table 6.3 demonstrates functional tests of strength for the elbow. Some of the more common functional elbow outcome measures include the **Mayo Elbow Performance Score** (eTool 6.2),[28,30] the **Disabilities of the Arm, Shoulder and Hand (DASH)** questionnaire (see eTool 5.7),[28,31] **QuickDASH**, and the **American Shoulder and Elbow Surgeons—Elbow (ASES-E)** scoring system (eTool 6.3).[32,33] Longo et al.,[34] Evans et al.,[35] and Nuttal et al.[28] outline many of the functional elbow questionnaires available.

Special Tests

An examiner should perform only those special tests that have relevance or will help to confirm the diagnosis. If the history has not indicated any trauma or repetitive movement that could be associated with problems, the examiner, depending on the age of the patient, may want to include some of the nerve root compression tests (see Chapter 3) to rule out the possibility of referred symptoms from the cervical spine or the possibility of a double crush injury.

For the reader who would like to review them, the reliability, validity, specificity, sensitivity, and odds ratios of some of the special tests used in the elbow joint are available in eAppendix 6.1.

TABLE **6.2**

Nerve Injuries About the Elbow

Nerve	Motor Loss	Sensory Loss	Functional Loss
Median nerve (C6 to C8, T1)	Pronator teres Flexor carpi radialis Palmaris longus Flexor digitorum superficialis Flexor pollicis longus Lateral half of flexor digitorum profundus Pronator quadratus Thenar eminence Lateral two lumbricals	Palmar aspect of hand with thumb, index, middle, and lateral half of ring finger Dorsal aspect of distal third of index, middle, and lateral half of ring finger	Pronation weak or lost Weak wrist flexion and abduction Radial deviation at wrist lost Inability to oppose or flex thumb Weak thumb abduction Weak grip Weak or no pinch (ape hand deformity)
Anterior interosseous nerve (branch of median nerve)	Flexor pollicis longus Lateral half of flexor digitorum profundus Pronator quadratus Thenar eminence Lateral two lumbricals	None	Pronation weak especially at 90° elbow flexion Weak opposition and flexion of thumb Weak finger flexion Weak pinch (no tip-to-tip)
Ulnar nerve (C7 to C8, T1)	Flexor carpi ulnaris Medial half of flexor digitorum profundus Palmaris brevis Hypothenar eminence Adductor pollicis Medial two lumbricals All interossei	Dorsal and palmar aspect of little and medial half of ring finger	Weak wrist flexion Loss of ulnar deviation at wrist Loss of distal flexion of little finger Loss of abduction and adduction of fingers Inability to extend second and third phalanges of little and ring fingers (benediction hand deformity) Loss of thumb adduction
Radial nerve (C5 to C8, T1)	Anconeus Brachioradialis Extensor carpi radialis longus and brevis Extensor digitorum Extensor pollicis longus and brevis Abductor pollicis longus Extensor carpi ulnaris Extensor indices Extensor digiti minimi	Dorsum of hand (lateral two-thirds) Dorsum and lateral aspect of thumb Proximal two-thirds of dorsum of index, middle, and half ring finger	Loss of supination Loss of wrist extension (wrist drop) Inability to grasp Inability to stabilize wrist Loss of finger extension Inability to abduct thumb
Posterior interosseous nerve (branch of radial nerve)	Extensor carpi radialis brevis Extensor digitorum Extensor pollicis longus and brevis Abductor pollicis longus Extensor carpi ulnaris Extensor indices Extensor digiti minimi	None	Weak wrist extension Weak finger extension Difficulty stabilizing wrist Difficulty with grasp Inability to abduct thumb

Tests for Ligamentous Instability

These tests are designed to test for valgus and varus instability in the elbow.

⚠ *Chair (or Standing) Push-up Test.*[3,6,8,16,38,39] The patient is seated in a chair with arms so elbows are at 90°. The patient is asked to push up on the arms of the chair with his or her hands with the forearms fully supinated into standing. If the patient's symptoms are reproduced, the patient becomes apprehensive, medial pain results, *or* the radial head dislocates as the elbow extends,[4] the test is positive for injury to the posterior band of the medial collateral ligament and there is posterolateral rotary instability (Fig. 6.24). If lateral pain results, it is probably lateral epicondylitis.[1]

⚠ *Gravity-Assisted Varus Stress Test.*[39,40] The patient stands with the arm abducted to 90° and in neutral rotation (i.e., thumb facing forward). The patient is then asked to flex and extend the elbow while keeping the hand and shoulder in the same position (Fig. 6.25). The

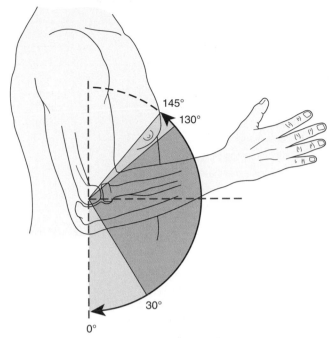

Fig. 6.20 Normal range of elbow flexion is approximately 0° to 145°. However, the functional arc of motion is somewhat less, and most activities can be performed with flexion of 30° to 130°. (Redrawn from Regan WD, Morrey BF: The physical examination of the elbow. In Morrey BF, editor: *The elbow and its disorders,* ed 2, Philadelphia, 1993, WB Saunders, p 81.)

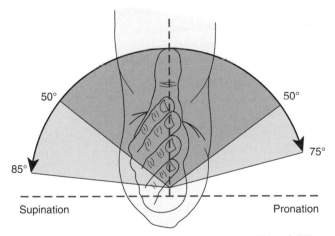

Fig. 6.21 Pronation and supination motions average 75° and 85°, respectively. Most activities of daily living, however, can be accomplished with 50° of each motion. (Redrawn from Regan WD, Morrey BF: The physical examination of the elbow. In Morrey BF, editor: *The elbow and its disorders,* ed 2, Philadelphia, 1993, WB Saunders, p 81.)

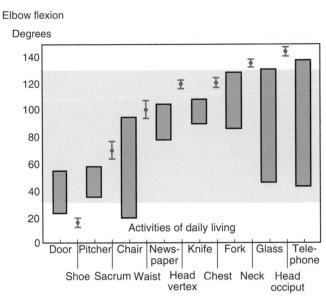

Fig. 6.22 The arc and position of elbow flexion required to accomplish fifteen daily activities. Most of these activities are accomplished within a flexion range of 30° to 130°. (Modified from Morrey BF, Askew LJ, Chao EY: A biomechanical study of normal functional elbow motion, *J Bone Joint Surg Am* 63:873, 1981.)

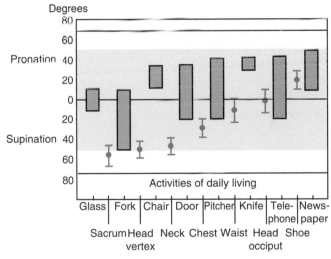

Fig. 6.23 Fifteen activities of daily living accomplished with pronation and supination of up to 50° each. (Modified from Morrey BF, Askew LJ, Chao EY: A biomechanical study of normal functional elbow motion, *J Bone Joint Surg Am* 63:874, 1981.)

position allows gravity to apply a varus stress while doing the elbow flexion and extension motion.

☑ *Lateral Pivot Shift Test of the Elbow.*[3,41] The patient lies supine with the arm to be tested overhead. The examiner grasps the patient's wrist and forearm with the elbow extended and the forearm fully supinated.[42] The patient's elbow is then flexed while a valgus stress and axial compression is applied to the elbow while maintaining supination (Fig. 6.26). This causes the radius (and ulna) to sublux off the humerus leading to a prominent radial head posterolaterally

and a dimple between the radial head and capitellum.[3,42] If the examiner continues flexing the elbow, at about 40° to 70° (see Fig. 6.26B), there is a sudden reduction (clunk) of the joint, which can be palpated, and a dimple in the skin can be seen proximal to the radial head.[4,43] If the patient is unconscious, subluxation and a clunk on reduction when the elbow is extended may occur, but these symptoms seldom present in the conscious patient who will show apprehension.[4]

☑ *Ligamentous Valgus Instability Test.* To test for valgus instability, the patient's arm is stabilized with one of the examiner's hands at the elbow and the other hand placed above the patient's wrist. An abduction or valgus force at

Key Tests Performed at the Elbow Depending on Suspected Pathology[a,36,37]

- **For ligamentous instability:**
  - ❷ Capitellar shear test
  - ⚠ Chair push-up test
  - ⚠ Gravity-assisted varus stress test
  - ✅ Lateral pivot shift test of the elbow
  - ✅ Ligamentous valgus instability test
  - ✅ Ligamentous varus instability test
  - ⚠ Milking maneuver
  - ✅ Moving valgus stress test
  - ❷ Posterolateral rotary apprehension test
  - ✅ Posterolateral rotary drawer test
  - ⚠ Prone push-up test
  - ⚠ Tabletop relocation test
  - ⚠ Trochlear shear test
  - ⚠ Valgus extension overload test
- **For muscle injury (third-degree strain):**
  - ⚠ Biceps crease interval
  - ⚠ Biceps squeeze test
  - ✅ Bicipital aponeurosis flex test
  - ⚠ Flexion initiation test
  - ⚠ Hook (distal biceps) test
  - ✅ Popeye sign (distal biceps tendon)
  - ⚠ Supination-pronation test
  - ⚠ TILT sign
  - ✅ Triceps squeeze test
- **For epicondylitis (epicondylalgia):**
  - ⚠ Cozen's test
  - ❷ Golfer's elbow test
  - ⚠ Kaplan's test
  - ❷ Maudsley's (middle finger) test
  - ⚠ Mill's test
  - ❷ Polk's test
  - ⚠ Tennis elbow shear test
- **For plica:**
  - ❷ Extension-supination plica test
  - ❷ Flexion-pronation plica test
  - ❷ Plica impingement test
  - ❷ Radiohumeral joint plica compression test
- **For posterior impingement:**
  - ⚠ Arm bar (posteromedial impingement) test
  - ❷ Extension impingement test
- **For joint dysfunction:**
  - ❷ Active radiocapitellar compression test
  - ❷ Radiohumeral joint distraction test
- **For fractures:**
  - ⚠ East Riding Elbow Rule (ER²)
  - ⚠ Montreal children's elbow test
- **For neurological dysfunction:**
  - ❷ Elbow pressure test
  - ❷ Maudsley's (middle finger) test
  - ✅ Pinch grip test (anterior interosseous branch of median nerve)
  - ⚠ Rule-of-nine (RON) test
  - ⚠ Scratch collapse test for ulnar, median and/or radial nerve
  - ❷ Test for pronator teres syndrome
  - ⚠ Tinel sign at elbow (ulnar nerve)
  - ✅ Wadsworth elbow flexion test (ulnar nerve)
  - ❷ Wartenberg sign

[a]See Chapter 1, Key for Classifying Special Tests.

TABLE 6.3

Functional Testing of the Elbow

Starting Position	Action	Functional Test[a]
Sitting	Bring hand to mouth lifting weight (elbow flexion)	Lift 2.3 kg–2.7 kg: Functional Lift 1.4 kg–1.8 kg: Functionally fair Lift 0.5 kg–0.9 kg: Functionally poor Lift 0 kg: Nonfunctional
Standing 90 cm from wall, leaning against wall	Push arms straight (elbow extension)	5–6 Repetitions: Functional 3–4 Repetitions: Functionally fair 1–2 Repetitions: Functionally poor 0 Repetitions: Nonfunctional
Standing, facing closed door	Open door starting with palm down (supination of arm)	5–6 Repetitions: Functional 3–4 Repetitions: Functionally fair 1–2 Repetitions: Functionally poor 0 Repetitions: Nonfunctional
Standing, facing closed door	Open door starting with palm up (pronation of arm)	5–6 Repetitions: Functional 3–4 Repetitions: Functionally fair 1–2 Repetitions: Functionally poor 0 Repetitions: Nonfunctional

[a]Younger patients should be able to lift more (2.7 kg to 4.5 kg) more often (6 to 10 repetitions). With age, weight and repetitions decrease.
Data from Palmer ML, Epler M: *Clinical assessment procedures in physical therapy*, Philadelphia, 1990, JB Lippincott, pp 109–111.

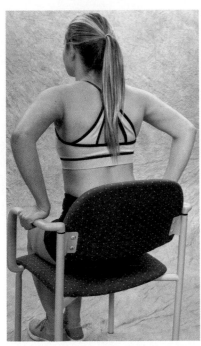

Fig. 6.24 Chair (or standing) push-up test for medial collateral ligament of the elbow.

the distal forearm is applied to test the medial collateral ligament (valgus instability) while the ligament is palpated (Fig. 6.27B).[3] Regan and Morrey advocate doing the valgus stress test with the humerus in full lateral rotation.[29] The examiner should note any laxity, decreased mobility, or altered pain that may be present compared with the uninvolved elbow. Anakwenze et al.[4] advocated doing the test in maximum medial rotation of the shoulder and elbow in pronation, thus locking the radiocapitellar joint. A valgus stress is then applied with the patient's elbow in 30° of flexion, as this is the position in which the medial (radial) collateral ligament is the primary stabilizer to valgus instability (Fig. 6.28).

✓ *Ligamentous Varus Instability Test.* With the patient's elbow slightly flexed (20° to 30°) and stabilized with the examiner's hand, an adduction or varus force is applied by the examiner to the distal forearm to test the lateral collateral ligament (varus instability) while the ligament is palpated (Fig. 6.27A). Normally, the examiner feels the ligament tense when stress is applied. Regan and Morrey advocated doing the varus stress test with the humerus in full medial rotation.[29] The examiner applies the force several times with increasing pressure while noting any alteration in pain or ROM. If excessive laxity is found when doing the test, or a soft end feel is felt, it indicates injury to the ligament (1°, 2°, or 3° sprain) and may, especially with a 3° sprain, indicate posterolateral joint instability. Posterolateral elbow instability is the most common pattern of elbow instability in which there is displacement of the ulna (accompanied by the radius) on the humerus, so the ulna supinates or laterally rotates away from or off the trochlea.[41]

⚠ *Milking Maneuver.*[3,8,16,41] The patient sits with the elbow flexed to 90° or more and the forearm

supinated. The examiner grasps the patient's thumb under the forearm and pulls it, imparting a valgus stress to the elbow (Fig. 6.29A). Reproduction of symptoms (i.e., apprehension, medial joint pain, gapping, instability) indicates a positive test and a partial tear of the medial collateral ligament. It has been suggested that abducting and laterally rotating the shoulder with the elbow at 70° and a valgus stress applied by the examiner's thumb can be used as part of the milking motion (Fig. 6.29B).[39,44]

✓ *Moving Valgus Stress Test.*[1,3,8,9,45] The patient lies supine or stands with the arm abducted and laterally rotated, and elbow flexed fully. While maintaining a valgus stress and holding the thumb, the examiner quickly extends the patient's elbow. Reproduction of the patient's pain between 120° and 70° indicates a positive test and a partial tear of the medial collateral ligament (Fig. 6.30). If medial pain is present at ≤60° (usually 10° to 40°), it is called the **Trochlear Shear Test** ⚠ and suggests a posteromedial chondral erosion.[46] If pain is more lateral and occurs around 45°, it is called the **Capitellar Shear Test**[46] ❓ and may indicate fracture of the capitellum.

❓ *Posterolateral Rotary Apprehension Test.*[3,41–43,47,48] The patient lies supine with the arm to be tested overhead. The elbow is supinated at the wrist, and a valgus stress is applied to the elbow while the examiner flexes the elbow. This movement (between 20° and 30° flexion) and stress cause the patient to be apprehensive that the elbow will dislocate, while reproducing the patient's symptoms. In the conscious patient, actual subluxation is rare. A positive test indicates posterolateral rotary instability (Fig. 6.31).

✓ *Posterolateral Rotary Drawer Test.*[3] The patient lies supine with the arm to be tested overhead and the elbow flexed 40° to 90° while the examiner holds the forearm and arm similar to doing a drawer test at the knee. As the humerus is stabilized and the radius and ulna are pushed posterolaterally, the radius and ulna rotate around an intact medial collateral ligament indicating a tear of the lateral collateral ligament and posterolateral instability at the elbow (Fig. 6.32). Apprehension or the presence of a dimple is considered to be a positive test.

⚠ *Prone Push-up Test.*[1,8,16,39,49] The patient, in prone, attempts to do a push-up starting with the elbow at 90° and arms abducted to more than shoulder width—first with the forearms maximally supinated (Fig. 6.33A) and then repeated with the forearms maximally pronated (Fig. 6.33B). The test is positive for posterolateral rotary instability if symptoms (i.e., pain and apprehension) occur when the forearms are supinated but not pronated. If pain occurs when the test is done with the forearm pronated, the pain most likely indicates lateral epicondylitis.[1]

⚠ *Tabletop Relocation Test.*[1,4,8,38,39,50] The patient is asked to stand in front of a table with the symptomatic arm placed over the table's lateral edge and elbow

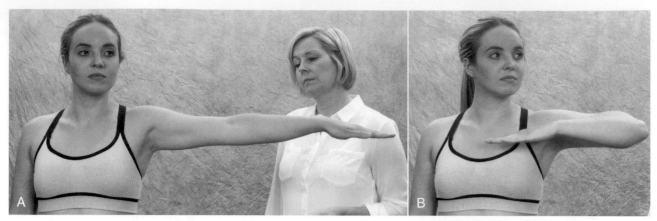

Fig. 6.25 Gravity-assisted varus stress test. (A) In extension. (B) In flexion.

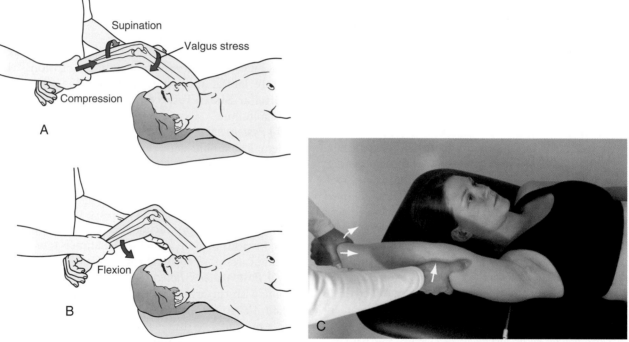

Fig. 6.26 Posterolateral pivot-shift apprehension test of the elbow. (A) The patient lies supine with the arm overhead. A mild supination force is applied to the forearm at the wrist. The patient's elbow is then flexed while a valgus stress and compression is applied to the elbow. (B) If the examiner continues flexing the elbow, at about 40° to 70°, a subluxation and a clunk on reduction when the elbow is extended may occur, but usually only in the unconscious patient. (C) Actual test with elbow positioned to resemble knee.

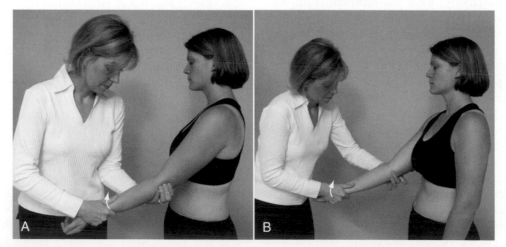

Fig. 6.27 Testing the collateral ligaments of the elbow. (A) Lateral collateral ligament. (B) Medial collateral ligament. Note the elbow is slightly flexed or "unlocked."

extended. First, the patient is asked to do a push-up (down phase) with the elbow pointed laterally maintaining the arm in supination by flexing the elbow (Fig. 6.34A). If the patient has posterolateral rotary instability, pain and apprehension will occur near 40° of flexion. Secondly, the movement is repeated while the examiner places a thumb over the radial head, pushing against the head to stabilize it, and when the patient does the "down" movement, the pain and apprehension are relieved (Fig. 6.34B). If the examiner removes the thumb, the pain and apprehension will return.

⚠ *Valgus Extension Overload Test.*[7] The patient is in standing. The examiner grasps the patient's test arm at the wrist with the patient's elbow in 20° to 30° of flexion. With the examiner's other hand at the patient's

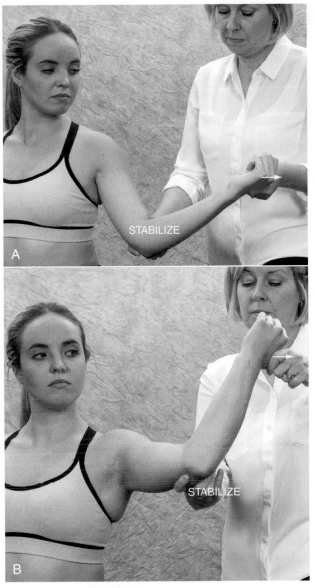

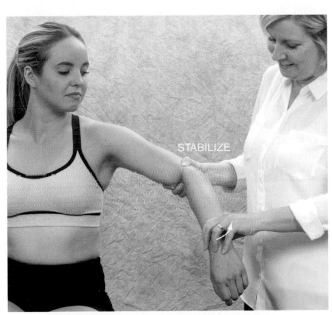

Fig. 6.28 Modified ligamentous valgus instability test.

Fig. 6.29 (A) Milking maneuver to test medial collateral ligament. (B) Modified milking maneuver in abduction.

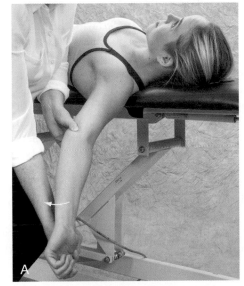

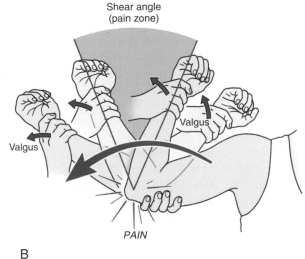

Fig. 6.30 (A) Moving valgus stress test in supine. (B) Schematic representation of the moving valgus stress test. The shear range refers to the range of motion that causes pain while the elbow is being extended with valgus stress. The shear angle is the point that causes maximum pain. (Used with permission of the Mayo Foundation for Medical Education and Research. All rights reserved.)

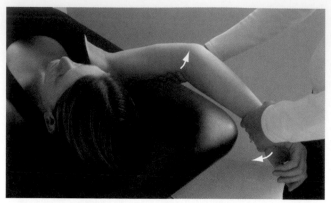

Fig. 6.31 Posterolateral rotary apprehension test.

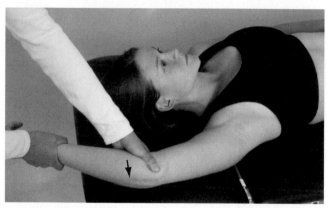

Fig. 6.32 Posterolateral rotary drawer test.

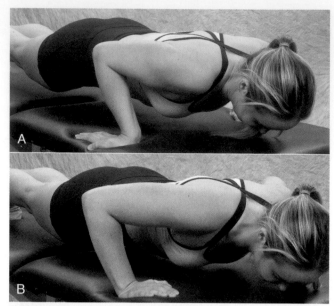

Fig. 6.33 Prone push-up test. (A) With forearms supinated. (B) With forearms pronated.

elbow, the examiner forcibly extends the elbow while applying a valgus stress (Fig. 6.35). The test is designed to replicate the symptoms caused by valgus extension overload stress (see Fig. 6.5) on the ulnar collateral ligament. Pain may also indicate pinching or entrapment of soft tissue in the posterior and medial olecranon fossa of the humerus.[8]

Tests for Muscle Injury (Third-Degree Strain)

Biceps Crease Interval.[8,51,52] The patient is seated. Starting with the patient's unaffected arm in flexion, the examiner extends the patient's elbow fully. A line is drawn across the flexion crease in the antecubital fossa. The examiner then lightly strokes the contour of the distal biceps back and forth along a central longitudinal line until the examiner can identify the point at which the distal biceps begins to turn most sharply toward the antecubital fossa and marks a transverse line at the distal cusp of the biceps. The examiner then measures the distance between the two transverse lines (Fig. 6.36). The distance is recorded as the **biceps crease interval (BCI)** and both arms are compared. The BCI is normally 4.8 cm ± 0.6 cm for both the dominant and non-dominant arm. If the BCI

is greater than 6.0 cm or the biceps crease ratio between the two arms is greater than 1.2, the test is positive for a distal biceps tendon rupture. The **biceps crease ratio** is a comparison of the BCI between the injured and non-injured arm.[8,52]

Biceps Squeeze Test.[49,53] The patient's elbow is flexed to between 60° and 80°. The examiner then squeezes the biceps muscle belly (Fig. 6.37). If the biceps tendon is ruptured, the patient's forearm will not supinate.

Bicipital Aponeurosis Flex Test.[54] When evaluating for the possibility of a distal biceps tendon rupture, it is also necessary to check for the integrity of the bicipital aponeurosis (Fig. 6.38). In some cases, the distal biceps may tear (3° strain) and the aponeurosis may remain intact, which may "hide" the rupture by supporting the biceps and allowing the biceps to have the appearance of normal length.[54] The test is performed with the patient seated with the elbow flexed to 75°. The patient is then asked to "make a fist" and actively flex the fingers and wrist with the forearm supinated (the examiner may offer isometric resistance to the patient's forearm with one hand). This action tenses the aponeurosis. While the aponeurosis is under tension, the examiner palpates the medial, lateral, then central parts of the antecubital fossa. If the bicipital aponeurosis is intact, a sharp thin edge of the aponeurosis will be felt **medially** (see Fig. 6.38). On the lateral side, the biceps tendon may be felt as a thick round structure. If the tendon has ruptured, there is a palpable gap between the two structures. Both arms should be compared.

Flexion Initiation Test.[52,55] The patient is seated with the test arm extended, forearm supinated, and holding a

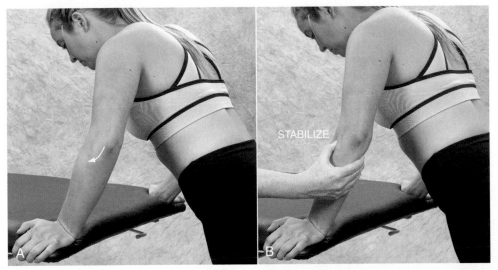

Fig. 6.34 Tabletop relocation test. (A) Push-up position as patient goes down with elbows pointed laterally. (B) Examiner stabilizes radial head as patient does "down" portion of push-up.

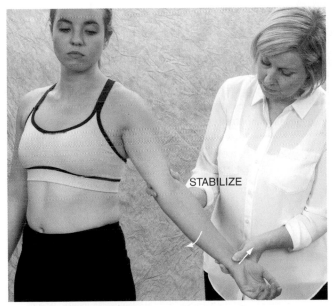

Fig. 6.35 Valgus extension overload test.

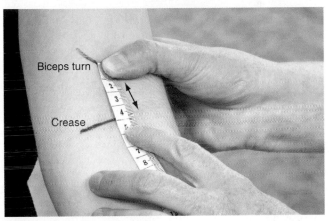

Fig. 6.36 Determining the biceps crease interval *(double-headed arrow)*.

4.5-kg (10-lb) weight in the hand. The patient is then asked to flex the elbow (Fig. 6.39). An inability to flex the elbow fully is a positive test for rupture of the distal biceps tendon.

Hook Test.[16,49,56] The patient abducts the shoulder to 90° with the elbow flexed to 90° and the arm supinated so that the thumb faces up (Fig. 6.40). The patient is then asked to actively supinate the forearm against resistance of the examiner. With the index finger of the other hand, the examiner attempts to "hook" underneath the biceps tendon, "hooking" from **lateral to medial**. If no cordlike structure can be hooked, the test is positive for a rupture of the distal biceps. Devereaux et al.[51] advocated

doing the **hook test**, the **passive forearm pronation test** and the **BCI test** in sequence, along with a thorough history, to confirm the distal biceps tendon rupture (3° strain).

Supination-Pronation Test.[8,16,57] The patient stands with both shoulders abducted to 90° and elbows flexed to 60° to 70°. The examiner stands in front of the patient and observes the contour of the biceps bilaterally as the patient actively supinates and pronates the forearm. If the distal biceps is intact, the shape of the biceps noticeably changes as the patient supinates (biceps moves proximally or rises; Fig. 6.41A) and pronates (biceps moves distally or falls; Fig. 6.41B). Lack of migration of the biceps muscle indicates a positive test. It has also been found that the same results occur if the test is done passively.[1,8,51] It may then be called the **passive forearm pronation test**[58], with the biceps muscle showing little movement on supination or pronation if the distal biceps tendon is ruptured.

⚠ *TILT Sign.*[59] The patient is seated with the elbow flexed to 90°. The examiner firmly palpates the radial tuberosity (where biceps inserts into the radius) just distal to the radial head (about 2.5 cm [1 inch] distal) while supinating and pronating the forearm. In reality, the tuberosity can only be palpated when the arm is in full pronation (Fig. 6.42). A positive test is indicated by tenderness over the lateral (radial) aspect of the tuberosity

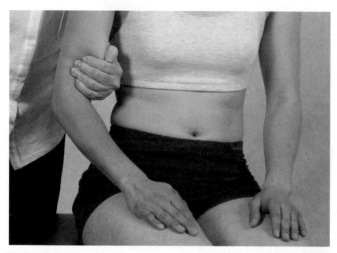

Fig. 6.37 Biceps squeeze test. Muscle is squeezed near insertion at the elbow.

(TILT) only in full arm pronation. This indicates a partial tear of the distal biceps tendon.

☑ *Triceps Squeeze Test.*[1,8] The patient is seated with the test forearm hanging comfortably over the back of the chair and the elbow is flexed to 90°. (The test may also be done in prone with the elbow at the edge of the examining table and forearm hanging down.) The examiner then squeezes the triceps muscle with both hands (Fig. 6.43). If the arm extends slightly without pain, the triceps tendon inserting into the olecranon is normal. If the movement is painful, the triceps tendon is partially torn. If no movement occurs or the movement is not painful, the triceps tendon is torn (3° strain).

Tests for Epicondylitis

Chronic overuse injury to the extensor (tennis elbow, or lateral epicondylitis) or flexor (golfer's elbow, or medial epicondylitis) tendons at the elbow result from repeated microtrauma to the tendon, leading to disruption and degeneration of the tendon's internal structure (tendinosus).[60] It appears to be a degenerative condition in which the tendon has failed to heal properly after repetitive microtrauma injury.[60,61]

When testing for epicondylitis, whether medial or lateral, the examiner must keep in mind that there may be referral of pain from the cervical spine or peripheral nerve involvement.[62] If the epicondylitis does not respond to treatment, the examiner would be wise to check for neurological pathology.

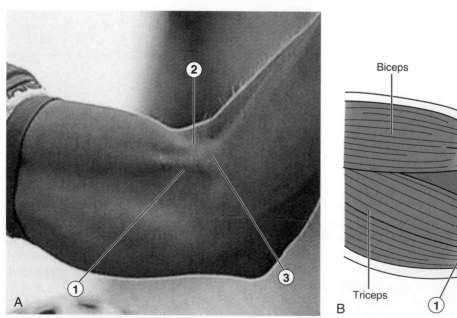

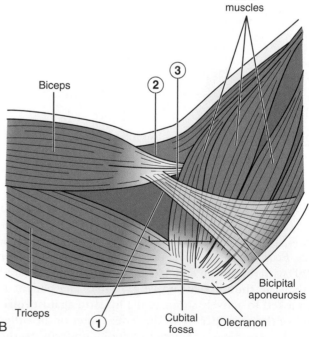

Fig. 6.38 Bicipital aponeurosis flex test. Photograph (A) and anatomic drawing (B) of the left elbow demonstrating the positioning for the bicipital aponeurosis flex test. *Location 1:* where the examiner palpates the sharp medial edge of the bicipital aponeurosis; *Location 2:* where the examiner palpates the rounder lateral edge of the distal biceps tendon; *Location 3:* the palpable "valley" or gap between the diverging medial edge of the distal biceps tendon and lateral edge of the bicipital aponeurosis. (Modified from El Maraghy A, Devereaux M: The bicipital aponeurosis flex test: evaluating the integrity of the bicipital aponeurosis and its implications for treatment of distal biceps tendon ruptures, *J Shoulder Elbow Surg* 22:908–914, 2013.)

⚠ *Kaplan's Test.*[8,63,64] The patient is seated with the elbow flexed to 90°. The examiner tests grip strength using a hand dynamometer and records the result. The examiner then applies a tennis elbow brace snugly about 3 cm (1.1 inch) below the elbow joint line over the bulk of the extensor muscles in the forearm (Fig. 6.44) and grip strength testing is repeated. If the grip strength increases with the brace and pain is decreased, the test is positive for lateral epicondylitis. Dorf et al.[64] noted that, in the presence of lateral epicondylitis, grip strength was less if tested

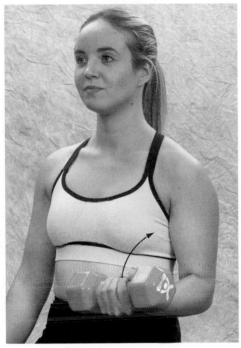

Fig. 6.39 Flexion initiation test.

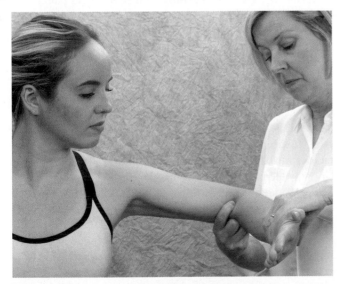

⊞ **Fig. 6.40** Hook test for distal biceps rupture at the elbow. It is important to do the "hook" from lateral to medial.

in extension as opposed to 90° flexion. Normally, there should be no difference in strength between extension and 90° flexion.

⚠ *Lateral Epicondylitis (Tennis Elbow or Cozen's) Test (Method 1).*[8] The patient's elbow is stabilized by the examiner's thumb, which rests on the patient's lateral epicondyle (Fig. 6.45). The patient is then asked to actively make a fist, pronate the forearm, and radially deviate and extend the wrist while the examiner resists the motion. A sudden severe pain in the area of the lateral epicondyle of the humerus is a positive sign. The epicondyle may be palpated to indicate the origin of the pain.

⚠ *Lateral Epicondylitis (Tennis Elbow or Mill's) Test (Method 2).*[8] While palpating the lateral epicondyle, the examiner passively pronates the patient's forearm, flexes the wrist fully, and extends the elbow (see Fig. 6.45). Pain over the lateral epicondyle of the humerus indicates a positive test. This maneuver also puts stress on the radial nerve and, in the presence of compression of the radial nerve, causes symptoms similar to those of tennis elbow.[65] Electrodiagnostic studies help differentiate the two conditions.

❓ *Lateral Epicondylitis (Tennis Elbow, Maudsley's or Middle Finger) Test (Method 3).*[8] The examiner resists extension of the third digit of the hand distal to the proximal interphalangeal joint, stressing the extensor digitorum muscle and tendon (see Fig. 6.45). A positive test is indicated by pain over the lateral epicondyle of the humerus. This same test may indicate a problem with the posterior interosseous nerve (**posterior interosseous nerve syndrome**), a branch of the radial nerve. In this case, there is weakness (but no pain) of resisted forearm supination and extension of the middle finger.

❓ *Medial Epicondylitis (Golfer's Elbow) Test.*[8] While the examiner palpates the patient's medial epicondyle, the patient's forearm is passively supinated and the examiner extends the elbow and wrist. A positive sign is indicated by pain over the medial epicondyle of the humerus.

❓ *Polk's Test.*[8,63,66] The patient is seated with the elbow flexed. The patient is asked to lift a 2.5-kg (5.5-lb) weight. The test is done in two parts. First, the patient attempts to lift the weight with the forearm pronated by flexing the elbow (Fig. 6.46A). If the pain is in the area of the lateral epicondyle, it is suggestive of lateral epicondylitis. Next, the patient is asked to repeat the movement with the forearm supinated (Fig. 6.46B). If the pain is in the area of the medial epicondyle, it is suggestive of medial epicondylitis. These motions also test the biceps (see flexion initiation test) and brachialis muscles.

⚠ *Tennis Elbow Shear Test (Medial Test).*[67] The patient is in sitting or standing. The examiner asks the patient to fully flex the elbow, pronate the forearm, and flex the wrist (Fig. 6.47A). The examiner then uses both hands to resist the patient's wrist flexion and forearm pronation while the patient quickly extends the elbow as if throwing a pitch

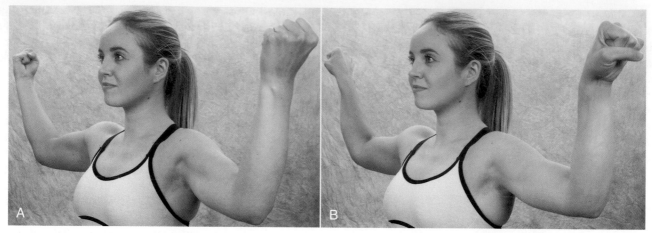

Fig. 6.41 Supination-pronation test for biceps. The examiner is watching the contour of the biceps change as the patient's forearm moves from supination to pronation. (A) In supination. (B) In pronation.

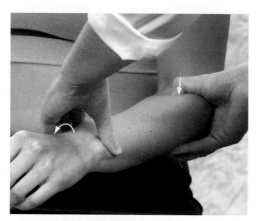

Fig. 6.42 TILT sign.

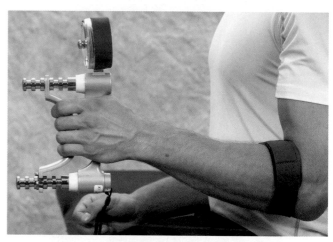

Fig. 6.44 Kaplan's test with tennis elbow splint.

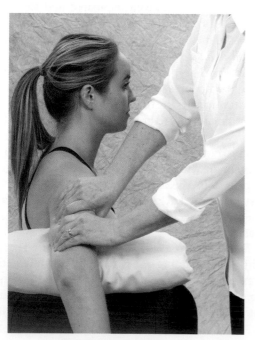

Fig. 6.43 Triceps squeeze test.

(Fig. 6.47B). The test is positive if it reproduces pain in the medial elbow at the common flexor-pronator origin.

Tests for Plica

? *Plica Impingement Test.*[49,68]   The examiner applies a valgus load to the elbow while passively flexing the elbow with the forearm held in pronation (Fig. 6.48A). Pain or snapping (more important) between 90° and 110° of flexion indicates a positive test for the anterior radiocapitellar plica (**flexion-pronation plica test ?**). To test the posterior radiocapitellar plica, the examiner applies a valgus load to the elbow while passively extending the elbow with the forearm held in supination (Fig. 6.48B; **extension-supination plica test ?**). Pain or a snap would indicate a positive test indicating a possible plica problem or radiocapitellar chondromalacia. If just pain occurs, it is unlikely to be a plica.

? *Radiohumeral Joint Plica Compression Test.*[69] The examiner stands facing the standing patient. The patient places his or her hands on the examiner's waist while the examiner holds and supports the patient's forearm with the palms while the patient's elbows are at 90°. The

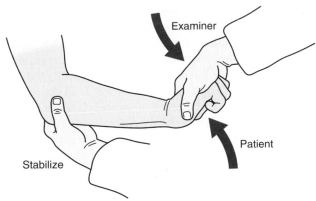

METHOD 1 Cozen's Test (Active)

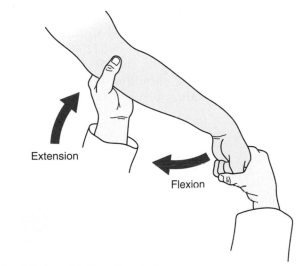

METHOD 2 Mill's Test (Passive)

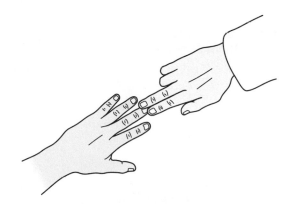

METHOD 3 Maudsley's (Middle Finger) Test (Active)

Fig. 6.45 Tests for tennis elbow.

examiner palpates the radiohumeral joint line using the index fingers. The examiner, while palpating and maintaining compression over the lateral joint line, moves the patient's elbows from 90° to full extension (Fig. 6.49). At the end of extension, the examiner determines how much pain was elicited and whether the palpating digit was able to remain within the radiohumeral indentation. If pain results and the finger is pushed out of the indentation, a possible hypertrophic plica is indicated.

Tests for Posterior Impingement

⚠ *Arm Bar Test (Posteromedial Impingement Test).*[8,9,49] The patient, while standing, rests the hand of the test arm on the examiner's shoulder with the elbow extended and shoulder medially rotated (thumb pointing downwards). The examiner pulls down on the olecranon or distal humerus to simulate forced extension (Fig. 6.50). Reproduction of pain, especially posteromedially along the olecranon, is a positive test for posterior impingement. The patient may also lack full extension.

❓ *Extension Impingement Test.*[8,9,49] The examiner applies a valgus stress to the elbow while quickly extending and flexing the elbow from 20° to 30° flexion to terminal extension repeatedly (Fig. 6.51). The test is then repeated without the valgus stress while the posteromedial olecranon is palpated for tenderness. This palpation differentiates tender impingement due to instability from pain over the medial olecranon without instability.

Tests for Joint Dysfunction

If the patient complains of pain in the elbow joint, especially on elbow movement, the examiner can perform two tests to differentiate between the radiohumeral and ulnohumeral joints. **To test the radiohumeral joint** ❓, the examiner positions the elbow joint at the position of pain and then radially deviates the wrist to compress the radial head against the humerus. The production of pain would be considered a positive test. **To test the ulnohumeral joint** ❓, the examiner again positions the elbow joint at the position of discomfort and causes compression of the ulnohumeral joint by ulnar deviation at the wrist.[13] Again, pain indicates a positive test.

❓ *Active Radiocapitellar Compression Test.*[9,49] The examiner applies an axial (compression) load to the elbow in full extension. It has been advocated by some that the compression should be applied with the elbow in 90° flexion as the radiocapitalar joint is in closed pack in 90° flexion, which causes more compression. The patient is asked to actively supinate and pronate the forearm while the compression is maintained (Fig. 6.52). Pain in the lateral compartment of the elbow is a positive test and may indicate an osteochondritis dissecans of the capitellum.

❓ *Radiohumeral Joint Distraction Test.*[69] The patient and examiner are in standing. The examiner grasps the patient's distal radius with a lumbrical grip (see Fig. 7.53F) and allows the dorsum of the patient's hand to rest under the examiner's forearm while the examiner stabilizes the distal humerus with the other hand (Fig. 6.53). The patient is then asked to extend the wrist against the examiner's forearm, applying as much resistance as possible. The examiner notes the amount of force generated and asks whether the patient's pain was produced and rates the pain intensity on a scale of 1 to 10. The patient relaxes and the examiner then applies and maintains a traction force along the line of the radius. While maintaining the traction, the patient is again asked to extend the wrist against the examiner's forearm. The examiner then again asks about pain generation and grades the pain. If the pain is less on the second test, the test indicates a possible loose body in the joint.

Tests for Fractures

⚠ *East Riding Elbow Rule (ER²).*[70] This test is designed to rule out the need for x-rays following an elbow injury. The test has two parts. For *Test One*, both of the patient's arms are exposed and the patient is asked to fully extend both elbows and the examiner compares the amount of extension in the two limbs. *Test Two* involves looking for swelling/bruising, and palpating the anterior forearm, the radial head, the medial epicondyle, and olecranon for tenderness. If any of the signs from the two tests are positive, the patient should be x-rayed.

⚠ *Montreal Children's Elbow Test (Index Test).*[71,72] The test is designed for children 18 years of age or under and involves two parts. For *Test One* (elbow extension test), both of the patient's arms are exposed and supinated. The patient is asked to extend the elbows fully and the examiner compares the amount of extension. *Test Two* involves palpating five areas of the elbow for tenderness: supracondylar region of the distal humerus, medial epicondyle, lateral condyle, olecranon, and radial head. The test is considered positive for possible fracture if any one or more of the six components of the two tests are positive. If all six components were negative, the test is negative. X-rays would be used to confirm if any of the six components are positive. The authors felt that if all six parts were negative, then a fracture was unlikely and x-rays would not be needed.

Tests for Neurological Dysfunction

☑ *Elbow Flexion Test (Wadsworth Elbow Flexion Test).* The patient is asked to fully flex the elbow with extension of the wrist and shoulder girdle abduction (90°) and depression,[73,74] and to hold this position for 3 to 5 minutes (Fig. 6.54). Ochi et al.[75] modified the test to include medial rotation of the shoulder, calling it the **shoulder internal (medial) rotation elbow flexion test** ⚠ (Fig. 6.55). They

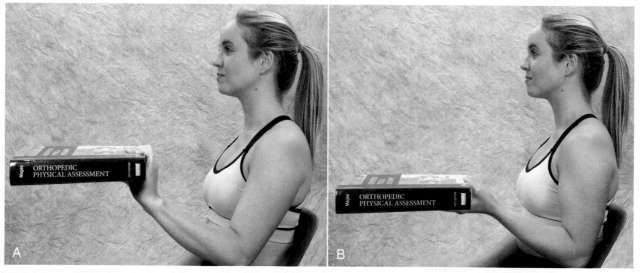

Fig. 6.46 Polk's test. (A) For lateral epicondylitis: with forearm pronated (palm down). (B) For medial epicondylitis: with forearm supinated (palm up).

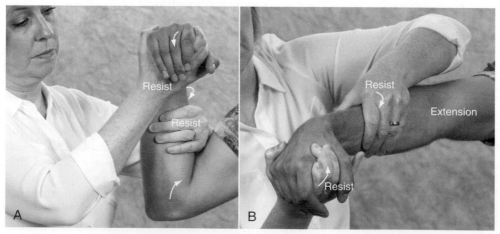

Fig. 6.47 Tennis elbow shear test. (A) Start position. (B) End position.

state that symptoms should develop in less than 5 seconds. Tingling or paresthesia in the ulnar nerve distribution of the forearm and hand indicates a positive test. The test helps to determine whether a cubital tunnel (ulnar nerve) syndrome is present (Fig. 6.56).

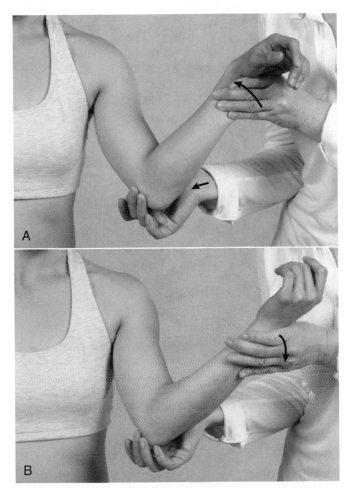

Fig. 6.48 Plica impingement tests. (A) Flexion-pronation plica testto test the anterior radiocapitellar plica. (B) Extension-supination plica test to test the posterior radiocapitellar plica.

The test may be modified by the examiner applying direct pressure over the ulnar nerve with the index and middle finger between the posteromedial olecranon and the medial epicondyle[76] (**elbow flexion compression test** or **cubital tunnel compression test** ⚠; Fig. 6.57).

❓ *Elbow Pressure Test.*[77] The examiner holds the patient's arm in 20° flexion with forearm supinated. The examiner then applies external pressure just proximal to the cubital tunnel for 60 seconds. A positive test is indicated by presence of worsening of numbness or paresthesia in the ulnar nerve distribution.

❓ *Maudsley's Test (Middle Finger Test).*[8] See Tests for Epicondylitis.

✓ *Pinch Grip Test.* The patient is asked to pinch the tips of the index finger and thumb together. Normally, there should be a tip-to-tip pinch ("OK" sign). If the patient is unable to pinch tip-to-tip and instead has an abnormal pulp-to-pulp pinch of the index finger and thumb, this is a positive sign for pathology to the anterior interosseous nerve, which is a branch of the median nerve (Fig. 6.58). This finding may indicate an entrapment of the anterior interosseous nerve as it passes between the two heads of the pronator teres muscle.[78] If there is hyperextension of the metacarpophalangeal joint of the thumb (**Jeanne sign**) when attempting the tip-to-tip test, it is an indication of loss of use of the adductor pollicis muscle which is supplied by the ulnar nerve.

⚠ *Rule-of-Nine (RON) Test.*[1,79-82] The test involves constructing nine equal size circles (or squares) on the anterior aspect of the forearm at the elbow (Fig. 6.59) and noting those circles where tenderness is elicited. Equal-size circles are drawn from the elbow crease and based on the width of the patient's fully extended elbow and fully supinated forearm; the distal extent of the circles is determined so that there are three rows and three columns of circles. The posterior interosseous nerve travels through the lateral column and the medial nerve passes

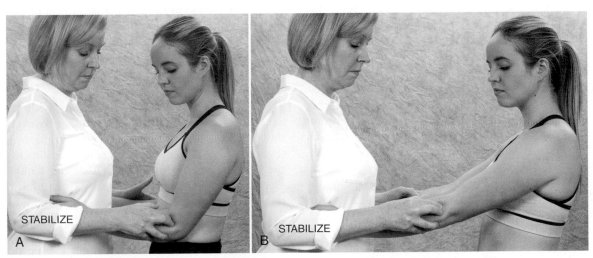

Fig. 6.49 Radiohumeral joint plica compression test. (A) In flexion. (B) In extension.

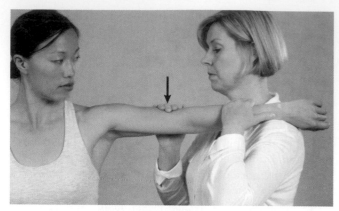

Fig. 6.50 Arm bar test for posterior impingement.

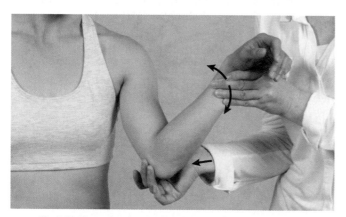

Fig. 6.51 Extension impingement test. Valgus stress shown.

through the middle column. No nerve passes through the medial column. If one palpates along the medial pathway of the median nerve, reproduction of pain or paresthesia within 30 seconds of compression indicates a positive test for **pronator syndrome**. The test is then called the **pronator compression test** ❓.[1]

⚠️ *Scratch Collapse Test for the Radial Nerve.*[83] The patient is in sitting with the upper arm by the side, elbow flexed to 90°, and the forearm and wrist in neutral. The examiner faces the patient, and applies an isometric force to resist the patient who attempts to do wrist extension and thumb/index finger extension (Fig. 6.60A). The amount of resistance by the examiner is just enough to "balance" the contractions of the patient. The patient then relaxes while the examiner strokes or scratches where the radial nerve moves from the posterior to the anterior compartment at the lateral elbow as it passes through the lateral intermuscular septum or fascia (see RON test) (Fig. 6.60B). Following the stroking, the examiner quickly tests the patient's wrist extension and thumb/index finger extension isometric strength again. If they are weak, it is a positive sign of radial neuropathy.

⚠️ *Scratch Collapse Test for the Ulnar and Median Nerves (MacKinnon's Scratch Collapse Test).*[16,84–86] The patient stands with the elbows flexed to 90° by the side (i.e., the shoulders in neutral at the side of the body and forearms and wrists in neutral), fingers in full extension, and the

patient's back not leaning against anything. The patient is asked to laterally rotate and abduct the forearms against isometric resistance provided by the examiner, which is a balanced force; the patient then relaxes (Fig. 6.61). The examiner then scratches along the course of the ulnar nerve at the elbow or anywhere along its path and then asks the patient to again resist the movement against isometric resistance for at least 2 to 3 seconds. If the patient shows weakness on the second isometric lateral rotation movement on the affected side, the test is considered positive for an ulnar nerve neuropathy.[87,88] It is important that the patient keep the elbows tight against the sides. If the patient starts to abduct the arms, the patient is trying too hard or the resisting force by the examiner is too great.[84,89]

A similar test may be used to test the median nerve in the forearm, especially if **anterior interosseous nerve syndrome, pronator syndrome,** or **carpal tunnel syndrome** are suspected.[86,90] In this case, the stroking is over the median nerve distribution. Davidge et al.[84] put forth the idea of a **"hierarchical" scratch collapse test**. The idea of the test was to try to determine where the nerve was compromised. For example, the ulnar nerve may be compromised in the cubital tunnel, when passing through flexor carpi ulnaris, in Guyon canal (antebrachial fascia), in the hand (deep motor branch of the ulnar nerve), in the Arcade of Struthers, at the brachial plexus (thoracic outlet), and parascapular muscles. If the examiner did the test at each site and sprayed ethyl chloride (i.e., freeze spray) over each site after finding a positive test, the test at that position would become negative. By testing each site, the examiner could determine where the problem is.

❓ *Test for Pronator Teres Syndrome.*[29] The patient sits with the elbow flexed to 90°. The examiner strongly resists pronation as the elbow is extended. Tingling or paresthesia in the median nerve distribution in the forearm and hand indicates a positive test.

⚠️ *Tinel Sign (at the Elbow).* The area of the ulnar nerve in the groove (between the olecranon process and medial epicondyle) is tapped. A positive sign is indicated by a tingling sensation in the ulnar distribution of the forearm and hand distal to the point of compression of the nerve (Fig. 6.62). The test indicates the point of regeneration of the sensory fibers of a nerve. The most distal point at which the patient feels the abnormal sensation represents the limit of nerve regeneration.

❓ *Wartenberg Sign.* The patient sits with his or her hands resting on the table. The examiner passively spreads the fingers apart and asks the patient to bring them together (i.e., adduct them) again. Inability to squeeze the little finger to the remainder of the hand indicates a positive test for ulnar neuropathy or cervical myelopathy.[29,87] As a modification, if the patient holds the fingers extended and adducted, and the little finger (i.e., fifth digit) spontaneously abducts due to weakness of the intrinsic muscle, it is called the **finger escape sign** and is associated with cervical myelopathy.[91]

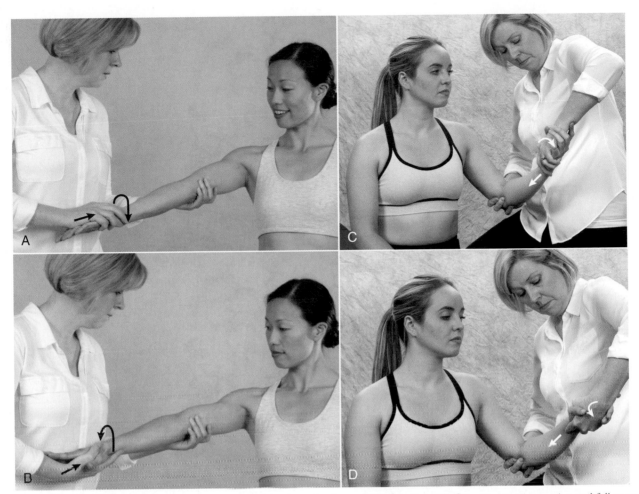

Fig. 6.52 Active radiocapitellar compression test. (A) Compression in supination and full extension. (B) Compression in pronation and full extension. (C) Compression in supination and 90° flexion. (D) Compression in pronation and 90° flexion.

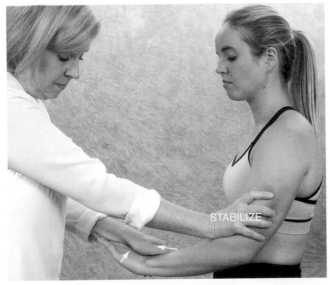

Fig. 6.53 Radiohumeral joint distraction test. The examiner stabilizes the humerus with the right hand while applying traction with the left hand. The patient pushes up into the examiner's arm.

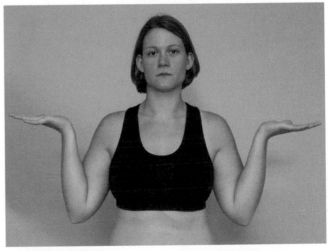

Fig. 6.54 Elbow flexion test for ulnar nerve pathology.

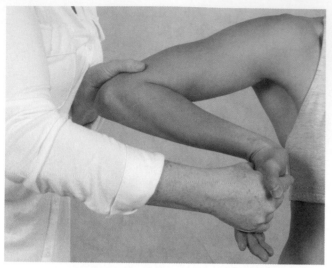

Fig. 6.55 Shoulder medial rotation elbow flexion test. Medial rotation of the shoulder, maximum elbow flexion, maximum forearm supination, and maximum wrist extension.

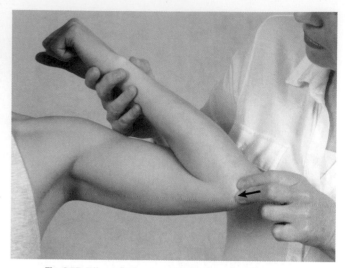

Fig. 6.57 Elbow flexion compression test for ulnar nerve.

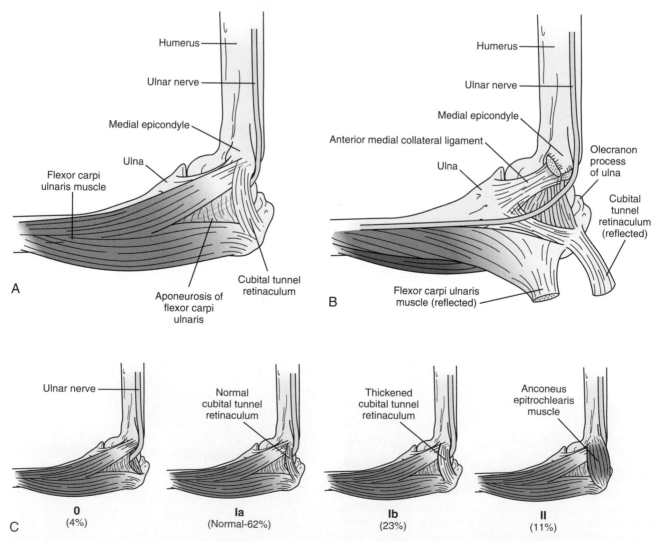

Fig. 6.56 Cubital tunnel. (A) Aponeurosis of flexor carpi ulnaris and retinaculum of cubital tunnel. (B) Aponeurosis and retinaculum reflected. Floor of tunnel formed by posterior and transverse components of medial collateral ligament and joint capsule. (C) Types of carpal tunnel. *0,* No retinaculum; *Ia,* normal retinaculum (CTR); *Ib,* thickened retinaculum; *II,* retinaculum replaced by muscle (i.e., anconeus epitrochlearis/accessory anconeus). (Redrawn from O'Driscoll SW, Horii E, Carmichael SW, Morrey BF: The cubital tunnel and ulnar neuropathy, *J Bone Joint Surg Br* 73(4):613–617, 1991.)

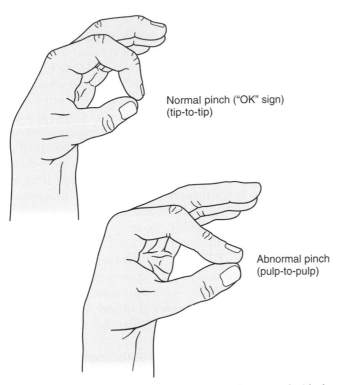

Normal pinch ("OK" sign)
(tip-to-tip)

Abnormal pinch
(pulp-to-pulp)

Fig. 6.58 Normal tip-to-tip pinch ("OK" sign) compared with the abnormal pulp-to-pulp pinch seen in anterior interosseous nerve syndrome.

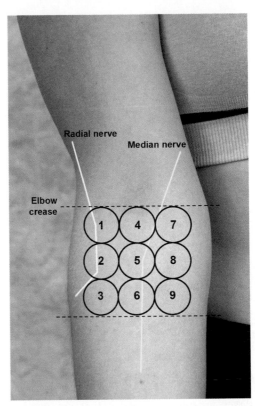

Fig. 6.59 Rule-of-nine test. Note pathway of radial (posterior interosseous) nerve and median nerve.

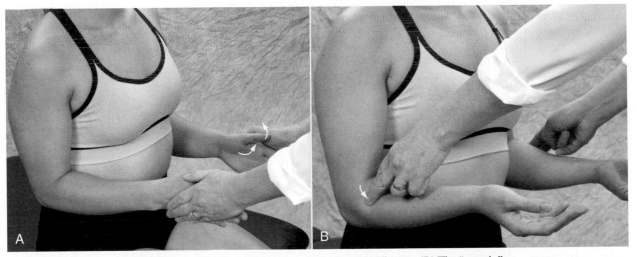

Fig. 6.60 Scratch collapse test for the radial nerve. (A) The test. (B) The "scratch."

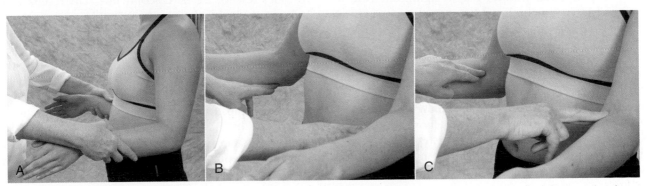

Fig. 6.61 Isometric scratch collapse test for the ulnar and median nerves. (A) The test—isometric lateral rotation. (B) Scratch along the ulnar nerve distribution. (C) Scratch along median nerve distribution.

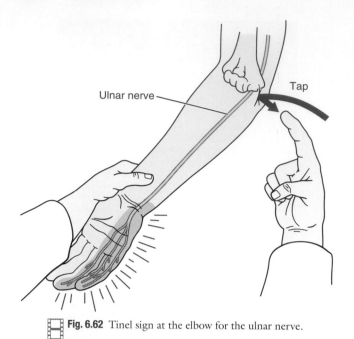

Fig. 6.62 Tinel sign at the elbow for the ulnar nerve.

Ulnar nerve

Tap

Reflexes and Cutaneous Distribution

The reflexes around the elbow that are often checked (Fig. 6.63) include the biceps (C5–C6), brachioradialis (C5–C6), and triceps (C7–C8). The examiner should also assess the dermatomes around the elbow and the cutaneous distribution of the various nerves, noting any differences (Figs. 6.64 and 6.65). When looking at the dermatomes, the examiner should realize there is a great deal of variability in the distribution patterns. Except for the T2 dermatome, which commonly ends at the elbow, all other dermatomes extend distally to the forearm, wrist, and hand; therefore, the elbow cannot be looked at in isolation when viewing dermatomes. Similarly, the peripheral nerves extend into the forearm, wrist, and hand, and so testing for sensory loss must involve the whole upper limb, not just the elbow. Pain may be referred to the elbow and surrounding tissues from the neck (often mimicking tennis elbow), the shoulder, or the wrist (Fig. 6.66; Table 6.4).

In the extremities, the neurological tissues (nerve roots and peripheral nerves) play a significant role in function. Injury, pinching, or stress to these structures can have dire consequences functionally for the patient. The next section is a review of the peripheral nerves and how and where they may be traumatized around the elbow.

Peripheral Nerve Injuries Around the Elbow[92–94]

Median Nerve (C6–C8, T1). In the elbow region, the median nerve proper can be injured by trauma (e.g., lacerations, fractures, dislocations), by systemic disease, and especially by compression and/or traction.[94–96]

The median nerve may also be pinched or compressed above the elbow as it passes under the **ligament of Struthers,** an anomalous structure found in approximately 1% of the population (Fig. 6.67).[97] The ligament runs from an abnormal spur on the shaft of the humerus to the medial epicondyle of the humerus. Because the brachial artery sometimes accompanies the nerve through this tunnel, it may also be compressed, resulting in possible vascular as well as neurological symptoms. In this case, the neurological involvement would include weakness of the pronator teres muscle and of those muscles affected by the pronator syndrome (see later discussion). The condition may also be called the **humerus supracondylar process syndrome.** Pressure in the ligament of Struthers area leads to motor loss (see Table 6.2) and sensory loss (see Fig. 7.123) of the median nerve. Initially, the patient complains of pain and paresthesia in the elbow and forearm; abnormality of motor function is secondary. With time, however, motor function is also affected, with wrist and finger flexion as well as thumb movements being most affected.

A second area of compression of the median nerve as it passes through the elbow occurs where it passes through the two heads of pronator teres (**pronator syndrome or proximal median nerve entrapment**).[80] In this case, the pronator teres remains normal, but the other muscles supplied by the median nerve (see Table 6.2) are affected, as is its sensory distribution. Pronation is possible, but weakness is evident as pronation is loaded. If the elbow is flexed to 90° and pronation is tested, noticeable weakness occurs, because in this position the action of the pronator teres is minimized.

Butlers and Singer[98] reported four possible ways of eliciting median nerve symptoms if the nerve is suffering from pathology:

- Resisted pronation with elbow and wrist flexion for 30 to 60 seconds
- Resisted elbow flexion and supination
- Resisted long finger flexion at the proximal interphalangeal joint
- Direct pressure over the proximal aspect of pronator teres during pronation

It is interesting to note that one of the tests is similar to Mill's test for lateral epicondylitis. The results should be compared with the good side, and production of the patient's symptoms is considered a positive test.

Anterior Interosseous Nerve. The anterior interosseous nerve, which is a branch of the median nerve, is sometimes pinched or entrapped as it passes between the two heads of the pronator teres muscle, leading to pain and functional impairment of the flexor pollicis longus, the lateral half of the flexor digitorum profundus, and the pronator quadratus muscles. The condition is called **anterior interosseous nerve syndrome** or **Kiloh-Nevin syndrome or sign** (Fig. 6.68)[80,99–101] and is characterized by

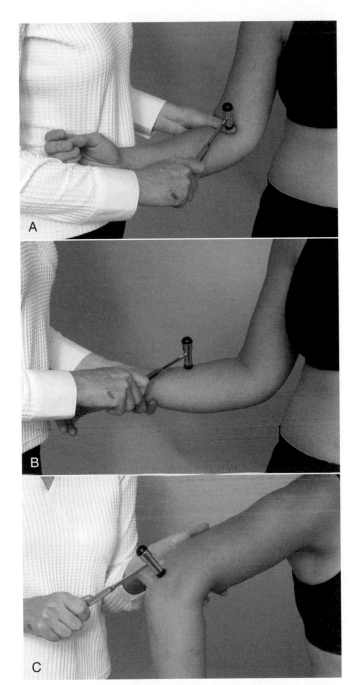

Fig. 6.63 Reflexes around the elbow. (A) Biceps (C5-6). (B) Brachioradialis (C5-6). (C) Triceps (C7-8).

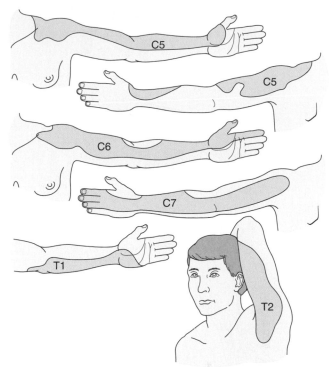

Fig. 6.64 Dermatomes around the elbow.

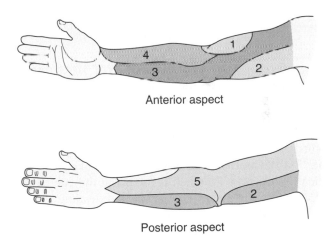

Fig. 6.65 Sensory nerve distribution around the elbow. *1,* Lower lateral cutaneous nerve of arm (radial); *2,* medial cutaneous nerve of arm; *3,* medial cutaneous nerve of forearm; *4,* lateral cutaneous nerve of forearm (musculocutaneous nerve); *5,* posterior cutaneous nerve of forearm (radial nerve).

a pinch deformity in which the patient is unable to make the **"OK" sign** with the thumb and index finger (see Fig. 6.58).[101] The deformity results from the paralysis of the flexors of the index finger and thumb. This leads to extension of the distal interphalangeal joint of the index finger and the interphalangeal joint of the thumb. The resulting pinch is pulp to pulp rather than tip to tip. It has been reported that the nerve may also be injured with a forearm fracture (Monteggia fracture).[102] With anterior interosseous syndrome, there is no sensory loss, because

the anterior interosseous nerve is a motor nerve; signs and symptoms of the condition are related to motor function.

Ulnar Nerve (C7–C8, T1). In the elbow region, the ulnar nerve is most likely to be injured, compressed, or stretched in the **cubital tunnel** (see Fig. 6.4A).[14,80,87,94,97,103–107] In fact, it is a common entrapment neuropathy, second only to carpal tunnel syndrome. The ulnar nerve may be injured or compressed as a result of swelling (e.g., trauma, pregnancy), osteophytes, arthritic diseases, trauma, or repeated microtrauma. This tunnel, which is relatively

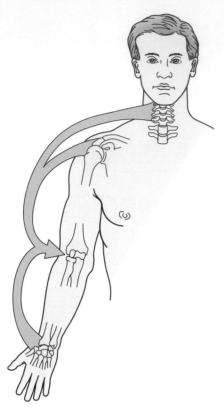

Fig. 6.66 Pain referred to the elbow. Referral is more likely from proximal areas rather than distal areas.

TABLE 6.4

Elbow Muscles and Referral of Pain

Muscles	Referral Pattern
Biceps	Upper shoulder (bicipital groove) to anterior elbow
Brachialis	Anterior arm, elbow to lateral thenar eminence
Triceps	Posterior shoulder, arm, elbow, and forearm to medial two fingers, medial epicondyle
Brachioradialis	Lateral epicondyle, lateral forearm to posterior web space between thumb and index finger
Anconeus	Lateral epicondyle area
Supinator	Lateral epicondyle and posterior web space between thumb and index finger
Pronator teres	Anterior forearm to wrist and part of anterior thumb
Extensor carpi ulnaris	Medial wrist
Extensor carpi radialis brevis	Posterior forearm to posterior wrist
Extensor carpi radialis longus	Lateral epicondyle to posterolateral wrist
Extensor indices	Posterior forearm to appropriate digit
Palmaris longus	Anterior forearm to palm
Flexor digitorum superficialis	Palm to appropriate digit
Flexor carpi ulnaris	Anteromedial wrist
Flexor carpi radialis	Anteromedial wrist

long, can compress the nerve as the nerve passes through the tunnel or between the two heads of the flexor carpi ulnaris muscle (**Osborne's band**).[84,89] Compression is altered as the elbow moves from extension (decreased) to flexion (increased), causing traction on the nerve, and is further enhanced if a significant cubitus valgus is present.[108,109] Symptoms therefore are more likely to occur when the elbow is flexed. It is usually in the cubital tunnel area that the ulnar nerve is affected, leading to tardy ulnar palsy. If the problem is the result of restriction in the cubital tunnel, direct pressure over the tunnel may reproduce or exacerbate the symptoms (see "Cubital Tunnel Compression Test").[94]

Tardy ulnar palsy implies that the symptoms of nerve injury come on long after the patient has been injured; this delayed reaction seems to be unique to the ulnar nerve. Although most common in adults, it has been reported in children, and in children the delay has been up to 29 months.[110] In adults, the possibility of a double crush injury (at cervical spine and elbow) should always be considered.

Injury to the ulnar nerve in the cubital tunnel affects the flexor carpi ulnaris and the ulnar half of the flexor digitorum profundus in the forearm, the hypothenar eminence in the hand (flexor digiti minimi, abductor digiti minimi, opponens digiti minimi, and adductor pollicis), the interossei, and the third and fourth lumbrical muscles (see Table 6.2). Commonly, patients cannot fully adduct the little finger and hold the finger

abducted and extended, because the denervated palmar interosseous muscle cannot oppose the abductor digiti minimi (see "**Wartenberg Sign**").[87] If there is loss of the hypothenar muscles and flattening of the palmar metacarpal arch, it is called **Masse's sign**. If there is an inability to flex the distal interphalangeal joints of the little and ring fingers (i.e., loss of flexor digitorum profundus), it is called **Pollock's sign**. Both indicate ulnar nerve involvement, as does clawing of the fourth and fifth digits (**benediction sign**, **preacher's sign**, or **Duchenne sign**) due to lumbrical paralysis of the fourth and fifth digits.[80,87] Although these muscles show weakness and atrophy over time, the earliest and most obvious symptoms are sensory, with pain and paresthesia in the medial elbow and forearm, and paresthesia in the ulnar sensory distribution of the hand (see Fig. 7.123).

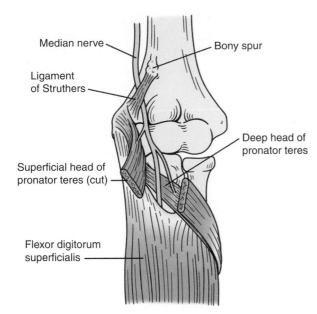

Fig. 6.67 Compression of the median nerve under ligament of Struthers and in pronator syndrome. In the pronator syndrome, the median nerve may be kinked against the flexor digitorum superficialis muscle or compressed by the forceful action or structural hypertrophy of the deep head of the pronator teres. Compression of the nerve above the elbow (ligament of Struthers) leads to weakness of the pronator teres, while this muscle is spared in the pronator syndrome, because the branches to the two heads of the pronator teres arise proximally to the muscle.

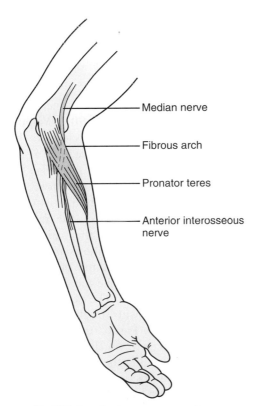

Fig. 6.68 Anterior interosseous syndrome.

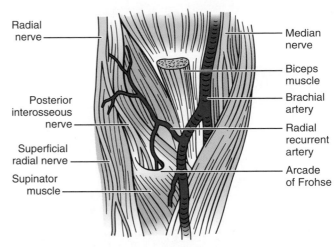

Fig. 6.69 Canal, or arcade, of Frohse.

Calfee et al.[111] recommended testing for a hypermobile ulnar nerve, which is reported to be found in over 30% of the population (**hypermobile ulnar nerve test ❓**). The patient maximally flexes the elbow with the forearm supinated. The examiner then places a finger on the proximal, posteromedial aspect of the medial epicondyle. The patient is asked to extend the elbow while the examiner holds the finger in place. If the ulnar nerve stays anterior to the examiner's finger, it is said to dislocate. If the nerve is below the examiner's finger, it is perched on the medial humeral epicondyle. If the nerve cannot be palpated, it is stable in the groove.

Radial Nerve (C5–C8, T1). The radial nerve may be injured near the elbow if there is a fracture of the shaft of the humerus. The nerve may be damaged as it winds around behind the humerus in the radial groove. Injury may occur at the time of the fracture, or the nerve may get caught in the callus of fracture healing. Because the radial nerve supplies all of the extensor muscles of the arm, only the triceps is spared with this type of injury, and even it may show some weakness. Symptoms include pain on resisted supination and pain on resisted extension of the middle finger (**Maudsley's sign**), which suggests compression of the nerve at the flexor digitorum superficialis arch.[92,112]

The major branch of the radial nerve in the forearm is the **posterior interosseous nerve,** which is given off in front of the lateral epicondyle of the humerus.[80,97,113] This branch may compress as it passes between the two heads of the supinator in the **arcade** or **canal of Frohse** (most common site for radial nerve compression[112]), a fibrous arch in the supinator muscle occurring in 30% of the population (Fig. 6.69). Compression can lead to functional involvement of the forearm extensor muscles (see Table 6.2) and functional wrist drop, and so the patient has difficulty or is unable to stabilize the wrist for proper hand function. Diagnosis of this condition is often delayed because there is no sensory deficit. Direct pressure over the supinator muscle while resisting supination may elicit weakness of supination or tenderness

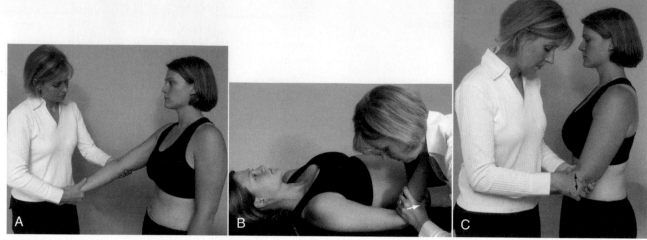

Fig. 6.70 Joint play movements of the elbow complex. (A) Radial and ulnar deviation of the ulna on the humerus. (B) Distraction of the olecranon process from the humerus. (C) Anteroposterior movement of the radius.

(**supinator compression test** ?).[94,114] This compression zone is one of five sites in the tunnel through which the radial nerve passes.[115] The nerve may also be compressed at the entrance to the radial tunnel anterior to the head of the radius, near where the nerve supplies brachioradialis and extensor carpi radialis longus (**leash of Henry**), between the ulnar half of the tendon of extensor carpi radialis brevis and its fascia, and at the distal border of supinator.[92,116,117] This condition, sometimes called **radial tunnel syndrome,** elicits pain with little muscle weakness and may mimic tennis elbow.[75,81,112,114,116,118–122] If the patient has a persistent form of tennis elbow, although radial tunnel pain is usually more distal,[114] a possible nerve lesion or cervical problem should be considered.[44,112]

A third area of pathology is compression of the superficial branch of the radial nerve as it passes under the tendon of the brachioradialis. This branch is sensory only, and the patient complains primarily of nocturnal pain along the dorsum of the wrist, thumb, and web space. Trauma, a tight cast, any swelling in the area, or forearm pronation with wrist flexion and ulnar deviation may cause the compression and produce paresthesia.[94] Direct pressure at the junction of extensor carpi radialis longus and brachioradialis may also reproduce the paresthesia or numbness.[94] The condition is referred to as **cheiralgia paresthetica** or **Wartenberg disease/sign.**[106]

Joint Play Movements

When examining the joint play movements (Fig. 6.70), the examiner must compare the injured side with the normal side.

Radial and ulnar deviations of the ulna and radius on the humerus are performed in a fashion similar to those in the collateral ligament tests but with less elbow flexion.

The examiner stabilizes the patient's elbow by holding the patient's humerus firmly and places the other hand above the patient's wrist, abducting and adducting the forearm (see Fig. 6.70A). The patient's elbow is almost straight (extended) during the movement, and the end feel should be bone-to-bone.

Joint Play Movements of the Elbow Complex

- Radial deviation of the ulna and radius on the humerus
- Ulnar deviation of the ulna and radius on the humerus
- Distraction of the olecranon from the humerus in 90° of flexion
- Anteroposterior glide of the radius on the humerus

To distract the olecranon from the humerus, the examiner flexes the patient's elbow to 90°. Wrapping both hands around the patient's forearm close to the elbow, the examiner then applies a distractive force at the elbow, ensuring that no torque is applied (see Fig. 6.70B). If the patient has a sore shoulder, counter-force should be applied with one hand around the humerus.

To test anteroposterior glide of the radius on the humerus, the examiner stabilizes the patient's forearm. The patient's arm is held between the examiner's body and arm. The examiner places the thumb of his or her hand over the anterior radial head while the flexed index finger is over the posterior radial head. The examiner then pushes the radial head posteriorly with the thumb and anteriorly with the index finger (see Fig. 6.70C). Commonly, posterior movement is easier to obtain with anterior movement in normal clients, being the result of the radial head returning to its normal position with a tissue stretch end feel. This movement must be performed with care, because it can be very painful as a result of pinching of the skin between the examiner's digits and the bone. In addition,

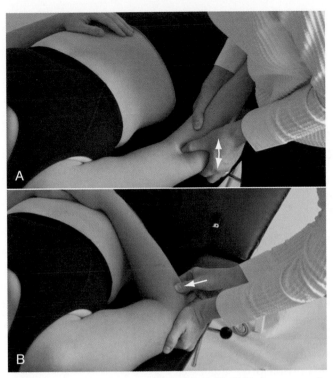

Fig. 6.71 Joint play of the head of the radius (method 2). Anteroposterior (A) and posteroanterior (B) glide of the radius.

pain may result from the force being applied even in the normal arm, so both sides must be compared.

The anterior and posterior glide of the radius may be tested in a slightly different way as well. To do anteroposterior glide of the head of the radius, the patient is placed in supine with the arm by the side. The examiner stands beside the patient, facing the patient's head, and holds the patient's arm slightly flexed by holding the hand between the examiner's thorax and elbow. The examiner places the thumbs over the head of the radius and carefully applies an anteroposterior pressure to the head of the radius, feeling the amount of movement and end feel. To do posteroanterior glide, the patient is in supine lying with the arm at the side and the hand resting on the stomach. The examiner places the thumbs over the posterior aspect of the radial head and carefully applies a posteroanterior pressure (Fig. 6.71).

Palpation

With the patient's arm relaxed, the examiner begins palpation on the anterior aspect of the elbow and moves to the medial aspect, the lateral aspect, and finally the posterior aspect (Fig. 6.72). The patient may sit or lie supine, whichever is more comfortable. The joint line is located about 2 cm below an imaginary line joining the two epicondyles.[6]

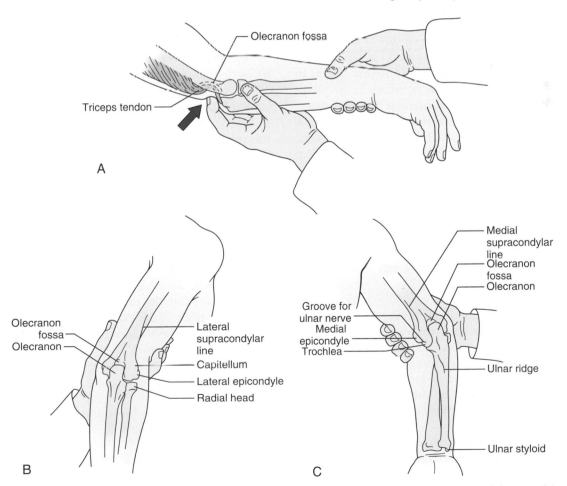

Fig. 6.72 Palpation around the elbow. (A) Olecranon fossa. (B) Posterolateral aspect of the elbow. (C) Posteromedial aspect of the elbow.

The examiner is looking for any tenderness, abnormality, change in temperature or in texture of the tissues, or abnormal bumps. As with all palpation, the injured side must be compared with the normal or uninjured side.

Anterior Aspect

Cubital Fossa. The fossa is bound by the pronator teres muscle medially, the brachioradialis muscle laterally, and an imaginary line joining the two epicondyles superiorly. Within the fossa, the biceps tendon, brachialis, and brachial artery may be palpated. After crossing the elbow joint, the **brachial artery** divides into two branches, the radial artery and the ulnar artery. The examiner must be aware of the brachial artery, because it has the potential to be injured as a result of severe trauma at the elbow (e.g., fracture, dislocation). Trauma to this area may lead to compartment syndromes, such as **Volkmann ischemic contracture.** The median and musculocutaneous nerves are also found in the fossa, but they are not palpable. Pressure on the median nerve may cause symptoms in its cutaneous distribution.

Coronoid Process, Head of Radius, and Radial Tuberosity. Within the cubital fossa, if the examiner palpates carefully so as not to hurt the patient, the coronoid process of the ulna and the head of the radius may be palpated. Palpation of the radial head is facilitated by supination and pronation of the forearm. The examiner may palpate the head of the radius from the posterior aspect at the same time by placing the fingers over the head on the posterior aspect and the thumb over it on the anterior aspect. In addition to the muscles previously mentioned, the biceps and brachialis muscles may be palpated for potential abnormality. If, on the anterior aspect, the examiner moves just distally to the radial head (about 1 inch [2.5 cm]), the radial tuberosity may be palpated when the arm is fully pronated. If the arm is then supinated, the tuberosity will disappear.[59] If the patient is complaining of pain and/or tenderness along the anteromedial humerus, radius, or ulna, especially after repeated stress, the examiner should palpate the specific area. This tenderness or pain may be due to periostitis resulting in **humeral shin splints** or "**forearm splints,**" which may be precursors to stress fractures.

Medial Aspect

Medial Epicondyle. Originating from the medial epicondyle are the **wrist flexor–forearm pronator** groups of muscles. Both the muscle bellies and their insertions into bone should be palpated. Tenderness over the epicondyle where the muscles insert is sometimes called **golfer's elbow** or **tennis elbow of the medial epicondyle** and may indicate epiphyseal injury in skeletally immature patients.

Medial (Ulnar) Collateral Ligament. This fan-shaped ligament may be palpated, because it extends from the medial epicondyle to the medial margin of the

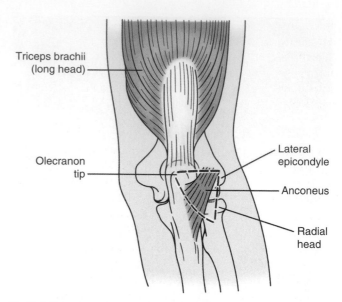

Fig. 6.73 Palpation of anconeus in triangle of olecranon tip, lateral epicondyle, and radial head.

coronoid process anteriorly and to the olecranon process posteriorly.

Ulnar Nerve. If the examiner moves posteriorly behind the medial epicondyle, the fingers will rest over the ulnar nerve in the cubital tunnel (proximal part). Usually, the nerve is not directly palpable, but pressure on the nerve often causes abnormal sensations in its cutaneous distribution. It is this nerve that is struck when someone hits his or her "funny bone."

Lateral Aspect

Lateral Epicondyle. The wrist extensor muscles originate from the lateral epicondyle, and their muscle bellies as well as their insertions into the epicondyle should be palpated. It is at this point of insertion of the common extensor tendon that lateral epicondylitis originates. Tenderness along the epicondyle in the skeletally immature may indicate an epiphyseal injury.[1] When palpating, the examiner should remember that the extensor carpi radialis longus muscle inserts above the epicondyle along a short ridge extending from the epicondyle to the humeral shaft. The examiner palpates the brachioradialis and supinator muscles on the lateral aspect of the elbow at the same time. If the examiner palpates the lateral epicondyle, the posterior radial head, and the olecranon tip, the anconeus "soft spot" will be found within this triangle (Fig. 6.73).[49] Pressure applied over the patient's lateral forearm about 3 to 5 cm (1.2 to 2 inches) distal to the elbow crease (over the supinator muscle) with the wrist in full supination will cause pain if there is pathology in the radial nerve.[80,101] (See RON test for radial nerve pathway.)

Lateral (Radial) Collateral Ligament. This cordlike ligament may be palpated as it extends from the lateral epicondyle of the humerus to the annular ligament and lateral surface of the ulna.

Annular Ligament. Distal to the lateral epicondyle, the annular ligament and head of the radius may be palpated if this has not previously been done. The palpation is facilitated by supination and pronation of the forearm.

Posterior Aspect

Palpation of posterior structures is shown in Fig. 6.72.

Olecranon Process and Olecranon Bursa. The olecranon process is best palpated with the elbow flexed to 90°. Tenderness along the distal and lateral aspect of the olecranon may be an indication of a stress fracture in throwing athletes.[7] If the elbow will not fully extend, the examiner should palpate the edges (especially the posteromedial tip) of the olecranon (normally smooth) for possible osteophytes.[7] If the examiner then grasps the skin overlying the process, the olecranon bursa can be palpated. Normally, it just feels like slippery tissue as the skin is moved. The examiner should note any synovial thickening, swelling, or the presence of any rice bodies, which are small seeds of fragmented fibrous tissue that can act as further irritants to the bursa should it be affected.

Triceps Muscle. The triceps muscle, which inserts into the olecranon process, should be palpated both at its insertion and along its length for any signs of abnormality.

Diagnostic Imaging

Plain Film Radiography

Common x-ray views of the elbow are outlined in the box below.

> **Common X-Ray Views of the Elbow (Depending on Pathology)**
>
> - Anteroposterior view (see Fig. 6.74A)
> - Lateral view at 90° flexion (see Fig. 6.74B)
> - Cubital tunnel view (see Fig. 6.79)
> - Anteroposterior internal oblique view (trauma) (Fig. 6.75B)
> - Anteroposterior external oblique view (trauma) (Fig. 6.75A)

Anteroposterior View. The examiner should note the relation of the epicondyles, trochlea, capitulum, radial head, radial tuberosity, coronoid process, and olecranon process (Fig. 6.74). Any bone spurs, osteochondral lesions, enthesopathy (i.e., disorders involving attachment of tendon or ligament to bone), loose bodies, calcification, myositis ossificans, joint space narrowing, or osteophytes should be identified.[44] A slight widening of the ulnohumeral joint (i.e., the **drop sign**) or posterior displacement of the radial head relative to the capitellum may be seen with posterolateral rotary instability. This may also be seen in the lateral view.[4] If the patient is a young child, the examiner should check the epiphyseal (growth) plate to see if it is normal for each bone. In the

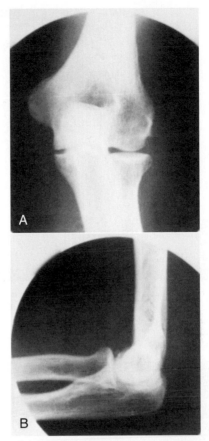

Fig. 6.74 Anteroposterior (A) and lateral (B) radiographs of the elbow.

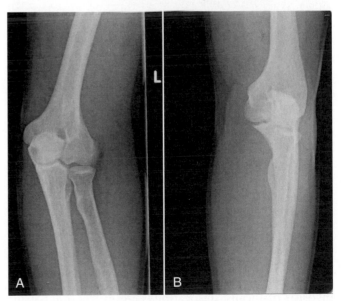

Fig. 6.75 (A) Anteroposterior external oblique view of the elbow. (B) Anteroposterior internal oblique view of the elbow.

upper limb, most growth in the humerus occurs at the shoulder and in the radius and ulna at the wrist.

Lateral View. The examiner should note the relation of the epicondyles, trochlea, capitulum, radial head, radial tuberosity, coronoid process, and olecranon

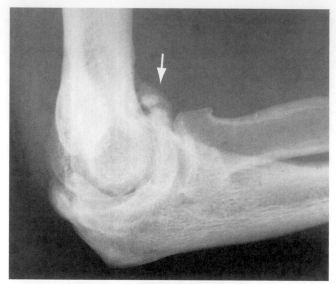

Fig. 6.76 Excessive ossification *(arrow)* after dislocation of elbow treated by early active use. (From O'Donoghue DH: *Treatment of injuries to athletes,* ed 4, Philadelphia, 1984, WB Saunders, p 232.)

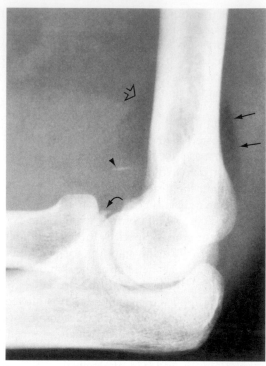

Fig. 6.78 Coronoid process fracture with hemarthrosis. The posterior fat pad *(arrows)* is shown clearly on this lateral view with the arm flexed to 90°, indicating joint effusion. The anterior fat pad *(open arrow)* is clearly visible. There is a fracture of the coronoid process *(curved arrow)* and a loose body *(arrowhead)*. (From Weissman BNW, Sledge CB: *Orthopedic radiology,* Philadelphia, 1986, WB Saunders, p 179.)

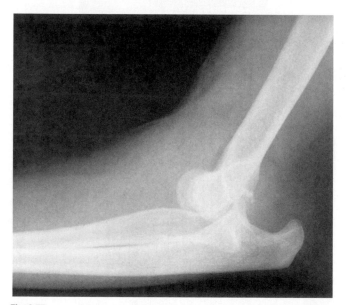

Fig. 6.77 Lateral film of a posterior dislocated elbow, showing the lower end of the humerus resting on the ulna in front of the coronoid. Note fragmentation of the coronoid. (From O'Donoghue DH: *Treatment of injuries to athletes,* ed 4, Philadelphia, 1984, WB Saunders, p 227.)

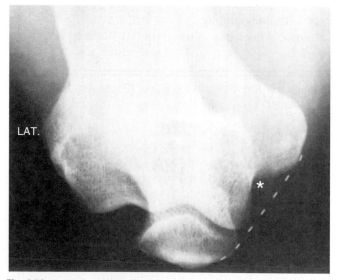

Fig. 6.79 Cubital tunnel. The ulnar nerve *(asterisk)* lies in a tunnel bridged by the arcuate ligament *(dashed line)*, which extends from the medial epicondyle to the olecranon process. *LAT,* Lateral.

process. As with the anteroposterior view, any loose bodies, calcifications in or around the joint (Fig. 6.76), myositis ossificans, dislocations (Fig. 6.77), joint space narrowing, or osteophytes should be noted. The presence of the fat-pad sign (Fig. 6.78) occurs with elbow joint effusion and may indicate, for example, a fracture, acute rheumatoid arthritis, infection, or osteoid osteoma.[123] A dislocation of the radial head may also cause an impaction defect to the capitellum (**Hill-Sachs lesion of the elbow**).[4] Plain radiographs may also be used to visualize the cubital tunnel (Fig. 6.79) and to measure the carrying angle (see Fig. 6.7).

Axial View. This view is taken with the elbow flexed to 45°. It shows the olecranon process and epicondyles. It is useful for showing osteophytes and loose bodies.[78]

Arthrography

Fig. 6.80 illustrates the views seen in normal elbow arthrograms. With the advent of magnetic resonance imaging (MRI), this technique is seldom used today.

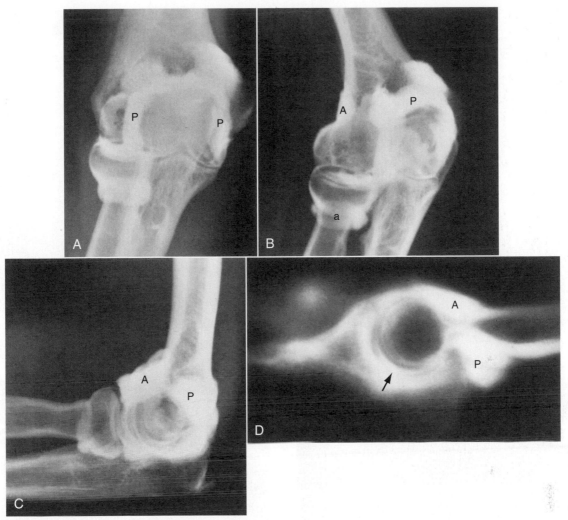

Fig. 6.80 Normal elbow arthrogram. Anteroposterior (A), external oblique (B), and lateral (C) views in extension show the normal annular *(a)*, anterior *(A)*, and posterior *(P)* recesses. (D) Lateral tomogram with the arm extended. The area of the trochlea that is devoid of cartilage *(arrow)* is shown. (From Weissman BNW, Sledge CB: *Orthopedic radiology,* Philadelphia, 1986, WB Saunders, p 178.)

Diagnostic Ultrasound Imaging

The elbow is especially well suited for ultrasound imaging because most of the structures that require viewing are relatively superficial. Ultrasound examination of the elbow can be performed from each of the four portions of the elbow. Different structures can be seen more clearly from a variety of angles, including anterior, medial, lateral, and posterior. Structures to be viewed include distal biceps tendon, brachialis tendon, common extensor and flexor tendons, lateral and medial collateral ligaments, triceps tendon, and median, ulnar, and radial nerves.[124–127]

Anterior View. The position used to examine the distal biceps brachii tendon is performed with the forearm supinated and the ultrasound transducer in the transverse axis just proximal to the elbow joint (Fig. 6.81). The cortex of the distal humerus will be seen inferiorly. The brachialis will also be seen inferiorly with the biceps brachii superior. In a normal muscle, the tissue will appear hypoechoic with some hyperechoic fibro-adipose separations (Fig. 6.82). By turning the transducer 90°, one

can then view the biceps tendon in its long axis (Fig. 6.83). The normal tendon will be long and fibrillar with uniform thickness (Fig. 6.84). If it is not possible to visualize the tendon using the anterior approach, then the tendon can also be seen from a lateral approach. The probe is placed longitudinally over the lateral arm with the forearm supinated and the elbow flexed to 90°. The transducer is actually in the short axis across the proximal radius in this position. The curved echogenic structure that can be seen is the radial head. As the forearm is pronated and supinated, the tendon of the biceps brachii can be seen moving dynamically. The radial head will also be seen rotating in this image.

The brachialis tendon can be seen deep to the biceps brachii tendon in the anterior arm. Along the anterior brachium, the transducer can be placed in the long axis. The coronoid and radial fossa may be seen as concavities in the distal humerus, with the brachialis overlying these depressions.

Lateral View. The common extensor tendon is viewed from the lateral side of the elbow with the transducer in

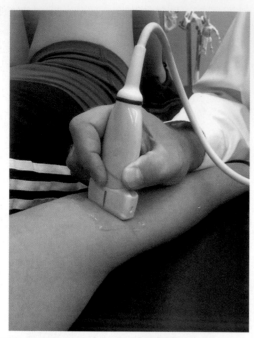

Fig. 6.81 Transverse view of anterior elbow proximal to elbow joint.

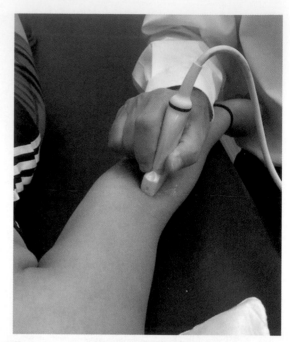

Fig. 6.83 Longitudinal view of anterior elbow proximal to elbow joint.

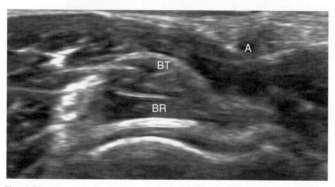

Fig. 6.82 Ultrasound of distal anterior elbow showing biceps brachii *(BT)*, brachialis *(BR)*, and brachial artery *(A)*.

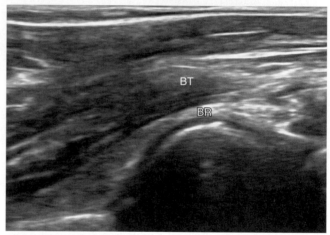

Fig. 6.84 Longitudinal image of biceps brachii *(BT)* in long axis superficial to the brachialis *(BR)*.

the long axis relative to the radius (Fig. 6.85). The hyperechoic radial head and the capitullum can be seen. Just off the lateral epicondyle, one will find the fibrillar common extensor tendon (Fig. 6.86). The common flexor tendon can be found on the medial elbow with the transducer placed in the long axis relative to the ulna. The common flexor tendon will be seen as hyperechoic and fibrillar just off the medial epicondyle, and will become hypoechoic muscle as one follows it further distally.

The lateral collateral ligament is not always easy to find. It is often difficult to differentiate the common extensor tendon from the lateral collateral ligament. If these structures are followed distally, the deeper radial collateral ligament will attach to the annular ligament immediately over the radial head while the common extensor tendon becomes more muscular superficially. The lateral collateral ligament can also be seen when the extensor carpi radialis brevis is torn.[128] If the transducer is placed over the lateral elbow and angled posteriorly from the distal humerus to

the ulna, the hyperechoic and fibrillary LUCL can be seen (Fig. 6.87).

The radial nerve can be seen laterally between the brachialis and the brachioradialis muscles. Placing the transducer in the short axis transversely will demonstrate hypoechoic fascicles surrounded by a hyperechoic epineurium.[128] The nerve can be followed proximally as it traverses the intermuscular fascia and follows the humerus. The nerve can also be followed in the long axis by turning the transducer 90°. Following distally, the nerve will branch into the deep branch entering the supinator muscle; the superficial branch will continue distally into the forearm.

Medial View. The medial elbow view is used primarily to examine the common flexor tendon and the ulnar collateral ligament. The elbow is placed near full extension or

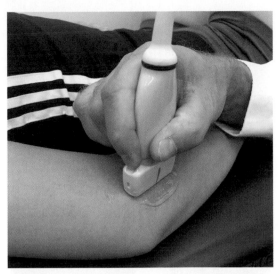

Fig. 6.85 Longitudinal view of common extensor tendon.

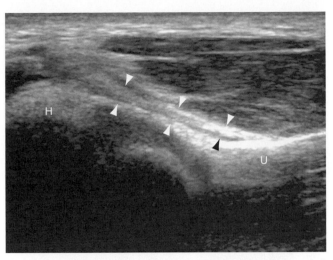

Fig. 6.87 Longitudinal view of lateral elbow demonstrating the lateral ulnar collateral ligament *(arrowheads)* from the humerus *(H)* to the ulna *(U)*. (From Jacobson JA: *Fundamentals of musculoskeletal ultrasound,* ed 3, Philadelphia, 2018, Elsevier.)

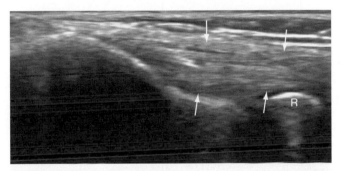

Fig. 6.86 Longitudinal image of common extensor tendon *(arrows)* in the forearm over the radial head *(R)*.

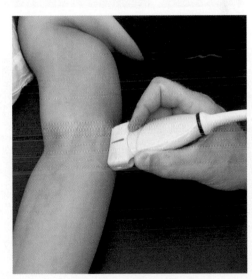

Fig. 6.88 Longitudinal view of ulnar collateral ligament on medial side of arm.

in slight flexion with the forearm in supination. The transducer is placed in the long axis with respect to the forearm to begin (Fig. 6.88). The bony contour of the medial epicondyle and the proximal ulna will be seen. Running between these two bony prominences is the common flexor tendon superficially and the ulnar collateral ligament deeper. The common flexor tendon is hyperechoic and fibrillary. It changes to a hypoechoic structure, however, as it runs distally to become muscular. The ulnar collateral ligament will be seen as hyperechoic and fibrillary (Fig. 6.89). One needs to be careful to stay perpendicular to the ligament as anisotropy may make the ligament appear less uniform. Ulnar collateral ligament thickness can vary from patient to patient; however, it has been shown that thickness increases in professional baseball players depending on their years of experience.[129]

Posterior View. The posterior view of the elbow visualizes the triceps tendon, the anconeus muscle, and the ulnar nerve. To examine the triceps tendon and the olecranon bursa, the elbow is flexed to 90° with arm resting on a table. The transducer is placed in the short axis and moved from the olecranon process to the myotendinous junction of the triceps muscle (Fig. 6.90). By toggling

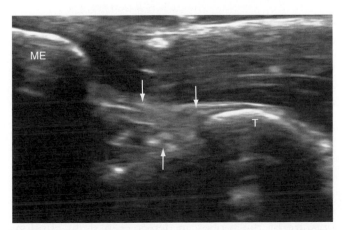

Fig. 6.89 Longitudinal image of ulnar collateral ligament *(arrows)*, medial epicondyle *(ME)*, and trochlea *(T)*. White dots are part of the bottom portion of tendon.

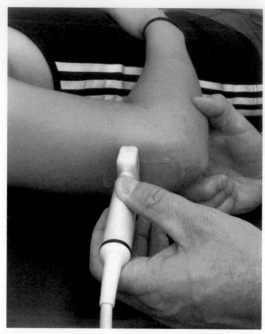

Fig. 6.90 Transverse view of posterior elbow joint and triceps tendon.

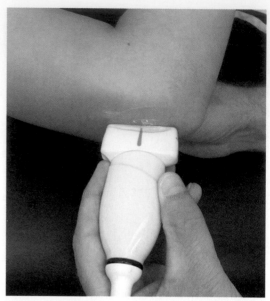

Fig. 6.92 Longitudinal view of posterior elbow and triceps tendon.

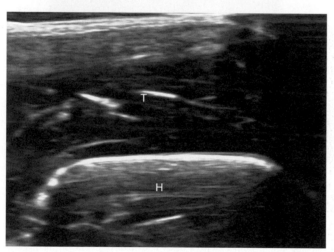

Fig. 6.91 Transverse image of posterior elbow including triceps tendon (T) and humeral surface (H).

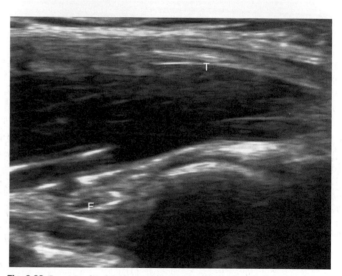

Fig. 6.93 Longitudinal image of posterior elbow flexed showing triceps muscle (T) and olecranon fossa with fat pad (F).

the ultrasound head, the examiner may be able to see the different components of the medial, lateral, and deep triceps tendinous compartments.[130] The tendon is usually fibrillar in nature (Fig. 6.91). By rotating the transducer 90°, the tendon can be viewed in its long axis (Fig. 6.92). The tendon should be clearly seen to be linear with some striations that are thought to be fat between tendon fibers.[128] If the tendon is followed distally, it can be seen over the top of the olecranon and superficial to the olecranon fossa (Fig. 6.93). Effusion in the elbow can be seen by flexing the elbow up to 45° which moves the fluid posteriorly into the olecranon recess. Gentle pressure by the probe can detect even slight effusions within the joint.

In select individuals, one may be able to find the anconeus epitrochlearis muscle, an accessory muscle located between the posterior aspect of the medial epicondyle of the humerus and the medial aspect of the olecranon. It may be too small to even be palpated, but can be seen as a small isolated ovoid mass forming the floor of the condylar groove just superficial to the ulnar nerve.[131]

The ulnar nerve can be seen at the medial side of the elbow. To find the ulnar nerve, the transducer is placed in the short axis over the posterior medial elbow, over the olecranon and the medial epicondyle (Fig. 6.94). The nerve can be seen as a hypoechoic structure within a hyperechoic nerve sheath. The patient may be asked to flex and extend the elbow while the examiner watches

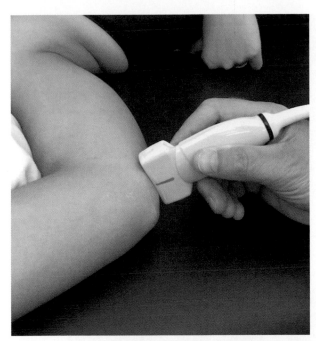

Fig. 6.94 Evaluation of the ulnar nerve (posteromedial aspect of arm).

for normal or abnormal translation of the ulnar nerve. Abnormal movement would include subluxation of the nerve over the medial epicondyle.

Magnetic Resonance Imaging

MRI is used to differentiate bone and soft tissues. Because of its high soft-tissue contrast, MRI, a noninvasive technique, is able to discriminate among bone marrow, cartilage, tendons, nerves, and vessels without the use of a contrast medium (Figs. 6.95 to 6.97).[132,133] The technique is used to demonstrate tendon ruptures, collateral ligament ruptures, cubital tunnel pathology, epicondylitis, and osteochondritis dissecans.[8,134–136]

Xerography

Fig. 6.98 illustrates the detailed borders of the various structures around the elbow.

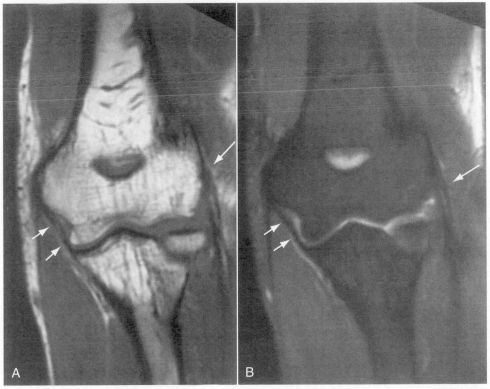

Fig. 6.95 Normal common extensor tendon and the medial collateral ligament (MCL) on magnetic resonance imaging. (A) Oblique coronal T1-weighted A spine echo and fat-saturated proton density. (B) Fast spin echo image demonstrates the normal, smooth, thin contour and low signal of the common extensor tendon *(long arrow)* and anterior bundle of the MCL *(short arrows)*. (From Schenk M, Dalinka MK: Imaging of the elbow: an update, *Orthop Clin North Am* 28:519, 1997.)

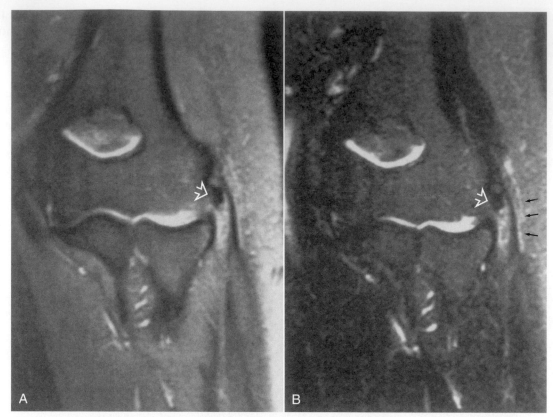

Fig. 6.96 Lateral epicondylitis tendinitis on magnetic resonance imaging. Oblique coronal fat-saturated proton density (A) and T2-weighted (B) fast spin echo images. Focal calcification within the common extensor tendon *(white arrow)*. There is a moderately increased signal within the tendon, without fiber disruption. Note the edema in the peritendinous tissues *(black arrows)*, suggesting active inflammation. (From Schenk M, Dalinka MK: Imaging of the elbow: an update, *Orthop Clin North Am* 28:524, 1997.)

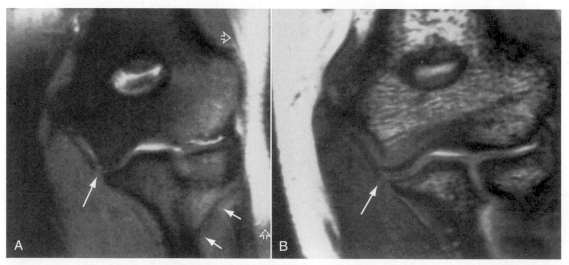

Fig. 6.97 (A and B) Medial collateral ligament (MCL) tear on magnetic resonance imaging. Surgically proven tear in an athlete who was injured 3 months before imaging and complained of persistent pain with throwing. Oblique coronal fat-saturated proton density image shows a complete tear of the anterior bundle at its distal attachment to the ulna *(long arrow)*. Note the lateral ulna collateral ligament inserting into the ulna *(short arrows)*. Also note the bright signal within the subcutaneous fat laterally *(open arrows)*, which is secondary to incomplete fat suppression and should not be mistaken for edema. Three-dimensional gradient echo image reformatted along the plane of the MCL also demonstrates the distal tear *(arrow)*. (From Schenk M, Dalinka MK: Imaging of the elbow: an update, *Orthop Clin North Am* 28:528, 1997.)

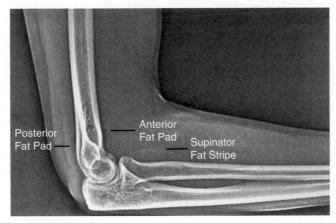

Fig. 6.98 Xerogram of the elbow demonstrating the fat pads and supinator fat stripe resulting from subtle radial head fracture. (From Berquist TH: Diagnostic radiographic techniques of the elbow. In Morrey BF, editor: *The elbow and its disorders*, Philadelphia, 1993, WB Saunders, p 106.)

PRÉCIS OF THE ELBOW ASSESSMENT[a]

NOTE: Suspected pathology will determine which *Special Tests* are to be performed.

History
Observation
Examination
 Active movements
  Elbow flexion
  Elbow extension
  Supination
  Pronation
  Combined movements (if necessary)
  Repetitive movements (if necessary)
  Sustained positions (if necessary)
 Passive movements (as in active movements, if necessary)
 Resisted isometric movements
  Elbow flexion
  Elbow extension
  Supination
  Pronation
  Wrist flexion
  Wrist extension
 Functional assessment
 Special tests
  For ligamentous instability:
   Chair push-up test
   Gravity-assisted varus stress test
   Lateral pivot shift test of the elbow
   Ligamentous valgus instability test
   Ligamentous varus instability test
   Milking maneuver
   Moving valgus stress test
   Posterolateral rotary drawer test
   Prone push-up test
   Tabletop relocation test
   Valgus extension overload test
  For muscle injury (third-degree strain):
   Biceps crease interval
   Biceps squeeze test
   Bicipital aponeurosis flex test
   Flexion initiation test
   Hook (distal biceps) test
   Popeye sign (distal biceps tendon)

   Supination-pronation test
   TILT sign
   Triceps squeeze test
  For epicondylitis (epicondylalgia):
   Cozen's test
   Golfer's elbow test
   Kaplan's test
   Maudsley's (middle finger) test
   Mill's test
   Polk test
   Tennis elbow shear test
  For fractures:
   East Riding Elbow Rule (ER[2])
   Montreal children's elbow test
  For joint dysfunction:
   Trochlea shear test
  For neurological dysfunction:
   Pinch grip test (anterior interosseous branch of median nerve)
   Rule-of-nine (RON) test
   Scratch collapse test for ulnar, median, and/or radial nerve
   Shoulder internal rotation elbow flexion test (ulnar nerve)
   Tinel sign at elbow (ulnar nerve)
   Wadsworth elbow flexion test (ulnar nerve)
 Reflexes and cutaneous distribution
  Reflexes
  Sensory scan
  Peripheral nerves
   Median nerve and branches
   Ulnar nerve
   Radial nerve and branches
 Joint play movements
  Radial deviation of ulna and radius on humerus
  Ulnar deviation of ulna and radius on humerus
  Distraction of olecranon process on humerus in 90° of flexion
  Anteroposterior glide of radius on humerus
 Palpation
 Diagnostic imaging

[a]The entire assessment may be done with the patient in sitting position. After any examination, the patient should be warned of the possibility that the assessment may exacerbate symptoms.

CASE STUDIES

When doing these case studies, the examiner should list the appropriate questions to ask the patient and should specify why they are being asked, what to look for and why, and what things should be tested and why. Depending on the patient's answers (and the examiner should consider numerous different responses), several possible causes of the patient's problem may become evident (examples are given in parentheses). The examiner should prepare a differential diagnosis chart (Table 6.5 is an example for question 1). The examiner can then decide how different diagnoses may affect the treatment plan.

1. A 16-year-old right-hand dominant male baseball pitcher comes to see you for elbow pain. One year ago, he had an ulnar nerve transposition which did well immediately after his surgery. When he started throwing, his numbness and tingling returned. He then had a second operation which was a partial triceps resection to decrease compression and irritation on the transposed ulnar nerve. He presents with medial elbow pain on palpation. He has 4/5 elbow and forearm strength. He does not presently have any numbness or tingling as he has not been throwing. Describe your assessment plan and your differential diagnosis.

2. A 17-year-old right-hand dominant female comes to see you three weeks after a posterior elbow dislocation and reduction following a fall from her horse. She did not incur any fractures with her accident. She comes to you in a sling. The referring physician has stated that her elbow is stable throughout her ROM now. Describe your assessment plan to evaluate her for initiation of treatment.

3. A 40-year-old male comes to see you following an injury to the right elbow. Three days ago, he was helping his brother move a 136-kg (300-lb) piece of angle iron from their father's barn. His brother accidently dropped his end causing the patient to have all the weight. He felt a "pop" and immediate pain in his right elbow. Since then, he has noticed swelling in his right anterior elbow. Yesterday, he started to notice a deformity and some ecchymosis. He has pain and cramping sensations with active elbow flexion ROM. Describe your assessment plan for this patient and your differential diagnosis (2° muscle strain vs. 3° rupture).

4. A 24-year-old woman comes to you complaining of pain in her right elbow on the medial side. The pain sometimes extends into the forearm and is often accompanied by tingling into the little finger and half of the ring finger. The pain and paresthesia are particularly bothersome when she plays recreational volleyball, which she enjoys very much. Describe your assessment plan for this patient (ulnar neuritis vs. medial epicondylitis).

5. A 52-year-old man is referred to you with a history of right elbow pain. He complains of tenderness over the lateral epicondyle. He informs you that he has not done any repetitive forearm activity and does not play tennis. He has some restriction of neck movement. Describe your assessment plan for this patient (cervical spondylosis vs. lateral epicondylitis).

6. A 26-year-old male football player is referred to you after surgery for a ruptured (third-degree strain) left biceps tendon at its insertion. His cast has been removed, and you have been asked to restore the patient to normal function. Describe your assessment plan for this patient.

7. Parents bring their 4-year-old daughter in to see you. They state that about 2 hours previously they were out shopping, and the mother was holding the little girl's arm. The little girl tripped, and the mother "yanked" her up as she fell. The little girl started to cry and would not move her elbow. Describe your assessment plan for this patient (radial head dislocation vs. ligamentous sprain).

8. A 46-year-old man comes to you complaining of diffuse left elbow pain. When he carries a briefcase for three or four blocks, his elbow becomes stiff and sore. When he picks up things with his left hand, the pain increases dramatically. Describe your assessment plan for this patient (lateral epicondylitis vs. osteoarthritis).

9. A 31-year-old man comes to you complaining of posterior elbow pain. He says he banged his elbow on the table 10 days earlier, and he has had posterior swelling for 8 or 9 days. Describe your assessment plan for this patient (olecranon bursitis vs. joint synovitis).

10. A 14-year-old female gymnast comes to you complaining of elbow pain. She explains she was doing a vault and bent her elbow backward, at which time she heard a snap. The injury occurred 1 hour earlier, and there is some swelling; she does not want to move the elbow. Describe your assessment plan for this patient (biceps tendon rupture vs. epiphyseal fracture).

TABLE **6.5**

Differential Diagnosis of Ulnar Neuritis and Medial Epicondylitis

	Ulnar Neuritis	Medial Epicondylitis
History	May follow repetitive activity May follow contused elbow May follow previously injured elbow Pain in forearm and into ulnar distribution of hand	Usually follows repetitive activity Pain in forearm, may radiate to wrist and may not follow normal dermatomal pattern
Observation	Normal	Normal
Active movements	Weakness of ulnar deviation Weakness of little and ring finger flexion	Slight pain on forearm pronation and wrist flexion
Passive movements	Normal, or pain may come on with elbow flexion and wrist flexion	Normal, but pain may occur with elbow extension and wrist extension
Resisted isometric movements	Weakness of ulnar deviation Weakness of little and ring finger flexion Pain on wrist flexion and pronation	Pain on wrist flexion with elbow extension Pain on pronation and wrist and finger flexion
Special tests	Tinel sign positive Wartenberg sign positive Elbow flexion test positive	Golfer's elbow test positive No paresthesia
Sensation	Paresthesia and pain in forearm, little finger, and half of ring finger	Pain in forearm, possibly to wrist

References

1. Smith MV, Lamplot JD, Wright RW, Brophy RH. Comprehensive review of the elbow physical examination. *J Am Acad Orthop Surg*. 2010;20(19):678–687.
2. Cohen MS, Bruno RJ. The collateral ligaments of the elbow: anatomy and clinical correlation. *Clin Orthop Relat Res*. 2001;383:123–130.
3. O'Driscoll SW. Acute, recurrent and chronic elbow instabilities. In: Norris TR, ed. *Orthopedic Knowledge Update 2: Shoulder and Elbow*. Rosemont, IL: American Academy of Orthopedic Surgeons; 2002.
4. Anakwenze OA, Kancherla VK, Iyengar J, et al. Posterolateral rotary instability of the elbow. *Am J Sports Med*. 2013;42(2):485–491.
5. Bozkurt M, Acar HI, Apaydin N, et al. The annular ligament: an anatomical study. *Am J Sports Med*. 2005;33:114–118.
6. Dutton M. *Orthopedic Examination, Evaluation and Intervention*. New York: McGraw-Hill; 2004.
7. Dugas JR. Valgus extension overload: diagnosis and treatment. *Clin Sports Med*. 2010;29(4):645–654.
8. Zwerus EL, Somford MP, Maissan F, et al. Physical examination of the elbow, what is the evidence? A systematic literature review. *Br J Sports Med*. 2017;51:1–9.
9. Redler LH, Watling JP, Ahmad CS. Five points on physical examination of the throwing athlete's elbow. *Am J Orthop*. 2015;44(1):13–18.
10. Sakata J, Nakamura E, Suzukawa M, et al. Physical risk factors for a medial elbow injury in junior baseball players – a prospective cohort study of 353 players. *Am J Sports Med*. 2016;45(1):135–143.
11. Noonan TJ, Thigpen CA, Bailey LB, et al. Humeral torsion as a risk factor for shoulder and elbow injury in professional baseball pitchers. *Am J Sports Med*. 2016;44(9):2214–2219.
12. Andrews JR, Wilk KE, Satterwhite YE, et al. Physical examination of the thrower's elbow. *J Orthop Sports Phys Ther*. 1993;17:296–304.
13. Petty NJ, Moore AP. *Neuromusculoskeletal Examination and Assessment*. London: Churchill Livingstone; 1990.
14. Palmer BA, Hughes TB. Cubital tunnel syndrome. *J Hand Surg Am*. 2010;35(1):153–163.
15. Beals RK. The normal carrying angle of the elbow. *Clin Orthop*. 1976;1190:194–196.
16. Hausman MR, Lang P. Examination of the elbow: current concepts. *J Hand Surg Am*. 2014;39:2534–2541.
17. Charton A. *The Elbow: The Rheumatological Physical Examination*. Orlando, FL: Grune & Stratton; 1986.
18. Kapandji AI. *The Physiology of the Joints, Upper Limb*. Vol 1. New York: Churchill Livingstone; 1970.
19. Dhillon MS, Gopinathan NR, Kumar V. Misconceptions about the three point bony relationship of the elbow. *Indian J Orthop*. 2014;48(5):453–457.
20. American Orthopaedic Association. *Manual of Orthopaedic Surgery*. Chicago: American Orthopaedic Association; 1972.
21. Tarr RR, Garfinkel AI, Sarmiento A. The effects of angular and rotational deformities of both bones of the forearm. *J Bone Joint Surg Am*. 1984;66:65–70.
22. Clarkson HM. *Musculoskeletal Assessment: Joint Range of Motion and Manual Muscle Strength*. Philadelphia: Lippincott Williams & Wilkins; 2000.
23. Askew LJ, An KN, Morrey BF, et al. Isometric elbow strength in normal individuals. *Clin Orthop*. 1987;222:261–266.
24. Ramsey ML. Distal biceps tendon injuries: diagnosis and management. *J Am Acad Orthop Surg*. 1999;7:199–207.
25. Morrey BF, An KN, Chao EYS. Functional evaluation of the elbow. In: Morrey BF, ed. *The Elbow and its Disorders*. Philadelphia: WB Saunders; 1993.
26. Alberta FG, El Attrache NS, Bissell S, et al. The development and validation of a functional assessment tool for the upper extremity in the overhead athlete. *Am J Sports Med*. 2010;38:903–911.
27. Domb BG, D JT, Alberta FG, et al. Clinical follow up of professional baseball players undergoing ulnar collateral ligament reconstruction using the new Kerlan-Jobe Orthopedic Clinic overhead athlete shoulder and elbow score (KJOC score). *Am J Sports Med*. 2010;38:1558–1563.
28. Nuttal D, Birch A. Trail II, et al. Assessing elbow assessment, past, present and future. *Shoulder Elbow*. 2010;2(1):43–54.
29. Regan WD, Morrey BF. The physical examination of the elbow. In: Morrey BF, ed. *The Elbow and its Disorders*. Philadelphia: WB Saunders; 1993.
30. Cusick MC, Bonnaig NS, Azar FM, et al. Accuracy and reliability of the Mayo elbow performance score. *J Hand Surg Am*. 2014;39(6):1146–1150.
31. Gummesson C, Atroshi I, Ekdahl C. The disabilities of the arm, shoulder and hand (DASH) outcome questionnaire: longitudinal construct validity and measuring self- related health change after surgery. *BMC Musculoskelet Disord*. 2003;4:11–17.
32. John M, Angst F, Awiszus F, et al. The American shoulder and elbow surgeons elbow questionnaire: cross-cultural adaptation in German and evaluation of its psychometric properties. *J Hand Ther*. 2010;23(3):301–314.
33. King GJW, Richards RR, Zuckerman JD, et al. A standardized method for assessment of elbow function. *J Shoulder Elbow Surg*. 1999;8:351–354.
34. Longo UG, Franceschi F, Loppini M, et al. Rating systems for evaluation of the elbow. *Br Med Bull*. 2008;87:131–161.
35. Evans JP, Smith CD, Fine NF, et al. Clinical rating systems in elbow research–a systematic review exploring trends and distributions of use. *J Shoulder Elbow Surg*. 2018;27(4):e98–e106.
36. Cook CE, Hegedus EJ. *Orthopedic Physical Examination Tests—An Evidence Based Approach*. Upper Saddle River, NJ: Pearson/Prentice Hall; 2008.

37. Cleland JA, Koppenhaver S. *Netter's Orthopedic Clinical Examination—An Evidence-Based Approach.* 2nd ed. Philadelphia: Saunders/Elsevier; 2011.

38. Regan W, Lapner PC. Prospective evaluation of two diagnostic apprehension signs for posterolateral instability of the elbow. *J Shoulder Elbow Surg.* 2006;15(3):344–346.

39. Karbach LE, Elfar J. Elbow instability: anatomy, biomechanics, diagnostic maneuvers, and testing. *J Hand Surg Am.* 2017;42:118–126.

40. Pollock JW, Brownhill J, Ferreira L, et al. The effect of anteromedial facet fractures of the coronoid and lateral collateral ligament injury on elbow stability and kinematics. *J Bone Joint Surg Am.* 2009;91(6):1448–1458.

41. O'Driscoll SW. Classification and evaluation of recurrent instability of the elbow. *Clin Orthop Relat Res.* 2000;370:34–43.

42. Mehta JA, Bain GI. Posterolateral rotary instability of the elbow. *J Am Acad Ortho Surg.* 2004;12:405–415.

43. O'Driscoll SW, Bell DF, Morrey BF. Posterolateral rotary instability of the elbow. *J Bone Joint Surg Am.* 1991;73:440–446.

44. Kane SF, Lynch JH, Taylor JC. Evaluation of elbow pain in adults. *Am Fam Physician.* 2014;89(8):649–657.

45. O'Driscoll SW, Lawton RM, Smith AM. The "moving valgus stress test" for medial collateral ligament tears of the elbow. *Am J Sports Med.* 2005;33:231–239.

46. Hassan SE, Osbahr DC. Ulnohumeral chondral and ligamentous overload. In: Dines J, Altchek DW, eds. *Elbow Ulnar Collateral Ligament Injury: A Guide to Diagnosis and Treatment.* New York: Springer; 2015.

47. Lee ML, Rosenwasser MP. Chronic elbow instability. *Orthop Clin North Am.* 1999;30:81–89.

48. Kalainov DM, Cohen MS. The posterolateral rotary instability of the elbow in association with lateral epicondylitis: a report to three cases. *J Bone Joint Surg Am.* 2005;87:1120–1125.

49. Hsu SH, Moen TC, Levine WN, et al. Physical examination of the athlete's elbow. *Am J Sports Med.* 2012;40:699–708.

50. Arvind CH, Hargeaves DG. Tabletop relocation test: a new clinical test for posterolateral rotary instability of the elbow. *J Shoulder Elbow Surg.* 2006;15(6):707–708.

51. Devereaux MW, ElMaraghy AW. Improving the rapid and reliable diagnosis of complete distal biceps tendon rupture: a nuanced approach to the clinical examination. *Am J Sports Med.* 2013;41(9):1998–2004.

52. ElMaraghy A, Devereaux M, Tsoi K. The biceps crease interval for diagnosing complete distal biceps tendon ruptures. *Clin Orthop Relat Res.* 2008;466:2255–2262.

53. Ruland RT, Dunbar RP, Bowen JD. The biceps squeeze test for diagnosis of distal biceps tendon ruptures. *Clin Orthop Relat Res.* 2005;437:128–131.

54. ElMaraghy A, Devereaux M. The "bicipital aponeurosis flex test: evaluating the integrity of the bicipital aponeurosis and its implications for treatment of distal biceps tendon ruptures. *J Shoulder Elbow Surg.* 2013;22(7):908–914.

55. Ross G. Improved clinical diagnosis of distal biceps tendon rupture: the flexion initiation test. Available at: http://www.aaos.org/wordhtml/anmt2004/poster/p260.htm

56. O'Driscoll SW, Goncalves LB, Dietz P. The hook test for distal biceps tendon avulsion. *Am J Sports Med.* 2007;35:1865–1869.

57. Metzman LS, Tivener KA. The supination–pronation test for distal biceps tendon rupture. *Am J Orthop (Belle Mead NJ).* 2015;44(10):E361–E364.

58. Harding WG. A new clinical test for avulsion of the insertion of the biceps tendon. *Orthopedics.* 2005;28(1):27–29.

59. Shim SS, Strauch RJ. A novel clinical test for partial tears of the distal biceps brachii tendon: the TILT sign. *Clin Anat.* 2018;31(2):301–303.

60. Kraushaar BS, Nirschl RP. Tendinosis of the elbow (tennis elbow). *J Bone Joint Surg Am.* 1999;81:259–278.

61. Johnstone AJ. Tennis elbow and upper limb tendinopathies. *Sports Med Arthro Rev.* 2000;8:69–79.

62. Vaquero-Piaco A, Barco R, Antuna SA. Lateral epicondylitis of the elbow. *EFFORT Open Rev.* 2018;1:391–397.

63. Evans RC. *Illustrated Orthopedic Physical Assessment.* St. Louis: Mosby/Elsevier; 2009.

64. Dorf ER, Chhabra AB, Golish SR, et al. Effect of elbow position on grip strength in the evaluation of lateral epicondylitis. *J Hand Surg Am.* 2007;32(6):882–886.

65. Roles NC, Maudsley RH. Radial tunnel syndrome: resistant tennis elbow as a nerve entrapment. *J Bone Joint Surg Br.* 1972;54:499–508.

66. Polkinghorn BS. A novel method for assessing elbow pain resulting from epicondylitis. *J Chiropr Med.* 2002;1(3):117–121.

67. Smith A, O'Driscoll SW. Diagnosing medial elbow pain in throwers. *Musculoskeletal Med.* 2005;22(6):305–316.

68. Jonely H, Brismee JM, Lutton D. A clinical test for diagnosis of humeroradial joint lesions in the presence of lateral elbow pain: single-case design with arthroscopic confirmation. *Int J Clin Med.* 2018;9:162–174.

69. Antuna SA, O'Driscoll SW. Snapping plica associated with radiocapitellar chondromalacia. *Arthroscopy.* 2001;17:491–495.

70. Arundel D, Williams P, Townend W. Deriving the East Riding Elbow Rule (ER²): a maximally sensitive decision tool for elbow injury. *Emerg Med J.* 2014;31:380–383.

71. Dubrovsky AS, Mok E, Lau SY, Al Humaidan M. Point tenderness at 1 of 5 locations and limited elbow extension identify significant injury in children with acute elbow trauma: a study of diagnostic accuracy. *Am J Emerg Med.* 2015;33:229–233.

72. Dubrovsky AS, Al Humaidan M, Lau S. Pediatric elbow fractures: diagnostic accuracy of the combination of point tenderness with the elbow extension test. *Pediatr Child Health.* 2014;19(6):e100.

73. Buehler MJ, Thayer DT. The elbow flexion test: a clinical test for the cubital tunnel syndrome. *Clin Orthop.* 1988;233:213–216.

74. Butler DS. *Mobilisation of the Nervous System.* Melbourne: Churchill Livingstone; 1991.

75. Ochi K, Horiuchi Y, Tanabe A, et al. Shoulder internal rotation elbow flexion test for diagnosing cubital tunnel syndrome. *J Shoulder Elbow Surg.* 2012;21:777–781.

76. Novak CB, Lee GW, Mackinnon SE, et al. Provocative testing for cubital tunnel syndrome. *J Hand Surg Am.* 1994;19:817–820.

77. Goldman SB, Brininger TL, Schrader JW, Koceja DM. A review of clinical tests and signs for the assessment of ulnar neuropathy. *J Hand Ther.* 2009;22:209–220.

78. Bigg-Wither G, Kelly P. Diagnostic imaging in musculoskeletal physiotherapy. In: Refshauge K, Gass E, eds. *Musculoskeletal Physiotherapy: Clinical Science and Practice.* Oxford: Butterworth-Heinemann; 1995.

79. Loh YC, Lam WL, Stanley JK, Soames RW. A new clinical test for radial tunnel syndrome–the Rule-of-Nine test: a cadaveric study. *J Orthop Surg.* 2004;12(1):83–86.

80. Strohl AB, Zelouf DS. Ulnar tunnel syndrome, radial tunnel syndrome, anterior interosseous nerve syndrome and pronator syndrome. *J Am Acad Orthop Surg.* 2017;25(1):e1–e10.

81. Moradi A, Ebrahimzadeh MH, Jupiter JB. Radial tunnel syndrome, diagnostic and treatment dilemma. *Arch Bone Jt Surg.* 2015;3(3):156–162.

82. Dang AC, Rodner CM. Unusual compression neuropathies of the forearm, part II: median nerve. *J Hand Surg Am.* 2009;34(10):1915–1920.

83. Hagert E, Hagert C-G. Upper extremity nerve entrapments: the axillary and radial nerves – clinical diagnosis and surgical treatment. *Plast Reconstr Surg.* 2014;134(1):71–80.

84. Davidge KM, Gontre G, Tang D, et al. The "hierarchical" scratch collapse test for identifying multilevel ulnar nerve compression. *Hand (N Y).* 2015;10(3):388–395.

85. Cebron U, Curtin CM. The scratch collapse test: a systematic review. *J Plast Reconstr Aesthetic Surg.* 2018;71(12):1693–1703.

86. Jimenez I, Delgado PJ. The scratch collapse test in the diagnosis of compression of the median nerve in the proximal forearm. *J Hand Surg Eur.* 2017;42(9):937–940.

87. Kroonen LT. Cubital tunnel syndrome. *Orthop Clin North Am.* 2012;43:475–486.

88. Cheng CJ, Mackinnon-Patterson B, Beck JL, et al. Scratch collapse test for evaluation of carpal and cubital tunnel syndrome. *J Hand Surg Am.* 2008;33:1518–1524.

89. Brown JM, Mokhtee D, Evangelista MS, Mackinnon SE. Scratch collapse test localizes Osborne's band as the point of maximum nerve compression in cubital tunnel syndrome. *Hand (N Y).* 2010;5(2):141–147.

90. Makanji HS, Becker SJ, Mudgal CS, et al. Evaluation of the scratch collapse test in the diagnosis of carpal tunnel syndrome. *J Hand Surg Eur.* 2014;39(2):181–186.

91. Ono K, Ebara S, Fuji T, et al. Myelopathy hand. New clinical signs of cervical cord damage. *J Bone Joint Surg Br.* 1987;69(2):215–219.

92. Kumar SD, Bourke G. Nerve compression syndromes at the elbow. *Orthop Trauma.* 2016;30(4):355–362.

93. Floranda EE, Jacobs BC. Evaluation and treatment of upper extremity nerve entrapment syndromes. *Prim Care.* 2013;40(4):925–943.

94. Popinchalk SP, Schaffer AA. Physical examination of upper extremity compression neuropathies. *Orthop Clin North Am.* 2012;43:417–430.

95. Limb D, Hodkinson SL, Brown RF. Median nerve palsy after posterolateral elbow dislocation. *J Bone Joint Surg Br.* 1994;76:987–988.

96. Conrad RW, Spinner RJ. Snapping brachialis tendon associated with median neuropathy. *J Bone Joint Surg Am.* 1995;77:1891–1893.

97. Spinner M, Spencer PS. Nerve compression lesions of the upper extremity: a clinical and experimental review. *Clin Orthop.* 1974;104:46–67.

98. Butlers KP, Singer KM. Nerve lesions of the arm and elbow. In: De Lee JC, Drez D, eds. *Orthopedic Sports Medicine: Principles and Practice.* Philadelphia: WB Saunders; 1994.

99. Rask MR. Anterior interosseous nerve entrapment (Kiloh-Nevin Syndrome). *Clin Orthop.* 1979;142:176–181.

100. Wiens E, Lau SCK. The anterior interosseous nerve syndrome. *Can J Surg.* 1978;21:354–357.

101. Rodner CM, Tinsley BA, O'Malley MP. Pronator syndrome and anterior interosseous nerve syndrome. *J Am Acad Orthop Surg.* 2013;21(5):268–275.

102. Engher WD, Keene JS. Anterior interosseous nerve palsy associated with a Monteggia fracture. *Clin Orthop.* 1983;174:133–137.

103. O'Driscoll SW, Horii E, Carmichael SW, et al. The cubital tunnel and ulnar neuropathy. *J Bone Joint Surg Br.* 1991;73:613–617.

104. McPherson SA, Meals RA. Cubital tunnel syndrome. *Orthop Clin North Am.* 1992;23:111–123.

105. Wadsworth TG. The external compression syndrome of the ulnar nerve at the cubital tunnel. *Clin Orthop.* 1977;124:189–204.

106. Pecina MM, Krmpotic-Nemanic J, Markiewitz AD. *Tunnel Syndromes.* Boca Raton, FL: CRC Press; 1991.

107. Khoo D, Carmichael SW, Spinner RJ. Ulnar nerve anatomy and compression. *Orthop Clin North Am.* 1996;27:317–338.

108. Gelberman RH, Eaton R, Urbaniak JR. Peripheral nerve compression. *J Bone Joint Surg Am.* 1993;75:1854–1878.

109. Apfelberg DB, Larsen SJ. Dynamic anatomy of the ulnar nerve by the deep flexor-pronator aponeurosis. *Plast Reconstr Surg.* 1973;51:79–81.

110. Holmes JC, Hall JE. Tardy ulnar nerve palsy in children. *Clin Orthop.* 1978;135:128–131.

111. Calfee RP, Manske PR, Gelberman RH, et al. Clinical assessment of the ulnar nerve at the elbow: reliability of instability testing and the association of hypermobility with clinical symptoms. *J Bone Joint Surg Am.* 2010;92:2801–2808.

112. Thurston A. Radial tunnel syndrome. *Orthop Trauma.* 2013;27(6):403–408.

113. Wadsworth TG. *The Elbow.* New York: Churchill Livingstone; 1982.

114. Dang AC, Rodner CM. Unusual compression neuropathies of the forearm, part I: radial nerve. *J Hand Surg Am.* 2009;34(10):1906–1914.

115. Clavert P, Lutz JC, Adam P, et al. Frohse's arcade is not the exclusive compression site of the radial nerve in its tunnel. *Orthop Traumatol Surg Res.* 2009;95(2):114–118.

116. Plancher KD, Peterson RK, Steichen JB. Compressive neuropathies and tendinopathies in the athletic elbow and wrist. *Clin Sports Med.* 1996;15:331–372.

117. Weinstein SM, Herring SA. Nerve problems and compartment syndromes in the hand, wrist and forearm. *Clin Sports Med.* 1992;11:161–188.

118. Lutz FR. Radial tunnel syndrome: an etiology of chronic lateral elbow pain. *J Orthop Sports Phys Ther.* 1991;14:14–17.

119. Ferlec DC, Morrey BF. Evaluation of the painful elbow: the problem elbow. In: Morrey BF, ed. *The Elbow and its Disorders.* Philadelphia: WB Saunders; 1993.

120. Lister GD, Belsole RB, Kleinert HE. The radial tunnel syndrome. *J Hand Surg.* 1979;4:52–59.

121. Van Rossum J, Buruma OJ, Kamphuisen HA, et al. Tennis elbow: a radial tunnel syndrome? *J Bone Joint Surg Br.* 1978;60:197–198.

122. Naam NH, Nemani S. Radial tunnel syndrome. *Orthop Clinics North Am.* 2012;43(4):529–536.

123. Quinton DN, Finlay D, Butterworth R. The elbow fat pad sign: brief report. *J Bone Joint Surg Br.* 1987;69:844–845.

124. Deniel A, Causeret A, Moser T, et al. Entrapment and traumatic neuropathies of the elbow and hand: an imaging approach. *Diagn Interv Imaging.* 2015;96(12):1261–1278.

125. De Maeseneer M, Brigido MK, Antic M, et al. Ultrasound of the elbow with emphasis on detailed assessment of ligaments, tendons, and nerves. *Eur J Radiol.* 2015;84(4):671–681.

126. De Maeseneer M, Marcelis S, Cattrysse E, et al. Ultrasound of the elbow: a systematic approach using bony landmarks. *Eur J Radiol.* 2012;81(5):919–922.

127. Miller TT, Reinus WR. Nerve entrapment syndromes of the elbow, forearm, and wrist. *AJR Am J Roentgenol.* 2010;195:585–594.

128. Bianchi S, Martinoli C. Elbow. In: Bianchi S, Martinoli C, eds. *Ultrasound of the Musculoskeletal System.* New York: Springer; 2007.

129. Atanda A, Buckley PS, Hammoud S, et al. Early anatomic changes of the ulnar collateral ligament identified by stress ultrasound of the elbow in young professional baseball pitchers. *Am J Sports Med.* 2015;43(12):2943–2949.

130. Tagliafico A, Gandolfo N, Michaud J, et al. Ultrasound demonstration of distal triceps tendon tears. *Eur J Radiol.* 2012;81(6):1207–1210.

131. Tagliafico AS, Bignotti B, Martinoli C. Elbow US. Anatomy, variants, and scanning technique. *Radiology.* 2015;275(3):636–650.

132. Herzog RJ. Efficacy of magnetic resonance imaging of the elbow. *Med Sci Sports Exerc.* 1994;26:1193–1202.

133. Miller TT. Imaging of elbow disorders. *Orthop Clin North Am.* 1999;30:21–36.

134. Fritz RC, Brody GA. MR imaging of the wrist and elbow. *Clin Sports Med.* 1995;14:315–352.

135. Schenk M, Dalinka MK. Imaging of the elbow: an update. *Orthop Clin North Am.* 1997;28:517–535.

136. Tuite MJ, Kijowski R. Sports related injuries of the elbow: an approach to MRI interpretation. *Clin Sports Med.* 2006;25:387–408.

137. Hawksworth CR, Freeland P. Inability to fully extend the injured elbow: an indicator of significant injury. *Arch Emerg Med.* 1991;8(4):253–256.

138. Docherty MA, Schwab RA, Ma OJ. Can elbow extension be used as a test of clinically significant injury? *Southern Med J.* 2002;95:539–541.

139. Irshad F, Shaw NJ, Gregory RJ. Reliability of fat pad sign in radial head/neck fractures of the elbow. *Injury.* 1997;28:433–435.

140. Patla CE, Paris SV. Reliability of interpretation of the Paris classification of normal end-feel for elbow flexion and extension. *J Man Manip Ther.* 1993;1:60–66.

141. Smidt N, van der Windt DA, Assendelft WJ, et al. Intraobserver reproducibility of the assessment of severity of complaints, grip strength, and pressure pain threshold in patients with lateral epicondylitis. *Arch Phys Med Rehabil.* 2002;83:1145–1150.

142. Stratford PW, Norman GR, McIntosh JM. Generalizability of grip strength measurements in patients with tennis elbow. *Phys Ther.* 1989;69:276–281.

143. Overend TJ, Wupri-Fearn JL, Kramer JF, et al. Reliability of a patient-rated forearm evaluation questionnaire for patients with lateral epicondylitis. *J Hand Ther.* 1999;12:31–37.

CHAPTER 7

Forearm, Wrist, and Hand

The hand and wrist are the most active and intricate parts of the upper extremity. Because of this and their complexity, they are vulnerable to injury, which can lead to large functional difficulties because of their role in eating, grooming and other activities of daily living (ADLs), and they do not respond well to serious trauma. Their mobility is enhanced by a wide range of movement at the shoulder and complementary movement at the elbow. The 28 bones, numerous articulations, and 19 intrinsic and 20 extrinsic muscles of the wrist and hand provide a tremendous variability of movement. In addition to being an expressive organ of communication, the hand has a protective role and acts as both a motor and a sensory organ, providing information on such things as temperature, thickness, texture, depth, and shape as well as the motion of an object. It is this sensual acuity that enables the examiner to accurately examine and palpate during an assessment.

The assessment of the hand and wrist should be performed with two objectives in mind. First, the injury or lesion should be assessed as accurately as possible to ensure proper treatment. Second, the examiner should evaluate the remaining function to determine whether the patient will have any incapacity in everyday life.

Although the joints of the forearm, wrist, and hand are discussed separately, they do not act in isolation but rather as functional groups. The position of one joint influences the position and action of the other joints. For example, if the wrist is flexed, the interphalangeal joints do not fully flex, primarily because of passive insufficiency of the finger extensors and their tendons. Each articulation depends on balanced forces for proper positioning and control. If this balance or equilibrium is not present because of trauma, nerve injury, or other factors, the loss of counterbalancing forces results in deformities. In addition, the entire upper limb should be considered a kinetic chain that enables the hand to be properly positioned. The actions of the shoulder, elbow, and wrist joints enable the hand to be placed on almost any area of the body.

Applied Anatomy

The **distal radioulnar joint** (DRUJ) is a uniaxial pivot joint that has 1° of freedom.[1] Although the radius moves over the ulna, the ulna does not remain stationary. The radius moves back and laterally during pronation and forward and medially during supination in relation to the ulna. The resting position of the joint is 10° of supination, and the close packed position is 5° of supination. The capsular pattern of the DRUJ is full range of motion (ROM) with pain at the extreme of rotation.

Distal Radioulnar Joint

Resting position:	10° of supination
Close packed position:	5° of supination
Capsular pattern:	Full range of motion, pain at extremes of rotation

---

The **radiocarpal (wrist) joint** is a biaxial ellipsoid joint.[1,2] The radius articulates with the scaphoid and lunate. The distal radius is not straight but is angled toward the ulna (15° to 20°), and its posterior margin projects more distally to provide a "buttress effect."[3] The lunate and triquetrum also articulate with the triangular cartilaginous disc (**triangular fibrocartilage complex [TFCC]**) (Figs. 7.1 and 7.2), which sits between the ulna and the lunate and triquetrum.[4] The TFCC is made up of the ulnolunate and ulnotriquetral ligament, the extensor carpi ulnaris tendon and its sheath, the ulnar capsule, the anterior and posterior radioulnar ligaments, the ulnomeniscal homolog (i.e., an organ corresponding to another organ in function and make up) and the triangular fibrocartilaginous disc,[4–7] and it is thicker in **ulnar negative** (i.e., **short ulna**) wrists.[4,8] The DRUJ (Fig. 7.3) is stabilized by the TFCC, extensor carpi ulnaris, interosseous ligament, pronator quadratus and other forearm muscles.[4] In the **ulnar neutral wrist**, the axial load across the TFCC is about 18%.[9] The disc extends from the ulnar side of the distal radius and attaches to the ulna at the base of the ulnar styloid process. The disc adds stability to the ulnocarpal articulations and the DRUJ.[5,8,10] The anterior part of the TFCC is tight on pronation and prevents posterior displacement of the ulna while the posterior part is tight on supination and prevents anterior displacement of the ulna. Forced ulnar deviation (e.g., swinging a bat or racquet) increases the load on the TFCC.[5,8,10] The TFCC creates a close relationship between the ulna and carpal

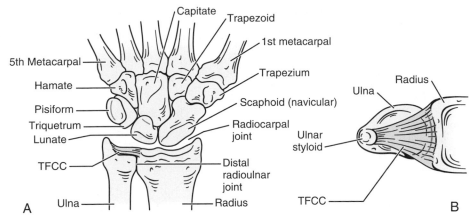

Fig. 7.1 Bones and triangular fibrocartilage complex *(TFCC)*. (A) Palmar view. (B) End view of TFCC and radius and ulna.

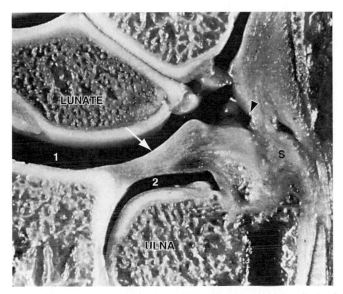

Fig. 7.2 Articulations of the wrist: specific compartments. Ulnar limit of the radiocarpal compartment (coronal section). Note the extent of this compartment *(1)*, its relationship to the inferior radioulnar compartment *(2)*, the intervening triangular fibrocartilage *(arrow)*, and the prestyloid recess *(arrowhead)*, which is intimate with the ulnar styloid *(s)*. (From Resnick D, Kransdorf MJ: *Bone and joint imaging*, Philadelphia, 2005, WB Saunders, p 27.)

Radiocarpal (Wrist) Joint

Resting position:	Neutral with slight ulnar deviation
Close packed:	Extension with radial deviation
Capsular pattern:	Flexion and extension equally limited (works with midcarpal joints)

The stability of the carpals (wrist) is primarily maintained by a complex configuration of ligaments and bones (Fig. 7.4).[15] The ligaments stabilizing the scaphoid, lunate, and triquetrum are the most important.[16] Of these ligaments, the radioscapholunate ligament, the scapholunate and the lunotriquetral ligaments are the most important intrinsic ligaments and are the ligaments most commonly disrupted.[17-19] These ligaments are most likely to be injured with a pronated fall on outstretched hand (FOOSH) injury (i.e., wrist extension, ulnar deviation, and intercarpal supination).[16,20] The scaphoid acts as a strut transmitting movements of the distal carpal row to the proximal carpal row. The scaphoid, lunate, and triquetrum are described as an **intercalated segment**.[21] The scapholunate interosseous ligament is the primary stabilizer of the scapholunate joint and if injured (3° sprain), the result is dynamic instability but not static instability, which only occurs when secondary ligamentous supports are also injured.[21] The bones of the intercalated segment work together with movement of one bone affecting the movement of the other two because of their ligament attachments. For example, during radial deviation, the scaphoid flexes, causing the lunate to flex because of the scapholunate ligament. However, excessive flexion of the lunate is restricted by the lunotriquetral ligament. As the triquetrum is linked to the distal carpal row by the triquetrocapitate ligament, there is an extension moment in the wrist with radial deviation.[22] Lunotriquetral injuries are more likely to occur with wrist extension, radial deviation, and intercarpal supination.[16] The palmar ligaments are much stronger than the dorsal ligaments. The palmar extrinsic ligaments control the movement of the wrist and scaphoid

bones and binds together and stabilizes the distal ends of the radius and ulna.[11,12] With the triangular disc in place and a neutral ulna, the radius bears 60% of the load and the ulna, through the triangular disc, bears 40%. If the disc is removed, the radius transmits 95% of the axial load and the ulna transmits 5%.[13] Therefore, the triangular cartilaginous disc acts as a cushion for the wrist joint and as a major stabilizer of the DRUJ.[3,14] The most common mechanism of injury to the TFCC is forced extension and pronation.

The distal end of the radius is concave and the proximal row of carpals is convex, but the curvatures are not equal. The joint has 2° of freedom, and the resting position is neutral with slight ulnar deviation. The close packed position is extension with radial deviation, and the capsular pattern is equal limitation of flexion and extension.

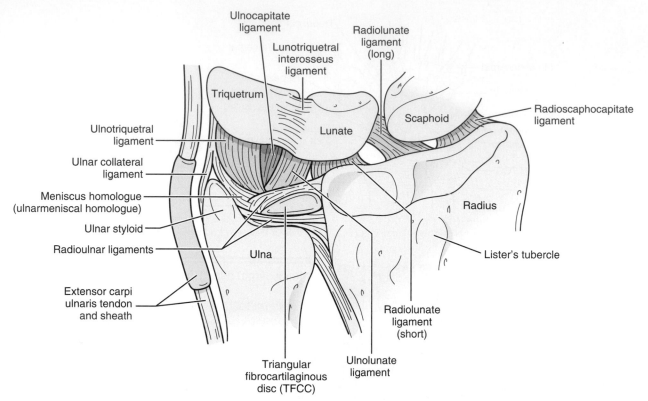

Fig. 7.3 Distal radioulnar joint anatomy. The triangular fibrocartilage complex *(TFCC)* is made up of the ulnar collateral ligament, meniscus homologue, triangular disc, and the radioulnar ligaments formed of the triangular ligament styloid band and the triangular ligament foveal band.

with the radioscapholunate ligament acting as a sling for the scaphoid.[17] This ligament—along with the radiolunate ligament—allows the scaphoid to rotate around them, and both stabilize the scaphoid at the extremes of motion.[17] On the ulnar side, the ligaments (i.e., palmar lunotriquetral, capitotriquetral, dorsal intercarpal, and the fibrocartilaginous disc) control the triquetrum.

The **intercarpal joints** include the joints between the individual bones of the proximal row of carpal bones (i.e., scaphoid, lunate, and triquetrum) and the joints between the individual bones of the distal row of carpal bones (i.e., trapezium, trapezoid, capitate, and hamate). Perilunate injuries involve the lunate and its relation with the other carpals as well as the radius and ulna.[23] They are bound together by small intercarpal ligaments (i.e., dorsal, palmar, and interosseous), which allow only a slight amount of gliding movement between the bones. The close packed position is extension, and the resting position is neutral or slight flexion.

The **pisotriquetral joint** is considered separately, because the pisiform sits on the triquetrum and does not take a direct part in the other intercarpal movements. Interestingly, the flexor carpi ulnaris inserting into the pisiform and hamate via the pisohamate ligament is the only muscle to insert into any of the wrist carpals. Thus, the examiner should understand carpal motion is primarily determined by passive forces, joint surface configurations, ligaments and load, and active forces only act indirectly.[24]

The **midcarpal joints** form a compound articulation between the proximal and distal rows of carpal bones with the exception of the pisiform bone. On the medial side, the scaphoid, lunate, and triquetrum articulate with the capitate and hamate, forming a compound sellar (saddle-shaped) joint. On the lateral aspect, the scaphoid articulates with the trapezoid and trapezium, forming another compound sellar joint. As with the intercarpal joints, these articulations are bound together by dorsal and palmar ligaments; however, there are no interosseous ligaments between the proximal and distal rows of bones. The distal row of carpals (i.e., the hamate, capitate, trapezoid and trapezium) are bound together by strong interosseous ligaments that limit motion between them and the metacarpals.[21] Therefore, greater movement exists at the midcarpal joints than between the individual bones of the two rows of the intercarpal joints. The close packed position of these joints is extension with ulnar deviation, and the resting position is neutral or slight flexion with ulnar deviation.

Intercarpal Joints

Resting position:	Neutral or slight flexion
Close packed position:	Extension
Capsular pattern:	None

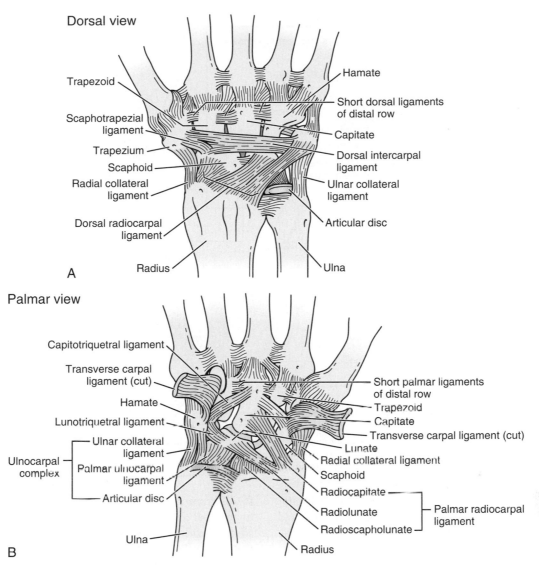

Dorsal view

- Trapezoid
- Scaphotrapezial ligament
- Trapezium
- Scaphoid
- Radial collateral ligament
- Dorsal radiocarpal ligament
- Radius

- Hamate
- Short dorsal ligaments of distal row
- Capitate
- Dorsal intercarpal ligament
- Ulnar collateral ligament
- Articular disc
- Ulna

A

Palmar view

- Capitotriquetral ligament
- Transverse carpal ligament (cut)
- Hamate
- Lunotriquetral ligament
- Ulnocarpal complex
  - Ulnar collateral ligament
  - Palmar ulnocarpal ligament
  - Articular disc
- Ulna

- Short palmar ligaments of distal row
- Trapezoid
- Capitate
- Transverse carpal ligament (cut)
- Lunate
- Radial collateral ligament
- Scaphoid
- Radiocapitate
- Radiolunate
- Radioscapholunate
- Palmar radiocarpal ligament
- Radius

B

Fig. 7.4 Ligaments of the wrist. (A) Dorsal aspect of the right wrist. (B) Palmar aspect of the right wrist. The transverse carpal ligament has been cut and reflected to show the underlying ligaments. (Redrawn from Neumann DA: Kinesiology of the musculoskeletal system—foundations for physical rehabilitation, St Louis, 2002, CV Mosby, pp 178–179.)

Midcarpal Joints	
Resting position:	Neutral or slight flexion with ulnar deviation
Close packed position:	Extension with ulnar deviation
Capsular pattern:	Equal limitation of flexion and extension (works with radiocarpal joints)

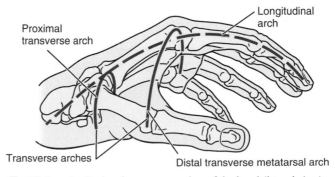

Fig. 7.5 Longitudinal and transverse arches of the hand (lateral view).

The **proximal transverse arch** (Fig. 7.5) that forms the carpal tunnel is formed by the distal row of carpal bones. In this relatively rigid arch, the capitate bone acts as a central keystone structure.[25]

At the thumb, the **carpometacarpal joint** is a sellar joint that has 3° of freedom, whereas the second to fifth carpometacarpal joints are plane joints.[26] The capsular pattern of the carpometacarpal joint of the thumb is abduction most limited, followed by extension. The resting position is midway between abduction and adduction and midway between flexion and extension. The close packed position of the carpometacarpal joint of the thumb is full opposition. For the second to fifth carpometacarpal

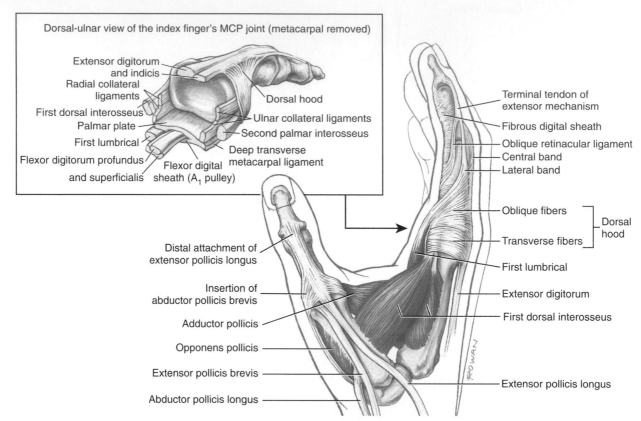

Fig. 7.6 A lateral view of the muscles, tendons, and extensor mechanism of the right hand. The illustration in the box highlights the anatomy associated with the metacarpophalangeal joint of the index finger. *MCP*, Metacarpophalangeal. (From Neumann DA: *Kinesiology of the musculoskeletal system—foundations for physical rehabilitation*, ed 2, St Louis, 2010, CV Mosby, p 269.)

joints, the capsular pattern of restriction is equal limitation in all directions. The bones of these joints are held together by dorsal and palmar ligaments. In addition, the thumb articulation has a strong lateral ligament extending from the lateral side of the trapezium to the radial side of the base of the first metacarpal, and the medial four articulations have an interosseous ligament similar to that found in the carpal articulation.

Carpometacarpal Joints

Resting position:	Thumb, midway between abduction and adduction, and midway between flexion and extension
	Fingers, midway between flexion and extension
Close packed position:	Thumb, full opposition
	Fingers, full flexion
Capsular pattern:	Thumb, abduction, extension
	Fingers, equal limitation in all directions

The carpometacarpal articulations of the fingers allow only gliding movement. The second and third carpometacarpal joints tend to be relatively immobile and are the primary "stabilizing" joints of the hand, whereas the fourth and fifth joints are more mobile to allow the hand to adapt to different shaped objects during grasping. The carpometacarpal articulation of the thumb is unique in that it allows flexion, extension, abduction, adduction, rotation, and circumduction. It is able to do this because the articulation is saddle shaped. Because of the many movements possible at this joint, the thumb is able to adopt any position relative to the palmar aspect of the hand.[26]

The plane **intermetacarpal joints** have only a small amount of gliding movement between them and do not include the thumb articulation. They are bound together by palmar, dorsal, and interosseous ligaments.

The **metacarpophalangeal joints** are condyloid joints. The collateral ligaments of these joints are tight on flexion and relaxed on extension. These articulations are also bound by palmar ligaments and deep transverse metacarpal ligaments. The **dorsal** or **extensor hood** (Fig. 7.6) reinforces the dorsal aspect of the metacarpophalangeal joints while **volar** or **palmar plates** reinforce the palmar aspect (see Fig. 7.6).[3] The flexor tendons and finger annular pulleys are key anatomical structures for the complex grasping function of the hand.[27] The pulleys orient the force of the flexor tendons and convert linear translation into rotation at the interphalangeal joints and prevent bowstringing.[27] Each joint has 2° of freedom. The first metacarpophalangeal joint has 3° of freedom, thus facilitating the movement of the carpometacarpal joint of the

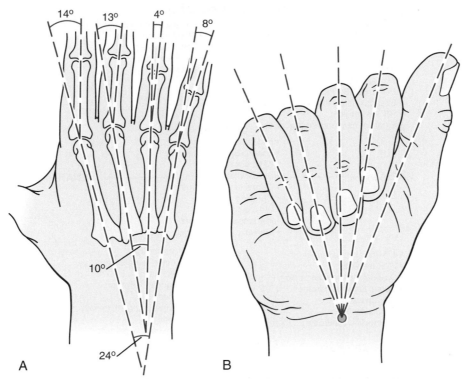

Fig. 7.7 Alignment of the fingers. (A) Normal physiological alignment. (B) Oblique flexion of the last four digits. Only the index ray flexes toward the median axis. When the last four digits are flexed separately at the metacarpophalangeal and proximal interphalangeal joints, their axes converge toward the scaphoid tubercle. (Redrawn from Tubiana R: *The hand*, Philadelphia, 1981, WB Saunders, p 22.)

thumb.[26] The close packed position of the first metacarpophalangeal joint is maximum opposition, and the close packed position for the second through the fifth metacarpophalangeal joints is maximum flexion.[28] The resting position of the metacarpophalangeal joints is slight flexion, whereas the capsular pattern is more limitation of flexion than extension.

Metacarpophalangeal Joints	
Resting position:	Slight flexion
Close packed position:	Thumb, full opposition
	Fingers, full flexion
Capsular pattern:	Flexion, extension

The **distal transverse arch** (see Fig. 7.5) passes through the metacarpophalangeal joints and has greater mobility than the proximal transverse arch, allowing the hand to form or fit around different objects. The second and third metacarpophalangeal joints form the stable portion of the arch while the fourth and fifth metacarpophalangeal joints form the mobile portion (see Fig. 7.39).[25]

The **longitudinal arch** follows the more rigid portion of the hand running from the carpals to the carpometacarpal joints providing longitudinal stability to the hand. The second and third metacarpophalangeal joints are the keystone to both the distal transverse arch and the distal longitudinal arch.[25]

The **interphalangeal joints** are uniaxial hinge joints, each having 1° of freedom (flexion and extension). The close packed position of the proximal interphalangeal joints and distal interphalangeal joints is full extension; the resting position is slight flexion. The capsular pattern of these joints in flexion is more limited than extension. The bones of these joints are bound together by a fibrous capsule and by the palmar and collateral ligaments. During flexion, there is some rotation in these joints so that the pulp of the fingers faces more fully the pulp of the thumb. If the metacarpophalangeal joints and the proximal interphalangeal joints of the fingers are flexed, they converge toward the scaphoid tubercle (Fig. 7.7). This is sometimes referred to as a **cascade sign.** If one or more fingers do not converge, it usually indicates trauma (e.g., fracture) to the digits that has altered their normal alignment.

Interphalangeal Joints	
Resting position:	Slight flexion
Close packed position:	Full extension
Capsular pattern:	Flexion, extension

Patient History

The assessment of the forearm, wrist, and hand often takes longer than that of other joints of the body because of the importance of the hand to everyday function and

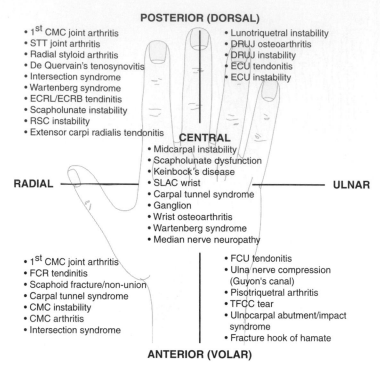

POSTERIOR (DORSAL)

• 1st CMC joint arthritis
• STT joint arthritis
• Radial styloid arthritis
• De Quervain's tenosynovitis
• Intersection syndrome
• Wartenberg syndrome
• ECRL/ECRB tendinitis
• Scapholunate instability
• RSC instability
• Extensor carpi radialis tendonitis

• Lunotriquetral instability
• DRUJ osteoarthritis
• DRUJ instability
• ECU tendonitis
• ECU instability

CENTRAL
• Midcarpal instability
• Scapholunate dysfunction
• Keinbock's disease
• SLAC wrist
• Carpal tunnel syndrome
• Ganglion
• Wrist osteoarthritis
• Wartenberg syndrome
• Median nerve neuropathy

RADIAL — ULNAR

• 1st CMC joint arthritis
• FCR tendinitis
• Scaphoid fracture/non-union
• Carpal tunnel syndrome
• CMC instability
• CMC arthritis
• Intersection syndrome

• FCU tendonitis
• Ulna nerve compression (Guyon's canal)
• Pisotriquetral arthritis
• TFCC tear
• Ulnocarpal abutment/impact syndrome
• Fracture hook of hamate

ANTERIOR (VOLAR)

Fig. 7.8 Wrist pathology listed by site of pain.[29–31] *CMC*, Carpometacarpal; *DRUJ*, distal radioulnar joint; *ECRB*, extensor carpi radialis brevis; *ECRL*, extensor carpi radialis longus; *ECU*, extensor carpi ulnaris; *FCR*, flexor carpi radialis; *FCU*, flexor carpi ulnaris; *RSC*, radioscapulocapitate; *SLAC*, scapholunate advanced collapse; *STT*, scaphotrapezial trapezoid; *TFCC*, triangular fibrocartilage complex. (Modified from Newton AW, Hawkes DH, Bhalaik V: Clinical examination of the wrist, *Orthop Trauma* 31(4):237–247, 2017.)

because of the many structures and joints involved (Fig. 7.8). Palpation of the various bones and their overlying tendons and ligaments can play a significant role in differentiating which structures are at fault.

To properly examine the forearm, wrist, and hand, the examiner should face the patient across a table so that the examiner can talk, observe and move the joints and the structures being assessed while watching the patient's reactions to the movements. This position also allows the patient to rest his or her elbow and arm on the examining table during the assessment.[31]

In addition to the questions listed under the "Patient History" section in Chapter 1, the examiner should obtain the following information from the patient:

1. *What is the patient's age?* Certain conditions are more likely to occur at different ages. For example, arthritic changes are most commonly seen in patients who are older than 40 years of age.[32] Kienbock's disease is more likely to be seen in males between 20 and 40 years of age.[5]

2. *What is the patient's occupation? Have there been any increased physical demands on the wrist?* Certain occupations are more likely to affect the wrist and hand. For example, typists are more likely to suffer repetitive strain injuries, and automobile mechanics are more likely to suffer traumatic injuries.

3. *What was the mechanism of injury?*[32,33] For example, a FOOSH injury may lead to a lunate dislocation,

Colles fracture, scaphoid fracture, injury to the TFCC, or extension of the fingers may cause dislocation of the fingers. Which side of the hand did the patient fall on? Flexion and supination injuries usually affect the radial side of the wrist while extension and pronation injuries affect the ulnar side of the wrist.[34] A rotational force applied to the wrist or near it may lead to a Galeazzi fracture, which is a fracture of the radius and dislocation of the distal end of the ulna. Compressive overload of the ulnar head onto the lunate and triquetrum can lead to **ulnocarpal impaction** causing pain when the arm is pronated (e.g., pushing a shopping cart).[5] If the wrist is in extension and ulnar deviation, impaction at the thenar eminence forces the hand into supination as the forearm pronates injuring the scapholunate interosseous ligament resulting in instability or fracture (Fig. 7.9).[35] This mechanism is seen in gymnastics in which the physis may close prematurely or hypertrophic posterior carpal synovitis may occur due to overuse.[35] Racquet sports, golf, baseball, and tennis can lead to a fracture of the hook of hamate (Fig. 7.10; also see Fig. 7.176), which, like the scaphoid, may not heal.[9] **Hypothenar hammer syndrome** is a vascular injury to the ulnar artery due to repetitive blunt trauma to the hypothenar eminence (i.e., using the palm as a hammer!). The TFCC may be injured from repetitive load bearing and rotational

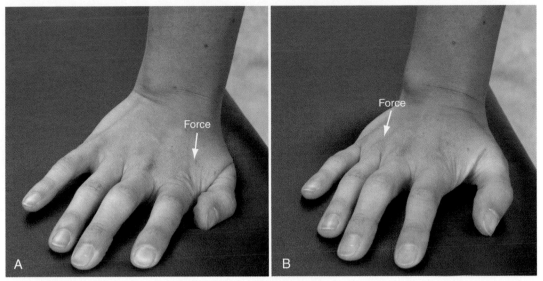

Fig. 7.9 The position of the hand on the forearm at the time of impact load (FOOSH injury) determines the location of tension forces. (A) Impaction on thenar eminence. (B) Impaction on hypothenar eminence. *FOOSH*, Fall on outstretched hand.

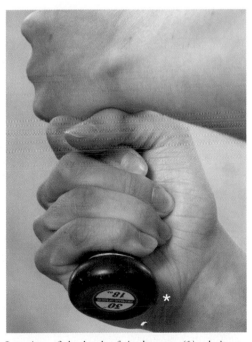

Fig. 7.10 Location of the hook of the hamate *(*)* relative to end of a baseball bat.

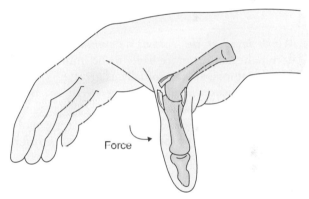

Fig. 7.11 Mechanism of injury resulting in a skier's thumb (also called gamekeeper's thumb or tear of the ulnar collateral ligament of the thumb). The ulnar collateral ligament of the metacarpophalangeal joint is disrupted by an abduction force. (From Dugan SA, Abreu Sosa SM: Ulnar collateral ligament sprain. In Frontera WR, Silver JK, Rizzo TD, editors: *Essentials of physical medicine and rehabilitation*, ed 4, Philadelphia, 2019, Elsevier. Reprinted from Mellion MB: *Office sports medicine*, ed 2, Philadelphia, 1996, Hanley & Belfus, p 228.)

Normal Functional Wrist Movement

For normal functional wrist movement, an individual should have:
- 40° flexion
- 40° extension
- 15° radial deviation
- 20° ulnar deviation

---

stresses (i.e., hyperpronation).[6,9] Skier's or gamekeeper's thumb involves injury to the ulnar collateral ligament (UCL) between the first metacarpal and the proximal phalanx of the thumb (Fig. 7.11).[36–39]

4. *What tasks is the patient able or unable to perform?* For example, is there any problem with buttoning, dressing, tying shoelaces, or any other everyday activity? This type of question gives an indication of the patient's functional limitations. Although normal actual ROM is greater than that usually needed for normal functional activity, functionally at the wrist, the patient should have about 40° flexion, 40° extension, 15° radial deviation and 20° ulnar deviation.[34]

5. *When did the injury or onset occur, and how long has the patient been incapacitated?* These questions are not necessarily the same; for instance, a burn may occur at a certain time, but incapacity may not occur until hypertrophic scarring appears. The wrist is commonly injured by weight bearing (e.g., gymnastics), by rotational stress combined with ulnar deviation (e.g., hitting a racquet), by twisting, and by impact loading (FOOSH injury).[33,40]

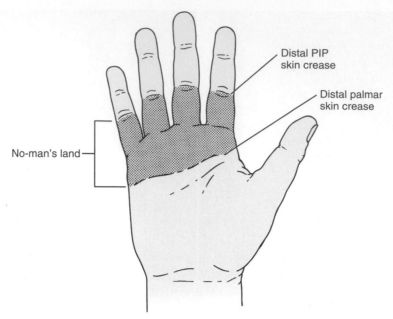

Fig. 7.12 Surgical "no-man's land" (palmar view). *PIP,* Proximal interphalangeal.

6. *Which hand is the patient's dominant hand?* The dominant hand is more likely to be injured, and the functional loss, at least initially, is greater.

7. *Has the patient injured the forearm, wrist, or hand previously?* Was it the same type of injury? Was the mechanism of injury the same? If so, how was it treated?

8. *Which part of the forearm, wrist, or hand is injured?* If the flexor tendons (which are round, have synovial sheaths, and have a longer excursion than the extensor tendons) are injured, they respond much more slowly to treatment than do extensor tendons (which are flat or ovoid). Within the hand, there is a surgical "no-man's land" (Fig. 7.12), which is a region between the distal palmar crease and the midportion of the middle phalanx of the fingers. Damage to the flexor tendons in this area requires surgical repair and usually lead to the formation of adhesive bands that restrict gliding. In addition, the tendons may become ischemic, being replaced by scar tissue. Because of this, the prognosis after surgery in this area is poor.

9. *Does pain or abnormal sensation (e.g., tingling, pins and needles) predominate?* In the hand and fingers, the examiner must take the time to differentiate exactly where the symptoms are to differentiate peripheral nerve neuropathy, nerve root symptoms, and other painful localized conditions.[41,42] What does the patient do if symptoms are worse? In the case of a nerve injury, certain fingers may be affected by different peripheral nerves causing part of the hand to "go to sleep" (i.e., tingling and numbness). To relieve the numbness, the patient often shakes or flicks the wrist and hand several times. This has been called the **flick sign.**[43,44] In older patients, insidious onset

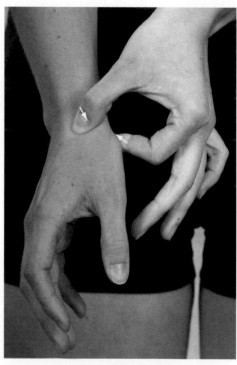

Fig. 7.13 Clamp sign for scaphoid injury.

of symptoms in the hand may be coming from the cervical spine.[34]

10. *Where is it painful?* The patient may describe a large or small area which may indicate injury to a specific structure or several structures. For example, if the patient grasps the scaphoid anteriorly and posteriorly (the **clamp sign**) (Fig. 7.13), saying that is where the pain is, the examiner might suspect a scaphoid fracture, avascular necrosis of the scaphoid, or injury to the scapholunate joint or ligaments.[34]

Observation

While observing the patient and viewing the forearms, wrists, and hands from both the anterior and posterior aspects, the examiner should note the patient's willingness and ability to use the hand doing activities such as removing a jacket, opening a door, weight-bearing on armrests while sitting down or standing up, taking something out of a pocket, and writing.[5] In some cases, a hand diagram (Fig. 7.14), that can be completed by the patient and/or the examiner, can be used to delineate different signs and symptoms with markings or colors which may help with the diagnosis.[45,46] For example, with carpal tunnel syndrome, a **Katz scoring system** of hand diagrams may sometimes be used for a diagnosis.[45–47]

Normally, when the hand is in the resting position and the wrist is in the normal position, the fingers are progressively more flexed as one moves from the radial side of the hand to the ulnar side. Loss of this normal attitude may be caused by pathology affecting the hand, such as a lacerated tendon, or by a contracture, such as Dupuytren contracture.

The bone and soft-tissue contours of the forearm, wrist, and hand should be compared for both upper limbs, and any deviation should be noted. For example, excessive prominence of the distal ulna (Fig. 7.15) compared to the other side may indicate disruption of the DRUJ. The cosmetic appearance of the hand is very important to some patients. The examiner should note the patient's reaction to the appearance of the hand and be prepared to provide a cosmetic evaluation. This evaluation should always be included with the more important functional assessment. The posture of the hand at rest often demonstrates common deformities. Are the normal skin creases present? Skin creases occur because of movement at the various joints. The examiner should note any muscle wasting on the thenar eminence (median nerve), first dorsal interosseous muscle (C7 nerve root), or hypothenar eminence (ulnar nerve) that may be indicative of peripheral nerve or nerve root injury.

Any localized swellings (e.g., ganglion) that are seen on the dorsum of the hand should be recorded (Fig. 7.16).[48] In the wrist and hand, effusion and synovial thickening are most evident on the dorsal and radial aspects. Swelling of the metacarpophalangeal and interphalangeal joints is most obvious on the dorsal aspect.

The dominant hand tends to be larger than the nondominant hand. If the patient has an area on the fingers that lacks sensation, this area is avoided when the patient lifts or identifies objects, and the patient uses another finger instead with normal sensitivity. Therefore, the examiner should watch for abnormal or different patterns of movement, which may indicate adaptations or modifications necessitated by the presence of pathology.

Any vasomotor, sudomotor, pilomotor, and trophic changes should be recorded. These changes may be

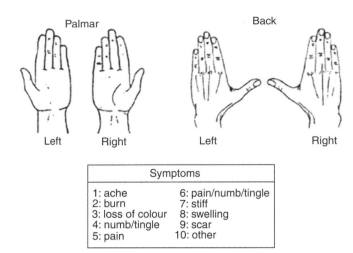

Fig. 7.14 Hand symptom diagram. (Modified from Bonauto DK, Silverstein B, Fan ZJ, et al: Evaluation of a symptom diagram for identifying carpal tunnel syndrome, *Occup Med* 58(8):561–566, 2008.)

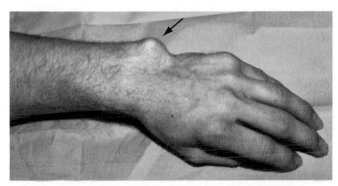

Fig. 7.15 Prominence of the distal ulna *(arrow)*, indicating distal radioulnar joint disruption. (From Skirven TM, Osterman AL, Fedorczyk J, Amadio PC: *Rehabilitation of the hand and upper extremity*, ed 6, St Louis, 2011, Elsevier.)

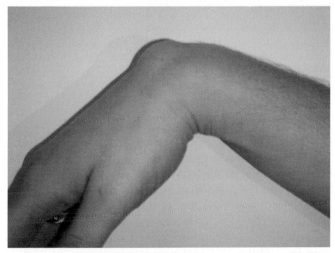

Fig. 7.16 Ganglion or small cystic swelling on the dorsum of the right hand just distal to the wrist joint.

indicative of a peripheral nerve injury, peripheral vascular disease, diabetes mellitus, Raynaud disease, or reflex neurovascular syndromes (also called **complex regional pain syndrome,** *reflex sympathetic dystrophy, causalgia,*

TABLE 7.1

Budapest Diagnostic Criteria for Complex Regional Pain Syndrome[50–52]

1. Continuing pain, which is disproportionate to any inciting event

2. Must report at least one symptom in three of the four following categories:
   - *Sensory*: reports of hyperesthesia (excessive skin sensitivity) and/or allodynia (central pain sensitization)
   - *Vasomotor (affects blood vessels)*: reports of temperature asymmetry and/or skin color changes and/or skin color asymmetry
   - *Sudomotor (affects sweat glands) or edema*: reports of edema and/or sweating changes and/or sweating asymmetry
   - *Motor or trophic (changes in soft tissue due to interruption of nerve supply leading to accumulation of fibrous tissue)*: reports of decreased range of motion and/or motor dysfunction (weakness, tremor, dystonia [repetitive muscle contractions or fixed postures]) and/or trophic changes (hair, nail, skin)

3. Must display at least one sign at time of evaluation in two or more of the following categories:
   - *Sensory*: evidence of hyperalgesia (enhanced pain response) (to pinprick) and/or allodynia (to light touch and/or deep somatic pressure and/or joint movement)
   - *Vasomotor*: evidence of temperature asymmetry and/or skin color changes and/or asymmetry
   - *Sudomotor or edema*: evidence of edema and/or sweating changes and/or sweating asymmetry
   - *Motor or trophic*: evidence of decreased range of motion and/or motor dysfunction (weakness, tremor, dystonia) and/or trophic changes (hair, nail, skin)

4. There is no other diagnosis that better explains the signs and symptoms

Modified from Harden RN, Bruehl S, Perez RS, et al: Validation of proposed diagnostic criteria (the "Budapest Criteria") for complex regional pain syndrome, *Pain* 150(2):268–274, 2010.

shoulder-hand syndrome, and *Sudeck atrophy*), which can be initiated by minor trauma, fracture, immobilization, stroke or surgery and is most prevalent in the upper limb.[49] The clinical signs and symptoms of complex regional pain syndrome affect the limb involved in a "glove" or "stocking" distribution (see Fig. 7.37), which is different from peripheral nerve distribution and the pain is often out of proportion to the injury. The changes seen in complex regional pain syndrome could include loss of hair on the hand, brittle fingernails, increase or decrease in sweating of the palm, shiny skin, radiographic evidence of osteoporosis, or any difference in temperature between the two limbs. Table 7.1 illustrates the **Budapest Diagnostic Criteria for Complex Regional Pain Syndrome.**[51–57]

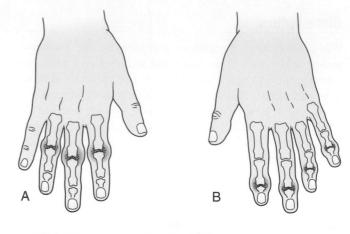

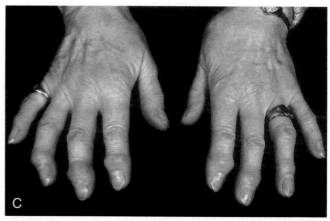

Fig. 7.17 (A) Bouchard nodes. (B) Heberden nodes. (C) Osteoarthritis of both hands. Note the large swellings of the distal interphalangeal joints (Heberden nodes) associated with some inflammation, and the earlier changes in the proximal interphalangeal joints (Bouchard nodes). (C, From Creamer P, Kidd BL, Conaghan PG: Osteoarthritis and related disorders. In Waldman SD, editor: *Pain management*, ed 2, Philadelphia, 2011, Elsevier.)

The examiner should note any hypertrophy of the fingers. Hypertrophy of the bone may be seen in Paget disease, neurofibromatosis, or arteriovenous fistula. The examiner should also look for a **carpal or metacarpal boss**, which is seen with arthritis and is hard swelling on the dorsum (i.e., back) of the hand as a bone spur forms at the base of the carpometacarpal joints of the index and middle finger or over the capitate and trapezoid. It is only of concern if painful and usually is seen in young adults (aged 20 to 40 years).[58–60]

The presence of Heberden or Bouchard nodes (Fig. 7.17) should be recorded. Heberden nodes appear on the dorsal surface of the distal interphalangeal joints and are associated with osteoarthritis. Bouchard nodes are on the dorsal surface of the proximal interphalangeal joints.[61] They are often associated with gastrectasis and osteoarthritis.

Skin color changes can give an indication of the state of the vascular system to the hand. Hyperemia may be the result of infection while dry and shiny skin may indicate systemic disease.[5,62]

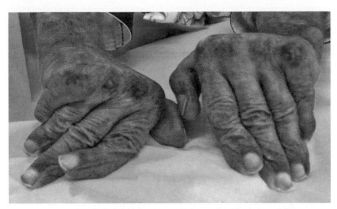

Fig. 7.18 Ulnar drift at the metacarpophalangeal joints especially in the right hand. (From Dall'Era M, Wofsy D: Clinical features of systemic lupus erythematosus. In Firestein GS, Budd RC, Gabriel SE, et al, editors: *Kelley and Firestein's textbook of rheumatology*, ed 10, Philadelphia, 2017, Elsevier.)

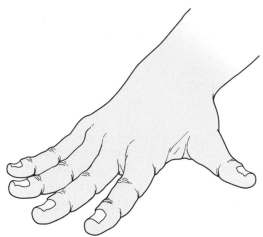

Fig. 7.19 Spoon-shaped nails.

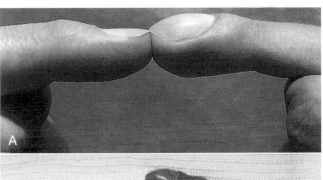

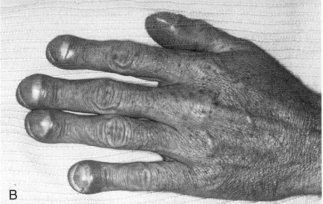

Fig. 7.20 Nail clubbing. (A) Close-up side view of clubbing on the right in comparison to normal on the left. (B) Dorsal view. (A, From Zipes DB, Libby P, Bonow RO, Braunwald E: *Braunwald's heart disease: a textbook of cardiovascular medicine*, ed 7, Philadelphia, 2005, Saunders; B, From Avidan AY, Kryger M: Physical examination in sleep medicine. In Kryger M, Roth T, Dement WC, editors: *Principles and practice of sleep medicine*, ed 6, Philadelphia, 2017, Elsevier. Courtesy Dr. Meir H. Kryger.)

Any ulcerations may indicate neurological or circulatory problems. Any alteration in the color of the limb with changes in position may indicate a circulatory problem.

The examiner should note any rotational or angulated deformities of the fingers or wrist, which may be indicative of previous fracture. The nail beds are normally parallel to one another. The fingers, when extended, are slightly rotated toward the thumb to aid pinch. **Ulnar drift** (Fig. 7.18) may be seen in rheumatoid arthritis, owing to the shape of the metacarpophalangeal joints and the pull of the long tendons.

The presence of any wounds or scars should be noted because they may indicate recent surgery or past trauma. If wounds are present, are they new or old? Are they healing properly? Is the scar red (new) or white (old)? Is the scar mobile or adherent? Is it normal, hypertrophic, or keloid? Palmar scars may interfere with finger extension. Web space scars or **congenital webbing** (i.e., **syndactyly**) may interfere with finger separation and metacarpophalangeal joint flexion.

The examiner should take time to observe the fingernails. **"Spoon-shaped" nails** (Fig. 7.19) are often the result of fungal infection, anemia, iron deficiency, long-term diabetes, local injury, developmental abnormality, chemical irritants, or psoriasis. They may also be a congenital or hereditary trait. **"Clubbed" nails** (Fig. 7.20) may result from hypertrophy of the underlying soft tissue or respiratory or cardiac problems, such as chronic obstructive pulmonary disease, severe emphysema, congenital heart defects, or cor pulmonale.[62] Table 7.2 shows other pathological processes that may affect the fingernails.

Common Hand and Finger Deformities

Ape Hand Deformity. Wasting of the thenar eminence of the hand occurs as a result of a median nerve palsy, and the thumb falls back in line with the fingers as a result of the pull of the extensor muscles. The patient is also unable to oppose or flex the thumb (Fig. 7.21).

Bishop's Hand or Benediction Hand Deformity (Duchene's Sign). Wasting of the hypothenar muscles of the hand, the interossei muscles, and the two medial lumbrical muscles occurs because of ulnar nerve palsy (Fig. 7.22). There is hyperextension of the metacarpophalangeal joint and flexion of the interphalangeal joints.[63,64] If the wrist flexes with metacarpophalangeal extension when the extrinsic

TABLE **7.2**

Glossary of Nail Pathology

Condition	Description	Occurrence
Beau lines	Transverse lines or ridges marking repeated disturbances of nail growth	Systemic diseases, toxic or nutritional deficiency states of many types, trauma (from manicuring)
Defluvium unguium (onychomadesis)	Complete loss of nails	Certain systemic diseases, such as scarlet fever, syphilis, leprosy, alopecia areata, exfoliative dermatitis
Diffusion of lunula unguis	"Spreading" of lunula	Dystrophies of the extremities
Eggshell nails	Nail plate thin, semitransparent bluish-white with a tendency to curve upward at the distal edge	Syphilis
Fragilitas unguium	Friable or brittle nails	Dietary deficiency, local trauma
Hapalonychia	Nails very soft, split easily	Following contact with strong alkalis; endocrine disturbances, malnutrition, syphilis, chronic arthritis
Hippocratic nails	"Watch-glass nails" associated with "drumstick fingers"	Chronic respiratory and circulatory diseases, especially pulmonary tuberculosis; hepatic cirrhosis
Koilonychia	"Spoon nails"—nails are concave on the outer surface	Dysendocrinisms (acromegaly), trauma, dermatoses, syphilis, nutritional deficiencies, hypothyroidism
Leukonychia	White spots or striations or rarely the whole nail may turn white (congenial type)	Local trauma, hepatic cirrhosis, nutritional deficiencies, and many systemic diseases
Mees' lines	Transverse white bands	Hodgkin's granuloma, arsenic and thallium toxicity, high fevers, local nutritional derangement
Moniliasis of nails	Infections (usually paronychial) caused by yeast forms (*Candida albicans*)	Occupational (common in food-handlers, dentists, dishwashers, and gardeners)
Onychatrophia	Atrophy or failure of development of nails	Trauma, infection, dysendocrinism, gonadal aplasia, and many systemic disorders
Onychauxis	Nail plate is greatly thickened	Mild persistent trauma, systemic diseases, such as peripheral stasis, peripheral neuritis, syphilis, leprosy, hemiplegia; or at times may be congenital
Onychia	Inflammation of the nail matrix causing deformity of the nail plate	Trauma, infection, many systemic diseases
Onychodystrophy	Any deformity of the nail plate, nail bed, or nail matrix	Many diseases, trauma, or chemical agents (poisoning, allergy)
Onychogryphosis	"Claw nails"—extreme degree of hypertrophy, sometimes with horny projections arising from the nail surface	May be congenital or related to many chronic systemic diseases (see Onychauxis)
Onycholysis	Loosening of the nail plate beginning at the distal or free edge	Trauma, injury by chemical agents, many systemic diseases
Onychomadesis	Shedding of all the nails (defluvium unguium)	Dermatoses, such as exfoliative dermatitis, alopecia areata, psoriasis, eczema, nail infection, severe systemic diseases, arsenic poisoning
Onychophagia	Nail biting	Neurosis
Onychorrhexis	Longitudinal ridging and splitting of the nails	Dermatoses, nail infections, many systemic diseases, senility, injury by chemical agents, hyperthyroidism
Onychoschizia	Lamination and scaling away of nails in thin layers	Dermatoses, syphilis, injury by chemical agents
Onychotillomania	Alteration of the nail structures caused by persistent neurotic picking of the nails	Neurosis
Pachyonychia	Extreme thickening of all the nails; the nails are more solid and more regular than in onychogryphosis	Usually congenital and associated with hyperkeratosis of the palms and soles
Pterygium unguis	Thinning of the nail fold and spreading of the cuticle over the nail plate	Associated with vasospastic conditions, such as Raynaud phenomenon and occasionally with hypothyroidism

From Berry TJ: *The hand as mirror systemic disease*, Philadelphia, 1963, FA Davis.

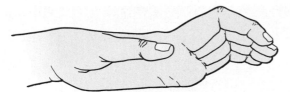

Fig. 7.21 Ape hand deformity.

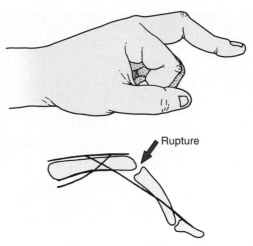

Rupture

Fig. 7.23 Boutonnière deformity. Note the flexion deformity at the proximal interphalangeal joint.

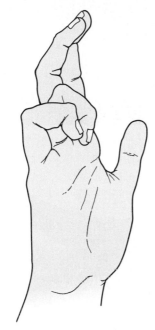

Fig. 7.22 Bishop's hand or benediction hand deformity.

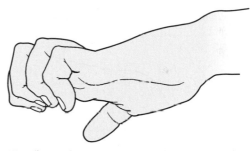

Fig. 7.24 Claw fingers (intrinsic minus hand). Fingers are hyperextended at the metacarpophalangeal joints and flexed at the interphalangeal joints.

extensors contract, it is a positive sign called the **André-Thomas sign**.[64]

Boutonnière Deformity. Extension of the metacarpophalangeal and distal interphalangeal joints and flexion of the proximal interphalangeal joint (primary deformity) are seen with this deformity. The deformity is the result of a rupture of the central tendinous slip of the extensor hood and is most common after trauma or in rheumatoid arthritis (Fig. 7.23).

Carpal (Carpometacarpal) Bossing. This deformity is an overgrowth of hard bone on the posterior aspect of the hand where the index and/or middle finger meets the trapezoid and capitate bones.[59,60] It is an indication of arthritis and can be seen on x-ray. Unless it causes pain, it is usually left alone.

Claw Fingers. This deformity results from the loss of intrinsic muscle action and the overaction of the extrinsic (long) extensor muscles on the proximal phalanx of the fingers. The metacarpophalangeal joints are hyperextended, and the proximal and distal interphalangeal joints are flexed (Fig. 7.24). If intrinsic function is lost, the hand is called an **intrinsic minus hand.** The normal cupping of

the hand is lost, both the longitudinal and the transverse arches of the hand (see Fig. 7.5) disappear, and there is intrinsic muscle wasting. The deformity is most often caused by a combined median and ulnar nerve palsy. If there is flattening of the dorsal transverse metatarsal arch (see Fig. 7.5) and the hand appears flattened, it is called **Masse's sign ❓** and is the result of hypothenar muscle paralysis.[63,64]

Dinner Fork Deformity. This deformity is seen with a malunion distal radial fracture (Colles fracture) with the distal radial fragment angulated posteriorly (Fig. 7.25).

Drop-Wrist Deformity. The extensor muscles of the wrist are paralyzed as a result of a radial nerve palsy, and the wrist and fingers cannot be actively extended by the patient (Fig. 7.26).

Dupuytren Contracture/Disease. This progressive disease of genetic origin results in contracture of the palmar fascia.[65] There is a fixed flexion deformity of the metacarpophalangeal and proximal interphalangeal joints (Fig. 7.27). Dupuytren contracture is usually seen in the ring or little finger, and the skin is often adherent to the fascia. It affects men more often than women and is usually seen in the 50- to 70-year-old age group.[66]

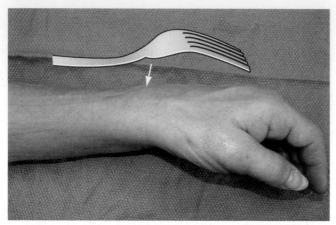

Fig. 7.25 Displaced distal radial fracture with a classic "silver fork" or "dinner fork" deformity. Note the pronation and dorsal angulation of the hand on the forearm. (From Green JB, Deveikas C, Ranger HE, et al: Hand, wrist, and digit injuries. In Magee DJ, Zachazewski JE, Quillen WS, Manske RC, editors: *Pathology and intervention in musculoskeletal rehabilitation*, ed 2, St. Louis, 2016, Elsevier.)

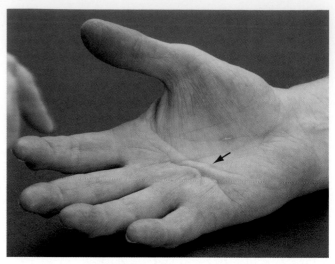

Fig. 7.27 Dupuytren's contracture.

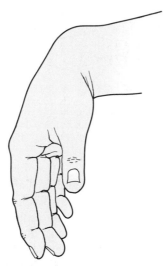

Fig. 7.26 Drop-wrist deformity.

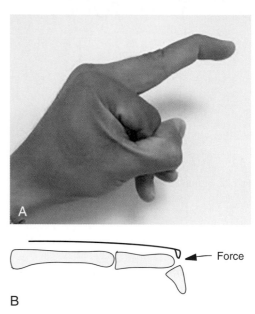

Fig. 7.28 Mallet finger. (A) Patient actively attempting to extend distal phalanx. (B) Mechanism of injury. Tendon is ruptured or avulsed from bone. (A, from Kreger VC, Canders CP: A man who is unable to extend his middle finger, *Visual J Emerg Med* 7:40–41, 2017.)

Extensor Plus Deformity. This deformity is caused by adhesions or shortening of the extensor communis tendon proximal to the metacarpophalangeal joint. It results in the inability of the patient to simultaneously flex the metacarpophalangeal and proximal interphalangeal joints, although they may be flexed individually.

Mallet Finger.[67] A mallet finger deformity is the result of a rupture or avulsion of the extensor tendon where it inserts into the distal phalanx of the finger. The distal phalanx rests in a flexed position (Fig. 7.28).

Myelopathy Hand. This deformity is a dysfunction of the hand caused by cervical spinal cord pathology in conjunction with cervical spondylosis. The patient shows an inability to extend and adduct the ring and little finger and sometimes the middle finger, especially rapidly, despite good function of the wrist, thumb, and index finger. In addition, the patient shows an exaggerated triceps reflex and positive pathological reflexes (e.g., Hoffman reflex).[68]

Pitres-Testus Sign. The Pitres-Testus ❓ sign is evident when the patient is asked to shape the hand in the form of a cone (modified cylinder grasp) and cannot do so because of loss of hypothenar muscles due to ulnar nerve neuropathy.[64]

Polydactyly and Triphalangism. Polydactyly is a congenital anomaly characterized by the presence of more than the normal number of fingers or, in the case of the foot, toes (Fig. 7.29A). Triphalangism implies there are three phalanges instead of the normal two as would be seen in the thumb.[69]

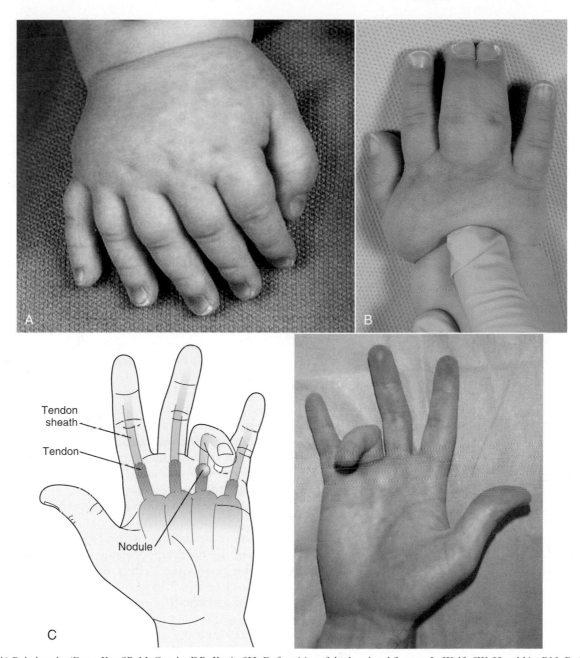

Fig. 7.29 (A) Polydactyly. (From Kay SP, McCombe DB, Kozin SH: Deformities of the hand and fingers. In Wolfe SW, Hotchkiss RN, Pederson WC, et al, editors: *Green's operative hand surgery*, ed 7, Philadelphia, 2017, Elsevier. Courtesy Shriners Hospital for Children, Philadelphia.) (B) Syndactyly. (From Hovius SER, van Nieuwenhoven CA: Congenital hand IV: syndactyly, synostosis, polydactyly, camptodactyly, and clinodactyly. In Chang J, Neligan PC, editors: *Plastic surgery: Volume 6: hand and upper extremity*, ed 2, St. Louis, 2018, Elsevier.) (C) Trigger finger. (From Silverstein JA, Moeller JL, Hutchinson MR: Common issues in orthopedics. In Rakel RE, Radel DP, editors: *Textbook of family medicine*, ed 9, Philadelphia, 2016, Elsevier.)

Prominent Ulnar Head.[58] A prominent ulnar head may indicate DRUJ pathology (e.g., posterior dislocation), ulnar side carpal pathology (e.g., subluxation and pronation of ulnar carpals), or TFCC pathology (see Fig. 7.15). In rheumatoid arthritis, this is known as **ulnar caput syndrome.** If there is no pathology present, it tends to occur in wrists where there is radial shortening with no tilt and is common in congenital **ulnar plus wrists.**[58]

Shoulder Sign of the Thumb. Subluxation of the carpometacarpal joint of the thumb may occur in arthritis and

if the subluxation is more than 2 to 3 mm, there will be a slight step at the joint. The step is sometimes called the **"shoulder sign"** (Fig. 7.30).[34,70] If axial loading is applied through the first carpometacarpal joint, pain and crepitus may be felt.[70]

Swan Neck Deformity. This deformity usually involves only the fingers. There is flexion of the metacarpophalangeal and distal interphalangeal joints, but the real deformity is extension of the proximal interphalangeal joint. The condition is a result of contracture of the intrinsic

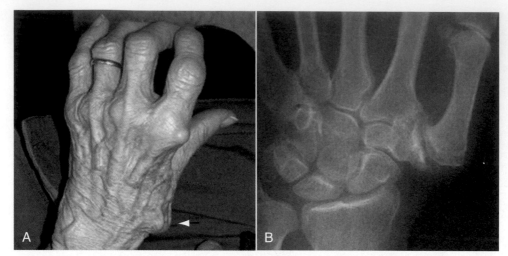

Fig. 7.30 First carpometacarpal arthritis. (A) Radial subluxation of the base of the first metacarpal giving the "shoulder sign" *(arrow)*. (B) Anteroposterior radiograph of the same hand. (From Young D, Papp S, Giachino A: Physical examination of the wrist, *Hand Clin* 26(1):21–36, 2010.)

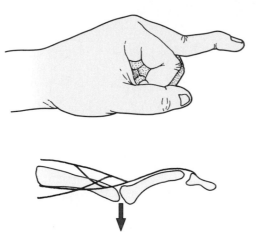

Fig. 7.31 Swan neck deformity. Note the hyperextension at the proximal interphalangeal joint.

muscles or tearing of the volar plate and is often seen in patients with rheumatoid arthritis or following trauma (Fig. 7.31).

Syndactyly. This deformity is a congenital condition in which some fingers (or toes in the feet) are wholly or partially united, joined, or webbed (Fig. 7.29B).[70] In the hand, if present, webbing is most common between the ring and middle finger (57%); ring and little finger (27%); index and middle finger (14%); and thumb and index finger (3%).[71]

Trigger Finger.[72] Also known as digital tenovaginitis stenosans, this deformity is the result of a thickening of the flexor tendon sheath (Notta's nodule), which causes sticking of the tendon when the patient attempts to flex the finger (Fig. 7.29C). A low-grade inflammation of the proximal fold of the flexor tendon leads to swelling and constriction (stenosis) in the digital flexor tendon. When the patient attempts to flex the finger, the tendon sticks, and the finger "let's go," often with

a snap. As the condition worsens, eventually the finger will flex but not let go, and it will have to be passively extended until finally a fixed flexion deformity occurs. The condition is more likely to occur in middle-aged women, whereas **"trigger thumb"** with a flexion deformity of the interphalangeal joint is more common in young children.[73] The condition usually occurs in the third or fourth finger. In adults, it is most often associated with rheumatoid arthritis and tends to be worse in the morning.

Ulnar Drift. This deformity, which is commonly seen in patients with rheumatoid arthritis but can occur with other conditions, results in ulnar deviation of the digits because of weakening of the capsuloligamentous structures of the metacarpophalangeal joints and the accompanying "bowstring" effect of the extensor communis tendons (see Fig. 7.18).

Ulnar Variance. The relationship of the distal articular surface of the ulna to the articular surface of the radius. It is positive if the ulna is more distal than the radius. It is negative (i.e., ulnar negative) if the ulna is shorter than the articular surface of the radius. It can be measured clinically with the shoulder abducted to 90°, elbow flexed to 90°, forearm in neutral and wrist and hand in neutral. The examiner then puts his or her nail beds at 90° to the long axis of the patient's forearm with one nail bed against the radial styloid and one against the ulnar styloid (Fig. 7.32). The level of the two landmarks gives a measure of **clinical ulnar variance** (measured from the styloid) as opposed to **true ulnar variance** (referenced from the ulnar head on x-ray).[70] **Neutral ulnar variance** means the articular surfaces of the radius and ulna are equal. It becomes more positive in pronation and during power grips. It decreases in supination. If it is negative, greater loads pass through the radius. It is more common to measure ulnar variance on x-ray if the examiner thinks the variance is not normal (see Fig. 7.142).

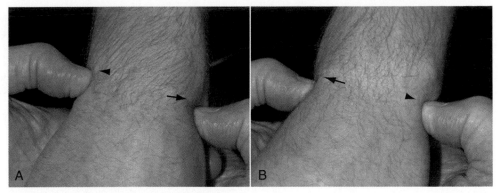

Fig. 7.32 Clinical ulnar variance. (A) Right wrist with normal clinical ulnar variance. (B) Left wrist with increased clinical ulnar variance after distal radius malunion (shortening). (From Young D, Papp S, Giachino A: Physical examination of the wrist, *Hand Clin* 26(1):21–36, 2010.)

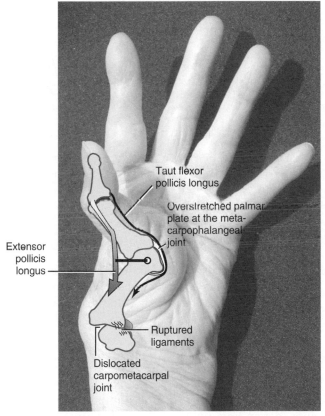

Fig. 7.33 Palmar view showing the pathomechanics of a common zig-zag deformity of the thumb caused by rheumatoid arthritis. The thumb metacarpal dislocates laterally at the carpometacarpal joint, causing hyperextension at the metacarpophalangeal joint. The interphalangeal joint remains partially flexed owing to the passive tension in the stretched and taut flexor pollicis longus. Note that the "bowstringing" of the tendon of the extensor pollicis longus across the metacarpophalangeal joint creates a large extensor moment arm, thereby magnifying the mechanics of the deformity. (From Neumann DA: *Kinesiology of the musculoskeletal system—foundations for physical rehabilitation,* St Louis, 2002, CV Mosby, p 237.)

Zigzag Deformity of the Thumb. The thumb is flexed at the carpometacarpal joint and hyperextended at the metacarpophalangeal joint (Fig. 7.33). The deformity is associated with rheumatoid arthritis. A "Z" deformity is due to hypermobility and may be familial (Fig. 7.34).

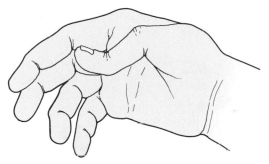

Fig. 7.34 "Z" deformity of the thumb.

Other Physical Findings

The hand is the terminal part of the upper limb. Many pathological conditions manifest themselves in this structure and may lead the examiner to suspect pathological conditions elsewhere in the body. It is important for the examiner to take the time to view the hands when assessing any joint, especially if an abnormal pattern is presented or the history gives an indication that more than one joint may be involved. For example, if a patient presents with insidious neck pain and demonstrates nail changes that indicate psoriasis, the examiner should consider the possibility of psoriatic arthritis affecting the cervical spine as well as the hand. Some conditions involving the hand include the following:

1. Generalized or continued body exposure to radiation produces brittle nails, longitudinal nail ridges, skin keratosis (thickening), and ulceration.
2. The Plummer-Vinson syndrome produces spoon-shaped nails (see Fig. 7.19). This condition is a dysphagia with atrophy in the mouth, pharynx, and upper esophagus.
3. Psoriasis may cause scaling, deformity, and fragmentation and detachment of the nails. Psoriasis may lead to psoriatic arthritis affecting spinal and peripheral joints.
4. Hyperthyroidism produces nail atrophy and ridging with warm, moist hands.

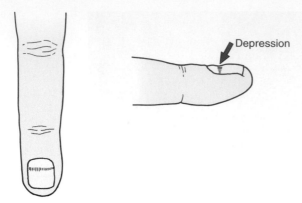

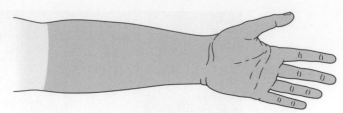

Fig. 7.37 "Opera glove anesthesia," showing area of abnormal sensation.

Fig. 7.35 Beau lines.

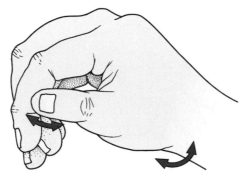

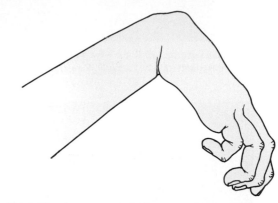

Fig. 7.38 Deformity seen with Volkmann ischemic contracture. Note clawed fingers.

Fig. 7.36 "Pill rolling hand," seen in Parkinson disease.

5. Vasospastic conditions produce a thin nail fold and pterygium (abnormal extension) of the cuticle.
6. Trauma to the nail bed, toxic radiation, acute illness, prolonged fever, avitaminosis, and chronic alcoholism produce transverse lines, or Beau lines, in the nails (Fig. 7.35).
7. Many arterial diseases produce a lack of linear growth with thick, dark nails.
8. Lues (syphilis) produces a hypertrophic overgrowth of the nail plate. The nails break and crumple easily.
9. Chronic respiratory disorders produce clubbing of the nails (see Fig. 7.20).
10. Subacute bacterial endocarditis may produce Osler nodes, which are small, tender nodes in the finger pads.
11. Congenital heart disease may produce cyanosis and nail clubbing.
12. Neurocirculatory aesthesia (loss of strength and energy) produces cold, damp hands.
13. Parkinson disease produces a typical hand tremor known as "pill rolling hand" (Fig. 7.36).
14. Causalgic states produce a painful, swollen, hot hand.
15. "Opera glove" anesthesia is seen in hysteria, leprosy, diabetes, or complex regional pain syndrome. It is a condition in which there is numbness from the elbow to the fingers (Fig. 7.37).
16. Raynaud disease produces a cold, mottled, painful hand. It is an idiopathic vascular disorder

characterized by intermittent attacks of pallor and cyanosis of the extremities brought on by cold or emotion.
17. Rheumatoid arthritis produces a warm, wet hand as well as joint swelling, dislocations or subluxations, and ulnar deviation or drift of the wrist (see Fig. 7.18).
18. The deformed hand of Volkmann ischemic contracture is one that is very typical for a compartment syndrome after a fracture or dislocation of the elbow (Fig. 7.38).[74]

Examination

The examination of the forearm, wrist, and hand may be very extensive, or it may be limited to one or two joints, depending on the area and degree of injury. Regardless, because of its functional importance, the examiner must take extra care when examining this area. Not only must clinical limitations be determined, but functional limitations brought on by trauma, nerve injuries, or other factors must be carefully considered to have an appropriate outcome functionally, cosmetically, and clinically.

Because there are so many joints, bones, muscles, and ligaments involved, the examiner must develop a working knowledge of all of these tissues and how they interact with one another. The examiner should remember that adduction of the hand (ulnar deviation) is greater

Outline of Physical Findings of the Hand

I. Variations in size and shape of hand

A. *Large, blunt fingers (spade hand)*
   1. Acromegaly
   2. Hurler's disease (gargoylism)

B. *Gross irregularity of shape and size*
   1. Paget disease of bone
   2. Maffucci's syndrome
   3. Neurofibromatosis

C. *Spider fingers, slender palm (arachnodactyly)*
   1. Hypopituitarism
   2. Eunuchism
   3. Ehlers-Danlos syndrome, pseudoxanthoma elasticum
   4. Tuberculosis
   5. Asthenic habitus
   6. Osteogenesis imperfecta

D. *Sausage-shaped phalanges*
   1. Rickets (beading of joints)
   2. Granulomatous dactylitis (tuberculosis, syphilis)

E. *Spindliform joints (fingers)*
   1. Early rheumatoid arthritis
   2. Systemic lupus erythematosus
   3. Psoriasis
   4. Rubella
   5. Boeck's sarcoidosis
   6. Osteoarthritis

F. *Cone-shaped fingers*
   1. Pituitary obesity
   2. Fröhlich's dystrophy

G. *Unilateral enlargement of hand*
   1. Arteriovenous aneurysm
   2. Maffucci's syndrome

H. *Square, dry hands*
   1. Cretinism
   2. Myxedema

I. *Single, widened, flattened distal phalanx*
   1. Sarcoidosis

J. *Shortened fourth and fifth metacarpals (bradymetacarpalism)*
   1. Pseudohypoparathroidism
   2. Pseudopseudohypoparathyroidism

K. *Shortened, incurved fifth finger (symptom of Du Bois)*
   1. Mongolism
   2. "Behavioral problem"
   3. Gargoylism (broad, short, thick-skinned hand)

L. *Malposition and abduction, fifth finger*
   1. Turner's syndrome (gonadal dysgenesis, webbed neck, etc.)

M. *Syndactylism*
   1. Congenital malformations of the heart, great vessels
   2. Multiple congenital deformities
   3. Laurence-Moon-Biedl syndrome
   4. In normal individuals as an inherited trait

N. *Clubbed fingers*
   1. Subacute bacterial endocarditis
   2. Pulmonary causes
      a. Tuberculosis
      b. Pulmonary arteriovenous fistula
      c. Pulmonic abscess
      d. Pulmonic cysts
      e. Bullous emphysema
      f. Pulmonary hypertrophic osteoarthropathy
      g. Bronchogenic carcinoma
   3. Alveolocapillary block
      a. Interstitial pulmonary fibrosis
      b. Sarcoidosis
      c. Beryllium poisoning
      d. Sclerodermatous lung
      e. Asbestosis
      f. Miliary tuberculosis
      g. Alveolar cell carcinoma
   4. Cardiovascular causes
      a. Patent ductus arteriosus
      b. Tetralogy of Fallot
      c. Taussig-Bing complex
      d. Pulmonic stenosis
      e. Ventricular septal defect
   5. Diarrheal states
      a. Ulcerative colitis
      b. Tuberculous enteritis
      c. Sprue
      d. Amebic dysentery
      e. Bacillary dysentery
      f. Parasitic infestation (gastrointestinal tract)
   6. Hepatic cirrhosis
   7. Myxedema
   8. Polycythemia
   9. Chronic urinary tract infections (upper and lower)
      a. Chronic nephritis
   10. Hyperparathyroidism (telescopy of distal phalanx)
   11. Pachydermoperiostosis (syndrome of Touraine, Solente, and Golé)

O. *Joint disturbances*
   1. Arthritides
      a. Osteoarthritis
      b. Rheumatoid arthritis
      c. Systemic lupus erythematosus
      d. Gout
      e. Psoriasis
      f. Sarcoidosis
      g. Endocrinopathy (acromegaly)
      h. Rheumatic fever
      i. Reiter's syndrome
      j. Dermatomyositis
   2. Anaphylactic reaction-serum sickness
   3. Scleroderma

II. Edema of the hand

A. *Cardiac disease (congestive heart failure)*

B. *Hepatic disease*

C. *Renal disease*
   1. Nephritis
   2. Nephrosis

D. *Hemiplegic hand*

E. *Syringomyelia*

F. *Superior vena caval syndrome*
   1. Superior thoracic outlet tumor
   2. Mediastinal tumor or inflammation
   3. Pulmonary apex tumor
   4. Aneurysm

Continued

Outline of Physical Findings of the Hand—cont'd

G. *Generalized anasarca, hypoproteinemia*
H. *Postoperative lymphedema (radical breast amputation)*
I. *Ischemic paralysis (cold, blue, swollen, numb)*
J. *Lymphatic obstruction*
  1. Lymphomatous masses in axilla
K. *Axillary mass*
  1. Metastatic tumor, abscess, leukemia, Hodgkin's disease
L. *Aneurysm of ascending or transverse aorta, or of axillary artery*
M. *Pressure on innominate or subclavian vessels*
N. *Raynaud disease*
O. *Myositis*
P. *Cervical rib*
Q. *Trichiniasis*
R. *Scalenus anterior syndrome*
III. Neuromuscular effects
A. *Atrophy*
  1. Painless
    a. Amyotrophic lateral sclerosis
    b. Charcot-Marie-Tooth peroneal atrophy
    c. Syringomyelia (loss of heat, cold, and pain sensation)
    d. Neural leprosy
  2. Painful
    a. Peripheral nerve disease
      1. Radial nerve (wrist drop)
        a. Lead poisoning, alcoholism, polyneuritis, trauma
        b. Diphtheria, polyarteritis, neurosyphilis, anterior poliomyelitis
      2. Ulnar nerve (benediction palsy)
        a. Polyneuritis, trauma
      3. Median nerve (claw hand)
        a. Carpal tunnel syndrome
          1. Rheumatoid arthritis
          2. Tenosynovitis at wrist
          3. Amyloidosis
          4. Gout
          5. Plasmacytoma
          6. Anaphylactic reaction
          7. Menopause syndrome
          8. Myxedema
B. *Extrinsic pressure on the nerve (cervical, axillary, supraclavicular, or brachial)*
  1. Pancoast tumor (pulmonary apex)
  2. Aneurysms of subclavian arteries, axillary vessels, or thoracic aorta
  3. Costoclavicular syndrome
  4. Superior thoracic outlet syndrome
  5. Cervical rib
  6. Degenerative arthritis of cervical spine
  7. Herniation of cervical intervertebral disc
C. *Shoulder-hand syndrome*
  1. Myocardial infarction
  2. Pancoast tumor
  3. Brain tumor
  4. Intrathoracic neoplasms
  5. Discogenetic disease

  6. Cervical spondylosis
  7. Febrile panniculitis
  8. Senility
  9. Vascular occlusion
  10. Hemiplegia
  11. Osteoarthritis
  12. Herpes zoster
D. *Ischemic contractures (sensory loss in fingers)*
  1. Tight plaster cast applications
E. *Polyarteritis nodosa*
F. *Polyneuritis*
  1. Carcinoma of lung
  2. Hodgkin's disease
  3. Pregnancy
  4. Gastric carcinoma
  5. Reticuloses
  6. Diabetes mellitus
  7. Chemical neuritis
    a. Antimony, benzene, bismuth, carbon tetrachloride, heavy metals, alcohol, arsenic, lead, gold, emetine
  8. Ischemic neuropathy
  9. Vitamin B deficiency
  10. Atheromata
  11. Arteriosclerosis
  12. Embolic
G. *Carpodigital (carpopedal spasm) tetany*
  1. Hypoparathyroidism
  2. Hyperventilation
  3. Uremia
  4. Nephritis
  5. Nephrosis
  6. Rickets
  7. Sprue
  8. Malabsorption syndrome
  9. Pregnancy
  10. Lactation
  11. Osteomalacia
  12. Protracted vomiting
  13. Pyloric obstruction
  14. Alkali poisoning
  15. Chemical toxicity
    a. Morphine, lead, alcohol
H. *Tremor*
  1. Parkinsonism
  2. Familial disorder
  3. Hypoglycemia
  4. Hyperthyroidism
  5. Wilson's disease (hepatolenticular degeneration)
  6. Anxiety
  7. Ataxia
  8. Athetosis
  9. Alcoholism, narcotic addiction
  10. Multiple sclerosis
  11. Chorea (Sydenham's, Huntington's)

Modified from Berry TJ: *The hand as a mirror of systemic disease*, Philadelphia, 1963, FA Davis.

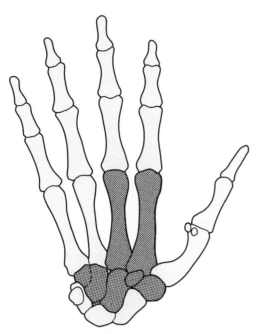

Fig. 7.39 Palmar view of hand, showing stable segment *(stippled areas)*.

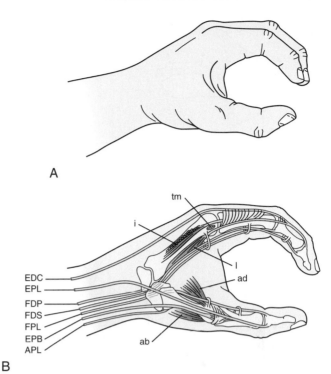

A

B

Fig. 7.40 Position of function of the hand. (A) Normal view. (B) The hand is in the position of function. Notice in particular that a very small amount of motion in the thumb and fingers is useful motion in that it can be used in pinch and grasp. Notice the close relation of the tendons to bone. The flexor tendons are held close to bone by a pulley-like thickening of the flexor sheath as represented schematically. With the hand in this position, intrinsic and extrinsic musculature is in balance, and all muscles are acting within their physiological resting length. *ab,* Abductor pollicis brevis; *ad,* adductor pollicis brevis; *APL,* abductor pollicis longus; *EDC,* extensor digitorum communis; *EPB,* extensor pollicis brevis; *EPL,* extensor pollicis longus; *FDP,* flexor digitorum profundus; *FDS,* flexor digitorum sublimis; *FPL,* flexor pollicis longus; *i,* interossei; *l,* lumbrical; *tm,* transverse metacarpal ligament. (B, Redrawn from O'Donoghue DH: *Treatment of injuries to athletes,* Philadelphia, 1984, WB Saunders, p 287.)

than abduction (radial deviation) because of shortness of the ulnar styloid process. Supination of the forearm is stronger than pronation, whereas abduction has a greater ROM in supination than pronation. Adduction and abduction ROM is minimal when the wrist is fully extended or flexed. Both flexion and extension at the fingers are maximal when the wrist is in a neutral position (not abducted or adducted); flexion and extension of the wrist are minimal when the wrist is in pronation.

The wrist and hand have both a fixed (stable) and a mobile segment. The fixed segment consists of the distal row of carpal bones (trapezium, trapezoid, capitate, and hamate) and the second and third metacarpals. This is the **stable segment** of the wrist and hand (Fig. 7.39), and movement between these bones is less than that between the bones of the mobile segment. This arrangement allows stability without rigidity, enables the hand to move more discretely and with suppleness, and enhances the function of the thumb and fingers when they are used for power and/or precision grip. The **mobile segment** is made up of the five phalanges and the first, fourth, and fifth metacarpal bones.

The **functional position** of the wrist is extension to between 20° and 35° with ulnar deviation of 10° to 15°.[28] This position, sometimes called the **position of rest,** minimizes the restraining action of the long extensor tendons and allows complete flexion of the finger; thus, the greatest power of grip occurs when the wrist is in this position (Fig. 7.40). In this position, the pulps of the index finger and thumb come into contact to facilitate thumb-finger action. The position of **wrist immobilization** (Fig. 7.41) is further extension than is seen in the position of rest with the metacarpophalangeal joints more flexed and the

interphalangeal joints extended. In this way, when the joints are immobilized, the potential for contracture is kept to a minimum.

During extension at the wrist (Fig. 7.42), most of the movement occurs in the radiocarpal joint (approximately 40°) and less occurs in the midcarpal joint (approximately 20°).[26] The motion of extension is accompanied by slight radial deviation and pronation of the forearm. During wrist flexion (see Fig. 7.42), most of the movement occurs in the midcarpal joint (approximately 40°) and less occurs in the radiocarpal joint (approximately 30°).[26] This movement is accompanied by slight ulnar deviation and supination of the forearm. Radial deviation occurs primarily between the proximal and distal rows of carpal bones (0° to 20°) with the proximal row moving toward the ulna and the distal row moving radially. Ulnar deviation occurs primarily at the radiocarpal joint (0° to 37°).[28]

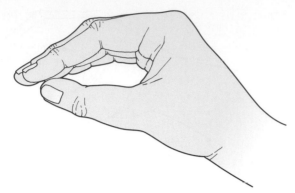

Fig. 7.41 Position of immobilization.

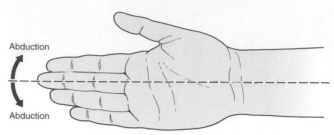

Fig. 7.43 Axis or reference position of the hand. The middle finger provides a central reference from which the other fingers abduct and adduct.

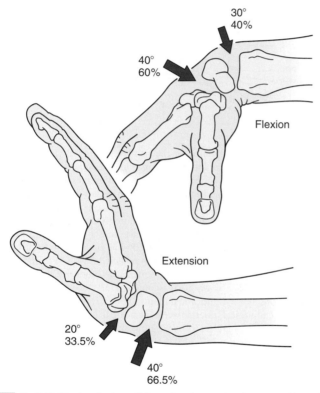

Fig. 7.42 During flexion of the wrist, the motion is more midcarpal and less radiocarpal. During extension of the wrist, the motion is more radiocarpal and less midcarpal. (Modified from Sarrafian SK, Melamed JL, Goshgarian GM: Study of wrist motion in flexion and extension, *Clin Orthop* 126:156, 1977.)

Active Movements

Active movements are sometimes referred to as *physiological movements*. If there is pathology to only one area of the hand or wrist, only that area needs to be assessed, provided the examiner is satisfied that the pathology is not affecting or has not affected the function of the other areas of the forearm, wrist, and hand. For example, if the patient has suffered a FOOSH injury to the wrist, the examiner spends most of the examination looking at the wrist. However, because positioning of the wrist can affect the function of the rest of the hand and forearm, the examiner must determine the functional effect of the injury to these other areas. If the injury is chronic, adaptive changes may have occurred in adjacent joints. In addition, when asking the patient to do specific movements, the examiner should watch for any compensatory movements. For example, if the patient is asked to maximally supinate the forearm, the patient may inadvertently laterally rotate the shoulder in the attempt to increase supination range.[34]

Examination is accomplished with the patient in the sitting position. As always, the most painful movements are done last. When the examiner is determining the movements of the hand, the middle finger is considered to be midline (Fig. 7.43). Wrist flexion decreases as the fingers are flexed just as finger flexion decreases as the wrist flexes, and movements of flexion and extension are limited, usually by the antagonistic muscles and ligaments. In addition, pathology to structures other than the joint may restrict ROM (e.g., muscle spasm, tight ligaments/capsules). If the examiner suspects these structures, passive movement end feels will help differentiate the problem. The patient should actively perform the various movements. Initially, the active movements of the forearm, wrist, and hand may be performed in a "scanning" fashion by having the patient make a fist and then open the hand wide. As the patient does these two movements, the examiner notes any restrictions, deviations, or pain. Depending on the results, the examiner can then do a detailed examination of the affected joints. This detailed examination is initiated by selection of the appropriate active movements to be performed, keeping in mind the effect one joint can have on others.

Active pronation and supination of the forearm and wrist are approximately 85° to 90°, although there is variability between individuals and it is more important to compare the movement with that of the normal side. Approximately 75° of supination or pronation occurs in the forearm articulations. The remaining 15° is the result of wrist action. Full pronation and full supination will tighten the anterior or posterior parts of the TFCC respectively and stabilize the DRUJ.[58] If full pronation or supination is not attainable, the stabilizers at the distal ulna may be affected.[58] If the patient complains of pain on supination, the examiner can differentiate between the DRUJ and the radiocarpal joints by passively supinating the radius on the ulna with no stress on the radiocarpal joint. If this passive movement is painful, the problem is in the DRUJ, not the radiocarpal joints. The normal end feel of both movements is tissue stretch, although in thin patients the end feel of pronation may be bone-to-bone.

Active Movements of the Forearm, Wrist, and Hand

- Pronation of the forearm (85°–90°)
- Supination of the forearm (85°–90°)
- Wrist abduction or radial deviation (15°)
- Wrist adduction or ulnar deviation (30°–45°)
- Wrist flexion (80°–90°)
- Wrist extension (70°–90°)
- Finger flexion (MCP, 85°–90°; PIP, 100°–115°; DIP, 80°–90°)
- Finger extension (MCP, 30°–45°; PIP, 0°; DIP, 20°)
- Finger abduction (20°–30°)
- Finger adduction (0°)
- Thumb flexion (CMC, 45°–50°; MCP, 50°–55°; IP, 85°–90°)
- Thumb extension (MCP, 0°; IP, 0°–5°)
- Thumb abduction (60°–70°)
- Thumb adduction (30°)
- Opposition of little finger and thumb (tip-to-tip)
- Combined movements (if necessary)
- Repetitive movements (if necessary)
- Sustained positions (if necessary)

CMC, Carpometacarpal; *DIP*, distal interphalangeal; *IP*, interphalangeal, *MCP*, metacarpophalangeal; *PIP*, proximal interphalangeal.

Radial and ulnar deviations of the wrist are 15° and 30° to 45°, respectively. The normal end feel of these movements is bone to bone.

Wrist flexion is 80° to 90°; **wrist extension** is 70° to 90°. The end feel of each movement is tissue stretch. Midcarpal instability may be evident on ulnar deviation. Normally, with radial deviation, the proximal carpal row flexes and the scaphoid moves out of the way to allow the trapezoid and trapezium to move in a radial direction. With ulnar deviation, the proximal row of carpals extends, the triquetrum moves out of the way and the hamate moves in an ulnar direction. These movements allow the distance between the capitate and radius to remain constant.[24] If there is midcarpal instability as the wrist is taken into ulnar deviation, the proximal row of carpals stays flexed longer and then audibly snaps or clunks into dorsiflexion (known as a **"catch up clunk"**).[16,75,76] Instability at the radiocarpal and midcarpal joints involving groups of bones may be called **carpal instability nondissociative (CIND).** If there is instability of one bone relative to the other bones in the same row, it may be called **carpal instability dissociative (CID).**[77] Pain in the forearm, about 4 cm (1.5 inches) above the wrist may indicate **intersection syndrome**, which results in pain, swelling, and crepitus on the radial side of the arm where the muscle bodies of abductor pollicis longus and extensor pollicis brevis cross over the tendons of the extensor carpi radialis longus and brevis.[5,29,78]

Flexion of the fingers occurs at the metacarpophalangeal joints (85° to 90°), followed by the proximal interphalangeal joints (100° to 115°) and the distal interphalangeal joints (80° to 90°). This sequence enables the hand to grasp large and small objects. **Extension** occurs at the metacarpophalangeal joints (30° to 45°), the proximal interphalangeal joints (0°), and the distal interphalangeal joints (20°). Hyperextension at the proximal interphalangeal joints can lead to a swan neck deformity. This hyperextension is usually prevented by the volar plates.[3] The end feel of finger flexion and extension is tissue stretch. **Finger abduction** occurs at the metacarpophalangeal joints (20° to 30°); the end feel is tissue stretch. **Finger adduction** (0°) occurs at the same joint.

The digits are medially deviated slightly in relation to the metacarpal bones (see Fig. 7.7). When the fingers are flexed, they should point toward the scaphoid tubercle; this is known as the **Cascade sign**. In addition, the metacarpals are at an angle to each other. These positions increase the dexterity of the hand and oblique flexion of the medial four digits but contribute to deformities (e.g., ulnar drift) in conditions such as rheumatoid arthritis.

Thumb flexion occurs at the carpometacarpal joint (45° to 50°), the metacarpophalangeal joint (50° to 55°), and the interphalangeal joint (80° to 90°). It is associated with medial rotation of the thumb as a result of the saddle shape of the carpometacarpal joint. **Extension of the thumb** occurs at the interphalangeal joint (0° to 5°); it is associated with lateral rotation. Flexion and extension take place in a plane parallel to the palm of the hand. **Thumb abduction** is 60° to 70°; **thumb adduction** is 30°. These movements occur in a plane at right angles to the flexion–extension plane.[28] The thumb is controlled by three nerves, a situation that is unique among the digits. The radial nerve controls extension and opening of the thumb as it does for the other digits. The ulnar nerve controls adduction, produces closure of pinch, and gives power to the grip; the median nerve controls flexion and opposition, producing precision with any grip.[3] The intrinsic muscles are stronger than the extrinsic muscles of the thumb; the opposite is true for the fingers.[3]

If the history has indicated that combined or repetitive movements and/or sustained postures have resulted in symptoms, these movements should also be tested. For example, the **dart throwing action** (i.e., supination–radial deviation–extension [Fig. 7.44A] to pronation–ulnar deviation–flexion [Fig. 7.44B]) is a motion that the scaphotrapezial trapezoid joint complex is stressed in the first position and the ulnotriquetral joints are stressed in the second position.[31]

The examiner must be aware that active movements may be affected because of neurological as well as contractile tissue problems. For example, the median nerve is sometimes compressed as it passes through the carpal tunnel (Fig.

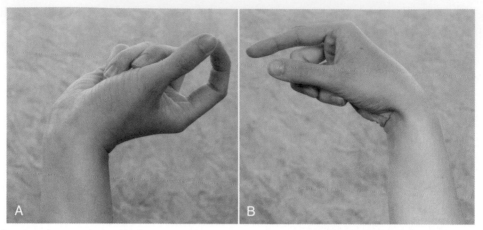

Fig. 7.44 The dart throwing movement. (A) Start: supination–radial deviation–extension. (B) End: pronation–ulnar deviation–flexion.

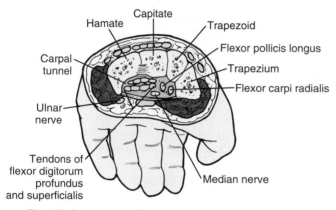

Fig. 7.45 Cross section of the wrist showing the carpal tunnel.

7.45), affecting its motor and sensory distribution in the hand and fingers. The condition is referred to as **carpal tunnel syndrome.** If the examiner asks the patient to squeeze the thumb and little finger together, normally a "dimple" appears on the side of the hypothenar eminence (Fig. 7.46). If the deep branch of the ulnar nerve in the hand has been injured, the dimple (which is caused by contraction of the palmaris brevis) will not appear due to palmaris brevis paralysis. This is called the **palmaris brevis sign.** Similarly, patients have an inability to flex the distal phalanx of the little finger if ulnar neuropathy is present. This is sometimes called the **fingernail sign.**[64]

If the patient does not have full active ROM and it is difficult to measure ROM because of swelling, pain, or contracture, the examiner can use a ruler or tape measure to record the distance from the fingertip to one of the palmar creases (Fig. 7.47).[79] This measurement provides baseline data for any effect of treatment. It is important to note on the chart which crease was used in the measurement. The majority of functional activities of the hand require that the fingers and thumb to open at least 5 cm (2 inches), and the fingers should be able to flex within 1 to 2 cm (0.4 to 0.8 inch) of the distal palmar crease.[80]

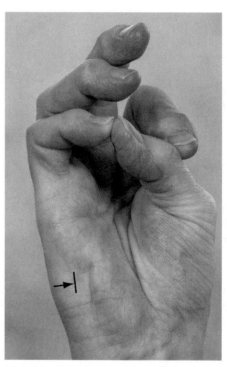

Fig. 7.46 A "dimple" appears on the side of the hypothenar eminence when squeezing the thumb and little finger together.

Passive Movements

If, when watching the patient perform the active movements, the examiner believes the ROM is full, overpressure can be gently applied to test the end feel of the joint in each direction. If the movement is not full, for example, the patient cannot lay the hand flat on a flat surface or cannot put the hands palm to palm as in "saying his or her prayers," passive movements must be carefully performed by the examiner to test the end feel. Normally the end feel between bones is tissue stretch while a more springy end feel indicates soft tissue obstruction or carpal malalignment while a hard end feel is more related to arthritis.[5] If there is limitation of wrist flexion with

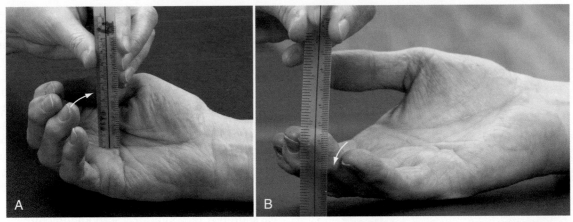

Fig. 7.47 A, Gross flexion is measured as the distance between fingertips and proximal palmar crease. B, Gross extension is measured as the distance between fingertips and dorsal plane.

a springy end feel, the examiner should evaluate the **scapulolunate interval** (see Fig. 7.158). If the scapulolunate joint is unstable, the lunate will extend posteriorly and slides anteriorly which decreases the space in the carpal tunnel. This posteriorly facing lunate is referred to as **dorsal intercalated segment instability (DISI)**.[5] If left untreated, the capitate will become wedged between the scaphoid and lunate. If passive extension is limited, the problem is probably on the ulnar side of the wrist and the **lunotriquetral interval** may be affected and the lunotriquetral ligament injured. In this case, the injury may progress to a **volar (anterior) intercalated segmental instability (VISI)**.

Passive Movements of the Forearm, Wrist, and Hand and Normal End Feel

- Pronation (tissue stretch)
- Supination (tissue stretch)
- Radial deviation (bone-to-bone)
- Ulnar deviation (bone-to-bone)
- Wrist flexion (tissue stretch)
- Wrist extension (tissue stretch)
- Finger flexion (tissue stretch)
- Finger extension (tissue stretch)
- Finger abduction (tissue stretch)
- Thumb flexion (tissue stretch)
- Thumb extension (tissue stretch)
- Thumb abduction (tissue stretch)
- Thumb adduction (tissue approximation)
- Opposition (tissue stretch)

The examiner should palpate for movement between the scaphoid, lunate, and triquetrum. Normally when the scaphoid moves anteriorly, the triquetrum moves posteriorly.[5] At the same time, the examiner must watch for the presence of a capsular pattern. The passive movements are the same as the active movements, and the examiner must remember to test each individual joint.

The capsular pattern of the DRUJ is full ROM with pain at the extremes of supination and pronation. At the wrist, the capsular pattern is equal limitation of flexion and extension. At the metacarpophalangeal and interphalangeal joints, the capsular pattern is flexion more limited than extension. At the trapeziometacarpal joint of the thumb, the capsular pattern is abduction more limited than extension.

In some cases, the examiner may want to test the length of the long extensor and flexor muscles of the wrist (Fig. 7.48). If the length of the muscles is normal, the passive range on testing is full and the end feel is the normal joint tissue stretch. If the muscles are tight, the end feel is muscle stretch, which is not as "stretchy" as tissue or capsular stretch, and the ROM is restricted.

To test the length of the long wrist extensors, the patient is placed in supine lying with the elbow extended. The examiner passively flexes the fingers and then flexes the wrist.[81] If the muscles are tight, wrist flexion is restricted.

To test the length of the long wrist flexors, the patient is placed in supine lying with the elbow extended. The examiner passively extends the fingers and then extends the wrist.[81] If the muscles are tight, wrist extension is limited.

Conjunct rotation can be tested by **folding and fanning the hand** (Fig. 7.49). To do this, the examiner holds the scaphoid and trapezium with the index and middle finger of one hand and the pisiform and hamate of the other hand while the capitate is held with the thumbs on the dorsum of the hand. The examiner then folds and fans the hand feeling the passive movement.[82]

Resisted Isometric Movements

As with the active movements, the resisted isometric movements to the forearm, wrist, and hand are done with the patient in the sitting position. Not all resisted isometric movements need to be tested, but the examiner must keep in mind that the actions of the fingers and thumb and the wrist are controlled by extrinsic muscles (wrist, fingers, thumb) and intrinsic muscles (fingers, thumb), so injury

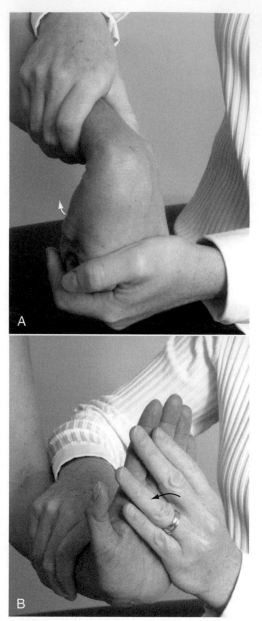

Fig. 7.48 Testing the length of the long extensor (A) and flexor (B) muscles of the wrist.

affecting these structures requires testing of the appropriate muscles. The movements must be isometric and must be performed in the neutral position (Figs. 7.50 and 7.51). For example, if resisted isometric radial abduction of the thumb causes pain on the ulnar side of the wrist, the pain may be due to tendinitis of the extensor carpi ulnaris muscle (i.e., **extensor carpi ulnaris synergy test**) as it acts with flexor carpi ulnaris to synergistically stabilize the wrist.[34] If the history has indicated that concentric, eccentric, or econcentric movements have caused symptoms, these different types of resisted movement should be tested, but only after the movements have been tested isometrically. For example, resisted supination with pain in the anatomical snuff box may indicate a scaphoid fracture.[83]

Table 7.3 shows the muscles (Fig. 7.52; see Fig. 6.18) and their actions for differentiation during resisted isometric testing. If measured by test instruments, the strength ratio of wrist extensors to wrist flexors is approximately 50%, whereas the strength ratio of ulnar deviators to radial deviators is approximately 80%. The greatest torque is produced by the wrist flexors, followed by the radial deviators, ulnar deviators, and finally the wrist extensors.[84]

Resisted Isometric Movements of the Forearm, Wrist, and Hand

- Pronation of the forearm
- Supination of the forearm
- Wrist abduction (radial deviation)
- Wrist adduction (ulnar deviation)
- Wrist flexion
- Wrist extension
- Finger flexion
- Finger extension
- Finger abduction
- Finger adduction
- Thumb flexion
- Thumb extension
- Thumb abduction
- Thumb adduction
- Opposition of the little finger and thumb

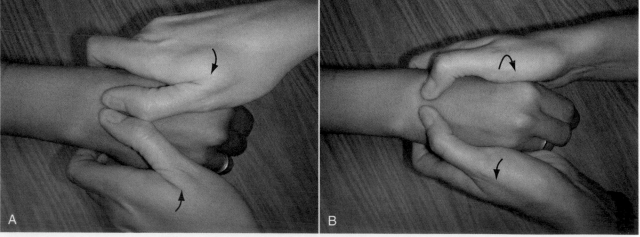

Fig. 7.49 (A) Fanning of the hand. (B) Folding of the hand.

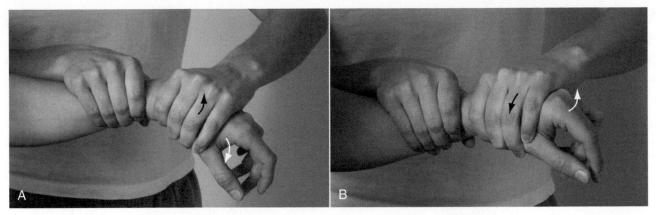

Fig. 7.50 Resisted isometric movements of the wrist. (A) Flexion. (B) Extension.

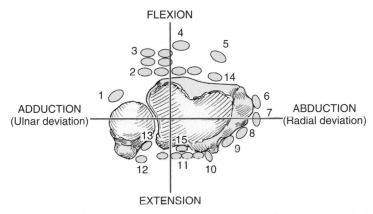

Fig. 7.51 Muscles and their actions at the wrist. *1*, Flexor carpi ulnaris; *2*, flexor digitorum profundus; *3*, flexor digitorum superficialis; *4*, palmaris longus; *5*, flexor carpi radialis; *6*, abductor pollicis longus; *7*, extensor pollicis brevis; *8*, extensor carpi radialis longus; *9*, extensor carpi radialis brevis; *10*, extensor pollicis longus; *11*, extensor digitorum; *12*, extensor digiti minimi; *13*, extensor carpi ulnaris; *14*, flexor pollicis longus; *15*, extensor indices.

TABLE 7.3

Muscles of the Forearm, Wrist, and Hand: Their Actions, Nerve Supply, and Nerve Root Derivation

Action	Muscles Acting	Nerve Supply	Nerve Root Deviation
Supination of forearm	1. Supinator	Posterior interosseous (radial)	C5, C6
	2. Biceps brachii	Musculocutaneous	C5, C6
Pronation of forearm	1. Pronator quadratus	Anterior interosseous (median)	C8, T1
	2. Pronator teres	Median	C6, C7
	3. Flexor carpi radialis	Median	C6, C7
Extension of wrist	1. Extensor carpi radialis longus	Radial	C6, C7
	2. Extensor carpi radialis brevis	Posterior interosseous (radial)	C7, C8
	3. Extensor carpi ulnaris	Posterior interosseous (radial)	C7, C8
Flexion of wrist	1. Flexor carpi radialis	Median	C6, C7
	2. Flexor carpi ulnaris	Ulnar	C7, C8
	3. Palmaris longus[a]	Median	C6, C7
Ulnar deviation of wrist	1. Flexor carpi ulnaris	Ulnar	C7, C8
	2. Extensor carpi ulnaris	Posterior interosseous (radial)	C7, C8
Radial deviation of wrist	1. Flexor carpi radialis	Median	C6, C7
	2. Extensor carpi radialis longus	Radial	C6, C7
	3. Abductor pollicis longus	Posterior interosseous (radial)	C7, C8
	4. Extensor pollicis brevis	Posterior interosseous (radial)	C7, C8

TABLE 7.3

Muscles of the Forearm, Wrist, and Hand: Their Actions, Nerve Supply, and Nerve Root Derivation—cont'd

Action	Muscles Acting	Nerve Supply	Nerve Root Deviation
Extension of fingers	1. Extensor digitorum communis	Posterior interosseous (radial)	C7, C8
	2. Extensor indices (second finger)	Posterior interosseous (radial)	C7, C8
	3. Extensor digiti minimi (little finger)	Posterior interosseous (radial)	C7, C8
Flexion of fingers	1. Flexor digitorum profundus	Anterior interosseous (median)	C8, T1
		Anterior interosseous (median): lateral two digits	C8, T1
		Ulnar: medial two digits	C8, T1
	2. Flexor digitorum superficialis	Median	C7, C8, T1
	3. Lumbricals	First and second: median; third and fourth: ulnar (deep terminal branch)	C8, T1 C8, T1
	4. Interossei	Ulnar (deep terminal branch)	C8, T1
	5. Flexor digiti minimi (little finger)	Ulnar (deep terminal branch)	C8, T1
Abduction of fingers (with fingers extended)	1. Dorsal interossei	Ulnar (deep terminal branch)	C8, T1
	2. Abductor digiti minimi (little finger)	Ulnar (deep terminal branch)	C8, T1
Adduction of fingers (with fingers extended)	1. Palmar (dorsal) interossei	Ulnar (deep terminal branch)	C8, T1
Extension of thumb	1. Extensor pollicis longus	Posterior interosseous (radial)	C7, C8
	2. Extensor pollicis brevis	Posterior interosseous (radial)	C7, C8
	3. Abductor pollicis longus	Posterior interosseous (radial)	C7, C8
Flexion of thumb	1. Flexor pollicis brevis	Superficial head: median (lateral terminal branch)	C8, T1
		Deep head: ulnar	C8, T1
	2. Flexor pollicis longus	Anterior interosseous (median)	C8, T1
	3. Opponens pollicis	Median (lateral terminal branch)	C8, T1
Abduction of thumb	1. Abductor pollicis longus	Posterior interosseous (radial)	C7, C8
	2. Abductor pollicis brevis	Median (lateral terminal branch)	C8, T1
Adduction of thumb	1. Adductor pollicis	Ulnar (deep terminal branch)	C8, T1
Opposition of thumb and little finger	1. Opponens pollicis	Median (lateral terminal branch	C8, T1
	2. Flexor pollicis brevis	Superficial head: median (lateral terminal branch)	C8, T1
	3. Abductor pollicis brevis	Median (lateral terminal branch)	C8, T1
	4. Opponens digiti minimi	Ulnar (deep terminal branch)	C8, T1

aFound in 87% of limbs.[34]

Functional Assessment (Grip)

Having completed the basic movement testing of active, passive, and resisted isometric movements, the examiner then assesses the patient's functional active movements. Functionally, the thumb is the most important digit. Because of its relation with the other digits, its mobility, and the force it can bring to bear, its loss can affect hand function greatly. The index finger is the second most important digit because of its musculature, its strength, and its interaction with the thumb. Its loss greatly affects lateral and pulp-to-pulp pinch and power grip. In flexion, the middle finger is strongest, and it is important for both precision and power grips. The ring finger has the least functional role in the hand. The little finger, because of its peripheral position, greatly enhances power grip, affects the capacity of the hand, and holds objects against the hypothenar eminence.[3] In terms of **functional impairment,** the loss of thumb function affects about 40% to 50% of hand function. The loss of index finger function accounts for about 20% of hand function; the middle finger, about 20%; the ring finger, about 10%; and the little finger, about 10%. Loss of the hand accounts for about 90% loss of upper limb function.[85]

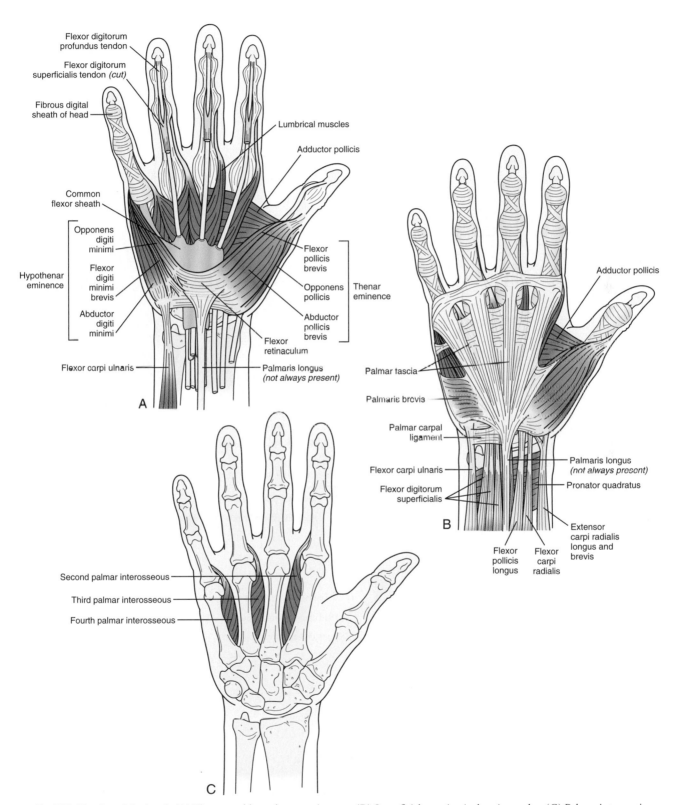

Fig. 7.52 Muscles of the hand. (A) Thenar and hypothenar eminences. (B) Superficial anterior (palmar) muscles. (C) Palmar interossei.

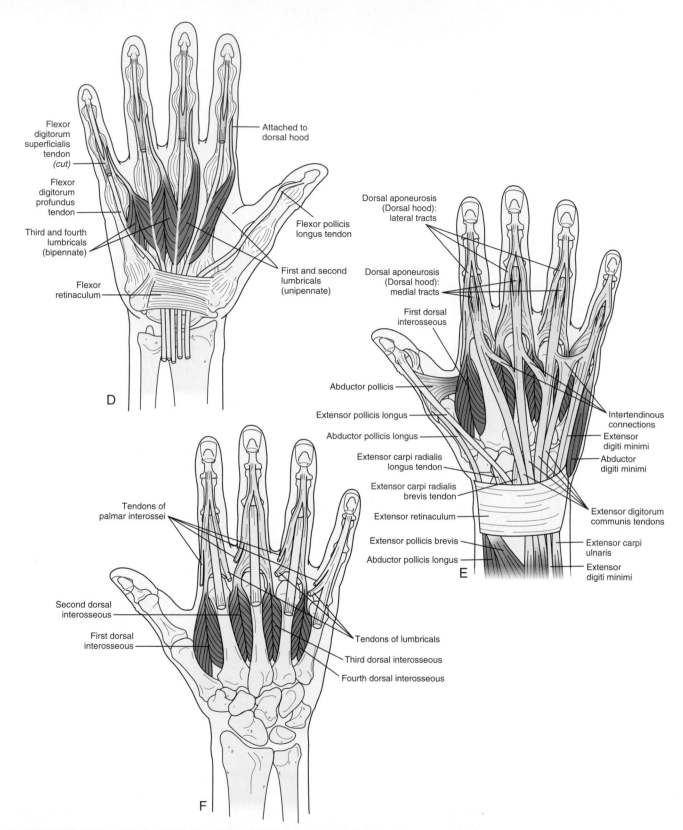

Flexor digitorum superficialis tendon *(cut)*

Flexor digitorum profundus tendon

Third and fourth lumbricals (bipennate)

Flexor retinaculum

Attached to dorsal hood

Flexor pollicis longus tendon

First and second lumbricals (unipennate)

D

Dorsal aponeurosis (Dorsal hood): lateral tracts

Dorsal aponeurosis (Dorsal hood): medial tracts

First dorsal interosseous

Abductor pollicis

Extensor pollicis longus

Abductor pollicis longus

Extensor carpi radialis longus tendon

Extensor carpi radialis brevis tendon

Extensor retinaculum

Extensor pollicis brevis

Abductor pollicis longus

Intertendinous connections

Extensor digiti minimi

Abductor digiti minimi

Extensor digitorum communis tendons

Extensor carpi ulnaris

Extensor digiti minimi

E

Tendons of palmar interossei

Second dorsal interosseous

First dorsal interosseous

Tendons of lumbricals

Third dorsal interosseous

Fourth dorsal interosseous

F

Fig. 7.52, cont'd (D) Lumbricals. (E) Muscles of the posterior (dorsal) hand. (F) Deep posterior muscles. Note: For forearm muscles, see Fig. 6.18.

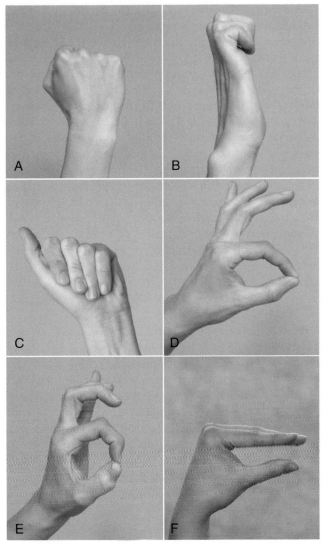

Fig. 7.53 Parts of a functional wrist and hand scan. (A) Standard fist (power grip). (B) Hook grasp fist. (C) Straight fist. (D) Pulp-to-pulp pinch. (E) Tip-to-tip pinch. (F) Lumbrical grip.

Functional Wrist and Hand Scan

- Wrist flexion and extension
- Wrist ulnar and radial deviation
- Making a standard fist
- Making a hook grasp
- Making a straight fist
- Pulp-to-pulp thumb to all fingers pinch
- Tip-to-tip thumb to all fingers pinch

Hand function can be quickly assessed by performing a number of movements to test overall function of the wrist and hand (functional hand and wrist scan) (Fig. 7.53).

Although the wrist, hand, and finger joints have the ability to move through a relatively large ROM, most functional daily tasks do not require full ROM. The optimum functional ROM at the wrist is approximately 10° flexion to 35° extension along with 10° of radial deviation and 15° of ulnar deviation.[86–89] Normally, the wrist is held in slight extension (10° to 15°) and slight ulnar deviation and is stabilized in this position to provide maximum function for the fingers and thumb. Excessive radial deviation, like ulnar drift of the fingers, can affect grip strength adversely.[90] Functional flexion at the metacarpophalangeal and proximal interphalangeal joints is approximately 60°. Functional flexion at the distal interphalangeal joint is approximately 40°. For the thumb, functional flexion at the metacarpophalangeal and interphalangeal joints is approximately 20°.[80] Within these ROMs, the hand is able to perform most of its grip[28,91] and other functional activities.

Stages of Grip

1. Opening of the hand, which requires the simultaneous action of the intrinsic muscles of the hand and the long extensor muscles
2. Positioning and closing of the fingers and thumb to grasp the object and adapt to the object's shape, which involves intrinsic and extrinsic flexor and opposition muscles
3. Exerted force, which varies depending on the weight, surface characteristics, fragility, and use of the object, again involving the extrinsic and intrinsic flexor and opposition muscles
4. Release, in which the hand opens to let go of the object, involving the same muscles as for opening of the hand

Estimated Use of Grips for Activities of Daily Living[91,93,94]

- 20% Pulp-to-pulp pinch:	20%
- Three-lateral pinch:	20%
- Five-finger pinch:	15%
- Fist grip:	15%
- Cylinder grip:	14%
- Three-fingered (thumb, index finger, middle finger) pinch:	10%
- Spherical grip:	4%
- Hook grip:	2%

The thumb, although not always used in gripping, adds another important dimension when it is used. It gives stability and helps control the direction in which the object moves. Both of these factors are necessary for precision movements. The thumb also increases the power of a grip by acting as a buttress, resisting the pressure of an object held between it and the fingers.

The nerve distribution and the functions of the digits also present interesting patterns. Flexion and sensation of the ulnar digits are controlled by the ulnar nerve and are more related to power grip. Flexion and sensation of the radial digits are controlled by the median nerve and are more related to precision grip. The muscles of the thumb, often used in both types of grip, are supplied by both nerves. In all cases of gripping, opening of the hand or release of grip depends on the radial nerve.

Power Grip. A power grip requires firm control and gives greater flexor asymmetry to the hand (Fig. 7.54). During power grip, an example of which is the standard **fist grip**, the ulnar side of the hand works with the radial side to give stronger stability. The ulnar digits tend to work together to provide support and static control.[3,28,91,92] This grip is used whenever strength or force is the primary consideration. With this grip, the digits maintain the object against the palm; the thumb

may or may not be involved, and the extrinsic (forearm) muscles are more important. The combined effect of joint position brings the hand into line with the forearm. For a power grip to be formed, the fingers are flexed and the wrist is in ulnar deviation and slightly extended. Examples of power grips include the **hook grasp,** in which all or the second and third fingers are used as a hook controlled by the forearm flexors and extensors. The hook grasp may involve the interphalangeal joints only or the interphalangeal and metacarpophalangeal joints (the thumb is not involved). In the **cylinder grasp,** a type of **palmar prehension,** the thumb is used, and the entire hand wraps around an object. With the **fist grasp,** or **digital palmar prehension,** the hand moves around a narrow object. Another type of power grip is the **spherical grasp,** another type of palmar prehension, in which there is more opposition and the hand moves around the sphere. **Crimp grip** (Fig. 7.55) is also a power grip, commonly used by climbers, that can result in a rupture of one of the flexor tendons.[27]

Precision or Prehension Grip. The precision grip is an activity limited mainly to the metacarpophalangeal joints and involves primarily the radial side of the hand (Fig. 7.56).[28,91,92] This grip is used whenever accuracy and precision are required. The radial digits (index and long fingers) provide control by working in concert with the thumb to form a "dynamic tripod" for precision handling.[3] With precision grips, the thumb and fingers are used and the palm may or may not be involved; there is pulp-to-pulp contact between the thumb and fingers, and

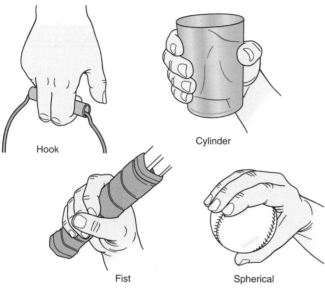

Fig. 7.54 Types of power grips.

Hook

Cylinder

Fist

Spherical

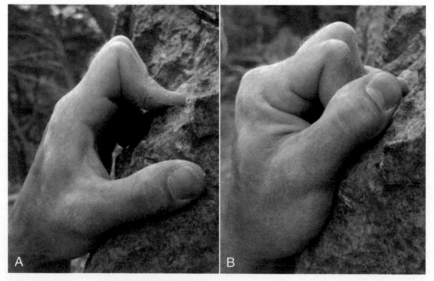

Fig. 7.55 Pulley injuries caused by the crimp grip. (A) The crimp grip is very useful when faced with small flat ledges in the rocks during rock climbing. It consists of a hyperextended distal interphalangeal, flexed proximal interphalangeal, and discrete flexion of the metacarpophalangeal. (B) Sometimes, for additional strength the thumb is locked over the dorsal side of the second finger's P3. (From Lapegue F, Andre A, Brun C, et al: Traumatic flexor tendon injuries, *Diagn Interv Imaging* 96:1279–1292, 2015.)

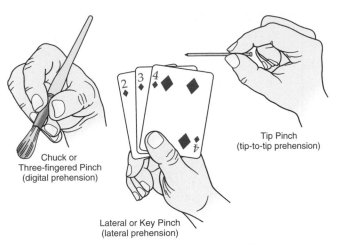

Fig. 7.56 Types of precision grips or pinches.

Chuck or
Three-fingered Pinch
(digital prehension)

Tip Pinch
(tip-to-tip prehension)

Lateral or Key Pinch
(lateral prehension)

the thumb opposes the fingers. The intrinsic muscles are more important in precision than in power grips. Thus, if an ulnar or median nerve lesion is suspected, specific questions should focus on activities that are controlled by the intrinsics and ulnar or median nerve (e.g., buttoning buttons, opening bottles, difficulty typing).[63] The thumb is essential for precision grips, because it provides stability and control of direction and can act as a buttress, providing power to the grip.[3] There are three types of **pinch grip.** The first is called a **three-point chuck,** three-fingered, or **digital prehension,** in which palmar pinch, or subterminal opposition, is achieved. With this grip, there is pulp-to-pulp pinch, and opposition of the thumb and fingers is necessary (e.g., holding a pencil). This grip is sometimes called a **precision grip with power.** The second pinch grip is termed **lateral key, pulp-to-side pinch, lateral prehension,** or **subterminolateral opposition.** The thumb and lateral side of the index finger come into contact. No opposition is needed. An example of this movement is holding keys or a card. The third pinch grip is called the **tip pinch, tip-to-tip prehension,** or **terminal opposition.** With this positioning, the tip of the thumb is brought into opposition with the tip of another finger. This pinch is used for activities requiring fine coordination rather than power.

Testing Grip Strength

When testing grip strength using the grip dynamometer, the examiner should use the five adjustable hand spacings in consecutive order with the patient grasping the dynamometer with maximum force (Fig. 7.57). Both hands are tested alternately, and each force is recorded.[95,96] Care must be taken to ensure that the patient does not fatigue. The results normally form a bell curve (Fig. 7.58) with the greatest strength readings at the middle (second and third) spacings and the weakest at the beginning and at the end. There should be a 5% to 10% difference between the dominant and nondominant hands.[97] With injury, the

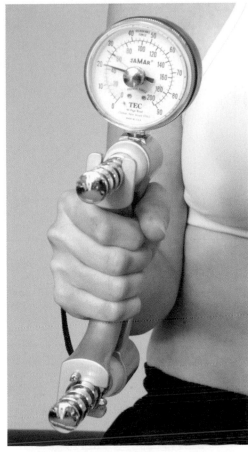

Fig. 7.57 Jamar dynamometer. Arm should be held at the patient's side with elbow flexed at approximately 90° when grip is measured.

bell curve should still be present, but the force exerted is less. If the patient does not exert maximum force for each test, the typical bell curve will not be produced, nor will the values obtained be consistent. Discrepancies of more than 20% in a test-retest situation indicate that the patient is not exerting maximal force.[96,98] Usually, the mean value of three trials is recorded, and both hands are compared.[80] Table 7.4 gives normal values by age group and gender.

Testing Pinch Strength

The strength of the pinch may be tested with the use of a pinch meter (Fig. 7.59). Average values are given for pulp-to-pulp pinch of each finger with the thumb (Table 7.5), lateral prehension (Table 7.6), and pulp-to-pulp pinch (Table 7.7) for different occupational levels. Normally, the mean value of three trials is recorded, and both hands are compared.

Other Functional Testing Methods

In addition to testing grip and pinch strength, the examiner may want to perform a full functional assessment of the patient.[99] eTools 7.1 and 7.2 give examples of functional assessment forms for the hand. These forms are

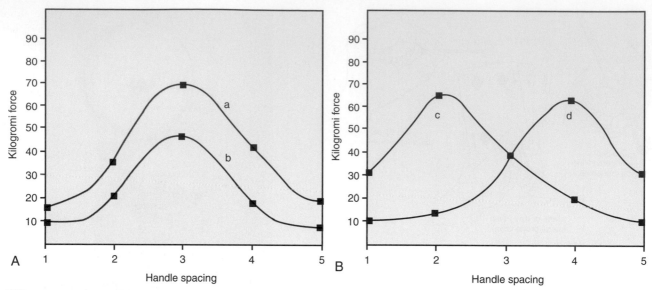

Fig. 7.58 (A) The grip strengths of a patient's uninjured hand *(a)* and injured hand *(b)* are plotted. Despite the patient's decrease in grip strength because of injury, *curve b* maintains a bell-shaped pattern and parallels that of the normal hand. These curves are reproducible in repeated examinations with minimal change in values. A great fluctuation in the size of the curve or absence of a bell-shaped pattern casts doubt on the patient's compliance with the examination and may indicate malingering. (B) If the patient has an exceptionally large hand, the curve shifts to the right *(d)*; with a very small hand, the curve shifts to the left *(c)*. In both cases, the bell-shaped pattern is maintained. (Redrawn from Aulicino PL, DuPuy TE: Clinical examination of the hand. In Hunter J, Schneider LH, Mackin EJ, et al, editors: *Rehabilitation of the hand: surgery and therapy*, St Louis, 1990, CV Mosby, p 45.)

TABLE **7.4**

Normal Values by Age Group (Years) and Gender for Combined Right- and Left-Hand Grip Strength (kg)

	AGES 15–19		AGES 20–29		AGES 30–39		AGES 40–49		AGES 50–59		AGES 60–69	
	Male	Female	Male	Female	Male	Female	Male	Female	Male	Female	Male	Female
Excellent	≥113	≥71	≥124	≥71	≥123	≥73	≥119	≥73	≥110	≥65	≥102	≥60
Above average	103–112	64–70	113–123	65–70	113–122	66–72	110–118	65–72	102–109	59–64	93–101	54–59
Average	95–102	59–63	106–112	61–64	105–112	61–65	102–109	59–64	96–101	55–58	86–92	51–53
Below average	84–94	54–58	97–105	55–60	97–104	56–60	94–101	55–58	87–95	51–54	79–85	48–50
Poor	≤83	≤53	≤96	≤54	≤96	≤55	≤93	≤54	≤86	≤50	≤78	≤47

Modified from Canadian Standardized Test of Fitness: *Operations Manual, Ottawa, Fitness and Amateur Sport,* Canada, 1986, p 36.

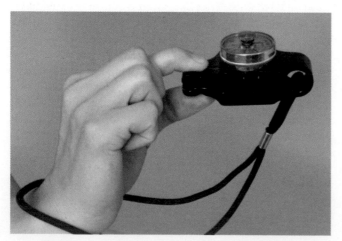

Fig. 7.59 Commercial pinch meter to test pinch strength.

TABLE **7.5**

Average Strength of Chuck (Pulp-to-Pulp) Pinch with Separate Digits (100 Subjects)

	PULP-TO-PULP PINCH (KG)			
	MALE HAND		FEMALE HAND	
Digit	Major	Minor	Major	Minor
II	5.3	4.8	3.6	3.3
III	5.6	5.7	3.8	3.4
IV	3.8	3.6	2.5	2.4
V	2.3	2.2	1.7	1.6

From Hunter J, Schneider LH, Mackin EJ, et al, editors: *Rehabilitation of the hand: surgery and therapy*, St Louis, 1990, CV Mosby, p 115.

TABLE **7.6**

Average Strength of Lateral Prehension Pinch by Occupation (100 Subjects)

| | LATERAL PREHENSION PINCH (KG) | | | |
| | MALE HAND | | FEMALE HAND | |
Occupation	Major	Minor	Major	Minor
Skilled	6.6	6.4	4.4	4.3
Sedentary	6.3	6.1	4.1	3.9
Manual	8.5	7.7	6.0	5.5
Average	7.5	7.1	4.9	4.7

From Hunter J, Schneider LH, Mackin EJ, et al, editors: *Rehabilitation of the hand: surgery and therapy*, St Louis, 1990, CV Mosby, p 114.

TABLE **7.7**

Average Strength of Chuck (Pulp-to-Pulp) Pinch by Occupation (100 Subjects)

| | PULP-TO-PULP PINCH (KG) | | | |
| | MALE HAND | | FEMALE HAND | |
Occupation	Major	Minor	Major	Minor
Skilled	7.3	7.2	5.4	4.6
Sedentary	8.4	7.3	4.2	4.0
Manual	8.5	7.6	6.1	5.6
Average	7.9	7.5	5.2	4.9

From Hunter J, Schneider LH, Mackin EJ, et al, editors: *Rehabilitation of the hand: surgery and therapy*, St Louis, 1990, CV Mosby, p 114.

not numerical scoring charts, but they do include some functional aspects. Buchanan et al.[100] found the most important questions to ask patients with wrist injuries, especially fractures, were questions related to severity of pain, ability to open food packets, cut meat, and perform household chores or usual occupation. Levine et al.[101] have developed a severity questionnaire including a functional component to measure severity of symptoms and functional disability for a nerve—in this case, the median nerve in the carpal tunnel (eTool 7.3). Chung et al.[102] have developed a very comprehensive hand outcomes questionnaire—the **Michigan Hand Outcomes Questionnaire**—which gives the patient's evaluation of his or her outcome based on overall hand function, ADLs, pain, work performance, esthetics, and patient satisfaction (eTool 7.4).[103] Likewise, Dias et al.[104] have developed the **Patient Evaluation Measure (PEM) Questionnaire** (eTool 7.5).[105–107] The **Mayo Wrist Score**,[108] the **Disability of Shoulder, Arm, and Hand (DASH)**[109–111] (see eTool 5.7), and the **Patient Rated Wrist and Hand Evaluation Form**[112] are examples of other useful functional outcome measures.[99,110,113,114] Table 7.8 provides a functional testing method. These strength values would be considered normal for an average population. They would be considered low for an athletic population or for persons in occupations subjecting the forearm, wrist, and hand to high repetitive loads.

Functional coordinated movements may be tested by asking the patient to perform simple activities, such as fastening a button, tying a shoelace, or tracing a diagram. Different prehension patterns are used regularly during daily activities.[94]

These tests may also be graded on a four-point scale.[95] This scale is particularly suitable if the patient has difficulty with one of the subtests, and the subtests can be scale-graded:

- Unable to perform task: 0
- Completes task partially: 1
- Completes task but is slow and clumsy: 2
- Performs task normally: 3

There have also been upper limb physical performance tests developed for athletes including the **Closed Kinetic Chain Upper Extremity Stability Test (CKCUEST)**[115–118] (eTool 7.6) (see Chapter 5); the two-handed shotput; the unilateral seated shotput; the medicine ball throw; the modified push-up; and the one-arm hop test.[116] Although most of these functional tests primarily stress the shoulder, the elbow, forearm, wrist, and hand are also stressed by the loaded dynamic movement.

As part of the functional assessment, manual dexterity tests may be performed. Many standardized tests have been developed to assess manual dexterity and coordination. If comparison with other subjects is desired, the examiner must ensure that the patient is compared with a similar group of patients in terms of age, disability, and occupation. Each of these tests has its supporters and detractors. Some of the more common tests include the ones that follow.

Jebson-Taylor Hand Function Test. This easily administered test involves seven functional areas: (1) writing; (2) card turning; (3) picking up small objects; (4) simulated feeding; (5) stacking; (6) picking up large, light objects; and (7) picking up large, heavy objects. The subtests are timed for each limb. This test primarily measures gross coordination, assessing prehension and manipulative skills with functional tests. It does not test bilateral integration.[80,119–121] Anyone wishing to perform the test should consult the original article[122] for details of administration.

Minnesota Rate of Manipulation Test. This test involves five activities: (1) placing; (2) turning; (3) displacing; (4) one-hand turning and placing; and (5) two-hand turning and placing. The activities are timed for both limbs and compared with normal values. The test primarily measures gross coordination and dexterity.[80,119,120]

Purdue Pegboard Test. This test measures fine coordination with the use of small pins, washers, and collars. The assessment categories of the test are: (1) right hand; (2) left hand; (3) both hands; (4) right, left, and

TABLE **7.8**

Functional Testing of the Wrist and Hand

Starting Position	Action	Functional Test
1. Forearm supinated, resting on table	Wrist flexion	Lift 0 lbs: Nonfunctional Lift 1–2 lbs: Functionally poor Lift 3–4 lbs: Functionally fair Lift 5+ lbs: Functional
2. Forearm pronated, resting on table	Wrist extension lifting 1–2 lbs	0 Repetitions: Nonfunctional 1–2 Repetitions: Functionally poor 3–4 Repetitions: Functionally fair 5+ Repetitions: Functional
3. Forearm between supination and pronation, resting on table	Radial deviation lifting 1–2 lbs	0 Repetitions: Nonfunctional 1–2 Repetitions: Functionally poor 3–4 Repetitions: Functionally fair 5+ Repetitions: Functional
4. Forearm between supination and pronation, resting on table	Thumb flexion with resistance from rubber band[a] around thumb	0 Repetitions: Nonfunctional 1–2 Repetitions: Functionally poor 3–4 Repetitions: Functionally fair 5+ Repetitions: Functional
5. Forearm resting on table, rubber band around thumb and index finger	Thumb extension against resistance of rubber band[a]	0 Repetitions: Nonfunctional 1–2 Repetitions: Functionally poor 3–4 Repetitions: Functionally fair 5+ Repetitions: Functional
6. Forearm resting on table, rubber band around thumb and index finger	Thumb abduction against resistance of rubber band[a]	0 Repetitions: Nonfunctional 1–2 Repetitions: Functionally poor 3–4 Repetitions: Functionally fair 5+ Repetitions: Functional
7. Forearm resting on table	Thumb adduction, lateral pinch of piece of paper	Hold 0 seconds: Nonfunctional Hold 1–2 seconds: Functionally poor Hold 3–4 seconds: Functionally fair Hold 5+ seconds: Functional
8. Forearm resting on table	Thumb opposition, pulp-to-pulp pinch of piece of paper	Hold 0 seconds: Nonfunctional Hold 1–2 seconds: Functionally poor Hold 3–4 seconds: Functionally fair Hold 5+ seconds: Functional
9. Forearm resting on table	Finger flexion, patient grasps mug or glass using cylindrical grasp and lifts off table	0 Repetitions: Nonfunctional 1–2 Repetitions: Functionally poor 3–4 Repetition: Functionally fair 5+ Repetitions: Functional
10. Forearm resting on table	Patient attempts to put on rubber glove keeping fingers straight	21+ seconds: Nonfunctional 10–20 seconds: Functionally poor 4–8 seconds: Functionally poor 2–4 seconds: Functional
11. Forearm resting on table	Patient attempts to pull fingers apart (finger abduction) against resistance of rubber band[a] and holds	Hold 0 seconds: Nonfunctional Hold 1–2 seconds: Functionally poor Hold 3–4 seconds: Functionally fair Hold 5+ seconds: Functional
12. Forearm resting on table	Patient holds piece of paper between fingers while examiner pulls on paper	Hold 0 seconds: Nonfunctional Hold 1–2 seconds: Functionally poor Hold 3–4 seconds: Functionally fair Hold 5+ seconds: Functional

[a]Rubber band should be at least 1 cm wide.
Data from Palmer ML, Epler M: *Clinical assessment procedures in physical therapy*, Philadelphia, 1990, JB Lippincott, pp 140–144.

both; and (5) assembly. The subtests are timed and compared with normal values based on gender and occupation.[80,119,120]

Crawford Small Parts Dexterity Test. This test measures fine coordination, including the use of tools such as tweezers and screwdrivers to assemble things, to adjust equipment, and to do engraving.[80,119]

Simulated Activities of Daily Living Examination. This test consists of nineteen subtests, including standing, walking, putting on a shirt, buttoning, zipping, putting on gloves, dialing a telephone, tying a bow, manipulating safety pins, manipulating coins, threading a needle, unwrapping a Band-Aid, squeezing toothpaste, and using a knife and fork. Each subtask is timed.[94]

Moberg's Pickup Test. An assortment of 9 or 10 objects (e.g., bolts, nuts, screws, buttons, coins, pens, paper clips, keys) is used. The patient is timed for the following tests:
1. Putting objects in a box with the affected hand
2. Putting objects in a box with the unaffected hand
3. Putting objects in a box with the affected hand with eyes closed

The examiner notes which digits are used for prehension. Digits with altered sensation are less likely to be used. The test is used for median or combined median and ulnar nerve lesions.[123]

Box and Block Test. This is a test for gross manual dexterity in which 150 blocks, each measuring 2.5 cm (1 inch) on a side, are used. The patient has 1 minute in which to individually transfer the blocks from one side of a divided box to the other. The number of blocks transferred is given as the score. Patients are given a 15 second practice trial before the test.[121]

Nine-Hole Peg Test. This test is used to assess finger dexterity. The patient places nine 3.2-cm (1.3-inch) pegs in a 12.7 × 12.7-cm (5 × 5-inch) board and then removes them. The score is the time taken to do this task. Each hand is tested separately.[121]

Special Tests

For the forearm, wrist, and hand, no special tests exist that are commonly done with each assessment. Depending on the history, observation, and examination to this point, certain special tests may be performed. In the latest literature, the authors have tended to divide wrist problems into two groups—radial side problems and ulnar side problems. It is important to understand that this does not mean that problems on one side do not affect the other side—they do, but dividing the problems this way helps the examiner focus and makes the assessment of the wrist and hand more systematic. The examiner picks the appropriate test or tests to help confirm the diagnosis. Ideally, when doing special tests, the examiner should start with the uninjured side of the body (i.e., the opposite limb) as that tells the patient what to do in the test, establishes a baseline for the examiner, and

decreases patient apprehension.[58] However, as with all special tests, the examiner must keep in mind that they are confirming tests. When they are positive, they are highly suggestive that the problem exists, but if they are negative, they do not rule out the problem. This is especially true for the tests of neurological dysfunction. Many of the special tests in this section are similar to joint play movements described in that section. The examiner may use either the special test or joint play movement to test for the relationship between the bones of the wrist and DRUJ.

For the reader who would like to review them, the reliability, validity, specificity, sensitivity, and odds ratios of some of the special tests used in the forearm, wrist, and hand are available in eAppendix 7.1.

General Tests for Wrist Pain

❓ ***Carpal Shake Test.***[34] The examiner grasps the patient's distal forearm and passively extends and flexes ("shakes") the patient's wrist (Fig. 7.60). Lack of pain, resistance or complaint indicates there is likely nothing wrong with the wrist.

⚠️ ***Sitting Hands (Press) Test.***[126,127] The patient places both hands on the arms of a stable chair and pushes off, suspending the body while using only the hands for support (Fig. 7.61). This test places a great deal of stress (axial ulnar load) at the wrist (and elbow; see elbow instability tests in Chapter 6) and is too difficult for the patient to do in the presence of significant wrist synovitis or wrist pathology.

❓ ***Windmill Test.***[34] The examiner grasps the patient's forearm and passively and rapidly rotates ("windmills the wrist") the patient's wrist in a circular fashion. Lack of pain, resistance, or complaint indicates there is nothing wrong with the wrist.

Tests for Bone, Ligament, Capsule, and Joint Instability

Carpal instability is the result of loss of normal bony alignment of the carpal bones and/or the radioulnar joint along with ligament damage so that there is a loss of balance between these joints resulting in altered biomechanics, changes in ROM, and pain. There are intrinsic ligaments connecting the different carpals and extrinsic ligaments that attach the carpals to the radius and ulna, and others that attach the carpals to the metacarpals. Functionally, the two most important intrinsic ligaments are the **scapulolunate ligament** and the **ulnotriquetral ligament**. With dynamic instability, malalignment occurs only under certain loads and certain positions while static instability is always present regardless of the load. The classifications of instability vary in the literature but there is most agreement with four types of carpal instabilities seen on x-ray:[128,129]

1. **Dorsiflexed intercalated (lunate) segment instability (DISI).** This is the most common and occurs when one falls on the thenar eminence of the hand

---

Key Tests Performed at the Forearm, Wrist, and Hand Depending on Suspected Pathology[a,124,125]

- *General tests for wrist pain:*
  - ❷ Carpal shake test
  - ⚠ Sitting hands (press) test
  - ❷ Windmill test
- *For bone, ligament, capsule, and joint instability:*
  - ❷ Anterior-posterior drawer test (Fisk's forward shift test—modified)
  - ❷ Axial load test
  - ❷ Catch-up clunk test
  - ⚠ Derby relocation test
  - ⚠ Distal radioulnar joint stability (ballottement) test
  - ❷ Dorsal capitate displacement apprehension test
  - ❷ Finger extension (shuck) test
  - ❷ Gripping rotary impaction test (GRIT)
  - ⚠ Kleinman's shear test
  - ⚠ Ligamentous instability test (fingers)
  - ❷ Linscheid squeeze test
  - ⚠ Lunotriquetral ballottement (Reagan's) test
  - ⚠ Lunotriquetral compression test
  - ⚠ Murphy's sign
  - ❷ Piano keys (DRUJ) test
  - ⚠ Pisiform boost test
  - ⚠ Pisotriquetral grind test
  - ❷ Pivot shift test of midcarpal joint
  - ❷ Prosser's relocation test
  - ⚠ Radioulnar shift test
  - ⚠ Scaphoid compression test
  - ⚠ Scapulolunate ligament test
  - ⚠ Steinberg sign
  - ❷ Supination lift test
  - ❷ Test for tight retinacular ligament
  - ❷ Testing ligaments of the TFCC
  - ❷ Thumb grind test
  - ⚠ Thumb ulnar collateral ligament laxity or instability test
  - ❷ Traction-shift (grind) test of thumb
  - ❷ Triangular fibrocartilage complex load test (Sharpey's test)
  - ❷ Triquetral lift maneuver
  - ✓ Ulnar fovea sign (ulnar snuff box) test
  - ❷ Ulnar impaction (grind) test
  - ⚠ Ulnar styloid triquetral impaction (USTI) provocation test
  - ⚠ Ulnocarpal stress test
  - ✓ Ulnomeniscotriquetral dorsal glide test
  - ⚠ Walker-Murdoch sign

- ✓ Watson (scaphoid shift) test
- ❷ Wrist hanging test
- *For tendons and muscles:*
  - ❷ Boyes test
  - ❷ Bunnel-Littler test
  - ⚠ Extensor carpi ulnaris synergy test
  - ✓ Finkelstein (Eichhoff) test
  - ❷ Lindburg's sign
  - ⚠ Sweater finger sign
  - ❷ Test for extensor hood rupture
  - ⚠ Wrist hyperflexion and abduction of thumb (WHAT) test
- *For neurological dysfunction:*
  - ⚠ Abductor pollicis brevis weakness
  - ❷ André-Thomas sign
  - ✓ Carpal compression test
  - ❷ Closed fist sign
  - ⚠ Crossed finger test
  - ❷ Dellon's moving two-point discrimination test
  - ❷ Egawa's sign
  - ⚠ Finger flexion sign
  - ⚠ First dorsal interossei screening test
  - ⚠ Flick maneuver
  - ⚠ Froment's "paper" sign
  - ✓ Hand elevation test
  - ❷ Nail file sign
  - ❷ Ninhydrin sweat test
  - ⚠ Okutsu test
  - ✓ Phalen's (wrist flexion) test
  - ⚠ Pollock sign
  - ⚠ Reverse Phalen's (prayer) test
  - ⚠ Scratch collapse test
  - ❷ Square wrist sign
  - ⚠ Tethered median nerve stress test
  - ⚠ Tinel sign at wrist
  - ❷ Tourniquet test
  - ✓ Weber's (Moberg's) two-point discrimination test
  - ⚠ Wrinkle (shrivel) test
- *For circulation and swelling:*
  - ✓ Allen test
  - ✓ Digital blood flow
  - ✓ Figure-of-eight measurement for swelling
  - ✓ Hand volume test

DRUJ, Distal radioulnar joint; *TFCC*, triangular fibrocartilage complex.
[a]The authors recommend these tests be learned by the clinician to facilitate a diagnosis. See Chapter 1, Key for Classifying Special Tests.

---

with the wrist in pronation and extended.[128] If the **scapholunate gap** is greater than 4 mm, it indicates the scapholunate ligament has been torn (see Fig. 7.158).[128] The gap is sometimes called the **Terry Thomas sign.**

2. **Volar flexed intercalated (lunate) segment instability (VISI)**
3. **Ulnar translocation** (proximal row is ulnarly deviated relative to radius)
4. **Dorsal translocation** (carpals are subluxed in a posterior [dorsal] direction secondary to fracture)

The reader is referred to other sources for detailed discussion on types of wrist instability—some based on radiological findings, others on motion patterns.[10,21,24,129,130]

Many of the tests for wrist ligaments and joint instability are provocative tests that are designed to stress different pairs or groups of carpals resulting in the patient's symptoms.[131] Many of these tests do not have high reliability or validity and only really become effective in the hands of an examiner who has a good knowledge of the anatomy of the area, how the bones interact with each other, and what happens when ligaments are injured.[131]

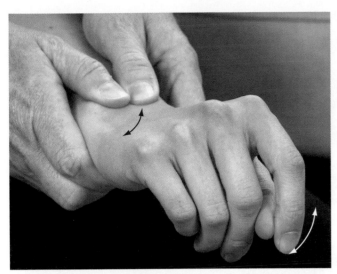

Fig. 7.60 Carpal shake test.

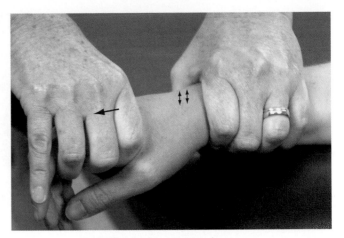

Fig. 7.62 Anterior-posterior drawer test.

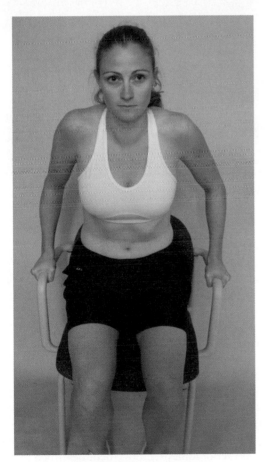

Fig. 7.61 Sitting hands test.

❷ Anterior-Posterior Drawer Test.[58] The patient sits with the forearm midway between supination and pronation (i.e., thumb faces up). The examiner holds the patient's forearm with one hand just proximal to the DRUJ and the other hand is around the metacarpal heads (Fig. 7.62). With the distal hand, the examiner applies axial traction and while applying slight traction, an anteroposterior

(AP) force is applied to the radiocarpal and midcarpal joints. Normally, the translation is about 1 cm (0.4 inch). The test is similar to the anterior–posterior glide in joint play except in this case, two rows of carpals are tested. In joint play, each row of carpals is tested separately. If there is pathology in the wrist, muscle spasm will limit the amount of translation. This pseudostability (i.e., lack of movement) is equivalent to apprehension in other joints. The test has also been called the **Fisk's Forward Shift Test—Modified.**[58]

❷ Axial Load Test. The patient sits while the examiner stabilizes the patient's wrist with one hand. With the other hand, the examiner carefully grasps the patient's thumb and applies axial compression. Pain and/or crepitation indicate a positive test for a fracture of metacarpal or adjacent carpal bones or joint arthrosis. A similar test may be performed for the fingers. If the wrist is then ulnarly deviated and the axial compression repeated, and pain occurs, it may indicate a TFCC problem or **ulnar impingement syndrome**.

❷ Catch-Up Clunk Test.[132] The patient has the forearm in pronation while radially and ulnarly deviating the wrist. Normally, during this movement, the proximal row of carpals rotates from flexion to extension while the distal row translates from anterior (palmar) to posterior when going from radial deviation to ulnar deviation. If there is midcarpal or radiocarpal instability during the movement from radial deviation to ulnar deviation, the proximal row remains flexed and the distal row remains anteriorly and takes longer to translate. As the soft tissue restraints become tighter, there is a sudden "catch-up" of the proximal row into extension and the distal row posteriorly often accompanied by a "clunk" indicating a positive test.

⚠ Derby Relocation Test.[5,30,133] This test assesses the integrity of the lunotriquetral interval and is used to assess for peritriquetral and triquetrolunate injuries. The patient is first asked "does the wrist feel unstable or loose?" (i.e., the question). This is then followed by three tests. If the findings of the tests are positive, including "yes" to the question, the overall test is considered positive. For *Test*

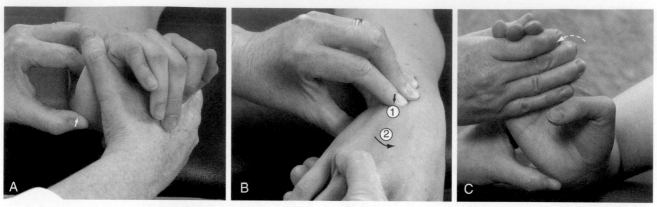

Fig. 7.63 Derby relocation test. (A) Test one. (B) Test two. (C) Test three.

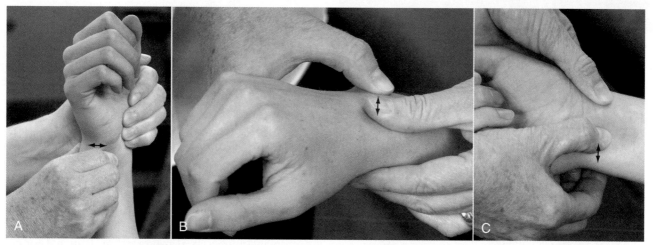

Fig. 7.64 Distal radioulnar joint stability (ballottement) test. (A) Forearm in neutral. (B) Forearm in pronation. (C) Forearm in supination.

One, the patient is seated with the arm resting on a table and elbow flexed to 90° and the wrist pronated, extended and radially deviated. The examiner places a thumb on the anterior aspect of the patient's pisiform and applies a posteriorly directed force while bringing the patient's wrist into neutral (Fig. 7.63A). In this position, a positive response is resolution of the subjective instability and improvement and/or grip strength can be maintained longer. For *Test Two*, the examiner then moves the patient's wrist until the patient's subjective feeling of wrist instability returns and the wrist is then pronated, radially deviated and in neutral flexion. The examiner then applies a posterior to anterior directed force to the dorsum of the patient's triquetrum while ulnarly deviating the patient's wrist (Fig. 7.63B). A positive test is pain with the wrist in ulnar deviation. For *Test Three*, the examiner moves the wrist until the subjective instability returns. The wrist is again pronated, radially deviated and in neutral flexion. The examiner places his or her thumb onto the anterior aspect of the patient's pisiform and applies a posteriorly directed force while ulnarly deviating the patient's wrist (Fig. 7.63C). A positive test is less pain with the wrist ulnar deviation than was experienced in test two.

⚠ *Distal Radioulnar Joint Stability (Ballottement) Test.*[5,30] The DRUJ is tested with the forearm in neutral (Fig. 7.64A), full pronation (Fig. 7.64B) and finally full supination (Fig. 7.64C) with the elbow at 90°. The distal ulna is stabilized about 4 cm (1.5 inches) above the wrist by the examiner with one hand to avoid structures that may cause pain while the other hand is placed around the patient's palm. In each of the above three positions, the joint is glided anteriorly and posteriorly, allowing it to spring back to neutral each time to determine the amount of movement and whether the movement is painful. The wrist can then be radially deviated to see if stability increases (due to TFCC injury). If the TFCC is torn, stability will not improve. This test is similar to the anterior–posterior joint play movement described in the joint play section.

❓ *Dorsal Capitate Displacement Apprehension Test.* This test is used to determine the stability of the capitate in its relation to the lunate.[5,134] The patient sits facing the examiner. The examiner holds the forearm (i.e., radius and ulna) with one hand. The thumb of the examiner's other hand is placed over the palmar aspect of the capitate while the fingers of that hand hold the patient's hand in neutral (no flexion or extension; no radial or ulnar deviation) and

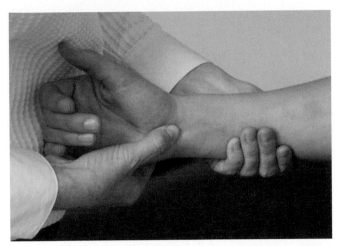

Fig. 7.65 Dorsal capitate displacement apprehension test. Note the position of the examiner's thumb over the capitate to push it posteriorly.

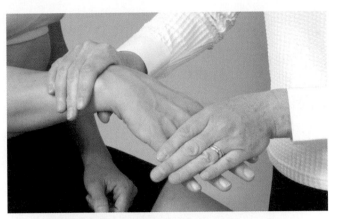

Fig. 7.66 Finger extension or "shuck" test.

applies a counter pressure when the examiner pushes the capitate posteriorly with the thumb (Fig. 7.65). The test may also be done similar to a joint play movement with the patient's lunate being stabilized with the thumb and index finger of one hand of the examiner while the thumb and index finger of the other hand glide the capitate anteriorly and posteriorly. The amount of movement is compared with the other limb.[5] Reproduction of the patient's symptoms, apprehension, or pain indicates a positive test for capitolunate instability.[135] A click or snap may also be heard when pressure is applied.

❓ *Finger Extension or "Shuck" Test*.[136,137] The patient is placed in sitting. The examiner holds the patient's wrist flexed and asks the patient to actively extend the fingers against resistance-loading the radiocarpal joints. Pain would indicate a positive test for radiocarpal or midcarpal instability, scaphoid instability, inflammation, or Kienböck disease (Fig. 7.66).

❓ *Gripping Rotary Impaction Test (GRIT)*.[129,131,138] Using a standard grip dynamometer (see Fig. 7.57), the patient's grip strength is tested with the arm in neutral, supinated, and then pronated, with both arms being tested. The GRIT ratio is calculated by dividing the supinated grip strength by the pronated grip strength. A GRIT greater than 1.0 is considered positive for lunate cartilage damage when it is accompanied by pain.

⚠ *Kleinman's Shear Test*.[6,30,34] This test is used to assess instability of the lunotriquetral joint. The examiner holds the patient's wrist in the neutral position with the patient's forearm supinated. With the same hand, the examiner places a finger over the posterior surface of the lunate. With the thumb of the other hand, the examiner applies a posteriorly directed force to the pisiform (and the triquetrum) while stabilizing the lunate or while pushing the lunate anteriorly (Fig. 7.67). Reproduction of the patient's symptoms is a positive test. The test is similar to joint play between the joints as described in Kaltenborn's carpal mobilization (see Joint Play Movements section, later).

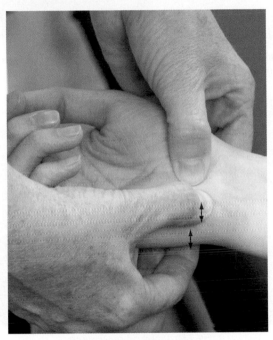

Fig. 7.67 Kleinman's shear test.

⚠ *Ligamentous Instability Test for the Fingers* The examiner stabilizes the test finger with one hand proximal to the joint to be tested. With the other hand, the examiner grasps the finger distal to the joint to be tested. The examiner's distal hand is then used to apply a varus or valgus stress to the joint (proximal or distal interphalangeal) to test the integrity of the collateral ligaments (Fig. 7.68). The results are compared for laxity with those of the uninvolved hand, which is tested first.

❓ *Linscheid Squeeze Test*.[30,126,139] This test is used to detect ligamentous instability of the second and third carpometacarpal joints. The examiner supports the metacarpal shafts with one hand. With the other hand, the examiner pushes the metacarpal heads dorsally, then palmarly (Fig. 7.69). Pain localized to the second or third carpometacarpal joints is a positive test.

⚠ *Lunotriquetral Ballottement Test (Reagan's Test, Reagan's Shuck Test, Masquelet's Ballottement Test, Lunotriquetral Shuck Test)*. This test is used to determine the integrity of the

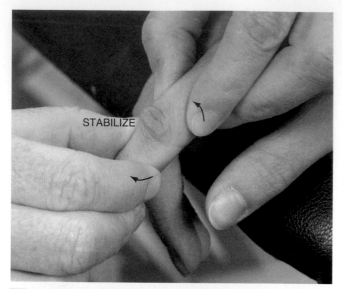

Fig. 7.68 Ligamentous instability test for the fingers. Varus stress applied to proximal interphalangeal joint.

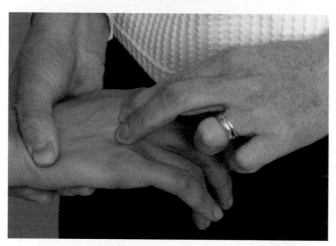

Fig. 7.69 Linscheid squeeze test.

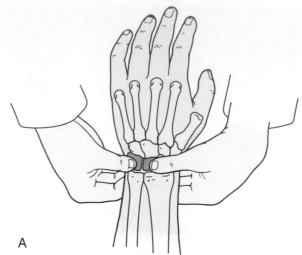

A

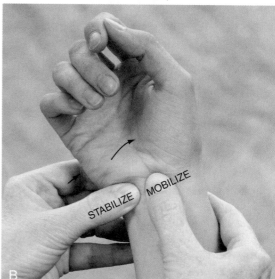

B

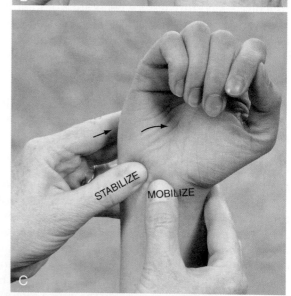

C

lunotriquetral ligament.[18,22] The patient is seated with the elbow flexed in neutral rotation and forearm resting on the examining table. The examiner grasps the pisotriquetrum (i.e., the pisiform and triquetrum) between the thumb and second finger of one hand and the lunate with the thumb and second finger of the other hand (Fig. 7.70A). The examiner then moves the lunate up and down (anteriorly and posteriorly), noting any laxity, crepitus, or pain, which indicates a positive test for lunotriquetral instability by comparing with the uninjured side. The **lunotriquetral shear test** ❓ (also called the **pisotriquetral shear test**) is similar except the examiner's thumb of the opposite hand loads the pisotriquetral joint, applying a shearing force to the lunotriquetral joint while moving the radiocarpal joint from ulnar (Fig. 7.70B) to radial deviation (Fig. 7.70C).[5,18,35,131,140,141] The test is similar to a joint play movement between the lunate and triquetrum.[18,142,143]

Fig. 7.70 (A) Lunotriquetral ballottement test (Reagan's test) for lunotriquetral interosseous ligament dissociations. One hand stabilizes the lunate and the other hand moves the triquetrum. (B) Lunotriquetral shear test in ulnar deviation. (C) Lunotriquetral shear test in radial deviation.

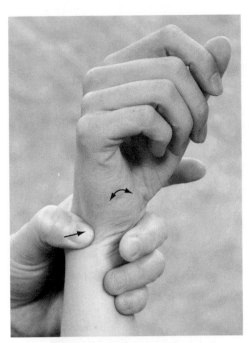

Fig. 7.71 Lunotriquetral compression test.

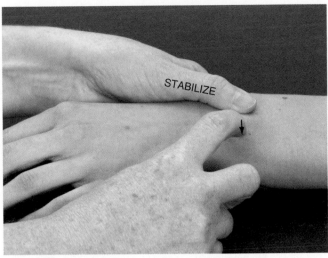

Fig. 7.72 "Piano keys" test (DRUJ test).

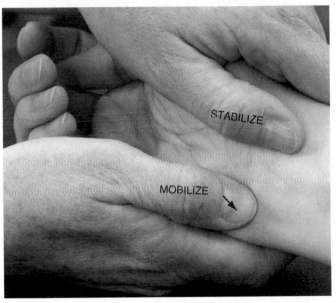

Fig. 7.73 Pisiform boost test.

⚠ *Lunotriquetral Compression Test.*[6,35,70] This test loads the lunotriquetral joint in an ulnar to radial direction eliciting pain with instability or degenerative joint disease. The examiner's thumb applies a hard radially directed pressure on the triquetrum in a rocking manner just distal to the ulnar styloid at the **"ulnar snuff box"** between the tendons of flexor carpi ulnaris and extensor carpi ulnaris (Fig. 7.71). Pain indicates a positive test for lunotriquetral pathology.

⚠ *Murphy's Sign.* The patient is asked to make a fist. If the head of the third metacarpal is level with the second and fourth metacarpals, the sign is positive and can be indicative of a lunate dislocation.[144] Normally, the third metacarpal would project beyond (i.e., further distally) the second and fourth metacarpals.

❓ *"Piano Keys" Test (Distal Radioulnar Joint Test [DRUJ test]).*[34] The patient sits with patient's arm in pronation. The examiner stabilizes the patient's arm with one hand so that the examiner's index finger can push down on the distal ulna. The examiner's other hand supports the patient's hand and radius. The examiner pushes down on the distal ulna, as one would push down on a piano key, pushing the ulnar head anteriorly while the pisiform is stabilized with a posteriorly directed force (Fig. 7.72). The results are compared with the nonsymptomatic side. A positive test is indicated by a difference in mobility and the production of pain and/or tenderness. A positive test is demonstrated by the ulnar head springing back into position (like a piano key) when the force is released and indicates instability of the DRUJ.[6,30,31,33,131]

⚠ *Pisiform Boost Test.*[34] The examiner applies a posteriorly (dorsally) directed pressure over the pisiform which lifts the triquetrum (Fig. 7.73). If pain, crepitus or clicking occur, it suggests pathology of the support structures on the ulnar side of the wrist.

⚠ *Pisotriquetral Grind Test.*[30,58,70] The examiner holds the patient's hand in one hand with the patient's wrist in flexion and palpates the pisiform moving it medially and laterally while flexing (more movement) (Fig. 7.74A) and extending the wrist (less movement because of the tightness of flexor carpi ulnaris) (Fig. 7.74B). The examiner may also apply compression to the pisiform while doing the movement. Crepitus or pain indicates pisotriquetral degenerative joint disease.[70] The test is the same as the joint play of the pisiform except in this case, the wrist is flexed and extended while doing the movement.

The examiner should be aware that normally the pisotriquetral joint is stabilized by the pisohamate ligament, the pisometacarpal ligament, the flexor carpi ulnaris, the ulnar pisotriquetral ligament, abductor digiti minimi, and extensor and flexor retinaculum. Increased motion in the pisiform may lead to ulnar nerve symptoms because the pisiform forms the ulnar border of the Guyan's canal.[141]

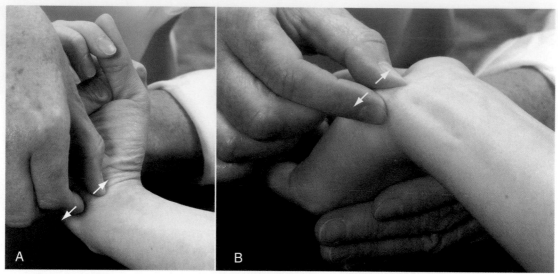

Fig. 7.74 Pisotriquetral grind test. (A) With wrist flexion. (B) With wrist extension.

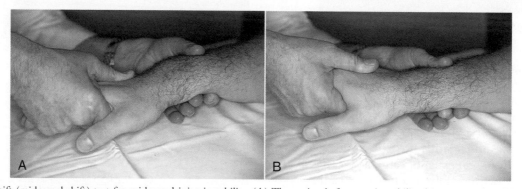

Fig. 7.75 Pivot shift (midcarpal shift) test for midcarpal joint instability. (A) The patient's forearm is stabilized in pronated position at 15° of ulnar deviation and by directing pressure palmarly over the distal capitate to reproduce the palmar translation. (B) The wrist is axially loaded and ulnarly deviated. A positive test is one that reproduces the patient's clunk and pain. The midcarpal shift test should be performed on the contralateral wrist for comparison. Many patients with generalized ligamentous laxity demonstrate bilateral midcarpal laxity as well. (From Lichtman DM, Reardon RS: Midcarpal instability. In Slutsky D, editor: *Principles and practice of wrist surgery*, Philadelphia, 2010, Elsevier.)

❓ *Pivot Shift Test of the Midcarpal Joint (Lichtman, Midcarpal Shift, or Catch-Up Clunk Test).*[31,35,58,70,145] The patient is seated with the elbow flexed to 90° and resting on a firm surface and the hand fully supinated. The examiner stabilizes the pronated forearm in 15° ulnar deviation with one hand and with the other hand takes the patient's hand into full radial deviation with the wrist in neutral and applies an anteriorly directed load through the capitate noting the amount and ease of translation (Fig. 7.75A).[34] While the examiner maintains the patient's hand position and applies an axial load, the patient's hand is taken into full passive ulnar deviation (Fig. 7.75B). A positive test results if a painful "catch-up" clunk occurs as the capitate "shifts" away from the lunate (i.e., the distal row of carpals snap back together in normal physiological position), indicating injury to the anterior capsule and interosseous ligaments.[3,58,146] The clunk represents an abrupt change of the proximal carpal row from flexion to extension as the capitate engages the lunate and the hamate engages the triquetrum under compressive load.[34] The examiner

can then stabilize the pisiform by direct pressure and with the same movement, the active clunk will disappear because stabilizing the pisiform rotates the proximal carpal row out of its flexed position, re-engaging the normal midcarpal joint contact forces.[147]

❓ *Prosser's Relocation Test.*[34] The examiner grasps the patient's forearm for stabilization. With the other hand placed over the proximal carpal row, the examiner pronates the forearm and glides the proximal carpals posteriorly gliding the carpals on the ulna (see Fig. 7.134). The test is positive if wrist pain is decreased as the maneuver relocates the proximal carpals into alignment with the ulna. This test is the same as joint play at the radiocarpal joint.

⚠ *Radioulnar Shift Test.*[5] There are two parts to this test. The normal unaffected side is tested first. *Test One* is used to test the anterior radioulnar ligaments. The patient's arm is in pronation while the examiner stabilizes the patient's distal ulna and the ulnar carpal column (i.e., ulna, trapezoid, hamate) while using the other hand to

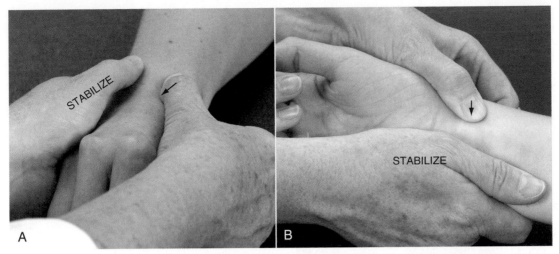

Fig. 7.76 (A) Radioulnar shift test in pronation (testing anterior radioulnar ligaments). (B) Radioulnar shift test in supination (testing posterior radioulnar ligaments).

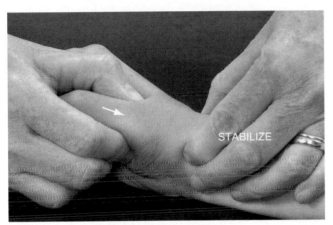

Fig. 7.77 Scaphoid compression test.

anteriorly translate the distal radius noting the amount of movement and end feel, which is compared with the normal side (Fig. 7.76A). *Test Two* is used to test the posterior radioulnar ligaments. The patient's arm is in supination, the examiner again stabilizes the patient's ulna and ulnar carpal column, and with the other hand, posteriorly translates the distal radius (Fig. 7.76B). As with the first test, in the presence of pathology, the amount of movement will increase, and there will be a soft end feel.[5] This is compared with the normal side.

⚠ *Scaphoid Compression Test.*[146,148] The patient is seated and the examiner holds the patient's forearm with one hand. With the other hand, the examiner grasps the patient's thumb and applies a longitudinal compression pressure along the thumb metacarpal towards the carpals (i.e., trapezium and scaphoid) (Fig. 7.77). If the scaphoid is fractured, the maneuver will cause pain.

⚠ *Scapulolunate Ligament Test.*[35] The patient is asked to flex the wrist fully and while holding that position, extend the fingers maximally (Fig. 7.78). This action pushes the capitate against the scaphoid and lunate increasing tension on the scapulolunate ligament. Pain indicates a positive test. The examiner should watch to ensure the wrist does not extend when the fingers extend.

⚠ *Steinberg Sign.* The patient is asked to fold the thumb into a closed fist (Fig. 7.79). The test is positive if the thumb tip extends beyond the palm of the hand. It is used to test for hypermobility and in the clinical evaluation of patients with Marfan syndrome.

❓ *Supination Lift Test.*[149] This test is used to determine pathology in the TFCC (also called the *triangular cartilaginous disc*). The patient is seated with elbows flexed to 90° and forearms supinated. The patient is asked to place the palms flat on the underside of a heavy table (or flat against the examiner's hands). The patient is then asked to lift the table (or push up against the resisting examiner's hands). Localized pain on the ulnar side of the wrist and difficulty applying the force are positive indications for a dorsal TFCC tear. Pain on forced ulnar deviation causing ulnar impaction is a symptom of TFCC tears (Fig. 7.80).

❓ *Test for Tight Retinacular (Collateral) Ligaments (Haines-Zancolli Test).*[150] This test tests the structures around the proximal interphalangeal joint. The proximal interphalangeal joint is held in a neutral position while the distal interphalangeal joint is flexed by the examiner (Fig. 7.81). If the distal interphalangeal joint does not flex, the retinacular (collateral) ligaments or proximal interphalangeal capsule are tight. If the proximal interphalangeal joint is flexed and the distal interphalangeal joint flexes easily, the retinacular ligaments are tight and the capsule is normal. During the test, the patient remains passive and does no active movements.

❓ *Testing the Ligaments of the TFCC.*[35] This test is divided into two parts. *Test One* tests the posterior (dorsal) deep fibers of the TFCC. The patient's forearm is placed in full supination which brings the deep fibers under tension, and keeps the fossa of the radius from translating on to the seat of the ulna. With the patient's forearm in supination, the examiner places four fingers on the palmar

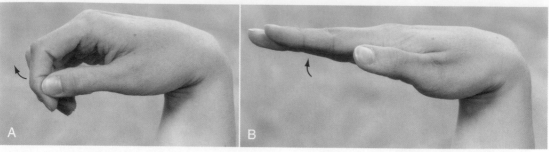

Fig. 7.78 Scapulolunate ligament test. (A) Start position. (B) End position. Note how wrist has slightly extended when fingers extend.

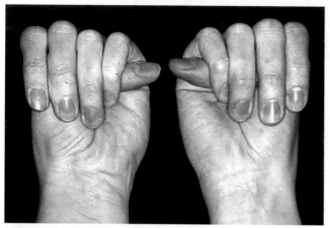

Fig. 7.79 Positive Steinberg sign. (From Bilodeau JE: Retreatment of a patient with Marfan syndrome and severe root resorption, *Am J Orthod Dentofacial Orthop* 137(1):123–134, 2010.)

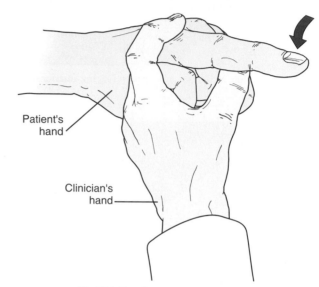

Fig. 7.81 Test for retinacular ligaments.

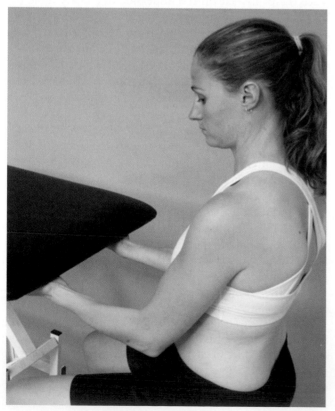

Fig. 7.80 Supination lift test.

surface of the distal radius and prepares to pull the radius forward. At the same time, the examiner places the thumb of the opposite arm on the posterior aspect of the distal ulna with the fingers of the same hand supporting the distal ulna on its anterior surface (Fig. 7.82A). The examiner pushes the ulna away with the thumb while pulling the radius toward the examiner. A positive test is pain. *Test Two* tests the anterior (palmar) deep fibers of the TFCC. The examiner places the patient's forearm in full pronation which tightens the deep anterior fibers. The ulna is then pushed away by the examiner using the thumb while the radius is pulled toward the examiner with the fingers (Fig. 7.82B). Pain is a positive test.

❓ *Thumb Grind Test.* The examiner holds the patient's hand with one hand and grasps the patient's thumb below the metacarpophalangeal joint with the other hand. The examiner then applies axial compression and rotation to the metacarpophalangeal joint (Fig. 7.83). If pain is elicited, the test is positive and indicative of degenerative joint disease in the metacarpophalangeal or metacarpotrapezial joint.[98,151] Axial compression with rotation to any of the wrist and hand joints may also indicate positive tests to those joints for the same condition.

⚠ *Thumb Ulnar Collateral Ligament Laxity or Instability Test.*[31,36] The patient sits while the examiner stabilizes

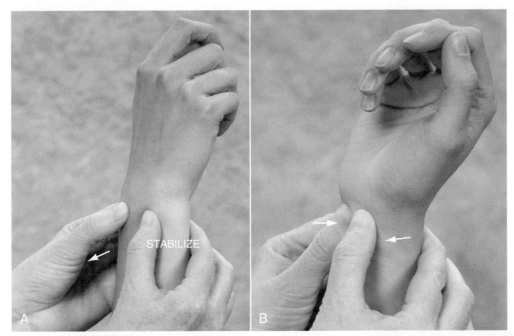

Fig. 7.82 Testing the triangular fibrocartilage complex ligaments. *Arrows* show direction of movement. (A) In supination. (B) In pronation.

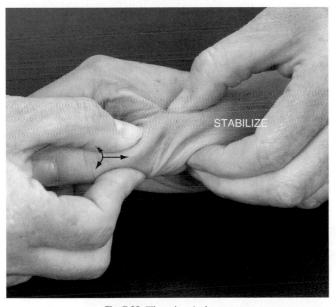

Fig. 7.83 Thumb grind test.

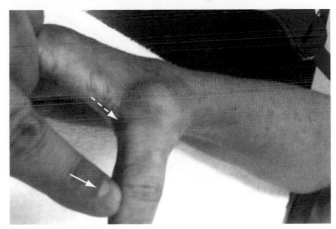

Fig. 7.84 Laxity of the ulnar collateral ligament *(dashed arrow)*. *Solid arrow* shows examiner's thumb pushing patient's thumb back. (Modified from Pitts G, Willoughby J, Cummings B, Uhl TL: Rehabilitation of wrist and hand injuries. In Andrews JR, Harrelson GL, Wilk KE, ed: *Physical rehabilitation of the injured athlete,* ed 4, Philadelphia, 2012, Saunders.)

the patient's hand with one hand and takes the patient's thumb into extension with the other hand. While holding the thumb in extension, the examiner applies a valgus stress to the metacarpophalangeal joint of the thumb, stressing the UCL and accessory collateral ligament (Fig. 7.84). If the valgus movement is greater than 30° to 35°, it indicates a complete tear of the ulnar collateral and accessory collateral ligaments.[152] If the ligament is only partially torn, the laxity would be less than 30° to 35°. In this case, laxity would still be greater than the unaffected side (normal laxity in extension is about 15°) but not as much as with a complete tear. To test the collateral ligament in isolation, the carpometacarpal joint is flexed to 30° and a valgus stress is applied.[153] This is a test for gamekeeper's

or skier's thumb (see Fig. 7.11).[36–39,154] Functional movements that may cause the same impaction pain include putting hand in back pocket, repetitive page turning, and distal supinated hand on stick (e.g., hockey, lacrosse).[70]

❓ *Traction-Shift (Grind) Test of the Thumb.*[29,31] With the patient's forearm and wrist supported by the examiner with one hand, the examiner's other hand grasps the head of the patient's first metacarpal, applies traction to the metacarpal, and extends the patient's thumb. At the same time, the examiner's thumb applies pressure to the dorsal aspect of the base of the first metacarpal (Fig. 7.85). A positive test is indicated by crepitus and pain, and is an indication of arthritis. The traction being applied is the same as in the joint play section.

❓ *Triangular Fibrocartilage Complex Load Test (Sharpey's Test).*[58,126] The examiner holds the patient's forearm with one hand and the patient's hand with the other hand. The examiner then axially loads and ulnarly deviates the wrist while moving it dorsally and palmarly or by rotating the forearm. A positive test is indicated by pain, clicking, or crepitus in the area of the TFCC or ulnocarpal abutment.

❓ *Triquetral Lift Maneuver.*[70] The patient's arm is placed in full pronation. The examiner resists the posterior movement of the triquetrum as the wrist moves from ulnar to radial deviation by placing a thumb over the dorsal aspect of the triquetrum to resist its posterior movement (Fig. 7.86). Resisting the posterior movement stresses the lunotriquetral joint and the triquetrohamate joint and causes pain if instability is present.

☑ *Ulnar Fovea Sign (Ulnar Snuff Box) Test.*[5,6,30,34,59] The test is used to differentiate between ulnotriquetral ligament tear, lunotriquetral instability, triquetrum/hamate pathology, or foveal disruption. The patient stands or sits

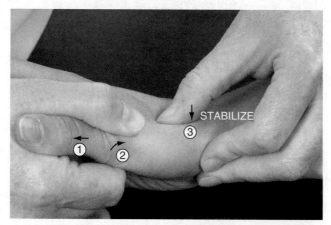

Fig. 7.85 Traction-shift (grind) test of the thumb.

and the patient's wrist and forearm are in neutral. The examiner presses a thumb or finger into the interval or depression (**fovea** or **ulnar snuff box**) between the ulnar styloid process and the flexor carpi ulnaris tendon on the triquetrum between the anterior surface of the ulnar head and the pisiform directing the force against the lunate (Fig. 7.87). The test is considered positive if the patient's pain is replicated or the area is very tender compared to the unaffected side.[155] The pain is believed to be due to distal radioulnar ligaments and ulnotriquetral ligament. Ulnotriquetral ligament tears are commonly associated with a stable DRUJ and fovea disruptions of the TFCC are associated with an unstable DRUJ.[155,156] Crepitus while doing the test with the wrist moving from ulnar to radial deviation is called a positive **Linscheid squeeze test** (see Fig. 7.69).[30]

❓ *Ulnar Impaction (Ulnar Grind) Test (TFCC Compression Test).*[70,82,131] This test is used if the distal ulnar head or styloid impinge on the lunate when ulnar deviation occurs. The patient is seated with the elbow flexed to 90° and the wrist in ulnar deviation. The examiner holds the patient's forearm with one hand and then applies an axial compression force through the fourth and fifth metacarpals (Fig. 7.88). A positive test is indicated by pain and may be related to a central tear of the TFCC or **ulnar impaction syndrome**.

⚠ *Ulnar Styloid Triquetral Impaction (USTI) Provocation Test.*[70,132] The patient is seated. The examiner holds the patient's elbow in one hand while the patient's wrist is extended and ulnarly deviated, and the forearm pronated (Fig. 7.89A). The test can be positioned in various degrees of wrist flexion and extension.[58] While maintaining extension and ulnar deviation, the forearm is supinated (Fig. 7.89B). Pain at the ulnar styloid indicates a

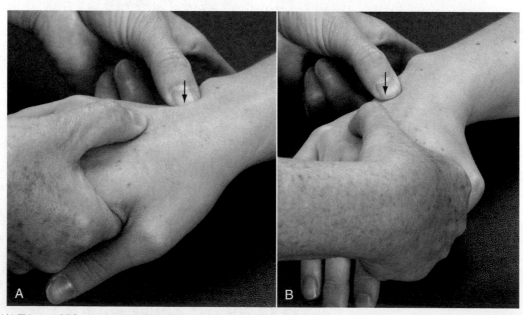

Fig. 7.86 (A) Triquetral lift maneuver in ulnar deviation (start position). (B) Triquetral lift maneuver in radial deviation (end position).

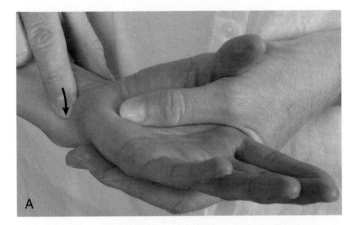

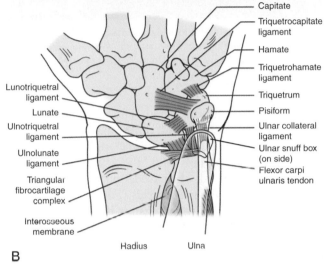

Fig. 7.87 Ulnar fovea sign (ulnar snuff box) test. (A) Area of palpation. (B) Anatomical area of palpation *(line art)*.

positive test for pathological impaction (i.e., ulnar impaction syndrome).

⚠ *Ulnocarpal Stress Test (Nakmura's Ulnar Stress Test).*[6,30,31] The patient sits with the test elbow at 90°, neutral forearm rotation and maximum ulnar deviation of the wrist. The examiner applies an axial load while passively supinating and pronating the ulnarly deviated wrist (Fig. 7.90). The test will be positive in anyone having ulnar-sided wrist pathology (e.g., ulnocarpal abutment syndrome [i.e., ulnar impaction syndrome], TFCC injuries, lunotriquetral injuries, or arthritis).[6]

✅ *Ulnomeniscotriquetral Dorsal Glide Test* The patient sits or stands with the arm pronated. The examiner places a thumb over the ulna dorsally and places the proximal

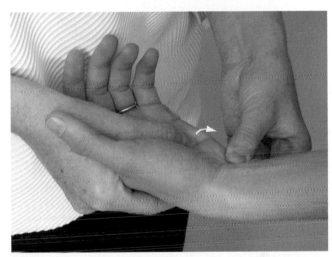

Fig. 7.88 Ulnar impaction test.

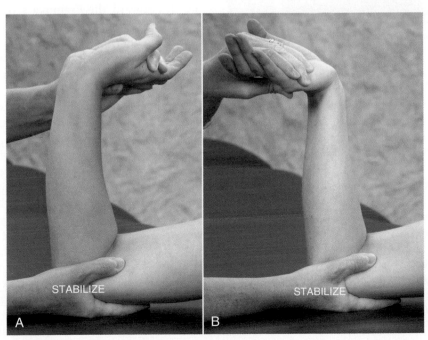

Fig. 7.89 Ulnar styloid triquetral impaction provocation test. (A) In pronation. (B) In supination.

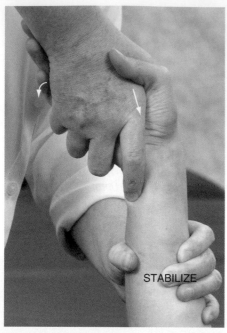

Fig. 7.90 Ulnocarpal stress (Nakmura's ulnar stress) test.

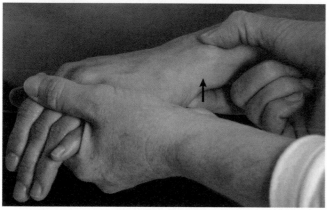

Fig. 7.91 Ulnomeniscotriquetral dorsal glide test.

interphalangeal joint of the index finger of the same hand over the pisotriquetral complex anteriorly. While stabilizing the ulna, the examiner applies a posteriorly directed force through the pisotriquetral complex stressing the TFCC (Fig. 7.91). Excessive laxity or pain when the posteriorly directed force is applied indicates a positive test for TFCC pathology.[131,157]

⚠ *Walker-Murdoch Sign.* The patient is asked to grip his or her wrist with the opposite hand (Fig. 7.92). If the thumb and fifth finger of the gripping hand overlap with each other, the test is positive. Like the Steinberg sign, this sign is used to help diagnose patients with Marfan syndrome. If the Steinberg and the Walker-Murdoch signs are both positive and there is hypermobility (see Beighton Score), there is a 90% chance the patient has Marfan syndrome.

☑ *Watson (Scaphoid Shift, Kirk Watson, Radial Stress) Test.*[21,31,34,58,70,158–160] For this provocative test or maneuver, the patient sits with the elbow resting on

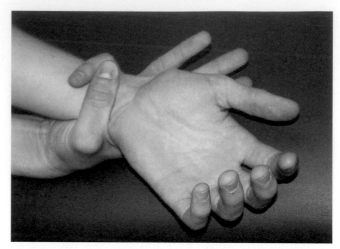

Fig. 7.92 Positive Walker-Murdoch sign. (From Jones KL, Jones MC, Del Campo M: *Smith's recognizable patterns of human malformation,* ed 7, Philadelphia, 2013, Elsevier. Courtesy Dr. Lynne M. Bird, Rady Children's Hospital, San Diego.)

the table and forearm pronated. The examiner faces the patient. The test is first done on the unaffected side for comparison. Ideally, the patient is relaxed before the test is attempted. With one hand, the examiner takes the patient's wrist into full ulnar deviation and slight extension while holding the metacarpals. The examiner presses the thumb of the other hand against the patient's scaphoid tubercle on the palmar side of the wrist to prevent it from moving toward the palm while the examiner's fingers provide a counter pressure on the dorsum of the forearm (Fig. 7.93A). Correct placement of the thumb on the scaphoid tubercle is determined by moving the patient's wrist from ulnar to radial deviation. During the deviation movement, the examiner should feel the scaphoid flex toward the examiner's thumb.[29] With the first hand, the examiner radially deviates and slightly flexes the patient's hand (Fig. 7.93B) while maintaining pressure on the scaphoid tubercle. This creates a subluxation stress if the scaphoid and the scapholunate joint are unstable and the scapholunate ligament is torn. If the scaphoid (and lunate) are unstable, the dorsal pole of the scaphoid subluxes or "shifts" over the dorsal rim of the radius and the patient complains of pain, indicating a positive test.[19,40,143,161] If the scaphoid subluxes with the thumb pressure, when the thumb is removed, the scaphoid commonly returns to its normal position with a "thunk" but no pain. If the ligamentous tissue is intact, the scaphoid normally moves forward, pushing the thumb forward with it. The test may also be used if a scaphoid fracture is suspected. In this case, pain occurs without the "thunk." A gritty sensation or clicking may indicate arthritis.[70] It should be pointed out that a clunk without pain may be normal in wrists without pathology if hypermobility is present at the joint.[21]

The test done actively by the patient doing the radial deviation is called the **scaphoid stress (compression)**

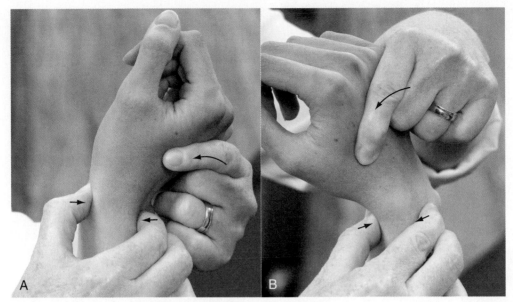

Fig. 7.93 Watson (scaphoid shift, Kirk Watson, radial stress) test. (A) Start position. (B) End position.

test or **scaphoid thrust test**.[34,159] Tenderness on palpating the scaphoid tubercle (**scaphoid tubercle tenderness test**), inside the anatomic snuff box (ASB) (**ASB tenderness test**), and the **scaphoid compression test** are suggestive of a scaphoid fracture.[146]

❓ *Wrist Hanging Test*.[70,108] The patient is asked to hang the wrist over the end of a table with the forearm supinated. If this action causes discomfort in the wrist, there may be capitolunate instability.

Tests for Tendons and Muscles

❓ *Boyes Test*.[162,163] This test also tests the central slip of the extensor hood. The examiner holds the finger to be examined in slight extension at the proximal interphalangeal joint. The patient is then asked to flex the distal interphalangeal joint. If the patient is unable or has difficulty flexing the distal interphalangeal joint, it is considered a positive test.

❓ *Bunnel-Littler (Finochietto-Bunnel) Test*. This test tests the structures around the metacarpophalangeal joint. The metacarpophalangeal joint is held slightly extended while the examiner moves the proximal interphalangeal joint into flexion, if possible (Fig. 7.94).[164] If the test is positive (which is indicated by inability to flex the proximal interphalangeal joint), there is a tight intrinsic muscle or contracture of the joint capsule. If the metacarpophalangeal joints are slightly flexed, the proximal interphalangeal joint flexes fully if the intrinsic muscles are tight, but it does not flex fully if the capsule is tight. The patient remains passive during the test. This test is also called the **intrinsic-plus test**.[3]

⚠ *Extensor Carpi Ulnaris Synergy Test*.[165] This test is used to diagnose extensor carpi ulnaris tendinitis. The patient sits with the arm supported on a table with the elbow flexed 90° and the wrist in neutral. The examiner grasps the patient's thumb and long fingers with one hand and

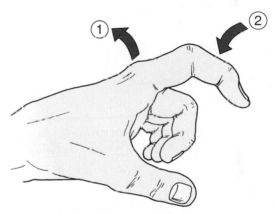

Fig. 7.94 Positioning for the Bunnel-Littler test.

palpates the extensor carpi ulnaris tendon with the other hand. The patient then isometrically abducts the thumb against resistance.[166] The extensor carpi ulnaris and flexor carpi ulnaris will contract to stabilize the wrist (Fig. 7.95). Pain along the dorsal ulnar aspect of the wrist is considered a positive test. In addition, the examiner should be aware that the extensor carpi ulnaris tendon may dislocate or sublux close to the ulnar styloid. The patient's wrist should be put in extension and pronation, and the examiner palpates the tendon while the patient moves the wrist into flexion and supination. As the wrist moves toward the second position, the examiner palpates the tendon to see if it subluxes.

✓ *Finkelstein (Eichhoff) Test*. The Finkelstein test[29,167] is used to determine the presence of de Quervain or Hoffmann disease, a paratenonitis in the thumb.[72] The patient makes a fist with the thumb inside the fingers (Fig. 7.96). The examiner stabilizes the forearm and deviates the wrist toward the ulnar side. A positive test is indicated by pain over the abductor pollicis longus and extensor

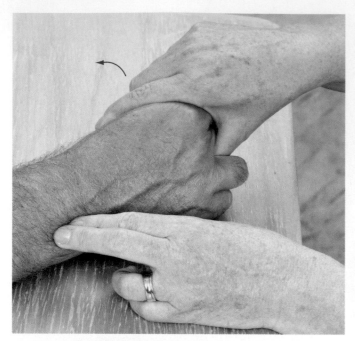

Fig. 7.95 Extensor carpi ulnaris synergy test.

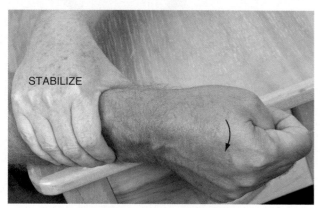

Fig. 7.96 Finkelstein (Eichhoff) test.

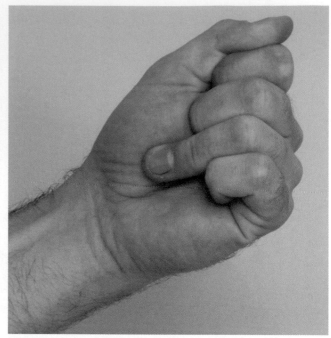

Fig. 7.97 Sweater finger sign. Rupture of the flexor profundus tendon in the ring finger of a football player (finger does not flex at the distal interphalangeal joint when making a fist).

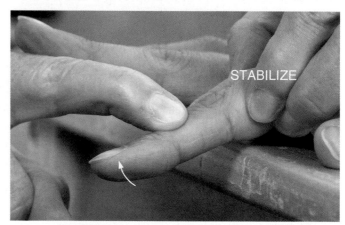

Fig. 7.98 Testing for rupture of the extensor hood.

pollicis brevis tendons at the wrist and is indicative of a paratenonitis of these two tendons. Because the test can cause some discomfort in normal individuals, the examiner should compare the pain caused on the affected side with that of the normal side. Only if the patient's symptoms are produced is the test considered positive.

❓ *Linburg's Sign.* The patient flexes the thumb maximally onto the hypothenar eminence and actively extends the index finger as far as possible. If limited index finger extension and pain are noted, the sign is positive for paratenonitis at the interconnection between flexor pollicis longus and flexor indices (an anomalous tendon condition seen in 10%–15% of hands).[142,168]

⚠ *Sweater (Jersey/Rugby) Finger Sign.* The patient is asked to make a fist. If the distal phalanx of one of the fingers does not flex, the sign is positive for a ruptured flexor digitorum profundus tendon (Fig. 7.97). It occurs most often to the ring finger[27] and can occur when the patient

grasps something using only the fingers to hold something. It is primarily seen in football and rock climbing.

❓ *Test for Extensor Hood Rupture.*[162] The finger to be examined is flexed to 90° at the proximal interphalangeal joint over the edge of a table. The finger is held in position by the examiner. The patient is asked to carefully extend the proximal interphalangeal joint while the examiner palpates the middle phalanx (Fig. 7.98). A positive test for a torn central extensor hood is the examiner's feeling little pressure or resistance from the middle phalanx while the distal interphalangeal joint is extending.

⚠ *Wrist Hyperflexion and Abduction of the Thumb Test (WHAT).*[29,31] The patient is asked to maximally flex the wrist and while holding that position abducts the thumb against the resistance of the examiner (Fig. 7.99).

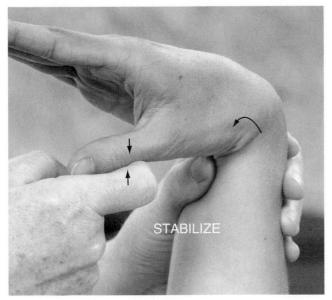

Fig. **7.99** Wrist hyperflexion and abduction of the thumb (WHAT) test.

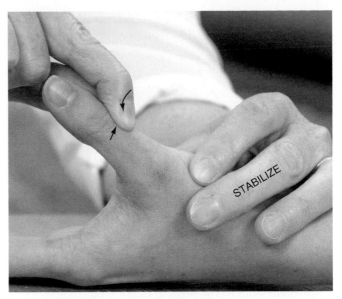

Fig. **7.100** Testing for abductor pollicis brevis weakness.

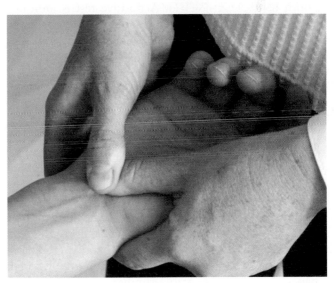

Fig. **7.101** Carpal compression (Durkan carpal compression/pressure provocation) test.

Reproduction of the patient's symptoms (i.e., pain, crepitus) is a positive test for tendinitis of the extensor pollicis brevis and abductor pollicis longus (de Quervain disease or tenosynovitis).

Tests for Neurological Dysfunction

Tests for neurological dysfunction are highly suggestive of a particular nerve lesion if they are positive, but they do not rule out the problem if they are negative. In fact, they may be negative 50% of the time, or more, when the condition actually exists with the symptoms varying during the day and daily, and the symptoms complained of by the patient are often outside the "normal" peripheral nerve territory.[42,66] Thus, diagnostic criteria for entrapment neuropathies, regardless of where they occur in the body may vary.[66] Electrodiagnostic tests are more conclusive but not infallible.[169–172] Keith et al.[42] noted that clinical tests by themselves are not reliable, but when symptoms, clinical tests, and electrodiagnosis are combined, the diagnosis is more reliable.

⚠ *Abductor Pollicis Brevis Weakness.*[43,173] The examiner faces the patient who is seated with the arm supinated on the table. The examiner passively abducts the patient's thumb fully (Fig. 7.100). The examiner asks the patient to hold the position while the examiner tries to push the thumb's interphalangeal joint posteriorly toward the metacarpophalangeal joint of the index (second) finger noting any weakness. Both sides are compared. Any weakness is noted and indicates either injury to the muscle or the median nerve which is its nerve supply.

❓ *André-Thomas Sign.*[64] In patients with ulnar nerve pathology and the loss of the lumbricals, clawing of the fourth and fifth fingers (**Benediction sign**—see Fig. 7.22) is made worse by the unconscious attempt by the patient to extend the fingers with tenodesis of the extensor digitorum communis by flexion of the wrist.

☑ *Carpal Compression Test (Durkan Carpal Compression Test, Pressure Provocation Test).*[31,34,43,174–183] The examiner holds the supinated wrist in both hands and applies direct, even pressure over the median nerve in the carpal tunnel for 30 to 60 seconds (some say 1 to 2 minutes) (Fig. 7.101). Production of the patient's symptoms is considered to be a positive test for carpal tunnel syndrome and median nerve involvement (see Fig. 7.123). This test is a modification of the reverse Phalen's test. The test may also involve flexing the wrist to 60° before applying the pressure (called the **wrist flexion and carpal compression test**) and whether symptoms are relieved when the examiner lets go (it may take a few minutes for the symptoms to be relieved).[178,184] The wrist flexion is felt to make the test more sensitive.

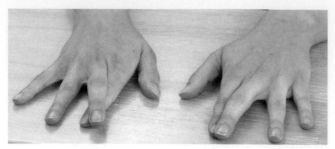

Fig. 7.102 Crossed finger test.

❓ *Closed Fist Sign (Berger Test, Lumbrical Provocation Test).* [43,44,180,182,185,186] The patient makes a tight fist and holds it for 60 seconds. A positive test is indicated by numbness or tingling in the median nerve distribution (see Fig. 7.123). It has been shown that during finger flexion, the lumbricals move into the carpal tunnel, which could contribute to the median nerve symptoms. [187]

⚠ *Crossed Finger Test.* [64,188] The examiner asks the patient to cross the middle finger over the index finger of both hands (Fig. 7.102). A positive test is indicated by an inability to cross the fingers, indicating ulnar nerve involvement (i.e., the interossei are affected).

❓ *Dellon's Moving Two-Point Discrimination Test.* This test is used to predict functional recovery; it measures the quickly adapting mechanoreceptor system. [91] The test is similar to Weber's two-point discrimination test except that the two points are moved during the test. This test is best for hand sensation related to activity and movement. The examiner moves two blunt points from proximal to distal along the long axis of the limb or digit, starting with a distance of 8 mm between the points. The distance between the points is increased or decreased, depending on the response of the patient, until the two points can no longer be distinguished. During the test, the patient's eyes are closed and the hand is cradled in the examiner's hand. The two smooth points, whether a paper clip, a two-point discriminator, or calipers, are gently placed longitudinally. There should be no blanching of the skin indicating too much pressure when the points are applied. The patient is asked whether one or two points are felt. If the patient is hesitant to respond or becomes inaccurate, the patient is required to respond accurately 7 or 8 of 10 times before the distance is narrowed and the test repeated. [80,123,189,190]

Normal discrimination distance recognition is 2 to 5 mm. [191] The values obtained for this test are slightly lower than those obtained for Weber's static two-point discrimination test. [189] Although the entire hand may be tested, it is more common to test only the anterior digital pulp.

❓ *Egawa's Sign.* The patient flexes the middle digit at the metacarpophalangeal joint and then alternately deviates the finger radially and ulnarly (i.e., abducts both ways) (Fig. 7.103). If the patient is unable to do this, the interossei are affected. A positive sign is indicative of ulnar nerve palsy.

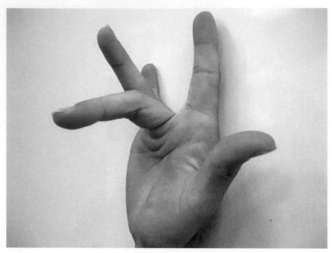

Fig. 7.103 Testing for Egawa's sign. (From Goldman SB, Brininger TL, Schrader JS, Koceja DM: A review of clinical tests and signs for the assessment of ulnar neuropathy, *J Hand Ther* 22(3):209–220, 2009.)

⚠ *Finger Flexion Sign.* [64] The patient sits with both arms on a table with forearms and wrists in neutral. The examiner places a piece of paper between the middle and ring fingers of both hands and asks the patient to prevent the pieces of paper from being pulled away distally by the examiner (Fig. 7.104). Normally, both sides are equal. In the presence of interosseous muscle weakness, the metacarpophalangeal joints will flex to compensate indicating ulnar nerve involvement.

⚠ *First Dorsal Interossei Screening Test.* [64] The patient places the radial aspects of the index fingers of both hands together in abduction and then the patient pushes the index fingers together. If the test is positive, the involved index finger will be overpowered by the uninvolved side and will be pushed into adduction (Fig. 7.105).

⚠ *Flick Maneuver.* [178,192,193] The patient is seated or standing and complains of paresthesia in the hand in the median nerve distribution (see Fig. 7.123). The patient is asked to vigorously shake the hands or "flick" the wrists (Fig. 7.106). A resolution of the symptoms after flicking or shaking the hands is considered a positive test for median nerve pathology primarily in the carpal tunnel.

⚠ *Froment's "Paper" Sign.* The patient attempts to grasp a piece of paper between the thumb and index finger (Fig. 7.107). [194] When the examiner attempts to pull away the paper, the terminal phalanx of the patient's thumb flexes because of paralysis of the adductor pollicis muscle, indicating a positive test for anterior interosseous nerve involvement. [64] It has been recommended to do the test in slight wrist flexion which will help eliminate substitution using extensor pollicis longus. If, at the same time, the metacarpophalangeal joint of the thumb hyperextends, the hyperextension is noted as a positive **Jeanne's sign**. [98] Both tests, if positive, are indicative of ulnar nerve paralysis.

✓ *Hand Elevation Test.* [195,196] The patient raises both hands over the head and maintains the position for at

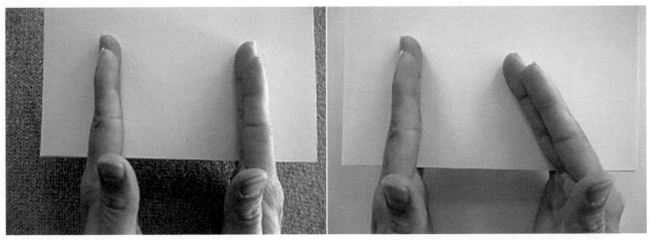

Fig. 7.104 Finger flexion sign. (From Goldman SB, Brininger TL, Schrader JS, Koceja DM: A review of clinical tests and signs for the assessment of ulnar neuropathy, *J Hand Ther* 22(3):209–220, 2009.)

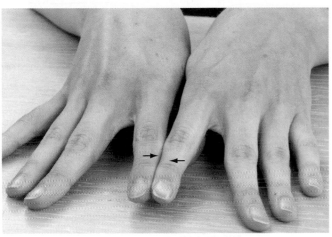

Fig. 7.105 First dorsal interossei screening test.

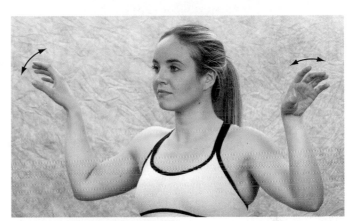

Fig. 7.106 Flick maneuver.

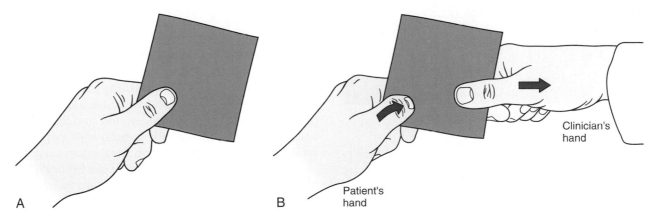

Fig. 7.107 Froment's "paper" sign. (A) Start position. (B) Thumb flexes when paper is pulled away (positive test).

least 3 minutes (Fig. 7.108). A positive test is indicated if symptoms are reproduced in the median nerve distribution (see Fig. 7.123) in less than 2 minutes.

❓ *Nail File Sign.*[64] The patient is asked to make a hook grasp as if he or she was going to file his or her nails (see Fig. 7.53B). The examiner places his or her index finger along the anterior surface of the patient's ring and little finger leaving the distal interphalangeal joints free to flex

(Fig. 7.109). Strength of the ring and little finger is compared to the other hand. A positive test of muscle weakness indicates possible ulnar nerve involvement.

❓ *Ninhydrin Sweat Test* The patient's hand is cleaned thoroughly and wiped with alcohol. The patient then waits 5 to 30 minutes with the fingertips not in contact with any surface. This allows time for the sweating process to ensue. After the waiting period, the fingertips

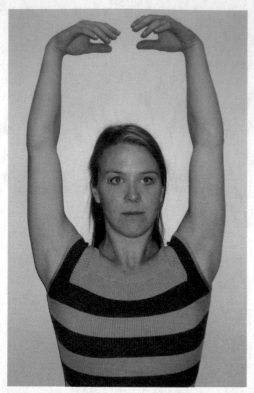

Fig. 7.108 Hand elevation test for median nerve.

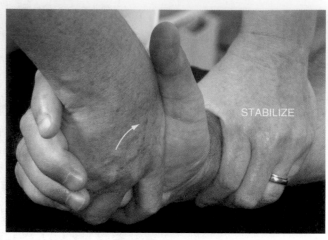

Fig. 7.110 Okutsu test.

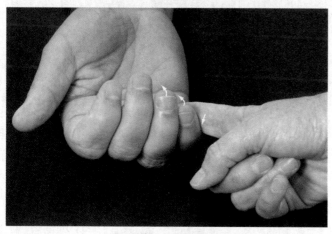

Fig. 7.109 Nail file sign.

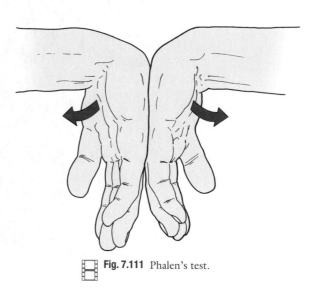

Fig. 7.111 Phalen's test.

are pressed with moderate pressure against good-quality bond paper that has not been touched. The fingertips are held in place for 15 seconds and traced with a pencil. The paper is then sprayed with triketohydrindene (Ninhydrin) spray reagent and allowed to dry (24 hours). The sweat areas stain purple. If the change in color (from white to purple) does not occur, it is considered a positive test for a nerve lesion.[123,197] The reagent must be fixed if a permanent record is required.

⚠ *Okutsu Test.*[198] The examiner grasps the patient's relaxed hand in a "shaking hands" position with the patient's metacarpophalangeal and interphalangeal joints of the thumb in extension while the wrist is moved into radial deviation and held for one minute (Fig. 7.110).

Development of median nerve neurological signs is considered a positive test.

✓ *Phalen's (Wrist Flexion) Test.*[177,179,182,183,199,200] The examiner flexes the patient's wrists maximally and holds this position for 1 minute by pushing the patient's wrists together (Fig. 7.111).[5] A positive test is indicated by tingling in the thumb, index finger, and middle and lateral half of the ring finger, and is indicative of carpal tunnel syndrome caused by pressure on the median nerve.[201]

⚠ *Pollock Sign.*[202] This is a test of the flexor digitorum profundus muscle following an ulnar nerve injury. The examiner asks the patient to hook the little finger of both hands (Fig. 7.112). The patient is then asked to pull the two fingers apart while trying to keep the distal phalanges flexed. If the flexor digitorum profundus muscle is weak due to ulnar nerve injury, the distal and middle phalanges on the affected side will extend.

⚠ *Reverse Phalen's (Prayer) Test.* The examiner extends the patient's wrist while asking the patient to grip the examiner's hand. The examiner then applies direct pressure over the carpal tunnel for 1 minute. The test is also described by having the patient put both hands together and bringing the hands down toward the waist while keeping the palms in full contact, causing extension of the wrist. Doing the test this way does not put as much pressure on the carpal tunnel. A positive test produces the same symptoms as those seen in Phalen's test and is indicative of pathology of the median nerve.[142]

▲ *Scratch Collapse Test for Median or Ulnar Nerve.*[203,204] This test is used to test for peripheral nerve neuropathy, specifically the median (carpal tunnel syndrome) at the wrist or ulnar nerve (cubital tunnel syndrome) at the elbow.[203] The patient stands with the elbows flexed to 90° and wrist in neutral so as to resist shoulder medial rotation. The examiner isometrically attempts to medially rotate the patient's arms while the patient resists with lateral rotation. The examiner then scratches the patient's skin over the area of nerve compression (median nerve—anterior wrist/ulnar nerve—posteromedial elbow) and then quickly has the patient resist isometric medial rotation of the shoulder again (see Fig. 6.61). If the patient has allodynia due to a compression neuropathy, a brief loss of resisted lateral rotation strength will occur. Other authors have described the same test for the long thoracic nerve,[187] peroneal nerve,[70] axillary nerve, and radial nerve. The sensitivity of the test for carpal tunnel syndrome is about 32%.[204–206]

❓ *Square Wrist Sign.*[43,44,181,200,207] The examiner measures the anterior-posterior and medial-lateral dimension of the wrist at the distal wrist crease using a caliper (Fig. 7.113). If the anterior-posterior dimension divided by the medial-lateral dimension is greater than 0.70, it indicates an increased possibility of development of carpal tunnel syndrome.

▲ *Tethered Median Nerve Stress Test.*[208] For the tethered median nerve stress test (TMNST), the patient stands or sits with the elbow flexed and forearm supinated with wrist in slight extension. The examiner then hyperextends the index finger at the distal interphalangeal joint (Fig. 7.114). If anterior radiating forearm pain is felt, the test is considered positive for median nerve pathology.[208] Positive results are more likely in chronic conditions.[209,210]

▲ *Tinel Sign (at the Wrist) (Hoffman-Tinel Sign).*[167,173,182,183,200,211] The examiner taps over the carpal tunnel at the wrist (Fig. 7.115). A positive test causes tingling or paresthesia

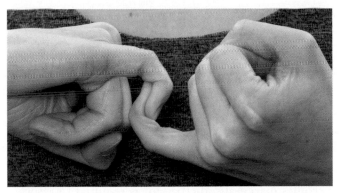

Fig. 7.112 Pollock sign.

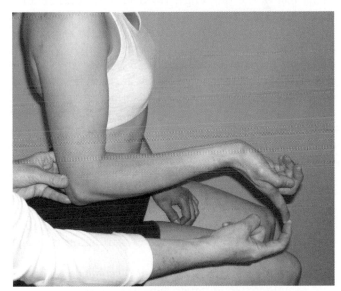

Fig. 7.114 Tethered median nerve stress test.

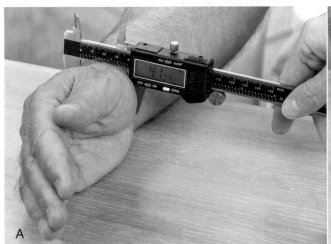
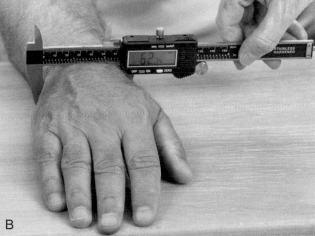

Fig. 7.113 Square wrist sign using caliper. (A) Anterior-posterior dimension. (B) Medial-lateral dimension.

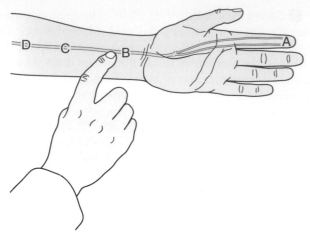

Fig. 7.115 Tinel sign at the wrist. Light percussion is applied along nerve starting at "A" and progressing proximally. The point at which paresthesia is elicited is the level of axonal regrowth.

into the thumb, index finger (forefinger), and middle and lateral half of the ring finger (median nerve distribution). Tinel sign at the wrist is indicative of a carpal tunnel syndrome. The tingling or paresthesia must be felt distal to the point of pressure for a positive test. The test gives an indication of the rate of regeneration of sensory fibers of the median nerve. The most distal point at which the abnormal sensation is felt represents the limit of nerve regeneration. Some authors[173,182] have advocated using a reflex hammer to provide the mechanical percussion and if there is a visible "motor jerk," the test is positive for motor axons of the ulnar nerve being affected.

? Tourniquet Test (Gilliat Test).[43,180–182,212–214] A tourniquet is applied to the patient's upper arm in the normal manner and inflated above the patient's systolic pressure for 1 to 2 minutes. A positive test is indicated by tingling or numbness in the median nerve distribution (see Fig. 7.123).

✓ Weber's (Moberg's) Two-Point Discrimination Test.[183] The examiner uses a paper clip, two-point discriminator, or calipers (Fig. 7.116) to simultaneously apply pressure on two adjacent points in a longitudinal direction or perpendicular to the long axis of the finger; the examiner moves proximal to distal in an attempt to find the minimal distance at which the patient can distinguish between the two stimuli.[91] This distance is called the *threshold for discrimination*. Coverage values are shown in Fig. 7.117. The patient must concentrate on feeling the points and must not be able to see the area being tested. Only the fingertips need to be tested. The patient's hand should be immobile on a hard surface. For accurate results, the examiner must ensure that the two points touch the skin simultaneously. There should be no blanching of the skin, indicating too much pressure when the points are applied. The distance between the points is decreased or increased depending on the response of the patient. The starting distance between the points is one that the patient can easily distinguish

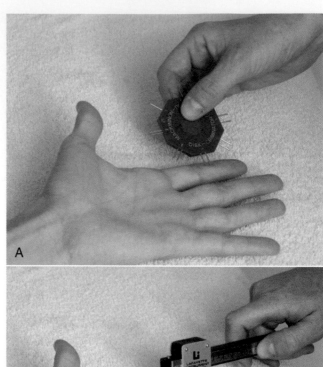
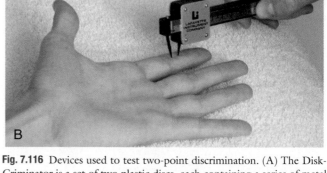

Fig. 7.116 Devices used to test two-point discrimination. (A) The Disk-Criminator is a set of two plastic discs, each containing a series of metal rods at varying intervals from 1 mm to 25 mm apart. This device evaluates both moving and static two-point discrimination. (B) Two-point esthesiometer.

(e.g., 15 mm). If the patient is hesitant to respond or becomes inaccurate, the patient is required to respond accurately on 7 or 8 of 10 trials before the distance is narrowed and the test repeated.[80,123,189,191] Normal discrimination distance recognition is less than 6 mm, but this varies from person to person. This test is best for hand sensation involving static holding of an object between the fingers and thumb and requiring pinch strength. Table 7.9 demonstrates some two-point discrimination normal values and distances required for certain tasks.

? Wrinkle (Shrivel) Test. The patient's fingers are placed in warm water for approximately 5 to 20 minutes. The examiner then removes the patient's fingers from the water and observes whether the skin over the pulp is wrinkled (Fig. 7.118). Normal fingers show wrinkling, but denervated ones do not. The test is valid only within the first few months after injury.[215–217] Absence of wrinkling is a sign of small fiber neuropathy and sympathetic function.

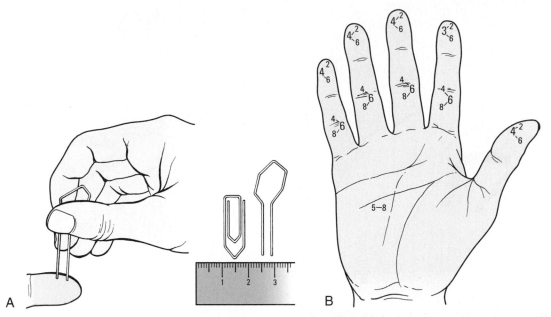

Fig. 7.117 Two-point discrimination. (A) Technique of performing the two-point discrimination test of Weber (after Moberg). (B) Values of discrimination in the Weber test in millimeters in the different zones of the palm. The largest figure indicates the average values, the other two figures the minimum and maximum values (after Moberg). (From Tubiana R: *The hand*, Philadelphia, 1981, WB Saunders, pp 645–646.)

TABLE **7.9**

Two-Point Discrimination Normal Values and Discrimination Distances Required for Certain Tasks

Normal	Less than 6 mm
Fair	6–10 mm
Poor	11–15 mm
Protective	1 point perceived
Anesthetic	0 points perceived
Winding a watch	6 mm
Sewing	6–8 mm
Handling precision tools	12 mm
Gross tool handling	Greater than 15 mm

Adapted from Callahan AD: Sensibility assessment for nerve lesions-in-continuity and nerve lacerations. In Hunter J, Schneider LH, Mackin EJ, et al, editors: *Rehabilitation of the hand and upper extremity*, St Louis, 2002, Mosby, p 233.

Tests for Circulation and Swelling

☑ *Allen Test.* The patient is asked to open and close the hand several times as quickly as possible and then squeeze the hand tightly (Fig. 7.119A).[201,218] The examiner's thumb and index finger are placed over the radial and ulnar arteries, compressing them (Fig. 7.119B). As an alternative technique, the examiner may use both hands, placing one thumb over each artery to compress the artery and placing the fingers on the posterior aspect of the arm for stability (Fig. 7.119D). The patient then opens the hand while pressure is maintained over the arteries. One artery is tested by releasing the pressure over that artery to see if the hand flushes (Fig. 7.119C). The other artery

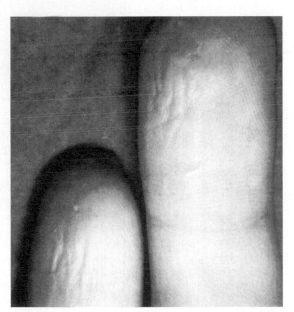

Fig. 7.118 The wrinkle test may be reliable for digital nerve sympathetic function if the fingers (in this case, the radial digital nerve of the fourth and fifth digits) are completely denervated. (From Waylett-Rendall J: Sensibility evaluation and rehabilitation, *Orthop Clin North Am* 19:48, 1988.)

is then tested in a similar fashion. The examiner may time how long it takes for the area to flush. The radial artery normally takes about 2.5 to 3.5 seconds to flush while the ulnar artery takes about 2 to 3 seconds.[34] Anything over 6 seconds is considered a positive test.[62] Both hands should be tested for comparison. This test determines the patency of the radial and ulnar arteries and determines which artery provides the major blood supply to the hand. Thrombosis of the ulnar artery may result from using the

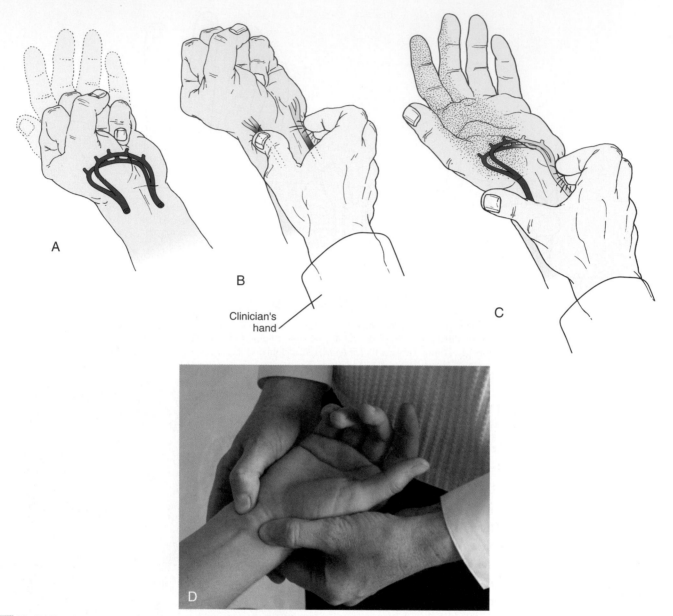

Fig. 7.119 Allen test. (A) The patient opens and closes the hand. (B) While the patient holds the hand closed, the examiner compresses the radial and ulnar arteries. (C) One artery (in this case, the radial artery) is then released, and the examiner notes the filling pattern of the hand until the circulation is normal. The process is then repeated for the ulnar artery. (D) Alternative hand hold applying pressure first on one side and release, and then repeated on the other side.

hand as a hammer by repeated impacts to the ulnar side of the hand (called **ulnar hammer** or **hypothenar hammer syndrome**).[34]

☑ *Digital Blood Flow.* To test distal blood flow, the examiner compresses the nail bed and notes the time taken for color to return to the nail (Fig. 7.120). Normally, when the pressure is released, color should return to the nail bed within 3 seconds. If return takes longer, arterial insufficiency to the fingers should be suspected. Comparison with the normal side gives some indication of restricted flow.

☑ *Figure of Eight Measurement.* Swelling of the hand and wrist may also be measured using a tape measure. The examiner places a mark on the distal aspect of the

ulnar styloid process as a starting point. The examiner then takes the tape measure across the anterior wrist to the most distal aspect of the radial styloid process (Fig. 7.121A). From there, the tape is brought diagonally across the back (dorsum) of the hand and over the fifth metacarpophalangeal joint line (Fig. 7.121B, palmar view; and 7.121C, dorsal view), across the anterior surface of the metacarpophalangeal joints (Fig. 7.121D) and then diagonally across the back of the hand to where the tape started (Fig. 7.121E).[219,220] Wrist swelling alone may be measured by measuring the circumference of the wrist just distal to the radial and ulnar styloids.[34]

The examiner may also measure around the proximal interphalangeal joints individually, around the

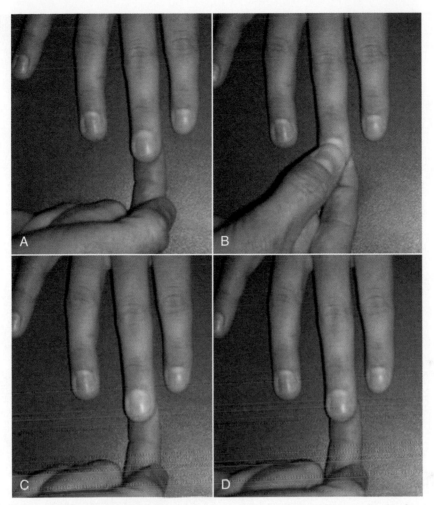

Fig. 7.120 Checking digital blood flow. (A) Starting position. (B) Compression on finger. (C) Immediately after pressure released. (D) Three seconds after pressure released. Note darker color of nail as blood flow returns.

metacarpophalangeal joints as a group, and/or around the palm and wrist. The values for both hands are compared.

✓ *Hand Volume Test.* If the examiner is concerned about changes in hand size, a volumeter (Fig. 7.122) may be used. This device can be used to assess change in hand size resulting from localized swelling, generalized edema, or atrophy.[119] Comparisons with the normal limb give the examiner an idea of changes occurring in the affected hand. Care must be taken when doing this test to ensure accurate readings. There is often a 10-mL difference between right and left hands and between dominant and nondominant hands. If swelling is the problem, differences of 30 to 50 mL can be noted.[80,221]

Reflexes and Cutaneous Distribution

Although it is possible to obtain reflexes from the tendons crossing the wrist, this is not commonly done. In fact, no deep tendon reflexes are routinely tested in the forearm, wrist, and hand. The only reflex that may be tested in the hand is Hoffman reflex, which is a pathological reflex. This reflex may be tested if an upper motor neuron lesion is suspected. To test the reflex, the examiner "flicks" the terminal phalanx of the index, middle, or ring finger. A positive test is indicated by reflex flexion of the distal phalanx of the thumb or a finger that was not "flicked."

The examiner must be aware of the sensory distribution of the ulnar, median, and radial nerves in the hand (Fig. 7.123) and must be prepared to compare peripheral nerve sensory distribution with nerve root sensory (dermatome) distributions for hypalgesia (i.e., decreased sensitivity to pain), tingling or numbness. As previously mentioned, there is variability in both distributions. However, it has been reported that each peripheral nerve of the upper limb has a "constant" area in the hand that is always affected if the nerve is injured. For the radial nerve, it is on the dorsum of the thumb near the apex of the anatomical snuff box; for the median nerve, it is the tip of the index finger; and for the ulnar nerve, it is the tip of the little finger.[222]

The median nerve gives off a sensory branch above the wrist before it passes through the carpal tunnel. This sensory branch supplies the skin of the palm (Fig. 7.124). Thus, most commonly, carpal tunnel syndrome does not

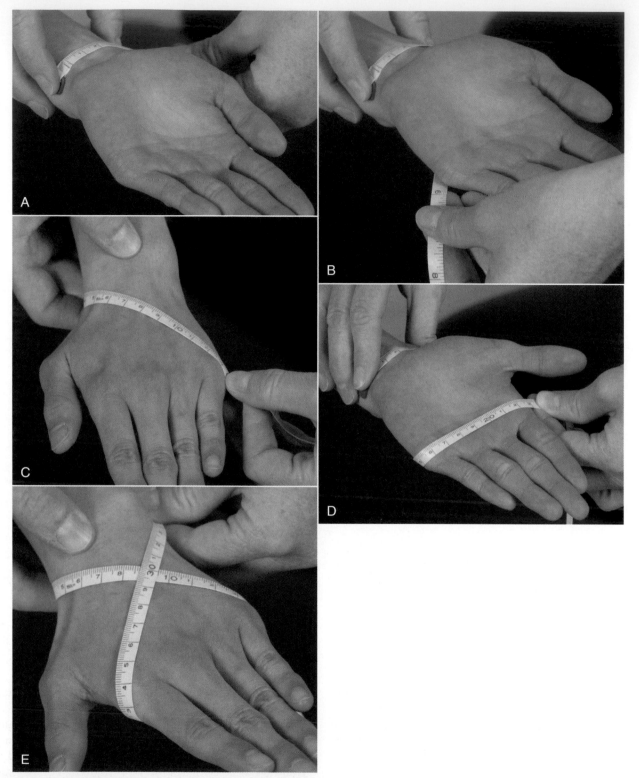

Fig. 7.121 Figure of 8 measurement for hand swelling. (A) Across wrist. (B) Across back of hand (supinated view). (C) Across back of hand (pronated view). (D) Across anterior metacarpal head. (E) Across back of hand to start point.

affect the median sensory distribution in the palm but results in altered sensation in the fingers.

Several sensation tests may be carried out in the hand. Table 7.10 illustrates the tests used and the sensation and nerve fibers tested. Pinprick is used to test for pain. Constant light touch, which is a component of fine discrimination, may be tested in the hand using a **Semmes-Weinstein** pressure esthesiometer (**Von Frey test**). ✓ This kit has 20 probes, each with different thicknesses of nylon monofilament (Fig. 7.125). The patient is

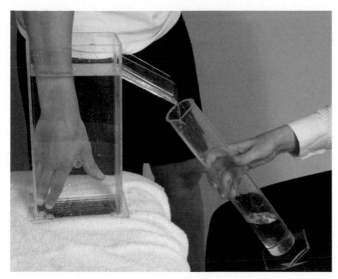

Fig. 7.122 Volumeter used to measure hand volume.

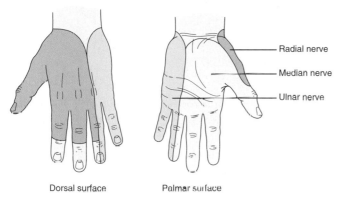

Dorsal surface   Palmar surface

Fig. 7.123 Peripheral nerve distribution in the hand.

- Radial nerve
- Median nerve
- Ulnar nerve

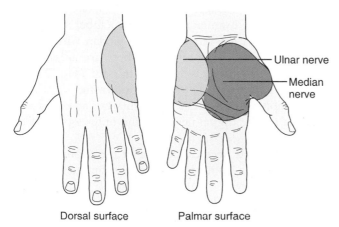

Dorsal surface   Palmar surface

- Ulnar nerve
- Median nerve

Fig. 7.124 Sensory distribution of branches of the ulnar and median nerves given off above the wrist.

TABLE **7.10**

Tests for Cutaneous Sensibility

Test	Sensation	Fiber/Receptor Type
Pin	Pain	Free nerve endings
Warm/cold	Temperature	Free nerve endings
Cotton wool	Moving touch	Quick adapting
Finger stroking	Moving touch	Quick adapting
Dellon's	Moving touch	Quick adapting
Tuning fork	Vibration	Quick adapting
Von Frey	Constant touch	Slow adapting
Weber's	Constant touch	Slow adapting
Pick-up	Constant touch	Slow adapting
Precision sensory grip	Constant touch	Slow adapting
Gross grip	Constant touch	Slow adapting

Modified from Dellon AL: The paper clip: light hardware to evaluate sensibility in the hand, *Contemp Orthop* 1:40, 1979.

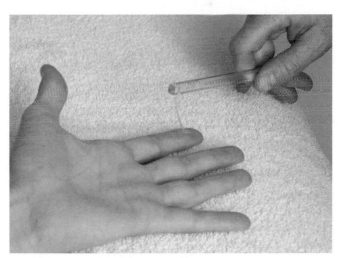

Fig. 7.125 The Semmes-Weinstein monofilament is applied perpendicular to the skin for 1 to 1.5 seconds, held in place for 1 to 1.5 seconds, and lifted for 1 to 1.5 seconds.

blindfolded or otherwise unable to see the hand, and each filament is applied perpendicularly to the finger with the smallest filament being used first. The filament is pushed against the finger until the filament bends. The next filament is then used, and so on until the patient feels one just before or just as it bends.[81,152] The test is repeated three times to ensure a positive result.[191] Normal values vary between probes 2.44 and 2.83 (Table 7.11). When doing the Semmes-Weinstein test, the hand and fingers are commonly divided into a grid (Fig. 7.126), and only one point (usually in the center) is tested in each square. It is primarily the palmar aspect of the hand that is tested.

Stereognosis or tactile gnosis, which is the ability to identify common objects by touch, should also be tested. Objects are placed in the patient's hand while the patient is blindfolded or otherwise unable to see the object. The time taken to recognize the object is noted. Normal subjects can usually name the object within 3 seconds of contact.[189]

TABLE **7.11**

Light Touch Testing Using Semmes-Weinstein Pressure Esthesiometer

Esthesiometer Probe Number	Calculated Pressure (g/mm²)	Interpretation
2.44–2.83	3.25–4.86	Normal light touch
3.22–4.56	11.1–47.3	Diminished light touch, point localization[a] intact
4.74–6.10	68.0–243.0	Minimal light touch, area localization[b] intact
6.10–6.65	243.0–439.0	Sensation but no localization sensibility

[a]Point localization: The dowel is in contact with the skin point stimulated.
[b]Area localization: The dowel is in contact with any point inside the zone of the area being tested (in the hand or foot).
From Omer GE: Report of the committee for evaluation of the clinical result in peripheral nerve injury, *J Hand Surg Am* 8:755, 1983.

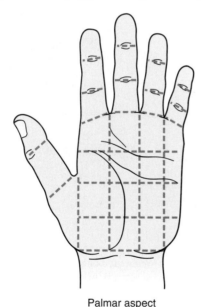

Palmar aspect

Fig. 7.126 Grid pattern used for recording results of light touch sensation testing.

Vibratory sense is tested using a 256-cps (high-frequency) or 30-cps (low-frequency) tuning fork. The patient, who cannot see the test site, indicates when vibration is felt as the examiner touches the skin with the vibrating tuning fork and whether the vibration feels the same. The score is the number of correct responses divided by the total number of presentations.[223]

To test moving touch, the examiner's fingers stroke the patient's finger. The patient notes whether the stroking was felt and what it felt like.

It must be remembered that pain may be referred to the wrist and hand from the cervical or upper thoracic

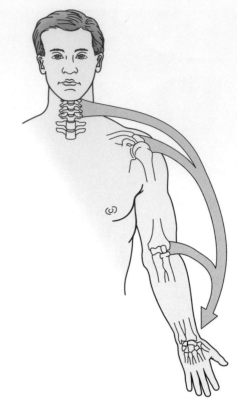

Fig. 7.127 Symptoms can be referred to the wrist and hand from the elbow, shoulder, and cervical spine.

spine, shoulder, and elbow. Seldom is wrist or hand pain referred up the limb (Fig. 7.127). Table 7.12 shows the muscles acting on the forearm, wrist, and hand and their pain referral patterns when injured.

The examiner can attempt a differential diagnosis of paresthesia in the hand if altered sensation is present. A comparison with a normal dermatome chart should be made, and the examiner should remember that there is a fair amount of variability and overlap with dermatomes (Fig. 7.128). In addition, there are areas of the hand where sensation is more important (Fig. 7.129). Abnormal sensation may mean the following:

1. Numbness in the thumb only may be caused by pressure on the digital nerve on the outer aspect of the thumb.
2. A "pins and needles" feeling in the thumb may be caused by a contusion of the thenar branch of the median nerve.
3. Paresthesia in the thumb and index finger may be caused by a C5 disc lesion or C6 nerve root palsy.
4. Paresthesia in the thumb, index finger, and middle finger may be caused by a C5 disc lesion, C6 nerve root palsy, or thoracic outlet syndrome.
5. Paresthesia of the thumb, index finger, middle finger, and half of the ring finger on the palmar aspect may be caused by an injury to the median nerve, possibly through the carpal tunnel; on the dorsal aspect, it could be caused by injury to the radial nerve.

TABLE 7.12

Forearm, Wrist, and Hand Muscles and Referral of Pain

Muscles	Referral Pattern
Brachioradialis	Lateral epicondyle, lateral forearm, and web space between thumb and index finger
Extensor carpi ulnaris	Medial side of dorsum of wrist
Extensor carpi radialis brevis	Middle of dorsum of wrist
Extensor carpi radialis longus	Lateral epicondyle, forearm, and lateral dorsum of hand
Extensor digitorum	Forearm, wrist to appropriate digit
Extensor indices	Dorsum of wrist to index finger
Palmaris longus	Anterior aspect of forearm to palm
Flexor carpi ulnaris	Anteromedial wrist into lateral palm
Flexor carpi radialis	Forearm to anterolateral wrist
Flexor digitorum superficialis	Palm into appropriate digit
Flexor pollicis longus	Thumb
Adductor pollicis	Anterolateral and posterolateral palm into thumb
Opponens pollicis	Anterolateral wrist into anterior thumb
Abductor digiti minimi	Dorsomedial surface of hand into little finger
Interossei	Into adjacent digit, and for first interossei, dorsum of hand

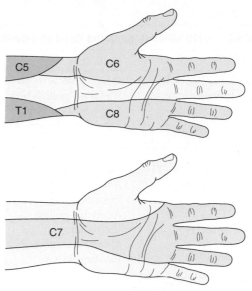

Fig. 7.128 Dermatomes of the hand. Note overlap at dermatomes. Both views are palmar.

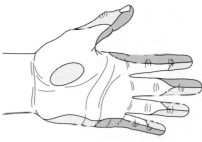

Fig. 7.129 Importance of hand sensation. *Darker areas* indicate where sensation is most important; *lighter areas,* where sensation is a little less important; and *white areas,* where sensation is least important. (Redrawn from Tubiana R: *The hand*, Philadelphia, 1981, WB Saunders, p 74.)

6. Numbness of the thumb and middle finger may be caused by a tumor of the humerus.
7. Paresthesia on all five digits in one or both hands may be caused by a thoracic outlet syndrome. If it is in both hands, it may be caused by a central cervical disc protrusion. The level of protrusion would be indicated by the distribution of the paresthesia.
8. Paresthesia of the index and middle fingers may be caused by a trigger finger or "stick" palsy, if it is on the palmar aspect, or by a C6 disc lesion or C7 nerve root palsy. On the dorsal aspect of the hand, it may be caused by a carpal exostosis or subluxation. Stick palsy is the result of an inordinate amount of pressure from a cane or crutches on the ulnar nerve as it passes through the palm.
9. Paresthesia of the index, middle, and ring fingers may be caused by a C6 disc lesion, C7 nerve root injury, or carpal tunnel syndrome.
10. Paresthesia of all four fingers may be caused by a C6 disc lesion or injury to the C7 nerve root.
11. Paresthesia of the middle finger only may be caused by a C6 disc lesion or C7 nerve root lesion.
12. Paresthesia of the middle and ring fingers may be caused by a C6 disc lesion, C7 nerve root lesion, or stick palsy.
13. Paresthesia of the middle, ring, and little fingers may be caused by a C7 disc lesion or C8 nerve root palsy. The same would be true if there were paralysis of the ring and little fingers. This paresthesia also may be the result of a thoracic outlet syndrome.
14. Paresthesia on the ulnar side of the ring finger and the entire little finger may be caused by pressure of the ulnar nerve at the elbow or in the palm.

Peripheral Nerve Injuries of the Forearm, Wrist, and Hand
Carpal Tunnel Syndrome (Median Nerve). The most common "tunnel" syndrome in the body is the carpal tunnel syndrome, in which the median nerve is compressed under the flexor retinaculum at the wrist (see Fig. 7.45).[177] This compression may follow trauma

TABLE **7.13**

Nerve Injuries (Neuropathy) about the Wrist and Hand

Nerve	Motor Loss	Sensory Loss	Functional Loss
Median nerve (C6–C8, T1; carpal tunnel)	Flexor pollicis brevis Abductor pollicis brevis Opponens pollicis Lateral two lumbricals	Palmar and dorsal thumb, index, middle and lateral half of ring finger If lesion above carpal tunnel, palmar sensation also affected	Thumb opposition Thumb flexion Weak or no pinch Weak grip
Ulnar nerve (C7, C8, T1; pisohamate canal)	Flexor digiti minimi Abductor digiti minimi Opponens digiti minimi Adductor pollicis Interossei Medial two lumbricals Palmaris brevis	Little finger, half of ring finger Palm often not affected	Thumb adduction Inability to extend PIP and DIP joints of fourth and fifth fingers Finger abduction Finger adduction Flexion of little finger

DIP, Distal interphalangeal; *PIP*, proximal interphalangeal.

TABLE **7.14**

The 6-Item Carpal Tunnel Syndrome Symptoms Scale

The following questions refer to your symptoms for a typical 24-hour period during the past 2 weeks. Mark one answer to each symptom.

How severe are the following symptoms in your hand?	None	Mild	Moderate	Severe	Very Severe
Pain at night	☐	☐	☐	☐	☐
Pain during daytime	☐	☐	☐	☐	☐
Numbness or tingling at night	☐	☐	☐	☐	☐
Numbness or tingling during daytime	☐	☐	☐	☐	☐
How often did the following symptoms in your hand wake you up at night?	**Never**	**Once**	**2 or 3 Times**	**4 or 5 Times**	**More Than 5 Times**
Pain	☐	☐	☐	☐	☐
Numbness or tingling	☐	☐	☐	☐	☐

From Atroshi I, Lyrén PE, Gummesson C: The 6-item CTS symptoms scale: a brief outcomes measure for carpal tunnel syndrome, *Qual Life Res* 18:347–358, 2009.

(e.g., a Colles fracture or lunate dislocation),[224] overuse of fingers and wrist (e.g., mobile phone keying, typing),[34] flexor tendon paratenonitis, hypertrophy of the lumbricals, a ganglion, arthritis (osteoarthritis or rheumatoid arthritis), or collagen disease. Different classification systems have been developed to determine the severity of the condition.[225,226] As many as 20% of pregnant women may experience median nerve symptoms because compression of the nerve as a result of fluid retention causing swelling in the carpal tunnel and the primary symptoms are motor loss.[227–229] With carpal tunnel syndrome, the symptoms, which are primarily distal to the wrist, are usually worse at night and include burning, tingling, pins and needles, and numbness into

the median nerve sensory distribution although it has been reported that many patients experience neurological symptoms outside the normal median nerve distribution (Table 7.13).[137,230] Table 7.14 outlines a six-item carpal tunnel syndrome symptoms scale.[231–234] In severe cases, pain may be referred to the forearm. Symptoms are often aggravated by wrist movements, and long-standing cases show atrophy and weakness of the thenar muscles (flexor and abductor pollicis brevis, opponens pollicis) and the lateral two lumbricals. The condition is most common in women (3×)[43] between 30 and 60 years of age, and, although it may occur bilaterally, it is seen most commonly in the dominant hand.[180] It is also commonly seen in younger patients who use their wrists a great deal in repetitive manual labor or are exposed to vibration.[235] Wainner et al.[175] developed a clinical prediction rule for diagnosing carpal tunnel syndrome. Because of the apparent connection between carpal tunnel syndrome and cervical lesions resulting in double crush syndromes, the examiner should take care to include cervical assessment if the history appears to warrant such inclusion.[236–238]

Clinical Prediction Rule for Carpal Tunnel Syndrome[175]

- Shaking hand(s) for symptom relief
- Wrist-ratio index >0.67
- Symptom severity scale >1.9
- Reduced median sensory field of digits (especially thumb)
- Age greater than 45 years

Guyon (Pisohamate) Canal (Ulnar Nerve). The ulnar nerve is sometimes compressed as it passes through the pisohamate, or Guyon canal (Fig. 7.130). The condition may also be called **ulnar tunnel syndrome,** because the nerve may be compressed in the wrist from trauma (acute or repetitive), a space occupying lesion, or vascular lesion.[228,239] The nerve may be compressed from trauma (e.g., fractured hook of hamate in racquet sports), use of crutches, or chronic pressure, as in people who cycle long distances while leaning on the handlebars or those who use pneumatic jackhammers. If the problem is in the Guyon canal, direct pressure over the canal may reproduce or exacerbate the symptoms (**Guyon canal compression test [cyclist's palsy**[34]**]**❓).[171] The ulnar nerve gives off two sensory branches above the wrist. These branches supply the palmar and dorsal aspects of the hand, as illustrated in Fig. 7.124, resulting in sensory symptoms alone[240] and do not pass through the Guyon canal. Therefore, if the ulnar nerve is compressed in the canal, only the fingers show an altered sensation, and the primary symptoms are motor loss (see Table 7.13).[228,240] Motor loss includes the muscles of the hypothenar eminence (flexor digiti minimi, abductor digiti minimi, and opponens digiti minimi), adductor pollicis, the interossei, medial two lumbricals, and palmaris brevis (Fig. 7.131).

Joint Play Movements

When assessing joint play movements, the examiner should remember that if the patient complains of instability or pain on wrist flexion, the lesion is probably in the midcarpal joints. If the patient complains of instability or pain on wrist extension, the lesion is probably in the radiocarpal joints, because it is in these joints that most of the movement occurs during these actions. If the patient complains of pain or instability

on supination and pronation, the lesion is probably in the ulnameniscocarpal joint or inferior radioulnar joint.

Joint Play Movements of the Hand

WRIST
- Long-axis extension (traction or distraction)
- Anteroposterior glide of the individual bones
- Side glide of bone rows
- Side tilt

INTERMETACARPAL JOINTS
- Anteroposterior glide

FINGERS
- Long-axis extension (traction or distraction)
- Anteroposterior glide
- Rotation
- Side glide

The amount of movement obtained by the joint play should be compared with that of the normal side and considered significant only if there is a difference between the two sides and there are other symptoms (e.g., pain, clunk, crepitus). Reproduction of the patient's symptoms would also give an indication of the joints at fault. Many of the joint play movements are similar to the special tests for wrist pain and tests for bone, ligament, capsule, and joint instability. The examiner would only need to do both if there is a need to help confirm the diagnosis.

Wrist

To perform **long-axis extension** at the wrist, the examiner stabilizes the radius and ulna with one hand (the patient's elbow may be flexed to 90°, and stabilization may be applied at the elbow if there is no pathology at the elbow) and places the other hand just distal to the wrist. The examiner then applies a longitudinal traction movement with the distal hand (Fig. 7.132).

AP glide is applied at the wrist in two positions. The examiner first places the stabilizing hand around the distal end of the radius and ulna just proximal to the radiocarpal joint and then places the other hand around the proximal row of carpal bones. If the examiner's hands are positioned properly, they should touch each other (Fig. 7.133). The examiner applies an AP gliding movement of the proximal row of carpal bones on the radius and ulna, testing the amount of movement and end feel. Then, the stabilizing hand is moved slightly distally (<1 cm) so that it is around the proximal row of carpal bones. The examiner places the mobilizing hand around the distal row of carpal bones. An AP gliding movement is applied to the distal row of carpal bones on the proximal row to test the

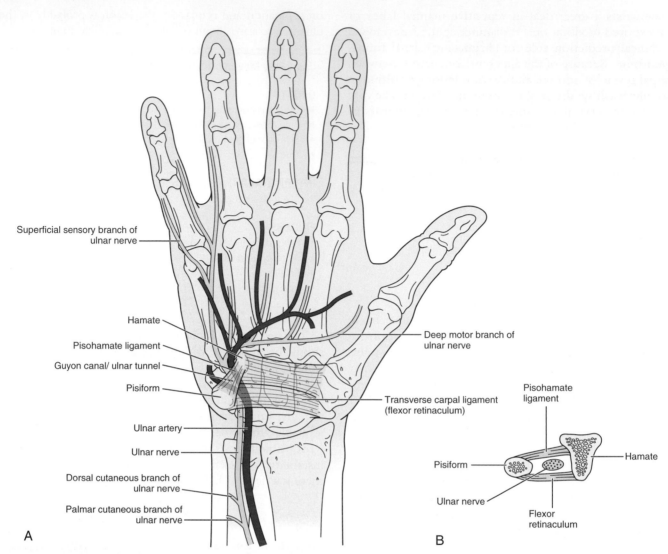

Superficial sensory branch of
ulnar nerve

Hamate

Pisohamate ligament

Guyon canal/ ulnar tunnel

Pisiform

Ulnar artery

Ulnar nerve

Dorsal cutaneous branch of
ulnar nerve

Palmar cutaneous branch of
ulnar nerve

Deep motor branch of
ulnar nerve

Transverse carpal ligament
(flexor retinaculum)

Pisohamate
ligament

Pisiform

Ulnar nerve

Hamate

Flexor
retinaculum

A

B

Fig. 7.130 Guyon canal. (A) Illustration showing the anatomy of the ulnar tunnel at the wrist. *H*, hamate, *P*, pisiform. (B) Section view showing position of nerve relative to pisohamate ligament and flexor retinaculum.

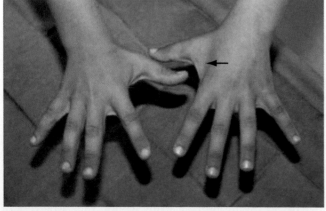

Fig. 7.131 First dorsal interosseous muscle wasting in the left hand *(arrow)*. (From Bachoura A, Jacoby SM: Ulnar tunnel syndrome, *Orthop Clin North Am* 43:467–474, 2012. Courtesy Dr. DG Efstathopoulos, KAT Accident Hospital, and Dr. ZT Kokkalis, Athens University Hospital, Athens, Greece.)

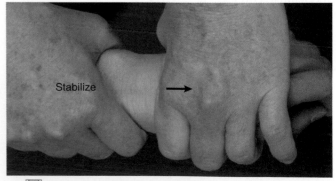

Stabilize

Fig. 7.132 Long-axis extension (traction) of the wrist.

amount of movement and end feel. These movements are sometimes called the **AP drawer tests** of the wrist.[3,70] If the examiner then moves the stabilizing hand slightly distally (<1 cm) again, the hand will be around the distal carpal bones. The mobilizing hand is then placed around the metacarpals, and an AP gliding movement is applied to the base of the metacarpals to test the amount of joint play and end feel.

Side glide is performed in a similar fashion, except that a side-to-side movement is performed instead of an AP movement. To perform **side tilting** of the carpals on the radius and ulna, the examiner stabilizes the radius and ulna by placing the stabilizing hand around the distal radius and ulna just proximal to the radiocarpal joint and the mobilizing hand around the patient's hand, and then radially and ulnarly deviating the hand on the radius and ulna (Fig. 7.134).

The joint play movements just described are general ones involving different "rows" of carpal bones. To check the joint play movements of the individual carpal bones, a procedure such as **Kaltenborn's technique** should be used. Kaltenborn[241] suggested 10 tests to determine the mobility of each of the carpal bones (see Fig. 7.67). The movement of each of the bones is determined in a sequential manner, and both sides are tested for comparison. These tests are sometimes referred to as **ballottement tests** or **shear tests** (Fig. 7.135).[3] The examiner may use Kaltenborn's order or any other order as long as each bone and its relationship to adjacent bones is tested individually for the amount of accessory movement and the end feel.[242] For example, some people start by testing the movement of the lunate relative to the radius, and then move to the capitate (relative to the lunate), followed by scaphoid-radius, scaphoid-trapezoid/trapezium, triquetrum-radius, and triquetrum-hamate. Pisiform may be tested individually. Pain on any of these joint play movements done in neutral, flexion, or extension could indicate pathology in the joint between the two bones.[82] As the examiner palpates the individual bones, a comparison is made with the individual bones of the uninjured wrist noting whether the movement of the bones are the same for both wrists and whether there are any other pathological findings (e.g., hypo- or hypermobility, pain, clunk, crepitus). It is especially important to compare the movement between the scaphoid and lunate (the scapholunate joint) and the lunate and the triquetrum (lunotriquetral joint) as these are the joints that are the most common traumatically injured wrist joints.[34] In both cases, the lunate is stabilized and the scaphoid or trapezoid is moved anteriorly and posteriorly around the lunate. If joint play is done between the scaphoid and lunate, it is called the **scapholunate ballottement test**. If done between the lunate and triquetrum, it is called the **lunotriquetral ballottement (Reagan's) test** (see Special Tests section earlier).

Kaltenborn's Individual Carpal Bone Mobilization

- Fixate the capitate, and move the trapezoid
- Fixate the capitate, and move the scaphoid
- Fixate the capitate, and move the lunate
- Fixate the capitate, and move the hamate
- Fixate the scaphoid, and move the trapezoid and trapezium
- Fixate the radius, and move the scaphoid
- Fixate the radius, and move the lunate
- Fixate the ulna, and move the triquetrum
- Fixate the triquetrum, and move the hamate
- Fixate the triquetrum, and move the pisiform

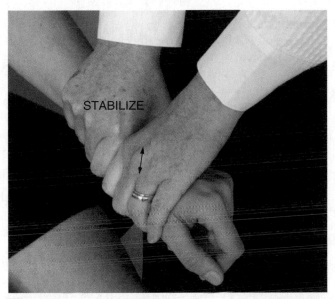

Fig. 7.133 Position for testing joint play movements of the wrist. Note that there is no gap between the web spaces of the two hands.

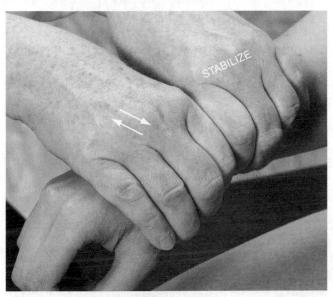

Fig. 7.134 Wrist side glide.

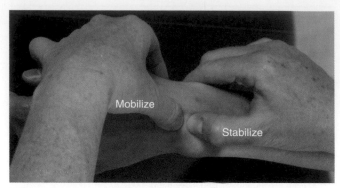

Fig. 7.135 Individual carpal bone shear tests. Anteroposterior shear (glide) of lunate on radius demonstrated.

Intermetacarpal Joints

To accomplish **AP glide** at the intermetacarpal joints, the examiner stabilizes one metacarpal bone and moves the adjacent metacarpal anteriorly and posteriorly in relation to the fixed bone to determine the amount of joint play and the end feel. The process is repeated for each joint (Fig. 7.136).

Fingers

The joint play movements for the fingers are the same for the metacarpophalangeal, proximal interphalangeal, and distal interphalangeal joints; the hand position of the examiner simply moves farther distally.

To perform **long-axis extension,** the examiner stabilizes the proximal segment or bone using one hand while placing the second hand around the distal segment or bone of the particular joint to be tested. With the mobilizing hand, the examiner applies a longitudinal traction to the joint (Fig. 7.137). If one was to apply axial compression to the first metacarpal (**grind test**), it may cause pain in the first carpometacarpal joint in the presence of degenerative arthritis in the joint.[34] This may be accompanied by subluxation of the joint in the chronic condition indicated by a step at the joint (i.e., **shoulder sign**) (see Fig. 7.30).

AP glide is accomplished by stabilizing the proximal bone with one hand. The mobilizing hand is placed around the distal segment of the joint, and the examiner applies an anterior and/or posterior movement to the distal segment, being sure to maintain the joint surfaces parallel to one another while determining the amount of movement and end feel (Fig. 7.138). A minimal amount of traction may be applied to bring about slight separation of the joint surfaces.

Rotation of the joints of the fingers is accomplished by stabilizing the proximal segment with one hand. With the other hand, the examiner applies slight traction to the joint to distract the joint surfaces and then rotates the distal segment on the proximal segment to determine the end feel and joint play (Fig. 7.139).

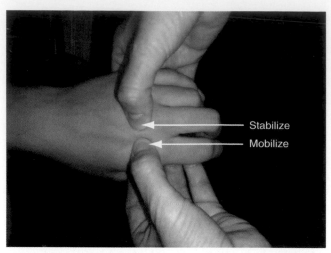

Fig. 7.136 Anteroposterior glide of the intermetacarpal joints.

To perform **side glide** joint play to the joints of the fingers, the proximal segment is stabilized with one hand. The examiner then applies slight traction to the joint with the mobilizing hand to distract the joint surfaces and then moves the distal segment sideways, keeping the joint surfaces parallel to one another to determine the joint play and end feel (Fig. 7.140).

Palpation

To palpate the forearm, wrist, and hand, the examiner starts proximally and works distally, first on the dorsal (posterior) surface and then on the anterior surface starting on the ulnar or radial side and the moving to the other side (Fig. 7.141). The muscles of the forearm are palpated first for any signs of tenderness or pathology.

Dorsal Surface

On the dorsal aspect, the examiner begins on the thumb (i.e., radial) side of the hand and palpates the radial styloid process, the anatomical "snuff box," the carpal bones, and the metacarpal bones and phalanges.

The styloid processes of the radius and ulna can be palpated on the medial and lateral sides of the arm. The examiner places the thumbs over the outside of the patient's thumb and over the outside of the patient's little finger and slides their thumbs up toward the elbow (i.e., proximally) until two hard structures are felt on the little finger side (i.e., ulnar styloid) and on the thumb side (i.e., radial styloid) (see Fig. 7.32). The examiner may also palpate distally from the radius and ulna until the thumb "falls into holes" or **fovea**, which indicates the distal ends of the two styloids. The examiner then notes the position of each styloid relative to each other. Normally, the radial styloid projects more distally than the ulnar styloid (see Fig. 7.32). The difference is called **clinical ulnar variance**. True ulnar variance would be measured from the head of the ulna on x-ray (Fig. 7.142).[34]

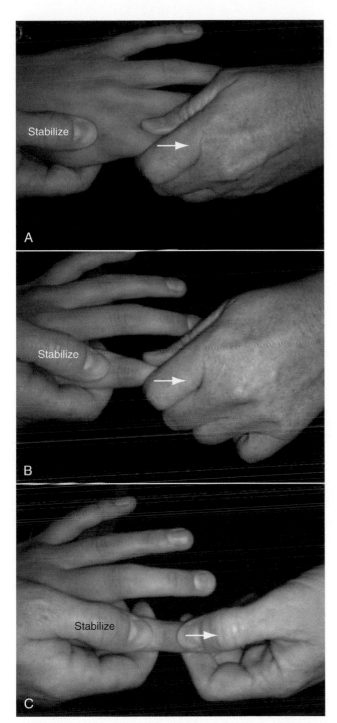

Fig. 7.137 Long axis extension (traction) of the joints of the fingers. (A) Metacarpophalangeal joint. (B) Proximal interphalangeal joint. (C) Distal interphalangeal joint.

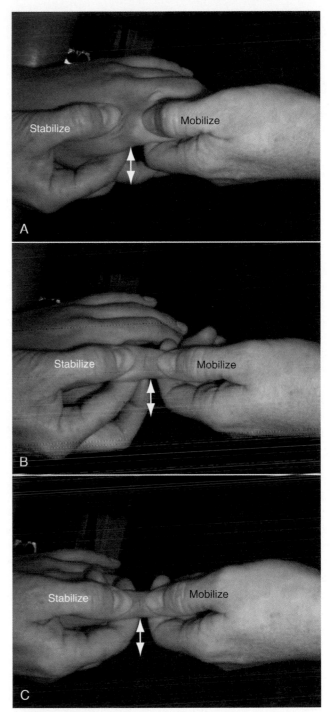

Fig. 7.138 Anteroposterior glide of the joints of the fingers. (A) Metacarpophalangeal joint. (B) Proximal interphalangeal joint. (C) Distal interphalangeal joint.

Anatomical Snuff Box. The anatomical snuff box is located between the tendons of extensor pollicis longus and extensor pollicis brevis on the lateral (radial) side of the wrist and can best be seen by having the patient actively extend the thumb. The waist of the scaphoid and radial styloid (proximally) may be easier to palpate in the anatomical snuff box if the wrist is ulnarly deviated (Fig. 7.143A).[58,70] The radial artery also runs through the anatomical snuff box.[8,62,78] The scaphoid bone may

be palpated inside the snuff box or along the **scaphoid tubercle**, which lies outside the extensor pollicis brevis, and more anterior and radial to the flexor carpi ulnaris when the wrist is radially deviated (Fig. 7.143B).[78] Tenderness in the anatomical snuff box, especially after a FOOSH injury, may indicate a fractured scaphoid, especially the anterior fragment or pole, necessitating diagnostic imaging.[146] If the wrist is radially deviated and the

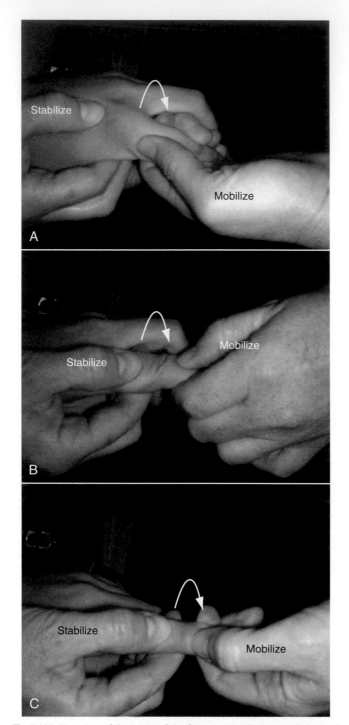

Fig. 7.139 Rotation of the joints of the fingers. (A) Metacarpophalangeal joint. (B) Proximal interphalangeal joint. (C) Distal interphalangeal joint.

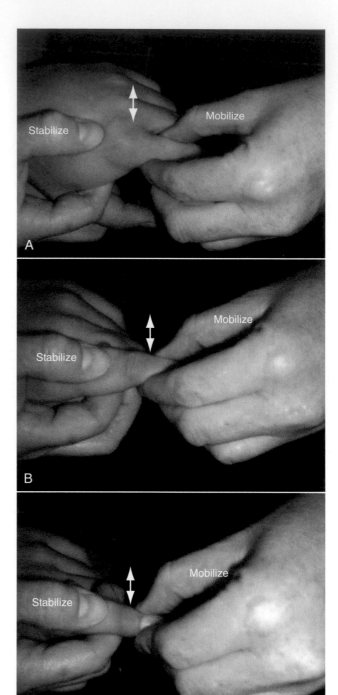

Fig. 7.140 Side glide of the joints of the fingers. (A) Metacarpophalangeal joint. (B) Proximal interphalangeal joint. (C) Distal interphalangeal joint.

radiopalmar aspect of the scaphoid is palpated (see Fig. 7.143B), the examiner will be palpating the scaphoid tubercle. It has been reported that this is a better test for a scaphoid fracture than palpating in the anatomical snuff box with the wrist in neutral.[146,243] In addition, if the examiner palpates the scaphoid tubercle but allows it to move into radial deviation, the tubercle will be felt to rotate anteriorly and become more prominent.[70] If

sufficient force is applied to the tubercle, radial deviation will not be possible.[70] If the examiner moves distal to the scaphoid tubercle, the trapezium will be felt. If the patient is asked to move the thumb actively, the examiner will feel the trapezium move while the scaphoid tubercle does not.[70] Proximal and medial to the scaphoid tubercle, the examiner will be able to feel the radial artery.[70] With the wrist in the anatomic position, proximal palpation is used to find the radial styloid on the lateral aspect. Moving distally over the scaphoid, the examiner will feel the scapho-trapezium joint and the trapezium. If the examiner has the patient put the small finger and thumb in opposition, the trapezium becomes more prominent. If the examiner has the patient then circumduct the thumb, it will be easier for the examiner to differentiate the trapezium from the first metacarpal.[34]

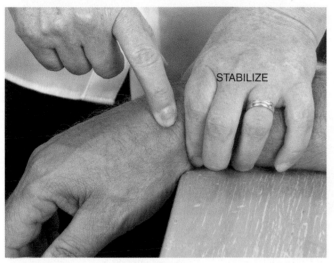

Fig. 7.141 Palpation of the wrist. The examiner stabilizes one or more bones while moving a distal bone or feeling the joint line.

Moving medially over the radius, the examiner comes to the **radial (Lister's) tubercle**, which is on the dorsal aspect of the radius at the level of the proximal extensor skin crease and lies directly in line with the third metacarpal.[62,244] The extensor pollicis longus tendon moves around the tubercle to enter the thumb, which gives it a different angle of pull from that of the extensor pollicis brevis. Inflammation of the extensor pollicis longus tendon is sometimes called **drummer's palsy**.[34] With the wrist still in the anatomic position, the ulnar styloid is palpated on the medial aspect of the wrist. Just distal to the ulnar styloid, the examiner may palpate an indentation or hole (fovea), which is sometimes called the "**ulnar snuff box**," on the medial (ulnar) side of the wrist (Fig. 7.143C). The ulnotriquetral ligament can be palpated within the border of the flexor carpi ulnaris tendon, the ulnar styloid, the anterior ulnar head, and the pisiform. Pressure applied to the ulnar snuff box applies pressure to the triquetrum causing pain, which may indicate involvement of the triquetrum, the triquetrohamate joint, the lunotriquetral joint, or the TFCC.[18,30,34] If the wrist is radially deviated, it will be easier to palpate the triquetrum as the proximal carpal row slides ulnarly with wrist radial deviation. On the dorsal surface of the ulna with the forearm pronated, the examiner can palpate the obvious styloid of the ulna (Fig. 7.144). It is the rounded prominence on the ulnar side of the wrist.[34] The ulnar

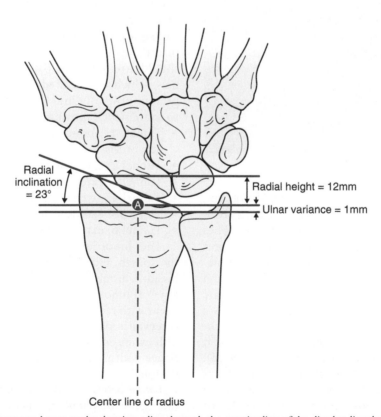

Fig. 7.142 True ulnar variance is measured on x-ray by drawing a line through the anterior line of the distal radius through the central reference point *(A)* perpendicular to its long axis. The variance is this distance between the radial line and the line along the distal cortical rim of the ulnar dome.

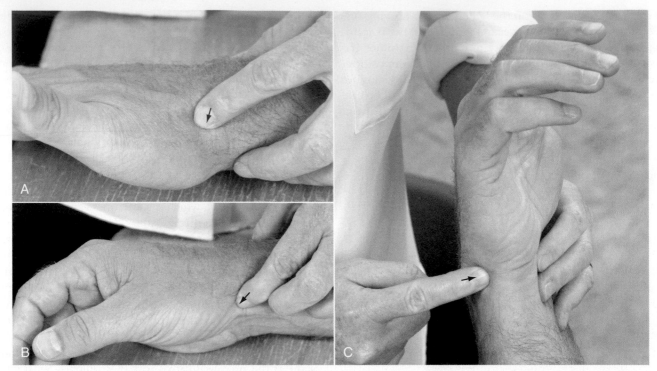

Fig. 7.143 Palpation of the (A) scaphoid in the anatomical snuff box, (B) scaphoid tubercle, (C) ulnar snuff box or fovea.

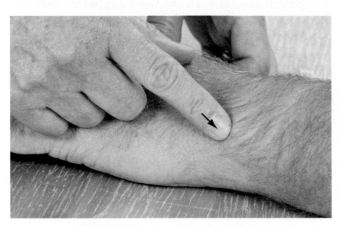

Fig. 7.144 Palpation of the ulnar styloid.

head should be the same size on both arms. If not, and one sticks out more than the other, it may indicate a problem with the DRUJ (see Fig. 7.15). The ulnar styloid lies slightly distal to it. The TFCC may be palpated as a soft mass between the ulnar styloid, pisiform, flexor carpi ulnaris, and the triquetrum, which supports the DRUJ and the lunate and triquetrum.[34,149] By continuing to palpate deeply and in a palmar direction, the **fovea**, which is a groove at the base of the ulnar styloid acting as an attachment point for the TFCC, may be palpated.[34] If tender, it may indicate injury to the TFCC (i.e., **ulnar fovea sign**). The radial styloid extends farther distally than the ulnar styloid. Tenderness along the abductor pollicis longus and extensor pollicis brevis may indicate tenosynovitis or **de Quervain's tenosynovitis.**[70] **Intersection syndrome**

(i.e., **peritendinitis crepitans**) is inflammation where the muscle bellies of abductor pollicis longus and extensor pollicis brevis underlie extensor carpi radialis longus and brevis resulting in crepitus and pain about 4 cm (1.6 inches) proximal to the tip of the radial styloid leading to **"squeaker's wrist."**[31] By palpating over the dorsum of the wrist, crossing the radius and ulna, the examiner should attempt to palpate the six extensor tendon tunnels, which are covered by the extensor retinaculum to prevent bowstringing[4] (noting any crepitus or restriction to movement), moving lateral to medial (see Fig. 7.51):

- Tunnel 1: abductor pollicis longus and extensor pollicis brevis
- Tunnel 2: extensor carpi radialis longus and brevis
- Tunnel 3: extensor pollicis longus
- Tunnel 4: extensor digitorum and extensor indices
- Tunnel 5: extensor digiti minimi
- Tunnel 6: extensor carpi ulnaris

The lunotriquetral joint can be palpated between the fourth and fifth extensor compartments one finger breadth distal to the DRUJ with the wrist in 30° flexion.[30] If lunotriquetral instability is present, a "click" may occur with radial to ulnar deviation.[30] The **lunotriquetral interval** is palpated posteriorly between the fourth and fifth extensor compartments about 1.3 cm (0.5 inch/one finger width) distal to the DRUJ with the wrist in 30° flexion.[6]

Carpal Bones. In the anatomical snuff box, the examiner can begin palpating the proximal row of carpal bones, starting with the scaphoid bone. When palpating the carpal bones, the examiner usually palpates them on the anterior and dorsal surfaces at the same time by applying AP joint play-like movements. The proximal row of carpal bones from lateral to medial (in the anatomic position) are the scaphoid, lunate, triquetrum (just below the ulnar styloid), and pisiform.

On the anterior aspect, the examiner should take care to ensure proper positioning of the lunate bone. If it dislocates or subluxes, it tends to move anteriorly into the carpal tunnel, which may lead to symptoms of carpal tunnel syndrome. The pisiform is often easier to palpate if the patient's wrist is flexed. The examiner may then palpate the pisiform where the flexor carpi ulnaris tendon inserts into it. Tenderness in the hollow between the pisiform and ulnar styloid may indicate TFCC pathology.[20]

Returning to the anatomical snuff box and moving distally, the examiner palpates the trapezium bone. The distal row of carpal bones from lateral to medial (in the anatomic position) is palpated individually: trapezium, trapezoid, capitate (distal to lunate and a slight indentation before the third metacarpal), and hamate (distal to triquetrum; the hook of the hamate on the anterior surface, which may be palpated proximal to the base of the fourth and fifth metacarpals[34]). If the examiner places the interphalangeal joint of the thumb over the patient's pisiform with the thumb facing the metacarpal head of the long (third) finger, the tip of the examiner's thumb will lie over the hook of the hamate (Fig. 7.145). The examiner should remember the ulnar nerve is found in the same area.[70] Tenderness in the posterior triquetral-hamate area is suggestive of midcarpal instability.[34] The hook of the hamate lies just distal to the pisiform (1 to 2 cm [0.4 to 0.8 inch] distal and radially) but as it is deep, it may be difficult to palpate.[4,62] The hamate is most commonly injured by direct trauma.[150,245] Guyon canal lies between the hook of the hamate and the pisiform (see Fig. 7.130).[62]

On the dorsal aspect, the examiner could begin palpation at the distal row of carpals. It is often easier to palpate the shafts of the metacarpals and move proximally until one feels a slight dip indicating the joint line between the base of the metacarpal and the carpal. If the examiner places a finger over the middle metacarpal and slides along it until the finger drops into a "hole" or depression, this depression is the capitate bone. Moving medially (hamate) and laterally (trapezoid, trapezium), the other bones of the distal row may be palpated again by making AP joint play-like movements. If the examiner then moves proximally from the capitate, the finger rests on the lunate. By flexing and extending the wrist, a lump which is the lunate will become prominent in flexion[70] in a recess (i.e., **crucifixion fossa**) about 1 cm (0.4 inch) distal to Lister's tubercle.[58,244] The recess disappears on flexion as the scaphoid and lunate come out from under

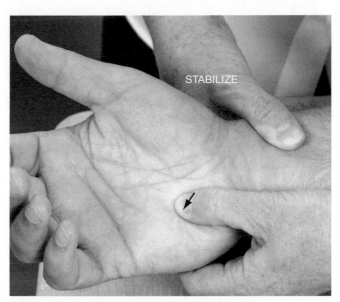

Fig. 7.145 Palpation of hook of hamate.

the radial overhang.[58] If the fossa cannot be palpated, it may be because of a ganglion (a soft mass) or **scaphoid dissociation** (subluxation).[58] The scaphoid dissociation is most painful in extension and radial deviation. The area between the lunate and the scaphoid tubercle is called the **scapulolunate interval** (seen on x-ray) (see Fig. 7.158) and it is where the scapholunate ligament is found.[34] Moving medially (triquetrum) and laterally (scaphoid), these carpals may be palpated.

Metacarpal Bones and Phalanges. The examiner returns to the trapezium bone and moves farther distally to palpate the first metacarpal joint of the thumb and the first metacarpal bone. Moving medially, the examiner palpates each metacarpal bone on the anterior and dorsal surface in turn. A similar procedure is carried out for the metacarpophalangeal and interphalangeal joints and the phalanges. These structures are also palpated on their medial and lateral aspects for tenderness, swelling, altered temperature, or other signs of pathology (Fig. 7.146).

Anterior Surface

Pulses. Proximally, the radial and ulnar pulses are palpated first. The radial pulse on the anterolateral aspect of the wrist on top of the radius is easiest to palpate and is the one most frequently used when taking a pulse. It runs between the tendons of flexor carpi radialis and abductor pollicis longus. The ulnar pulse may be palpated lateral to the tendon of flexor carpi ulnaris. It is more difficult to palpate because it runs deeper and lies under the pisiform and the palmar fascia.

Tendons. Moving across the anterior aspect, the examiner may be able to palpate the long flexor tendons (see Fig. 7.51) in a lateral-to-medial direction: flexor carpi radialis, flexor pollicis longus, flexor digitorum superficialis, flexor digitorum profundus, palmaris longus (if present), and flexor carpi ulnaris (inserts into pisiform). The palmaris longus (if present) lies over the tendons of the flexor digitorum superficialis, which lie over the tendons of the flexor digitorum profundus. The palmaris longus tendon may sometimes be used for tendon repairs or transfers.

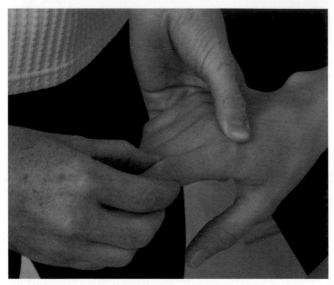

Fig. 7.146 Palpation of the proximal interphalangeal joint of the second finger.

Palmar Fascia and Intrinsic Muscles. The examiner should then move distally to palpate the palmar fascia and intrinsic muscles of the thenar and hypothenar eminences for indications of pathology.

Skin Flexion Creases. From an anatomic point of view, the examiner should note the various skin flexion creases of the wrist, hand, and fingers (Fig. 7.147). The flexion creases indicate lines of adherence between the skin and fascia with no intervening adipose tissue. The following creases should be noted:

1. The proximal skin crease of the wrist indicates the upper limit of the synovial sheaths of the flexor tendons.
2. The middle skin crease of the wrist indicates the wrist (radiocarpal) joint.
3. The distal skin crease of the wrist indicates the upper margin of the flexor retinaculum.
4. The radial longitudinal skin crease of the palm encircles the thenar eminence. (Palm readers refer to this line as the "life line.")
5. The proximal transverse line of the palm runs across the shafts of the metacarpal bones, indicating the superficial palmar arterial arch. (Palm readers refer to this line as the "head line.")
6. The distal transverse line of the palm lies over the heads of the second to fourth metacarpals. (Palm readers refer to this line as the "love line.")

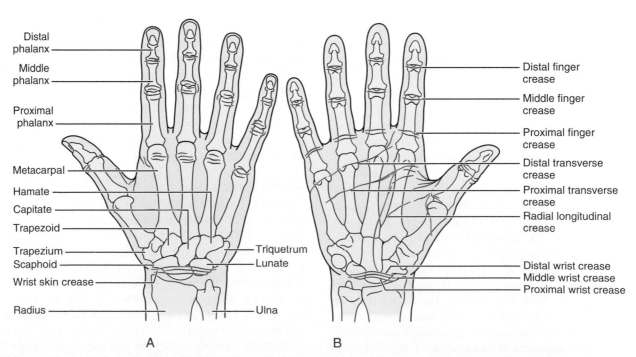

Fig. 7.147 Bony landmarks and skin creases of the hand and wrist. (A) Dorsal view. (B) Palmar view. (Adapted from Tubiana R: *The hand*, Philadelphia, 1981, WB Saunders, p 619.)

7. The proximal skin crease of the fingers is 2 cm (0.8 inch) distal to the metacarpophalangeal joints.

8. The middle skin crease of the fingers is made up of two lines and lies over the proximal interphalangeal joints.

9. The distal skin crease of the fingers lies over the distal interphalangeal joints.

10. On the flexor and extensor aspects, the skin creases over the proximal and distal interphalangeal joints lie proximal to the joint. On the extensor aspect, the metacarpophalangeal creases lie proximal to the joint; on the flexor aspect, they lie distal to the joint.

Arches. In addition, the examiner should ensure the viability of the arches of the hand (see Fig. 7.5). The carpal transverse arch is the result of the shape of the carpal bones, which in part forms the carpal tunnel. The flexor retinaculum forms the roof for the tunnel. The metacarpal transverse arch is formed by the metacarpal bones, and its shape can have great variability because of the mobility of these bones. This arch is most evident when the palm is cupped. The longitudinal arch is made of the carpal bones, metacarpal bones, and phalanges. The keystone of this arch is the metacarpophalangeal joints, which provide stability and support for the arch. Weakness or atrophy of the intrinsic muscles of the hand leads to a loss of these arches. The deformity is most obvious with paralysis of the median and ulnar nerve, which results in an **"ape hand" deformity**.

Diagnostic Imaging

Plain Film Radiography

A routine wrist series of x-rays involves the following views: AP, lateral, and scaphoid.[246] Motion views are sometimes taken, especially if instability is suspected.

Common X-Ray Views of the Forearm, Wrist, and Hand

- Anteroposterior/posteroanterior view
  ◦ Forearm (Fig. 7.149B)
  ◦ Wrist (in neutral) (Fig. 7.150B)
  ◦ Hand (Fig. 7.151)
  ◦ Digits (Fig. 7.152C)
- Lateral view
  ◦ Forearm (see Fig. 7.149A)
  ◦ Wrist (in neutral) (see Fig. 7.153B)
  ◦ Hand
  ◦ Digits (see Fig. 7.152A)
- Scaphoid view (see Fig. 7.155A)
- Carpal tunnel (axial) view (see Fig. 7.162)
- Clenched-fist view (see Fig. 7.163)
- Posteroanterior oblique view (Fig. 7.150A)
- Ulnar deviation of wrist
- Radial deviation of wrist
- Oblique view of digit (Fig. 7.152B)

Posteroanterior View.[247–249] The examiner should note the shape and position of the bones (Fig. 7.148), watching for any evidence of fractures (Fig. 7.153) or displacement, decrease in the joint spaces, or change in bone density, which may be caused by avascular necrosis. **True ulnar variance** is measured by drawing a line through the anterior line of the distal radius through the central reference point perpendicular to its long axis. The variance is the distance between the radial line and the line along the distal cortical rim of the ulnar dome (see Fig. 7.142).[248,250] The arcs of the wrist (called **Gilula's lines** or **arcs**) (Fig. 7.154), seen only on the AP view show the normal relation of the carpal bones in the AP view.[18,130,251] Instability is commonly suspected if the arcs are disrupted.[18] If avascular necrosis is present, there is rarefaction and increased density of the bone (i.e., increased whiteness) and possibly sclerosis (i.e., patchy appearance) of the bone. Avascular necrosis is often seen in the scaphoid bone (Figs. 7.155 and 7.156A) after a fracture or in the lunate in Kienböck disease (Fig. 7.156B).[121] In some cases, the TFCC may be visualized (Fig. 7.157). The AP view may also be used to show dislocations of the lunate (Fig. 7.158A), the distal ulna (Fig. 7.158B), the lunotriquetral relation (Fig. 7.158C), and ulnar variance (length of ulna in relation to radius).[252] Normally, the gap between the scaphoid and lunate is about 2 mm. Widening of the space (i.e., **Terry Thomas sign**) to greater than 4 mm may indicate scapholunate dissociation and is best seen in ulnar deviation.[130]

The AP view of the wrist and hand is also used to determine the skeletal age of a patient.[97] The left hand

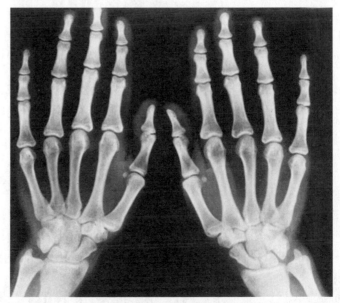

Fig. 7.148 Radiograph showing the bones of both hands. The thumb metacarpal is the shortest, and the index metacarpal is by far the longest. The first and second phalanges of the middle and ring fingers are longer than those of the index finger. Note the interlocking design of the carpometacarpal articulations and the saddle shape in opposing planes of the articular surfaces of the trapezium and the base of the first metacarpal. (From Tubiana R: *The hand*, Philadelphia, 1981, WB Saunders, p 21.)

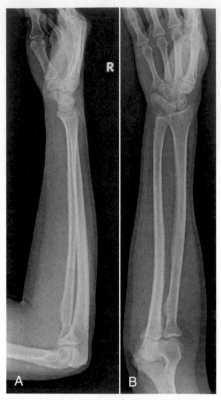

Fig. 7.149 Radiographic views of the forearm. (A) Lateral. (B) Posteroanterior.

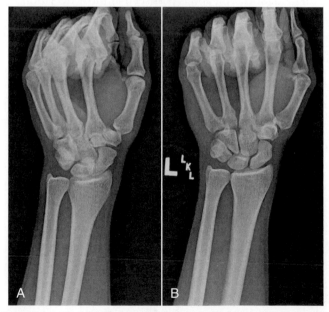

Fig. 7.150 Radiographic views of the wrist (in neutral). (A) Oblique. (B) Posteroanterior.

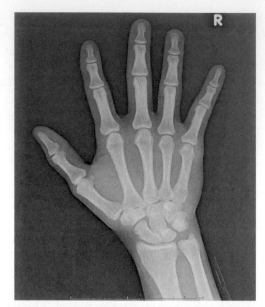

Fig. 7.151 Posteroanterior view of the hand.

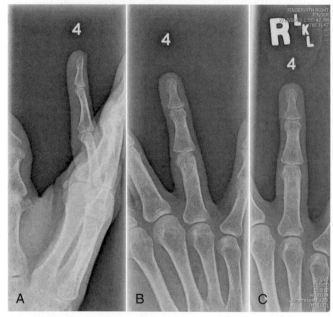

Fig. 7.152 Radiographic views of the digits. (A) Lateral. (B) Oblique. (C) Anteroposterior.

and wrist are used for study because they are thought to be less influenced by environmental factors. The method used in this technique is based on the fact that after an **ossification center** appears (Fig. 7.159), it changes its shape and size in a systematic manner as the ossification gradually spreads throughout the cartilaginous

parts of the skeleton. The wrist and hand are studied because several bones are available for overall comparison, including the carpal bones, the metacarpal growth plates (seen at the distal end of bone), and the phalangeal growth plates (seen at the proximal end of bone). The patient's hand is compared with standard plates[150] until one plate is found that best approximates that of the patient. There is one standard for males and another for females. In two-thirds of the population, skeletal age is no more than 1 year above or below chronologic age. Acceleration or retardation of 3 years or more is considered abnormal. At birth, none of the carpal bones is visible (see Fig. 1.19). This method may be

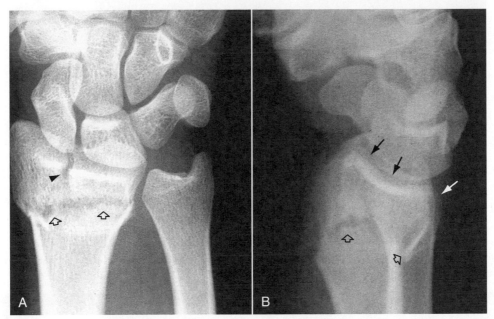

Fig. 7.153 Wrist fracture: Colles fracture. (A) Observe the transverse fracture of the distal portion of the radius *(open arrows)* with extension into the radiocarpal joint *(arrowhead)*. (B) In the lateral projection, dorsal angulation of the articular surface of the radius *(solid arrows)* is apparent and caused by compaction of bone dorsally. This injury is a three-part fracture. The ulnar styloid process is intact, and no evidence of subluxation of the distal portion of the ulna can be seen. (From Resnick D, Kransdorf MJ: *Bone and joint imaging*, Philadelphia, 2005, WB Saunders, p 851.)

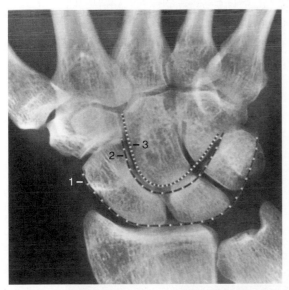

Fig. 7.154 Wrist arcs. Three arcuate lines, called Gilula lines or arcs, can normally be constructed along the carpal articular surfaces: *1,* Along the proximal margins of the scaphoid, lunate, and triquetrum; *2,* along the distal aspects of these bones; *3,* along the proximal margins of the capitate and hamate. (From Weissman BNW, Sledge CB: *Orthopedic radiology*, Philadelphia, 1986, WB Saunders, p 117.)

used up to age 20 when the bones of the hand and wrist have fused.

Lateral View. The examiner should note the shape and position of bones for any evidence of fracture and/or displacement (Fig. 7.160A). The lateral view is also useful in detecting swelling around the carpal bones and for measuring the relation of the scaphoid and lunate to the radius and metacarpals (Fig. 7.161).[252]

Scaphoid View. This view isolates the scaphoid to show a possible fracture (see Fig. 7.155A).

Carpal Tunnel (Axial) View. This view is used to show the margins of the carpal tunnel and is useful for determining fractures of the hook of hamate and trapezium (Fig. 7.162).

Clenched-Fist (Anteroposterior) View. This view is sometimes useful to show increased gapping between the carpal bones, indicating instability (Fig. 7.163).[253]

Arthrography

If the history and clinical assessment suggest a ligament or fibrocartilage problem of the wrist, arthrography can help to confirm the diagnosis (Fig. 7.164). Arthrograms, especially of the wrist, can demonstrate compartment communication, tendon sheaths, synovial irregularity, loose bodies, and cartilage abnormalities.

Diagnostic Ultrasound Imaging

Anterior/Volar Wrist. One of the main areas to view on the anterior (volar) wrist is the carpal tunnel. Bony landmarks play a key in finding this location. In the proximal portion of the carpal tunnel, the scaphoid and the pisiform

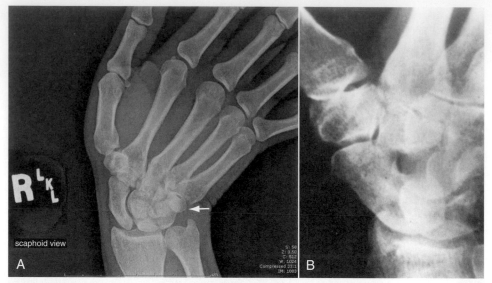

Fig. 7.155 Radiographs of the normal scaphoid. (A) Scaphoid view. Note the ulnar styloid and the location of the ulnar snuff box *(arrow)*. (B) Lateral view. (B, From Tubiana R: *The hand*, Philadelphia, 1981, WB Saunders, p 659.)

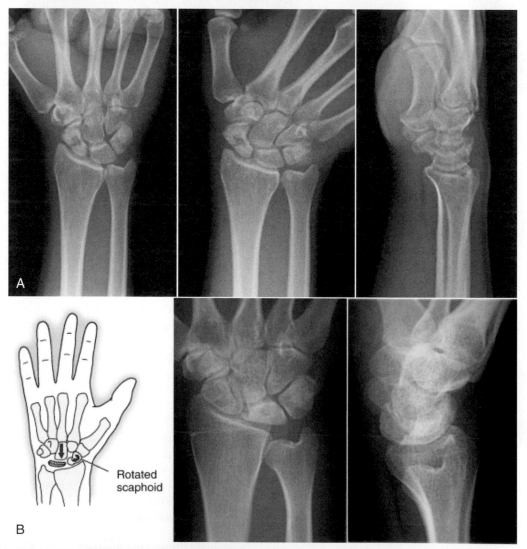

Fig. 7.156 (A) Preoperative radiographs demonstrate a scaphoid waist nonunion with proximal pole sclerosis consistent with avascular necrosis. Distal fragment cystic changes and a humpback deformity are evident. The radiolunate angle remains normal, and arthritic changes are absent. *A-left,* Neutral position. *A-middle,* Ulnar deviation. *A-right,* Lateral view. (A, From Kazmers NH, Thibaudeau S, Levin LS: A scapholunate ligament–sparing technique utilizing the medial femoral condyle corticocancellous free flap to reconstruct scaphoid nonunions with proximal pole avascular necrosis, *J Hand Surg Am* 41(9):e309-e315, 2016.) (B) In stage IIIB Kienböck disease, there is collapse of the lunate and rotation of the scaphoid, creating a dorsal intercalated segment instability pattern. This is often combined with proximal capitate migration. Posteroanterior and lateral radiographs demonstrate collapse of the lunate, flexion of the scaphoid, and proximal migration of the capitate. *B-left,* Diagrammatic view. *B-middle,* Neutral position. *B-right,* Lateral view. (B, From Lauder AJ, Waitayawinyu T: Carpal avascular necrosis: Kienböck disease and Preiser disease. In Trumble TE, Rayan GM, Budoff JE et al, eds: *Principles of hand surgery and therapy,* ed 3, Philadelphia, 2017, Elsevier, pp 490-508.)

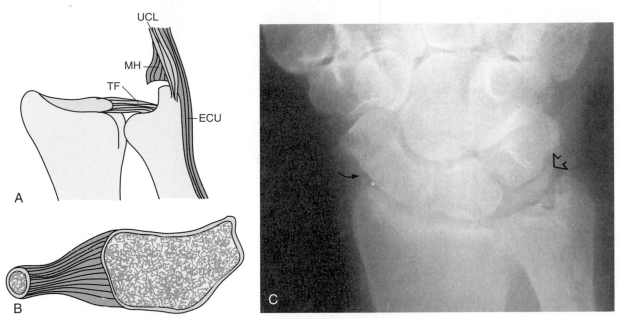

Fig. 7.157 Triangular fibrocartilage complex (TFCC). (A) This complex includes the triangular fibrocartilage *(articular disc, TF)*, the meniscus homolog *(MH)*, the ulnar collateral ligament *(UCL)*, and the dorsal and volar radioulnar ligaments (not shown). The extensor carpi ulnaris tendon *(ECU)* is shown. (B) The triangular fibrocartilage *(dotted area)* attaches to the ulnar border of the radius and the distal ulna. The triangular shape is evident on this transverse section through the radius and ulnar styloid. The volar aspect of the wrist is at the top. (C) Chondrocalcinosis. There is heavy calcification of the articular cartilage *(curved arrow)* and the area of the TFCC *(open arrow)*. (From Weissman BNW, Sledge CB: *Orthopedic radiology*, Philadelphia, 1986, WB Saunders, p 115.)

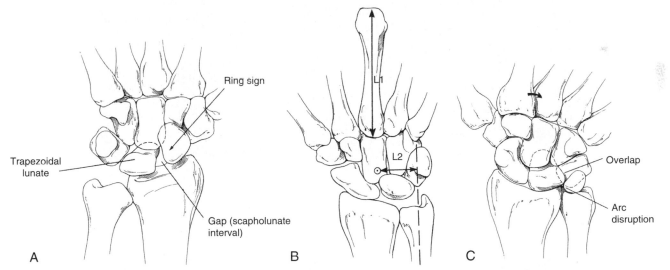

Fig. 7.158 (A) Scapholunate dissociation. The scaphoid is palmar flexed, producing a cortical ring sign. A gap is present between the scaphoid and the lunate. The lunate appears trapezoidal. (B) Ulnar translocation can be identified radiographically from the ratio of the distance between the center of the capitate and a line along the longitudinal axis of the ulna *(L2)* divided by the length of the third metacarpal *(L1)*. In normal wrists, this ratio is 0.30 ± 0.03; it is decreased in wrists with ulnar translocation. (C) Lunatotriquetral instability. Shortened scaphoid and cortical ring sign are present without scapholunate widening. Lunate appears triangular. Lunatotriquetral widening is not present. (© 1993 American Academy of Orthopaedic Surgeons. Reprinted from the Journal of the American Academy of Orthopaedic Surgeons: A Comprehensive Review, 1[1], pp 14–15, with permission.)

bone on the medial and lateral wrist, respectively, are key landmarks to find. To begin, the transducer should be placed along the proximal carpal tunnel in the short axis (Fig. 7.165). The median nerve described below, as well as the flexor carpi radialis, the flexor digitorum superficialis, and the tendons of the flexor digitorum profundus, can be viewed. In Fig. 7.166, one can see the radius and

ulna as well as the median nerve *(arrowheads)*, flexor carpi radialis *(F)*, palmaris longus *(P)*, and the radial artery *(r)*. Once each of these structures are found, dynamic evaluation can be performed by having the patient flex and extend each finger.

The next structure that can be viewed on the anterior portion of the wrist is the median nerve. To begin, the

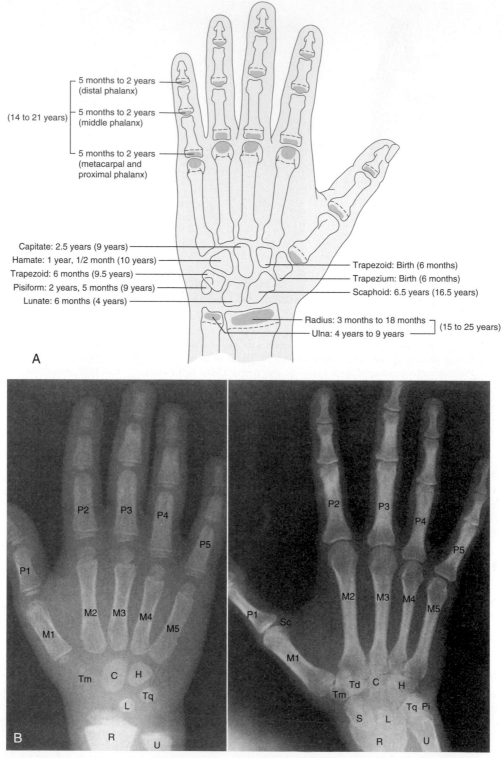

Fig. 7.159 Ossification centers of the hand. (A) Dates of appearance of ossification centers are shown with dates of fusion in parentheses. Note the different proximal and distal locations of growth plates. (B) Radiographs of the hand and wrist of a 4- to 5-year-old boy or 3- to 4-year-old girl *(left)* and of an adult *(right)*. *C,* Capitate; *H,* hamate; *L,* lunate; *M,* metacarpal; *P,* phalanx; *Pi,* pisiform; *R,* radius; *S,* scaphoid; *Td,* trapezoid; *Tm,* trapezium; *Tq,* triquetrum; *U,* ulna. (A, Redrawn from Tubiana R: *The hand*, Philadelphia, 1981, WB Saunders, p 11. B, From Liebgott B: *The anatomical basis of dentistry*, St Louis, 1986, CV Mosby.)

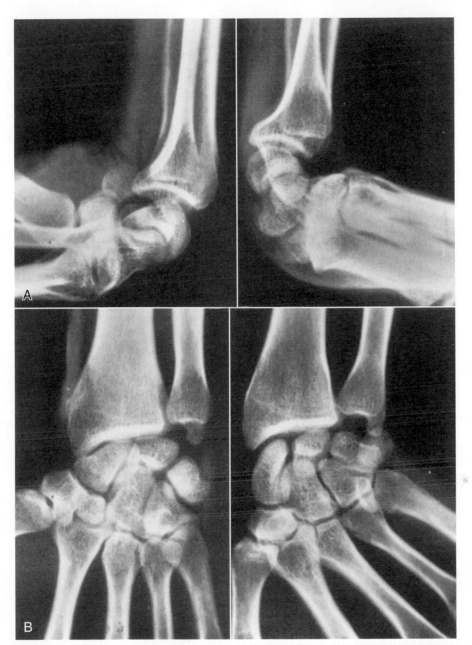

Fig. 7.160 (A) Lateral radiographs showing wrist flexion *(left)* and extension *(right)*. (B) Posteroanterior views of wrist in radial *(left)* and ulnar *(right)* deviation. Note the change in the form of the lunate, indicating a slipping toward the front in the radial slant and toward the rear in the ulnar slant. (From Tubiana R: *The hand*, Philadelphia, 1981, WB Saunders, p 655.)

transducer is placed in the short transverse axis along the anterior wrist along the wrist crease. As before, nerves viewed in the short axis will appear as "honeycomb" hypoechoic fascicles surrounded by hyperechoic epineurium connective tissue (see Fig. 7.166). The median nerve at this site will be surrounded by hyperechoic tendon structures of the forearm and finger flexors that run with the nerve under the carpal tunnel. The shape of the median nerve changes as it runs distally. It appears oval in the initial segment and becomes flatter shaped at the level of the hook of the hamate.[254] From this point, the nerve can be followed slightly further distally into the carpal tunnel where the thin flexor retinaculum will be

seen superior to the nerves and tendons. If continuing just a little bit further, the palmar cutaneous branch of the median nerve may be picked up superficial to the flexor retinaculum. This branch off of the median nerve occurs proximal to the retinaculum and courses superficially to the flexor carpi radialis tendon above the retinaculum.

The transducer can be turned 90° to view the nerve in long axis (Fig. 7.167). The nerve is much easier seen in this view as its echogenicity is clearly different from other surrounding structures. Nerve fascicles can clearly be seen as the nerve runs distally along the forearm (Fig. 7.168). A nerve compression can be seen by enlargement of the nerve diameter at the compression site and

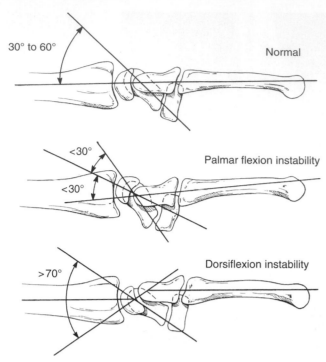

Fig. 7.161 Scapholunate angle measurement in normal wrist and in carpal instability. (© 1993 American Academy of Orthopaedic Surgeons. Reprinted from the Journal of the American Academy of Orthopaedic Surgeons: A Comprehensive Review, 1[1], p 14, with permission.)

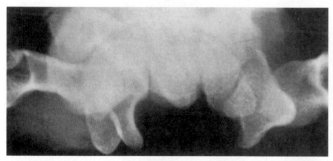

Fig. 7.162 Carpal tunnel or axial radiographic view. (From Tubiana R: *The hand*, Philadelphia, 1981, WB Saunders, p 662.)

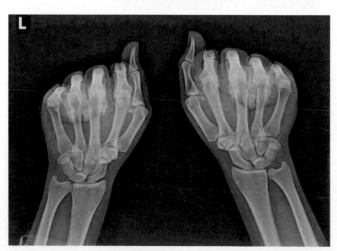

Fig. 7.163 Clenched-fist view.

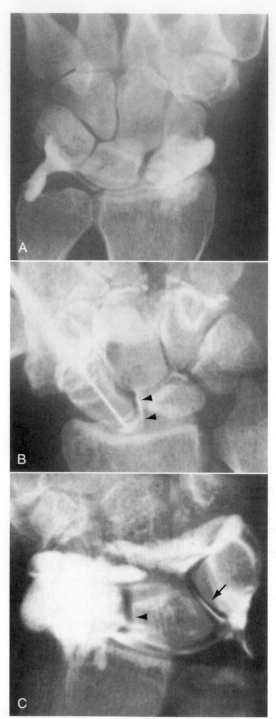

Fig. 7.164 (A) Posteroanterior view of the wrist after a normal radiocarpal joint arthrogram. Contrast remains confined to the radiocarpal space. (B) After a radiocarpal joint space injection, contrast tracks *(arrowheads)* through a disrupted scapholunate ligament to fill the midcarpal and carpometacarpal joint spaces. (C) After a radiocarpal joint space arthrogram, the scapholunate ligament is intact because contrast has not yet filled the scapholunate space *(arrowhead);* however, contrast tracks through the lunotriquetral joint space *(arrow)* as a result of lunotriquetral ligament disruption. (From Lightman DM: *The wrist and its disorders*, Philadelphia, 1988, WB Saunders, p 89.)

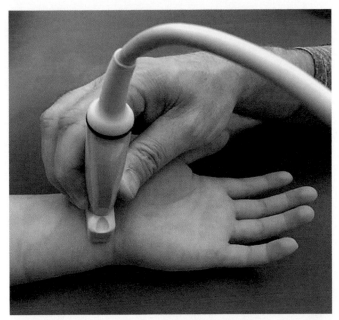

Fig. 7.165 Transverse view of carpal tunnel at the anterior wrist joint.

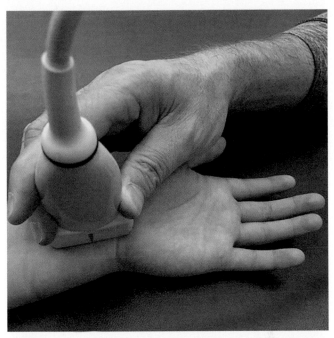

Fig. 7.167 Longitudinal view of carpal tunnel at the anterior wrist joint.

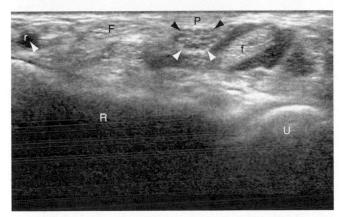

Fig. 7.166 Transverse view of carpal tunnel demonstrating radius *(R)*, ulna *(U)*, median nerve *(arrowheads)*, flexor carpi radialis *(F)*, palmaris longus *(P)*, and the radial artery *(r)*. (From Jacobson JA: *Fundamentals of musculoskeletal ultrasound*, ed 2, Philadelphia, 2013, Elsevier, p 117.)

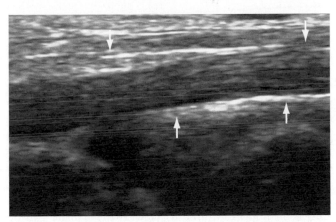

Fig. 7.168 Longitudinal view of carpal tunnel demonstrating the median nerve running proximal to distal. In this view the median nerve appears hyperechoic through its length in the field of view *(arrows)*.

proximally with echotexture changes.[255] A normal median nerve on ultrasonography has been shown to have average cross-sectional area at the wrist of 9 mm², however, this has been shown to increase to 14 mm² in those with carpal tunnel syndrome. Higher measurements are associated with abnormal nerve conduction velocity studies.[256] As the size of the nerve varies, one should carefully note at what level the measurements are taken as they can differ from proximal to distal locations. To ensure reliability, the measurement should be taken at the level of the distal radius or pisiform.[257,258]

The flexor tendons can be viewed beginning at the wrist crease and then followed either proximally or distally. The superficialis and profundus muscles are surrounding the median nerve at the wrist crease. The flexor digitorum tendons will travel under the carpal tunnel and are enveloped by a synovial sheath that are sonographically depicted as thin echogenic fluid-filled structures. However, the palmaris longus runs superficial to the carpal tunnel near midline of the wrist and the flexor carpi ulnaris runs superficial and on the ulnar side of the wrist.

Specifically, along the radial side of the anterior wrist the scaphoid, flexor carpi radialis tendon, and radial artery can be viewed. With the transducer in the long axis just lateral to the median nerve (Fig. 7.169), the flexor carpi radialis can be seen attaching to the second and third metacarpal. In this plane, the tendon will be hypoechoic and in a fibular pattern. In this same plane, the distal radius and scaphoid will be seen as hyperechoic bone contours (Fig. 7.170). If the scaphoid can be seen clearly, an irregularity of the bony surface may be indicative of

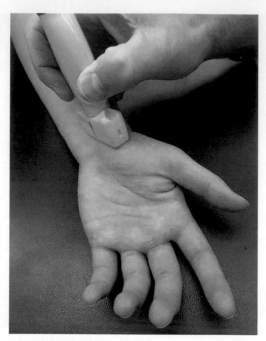

Fig. 7.169 Longitudinal view of the radial side of the anterior surface of the wrist.

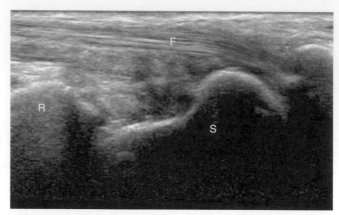

Fig. 7.170 Longitudinal view over the radial side of wrist and base of thumb showing flexor carpi radialis tendon *(F)*, scaphoid *(S)*, and radius *(R)*. (From Jacobson JA: *Fundamentals of musculoskeletal ultrasound*, ed 2, Philadelphia, 2013, Elsevier, p 119.)

a scaphoid fracture. Turning the transducer 90° to the short axis, the radial artery and vein can be seen just radial to the flexor carpi radialis.

Lastly, the ulnar aspect of the anterior wrist can view ulnar nerve, artery, and vein. While in short axis, the transducer is moved in the ulnar direction until the pisiform bone can be seen. The ulnar nerve will be seen between the pisiform and the ulnar artery. Like the median nerve described earlier, it will be a bunch of hypoechoic nerve fascicules surrounded by hyperechoic connective tissue. Moving distally, the hook of the hamate may be seen. This is an important area to view as the hamate can be fractured during falls, golfing, or batting. These injuries can cause compression to nerves and arteries around the hamate. In the short axis, the branches of the ulnar nerve course around the hamate (deep motor on ulnar side, and sensory branch superficial to hamate). Evaluation of the ulnar nerve can be completed in the long axis view of the anterior side of the wrist (Fig. 7.171). In this view, the hook of hamate and ulnar can never be seen simultaneously (Fig. 7.172).

Posterior/Dorsal Wrist. There are numerous structures that can be viewed along the dorsal wrist. To begin, the dorsal wrist tendons, including the long extensor and abductor tendons in the dorsal compartments, can be seen (Fig. 7.173). The initial landmark to find on the dorsal wrist is Lister tubercle. It will be seen near the midline as a hyperechoic bony structure. With the transducer in the short axis, move ulnarly to the tubercle to find the extensor pollicus longus, the extensor indicis, and multiple tendons of the extensor digitorum, and finally the extensor digiti minimi (Fig. 7.174). The final tendon that will be seen in

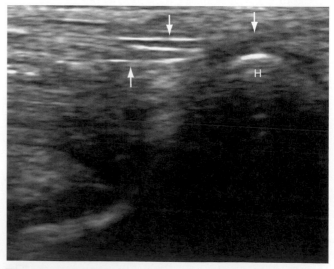

Fig. 7.171 Longitudinal view of ulnar side of wrist over hook of hamate.

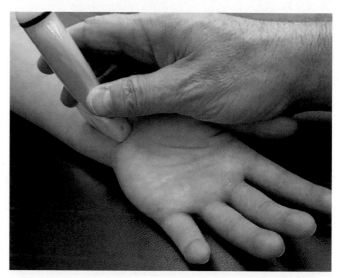

Fig. 7.172 Longitudinal view of ulnar side of wrist demonstrating the hook of hamate *(H)* and the ulnar nerve *(arrows)*.

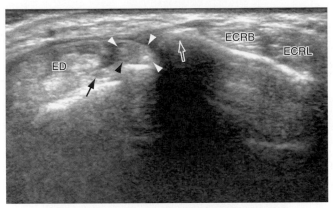

Fig. 7.174 Transverse view of dorsal proximal wrist demonstrating Lister tubercle *(arrow)*, extensor digitorum *(ED)*, extensor carpi radialis brevis *(ECRB)*, and extensor carpi radialis longus *(ECRL)*. (From Jacobson JA: *Fundamentals of musculoskeletal ultrasound*, ed 2, Philadelphia, 2013, Elsevier, p 122.)

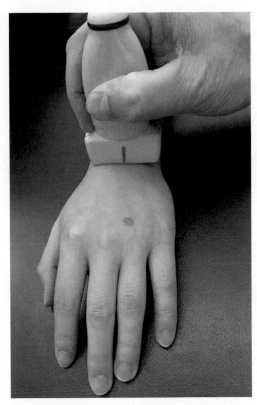

Fig. 7.173 Transverse view of dorsal proximal wrist.

the ulnar direction is the extensor carpi ulnaris. Moving radially will bring into view the extensor carpi radialis brevis and then longus (see Fig. 7.174). Turning the transducer to the long axis, these tendons can all be seen as they travel proximally into the forearm. Tendons can be evaluated dynamically to improve visualization of tendon end retraction as well as tendon subluxation or dislocation.[259,260]

Tendinosis can be seen as variable areas of decreased echogenicity and thickening of the tendon with sheath effusion. Frank tears are identified by seeing complete or partial discontinuity in the tendon fibers often with fluid interposed.[260]

The TFCC is found on the ulnar side of the dorsal wrist situated between the carpals and the ulna.

Ulnar Side. A common injury to the thumb is injury to the UCL of the metacarpophalangeal joint commonly known as **gamekeeper's or skier's thumb**. This injury is caused by a forceful hyperabduction of the thumb, which commonly occurs during contact sports or from a ski pole (see Fig. 7.11). The ligament that is injured will appear hyperechoic and swollen. The smaller "hockey stick" transducer (Fig. 7.175) will be used and placed in long axis along the ulnar side of the first metacarpophalangeal

joint. A **Stener lesion** occurs when a full-thickness tear occurs and the torn end is retracted and displaced under the adductor aponeurosis. The Stener lesion has been described as a "yo-yo on a string" appearance with the string representing the adductor aponeurosis and the yo-yo representing the balled up and proximally retracted UCL.[261,262] Dynamic evaluation of the thumb UCL in the long axis provides visualization of the ligament and adductor aponeurosis.[263,264]

Radial Side. Radial side ligament injuries are much less common than the ulnar side. However, due to the force required to injure the thumb radial collateral ligament, lesions on this side of the hand result in joint instability and progressive instability. The appearance on ultrasound is very similar to UCLs.[265]

Computed Tomography
Computed tomography can be used to visualize bones and soft tissue; by making computer-assisted "slices," it allows tissues to be better visualized (Fig. 7.176).

Magnetic Resonance Imaging
Magnetic resonance imaging is a noninvasive technique that is useful for visualizing the soft tissues of the wrist and hand and provides the best means of delineating the soft tissues (primarily ligaments and the TFCC), as well as showing instability problems and bone.[266–270] For example, it can show swelling of the median nerve in carpal tunnel syndrome, tears in the triangular fibrocartilage (Fig. 7.177), and thickening of tendon sheaths (Fig. 7.178).

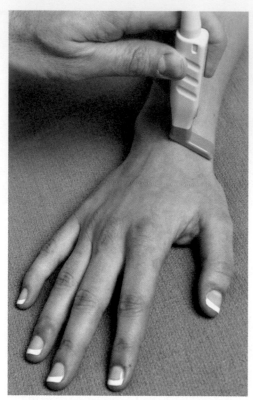

Fig. 7.175 "Hockey stick" transducer. (From Jacobson JA: *Fundamentals of musculoskeletal ultrasound*, ed 3, Philadelphia, 2018, Elsevier.)

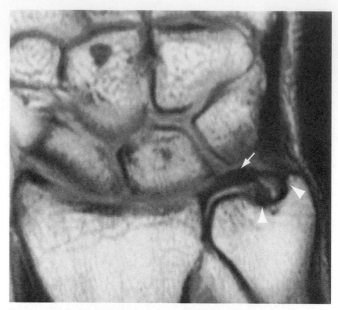

Fig. 7.177 Triangular fibrocartilage complex: Normal appearance. On a coronal intermediate-weighted (TR/TE, 2000/20) spin echo magnetic resonance image, observe the low-signal intensity of the triangular fibrocartilage *(arrow)* with bifurcated bands of low-signal intensity *(arrowheads)* attaching to or near the styloid process of the ulna. The scapholunate and lunotriquetral interosseous ligaments are not well seen on this image. Note the two bone islands, which appear as foci of low-signal intensity, in the lunate and capitate. (From Resnick D, Kransdorf MJ: *Bone and joint imaging*, Philadelphia, 2005, WB Saunders, p 907. Courtesy AG Bergman, MD, Stanford, CA.)

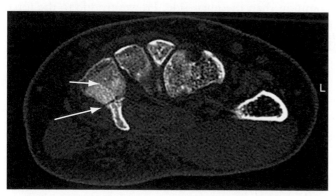

Fig. 7.176 Hook of hamate fracture shown *(large white arrow)* and a nutrient vessel is seen in the body of hamate *(small white arrow)* on an axial computed tomography image. (From Sahu A, Pang CL, Lynch J, Suresh P: A review of radiological imaging in the hand and wrist, *Orthop Trauma* 28[3]:177, 2014.)

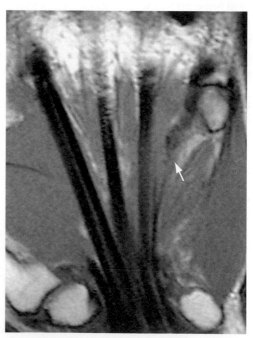

Fig. 7.178 Tendon rupture. Coronal T1-weighted (TR/TE, 500/14) spin echo from magnetic resonance image of the hand shows rupture of the flexor tendon of the little finger. The free edge of the thickened, retracted, ruptured tendon *(arrow)* is well seen. (From Resnick D, Kransdor MJ: *Bone and joint imaging*, Philadelphia, 2005, WB Saunders, p 913.)

PRÉCIS OF THE FOREARM, WRIST, AND HAND ASSESSMENT[a]

NOTE Suspected pathology will determine which *Special Tests* are to be performed.

History (sitting)
Observation (sitting)
Examination (sitting)
Active movements
  Pronation of the forearm
  Supination of the forearm
  Wrist flexion
  Wrist extension
  Radial deviation of wrist
  Ulnar deviation of wrist
  Finger flexion (at MCP, PIP, and DIP joints)
  Flexion extension (at MCP, PIP, and DIP joints)
  Finger abduction
  Finger adduction
  Thumb flexion
  Thumb extension
  Thumb abduction
  Thumb adduction
  Opposition of the thumb and little finger
Passive movements (as in active movements)
Resisted isometric movements (as in active movements, in the neutral position)
Functional testing
  Functional grip tests
  Pinch tests
  Coordination tests
Special tests (sitting)
  General tests for wrist pain:
    Sitting hands (press) test
  For bone, ligament, capsule, and joint instability:
    Derby relocation test
    Distal radioulnar joint stability (ballottement) test
    Kleinman's shear test
    Ligamentous instability test (fingers)
    Lunotriquetral ballottement (Reagan's) test
    Lunotriquetral compression test
    Murphy's sign
    Pisiform boost test
    Pisotriquetral grind test
    Radioulnar shift test
    Scaphoid compression test
    Scapulolunate ligament test
    Thumb ulnar collateral ligament laxity or instability test
    Ulnar fovea sign (ulnar snuff box) test
    Ulnar styloid triquetral impaction (USTI) provocation test
    Ulnocarpal stress test
    Ulnomeniscotriquetral dorsal glide test
    Watson (scaphoid shift) test

For tendons and muscles:
  Extensor carpi ulnaris synergy test
  Finkelstein (Eichhoff) test
  Sweater finger sign
  Wrist hyperflexion and abduction of thumb (WHAT) test
For neurological dysfunction:
  Abductor pollicis brevis weakness
  Carpal compression test
  Crossed finger test
  Finger flexion sign
  First dorsal interossei screening test
  Flick maneuver
  Froment's paper sign
  Hand elevation test
  Okutsu test
  Phalen's (wrist flexion) test
  Pollock sign
  Reverse Phalen's (prayer) test
  Scratch collapse test
  Tethered median nerve stress test
  Tinel sign at wrist
  Weber's (Moberg's) two-point discrimination test
  Wrinkle (shrivel) test
For circulation and swelling:
  Allen test
  Digital blood flow
  Figure of eight measurement for swelling
  Hand volume test
Reflexes and cutaneous distribution (sitting)
  Reflexes
  Sensory scan
  Nerve injuries
  Median nerve
  Ulnar nerve
  Radial nerve
Joint play movements (sitting)
  Long-axis extension at the wrist and fingers (MCP, PIP, and DIP joints)
  Anteroposterior glide at the wrist and fingers (MCP, PIP, and DIP joints)
  Side glide at the wrist and fingers (MCP, PIP, and DIP joints)
  Side tilt at the wrist
  Anteroposterior glide at the intermetacarpal joints
  Rotation at the MCP, PIP, and DIP joints
  Individual carpal bone mobility
Palpation (sitting)
Diagnostic imaging

[a]After any examination, the patient should be warned of the possibility of exacerbation of symptoms as a result of the assessment.
DIP, Distal interphalangeal; *MCP,* metacarpophalangeal; *PIP,* proximal interphalangeal.

CASE STUDIES

When doing these case studies, the examiner should list the appropriate questions to be asked and why they are being asked, what to look for and why, and what things should be tested and why. Depending on the answers of the patient (and the examiner should consider different responses), several possible causes of the patient's problem may become evident (examples are given in parentheses). A differential diagnosis chart should be made up. The examiner can then decide how different diagnoses may affect the treatment plan. For example, a 26-year-old man comes to you complaining of pain and clicking in his wrist. He is a carpenter, and it especially bothers him when he uses a screwdriver. See Table 7.15 for an example of a differential diagnosis chart for this patient.

1. A 22-year-old female comes to see you for stiffness in her wrist. She had arthroscopic debridement of a cyst in her radial side carpals four months ago. She was sent to occupational therapy at that time for about a month for rehabilitation at which time she regained some of her motion into wrist flexion, ulnar and radial deviation but consistently had difficulties with wrist extension. She now has good strength in all planes, but continues to feel tightness and stiffness when moving into wrist extension. Describe your assessment of this to determine if it is caused by contractile or inert tissues. Describe possible causes for this stiffness and your differential diagnosis for her issues.

2. A 31-year-old pregnant woman complains of pain in the right hand with a duration of 3 months. The pain awakens her at night and is relieved only by vigorous rubbing of her hand and motion of the fingers and wrist. There is some tingling in the index and middle fingers. Describe your assessment for this patient (carpal tunnel syndrome vs. lunate subluxation).

3. An 18-year-old man comes to you after suffering a right scaphoid fracture. He has been in a cast for 12 weeks, and clinical union has been achieved. Describe your assessment for this patient.

4. A 16-year-old girl comes to you complaining of thumb pain. She was skiing during the weekend and fell, landing on her ski pole. She hurt her thumb when she fell. Describe your assessment for this patient (ulnar collateral ligament sprain vs. Bennett fracture).

5. A 48-year-old man comes to you complaining of a painful hand. He happened to hit it against a metal door jamb as he was going outside. During the next few days, the hand became swollen and painful, and he has become very protective of it. Describe your assessment of this patient (Sudeck atrophy vs. hand aneurysm).

6. A 52-year-old woman who has rheumatoid arthritis comes to you because her hands hurt and she has difficulty doing things functionally. Describe your assessment of this patient.

7. A 14-year-old boy comes to you complaining of wrist pain with swelling on the dorsum of the hand. He says he tripped and fell on the outstretched hand. He states the wrist hurt, the pain decreased, and then the swelling came on over 2 or 3 days. Describe your assessment of this patient (scaphoid fracture vs. ganglion).

8. A 28-year-old man was in an industrial accident and lacerated the flexor tendons in the palm of his hand. Describe your assessment of this patient.

9. A 37-year-old woman comes to you complaining of pain and grating on the radial side of the wrist. Describe your assessment of this patient (cartilaginous disc vs. scaphoid fracture).

10. A 72-year-old woman comes to you with a left Colles fracture. Describe your assessment of this patient.

TABLE **7.15**

Differential Diagnosis of Wrist Cartilaginous Disc and Degenerative Osteoarthritis

	Wrist Cartilaginous Disc	Degenerative Osteoarthritis
Mechanism of injury	Compression and pronation	Vibration, repetitive compression
Age affected	25 years and older	35 years and older
Active movement	Pain on compression and pronation Limited wrist extension more than flexion	Limited wrist flexion and extension
Passive movement	Pain on extension overpressure Pain on compression and pronation Tissue stretch end feel	Capsular pattern of wrist End feel is soft early, hard later
Resisted isometric movement	Pain on pronation	Possibly weak on wrist movements
Special tests	None	None
Reflexes and sensory distribution	Normal	Normal
Joint play	Pain on anteroposterior glide of radiocarpal joint	Pain on anteroposterior glide of radiocarpal and midcarpal joints
Palpation	Pain over lunate	Pain over affected carpal bones

References

1. Chidgey JK. The distal radioulnar joint: problems and solutions. *J Am Acad Orthop Surg*. 1995;3:95–109.
2. Berger RA. The anatomy and basic biomechanics of the wrist joint. *J Hand Surg*. 1996;9:84–93.
3. Tubiana R, Thomiene JM, Mackin E. *Examination of the Hand and Wrist*. St Louis: CV Mosby; 1996.
4. Eathorne SW. The wrist: clinical anatomy and physical examination – an update. *Prim Care*. 2005;32(1):17–33.
5. Porretto-Loehrke A, Schuh C, Szekeres M. Clinical manual assessment of the wrist. *J Hand Ther*. 2016;29(2):123–135.
6. Sachar K. Ulnar-sided wrist pain: evaluation and treatment of triangular fibrocartilage complex tears, ulnocarpal impaction syndrome, and lunotriquetral ligament tears. *J Hand Surg Am*. 2008;33(9):1669–1679.
7. Cody ME, Nakamura DT, Small KM, Yoshioka H. MR imaging of the triangular fibrocartilage complex. *Magn Reson Imaging Clin North Am*. 2015;23(3):393–403.
8. Alsousou J, Bhalaik V. Anatomy and approaches of the wrist. *Orthop Trauma*. 2017;31(4):229–236.
9. Henderson CJ, Kobayashi KM. Ulnar-sided wrist pain in the athlete. *Ortho Clin North Am*. 2016;47(4):789–798.
10. Heire P, Temperley D, Murali R. Radiological imaging of the wrist joint. *Orthop Trauma*. 2017;31(4):248–256.
11. Halikis MN, Taleisnik J. Soft-tissue injuries of the wrist. *Clin Sports Med*. 1996;15:235–259.
12. Gan BS, Richards RS, Roth JH. Arthroscopic treatment of triangular fibrocartilage tears. *Orthop Clin North Am*. 1995;26:721–729.
13. Palmer AD, Werner FW. The triangular fibrocartilage complex of the wrist: anatomy and function. *J Hand Surg Am*. 1981;6:153–162.
14. Palmer AK, Werner FW. Biomechanics of the distal radioulnar joint. *Clin Orthop*. 1984;187:26–35.
15. Berger RA. The anatomy of the ligaments of the wrist and distal radioulnar joints. *Clin Orthop Relat Res*. 2001;383:32–40.
16. Rettig AC. Athletic injuries of the wrist and hand. Part I: traumatic injuries of the wrist. *Am J Sports Med*. 2003;31:1038–1048.
17. Steinberg BD, Plancher KD. Clinical anatomy of the wrist and elbow. *Clin Sports Med*. 1995;14:299–313.
18. Shin AY, Battaglia MJ. Bishop AT: Lunotriquetral instability: diagnosis and treatment. *J Am Acad Orthop Surg*. 2000;8:170–179.
19. Taleisnik J. Carpal instability. *J Bone Joint Surg Am*. 1988;70:1262–1268.
20. Mayfield JK, Johnson RP, Kilcoyne RK. Carpal dislocations: pathomechanics and progressive perilunar instability. *J Hand Surg Am*. 1980;5:226–241.
21. Sen S, Talwalkar S. Acute and chronic scapholunate ligament instability. *Orthop Trauma*. 2017;31(4):266–273.
22. Odak S, Murali SR. Luno-triquetral dissociation – a review of the current literature. *Orthop Trauma*. 2017;31(4):279–281.
23. Kozin SH. Perilunate injuries: diagnosis and treatment. *J Am Acad Orthop Surg*. 1998;6:112–120.
24. Carlsen BT, Shin AY. Wrist instability. *Scand J Surg*. 2008;97(4):324–332.
25. Neumann DA. *Kinesiology of the Musculoskeletal System*. ed 2. St Louis: CV Mosby; 2010.
26. Sarrafian SK, Melamed JL, Goshgarian GM. Study of wrist motion in flexion and extension. *Clin Orthop*. 1977;126:153–159.
27. Lapegue F, Andre A, Brun C, et al. Traumatic flexor tendon injuries. *Diagn Interv Imaging*. 2015;96:1279–1292.
28. Kapandji IA. *The Physiology of Joints*. vol. 1. New York: Churchill Livingstone; 1970.
29. Sauve PS, Rhee PC, Shin AY, Lindau T. Examination of the wrist: radial–sided wrist pain. *J Hand Surg Am*. 2014;39(10):2089–2092.
30. Rhee PC, Sauve PS, Lindau T, Shin AY. Examination of the wrist: ulnar-sided wrist pain due to ligamentous injury. *J Hand Surg Am*. 2014;39(9):1859–1862.
31. Newton AW, Hawkes DH, Bhalaik V. Clinical examination of the wrist. *Orthop Trauma*. 2017;31(4):237–247.
32. Nagle DJ. Evaluation of chronic wrist pain. *J Am Acad Orthop Surg*. 2000;8:45–55.
33. Rettig AC. Wrist injuries: avoiding diagnostic pitfalls. *Phys Sportsmed*. 1994;22:33–39.
34. Skirven TM, Osterman AL, Fedorczyk J, Amadio PC. *Rehabilitation of the Hand and Upper Extremity*. ed 6. St Louis: Elsevier; 2011.
35. Kleinman WB. Physical examination of the wrist: useful provocative maneuvers. *J Hand Surg Am*. 2015;40(7):1486–1500.
36. Tsiouri C, Hayton MJ, Baratz M. Injury to the ulnar collateral ligament of the thumb. *Hand*. 2009;4(1):12–18.
37. Neuman DA, Bielefeld T. The carpometacarpal joint of the thumb: stability, deformity and therapeutic intervention. *J Orthop Sports Phys Ther*. 2003;33(7):386–399.
38. Gomez CL, Gondolbeau AM, Marti RM, et al. The role of the carpometacarpal ligaments of the thumb in stability and the development of osteoarthritis lesions: an anatomical study. *Acta Orthop Belg*. 2015;83:449–457.
39. Hinke DH, Erickson SJ, Chamoy L, Timins ME. Ulnar collateral ligament of the thumb: MR findings in cadavers, volunteers, and patients with ligamentous injury (gamekeeper's thumb). *AJR Am J Roentgenol*. 1994;163(6):1431–1434.
40. Burton RI, Eaton RG. Common hand injuries in the athlete. *Orthop Clin North Am*. 1975;4:309–338.
41. Gonzalez-Iglesias J, Huijbregts P, Fernandez-de-las-Panas C, et al. Differential diagnosis and physical therapy management of a patient with radial wrist pain of 6 months duration: a case report. *J Orthop Sports Phys Ther*. 2010;40:361–368.
42. Keith MW, Masear V, Chung K, et al. Diagnosis of carpal tunnel syndrome. *J Am Acad Orthop Surg*. 2009;17:389–396.
43. D'Arcy CA, McGee S. Does this patient have carpal tunnel syndrome? *JAMA*. 2000;283(23):3110–3117.
44. Rowell RM. Your patient has wrist/hand pain and paresthesia – does she have carpal tunnel syndrome? *J Am Chiropractic Assoc*. 2013:7–11.
45. Calfee RP, Dale AM, Ryan D, et al. Performance of simplified scoring systems for hand diagrams in carpal tunnel syndrome screening. *J Hand Surg Am*. 2012;37(1):10–17.
46. Bonauto DK, Silverstein BA, Fan ZJ, et al. Evaluation of a symptom diagram for identifying carpal tunnel syndrome. *Occup Med*. 2008;58(8):561–566.
47. Katz JN, Stirrat CR. A self-administered hand diagram for the diagnosis of carpal tunnel syndrome. *J Hand Surg Am*. 1990;15(2):360–363.
48. Thornburg LE. Ganglions of the hand and wrist. *J Am Acad Orthop Surg*. 1999;7:231–238.
49. Birklein F, O'Neill D, Schlereth T. Complex regional pain syndrome: an optimistic perspective. *Neurology*. 2015;84(1):89–96.
50. Maihöfner C, Seifert F, Markovic K. Complex regional pain syndromes: new pathophysiological concepts and therapies. *Eur J Neurol*. 2010;17(5):649–660.
51. GalveVilla M, Rittig-Rasmussen B, Moeller Schear Mikklesen L, Groendahl Poulsen A. Complex regional pain syndrome. *Man Ther*. 2016;26:223–230.
52. Marinus J, Moseley GL, Birklein F, et al. Clinical features and pathophysiology of complex regional pain syndrome. *Lancet Neurol*. 2011;10(7):637–648.
53. Birklein F. Complex regional pain syndrome. *J Neurol*. 2005;252(2):131–138.
54. Harden RN, Bruehl S, Perez RS, et al. Validation of proposed diagnostic criteria (the "Budapest Criteria") for complex regional pain syndrome. *Pain*. 2010;150(2):268–274.
55. Birklein F, Dimova V. Complex regional pain syndrome - up-to-date. *PAIN Reports*. 2017;2(6):3624.
56. Harden RN, Bruehl S, Stanton-Hicks M, Wilson PR. Proposed new diagnostic criteria for complex regional pain syndrome. *Pain Med*. 2007;8(4):326–331.
57. Bruehl S, Harden RN, Galer BS, et al. External validation of IASP diagnostic criteria for complex regional pain syndrome and proposed research diagnostic criteria. International Association for the Study of Pain. *Pain*. 1999;81(1-2):147–154.
58. Reddy RS, Compson J. Examination of the wrist – soft tissue, joints and special tests. *Curr Orthop*. 2005;19:180–189.
59. Poh F. Carpal boss in chronic wrist pain and its association with partial osseous coalition and osteoarthritis – a case report with focus on MRI findings. *Indian J Radiol Imaging*. 2015;25(3):276–279.
60. Vieweg H, Radmer S, Fensow R, Tabibzada AM. Diagnosis and treatment of symptomatic carpal bossing. *J Clin Diagn Res*. 2015;9(10):RC01–RC03.
61. Altman R, Alarcon G, Appelrouth D, et al. The American College of Rheumatology criteria for the classification and reporting of osteoarthritis of the hand. *Arthritis Rheum*. 1990;33(11):1601–1610.
62. Dincer F, Sumat G. *Physical Examination of the Hand*. In Duruöz MT, ed. *Hand Function: A Practical Guide To Assessment*. New York: Springer Science; 2014.
63. Palmer BA, Hughes TB. Cubital tunnel syndrome. *J Hand Surg Am*. 2010;35(1):153–163.
64. Goldman SB, Brininger TL, Schrader JS, Koceja DM. A review of clinical tests and signs for the assessment of ulnar neuropathy. *J Hand Ther*. 2009;22(3):209–220.
65. Black EM, Blazar PE. Dupuytren disease: an evolving understanding of an age-old disease. *J Am Acad Orthop Surg*. 2011;19:746–757.
66. Schmid AB, Nee RJ, Coppieters MW. Reappraising entrapment neuropathies - mechanisms, diagnosis and management. *Man Ther*. 2013;18(6):449–457.
67. Bendre AA, Hartigan BJ, Kalainov DM. Mallet finger. *J Am Acad Ortho Surg*. 2005;13:336–344.
68. Ono K, Ebara S, Fuji T, et al. Myelopathy hand-new clinical signs of cervical cord damage. *J Bone Joint Surg Br*. 1987;69:215–219.
69. Brown JA, Lichtman DM. Midcarpal instability. *Hand Clin*. 1987;3:135–140.
70. Young D, Papp S, Giachino A. Physical examination of the wrist. *Hand Clin*. 2010;26(1):21–36.
71. Flatt AE. Webbed fingers. *Proc (Bayl Univ Med Cent)*. 2005;18:26–387.
72. Johnstone AJ. Tennis elbow and upper limb tendinopathies. *Sports Med Arthro Rev*. 2000;8:69–79.
73. Shah AS, Bae DS. Management of pediatric trigger thumb and trigger finger. *J Am Acad Orthop Surg*. 2012;20:206–213.

74. Prasarn ML, Ouellette EA. Acute compartment syndrome of the upper extremity. *J Am Acad Orthop Surg.* 2011;19:49–58.

75. Cowell HR. Polydactyly, triphalangism of the thumb, and carpal abnormalities in the family. *Clin Orthop Relat Res.* 2005;434:16–25.

76. Lichtman DM, Schneider JR, Swafford AR, et al. Ulnar midcarpal instability—clinical and laboratory analysis. *J Hand Surg Am.* 1981;6:515–523.

77. Wolfe SW, Garcia-Elias M, Kitay A. Carpal instability nondissociative. *J Am Acad Orthop Surg.* 2012;20(9):575–585.

78. Sobel AD, Shah KN, Katarincic JA. The imperative nature of physical exam in identifying pediatric scaphoid fractures. *J Pediatr.* 2016;177:323–323.

79. Wadsworth CT. Wrist and hand examination and interpretation. *J Orthop Sports Phys Ther.* 1983;5:108–120.

80. Blair SJ, McCormick E, Bear-Lehman J, et al. Evaluation of impairment of the upper extremity. *Clin Orthop.* 1987;221:42–58.

81. Clarkson HM. *Musculoskeletal Assessment—Joint Range of Motion and Manual Muscle Strength.* Philadelphia: Lippincott Williams & Wilkins; 2000.

82. Dutton M. *Orthopedic Examination, Evaluation and Intervention.* New York: McGraw Hill; 2004.

83. Waizenegger M, Barton NJ, Davis TR, Wastie ML. Clinical signs in scaphoid fractures. *J Hand Surg Br.* 1994;19(6):743–747.

84. Vanswearingen JM. Measuring wrist muscle strength. *J Orthop Sports Phys Ther.* 1983;4:217–228.

85. Hume MC, Gellman H, McKellop H, et al. Functional range of motion of the joints of the hand. *J Hand Surg Am.* 1990;15:240–243.

86. Brumfield RH, Champoux JA. A biomechanical study of normal functional wrist motion. *Clin Orthop.* 1984;187:23–25.

87. Ryu JY, Cooney WP, Askew JL, et al. Functional range of motion of the wrist joint. *J Hand Surg.* 1991;16:409–419.

88. Palmer AK, Werner FW, Murphy D, et al. Functional wrist motion: a biomechanical study. *J Hand Surg Am.* 1985;10:39–46.

89. Nelson DL. Functional wrist motion. *Hand Clin.* 1997;13:83–92.

90. Lamereaux L, Hoffer MM. The effect of wrist deviation on grip and pinch strength. *Clin Orthop.* 1995;314:152–155.

91. Tubiana R. *The Hand.* Philadelphia: WB Saunders; 1981.

92. Reid DC. *Functional Anatomy and Joint Mobilization.* Edmonton: University of Alberta Press; 1970.

93. Sollerman C, Sperling L. Evaluation of activities of daily living function—especially hand function. *Scand J Rehab Med.* 1978;10:139–145.

94. McPhee SD. Functional hand evaluations: a review. *Am J Occup Ther.* 1987;41:158–163.

95. Bechtal CD. Grip test: the use of a dynamometer with adjustable handle spacing. *J Bone Joint Surg Am.* 1954;36:820–832.

96. Mathiowetz V, Weber K, Volland G, et al. Reliability and validity of grip and pinch strength evaluations. *J Hand Surg Am.* 1984;9:222–226.

97. Hansman CF, Mresh MM. Appearance and fusion of ossification centers in the human skeleton. *Am J Roentgenol.* 1962;88:476–482.

98. Aulicino PL, DuPuy TE. Clinical examination of the hand. In: Hunter J, Schneider LH, Mackin EJ, et al., eds. *Rehabilitation of the Hand: Surgery And Therapy.* St Louis: CV Mosby; 1990.

99. Sambandam SN, Priyanka P, Gul A, Ilango B. Critical analysis of outcome measures used in the assessment of carpal tunnel syndrome. *Int Orthop.* 2008;32(4):497–504.

100. Buchanan D, Prothero D, Field J. Which are the most relevant questions in the assessment of outcome after distal radial fractures? *Adv Orthop.* 2015;2015:460589.

101. Levine DW, Simmons BP, Koris MJ, et al. A self-administered questionnaire for the assessment of severity of symptoms and functional status in carpal tunnel syndrome. *J Bone Joint Surg Am.* 1993;75:1585–1592.

102. Chung KC, Pillsbury MS, Walter MR, et al. Reliability and validity testing of the Michigan hand outcomes questionnaire. *J Hand Surg Am.* 1998;23:575–587.

103. Wehrli M, Hensler S, Schindele S, et al. Measurement properties of the Brief Michigan Hand Outcomes Questionnaire in patients with Dupuytren contracture. *J Hand Surg Am.* 2016;41(9):896–902.

104. Dias JJ, Bhowal B, Wildin CJ, et al. Assessing the outcome of disorders of the hands—is the patient evaluation measure reliable, responsive, and without bias? *J Bone Joint Surg Br.* 2001;83:235–240.

105. Forward DP, Sithole JS, Davis TR. The internal consistency and validity of the patient evaluation measure for outcomes assessment in distal radial fractures. *J Hand Surg Eur.* 2007;32(3):262–267.

106. Hobby JL, Watts C, Elliot D. Validity and responsiveness of the patient evaluation measure as an outcome measure for carpal tunnel syndrome. *J Hand Surg Br.* 2005;30(4):350–354.

107. Dias JJ, Rajan RA, Thompson JR. Which questionnaire is best? The reliability, validity and ease of use of the patient evaluation measure, the disabilities of the arm, shoulder and hand, and the Michigan Hand Outcome measure. *J Hand Surg Eur.* 2008;33(1):9–17.

108. Apergis EP. The unstable capitolunate and radiolunate joints as a source of wrist pain in young women. *J Hand Surg Br.* 1996;21(4):501–506.

109. Kwok IH, Leung F, Yuen G. Assessing results after distal radius fracture treatment: a comparison of objective and subjective tools. *Geriatr Orthop Surg Rehabil.* 2011;2(4):155–160.

110. Dacombe PJ, Amirfeyz R, Davis T. Patient-reported outcome measures for hand and wrist trauma: is there sufficient evidence of reliability, validity and responsiveness? *Hand (N Y).* 2016;11(1):11–21.

111. Souer JS, Lozano-Calderon SA. Ring D: Predictors of wrist function and health status after operative treatment of fractures of the distal radius. *J Hand Surg Am.* 2008;33(2):157–163.

112. MacDermid JC, Turgeon T, Richards RS, et al. Patient rating of wrist pain and disability: a reliable and valid measurement tool. *J Orthop Trauma.* 1998;12(8):577–586.

113. Slutsky DJ. Outcomes assessment in wrist surgery. *J Wrist Surg.* 2013;2(1):1–4.

114. MacDermid JC. Patient reported outcomes: state-of-the-art hand surgery and future applications. *Hand Clin.* 2014;30(3):293–304.

115. Goldbeck TG, Davies GJ. Test-retest reliability of the closed kinetic chain–upper extremity stability test: a clinical field test. *J Sports Rehab.* 2000;9:35–43.

116. Tucci HT, Martins J, de Carvalho Sposito G, et al. Closed kinetic chain upper extremity stability test (CKCUES test): a reliability study in persons with and without shoulder impingement syndrome. *BMC Musculoskelet Disord.* 2014;15:1–9.

117. de Oliveira VM, Pitangui AC, Nascimento VY, et al. Test-retest reliability of the closed kinetic chain upper extremity stability test (CKCUEST) in adolescents: reliability of CKCUEST in adolescents. *Int J Sports Phys Ther.* 2017;12(1):125–132.

118. Tarara DT, Fogaca LR, Taylor JB, Hegedus EJ. Clinician-friendly physical performance tests in athletes part 3: a systemic review of measurement properties and correlations to injury for tests in the upper extremity. *Br J Sports Med.* 2016;50(9):545–551.

119. Fess EE. Documentation: essential elements of an upper extremity assessment battery. In: Hunter J, Schneider LH, Mackin EJ, et al., eds. *Rehabilitation of the Hand: Surgery and Therapy.* St Louis: CV Mosby; 1990.

120. Baxter-Petralia PL, Blackmore SM, McEntee PM. Physical capacity evaluation. In: Hunter J, Schneider LH, Mackin EJ, et al., eds. *Rehabilitation of the Hand: Surgery and Therapy.* St Louis: CV Mosby; 1990.

121. Beckenbaugh RD, Shives TC, Dobyns JH, et al. Kienböck's disease: the natural history of Kienböck's disease and consideration of lunate fractures. *Clin Orthop.* 1980;149:98–106.

122. Jebsen RH, Taylor N, Trieschmann RB, et al. An objective and standardized test of hand function. *Arch Phys Med Rehabil.* 1969;50:311–319.

123. Callahan AD. Sensibility testing. In: Hunter J, Schneider LH, Mackin EJ, et al., eds. *Rehabilitation of the Hand: Surgery and Therapy.* St Louis: CV Mosby; 1990.

124. Cleland JA, Koppenhaver S. *Netter's Orthopedic Clinical Examination—An Evidence Based Approach.* ed 2. Philadelphia: Saunders/Elsevier; 2011.

125. Cook CE, Hegedus EJ. *Orthopedic Physical Examination Tests—An Evidence Based Approach.* Upper Saddle River, NJ: Prentice Hall/Pearson; 2008.

126. Skirven T. Clinical examination of the wrist. *J Hand Surg.* 1996;9:96–107.

127. Lester B, Halbrecht J, Levy IM, et al. "Press test" for office diagnosis of triangular fibrocartilage complex tears of the wrist. *Ann Plast Surg.* 1995;35:41–45.

128. Muminagic S, Kapidzic T. Wrist instability after injury. *Mater Sociomed.* 2012;24(2):121–124.

129. Lee DJ, Elfar JC. Carpal ligament injuries, pathomechanics and classification. *Hand Clin.* 2015;31(3):389–398.

130. De Filippo M, Sudberry JJ, Lombardo E, et al. Pathogenesis and evolution of carpal instability: imaging and topography. *Acta Biomed.* 2006;77:168–180.

131. Prosser R, Harvey L, LaStayo P, et al. Provocative wrist tests and MRI are of limited diagnostic value for suspected wrist ligament injuries: a cross-sectional study. *J Physiother.* 2011;57(4):247–253.

132. Young D, Papp S, Giachimo A. Physical examination of the wrist. *Orthop Clin North Am.* 2007;38:149–165.

133. Christodoulou Bainbridge LC. Clinical diagnosis of triquetrolunate ligament injuries. *J Hand Surg Br.* 1999;24(5):598–600.

134. Johnson RP, Carrera GP. Chronic capitolunate instability. *J Bone Joint Surg Am.* 1986;68:1164–1176.

135. Salva-Coll G, Garcia-Elias M, Hagert E. Scapholunate instability: proprioception and neuromuscular control. *J Wrist Surg.* 2013;2(2):136–140.

136. Nguyen DT, McCue FC, Urch SE. Evaluation of the injured wrist on the field and in the office. *Clin Sports Med.* 1998;17:421–432.

137. Broekstra DC, Lanting R, Werker PM, van den Heuval ER. Intra-and inter-observer agreement on diagnosis of Dupuytren disease, measurements of severity of contracture, and disease extent. *Man Ther.* 2015;20(4):580–586.

138. Lastayo P, Weiss S. The GRIT: a quantitative measure of ulnar impaction syndrome. *J Hand Ther.* 2001;14(3):173–179.

139. Beckenbaugh RD. Accurate evaluation and management of the painful wrist following injury. *Orthop Clin North Am.* 1984;15:289–306.

140. Kleinman WB. The lunotriquetral shuck test. *Am Soc Surg Hand Corr News.* 1985;51.

141. Shulman BS, Rettig M, Sapienza A. Management of pisotriquetral instability. *J Hand Surg Am.* 2018;43(1):54–60.

142. Post M. *Physical Examination of the Musculoskeletal System*. Chicago: Year Book Medical; 1987.

143. Taliesnik J. Soft tissue injuries of the wrist. In: Strickland JW, Rettig AC, eds. *Hand Injuries in Athletes*. Philadelphia: WB Saunders; 1992.

144. Booher JM, Thibodeau GA. *Athletic Injury Assessment*. St Louis: CV Mosby; 1989.

145. Lichtman DM, Reardon RS. Midcarpal instability. In: Slutsky D, ed. *Principles and Practice of Wrist Surgery*. Philadelphia: Elsevier; 2010.

146. Burrows B, Moreira P, Murphy C, et al. Scaphoid fractures: a higher order analysis of clinical tests and application of clinical reasoning strategies. *Man Ther*. 2014;19(5):372–378.

147. Niacaris T, Ming BW, Lichtman DM. Midcarpal instability – a comprehensive review and update. *Hand Clin*. 2015;31:487–493.

148. Chen SC. The scaphoid compression test. *J Hand Surg Br*. 1989;14:323–325.

149. Buterbaugh GA, Brown TR, Horn PC. Ulnar-sided wrist pain in athletes. *Clin Sports Med*. 1998;17:567–583.

150. Murray PM, Cooney WP. Golf-induced injuries of the wrist. *Clin Sports Med*. 1996;15:85–109.

151. Swanson A. Disabling arthritis at the base of the thumb: treatment by resection of the trapezium and flexible implant arthroplasty. *J Bone Joint Surg Am*. 1972;54:456–471.

152. Heyman P, Gelberman RH, Duncan K, et al. Injuries of the ulnar collateral ligament of the thumb metacarpophalangeal joint. *Clin Orthop*. 1993;292:165–171.

153. Heyman P. Injuries to the ulnar collateral ligament of the thumb metacarpophalangeal joint. *J Am Acad Orthop Surg*. 1997;5:224–229.

154. Tang P. Collateral ligament injuries of the thumb metacarpophalangeal joint. *J Am Acad Orthop Surg*. 2011;19:287–296.

155. Tay SC, Tomita K, Berger RA. The "ulnar fovea sign" for defining ulnar wrist pain: an analysis of sensitivity and specificity. *J Hand Surg Am*. 2007;32:438–444.

156. Sachar K. Ulnar-sided wrist pain: evaluation and treatment of triangular fibrocartilage complex tears, ulnocarpal impaction syndrome and lunotriquetral ligament tears. *J Hand Surg Am*. 2012;37:1489–1500.

157. LaStayo P, Howell J. Clinical provocation tests used in evaluating wrist pain: a descriptive study. *J Hand Ther*. 1995;8:10–17.

158. Watson HK, Ballet FL. The SLAC wrist: scapulolunate advanced collapse pattern of degenerative arthritis. *J Hand Surg Am*. 1984;9:358–365.

159. Lane LB. The scaphoid shift test. *J Hand Surg*. 1993;18(2):366–368.

160. Wolfe SW, Crisco JJ. Mechanical evaluation of the scaphoid shift test. *J Hand Surg Am*. 1994;19(5):762–7658.

161. Watson HK, Ashmead D, Makhlouf MV. Examination of the scaphoid. *J Hand Surg Am*. 1988;13:657–660.

162. Elson RA. Rupture of the central slip of the extensor hood of the finger: a test for early diagnosis. *J Bone Joint Surg Br*. 1986;68:229–231.

163. Boyes J. *Bunnell's Surgery of the Hand*. Philadelphia: JB Lippincott; 1970.

164. Hoppenfeld S. *Physical Examination of the Spine and Extremities*. New York: Appleton-Century-Crofts; 1976.

165. Ruland RT, Hogan CJ. The ECU synergy test: an aid to diagnose ECU tendonitis. *J Hand Surg Am*. 2008;33(10):1777–1782.

166. Campbell D, Campbell R, O'Connor P, Hawkes R. Sports-related extensor carpi ulnaris pathology: a review of functional anatomy, sports injury and management. *Br J Sports Med*. 2013;47(17):1105–1111.

167. Finkelstein H. Stenosing tendovaginitis at the radial styloid process. *J Bone Joint Surg*. 1930;12:509.

168. Linburg RM, Comstock BE. Anomalous tendon slips from the flexor pollicis longus to the flexor digitorum profundus. *J Hand Surg Am*. 1979;4:79–83.

169. Golding DN, Rose DM, Selvarajah K. Clinical tests for carpal tunnel syndrome: an evaluation. *Br J Rheum*. 1986;25:388–390.

170. Gunnarsson LG, Amilon A, Hellstrand P, et al. The diagnosis of carpal tunnel syndrome-sensitivity and specificity of some clinical and electrophysiological tests. *J Hand Surg Br*. 1997;22:34–37.

171. Popinchalk SP, Schaffer AA. Physical examination of upper extremity compressive neuropathies. *Orthop Clin North Am*. 2012;43:417–430.

172. Fowler JR, Cipolli W, Hanson T. A comparison of three diagnostic tests for carpal tunnel syndrome using latent class analysis. *J Bone Joint Surg Am*. 2015;97(23):1958–1961.

173. Kuhlman KA, Hennessey WJ. Sensitivity and specificity of carpal tunnel syndrome signs. *Am J Phys Med Rehabil*. 1997;76(6):451–457.

174. Durkan JA. A new diagnostic test for carpal tunnel syndrome. *J Bone Joint Surg Am*. 1991;73:535–538.

175. Wainner RS, Fritz JM, Irrgang JJ, et al. Development of a clinical prediction rule for the diagnosis of carpal tunnel syndrome. *Arch Phys Med Rehabil*. 2005;86:609–618.

176. Almasi-Doghaee M, Boostani R, Saeedi M, et al. Carpal compression, Phalen's and Tinel's test: which one is more suitable for carpal tunnel syndrome? *Iran J Neurol*. 2016;15(3):173–174.

177. Calandruccio JH, Thompson NB. Carpal tunnel syndrome: making evidence-based treatment decisions. *Orthop Clin North Am*. 2018;49(2):223–229.

178. Massy-Westropp N, Grimmer K, Bain G. A systematic review of the clinical diagnostic tests for carpal tunnel syndrome. *J Hand Surg Am*. 2000;25(1):120–127.

179. Valdes K, LaStayo P. The value of provocative tests for the wrist and elbow: a literature review. *J Hand Ther*. 2013;26(1):32–43.

180. Cranford CS, Ho JY, Kalainov DM, Hartigan BJ. Carpal tunnel syndrome. *J Am Acad Orthop Surg*. 2007;15(9):537–548.

181. Aroori S, Spence RA. Carpal tunnel syndrome. *Ulster Med J*. 2008;77(1):6–17.

182. De Smet L. Value of some clinical provocative tests in carpal tunnel syndrome: do we need electrophysiology and can we predict the outcome? *Hand Clin*. 2003;19:387–391.

183. Slater RR. Carpal tunnel syndrome: current concepts. *J South Orthop Assoc*. 1999;8(3):203–213.

184. Tetro AM, Evanoff BA, Hollstein SB, et al. A new provocative test for carpal tunnel syndrome: assessment of wrist flexion and nerve compression. *J Bone Joint Surg Br*. 1998;80:493–498.

185. Karl AI, Carney ML, Kaul MP. The lumbrical provocation test in subjects with median inclusive paresthesia. *Arch Phys Med Rehabil*. 2001;82(7):935–937.

186. Yii NW, Elliot D. A study of the dynamic relationship of the lumbrical muscles and the carpal tunnel. *J Hand Surg Br*. 1994;19(4):439–443.

187. Cobb TK, An KN, Cooney WP, Berger RA. Lumbrical muscle incursion into the carpal tunnel during finger flexion. *J Hand Surg Br*. 1994;19(4):434–438.

188. Earle AS, Vlastou C. Crossed fingers and other tests of ulnar nerve motor function. *J Hand Surg*. 1980;5(6):560–565.

189. Jones LA. The assessment of hand function: a critical review of techniques. *J Hand Surg Am*. 1989;14:221–228.

190. Dellon AL, Kallman CH. Evaluation of functional sensation in the hand. *J Hand Surg Am*. 1983;8:865–870.

191. Omer GE. Report of the Committee for Evaluation of the Clinical Result in Peripheral Nerve Injury. *J Hand Surg Am*. 1983;8:754–759.

192. Hansen PA, Micklesen P, Robinson LR. Clinical utility of the flick maneuver in diagnosing carpal tunnel syndrome. *Am J Phys Med Rehabil*. 2004;83:363–367.

193. Pryse-Phillips WE. Validation of a diagnostic sign in carpal tunnel syndrome. *J Neurol Neurosurg Psychiatry*. 1984;47(8):870–872.

194. Moldaver J. Tinel's sign. its characteristics and significance. *J Bone Joint Surg Am*. 1978;60:412–414.

195. Ahn DS. Hand elevation: a new test for carpal tunnel syndrome. *Ann Plast Surg*. 2001;46:120–124.

196. Ma H, Kim I. The diagnostic assessment of hand elevation test in carpal tunnel syndrome. *J Korean Neurosurg Soc*. 2012;52:472–475.

197. Stromberg WB, McFarlane RM, Bell JL, et al. Injury of the median and ulnar nerves: 150 cases with an evaluation of Moberg's ninhydrin test. *J Bone Joint Surg Am*. 1961;43:717–730.

198. Yoshida A, Okutsu I, Hamanaka I. A new diagnostic provocation test for carpal tunnel syndrome: Okutsu test. *Hand Surg*. 2010;15(2):65–69.

199. MacDermid JC, Wessel J. Clinical diagnosis of carpal tunnel syndrome: a systematic review. *J Hand Surg*. 2004;17:309–319.

200. Radecki P. A gender specific wrist ratio and the likelihood of a median nerve abnormality at the carpal tunnel. *Am J Phys Med Rehabil*. 1994;73(3):157–162.

201. *American Society for Surgery of the Hand: The Hand: Examination and Diagnosis*. Aurora, CO: American Society for Surgery of the Hand; 1978.

202. Goloborod'ko SA. New clinical motor test for cubital tunnel syndrome. *J Hand Ther*. 2012;25(4):422–424.

203. Cheng CJ, Mackinnon-Patterson B, Beck JL, Mackinnon SE. Scratch collapse test for evaluation of carpal and cubital tunnel syndrome. *J Hand Surg Am*. 2008;33(9):1518–1524.

204. Blok RD, Becker SJ, Ring DC. Diagnosis of carpal tunnel syndrome: interobserver reliability of the blinded scratch-collapse test. *J Hand Microsurg*. 2014;6(1):5–7.

205. Huynh MN, Karir A, Bennett A. Scratch collapse test for carpal tunnel syndrome: a systematic review and meta-analysis. *Plast Reconstr Surg Glob Open*. 2018;6(9):e1933.

206. Simon J, Lutsky K, Maltenfort M, Beredjiklian PK. The accuracy of the scratch collapse test performed by blinded examiners on patients with suspected carpal tunnel syndrome assessed by electrodiagnostic studies. *J Hand Surg Am*. 2017;42(5):386. e1–386.e5.

207. Shiri R. A square-shaped wrist as a predictor of carpal tunnel syndrome: a meta-analysis. *Muscle Nerve*. 2015;52(5):709–713.

208. LaBan MM, Mackenzie JR, Zemenick GA. Anatomic observations in carpal tunnel syndrome as they relate to the tethered median nerve stress test. *Arch Phys Med Rehabil*. 1989;70:44–46.

209. LaBan MM, Friedman NA, Zemenick GA. "Tethered" median nerve stress test in chronic carpal tunnel syndrome. *Arch Phys Med Rehabil*. 1986;67:803–804.

210. Raudino F. Tethered median nerve stress test in the diagnosis of carpal tunnel syndrome. *Electromyogr Clin Neurophysiol*. 2000;40:57–60.

211. Kuschner SH, Ebramzadeh E, Johnson D, et al. Tinel's sign and Phalen's test in carpal tunnel syndrome. *Orthopedics*. 1992;15:1297–1302.

212. Thungen T, Sadowski M, El Kazzi W, Schuind F. Value of Gilliatt's pneumatic tourniquet test for diagnosis of carpal tunnel syndrome. *Chir Main*. 2012;31(3):152–156.

213. De Smet L. Recurrent carpal tunnel syndrome. Clinical testing indicating incomplete section of the flexor retinaculum. *J Hand Surg Br.* 1993;18(2):189.

214. Gilliat RW, Wilson TG. A pneumatic-tourniquet test in the carpal-tunnel syndrome. *Lancet.* 1953;265(6786):595–597.

215. O'Riain S. Shrivel test: a new and simple test of nerve function in the hand. *Br Med J.* 1973;3:615–616.

216. Tindall A, Dawood R, Povlsen B. Case of the month: the skin wrinkle test: a simple nerve injury test for pediatric and uncooperative patients. *Emerg Med J.* 2006;23(11):883–886.

217. Wilder-Smith EP. Stimulated skin wrinkling as an indicator of limb sympathetic function. *Clin Neurophysiol.* 2015;126(1):10–16.

218. Allen EV. Thromboangiitis obliterans: methods of diagnosis of chronic occlusive arterial lesions distal to the wrist with illustrative cases. *Am J Med Sci.* 1929;178:237–244.

219. Pellecchia GL. Figure of eight method of measuring hand size: reliability and concurrent validity. *J Hand Ther.* 2003;16:300–304.

220. Leard JS, Breglio L, Fraga L, et al. Reliability and concurrent validity of the figure-of-eight method of measuring hand size in patients with hand pathology. *J Orthop Sports Phys Ther.* 2004;34:335–340.

221. Bell-Krotoski JA, Breger DE, Beach RB. Application of biomechanics for evaluation of the hand. In: Hunter J, Schneider LH, Mackin EJ, et al., eds. *Rehabilitation of the Hand: Surgery and Therapy.* St Louis: CV Mosby; 1990.

222. Halpern JS. Upper extremity peripheral nerve assessment. *J Emerg Nurs.* 1989;15:261–265.

223. Trombly CA, Scott AD. Evaluation of motor control. In: Trombly CA, ed. *Occupational Therapy for Physical Dysfunction.* Baltimore: Williams & Wilkins; 1989.

224. Tosti R, Ilyas AM. Acute carpal tunnel syndrome. *Orthop Clin North Am.* 2012;43(4):459–465.

225. Bland JD. A neurophysiological grading scale for carpal tunnel syndrome. *Muscle Nerve.* 2000;23:1280–1283.

226. El-Magzoub S, Mustafa ME, Abdalla SF. Neurophysiologic pattern and severity grading scale of carpal tunnel syndrome in Sudanese patients. *J Neurol Neurosci.* 2017;8(4):213–221.

227. Lai WK, Chiu YT, Law WS. The deformation and longitudinal excursion of median nerve during digits movement and wrist extension. *Man Ther.* 2014;19:608–613.

228. Bachoura A, Jacoby SM. Ulnar tunnel syndrome. *Orthop Clin North Am.* 2012;43:467–474.

229. Osterman M, Ilyas AM, Matzon JL. Carpal tunnel syndrome in pregnancy. *Orthop Clin North Am.* 2012;43(4):515–520.

230. Wilder-Smith EP, Ng ES, Chan YH, Therimadasamy AK. Sensory distribution indicates severity of median nerve damage in carpal tunnel syndrome. *Clin Neurophysiol.* 2008;119:1619–1625.

231. Atroshi I, Lyren P-E, Gummesson C. The 6-item CTS symptoms scale: a brief outcomes measure for carpal tunnel syndrome. *Qual Life Res.* 2009;18:347–358.

232. Craw JR, Church DJ, Hutchison RL. Prospective comparison of the six-item carpal tunnel symptoms scale and portable nerve conduction testing in measuring the outcomes of treatment of carpal tunnel syndrome with steroid injection. *Hand (N Y).* 2015;10(1):49–53.

233. Duckworth AD, Jenkins PJ, McEachan JE. Diagnosing carpal tunnel syndrome. *J Hand Surg Am.* 2014;39(7):1403–1407.

234. Atroshi I, Lyren PE, Ornstein E, Gummesson C. The six-item CTS symptoms scale and palmer pain scale in carpal tunnel syndrome. *J Hand Surg Am.* 2011;36(5):788–794.

235. Szabo RM, Madison M. Carpal tunnel syndrome. *Orthop Clin North Am.* 1992;23:103–109.

236. Murray-Leslie CF, Wright V. Carpal tunnel syndrome, humeral epicondylitis and the cervical spine: a study of clinical and dimensional relations. *Br Med J.* 1976;1:1439–1442.

237. Hurst LC, Weissberg D, Carroll RE. The relationship of the double crush to carpal tunnel syndrome. *J Hand Surg Br.* 1985;10:202–204.

238. Massey EW, Riley TL, Pleet AB. Co-existent carpal tunnel syndrome and cervical radiculopathy (double crush syndrome). *South Med J.* 1981;74:957–959.

239. Strohl AB, Zelouf DS. Ulnar tunnel syndrome, radial tunnel syndrome, anterior interosseous nerve syndrome and pronator syndrome. *J Am Acad Orthop Surg.* 2017;25(1):e1–e10.

240. Xing SG, Tang JB. Entrapment neuropathy of the wrist, forearm and elbow. *Clin Plast Surg.* 2014;41(3):561–588.

241. Kaltenborn FM. *Mobilization of the Extremity Joints.* Oslo: Olaf Norlis Bokhandel; 1980.

242. Staes FF, Banks KJ, DeSmet L, et al. Reliability of accessory motion testing at the carpal joints. *Man Ther.* 2009;14:292–298.

243. Freeland P. Scaphoid tubercle tenderness: a better indicator of scaphoid fractures? *Arch Emerg Med.* 1989;6(1):46–50.

244. Reddy RS, Compson J. Examination of the wrist – surface anatomy and the carpal bones. *Curr Orthop.* 2005;19:171–179.

245. Bishop AT, Beckenbaugh RD. Fracture of the hamate bone. *J Hand Surg Am.* 1988;13:135–139.

246. Peterson JJ, Bancroft LW. Injuries of the fingers and thumb in the athlete. *Clin Sp Med.* 2006;25:527–542.

247. Schuind FA, Linscheid RL, An KN, et al. A normal database of posteroanterior roentgenographic measurements of the wrist. *J Bone Joint Surg Am.* 1992;74:1418–1429.

248. Medoff RJ. Essential radiographic evaluation for distal radius fractures. *Hand Clin.* 2005;21(3):279–288.

249. Feipel V, Rinnen D, Rooze M. Postero-anterior radiography of the wrist: normal database of carpal measurements. *Surg Radiol Anat.* 1998;20(3):221–226.

250. Cha S-M, Shin H-D, Kim K-C. Positive or negative ulnar variance after ulnar shortening of ulnar impaction syndrome: a retrospective study. *Clin Orthop Surg.* 2012;4(3):216–220.

251. Reisler T, Therattil PJ, Lee ES. Perilunate dislocation. *Eplasty.* 2015;15:ic9.

252. Bednar JM, Osterman AL. Carpal instability: evaluation and treatment. *J Am Acad Orthop Surg.* 1993;1:10–17.

253. Weiss AP, Akelman E. Diagnostic imaging and arthroscopy for chronic wrist pain. *Orthop Clin North Am.* 1995;26:759–767.

254. Olchowy C, Solinski D, Lasecki M, et al. Wrist ultrasound examination – scanning technique and ultrasound anatomy. Part 2: ventral wrist. *J Ultrason.* 2017;17(69):123–128.

255. Starr HM, Sedgley MD, Means KR, Murphy MS. Ultrasonography for hand and wrist conditions. *J Am Acad Orthop Surg.* 2016;24(8):544–554.

256. Wiesler ER, Chloros GD, Cartwright MS, et al. The use of diagnostic ultrasound in carpal tunnel syndrome. *J Hand Surg Am.* 2006;31(5):726–732.

257. Sofka CM. Ultrasound of the hand and wrist. *Ultrasound Q.* 2014;30(3):184–192.

258. Chen P, Maklad N, Radwine M, et al. Dynamic high-resolution sonograph of the carpal tunnel. *Am J Roentgenol.* 1997;168(2):533–537.

259. Chiavaras MM, Jacobson JA, Yablon CM, et al. Pitfalls in wrist and hand ultrasound. *Am J Roentgenol.* 2014;203(3):531–540.

260. Daenen B, Houben G, Bauduin E, et al. Sonography in wrist tendon pathology. *J Clin Ultrasound.* 2004;32(9):462–469.

261. Haramati N, Hiller N, Dowdle J, et al. MRI of the Stener lesion. *Skeletal Radiol.* 1995;24(7):515–518.

262. Shroeder NS, Goldfarb CA. Thumb ulnar collateral and radial collateral ligament injuries. *Clin Sports Med.* 2015;34(1):117–126.

263. Jones MH, England SJ, Muwanga CL, Hildreth T. The use of ultrasound in the diagnosis of injuries of the ulnar collateral ligament of the thumb. *J Hand Surg Br.* 2000;25(1):29–32.

264. Melville DM, Jacobson JA, Fessell DP. Ultrasound of the thumb ulnar collateral ligament: techniques and pathology. *Am J Roentgenol.* 2014;202(2):W168.

265. Ebrahim FS, De Maeseneer M, Jager T, et al. Ultrasound diagnosis of UCL tears of the thumb and Stener lesions: technique, pattern-based approach, and differential diagnosis. *Radiographics.* 2006;26:1007–1020.

266. Siegel S, White LM, Brahme S. Magnetic resonance imaging of the musculoskeletal system—the wrist. *Clin Orthop Relat Res.* 1996;332:281–300.

267. Bencardino JT, Rosenberg ZS. Sports related injuries of the wrist: an approach to MRI interpretation. *Clin Sports Med.* 2006;25:409–432.

268. Coggins CA. Imaging of the ulnar-sided wrist pain. *Clin Sports Med.* 2006;25:505–526.

269. Sahu A, Pang CL, Lynch J, Suresh P. A review of radiological imaging in the hand and wrist. *Orthop Trauma.* 2014;28(3):172–186.

270. Ringler MD. MRI of wrist ligaments. *J Hand Surg Am.* 2013;38(10):2034–2046.

271. MacDermid JC, Doherty T. Clinical and electrodiagnostic testing of carpal tunnel syndrome. A narrative review. *J Orthop Sport Phys Ther.* 2004;34(10):565–588.

272. Makanji HS, Becker SJ, Mudgal CS, et al. Evaluation of the scratch collapse test for the diagnosis of carpal tunnel syndrome. *J Hand Surg Eur.* 2014;39(2):181–186.

273. Grover R. Clinical assessment of scaphoid injuries and the detection of fractures. *J Hand Surg Br.* 1996;21:341–343.

274. Desrosiers J, Bravo G, Hebert R, et al. Validation of the box and block test as a measure of dexterity of elderly people: reliability, validity, and norms studies. *Arch Phys Med Rehabil.* 1994;75(7):751–755.

275. Connell LA, Tyson SF. Clinical reality of measuring upper-limb ability in neurological conditions: a systematic review. *Arch Phys Med Rehabil.* 2012;93:221–228.

276. Priganc VW, Henry SM. The relationship among five common carpal tunnel syndrome tests and the severity of carpal tunnel syndrome. *J Hand Ther.* 2003;16:225–236.

277. Szabo RM, Slater RR, Farver TB, et al. The value of diagnostic testing in carpal tunnel syndrome. *J Hand Surg Am.* 1999;24(4):704–714.

278. Modelli M, Passero S, Giannini F. Provocative tests in different stages of carpal tunnel syndrome. *Clin Neurol Neurosurg.* 2001;103:170–183.

279. Del Pino JG, Delgado-Martinez AD, Gonzalez I, et al. Value of the carpal compression test in the diagnosis of carpal tunnel syndrome. *J Hand Surg Br.* 1997;20:38–41.

280. Fertl E, Wober C, Zeitlhofer J. The serial use of two provocative tests in the clinical diagnosis of carpal tunel syndrome. *Acta Neurol Scand.* 1998;98(5):328–332.

281. Farrell K, Johnson A, Duncan H, et al. The intertester and intratester reliability of hand volumetrics. *J Hand Ther.* 2003;16(4):292–299.

282. Doods RL, Nielsen KA, Shirley AG, et al. Test-retest reliability of the commercial volumeter. *Work.* 2004;22(2):107–110.

283. Jung HY, Kong MS, Lee SH, et al. Prevalence and related characteristics of carpal tunnel syndrome among orchardists in the Gyeongsangna-do Region. *Ann Rehabil Med.* 2016;40(5):902–914.

284. Choa RM, Parvizi N, Giele HP. A prospective case-control study to compare the sensitivity and specificity of the grind and traction-shift (subluxation-relocation) clinical tests in osteoarthritis of the thumb carpometacarpal joint. *J Hand Surg Eur.* 2014;39(3):282–285.

285. MacDermid JC, Kramer JF, Woodbury MG, et al. Interrater reliability of pinch and grip strength measurements in patients with cumulative trauma disorders. *J Hand Surg.* 1994;7:10–14.

286. Haward BM, Griffin MJ. Repeatability of grip strength and dexterity tests and the effects of age and gender. *Int Arch Occup Environ Health.* 2002;75(1–2):111–119.

287. Schreuders TA, Roebroeck ME, Goumans J, et al. Measurement error in grip and pinch force measurements in patients with hand injuries. *Phys Ther.* 2003;83:806–815.

288. Brown A, Cramer LD, Eckhaus D, et al. Validity and reliability of the Dexter hand evaluation and therapy system in hand-injured patients. *J Hand Ther.* 2000;25:37–45.

289. Turgut AC, Tubbs RS, Turgut M, Hoffman Paul. (1884-1962 AD) and Jules Tinel (1879-1952 AD), and their legacy to neuroscience: the Hoffman-Tinel sign. *Childs Nerv System.* 2019;35:733–734.

290. Agre JC, Magness JL, Hull SZ, et al. Strength testing with a portable dynamometer: reliability for upper and lower extremities. *Arch Phys Med Rehabil.* 1987;68:454–458.

291. Karl AI, Carney ML, Kaul MP. The lumbrical provocation test in subjects with median inclusive paresthesia. *Arch Phys Med Rehabil.* 2001;82(7):935–937.

292. Prosser R, Herbert R, LaStayo P. Current practice in the diagnosis and treatment of carpal instability - results of a survey of Australian hand therapists. *J Hand Ther.* 2007;20:239–243.

293. Wiederien RC, Feldman TD, Heusel LD, et al. The effect of the median nerve compression test on median nerve conduction across the carpal tunnel. *Electromyogr Clin Neurophysiol.* 2002;42(7):413–421.

294. Chung KC, Pillsbury MS, Walters MR, et al. Reliability and validity testing of the Michigan Hand Outcomes Questionnaire. *J Hand Surg Am.* 1998;23(4):575–587.

295. Chung KC, Hamill JB, Walters MR, et al. The Michigan Hand Outcomes Questionnaire (MHQ): assessment of responsiveness to clinical change. *Ann Plast Surg.* 1999;42(6):619–622.

296. Feinstein WK, Lichtman DM, Noble PC, et al. Quantitative assessment of the midcarpal shift test. *J Hand Surg Am.* 1999;24(5):977–983.

297. Desrosiers J, Rochette A, Hebert R, et al. The Minnesota Manual Dexterity Test: reliability, validity and reference values studies with healthy elderly people. *Can J Occup Ther.* 1997;64(5):270–276.

298. Ruengsakulrach P, Brooks M, Hare DL, et al. Preoperative assessment of hand circulation by means of Doppler ultrasonography and the modified Allen test. *J Thorac Cardiovasc Surg.* 2001;121(3):526–531.

299. Bovend'Eerdt TJ, Dawes H, Johansen-Berg H, et al. Evaluation of the Modified Jebsen Test of Hand Function and the University of Maryland Arm Questionnaire for Stroke. *Clin Rehabil.* 2004;18(2):195–202.

300. MacDermid JC, Kramer JF, McFarlane RM, et al. Inter-rater agreement and accuracy of clinical tests used in diagnosis of carpal tunnel syndrome. *Work.* 1997;8:37–44.

301. Buch-Jaeger N, Foucher G. Correlation of clinical signs with nerve conduction tests in the diagnosis of carpal tunnel syndrome. *J Hand Surg Br.* 1994;19(6):720–724.

302. Smith YA, Hong E, Presson C. Normative and validation studies of the Nine-hole Peg Test with children. *Percept Mot Skills.* 2000;90:823–843.

303. Waeckerle JF. A prospective study identifying the sensitivity of radiographic findings and the efficacy of clinical findings in carpal navicular fractures. *Ann Emerg Med.* 1987;16(7):733–777.

304. Marx RG, Hudak PL, Bombardier C, et al. The reliability of physical examination for carpal tunnel syndrome. *J Hand Surg Br.* 1998;23(4):499–502.

305. Katz JN, Larson MG, Sabra A, et al. The carpal tunnel syndrome: diagnostic utility of the history and physical examination findings. *Channels Int Med.* 1990;112:321–327.

306. Gellman H, Gellman RH, Tan AM, et al. Carpal tunnel syndrome—an evaluation of the provocative diagnostic tests. *J Bone Jone Surg Am.* 1980;68:735–737.

307. Heller L, Ring H, Costeff H, et al. Evaluation of Tinel's and Phalen's sign in diagnosis of the carpal tunnel syndrome. *Eur Neurol.* 1986;25:40–42.

308. Williams TM, Mackinnon SE, Novak CB. Verification of the pressure provocative test in carpal tunnel syndrome. *Ann Plast Surg.* 1992;29:8–11.

309. Fong PW, Ng GY. Effect of wrist positioning on the repeatability and strength of power grip. *Am J Occup Ther.* 2001;55(2):212–216.

310. Reddon JR, Gill DM, Gauk SE, et al. Purdue Pegboard: test-retest estimates. *Percept Mot Skills.* 1988;66(2):503–506.

311. Desrosiers J, Hebert R, Bravo G, et al. The Purdue Pegboard Test: normative data for people aged 60 and over. *Disabil Rehabil.* 1995;17(5):217–224.

312. Gallus J, Mathiowetz V. Test-retest reliability of the Purdue Pegboard for persons with multiple sclerosis. *Am J Occup Ther.* 2003;57(1):108–111.

313. Buddenberg LA, Davis C. Test-retest reliability of the Purdue Pegboard Test. *Am J Occup Ther.* 2000;54(5):555–558.

314. Lee P, Liu CH, Fan CW, et al. The test-retest reliability and the minimal detectable change of the Purdue pegboard test in schizophrenia. *J Formos Med Assoc.* 2013;112(6):332–337.

315. Sharar RB, Kizony R, Nota A. Validity of the Purdue Pegboard Test in assessing patients after traumatic hand injury. *Work.* 1998;11:315–320.

316. Esberger DA. What value the scaphoid compression test? *J Hand Ther Br.* 1994;19(6):748–749.

317. Parvizi J, Wayman J, Kelly P, Moran CG. Combining the clinical signs improves diagnosis of scaphoid fractures. A prospective study with follow-up. *J Hand Surg Br.* 1998;23(3):324–327.

318. Powell JM, Lloyd GJ, Rintoul RF. New clinical test for fracture of the scaphoid. *Can J Surg.* 1988;31:237–238.

319. Rahman S. A squared-shaped wrist as a predictor of carpal tunnel syndrome: a meta-analysis. *Muscle Nerve.* 2015;52(5):709–713.

320. Novak CB, Lee GW, Mackinnon SE, et al. Provocative testing for cubital tunnel syndrome. *J Hand Surg Am.* 1994;19:817–820.

321. Kingery WS, Park KS, Wu PB, et al. Electromyographic motor Tinel's sign in ulnar mononeuropathies at the elbow. *Am J Phys Med Rehabil.* 1995;74(6):419–426.

322. Schmauss D, Pohlmann S, Lohmeyer JA, et al. Clinical tests and magnetic resonance imaging have limited diagnostic value for triangular fibrocartilaginous complex lesions. *Arch Orthop Trauma Surg.* 2016;136(6):873–880.

323. Bohannon RW, Andrews AW. Interrater reliability of hand-held dynamometry. *Phys Ther.* 1987;67:931–933.

324. Wadsworth CT, Krishnan R, Sear M, et al. Intrarater reliability of manual muscle testing in hand-held dynametric muscle testing. *Phys Ther.* 1987;7:1342–1347.

325. Rheault W, Beal JL, Kubic KR, et al. Intertester reliability of the hand-held dynamometer for wrist flexion and extension. *Arch Phys Med Rehabil.* 1989;70:907–910.

326. Goubau JF, Goubau L, Van Tongel A, et al. The wrist hyperflexion and abduction of the thumb test (WHAT): a more sensitive and specific test to diagnose de Quervain tenosynovitis than the Eichoff's test. *J Hand Surg Eur.* 2014;39(3):286–292.

CHAPTER 8

Thoracic (Dorsal) Spine

Assessment of the thoracic spine involves examination of the part of the spine that is most rigid because of the associated rib cage. The rib cage in turn provides protection for the heart, lungs, and other vital organs. Normally, the thoracic spine, being one of the primary curves, exhibits a mild **kyphosis** (posterior curvature); the cervical and lumbar sections, being secondary curves, exhibit a mild **lordosis** (anterior curvature). When the examiner assesses the thoracic spine, it is essential that the cervical and/or lumbar spines be evaluated at the same time (Fig. 8.1; see Fig. 3.7).

Because the spine and ribs protect vital organs (e.g., heart, lungs, and viscera), it is important that the examiner be able to differentiate problems with the vital organs (see Chapter 17) from mechanical problems occurring in the thoracic spine and ribs. These include cardiac, pulmonary, gastrointestinal, and renal problems. Finally, when assessing the thoracic spine, the examiner should be aware that movements in the shoulder may give the appearance of movement in the thoracic spine and vice versa, and that rib movement and pathology can affect shoulder movement.

Applied Anatomy

The **costovertebral joints** are synovial plane joints located between the ribs and the vertebral bodies (Fig. 8.2). There are 24 of these joints, and they are divided into two parts. Ribs 1, 10, 11, and 12 articulate with a single vertebra. The other articulations have no intra-articular ligament that divides the joint into two parts, so each of ribs 2 through 9 articulates with two adjacent vertebrae and the intervening intervertebral disc. The main ligament of the costovertebral joint is the radiate ligament, which joins the anterior aspect of the head of the rib radiating to the sides of the vertebral bodies and disc in between. For ribs 10, 11, and 12, it attaches only to the adjacent vertebral body. The intra-articular ligament divides the joint and attaches to the disc.

The **costotransverse joints** are synovial joints found between the ribs and the transverse processes of the vertebra of the same level for ribs 1 through 10 (see Fig. 8.2). Because ribs 11 and 12 do not articulate with the

transverse processes, this joint does not exist for these two levels. The costotransverse joints are supported by three ligaments. The superior costotransverse ligament runs from the lower border of the transverse process above to the upper border of the rib and its neck. The costotransverse ligament runs between the neck of the rib and the transverse process at the same level. The lateral costotransverse ligament runs from the tip of the transverse process to the adjacent rib.

The **costochondral joints** lie between the ribs and the costal cartilage (Fig. 8.3). The **sternocostal joints** are found between the costal cartilage and the sternum. Joints 2 through 6 are synovial, whereas the first costal cartilage is united with the sternum by a synchondrosis. Where a rib articulates with an adjacent rib or costal cartilage (ribs 5 through 9), a synovial interchondral joint exists.

As in the cervical and lumbar spines, the two **apophyseal** or **facet joints** (also called the **zygapophyseal joints**) make up the main trijoint complex along with the disc between the vertebrae. The superior facet of the T1 vertebra is similar to a facet of the cervical spine. Because of this, T1 is classified as a **transitional vertebra.** The superior facet faces up and back; the inferior facet faces down and forward. The T2 to T11 superior facets face up, back, and slightly laterally; the inferior facets face down, forward, and slightly medially changing from a 45° to 60° inclination (T2-T3) to 90° inclination (T4-T9) (Fig. 8.4). This shape enables slight rotation in the thoracic spine. In fact, the facet joints limit flexion and anterior translation and facilitate rotation.[1] Thoracic vertebrae T11 and T12 are classified as transitional, and the facets of these vertebrae become positioned in a way similar to those of the lumbar facets. The superior facets of these two vertebrae face up, back, and more medially; the inferior facets face forward and slightly laterally. The ligaments between the vertebral bodies include the ligamentum flavum, the anterior and posterior longitudinal ligaments, the interspinous and supraspinous ligaments, and the intertransverse ligament. These ligaments are found in the cervical, thoracic, and lumbar spine. The close packed position of the facet joints in the thoracic spine is extension.

Facet Joints of the Thoracic Spine

Resting position:	Midway between flexion and extension
Close packed position:	Full extension
Capsular pattern:	Side flexion and rotation equally limited, extension

Within the thoracic spine, there are 12 vertebrae, which diminish in size from T1 to T3 and then increase progressively in size to T12. These vertebrae are distinctive in having facets on the body and transverse processes for articulation with the ribs. The spinous processes of these vertebrae face obliquely downward (Fig. 8.5). T7 has the greatest spinous process angulation, whereas the upper three thoracic vertebrae have spinous processes that project directly posteriorly. In other words, the spinous process of these vertebrae is

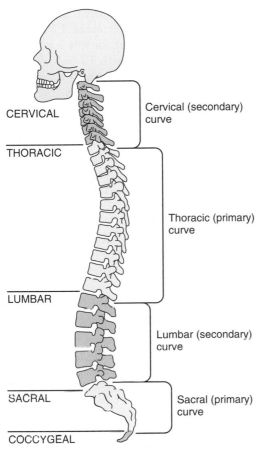

Fig. 8.1 The articulated spine.

CERVICAL — Cervical (secondary) curve

THORACIC — Thoracic (primary) curve

LUMBAR — Lumbar (secondary) curve

SACRAL — Sacral (primary) curve

COCCYGEAL

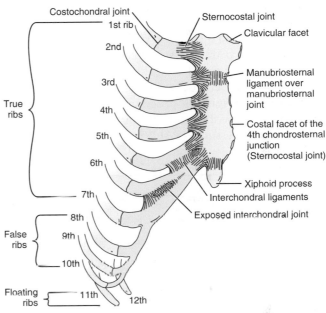

Fig. 8.3 Anterior view of the part of the thoracic wall highlights the manubriosternal joint, sternocostal joints with costochondral and chondrosternal joints, and interchondral joints. The ribs are removed on the left side to expose the costal facets. (Modified from Neumann DA: *Kinesiology of the musculoskeletal system—foundations for physical rehabilitation*, St. Louis, 2002, CV Mosby, p 370.)

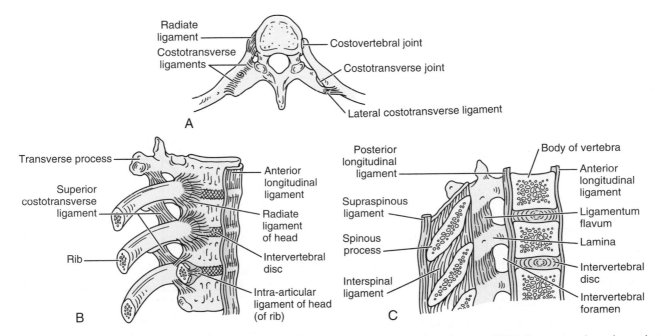

Fig. 8.2 Joints and ligaments of the thoracic vertebrae and ribs. (A) Superior view. (B) Anterolateral aspect. (C) Median section through vertebra.

on the same plane as the transverse processes of the same vertebrae.

T4 to T6 vertebrae have spinous processes that project downward slightly. In this case, the tips of the spinous processes are on a plane halfway between their own transverse processes and the transverse processes of the vertebrae below. For T7, T8, and T9 vertebrae, the spinous processes project downward, the tip of the spinous processes being on a plane of the transverse processes of the vertebrae below. For the T10 spinous process, the arrangement is similar to that of the T9 spinous process (i.e., the spinous process is level with the transverse process of the vertebra below). For T11, the arrangement is similar to that of T6 (i.e., the spinous process is halfway between the two transverse processes of the vertebra), and T12 is similar to T3 (i.e., the spinous process is level with the transverse process of the same vertebra). The location of the spinous processes becomes important if the examiner wishes to perform posteroanterior central vertebral pressures (PACVPs). For example, if the

examiner pushes on the spinous process of T8, the body of T9 also moves. In fact, the vertebral body of T8 probably arcs backward slightly, whereas T9 will move in an anterior direction. T7 is sometimes classified as a transitional vertebra, because it is the point at which the lower limb axial rotation alternates with the upper limb axial rotation (Fig. 8.6).

The ribs, which help to stiffen the thoracic spine, articulate with the demifacets on vertebrae T2 to T9. For T1 and T10, there is a whole facet for ribs 1 and 10, respectively. The first rib articulates with T1 only, the second rib articulates with T1 and T2, the third rib articulates with T2 and T3, and so on. Ribs 1 through 7 articulate with the sternum directly and are classified as **true ribs** (see Fig. 8.3). Ribs 8 through 10 join directly with the costocartilage of the rib above and are classified as **false ribs.** Ribs 11 and 12 are classified as **floating ribs** because they do not attach to either the sternum or the costal cartilage at their distal ends. Ribs 11 and 12 articulate only with the bodies of the T11 and T12 vertebrae, not with the transverse processes of the vertebrae nor with the costocartilage of the rib above. The ribs are held by ligaments to the body of the vertebra and to the transverse processes of the same vertebrae. Some of these ligaments also bind the rib to the vertebra above.

At the top of the rib cage, the ribs are relatively horizontal. As the rib cage descends, they run more and more obliquely downward. By the 12th rib, the ribs are more vertical than horizontal. With inspiration, the ribs are pulled up and forward; this increases the anteroposterior diameter of the ribs. The first six ribs increase the anteroposterior dimension of the chest, mainly by rotating around their long axes. Rotation downward of the rib neck is associated with depression, whereas rotation upward of the same portion is associated with elevation. These movements are known as a **pump handle action** and are accompanied by elevation of the manubrium sternum upward and forward (Fig. 8.7A).[2–4] Ribs 7 through 10 mainly increase in lateral,

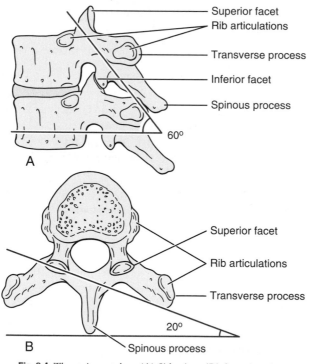

Fig. 8.4 Thoracic vertebra. (A) Side view. (B) Superior view.

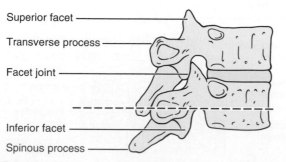

Fig. 8.5 Spinous process of one thoracic vertebra at level of body of vertebra below (T7–T9).

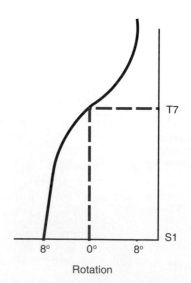

Fig. 8.6 Axial rotation of the spine going from left to right on heel strike.

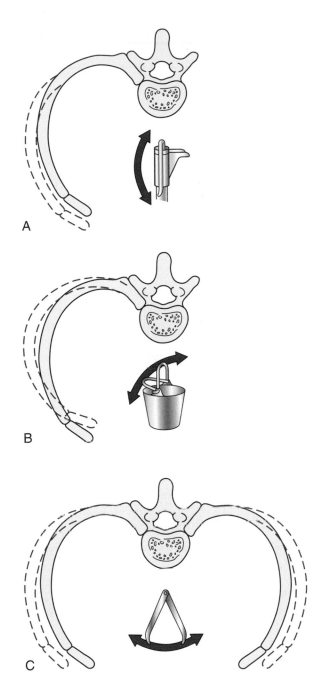

Fig. 8.7 Actions of the ribs. (A) Pump handle action (T1–T6). (B) Bucket-handle action (T7–T10). (C) Caliper action (T11–T12). (A and B, Modified from Williams P, Warwick R, editors: *Gray's anatomy*, ed 37, Edinburgh, 1989, Churchill Livingstone, p 498.)

or transverse, dimension. To accomplish this, the ribs move upward, backward, and medially to increase the infrasternal angle, or they move downward, forward, and laterally to decrease the angle. These movements are known as a **bucket-handle action.** This action is also performed by ribs 2 through 6 but to a much less degree (Fig. 8.7B). The lower ribs (ribs 8 through 12) move laterally, in what is known as a **caliper action,** to increase lateral diameter (Fig. 8.7C).[3] The ribs are quite elastic in children, but they become increasingly brittle with age. In the anterior half of the chest, the ribs are subcutaneous; in the posterior half, they are covered by muscles.

Patient History

A thorough and complete history should include past and present problems. By listening carefully, the examiner is often able to identify the patient's problem, develop a working diagnosis, and then use the observation and examination to confirm or refute the impressions established from the history. All information concerning the present pain and its site, nature, and behavior is important. If any part of the history implicates the cervical or lumbar spine, the examiner must include these areas in the assessment as well.

> **Clinical Note**
>
> In the thoracic spine, because of the many internal organs surrounded by the ribs and spine, the potential for red flags from other systemic problems (see Table 8.1) must always be kept in mind and cleared so that one is confident that he or she, as the examiner, is dealing with a musculoskeletal issue.[5] If not, consideration should be given to referral to the appropriate health care provider.[6]

In addition to the questions listed under the "Patient History" section in Chapter 1, the examiner should obtain the following information from the patient:

1. *What are the patient's age and occupation?* For example, conditions such as Scheuermann's disease typically occur in young people between 13 and 16 years of age. Idiopathic scoliosis is most commonly seen in adolescent females.

2. *What was the mechanism of injury?* Most commonly, rib injuries are caused by trauma. Thoracic spine problems may result from disease processes (e.g., scoliosis) and may have an insidious onset. Pain from true thoracic trauma tends to be localized to the area of injury. Facet syndromes present as stiffness and local pain, which can be referred.[7,8]

3. *What are the details of the present pain and other symptoms? What are the sites and boundaries of the pain?* Have the patient point to the location or locations. Is one spot picked or does the patient identify an area? Is there any radiation of pain? Is the pain present at night, at rest, with activity?[5] The examiner should remember that many of the abdominal structures, such as the stomach, liver, and pancreas, may refer pain to the thoracic region (see Tables 8.1 and 8.2 for thoracic spine and rib cage red flags and chest pain patterns). It should be remembered that thoracic spine pain and visceral pain can mimic each other. With thoracic disc lesions, because of the rigidity of the thoracic spine, active movements do not often show the characteristic pain pattern, and sensory and strength deficits are difficult if not impossible to detect.[9] Thoracic root involvement or spondylosis usually causes pain that follows the path of the ribs or a deep, "through-the-chest" pain. Costovertebral, and costotransverse joints, and ribs commonly refer pain

▼ TABLE **8.1**

Thoracic Spine and Rib Cage Red Flags

Condition	Red Flags
Myocardial infarction	Chest pain Pallor, sweating, dyspnea, nausea, or palpitations Presence of risk factors: previous history of coronary heart disease, hypertension, smoking, diabetes, and elevated blood serum cholesterol (>240 mg/dL) Men aged over 40 years and women aged over 50 years Symptoms lasting greater than 30 minutes and not relieved with sublingual nitroglycerin
Stable angina pectoris	Chest pain or pressure that occurs with predictable levels of exertion (if not, suspect unstable angina pectoris) Symptoms are also predictably alleviated with the rest or sublingual nitroglycerin (if not, suspect unstable angina pectoris)
Pericarditis	Sharp or stabbing chest pain that may be referred to the lateral neck or either shoulder Increased pain with left side lying Relieved with forward lean while sitting (supporting arms on knees or a table)
Pulmonary embolus	Chest, shoulder, or upper abdominal pain Dyspnea
Pleurisy	Severe, sharp knife-like pain with inspiration History of a recent or coexisting respiratory disorder (e.g., infection, pneumonia, tumor, or tuberculosis)
Pneumothorax	Chest pain that is intensified with inspiration, ventilation, or expanding rib cage Recent bout of coughing or strenuous exercise or trauma Hyperresonance upon percussion Decreased breath sounds
Pneumonia	Pleuritic pain that may be referred to shoulder Fever, chills, headache, malaise, or nausea Productive cough
Cholecystitis	Colicky pain in the right upper abdominal quadrant with accompanying right scapula pain Symptoms may worsen with ingestion of fatty foods Symptoms unaffected by activity or rest
Peptic ulcer	Dull, gnawing pain, or burning sensation in the epigastrium, mid back, or supraclavicular regions Symptoms relieved with food Localized tenderness at the right epigastrium Constipation, bleeding, vomiting, tarry colored stools, and coffee ground emeses
Pyelonephritis	Recent or coexisting urinary tract infection Enlarged prostate Kidney stone or past kidney stone
Nephrolithiasis (kidney stones)	Sudden, severe back or flank pain Chills and fever Nausea or vomiting Renal colic Symptoms of urinary tract infection Reside in hot and humid environment Past episode(s) of kidney stone(s)

From Dutton M: *Dutton's orthopedic examination, evaluation and intervention*, ed 3, New York, 2012, McGraw Hill, p 1247.

along the rib. Progressive abdominal pain preceding nausea, vomiting, diarrhea, fever, and loss of appetite in children is suggestive of acute appendicitis.[6] There may also be localized tenderness on the right side, muscle guarding, tachycardia, and rebound tenderness.[6]

4. *Does the pain occur on inspiration, expiration, or both?* Pain related to breathing may signal pulmonary problems or may be related to movement of the ribs. Pain referred around the chest wall tends to be costovertebral in origin. Does the patient have any difficulty in breathing? If a breathing problem exists, it may be caused by a structural deformity (e.g., scoliosis); thoracic trauma, such as disc lesions, fractures, or contusions; or thoracic pathology, such as pneumothorax, pleurisy, tumors, or pericarditis.

▼ TABLE **8.2**

▼ **Chest Pain Patterns**

Origin of Pain	Site of Referred Pain	Type of Disorder
Substernal or retrosternal	Neck, jaw, back, left shoulder and arm, and abdomen	Angina
Substernal, anterior chest	Neck, jaw, back, and bilateral arms	Myocardial infarction
Substernal or above the sternum	Neck, upper back, upper trapezius, supraclavicular area, left arm, and costal margin	Pericarditis
Anterior chest (thoracic aneurysm); abdomen (abdominal aneurysm)	Posterior thoracic, chest, neck, shoulders, interscapular, or lumbar region	Dissecting aortic aneurysm
Variable	Variable, depending on structures involved	Musculoskeletal
Costochondritis (inflammation of the costal cartilage): sternum and rib margins	Abdominal oblique trigger points: pain referred up into the chest area	
Upper rectus abdominis trigger points (left side), pectoralis, serratus anterior, and sternalis muscles: precordial pain	Pectoralis trigger points: pain referred down medial bilateral arms along ulnar nerve distribution (fourth and fifth fingers)	
Precordium region (upper central abdomen and diaphragm)	Sternum, axillary lines, and either side of vertebrae; lateral and anterior chest wall; occasionally to one or both arms	Neurological
Substernal, epigastric, and upper abdominal quadrants	Around chest area, shoulders, and upper back region	Gastrointestinal
Within breast tissue; may be localized in pectoral and supraclavicular regions	Chest area, axilla, mid back, and neck, and posterior shoulder girdle	Breast pain
Commonly substernal and anterior chest region	No referred pain	Anxiety

From Dutton M: *Dutton's orthopedic examination, evaluation and intervention*, ed 3, New York, 2012, McGraw Hill, p 1246.

5. *Is the pain deep, superficial, shooting, burning, or aching?* Thoracic nerve root pain is often severe and is referred in a sloping band along an intercostal space. Pain between the scapulae may be the result of a cervical lesion. It has been reported that any symptoms above a line joining the inferior angles of the scapula should be considered of cervical origin until proven otherwise, especially if there is no history of trauma.[10]

6. *Is the pain affected by coughing, sneezing, or straining?* Dural pain is often accentuated by these maneuvers.

7. *Which activities aggravate the problem?* Active use of the arms sometimes irritates a thoracic lesion. Pulling and pushing activities can be especially bothersome to a patient with thoracic problems. Costal pain is often elicited by breathing and/or overhand arm motion.

8. *Which activities ease the problem?* For example, bracing the arms often makes breathing easier because this facilitates the action of the accessory muscles of respiration.

9. *Is the condition improving, becoming worse, or staying the same?*

10. *Does any particular posture bother the patient?* Can the patient comfortably lie supine? Prone? On side? Sit? Stand? Pathology in the thoracic spine often does not enable the patient to assume different postures comfortably. For example, sitting upright into full extension may be painful for those with facet pathology; forward flexed postures may be painful in those with anterior vertebral compression fractures and could add to the deformity.

11. *Is there any paresthesia or other abnormal sensation that may indicate a disc lesion or radiculopathy?*

12. *Are the patient's symptoms referred to the legs, arms, or head and neck?* If so, it is imperative that the examiner assess these areas as well. For example, shoulder movements may be restricted with thoracic spine or rib problems. Any positive responses to this question may indicate a neurological exam going over sensory testing, nerve root testing, neurological screening, and upper motor neuron reflexes is also necessary.

13. *Does the patient have any problems with digestion?* Pain may be referred to the thoracic spine or ribs from pathological conditions within the thorax or abdomen. Visceral pain tends to be vague, dull, and indiscrete and may be accompanied by nausea and sweating. It tends to follow dermatome patterns in its referral. For example, cardiac pain is referred to the shoulder (C4) and posteriorly to T2. Stomach

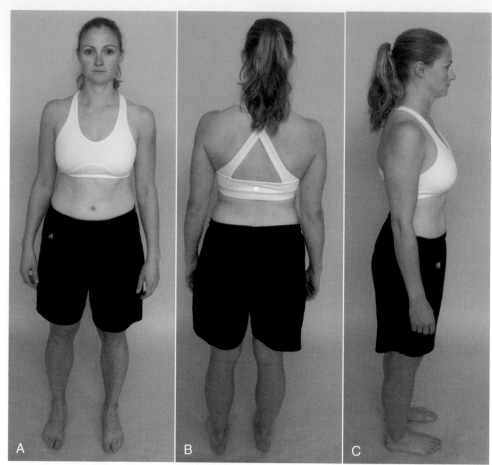

Fig. 8.8 Normal posture. (A) Front view. (B) Posterior view. (C) Side view.

pain is referred to T6–T8 posteriorly. Ulcers may be referred to T4–T6 posteriorly.[7]

14. *Is the skin in the thorax area normal?* Conditions, such as herpes zoster, can cause unilateral, spontaneous pain. In the observation, the examiner should watch for erythema and grouped vesicles.[9]

15. *Have there been previous examinations for other systemic problems?* Does the patient have a history of heart problems? High blood pressure? Diabetes? Fever? Being bedridden? Difficulty breathing? Receiving a blow to the chest? All these questions are related to possible problems beyond the musculoskeletal system.

Observation

The patient must be suitably undressed so that the body is exposed as much as possible. In the case of a female, the bra is often removed to provide a better view of the spine and rib cage. The patient is usually observed first standing and then sitting.

As with any observation, the examiner should note any alteration in the overall spinal posture (see Chapter 15), because it may lead to problems in the thoracic spine. It is important to observe the total body posture from the head to the toes and look for any deviation from normal (Fig. 8.8). Thus one looks for symmetry in the spinal curves and any compensation, any deviations, shoulder and pelvic levels, scapular position, limb position, muscle bulk and tone, gait, weight transfer when moving, and motion patterns (e.g., lifting arms over head, sit to stand, side lying to sitting). Posteriorly, the medial edge of the spine of the scapula should be level with the T3 spinous process, whereas the inferior angle of the scapula is level with the T7–T9 spinous process, depending on the size of the scapula. The medial border of the scapula is parallel to the spine and approximately 5 cm lateral to the spinous processes.

Kyphosis

Kyphosis is a condition that is most prevalent in the thoracic spine (Fig. 8.9). The examiner must ensure that a kyphosis is actually present, remembering that a slight kyphosis, or posterior curvature, is normal and is found in every individual. Normal kyphosis in the thoracic spine is 20° to 40° and will depend on age (increases) and sex, although the actual degrees has been questioned.[11] Hyperkyphosis is a kyphotic angle of greater than 40°

commonly measured by the Cobb method (see Fig. 8.70) on a lateral x-ray measuring between T4 and T12.[12] After age 40, the thoracic kyphosis tends to increase and the increase is higher in females.[11,12] In addition, some people have "flat" scapulae, which give the appearance of an

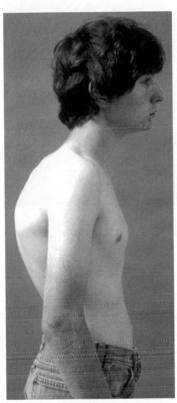

Fig. 8.9 A 16-year-old boy with 70° kyphosis and midthoracic pain. (From Johnston CE: Kyphosis. In Herring JA, editor: *Tachdjian's pediatric orthopaedics*, ed 5, Philadelphia, 2014, Saunders.)

excessive kyphosis, as does winging of the scapulae. The examiner must ensure that it is actually the spine that has the excessive curvature. Types of kyphotic deformities are shown in Fig. 8.10 and listed as follows[13]:

1. **Round back** is decreased pelvic inclination (20°) with a thoracolumbar or thoracic kyphosis (Fig. 8.11). Most forms of kyphosis seen show a decreased pelvic inclination. To compensate and maintain the body's center of gravity a structural kyphosis, usually caused by tight soft tissues from prolonged postural change or by a growth disturbance, results, causing a round back deformity.

2. **Scheuermann's disease** is the most common structural kyphosis in adolescents but can occur in adults. Its etiology is unknown.[14]

3. **Hump back** is a localized, sharp, posterior angulation called a **gibbus**.[12] This kyphotic deformity is usually structural and often results from an anterior wedging of the body of one or two thoracic vertebrae. The wedging may be caused by a compression fracture, tumor, or bone disease. The pelvic inclination is usually normal (30°).

4. **Flat back** is decreased pelvic inclination (20°) with a mobile spine. This kyphotic deformity is similar to round back, except that the thoracic spine remains mobile and is able to compensate throughout its length for the altered center of gravity caused by the decreased pelvic inclination. Therefore, although a kyphosis is or should be present, it does not have the appearance of an excessive kyphotic curve.

5. **Dowager's hump**[12] results from postmenopausal osteoporosis. Because of the osteoporosis, anterior wedge fractures occur to several vertebrae, usually in the upper to middle thoracic spine, causing a structural scoliosis that also contributes to a decrease in height.

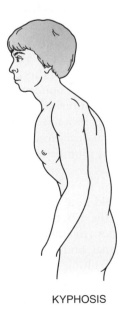
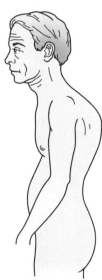
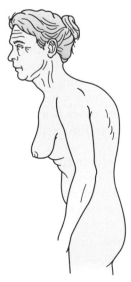

KYPHOSIS   GIBBUS   DOWAGER'S HUMP

Fig. 8.10 Kyphotic deformities.

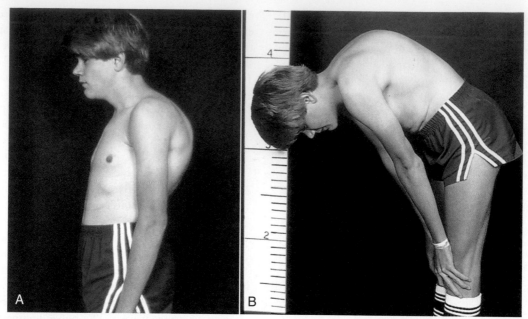

Fig. 8.11 (A) Severe kyphosis of the thoracic spine secondary to vertebral wedging in a patient with glycogen storage disease. To stand upright, the patient must increase his lumbar lordosis and thrust his head forward to center it above the pelvis. (B) The kyphotic deformity is accentuated on forward bending. (From Deeney VF, Arnold J: Orthopedics. In Zitelli BJ, McIntire SC, Nowalk AJ, editors: *Zitelli and Davis' atlas of pediatric physical diagnosis*, ed 7, Philadelphia, 2018, Elsevier.)

Scoliosis

Scoliosis is a deformity in which there are one or more lateral curvatures of the lumbar or thoracic spine; it is this spinal deformity that was suffered by the "Hunchback of Notre Dame." (In the cervical spine, the condition is called **torticollis.**) The curvature may occur in the thoracic spine alone, in the thoracolumbar area, or in the lumbar spine alone (Fig. 8.12). Scoliosis may be nonstructural (i.e., relatively easily correctable once the cause is determined) or structural. Poor posture, hysteria, nerve root irritation, inflammation in the spine area, leg length discrepancy, or hip contracture can cause nonstructural scoliosis. Structural changes may be genetic, idiopathic, or caused by some congenital problem, such as a wedge vertebra, hemivertebra, or failure of vertebral segmentation. In other words, there is a structural change in the bone, and normal flexibility of the spine is lost.[15]

A number of curve patterns may be present with scoliosis (Fig. 8.13).[15] The curve patterns are designated according to the level of the apex of the curve (Table 8.3). A right thoracic curve has a convexity toward the right, and the apex of the curve is in the thoracic spine. With a cervical scoliosis, or torticollis, the apex is between C1 and C6. For a cervicothoracic curve, the apex is at C7 or T1. For a thoracic curve, the apex is between T2 and T11. The thoracolumbar curve has its apex at T12 or L1. The lumbar curve has an apex between L2 and

L4, and a lumbosacral scoliosis has an apex at L5 or S1. The involvement of the thoracic spine results in a very poor cosmetic appearance or greater visual defect as a result of deformation of the ribs along with the spine. The deformity can vary from a mild rib hump to a severe rotation of the vertebrae, causing a rib deformity called a **razorback spine.**

With a structural scoliosis, the vertebral bodies rotate to the convexity of the curve and become distorted.[16] If the thoracic spine is involved, this rotation causes the ribs on the convex side of the curve to push posteriorly, causing a rib "hump" and narrowing the thoracic cage on the convex side. As the vertebral body rotates to the convex side of the curve, the spinous process deviates toward the concave side. The ribs on the concave side move anteriorly, causing a "hollow" and a widening of the thoracic cage on the concave side (Fig. 8.14). Lateral deviation may be more evident if the examiner uses a plumb bob (plumb line) from the C7 spinous process or external occipital protuberance (Fig. 8.15).

The examiner should note whether the ribs are symmetric and whether the rib contours are normal and equal on the two sides. In idiopathic scoliosis, the rib contours are not normal, and there is asymmetry of the ribs. Muscle spasm resulting from injury may also be evident. The bony and soft-tissue contours should be observed for equality on both sides or for any noticeable difference.

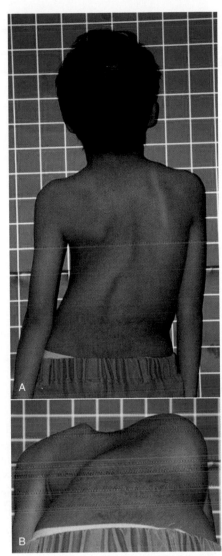

Fig. 8.12 Idiopathic scoliosis. (A) Postural deformity caused by idiopathic thoracolumbar scoliosis. (B) Asymmetry of posterior thorax accentuated with patient flexed. Note "hump" on the right and "hollow" on the left. (From Zhou C, Liu L, Song Y et al: Two-stage vertebral column resection for severe and rigid scoliosis in patients with low body weight, *Spine J* 13[5]:481-486, 2013.)

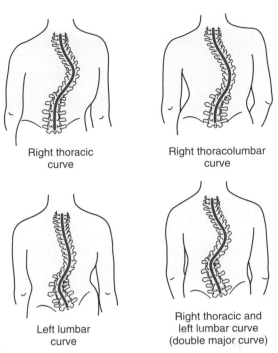

Fig. 8.13 Examples of scoliosis curve patterns.

The examiner should note whether the patient sits up properly with the normal spinal curves present (Fig. 8.16A); whether the tip of the ear, tip of the acromion process, and high point of the iliac crest are in a straight line as they should be; and whether the patient sits in a slumped position (i.e., sag sitting, as in Fig. 8.16B).

The skin should be observed for any abnormality or scars (Fig. 8.17). If there are scars, are they a result of surgery or trauma? Are they new or old scars? If from surgery, what was the purpose of the surgery?

Breathing

As part of the observation, the examiner should note the patient's breathing pattern. Children tend to breathe abdominally, whereas women tend to do upper thoracic breathing. Men tend to be upper and lower thoracic breathers. In the aged, breathing tends to be in the lower thoracic and abdominal regions (Fig. 8.18). The examiner should note the quality of the respiratory movements as well as the rate, rhythm, and effort required to inhale and exhale. The examiner should also note whether the patient is using the primary muscles of respiration and/or the accessory muscles of respiration, because this will help to indicate the ease of the patient's breathing (Table 8.4). In addition, the presence of any coughing or noisy or abnormal breathing patterns should be noted. Because the chest wall movement that occurs during breathing displaces the pleural surfaces, thoracic muscles, nerve and ribs, pain is accentuated by breathing and coughing if any one of these structures is injured.

Chest Deformities

In addition to rib movements during breathing, the examiner should note the presence of any chest deformities. The more common deformities are shown in Fig. 8.19 and are listed as follows:

1. With a **pigeon chest** (pectus carinatum) deformity, the sternum projects forward and downward like the

TABLE **8.3**

Curve Patterns and Prognosis in Idiopathic Scoliosis

	CURVE PATTERN				
	Primary Lumbar	**Thoracolumbar**	**Combined Thoracic and Lumbar**	**Primary Thoracic**	**Cervicothoracic**
Incidence (%)	23.6	16	37	22.1	31.3
Average age curve noted (year)	13.25	14	12.3	11.1	15.3
Average age curve stabilized (year)	14.5	16	15.5	16.1	16.3
Extent of curve	T11–L3	T6 or T7–L1 or L1, L2	Thoracic, T6–T10 Lumbar, T11–L4	T6–T11	C7 or T1–T4 or T5
Apex of curve	L1 or L2	T11 or L2	Thoracic, T7 or T8 Lumbar, L2	T8 or T9 (rotation extreme, convexity usually to right)	T3
Average angular value at maturity (degrees) Standing	36.8	42.7	Thoracic, 51.9; lumbar, 41.4	81.4	34.6
Supine	29.1	35	Thoracic, 41.4; lumbar, 37.7	73.8	32.2
Prognosis	Most benign and least deforming of all idiopathic curves	Not severely deforming Intermediate between thoracic and lumbar curves	Good Body usually well aligned, curves even if severe tend to compensate each other High percentage of very severe scoliosis if onset before age of 10 years	Worst Progresses more rapidly, becomes more severe, and produces greater clinical deformity than any other pattern Five years of active growth during which curve could increase	Deformity unsightly Poorly disguised because of high shoulder, elevated scapula, and deformed thoracic cage

Adapted from Ponseti IV, Friedman B: Prognosis in idiopathic scoliosis. *J Bone Joint Surg Am* 32(2):381–395, 1950.

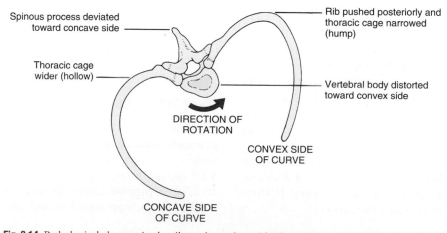

Fig. 8.14 Pathological changes in the ribs and vertebra with idiopathic scoliosis in the thoracic spine.

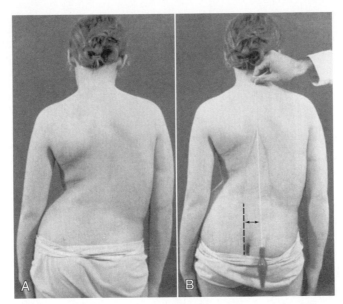

Fig. 8.15 Right thoracic idiopathic scoliosis (posterior view). (A) The left shoulder is lower, and the right scapula is more prominent. Note the decreased distance between the right arm and the thorax with the shift of the thorax to the right. The left iliac crest appears higher, but this results from the shift of the thorax with fullness on the right and elimination of the waistline; the "high" hip is only apparent, not real. (B) Plumb line dropped from the prominent vertebra of C7 (vertebra prominens) measures the decompensation of the thorax over the pelvis. The distance from the vertical plumb line to the gluteal cleft is measured in centimeters and is recorded along with the direction of deviation. If there is a cervical or cervicothoracic curve, the plumb should fall from the occipital protuberance (inion). (From Moe JH, Winter RB, Bradford DS, et al: *Scoliosis and other spinal deformities*, Philadelphia, 1978, WB Saunders, p 14.)

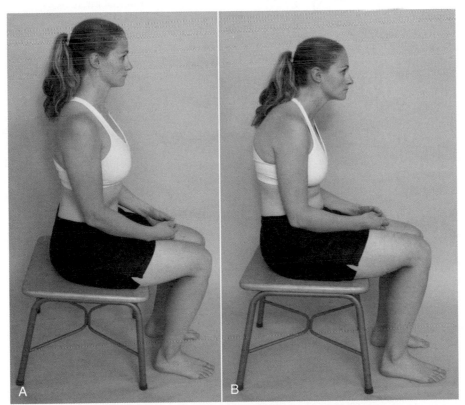

Fig. 8.16 Sitting posture. (A) Normal position. (B) Sag sitting.

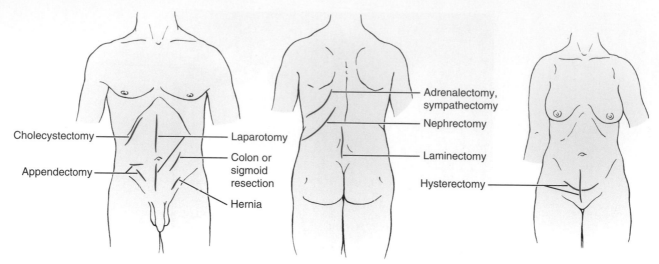

Fig. 8.17 Common surgical scars of the abdomen and thorax. (Redrawn from Judge RD, Zuidema GD, Fitzgerald FT: *Clinical diagnosis: a physiologic approach*, Boston, 1982, Little Brown, p 295.)

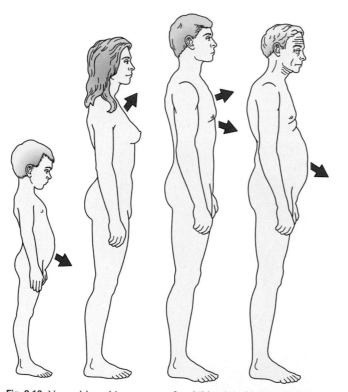

Fig. 8.18 Normal breathing patterns for child, adult female, adult male, and elderly person.

TABLE 8.4

Muscles of Respiration

	Primary	Secondary
Inspiration	Diaphragm Levator costorum External intercostals Internal intercostals (anterior)	Scaleni Sternocleidomastoid Trapezius Serratus anterior and posterior Pectoralis major Pectoralis minor Subclavius
Both		Latissimus dorsi
Expiration	Internal obliques External obliques Rectus abdominis Transverse abdominis Transversus thoracis Transverse intercostals Internal intercostals (posterior)	Serratus posterior inferior Quadratus lumborum Iliocostalis lumborum

heel of a boot, increasing the anteroposterior dimension of the chest. This congenital deformity impairs the effectiveness of breathing by restricting ventilation volume.

2. The **funnel chest** (pectus excavatum) is a congenital deformity that results from the sternum's being pushed posteriorly by an overgrowth of the ribs.[17] The anteroposterior dimension of the chest is decreased, and the heart may be displaced. On inspiration, this deformity causes a depression of the sternum that affects respiration and may result in kyphosis.

3. With the **barrel chest** deformity, the sternum projects forward and upward so that the anteroposterior diameter is increased. It is seen in pathological conditions, such as emphysema.

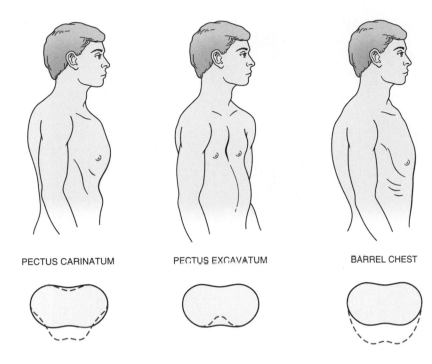

PECTUS CARINATUM   PECTUS EXCAVATUM   BARREL CHEST

Fig. 8.19 Chest deformities. Lower vertical views show change in chest wall contours with deformity.

Examination

Although the assessment is primarily of the thorax and thoracic spine, if the history, observation, or examination indicates symptoms into or from the neck, upper limb, or lumbar spine and lower limb, these structures must be examined as well using an upper or lower scanning examination. If any signs or symptoms are elicited in the scanning exam, more detailed examination of the cervical or lumbar spine may be performed. Therefore the examination of the thoracic spine may be an extensive one. Unless there is a history of specific trauma or injury to the thoracic spine or ribs, the examiner must be prepared to assess more than that area alone. If a problem is suspected above the thoracic spine, the scanning examination of the cervical spine and upper limb (as described in Chapter 3) should be performed. If a problem is suspected below the thoracic spine, the scanning examination of the lumbar spine (as described in Chapter 9), lower limb especially the hip (Chapter 11) and pelvis (Chapter 10), and shoulder (Chapter 5) should be performed. Added to this is the potential of issues with the other "systems" protected by the thoracic spine and rib cage. Only examination of the thoracic spine is described here.

Active Movements

The active movements of the thoracic spine are usually done with the patient standing. Movement in the thoracic spine is limited by the rib cage and the long spinous processes of the thoracic spine. When assessing the thoracic spine, the examiner should be sure to note whether the movement occurs in the spine or in the hips. A patient can touch the toes with a completely rigid spine if there is sufficient range of motion (ROM) in the hip joints. Likewise, tight hamstrings may alter the results. The movements may be done with the patient sitting, in which case the effect of hip movement is eliminated or decreased. Similarly, shoulder motion may be restricted if the upper thoracic segments or ribs are hypomobile.[1] As with any examination, the most painful movements are done last. The active movements to be carried out in the thoracic spine are shown in Fig. 8.20.

Active Movements of the Thoracic Spine

- Forward flexion (20°–45°)
- Extension (25°–45°)
- Side flexion, left and right (20°–40°)
- Rotation, left and right (35°–50°)
- Costovertebral expansion (3–7.5 cm)
- Rib motion (pump handle, bucket handle, and caliper)
- Combined movements (if necessary)
- Repetitive movements (if necessary)
- Sustained postures (if necessary)

Forward Flexion

The normal ROM of forward flexion (forward bending) in the thoracic spine is 20° to 45° (Fig. 8.21). Because the ROM at each vertebra is difficult to measure, the examiner can use a tape measure to derive an indication of overall movement (Fig. 8.22). The examiner first measures the length of the spine from the C7 spinous process to the T12 spinous process with the patient in the

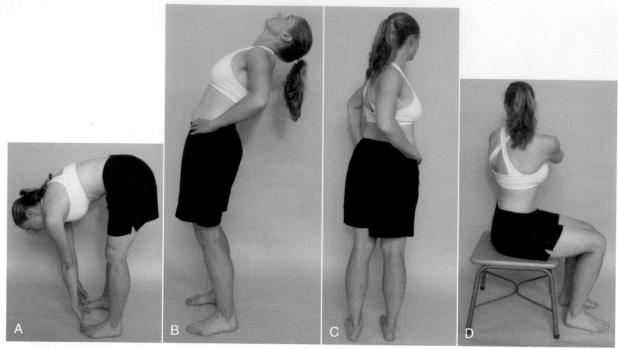

Fig. 8.20 Active movements. (A) Forward flexion. (B) Extension. (C) Rotation (standing). (D) Rotation (sitting).

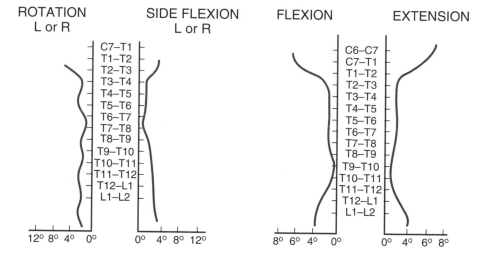

Fig. 8.21 Average range of motion in the thoracic spine. (Adapted from Grieve GP: *Common vertebral joint problems*, Edinburgh, 1981, Churchill Livingstone, pp 41–42.)

ROTATION L or R — C7–T1, T1–T2, T2–T3, T3–T4, T4–T5, T5–T6, T6–T7, T7–T8, T8–T9, T9–T10, T10–T11, T11–T12, T12–L1, L1–L2 — 12° 8° 4° 0°

SIDE FLEXION L or R — 0° 4° 8° 12°

FLEXION — C6–C7, C7–T1, T1–T2, T2–T3, T3–T4, T4–T5, T5–T6, T6–T7, T7–T8, T8–T9, T9–T10, T10–T11, T11–T12, T12–L1, L1–L2 — 8° 6° 4° 0°

EXTENSION — 0° 4° 6° 8°

normal standing posture. The patient is then asked to bend forward, and the spine is again measured. A 2.7-cm (1.1-inch) difference in tape measure length is considered normal.

If the examiner wishes, the spine may be measured from the C7 to S1 spinous process with the patient in the normal standing position. The patient is then asked to bend forward, and the spine is again measured. A 10-cm (4-inch) difference in tape measure length is considered normal. In this case, the examiner is measuring movement in the lumbar spine as well as in the thoracic spine; most movement, approximately 7.5 cm (3 inches), occurs between T12 and S1.

A third method of measuring spinal flexion is to ask the patient to bend forward and try to touch the toes while keeping the knees straight. The examiner then measures from the fingertips to the floor and records the distance. The examiner must keep in mind that with this method, in addition to the thoracic spine movement, the movement may also occur in the lumbar spine and hips; in fact, movement could occur totally in the hips.

Each of these methods is indirect. To measure the ROM at each vertebral segment, a series of radiographs would be necessary. The examiner can decide which method to use. However, it is of primary importance to note on the patient's chart how the measuring was done and which reference points were used.

While the patient is flexed forward, the examiner can observe the spine from the "skyline" view (Fig. 8.23). With nonstructural scoliosis, the scoliotic curve disappears on forward flexion; with structural scoliosis, it remains. With the skyline view, the examiner is looking for a hump on one side (convex side of curve) and a hollow (concave side of curve) on the other. This "hump and hollow" sequence is caused by vertebral rotation in idiopathic scoliosis, which pushes the ribs and muscles out on one side and causes the paravertebral valley on the opposite side. The vertebral rotation is most evident in the flexed position.

When the patient flexes forward, the thoracic spine should curve forward in a smooth, even manner with no rotation or side flexion (Fig. 8.24). The examiner should look for any apparent tightness or sharp angulation, such as a gibbus, when the movement is performed. If the patient has an excessive kyphosis to begin with, very little forward flexion movement occurs in the thoracic spine. McKenzie[10] advocates doing flexion while sitting to decrease pelvic and hip movements. The patient then slouches forward flexing the thoracic

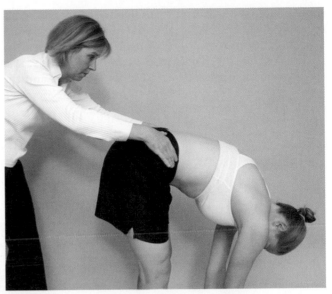

Fig. 8.23 Examiner performing skyline view of spine for assessment of scoliosis.

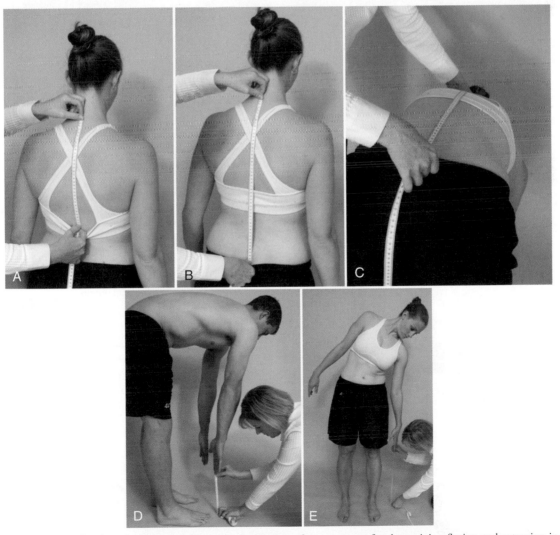

Fig. 8.22 Tape measurements for thoracic spine movement. (A) Positioning of tape measure for determining flexion and extension in the thoracic spine. (B) Positioning of tape measure for determining flexion or extension in the thoracic and lumbar spines combined. (C) Forward flexion measurement of thoracic and lumbar spines. (D) Forward flexion measurement of thoracic and lumbar spines and hips (fingertips to floor). (E) Side flexion measurement (fingertips to floor).

spine. The patient can put the hands around the neck to apply overpressure at the end of flexion. If symptoms arise from forward flexion on the spine with the neck flexed by the hands, the examiner should repeat the movement with the neck slightly extended and the hands removed. This will help to differentiate between cervical and thoracic pain.

During flexion and extension of the thoracic spine, the facet joints and ribs also move. During flexion, the ribs roll forward, their anterior aspect drops, and the facet joints glide superiorly (Fig. 8.25A). During extension, the opposite occurs with the ribs rolling backward, their anterior aspect elevates, and the facet joints glide inferiorly (Fig. 8.25B).[18]

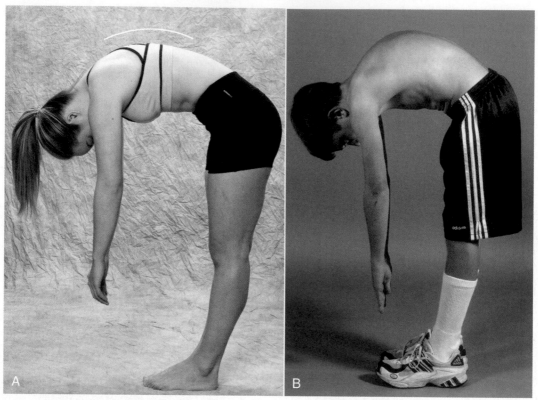

Fig. 8.24 Side view in forward bending position for assessment of kyphosis. (A) Normal thoracic roundness is demonstrated with a gentle curve to the whole spine. (B) Limited forward bending with increased kyphosis in a boy with juvenile ankylosing spondylitis. (B, From Herring JA: Arthritis. In Herring JA, editor: *Tachdjian's pediatric orthopaedics*, ed 5, Philadelphia, 2014, Saunders.)

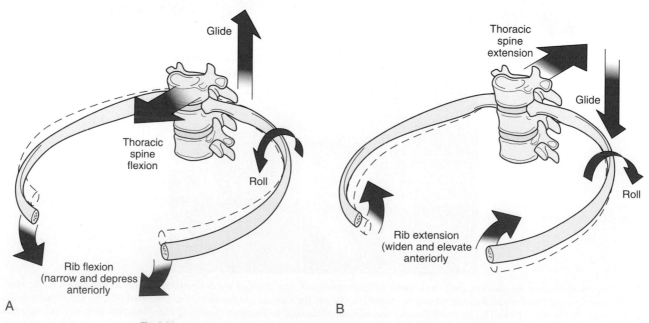

Fig. 8.25 Movement of ribs and facet joints during (A) flexion and (B) extension.

Extension

Extension (backward bending) in the thoracic spine is normally 25° to 45°. At a minimum, the normal kyphotic posture of the thoracic spine should disappear on active and passive extension with the spine becoming straight. If it does not, then there is hypomobility in one or more segments. Because this movement occurs over 12 vertebrae, the movement between the individual vertebrae is difficult to detect visually. As with flexion, the examiner can use a tape measure and obtain the distance between the same two points (the C7 and T12 spinous processes). Again, a 2.5-cm (1-inch) difference in tape measure length between standing and extension is considered normal. McKenzie[10] advocated having the patient place the hands in the small of the back to add stability while performing the backward movement or to do extension while sitting or prone lying (sphinx position).

As the patient extends, the thoracic curve should curve backward or at least straighten in a smooth, even manner

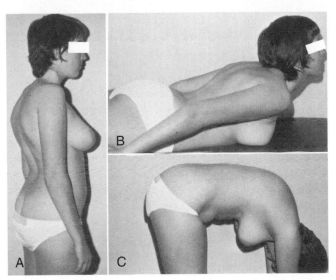

Fig. 8.26 Kyphosis and lordosis. (A) On physical examination, definite increases in thoracic kyphosis and lumbar lordosis are visualized. (B) Thoracic kyphosis does not fully correct on thoracic extension. (C) Lumbar lordosis, on the other hand, usually corrects on forward bending; in this case, some lordosis remains. (From Moe JH, Winter RB, Bradford DS, et al: *Scoliosis and other spinal deformities*, Philadelphia, 1978, WB Saunders, p 339.)

with no rotation or side flexion. Lee[19] advocates asking the patient to fully forward flex the arms during extension to facilitate extension. The examiner should look for any apparent tightness or angulation when the movement is performed. If the patient shows excessive kyphosis (Fig. 8.26), the kyphotic curvature remains on extension; that is, the thoracic spine remains flexed, whether the movement is tested while the patient is standing or lying prone (see Fig. 8.26).

If extension is tested in prone lying, the normal thoracic kyphosis should, for the most part, disappear. If there is a structural kyphosis, the kyphotic curve will remain on extension. McKenzie[10] advocated doing prone extension by using a modified push-up straightening the arms and allowing the spine to "sag down" toward the bed (Fig. 8.27).

Side Flexion

Side (lateral) flexion is approximately 20° to 40° to the right and left in the thoracic spine. The patient is asked to run the hand down the side of the leg as far as possible without bending forward or backward. The examiner can then estimate the angle of side flexion or use a tape measure to determine the length from the fingertips to the floor and compare it with that of the other side (see Fig. 8.22E). Normally, the distances should be equal. In either case, the examiner must remember that movement in the lumbar spine as well as in the thoracic spine is being measured. As the patient bends sideways, the spine should curve sideways in a smooth, even, sequential manner. The examiner should look for any tightness or abnormal angulation, which may indicate hypomobility or hypermobility at a specific segment when the movement is performed. If, on side flexion, the ipsilateral paraspinal muscles tighten or their contracture is evident (**Forestier's bowstring sign**), ankylosing spondylitis or pathology causing muscle spasm should be considered.[20] In reality, side flexion cannot occur without rotation so both occur together (called rotation by some) and in the same direction, especially as one nears and reaches end range.[21]

Rotation

Rotation in the thoracic spine is approximately 35° to 50° and is the primary movement in the thoracic spine.[22] The patient is asked to cross the arms in front or place

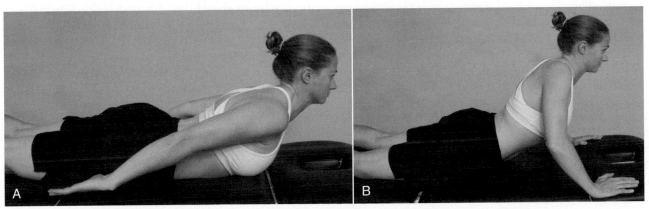

Fig. 8.27 Thoracic extension in prone lying. (A) Prone extension. (B) McKenzie prone extension.

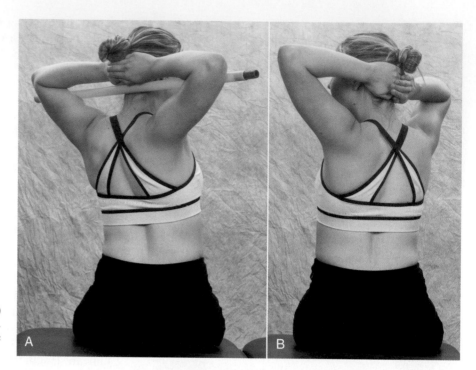

Fig. 8.28 Trunk (thoracic spine) rotation. (A) Using a pole to eliminate shoulder movement. (B) Placing hands behind head to eliminate shoulder movement.

the hands on opposite shoulders and then rotate to the right and left while the examiner looks at the amount of rotation, comparing both ways. The examiner must also ensure that the patient does not add shoulder movement (i.e., protraction of the scapula on one side, retraction on the other side) to give the appearance of more rotation in the thoracic spine. It has been advocated that the patient, while seated, hold a pole or bar across the shoulders held by the arms when doing the rotation (Fig. 8.28A) or place the hands behind the head (Fig. 8.28B). This eliminates shoulder movement which could potentially give the appearance of increased trunk rotation. When doing the rotation, the examiner watches to see how much movement occurs in each **thoracic ring** (a thoracic ring is made up of two vertebrae, the adjacent two ribs and their attachments into the sternum, the intervertebral disc and the costal cartilage and sternum, so there are 10 thoracic rings). Because of the shape of the facets, there is more rotation in the upper thoracic spine than the lower thoracic spine. The examiner must remember that movement in the lumbar spine and hips as well as in the thoracic spine is occurring. To eliminate or decrease the amount of the hip movement, rotation may be done in sitting.

When doing the rotation, the examiner should watch and palpate the movement of the vertebra and ribs as the movement is different on both sides (Fig. 8.29). For example, with right rotation, the T5 vertebra rotates and side flexes to the right and translates to the left relative to T6 while at the same time, the right sixth rib posteriorly rotates and translates anteromedially relative to the T6 transverse process and the right sixth rib rotates anteriorly and translates posterolaterally relative to the T6 transverse

process (Fig. 8.30).[21-23] The examiner, when palpating the thoracic ring, is looking for incorrect alignment, improper thoracic ring movement, and loss of movement control. If any of these are present, then a **nonoptimal load transfer (NOLT)** may be occurring and will need correction.[22] The correction may involve mobilization techniques to the costovertebral or costotransverse joints, or stabilization techniques for the thoracic spine muscles.

If the history indicated that repetitive motion, sustained postures, or combined movements caused aggravation of symptoms, then these movements should also be tested, but only after the original movements of flexion, extension, side flexion, and rotation have been completed. Combined movements that may be tested in the thoracic spine include forward flexion and side bending, backward bending and side flexion, and lateral bending with flexion and lateral bending with extension. Any restriction of motion, excessive movement (hypermobility) or curve abnormality should be noted. These movements would be similar to the H and I test described in the lumbar spine (see Chapter 9).

Costovertebral Expansion

Costovertebral joint movement is usually determined by measuring chest expansion (Fig. 8.31). The examiner places the tape measure around the chest at the level of the fourth intercostal space. The patient is asked to exhale as much as possible, and the examiner takes a measurement. The patient is then asked to inhale as much as possible and hold the breath while the second measurement is taken. The normal difference between inspiration and expiration is 3 to 7.5 cm (1 to 3 inches).[5]

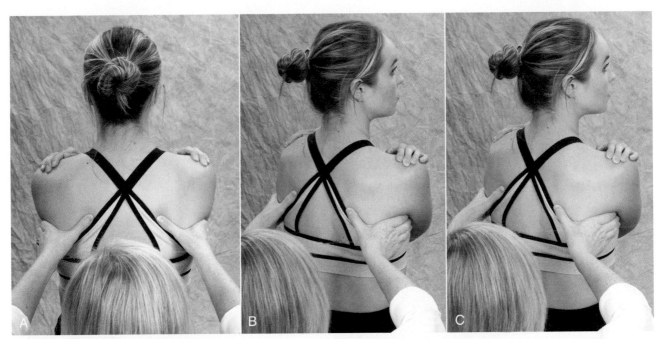

Fig. 8.29 Seated trunk rotation with thoracic ring palpation and correction. (A) Examiner's hand position for palpation of the 4th and 5th thoracic rings. The examiner performs the palpation using the distal end of the flat fingers; there should be no pressure posteriorly from the heel of the hand or palm. (B) The patient right rotates while the examiner notes the range of motion and any **nonoptimal load transfer** of the upper thoracic rings during the movement. The patient then returns to neutral. (C) Right rotation with correction of the 5th thoracic ring on the right and the 4th thoracic ring on the left showing facilitation of optimal biomechanics. Range of motion should increase resulting from this ring correction. (Concept from Lee LJ: The thoracic ring approach™—a whole person framework to assess and treat the thoracic spine and ribcage. In Magee DJ, Zachazewski JE, Quillen WS, Manske RC, editors: *Pathology and intervention in musculoskeletal rehabilitation,* ed 2, Philadelphia, 2016, Elsevier.)

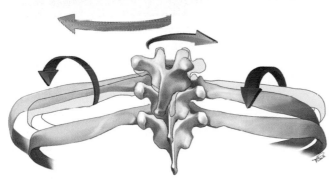

Fig. 8.30 Two "thoracic rings," with the upper thoracic ring depicting the osteokinematics that occur with right rotation. During right rotation, the vertebra rotates right, the right rib rotates posteriorly, and the left rib rotates anteriorly, and there is a left (i.e., contralateral) translation of the thoracic ring that can be palpated at the lateral aspect of the ring using the technique described in Fig. 8.29. (Copyright LJ Lee Physiotherapist Corp. From Lee LJ: The thoracic ring approach™— a whole person framework to assess and treat the thoracic spine and ribcage. In Magee DJ, Zachazewski JE, Quillen WS, Manske RC, editors: *Pathology and intervention in musculoskeletal rehabilitation,* ed 2, Philadelphia, 2016, Elsevier, p 448.)

A second method of measuring chest expansion is to measure at three different levels. If this method is used, the examiner must take care to ensure that the levels of measurement are noted for consistency. The levels are (1) under the axillae for apical expansion, (2) at the nipple line or xiphisternal junction for midthoracic expansion, and (3) at the T10 rib level for lower thoracic expansion. As before, the measurements are taken after expiration and inspiration.

After the measurement of chest expansion, it is worthwhile for the patient to take a deep breath and cough so that the examiner can determine whether this action causes or alters any pain. If it does, the examiner may suspect a respiratory-related problem or a problem increasing intrathecal pressure in the spine.

Evjenth and Gloeck[24] have noted a way to differentiate thoracic spine and rib pain during movement. If the patient has pain on flexion, the patient is returned to neutral and is asked to take a deep breath and hold it. While holding the breath, the patient flexes until pain is felt. At this point, the patient stops flexing and exhales. If further flexion can be accomplished after exhaling, the problem is more likely to be the ribs than the thoracic spine. Extension can be tested in a similar fashion.

Rib Motion

The patient is asked to lie supine. The examiner's hands are placed in a relaxed fashion over the upper chest. In this position, the examiner is feeling anteroposterior movement of the ribs (Fig. 8.32). As the patient inhales and exhales, the examiner should compare both sides to see whether the movement is equal. Any restriction or difference in motion should be noted. If a rib stops moving relative to the other ribs on inhalation, it is classified as a **depressed rib.** If a rib stops moving relative to the other ribs on exhalation, it is classified as an **elevated rib.** It must be remembered that restriction of one rib affects the adjacent ribs. If a depressed rib is implicated, it is usually

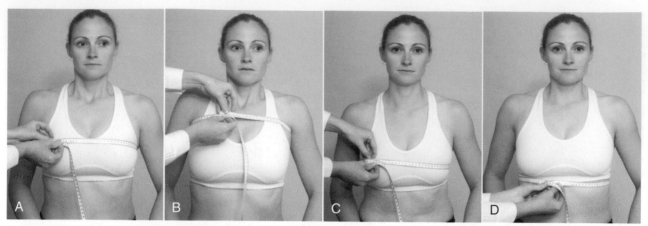

Fig. 8.31 Measuring chest expansion. (A) Fourth lateral intercostal space. (B) Axilla. (C) Nipple line. (D) Tenth rib.

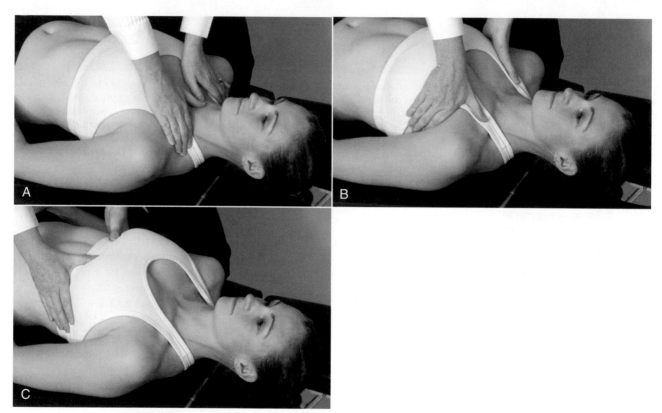

Fig. 8.32 Feeling rib movement. (A) Upper ribs. (B) Middle ribs. (C) Lower ribs.

the highest restricted rib that causes the greatest problem. If an elevated rib is present, it is usually the lowest restricted rib that causes the greatest problem although for both depressed and elevated rib the opposite may be true.[4,25] Rib springing or the presence of pain on stressing the rib joints will help to confirm the level that is hypomobile. The examiner then moves his or her hands down the patient's chest, testing the movement in the middle and lower ribs in a similar fashion.

To test lateral movement of the ribs, the examiner's hands are placed around the sides of the rib cage approximately 45° to the vertical axis of spine of the patient's body. The

examiner begins at the level of the axilla and works down the lateral aspect of the ribs, feeling the movement of the ribs during inspiration and expiration and noting any restriction.

Rib dysfunctions may be divided into structural, torsional, and respiratory (Table 8.5).[26] Structural rib dysfunctions are due to joint subluxation or dislocation. Torsional rib dysfunctions are due to thoracic vertebra dysfunction as a result of hypomobility or hypermobility. Respiratory rib dysfunctions are due to either hypomobility between the ribs (e.g., intercostal shortening) or hypomobility at the costotransverse or costovertebral joints.[26]

TABLE **8.5**

Rib Dysfunction

STRUCTURAL RIB DYSFUNCTION

Dysfunction	Rib Angle	Midaxillary Line	Intercostal Space	Anterior Rib
Anterior subluxation	Less prominent	Symmetric	Tender, often with intercostal neuralgia	More prominent
Posterior subluxation	More prominent	Symmetric	Tender, often with intercostal neuralgia	Less prominent
Superior first rib subluxation	Superior aspect of first rib elevated (5 mm)	Hypertonicity of the scalene muscles on the same side		Marked tenderness of the superior aspect
Anterior posterior rib compression	Less prominent	Prominent	Tender, often with intercostal neuralgia	Less prominent
Lateral compression	More prominent	Less prominent	Tender	More prominent
Laterally elevated	Tender	Prominent	Narrow above, wide below	Exquisitely tender at pectoral minor

TORSIONAL RIB DYSFUNCTION

Dysfunction	Rib Angle	Midaxillary Line	Intercostal Space
External rib torsion	Superior border prominent and tender	Symmetric	Wide above, narrow below
Internal rib torsion	Inferior border prominent and tender	Symmetric	Narrow above, wide below

RESPIRATORY RIB FUNCTION

Dysfunction	Rib Angle	Key Rib
Inhalation restriction	During inspiration the rib or group of ribs that cease rising	Top or superior rib
Exhalation restriction	During exhalation the rib or group of ribs that stop falling	Bottom or inferior rib

Modified from Bookhout MR: Evaluation of the thoracic spine and rib cage. In Flynn TW, editor: *The thoracic spine and rib cage*, Boston, 1996, Butterworth Heinemann, pp 163, 165, 166.

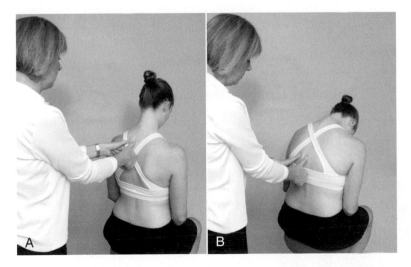

Fig. 8.33 Testing mobility of rib relative to thoracic vertebra. Note one thumb is on the transverse process of the vertebra and one thumb is on the rib. (A) Upper ribs. (B) Lower ribs.

To test the movement of the ribs relative to the thoracic spine, the patient is placed in a sitting position. The examiner places one thumb or finger on the transverse process and the thumb of the other hand just lateral to the tubercle of the rib. The patient is asked to forward flex the head (for the upper thoracic spine) and thorax (for lower thoracic spine) while the examiner feels the movement of the rib (Fig. 8.33). Normally, the rib rotates anteriorly and the rib tubercle stays at the same level as the transverse process on the forward movement. If the rib is hypermobile, the rib elevates relative to the transverse process. If the rib is hypomobile, its motion stops before the thoracic spine.[19] Extension may also be tested in a similar fashion, but the rib rotates posteriorly.

Passive Movements

Because passive movements in the thoracic spine are difficult to perform in a gross fashion, the movement between each pair of vertebrae may be assessed. With the patient sitting, the examiner places one hand on the patient's forehead or on top of the head (Fig. 8.34). With the other hand, the examiner palpates over and between the spinous processes of the lower cervical and upper thoracic spines (C5–T3) and feels for movement between the spinous processes while flexing (move apart) and extending (move together) the patient's head. Rotation (one side moves forward, the other moves back) and side flexion (one side moves apart, one side moves together) may be tested by rotating and side flexing the patient's head. To test the movement properly, the examiner places the middle finger over the spinous process of the vertebra being tested and the index and ring fingers on each side of it, between the spinous processes of the two adjacent vertebrae. The examiner should feel the movement occurring, assess its quality, and note whether the movement is hypomobile or hypermobile relative to the adjacent vertebrae. The hypomobility or hypermobility may be indicative of pathology.[25] Although an individual examiner may be able to differentiate passive movements in the thoracic spine, it has been reported that interrater reliability is poor.[27]

Passive Movements of the Thoracic Spine and Normal End Feel

- Forward flexion (tissue stretch)
- Extension (tissue stretch)
- Side flexion, left and right (tissue stretch)
- Rotation, left and right (tissue stretch)

If, when the spinous processes are palpated, one process appears to be out of alignment, the examiner can then palpate the transverse processes on each side and compare them with the levels above and below to determine whether the vertebra is truly rotated or side flexed. For example, if the spinous process of T5 is shifted to the right and if rotation has occurred at that level, the left transverse process would be more superficial posteriorly, whereas the right one would appear deeper. If the spinous process rotation was an anomaly, the transverse processes would be equal as would the ribs. Passive or active movement of the spine while palpating the transverse processes also helps to indicate abnormal movement when comparing both sides or when comparing one level to another. If the alignment is normal to begin with and becomes abnormal with movement, or if it is abnormal to begin with and becomes normal with movement, it indicates a functional asymmetry rather than a structural one. In general, a structural asymmetry would be evident if it remains through all movements.[26]

To test the movement of the vertebrae between T3 and T11, the patient sits with the fingers clasped behind the neck and the elbows together in front. The examiner places one hand and arm around the patient's elbows while palpating over and between the spinous processes, as previously described. The examiner then flexes and extends the spine by lifting and lowering the patient's elbows.

Side flexion and rotation of the trunk may be performed in a similar fashion to test these movements. The patient sits with the hands clasped behind the head. The examiner uses the thumb on one side of the spinous process and/or the index finger and/or the middle finger on the other side to palpate just lateral to the interspinous space. For side flexion, the examiner moves the patient into right side flexion and then left side flexion and by palpation compares the amount and quality of right and left movement including adjacent segments (Fig. 8.35A). For rotation, the examiner rotates the patient's shoulders to the right or left, comparing by palpation the amount and quality of movement of each segment as well as that of adjacent segments (Fig. 8.35B).[25]

Resisted Isometric Movements

Resisted isometric movements are performed with the patient in the sitting position. The examiner places one leg

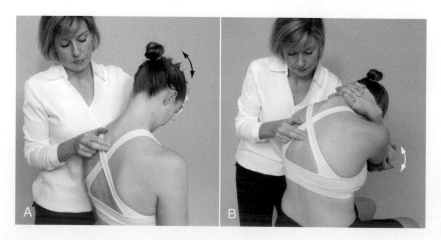

Fig. 8.34 Passive flexion/extension movement of the thoracic spine. (A) Upper thoracic spine. (B) Middle and lower thoracic spine. Note how the examiner uses her left hand/arm to control movement of the patient's head and shoulders.

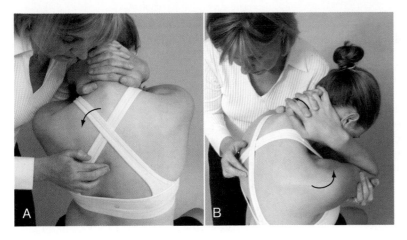

Fig. 8.35 (A) Passive side flexion of the thoracic spine. (B) Passive rotation of the thoracic spine. Note how the examiner uses her left hand/arm to control movement of the patient's head and shoulders.

behind the patient's buttocks and the upper limbs around the patient's chest and back (Fig. 8.36). The examiner then instructs the patient, "Don't let me move you," and isometrically tests the movements, noting any alteration in strength and occurrence of pain.

Resisted Isometric Movements of the Thoracic Spine

- Forward flexion
- Extension
- Side flexion, left and right
- Rotation, left and right

The thoracic spine should be tested in a neutral position, and the most painful movements are done last. Table 8.6 lists the muscles of the thoracic spine (Figs. 8.37 and 8.38), their actions, and their innervations. It must be remembered that the resisted isometric testing of the spine is in reality a very gross test, and subtle alterations in strength are almost impossible to detect. However, if the muscles being tested have been strained (1° or 2°), contraction of the muscle commonly produces pain. However, in some cases, the spine and thorax may have to be repositioned to isolate a particular muscle.

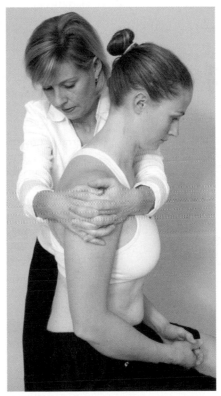

Fig. 8.36 Positioning for resisted isometric movements.

TABLE 8.6

Muscles of the Thorax and Abdomen: Their Actions and Nerve Root Derivation/Nerve Supply in the Thoracic Spine

Action	Muscles Acting	Nerve Root Derivation
Flexion of thoracic spine	1. Rectus abdominis	T6–T12
	2. External abdominal oblique (both sides acting together)	T7–T12
	3. Internal abdominal oblique (both sides acting together)	T7–T12, L1
Extension of thoracic spine	1. Spinalis thoracis	T1–T12
	2. Iliocostalis thoracis (both sides acting together)	T1–T12
	3. Longissimus thoracis (both sides acting together)	T1–T12
	4. Semispinalis thoracis (both sides acting together)	T1–T12
	5. Multifidus (both sides acting together)	T1–T12
	6. Rotatores (both sides acting together)	T1–T12
	7. Interspinalis	T1–T12

Continued

TABLE **8.6**

Muscles of the Thorax and Abdomen: Their Actions and Nerve Root Derivation/Nerve Supply in the Thoracic Spine—cont'd

Action	Muscles Acting	Nerve Root Derivation
Rotation and side flexion of thoracic spine	1. Iliocostalis thoracis (to same side)	T1–T12
	2. Longissimus thoracis (to same side)	T1–T12
	3. Intertransverse (to same side)	T1–T12
	4. Internal abdominal oblique (to same side)	T7–T12, L1
	5. Semispinalis thoracis (to opposite side)	T1–T12
	6. Multifidus (to opposite side)	T1–T12
	7. Rotatores (to opposite side)	T1–T12
	8. External abdominal oblique (to opposite side)	T7–T12
	9. Transverse abdominis (to opposite side)	T7–T12, L1
Elevation of ribs	1. Scalenus anterior (first rib)	C4–C6
	2. Scalenus medius (first rib)	C3–C8
	3. Scalenus posterior (second rib)	C6–C8
	4. Serratus posterior superior (second to fifth ribs)	2 to 5 intercostal
	5. Iliocostalis cervicis (first to sixth rib)	C6–C8
	6. Levatores costarum (all ribs)	T1–T12
	7. Pectoralis major (if arm fixed)	Lateral pectoral (C6, C7)
		Medial pectoral (C7, C8, T1)
	8. Serratus anterior (lower ribs if scapula fixed)	Long thoracic (C5–C7)
	9. Pectoralis minor (second to fifth ribs if scapula fixed)	Lateral pectoral (C6, C7)
		Medial pectoral (C7, C8)
	10. Sternocleidomastiod (if head fixed)	Accessory C2, C3
Depression of ribs	1. Serratus posterior inferior (lower four ribs)	T9–T12
	2. Iliocostalis lumborum (lower six ribs)	L1–L3
	3. Longissimus thoracis	T1–T12
	4. Rectus abdominis	T6–T12
	5. External abdominal oblique (lower five to six ribs)	T7–T12
	6. Internal abdominal oblique (lower five to six ribs)	T7–T12, L1
	7. Transverse abdominal (all acting to depress lower ribs)	T7–T12, L1
	8. Quadratus lumborum (twelfth rib)	T12, L1–L4
	9. Transverse thoracis	T1–T12
Approximation of ribs	1. Iliocostalis thoracis	T1–T12
	2. Intercostals (internal and external)	1 to 11 intercostal
	3. Diaphragm	Phrenic
Inspiration	1. External intercostals	1 to 11 intercostal
	2. Transverse thoracis (sternocostalis)	1 to 11 intercostal
	3. Diaphragm	Phrenic
	4. Sternocleidomastoid	Accessory C2, C3
	5. Scalenus anterior	C4–C6
	6. Scalenus medius	C3–C8
	7. Scalenus posterior	C6–C8
	8. Pectoralis major	Lateral pectoral (C5, C6)
		Medial pectoral (C7, C8, T1)
	9. Pectoralis minor	Lateral pectoral (C6, C7)
		Medial pectoral (C7, C8)
	10. Serratus anterior	Long thoracic (C5-C7)
	11. Latissimus dorsi	Thoracodorsal (C6, C8)
	12. Serratus posterior superior	2 to 5 intercostal
	13. Iliocostalis thoracis	T1–T12
Expiration	1. Internal intercostal	1 to 11 intercostal
	2. Rectus abdominis	T6–T12
	3. External abdominal oblique	T7–T12
	4. Internal abdominal oblique	T7–T12, LI
	5. Ilicostalis lumborum	L1–L3
	6. Longissimus	T1–L3
	7. Serratus posterior inferior	T9–TI2
	8. Quadratus lumborum	T12, L1–L4

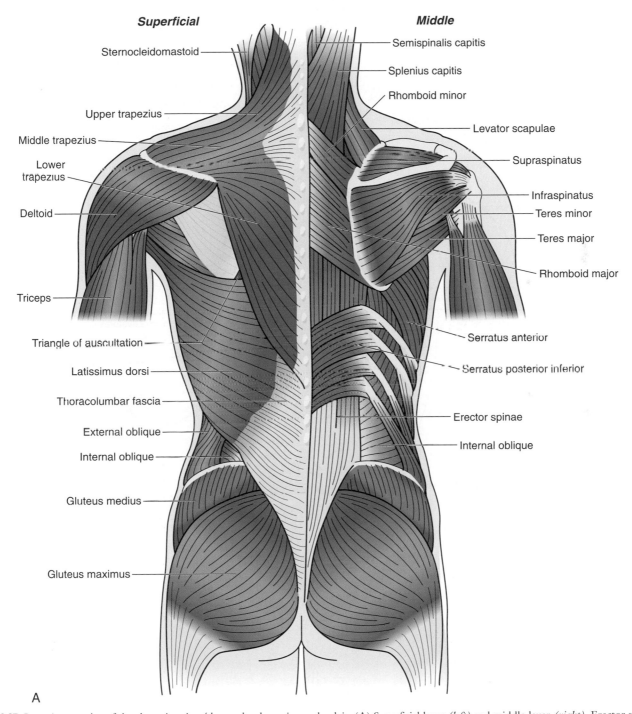

Superficial

Middle

Sternocleidomastoid

Upper trapezius

Middle trapezius

Lower trapezius

Deltoid

Triceps

Triangle of auscultation

Latissimus dorsi

Thoracolumbar fascia

External oblique

Internal oblique

Gluteus medius

Gluteus maximus

Semispinalis capitis

Splenius capitis

Rhomboid minor

Levator scapulae

Supraspinatus

Infraspinatus

Teres minor

Teres major

Rhomboid major

Serratus anterior

Serratus posterior inferior

Erector spinae

Internal oblique

A

Fig. 8.37 Posterior muscles of the thoracic spine/thorax, lumbar spine and pelvis. (A) Superficial layer *(left)* and middle layer *(right)*. Erector spinae consists of the iliocostalis, longissimus, and spinalis muscles.

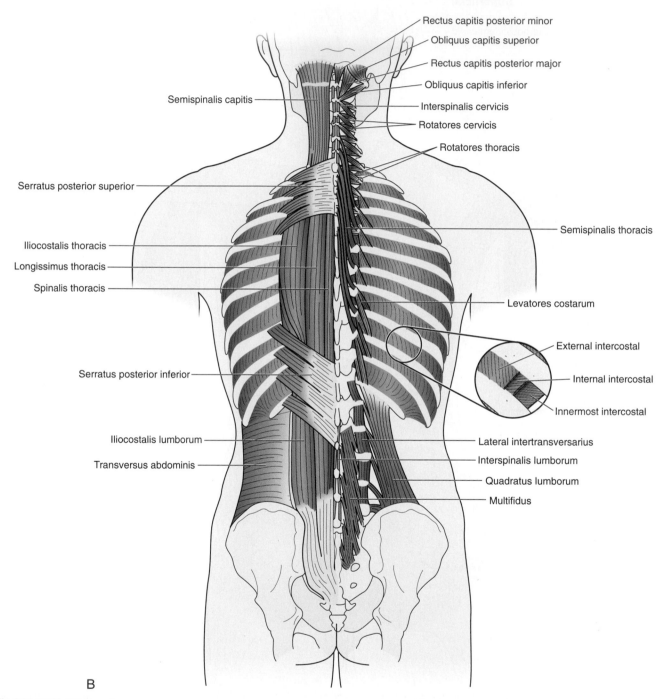

Rectus capitis posterior minor

Obliquus capitis superior

Rectus capitis posterior major

Obliquus capitis inferior

Interspinalis cervicis

Rotatores cervicis

Rotatores thoracis

Semispinalis capitis

Serratus posterior superior

Semispinalis thoracis

Iliocostalis thoracis

Longissimus thoracis

Spinalis thoracis

Levatores costarum

External intercostal

Internal intercostal

Innermost intercostal

Serratus posterior inferior

Iliocostalis lumborum

Transversus abdominis

Lateral intertransversarius

Interspinalis lumborum

Quadratus lumborum

Multifidus

B

Fig. 8.37 cont'd (B) Deep layer.

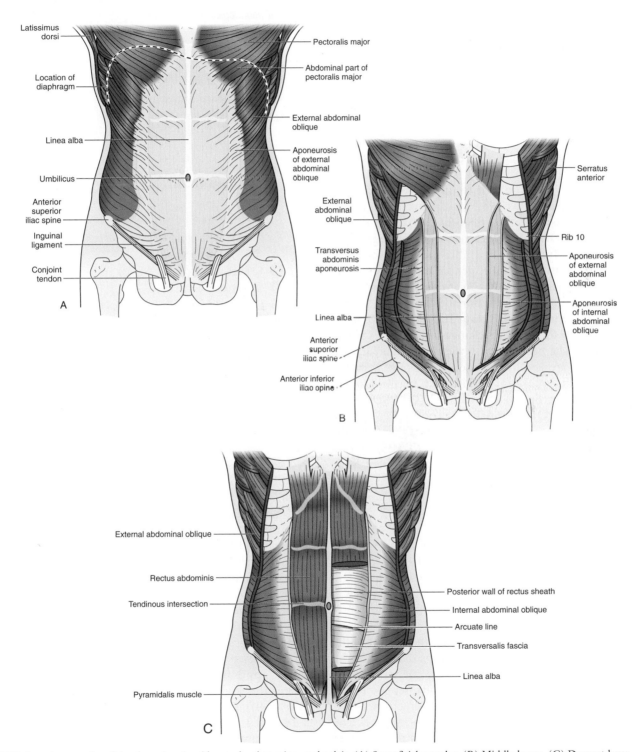

Fig. 8.38 Anterior muscles of the thoracic spine/thorax, lumbar spine, and pelvis. (A) Superficial muscles. (B) Middle layers. (C) Deepest layer.

Functional Assessment

When doing specific activities, the thoracic spine primarily plays a stabilization role. Therefore activities involving the cervical spine, lumbar spine, and shoulder may be impaired as a result of thoracic lesions. Functional activities involving these three areas should be reviewed or considered if functional impairment appears to be related to the thoracic spine or ribs. Activities such as lifting, rotating the thorax, or doing heavy work; any activity requiring stabilization of the thorax; or any activity increasing cardiopulmonary output are most likely to provoke thoracic symptoms.

Functional disability scales, such as the Oswestry Disability Questionnaire[28] (see Chapter 9), although designed for the lumbar spine, could be used to test functional capacity in the thoracic spine as well.[28–30] The Oswestry Disability Questionnaire is better suited for persistent severe disability.[29] The **Neck Disability Index,** although designed for the cervical spine (see Chapter 3), may be useful for upper thoracic complaints. Other more general outcome measures include the **Numeric Pain Rating Scale** (see Chapter 1) and the **Patient Specific Functional Scale** (see Chapters 3 and 12). The **Functional Rating Index** (eTool 8.1) has been designed to show clinical change in conditions affecting the spine, whether cervical, thoracic, or lumbar.[31] In addition, there are specific functional outcome measures related to specific spinal deformities such as the **Quality of Life Profile for Spinal Deformities (QLPSD),**[32] the **SRS-22 Patient Questionnaire** (eTool 8.2),[32–34] the **Spinal Appearance Questionnaire (SAQ),**[32,35,36] the **Trunk Appearance Perception Scale (TAPS)** (eTool 8.3),[32,36,37] and the **Walter Reed Visual Assessment Scale** (eTool 8.4).[38]

Special Tests

For the reader who would like to review them, the reliability, validity, specificity, sensitivity, and odds ratios of some of the special tests used in the thoracic spine are available in eAppendix 8.1.

Tests for Neurological Involvement

If the examiner suspects a problem with movement of the spinal cord, any of the neurodynamic tests that stretch the cord may be performed. These include the straight leg raising test and the Kernig sign (see Chapter 9). Either neck flexion from above or straight leg raising from below stretches the spinal cord within the thoracic spine. The following tests should be performed only if the examiner believes they are relevant.

❓ *First Thoracic Nerve Root Stretch.* The patient abducts the arm to 90° and flexes the pronated forearm to 90°.

Key Tests Performed on the Thoracic Spine Depending on Suspected Pathology[a39,40]

- *For neurological involvement:*
  - ✓ Slump test
  - ✓ Upper limb neurodynamic (tension) tests (ULNT)
- *For thoracic outlet syndrome:*
  - ❓ Adson maneuver
  - ❓ Costoclavicular syndrome test
  - ⚠ Cyriax release test
  - ⚠ Hyperabduction test (elevated arm stress test [EAST])
  - ⚠ Roos test
- *For rib mobility:*
  - ⚠ Deep breath and flexion test
  - ✓ First rib mobility
  - ✓ Rib spring test
- *For thoracic spine and sternal involvement:*
  - ⚠ Reflex hammer test
  - ❓ Schepelmann sign
  - ❓ Sternal compression test
- *For failed load transfer (kinetic chain instability):*
  - ❓ Prone arm lift (PAL) test
  - ❓ Sitting arm lift or single arm lift (SAL) test
- *For medical screening:*
  - ❓ Kehr's sign
  - ⚠ Murphy's percussion test

[a]The authors recommend these key tests be learned by the clinician to facilitate a diagnosis. See Chapter 1, Key for Classifying Special Tests.

No symptoms should appear in this position. The patient then fully flexes the elbow, putting the hand behind the neck/head (Fig. 8.39). This action stretches the ulnar nerve and T1 nerve root. Pain into the scapular area or arm is indicative of a positive test for T1 nerve root.[41] Care should be taken to ensure the patient does not forward flex the neck or forward flex the arm so that the stress is taken off the nerve root.

If the patient has upper limb symptoms that have become evident at the same time as thoracic symptoms, upper limb tension tests should also be considered to rule out referral of neurological symptoms from the thoracic spine.[42]

❓ *Passive Scapular Approximation.* The patient lies prone, stands, or sits while the examiner passively approximates the scapulae by lifting the shoulders up and back (Fig. 8.40). Pain in the scapular area may be indicative of a T1 or T2 nerve root problem on the side on which the pain is being experienced.[41,43]

✓ *Slump Test (Sitting Dural Stretch Test).* The patient sits on the examining table and is asked to "slump" so that the spine flexes and the shoulders sag forward while the

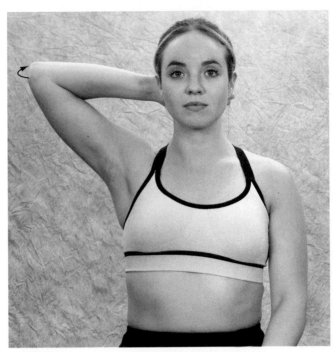

Fig. 8.39 First thoracic nerve root stretch. Elbow should be behind plane of head.

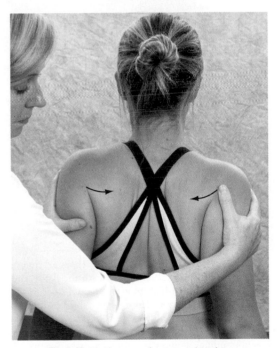

Fig. 8.40 Passive scapular approximation.

examiner holds the chin and head erect. The patient is asked if any symptoms are produced. If no symptoms are produced, the examiner flexes the patient's neck and holds the head down and shoulders slumped to see if symptoms are produced. If no symptoms are produced, the examiner passively extends one of the patient's knees to see if symptoms are produced. If no symptoms are produced, the examiner then passively dorsiflexes the foot of the

same leg to see if symptoms are produced (Fig. 8.41). The process is repeated with the other leg. Symptoms of sciatic pain or reproduction of the patient's symptoms indicates a positive test, implicating impingement of the dura and spinal cord or nerve roots.[44] Butler[45] and Lee[22] suggested that, when testing the thoracic spine while the patient is in the slump position, trunk rotation left and right should be added. Butler felt this maneuver increased the stress on the intercostal nerves. Lee[22] felt that the examiner should palpate the thoracic rings and look for any rings demonstrating any nonoptimal load transfer (i.e., excessive or asymmetrical compression, lateral translation or rotation, side flexion) as the patient moves into the slump position (Fig. 8.42). If the thoracic rings are normal, they will remain "stacked" (i.e., vertical) throughout the slump test.[22] The pain is usually produced at the site of the lesion in a positive test.

✓ *Upper Limb Neurodynamic (Tension) Test.* See Chapter 3 for a description of the upper limb neurodynamic (tension) test (ULNT4). Lee[22] suggests that if the examiner feels the ULTT tests are necessary, it is advisable to repeat the positive test while palpating the lateral border of the thoracic rings to feel for any lateral translation or any other nonoptimal load transfer (normally the lateral borders should be relatively vertically aligned) (Fig. 8.43). If the lateral translation is treated and the test repeated and the symptoms decrease, the affected thoracic ring should be included in the treatment.

Tests for Thoracic Outlet Syndrome
There are several special tests that the examiner may consider if thoracic outlet syndrome is suspected. Because all of the tests have questionable statistical value in terms of their reliability, the examiner should listen to the patient and use the test that best replicates the position or positions in which the patient has symptoms.

❓ *Adson Maneuver.* See Chapter 5 for a description of the test.

❓ *Costoclavicular Syndrome (Military Brace) Test.* See Chapter 5 for a description of the test.

⚠️ *Cyriax Release Test.* The patient is sitting with elbows flexed. The examiner stands behind the patient and grasps under the patient's forearms while the patient's forearms, wrists, and hands are in neutral (Fig. 8.44). The examiner then leans the patient's trunk backward approximately 15° and lifts the patient's shoulder girdle to end range holding the position for 3 minutes. The production of symptoms or the disappearance of neurological signs (**release phenomenon**) indicates a positive test.

❓ *Halstead Maneuver.* See Chapter 5 for a description of the test.

⚠️ *Roos Test (Elevated Arm Stress Test).* See Chapter 5 for a description of the test. The Roos test may also be used

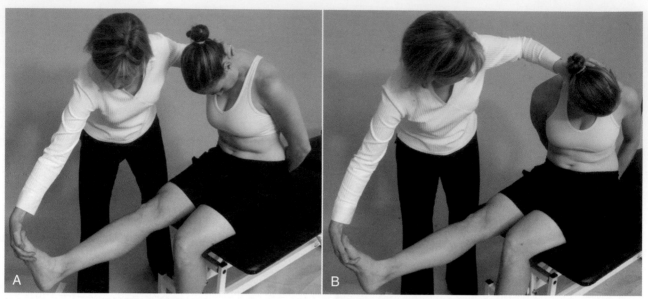

Fig. 8.41 Slump test. (A) Classic test. (B) Trunk rotation added to classic test.

to test the arterial portion of thoracic outlet syndrome (testing the radial artery) by positioning the patient in the same position but while looking for neurological signs, the radial pulse is also taken. If the pulse decreases when the patient is in the test position (called the **hyperabduction test** or **elevated arm stress test [EAST]** ⚠), it is considered a positive test for thoracic outlet syndrome.

❓ *Wright Test or Maneuver.* See Chapter 5 for a description of the test.

Tests for Rib Mobility
See Chapter 3.

⚠ *Deep Breath and Flexion Test.*[1] The test is used if a patient complains of pain on forward flexion. The patient is seated, sitting tall and the spine in neutral. The patient is asked to take a deep breath and hold it while forward flexing until pain is felt and stops at this point. The patient then slowly exhales and attempts further flexion. If the patient can forward flex further after exhaling, the source of the pain is more likely the ribs than the thoracic spine.

✓ *Rib Spring Test.*[1] The patient is in prone with the examiner on one side of the patient opposite the side to be tested (e.g., on the left to test the right side). The examiner then places the extended thumb and adjacent finger along the right rib to be tested (Fig. 8.45A). The examiner then applies a posteroanterior springing force to the rib. This action is the same as left rotation. The examiner then uses the ulnar border of the left hand or thumb over the left transverse process or right spinous process to block the vertebra from rotating (Fig. 8.45B). The examiner then repeats the springing action to the rib. If the second part of the test causes pain and the

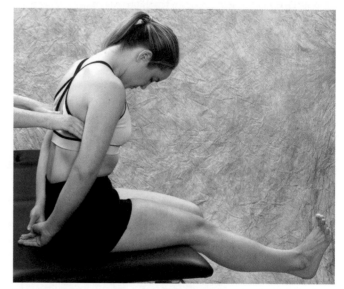

Fig. 8.42 Slump test for neurodynamic and thoracic ring function testing. The examiner spans several rings with the flat of the fingers to determine if nonoptimal load transfer (NOLT) occurs as the patient performs the slump test. The overall range of motion of the slump test (i.e., the amount of leg extension and ankle dorsiflexion) is noted, and all thoracic rings are palpated to identify any levels displaying nonoptimal alignment, biomechanics, or control during the slump test. Timing of NOLT relative to initiation of the slump movement is noted, and the rings displaying NOLT the earliest are corrected first while the slump test is repeated. The impact of the correction on leg extension and ankle dorsiflexion range of motion and on the patient's symptoms are then noted. If the NOLT is corrected and symptoms relieved when the slump test is repeated, it is the NOLT that is the primary problem or "driver." (Concept from Lee LJ: The thoracic ring approach™—a whole person framework to assess and treat the thoracic spine and ribcage. In Magee DJ, Zachazewski JE, Quillen WS, Manske RC, editors: *Pathology and intervention in musculoskeletal rehabilitation*, ed 2, Philadelphia, 2016, Elsevier.)

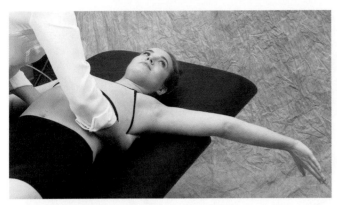

Fig. 8.43 Upper limb neurodynamic test for neurodynamic and thoracic ring function testing. The examiner performs the appropriate variation of the upper limb neurodynamic test *(ULNT1 shown in photo)* based on the patient's symptoms and restricted motion compared to the opposite side. Several thoracic rings are then palpated laterally while the test is repeated if positive. If lateral translation or other types of nonoptimal load transfer are found in one or more thoracic rings during the test, the examiner returns to the start position and performs a thoracic ring correction.[22] While maintaining optimal ring alignment, the test is repeated. A significant increase in range of motion at the elbow or wrist and/or decrease in symptoms supports that the thoracic ring(s) may be a driver for the restriction in the neurodynamic test. (Concept from Lee LJ: The thoracic ring approach™—a whole person framework to assess and treat the thoracic spine and ribcage. In Magee DJ, Zachazewski JE, Quillen WS, Manske RC, editors: *Pathology and intervention in musculoskeletal rehabilitation*, ed 2, Philadelphia, 2016, Elsevier.)

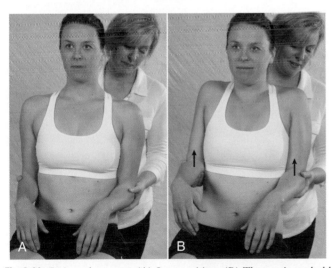

Fig. 8.44 Cyriax release test. (A) Start position. (B) Three-minute hold position.

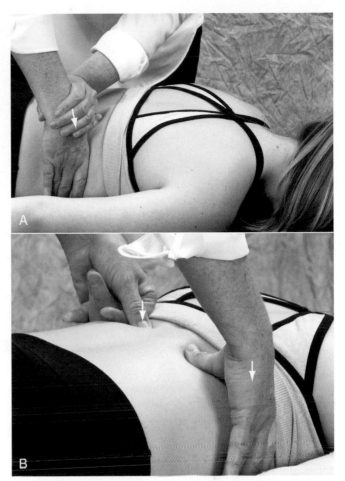

Fig. 8.45 Rib spring test. (A) The examiner places the extended thumb and adjacent (second) finger along the rib on the side to be tested (in this case, the right side is tested). (B) The examiner then uses the thumb of the left hand over the left transverse process, or over the right side of the spinous process to block the vertebra from rotating while a downward pressure is applied to the rib.

first does not, the problem is in the costovertebral or costotransverse joints. The amount and quality of movement occurring on both sides can be noted looking for hypomobility or hypermobility in relation to the others being tested.

Tests for Thoracic Spine and Sternal Involvement

⚠ *Reflex Hammer Test.*[1] This test is used if there has been trauma to the posterior elements of the thoracic

vertebra. The patient is seated, sitting tall. The examiner then taps over each spinous process to see if pain or muscle spasm is provoked (Fig. 8.46A). If so, a fracture may be suspected. One may also use a closed fist in place of the reflex hammer (Fig. 8.46B). In this case, it is called the **closed-fist percussion sign**.[18] The examiner may also percuss the paravertebral tissue which, if pathological, will go into spasm.[43]

❓ *Schepelmann Sign.*[43] The patient stands and elevates both hands over the head and then side flexes one way and then the other (Fig. 8.47). If pain occurs on the concave side, either the intercostals or the costovertebral or costotransverse joints on the concave side are affected. If pain occurs on the convex side, it may be a problem with the intercostals or lungs or there may be NOLT of the ribs.

❓ *Sternal Compression Test.*[43] The patient lies in relaxed supine. The examiner places the thenar eminence of one hand supported by the other over the sternum and applies a vertical force to the sternum (Fig. 8.48). A positive test is pain which may indicate a fracture or

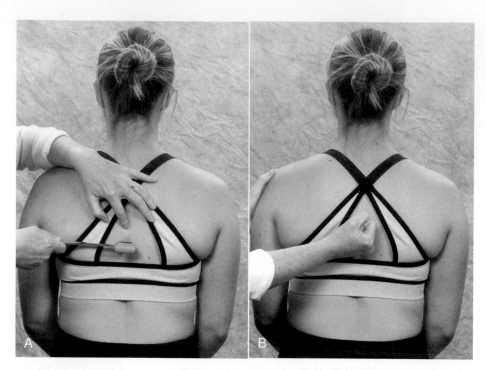

Fig. 8.46 (A) Reflex hammer test for spinous process of thoracic spine. (B) Closed fist percussion for spinous process of thoracic spine.

costochondritis. The examiner may also use the test to determine the flexibility of the sternum and ribs.

Tests for Failed Load Transfer (Kinetic Chain Instability or Loss of Movement Control)

These tests have been designed to demonstrate the transfer of load through the thoracic spine as part of the kinetic chain. The tests identify the site within the thorax where there are load transfer problems and where in the thoracic area stabilization does not occur during movement.

❓ *Prone Arm Lift Test.*[46] The prone arm lift (PAL) test is a modification of the sitting arm lift (SAL) test. It assesses the ability of the arm to take a load in a higher angle of shoulder flexion. This test is especially useful in people who do overhead activities or who complain of problems when they try to lift heavy loads or try to move the arm too quickly. The patient lies prone with the arms overhead at approximately 140° of flexion and fully supported on the bed. The patient is then asked to lift one arm 2 cm and then lower it (Fig. 8.49A). This is repeated with the other side. If one arm is heavier than the other, it is considered the positive side. The examiner can then proceed to do an assessment like the second part of the SAL test, palpating the ribs for abnormal translation, watching the movement of the scapula for scapular dyskinesia, ensuring that the head of the humerus remains centralized in the glenoid, and palpating the cervical spine for abnormal translation (Fig. 8.49B).

❓ *Sitting Arm Lift or Single Arm Lift Test.*[46] The patient sits on the bed with the hands resting on the thighs. The examiner asks the patient to lift one arm (the unaffected side first) into elevation through shoulder flexion with the arm straight and the thumb up. The patient then does the

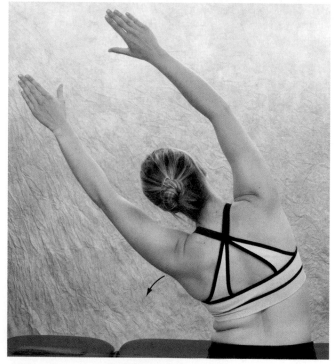

Fig. 8.47 Schepelmann sign.

same movement with the opposite side. The examiner asks the patient whether one arm feels heavier to lift than the other. The examiner notes whether any symptoms are produced and which arm requires more effort to lift. If one arm is heavier and requires more effort to lift, the first part of the test is considered positive. The patient is then asked to repeat the movement several times while the examiner palpates the ribs individually by placing the thumb on the spinous process and index finger along the rib, noting whether there is any translation of the rib, especially in the first 90° of movement (Fig. 8.50). Normally, when the patient lifts the arm, the muscles of the thorax are activated, stabilizing the thoracic spine so that there is no translation. A positive test for the second part of the test would be indicated by one or more of the thoracic rings (i.e., ribs or vertebrae) translating along any axis or rotating in any plane during the test. The examiner should note the level and direction of the loss of control. Normally what is seen is loss of rotational control with concurrent lateral translation either to the same side as the arm lift or to the contralateral side. This loss of control is usually seen between 0° and 90° of forward flexion.

The SAL test may also be used to demonstrate stability in the scapula, glenohumeral joint, and cervical spine. For the scapula, the examiner should watch the movement of the scapula to determine if there is any scapular dyskinesia indicating a loss of control. For the glenohumeral joint, the head of the humerus should remain centered in the glenoid fossa throughout the full forward flexion into elevation movement. To test the cervical spine, the examiner palpates the lateral aspect of the articular pillars of the cervical spine vertebra bilaterally while the patient does the movement. If there is translation of one vertebra relative to another when the patient does the SAL test, it indicates a lack of control of that individual segment.

Tests for Medical Screening

⚠ *Kehr's Sign.* Kehr's sign is pain referred from the diaphragm via the phrenic nerve to cause pain above the clavicle at the tip of the shoulder. It may be due to blood in the peritoneal cavity, injury to the spleen, renal calculi, or ruptured ectopic pregnancy.[47] Testing for the sign is pain when the patient is lying down with the legs elevated. The sign has also been called the **Saegesser's Sign** or **Phrenic-Point test**. In this case, the examiner, standing at the head of the patient, places the thumb of one hand on the right side of the neck between the sternocleidomastoid and scalenus anterior muscles. The examiner then directs pressure with the thumb backward toward the larynx and vertebral column (Fig. 8.51). This pressure will cause pain in the upper or lower part of the abdomen, usually in line with the lateral border of the rectus abdominis muscle on the side of the body on which the pressure was exerted.[48]

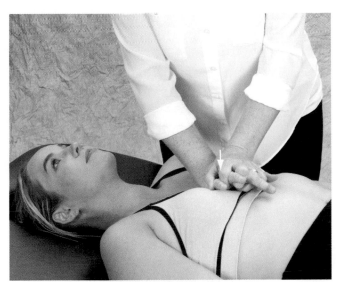

Fig. 8.48 Sternal compression test.

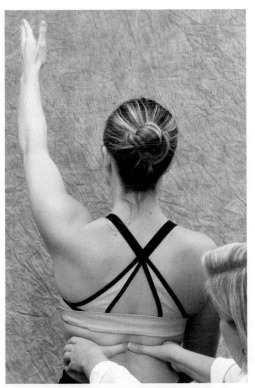

Fig. 8.50 Sitting arm lift or single arm lift test.

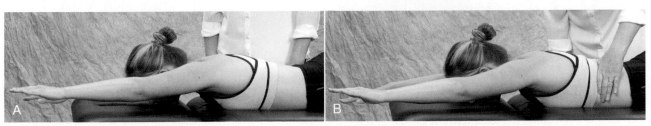

Fig. 8.49 (A) Prone arm lift test. (B) Prone arm lift test while palpating ribs.

⚠ *Murphy's Percussion Test (Costovertebral Angle Tenderness or Murphy's Sign).* This test is used to rule out kidney problems. The patient is in prone or sitting. The examiner places one hand over the costovertebral angle of the patient's back and with the other hand (in a fist) provides a percussive thump over the first hand (Fig. 8.52). The thump should be applied to both the right and left sides. A positive test is indicated by costovertebral tenderness or back/flank pain indicating renal involvement.[49]

Reflexes and Cutaneous Distribution

Within the thoracic spine, there is a great deal of overlap of the dermatomes (Fig. 8.53). The dermatomes tend to follow the ribs, and the absence of only one dermatome may lead to no loss of sensation. Pain may be referred to the thoracic spine from various abdominal organs (Fig. 8.54; Table 8.7). Although there are no reflexes to test in conjunction with the thoracic spine, the examiner would be wise to test the lumbar

reflexes—the patellar reflex (L3–L4), the medial hamstrings reflex (L5–S1), and the Achilles reflex (S1–S2)—because pathology in the thoracic spine can affect these reflexes.

Thoracic nerve root symptoms tend to follow the course of the ribs and may be referred as follows[50]:
- T10 to T11: Pain in epigastric area
- T5: Pain around nipple
- T7 to T8: Pain in epigastric area
- T10 to T11: Pain in umbilical area
- T12: Pain in the groin

Muscles of the thoracic spine may also refer pain into adjacent areas (Table 8.8).

Joint Play Movements

The joint play movements performed on the thoracic spine are specific ones that were developed by Maitland.[50] They are sometimes called *passive accessory intervertebral movements (PAIVMs)*. When testing joint play movements, the examiner should note any decreased ROM, muscle spasm, pain, or difference in end feel. The normal end feel is tissue stretch.

> **Joint Play Movements of the Thoracic Spine**
>
> - Posteroanterior central vertebral pressure (PACVP)
> - Posteroanterior unilateral vertebral pressure (PAUVP)
> - Transverse vertebral pressure (TVP)
> - Rib springing

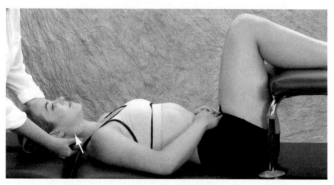

Fig. 8.51 Kehr's sign.

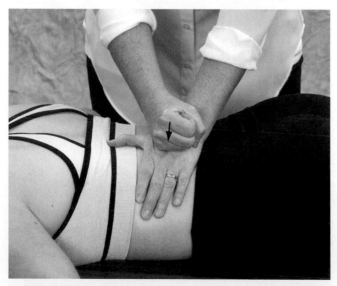

Fig. 8.52 Murphy's percussion test (costovertebral angle tenderness or Murphy's sign).

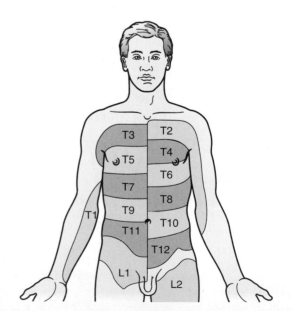

Fig. 8.53 The cutaneous areas (dermatomes) supplied by the thoracic nerve roots (after Foerster). By comparing both sides, the degree of overlapping and the area of exclusive supply of any individual nerve root may be estimated. (Adapted from Williams P, Warwick R, editors: *Gray's anatomy*, ed 37, Edinburgh, 1989, Churchill Livingstone, p 1150.)

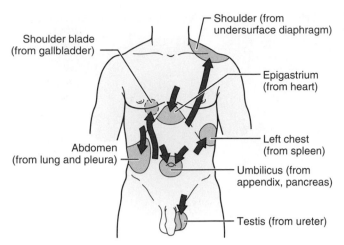

Shoulder blade
(from gallbladder)

Shoulder (from
undersurface diaphragm)

Epigastrium
(from heart)

Abdomen
(from lung and pleura)

Left chest
(from spleen)

Umbilicus (from
appendix, pancreas)

Testis (from ureter)

Fig. 8.54 Referred pain in the thorax and chest. (Modified from Judge RD, Zuidema GD, Fitzgerald FT: *Clinical diagnosis: a physiologic approach*, Boston, 1982, Little Brown, p 285.)

TABLE **8.7**

Differences in Pain Perception

Structure	Effective Stimulus[a]	Conscious Pain Perception
Skin	Discrete touch, prick, heat, cold	Precisely localized, superficial, burning, sharp
Chest wall (muscles, ribs, ligaments, parietal pleura)	Movement, deep pressure	Intermediate in localization and depth; aching, sharp, or dull
Thoracic viscera	Ischemia, distension, muscle spasm	Vague, diffuse, deep, aching, usually dull

[a]The effectiveness of a stimuli is heightened by the presence of inflammation.
From Levene D: *Chest pain: an integrated diagnostic approach*, Philadelphia, 1977, Lea & Febiger.

For the vertebral movements, the patient lies prone. The examiner palpates the thoracic spinous processes, starting at C6 and working down to L1 or L2. The occurrence of muscle spasm and/or pain on application of the vertebral pressure gives the examiner an indication of where the pathology may lie. However, the examiner must take care because the pain and/or muscle spasm at one level may be the result of compensation for a lesion at another level. For example, if one level is hypomobile as a result of trauma, another level may become hypermobile to compensate for the decreased movement at the traumatized level. It is probable that both the hypomobile and the hypermobile segments will cause pain and/or muscle spasm. It is then important to determine which joint complex is hypomobile and which is hypermobile, because the treatment for each is different. It has been found that

TABLE **8.8**

Thoracic Muscles and Referral of Pain

Muscles	Referral Pattern
Levator scapulae	Neck shoulder angle to posterior shoulder and along medial edge of scapula
Latissimus dorsi	Inferior angle of scapula to posterior shoulder; iliac crest
Rhomboids	Medial border of scapula
Trapezius	Upper thoracic spine to medial border of scapula
Serratus anterior	Lateral chest wall to lower medial border of scapula
Serratus posterior	Medial border of arm to medial two fingers
Serratus superior	Scapular area to posterior and anterior arm down to little finger
Multifidus	Adjacent to spinal column
Iliocostalis	Spinal column to line along medial border of scapula

this type of joint mobility testing showed good intraexaminer reliability as long as more than one vertebral level was assessed.[51]

Posteroanterior Central Vertebral Pressure

Some call this the **thoracic spring test**.[1] The examiner's hands, fingers, and thumbs are positioned as in Fig. 8.55A. The examiner then applies pressure to the spinous process through the thumbs, pushing the vertebra forward. Care must be taken to apply pressure slowly and with careful control, so that the movement, which is minimal, can be felt. This springing test may be repeated several times to determine the quality of the movement. The load applied to the spinous process is primarily taken up by the thoracic spine, although part of it is taken up by the rib cage.[52] Each spinous process is done in turn, starting at C6 and working down to L1 or L2. When doing this test, the examiner must keep in mind that the thoracic spinous processes are not always at the level of the same vertebral body. For example, the spinous processes of T1, T2, T3, and T12 are at the same levels as the T1, T2, T3, and T12 vertebral bodies, but the spinous processes of T7, T8, T9, and T10 are at the same levels as the T8, T9, T10, and T11 vertebral bodies, respectively.

Posteroanterior Unilateral Vertebral Pressure

The examiner's fingers are moved laterally away from the tip of the spinous process so that the thumbs rest on the

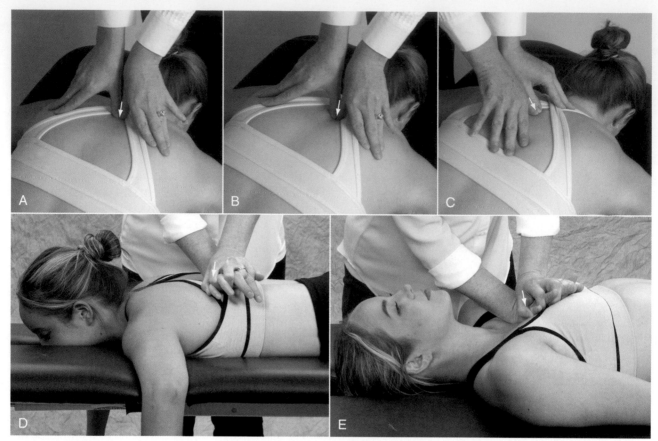

Fig. 8.55 Hand, finger, and thumb positions for joint play movements. (A) Posteroanterior central vertebral pressure (PACVP). (B) Posteroanterior unilateral vertebral pressure (PAUVP). (C) Transverse vertebral pressure (TVP). (D) Rib springing in prone using hypothenar eminence to spring ribs. (E) Rib springing in supine using hypothenar eminence to spring ribs.

appropriate lamina or transverse process of the thoracic vertebra (Fig. 8.56; see Fig. 8.55B). The same anterior springing pressure is applied as in the PACVP technique. Again, each vertebra is done in turn. The two sides should be examined and compared. It must be remembered that in the thoracic area, the spinous process is not necessarily at the same level as the transverse process on the same vertebra. For example, the T9 spinous process is at the level of the T10 transverse process. Therefore it is necessary to move the fingers up and out from the tip of the T9 spinous process to the T9 transverse process, which is at the level of the T8 spinous process. This difference does not hold true for the entire thoracic spine. It is also important to realize that a posteroanterior unilateral vertebral pressure (PAUVP) applies a rotary force to the vertebra; it therefore places a greater stress at the costotransverse joints because the ribs are also stressed where they attach to the vertebrae. A PAUVP applied to the right transverse process causes the vertebral body to rotate to the left.

Transverse Vertebral Pressure

The examiner's fingers are placed along the side of the spinous process, as shown in Figs. 8.55C and 8.56. The examiner then applies a transverse springing pressure to the side of the spinous process, feeling for the quality of movement. As before, each vertebra is assessed in turn, starting at C6 and working down to L1 or L2. Pressure should be applied to both sides of the spinous process to compare the movement. This technique also applies a rotary force to the vertebra but in the opposite direction to that caused by the PAUVP. A TVP applied to the right side of the spinous process causes the spinous process to rotate to the left and the vertebral body to rotate to the right.

The **individual apophyseal** joints may also be tested (Fig. 8.57). The patient is placed in a prone lying position with the thoracic spine in neutral. To test the superior glide at the apophyscal joint (i.e., to test the ability of the inferior articular process of the superior vertebra [e.g., T6] to glide superiorly on the superior articular process of the inferior vertebra [e.g., T7]), the examiner stabilizes the transverse process of the inferior vertebra (e.g., T7) with one thumb while the other thumb glides the inferior articular process of the superior vertebra (e.g., T6) superoanteriorly, noting the end feel and quality of the motion (see Fig. 8.57A).[19]

To test the inferior glide at the apophyseal joint (i.e., to test the ability of the inferior articular process of the superior vertebra [e.g., T6] to glide inferiorly on the superior articular process of the inferior vertebra [e.g., T7]), the examiner stabilizes the transverse process of the inferior vertebra (e.g., T7) with one thumb while the other thumb glides the inferior articular process of the superior vertebra (e.g., T6) inferiorly, noting the end feel and quality of the movement (see Fig. 8.57B).[19]

To test the costotransverse joints, the patient is placed in a prone lying position with the spine in neutral. The examiner stabilizes the thoracic vertebra by placing one thumb along or against the side of the transverse process. The other thumb is placed over the posterior and/or superior aspect of the rib just lateral to the tubercle. Some examiners may find it easier to cross thumbs. An anterior or inferior glide is applied to the rib, causing an anterior or inferior movement (Fig. 8.58).

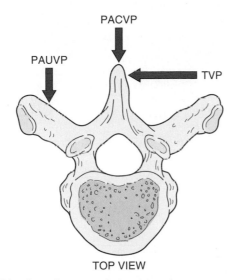

PACVP

PAUVP

TVP

TOP VIEW

Fig. 8.56 Direction of pressure during joint play movements. *PACVP,* Posteroanterior central vertebral pressure; *PAUVP,* posteroanterior unilateral vertebral pressure; *TVP,* transverse vertebral pressure.

Rib Springing

With the patient in relaxed prone or supine and the arms hanging over the plinth to protract the scapulae out of the way, the examiner places the hypothenar eminence of one hand supported by the other hand over several ribs starting at the top of the rib cage and working down and applies a vertical springing force to the ribs, noting any pain and the flexibility of the rib movement (Fig. 8.55D and E). The examiner can do the rib springing movements from above down and right to left, and in supine or prone comparing the rib movement. Care should be taken when doing this on older or osteoporotic patients, as the springing may cause a fracture.

See Chapter 3 for first rib mobility.

Palpation

As with any palpation technique, the examiner is looking for tenderness, muscle spasm, temperature alteration, swelling, or other signs that may indicate disease. Palpation should begin on the anterior chest wall, move around the lateral chest wall, and finish with the posterior structures (Fig. 8.59). Palpation is usually done with the patient sitting, although it may be done by combining the supine and prone lying positions. At the same time, the thorax may be divided into sections (Fig. 8.60) to give some idea, in charting, where the pathology may lie.

Anterior Aspect

Sternum. In the midline of the chest, the manubrium sternum, body of the sternum, and xiphoid process should be palpated for any abnormality or tenderness.

Ribs and Costal Cartilage. Adjacent to the sternum, the examiner should palpate the sternocostal and costochondral articulations, noting any swelling, tenderness, or abnormality. These "articulations" are sometimes sprained or subluxed, or a costochondritis (e.g., Tietze syndrome) may be evident. The ribs should be palpated as they extend

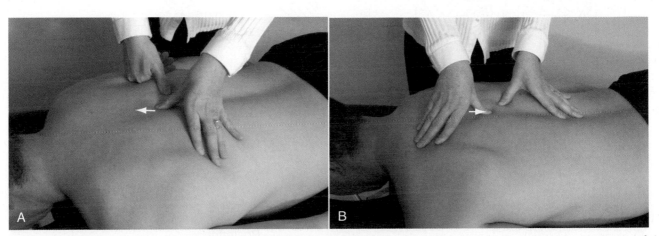

Fig. 8.57 (A) Superior glide of inferior facet of superior vertebra on inferior vertebra. (B) Inferior glide of inferior facet of superior vertebra on inferior vertebra.

around the chest wall with any potential pathology or crepitations (e.g., subcutaneous emphysema) noted.

Clavicle. The clavicle should be palpated along its length for abnormal bumps (e.g., fracture, callus) or tenderness.

Abdomen. The abdomen should be palpated for tenderness or other signs indicating pathology. The palpation is done in a systematic fashion, using the fingers of one hand to feel the tissues while the other hand is used to apply pressure. Palpation is carried out to a depth of 1 to 3 cm (0.5 to 1.5 inches) to reveal areas of tenderness and abnormal masses. When palpating, if the examiner places the hand on the abdomen away from the area of suspected pathology and palpates deeply and then quickly removes the hand, if pain is felt on release, it is called **rebound tenderness** and may indicate an inflamed peritoneum. Palpation is usually carried out using the four-quadrant or the nine-region system (Fig. 8.61). To palpate the **abdominal aortic pulse**, the patient is placed in crook lying with the abdominal muscles relaxed. The examiner palpates to the left of the navel (i.e., umbilicus or belly button) feeling for a pulse. Once the pulse is found, the examiner continues laterally until the pulse

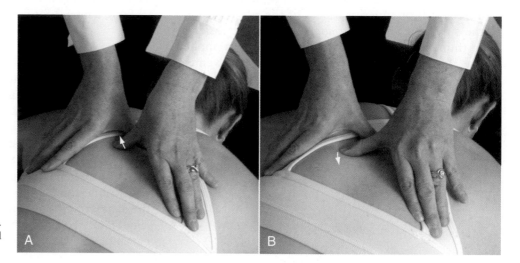

Fig. 8.58 Testing costotransverse joints. (A) Anterior glide with crossed thumbs. (B) Inferior glide.

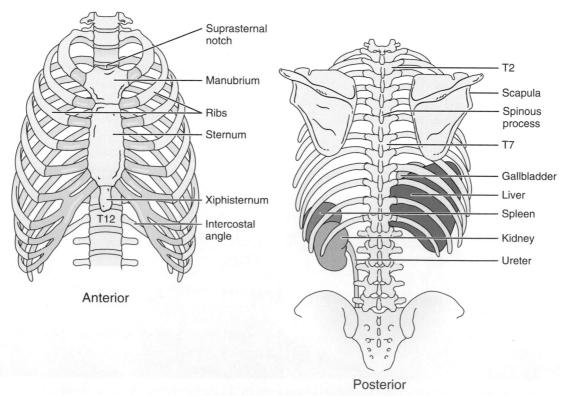

Anterior

Posterior

Fig. 8.59 Landmarks of the thoracic spine.

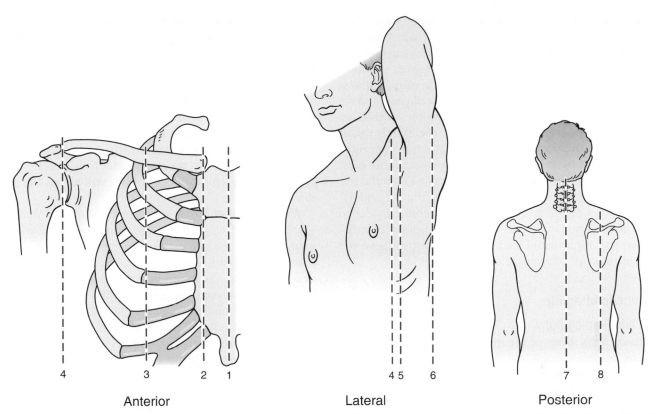

Fig. 8.60 Lines of reference in the thoracic area: *1*, midsternal line; *2*, parasternal line; *3*, midclavicular line; *4*, anterior axillary line; *5*, midaxillary line; *6*, posterior axillary line; *7*, midspinal (vertebral) line; *8*, midscapular line.

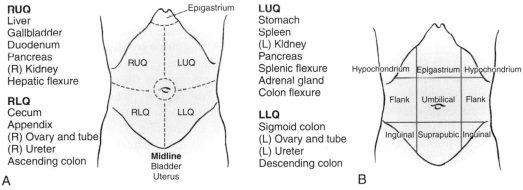

RUQ
Liver
Gallbladder
Duodenum
Pancreas
(R) Kidney
Hepatic flexure

RLQ
Cecum
Appendix
(R) Ovary and tube
(R) Ureter
Ascending colon

LUQ
Stomach
Spleen
(L) Kidney
Pancreas
Splenic flexure
Adrenal gland
Colon flexure

LLQ
Sigmoid colon
(L) Ovary and tube
(L) Ureter
Descending colon

Fig. 8.61 Superficial topography of the abdomen. (A) Four-quadrant system. *LLQ*, Left lower quadrant; *LUQ*, left upper quadrant; *RLQ*, right lower quadrant; *RUQ*, right upper quadrant. (B) Nine-regions system. (From Judge RD, Zuidema GD, Fitzgerald FT: *Clinical diagnosis: a physiologic approach*, Boston, 1982, Little Brown, p 284.)

is no longer detected. If the distance between the two points is greater than 2.5 cm (1 inch), the patient should be referred for follow-up for possible aortic damage (e.g., aneurysm).

Posterior Aspect

Scapula. The medial, lateral, and superior borders of the scapula should be palpated for any swelling or tenderness. The scapula normally extends from the spinous process of T2 to that of T7–T9. After the borders of the scapula have been palpated, the examiner palpates the posterior surface of the scapula. Structures palpated are the supraspinatus and infraspinatus muscles and the spine of the scapula.

Spinous Processes of the Thoracic Spine. In the midline, the examiner may posteriorly palpate the thoracic spinous processes for abnormality. The examiner then moves laterally approximately 2 to 3 cm (0.8 to 1.2 inches) to palpate the thoracic facet joints. Because of the overlying muscles, it is usually very difficult to palpate these joints, although the examiner may be able to palpate for muscle spasm and tenderness. Muscle spasm may also be elicited if some internal structures are injured. For example, pathology affecting the following structures can cause muscle spasm in the surrounding area: gallbladder (spasm on the right side in the area of the eighth and ninth costal cartilages), spleen (spasm at the level of ribs 9 through 11 on the left side), and kidneys (spasm at the level of ribs 11 and 12 on both sides at the level of the L3 vertebra). Evidence of positive findings with no comparable history of musculoskeletal origin could lead the examiner to believe the problem was not of a musculoskeletal origin.

Diagnostic Imaging

Plain Film Radiography

Common x-ray views of the thoracic spine are outlined in the box below.

Common X-Ray Views of the Thoracic Spine

- Anteroposterior view (routine) (Fig. 8.63)
- Lateral view (include ribs and sternum) (routine) (Fig. 8.66)
- Lateral view (arm overhead)
- Oblique view (include ribs and sternum) (Fig. 8.68)
- Swimmer's view (Fig. 8.69)

Anteroposterior View. With this view (Fig. 8.62), the examiner should note the following:

1. Any wedging of the vertebrae
2. Whether the disc spaces appear normal
3. Whether the ring epiphysis, if present, is normal
4. Whether there is a "bamboo" spine, indicative of ankylosing spondylitis (Fig. 8.64)
5. Any scoliosis (Fig. 8.65)
6. Malposition of heart and lungs
7. Normal symmetry of the ribs

Lateral View. The examiner should note the following:

1. A normal mild kyphosis
2. Any wedging of the vertebrae, which may be an indication of structural kyphosis resulting from conditions such as Scheuermann's disease or wedge fracture from trauma or osteoporosis (Fig. 8.67). Scheuermann's disease is radiologically defined as an anterior kyphosis in which there is a 5° or greater anterior wedging of at least three consecutive vertebral bodies.[14]
3. Whether the disc spaces appear normal
4. Whether the ring epiphysis, if present, is normal

5. Whether there are any **Schmorl's nodules,** indicating herniation of the intervertebral disc into the vertebral body
6. Angle of the ribs
7. Any osteophytes

Diffuse Idiopathic Skeletal Hyperostosis. This condition of unknown etiology is indicated by ossification along the anterolateral aspect of at least four contiguous vertebrae leading to back pain and spinal stiffness. It is most common in the thoracic spine, followed by cervical and lumbar spines. It does not involve the sacroiliac joints.

Measurement of Spinal Curvature for Scoliosis. With the Cobb method (Fig. 8.70), an anteroposterior view is used.[15,53,54] A line is drawn parallel to the superior cortical plate of the proximal end vertebra and to the inferior cortical plate of the distal end vertebra. A perpendicular line is erected to each of these lines, and the angle of intersection of the perpendicular lines is the angle of spinal curvature resulting from scoliosis. Such techniques have led the Scoliosis Research Society to classify all forms of scoliosis according to the degree of curvature: group 1: 0° to 20°; group 2: 21° to 30°; group 3: 31° to 50°; group 4: 51° to 75°; group 5: 76° to 100°; group 6: 101° to 125°; and group 7: 126° or greater.[16] Other noninvasive methods of measuring the curve have been advocated. However, the examiner should use the same method each time for consistency and reliability.[55,56]

The rotation of the vertebrae may also be estimated from an anteroposterior view (Fig. 8.71). This estimation is best done by the **pedicle method,** in which the examiner determines the relation of the pedicles to the lateral margins of the vertebral bodies. The vertebra is in neutral position when the pedicles appear to be at equal distance from the lateral margin of the peripheral bodies on the film. If rotation is evident, the pedicles appear to move laterally toward the concavity of the curve.

Computed Tomography

Computed tomography is of primary use in evaluating the bony spine, the spinal contents, and the surrounding soft tissues in cross-sectional views.

Magnetic Resonance Imaging

Magnetic resonance imaging (MRI) is a noninvasive technique that is useful for delineating soft tissue, including herniated discs and intrinsic spinal cord lesions, as well as bony tissue (Fig. 8.72). However, MRI should be used only to confirm a clinical diagnosis, because conditions such as disc herniation have been demonstrated on MRI in the absence of clinical symptoms.[57,58]

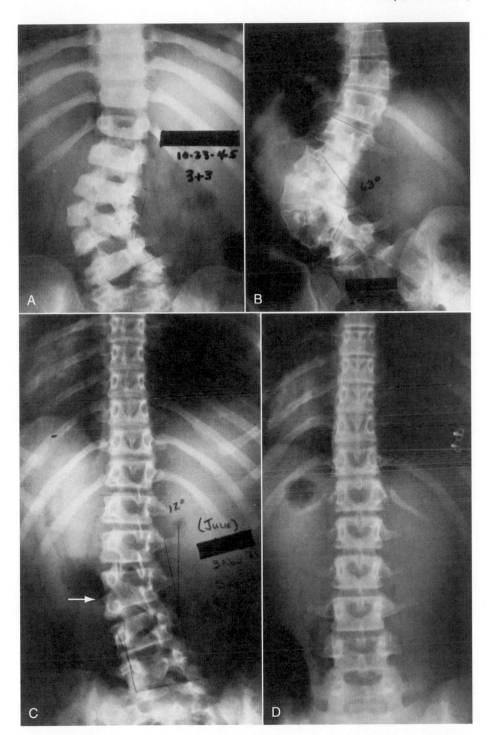

Fig. 8.62 Structural scoliosis caused by congenital defect. (A) Left midlumbar and right lumbosacral hemivertebrae in a 3-year-old child (example of hemimetameric shift). (B) A first cousin also demonstrates a midlumbar hemivertebra as well as asymmetric development of the upper sacrum. (C) This girl has a semisegmented hemivertebra *(arrow)* in the midlumbar spine with a mild 12° curve. (D) Her identical twin sister showed no congenital anomalies of the spine. (From Moe JH, Winter RB, Bradford DS, et al: *Scoliosis and other spinal deformities*, Philadelphia, 1978, WB Saunders, p 134.)

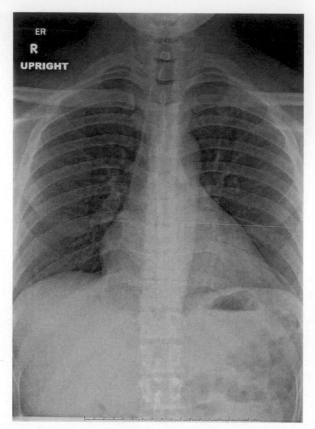

Fig. 8.63 Anteroposterior view of the thoracic spine.

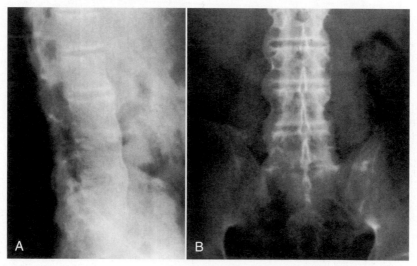

Fig. 8.64 Ankylosing spondylitis of spine. Note the bony encasement of vertebral bodies on the lateral view (A) and the bamboo effect on the anteroposterior view (B). (From Gartland JJ: *Fundamentals of orthopedics*, Philadelphia, 1979, WB Saunders, p 147.)

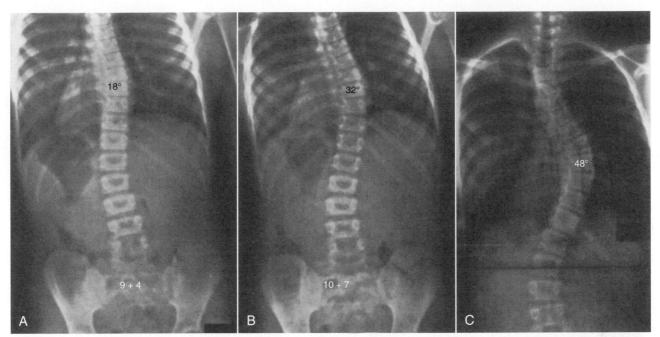

Fig. 8.65 The natural history of idiopathic scoliosis. (A) Note the mild degree of vertebral rotation and curvature and the imbalance of the upper torso. (B) Note the rather dramatic increase in curvature and the increased rotation of the apical vertebrae 1 year later. (C) Further progression of the curvature has occurred, and the opportunity for brace treatment has been missed. (From Bunnel WP: Treatment of idiopathic scoliosis, *Orthop Clin North Am* 10:813–827, 1979.)

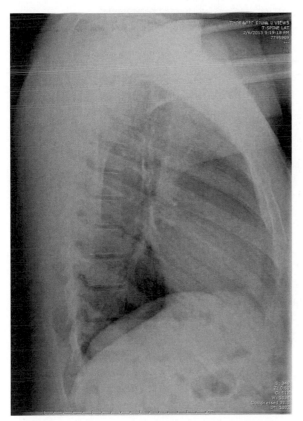

Fig. 8.66 Lateral view of the thoracic spine (including ribs).

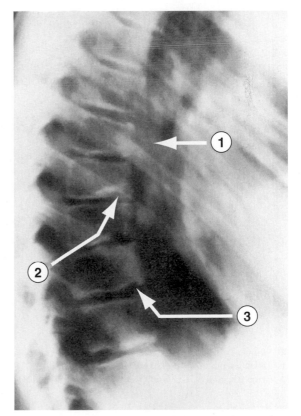

Fig. 8.67 A classic x-ray appearance of the spine in a patient with Scheuermann disease. Note the wedged vertebra *(1)*, Schmorl nodules *(2)*, and marked irregularity of the vertebral end plates *(3)*. (From Moe JH, Bradford DS, Winter RB, et al: *Scoliosis and other spinal deformities*, Philadelphia, 1978, WB Saunders, p 332.)

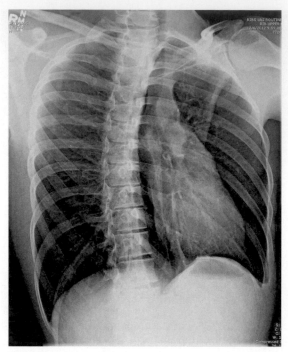

Fig. 8.68 Oblique view of the thoracic spine (including ribs and sternum).

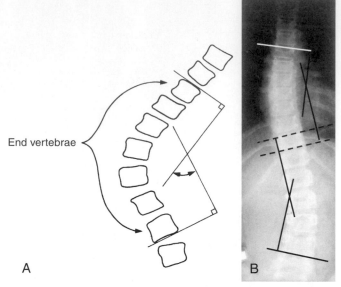

Fig. 8.70 (A) Cobb method of measuring scoliotic curve. (B) Measurement of idiopathic scoliosis (Cobb method). This 10-year-old girl has a T4–T11 right spinal curvature of 20° and a T11–L4 left spinal curvature of 27°. Note that T11 is included in both curve measurements. Minimal rotation occurs in the thoracic region and essentially none in the lumbar segment. (B, From Ozonoff MB: *Pediatric orthopedic radiology*, ed 2, Philadelphia, 1992, WB Saunders.)

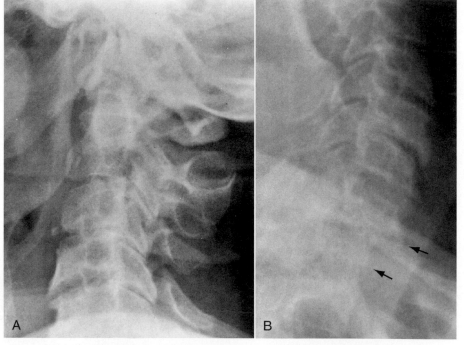

Fig. 8.69 Swimmer's projection in demonstration of the cervicothoracic junction. (A) Initial lateral radiograph includes only the first five cervical vertebrae. There is a small fracture from the anterior inferior margin of C3. (B) A swimmer's projection clearly demonstrates dislocation at C7–T1 *(arrows)*. (From Adam A, Dixon AK, editors: *Grainger & Allison's diagnostic radiology: a textbook of medical imaging*, ed 5, Edinburgh, 2008, Churchill Livingstone/Elsevier.)

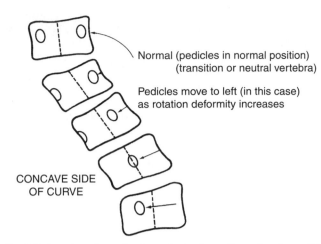

Fig. 8.71 Rotation of vertebra in scoliosis. On radiography, the pedicles appear to be off center as the curve progresses.

Normal (pedicles in normal position)
(transition or neutral vertebra)

Pedicles move to left (in this case)
as rotation deformity increases

CONCAVE SIDE
OF CURVE

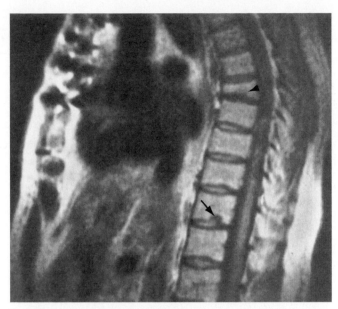

Fig. 8.72 Osteoporotic compression fracture of thoracic spine. Midline sagittal T1-weighted magnetic resonance image (SE 500/30) shows compression fracture of upper thoracic vertebral body *(arrowhead)*, indicated by anterior wedging. Marrow signal intensity is maintained *(arrowhead)*. Schmorl nodule is incidentally noted at a lower level *(arrow)*. (From Bassett LW, Gold RH, Seeger LL: *MRI atlas of the musculoskeletal system*, London, 1989, Martin Dunitz, p 49.)

PRÉCIS OF THE THORACIC SPINE ASSESSMENT[a]

NOTE: Suspected pathology will determine which *Special Tests* are to be performed.
History
Observation (standing)
Examination
  Active movements (standing or sitting)
    Forward flexion
    Extension
    Side flexion (left and right)
    Rotation (left and right)
    Combined movements (if necessary)
    Repetitive movements (if necessary)
    Sustained postures (if necessary)
  Passive movements (sitting)
    Forward flexion
    Extension
    Side flexion (left and right)
    Rotation (left and right)
  Resisted isometric movements (sitting)
    Forward flexion
    Extension
    Side flexion (left and right)
    Rotation (left and right)
  Functional assessment
  Special tests (sitting)
    Adson test

    Costoclavicular maneuver
    Cyriax release test
    Deep breath and flexion test
    Hyperabduction test (elevated arm stress test [EAST])
    Murphy's percussion test
    Reflex hammer test
    Roos test
    Slump test
  Reflexes and cutaneous distribution (sitting)
    Reflex testing
    Sensation scan
  Special tests (prone lying)
    Rib spring test
  Joint play movements (prone lying)
    Posteroanterior central vertebral pressure (PACVP)
    Posteroanterior unilateral vertebral pressure (PAUVP)
    Transverse vertebral pressure (TVP)
    Rib springing
  Palpation (prone lying)
  Special tests (supine lying)
    First rib mobility
    Rib springing
    Upper limb neurodynamic (tension) test 4 (ULNT4)
  Palpation (supine lying)
  Diagnostic imaging

After any assessment, the patient should be warned of the possibility of exacerbation of symptoms as a result of assessment.
[a]The précis is shown in an order that limits the amount of movement that the patient has to do but ensures that all necessary structures are tested.

TABLE **8.9**

Differential Diagnosis of Ankylosing Spondylitis and Thoracic Spinal Stenosis

	Ankylosing Spondylitis	Thoracic Spinal Stenosis
History	Morning stiffness Intermittent aching pain Male predominance Sharp pain → ache Bilateral sacroiliac pain may refer to posterior thigh	Intermittent aching pain Pain may refer to both legs with walking (neurogenic intermittent claudication)
Active movements	Restricted	May be normal
Passive movements	Restricted	May be normal
Resisted isometric movements	Normal	Normal
Special tests	None	Bicycle test of van Gelderen may be positive Stoop test may be positive
Reflexes	Normal	May be affected in long-standing cases
Sensory deficit	None	Usually temporary
Diagnostic imaging	Plain films are diagnostic	Computed tomography scans are diagnostic

CASE STUDIES

When doing these case studies, the examiner should list the appropriate questions to be asked and why they are being asked, what to look for and why, and what things should be tested and why. Depending on the answers of the patient (and the examiner should consider different responses), several possible causes of the patient's problems may be evident (examples are given in parentheses). If so, a differential diagnosis chart (see Table 8.9 as an example) should be made up. The examiner can then decide how different diagnoses may affect the treatment plan.

1. A 16-year-old high school female comes to see you with a 2-week history of mid to low back pain following starting volleyball practice. She can practice but usually about halfway through a 2-hour practice, she has significant back pain. It is worse with running and setting and seems to be better when she is sitting slumped. She has full strength of her trunk and extremities. There are no radicular symptoms. She does have point tenderness to palpation of the transverse and spinous processes around T10. Symptoms are increased when she actively or passively extends her spine past neutral. Give your assessment plan and differential diagnosis.

2. A 72-year-old female is seeing you for mid back pain following a recent fall down a stair at home. She was carrying laundry down to her basement bathroom and accidently missed the last step and fell. She noticed immediate pain in her mid back that has not resolved. Spinal extension aggravates her symptoms. She is having difficulty sleeping due to pain while laying on her back. She appears to have some increased kyphosis in the upper to mid thoracic spine area. She also has point

tenderness to spinous process of T7 and T8. She has not yet had diagnostic imaging. Give your assessment plan and differential diagnosis.

3. A 52-year-old male comes to see you for left shoulder and upper back pain. He has a history of high blood pressure and a family history of cardiac disease. During exercise in the last two weeks, he has felt shortness of breath and has also felt some slight left neck, jaw, upper back, and arm pain that increases with his exercise intensity. He states that he wonders sometimes if he is a hypochondriac and is usually hesitant to seek medical help. You are unable to find any palpable pain, and he seems to be in no distress at the moment. He has full shoulder and trunk mobility. You assess his blood pressure, and it is rather high at 170/100 while resting. Describe your assessment plan and differential diagnosis.

4. A 17-year-old, male, right-hand dominant baseball player comes to see you for lower to mid back pain on the left following "getting beaned" by a baseball in a recent game. He bats right and turned to his right to get away from the wild pitch. He has a large area of discoloration in the

CASE STUDIES—cont'd

left lower back area near ribs T9–12. He is also tender to palpation of that area. The area feels somewhat enlarged and swollen. He also reported a rebound type pain when palpating the ribs in that area. You are somewhat concerned as you know that the spleen lies directly under these ribs in this location. Describe your assessment plan and your differential diagnosis.

5. A 33-year-old patient comes to you complaining of stiffness in the lower spine that is extending into the thoracic spine. Describe your assessment plan for this patient (ankylosing spondylitis vs. thoracic spinal stenosis).

6. A 14-year-old boy presents complaining of a severe aching pain in the mid-dorsal spine of several weeks' duration. He is neurologically normal. X-rays reveal a narrowing and anterior wedging at T5 with a Schmorl nodule into T4. Describe your assessment plan for this patient (kyphosis vs. Scheuermann disease).

7. A 23-year-old woman has a structural scoliosis with a single C curve having its apex at T7.

Describe your assessment plan before beginning treatment. How would you measure the curve and the amount of rotation?

8. A 38-year-old woman comes to your clinic complaining of chest pain with tenderness at the costochondral junction of two ribs on the left side. Describe your assessment plan for this patient (Tietze syndrome vs. rib hypomobility).

9. A 26-year-old male ice hockey player comes to you complaining of back pain that is referred around the chest. He explains that he was "boarded" (hit between another player and the boards). He did not notice the pain and stiffness until the next day. He has had the problem for 2 weeks. Describe your assessment plan for this patient (rib hypomobility vs. ligament sprain).

10. A 21-year-old female synchronized swimmer comes to you complaining of pain in her side. She says she was kicked when she helped boost another athlete out of the water 5 days ago. Describe your assessment plan for this patient (rib fracture vs. rib hypomobility).

References

1. Dutton M. *Dutton's Orthopedic Examination, Evaluation and Intervention*. 4th ed. New York: McGraw-Hill Education; 2017.
2. Williams P, Warwick R, eds. *Gray's Anatomy*. 36th ed. British, Edinburgh: Churchill Livingstone; 1980.
3. MacConaill MA, Basmajian JV. *Muscles and Movements: A Basis for Human Kinesiology*. Baltimore: Williams & Wilkins; 1969.
4. Mitchell FL, Moran PS, Pruzzo NA. *An Evaluation and Treatment Manual of Osteopathic Muscle Energy Procedures*. Valley Park, MO: Mitchell, Moran & Pruzzo, Assoc; 1979.
5. Michael AL, Newman J, Rao AS. The assessment of thoracic pain. *Orthop Trauma*. 2009;24:63–73.
6. Hijaz NM, Friesen CA. Managing acute abdominal pain in pediatric patients: current perspectives. *Pediatric Health Med Ther*. 2017;8:83–91.
7. Henderson JM. Ruling out danger: differential diagnosis of thoracic spine. *Phys Sportsmed*. 1992;20:124–132.
8. Dreyfuss P, Tibiletti C, Dreyer SJ. Thoracic zygapophyseal joint pain patterns: a study in normal volunteers. *Spine*. 1994;19:807–811.
9. Ombregt L, Bisschop P, ter Veer HJ, et al. *A System of Orthopedic Medicine*. London: WB Saunders; 1995.
10. McKenzie RA. *The Cervical and Thoracic Spine: Mechanical Diagnosis and Therapy*. Waikanae, New Zealand: Spinal Publications; 1981.
11. Fon G, Pitt MJ, Thies AC. Thoracic kyphosis: range in normal subjects. *Am J Roentgenol*. 1980;134(5):979–983.
12. Katzman WB, Wanek L, Shepherd JA, et al. Age-related hyperkyphosis: its causes, consequences

and management. *J Orthop Sports Phys Ther*. 2010;40:352–360.
13. Wiles P, Sweetnam R. *Essentials of Orthopaedics*. London: JA Churchill; 1965.
14. Wood KB, Melikian R, Villamil F. Adult Scheuermann kyphysis: evaluation, management and new developments. *J Am Acad Orthop Surg*. 2012;20:113–121.
15. Keim HA. Scoliosis. *Clin Symposia*. 1973;25:1–25.
16. Keim HA. *The Adolescent Spine*. New York: Springer-Verlag; 1982.
17. Sutherland ID. Funnel chest. *J Bone Joint Surg Br*. 1958;40:244–251.
18. Reiman MP. *Orthopedic Clinical Examination*. Champaign, Il: Human Kinetics; 2016.
19. Lee D. *Manual Therapy for the Thorax—A Biomechanical Approach*. Delta, BC: DOPC; 1994.
20. Evans RC. *Illustrated Essentials in Orthopedic Physical Assessment*. St Louis: CV Mosby; 1994.
21. Lee DG. Rotational instability of the mid-thoracic spine: assessment and management. *Man Ther*. 1996;1(5):234–241.
22. Lee LJ. The thoracic ring approach™ — a whole person framework to assess and treat the thoracic spine and ribcage. In: Magee DJ, Zachazewski JE, Quillen WS, Manske RC, eds. *Pathology and Intervention in Musculoskeletal Rehabilitation*. 2nd ed. Philadelphia: Elsevier; 2016.
23. Lee DG. Biomechanics of the thorax: a clinical mode of in vivo function. *J Man Manip Ther*. 1993;1:13–21.
24. Evjenth O, Gloeck C. *Symptoms Localization in the Spine and the Extremity Joints*. Minneapolis: OPTP; 2000.
25. Stoddard A. *Manual of Osteopathic Technique*. London: Hutchinson Medical Publications; 1959.

26. Bookhout MR. Evaluation of the thoracic spine and rib cage. In: Flynn TW, ed. *The Thoracic Spine and Rib Cage*. Boston: Butterworth-Heinemann; 1996.
27. Walker BF, Koppenhaver L, Tomski N, Hebert JJ. Interrater reliability of motion palpation in the thoracic spine. *Evid Based Complement Alternat Med*. Vol 2015:6. Article ID I815407.
28. Fairbank JC, Pynsent PD. The Oswestry disability index. *Spine*. 2000;25:2940–2953.
29. Roland M, Fairbank J. The Roland-Morris disability questionnaire and the Oswestry disability questionnaire. *Spine*. 2000;25:3115–3124.
30. Fairbank JC, Couper J, Davies JB, et al. The Oswestry low back pain disability questionnaire. *Physiotherapy*. 1980;66:271–273.
31. Feise RJ, Menke JM. Functional rating index: a new valid and reliable instrument to measure the magnitude of clinical change in spinal conditions. *Spine*. 2001;26:78–87.
32. Matamalas A, Bago J, D'Agata E, Pellise F. Body image in idiopathic scoliosis: a comparison of psychometric properties between four patient-reported outcome instruments. *Health Qual Life Outcomes*. 2014;12:81–89.
33. Brewer P, Berryman F, Baker D, et al. Analysis of the scoliosis research society–22 questionnaire scores: is there a difference between a child and parent and does physician review change that? *Spine Deformity*. 2014;2:34–39.
34. Asher M, Min Lai S, Burton D, Manna B. The reliability and concurrent validity of the scoliosis research society–22 patient questionnaire for idiopathic scoliosis. *Spine*. 2003;28(1):63–69.

35. Sanders JO, Harrast JJ, Tuklo TR, et al. The spinal appearance questionnaire – Results of reliability, validity, and responsiveness testing in patients with idiopathic scoliosis. *Spine*. 2007;32(24):2719–2722.

36. Thielsch MT, Wetterkamp M, Boertz P, et al. Reliability and validity of the spinal appearance questionnaire (SAQ) and the trunk appearance perception scale (TAPS). *J Orthop Surg Res*. 2018;13(1):274–283.

37. Bago J, Sanchez-Raya J, Perez-Grueso FJ, Climent JM. The trunk appearance perception scale (TAPS): a new tool to evaluate subjective impression of trunk deformity in patients with idiopathic scoliosis. *Scoliosis*. 2010;5:6–15.

38. Pineda S, Bago J, Gilperez C, Climent JM. Validity of the Walter Reed Visual Assessment Scale to measure subjective perception of spine deformity in patients with idiopathic scoliosis. *Scoliosis*. 2006;1:18–26.

39. Cook CE, Hegedus EJ. *Orthopedic Physical Examination Tests—An Evidence Based Approach*. Upper Saddle River, NJ: Prentice Hall/Pearson; 2008.

40. Cleland JA, Koppenhaver S. *Netter's Orthopedic Clinical Examination—An Evidence Based Approach*. 2nd ed. Philadelphia: Saunders/Elsevier; 2011.

41. Cyriax J. *Textbook of Orthopaedic Medicine. Diagnosis of Soft Tissue Lesions*. vol. 1. London: Bailliere Tindall; 1982.

42. Wilke A, Wolf U, Lageard P, et al. Thoracic disc herniation: a diagnostic challenge. *Man Ther*. 2000;5:181–184.

43. Evans RC. *Illustrated Orthopedic Physical Assessment*. 3rd ed. St Louis: Elsevier; 2009.

44. Maitland GD. The slump test: examination and treatment. *Aust J Physiother*. 1985;31:215–219.

45. Butler DS. *Mobilization of the Nervous System*. Melbourne: Churchill Livingstone; 1991.

46. Lee L-J, Lee D. The thoracic spine and ribs. In: Magee DJ, Zachazewski J, Quillen W, eds. *Musculoskeletal Rehabilitation—Pathology and Intervention*. St Louis: Elsevier; 2009.

47. Soyuncu S, Bektas F, Cete Y. Traditional Kehr's sign: left shoulder pain related to splenic abscess. *Turkish J Trauma Emerg Surg*. 2012;18(1):87–88.

48. Heslop JH. Saegesser's sign or the phrenic-point test. *Lancet*. 1956;271(6954):1184–1185.

49. Lonnemann ME, Burke-Doe A. Special tests for medical screening. In: Placzek, Boyce D, eds. *Orthopedic Physical Therapy Secrets*. 3rd ed. Philadelphia: Elsevier; 2017.

50. Maitland GD. *Vertebral Manipulation*. London: Butterworths; 1973.

51. Heiderscheit B, Boissonnault W. Reliability of joint mobility and pain assessment of the thoracic spine and rib cage in asymptomatic individuals. *J Man Manip Ther*. 2008;16(4):210–216.

52. Edmondston SJ, Allison GT, Althorpe BM, et al. Comparison of rib cage and posteroanterior thoracic spine stiffness: an investigation of the normal response. *Man Ther*. 1999;4:157–162.

53. Adam CJ, Izatt MT, Harvey JR, et al. Variability in Cobb angle measurements using reformatted computerized tomography scans. *Spine*. 2005;50:1664–1669.

54. Loder RT, Spiegel D, Gutknecht S, et al. The assessment of intraobserver and interobserver error in measurement of noncongenital scoliosis in children = 10 years of age. *Spine*. 2004;29:2548–2553.

55. Pearsall DJ, Reid JG, Hedden DM. Comparison of three noninvasive methods for measuring scoliosis. *Phys Ther*. 1992;72:648–657.

56. Pun WK, Luk KD, Lee W, et al. A simple method to estimate the rib hump in scoliosis. *Spine*. 1987;12:342–345.

57. Wood KB, Garvey TA, Gundry C, et al. Magnetic resonance imaging of the thoracic spine. *J Bone Joint Surg Am*. 1995;77:1631–1638.

58. Wood KB, Blair JM, Aepple DM, et al. The natural history of asymptomatic thoracic disc herniations. *Spine*. 1997;22:525–530.

59. Cote P, Kreitz BG, Cassidy JD, et al. A study of the diagnostic accuracy and reliability of the scoliometer and Adam's forward bend test. *Spine*. 1998;23(7):796–803.

60. Karachalios T, Sofianos J, Roidis N, et al. Ten-year follow-up evaluation of a school screening program for scoliosis. *Spine*. 1999;24(22):2318–2324.

61. Langdon J, Way A, Heaton S, Bernard J, Molloy S. Vertebral compression fractures new clinical signs to aid diagnosis. *Ann R Coll Surg Engl*. 2010;92(2):163–166.

62. Ueda T, Ishida E. Indirect Fist Percussion of the Liver Is a More Sensitive Technique for Detecting Hepatobiliary Infections than Murphy's Sign. *Curr Gerontol Geriatr Res*. 2015;2015:431638.

63. Philip K, Lwe P, Matyas TA. The inter-therapist reliability of the slump test. *Austr J Phys Ther*. 1989;35(2):89–94.

64. Urban LM, MacNeil BJ. Diagnostic accuracy of the slump test for identifying neuropathic pain in the lower limb. *J Orthop Sports Phys Ther*. 2015;45(8):596–603.

65. Majlesi J, Togay H, Unalan H, Toprak S. The sensitivity and specificity of the slump and the straight leg raising tests in patients with lumbar disc herniation. *J Clin Rheumatol*. 2008;14(2):87–91.

66. Stankovic R, Johnell O, Maly P, Willner S. Use of lumbar extension, slump test, physical and neurological examination in the evaluation of patients with suspected herniated nucleus pulposus: a prospective clinical study. *Man Ther*. 1999;4(1):25–32.

67. Bridwell KH, Cats-Baril W, Harrast J, et al. The validity of the SRS-22 instrument in an adult spinal deformity population compared with the Oswestry and SF-12: a study of response distribution, concurrent validity, internal consistency and reliability. *Spine*. 2005;30(4):455–461.

CHAPTER 9

Lumbar Spine

Back pain is one of the great human afflictions. Almost anyone born today in Europe or North America has a great chance of suffering a disabling back injury regardless of occupation.[1] The lumbar spine supports the upper body and transmits the weight of the upper body to the pelvis and lower limbs. Because of the strategic location of the lumbar spine, this structure should be included in any examination of the spine as a whole (i.e., posture) or in any examination of the hip or sacroiliac joints. Unless there is a definite history of trauma, determining whether an injury originates in the lumbar spine, sacroiliac joints, or hip joints is often difficult; therefore all three should be examined in a sequential fashion.

Applied Anatomy

There are 10 (five pairs) facet joints (also called *apophyseal* or *zygoapophyseal joints*) in the lumbar spine (Fig. 9.1).[2] These diarthrodial joints consist of superior and inferior facets and a capsule. The facets are located on the vertebral arches. With a normal intact disc, the facet joints carry about 20% to 25% of the axial load, but this may reach 70% with degeneration of the disc. The facet joints also provide 40% of the torsional and shear strength.[3] Injury, degeneration, or trauma to the **motion segment** (the facet joints and disc) may lead to **spondylosis**[4] (degeneration of the intervertebral disc), **spondylolysis**[5] (a defect in the pars interarticularis or the arch of the vertebra), **spondylolisthesis**[5] (a forward displacement of one vertebra over another), or **retrolisthesis** (backward displacement of one vertebra on another). The superior facets, or articular processes, face medially and backward and in general are concave; the inferior facets face laterally and forward and are convex (Fig. 9.2). There are, however, abnormalities, or **tropisms,** that can occur in the shape of the facets, especially at the L5–S1 level (Figs. 9.3 and 9.4).[6] In the lumbar spine, the transverse processes are virtually at the same level as the spinous processes.

These posterior facet joints direct the movement that occurs in the lumbar spine. Because of the shape of the facets, rotation in the lumbar spine is minimal and is accomplished only by a shearing force. Side flexion, extension, and flexion can occur in the lumbar spine, but the facet joints control the direction of movement. The close packed position of the facet joints in the lumbar spine is extension. Normally, the facet joints carry only a small amount of weight; however, with increased extension, they begin to have a greater weight-bearing function. The resting position is midway between flexion and extension. The capsular pattern is side flexion and rotation equally limited, followed by extension. However, if only one facet joint in the lumbar spine has a capsular restriction, the amount of observable restriction is minimal. The first sacral segment is usually included in discussions of the lumbar spine, and it is at this joint that the fixed segment of the sacrum joins with the mobile segments of the lumbar spine. In some cases the S1 segment may be mobile. This occurrence is called **lumbarization** of S1, and it results in a sixth "lumbar" vertebra. At other times, the fifth lumbar segment may be fused to the sacrum or ilium, resulting in a **sacralization** of that vertebra. Sacralization results in four mobile lumbar vertebrae. These abnormal segments are sometimes called transitional vertebra.[7]

Lumbar Spine

Resting position:	Midway between flexion and extension
Close packed position:	Full extension
Capsular pattern:	Side flexion and rotation equally limited, extension

---

The main ligaments of the lumbar spine are the same as those in the lower cervical and thoracic spine excluding the ribs. These ligaments include the anterior and posterior longitudinal ligaments, the ligamentum flavum, the supraspinous and interspinous ligaments, and the intertransverse ligaments (Fig. 9.5). In addition, there is an important ligament unique to the lumbar spine and pelvis—the iliolumbar ligament (Fig. 9.6), which connects the transverse process of L5 to the posterior ilium.[8] This ligament helps to stabilize L5 with the ilium and to prevent anterior displacement of L5.[9]

The intervertebral discs make up approximately 20% to 25% of the total length of the vertebral column. The function of the intervertebral disc is to act as a shock absorber, distributing and absorbing some of the load applied to the spine, to hold the vertebrae together and allow movement between the bones, to separate the vertebra as part of a **functional segmental unit** (Fig. 9.7; Table 9.1) acting in concert with the facet joints and, by separating the vertebrae, to allow the free passage of the nerve roots out from the spinal cord through the intervertebral foramina. With age, the percentage of spinal length attributable to the discs decreases as a result of disc degeneration and loss of hydrophilic action in the disc.

The **annulus fibrosus,** the outer laminated portion of the disc, consists of three zones: (1) an outer zone made up of fibrocartilage (classified as **Sharpey's fibers**) that attaches to the outer or peripheral aspect of the vertebral body and contains increasing numbers of cartilage cells in the fibrous strands with increasing depth, (2) an intermediate zone made up of another layer of fibrocartilage, and (3) an inner zone primarily made up of fibrocartilage and containing the largest number of cartilage cells.[10] The annulus fibrosus contains 20 concentric, collar-like rings of collagenous fibers that crisscross each other to increase their strength and accommodate torsional movements (Fig. 9.8).[11]

The **nucleus pulposus** is well developed in both the cervical and lumbar spines. At birth, it is made up of a hydrophilic mucoid tissue, which is gradually replaced by fibrocartilage. With increasing age, the nucleus pulposus increasingly resembles the annulus fibrosus.[12–14] The water-binding capacity of the disc decreases with age, and degenerative changes (spondylosis) begin to occur after the second decade of life. Initially, the disc contains approximately 85% to 90% water, but the amount decreases to 65% with age.[15] In addition, the disc contains a high proportion of mucopolysaccharides, which cause the disc to act as an incompressible fluid. However, these mucopolysaccharides decrease with age and are replaced with collagen. The nucleus pulposus lies slightly posterior to the center of rotation of the disc in the lumbar spine.

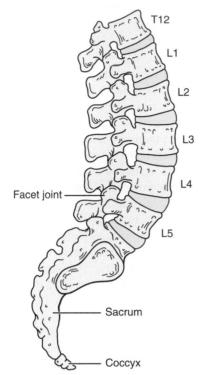

Fig. 9.1 Lateral view of the lumbar spine.

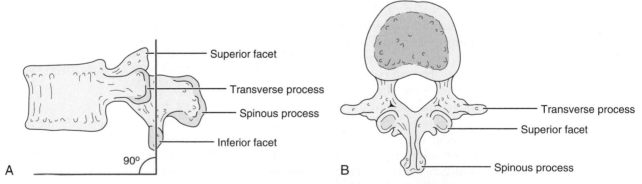

Fig. 9.2 Lumbar vertebra. (A) Side view. (B) Superior view.

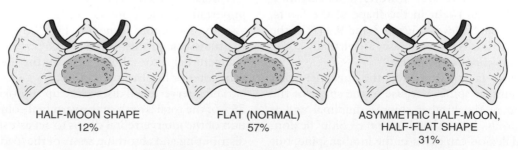

HALF-MOON SHAPE
12%

FLAT (NORMAL)
57%

ASYMMETRIC HALF-MOON, HALF-FLAT SHAPE
31%

Fig. 9.3 Facet anomalies (tropisms) at L5–S1.

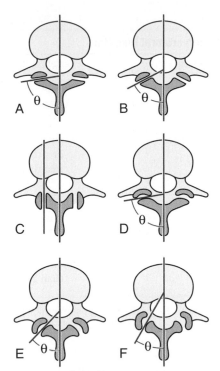

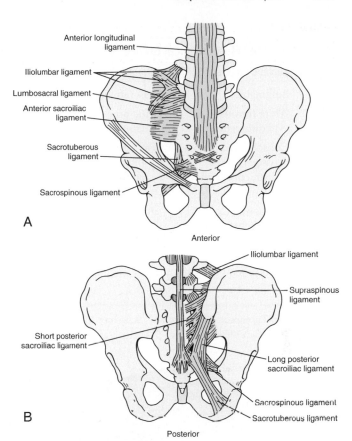

Fig. 9.6 Ligaments of the sacrum, coccyx, and some in the lumbar spine. (A) Anterior view. (B) Posterior view.

Fig. 9.4 The varieties of orientation and curvature of the lumbar zygapophyseal joints. (A) Flat joints oriented close to 90° to the sagittal plane. (B) Flat joints orientated at 60° to the sagittal plane. (C) Flat joints orientated parallel (0°) to the sagittal plane. (D) Slightly curved joints with an average orientation close to 90° to the sagittal plane. (E) "C"-shaped joints orientated at 45° to the sagittal plane. (F) "J"-shaped joints orientated at 30° to the sagittal plane. (Redrawn from Bogduk N, Twomey LT: *Clinical anatomy of the lumbar spine*, New York, 1987, Churchill Livingstone, p 26.)

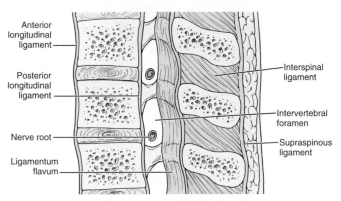

Fig. 9.5 Ligaments of the lumbar spine.

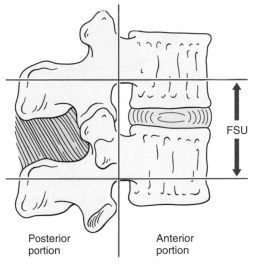

Fig. 9.7 Functional segmental unit *(FSU)* (three-joint complex) in the lumbar spine. Such a complex may also be seen in the cervical and thoracic spines.

The shape of the disc corresponds to that of the body to which it is attached. The disc adheres to the vertebral body by means of the cartilaginous end plate. The end plates consist of thin layers of cartilage covering the majority of the inferior and superior surfaces of the vertebral body. The cartilaginous end plates are approximately 1 mm thick and allow fluid to move between the disc and the vertebral body. The discs are primarily avascular, with only the periphery receiving a blood supply. The remainder of the disc receives nutrition by diffusion, primarily through the cartilaginous end plate. The end plate serves

as a biologic filter, which restricts both the movement of large molecules into the disc and also the expulsion of water from the nucleus when the disc is compressed.[16] Until the age of 8 years, the intervertebral discs have some vascularity; with age, however, this vascularity decreases.

The intervertebral disc usually has no nerve supply, although the peripheral posterior aspect of the annulus

TABLE **9.1**

Description of the Morphological Grades of the Human Functional Segmental Intervertebral Disc Unit

Grade	Nucleus Pulposus (NP)	Annulus Fibrosus (AF)	Cartilaginous End Plate	Vertebral Body
I	Bulging gel	Discrete fibrous lamellae	Hyaline, uniformly thick	Margins rounded
II	White fibrous tissue peripherally	Mucinous material between lamellae	Thickness irregular	Margins pointed
III	Consolidated fibrous tissue (loss of distraction between NP and AF)	Extensive mucinous infiltration; loss of annular-nuclear demarcation	Focal defects in cartilage	Early chondrophytes or osteophytes at margins
IV	Horizontal clefts parallel to end plate; fissures	Focal disruptions	Fibrocartilage extending from subchondral bone (Schmorl's nodules) Irregularity and focal sclerosis in subchondral bone	Osteophytes less than 2 mm
V	Clefts extend through nucleus and annulus		Diffuse sclerosis Schmorl's nodules	Osteophytes greater than 2 mm

Modified from Thompson JP, Pearce RH, Schechter MT, et al: Preliminary evaluation of a scheme for grading the gross morphology of the human intervertebral disc, *Spine* 15(5):412, 1990.

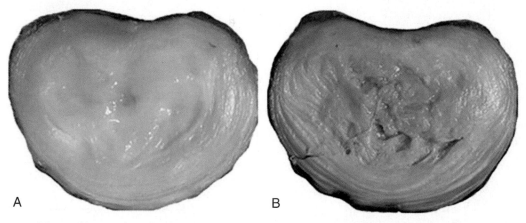

Fig. 9.8 Gross features of the aged human discs. Axial sections of young (16 years) (A) and aged (55 years) (B) lumbar discs. Old discs exhibit an overall loss of hydration, loss of demarcation between the annulus fibrosus and nucleus pulposus boundary, and tissue discoloration (old disc more yellowish). Average lumbar disc cross-sectional diameter is 45 to 55 mm for humans. (From Vo NV, Hartman RA, Patil PR, et al: Molecular mechanisms of biological aging in intervertebral discs, *J Orthop Res* 34:1292, 2016. Courtesy Dr. Ian Stokes.)

fibrosus may be innervated by a few nerve fibers from the sinuvertebral nerve.[17,18] The lateral aspects of the disc are innervated peripherally by the branches of the anterior rami and gray rami communicants. The pain-sensitive structures around the intervertebral disc are the anterior longitudinal ligament, posterior longitudinal ligament, vertebral body, nerve root, and cartilage of the facet joint.

With the movement of fluid vertically through the cartilaginous end plate, the pressure on the disc decreases as the patient assumes the natural lordotic posture in the lumbar spine. Direct vertical pressure on the disc can cause the disc to push fluid into the vertebral body. If the pressure is great enough, defects may occur in the cartilaginous end plate, resulting in **Schmorl's nodules,** which are herniations of the nucleus pulposus into the vertebral body (Fig. 9.9). These are found in 20% to 30% of individuals.[19] Normally, an adult is 1 to 2 cm (0.4 to 0.8 inch) taller in the morning than in the evening (20% diurnal variation).[3,20] This change results from fluid movement in and out of the disc during the day through the cartilaginous end plate. This fluid shift acts as a pressure safety valve to protect the disc.

If there is an injury to the disc, four problems can result, all of which can cause symptoms.[21] There may be a **protrusion** of the disc, in which the disc bulges posteriorly without rupture of the annulus fibrosus. In the case of a disc **prolapse,** only the outermost fibers of the annulus fibrosus contain the nucleus. With a disc **extrusion,** the annulus fibrosus is perforated, and discal material (part of the nucleus pulposus) moves into the epidural

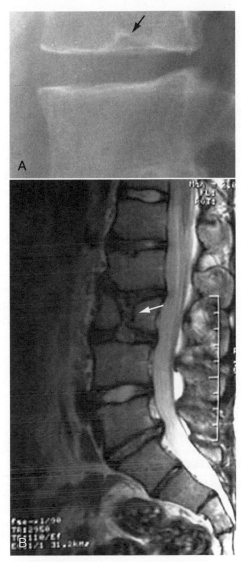

space. The fourth problem is a **sequestrated** disc, or a formation of discal fragments from the annulus fibrosus and nucleus pulposus outside the disc proper (Fig. 9.10).[22] These injuries can result in pressure on the spinal cord itself (upper lumbar spine), leading to a myelopathy; pressure on the cauda equina, leading to **cauda equina syndrome** (saddle anesthesia [Fig. 9.11] bowel/bladder dysfunction);[23] or pressure on the nerve roots (most common). The amount of pressure on the neurological tissues determines the severity of the neurological deficit.[24] The pressure may be the result of the disc injury itself or may occur in combination with the inflammatory response to the injury. Saal has outlined favorable, unfavorable, and neutral factors in relation to a positive prognosis for a nonoperative lumbar disc herniation (Table 9.2).[21]

Within the lumbar spine, different postures can increase pressure on the intervertebral disc (Fig. 9.12). This information is based on the work of Nachemson and colleagues,[25,26] who performed studies of intradiscal pressure changes in the L3 disc with changes in posture. The pressure in the standing position is classified as the norm; the values given are increases or decreases above or below this norm that occur with the change in posture.

Fig. 9.9 (A) X-ray of Schmorl's nodes *(arrow)*. Note the sharply defined dome-like densities arising from the end plate in these two adjacent vertebrae. (B) Magnetic resonance image of Schmorl's nodes going through the cartilaginous end plate *(arrow)*. (A, From Adam A, Dixon AK, Grainger RG, Allison DJ: *Grainger & Allison's diagnostic radiology*, ed 5, Edinburgh, 2007, Churchill Livingstone; B, From Slotkin JR, Mislow JMK, Day AL, Proctor MR: Pediatric disk disease, *Neurosurg Clin North Am* 18[4]:659–667, 2007.)

Activity and Percentage Increase in Disc Pressure at L3

• Coughing or straining:	5%–35%
• Laughing:	40%–50%
• Walking:	15%
• Side bending:	25%
• Small jumps:	40%
• Bending forward:	150%
• Rotation:	20%
• Lifting a 20-kg weight with the back straight and knees bent:	73%
• Lifting a 20-kg weight with the back bent and knees straight:	169%

In the lumbar spine, the nerve roots exit through relatively large intervertebral foramina; as in the thoracic

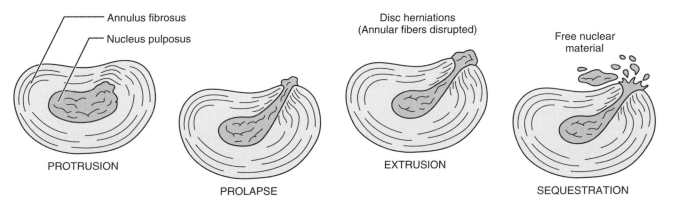

Annulus fibrosus
Nucleus pulposus

Disc herniations
(Annular fibers disrupted)

Free nuclear material

PROTRUSION

PROLAPSE

EXTRUSION

SEQUESTRATION

Fig. 9.10 Types of disc herniations.

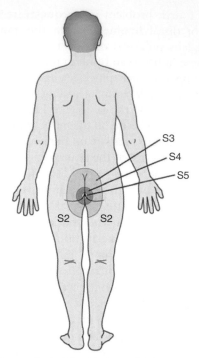

Fig. 9.11 Saddle anesthesia. The S3, S4, and S5 nerves provide sensory innervation to the inner thigh, perineum, and rectum.

spine, each root is named for the vertebra above it (in the cervical spine, the nerve roots are named for the vertebra below). For example, the L4 nerve root exits between the L4 and L5 vertebrae. Because of the course of the nerve root as it exits, the L4 disc (between L4 and L5) only rarely compresses the L4 nerve root; it is more likely to compress the L5 nerve root (Fig. 9.13).

In general, the L5–S1 segment is the most common site of problems in the vertebral column because this level bears more weight than any other vertebral level. The center of gravity passes directly through this vertebra, which is of benefit because it may decrease the shearing stresses to this segment. There is a transition from the mobile segment, L5, to the stable or fixed segment of the sacrum (S1), which can increase the stress on this area. Because the angle between L5 and S1 is greater than the angles between the other vertebrae, this joint has a greater chance of having stress applied to it. Another factor that increases the amount of stress on this area is the relatively greater amount of movement that occurs at this level compared with other levels of the lumbar spine.

TABLE 9.2

Prognostic Factors for Positive Outcome With Nonoperative Care for Lumbar Disc Herniation

Favorable Factors	Unfavorable Factors	Neutral Factors	Questionable Factors
• Absence of crossed SLR • Spinal motion in extension that does not reproduce leg pain • Large extrusion or sequestration • Relief of >50% reduction in leg pain within the first 6 weeks of onset • Positive response to corticosteroid treatment • Limited psychosocial issues • Self-employed • Motivated to recover and return to function • Educational level >12 years • Good fitness level • Motivated to exercise and participate in recovery • Absence of spinal stenosis • Progressive return from neurological deficit within the first 12 weeks	• Positive crossed SLR • Leg pain produced in spinal extension • Subligamentous contained LDH • Lack of >50% reduction in leg pain within the first 6 weeks of onset • Negative response to corticosteroid treatment • Overbearing psychosocial issues • Worker's compensation • Unmotivated to return to function • Educational level <12 years • Illiteracy • Unreasonable expectation of recovery time frames • Poorly motivated and passive in recovery process • Concomitant spinal stenosis • Progressive neurological deficit • Cauda equina syndrome	• Degree of SLR • Response to bed rest • Response to passive care • Gender • Age • Degree of neurological deficit (except progressive deficit and cauda equina syndrome)	• Actual size of LDH • Canal position of LDH • Spinal level of LDH • Multilevel disc abnormalities • LDH material

LDH, Lumbar disc herniation; *SLR,* straight leg raise.
Modified from Saal JA: Natural history and nonoperative treatment of lumbar disc herniation, *Spine* 21(24S):7S, 1996.

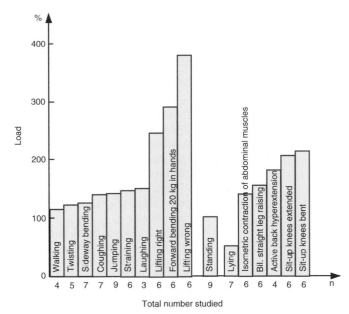

Fig. 9.12 Mean change in load on L3 disc with various activities compared with upright standing. (From Nachemson A, Elfstrom C: Intravital dynamic pressure measurements in lumbar discs, *Scand J Rehabil Med* [Suppl. 1]:31, 1970.)

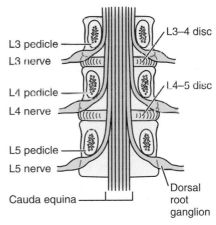

Fig. 9.13 A coronal schematic view of the exiting lumbar spinal nerve roots. Note that the exiting root takes the name of the vertebral body under which it travels into the neural foramen. Because of the way the nerve roots exit, L4–L5 disc pathology usually affects the L5 root rather than the L4 root. (Redrawn from Borenstein DG, Wiesel SW, Boden SD: *Low back pain: medical diagnosis and comprehensive management*, Philadelphia, 1995, WB Saunders, p 5.)

Patient History

Problems of the lumbar spine are difficult to diagnose; in fact, diagnosing pain due to a disc is primarily a diagnosis of exclusion.[27] That being said, the examiner must first clear any red flags to serious spinal pathology and, as the examination progresses, watch for any yellow flags that increase the risk of developing chronic pain and long-term disability.[28] Individual red flags do not necessarily mean serious pathology, but they should still be checked.[28] In addition, the examiner must be aware that visceral tissues are adjacent to the lumbar spine and pelvis and therefore must be considered in any assessment of the area, especially in the history, similar to the thoracic spine.[29,30] Most of the examination commonly revolves around differentiating symptoms of a herniated disc (or space-occupying lesion), which refers radicular symptoms into the leg from other conditions (e.g., inflammatory reaction, sprains, strains, facet syndrome) more likely to cause localized pain.[31] If there are no radicular symptoms below the knee, it often becomes difficult for the examiner to determine where in the spine the problem is or, for that matter, whether the problem is truly in the lumbar spine or coming from problems in the pelvic joints, primarily the sacroiliac joints, the hips, or visceral disorders (Table 9.3). Waddell pointed out that in only about 15% of cases can a definitive diagnosis as to the pathology of back pain be made.[3] Hall broke low back pain into four categories—two of which are **back pain dominant** and two of which are **leg pain dominant** (Table 9.4).[32] Pattern 1 suggests disc involvement, whereas pattern 2 suggests facet joint involvement. Pattern 3 suggests nerve root involvement (primarily by a disc or some other space-occupying lesion or an injury accompanied by inflammatory swelling), and pattern 4 suggests neurogenic intermittent claudication (pressure on the cauda equina). Thus, only by taking a careful history followed by a detailed examination is the examiner able to determine the cause of the problem.[33–35] Even then, some doubt may remain.

In addition to the questions listed in the "Patient History" section of Chapter 1, the examiner should obtain the following information from the patient while also watching for potential red and yellow flags:

1. *What is the patient's age?*[36] Different conditions affect patients at different ages. For example, disc problems usually occur between the ages of 15 and 40 years, and ankylosing spondylitis is evident between 18 and 45 years. Osteoarthritis and spondylosis are more evident in people older than 45 years of age, and malignancy of the spine is most common in people older than 50 years of age.

2. *What is the patient's occupation?*[3,37] Back pain tends to be more prevalent in people with strenuous occupations,[38] although it has been reported that familial influences have an effect as well as occupation.[39,40] For example, truck drivers (vibration) and warehouse workers have a high incidence of back injury.[41] Patients who have chronic low back pain develop a **deconditioning syndrome,** which compounds the problem as it leads to decreased muscle strength, impaired motor control, and decreased coordination and postural control.[42] An important question regards how active the patient is at work (usual job, light duties, full time, frequent days off because of back pain, unemployed because of back, or retired).

3. *What is the patient's sex?* Lower back pain has a higher incidence in women. Female patients should be asked

TABLE **9.3**

Differential Diagnosis of Low Back Pain

Mechanical Spine Etiologies	NONMECHANICAL ETIOLOGIES	
	Spinal Disorders	Visceral Disorders
Lumbar strain or sprain[a]	Neoplasia	Pelvic organs
Degenerative disease	• Metastatic carcinoma	• Prostatitis
• Discs (spondylosis)	• Multiple myeloma	• Endometriosis
• Facet joints[b]	• Lymphoma and leukemia	• Pelvic inflammatory disease
• Diffuse idiopathic skeletal hyperostosis[b]	• Primary spinal cord or vertebral tumor	Renal disease
Spondylolysis[b,c]	• Retroperitoneal tumors	• Nephrolithiasis
Spondylolisthesis[d]	Infection	• Pyelonephritis
Intervertebral disc herniation	• Osteomyelitis	• Perinephric abscess
Spinal stenosis	• Septic discitis	Vascular disease
Fracture	• Paraspinal or epidural abscess	• Abdominal aortic aneurysm
• Traumatic	• Herpes zoster (shingles)	• Aortoiliac disease
• Osteoporotic	Inflammatory arthritis	Gastrointestinal disease
Congenital disease	• Ankylosing spondylitis	• Pancreatitis
• Severe kyphosis	• Reiter's syndrome	• Cholecystitis
• Severe scoliosis	• Psoriatic spondylitis	• Perforated bowel
• Transitional vertebrae	• Inflammatory bowel disease	
Internal disc disruption (discogenic pain)[b]	Paget's disease	
	Scheuermann's disease (osteochondrosis)	

[a]Lumbar strains or sprains can be considered due to a nonspecific (idiopathic) musculoligamentous etiology.
[b]The relationship between symptoms and objective findings for these conditions is not clearly established.
[c]Spondylolysis is a defect in the pars interarticularis without vertebral slippage.
[d]Spondylolisthesis is anterior displacement of one vertebra, typically L5, over the one beneath it.
Modified from Atlas SJ, Nardin RA: Evaluation and treatment of low back pain: an evidence-based approach to clinical care, *Muscle Nerve* 27:267, 2003.

about any changes that occur with menstruation, such as altered pain patterns, irregular menses, and swelling of the abdomen or breasts. Has the patient ever been diagnosed with osteoporosis? Knowledge of the date of the most recent pelvic examination is also useful. Ankylosing spondylitis is more common in men.

4. *What was the mechanism of injury?* Was major trauma (e.g., a car accident) involved? Lifting commonly causes low back pain (Tables 9.5 and 9.6). This is not surprising when one considers the forces exerted on the lumbar spine and disc. For example, a 77-kg (170-lb) man lifting a 91-kg (200-lb) weight approximately 36 cm (14 inches) from the intervertebral disc exerts a force of 940 kg (2072 lb) on that disc. The force exerted on the disc can be calculated as roughly 10 times the weight being lifted. Pressure on the intervertebral discs varies depending on the position of the spine. Nachemson and colleagues showed that pressure on the disc can be decreased by increasing the supported inclination of the back rest (e.g., an angle of 130° decreases the pressure on the disc by 50%).[25,26] Using the arms for support can also decrease the pressure on the disc. When one is standing, the disc pressure is approximately 35% of the pressure that occurs in the relaxed sitting position. The examiner should also keep in mind that stress on the lower back tends to be 15% to 20% higher in men than in women because men are taller and their weight is distributed higher in the body.

5. *How long has the problem bothered the patient?* Acute back pain lasts 3 to 4 weeks. Subacute back pain lasts up to 12 weeks. Chronic pain is any pain lasting longer than 3 months. Waddell has outlined predictors (yellow flags) of chronicity with back pain patients.[3,43]

Predictors of Chronicity Within the First 6 to 8 Weeks (Yellow Flags)[3]

- Nerve root pain or specific spinal pathology
- Reported severity of pain at the acute stage
- Beliefs about pain being work related
- Psychological distress
- Psychosocial aspects of work
- Compensation
- Time off work
- The longer someone is off work with back pain, the lower the probability that he or she will return to work

TABLE **9.4**

Patterns of Back Pain

	Pattern	Where Pain Is Worst	Aggravating Movement	Relieving Movement	Onset	Duration	Probable Cause
Back-dominant pain/ mechanical cause	1	Back/buttocks (>90% back pain) Myotomes seldom affected Dermatomes not affected	Flexion Stiff in morning	Extension	Hours to days	Days to months (sudden or slow)	Disc involvement (minor herniation, spondylosis), sprain, strain
	2	Back/buttocks Myotomes seldom affected Dermatomes not affected	Extension/rotation	Flexion	Minutes to hours	Days to weeks (sudden)	Facet joint involvement, strain
Leg-pain dominant/ nonmechanical cause	3	Leg (usually below knee) Myotomes commonly affected (especially in chronic cases) Pain in dermatomes	Flexion	Extension	Hours to days	Weeks to months	Nerve root irritation (most likely cause—disc herniation)
	4	Leg (usually below knee; may be bilateral) Myotomes commonly affected (especially in chronic cases) Pain in dermatomes	Walking(extension)	Rest (sitting) and/or postural change	With walking	?	Neurogenic intermittent claudication (stenosis)

Modified from Hall H: A simple approach to back pain management, *Patient Care* 15:77–91, 1992.

6. *Where are the sites and boundaries of pain?* Have the patient point to the location or locations. Note whether the patient indicates a specific joint or whether the pain is more general. The more specific the pain, the easier it is to localize the area of pathology. Unilateral pain with no referral below the knee may be caused by injury to muscles (strain) or ligaments (sprain), the facet joint, or, in some cases, the sacroiliac joints. This is called **mechanical low back pain** (in older books, it is called "lumbago"). With each of these injuries, there is seldom if ever peripheralization of the symptoms. The symptoms tend to stay centralized in the back. If the muscles and ligaments are affected, movement will decrease and pain will increase with repeated movements.

If the pain extends to the hip, the hip must be cleared by examination. With facet joint problems, the range of motion (ROM) remains the same (it may be restricted from the beginning), as does the pain with repeated movements. Pain on standing that improves with walking and pain on forward flexion with no substantial muscle tenderness suggests disc involvement.[44] The sacroiliac joints will show pain when pain-provoking (stress) tests are used. A minor disc injury (protrusion) may show the same symptoms, but the pain is more likely to be bilateral if it is a central protrusion, spondylolisthesis, spinal stenosis, or metastases.[45,46] Dural pain is extra segmental and felt over a larger area (e.g., it may spread upward to the chest or down both thighs to the ankles),

TABLE **9.5**

Some Implications of Painful Reactions

Activity	Reaction of Pain	Possible Structural and Pathological Implications
Lying sleeping	↓	Decreased compressive forces—low intradiscal pressures Absence of forces produced by muscle activity
	↑	Change of position—noxious mechanical stress Decreased mechanoreceptor input Motor segment "relaxed" into a position compromising affected structure Poor external support (bed) Nonmusculoskeletal cause
First rising (stiffness)	↑	Nocturnal imbibition of fluid, disc volume greatest Mechanical inflammatory component (apophyseal joints) Prolonged stiffness, active inflammatory disease (e.g., ankylosing spondylitis)
Sitting	↑	Compressive forces High intradiscal pressure
With extension	↓	Intradiscal pressure reduced Decreased paraspinal muscle activity
	↑	Greater compromise of structures of lateral and central canals Compressive forces on lower apophyseal joints
With flexion	↓	Little compressive load on lower apophyseal joints Greater volume lateral and central canals Reduced disc bulge posteriorly
	↑	Very high intradiscal pressures Increased compressive loads upper and mid apophyseal joints Mechanical deformation of spine
Prolonged sitting	↑	Gradual creep of tissues
Sitting to standing	↑	Creep, time for reversal, difficulty in straightening up Extension of spine, increase disc bulge posteriorly

Walking	↑	Shock loads greater than body weight
		Compressive loads (vertical creep)
		Leg pain
		  Neurogenic claudication
		  Vascular claudication

Driving	↑	Sitting: compressive forces Vibration: vibro creep repetitive loading, decreased hysteresis loading, decreased hysteresis Increased dural tension sitting with legs extended Short hamstrings: pull lumbar spine into greater flexion
Coughing, sneezing, straining	↑	Increased pressure subarachnoid space (increased blood flow, Batson plexus, compromises space in lateral and central canal) Increased intradiscal pressure Mechanical "jarring" of sudden uncontrolled movement

From Jull GA: Examination of the lumbar spine. In Grieve GP, editor: *Modern manual therapy of the vertebral column*, Edinburgh, 1986, Churchill Livingstone, p 553.

whereas radicular pain is usually restricted to one dermatome.[46] Pressure on a nerve root sheath by a disc lesion will usually result in pain followed by paresthesia. If any paresthesia is painless, a disc problem is unlikely and conditions such as cord compression, diabetes, pernicious anemia, or multiple sclerosis should be considered.[46] If the patient indicates pain in the upper lumbar/lower thoracic spine, the examiner should be alert to the fact that disc lesions in this area are rare but that serious disorders unrelated to activity (e.g., septic or rheumatic inflammation, tumors, metabolic disorders) are often found in this area.[46]

TABLE **9.6**

Some Mechanisms of Musculoskeletal Pain

Behavior of Pain	Possible Mechanisms
Constant ache	Inflammatory process, venous hypertension
Pain on movement	Noxious mechanical stimulus (stretch, pressure, crush)
Pain accumulates with activity	Repeated mechanical stress Inflammatory process Degenerative disc—hysteresis decreased, less protection from repetitive loading
Pain increases with sustained postures	Fatigue of supporting muscles Gradual creep of tissues may stress affected part of motor unit
Latent nerve root pain	Movement has produced an acute and temporary neurapraxia

From Jull GA: Examination of the lumbar spine. In Grieve GP, editor: *Modern manual therapy of the vertebral column*, Edinburgh, 1986, Churchill Livingstone, p 553.

"Mechanical" Low Back Pain[3]

- Pain is usually cyclic
- Low back pain is often referred to the buttocks and thighs
- Morning stiffness or pain is common
- Start pain (i.e., when starting movement) is common
- There is pain on forward flexion and often also on returning to the erect position
- Pain is often produced or aggravated by extension, side flexion, rotation, standing, walking, sitting, and exercise in general
- Pain usually becomes worse over the course of the day
- Pain is relieved by a change of position
- Pain is relieved by lying down, especially in the fetal position

7. *Is there any radiation of pain? Is the pain centralizing or peripheralizing* (Fig. 9.14)?[47,48] **Centralization** implies that the pain is moving toward or is centered in the lumbar spine.[49–52] **Peripheralization** implies the pain is being referred or is moving into the limb. If so, it is helpful for the examiner to remember and correlate this information with dermatome findings when sensation is being evaluated. With regard to the lumbar spine, the examiner must be careful not to consider every back problem a disc problem. It has been reported that disc problems account for only about 5% of patients with low back pain.[53] Some authors feel the only definitive clinical diagnosis of a disc problem is neurological pain extending below the knee.[32] This means that although there may be pain in the back and in the leg, the leg pain is dominant.[3] Pain on the anterolateral aspect of the leg is highly suggestive of L4 disc problems, whereas, if the history indicates that a disc may be injured, pain radiating to the posterior

aspect of the foot suggests L5 disc problems.[54] Pain radiating into the leg below the knee is highly suggestive of a disc lesion, but isolated back or buttock pain does not rule out the disc. Minor injuries, such as protrusion of the disc, may result only in back or buttock pain.[54] Such an injury makes diagnoses more difficult because such pain may also result from muscle or ligament injury or from injury or degeneration to the adjacent facet joints.

Lumbar and sacroiliac pain tends to be referred to the buttock and posterior leg (and sometimes to the lateral aspect of the leg). Hip pain tends to be in the groin and anterior thigh although it may be referred to the knee (usually medial side). The hip can be ruled out later in the examination by the absence of a hip capsular pattern and a negative sign of the buttock.[55] The examiner must also determine whether the musculoskeletal system is involved or whether the pain is being referred from another structure or system (e.g., abdominal organs). Abnormal signs and symptoms or red flags (see Table 1.1) would lead the examiner to consider causes other than the musculoskeletal system.

8. *Is the pain deep? Superficial? Shooting? Burning? Aching?* Questions related to the depth and type of pain often help to locate the structure injured and the source of pain.

9. *Is the pain improving? Worsening? Staying the same?* The answers to these questions indicate whether the condition is settling down and improving, or they may indicate that the condition is in the inflammation phase (acute) or in the healing phase. Does the patient complain of more pain than the injury would suggest should occur? If so, psychosocial testing may be appropriate.

10. *Is there any increase in pain with coughing? Sneezing? Deep breathing? Straining? Laughing?* All of these actions increase the **intrathecal pressure** (the pressure inside the covering of the spinal cord) and would indicate the problem is in the lumbar spine and affecting the neurological tissue.[28]

11. *Are there any postures or actions that specifically increase or decrease the pain or that cause difficulty?*[47,56] What is the relationship between the pain and activity?[46] For example, if sitting increases the pain and other symptoms, the examiner may suspect that sustained flexion is causing mechanical deformation of the spine or increasing the intradiscal pressure.[57] Classically, disc pathology causes increased pain on sitting, lifting, twisting, and bending.[58] It is the most common space-occupying lesion in the lumbar spine; therefore it is the most common cause of radiating pain below the knee. If standing increases the pain and other symptoms, the examiner may suspect that extension, especially relaxed standing, is the cause. If walking increases the pain and other symptoms, extension is probably causing the mechanical

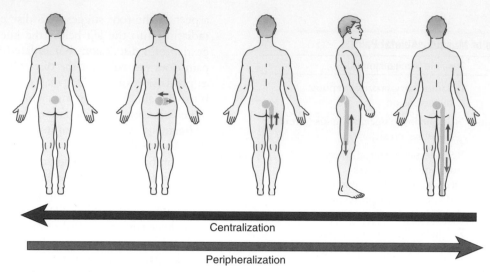

Centralization

Peripheralization

Fig. 9.14 Centralization of pain is the progressive retreat of the most distal extent of referred or radicular pain toward the lumbar midline. Peripheralization of pain moves in the opposite direction.

deformation, because walking accentuates extension. If lying (especially prone lying) increases the pain and other symptoms, extension may be the cause. Persistent pain or progressive increases in pain while the patient is in the supine position may lead the examiner to suspect a neurogenic or space-occupying lesion, such as an infection, swelling, or tumor. It is important to remember that pain may radiate to the lumbar spine from pathological conditions in other areas as well as from direct mechanical problems. For example, tumors of the pancreas refer pain to the low back. Stiffness or pain after rest may indicate ankylosing spondylitis or Scheuermann disease. Pain from mechanical breakdown tends to increase with activity and decrease with rest. Discogenic pain increases if the patient maintains a single posture (especially flexion) for a long period. Pain arising from the spine is almost always influenced by posture and movement.

The pelvis is the key to proper back posture. Ideally, an individual should be able to stand with the pelvis in neutral. In this position, the anterosuperior iliac spines (ASISs) are one to two finger widths lower than the posterosuperior iliac spines (PSISs). For the pelvis to "sit" properly on the femora, the abdominal, hip flexor, hip extensor, and back extensor muscles must be strong, supple, and "balanced" (Fig. 9.15). Any deviation in the normal alignment should be noted and recorded. For example, shoe heel height can modify the pelvic angle and lumbar curve, thus altering the stress on the spine.[59]

12. *Is the pain worse in the morning or evening? Does the pain get better or worse as the day progresses? Does the pain wake you up at night?* For example, osteoarthritis of the facet joints leads to morning stiffness, which in turn is relieved by activity.

13. *Which movements hurt? Which movements are stiff?* How does the patient move when walking? When

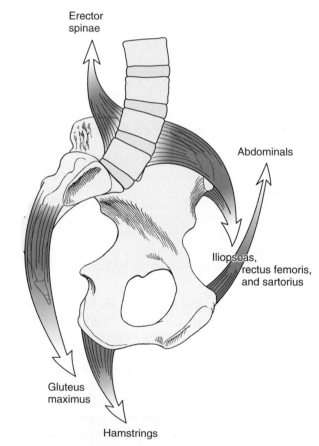

Fig. 9.15 Muscles "balancing" the pelvis. (Modified from Dyrek DA, Micheli LJ, Magee DJ: Injuries to the thoracolumbar spine and pelvis. In Zachazewski JE, Magee DJ, Quillen WS, editors: *Athletic injuries and rehabilitation*, Philadelphia, 1996, WB Saunders, p 470.)

sitting? When getting up from sitting? Table 9.7 demonstrates some of the causes of mechanical low back pain and their symptoms. The examiner must help the patient differentiate between true pain and discomfort that is caused by stretching. **Postural,**

TABLE **9.7**

Differential Diagnosis of Mechanical Low Back Pain

	Muscle Strain	Herniated Nucleus Pulposus	Osteoarthritis	Spinal Stenosis	Spondylolisthesis	Scoliosis
Age (years)	20–40	30–50	>50	>60	20	30
Pain pattern						
Location	Back (unilateral)	Back, leg (unilateral)	Back (unilateral)	Leg (bilateral)	Back	Back
Onset	Acute	Acute (prior episodes)	Insidious	Insidious	Insidious	Insidious
Standing	↑	↓	↑	↑	↑	↑
Sitting	↓	↑	↓	↓	↓	↓
Bending	↑	↑	↓	↓	↑	↑
Straight leg raise	–	+	–	+(stress)	–	–
Plain x-ray	–	–	+	+	+	+

From Borenstein DG, et al: *Low back pain: medical diagnosis and comprehensive management*, Philadelphia, 1995, WB Saunders, p 189.

or **static, muscles** (e.g., iliopsoas) tend to respond to pathology with tightness in the form of spasm or adaptive shortening; **dynamic,** or **phasic, muscles** (e.g., abdominals) tend to respond with atrophy. Pathology affecting both or one of the types of muscles can lead to segmental instability between the vertebra and possibly a **pelvic crossed syndrome** (discussed later). Does the patient describe a **painful arc** of movement on forward or side flexion? Painful arc in this case means that there is pain in only part of the ROM being attempted. If so, it may indicate a disc protrusion with a nerve root riding over the bulge or instability in part of the ROM.[56] Patients with lumbar instability or lumbar muscle spasm have trouble moving to the seated position, whereas those with discogenic pain usually have pain in flexion (e.g., sitting) and the pain may increase the longer they are seated. If pain is not aggravated by activity or relieved by rest, a non–activity-related problem possibly involving the visceral tissue should be considered.[46] Unilateral pain in the upper sacroiliac region or in the groin on extension may indicate injury to the iliolumbar ligaments.

14. *Is paresthesia (a "pins and needles" feeling) or anesthesia present?* A patient may experience a sensation or a lack of sensation if there is pressure on a nerve root. Paresthesia occurs if pressure is relieved from a nerve trunk, whereas if the pressure is on the nerve trunk, the patient experiences a numb sensation. Does the patient experience any paresthesia or tingling and numbness in the extremities, perineal (saddle) area, or pelvic area? Abnormal sensations in the perineal area often have associated micturition (urination) problems. These symptoms may indicate a myelopathy and are considered by many

to be an emergency surgical situation because of potential long-term bowel and bladder problems if the pressure on the spinal cord is not relieved as soon as possible.[60,61] The examiner must remember that the adult spinal cord ends at the bottom of the L1 vertebra and becomes the cauda equina within the spinal column. The nerve roots extend in such a way that it is rare for the disc to pinch on the nerve root of the same level. For example, the L5 nerve root is more likely to be compressed by the L4 intervertebral disc than by the L5 intervertebral disc (Fig. 9.16). The nerve root is seldom compressed by the disc at the same level except when the protrusion is more lateral.

15. *Has the patient noticed any weakness or decrease in strength? Has the patient noticed that his or her legs have become weak while walking or climbing stairs?* This may be the result of an injury to the muscles themselves, their nerve supply, or reflex inhibition caused by pain.[35,62]

16. *What is the patient's usual activity or pastime? Before the injury, did the patient modify or perform any unusual repetitive or high-stress activity?* Such questions help the examiner to determine whether the cause of injury was macrotrauma, microtrauma, or a combination of both.

17. *Which activities aggravate the pain? Is there anything in the patient's lifestyle that increases the pain?* Many common positions assumed by patients are similar to those in some of the provocative special tests. For example, getting into and sitting in a car is similar to the slump test and straight leg raise test. Long sitting in bed is a form of straight leg raise. Reaching up into a cupboard can be similar to an upper limb tension test. A word of caution: There can be 10° to 20° of difference in

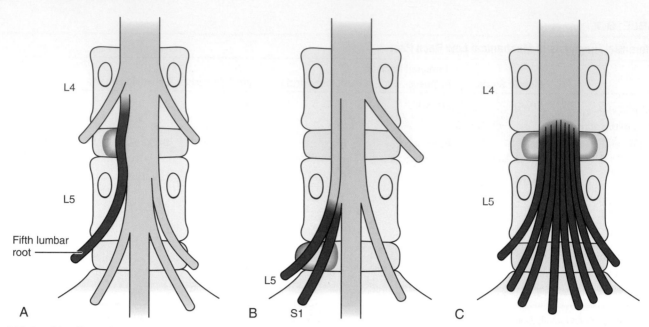

Fig. 9.16 Possible effects of disc herniation. (A) Herniation of the L4–L5 disc compresses the fifth lumbar root. (B) Large herniation of the L5–S1 disc compromises not only the nerve root crossing it (first sacral nerve root) but also the nerve root emerging through the same foramen (fifth lumbar nerve root). (C) Massive central sequestration of the L4–L5 disc involves all of the nerve roots in the cauda equina and may result in bowel and bladder paralysis. (Redrawn from MacNab I: *Backache*, Baltimore, 1977, Williams & Wilkins, pp 96–97.)

straight leg raise while lying and sitting because of the change in lordosis and position of the pelvis.[3]

18. *Which activities ease the pain?* If there are positions that relieve the pain, the examiner should use an understanding of anatomy to determine which tissues would have stress taken off them in the pain-relieving postures; these postures may later be used as resting postures during the treatment.

19. *What is the patient's sleeping position? Does the patient have any problems sleeping? What type of mattress does the patient use (hard, soft)?* The best sleeping position is in side lying with the legs bent in a semifetal position. If the patient lies prone, the lumbar spine often falls into extension, thus increasing the stress on the posterior elements of the vertebrae. In supine lying, the spine tends to flatten out, decreasing the stress on the posterior elements.

20. *Does the patient have any difficulty with micturition?* If so, the examiner should proceed with caution, because the condition may involve more than the lumbar spine (e.g., a myelopathy, cauda equina syndrome, tabes dorsalis, tumor, multiple sclerosis). Conversely, these symptoms may result from a disc protrusion or spinal stenosis with minimal or no back pain or sciatica. A disc derangement can cause total urinary retention; chronic, long-standing partial retention; vesicular irritability; or the loss of desire or awareness of the necessity to void.

21. *Are there any red flags that the examiner should be aware of, such as a history of cancer, sudden weight loss*

for no apparent reason, immunosuppressive disorder, infection, fever, or bilateral leg weakness?

22. *Is the patient receiving any medication?* For example, the long-term use of steroid therapy can lead to osteoporosis. Also, if the patient has taken medication just before the assessment, the examiner may not get a true reading of the pain.

23. *Is the patient able to cope during daily activities?* Psychosocial issues often play a role in low back pain, especially if it is chronic.[63–66] Waddell et al.[67] defined nonorganic signs (**Waddell's signs**) as those seen in patients who need a more intense psychosocial examination (see the section titled "Functional Assessment," further on). It is normal for people suffering prolonged pain to exhibit altered psychosocial behaviors; these are subject to wide individual differences and the effects of learning.[68] Fear-avoidance questionnaires, especially that of Waddell et al.[69] titled **Fear-Avoidance Beliefs Questionnaire (FABQ)** (eTool 9.1); the **Tampa Bay Scale of Kinesiophobia**[70–75] (eTool 9.2); and Linton and Hallden's **Acute Low Back Pain Screening Questionnaire**[76] (eTool 9.3) are becoming more commonly used in lumbar examinations.[77–83] The **New Zealand Acute Low Back Pain Guide** and the **New Zealand Guide to Assessing Psychosocial Yellow Flags in Acute Low Back Pain**[84] outline yellow flags that indicate psychosocial barriers for recovery, with questions related to attitudes and beliefs about back

TABLE **9.8**

Indications of Serious Spinal Pathology

Red Flags	Cauda Equina Syndrome/Widespread Neurological Disorder	Inflammatory Disorders (Ankylosing Spondylitis and Related Disorders)
• Presentation age <20 years or onset >55 years • Violent trauma, such as a fall from a height or a car accident • Constant, progressive, nonmechanical pain • Thoracic pain • Previous history of immune system failure, carcinoma, use of systemic steroids, drug abuse • Weight loss (unexpected) (i.e., >4.5 kg [10 lb] over preceding 6 months) • Systematically unwell • Persisting severe restriction of lumbar flexion • Widespread neurological abnormalities (e.g., bilateral symptoms, loss of bowel and bladder control) • Structural deformity • Investigations when required erythrocyte sedimentation rate (ESR) >25; plain x-ray: vertebral collapse or bone destruction • Blood in urine or stools • History of osteoporosis • Corticosteroid use • Fever/chills—infection • Immunosuppression	• Difficulty with micturition • Loss of anal sphincter tone or fecal incontinence • Saddle anesthesia about the anus, perineum, or genitals • Widespread (>1 nerve root) or progressive motor weakness in the legs or gait disturbance • Sensory level	• Gradual onset before age 40 years • Marked morning stiffness • Persisting limitation of spinal movements in all directions • Peripheral joint involvement • Iritis, skin rashes (psoriasis), colitis, urethral discharge • Family history • Morning stiffness >1 hour

Modified from Waddell G: *The back pain revolution*, New York, 1998, Churchill Livingstone, p 12.

pain, behavior, compensation issues, diagnosis and treatment, emotions, family, and work.[68] These yellow flags should be seen as factors that can be influenced positively to facilitate recovery and reduce work loss and long-term disability.[68] Their presence shows an increased risk of developing chronic pain and long-term disability.[28] Haggman et al.[85] felt that two questions were particularly significant to ask the patient in screening for depressive symptoms: (1) "During the past month, have you often been bothered by feeling down, depressed, or hopeless?" and (2) "During the past month, have you been bothered by little interest or pleasure in doing things?"[44,86] If the answers to these questions are positive, the patient should be monitored closely; if progress does not occur, then further psychological follow-ups should be considered.[87] Does the patient have trouble with work, leisure activities, washing, or dressing? How far can the patient walk before the pain begins?[88] What is the patient's level of disability? Disability implies the effect of the pathology on activity, not pain. Thus disability testing commonly revolves around activities of daily living (ADLs) and functional activities. This question may be tied in with the use of the questions in the functional assessment discussed later.

Psychosocial Yellow-Flag Barriers to Recovery[68]

- Belief that pain and activity are harmful
- "Sickness behaviors" (such as extended rest)
- Low or negative moods, social withdrawal
- Treatment that does not fit best practice
- Problems with claim and compensation
- History of back pain, time off, other claims
- Problems at work, poor job satisfaction
- Heavy work, unsociable hours
- Overprotective family or lack of support

Finally, the examiner must be aware that although, in most cases, people who have low back pain have simple mechanical back problems or have nerve root problems involving the disc, there is always the possibility of non-musculoskeletal causes (e.g., kidney stones, abdominal aortic aneurysm, pancreatic problems) or serious spinal pathology (e.g., tumors).[27,44] Waddell outlined signs and symptoms that would lead the examiner to conclude that more serious pathology is present in the lumbar spine (Table 9.8).[3,89]

Observation

The patient must be suitably undressed. Males must wear only shorts, and females must wear only a bra and shorts. While doing the observation, the examiner should note the patient's willingness to move and the pattern of movement. The patient should be observed for the following traits, first in the standing and then in the sitting position.

Body Type

There are three general body types (see Fig. 15.19): **ectomorphic**—thin body build, characterized by relative prominence of structures developed from the embryonic ectoderm; **mesomorphic**—muscular or sturdy body build, characterized by relative prominence of structures developed from the embryonic mesoderm; and **endomorphic**—heavy (fat) body build, characterized by relative prominence of structures developed from the embryonic endoderm.

Gait

Does the gait appear to be normal when the patient walks into the examination area, or is it altered in some way? If it is altered, the examiner must take time to find out whether the problem is in the limb or whether the gait is altered to relieve symptoms in the spine or elsewhere.

Attitude

What is the patient's appearance? Is the patient tense, bored, lethargic, healthy looking, emaciated, or over weight?

Total Spinal Posture

The patient should be examined in the habitual relaxed posture (see Chapter 15) that he or she would usually adopt. With acute back pain, the patient presents with some degree of antalgic (painful) posturing. Usually, a loss of lumbar lordosis is present, and there may be a lateral shift or scoliosis. This posturing is involuntary and often cannot be reduced because of the muscle spasm.[90,91]

The patient should be observed anteriorly, laterally, and posteriorly, looking for symmetry (Fig. 9.17). During the observation, the examiner should pay particular attention to whether the patient holds the pelvis "in neutral" naturally; if not, is he or she able to achieve the "neutral pelvis" position in standing (normal lordotic curve with the ASISs being slightly lower [one to two finger widths] than the PSISs)? Many people with back pain are unable to maintain a **neutral pelvis** position. Three questions should be considered when one is

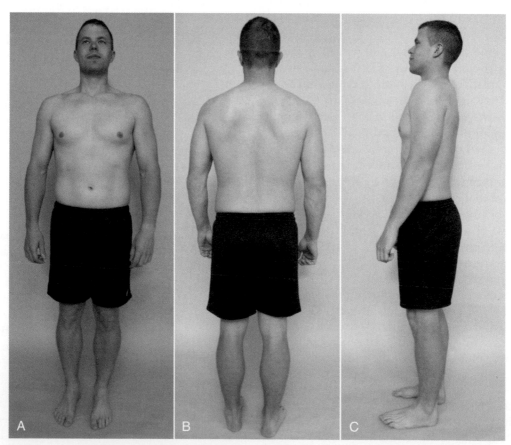

Fig. 9.17 Views of the patient in the standing position. (A) Anterior view. (B) Posterior view. (C) Lateral view.

looking for a neutral pelvis and whether the pelvis can be stabilized:

1. Can the patient get into the neutral pelvis position? If not, what is restricting the movement or what muscles are weak so the position cannot be attained?
2. Can the patient hold (i.e., stabilize) the neutral pelvis statically? If not, what muscles need to be strengthened?
3. Can the patient hold (i.e., stabilize) the neutral pelvis when moving dynamically? If not, which muscles are weak and/or not functioning correctly (i.e., functioning isometrically, concentrically, or eccentrically)?

These questions will help the examiner to determine if the pelvis (and lumbar spine) can be stabilized during different movements or positions so that other muscles originating from the pelvis can function properly. For example, side lying hip abduction should be able to be performed in the frontal plane with the lower limbs, pelvis, trunk, and shoulder aligned in the frontal plane (**active hip abduction test** ☑) (Fig. 9.18).[92] If the leg wobbles, the pelvis tips, the shoulders or trunk rotate, the hip flexes, or the abducted limb rotates medially or laterally, it is an indication of lack of movement control and lack of muscle strength and balance. This concept is related to spine and **core stability**, in which the muscles of the trunk and pelvis function to stabilize the lower spine, pelvis, and hips along with proprioceptive feedback from mechanoreceptors to stabilize the area statically and dynamically.[93–95]

Anteriorly, the head should be straight on the shoulders and the nose should be in line with the manubrium, sternum, and xiphisternum or umbilicus. The shoulders and clavicle should be level and equal, although the dominant side may be slightly lower. The waist angles should be equal. Does the patient show a lateral shift or list (Fig. 9.19)? Such a shift may be straight lateral movement or it may be a **structural scoliosis** (rotation involved). The straight shift is more likely to be caused by mechanical dysfunction and muscle spasm (**functional scoliosis**) and is likely to disappear on lying down or hanging.[3,96] True structural scoliosis commonly has compensating curves and does not change with lying down or hanging. The arbitrary "high" points on both iliac crests should be the same height. If they are not, the possibility of unequal leg length should be considered. The difference in height would indicate a functional limb length discrepancy. This discrepancy could be caused by altered bone length, altered mechanics (e.g., pronated foot on one side), or joint dysfunction (Table 9.9). The ASISs should be level. The patellae should point straight ahead. The lower limbs should be straight and not in genu varum or genu valgum. The heads of the fibulae should be level. The medial malleoli should be level, as should the lateral malleoli. The medial longitudinal arches of the feet should be evident, and the feet should angle out equally. The arms should be an equal distance from the trunk and equally medially or laterally rotated. Any protrusion or depression of the sternum, ribs, or costal cartilage, as well as any bowing of bones should be noted. The bony or soft tissue contours should be equal on both sides.

From the side, the examiner should look at the head to ensure that the earlobe is in line with the tip of the shoulder (acromion process) and the arbitrary high point of the iliac crest. Each segment of the spine should have a normal curve. Are any of the curves exaggerated or

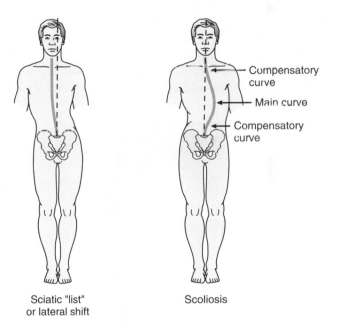

Sciatic "list" or lateral shift   Scoliosis

Fig. 9.19 Lateral shift or list.

TABLE **9.9**

Functional Limb Length Difference

Joint	Functional Lengthening	Functional Shortening
Foot	Supination	Pronation
Knee	Extension	Flexion
Hip	Lowering Extension Lateral rotation	Lifting Flexion Medial rotation
Sacroiliac	Anterior rotation	Posterior rotation

From Wallace LA: Lower quarter pain: mechanical evaluation and treatment. In Grieve GP, editor: *Modern manual therapy of the vertebral column*, Edinburgh, 1986, Churchill Livingstone, p 467.

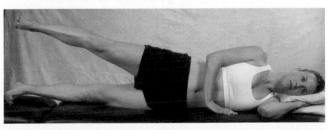

Fig. 9.18 Active hip abduction test. Note how the shoulders, trunk, pelvis, and lower limbs are all in alignment in a negative test.

decreased? Is the anterior **pelvic tilt** normal? (Normal values are 10° to 13° on x-ray.) Is excessive lordosis present? Is there a kyphosis (usually in the cervical or thoracic spine)? Do the shoulders droop forward? Normally, with a neutral pelvis, the ASISs are slightly lower (one to two finger widths) than the PSISs. Are the knees straight, flexed, or in recurvatum (hyperextended)? Normally, if a person has the correct pelvic tilt, he or she would stand with the knees slightly flexed or "unlocked." The gluteus maximus and hamstrings work with the abdominals to produce posterior pelvic tilt while the iliopsoas and rectus femoris work with the erector spinae to produce anterior pelvic tilt.

From behind, the examiner should note the level of the shoulders, spines and inferior angles of the scapula as well as any deformities (e.g., a Sprengel deformity). Any lateral spinal curve (scoliosis) should be noted, along with the presence of excess hair in the midline (Fig. 9.20). Eighty percent of occult **spinal dysraphism** (i.e., incomplete fusion of the spinal neural tube) show excessive midline hair.[46] If the scoliotic curve is due to a disc herniation, the herniation usually occurs on the convex side of the curve.[97] The waist angles should be equal from the posterior aspect, as they were from the anterior aspect with the iliac crests level with the spinous process of L4. The PSISs should be level. The examiner should

note whether the PSISs are higher or lower than the ASISs and should also note the patient's ability to maintain a neutral pelvis. The gluteal folds and knee joints should be level. The Achilles tendons and heels should appear to be straight. Marked wasting of the calves, hamstrings, and/or buttocks can occur with L1 or S1 root palsies.[46] The examiner should note whether there is any protrusion of the ribs. Any deviation in the normal spinal postural alignment should be noted and recorded. The various possible sources of pathology related to posture are discussed in Chapter 15.

Janda and Jull described a lumbar or **pelvic crossed syndrome** (Fig. 9.21) to show the effect of muscle imbalance on the ability of a patient to hold and maintain a neutral pelvis.[98] With this syndrome, they hypothesized that there was a combination of weak long muscles and short strong muscles that resulted in an imbalance pattern leading to low back pain.[99] They felt that only by treating the different groups appropriately could the back pain be relieved. The weak and long inhibited muscles were the abdominals and gluteus maximus, whereas the strong and tight (shortened) muscles were the hip flexors (primarily the iliopsoas) and the back extensors. The imbalance pattern promotes increased lumbar lordosis because of the forward pelvic tilt and hip flexion contracture and overactivity of the hip flexors, which are compensating for the weak abdominals. The weak gluteals result in increased

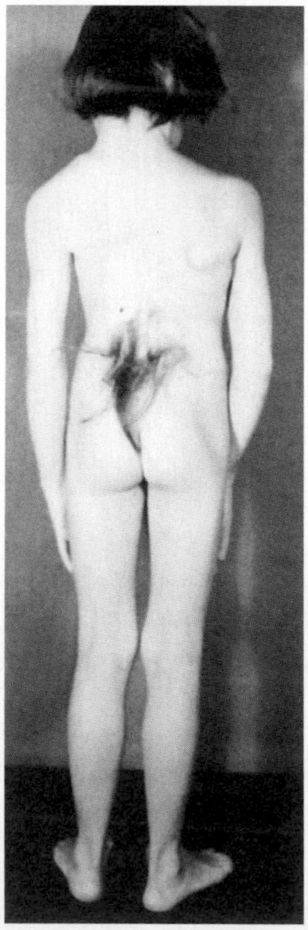

Fig. 9.20 Congenital scoliosis and a diastematomyelia in a 9-year-old girl. This type of hairy patch strongly indicates a congenital maldevelopment of the neural axis. (From Rothman RH, Simeone FA: *The spine*, Philadelphia, 1982, WB Saunders, p 371.)

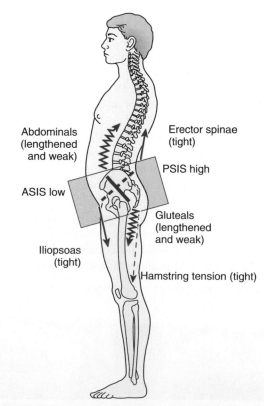

Fig. 9.21 The pelvic crossed syndrome as described by Janda and Jull. *ASIS,* Anterior superior iliac spine; *PSIS,* posterior superior iliac spine.

activity in the hamstrings and erector spinae as compensation to assist hip extension. Interestingly, although the long spinal extensors show increased activity, the short lumbar muscles (e.g., multifidus, rotatores) show weakness. Also, the hamstrings show tightness as they attempt to pull the pelvis backward to compensate for the anterior rotation caused by the tight hip flexors. Weakness of the gluteus medius results in increased activity of the quadratus lumborum and tensor fasciae latae on the same side. This syndrome is often seen in conjunction with the **upper crossed syndrome** (see Chapter 3). The two syndromes together are called the **layer syndrome**.[98]

Markings

A "faun's beard" (tuft of hair) may indicate a dysraphism (e.g., spina bifida occulta or diastematomyelia) (see Fig. 9.20).[100] Café-au-lait spots may indicate neurofibromatosis or collagen disease (Fig. 9.22). Unusual skin markings or the presence of skin lesions in the midline may lead the examiner to consider the possibility of underlying neural and mesodermal anomalies. Musculoskeletal anomalies tend to form at the same time embryologically. Thus if the examiner finds one anomaly, he or she must consider the possibility of other anomalies.

Step Deformity

A step deformity in the lumbar spine may indicate a spondylolisthesis. The "step" occurs because the spinous process of one vertebra becomes prominent when either the vertebra above (for example, spondylitic spondylolisthesis) or the affected vertebra (e.g., spondylolytic spondylolisthesis) slips forward on the one below (Fig. 9.23).

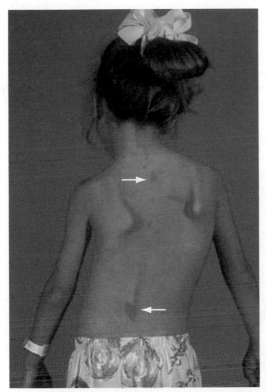

Fig. 9.22 Neurofibromatosis with scoliosis. Note the café-au-lait spots *(arrows)* on the back. (From Diab M: Physical examination in adolescent idiopathic scoliosis, *Neurosurg Clin North Am* 18[2]:229–236, 2007.)

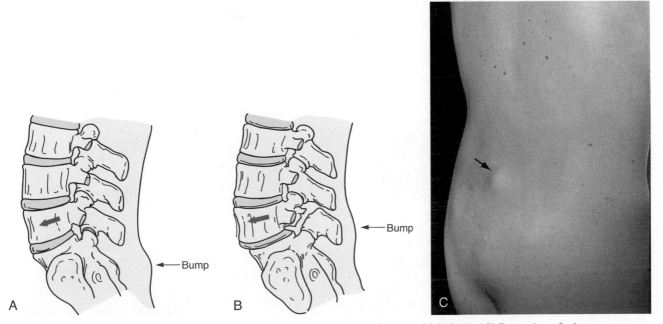

Fig. 9.23 Step deformity in the lumbar spine. (A) Caused by spondylosis. (B) Caused by spondylolisthesis. (C) Protrusion of spinous process caused by step deformity *(arrow)*.

Examination

When the lumbar spine is being assessed, the examiner must remember that referral of symptoms or the presence of neurological symptoms often makes it necessary to "clear" or rule out the lower limb pathology. Many of the symptoms that occur in the lower limb may originate in the lumbar spine. Unless there is a history of definitive trauma to a peripheral joint, a screening or scanning examination must accompany assessment of that joint to rule out problems within the lumbar spine referring symptoms to that joint. It is often helpful at this stage to ask the patient to demonstrate the movements that produce

or have produced the pain. After asking the patient to do this, the examiner must allow time for symptoms to disappear before completing the examination.

Active Movements

Active movements are performed with the patient standing (Fig. 9.24). The examiner is looking for differences in ROM and the patient's willingness to do the movement. The ROM taking place during the active movement is normally the summation of the movements of the entire lumbar spine, not just movement at one level, along with hip movement. The most painful movements are done

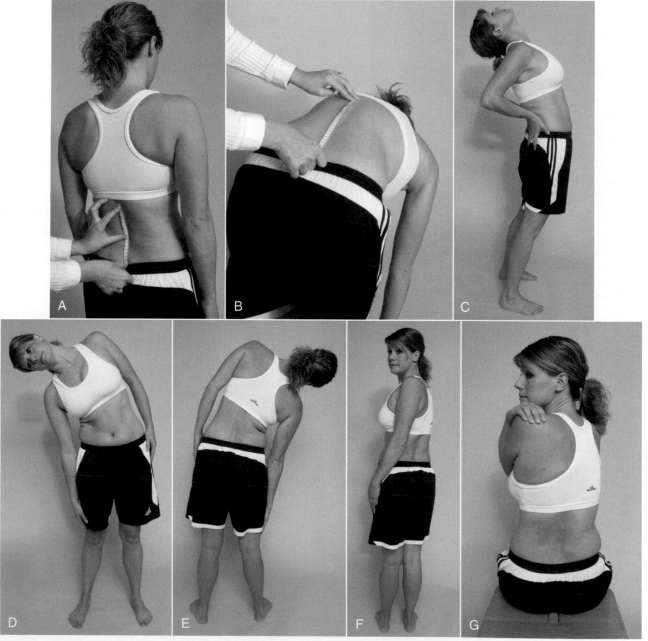

Fig. 9.24 Active movements of the lumbar spine. (A and B) Forward flexion being measured with a tape measure. (C) Extension. (D) Side flexion (anterior view). (E) Side flexion (posterior view). (F) Rotation (standing). (G) Rotation (sitting).

last. If the problem is mechanical, at least one or more of the movements will be painful.[34]

Active Movements of the Lumbar Spine

- Forward flexion (40°–60°)
- Extension (20°–35°)
- Side (lateral) flexion, left and right (15°–20°)
- Rotation, left and right (3°–18°)
- Sustained postures (if necessary)
- Repetitive motion (if necessary)
- Combined movements (if necessary)

While the patient is doing the active movements, the examiner looks for limitation of movement and its possible causes, such as pain, spasm, stiffness, or blocking including a painful arc in part of the movement as pathognomonic (i.e., a specific characteristic) of a disc lesion.[46] The painful arc may occur during the movement or on the return to neutral. As the patient reaches the full range of active movement, passive overpressure may be applied, but only if the active movements appear to be full and pain free. The overpressure must be applied with extreme care because the upper body weight is already being applied to the lumbar joints by virtue of their position and gravity. If the patient reports that a sustained position increases the symptoms, then the examiner should consider having the patient maintain the position (e.g., flexion) at the end of the ROM for 10 to 20 seconds to see whether symptoms increase. Likewise, if repetitive motion or combined movements have been reported in the history as causing symptoms, these movements should be performed as well, but only after the patient has completed the basic movements.

The greatest motion in the lumbar spine occurs between the L4 and L5 vertebrae and between L5 and S1. There is considerable individual variability in the ROM of the lumbar spine (Fig. 9.25).[101–105] In reality, little obvious movement occurs in the lumbar spine, especially in the individual segments, because of the shape of the facet joints, tightness of the ligaments, presence of the intervertebral discs, and size of the vertebral bodies.

For flexion (forward bending), the maximum ROM in the lumbar spine is normally 40° to 60°. The examiner must differentiate the movement occurring in the lumbar spine from that occurring in the hips or thoracic spine. Some patients can touch their toes by flexing the hips, even if no movement occurs in the spine. On forward flexion, the lumbar spine should move from its normal lordotic curvature to at least a straight or slightly flexed curve (Fig. 9.26).[106] If this change in the spine does not occur, there is probably some hypomobility in the lumbar spine resulting from either tight structures or muscle spasm (e.g., the erector spinae). The degree of injury also has an effect. For example, the more severely a disc is injured (e.g., if sequestration has occurred rather than a protrusion), the greater the limitation of movement.[107] With disc degeneration, intersegmental motion may increase as disc degeneration increases up to a certain point and follows the Kirkaldy-Willis description of degenerative changes in the disc.[108] This author divided the changes into three stages: dysfunctional, unstable, and stable. During the first two phases, intersegmental motion increases in flexion, rotation, and side flexion[109] and then decreases in the final stabilization phase. During the unstable phase, it is often possible to see an instability "jog" during one or more movements, especially flexion, returning to neutral from flexion, or side flexion.[110,111] An **instability jog** is a sudden movement shift or "rippling" of the muscles during active movement, indicating an unstable segment.[106,112] Similarly, muscle twitching during movement or complaints of something "slipping out" during lumbar spine movement may indicate instability.[113] If the patient bends one or both knees

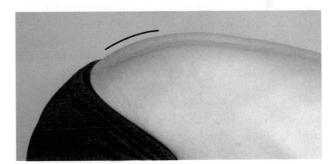

Fig. 9.26 On forward flexion, the lumbar curve should normally flatten or go into slight flexion, as shown.

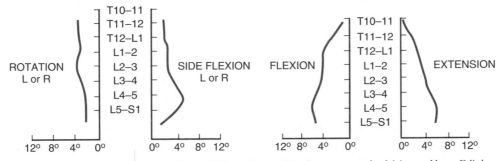

Fig. 9.25 Average range of motion in the lumbar spine. (Adapted from Grieve GP: *Common vertebral joint problems*, Edinburgh, 1981, Churchill Livingstone.)

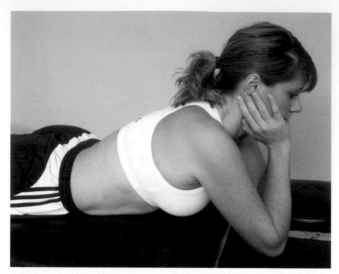

Fig. 9.27 The sphinx position.

on forward flexion, the examiner should watch for nerve root symptoms or tight hamstrings, especially if spinal flexion is decreased when the knees are straight. If tight hamstrings or nerve root symptoms are suspected, the examiner should perform suitable tests (see "Special Tests," later) to determine if the hamstrings or nerve root restriction (see "Knee Flexion Test," later) are the cause of the problem. When he or she is returning to the upright posture from forward flexion, the patient with no back pain first rotates the hips and pelvis to about 45° of flexion; during the last 45° of extension, the low back resumes its lordosis. Commonly, in patients with back pain, most movement occurs in the hips, accompanied by knee flexion and sometimes with hand support working up the thighs.[114] As with the thoracic spine, the examiner may use a tape measure to determine the increase in spacing of the spinous processes on forward flexion. Normally, the measurement should increase 7 to 8 cm (2.8 to 3.1 inches) if it is taken between the T12 spinous process and S1 (see Fig. 9.24A and B). The examiner should note how far forward the patient is able to bend (i.e., to midthigh, knees, midtibia, or floor) and compare this finding with the results of straight leg raising tests (see "Special Tests," later). Straight leg raising, especially if bilateral, is essentially the same movement done passively except that it is a movement occurring from below upward instead of from above downward.

During the active movements, especially during flexion or extension, the examiner should watch for a **painful arc.** The pain seen in a lumbar painful arc tends to be neurologically based (i.e., it is lancinating or lightening like); but it may also be caused by instability. If it does occur on movement in the lumbar spine, it is likely that a space-occupying lesion (most probably a small herniation of the disc) is pinching the nerve root in part of the range as the nerve root moves with the motion.[96]

Maigne described an active movement flexion maneuver to help confirm lumbar movement and control.[90] In

the **happy round maneuver,** the patient bends forward and places the hands on a bed or on the back of a chair. The patient then attempts to arch or hunch the back. Most patients with lumbar pathology are unable to sustain the hunched position.

Extension (backward bending) is normally limited to 20° to 35° in the lumbar spine. While performing the movement, the patient is asked to place the hands in the small of the back to help stabilize the back. Bourdillon and Day have advocated doing this movement in the prone position to hyperextend the spine.[115] They called the resulting position the **sphinx position.** The patient hyperextends the spine by resting on the elbows with the hands holding the chin (Fig. 9.27), allowing the abdominal wall to relax. The position is held for 10 to 20 seconds to see if symptoms occur or, if symptoms present, to see whether they become worse. Dobbs et al.[116] advocated holding the extension for up to a minute and then repeating the test but combining extension and side flexion. If the patient is over 50 years old, symptoms are produced to the same side as the side flexion and symptoms radiate below the gluteal fold, the test is positive for lumbar spinal stenosis. The authors called this the **Modified Extension Test (MExT)** ⚠.[116] They also advocated that the patient remain in the clinic for 10 minutes after the test to make sure that no immediate adverse effects had occurred.

Side (lateral) flexion or side bending is approximately 15° to 20° in the lumbar spine. The patient is asked to run the hand down the side of the leg and not to bend forward or backward while performing the movement. The examiner can then eyeball the movement and compare it with that of the other side. The distance from the fingertips to the floor on both sides may also be measured, noting any difference. In the spine, the movement of side flexion is a **coupled movement** with rotation. Because of the position of the facet joints, both side flexion and rotation occur together, although the amount of movement and its direction may not be the same. Table 9.10 shows how different authors interpret the coupled movement in the spine. As the patient side flexes, the examiner should watch the lumbar curve. Normally the lumbar curve is smooth on side flexion, and there should be no obvious sharp angulation at only one level. If angulation does occur, it may indicate hypomobility below the level or hypermobility above the level in the lumbar spine (Fig. 9.28). Mulvein and Jull advocated having the patient do a lateral shift (Fig. 9.29) in addition to side flexion.[117] Their viewpoint is that lateral shift in the lumbar spine focuses the movement more in the lower spine (L4–S1) and helps to eliminate the compensating movements in the rest of the spine.

Rotation in the lumbar spine is normally 3° to 18° to the left or right, and it is accomplished by a shearing movement of the lumbar vertebrae on each other. Although the patient is usually in the standing position, rotation may be performed while sitting to eliminate pelvic and hip movement. If the patient stands, the examiner

TABLE **9.10**

Coupled Movements (Side Flexion and Rotation) Believed to Occur in the Spine in Different Positions (Note the Differences)

Author	In Neutral	In Flexion	In Extension
MacConnaill		Ipsilateral	Contralateral
Farfan		Contralateral	Contralateral
Kaltenborn		Ipsilateral	Ipsilateral
Grieve		Ipsilateral	Contralateral
Fryette	Contralateral	Ipsilateral	Ipsilateral
Pearcy		Ipsilateral (L5–S1) Contralateral (L4, 5)	
Oxland		Ipsilateral (L5–S1)[a] Contralateral (L5–S1)[b]	

[a]If side flexion is induced first.
[b]If rotation is induced first.
Ipsilateral implies both movements occur in the same direction, contralateral implies they occur in opposite directions.

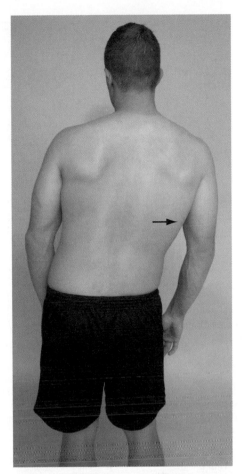

Fig. 9.29 Lumbar lateral shift.

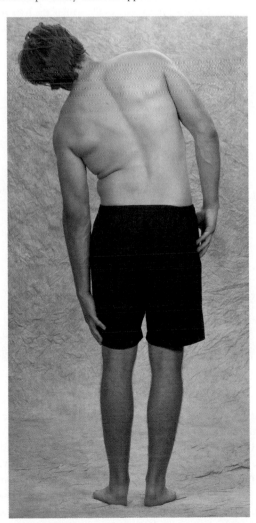

Fig. 9.28 Lateral (side) flexion. Note that the lower lumbar spine stays straight and the upper lumbar and lower thoracic spine side flexes, although the curve is not a smooth one.

must take care to watch for this accessory movement and try to eliminate it by stabilizing the pelvis.

If a movement such as side flexion toward the painful side increases the symptoms, the lesion is probably intraarticular, because the muscles and ligaments on that side are relaxed. If a disc protrusion is present and lateral to the nerve root, side flexion to the painful side increases the pain and radicular symptoms on that side. If a movement (such as side flexion away from the painful side) alters the symptoms, the lesion may be articular or muscular in origin, or it may be a disc protrusion medial to the nerve root (Fig. 9.30).

McKenzie advocated repeating the active movements, especially flexion and extension, 10 times to see whether the movement increased or decreased the symptoms.[47] He also advocated, as did Mulvein and Jull,[117] a sidegliding movement in which the head and feet remain in position and the patient shifts the pelvis to the left and to the right.

If the examiner finds that side flexion and rotation have been equally limited and extension has been limited to a lesser extent, a capsular pattern may be suspected. A capsular pattern in one lumbar segment, however, is difficult to detect.

Because back injuries rarely occur during a "pure" movement (such as flexion, extension, side flexion, or rotation),

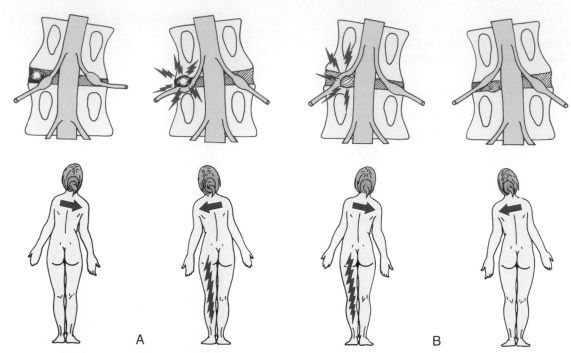

Fig. 9.30 Patients with herniated disc problems may sometimes list to one side. This is a voluntary or involuntary mechanism to alleviate nerve root irritation. The list in some patients is toward the side of the sciatica; in others, it is toward the opposite side. A reasonable hypothesis suggests that when the herniation is lateral to the nerve root (A), the list is to the side opposite the sciatica because a list to the same side would elicit pain. Conversely, when the herniation is medial to the nerve root (B), the list is toward the side of the sciatica because tilting away would irritate the root and cause pain. (Redrawn from White AA, Panjabi MM: *Clinical biomechanics of the spine*, ed 2, Philadelphia, 1990, JB Lippincott, p 415.) (© Augustus A. White III and MM Panjabi.)

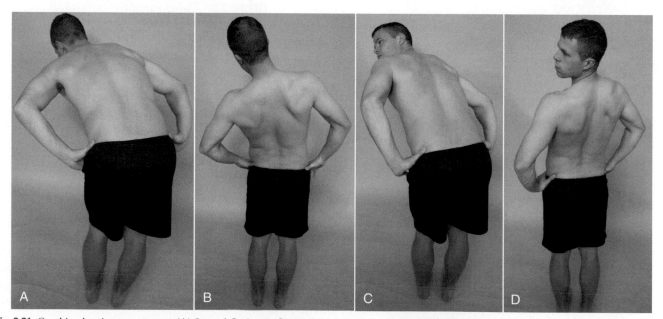

Fig. 9.31 Combined active movements. (A) Lateral flexion in flexion. (B) Lateral flexion in extension. (C) Rotation and flexion. (D) Rotation and extension.

it has been advocated that **combined movements** of the spine should be included in the examination.[118,119] The examiner may want to test the following more habitual combined movements: lateral flexion in flexion, lateral flexion in extension, flexion and rotation, and extension and rotation. These combined movements (Fig. 9.31) may cause signs and symptoms different from those produced by single-plane movements and are definitely indicated if the patient has shown that a combined movement is what causes the symptoms. For example, if the patient is suffering from a facet syndrome, combined extension and rotation is the movement most likely to exacerbate symptoms.[120] Other symptoms that would indicate facet involvement include absence of radicular signs or neurological deficit,

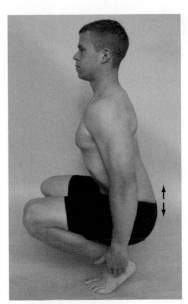

Fig. 9.32 Quick test.

hip and buttock pain, and sometimes leg pain above the knee, no paresthesia, and low back stiffness.[121,122]

While the patient is standing, the examiner may perform a **quick test** of the lower peripheral joints (Fig. 9.32) provided that the examiner believes that the patient will be able to do the test. The patient squats down as far as possible, bounces two or three times, and returns to the standing position. This action quickly tests the ankles, knees, and hips as well as the sacrum for any pathological condition. If the patient can fully squat and bounce without any signs or symptoms, these joints are probably free of pathology related to the complaint. However, this test should be used only with caution and should not be done with patients suspected of having arthritis or pathology in the lower limb joints, pregnant patients, or older patients who exhibit weakness and hypomobility. If this test is negative, there is no need to test the peripheral joints (peripheral joint scan) with the patient lying down.

The patient is then asked to balance on one leg and to go up and down on the toes four or five times. This is, in effect, a **modified Trendelenburg test.** While the patient does this, the examiner watches for the **Trendelenburg sign** (Fig. 9.33). A positive Trendelenburg sign is shown by the non–stance side ilium dropping down instead of elevating, as it normally would when a person is standing on one leg. A weak gluteus medius muscle or a coxa vara (abnormal shaft-neck angle of the femur) on the stance leg side may produce a positive sign. If the patient is unable to complete the movement by going up and down on the toes, the examiner should suspect an S1 nerve root lesion. Both legs are tested.

McKenzie advocated doing flexion movements with the patient in the supine position as well.[47] In the standing position, flexion in the spine takes place from above downward, so pain at the end of the ROM indicates that L5–S1 is affected. When the patient is in the supine position with the knees being lifted to the chest, flexion takes place from below upward, so that pain at the beginning of movement indicates that L5–S1 is affected. It is well to remember that greater stretch is placed on L5–S1 when the patient is in the lying position.

During the observation stage of the assessment, the examiner will have noted any changes in functional limb length (see Table 9.9). Wallace developed a method for measuring **functional leg length.**[123] The patient is first assessed in a relaxed stance. In this position, the examiner palpates the ASISs and the PSISs, noting any asymmetry. The examiner then places the patient in a symmetric stance, ensuring that the subtalar joint is in the neutral position (see Chapter 13), the toes are straight ahead, and the knees are extended. The ASISs and PSISs are again assessed for asymmetry. If differences are still noted, the examiner should check for structural leg length differences (see Chapters 10 and 11), sacroiliac joint dysfunction, or weak gluteus medius or quadratus lumborum (Fig. 9.34). The pelvis may also be leveled with the use of calibrated blocks or cards so that the functional length difference can be recorded.

Passive Movements

Passive movements are difficult to perform in the lumbar spine because of the weight of the body. If active movements are full and pain free, overpressure can be attempted with care. However, it is safer to check the end feel of the individual vertebrae in the lumbar spine during the assessment of joint play movements. The end feel is the same, but the examiner has better control of the patient and is less likely to overstress the joints.

Passive Movements of the Lumbar Spine and Normal End Feel

- Flexion (tissue stretch)
- Extension (tissue stretch)
- Side flexion (tissue stretch)
- Rotation (tissue stretch)

Resisted Isometric Movements

Resisted isometric muscle strength of the lumbar spine is first tested in the neutral position. The patient is seated. The contraction must be resisted and isometric so that no movement occurs (Fig. 9.35). Because of the strength of the trunk muscles, the examiner should say, "Don't let me move you," so that movement is minimized. The examiner tests flexion, extension, side flexion, and rotation. Fig. 9.36 shows the axes of movement of the lumbar spine. The lumbar spine should be in a neutral position, and the painful movements should be done last. The examiner should keep in mind that strong abdominal muscles help to reduce the load on the lumbar spine by approximately 30% and on the thoracic spine by approximately 50% as a result of the increased intrathoracic and intra-abdominal pressures caused by the contraction

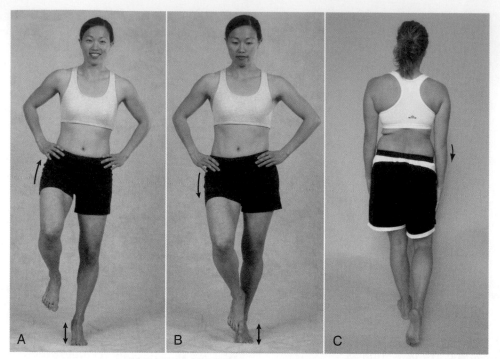

Fig. 9.33 Trendelenburg and S1 nerve root test. (A) Negative Trendelenburg test (hip hikes) while doing S1 test (up and down on toes). (B) Positive Trendelenburg test (hip drops) while doing the S1 test. If the patient cannot go up on his or her toes, it would indicate a positive S1 test. (C) Posterior view. Positive Trendelenburg test for a weak right gluteus medius.

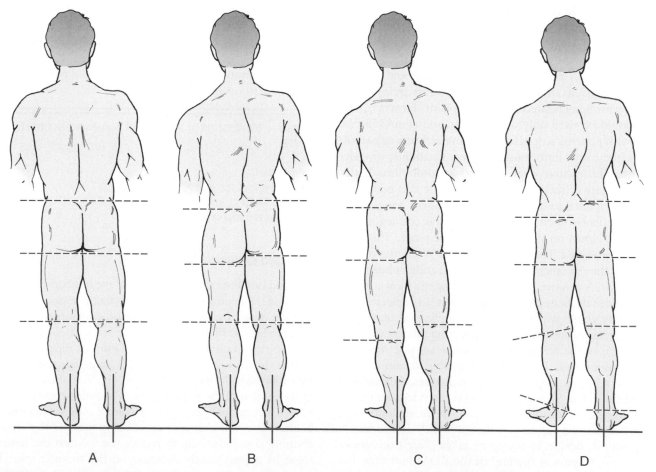

Fig. 9.34 Effect of different leg lengths and posture. Note the presence of scoliosis on the side with the "short" limb. (A) Normal. (B) Short left femur. (C) Short left tibia. (D) Pronation of left foot.

of these muscles. Table 9.11 lists the muscles acting on the lumbar vertebrae (Fig. 9.37; see also Figs. 8.37 and 8.38).

Resisted Isometric Movements of the Lumbar Spine

- Forward flexion
- Extension
- Side flexion (left and right)
- Rotation (left and right)
- Dynamic abdominal endurance
- Double straight leg lowering
- Dynamic extensor endurance
- Isotonic horizontal side support
- Internal/external abdominal oblique test

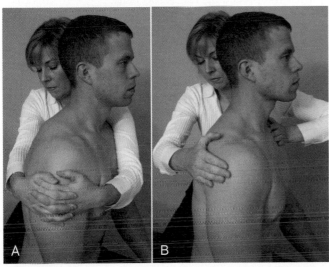

Fig. 9.35 Positioning for resisted isometric movements of the lumbar spine. (A) Flexion, extension, and side flexion. (B) Rotation to right.

Provided that neutral isometric testing is normal or only causes a small amount of pain, the examiner can go on to other tests that will place greater stress on the muscles. These tests are often dynamic and provide both concentric and eccentric work for the muscles supporting the spine. With all of the following tests, the examiner should make sure that the patient can hold a neutral pelvis. If there is excessive movement of the ASISs (supine) or PSISs (prone) when doing the test, the patient should not be allowed to do them. In normal individuals, the ASISs or PSISs should not move while the tests are being done. Motivation may also affect the results.[124]

Dynamic Abdominal Endurance Test.[125–127] This test checks the endurance of the abdominals. The patient is supine with the hips at 45°, knees at 90°, and hands at sides. A line is drawn 8 cm (for patients over 40 years of age) or 12 cm (for patients under 40 years of age) distal to the fingers. The patient tucks in his or her chin and curls the trunk to touch the line with the fingers (Fig. 9.38) and repeats as many curls as possible using a cadence of 25 repetitions per minute. The number of repetitions possible before cheating (holding breath, altered mechanics) or fatigue occurs is recorded as the score. The test may also be done as an isometric test (Fig. 9.39) by assuming the end position and holding it. The grading for this **isometric abdominal test** would be as follows[128–130].

- Normal (5) = Hands behind neck until scapulae clear table (20- to 30-second hold)
- Good (4) = Arms crossed over chest until scapulae clear table (15- to 20-second hold)
- Fair (3) = Arms straight until scapulae clear table (10- to 15-second hold)

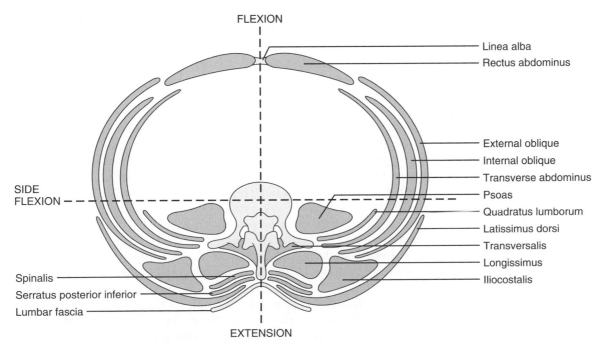

FLEXION

Linea alba
Rectus abdominus

External oblique
Internal oblique
Transverse abdominus
Psoas
Quadratus lumborum
Latissimus dorsi
Transversalis
Longissimus
Iliocostalis

SIDE FLEXION

Spinalis
Serratus posterior inferior
Lumbar fascia

EXTENSION

Fig. 9.36 Diagram of relations of the lumbar spine showing movement.

TABLE **9.11**

Muscles of the Lumbar Spine: Their Actions and Nerve Root Derivations

Action	Muscles Acting	Nerve Root Derivation
Forward flexion	1. Psoas major	L1–L3
	2. Rectus abdominis	T6–T12
	3. External abdominal oblique	T7–T12
	4. Internal abdominal oblique	T7–T12, L1
	5. Transversus abdominis	T7–T12, L1
	6. Intertransversarii	L1–L5
Extension	1. Latissimus dorsi	Thoracodorsal (C6–C8)
	2. Erector spinae	L1–L3
	Iliocostalis lumborum	L1–L3
	Longissimus thoracis	L1–L5
	3. Transversospinalis	L1–L5
	4. Interspinales	L1–L5
	5. Quadratus lumborum	T12, L1–L4
	6. Multifidus	L1–L5
	7. Rotatores	L1–L5
	8. Gluteus maximus	L1–L5
Side flexion	1. Latissimus dorsi	Thoracodorsal (C6–C8)
	2. Erector spinae	L1–L3
	Iliocostalis lumborum	L1–L3
	Longissimus thoracis	L1–L5
	3. Transversalis	L1–L5
	4. Intertransversarii	L1–L5
	5. Quadratus lumborum	T12, L1–L4
	6. Psoas major	L1–L3
	7. External abdominal oblique	T7–T12
Rotation[a]	1. Transversalis	L1–L5
	2. Rotatores	L1–L5
	3. Multifidus	L1–L5

[a]Very little rotation occurs in the lumbar spine because of the shape of the facet joints. Any rotation would be a result of shearing movement.

- Poor (2) = Arms extended toward knees until tops of scapulae lift from table (1- to 10-second hold)
- Trace (1) = Unable to raise more than head off table

McGill[131] advocated doing the isometric test by starting with the patient resting against a back rest angled at 60° from the horizontal with the hips and knees flexed to 90°, the arms folded across the chest, and the hands on opposite shoulders (Fig. 9.40). The patient's feet are held securely and the back rest is lowered away from the patient's back while the patient maintains the 60° position as long as possible.

Dynamic Extensor Endurance Test.[125,127,132,133] This test is designed to test the strength of iliocostalis lumborum (erector spinae) and multifidus. The patient is placed prone with the hips and iliac crests resting on the end of the examining table and the hips and pelvis stabilized with straps (Fig. 9.41). Initially the patient's hands support the upper body in 30° flexion on a chair or bench (see Fig. 9.41A). Keeping the spine straight, the examiner instructs the patient to extend the trunk to neutral and then lower the head to the start position. During the exercise, the patient's arms are crossed at the chest. The cadence is 25 repetitions per minute. The number of repetitions possible before cheating (holding breath, altered mechanics) or fatigue occurs is recorded as the score. The test may also be done isometrically, and the examiner times how long the patient can hold the contraction without pelvic or spinal movement. This test may also be done with the patient beginning in the prone position and extending the spine if the preceding test is too hard.[134,135] In this case, the patient can start with the hands by the side, moving the hands in the small of the back, and finally moving the hands behind the head for increasing difficulty. The test, if done isometrically **(isometric extensor test)** (Fig. 9.42), would be graded as follows[128–130]:

- Normal (5) = With hands clasped behind the head, extends the lumbar spine, lifting the head, chest, and ribs from the floor (20- to 30-second hold)
- Good (4) = With hands at the side, extends the lumbar spine, lifting the head, chest, and ribs from the floor (15- to 20-second hold)
- Fair (3) = With hands at the side, extends the lumbar spine, lifting the sternum off the floor (10- to 15-second hold)
- Poor (2) = With hands at the side, extends the lumbar spine, lifting the head off the floor (1- to 10-second hold)
- Trace (1) = Only slight contraction of the muscle with no movement

Biering and Sorensen described a similar test **(Biering-Sorensen fatigue test)** in which the subject had arms by the side; then the time for which the patient was able to hold the straight position before fatigue was recorded (i.e., the patient could not hold the position).[127,136,137] The start position is the same as for the dynamic test. Table 9.12 shows normative data from several authors.

Double Straight Leg Lowering Test.[134,135,141] (Note: This test checks the abdominals. It should be performed only if the patient receives a "normal" grade in the dynamic abdominal endurance test or the abdominal isometric test.) This is an abdominal eccentric test that can place a great deal of stress on the spine, so the examiner must make sure that the patient is able to hold a neutral pelvis before doing the exercise. It also causes greater abdominal activation than curl-ups.[142] The patient lies supine and flexes the hips to 90° (Fig. 9.43A) and then straightens the knees (Fig. 9.43B). The patient then positions the pelvis in neutral (i.e., the PSISs are slightly superior to the ASISs) by doing a posterior pelvic tilt and holding the spinous processes tightly against the examining table. The straight legs are eccentrically lowered

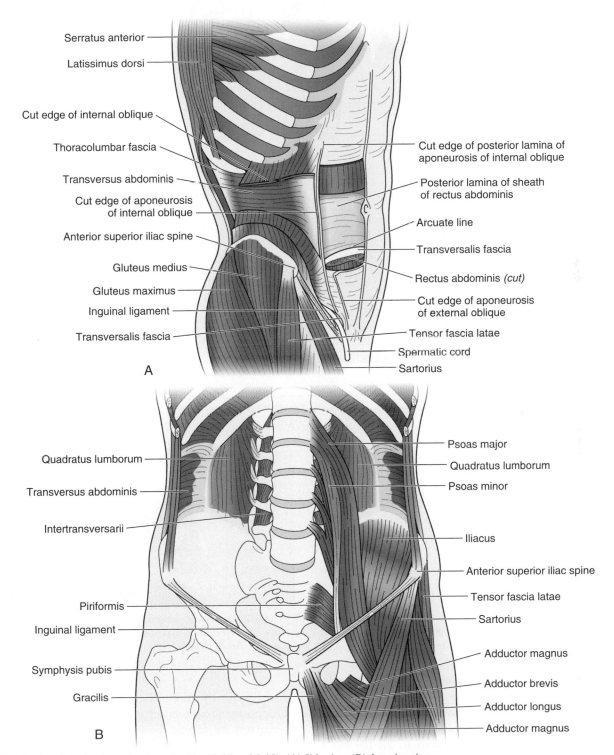

Serratus anterior

Latissimus dorsi

Cut edge of internal oblique

Thoracolumbar fascia

Transversus abdominis

Cut edge of aponeurosis
of internal oblique

Anterior superior iliac spine

Gluteus medius

Gluteus maximus

Inguinal ligament

Transversalis fascia

Cut edge of posterior lamina of
aponeurosis of internal oblique

Posterior lamina of sheath
of rectus abdominis

Arcuate line

Transversalis fascia

Rectus abdominis *(cut)*

Cut edge of aponeurosis
of external oblique

Tensor fascia latae

Spermatic cord

Sartorius

A

Quadratus lumborum

Transversus abdominis

Intertransversarii

Piriformis

Inguinal ligament

Symphysis pubis

Gracilis

Psoas major

Quadratus lumborum

Psoas minor

Iliacus

Anterior superior iliac spine

Tensor fascia latae

Sartorius

Adductor magnus

Adductor brevis

Adductor longus

Adductor magnus

B

Fig. 9.37 Muscles of the lumbar spine (see also Figs. 8.37 and 8.38). (A) Side view. (B) Anterior view.

Continued

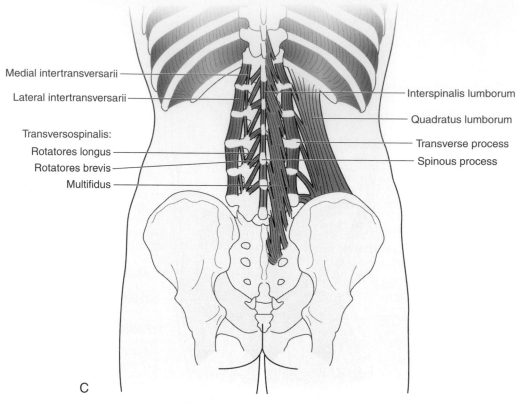

Medial intertransversarii

Lateral intertransversarii

Transversospinalis:
Rotatores longus
Rotatores brevis
Multifidus

Interspinalis lumborum

Quadratus lumborum

Transverse process

Spinous process

C

Fig. 9.37, cont'd (C) Posterior view.

(Fig. 9.43C). As soon as the ASISs start to rotate forward, the test is stopped, the angle is measured (plinth-to-thigh angle), and the knees are bent. The test must be done slowly, and the patient must not hold his or her breath. The grading of the test is as follows[129]:

- Normal (5) = Able to reach 0° to 15° from table before pelvis tilts
- Good (4) = Able to reach 16° to 45° from table before pelvis tilts
- Fair (3) = Able to reach 46° to 75° from table before pelvis tilts
- Poor (2) = Able to reach 75° to 90° from table before pelvis tilts
- Trace (1) = Unable to hold pelvis in neutral at all

Internal/External Abdominal Obliques Test.[134,135] This test checks the combined action of the internal oblique muscle of one side and the external oblique muscle on the opposite side. The patient is in the supine position with hands by the side. The patient is asked to lift the head and shoulder on one side and reach over and touch the fingernails of the other hand (Fig. 9.44A). The examiner counts the number of repetitions the patient performs. The patient's feet should not be supported and the patient should breathe normally. The test can be made

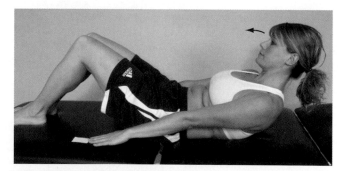

Fig. 9.38 Dynamic abdominal endurance test. The patient tucks in the chin and curls up the trunk, lifting the trunk off the bed. Ideally, the scapula should clear the bed.

more difficult by asking the patient to put the hands on the opposite shoulders across the chest (Fig. 9.44B) and do the test by taking the elbow toward where the fingers would have rested beside the body or, more difficult still, by putting the hands behind the head and taking the elbows toward the position where the fingernails would have rested beside the body (Fig. 9.44C). The grading of the test, if done isometrically **(isometric internal/external abdominal oblique test),** would be as follows[129]:

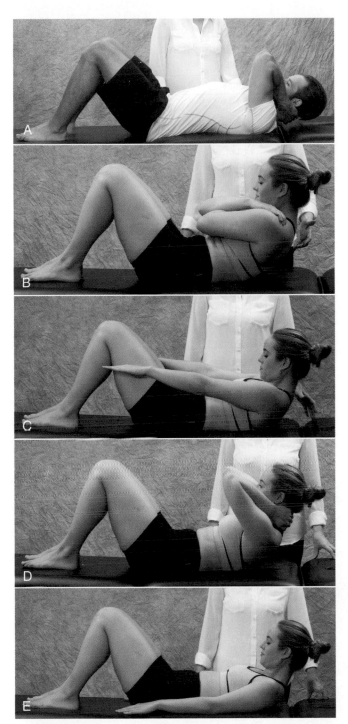

Fig. 9.39 Isometric abdominal test. (A) Hands behind neck. (B) Arms crossed over chest, scapulae off table. (C) Arms straight, scapulae off table. (D) Hands behind head, top of scapulae off table. (E) Arms straight, only head off table.

- Normal (5) = Flexes and rotates the lumbar spine fully with hands behind head (20- to 30-second hold)
- Good (4) = Flexes and rotates the lumbar spine fully with hands across chest (15- to 20-second hold)
- Fair (3) = Flexes and rotates the lumbar spine fully with arms reaching forward (10- to 15-second hold)

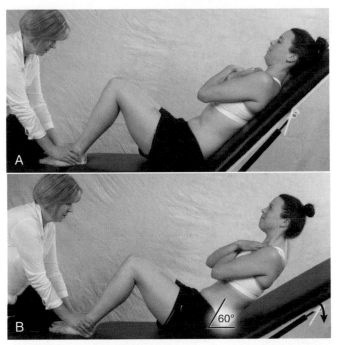

Fig. 9.40 McGill's isometric abdominal test. (A) Start position: back rest at 60°. (B) Hold position.

- Poor (2) = Unable to flex and rotate fully
- Trace (1) = Only slight contraction of the muscle with no movement
- (0) = No contraction of the muscle

Dynamic Horizontal Side Support (Side Bridge) Test.[143] This movement tests the quadratus lumborum muscle. The patient is in a side lying position, resting the upper body on his or her elbow (Fig. 9.45A). To begin, the patient side lies and flexes the knees to 90°. The examiner asks the patient to lift the pelvis off the examining table (Fig. 9.45B) and straighten the spine. The patient should not roll forward or backward when doing the test. The patient repeats the movement as many times as possible in a dynamic test or holds for as long as possible in an isometric test. In younger, more fit patients, the test can be made more difficult by having the legs straight and asking the patient to lift the knees and pelvis off the examining table with the feet as the base so that the whole body is straight (Fig. 9.45C). As an isometric test, the test would be graded as follows:

- Normal (5) = Able to lift pelvis off examining table and hold spine straight (10- to 20-second hold)
- Good (4) = Able to lift pelvis off examining table but has difficulty holding spine straight (5- to 10-second hold)
- Fair (3) = Able to lift pelvis off examining table and cannot hold spine straight (<5-second hold)
- Poor (2) = Unable to lift pelvis off examining table

McGill reported that the side bridge should be able to be held 65% of the extensor time for men and 39% for women and 99% of the flexor time for men and 79% for

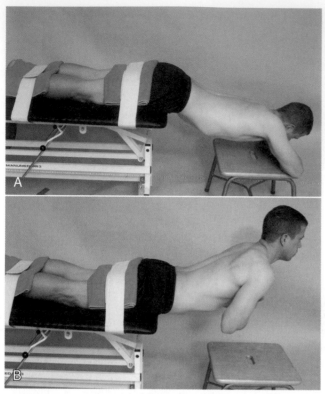

Fig. 9.41 Dynamic extensor endurance test. (A) Starting position. (B) End position.

TABLE 9.12

Normative Data for Biering-Sorensen Fatigue Test From Three Author Groups

Study	Values
Demoulin et al.[138]	Healthy males: 198 seconds Prior low back pain males: 176 seconds Current low back pain males: 163 seconds Healthy females: 197 seconds Prior low back pain females: 210 seconds Current low back pain females: 177 seconds
McGill et al.[139]	Males: 164 ± 51 seconds Females: 189 ± 60 seconds
Simmonds et al.[140]	Healthy pain-free subjects: 77.76 ± 36.63 (trial 1) 72.73 ± 29.79 (trial 2) Low back pain subjects: 39.55 ± 36.31 (trial 1) 36.64 ± 33.32 (trial 2)

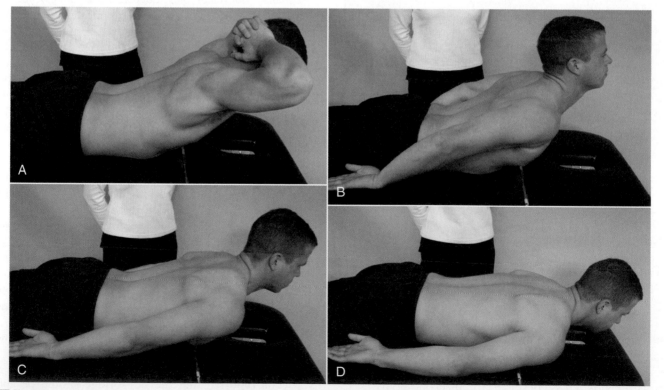

Fig. 9.42 Isometric extensor test. (A) Hands behind head, lift head, chest, and ribs off bed. (B) Hands at side, lift head, chest, and ribs off bed. (C) Hands at side, lift sternum off bed. (D) Hands at side, lift head off bed.

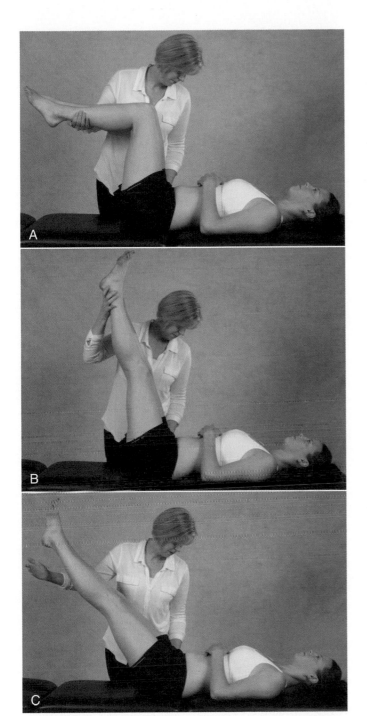

Fig. 9.43 Double straight leg lowering test. (A) Flexing hips to 90°. (B) Start position with knees straight. (C) Example of leg lowering. Note how the examiner is watching for anterior pelvic rotation, which would indicate an inability to hold a neutral pelvis.

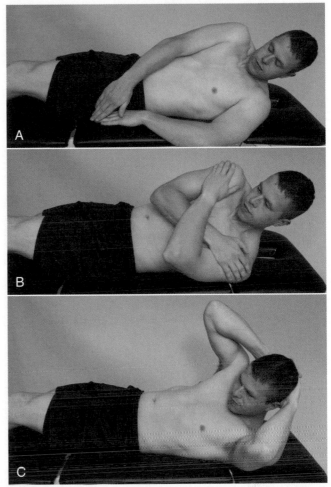

Fig. 9.44 Internal/external abdominal oblique test. (A) Test position with hands at side. (B) Test position with hands on shoulders. (C) Test position with hands behind head.

women.[139] Two other variations of testing bridging may be found in the section titled "Special Tests," later (prone and supine bridge tests) further on.

Back Rotators/Multifidus Test. This test checks the ability of the lumbar rotators and multifidus to stabilize the trunk during dynamic extremity movement. The patient assumes the quadruped position (Fig. 9.46A) and is asked

to hold the "neutral pelvis" position and breathe normally. The patient is then asked to do the following movements (Fig. 9.46B–D):

1. Single straight arm lift and hold
2. Single straight leg lift and hold
3. Contralateral straight arm and straight leg lift and hold
   The scoring for the test would be as follows:

- Normal (5) = Able to do contralateral arm and leg, both sides, while maintaining neutral pelvis (20- to 30-second hold)
- Good (4) = Able to maintain neutral pelvis while doing single leg lift but not able to hold neutral pelvis when doing contralateral arm and leg (20-second hold)
- Fair (3) = Able to do single arm lift and maintain neutral pelvis (20-second hold)
- Poor (2) = Unable to maintain neutral pelvis while doing single arm lift

If tested isokinetically, the back extensors are stronger than the flexors. Men produce a force equal to

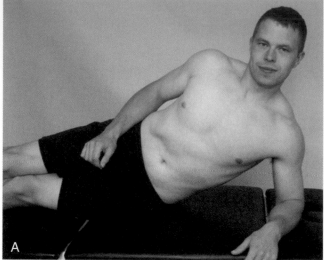

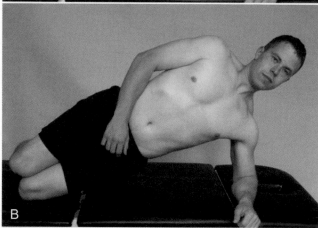

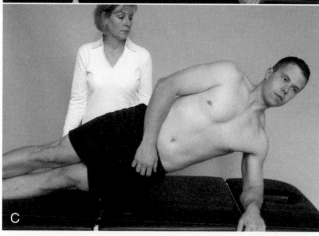

Fig. 9.45 Dynamic horizontal side support. (A) Start position. (B) Lifting pelvis off bed using knees as support. (C) Lifting pelvis off bed using feet and ankles as support.

approximately 65% of body weight in flexion, whereas women produce approximately 65% to 70% of their body weight in flexion. In extension, men produce approximately 90% to 95% of their body weight and women produce 80% to 95% of their body weight, depending on the

speed tested. In rotation, men produce approximately 55% to 65% of their body weight, whereas women produce approximately 40% to 55% of their body weight, depending on the speed tested.[144]

Peripheral Joint Scanning Examination

After the resisted isometric movements of the lumbar spine have been completed, if the examiner did not use the quick test to test the peripheral joints or is unsure of the findings or whether the peripheral joints are involved, the peripheral joints should be quickly scanned to rule out obvious pathology in the extremities. Any deviation from normal should lead the examiner to do a detailed examination of that joint. The following joints are scanned.[145]

Lower Limb Scanning Examination

- Sacroiliac joints
- Hip joints
- Knee joints
- Ankle joints
- Foot joints

Sacroiliac Joints

With the patient standing, the examiner palpates the PSIS on one side with one thumb and one of the sacral spines with the other thumb. The patient then fully flexes the hip on that side, and the examiner notes whether the PSIS drops as it normally should or whether it elevates, indicating fixation of the sacroiliac joint on that side (Fig. 9.47). The examiner then compares the other side. The examiner next places one thumb on one of the patient's ischial tuberosities and one thumb on the sacral apex. The patient is then asked to flex the hip on that side again. If the movement is normal, the thumb on the ischial tuberosity moves laterally. If the sacroiliac joint on that side is fixed, the thumb moves up. The other side is then tested for comparison. This test has also been called the *Gillet's* or the *sacral fixation test* (see Chapter 10).

Hip Joints

These joints are actively moved through flexion, extension, abduction, adduction, and medial and lateral rotation in as full a ROM as possible. Any pattern of restriction or pain should be noted. As the patient flexes the hip, the examiner may palpate the ilium, sacrum, and lumbar spine to determine when movement begins at the sacroiliac joint on that side and at the lumbar spine during the hip movement. The two sides should be compared.

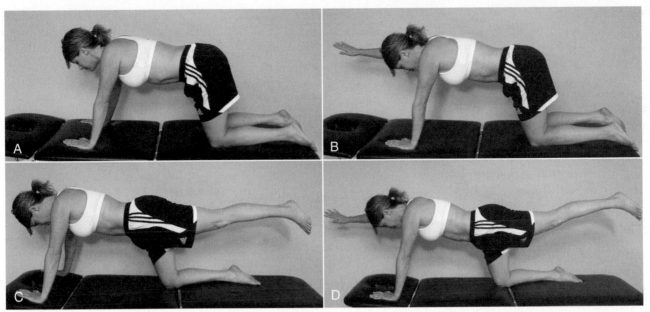

Fig. 9.46 Back rotators/multifidus test. (A) Start position. (B) Single straight arm lift. (C) Single straight leg lift. (D) Contralateral straight arm and leg lift.

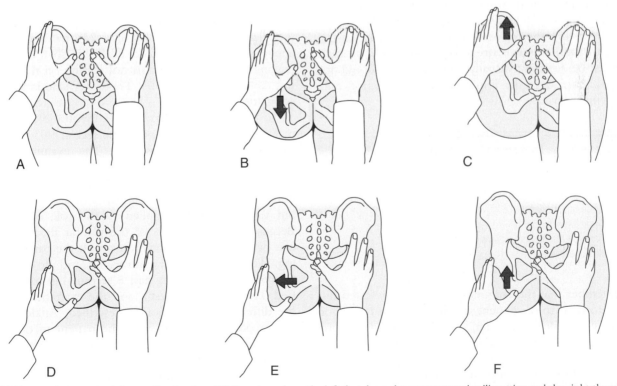

Fig. 9.47 Tests to demonstrate left sacroiliac fixation. (A) Examiner places the left thumb on the posterosuperior iliac spine and the right thumb over one of the sacral spinous processes. (B) With normal movement, the examiner's left thumb moves downward as the patient raises the left leg with full hip flexion. (C) If the joint is fixed, the examiner's left thumb moves upward as the patient raises the left leg. (D) The examiner places the left thumb over the ischial tuberosity and the right thumb over the apex of the sacrum. (E) With normal movement, the examiner's left thumb moves laterally as the patient raises the left leg with full hip flexion. (F) If the joint is fixed, the examiner's left thumb moves slightly upward as the patient raises the left leg. (Modified from Kirkaldy-Willis WH: *Managing low back pain*, New York, 1983, Churchill Livingstone, p 94.)

Knee Joints

The patient actively moves the knee joints through as full a range of flexion and extension as possible. Any restriction of movement or abnormal signs and symptoms should be noted.

Foot and Ankle Joints

Plantar flexion, dorsiflexion, supination, and pronation of the foot and ankle as well as flexion and extension of the toes are actively performed through a full ROM. Again, any alteration in signs and symptoms should be noted.

Myotomes

Having completed the scanning examination of the peripheral joints, the examiner next tests the patient's muscle power for possible neurological weakness (Table 9.13).[145] With the patient lying supine, the myotomes are assessed individually (Fig. 9.48). When myotomes are being tested (Table 9.14), the examiner should place the test joint or joints in a neutral or resting position and then apply a resisted isometric pressure. The contraction should be held for at least 5 seconds so as to show any weakness. If feasible, the examiner should test the two sides simultaneously to provide a comparison. The simultaneous bilateral comparison is not possible for movements involving the hip and knee joints because of the weight of the limbs and stress to the low back, so each side must be done individually. The examiner should not apply pressure over the joints because this action may mask symptoms.

Myotomes of the Lumbar and Sacral Spines

- L2: Hip flexion
- L3: Knee extension
- L4: Ankle dorsiflexion
- L5: Great toe extension
- S1: Ankle plantar flexion, ankle eversion, hip extension
- S2: Knee flexion

Remember that the examiner has previously tested the S1 myotome with the patient standing and has tested for a positive Trendelenburg sign (modified Trendelenburg test). These movements are repeated here only if the examiner is unsure of the result and wants to test again. The ankle movements should be tested with the knee flexed approximately 30°, especially if the patient complains of sciatic pain, because full dorsiflexion is considered a provocative maneuver for stretching neurological tissue. Likewise, the extended knee increases the stretch

on the sciatic nerve and may result in false signs, such as weakness resulting from pain rather than from pressure on the nerve root. Rainville et al.[146] have recommended testing the L3 and L4 nerve roots at the same time by doing a **single leg sit-to-stand** test to check for unilateral quadriceps weakness (Fig. 9.49). The patient can hold the examiner's hands for balance.

If the patient is in extreme pain, all tests with the patient in the supine position should be completed before the patient is tested prone. This reduces the amount of movement the patient must do, thus decreasing the patient's discomfort. Ideally, all tests in the standing position should be performed first, followed by tests in the sitting, supine, side-lying, and prone positions. This procedure is shown in the précis at the end of the chapter.

To test hip flexion (L2 myotome), the examiner flexes the patient's hip to 30° to 40°. The examiner then applies a resisted force into extension proximal to the knee while ensuring that the heel of the patient's foot is not resting on the examining table (see Fig. 9.48A). The other side is then tested for comparison. To prevent excessive stress on the lumbar spine, the examiner must ensure that the patient does not increase the lumbar lordosis while doing the test and that only one leg at a time is tested.

To test knee extension or the L3 myotome, the examiner flexes the patient's knee to 25° to 35° and then applies a resisted flexion force at the midshaft of the tibia, making sure that the heel is not resting on the examining table (see Fig. 9.48B). The other side is tested for comparison.

To test ankle dorsiflexion (L4 myotome), the examiner asks the patient to place the feet at 90° relative to the leg (plantigrade position). The examiner applies a resisted force to the dorsum of each foot and compares the two sides (see Fig. 9.48C). Ankle plantar flexion (S1 myotome) is compared in a similar fashion, but the resistance is applied to the sole of the foot. Because of the strength of the plantar flexor muscles, it is better to test this myotome with the patient standing. The patient slowly moves up and down on the toes of each foot (for at least 5 seconds) in turn **(modified Trendelenburg test),** and the examiner compares the differences as previously described. Ankle eversion (S1 myotome) is tested with the patient in the supine position and the examiner applies a force to move the foot into inversion (see Fig. 9.48D).

Toe extension (L5 myotome) is tested with the patient holding both big toes in a neutral position. The examiner applies resistance to the nails of both toes and compares the two sides (see Fig. 9.48E). It is imperative that the resistance be isometric, so the amount of force in this

TABLE **9.13**

Lumbar Root Syndromes

Root	Dermatome	Muscle Weakness	Reflexes/Special Tests Affected	Paresthesias
L1	Back, over trochanter, groin	None	None	Groin, after holding posture, which causes pain
L2	Back, front of thigh to knee	Psoas, hip adductors	None	Occasionally front of thigh
L3	Back, upper buttock, front of thigh and knee, medial lower leg	Psoas, quadriceps—thigh wasting	Knee jerk sluggish, PKB positive, pain on full SLR	Inner knee, anterior lower leg
L4	Inner buttock, outer thigh, inside of leg, dorsum of foot, big toe	Tibialis anterior, extensor hallucis	SLR limited, neck-flexion pain, weak knee jerk; side flexion limited	Medial aspect of calf and ankle
L5	Buttock, back and side of thigh, lateral aspect of leg, dorsum of foot, inner half of sole and first, second, and third toes	Extensor hallucis, peroneals, gluteus medius, ankle dorsiflexors, hamstrings—calf wasting	SLR limited to one side, neck-flexion pain, ankle jerk decreased, crossed-leg raising—pain	Lateral aspect of leg, medial three toes
S1	Buttock, back of thigh, and lower leg	Calf and hamstrings, wasting of gluteals, peroneals, plantar flexors	SLR limited	Lateral two toes, lateral foot, lateral leg to knee, plantar aspect of foot
S2	Same as S1	Same as S1 except peroneals	Same as S1	Lateral leg, knee, heel
S3	Groin, inner thigh to knee	None	None	None
S4	Perineum, genitals, lower sacrum	Bladder, rectum	None	Saddle area, genitals, anus, impotence

PKB, Prone knee bending; *SLR*, straight leg raising.
Manipulation and traction are contraindicated if S4 or massive posterior displacement causes bilateral sciatica and S3 pain.

case is less than that applied during knee extension, for example.

Hip extension (S1 myotome) is tested with the patient lying prone. This test must be done only if the patient is unable to do plantar flexion testing in standing or ankle eversion. The knee is flexed to 90°. The examiner then lifts the patient's thigh slightly off the examining table while stabilizing the leg. A downward force is applied to the patient's posterior thigh with one hand while the other hand ensures that the patient's thigh is not resting on the table (see Fig. 9.48F).

Knee flexion (S1–S2 myotomes) is tested in the same position (prone) with the knee flexed to 90°. An extension isometric force is applied just above the ankle (see Fig. 9.48G). Although it is possible to test both knee flexors at the same time, it is not advisable to do this because the stress on the lumbar spine would be too great.

Functional Assessment

Injury to the lumbar spine can greatly affect the patient's ability to function. Activities such as standing, walking, bending, lifting, traveling, socializing, dressing, and sexual intercourse can be affected. Numerical scoring tables may be used to determine the degree of pain caused by lumbar spine pathology or disability. When one of these scales is being selected, care must be taken to make sure that it measures the disability from the patient's perspective.[147–150] Examples are the the **Oswestry Disability Index**[151–153] (eTool 9.4); the **Quebec Back Pain Disability Scale**[154,155] (eTool 9.5); the **Hendler 10-Minute Screening Test for Chronic Back Pain Patients** (eTool 9.6)[149,152,156]; and the **Back Pain Attitudes Questionnaire (Back-PAQ)**,[70,75,157] which was developed as a 34-item questionnaire and also as another with only 10 items. The 10-item questionnaire was felt to be suitable as a screening tool and an outcome

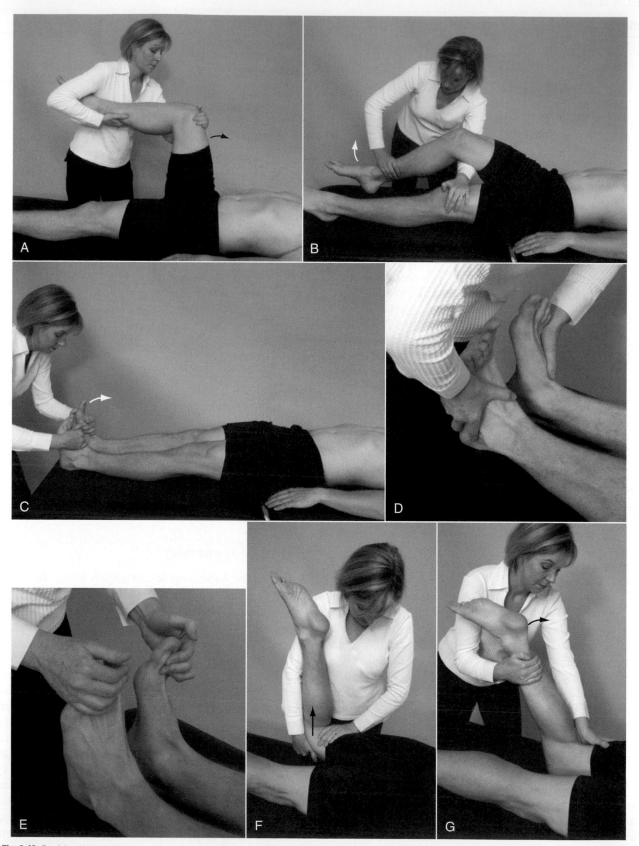

Fig. 9.48 Positioning to test myotomes. (A) Hip flexion (L2). (B) Knee extension (L3). (C) Foot dorsiflexion (L4). (D) Ankle eversion (S1). (E) Extension of the big toe (L5). (F) Hip extension (S1). (G) Knee flexion (S1–S2).

TABLE **9.14**

Myotomes of the Lower Limb

Nerve Root	Test Action	Muscles
L1–L2	Hip flexion	Psoas, iliacus, sartorius, gracilis, pectineus, adductor longus, adductor brevis
L3	Knee extension	Quadriceps, adductor longus, magnus, and brevis
L4	Ankle dorsiflexion	Tibialis anterior, quadriceps, tensor fasciae latae, adductor magnus, obturator externus, tibialis posterior
L5	Toe extension	Extensor hallucis longus, extensor digitorum longus, gluteus medius and minimus, obturator internus, semimembranosus, semitendinosus, peroneus tertius, popliteus
S1	Ankle plantar flexion Ankle eversion	Gastrocnemius, soleus, gluteus maximus, obturator internus, piriformis, biceps femoris, semitendinosus, popliteus, peroneus longus and brevis, extensor digitorum brevis
S2	Hip extension Knee flexion	Biceps femoris, piriformis, soleus, gastrocnemius, flexor digitorum longus, flexor hallucis longus, intrinsic foot muscles
S3	Knee flexion	Intrinsic foot muscles (except abductor hallucis, flexor hallucis brevis, flexor digitorum brevis, extensor digitorum brevis)

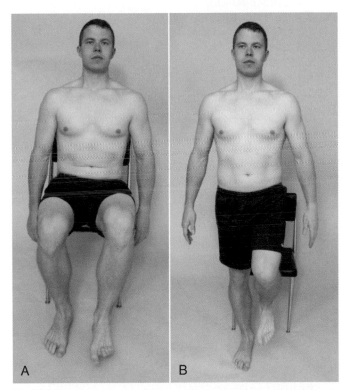

Fig. 9.49 Single leg sit-to-stand test. (A) Start position. Note patient's left leg is off the floor. (B) End position.

measurement tool.[157] The Keele University **STart Back Screening Tool** was designed to group patients into risk groups reflecting the severity of their back problems.[158] It has been reported that the Hendler test helps to differentiate organic from functional low back pain.[159] The Oswestry Disability Index is a good functional scale because it deals with ADLs and therefore is based on the patient's response and concerns affecting daily life. It is the most commonly used functional back scale. The disability index is calculated by dividing the total score (each section is worth from 1 to 6 points) by the number of sections answered and multiplying by 100. The **Roland-Morris Disability Questionnaire** is short and simple; it is suitable for following up on progress in clinical settings and for combining with other measures of function (e.g., work disability) (eTool 9.7).[160–162] Several of the tests are related to pain and the patient's perception of the pain relative to the injury[81–83,163] (see item 23 in the section labeled "Patient History," earlier). Other numerical back pain scales include the **Functional Rating Index**,[164,165] the **Dallas Pain Questionnaire**,[166] the **Million Index**,[167] the **Japanese Orthopedic Association Scale**,[168] the **Iowa Low Back Rating Scale**,[169] the **Bournemouth Questionnaire**,[170,171] the **Scoliosis Research Society Form** (SRS-22 for those with spinal deformity),[172–174] the **Lumbar Spinal Stenosis Questionnaire**,[175] and the **Aberdeen Back Pain Scale**.[176] Thomas provides a good review of these and other scales.[149] Lehman and colleagues developed a rating scale for lumbar dysfunction (eTool 9.8) that includes assessment criteria, physician criteria, and, perhaps more importantly, patient criteria for determining the degree of dysfunction.[169] These criteria can be evaluated during the normal assessment for the patient.

Waddell and colleagues developed a series of tests to differentiate between organic and nonorganic back pain (**Waddell's signs**).[52,67,177,178] Each test counts +1 if positive or 0 if negative:

1. Superficial skin tenderness to light pinch over wide area of lumbar spine
2. Deep tenderness over a wide area, often extending to the thoracic spine, sacrum, or pelvis
3. Low back pain on axial loading of the spine in standing

4. Straight leg raising test positive when specifically tested but not when patient is seated with knee extended to test Babinski reflex
5. Abnormal neurological (motor or sensory) patterns
6. Overreaction

Positive findings of +3 or more should be investigated for a nonorganic cause; these patients may also have social and psychological components to their complaint.[3,179,180]

Waddell also described a simple clinical functional capacity evaluation (eTool 9.9)[3] that examiners may find useful for testing patients.[181]

Simmonds et al.[140] came up with several functional tests or physical performance measures that they felt would be useful and discriminate between individuals with and without low back pain:

- **Timed 15-m (50-ft) walk:**[127] Patient walks 7.5 m (25 ft) as fast as he or she can, turns, and returns to the starting position while being timed.
- **Loaded reach test:**[127] Patient stands next to a wall, which has a meter ruler at shoulder height. The patient reaches forward with a weight at shoulder height as far as he or she can while keeping the heels on the floor. The weight should not exceed a maximum of 5% of body weight or 4.5 kg (9.9 lb).
- **Repeated sit-to-stand:**[127] This timed test involves the patient starting by sitting in a chair. The patient then stands fully and returns to sitting, repeating the sequence 10 times as fast as possible. The average value of two trials is used as the time.
- **Repeated trunk flexion:**[182] This timed test involves the patient starting in a standing position and then flexing forward as far as possible and returning to the upright posture as fast as tolerable, repeating the motion 10 times. The average value of two trials is used as the time.
- **Biering-Sorensen fatigue test:** Described previously under "Resisted Isometric Movements."

Special Tests

Special tests should always be considered as an integral part of a much larger examination process.[183] They should never be used in isolation.[184] Many of the special tests in the lumbar spine are purported to have poor diagnostic value.[127,185] Because these are clinical tests and commonly depend on the skill of the examiner, many of them show low reliability and validity or have not been studied at all.[186–190] Thus, the icons are graded primarily on clinical experience.

For the reader who would like to review them, the reliability, validity, specificity, sensitivity, and odds ratios of some of the special tests used in the lumbar spine are available in eAppendix 9.1.

When the examiner performs special tests in the lumbar assessment, the straight leg raising test, the prone knee bending (PKB) test, and the slump test should always be done, especially if there are neurological symptoms. The other tests need be done only if the examiner believes they are relevant or to confirm a diagnosis.

Key Tests Performed on the Lumbar Spine Depending on Suspected Pathology[a]

- **For neurological dysfunction:**
  - ✓ Centralization/peripheralization
  - ⚠ Cross straight leg raise test
  - ⚠ Femoral nerve traction test
  - ⚠ Prone knee bending test or variant
  - ✓ Slump test or variant
  - ✓ Straight leg raise or variant
- **For lumbar instability:**
  - ❓ H and I test
  - ✓ Passive lumbar extension test
  - ❓ Posterior shear test
  - ⚠ Prone hip extension test
  - ❓ Prone segmental instability test
  - ❓ Specific lumbar torsion test
  - ⚠ Test for anterior lumbar spine instability
  - ⚠ Test for posterior lumbar spine instability
- **For joint dysfunction:**
  - ❓ Bilateral straight leg raise test
  - ⚠ Clinical prediction rule for facet (zygapophyseal) joint involvement
  - ⚠ One-leg standing (stork standing) lumbar extension test
  - ⚠ Quadrant test
- **For muscle tightness:**
  - ✓ 90–90 straight leg raise test
  - ⚠ Ober test
  - ⚠ Rectus femoris test
  - ⚠ Thomas test
- **For muscle dysfunction:**
  - ✓ Prone bridge test
  - ⚠ Supine bridge test
- **Other tests:**
  - ⚠ Gower's sign
  - ❓ Heel-tap test
  - ❓ Sign of the buttock

[a]See Chapter 1, "Key for Classifying Special Tests."

Tests for Neurological Dysfunction (Neurodynamic Tests)

Neurodynamic tests check the mechanical movement of the neurological tissues as well as their sensitivity to mechanical stress or compression.[191,192] These neurodynamic tests, along with relevant history and decreased ROM, are considered by some to be the most important physical signs of disc herniation,[193] regardless of the degree of disc injury. Most of the special tests for neurological involvement are progressive or sequential. The patient is positioned, and one maneuver is tried; if no symptoms result, a second provocative, enhancing, or sensitizing maneuver is then carried out, and so on, while the examiner watches to see if the patient's symptoms are reproduced. The order in which these maneuvers are done also makes a difference. For example, with straight leg raising, the results are different if the hip is flexed with the knee extended than if the hip is flexed with the knee first flexed and then extended after the hip is in position.

Because of **tension points,** the neurological tissues move in different directions (Fig. 9.50) depending on where the stress is applied[192,194]; the direction and amount of movement vary depending on where movement is initiated.[195] For example, when doing the straight leg raising test, movement is toward the hip; with dorsiflexion as a sensitizing maneuver, the neurological tissue moves toward the ankle. If knee extension is performed in the slump test, the neurological tissue moves toward the knee.[191] This movement in different directions or in convergence toward the joint being moved can produce different symptoms depending on where and in what

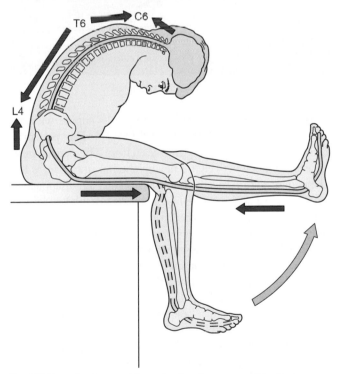

Fig. 9.50 Postulated neurobiomechanics that occur with slump movement. The approximate points C6, T6, L4, and the knee are where the neural tissue does not move in relation to the movements of the spinal canal. It is important to understand, however, that movement of neurological tissue is toward the joint where movement was initiated. (Modified from Butler DS: *Mobilisation of the nervous system*, Melbourne, 1991, Churchill Livingstone, pp 41–42.)

direction the movement occurs. The neurological tissue may move in one direction for one part of the test and in another for the next part of the test. Pathology may restrict this normal movement. Tension points are areas where there is minimal movement of the neurological tissue. According to Butler,[192] these areas are C6, the elbow, the shoulder, T6, L4, and the knee. It is important to realize, however, that the amount of tension placed on these points depends on the position of the extremity.

For a neurodynamic test to be positive, it must reproduce the patient's symptoms. Because these are provocative tests designed to put stress on the neurological tissue, they often cause discomfort or pain, which may be bilateral. However, if the patient's symptoms are not reproduced, the test should be considered negative. As a second check for a positive test, the symptoms that have been produced may be increased or decreased by adding or taking away the sensitizing parts (i.e., sensitizing tests such as neck flexion, foot dorsiflexion) of the test.[196,197]

The examiner has no need to do all or most of the neurodynamic tests listed. Some examiners will find one method more effective, others will find other tests more effective. The examiner should develop the skill to do two or three tests effectively and develop an understanding of how the neurological tissue is being stretched and which neurological tissue in particular is demonstrating signs and symptoms.

⚠ *Babinski Test.* The examiner runs a pointed object along the plantar aspect of the patient's foot.[198] A positive Babinski test or pathological reflex suggests an upper motor neuron lesion if the reflex is present on both sides; it may be evident in lower motor neuron lesions if it is seen on only one side. The reflex is demonstrated by extension of the big toe and abduction (splaying) of the other toes. In an infant up to a few weeks old, a positive test is normal.

❓ *"Bowstring" Test (Cram Test or Popliteal Pressure Sign).* The examiner carries out a straight leg raising test, and pain results (Fig. 9.51).[22,199] While maintaining the thigh in the same position, the examiner flexes the knee slightly (20°), reducing the symptoms. Thumb or finger pressure is then applied to the popliteal area to reestablish the painful radicular symptoms. The test indicates tension or pressure on the sciatic nerve and is a modification of the straight leg raising test.

The test may also be done in the sitting position with the examiner passively extending the knee to produce pain. The examiner then slightly flexes the knee so that the pain and symptoms disappear. The examiner holds this slightly flexed position by clasping the patient's leg between the examiner's knees. The examiner then presses the fingers of both hands into the popliteal space. Pain resulting from these maneuvers indicates a positive test and pressure or tension on the sciatic nerve. In this case, the test is called the **sciatic tension test** or **Deyerle's sign.**[68,200,201]

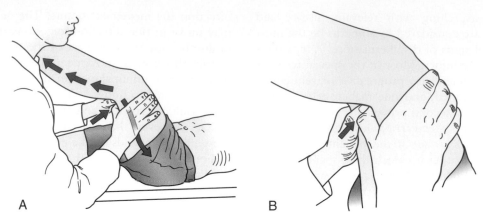

Fig. 9.51 Bowstring sign. (A) The examiner does a straight leg raise test. If a positive test results, the examiner relieves the pain by flexing the knee slightly. (B) The examiner then pushes into the popliteal space to increase the stress on the sciatic nerve, looking for a return of the same symptoms that present with the straight leg raise test.

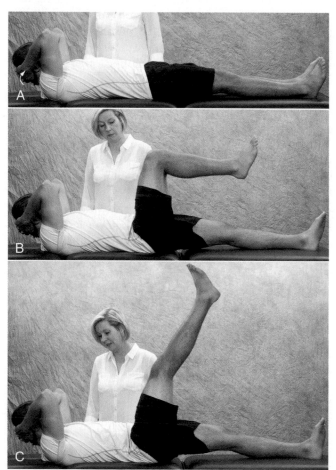

Fig. 9.52 Brudzinski-Kernig test. (A) In the Brudzinki portion of the test, the patient lies supine and elevates the head from the table. (B) When the head is lifted in a positive test, the patient complains of neck and low back discomfort and attempts to relieve the meningeal irritation by involuntary flexion of the knees and hips. (C) In the Kernig portion of the test, the patient lies supine with the hip and knee flexed to 90°, as in (B). The patient then extends the knee. If the patient complains of pain in the lower back, neck, or head on knee extension, it is suggestive of meningeal irritation. Returning to knee flexion will relieve the pain.

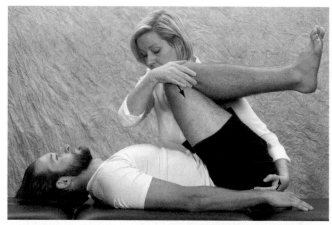

Fig. 9.53 Compression test.

❓ *Brudzinski-Kernig Test.* The patient is supine with the hands cupped behind the head.[200,202–204] The patient is instructed to flex the head onto the chest. The patient raises the extended leg actively by flexing the hip until pain is felt. The patient then flexes the knee, and if the pain disappears, it is considered a positive test. The mechanics of the Brudzinski-Kernig test are similar to those of the straight leg raising test except that the patient performs the movements actively (Fig. 9.52). Pain is a positive sign and may indicate meningeal irritation, nerve root involvement, or dural irritation. Brudzinski originally described the neck flexion aspect of the test, and Kernig described the hip flexion component. The two parts of the test may be done individually, in which case they are described as the test of the original author.

❓ *Compression Test.*[96] The patient lies supine with the hips and knees flexed. The hips are flexed until the PSISs start to move backward (usually about 100° hip flexion). The examiner then applies direct pressure against the patient's knees or buttocks applying axial compression to the spine (Fig. 9.53). If radicular pain into the posterior leg is produced, the test is thought to be positive for a possible disc herniation.

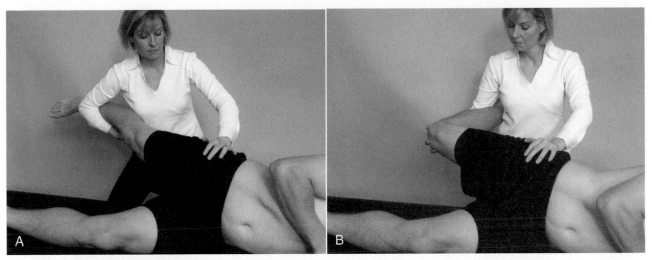

Fig. 9.54 Femoral nerve traction test. (A) The hip and knee are extended. (B) Then the knee is flexed.

⚠️ *Femoral Nerve Traction Test.* The patient lies on the unaffected side with the unaffected limb flexed slightly at the hip and knee (Fig. 9.54).[205] The patient's back should be straight, not hyperextended. The patient's head should be slightly flexed. The examiner grasps the patient's affected or painful limb and extends the knee while gently extending the hip approximately 15°. The patient's knee is then flexed on the affected side; this movement further stretches the femoral nerve. The test is positive if neurological pain radiates down the anterior thigh.

This is also a traction test for the nerve roots at the midlumbar area (L2–L4). As with the straight leg raising test, there is also a contralateral positive test. That is, when the test is performed, the symptoms occur in the opposite limb. This is called the **crossed femoral stretching test.**[206] Pain in the groin and hip that radiates along the anterior medial thigh indicates an L3 nerve root problem; pain extending to the midtibia indicates an L4 nerve root problem.

This test is similar to Ober's test for a tight iliotibial band, so the examiner must be able to differentiate between the two conditions. If the iliotibial band is tight, the test leg does not adduct but remains elevated away from the table as the tight tendon riding over the greater trochanter keeps the leg abducted. Femoral nerve injury presents with a different history, and the referred pain (anteriorly) tends to be stronger.

❓ *Flip Sign.* While the patient is sitting, the examiner extends the patient's knee and looks for symptoms. The patient is then placed supine, and a unilateral straight leg raising test is performed. For the sign to be positive, both tests must cause pain in the sciatic nerve distribution. If only one test is positive, the examiner should suspect problems in the lower lumbar spine. This is a combination of the classic Lasègue test and the sitting root test.

❓ *Gluteal Skyline Test.* The patient is relaxed in a prone position with the head straight and arms by the sides.[207] The examiner stands at the patient's feet and observes the buttocks from the level of the buttocks. The affected gluteus maximus muscle appears flat as a result of atrophy. The patient is asked to contract the gluteal muscles. The affected side may show less contraction, or it may be atonic and remain flat. If this occurs, the test is positive and may indicate damage to the inferior gluteal nerve or pressure on the L5, S1, or S2 nerve roots.

❓ *Knee Flexion Test.*[208] The patient, who has complained of sciatica, is in a standing position. The patient is asked to bend forward to touch the toes. If the patient bends the knee on the affected side while forward flexing the spine, the test is positive for sciatic nerve root compression. Likewise, if the patient is not allowed to bend the knee, spinal flexion is decreased.

❓ *Naffziger Test.*[28] The patient lies supine while the examiner gently compresses the jugular veins (which lie beside the carotid artery) for approximately 10 seconds (Fig. 9.55). The patient's face flushes, and then the patient is asked to cough. If coughing causes pain in the low back, the spinal theca is being compressed, leading to an increase in intrathecal pressure. The theca is the covering (pia mater, arachnoid mater, and dura mater) around the spinal cord.

⚠️ *Oppenheim Test.* The examiner runs a fingernail along the crest of the patient's tibia.[198] A negative Oppenheim test is indicated by no reaction or no pain. A positive test is indicated by a positive Babinski sign (positive pathological reflex) and suggests an upper motor neuron lesion.

⚠️ *Prone Knee Bending (Nachlas) Test.* The patient lies prone while the examiner passively flexes the knee as far as possible so that the patient's heel rests against the buttock.[209-211] At the same time, the examiner should ensure that the patient's hip is not rotated. If the examiner is unable to flex the patient's knee past 90° because of a pathological condition in the knee, the test may be performed by passive extension of the hip while the knee is flexed as much as possible. Unilateral neurological pain in

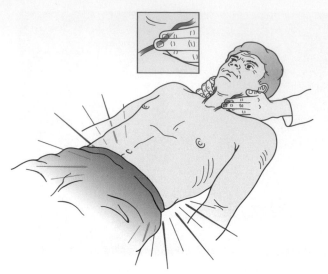

Fig. 9.55 Naffziger test. This test may be done while the patient is standing or lying down. The examiner applies bilateral compression to the jugular veins, which is hypothesized to increase cerebral spinal fluid pressure. This increased pressure in the subarachnoid space in the root canal may cause back or leg pain by irritating a local mechanical or inflammatory condition.

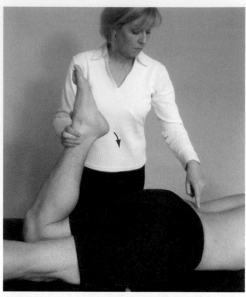

Fig. 9.56 Basic prone knee bending (PKB1) test, which stresses the femoral nerve and L2–L4 nerve root. The examiner is pointing to where pain in the lumbar spine may be expected with a positive test.

the lumbar area, buttock, or posterior thigh or sometimes the anterior thigh may indicate an L2 or L3 nerve root lesion (Fig. 9.56).

This test also stretches the femoral nerve. Pain in the anterior thigh indicates tight quadriceps muscles or stretching of the femoral nerve. A careful history and pain differentiation can help to delineate the problem. If the rectus femoris is tight, the examiner should remember that taking the heel to the buttock may cause anterior torsion to the ilium, which could lead to sacroiliac or lumbar pain. The flexed knee position should be maintained for 45 to 60 seconds. Butler has suggested modifications of the PKB test to stress individual peripheral nerves[192] (Table 9.15 and Fig. 9.57).

⚠ *Sitting Root Test.* This test is a modification of the slump test. The patient sits with a flexed neck. The knee is actively extended while the hip remains flexed at 90°. Increased pain indicates tension on the sciatic nerve. This test is sometimes used to catch the patient unaware. In this case, the examiner passively extends the knee while pretending to examine the foot. Davis et al.[212] reported that pain should occur before there is 22° of knee extension remaining for the test to be positive if knee extension is the last part of the test performed. Patients with true sciatic pain arch backward and complain of pain into the buttock, posterior thigh, and calf when the leg is straightened, indicating a positive test.[213] The **Bechterewis test** follows a similar pattern.[214] The patient is asked to extend one knee at a time. If no symptoms result, the patient is asked to extend both legs simultaneously. Symptoms in the back or leg indicate a positive response.[215]

✓ *Slump Test.* The slump test has become the most common neurological test for the lower limb. The patient is seated on the edge of the examining table with the legs supported, the hips in neutral position (i.e., no rotation, abduction, or adduction), and the hands behind the back (Fig. 9.58). The examination is performed in sequential steps. First, the patient is asked to "slump" the back into thoracic and lumbar flexion. The examiner maintains the patient's chin in the neutral position to prevent neck and head flexion. The examiner then uses one arm to apply overpressure across the shoulders to maintain flexion of the thoracic and lumbar spines. While this position is held, the patient is asked to actively flex the cervical spine and head as far as possible (i.e., chin to chest). The examiner then applies overpressure to maintain flexion of all three parts of the spine (cervical, thoracic, and lumbar) using the hand of the same arm to maintain overpressure in the cervical spine. With the other hand, the examiner then holds the patient's foot in maximum dorsiflexion. While the examiner holds these positions, the patient is asked to actively straighten the knee as much as possible. The test is repeated with the other leg and then with both legs at the same time. If the patient is unable to fully extend the knee because of pain, the examiner releases the overpressure to the cervical spine and the patient actively extends the neck. If the knee extends further, the symptoms decrease with neck extension, or if the positioning of the patient increases the patient's symptoms, then the test is considered positive for increased tension in the neuromeningeal tract.[216–219] Some clinicians modify the test to make the knee extension of the test passive. Once the patient is positioned with the three parts of the spine in flexion, the examiner first passively extends the knee. If symptoms do not result, then the examiner passively dorsiflexes the foot. A positive test would indicate the same lesion.

TABLE **9.15**

Prone Knee Bending Test and Its Modification

	Basic Prone Knee Bending (PKB1)	Prone Knee Bending (PKB2)	Prone Knee Extension (PKE)
Cervical spine	Rotation to test side	Rotation to test side	—
Thoracic and lumbar spine	Neutral	Neutral	Neutral
Hip	Neutral	Extension, adduction	Extension, abduction, lateral rotation
Knee	Flexion	Flexion	Extended
Ankle	—	—	Dorsiflexion
Foot	—	—	Eversion
Toes	—	—	—
Nerve bias	Femoral nerve, L2–L4 nerve root	Lateral femoral cutaneous nerve	Saphenous nerve

Data from Butler DA: *Mobilisation of the nervous system*, Melbourne, 1991, Churchill Livingstone.

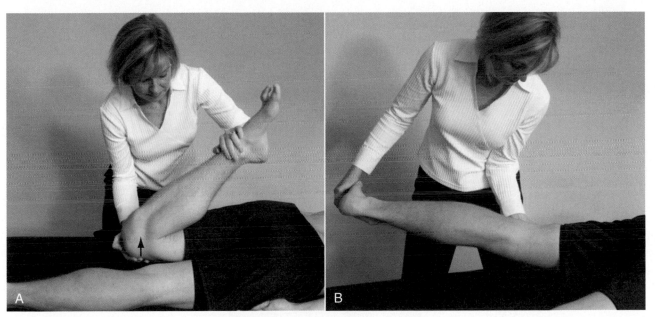

Fig. 9.57 Modifications to the prone knee bending (PKB) test to stress specific nerve. (A) PKB2 (lateral femoral cutaneous nerve). (B) Prone knee extension (saphenous nerve). See Table 9.15 for movements at each joint.

Butler advocated doing bilateral knee extension in the slump position.[192] Any asymmetry in the amount of knee extension is easier to note this way. Also, the effect of releasing neck flexion on the patient's symptoms should be noted. Butler has also suggested modifications to the slump test to stress individual nerves (Table 9.16 and Fig. 9.59).[192] In hypermobile patients, more hip flexion (more than 90°), as well as hip adduction and medial rotation may be required to elicit a positive response.[192] It is important that if symptoms are produced in any phase of the sequence, the provocative maneuvers are stopped to prevent undue discomfort to the patient.

When doing the slump test, the examiner is looking for reproduction of the patient's pathological symptoms, not just the production of symptoms.[220] The test does place stress on certain tissues, so some discomfort or pain is not necessarily symptomatic for the problem. For example, nonpathological responses include pain or discomfort in the area of T8–T9 (in 50% of normal patients), pain or discomfort behind the extended knee and hamstrings, symmetric restriction of knee extension, symmetric restriction of ankle dorsiflexion, and symmetric increased range of knee extension and ankle dorsiflexion on release of neck flexion.[192]

☑ *Straight Leg Raising Test (Lasègue's Test).* The straight leg raising test (Fig. 9.60) is done with the patient completely relaxed.[28,221–228] It is one of the most common neurological tests of the lower limb. It is a passive test, and each leg is tested individually with the normal leg being tested first. With the patient in the supine position, the hip medially rotated and adducted to neutral and the knee extended, the examiner flexes the hip until

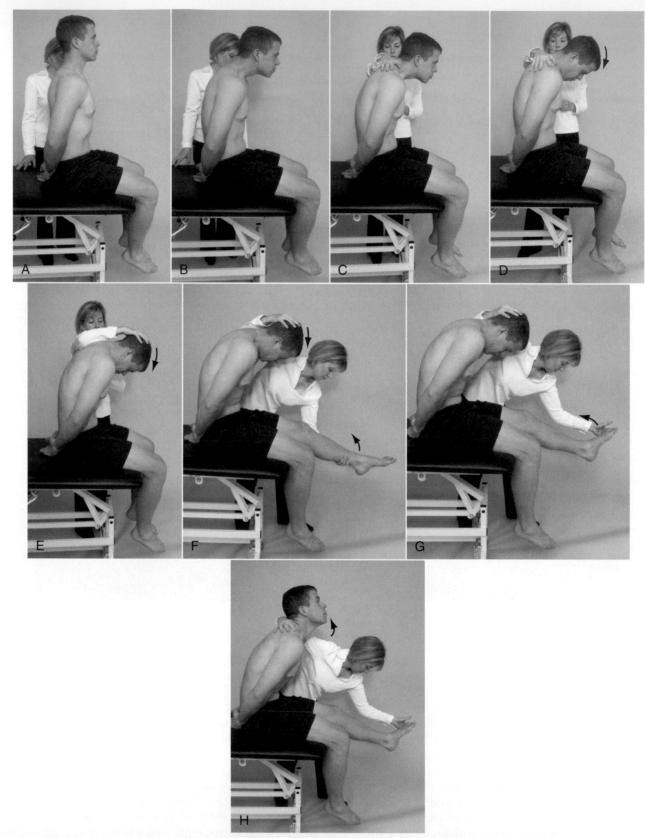

Fig. 9.58 Sequence of subject postures in the slump test. (A) Patient sits erect with hands behind back. (B) Patient slumps lumbar and thoracic spine while either patient or examiner keeps the head in neutral. (C) Examiner pushes down on shoulders while patient holds head in neutral. (D) Patient flexes head. (E) Examiner carefully applies overpressure to cervical spine. (F) Examiner extends patient's knee while holding the cervical spine flexed. (G) While holding the knee extended and cervical spine flexed, the examiner dorsiflexes the foot. (H) Patient extends head, which should relieve any symptoms. If symptoms are reproduced at any stage, further sequential movements are not attempted.

TABLE **9.16**

Slump Test and Its Modifications

	Slump Test (ST1)	Slump Test (ST2)	Side-Lying Slump Test (ST3)	Long Sitting Slump Test (ST4)
Cervical spine	Flexion	Flexion	Flexion	Flexion, rotation
Thoracic and lumbar spine	Flexion (slump)	Flexion (slump)	Flexion (slump)	Flexion (slump)
Hip	Flexion (90°+)	Flexion (90°+), abduction	Flexion (20°)	Flexion (90°+)
Knee	Extension	Extension	Flexion	Extension
Ankle	Dorsiflexion	Dorsiflexion	Plantar flexion	Dorsiflexion
Foot	—	—	—	—
Toes	—	—	—	—
Nerve bias	Spinal cord, cervical and lumbar nerve roots, sciatic nerve	Obturator nerve	Femoral nerve	Spinal cord, cervical and lumbar nerve roots, sciatic nerve

Data from Butler DA: *Mobilisation of the nervous system*, Melbourne, 1991, Churchill Livingstone.

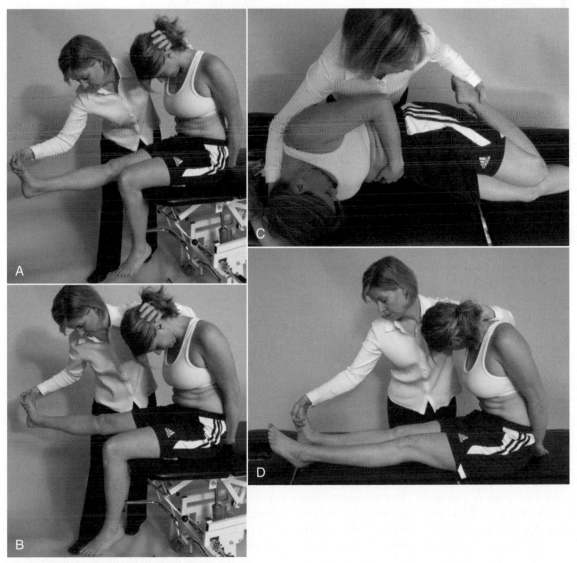

Fig. 9.59 Modifications of the slump test (ST) to stress specific nerve. (A) Basic ST1 test (spinal cord, nerve roots). (B) ST2 (obturator nerve). (C) ST3 (femoral nerve). (D) ST4 (spinal cord, nerve roots). See Table 9.16 for movements at each joint.

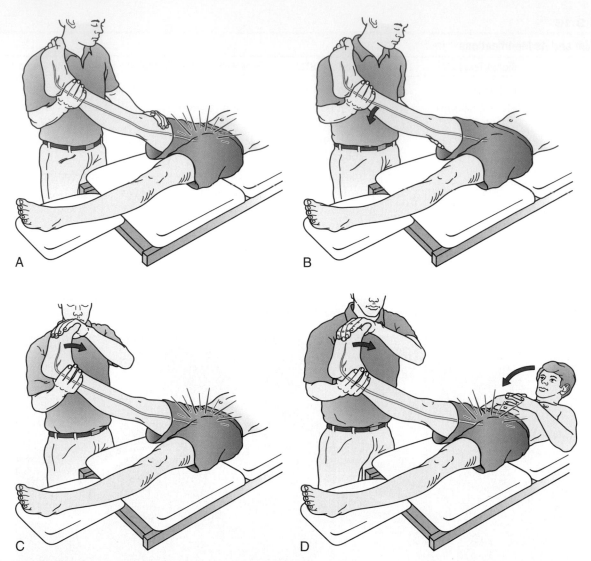

Fig. 9.60 Straight leg raising. (A) Radicular symptoms are precipitated on the same side with straight leg raising. (B) The leg is lowered slowly until pain is relieved. (C) The foot is then dorsiflexed, causing a return of symptoms; this indicates a positive test. (D) To make the symptoms more provocative, the neck can be flexed by lifting the head at the same time as the foot is dorsiflexed.

the patient complains of pain or tightness in the back or back of the leg.[192] If the pain is primarily back pain, it is more likely a disc herniation from pressure on the anterior theca of the spinal cord,[229] or the pathology causing the pressure is more central. "Back pain only" patients who have a disc prolapse have smaller, more central prolapses.[229] If pain is primarily in the leg, it is more likely that the pathology causing the pressure on neurological tissues is more lateral. Disc herniations or pathology causing pressure between the two extremes are more likely to cause pain in both areas.[230] The examiner then slowly and carefully drops the leg back (extends it) slightly until the patient feels no pain or tightness. The patient is then asked to flex the neck so the chin is on the chest, or the examiner may dorsiflex the patient's foot, or both actions may be done simultaneously. Most commonly, foot dorsiflexion is done first. Both of these maneuvers are considered to be provocative or sensitizing tests for neurological

tissue. Table 9.17 and Fig. 9.61 show modifications of the straight leg raising test that can be used to stress different peripheral nerves to a greater degree; these are referred to as straight leg raising tests with a particular nerve bias. It has been suggested that SLR3 be done in the side-lying position and that the ankle dorsiflexion should occur first, followed by hip flexion, as the hip flexion increases the mechanical loading of the sural nerve at the ankle with the nerve tethered distally by the dorsiflexion.[231]

The neck flexion movement has also been called the **Hyndman's sign, Brudzinski's sign, Lindner's sign,** and **Soto-Hall test.** If the examiner desires, neck flexion may be done by itself as a passive movement (passive neck flexion). Tension in the cervicothoracic junction is normal and should not be considered a production of symptoms. If lumbar, leg, or arm symptoms are produced, the neurological tissue is involved. The ankle dorsiflexion movement has also been called the **Bragard's**

TABLE **9.17**

Straight Leg Raising Test and Its Modifications

	SLR (Basic)	SLR2	SLR3	SLR4	Cross (Well Leg) SLR5
Hip	Flexion and adduction	Flexion	Flexion	Flexion and medial rotation	Flexion
Knee	Extension	Extension	Extension	Extension	Extension
Ankle	Dorsiflexion	Dorsiflexion	Dorsiflexion	Plantar flexion	Dorsiflexion
Foot	—	Eversion	Inversion	Inversion	—
Toes	—	Extension	—	—	—
Nerve bias	Sciatic nerve and tibial nerve	Tibial nerve	Sural nerve	Common peroneal nerve	Nerve root (disc prolapse)

SLR, Straight leg raising.
Data from Butler DA: *Mobilisation of the nervous system*, Melbourne, 1991, Churchill Livingstone.

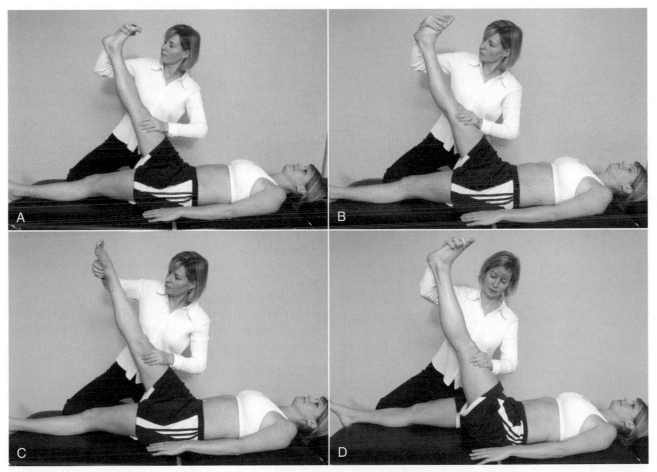

Fig. 9.61 Modifications to straight leg raising (SLR) to stress specific nerve. (A) Basic SLR and SLR2 (sciatic and tibial nerves). (B) SLR3 (sural nerve). (C) SLR4 (common peroneal nerve). (D) SLR5 (intervertebral disc and nerve root). See Table 9.17 for movements at each joint.

test. Pain that increases with neck flexion, ankle dorsiflexion, or both indicates stretching of the dura mater of the spinal cord or a lesion within the spinal cord (e.g., disc herniation, tumor, meningitis). Pain that does not increase with neck flexion may indicate a lesion in the hamstring area (tight hamstrings) or in the lumbosacral or sacroiliac joints. The **Sicard's test** involves straight leg raising and then extension of the big toe instead of

foot dorsiflexion. The **Turyn's test** involves only extension of the big toe.[232]

With unilateral straight leg raising, the nerve roots, primarily the L5, S1, and S2 nerve roots (sciatic nerve), are normally completely stretched at 70°, having an excursion of approximately 2 to 6 cm (0.8 to 2.4 inches).[226] Pain after 70° is probably joint pain from the lumbar area (e.g., facet joints) or sacroiliac joints (Fig. 9.62). However, if the examiner suspects hamstring tightness, the hamstrings must also be cleared by examination (see Chapter 11). The examiner should compare the two legs for any differences. Although the sciatic nerve roots are commonly stretched at 70° hip flexion, the ROM for straight leg raising and the stress placed on the neurological tissue vary greatly from person to person. For example, patients who are very hypermobile (e.g., gymnasts, synchronized swimmers) may not show a positive straight leg raising test until 110° to 120° of hip flexion even in the presence of nerve root pathology. It is more important to compare left and right sides for symptoms before deciding whether a lesion is caused by stretching of the neurological tissue or arises from the joints or other soft tissues.

During the unilateral straight leg raising test, tension develops in a sequential manner. It first develops in the greater sciatic foramen, then over the ala of the sacrum, next in the area where the nerve crosses over the pedicle, and finally in the intervertebral foramen. The test causes traction on the sciatic nerve, lumbosacral nerve roots, and dura mater. Adhesions within these areas may result from herniation of the intervertebral disc or extradural or meningeal irritation. Pain comes from the dura mater, nerve root, adventitial sheath of the epidural veins, or synovial facet joints. The test is positive if pain extends from the back down into the leg in the sciatic nerve distribution.

A central protrusion of an intervertebral disc (L4 or L5 disc affecting nerve roots from L4 down to S3) leads to pain primarily in the back with the possibility of bowel and bladder symptoms; a protrusion in the intermediate area causes pain in the posterior aspect of the lower limb and low back; and a lateral protrusion causes pain primarily in the posterior leg with pain below the knee. Having said this, however, the examiner must realize that the intervertebral disc is only one cause of back pain.

For patients who have difficulty lying supine, a **modified straight leg raising test** has been suggested.[233] The patient is in a side-lying position with the test leg uppermost and the hip and knee at 90°. The lumbosacral spine is in neutral but may be positioned in slight flexion or extension if this is more comfortable for the patient. The examiner then passively extends the patient's knee (Fig. 9.63), noting pain, resistance, and reproduction of the patient's symptoms for a positive test. The knee position (amount of flexion remaining) on the affected side is compared with that on the good side.

The examiner should then test both legs simultaneously (**bilateral straight leg raising** ❓; Fig. 9.64). This test must be done with care, because the examiner is lifting the weight of both lower limbs and thereby placing a large stress on the examiner's lumbar spine. With the patient relaxed in the supine position and knees extended, the examiner lifts both of the legs by flexing the patient's hips until the patient complains of pain or tightness. Because both legs are lifted the pelvis

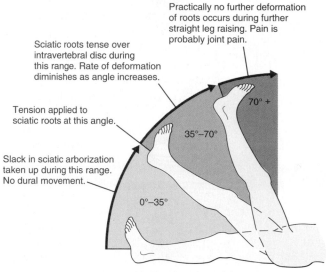

Practically no further deformation of roots occurs during further straight leg raising. Pain is probably joint pain.

Sciatic roots tense over intravertebral disc during this range. Rate of deformation diminishes as angle increases.

Tension applied to sciatic roots at this angle.

Slack in sciatic arborization taken up during this range. No dural movement.

70° +

35°–70°

0°–35°

Fig. 9.62 Dynamics of single straight leg raising test in most people. (Modified from Fahrni WS: Observations on straight leg raising with special reference to nerve root adhesions, *Can J Surg* 9:44, 1966.)

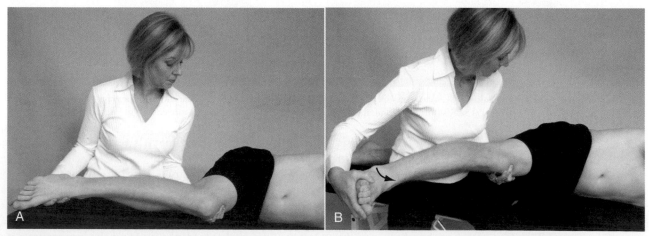

Fig. 9.63 Modified straight leg raising for patients who cannot lie supine. (A) Starting position with knee flexed to 90°. (B) Knee is extended as far as possible.

is not stabilized (as it would be by one leg in unilateral straight leg raise), so on hip flexion the pelvis is freer to rotate, thereby decreasing the stress on the neurological tissue. If the test causes pain before 70° of hip flexion, the lesion is probably in the sacroiliac joints; if the test causes pain after 70°, the lesion is probably in the lumbar spine area.

With the unilateral straight leg raising test, 80° to 90° of hip flexion is normal. If one leg is lifted and the patient complains of pain on the opposite side, it is an indication of a space-occupying lesion (e.g., a herniated disc, inflammatory swelling). This finding of pain when the examiner is testing the opposite (good) leg may be called the **well leg raising test of Fajersztajn** (Fig. 9.65), a **prostrate leg raising test,** a **sciatic phenomenon, Lhermitt's test,** or the **crossover sign** ⚠.[28,213,226,234] It typically indicates a rather large intervertebral disc protrusion, usually medial to the nerve root (see Fig. 9.65), and a poor prognosis for conservative treatment.[228,235]

The test causes stretching of the ipsilateral as well as the contralateral nerve root, pulling laterally on the dural sac. A positive Lasègue's test and crossover sign can also indicate the degree of disc injury. For example, both are limited to a greater degree if sequestration of the disc occurs.[107] If the examiner finds this test positive, careful questioning about bowel and bladder symptoms is a necessity. Many, but not all, patients with a central protrusion are candidates for surgery, especially if there are bowel and bladder symptoms.

❷ _Valsalva Maneuver._ The seated patient is asked to take a breath, hold it, and then bear down as if evacuating the bowels (Fig. 9.66). If pain increases, it indicates increased intrathecal pressure. The symptoms may be accentuated by having the patient first flex the hip to a position just short of that causing pain.[226]

Tests for Lumbar Instability

Lumbar instability implies that during movement, the patient loses the ability to control the movement for a brief time (milliseconds), or it may mean the segment is structurally unstable. The brief loss of control often results in a painful catch, apprehension, or an **instability jog** (sudden shift of movement in part of the ROM).[108,236] Pope called this "loss of control in the neutral spine."[237] It commonly occurs with spondylosis owing to degeneration of the disc.[237,238] Structural instability primarily results from spondylolisthesis; the following tests are designed to test for structural instability and aberrant movement patterns.[239–241]

❷ _Farfan Torsion Test._[39,45] This nonspecific test stresses the facet joints, joint capsule, supraspinous and interspinous ligaments, neural arch, the longitudinal ligaments, and the disc. The patient lies prone. The examiner stabilizes the ribs and spine (at about T12) with one hand and places the other hand under the anterior aspect of the ilium. The examiner then pulls the ilium backward (Fig. 9.67) causing the spine to be rotated on the opposite side producing torque on the opposite side. The test is said

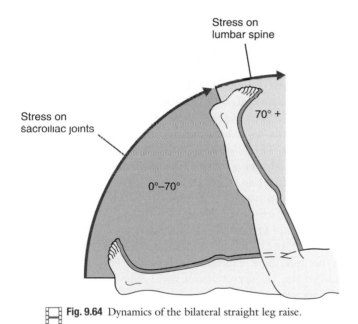

Fig. 9.64 Dynamics of the bilateral straight leg raise.

Stress on lumbar spine

Stress on sacroiliac joints

70° +

0°–70°

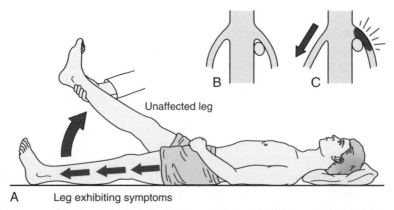

Unaffected leg

B

C

A Leg exhibiting symptoms

Fig. 9.65 Well leg raising test of Fajersztajn. (A) Movement of nerve roots occurs when the leg on the opposite side is raised. (B) Position of disc and nerve root before opposite leg is lifted. (C) When the leg is raised on the unaffected side, the roots on the opposite side slide slightly downward and toward the midline. In the presence of a disc lesion, this movement increases the root tension, resulting in radicular signs in the affected leg, which remains on the table. (Modified from DePalma AF, Rothman RH: _The intervertebral disc,_ Philadelphia, 1970, WB Saunders.)

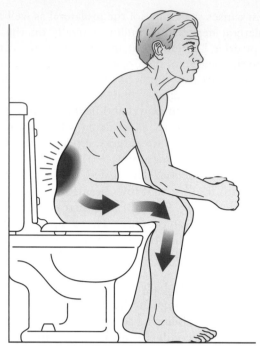

Fig. 9.66 The Valsalva maneuver. Increased intrathecal pressure leads to symptoms in the sciatic nerve distribution in a positive test.

to be positive if it reproduces all or some of the patient's symptoms. The other side is tested for compression.

❓ _H and I Stability Tests._[96,113] This set of movements tests for muscle spasm and can be used to detect instability. The H and I monikers relate to the movements that occur (Fig. 9.68).

The first part of the test is the **"H"** movement. The patient stands in the normal resting position, which would be considered the center of the **"H"**. The pain-free side is tested first. The patient is asked, with guidance from the clinician, to side flex as far as possible (the side of the **"H"**). While in this position, the patient is then asked to flex (the front of the **"H"**) and then move into extension (the back of the **"H"**). If flexion was more painful than extension, then extension would be done before flexion. The patient then returns to neutral and repeats the movements to the other side. The clinician may stabilize the pelvis with one hand and guide the movement with the other hand on the shoulder.

The second part of the test is the **"I"** movement. The patient stands in the normal resting position, which would be considered the center of the **"I"**. Pain-free movement (flexion or extension) is tested first. With guidance from the clinician, the patient is asked to forward flex (or extend) the lumbar spine until the hips start to move (top part of the **"I"**). Once in flexion, the patient is guided into side bending (to the pain-free side first **"I"**), followed by return to neutral and then side bending to the opposite side. The patient then returns to neutral standing and does the opposite movement (extension in this case) followed by side bending.

If a hypomobile segment is present, at least two of the movements (the movements into the same quadrant [for

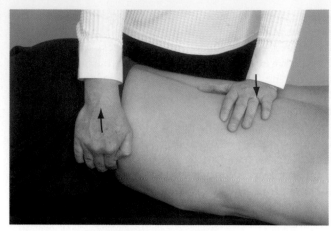

Fig. 9.67 Farfan torsion test.

example, the top right of the "H" and "I"]) would be limited. If instability is present, one quadrant will again be affected, but only by one of the moves (i.e., by the "H" movement or the "I" movement—not both). For example, if the patient had spondylolisthesis instability in anterior shear (a component of forward flexion) and the "I" is attempted, the shear or slip occurs on forward flexion, and there is little movement during the attempted side bending or flexion. If the "H" is attempted, the side bending is normal, and the following forward flexion is full because the shear occurs in the second phase. So, in this case, the "I" movement is limited but not the "H" movement. This test is primarily for structural instability, but an instability jog may be evident during one of the movements if loss of control occurs. In this case, the end range is commonly normal, but loss of control occurs somewhere in the available ROM.

❓ _Lateral Lumbar Spine Stability Test._[113] The patient is placed in the side-lying position with the lumbar spine in neutral. The examiner places the forearm over the side of the thorax at about the L3 level as an example. The examiner then applies a downward pressure to the transverse process of L3, which produces a shear to the side on which the patient is lying for vertebra below L3 and a relative lateral shear in the opposite direction to the segments above L3 (Fig. 9.69). The production of the patient's symptoms indicates a positive test.

✓ _Passive Lumbar Extension Test._[242–244] The patient lies prone and relaxed. The examiner passively lifts and extends both extremities at the same time to about 1 ft (30 cm) from the bed. While maintaining the extension, the examiner gently pulls the legs (Fig. 9.70). The test is considered positive if, in the extended position, the patient complains of strong pain in the lumbar region, very heavy feeling in the low back, or it feels like the low back is "coming off" and the pain disappears when the legs are lowered to the start position. Numbness or prickling sensation are not positive signs.

❓ _Pheasant Test._ The patient lies prone. With one hand, the examiner gently applies pressure to the

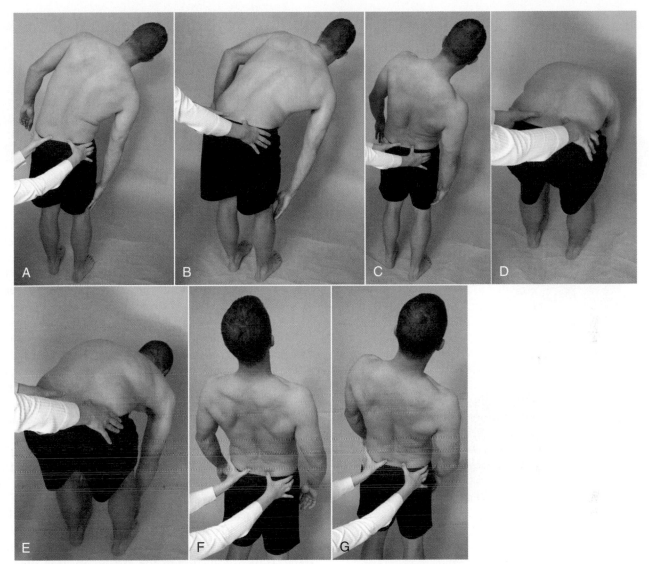

Fig. 9.68 H and I stability tests. (A) H test, side flexion. (B) H test, side flexion followed by forward flexion. (C) H test, side flexion followed by extension. (D) I test, forward flexion. (E) I test, forward flexion and side flexion. (F) I test, extension. (G) I test, extension and side flexion.

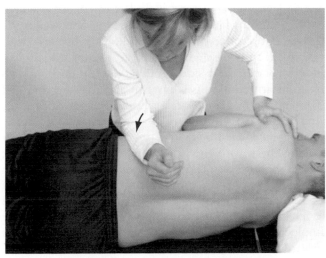

Fig. 9.69 Lateral lumbar spine stability test.

posterior aspect of the lumbar spine. With the other hand, the examiner passively flexes the patient's knees until the heels touch the buttocks (Fig. 9.71). If this hyperextension of the spine causes the patient to feel pain in the leg, the test is considered positive and indicates an unstable spinal segment.[245]

⏺ *Posterior Shear Test.*[246] The patient stands with arms across the lower abdomen. The examiner stands at the side of the patient so that the dominant hand is placed over the patient's crossed arms while the heel of the nondominant hand is placed on the patient's individual spinous processes for stabilization. The examiner then produces a posterior directed force through the patient's arms and abdomen and an anterior force with the other hand on the individual spinous processes (Fig. 9.72). Provocation of symptoms indicates a positive test.

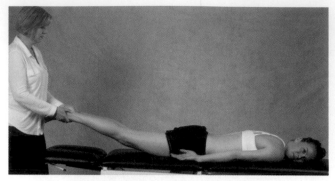

Fig. 9.70 Passive lumbar extension test.

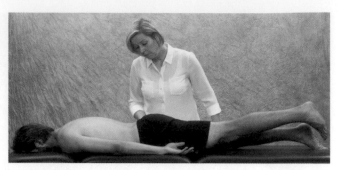

Fig. 9.73 Prone hip extension test. Note how examiner watches for movement in the lumbar spine and pelvis.

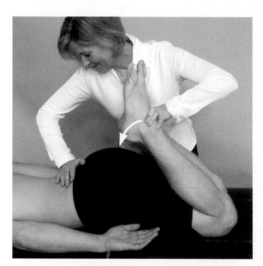

Fig. 9.71 Pheasant test.

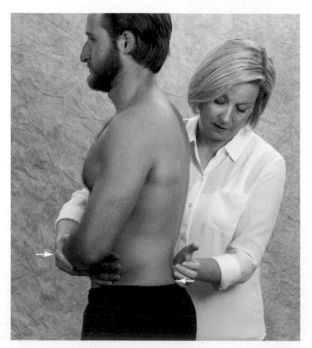

Fig. 9.72 Posterior shear test.

Prone Hip Extension Test.[247] The patient lies prone with the examiner by the side at the level of the patient's hip. Starting with the "good" leg, the patient is asked to extend the hip about 20 cm (8 inches) off the table (Fig. 9.73). While the patient lifts the leg, the examiner observes (or palpates), watching for one of four abnormal lumbo-pelvic motion patterns: (1) rotation of the lumbar spine so that the spinous processes move toward the side of hip extension; (2) a lateral shift of the lumbar spine toward the side of hip extension; (3) extension of the lumbar spine; or (4) the pelvic girdle raises off the table. The test is then repeated with the affected leg. If the spine and pelvis do not move, the test is negative for abnormal lumbopelvic motion and microinstability in the lumbar spine.

Prone Segmental Instability (PIT) Test. The patient lies prone with the body on the examining table and the legs over the edge resting on the floor (Fig. 9.74). The examiner applies pressure to the posterior aspect of the lumbar spine while the patient rests in this position. The patient then lifts the legs off the floor, and the examiner again applies posterior compression to the lumbar spine. If pain is elicited in the resting position only, the test is positive, because the muscle action masks the instability.[246,248–250]

Specific Lumbar Spine Torsion Test.[96,113] This test stresses specific levels of the lumbar spine. To do this, the specific level must be rotated and stressed. An example would be testing the integrity of left rotation on L5-S1. The patient is placed in a right side-lying position with the lumbar spine in slight extension (slight lordosis). To achieve rotation and side bending, the examiner grasps the right arm and pulls it upward and forward at a 45° angle until movement is felt at the L5 spinous process. This "locks" all the vertebrae above L5. The examiner then stabilizes the L5 spinous process by holding the left shoulder back with the examiner's elbow while rotating the pelvis and sacrum forward until S1 starts to move (Fig. 9.75) with the opposite hand. Minimal movement should occur, and a normal capsular tissue stretch should be felt when L5-S1 is stressed by carefully pushing the shoulder back with the elbow and rotating the pelvis forward with the other arm/hand. This test position is a common position used to manipulate the spine, so the

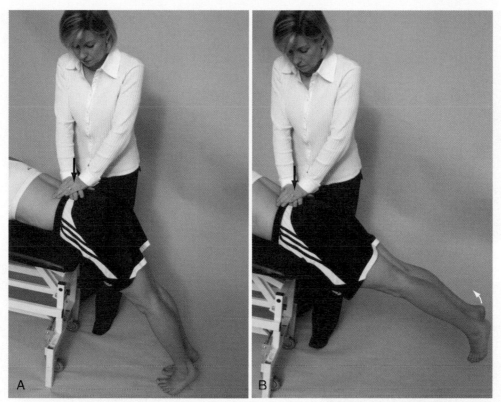

Fig. 9.74 Prone segmental instability test. (A) Toes on floor. (B) Feet lifted off floor.

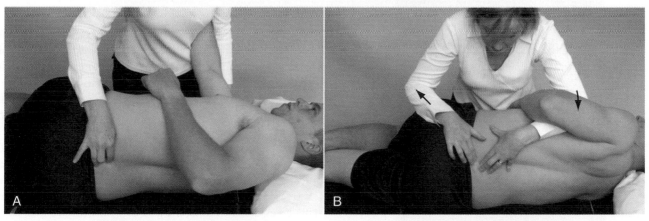

Fig. 9.75 Specific lumbar spine torsion test (to L5–S1). (A) Start position. (B) Final position.

examiner should take care not to overstress the rotation during assessment. In some cases, when doing the test, the examiner may hear a "click" or "pop." This is the same pop or click that would be heard with a manipulation.

⚠ *Test of Anterior Lumbar Spine Instability.*[113] The patient is placed in the side-lying position with the hips flexed to 70° and knees flexed. The examiner palpates the desired spinous processes (e.g., L4–L5). By pushing the patient's knees posteriorly with the body along the line of the femur, the examiner can feel the relative movement of the L5 spinous process on L4 (Fig. 9.76). Normally there should be little or no movement. Other levels of the spine may be tested in a similar fashion. A problem with the test is that the examiner should ensure that the posterior

ligaments of the spine are relatively loose or relaxed. This can be controlled by altering the amount of hip flexion. With greater hip flexion, the posterior ligaments tighten more from the bottom (sacrum) up.

⚠ *Test of Posterior Lumbar Spine Instability.*[113] The patient sits on the edge of the examining table. The examiner stands in front of the patient. The patient places the pronated arms with elbows bent on the anterior aspect of the examiner's shoulders. The examiner puts both hands around the patient so the fingers rest over the lumbar spine and with the heels of the hands gently pull the lumbar spine into full lordosis. To stress L5 on S1, the examiner stabilizes the sacrum with the fingers of both hands and asks the patient to push through the forearm

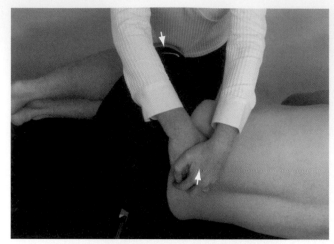

Fig. 9.76 Test of anterior lumbar spine stability.

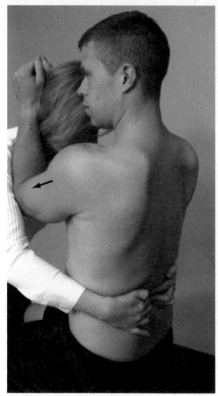

Fig. 9.77 Test of posterior lumbar spine instability.

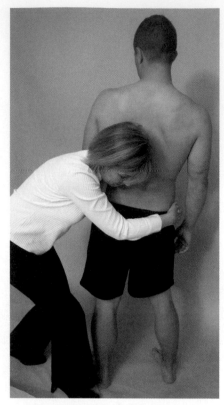

Fig. 9.78 McKenzie's side glide test.

while maintaining the lordotic posture (Fig. 9.77). This produces a posterior shear of L5 on S1. Other levels of the spine may be tested in a similar fashion.

Tests for Joint Dysfunction

⚠️ *Clinical Prediction Rule for Facet (Zygapophyseal) Joint Involvement.*[251] Indicators of facet joint pain include (1) localized unilateral back pain; (2) replication/aggravation of pain by unilateral pressure over facet joint or transverse process; (3) lack of nerve root symptoms; (4) if referred, pain does not extend beyond the knee; (5) pain is eased in flexion; (6) reduced movement on side of facet joint pain;

(7) unilateral muscle spasm over facet joint; and (8) pain on extension and extension with lateral flexion or rotation to same side. Any of the indicators may indicate facet joint involvement and the more indicators present, the higher the likelihood that the facet joints are involved.

❓ *McKenzie's Side Glide Test.* The patient stands with the examiner standing to one side. The examiner grasps the patient's pelvis with both hands and places a shoulder against the patient's lower thorax. Using the shoulder as a block, the examiner pulls the pelvis toward the examiner's body (Fig. 9.78). The position is held for 10 to 15 seconds, and then the test is repeated on the opposite side.[47,215] If the patient has an evident scoliosis, the side to which the scoliosis curves should be tested first. A positive test is indicated by increased neurological symptoms on the affected side. It also indicates whether the symptoms are actually causing the scoliosis.

❓ *Milgram's Test.* The patient lies supine and actively lifts both legs simultaneously off the examining table 5 to 10 cm (2 to 4 inches), holding this position for 30 seconds. The test is positive if the limbs or affected limb cannot be held for 30 seconds or if symptoms are reproduced in the affected limb.[214,215] This test should always be performed with caution because of the high stress load placed on the lumbar spine.

⚠️ *One-Leg Standing (Stork Standing) Lumbar Extension Test.* The patient stands on one leg and extends the spine while balancing on the leg (Fig. 9.79). The test is repeated with the patient standing on the opposite leg. A positive test is indicated by pain in the back and

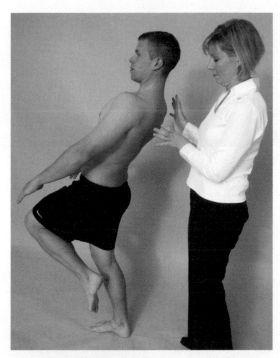

Fig. 9.79 One-leg standing lumbar extension test.

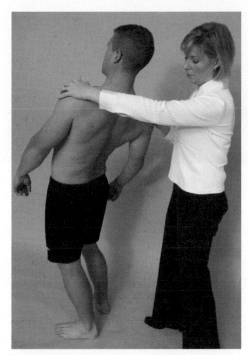

Fig. 9.80 Quadrant test for the lumbar spine.

is associated with a pars interarticularis stress fracture (spondylolisthesis). If the stress fracture is unilateral, standing on the ipsilateral leg causes more pain.[211,252–254] If rotation is combined with extension and pain results, this indicates possible facet joint pathology on the side to which rotation occurs.

? *Quadrant (Lumbar Quadrant, Extension Quadrant, Kemp's Test) Test.*[44,232,255] The patient stands with the examiner standing behind. The examiner may place a hand on the ipsilateral ilium to stabilize it. The patient extends the spine while the examiner controls the movement by holding the patient's shoulders. The examiner may use his or her shoulders to hold the occiput and take the weight of the head. Overpressure is applied in extension while the patient side flexes and rotates to the side of pain. The movement is continued until the limit of range is reached or until symptoms are produced (Fig. 9.80). The position causes maximum narrowing of the intervertebral foramen and stress on the facet joint to the side on which rotation occurs.[163] The test is positive if symptoms are produced.[256]

? *Schober Test.* The Schober test may be used to measure the amount of flexion occurring in the lumbar spine. A point is marked midway between the two PSISs ("dimples of the pelvis"), which is the level of S2; then, points 5 cm (2 inches) below and 10 cm (4 inches) above that level are marked. The distance between the three points is measured, the patient is asked to flex forward, and the distance is remeasured. The difference between the two measurements indicates the amount of flexion occurring in the lumbar spine. Little reported a modification of the Schober test to measure extension as well.[257]

After completion of the flexion movement, the patient extends the spine, and the distance between the marks is noted. Little also advocated using four marking points (one below the dimples and three above) with 10 cm (4 inches) between them.

? *Yeoman's Test.* The patient lies prone while the examiner stabilizes the pelvis and extends each of the patient's hips in turn with the knees extended. The examiner then extends each of the patient's legs in turn with the knee flexed. In both cases, the patient remains passive. A positive test is indicated by pain in the lumbar spine during both parts of the test.

Tests for Muscle Tightness

☑ *90–90 Straight Leg Raising Test.* See tests for tight hamstrings in Chapter 11.

⚠ *Ober's Test.* See tests for tight tensor fasciae latae in Chapter 11.

⚠ *Rectus Femoris Test.* See tests for tight rectus femoris in Chapter 11.

⚠ *Thomas Test.* See tests for tight iliopsoas in Chapter 11.

Tests for Muscle Dysfunction

? *Beevor Sign.* The patient lies supine. The patient flexes the head against resistance, coughs, or attempts to sit up with the hands resting behind the head.[214,258] The sign is positive if the umbilicus does not remain in a straight line when the abdominals contract, indicating pathology in the abdominal muscles (i.e., weakness or paralysis).

☑ *Prone Bridge Test (Plank Test, 4-Point Hold Test, Hover Test).*[259,260] This test is used to measure the endurance of

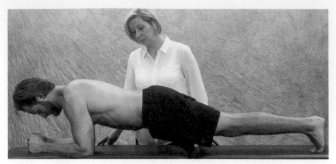

Fig. 9.81 Prone bridge (plank, four-point hold, hover) test. Note how examiner watches lumbar spine and pelvis.

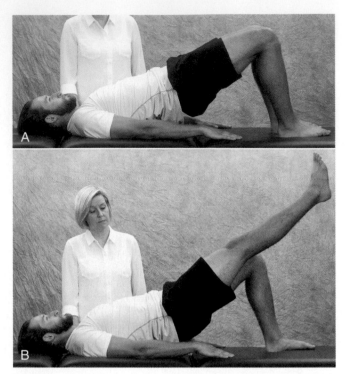

Fig. 9.82 Supine bridge test. (A) Patient "bridges," lifting the buttocks off the bed. (B) Patient extends one knee while in the bridged position.

the abdominal and back extensor muscles and the ability to maintain core stability. The patient assumes the elbow push-up position with feet together and hands shoulder width apart (Fig. 9.81). The patient then does a push-up while maintaining a straight line (plank) from the shoulders to the feet. The patient should be able to hold the position for at least 90 seconds (normal: 145 ± 71.5 seconds) with no shaking.[259] The examiner should watch for increased lumbar lordosis; signs of fatigue (shaking); or shoulder dipping, which would indicate fatigue and loss of control, so the test should be stopped.

⚠ *Supine Bridge Test.*[261] This test is used to measure core trunk stability and strength of the hip and spine extensors and the contralateral external oblique and ipsilateral internal oblique muscles. The patient lies supine with the hips at 45° and knees at 90°. The patient then "bridges" lifting the buttocks off the bed and maintains a straight line between the knees and shoulders with the pelvis held in neutral (Fig. 9.82A). The patient should be able to hold this plank position with no shaking for at least 90 seconds (normal: 170 ± 42.5 seconds).[262] The test can be made more difficult by asking the patient to extend one knee while in the bridged position (Fig. 9.82B).

Tests for Intermittent Claudication

Intermittent claudication implies arterial insufficiency to the tissues. It is most commonly evident when activity occurs because of the increased vascular demand of the tissues. There are two types of intermittent claudication—vascular and neurogenic. The vascular type is most commonly the result of arteriosclerosis, arterial embolism, or thrombo-angiitis obliterans and commonly manifests itself with symptoms in the legs. The neurogenic type is sometimes called **pseudoclaudication** or *cauda equina syndrome* and is commonly associated with spinal stenosis and its effect on circulation to the spinal cord and cauda equina.[263–268] The symptoms in this case may be manifested in the back or sciatic nerve distribution.

⚠ *Bicycle Test of van Gelderen.*[269] The patient is seated on an exercise bicycle and is asked to pedal against resistance. The patient starts pedaling while leaning backward to accentuate the lumbar lordosis (Fig. 9.83). If pain into the buttock and posterior thigh occurs, followed by tingling in the affected lower extremity, the first part of the test is positive. The patient is then asked to lean forward while continuing to pedal. If the pain subsides over a short period of time, the second part of the test is positive; if the patient sits upright again, the pain returns. The test determines whether the patient has neurogenic intermittent claudication.

❓ *Stoop Test.* The stoop test is performed to assess neurogenic intermittent claudication to determine whether a relation exists between neurogenic symptoms, posture, and walking.[270] When the patient with neurogenic intermittent claudication walks briskly, pain ensues in the buttock and lower limb within a distance of 50 m (165 ft). To relieve the pain, the patient flexes forward. These symptoms may also be relieved when the patient is sitting and flexing forward. If flexion does not relieve the symptoms, the test is negative. Extension may also be used to bring the symptoms back.

❓ *Treadmill Test.*[271,272] This test may also be used to determine if the patient has intermittent claudication. Two trials are conducted—one at 1.2 mph and one at the patient's preferred walking speed. The patient walks upright (no leaning forward or holding handrails is allowed) on the treadmill for 15 minutes or until the onset of severe symptoms (symptoms that would make the patient stop walking in usual life situations). Time to first symptoms, total ambulatory time, and precipitating symptoms are recorded.

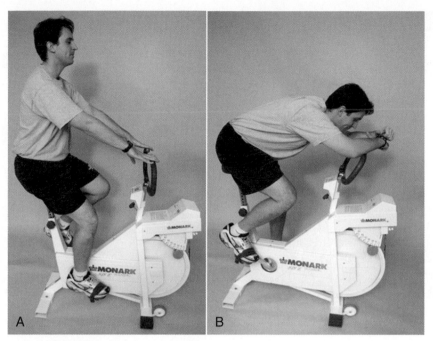

Fig. 9.83 Bicycle test of van Gelderen. (A) Sitting erect. (B) Sitting flexed.

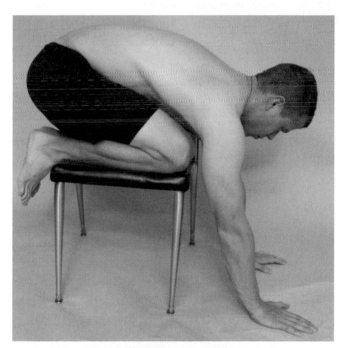

Fig. 9.84 Burns test.

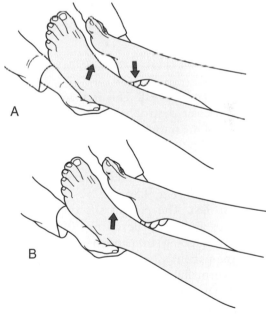

Fig. 9.85 Hoover test. (A) Normally, when the patient attempts to elevate one leg, the opposite leg pushes down as a counterbalance. (B) When the "weak" leg attempts to elevate but the opposite (asymptomatic) leg does not help by pushing down, at least some of the weakness is probably feigned.

Tests for Malingering

? Burns Test. The patient is asked to kneel on a chair and then bend forward to touch the floor with the fingers (Fig. 9.84). The test is positive for malingering if the patient is unable to perform the test or the patient overbalances.[215]

? Hoover Test. The patient lies supine. The examiner places one hand under each calcaneus while the patient's legs remain relaxed on the examining table (Fig. 9.85).[273–275]

The patient is then asked to lift one leg off the table, keeping the knees straight, as for active straight leg raising. If the patient does not lift the leg or the examiner does not feel pressure under the opposite heel, the patient is probably not really trying or may be a malingerer. If the lifted limb is weaker, however, pressure under the normal heel increases, because of the increased effort to lift the weak leg. The two sides are compared for differences.

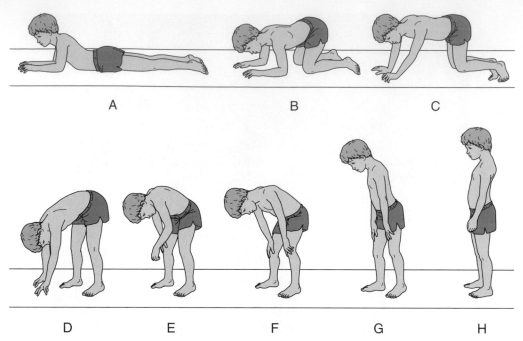

Fig. 9.86 Gower's sign. (A–C) First, the legs are pulled up under the body, and the weight is shifted to rest on the hands and feet. (D) The hips are then thrust in the air as the knees are straightened, and the hands are brought closer to the legs. (E–G) Finally, the trunk is slowly extended by the hands walking up the thighs. (H) The erect position is attained. (From Varma R, Williams SD: Neurology. In Zitelli BJ, McIntire SC, Nowalk AJ, editors: *Zitelli and Davis' atlas of pediatric physical diagnosis*, ed 7, Philadelphia, 2018, Elsevier.)

Other Tests

⚠ *Gower's Sign.*[239,243,276] This is a sign of any condition (e.g., muscular dystrophy) that may be associated with weakness of the muscles of the pelvic girdle on lower limbs. The sign is positive when the patient who has been lying, kneeling, or squatting uses his or her hands and arms to "walk up" his or her body due to lack of thigh or hip muscle strength (Fig. 9.86).

❓ *Heel-Tap Test.* The patient sits on the examining table with hips and knees flexed to 90°. The examiner explains what is going to happen (i.e., examiner will lightly tap the patient's heel) and that it may cause low back pain. Normally such a test would not cause pain (although it has been suggested to the patient that it will). If the patient complains of pain, the test is positive for nonorganic causes of back pain similar to Waddell's signs.

❓ *Sign of the Buttock.* The patient lies supine,[67] and the examiner performs a passive unilateral straight leg raising test. If there is unilateral restriction, the examiner then flexes the knee to see whether hip flexion increases. If the problem is in the lumbar spine or hamstrings, hip flexion increases when the knee is flexed. This finding indicates a negative sign of the buttock test. If hip flexion does not increase when the knee is flexed, it is a positive sign of the buttock test and indicates pathology in the buttock behind the hip joint, such as a bursitis, tumor, or abscess.[277] The patient should also exhibit a noncapsular pattern of the hip.

Reflexes and Cutaneous Distribution

After the special tests, the reflexes should be checked for differences between the two sides (Fig. 9.87) if one suspects neurological involvement in the patient's problem.

The deep tendon reflexes are tested with a reflex hammer with the patient's muscles and tendons relaxed. The patellar reflex may be performed with the patient sitting or lying, and the hammer strikes the tendon directly. To test the patellar reflex (L3–L4), the knee is flexed to 30° (supine lying) or 90° (sitting). The Achilles reflex (S1–S2) may be tested in prone, sitting, or kneeling position. To test the Achilles reflex, the ankle is at 90° or slightly dorsiflexed. The examiner must ensure that the patient's dorsiflexors are relaxed before performing the test; otherwise, the test will not work. This is done by passively dorsiflexing the foot and feeling for the "springing back" of the foot into plantar flexion. If this does not occur, the dorsiflexors are not relaxed.

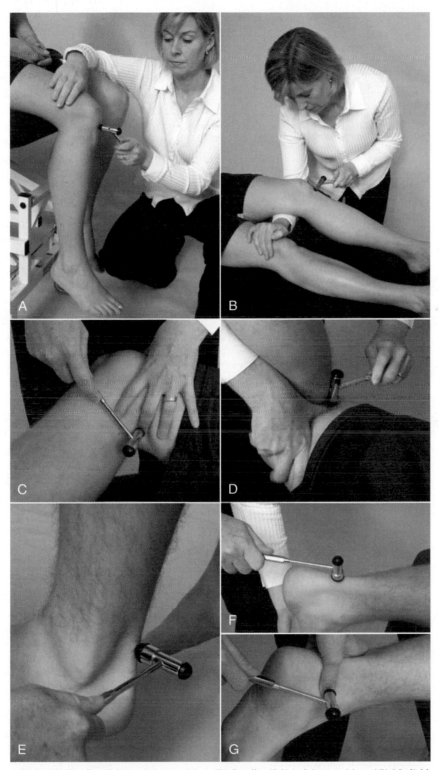

Fig. 9.87 Reflexes of the lower limb. (A) Patellar (L3) in sitting position. (B) Patellar (L3) in lying position. (C) Medial hamstrings (L5) in supine lying position. (D) Lateral hamstrings (S1, S2) in prone lying position. (E) Achilles (S1) in sitting position. (F) Achilles (S1) in kneeling position. (G) Posterior tibial (L4, L5) in prone lying position.

Reflexes of the Lumbar Spine

- Patellar (L3–L4)
- Medial hamstring (L5–S1)
- Lateral hamstring (S1–S2)
- Posterior tibial (L4–L5)
- Achilles (S1–S2)

TABLE **9.18**

Differential Diagnosis of Intermittent Claudication

	Vascular	Neurogenic
Pain	Related to exercise (e.g., walking); occurs at various sites simultaneously	Related to exercise (e.g., walking); sensations spread from area to area
Pulse	Absent after exercise	Present after exercise
Protein content of cerebrospinal fluid	Normal	Raised
Sensory change	Variable	Follows more specific dermatomes
Reflexes	Normal	Decreased but returns quickly

To test the hamstring reflex (semimembrinosus: L5, S1; and biceps femoris: S1–S2), the examiner places the thumb over the appropriate tendon and taps the thumbnail to elicit the reflex. Again, the knee should be slightly flexed with the hamstrings relaxed to perform the test.

Neurogenic intermittent claudication may cause the reflexes to be absent soon after exercise (Table 9.18).[278,279] If neurogenic intermittent claudication is suspected, it is necessary to test the reflexes immediately, because reflexes may return within 1 to 3 minutes after stopping the activity.

Another reflex that may be tested is the **superficial cremasteric reflex,** which occurs in males only (Fig. 9.88). The patient lies supine while the examiner strokes the inner side of the upper thigh with a pointed object. The test is negative if the scrotal sac on the tested side pulls up. Absence or reduction of the reflex bilaterally suggests an upper motor neuron lesion. A unilateral absence suggests a lower motor neuron lesion between L1 and L2. Absences have increased significance if they are associated with increased deep tendon reflexes.[280]

Two other superficial reflexes are the **superficial abdominal reflex** (Fig. 9.89) and the **superficial anal reflex.** To test the superficial abdominal reflex, the examiner uses a pointed object to stroke each quadrant of the abdomen of the supine patient in a triangular fashion around the umbilicus. Absence of the reflex (reflex movement of the skin) indicates an upper motor neuron lesion; unilateral absence indicates a lower motor neuron lesion from T7 to L2, depending on where the absence is noted, as a result of the segmental innervation. The examiner tests the superficial anal reflex by touching the perianal skin. A normal result is shown by contraction of the anal sphincter muscles (S2–S4).

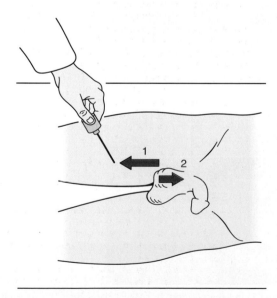

Fig. 9.88 Cremasteric reflex. *1,* The examiner runs a sharp object along the inner thigh. *2,* A negative reflex is indicated by the scrotum's rising on that side.

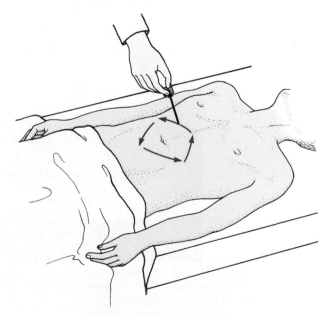

Fig. 9.89 Superficial abdominal reflex.

TABLE **9.19**

Peripheral Nerve Lesions

Nerve (Root Derivation)	Sensory Supply	Sensory Loss	Motor Loss	Reflex Change	Lesion
Lateral cutaneous nerve of thigh (L2–L3)	Lateral thigh	Lateral thigh; often intermittent	None	None	Lateral inguinal entrapment
Posterior cutaneous nerve of thigh (S1–S2)	Posterior thigh	Posterior thigh	None (sciatic nerve often involved too)	None (sciatic nerve often involved too)	Local (buttock) trauma Pelvic mass Hip fracture
Obturator nerve (L2–L4)	Medial thigh	Often none ± medial thigh	Thigh adduction	None	Pelvic mass
Femoral nerve (L2–L4)	Anteromedial thigh and leg	Anteromedial thigh and leg	Knee extension ± hip flexion	Diminished knee jerk	Retroperitoneal or pelvic mass Femoral artery aneurysm (or puncture) Diabetic mononeuritis
Saphenous branch of femoral nerve (L2–L4)	Anteromedial knee and medial leg	Medial leg	None (positive Tinel sign 5–10 cm above medial femoral epicondyle of knee)	None (positive Tinel sign 5–10 cm above medial femoral epicondyle of knee)	Local trauma Entrapment above medial femoral condyle
Sciatic nerve (L4–L5, S1)	Anterior and posterior leg Sole and dorsum of foot	Entire foot	Foot dorsiflexion Foot inversion ± plantar flexion ± knee flexion	Diminished ankle jerk	Pelvic mass Hip fracture Piriformis entrapment Misplaced buttock injection
Common peroneal nerve (division of sciatic nerve)	Anterior leg, dorsum of foot	None or dorsal foot	Foot dorsiflexion, inversion, and eversion (positive Tinel sign at lateral fibular neck)	None (positive Tinel sign at lateral fibular neck)	Entrapment pressure at neck of fibula Rarely, diabetes, vasculitis, leprosy

From Reilly BM: *Practical strategies in outpatient medicine*, Philadelphia, 1991, WB Saunders, p 928.

Finally, the examiner should perform one or more of the pathological reflex tests (see Table 1.32) used to determine upper motor lesions or pyramidal tract disease, such as the Babinski or Oppenheim tests (see "Special Tests," earlier). The presence of these reflexes indicates the possible presence of disease or upper motor neuron lesion, whereas their absence reflects the normal situation.

If neurological symptoms are found, the examiner must check the dermatome patterns of the nerve roots as well as the peripheral sensory distribution of the peripheral nerves (Table 9.19 and Fig. 9.90). Remember that dermatomes vary from person to person, and the accompanying representations are estimations only. The examiner tests for sensation by running relaxed hands over the back, abdomen, and lower limbs (front, sides, and back), being sure to cover all aspects of the leg and foot. If any difference between the sides is noted during this **sensation scan,** the examiner may then use a pinwheel, pin, cotton ball, or brush to map out the exact area of sensory difference and determine the peripheral nerve or nerve root affected.

Pain may be referred from the lumbar spine to the sacroiliac joint and down the leg as far as the foot. Seldom is pain referred up the spine (Fig. 9.91). Pain may be referred to the lumbar spine from the abdominal organs, the lower thoracic spine, and the sacroiliac joints. Muscles may also refer pain to the lumbar area (Table 9.20).[281]

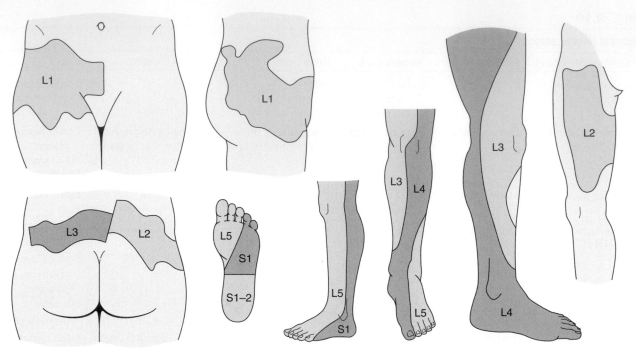

Fig. 9.90 Lumbar dermatomes.

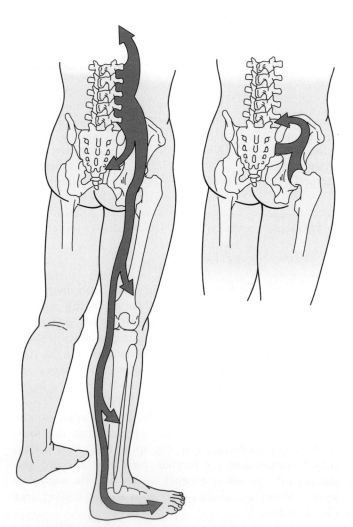

Fig. 9.91 Referral of pain from and to the lumbar spine.

TABLE **9.20**

Lumbar Muscles and Referral of Pain

Muscle	Referral Pattern
Iliocostalis lumborum	Below T12 ribs lateral to spine down to buttock
Longissimus	Beside spine down to gluteal fold
Multifidus	Lateral to spine, sacrum to gluteal cleft, posterior leg, and lower abdomen
Abdominals	Below xiphisternum and along anterior rib cage down along inguinal ligament to genitals
Serratus posterior inferior	Lateral to spine in T9–T12 posterior rib area

Data from Travell JG, Simons DG: *Myofascial pain and dysfunction: the trigger point manual*, Baltimore, 1983, Williams & Wilkins.

Peripheral Nerve Injuries of the Lumbar Spine

Lumbosacral Tunnel Syndrome. This syndrome involves compression of the L5 nerve root as it passes under the iliolumbar ligament in the iliolumbar canal (Fig. 9.92). The usual cause of compression is trauma (inflammation), osteophytes, or a tumor. Symptoms are primarily sensory (L5 dermatome) and pain. There is minimal or no effect on the L5 myotome.[282]

Joint Play Movements

The joint play movements have special importance in the lumbar spine, because they are used to determine the end

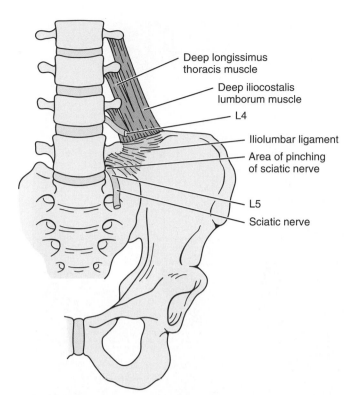

Fig. 9.92 Lumbosacral tunnel syndrome. This syndrome involves compression of the L5 nerve root as it passes under the iliolumbar ligament in the iliolumbar canal.

feel of joint movement as well as the presence of joint play. They are often used to replace passive movements in the lumbar spine, which are difficult to perform because of the need to move the heavy trunk or lower limbs. As the joint play movements are performed, the examiner should note any decreased ROM, pain, or difference in end feel.[283]

Joint Play Movements of the Lumbar Spine

- Flexion
- Extension
- Side flexion
- Posteroanterior central vertebral pressure (PACVP)
- Posteroanterior unilateral vertebral pressure (PAUVP)
- Transverse vertebral pressure (TVP)

Flexion, Extension, and Side Flexion

The movements tested during these motions are sometimes called **passive intervertebral movements (PIVMs).**[284] Flexion is accomplished with the patient in the side-lying position. The examiner flexes both of the patient's bent knees toward the chest by flexing the hips (Fig. 9.93A). While palpating between the spinous processes of the lumbar vertebrae with one hand (one finger on the spinous process, one finger above, and one finger below the process), the examiner passively flexes and

releases the patient's hips; the examiner's body weight is used to cause the movement. The examiner should feel the spinous processes gap or move apart on flexion. If this gapping does not occur between two spinous processes, or if it is excessive in relation to the other gapping movements, the segment is hypomobile or hypermobile, respectively. The results, however, will depend on the skill of the examiner as interrater reliability studies have shown only average reliability.[284]

Extension (Fig. 9.93B) and side flexion (Fig. 9.93C) are tested in a similar fashion, except that the movement is passive extension or passive side flexion rather than passive flexion. Side flexion is most easily accomplished by grasping the patient's uppermost leg and rotating the leg upward, which causes side flexion in the lumbar spine by tilting the pelvis. Hip pathology must be ruled out before this is performed.

Central, Unilateral, and Transverse Vertebral Pressure

These movements are sometimes called **passive accessory intervertebral movements (PAIVMs).** To perform the last three joint play movements, the patient lies prone.[285] The lumbar spinous processes are palpated beginning at L5 and working up to L1. If the examiner plans to test end feel over several occasions, the same examining table should be used to improve reliability.[286] Likewise, the patient should be positioned the same way each time. The greatest movement occurs with the spine in neutral.[287] Interrater reliability of these techniques is often low.[288]

The examiner positions the hands, fingers, and thumbs as shown in Fig. 9.93D, to perform **posteroanterior central vertebral pressure (PACVP).** Pressure is applied through the thumbs, with the vertebrae being pushed anteriorly (see Fig. 8.56). The examiner must apply the pressure slowly and carefully so that the feel of the movement can be recognized. In reality, the movement is minimal. This springing test may be repeated several times to determine the quality of the movement through the range available and the end feel.

To perform **posteroanterior unilateral vertebral pressure (PAUVP),** the examiner moves the fingers laterally away from the tip of the spinous process about 2.5 to 4.0 cm (1.0 to 1.5 inches) so that the thumbs rest on the muscles overlying the lamina or the transverse process of the lumbar vertebra (Fig. 9.93E). The same anterior springing pressure is applied as in the central pressure technique. This springing pressure causes a slight rotation of the vertebra in the opposite direction, which can be confirmed by palpating the spinous process while doing the technique. The two sides should be evaluated and compared.

To perform **transverse vertebral pressure (TVP),** the examiner's fingers are placed along the side of the spinous process of the lumbar spine (Fig. 9.93F). The examiner then applies a transverse springing pressure to the side of the spinous process, which causes the vertebra to rotate in the direction of the pressure, feeling for the quality of

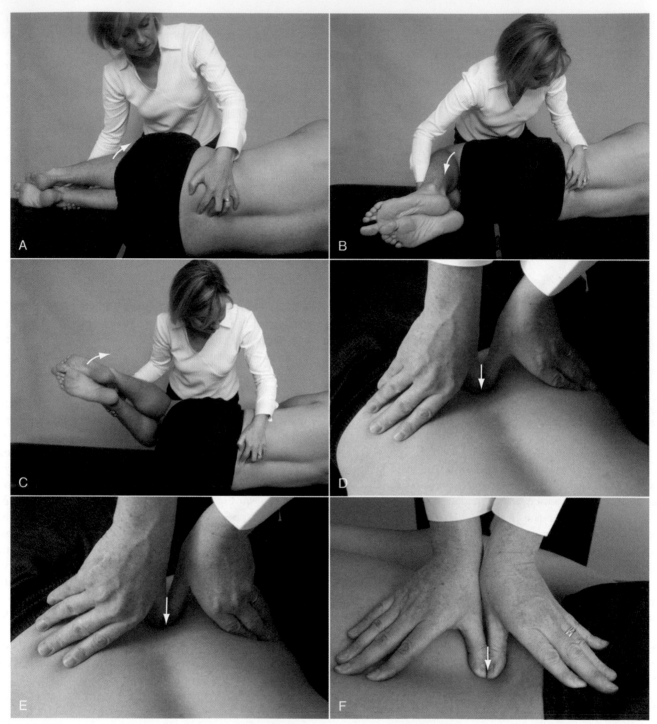

Fig. 9.93 Joint play movements of the lumbar spine. (A) Flexion. (B) Extension. (C) Side flexion. (D) Posteroanterior central vertebral pressure. (E) Posteroanterior unilateral vertebral pressure. (F) Transverse vertebral pressure.

movement. Pressure should be applied to both sides of the spinous process to compare the quality of movement through the range available and the end feel.

Palpation

If the examiner, having completed the examination of the lumbar spine, decides that the problem is in another joint, palpation should not be done until that joint is completely examined. However, when palpating the lumbar spine, any tenderness, altered temperature, muscle spasm, or other signs and symptoms that may indicate the source of pathology should be noted. If the problem is suspected to be in the lumbar spine area, palpation should be carried out in a systematic fashion, starting on the anterior aspect and working around to the posterior aspect.

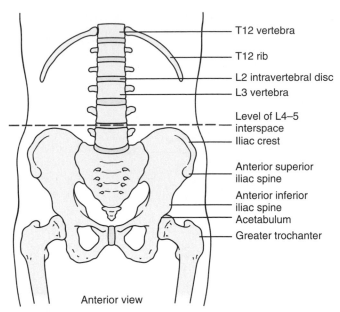

Fig. 9.94 Bony landmarks of the lumbar spine (anterior view).

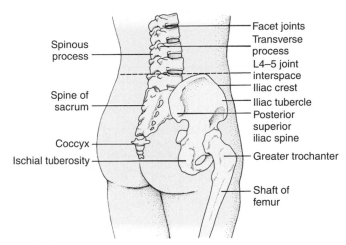

Fig. 9.95 Bony landmarks of the lumbar spine (posterior view).

Anterior Aspect

With the patient lying supine, the following structures are palpated anteriorly (Fig. 9.94).

Umbilicus. The umbilicus lies at the level of the L3–L4 disc space and is the point of intersection of the abdominal quadrants. It is also the point at which the aorta divides into the common iliac arteries. With some patients, the examiner may be able to palpate the anterior aspects of the L4, L5, and S1 vertebrae along with the discs and anterior longitudinal ligament with careful deep palpation. The abdomen may also be carefully palpated for symptoms (e.g., pain, muscle spasm) arising from internal organs. For example, the appendix is palpated in the right lower quadrant and the liver in the right upper quadrant; the kidneys are located in the left and right upper quadrants, and the spleen is found in the left upper quadrant.

Inguinal Area. The inguinal area is located between the ASIS and the symphysis pubis. The examiner should carefully palpate for symptoms of a hernia, abscess, infection (lymph nodes), or other pathological conditions in the area.

Iliac Crest. The examiner palpates the iliac crest from the ASIS, moving posteriorly and looking for any symptoms (e.g., hip pointer or apophysitis).

Symphysis Pubis. The examiner uses both thumbs to palpate the symphysis pubis. Standing at the patient's side, the examiner pushes both thumbs down onto the symphysis pubis so that the thumbs rest on the superior aspect of the pubic bones (see Fig. 10.16). In this way, one can ensure that the two pubic bones are level. The symphysis pubis and pubic bones may also be carefully palpated for any tenderness (e.g., osteitis pubis).

Posterior Aspect

The patient is then asked to lie prone, and the following structures are palpated posteriorly (Fig. 9.95).

Spinous Processes of the Lumbar Spine. The examiner palpates a point in the midline, which is on a line joining the high point of the two iliac crests. This point is the L4–L5 interspace. After moving down to the first hard mass, the fingers will be resting on the spinous process of L5. Moving toward the head, the interspaces and spinous processes of the remaining lumbar vertebrae can be palpated. In addition to looking for tenderness, muscle spasm, hypo- or hypermobility, and other signs of pathology, the examiner should watch for signs of a spondylolisthesis, which is most likely to occur at L4–L5 or L5–S1. A visible or palpable dip or protrusion from one spinous process to another may be evident, depending on the type of spondylolisthesis present. In addition, absence of a spinous process may be seen in a spina bifida. If the examiner moves laterally 2 to 3 cm (0.8 to 1.2 inches) from the spinous processes, the fingers will be resting over the lumbar facet joints. These joints should also be palpated for signs of pathology. Because of the depth of these joints, the examiner may have difficulty palpating them. However, pathology in this area results in spasm of the overlying paraspinal muscles, which can be palpated. Parkinson et al.[289] felt that the examiner should also palpate between the spinous process during a **sit-to-stand test** as they noted that the movement in the upper lumbar spine and lower lumbar spine was different and there were also gender differences during the movement.[289]

Sacrum, Sacral Hiatus, and Coccyx. If the examiner returns to the spinous process of L5 and moves caudally, the fingers will be resting on the sacrum. Like the lumbar spine, the sacrum has spinous processes, but they are much harder to distinguish because there are no interposing soft-tissue spaces between them. The S2 spinous process is at the level of a line joining the two

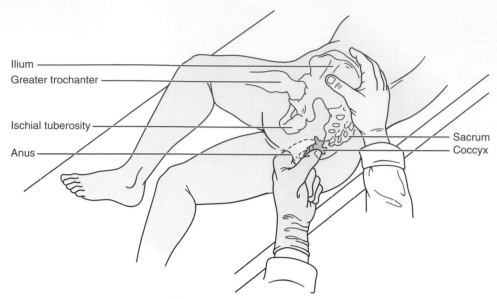

Fig. 9.96 Palpation of the coccyx.

PSISs ("posterior dimples"). Moving distally, the examiner's fingers may palpate the sacral hiatus, which is the caudal portion of the sacral canal. It has an inverted U shape and lies approximately 5 cm (2 inches) above the tip of the coccyx. The two bony prominences on each side of the hiatus are called the **sacral cornua** (see Fig. 10.70). As the examiner's fingers move farther distally, they eventually rest on the posterior aspect of the coccyx. Proper palpation of the coccyx requires a rectal examination using a surgical rubber glove (Fig. 9.96). The index finger is lubricated and inserted into the anus while the patient's sphincter muscles are relaxed. The finger is inserted as far as possible and then rotated so that the pulpy surface rests against the anterior surface of the coccyx. The examiner then places the thumb of the same hand against the posterior aspect of the sacrum. In this way, the coccyx can be moved back and forth. Any major tenderness (e.g., coccyodynia) should be noted.

Iliac Crest, Ischial Tuberosity, and Sciatic Nerve. Beginning at the PSISs, the examiner moves along the iliac crest, palpating for signs of pathology. Then, moving slightly distally, the examiner palpates the gluteal muscles for spasm, tenderness, or the presence of abnormal nodules. Just under the gluteal folds, the examiner should palpate the ischial tuberosities on both sides for any abnormality. As the examiner moves laterally, the greater trochanter of the femur is palpated. It is often easier to palpate if the hip is flexed to 90°. Midway between the ischial tuberosity and the greater trochanter, the examiner may be able to palpate the path of the sciatic nerve. The nerve itself is not usually palpable. Deep to the gluteal muscles, the piriformis muscle should also be palpated for potential pathology. This muscle is in a line dividing the PSIS of

the pelvis and greater trochanter of the femur from the ASIS and ischial tuberosity of the pelvis.

Diagnostic Imaging[290–300]

It is imperative when using diagnostic imaging, to correlate clinical findings with imaging findings, because many anomalies, congenital abnormalities, and aging changes may be present that are not related to the patient's problems and may be seen in asymptomatic individuals.[29,301]

Plain Film Radiography

Routine plane lumbosacral x-rays are most appropriate when risk factors of a vertebral fracture are present or if the patient has not improved after a course of conservative treatment (about 1 month).[29] In adults under 50 years of age with no signs or symptoms of systemic disease, imaging is not required.[302] For patients over 50 years of age, plain x-rays and laboratory tests can rule out most systemic diseases.[302]

Risk Factors for Vertebral Fractures[29]

- Age 50 years or older
- Significant trauma (external trauma or fall from a height)
- History of osteoporosis
- Corticosteroid use
- Substance abuse (higher rate of trauma)

Normally, anteroposterior and lateral views are taken.[303] In some cases, two lateral views may be taken, one that shows the whole lumbar spine, and one that focuses

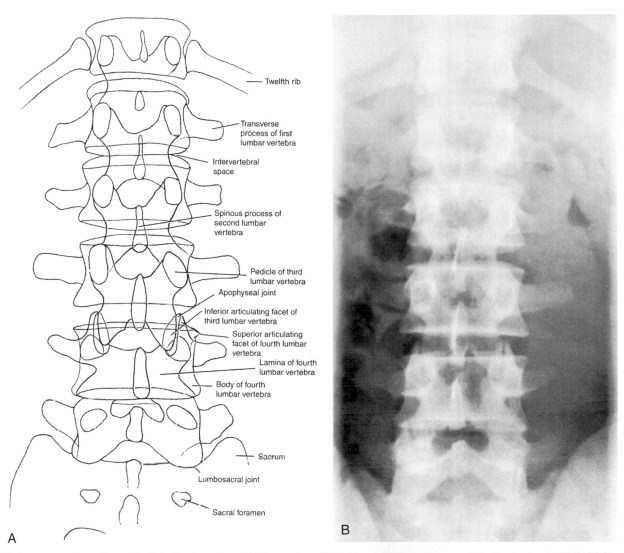

Twelfth rib

Transverse process of first lumbar vertebra

Intervertebral space

Spinous process of second lumbar vertebra

Pedicle of third lumbar vertebra

Apophyseal joint

Inferior articulating facet of third lumbar vertebra

Superior articulating facet of fourth lumbar vertebra

Lamina of fourth lumbar vertebra

Body of fourth lumbar vertebra

Sacrum

Lumbosacral joint

Sacral foramen

A

B

Fig. 9.97 Anteroposterior radiograph of the lumbar spine. (A) Film tracing. (B) Radiograph. (From Finneson BE: *Low back pain*, Philadelphia, 1973, JB Lippincott, pp 52–53.)

on the lower two segments. Oblique views are taken if spondylolysis or spondylolisthesis is suspected.[148]

Common X-Ray Views of the Lumbar Spine Depending on Pathology

- Anteroposterior view (Fig. 9.97)
- Lateral view (see Fig. 9.107)
- Oblique view (spondylosis, spondylolisthesis) (see Fig. 9.111)
- Lateral L5–S1 (coned) view (Fig. 9.98)
- Anteroposterior axial view
- Lateral view in flexion (Fig. 9.99A)
- Lateral view in extension (Fig. 9.99B)

Anteroposterior View. With this view (see Fig. 9.97), the examiner should note the following:
1. Shape of the vertebrae.
2. Any wedging of the vertebrae, possibly resulting from fracture (Fig. 9.100).

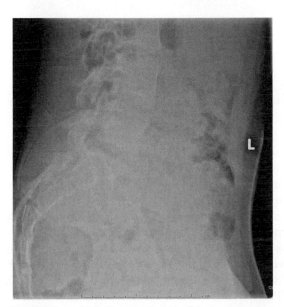

Fig. 9.98 Lateral L5–S1 (coned) view of the lumbar spine.

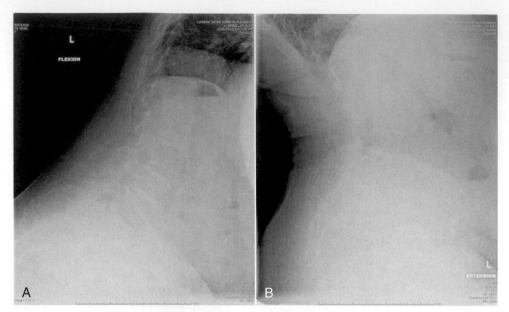

Fig. 9.99 Lateral view of the lumbar spine. (A) In flexion. (B) In extension.

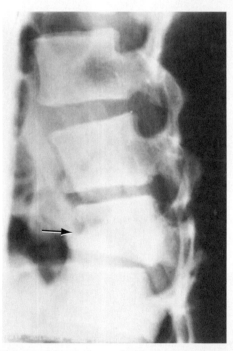

Fig. 9.100 Wedging *(arrow)* of a vertebral body. Some wedging may also be seen in the vertebra above.

3. Disc spaces. Do they appear normal, or are there height decreases, as occurs in spondylosis?
4. Are there any vertebral deformity, such as a hemivertebra or other anomalies (Figs. 9.101 to 9.104)?
5. Is a bamboo spine present, as seen in ankylosing spondylitis?
6. Is there any evidence of lumbarization of S1, making S1–S2 the first mobile segment rather than L5–S1? Lumbarization occurs in 2% to 8% of the population (Fig. 9.105).
7. Is there any evidence of sacralization of L5, making the L4–L5 level the first mobile segment rather than

L5–S1? This anomaly occurs in 3% to 6% of the population (Fig. 9.106).
8. Is there any evidence of spina bifida occulta, which occurs in 6% to 10% of the population (see Fig. 9.103)?
Lateral View. With this view (Fig. 9.107), the examiner should note the following:
1. Any evidence of spondylosis or spondylolisthesis, which occurs in 2% to 4% of the population (Fig. 9.108). The degree of slipping can be graded as shown in Fig. 9.109.[304] New grading or classification system involving lateral sacropelvic and spinopelvic balance have also been suggested.[305]
2. A normal lordosis. Do the intervertebral foramina appear normal?
3. Any wedging of the vertebrae.
4. Normal disc spacing.
5. Alignment of the vertebrae should be noted. Disruption of the curve may indicate spinal instability.
6. Any osteophyte formation or traction spurs (Fig. 9.110).[297,306] Traction spurs indicate an unstable lumbar intervertebral segment. A traction spur occurs approximately 1 mm from the disc border; an osteophyte occurs at the disc border with the vertebral body.
Oblique View. With the oblique view (Fig. 9.111), the examiner should look for any evidence of spondylolisthesis (sometimes referred to as a "Scottie dog decapitated") or spondylolysis (sometimes referred to as a "Scottie dog with a collar," Fig. 9.112).
Motion Views. In some cases, motion views may be used to demonstrate abnormal spinal motion or structural abnormalities. These are usually lateral views showing flexion and extension to demonstrate instability or spondylolisthesis (Fig. 9.113), but they may also include anteroposterior views with side bending.[196,307,308]

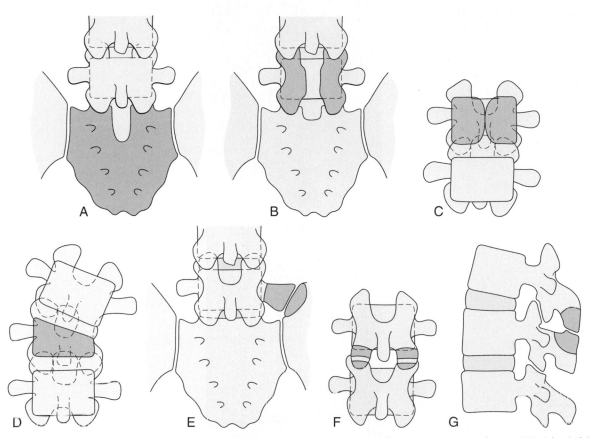

Fig. 9.101 Diagrammatic representation of the x-ray appearance of common anatomical anomalies in the lumbosacral spine. (A) Spina bifida occulta, S1. (B) Spina bifida, L5. (C) Anterior spina bifida ("butterfly vertebra"). (D) Hemivertebra. (E) Iliotransverse joint (transitional segments). (F) Ossicles of Oppenheimer. These are free ossicles seen at the tip of the inferior articular facets and are usually found at the level of L3. (G) "Kissing" spinous processes. (Redrawn from MacNab I: *Backache*, Baltimore, 1977, Williams & Wilkins, pp 14–15.)

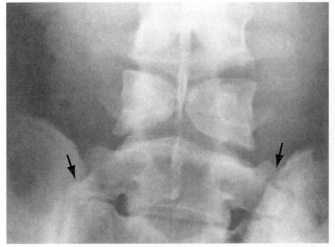

Fig. 9.102 Butterfly vertebra. Also note transitional segments *(large arrows).* (Modified from Jaeger SA: *Atlas of radiographic positioning: normal anatomy and developmental variants*, Norwalk, CT, 1988, Appleton & Lange, p 333.)

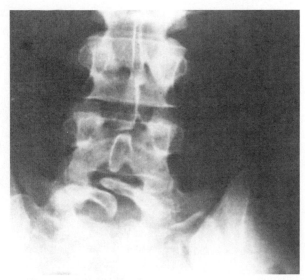

Fig. 9.103 Spina bifida occulta. (From Jaeger SA: *Atlas of radiographic positioning: normal anatomy and developmental variants*, Norwalk, CT, 1988, Appleton & Lange, p 317.)

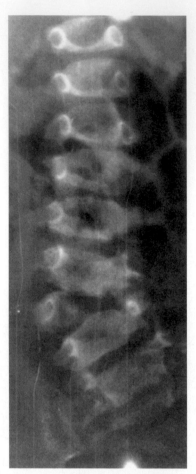

Fig. 9.104 Hemivertebra shown on an anteroposterior radiograph.

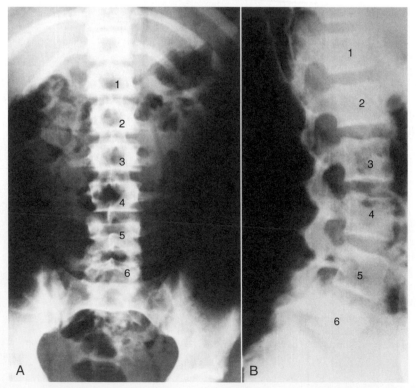

Fig. 9.105 Lumbarization of the S1 vertebra seen on anteroposterior (A) and lateral (B) radiographs.

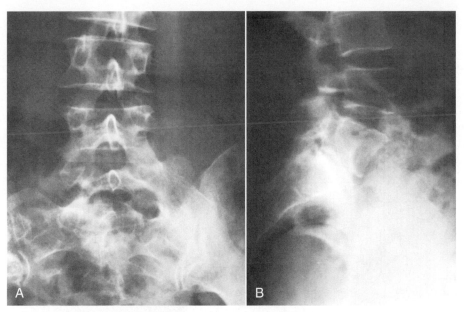

Fig. 9.106 Unilateral sacralization of the fifth lumbar vertebra. (A) Note the massive formation of sacral ala on the left side with a relatively normal transverse process on the right (anteroposterior view). (B) Lateral view showing the narrow disc space and the massive arches. (From O'Donoghue DH: *Treatment of injuries to athletes*, ed 4, Philadelphia, 1984, WB Saunders, p 403.)

Myelography

A myelogram—although seldom used today because of its complications and replacement by computed tomography (CT) scans and magnetic resonance imaging (MRI)—can confirm the presence of a protruding intervertebral disc, osteophytes, a tumor, or spinal stenosis (Figs. 9.114 to 9.116). The examiner must be careful of the side effects of myelograms, which include headache, stiffness, low back pain, cramps, and paresthesia in the lower limbs. Although side effects do occur, no permanent injuries have been noted.

Radionuclide Imaging (Bone Scans)

Bone scans are useful for detecting active bone disease processes and areas of high bone turnover. In children, the epiphyseal and metaphyseal areas of the long bones show increased uptake. In adults, only the metaphyseal area is so affected. Traumatic bone injuries, tumors, metabolic abnormalities (e.g., Paget disease), infection, and arthritis may be detected on bone scan.[149]

Diagnostic Ultrasound Imaging

Because low back pain is one of the most common forms of disability, diagnostic ultrasound imaging (DUSI) can be utilized to help not only diagnose the many causes of this problem, it has also been used to dynamically evaluate muscle contractile abilities. The methods used for these findings are described next.

Porter et al.[309] used early forms of pulsed ultrasound echoes to determine the spinal canal diameter by placing a transducer of the ultrasound in an oblique midsagittal plane 1 cm lateral to midline. It was determined that the canal diameter in those with low back pain was smaller than those without—1.44 cm compared with 1.61 cm. However, this method has not gained wide attention and requires techniques not normally used in today's age. Additionally, although spinal canal diameter may be a risk factor for low back pain, more recent studies have shown that it has no practical role in prediction or estimation of prognosis of low back pain in several populations including normal and workers with back pain.[310,311]

One of the more common uses of DUSI for the low back is to view the paraspinal muscles. Probably, the most common is the viewing of the lumbar multifidus. It is theorized that these muscles have a unique role in helping to provide up to two-thirds of lumbar stability, especially in the lower lumbar region.[312] The multifidus have been reported as one of the major muscle groups affected in those with low back pain. They have been shown to be round or oval, and symmetrical between sides, while increasing in size from cranial to caudal in healthy subjects.[62,313–316] Multifidus atrophy is a common finding (around 80%) in patients with chronic low back pain.[317] Lower back injury can result in lumbar muscle inhibition and loss of control, which may not recover spontaneously.[318]

Multifidus muscle size and body mass index (BMI) appear to have a positive correlation in both healthy adolescents and those suffering from low back pain, and those with low back pain had decreased cross section size

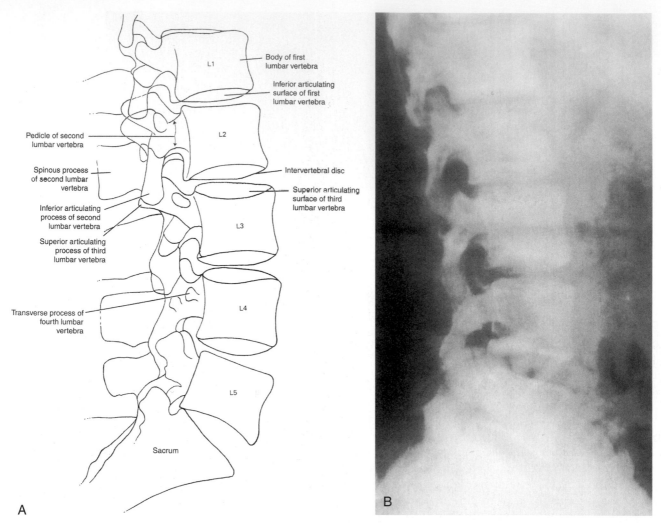

Fig. 9.107 Lateral radiograph of the lumbar spine. (A) Film tracing. (B) Radiograph. (From Finneson BE: *Low back pain*, Philadelphia, 1973, JB Lippincott, pp 54–55.)

compared to those without low back pain.[319,320] Previous studies have shown that the pattern of multifidus muscle atrophy is more localized at the specific level of injury and that there is a significant correlation between muscle atrophy and the capacity of creating voluntary isometric contractions of the muscle.[321]

One method to assess multifidus function is to measure the cross-sectional area. It is thought that this value will be a surrogate measurement for its force generation and activity level capacity.[322,323] To be able to evaluate the cross-sectional area of the multifidus, the patient should be in the prone position with a pillow under the abdomen. The image can be taken at any location; however, a convenient spot to image is the L5-S1 level. In order to identify the multifidus, a line connecting the iliac crests can be used to find L5-S1 level. The ultrasound transducer can be then placed in the sagittal plane parallel to the vertebra (Fig. 9.117). In this position, the facets can be viewed with multifidus muscle in between (Fig. 9.118). The transducer can then be turned transversely over the spinous process

(Fig. 9.119) and simultaneous measurements of right and left multifidus can be obtained (Fig. 9.120).

Muscle activation can also be measured by viewing dynamic contractions of the spinal muscles. DUSI can be used to view actual muscle contractions and measure muscle thickness in relaxed and contracted muscle tissue. The ability of patients with chronic low back pain to activate the multifidus at affected lumbar sections is reduced as evidenced by smaller increases in thickness of images during contraction compared to contralateral normal side muscle or compared to asymptomatic control subjects.[321,324]

Ultrasound of Abdominal Muscles. Ultrasound provides an excellent method for assessment and rehabilitation of the abdominal muscles and can be used to appraise the morphology and behavior of these muscles. These anterior stabilizing muscles are as important as the muscles of the back. Muscles that can be viewed include the oblique externus abdominis, the obliquus internus abdominis, the transverse abdominis, and the recuts abdominis and surrounding fascia.

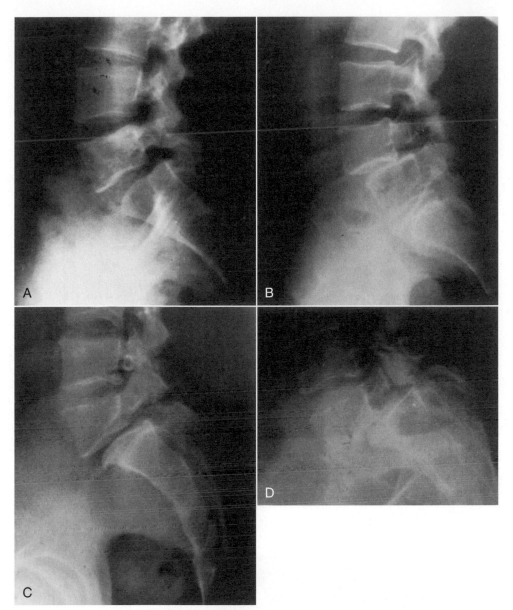

Fig. 9.108 Spondylolisthesis. (A) Grade 1: Arch defect in L5 with mild forward displacement of L5 on S1; backache but no gross disability. (B) Grade 2: More forward slipping between L4 and L5 with collapse of the intervertebral disc; definite symptomatic back with restriction of motion, muscle spasm, and curtailment of activities. (C) Grade 3: More extensive slipping combined with a wide separation at the arch defect and degenerative changes of the disc; grossly symptomatic. (D) Grade 4: Vertebrae slipped forward more than halfway; severe disability. (From O'Donoghue DH: *Treatment of injuries to athletes,* ed 4, Philadelphia, 1984, WB Saunders, p 402.)

When viewing the lateral abdominal wall, the clinician will image three layers of muscles separated by hyperechoic lines that are composed of intermuscular fascia (Fig. 9.121). These muscles are usually imaged in supine or hook lying with the knees flexed with the muscles relaxed (Fig. 9.122). However, due to the portability of modern ultrasound machines, images can be taken in other positions, such as quadruped,[325] sitting,[326,327] standing, and walking.[328,329] The transducer is placed transversely at various locations of the anterior abdominal wall. A standardized location has not yet been agreed upon. It is usually the middle abdominal region between the border of the 11th costal cartilage and the iliac crest along either the midaxillary or anterior axillary line.[330] These images can be captured during relaxation and during end of expiration. Although a range of transducer frequencies permits adequate visualization of the lateral abdominal muscles, a higher-frequency curvilinear transducer, with a diverging field of view, is ideal as it allows for a greater visualization of each muscle throughout its length. There is variation from person to person. The image of lateral abdominal muscles normally shows several muscle layers that are tapered in thickness toward their anterior border. The thickness is even throughout the middle of the muscle and generally curves laterally.

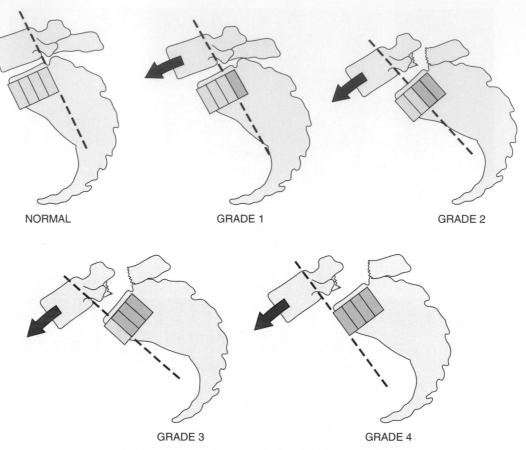

NORMAL   GRADE 1   GRADE 2

GRADE 3   GRADE 4

Fig. 9.109 Meyerding grading system for slipping in spondylolisthesis.

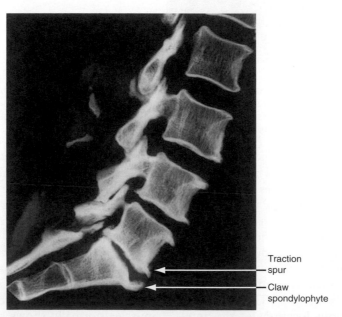

Traction spur

Claw spondylophyte

Fig. 9.110 Lateral radiograph of a thin-slice pathological section of lumbar spine. Note traction spur and claw spondylophyte. (From Rothman RH, Simeone FA: *The spine*, Philadelphia, 1982, WB Saunders, p 512.)

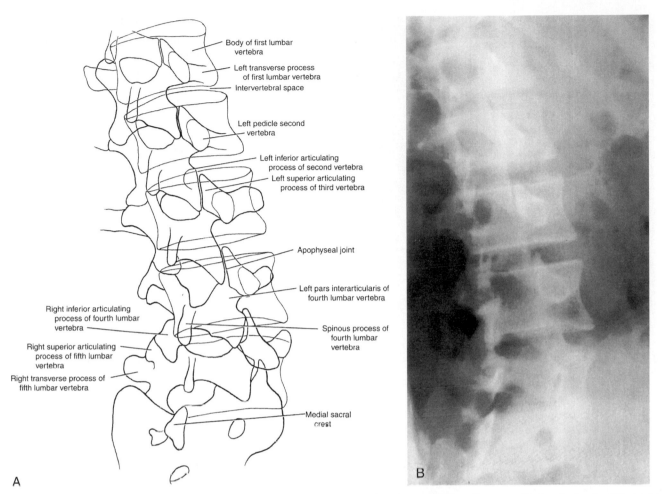

Body of first lumbar vertebra

Left transverse process of first lumbar vertebra

Intervertebral space

Left pedicle second vertebra

Left inferior articulating process of second vertebra

Left superior articulating process of third vertebra

Apophyseal joint

Left pars interarticularis of fourth lumbar vertebra

Right inferior articulating process of fourth lumbar vertebra

Spinous process of fourth lumbar vertebra

Right superior articulating process of fifth lumbar vertebra

Right transverse process of fifth lumbar vertebra

Medial sacral crest

A

B

Fig. 9.111 Left posterior oblique radiograph of the lumbar spine. (A) Film tracing. (B) Radiograph. (From Finneson BE: *Low back pain*, Philadelphia, 1973, JB Lippincott, pp 56–57.)

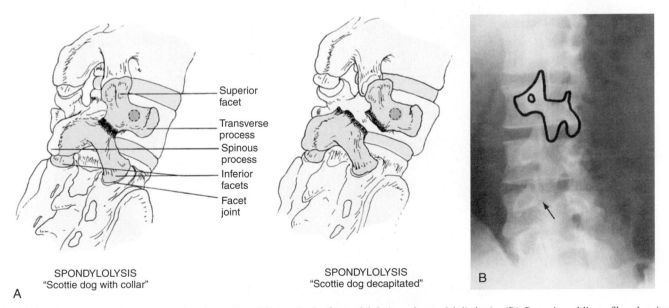

Superior facet

Transverse process

Spinous process

Inferior facets

Facet joint

SPONDYLOLYSIS
"Scottie dog with collar"

SPONDYLOLYSIS
"Scottie dog decapitated"

A

B

Fig. 9.112 (A) Diagrammatic representation (posterior oblique view) of spondylolysis and spondylolisthesis. (B) Posterior oblique film showing "Scottie dog" at L2. L4 shows Scottie dog with a "collar" *(arrow)*, indicating spondylolysis.

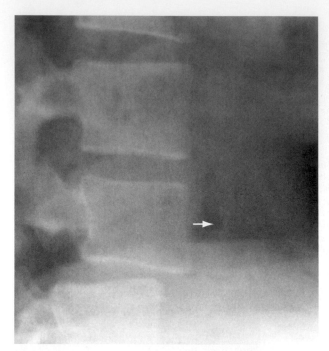

Fig. 9.113 Lumbar spine in flexion. Note forward slipping of one vertebra on the one below *(arrow)*.

The relative thickness of the abdominal muscles normally shows the rectus abdominis muscle as the thickest. It is the only abdominal muscle in which cross-sectional area may be measured and men have a larger cross-sectional area than females when normalized for body mass. The transverse abdominis is the thinnest.[331] The rectus abdominis muscle is a large muscle with the primary function of approximating the rig cage with the pelvis by producing a flexion moment in the sagittal plane.[332] When examining for homogeneity of abdominal muscle thickness, it has been reported that the upper portions of the lateral abdominal wall are generally thicker.[331,333]

Measurements of thickness of muscles vary based on location. It is predictable that the muscles would be thicker during expiration than during inspiration.[326,327,334,335] The measurements for assessment of thickness will depend on the intention of the evaluation in clinical practice such as either absolute or relative thickness values may be appropriate for assessment of thickness of adjacent muscle layers. Assessment of asymmetry in base line thickness values may be best represented as a percent difference between symptomatic and non-symptomatic sides. A change in muscle thickness is typically presented either as a percent change in muscle thickness or as muscle thickness during activity as a ratio to muscle thickness at rest.[336–338]

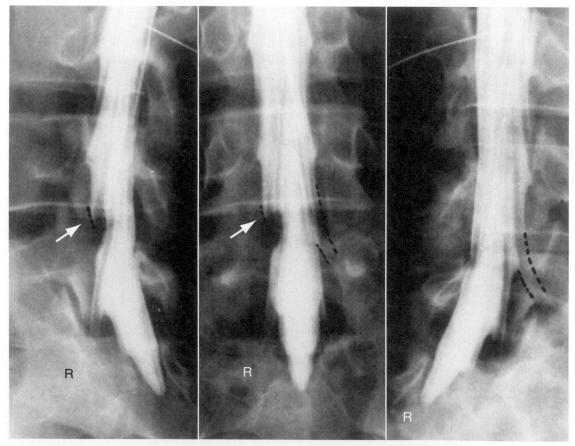

Fig. 9.114 Metrizamide myelograms illustrating a herniated disc at L4–L5 on the right. Note lack of filling of the nerve root sleeve and indentation *(arrow)* of the dural sac. (From Rothman RH, Simeone FA: *The spine*, Philadelphia, 1982, WB Saunders, p 550.)

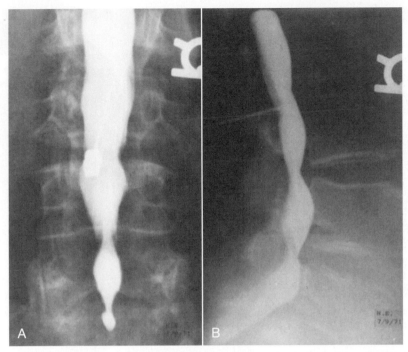

Fig. 9.115 Oil myelograms showing the characteristic appearance of chronic disc degeneration and spinal stenosis with diffuse posterior bulging of the annulus and osteophyte formation. (A) Symmetric wasting of the dye column is shown in the anteroposterior view. Note the hourglass configuration. (B) Indentation of the dye column of the annulus anteriorly and the buckled ligamentum flavum and facet joints posteriorly (lateral view). (From Rothman RH, Simeone FA: *The spine*, Philadelphia, 1982, WB Saunders, p 553.)

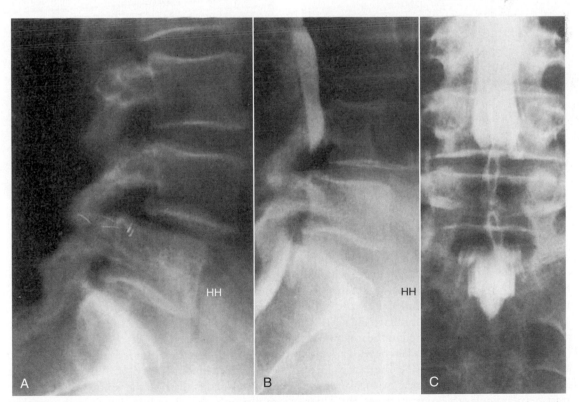

Fig. 9.116 Metrizamide myelograms showing stenotic block at the L4–L5 level as a result of degenerative spondylolisthesis and spinal stenosis at the L4–L5 level. (A) Note the 4-mm anterior migration of L4 on L5 caused by the degenerative spondylolisthesis. (B and C) The extensive block on the myelogram is caused by spinal stenosis. (From Rothman RH, Simeone FA: *The spine*, Philadelphia, 1982, WB Saunders, p 553.)

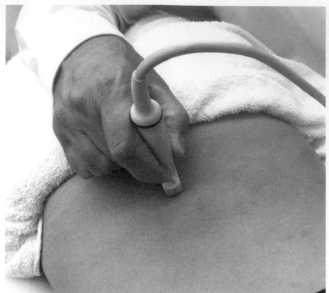

Fig. 9.117 Transducer placement for viewing a sagittal plane (long axis) image of the multifidus muscle.

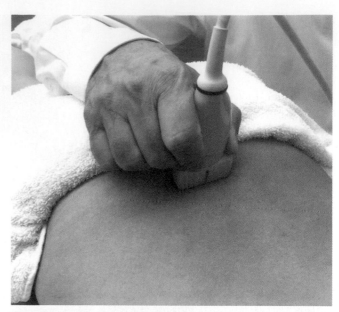

Fig. 9.119 Transducer placement for viewing a transverse (short axis) view of bilateral lumbar multifidus muscles.

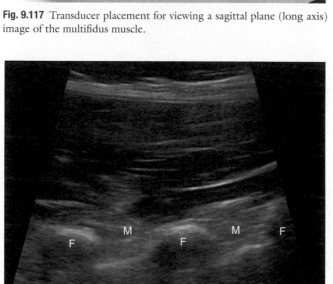

Fig. 9.118 Image of facet joints *(F)* and multifidus muscle *(M)* in between.

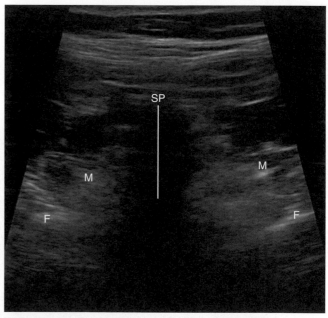

Fig. 9.120 Image of the bilateral multifidus muscles. Multifidus *(M)*, spinous process *(SP)*, facet joints *(F)*.

To determine the cross-sectional area of the rectus abdominis muscle, the patient is typically supine with the hips and knees flexed.[330] The image with a large transducer can generally be seen by placement immediately above the umbilicus and moving laterally from midline (Fig. 9.123), until the muscle cross section is centered in the image (Fig. 9.124).[331] Muscle cross-sectional area can be measured by outlining the muscle border just inside the fascial layer, while muscle thickness can be obtained by measurement of the greatest perpendicular thickness between the superficial to deep fascia.[330] Width can be measured from the most medial to the most lateral border of the muscle.[330]

Computed Tomography

A CT scan may be used to delineate a fracture or to show the presence of spinal stenosis caused by protrusion or a tumor, or if a bony abnormality is suspected (Figs. 9.125 to 9.128).[29] As with plain x-rays, results must be correlated with clinical findings, because the anatomical changes seen are often unassociated with the patient's symptoms.[301,339,340] This technique provides an axial projection of the spine, showing the anatomy of not only the spine but also the paravertebral muscles, vascular structures, and organs of the body cavity. In doing so, it shows more precisely the relation among the intervertebral discs, spinal canal, facet joints, and intervertebral foramina. It may be used to evaluate spinal stenosis, the shape of the spinal canal, epidural scarring (after surgery), facet joint arthritis, tumors, and trauma.[149,341,342] It may be used in conjunction with a water-soluble contrast medium (computer-assisted myelography) to further delineate the structures.

Magnetic Resonance Imaging

MRI is a noninvasive technique that can be used in several planes (transaxial, coronal, or sagittal) to delineate bony and soft tissues. This technique is commonly used to diagnose tumors, to view the spinal cord within the spinal canal, and to assess for syringomyelia, cord infarction, or traumatic injury.[149,343] The delineation of soft tissues is much greater with MRI than with CT.[344] For example, with MRI, the nucleus pulposus and the annulus fibrosis are easier to differentiate because of their different water contents, making it the preferred imaging modality

for disc disease and radiculopathy (Figs. 9.129 through 9.133).[27,29,345,346] As with other diagnostic imaging techniques, clinical findings must support what is seen before the structural abnormalities can be considered the source of the problem.[301,339,347–349] Up to 30% of asymptomatic patients with no history of low back pain show disc abnormalities.[27,350] Things to look for on MRI are disc height, presence or absence of annular tears, degenerative signs, and end plate changes.[27]

Discography[351]

For discography, radiopaque dye is injected into the nucleus pulposus. It is not a commonly used technique but may be used to see whether injection of dye reproduces the patient's symptoms, making it diagnostic (Fig. 9.134).

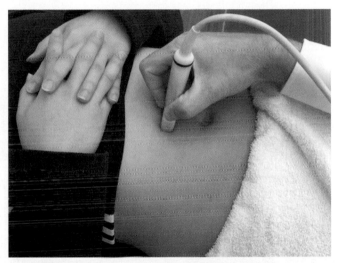

Fig. 9.123 Transducer placement to view bilateral rectus abdominis.

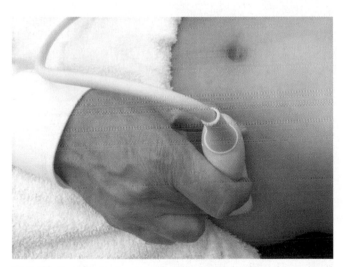

Fig. 9.121 Transducer placement for viewing the lateral abdominal wall.

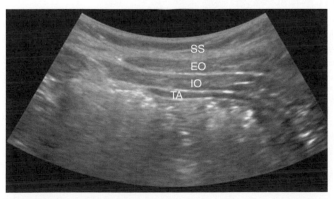

Fig. 9.122 Image of lateral abdominal wall, demonstrating superficial soft tissue *(SS)*, external oblique *(EO)* muscles, internal oblique *(IO)* muscles, and transverse abdominus *(TA)*.

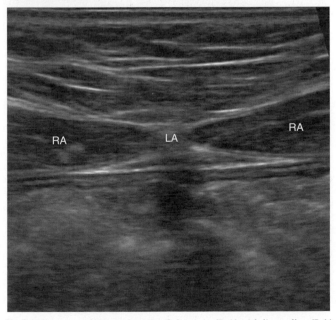

Fig. 9.124 Image of bilateral rectus abdominis *(RA)* with linea alba *(LA)* in between.

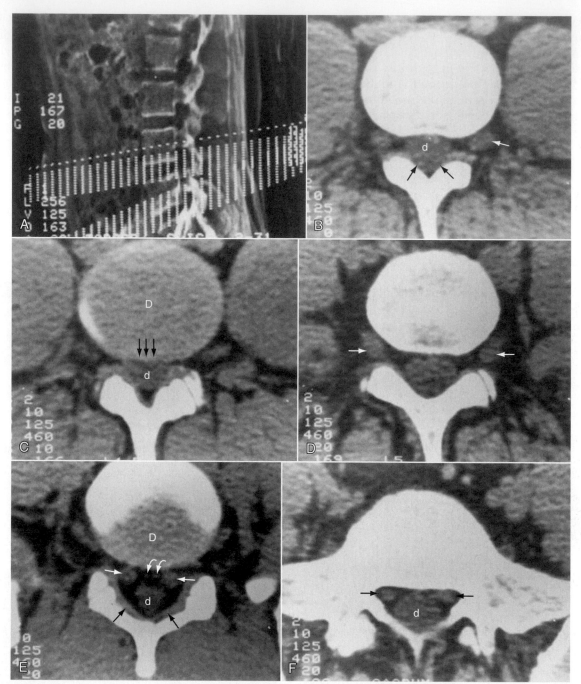

Fig. 9.125 Normal disc anatomy on computed tomography (CT). (A) Scout view. The chosen sections *(dashed lines)* can be planned and angled along the planes of the discs. (B) CT scan through the L4 vertebral body shows the neural foramina and the L4 nerve root ganglia *(white arrow indicates left ganglion)*. The dural sac *(d)* and ligamenta flava *(black arrows)* are shown. (C) CT scan through the L4–L5 disc (labeled *D*) shows very little fat between the posterior margin of the disc *(arrows)* and the dural sac *(d)*. The nerve roots are not clearly shown. (D) CT scan through the L5 vertebral body and foramina shows the L5 nerve root ganglia *(arrows)*. (E) CT scan through the L5–S1 disc space (labeled *D*) shows the L5 nerve roots *(straight white arrows)*, the dural sac *(d)*, and the ligamenta flava *(black arrows)*. Small epidural veins are noted *(curved arrows)*. (F) At the S1 level, the S1 nerve roots *(arrows)* and dural sac *(d)* are clearly visualized. (From Weissman BNW, Sledge CB: *Orthopedic radiology*, Philadelphia, 1986, WB Saunders, p 306.)

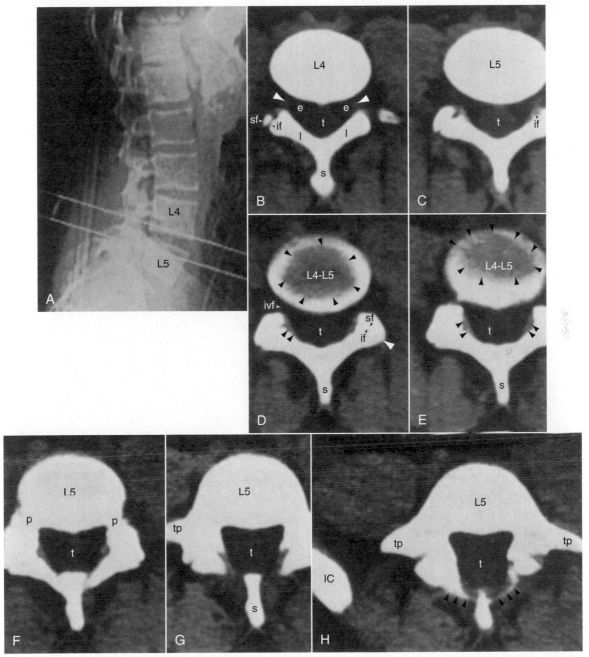

Fig. 9.126 Soft tissue detail of the L4–L5 intervertebral disc space on computed tomography (CT). (A) Lateral digital scout view obtained through the lumbosacral spine. The upper and lower scan limits through the L4–L5 region are designated with an electronic cursor. Scan collimation is 5 mm thick; incrementation is 3 mm (2-mm overlap). (B) Axial CT section of L4. The L4 root ganglia and spinal nerves are seen within the intervertebral foramina *(white arrowheads)* surrounded by abundant epidural fat *(e)*. The thecal sac *(t)* is bounded anterolaterally by fat in the lateral recess. The posterior arch of L4 consists of inferior facets *(if)*, laminae *(l)*, and spinous process *(s)*. The superior facet of L5 *(sf)* is just visible. (C) The next lower axial section demonstrates the L4–L5 facet articulations. The ligamentum flavum *(if)* is contiguous with the facet joint capsule. Again, the thecal sac *(t)* is readily apparent; it is slightly higher in density than the adjacent epidural fat. Note that without subarachnoid contrast media, the intrathecal contents cannot be discerned. (D) Axial CT section of the L4–L5 disc space. The disc *(multiple black arrowheads)* is a region of central hypodensity surrounded by the cortical margin of L4. The posterior arch of L4 projects below the disc level. The intervertebral foramina *(ivf)* have begun to close. The cartilaginous articular surfaces *(white arrowhead)* between superior *(sf)* and inferior *(if)* facets are poorly demonstrated with these window settings. The ligamentum flavum *(double black arrowheads)* is noted medial to the facet joints. *s,* Spinous process; *t,* thecal sac. (E) The next inferior CT section demonstrates the disc *(multiple arrowheads)* positioned somewhat more anteriorly, marginated posteriorly at this level by the posterosuperior cortical rim of the L5 body. The ligamentum flavum *(double arrowheads)* normally maintains a flat medial surface adjacent to the thecal sac *(t)*. The posterior arch of L4 and its spinous process *(s)* are still in view. (F) Axial CT section through the L5 body at the level of the pedicles *(p)*. The canal now completely encloses the thecal sac *(t)*. (G) Immediately below, only the spinous process *(s)* of the posterior arch of L4 is visible. The transverse process *(tp)* of L5 is noted. *t,* Thecal sac. (H) At the level of the iliac crest *(IC)*, the posterior arch of L5 *(small arrowheads)* has just begun to form. The transverse processes *(tp)* are quite large at this level. *t,* Thecal sac. (From LeMasters DL, Dowart RL: High-resolution, cross-sectional computed tomography of the normal spine, *Orthop Clin North Am* 16:359, 1985.)

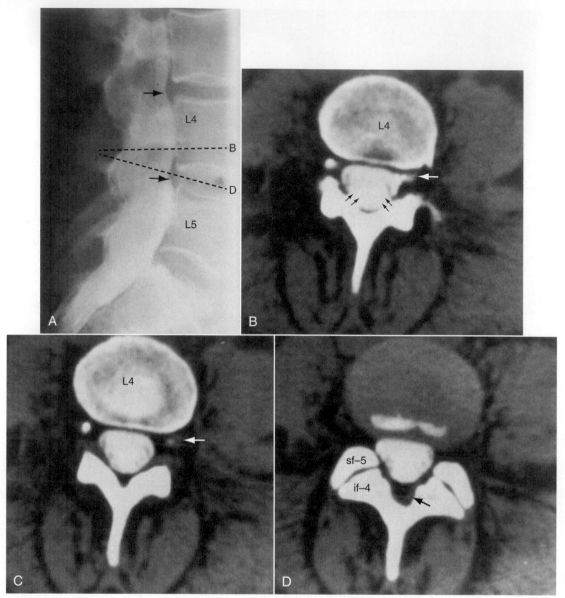

Fig. 9.127 Computed tomography (CT) anatomy of L4 nerve roots. (A) Lateral view during metrizamide myelography showing indentations on the anterior aspect of the contrast column *(arrows)* at L3–L4 and L4–L5 resulting from bulging intervertebral discs. The levels for subsequent CT sections B and D are marked. (B) CT section through the L4 vertebra and L4–L5 foramina 1 hour after a metrizamide myelogram. Contrast agent fills the left axillary pouch *(white arrow)* and the right nerve root sleeve. *Small arrows* indicate the filling defects produced by the remaining nerve roots. (C) CT section slightly more distal than B shows the L4 nerve root ganglia (left ganglion is indicated by *arrow*). (D) Section through the L4–L5 disc and the posterior inferior body of L4 shows an abnormally bulging disc without compression of the subarachnoid space. The ligamentum flavum on the left *(arrow)*, the superior facet of L5 *(sf-5)*, and the inferior facet of L4 *(if-4)* are indicated. (From Weissman BNW, Sledge CB: *Orthopedic radiology*, Philadelphia, 1986, WB Saunders, p 284.)

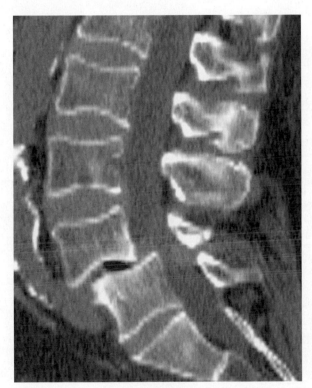

Fig. 9.128 Degenerative spondylolisthesis. Sagittal reformatted image derived from transverse CT scans of the lumbar spine shows degeneration at the L4–L5 level with a vacuum phenomenon. A grade II spondylolisthesis at the L4–L5 level results from osteoarthritis of the facet joints. (From Resnick D, Kransdorf MJ: *Bone and joint imaging*, Philadelphia, 2005, WB Saunders, p 146.)

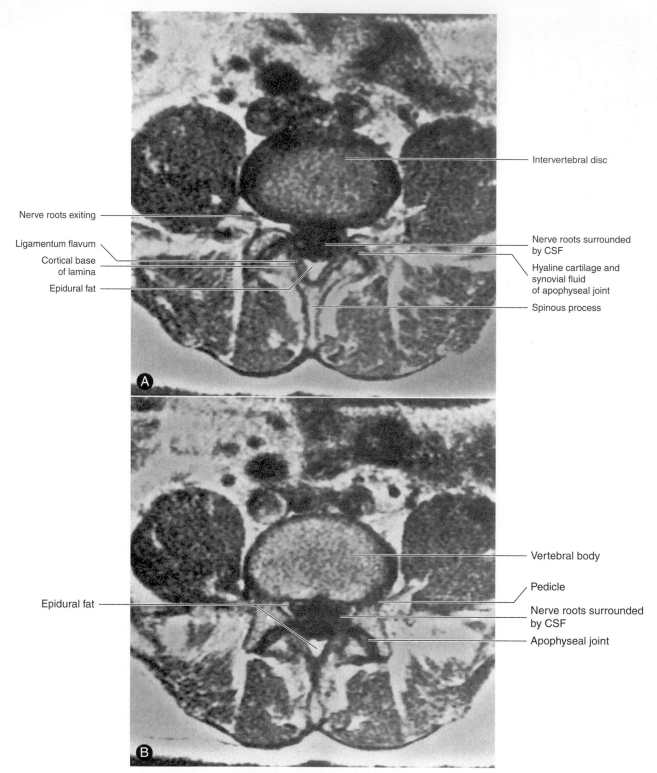

Intervertebral disc

Nerve roots exiting

Ligamentum flavum

Cortical base of lamina

Epidural fat

Nerve roots surrounded by CSF

Hyaline cartilage and synovial fluid of apophyseal joint

Spinous process

Epidural fat

Vertebral body

Pedicle

Nerve roots surrounded by CSF

Apophyseal joint

Fig. 9.129 Magnetic resonance imaging (MRI) of normal lumbar spine. (A) Level of neural canal. (B) Level of pedicle. *CSF*, Cerebrospinal fluid (From Bassett LW, Gold RH, Seeger LL: *MRI atlas of the musculoskeletal system*, London, 1989, Martin Dunitz, p 40.)

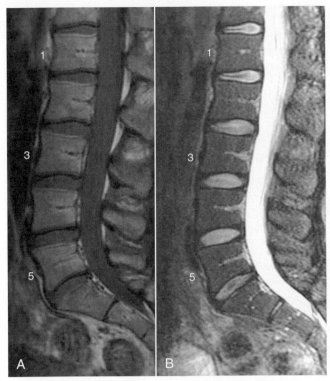

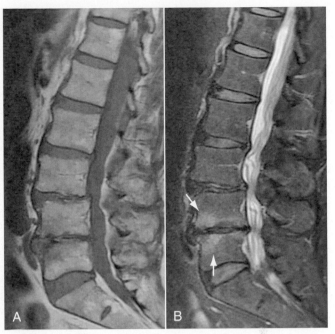

Fig. 9.130 Sagittal (A) T1-weighted and (B) fat-saturated T2-weighted fast spin echo sequences of the lumbar spine, showing normal disc spaces with normal disc and adjacent bone marrow signal. (From Majumdar S, Link TM, Steinbach LS, et al: Diagnostic tools and imaging methods in intervertebral disc degeneration, *Orthop Clin North Am* 42:503, 2011.)

Fig. 9.131 Sagittal T1-weighted and fat-saturated (A) T2-weighted fast spin echo (B) sequences of the lumbar spine demonstrate severe degenerative disc disease at L3/4 and L4/5 with disc height loss, disc desiccation, decreased signal, posterior disc bulges, and Modic type 1 reactive end-plate changes at L4/5 *(arrows)*. Note substantial spinal canal narrowing from L3–S1. (From Majumdar S, Link TM, Steinbach LS, et al: Diagnostic tools and imaging methods in intervertebral disk degeneration, *Orthop Clin North Am* 42:503, 2011.)

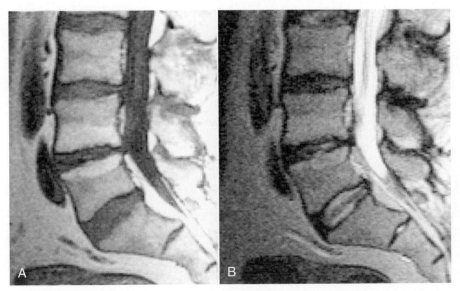

Fig. 9.132 Type II vertebral end plates. Sagittal T1-weighted (A) and T2-weighted (B) spin echo magnetic resonance images of the lumbar spine show signal intensity changes at the L4–L5 level that are typical of a type II end plate. The signal intensity of subchondral bone at this level is identical to that of fat. There is also evidence of degeneration of the intervertebral disc at this level, with a decrease in disc space height and loss of disc signal on the T2-weighted image. (From Resnick D, Kransdorf MJ: *Bone and joint imaging*, Philadelphia, 2005, WB Saunders, p 144.)

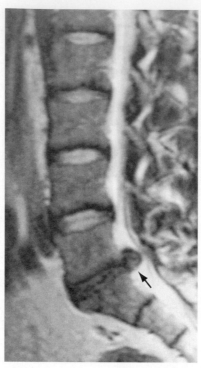

Fig. 9.133 Normal and abnormal intervertebral disc: sagittal T2-weighted (TR/TE, 3400/96) spin echo magnetic resonance imaging technique. In discs that are relatively normal (L1–L2, L3–L4, and L4–L5), a central portion of high signal intensity containing a horizontal line of low signal intensity is evident. In the disc (L2–L3) with mild intervertebral (osteo)chondrosis, minimal loss of signal intensity is shown, particularly in its anterior third. With severe intervertebral (osteo)chondrosis (L5–S1), the disc is of low signal intensity and diminished in height. A large posterior extruded disc *(arrow)* with low signal intensity is also evident. (From Resnick D, Kransdorf MJ: *Bone and joint imaging*, Philadelphia, 2005, WB Saunders, p 399.)

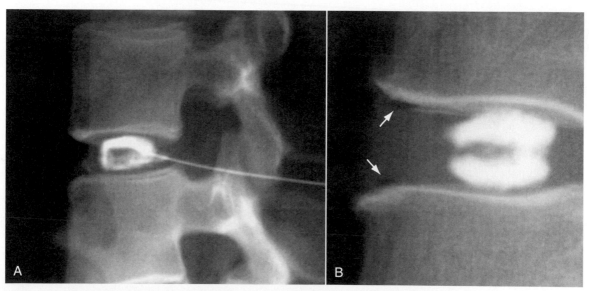

Fig. 9.134 Lumbar discography. (A) Lateral lumbar spine with discographic needle entry low in the posterior disc margin. Note the normal unilocular appearance of the nucleogram. (B) Normal bilocular appearance of the nucleogram. The anterior *arrows* identify anterior vacuum phenomena in the anulus fibrosus, consistent with peripheral annular tears that were asymptomatic at discography. (From Resnick D, Kransdorf MJ: *Bone and joint imaging*, Philadelphia, 2005, WB Saunders, p 164.)

PRÉCIS OF THE LUMBAR SPINE ASSESSMENT[a]

NOTE: Suspected pathology will determine which *Special Tests* are to be performed.

History (sitting)
Observation (standing)
Examination

Active movements (standing)
  Forward flexion
  Extension
  Side flexion (left and right)
  Rotation (left and right)
  Quick test (if possible)
  Trendelenburg test and S1 nerve root test (modified Trendelenburg test)
Passive movements (only with care and caution)
Peripheral joint scan (standing)
  Sacroiliac joints
Functional assessment
Special tests (standing)
  For lumbar instability:
    H and I test
  For joint dysfunction:
    One-leg standing (stork standing) lumbar extension test
    Quadrant test
  Other:
    Gower's sign
Resisted isometric movements (sitting)
  Forward flexion
  Extension
  Side flexion (left and right)
  Rotation (left and right)
Special tests (sitting)
  For neurological dysfunction:
    Slump test or one of its variants
  For lumbar instability:
    Test for anterior lumbar spine instability
    Test for posterior lumbar spine instability
Resisted isometric movements (supine lying)
  Dynamic abdominal endurance
  Double straight leg lowering
  Internal/external abdominal obliques test
Peripheral joint scan (supine lying)
  Hip joints (flexion, abduction, adduction, and medial and lateral rotation)
  Knee joints (flexion and extension)
  Ankle joints (dorsiflexion and plantar flexion)
  Foot joints (supination, pronation)
  Toe joints (flexion, extension)
Myotomes (supine lying)
  Hip flexion (L2)
  Knee extension (L3)
  Ankle dorsiflexion (L4)
  Toe extension (L5)

Ankle eversion or plantar flexion (S1)
Special tests (supine lying)
  For neurological dysfunction:
    Straight leg raise test or one of its variants
  For muscle tightness:
    90–90 straight leg raise test
    Rectus femoris test
    Thomas test
  For muscle dysfunction:
    Supine bridge test
  Other tests:
    Sign of the buttock
Reflexes and cutaneous distribution (anterior and side aspects)
Palpation (supine lying)
Resisted isometric movements (side lying)
  Horizontal side support
Special tests (side lying)
  For neurological dysfunction:
    Femoral nerve traction test
  For lumbar instability:
    Specific lumbar torsion test
  For muscle tightness:
    Ober test
Joint play movements (side lying)
  Flexion
Peripheral joint scan (prone lying)
  Hip joints (extension, medial and lateral rotation)
Myotomes (prone lying)
  Hip extension (S1)
  Knee flexion (S1, S2)
Resisted isometric movements
  Dynamic extension test
Special tests (prone lying)
  For neurological dysfunction:
    Prone knee bending test or one of its variants
  For lumbar instability:
    Passive lumbar extension test
    Prone hip extension test
    Prone segmental instability test
  For muscle dysfunction:
    Prone bridge test
Reflexes and cutaneous distribution (prone lying) (posterior aspect)
Joint play movements (prone lying)
  Posteroanterior central vertebral pressure (PACVP)
  Posteroanterior unilateral vertebral pressure (PAUVP)
  Transverse vertebral pressure (TVP)
Palpation (prone lying)
Resisted isometric movements (quadruped position)
  Back rotators/multifidus test
Diagnostic imaging

[a]The précis is shown in an order that limits the amount of movement that the patient has to do but ensures that all necessary structures are tested. After any examination, the patient should be warned of the possibility that symptoms may be exacerbated as a result of the assessment.

CASE STUDIES

When doing these case studies, the examiner should list the appropriate questions to ask and specify why they are being asked, what to look for and why, and what things should be tested and why. Depending on the patient's answers (and the examiner should consider different responses), several possible causes of the patient's problem may become evident (examples given in parentheses). The examiner should prepare a differential diagnosis chart and then decide how different diagnoses may affect the treatment plan. For example, an 18-year-old female synchronized swimmer was "boosting" another swimmer out of the water when she felt a sharp pain in her back. She found that she could no longer swim because of the pain. She demonstrated paresthesia on the dorsum of the foot and lateral aspect of the leg. Describe your assessment plan for this patient (acute disc herniation versus lumbar strain) (Table 9.21).

1. A 27-year-old female who is on disability due to Ehlers-Danlos syndrome is coming to see you for chronic sacroiliitis that is causing pain with all of her activities of daily living (ADLs) at home. She has pain with most transitional movement patterns and with prolonged standing or walking. Describe your assessment of this condition and list several significant issues that could complicate this case due to the underlying Ehler-Danlos syndrome.

2. A 54-year-old male soccer coach is coming to see you following L3–4 and L4–5 lumbar laminectomy surgery. He reports having had a very swift loss of dorsiflexion strength prior to surgery. His surgery occurred 2 weeks ago. He continues to wear his postsurgical back brace. Describe your assessment process for this patient and list three areas regarding your examination where caution should be taken.

3. A 23-year-old male comes to you complaining of a low backache. He works as a dishwasher, and although the pain has been present for 5 months, he has not missed any work. The pain gets worse as the day progresses and is relieved by rest. X-rays reveal some sclerosis in the area of the sacroiliac joints. Describe your assessment plan for this patient (ankylosing spondylitis vs. lumbar sprain).

4. A 36-year-old female comes to you complaining of a chronic backache of 6 months' duration. The pain has been gradually increasing in severity and is worse at rest and in the morning on arising from bed. When present, the pain is centered in her low back and radiates into her buttocks and posterior left thigh. Describe your assessment plan for this patient (lumbar stenosis vs. lumbar disc lesion).

5. A 13-year-old female gymnast comes to you complaining of low back pain. The pain increases when she extends the spine. Like most gymnasts, she is hypermobile in most of her joints. Describe your assessment plan for this patient (spondylolisthesis vs. lumbar sprain).

6. A 56-year-old male steelworker comes to you complaining of low back pain that was brought on when he slipped on ice and twisted his trunk while trying to avoid falling. The injury occurred 2 days earlier, and he has right-sided sciatica. X-rays show some lipping at L4–L5 and L5–S1 with slight narrowing of the L5 disc. He has difficulty bending forward. Describe your assessment plan for this patient (lumbar spondylosis vs. acute lumbar disc herniation).

7. A 28-year-old male had a laminectomy for a herniated L5 disc 2 days earlier. He is still an inpatient. Describe your assessment plan for this patient.

8. A 32-year-old male comes to you complaining of back pain and stiffness, especially with activity. He has a desk job and has no history of unusual activity. Describe your assessment plan for this patient (chronic lumbar sprain vs. lumbar spina bifida occulta).

9. A 39-year-old male electrician comes to you complaining of back pain after a motor vehicle accident in which he was hit from behind while stopped for a red light. The accident occurred 3 days earlier. Describe your assessment program for this patient (lumbar sprain vs. lumbar stenosis).

10. A 26-year-old female comes to you complaining of low back pain. She appears to have a functional leg length difference. Describe your assessment plan for this patient (lumbar sprain vs. congenital anomaly).

TABLE **9.21**

Differential Diagnosis of Lumbar Strain and Posterolateral Lumbar Disc Herniation at L5 to S1

	Lumbar Strain	Lumbar Disc (L5–S1)
History	Mechanism of injury: flexion, side flexion, and/or rotation under load or without control	Quick movement into flexion, rotation, side flexion, or extension (may or may not be under load)
Pain	In lumbar spine, may be referred into buttocks May increase with extension (muscle contraction) or flexion (stretch)	In lumbar spine with referral into posterior leg to foot (radicular pain) Increases with extension
Observation	Scoliosis may be present Muscle spasm	Scoliosis may be present Muscle guarding
Active movement	Pain especially on stretch (flexion, side flexion, and rotation) Pain on unguarded movement Limited ROM	Pain especially on extension and flexion Side flexion and rotation may be affected Limited ROM
Resisted isometric movement	Pain on muscle contraction (often minimal pain) Myotomes normal	Minimal pain unless large protrusion L5–S1 myotomes may be affected
Special tests	Neurological tests negative	SLR and slump test often positive
Sensation	Normal	L5–S1 dermatomes may be affected
Reflexes	Normal	L5–S1 reflexes may be affected
Joint play	Muscle guarding	Muscle guarding

ROM, Range of motion; *SLR*, straight leg raising.

References

1. Deyo RA, Phillips WR. Low back pain: a primary care challenge. *Spine*. 1996;21:2826–2832.
2. Frymoyer JW, Akeson W, Brandt K, et al. Clinical perspectives. In: Frymoyer JW, Gordon SL, eds. *New Perspectives in Low Back Pain*. Park Ridge, IL: American Academy of Orthopedic Surgeons; 1989.
3. Waddell G. *The Back Pain Revolution*. New York: Churchill Livingstone; 1998.
4. Beattie P. Current understanding of lumbar intervertebral disc degeneration: a review with emphasis upon etiology, pathophysiology, and lumbar magnetic resonance imaging findings. *J Orthop Sports Phys Ther*. 2008;38:329–340.
5. Hu SS, Tribus CB, Diab M, et al. Spondylolisthesis and spondylolysis. *J Bone Joint Surg Am*. 2008;90:656–671.
6. Taylor JR, Twomey LT. Structure and function of lumbar zygapophyseal (facet) joints. In: Boyling JD, Palastanga N, eds. *Grieve's Modern Manual Therapy: The Vertebral Column*. 2nd ed. Edinburgh: Churchill Livingstone; 1994.
7. Iwamoto J, Abe H, Tsukimura Y, et al. Relationship between radiographic abnormalities of lumbar spine and incidence of low back pain in high school and college football players: a prospective study. *Am J Sports Med*. 2004;32:781–786.
8. Fujiwana A, Tamai K, Yoshida H, et al. Anatomy of the iliolumbar ligament. *Clin Orthop Relat Res*. 2000;380:167–172.
9. Aihara T, Takahashi K, Yamagata M, et al. Does the iliolumbar ligament prevent anterior displacement of the fifth lumbar vertebra with defects of the pars? *J Bone Joint Surg Br*. 2000;82:846–850.

10. Kramer J. *Intervertebral Disk Disease: Causes, Diagnosis, Treatment and Prophylaxis*. Chicago: Year Book Medical; 1981.
11. Farfan HF. *Mechanical Disorders of the Low Back*. Philadelphia: Lea & Febiger; 1973.
12. Roughley PJ. Biology of intervertebral disc aging and degeneration – involvement of the extra cellular matrix. *Spine*. 2004;29(23):2691–2699.
13. Urban JP, Roberts S. Degeneration of the intervertebral disc. *Arthr Res Ther*. 2003;5(3):120–130.
14. da Silva Batista J, de Vasconcellos Fontes RB, Liberti EA. Aging and degeneration of the intervertebral disc: review of basic science. *Coluna/Columna*. 2015;14(2):144–148.
15. Coventry MB, Ghormley RK, Kernohan JW. The intervertebral disc: its microscopic anatomy and pathology. Part I: Anatomy, development and physiology; Part II: Changes in the intervertebral disc concomitant with age; Part III: Pathological changes in the intervertebral disc. *J Bone Joint Surg*. 1945;27:105 (Part I), 233 (Part II), 460 (Part III).
16. Rodriquez AG, Slichter CK, Acosta FL, et al. Human disc nucleus properties and vertebral endplate permeability. *Spine*. 2011;36(7):512–520.
17. Bogduk N. The innervation of the lumbar spine. *Spine*. 1983;8:286–293.
18. Edgar MA, Ghadially JA. Innervation of the lumbar spine. *Clin Orthop*. 1976;115:35–41.
19. Vernon-Roberts B, Moore RJ, Fraser RD. The natural history of age-related disc degeneration—the pathology and sequelae of tears. *Spine*. 2007;32:2797–2804.
20. Ledsome JR, Lessoway V, Susak LE, et al. Diurnal changes in lumbar intervertebral distance, measured using ultrasound. *Spine*. 1996;21:1671–1675.

21. Saal JA. Natural history and nonoperative treatment of lumbar disc herniation. *Spine*. 1996;21(24S):2S–9S.
22. Macnab I. *Backache*. Baltimore: Williams & Wilkins; 1977.
23. Spector LR, Madigan L, Rhyme A, et al. Cauda equina syndrome. *J Am Acad Orthop Surg*. 2008;16:471–479.
24. Takahashi K, Shima I, Porter RW. Nerve root pressure in lumbar disc herniation. *Spine*. 1999;24:2003–2006.
25. Nachemson A, Morris JM. In vivo measurements of intradiscal pressure. *J Bone Joint Surg Am*. 1964;46:1077–1092.
26. Nachemson A, Elfstrom C. Intravital dynamic pressure measurements in lumbar discs. *Scand J Rehabil Med*. 1970;(suppl 1):5–40.
27. Madigan L, Vaccaro AR, Spector LR, et al. Management of symptomatic lumbar degenerative disc disease. *J Am Acad Orthop Surg*. 2009;17:102–111.
28. Rubinstein SM, Van Tulder M. A best-evidence review of diagnostic procedures for neck and low-back pain. *Best Pract Res Clin Rheumatol*. 2008;22(3):471–482.
29. Atlas SJ, Nardin RA. Evaluation and treatment of low back pain: an evidence-based approach to clinical care. *Muscle Nerve*. 2003;27:265–284.
30. Kim I, Jeong S, Hong S, et al. External iliac artery rupture presenting with lumbar herniated disc. *J Emerg Med*. 2013;44(1):e131–e132.
31. Deyo RA, Rainville J, Kent DL. What can the history and physical examination tell us about low back pain? *J Am Med Assoc*. 1992;268:760–765.
32. Hall H. A simple approach to back pain management. *Patient Care*. 1992;15:77–91.
33. Walsh M. Evaluation of orthopedic testing of the low back for nonspecific low back pain. *J Manip Physiol Ther*. 1998;21:232–236.

34. Leboeuf-Yde C, Kyuik KO. Is it possible to differentiate people with or without low back pain on the basis of tests of lumbopelvic dysfunction? *J Manip Physiol Ther*. 2000;23:160–167.

35. Vroomen PC, de Krom MC, Knottnerus JA. Consistency of history taking and physical examination in patients with suspected lumbar nerve root involvement. *Spine*. 2000;25:91–97.

36. Frymoyer JW. Epidemiology. In: Frymoyer JW, Gordon SL, eds. *New Perspectives in Low Back Pain*. Park Ridge, IL: American Academy of Orthopedic Surgeons; 1989.

37. White AA. The 1980 symposium and beyond. In: Frymoyer JW, Gordon SL, eds. *New Perspectives in Low Back Pain*. Park Ridge, IL: American Academy of Orthopedic Surgeons; 1989.

38. Luoma K, Riihimaki H, Luukkonen R, et al. Low back pain in relation to lumbar disc degeneration. *Spine*. 2000;25:487–492.

39. Videman T, Battié MC. The influence of occupational on lumbar degeneration. *Spine*. 1999;24:1164–1168.

40. Richardson JK, Chung T, Schultz JS, et al. A familial predisposition toward lumbar disc injury. *Spine*. 1997;22:1487–1493.

41. Wilder DG, Pope MH, Frymoyer FW. The biomechanics of lumbar disc herniation and the effect of overload and instability. *J Spinal Dis*. 1988;1:16–32.

42. Luoto S, Taimela S, Hurri H, et al. Psychomotor speed and postural control in chronic low back pain patients: a controlled follow-up study. *Spine*. 1996;21:2621–2627.

43. Stewart J, Kempenaar L, Lanchlin D. Rethinking yellow flags. *Man Ther*. 2011;16:196–198.

44. Brodke DS, Ritter SM. Nonoperative management of low back pain and lumbar disc degeneration. *J Bone Joint Surg Am*. 2004;86:1810–1818.

45. Young S, Aprill C. Characteristics of a mechanical assessment for chronic lumbar facet joint pain. *J Man Manip Ther*. 2000;8:78–84.

46. Ombregt L. *A System of Orthopedic Medicine*. 3rd ed. Edinburgh: Churchill Livingstone; 2013.

47. McKenzie RA. *The Lumbar Spine: Mechanical Diagnosis and Therapy*. Waikanae, New Zealand: Spinal Publications; 1981.

48. Donelson R, Aprill C, Metcalf R, et al. A prospective study of centralization of lumbar and referred pain: a predictor of symptomatic discs and annular competence. *Spine*. 1997;22:1115–1122.

49. Long AL. The centralization phenomenon: its usefulness as a predictor of outcome in conservative treatment of chronic low back pain (a pilot study). *Spine*. 1995;20:2513–2521.

50. Aina A, May S, Clare H. The centralization phenomenon of spinal symptoms: a systematic review. *Man Ther*. 2004;9(3):134–143.

51. Skyttle L, May S, Petersen P. Centralization: its prognostic value in patients with referred symptoms and sciatica. *Spine*. 2005;30:E293–E299.

52. Yoo JU, McIver TC, Hiratzka J, et al. The presence of Waddell signs depends on age and gender, not diagnosis. *Bone Joint J*. 2018;100-B(2):219–225.

53. Mooney V. Where does the pain come from? *Spine*. 1987;12:754.

54. Vucetic N, Maattanen H, Svensson O. Pain and pathology in lumbar disc hernia. *Clin Orthop Relat Res*. 1995;320:65–72.

55. Greenwood MJ, Erhard RE, Jones DL. Differential diagnosis of the hip vs lumbar spine: five case reports. *J Orthop Sports Phys Ther*. 1998;27:308–315.

56. Stoddard A. *Manual of Osteopathic Practice*. New York: Harper & Row; 1970.

57. Lord MJ, Small JM, Dinsay JM, et al. Effects of sitting and standing. *Spine*. 1997;22:2571–2574.

58. Liss H, Liss D. History and past medical history. In: Cole AJ, Herring SA, eds. *The Low Back Pain Handbook*. Philadelphia: Hanley & Belfus; 1997.

59. Bendix T, Sorenson SS, Klausen K. Lumbar curve, trunk muscles, and line of gravity with different heel heights. *Spine*. 1984;9:223–227.

60. Shapiro S. Medical realities of cauda equina syndrome secondary to lumbar disc herniation. *Spine*. 2000;25:348–352.

61. Ahn UM, Ahn N, Buchowski JM, et al. Cauda equina syndrome secondary to lumbar disc herniation. *Spine*. 2000;25:1515–1522.

62. Hides JA, Stokes MH, Saide M, et al. Evidence of lumbar multifidus muscle wasting ipsilateral to symptoms in patients with acute/subacute low back pain. *Spine*. 1994;19:165–172.

63. Bishop A, Foster NE. Do physical therapists in the United Kingdom recognize psychosocial factors in patients with acute low back pain. *Spine*. 2005;30:1316–1322.

64. Antony MM, Bieling PJ, Cox BJ, et al. Psychometric properties of the 42-item and 21-item versions of the depression anxiety stress scales in clinical groups and a community sample. *Psych Assess*. 1998;10:176–181.

65. Brown TA, Chorpita BF, Korotitsch W, et al. Psychometric properties of the depression anxiety stress scales (DASS) in clinical samples. *Behav Res Ther*. 1997;35:79–89.

66. Lovibond PF, Lovibond SH. The structure of negative emotional states: comparison of the expression anxiety stress scales (DASS) with the Beck depression and anxiety inventories. *Behav Res Ther*. 1995;33:335–343.

67. Waddell G, McCulloch J, Kummel E. Nonorganic physical signs in low back pain. *Spine*. 1980;5:117–125.

68. Accident Compensation Corp. *New Zealand Acute Low Back Pain Guide*. Wellington, New Zealand: New Zealand Guidelines Groups; 2004.

69. Waddell G, Newton M, Henderson I, et al. A fear-avoidance questionnaire (FABQ) and the role of fear avoidance beliefs in chronic low back pain and disability. *Pain*. 1993;52:157–168.

70. Moran RW, Rushworth WM, Mason J. Investigation of four self-report instruments (FABT, TSK-HC, Back-PAQ, HC-PAIRS) to measure healthcare practitioners' attitudes and beliefs toward low back pain: reliability, convergent validity and survey of New Zealand osteopaths and manipulative physiotherapists. *Musculoskelet Sci Pract*. 2017;32:44–50.

71. Swinkels-Meewisse EJ, Swinkels RA, Verbeek AL, et al. Psychometric properties of the Tampa Scale for Kinesiophobia and the fear-avoidance beliefs questionnaire in acute low back pain. *Man Ther*. 2003;8(1):29–36.

72. Roelofs J, Goubert L, Peters ML, et al. The Tampa Scale for Kinesiophobia: further examination of psychometric properties in patients with chronic low back pain and fibromyalgia. *Eur J Pain*. 2004;8(5):495–502.

73. Weermeijer JD, Meulders A. Clinimetrics: Tampa scale for kinesiophobia. *J Physiother*. 2018;64(2):126.

74. Miller RP, Kori SH, Todd DD. The Tampa Scale: a measure of kinesiophobia. *Clin J Pain*. 1991;7(1):51–52.

75. Damsgard E, Fors T, Anke A, Roe C. The Tampa Scale of Kinesiophobia: a Rasch analysis of its properties in subjects with low back and more widespread pain. *J Rehabil Med*. 2007;39:672–678.

76. Linton SJ, Hallden K. Can we screen for problematic back pain? A screening questionnaire for predicting outcome in acute and subacute low back pain. *Clin J Pain*. 1998;14(3):209–215.

77. Vlaeyen JW, Kole-Snijders AM, Boeren RG, et al. Fear of movement/(re)injury in chronic low back pain and its relation to behavioral performance. *Pain*. 1995;62:363–372.

78. Asmundson GJ, Norton PJ, Norton GR. Beyond pain: the role of fear and avoidance of chronicity. *Clin Psych Rev*. 1999;19:97–119.

79. McCracken LM, Gross RT, Aikens J, et al. The assessment of anxiety and fear in persons with chronic pain: a comparison of instruments. *Behav Res Ther*. 1996;34:927–933.

80. Fritz JM, George SZ, Delitto A. The role of fear avoidance beliefs in acute low back: relationships with current and future disability and work status. *Pain*. 2001;94:7–15.

81. Crombez G, Vlaeyen JW, Heuts PH, et al. Pain-related fear is more disabling than pain itself: evidence on the role of pain related fear in chronic back pain disability. *Pain*. 1999;80:329–359.

82. Vlaeyen JW, Crombez G. Fear of movement/(re)injury, avoidance and pain disability in chronic low back pain patients. *Man Ther*. 1999;4:187–195.

83. Walsh DA, Radcliffe JC. Pain beliefs and perceived physical disability of patients with chronic low back pain. *Pain*. 2002;97:23–31.

84. New Zealand National Advisory Committee on Health and Disability and New Zealand Accident Compensation Corp. *Guide to Assessing Psychosocial Yellow Flags in Acute Low Back Pain*; 1997. Wellington, New Zealand.

85. Haggman S, Maher CG, Refshauge KM. Screening for symptoms of depression by physical therapists managing low back pain. *Phys Ther*. 2004;84:1157–1166.

86. Kroenke K, Spitzer RL, Williams JB. The patient health questionnaire-2: validity of a two-item depression screener. *Med Care*. 2003;41:1284–1292.

87. Grotle M, Brox JI, Veierod MB, et al. Clinical course and prognostic factors in acute low back pain: patients consulting primary care for the first time. *Spine*. 2005;30:976–982.

88. McGregor AH, Doré CJ, McCarthy ID, et al. Are subjective clinical findings and objective clinical tests related to motion characteristics of low back pain subjects? *J Orthop Sports Phys Ther*. 1998;28:370–377.

89. Sizer PS, Brismee JM, Cook C. Medical screening for red flags in the diagnosis and management of musculoskeletal spine pain. *Pain Pract*. 2007;7(1):53–71.

90. Maigne R. *Diagnosis and Treatment of Pain of Vertebral Origin*. Baltimore: Williams & Wilkins; 1996.

91. Evans RC. *Illustrated Essentials in Orthopedic Physical Assessment*. St Louis: Mosby; 1994.

92. Nelson-Wong E, Flynn T, Callaghan JP. Development of acute hip abduction as a screening test for identifying occupational low back pain. *J Orthop Sports Phys Ther*. 2009;39:649–657.

93. Reeves NP, Narendra KS, Cholewicki J. Spine stability: the six blind men and the elephant. *Clin Biomech*. 2007;22(3):266–274.

94. Reeves NP, Narendra KS, Cholewicki J. Spine stability lessons from balancing a stick. *Clin Biomech*. 2011;26:325–330.

95. Key J. 'The core': understanding it, and retraining its dysfunction. *J Bodywork Mov Ther*. 2013;17:541–559.

96. Meadows JT. *Orthopedic Differential Diagnosis in Physical Therapy: A Case Study Approach*. New York: McGraw-Hill; 1999.

97. Matsui H, Ohmori K, Kanamori M, et al. Significance of sciatic scoliotic list in operated patients with lumbar disc herniation. *Spine*. 1998;23:338–342.

98. Jull G, Janda V. Muscles and motor control in low back pain. In: Twomey LT, Taylor JR, eds. *Physical Therapy for the Low Back*. New York: Churchill Livingstone; 1987.

99. Schink MB. Muscle imbalance patterns associated with low back pain syndromes. In: Watkins RG, ed. *The Spine in Sports*. St Louis: Mosby; 1996.

100. Matson DD, Woods RP, Campbell JB, et al. Diastematomyelia (congenital clefts of the spinal cord). *Pediatrics*. 1950;6:98–112.

101. Allbrook D. Movements of the lumbar spinal column. *J Bone Joint Surg Br*. 1957;39:339–345.

102. Moll JMH, Wright V. Normal range of spinal mobility: an objective clinical study. *Ann Rheum Dis*. 1971;30:381–386.

103. Moll J, Wright V. Measurement of spinal movement. In: Jayson M, ed. *The Lumbar Spine and Back Pain*. New York: Grune & Stratton; 1976.

104. Pennal GF, Conn GS, McDonald G, et al. Motion studies of the lumbar spine. *J Bone Joint Surg Br*. 1972;54:442–452.

105. Tanz SS. Motion of the lumbar spine: a roentgenologic study. *Am J Roentgenol*. 1953;69:399–412.

106. Okawa A, Shinomiya K, Komori H, et al. Dynamic motion study of the whole lumbar spine by videofluoroscopy. *Spine*. 1998;23:1743–1749.

107. Vucetic N, Svensson O. Physical signs in lumbar disc hernia. *Clin Orthop Relat Res*. 1996;333:192–201.

108. Kirkaldy-Willis WH. *Managing Low Back Pain*. New York: Churchill-Livingstone; 1983.

109. Fujiwara A, Lim TH, An HS, et al. The effect of disc degeneration and facet joint osteoarthritis on the segmental flexibility of the lumbar spine. *Spine*. 2000;25:3036–3044.

110. Paris WV. Physical signs of instability. *Spine*. 1985;10:277–279.

111. Ogon M, Bender BR, Hooper DM, et al. A dynamic approach to spinal instability: part II hesitation and giving-way during interspinal motion. *Spine*. 1997;22:2859–2866.

112. Schneider G, Pearcy MJ, Bogduk N. Abnormal motion in spondylolytic spondylolisthesis. *Spine*. 2005;30:1159–1164.

113. Dobbs AC. Evaluation of instabilities of the lumbar spine. *Orthop Phys Ther Clin North Am*. 1999;8:387–400.

114. Porter JL, Wilkinson A. Lumbar-hip flexion motion: a comparative study between asymptomatic and chronic low back pain in 18 to 36 year old men. *Spine*. 1997;22:1508–1514.

115. Bourdillon JF, Day EA. *Spinal Manipulation*. London: Wm Heinemann Medical Books; 1987.

116. Dobbs R, May S, Hope P. The validity of a clinical test for the diagnosis of lumbar spinal stenosis. *Man Ther*. 2016;25:27–34.

117. Mulvein K, Jull G. Kinematic analyses of the lumbar lateral flexion and lumbar lateral shift movement techniques. *J Man Manip Ther*. 1995;3:104–109.

118. Edwards BC. Clinical assessment: the use of combined movements in assessment and treatment. In: Twomey LT, Taylor JR, eds. *Physical Therapy of The Low Back: Clinics in Physical Therapy*. Edinburgh: Churchill Livingstone; 1987.

119. Brown L. An introduction to the treatment and examination of the spine by combined movements. *Physiotherapy*. 1988;74:347–353.

120. Watkins RG. Lumbar spine injuries. In: Watkins RG, ed. *The Spine in Sports*. St Louis: Mosby; 1996.

121. Hourigan CL, Bassett JM. Facet syndrome: clinical signs, symptoms, diagnosis, and treatment. *J Manip Physiol Ther*. 1989;12:293–297.

122. Lippitt AB. The facet joint and its role in spine pain management with facet joint injections. *Spine*. 1984;9:746–750.

123. Wallace LA. Limb length difference and back pain. In: Grieve GP, ed. *Modern Manual Therapy of the Vertebral Column*. Edinburgh: Churchill Livingstone; 1986.

124. Moreau CE, Green BN, Johnson CD, et al. Isometric back extension endurance tests: a review of the literature. *J Manip Physiol Ther*. 2001;24:110–122.

125. Moreland J, Finch E, Stratord P, et al. Interrater reliability of six tests of trunk muscle function and endurance. *J Orthop Sports Phys Ther*. 1997;26:200–208.

126. Ito T, Shirado O, Suzuki H, et al. Lumbar trunk muscle endurance testing: an inexpensive alternative to a machine for evaluation. *Arch Phys Med Rehabil*. 1996;77(1):75–79.

127. May S, Littlewood C, Bishop A. Reliability of procedures used in the physical examination of nonspecific low back pain: a systematic review. *Aust J Physiother*. 2006;52(2):91–102.

128. Kendall F. *Muscles, Testing and Function*. 3rd ed. Baltimore: Williams & Wilkins; 1983.

129. Reese NB. *Muscle and Sensory Testing*. Philadelphia: WB Saunders; 1999.

130. Jorgensen K, Nicolaisen T. Trunk extensor endurance: determination and relation to low-back trouble. *Ergonomics*. 1987;30:259–267.

131. McGill S. *Low Back Disorders—Evidence-Based Prevention and Rehabilitation*. Champaign: Human Kinetics; 2002.

132. Ng JK, Richardson CA, Jull GA. Electromyographic amplitude and frequency changes in the iliocostalis lumborum and multifidus muscles during a trunk holding exercise. *Phys Ther*. 1987;77:954–961.

133. Moffroid MT. Endurance of trunk muscles in persons with chronic low back pain: assessment, performance, training. *J Rehab Res Train*. 1997;34:440–447.

134. Clarkson HM. *Musculoskeletal Assessment*. 2nd ed. Philadelphia: Lippincott Williams & Wilkins; 2000.

135. Reese NB. *Muscle and Sensory Testing*. Philadelphia: WB Saunders; 1999.

136. Biering-Sorensen F. Physical measurements as risk indicators for low back trouble over a one-year period. *Spine*. 1984;9:106–109.

137. Latimer J, Maher CG, Refchauge K, et al. The reliability and validity of the Biering-Sorenson test in asymptomatic subjects and subjects reporting current or previous nonspecific low back pain. *Spine*. 1999;24:2085–2090.

138. Demoulin C, Vanderthommen M, Duysens C, Crielaard CM. Spinal muscle evaluation using the Sorensen test: a critical appraisal of the literature. *Joint Bone Spine*. 2006;73(1):43–50.

139. McGill SM, Childs A, Liebenson C. Endurance times for low back stabilization exercises: clinical targets for testing and training from a normal database. *Arch Phys Med Rehabil*. 1999;80:941–944.

140. Simmonds MJ, Olson SL, Jones S, et al. Psychometric characteristics and clinical usefulness of physical performance tests in patients with low back pain. *Spine*. 1998;23:2412–2421.

141. Youdas JW, Garrett TR, Egan KS, et al. Lumbar lordosis and pelvic inclination in adults with chronic low back pain. *Phys Ther*. 2000;80:261–275.

142. Shields RK, Heiss DG. An electromyographic comparison of abdominal muscle synergies during curl and double straight leg lowering exercises with control of the pelvic position. *Spine*. 1999;22:1873–1879.

143. McGill SM. Low back exercises: evidence for improving exercise regimes. *Phys Ther*. 1998;78:754–765.

144. Smith SS, Mayer TG, Gatchel RJ, et al. Quantification of lumbar function: isometric and multispeed isokinetic trunk strength measures in sagittal and axial planes in normal subjects. *Spine*. 1985;10:757–764.

145. Cyriax J. Textbook for orthopaedic medicine. In: *Diagnosis of Soft Tissue Lesions*. Vol. I. London: Balliere Tindall; 1975.

146. Rainville J, Jouve C, Finno M, et al. Comparison of four tests of quadriceps strength in L3 or L4 radiculopathies. *Spine*. 2003;28(21):2466–2471.

147. Grotle M, Brox JI, Vollestad NK. Functional status and disability questionnaire: what do they assess? A systematic review of back specific outcome questionnaires. *Spine*. 2004;30:130–140.

148. Mayer TG. Assessment of lumbar function. *Clin Orthop*. 1987;221:99–109.

149. Thomas AM. The spine. In: Pynsent P, Fairbank J, Carr A, eds. *Outcome Measures in Orthopedics*. Oxford: Butterworth Heinemann; 1994.

150. Beurskens AJ, de Vet HC, Koke AJ, et al. Measuring the functional status of patients with low back pain. *Spine*. 1995;20:1018–1028.

151. Fairbank JC, Pynsent PB. The Oswestry disability index. *Spine*. 2000;25:2940–2953.

152. Fairbank JC, Cooper J, Davies JB, et al. The Oswestry low back pain disability questionnaire. *Physiotherapy*. 1980;66:271–273.

153. Frost H, Lamb SE, Stewart-Brown S. Responsiveness of a patient specific outcome measure compared with the Oswestry Disability Index v2.1 and Roland and Morris Disability Questionnaire for patients with subacute and chronic low back pain. *Spine*. 2008;33:2450–2457.

154. Kopec JA, Esdaile JM, Abrahamowicz M, et al. The Quebec Back Pain Disability Scale: measurement properties. *Spine*. 1995;20(3):341–352.

155. Davidson M, Keating JL. A comparison of five low back disability questionnaires: reliability and responsiveness. *Phys Ther*. 2002;82(1):8–24.

156. Borenstein DG, Wiesel SW, Boden SD. *Low Back Pain: Medical Diagnosis and Comprehensive Management*. Philadelphia: WB Saunders; 1995.

157. Darlow B, Perry M, Mathieson F, et al. The development and exploratory analysis of the Back Pain Attitudes Questionnaire (Back-PAQ). *BMJ Open*. 2014;4:e005251.

158. Robinson HS, Dagfinrud H. Reliability and screening ability of the StarT Back screening tool in patients with low back pain in physiotherapy practice, a cohort study. *BMC Musculoskelet Disord*. 2017;18:232–239.

159. Hendler N, Mollett A, Talo S, et al. A comparison between the minnesota multiphasic personality inventory and the mensana clinic back pain test for validating the complaint of chronic back pain. *J Occup Med*. 1988;30:98–102.

160. Roland M, Fairbank J. The Roland-Morris Disability Questionnaire and the Oswestry Disability Questionnaire. *Spine*. 2000;25:3115–3124.

161. Stratford PW, Binkley J, Solomon P, et al. Defining the minimum level of detectable change for the Roland-Morris questionnaire. *Phys Ther*. 1996;76:359–365.

162. Stratford PW, Riddle DL. A Roland Morris Disability Questionnaire target value to distinguish between functional and dysfunctional states in people with low back pain. *Physiother Can*. 2016;68(1):29–35.

163. Lyle MA, Manes S, McGuinness M, et al. Relationship of physical examination findings and self-reported symptoms severity and physical function in patients with degenerative lumbar conditions. *Phys Ther*. 2005;85:120–133.

164. Feise RJ, Menke JM. Functional rating index: a new valid and reliable instrument to measure the magnitude of clinical change in spinal conditions. *Spine*. 2001;26:78–87.

165. Chansirinukor W, Maher CG, Latimer J, et al. Comparison of the Functional Rating Index and the 18-item Roland-Morris Disability Questionnaire: responsiveness and reliability. *Spine*. 2005;30(1):141–145.

166. Lawlis GF, Cuencas R, Selby D, et al. The development of the Dallas Pain Questionnaire. *Spine*. 1989;14:511–516.

167. Million R, Hall W, Haavick-Nilsen K, et al. Assessment of the progress of the back pain patient. *Spine*. 1982;7:204–212.

168. Japanese Orthopedic Association. Assessment of treatment of low back pain. *J Jap Orthop Assoc.* 1986;60:909–911.

169. Lehmann TR, Brand RA, German TW. A low back rating scale. *Spine.* 1983;8:308–315.

170. Bolton JE, Breen AC. The Bournemouth questionnaire: a short-form comprehensive outcome measure. I. Psychometric properties in back pain patients. *J Manip Physiol Ther.* 1999;22:503–510.

171. Larsen K, Leboeuf-Yde C. The Bournemouth questionnaire: can it be used to monitor and predict treatment outcome in chiropractic patients with persistent low back pain? *J Manip Physiol Ther.* 2005;28:219–227.

172. Berven S, Deviren V, Demir-Deviren S, et al. Studies in the modified Scoliosis Research Society outcomes instrument in adults: validation, reliability and discriminatory capacity. *Spine.* 2004;28:2164–2169.

173. Haher TR, Group JM, Shin TM, et al. Results of the Scoliosis Research Society instrument for evaluation of surgical outcome in adolescent scoliosis: a multicentre study of 244 patients. *Spine.* 1999;24:1435–1440.

174. Bridwell KH, Cats-Baril W, Harrast J, et al. The validity of the SRS-22 instrument in an adult spinal deformity population compared with Oswestry and SF12. *Spine.* 2005;30:455–461.

175. Stucki G, Daltroy L, Lang MH, et al. Measurement properties of a self-administered outcome measure in lumbar spinal stenosis. *Spine.* 1996;21:796–803.

176. Williams NH, Wilkinson C, Russell IT. Extending the Aberdeen back pain scale to include the whole spine: a set of outcome measures for the neck, upper and lower back. *Pain.* 2001;94:261–274.

177. Novy DM, Collins HS, Nelson DV, et al. Waddell signs: distributional properties and correlates. *Acta Phys Med Rehabil.* 1998;79(7):820–822.

178. Weaver CS, Kvaal SA, McCracken L. Waddell signs as behavioral indicators of depression and anxiety in chronic pain. *J Back Musculoskel Rehabil.* 2003;17:21–26.

179. Burton AK, Tillotson KM, Main CJ, et al. Psychosocial predictors of outcome in acute and subacute low back trouble. *Spine.* 1995;20:722–728.

180. Gatchel RJ, Polatin PB, Mayer TG. The dominant role of psychosocial risk factors in the development of chronic low back pain disability. *Spine.* 1995;20:2702–2709.

181. Harding VR, Williams AC, Richardson PH, et al. The development of a battery of measures for assessing physical functioning of chronic pain patients. *Pain.* 1994;58:367–375.

182. Marras WS, Wongsamm PE. Flexibility and velocity of normal and impaired lumbar spine. *Arch Phys Med Rehabil.* 1986;67:213–217.

183. Andersson GB, Deyo RA. History and physical examination in patients with herniated lumbar discs. *Spine.* 1996;21(24S):10S–18S.

184. Cook C, Hegedus E. Diagnostic utility of clinical tests for spinal dysfunction. *Man Ther.* 2011;16:21–25.

185. Cook CE, Hegedus EJ. *Orthopedic Physical Examination Tests—An Evidence Based Approach.* Upper Saddle River, NJ: Prentice Hall/Pearson; 2008.

186. Hestbaek L, Leboeuf-Yde C. Are chiropractic tests for the lumbo-pelvic spine reliable and valid? A systematic critical literature review. *J Manip Physiol Ther.* 2000;23:258–266.

187. Deville WL, van der Windt DA, Dzaferagic A, et al. The test of Lasègue: systematic review of the accuracy in diagnosing herniated discs. *Spine.* 2000;25:1140–1147.

188. Strender LE, Sjoblom A, Sundell K, et al. Interexaminer reliability in physical examination of patients with low back pain. *Spine.* 1997;22:814–820.

189. McCarthy CJ, Gittins M, Roberts C, et al. The reliability of the clinical tests and questions recommended in international guidelines for low back pain. *Spine.* 2007;32:921–926.

190. Paatelma M, Karvonen E, Heiskanen J. Clinical perspective: how do clinical test results differentiate chronic and subacute low back pain patients from "non-patients"? *J Man Manip Ther.* 2009;17:11–19.

191. Shacklock M. Neurodynamics. *Physiotherapy.* 1995;81:9–16.

192. Butler DA. *Mobilisation of the Nervous System.* Melbourne: Churchill Livingstone; 1991.

193. Vucetic N, Astrand P, Guntner P, et al. Diagnosis and prognosis in lumbar disc herniation. *Clin Orthop Relat Res.* 1999;361:116–122.

194. Slater H, Butler DS, Shacklock MD. The dynamic central nervous system: examination and assessment using tension tests. In: Boyling JD, Palastanga N, eds. *Grieve's Modern Manual Therapy: The Vertebral Column.* 2nd ed. Edinburgh: Churchill Livingstone; 1994.

195. Ridehalgh C, Moore A, Hough A. Normative sciatic nerve excursion during a modified straight leg test. *Man Ther.* 2014;19(1):59–64.

196. Butler D, Gifford L. The concept of adverse mechanical tension in the nervous system. *Physiotherapy.* 1989;75:622–636.

197. Herrington L, Bendix K, Cornwall C, et al. What is the normal response to structural differentiation within the slump and straight leg raise tests? *Man Ther.* 2008;13:289–294.

198. Dommisse GF, Grobler L. Arteries and veins of the lumbar nerve roots and cauda equina. *Clin Orthop.* 1976;115:22–29.

199. Cram RH. A sign of sciatic nerve root pressure. *J Bone Joint Surg Br.* 1953;35:192–195.

200. Brudzinski J. A new sign of the lower extremities in meningitis of children (neck sign). *Arch Neurol.* 1969;21:217.

201. Deyerle WM, May VR. Sciatic tension test. *South Med J.* 1956;49:999–1005.

202. Wartenberg R. The signs of Brudzinski and of Kernig. *J Pediatr.* 1950;37:679–684.

203. Brody IA, Williams RH. The signs of Kernig and Brudzinski. *Arch Neurol.* 1969;21:215.

204. Kernig W. Concerning a little noted sign of meningitis. *Arch Neurol.* 1969;21:216.

205. Dyck P. The femoral nerve traction test with lumbar disc protrusion. *Surg Neurol.* 1976;6:163–166.

206. Kreitz BG, Coté P, Yong-Hing K. Crossed femoral stretching test: a case report. *Spine I.* 1996;21:1584–1586.

207. Katznelson A, Nerubay J, Level A. Gluteal skyline (G.S.L.): a search for an objective sign in the diagnosis of disc lesions of the lower lumbar spine. *Spine.* 1982;7:74–75.

208. Rask M. Knee flexion test and sciatica. *Clin Orthop.* 1978;134:221.

209. Herron LD, Pheasant HC. Prone knee-flexion provocative testing for lumbar disc protrusion. *Spine.* 1980;5:65–67.

210. Postacchini F, Cinotti G, Gumina S. The knee flexion test: a new test for lumbosacral root tension. *J Bone Joint Surg Br.* 1993;75:834–835.

211. Carlsson H, Rasmussen-Barr E. Clinical screening tests for assessing movement control in non-specific low-back pain. A systematic review of intra-and inter-observer reliability studies. *Man Ther.* 2013;18(2):103–110.

212. Davis DS, Anderson IB, Carson MC, et al. Upper limb neural tension and seated slump tests: the false positive rate among healthy young adults without cervical or lumbar symptoms. *J Man Manip Ther.* 2008;16:136–141.

213. Spengler DM. *Low Back Pain: Assessment and Management.* Orlando, FL: Grune & Stratton; 1982.

214. Hudgins WR. The crossed-straight-leg raising test. *N Engl J Med.* 1977;297:1127.

215. Palmer ML, Epler M. *Clinical Assessment Procedures In Physical Therapy.* Philadelphia: JB Lippincott; 1990.

216. Maitland GD. The slump test: examination and treatment. *Aust J Physiother.* 1985;31:215–219.

217. Philip K, Lew P, Matyas TA. The inter-therapist reliability of the slump test. *Aust J Physiother.* 1989;35:89–94.

218. Maitland GD. Negative disc exploration: positive canal signs. *Aust J Physiother.* 1979;25:129–134.

219. Fidel C, Martin E, Dankaerts W, et al. Cervical spine sensitizing maneuvers during the slump test. *J Man Manip Ther.* 1996;4:16–21.

220. Johnson EK, Chiarello CM. The slump test: the effects of head and lower extremity position on knee extension. *J Orthop Sports Phys Ther.* 1997;26:310–317.

221. Breig A, Troup JDG. Biomechanical considerations in straight-leg-raising test: cadaveric and clinical studies of the effects of medical hip rotation. *Spine.* 1979;4:242–250.

222. Charnley J. Orthopedic signs in the diagnosis of disc protrusion with special reference to the straight-leg-raising test. *Lancet.* 1951;1:186–192.

223. Edgar MA, Park WM. Induced pain patterns on passive straight-leg-raising in lower lumbar disc protrusion. *J Bone Joint Surg Br.* 1974;56:658–667.

224. Fahrni WH. Observations on straight-leg-raising with special reference to nerve root adhesions. *Can J Surg.* 1966;9:44–48.

225. Goddard BS, Reid JD. Movements induced by straight-leg-raising in the lumbosacral roots, nerves, and plexus and in the intrapelvic section of the sciatic nerve. *J Neurol Neurosurg Psychiatry.* 1965;28:12–18.

226. Scham SM, Taylor TKF. Tension signs in lumbar disc prolapse. *Clin Orthop.* 1971;75:195–204.

227. Urban LM. The straight-leg-raising test: a review. *J Orthop Sports Phys Ther.* 1981;2:117–133.

228. Wilkins RH, Brody IA. Lasègue's sign. *Arch Neurol.* 1969;21:219–220.

229. Summers B, Malhan K, Cassar-Pullicino V. Low back pain on passive straight leg raising: the anterior theca as a source of pain. *Spine.* 2005;30:342–345.

230. Shiqing X, Quanzhi Z, Dehao F. Significance of the straight-leg-raising test in the diagnosis and clinical evaluation of lower lumbar intervertebral disc protrusion. *J Bone Joint Surg Am.* 1987;69:517–522.

231. Coppieters MW, Crooke JL, Lawrenson PR, et al. A modified straight leg raise test to differentiate between sural nerve pathology and Achilles tendinopathy. A cross-sectional cadaver study. *Man Ther.* 2015;20(4):587–591.

232. Cipriano JJ. *Photographic Manual of Regional Orthopedic Tests.* Baltimore: Williams & Wilkins; 1985.

233. Hall T, Hepburn M, Elvey RL. The effect of lumbosacral posture on a modification of the straight leg raise test. *Physiotherapy.* 1993;79:566–570.

234. Woodhall R, Hayes GJ. The well-leg-raising test of Fajersztajn in the diagnosis of ruptured lumbar intervertebral disc. *J Bone Joint Surg Am.* 1950;32:786–792.

235. Khuffash B, Porter RW. Cross leg pain and trunk list. *Spine.* 1989;14:602–603.

236. Kotilainen K, Valtonen S. Clinical instability of the lumbar spine after microdiscectomy. *Acta Neurochir.* 1993;125:120–126.

237. Pope MH, Frymoyer JW, Krag MH. Diagnosing instability. *Clin Orthop Relat Res.* 1992;279:60–67.

238. Fritz JM, Erhard RE, Hagen BF. Segmental instability of the lumbar spine. *Phys Ther.* 1998;78:889–896.

239. Biely SA, Silfies SP, Smith SS, Hicks GE. Clinical observation of standing trunk movements: what do the aberrant movement patterns tell us? *J Orthop Sports Phys Ther.* 2014;44(4):262–272.

240. Teyhen DS, Flynn TW, Childs JD, et al. Fluoroscopic video to identify aberrant lumbar motions. *Spine.* 2007;32(7):E220–E229.

241. Wattananon P, Ebaugh D, Biely SA, et al. Kinematic characterization of clinically observed aberrant movement patterns in patients with non-specific low back pain: a cross-sectional study. *BMC Musculoskelet Disord18.* 2017;(1):455–467.

242. Kasai Y, Morishita K, Kawakita E, et al. A new evaluation method for lumbar spinal instability: passive lumbar extension test. *Phys Ther.* 2006;86:1661–1667.

243. Alqarni AM, Schneiders AG, Hendrick PA. Clinical tests to diagnose lumbar segmental instability: a systematic review. *J Orthop Sports Phys Ther.* 2011;41:130–140.

244. Ferrani S, Manni T, Bonetti F, et al. A literature review of clinical tests for lumbar instability in low back pain: validity and applicability in clinical practice. *Chiropr Man Ther.* 2015;23:14–26.

245. Kirkaldy-Willis WH. *Managing Low Back Pain.* Edinburgh: Churchill Livingstone; 1983.

246. Hicks GE, Fritz JM, Delitto A, McGill SM. Preliminary development of a clinical prediction rule for determining which patients with low back pain will respond to a stabilization exercise program. *Arch Phys Med Rehabil.* 2005;86(9):1753–1762.

247. Bruno PA, Goertzen DA, Millar DP. Patient-reported perception of difficulty as a clinical indicator of dysfunctional neuromuscular control during the prone extension test and active straight leg raise test. *Man Ther.* 2014;19(6):602–607.

248. Wadsworth CT, DeFabio RF, Johnson D. The spine. In: Wadsworth CT, ed. *Manual Examination and Treatment of the Spine and Extremities.* Baltimore: Williams & Wilkins; 1988.

249. Hicks GE, Fritz JM, Delitto A, et al. Interrater reliability of clinical examination measures for identification of lumbar segmental instability. *Arch Phys Med Rehabil.* 2003;84:1858–1864.

250. Ravenna MM, Hoffman SL, Van Dillen LR. Low interrater reliability of examiners performing the prone instability test: a clinical test for lumbar shear instability. *Arch Phys Med Rehabil.* 2011;92(6):913–919.

251. Wilde VE, Ford JJ, McMeeken JM. Indicators of lumbar zygapophyseal joint pain: survey of an expert panel with the Delphi Technique. *Phys Ther.* 2007;87(10):1348–1361.

252. Garrick JG, Webb DR. *Sports Injuries: Diagnosis and Management.* Philadelphia: WB Saunders; 1990.

253. Jackson DW, Ciullo JV. Injuries of the spine in the skeletally immature athlete. In: Nicholas JA, Hershmann EB, eds. *The Lower Extremity and Spine in Sports Medicine.* Vol 2. St Louis: Mosby; 1986.

254. Jackson DW, Wiltse LL, Dingeman RD, et al. Stress reactions involving the pars interarticularis in young athletes. *Am J Sports Med.* 1981;9:304–312.

255. Stuber K, Lerede C, Kristmanson K, et al. The diagnostic accuracy of the Kemp's test: a systematic review. *J Can Chiropr Assoc.* 2014;58(3):258–267.

256. Corrigan B, Maitland GD. *Practical Orthopedic Medicine.* London: Butterworths; 1985.

257. Little H. *The Neck and Back: The Rheumatological Physical Examination.* Orlando, FL: Grune & Stratton; 1986.

258. Post M. *Physical Examination of the Musculoskeletal System.* Chicago: Year Book Medical; 1987.

259. Bohannon RW, Steffl M, Glenney SS, et al. The prone bridge test: performance, validity, and reliability among older and younger adults. *J Body Mov Ther.* 2018;22(2):385–389.

260. Reece JD. *Development of a Prone Bridge Test As a Measurement of Abdominal Stability in Healthy Adults;* 2009. https://scholarsarchive.byu.edu/etd/1845.

261. Andrade JA, Figueiredo LC, Santos TR, et al. Reliability of transverse plane pelvic alignment measurement during the bridge test with unilateral knee extension. *Rev Bras Fisioter.* 2012;16(4):268–274.

262. Brumitt J, Matheson JW, Meira EP. Core stabilization exercise prescription, Part 1: current concepts in assessment and intervention. *Sports Health.* 2013;5(6):504–509.

263. Blou JN, Logue V. Intermittent claudication of the cauda equina. *Lancet* (May). 1961:1081–1085.

264. Dyck P, Pheasant HC, Doyle JB, et al. Intermittent cauda equina compression syndrome. *Spine.* 1977;2:75–81.

265. Floman Y, Wiesel SW, Rothman RH. Cauda equina syndrome presenting as a herniated lumbar disc. *Clin Orthop Relat Res.* 1980;147:234–237.

266. Wilson CB, Ehni G, Grollmus J. Neurogenic intermittent claudication. *Clin Neurosurg.* 1970;18:62–85.

267. Laslett M. Bilateral buttock pain caused by aortic stenosis: a case report of claudication of the buttock. *Man Ther.* 2000;5:227–233.

268. Kikuchi S, Watanabe E, Hasue M. Spinal intermittent claudication due to cervical and thoracic degenerative spine disease. *Spine.* 1996;21:313–318.

269. Dyck P, Doyle JB. "Bicycle test" of van Gelderen in diagnosis of intermittent cauda equina compression syndrome. *J Neurosurg.* 1977;46:667–670.

270. Dyck P. The stoop-test in lumbar entrapment radiculopathy. *Spine.* 1979;4:89–92.

271. Deen HG, Zimmerman RS, Lyons MK, et al. Use of an exercise treadmill to measure baseline functional status and surgical outcome in patients with severe spinal stenosis. *Spine.* 1998;23:244–248.

272. Tokuhashi Y, Matsuzaki H, Sano S. Evaluation of clinical lumbar instability using the treadmill. *Spine.* 1993;18:2321–2324.

273. Archibald KC, Wiechec F. A reappraisal of Hoover's test. *Arch Phys Med Rehabil.* 1970;51:234–238.

274. Arieff AJ, Tigay El, Kurtz JF, et al. The Hoover sign: an objective sign of pain and/or weakness in the back or lower extremities. *Arch Neurol.* 1961;5:673–678.

275. Hoover CF. A new sign for the detection of malingering and functional paresis of the lower extremities. *JAMA.* 1980;51:746–747.

276. Chang RF, Mubarak SJ. Pathomechanics of Gower's sign: a video analysis of a spectrum of Gower's maneuvers. *Clin Orthop Relat Res.* 2012;470(7):1987–1991.

277. Gurney B, Boissonault WG, Andrews R. Differential diagnosis of a femoral neck/head stress fracture. *J Orthop Sports Phys Ther.* 2006;36:80–88.

278. Dyck P, Pheasant HC, Doyle JB, et al. Intermittent cauda equina compression syndrome. *Spine.* 1977;2:75–81.

279. Joffe R, Appleby A, Arjona V. Intermittent ischemia of the cauda equina due to stenosis of the lumbar canal. *J Neurol Neurosurg Psychiatry.* 1966;29:315–318.

280. Hoppenfeld S. *Physical Examination of the Spine and Extremities.* New York: Appleton-Century-Crofts; 1976.

281. Travell JG, Simons DG. *Myofascial Pain and Dysfunction: The Trigger Point Manual.* Baltimore: Williams & Wilkins; 1983.

282. Pecina MM, Krmpotic-Nemanic J, Markiewitz AD. *Tunnel Syndromes.* Boca Raton, FL: CRC Press; 1991.

283. Haneline MT, Cooperstein R, Young M, et al. Spinal motion palpation: a comparison of studies that assessed intersegmental end feel vs excursion. *J Manip Physiol Ther.* 2008;31:616–626.

284. Inscoe EL, Witt PL, Gross MT, et al. Reliability in evaluating passive intervertebral motion of the lumbar spine. *J Man Manip Ther.* 1995;3:135–143.

285. Maitland GD. Examination of the lumbar spine. *Aust J Physiother.* 1971;17:5–11.

286. Latimer J, Holland M, Lee M, et al. Plinth padding and measures of posteroanterior lumbar stiffness. *J Manip Physiol Ther.* 1997;20:315–319.

287. Edmonston SJ, Allison GT, Gregg CD, et al. Effect of position on the posteroanterior stiffness of the lumbar spine. *Man Ther.* 1998;3:21–26.

288. Binkley J, Stratford PW, Gill C. Interrater reliability of lumbar accessory motion mobility testing. *Phys Ther.* 1995;75:786–795.

289. Parkinson S, Campbell A, Dankaerts W, et al. Upper and lower lumbar segments move differently during sit-to-stand. *Man Ther.* 2013;18(5):390–394.

290. Fullenlove TM, Williams AJ. Comparative roentgen findings in symptomatic and asymptomatic backs. *Radiology.* 1957;68:572–574.

291. Gillespie HW. The significance of congenital lumbosacral abnormalities. *Br J Radiol.* 1949;22:270–275.

292. Magora A, Schwartz A. Relation between the low back pain syndrome and x-ray findings. *Scand J Rehabil Med.* 1978;10:135–145.

293. Southworth JD, Bersack SR. Anomalies of the lumbosacral vertebrae in five hundred and fifty individuals without symptoms referable to the low back. *Am J Roentgenol.* 1950;64:624–634.

294. Tulsi RS. Sacral arch defect and low backache. *Australas Radiol.* 1974;18:43–50.

295. Willis TA. An analysis of vertebral anomalies. *Am J Surg.* 1929;6:163–168.

296. Willis TA. Lumbosacral anomalies. *J Bone Joint Surg Am.* 1959;41:935–938.

297. Macnab I. The traction spur: an indicator of segmental instability. *J Bone Joint Surg Am.* 1971;53:663–670.

298. Friberg O. Functional radiography of the lumbar spine. *Ann Med.* 1989;21:341–346.

299. Boden SD. The use of radiographic imaging studies in the evaluation of patients who have degenerative disorders of the lumbar spine. *J Bone Joint Surg Am.* 1996;78:114–124.

300. Kingston RS. Radiology of the spine. In: Watkins RG, ed. *The Spine in Sports.* St Louis: Mosby; 1996.

301. Boden SD, Wiesel SW. Lumbar spine imaging: role in clinical decision making. *J Am Acad Orthop Surg.* 1996;4:238–248.

302. Jarvik JG, Deyo RA. Diagnostic evaluation of low back pain with emphasis on imaging. *Ann Intern Med.* 2002;137:586–597.

303. Deyo RA, Bigos SJ, Maravilla KR. Diagnostic imaging procedures for the lumbar spine. *Ann Intern Med.* 1989;111:865–868.

304. Timon SJ, Gardner MJ, Wanich T, et al. Not all spondylolisthesis grading instruments are reliable. *Clin Orthop Relat Res.* 2005;434:157–162.

305. Li Y, Hresko MY. Radiographic analysis of spondylolisthesis and sagittal spinopelvic deformity. *J Am Acad Orthop Surg.* 2012;20(4):194–205.

306. Pate D, Goobar J, Resnick D, et al. Traction osteophytes of the lumbar spine: radiographic: pathologic correlation. *Radiology.* 1988;166:843–846.

307. Bigg-Wither G, Kelly P. Diagnostic imaging in musculoskeletal physiotherapy. In: Refshauge K, Gass E, eds. *Musculoskeletal Physiotherapy: Clinical Science and Practice.* Oxford: Butterworth Heinemann; 1995.

308. Wood KB, Popp CA, Transfeldt EE, et al. Radiographic evaluation of instability in spondylolisthesis. *Spine.* 1994;19:1697–1703.

309. Porter RW, Wicks M, Ottewell D. Measurement of the spinal canal by diagnostic ultrasound. *J Bone Joint Surg Br.* 1978;60B(4):481–484.

310. Battié MC, Hansson T, Bigos S, et al. B-scan ultrasonic measurement of the lumbar spinal canal as a predictor of industrial back pain complaints and extended work loss. *J Occup Med.* 1993;35(112):1250–1255.

311. Porter RW, Bewley B. A ten-year prospective study of vertebral canal size as a predictor of back pain. *Spine.* 1994;19(2):173–175.

312. Wilke HJ, Wolf S, Claes LE, et al. Stability increase of the lumbar spine with different muscle groups. A biomechanical in vitro study. *Spine*. 1995;20(2):192–198.

313. Bierry G, Kremer S, Kellner F, et al. Disorders of the paravertebral lumbar muscles: from pathology to cross-sectional imaging. *Skeletal Radiol*. 2008;37(11):967–977.

314. Hides JA, Cooper DH, Stwokes MJ. Diagnostic ultrasound imaging for measurement of the lumbar multifidus muscle in normal young adults. *Physiother Theory Pract*. 1992;8(1):19–26.

315. Stokes M, Rankin G, Newham DJ. Ultrasound imaging of lumbar multifidus muscle: normal reference ranges for measurements and practical guidance on the technique. *Man Ther*. 2005;10(2):116–126.

316. Hides JA, Richardson CA, Jull GA. Magnetic resonance imaging and ultrasonography of the lumbar multifidus muscle. Comparison of two different modalities. *Spine*. 1995;20(1):54–58.

317. Kader DR, Wardlaw D, Smith FW. Correlation between the MRI changes in the lumbar multifidus muscles and leg pain. *Clin Radiol*. 2000;55(2):145–149.

318. Hides JA, Richardson CA, Jull GA. Multifidus muscle recovery is not automatic after resolution of acute, first-episode low back pain. *Spine*. 1996;21(23):2763–2769.

319. Rahmani N, Kiani A, Mohseni-Bandpei MA, Abdollahi I. Multifidus muscle size in adolescents with and without back pain using ultrasonography. *J Body Mov Ther*. 2018;22(1):147–151.

320. Valentin S, Licka T, Elliott J. Age and side-related morphometric MRI evaluation of trunk muscles in people without back pain. *Man Ther*. 2015;20(1):90–95.

321. Wallwork TL, Stanton WR, Freke M, Hides JA. The effect of chronic low back pain on size and contraction of the lumbar multifidus muscle. *Man Ther*. 2009;14(5):496–500.

322. Kanehisa H, Ikegawa S, Fukunaga T. Comparison of muscle cross sectional area and strength between untrained women and men. *Eur J Appl Physiol Occup Physiol*. 1994;68(2):148–154.

323. Maughan RJ, Watson JS, Weir J. Strength and cross-sectional area of human skeletal muscle. *J Physiol*. 1983;338:37–49.

324. Zedka M, Prochazka A, Knight B, et al. Voluntary and reflex control of human back muscles during induced pain. *J Physiol*. 1999;520(2):591–604.

325. Critchley D, Coutts F. Abdominal muscle function in chronic low back pain patients: measurements with real-time ultrasound scanning. *Physiother*. 2002;88(6):322–332.

326. Ainscough-Potts AM, Morrissey MC, Critchley D. The response of the transverse abdominis and internal oblique muscles to different postures. *Man Ther*. 2006;11(1):54–60.

327. De Troyer A, Estenne M, Ninane V, et al. Transversus abdominis muscle function in humans. *J Appl Physiol*. 1990;68(3):1010–1016.

328. Bunce SM, Hough AD, Moore AP. Measurement of abdominal muscle thickness using M-mode ultrasound imaging during functional activities. *Man Ther*. 2004;9(1):41–44.

329. Bunce SM, Moore AP, Hough AD. M-mode ultrasound: a reliable measure of transversus abdominis thickness? *Clin Biomech*. 2002;17(4):315–317.

330. Teyhen DS, Gill NW, Whittaker JL, et al. Rehabilitative ultrasound imaging of the abdominal muscles. *J Orthop Sports Phys Ther*. 2007;37(8):450–466.

331. Rankin G, Stokes M, Newham DJ. Abdominal muscle size and symmetry in normal subjects. *Muscle Nerve*. 2006;34(3):320–326.

332. Cropper J. Regional anatomy and biomechanics. In: Flynn T, ed. *The Thoracic Spine and Rib Cage: Musculoskeletal Evaluation and Treatment*. Newton, MA: Butterworth-Heinemann; 1996.

333. Urquhart DM, Barker PJ, Hodges PW, et al. Regional morphology of the transverse abdominis and obliquus internus and externus abdominis muscles. *Clin Biomech*. 2005;20(3):233–241.

334. Misuri G, Colagrande S, Gorini M, et al. In vivo ultrasound assessment of respiratory function of abdominal muscles in normal subjects. *Eur Respir J*. 1997;10(12):2861–2867.

335. Strohl KP, Mead J, Banzett RB, et al. Regional differences in abdominal muscle activity during various maneuvers in humans. *J Appl Physiol Respir Environ Exerc Physiol*. 1981;51(6):1471–1476.

336. Kiesel KB, Uhl TL, Underwood FB, et al. Measurement of lumbar multifidus muscle contraction with rehabilitative ultrasound imaging. *Man Ther*. 2007;12(2):161–166.

337. Springer BA, Mielcarek BJ, Nesfield TK, Teyhan DS. Relationships among lateral abdominal muscles, gender, body mass index, and hand dominance. *J Orthop Sports Phys Ther*. 2006;36(5):289–297.

338. Teyhen DS, Miltenberger CE, Deiters HM, et al. The use of ultrasound imaging of the abdominal drawing-in maneuver in subjects with low back pain. *J Orthop Sports Phys Ther*. 2005;35(6):346–355.

339. Herzog RJ. The radiologic assessment for a lumbar disc herniation. *Spine*. 1996;21(24S):19S–38S.

340. Forristall RM, Marsh HO, Pay NT. Magnetic resonance imaging and contrast CT of the lumbar spine: comparison of diagnostic methods and correlation with surgical findings. *Spine*. 1988;13:1049–1054.

341. Lehman RA, Helgeson MD, Keeler KA, et al. Comparison of magnetic resonance imaging and computed tomography in predicting facet arthrosis in the cervical spine. *Spine*. 2008;34:65–68.

342. Masharawi Y, Kjaer P, Bendix T, et al. The reproducibility of quantitative measurements in lumbar magnetic resonance imaging of children from the general population. *Spine*. 2008;33(9):2094–2100.

343. Cousins JP, Haughton VM. Magnetic resonance imaging of the spine. *J Am Acad Orthop Surg*. 2009;17:22–30.

344. Fujiwara A, Tamai K, An HS, et al. The interspinous ligament of the lumbar spine: magnetic resonance images and their clinical significance. *Spine*. 2000;25:358–363.

345. Milette PC, Fontaine S, Lepanto L, et al. Differentiating lumbar disc protrusions, disc bulges and discs with normal contour but abnormal signal intensity: Magnetic resonance imaging with discographic correlations. *Spine*. 1999;24:44–53.

346. Saiffudin A, Braithwaite I, White J, et al. The value of lumbar spine magnetic resonance imaging in the demonstration of annular tears. *Spine*. 1998;23:453–457.

347. Ito M, Incorvaia KM, Yu SF, et al. Predictive signs of discogenic lumbar pain on magnetic resonance imaging with discography correlation. *Spine*. 1998;23:1252–1260.

348. Beattie PF, Meyers SP. Magnetic resonance imaging in low back pain: general principles and clinical issues. *Phys Ther*. 1998;78:738–753.

349. Raininko R, Manninen H, Battié MC, et al. Observer variability in the assessment of disc degeneration on magnetic resonance images of the lumbar and thoracic spine. *Spine*. 1995;20:1029–1035.

350. Boden SD, Davis DO, Dina TS, et al. Abnormal magnetic resonance scans of the lumbar spine in asymptomatic subjects: a prospective investigation. *J Bone Joint Surg*. 1990;72:403–408.

351. Bogduk N, Modic MT. Controversy: lumbar discography. *Spine*. 1996;21:402–404.

352. Magnussen L, Strand LI, Lygren H. Reliability and validity of the back performance scale: observing activity limitation in patients with back pain. *Spine*. 2004;29(8):903–907.

353. Strand LI, Anderson B, Lygren H, et al. Responsiveness to change of 10 physical tests used for patients with back pain. *Phys Ther*. 2011;91(3):404–415.

354. Demircan MN. Cramp finding: can it be used as a new diagnostic and prognostic factor in lumbar disc surgery? *Eur Spine J*. 2002;11:47–51.

355. Hanten WP, Dawson DD, Iwata M, et al. Craniosacral rhythm: reliability and relationships with cardiac and respiratory rates. *J Orthop Sports Phys Ther*. 1998;27(3):213–218.

356. Gilleard WL, Brown JM. An electromyographic validation of an abdominal muscle test. *Arch Phys Med Rehabil*. 1994;75:1002–1007.

357. Haladay DE, Denegar CR, Miller SJ, Challis J. Electromyographic and kinetic analysis of two abdominal muscle performance tests. *Physiother Theory Pract*. 2015;31(8):587–593.

358. Beattie P, Rothstein JM, Lamb RL. Reliability of the attraction method for measuring lumbar spine backward bending. *Phys Ther*. 1987;67(3):364–369.

359. Kippers V, Parker AW. Toe-touch test: a measure of its validity. *Phys Ther*. 1987;67(11):1680–1684.

360. Gross MT, Burns CB, Chapman SW, et al. Reliability and validity of rigid lift and pelvic leveling device method in assessing functional leg length inequality. *J Orthop Sports Phys Ther*. 1998;27(4):285–294.

361. Bayar B, Bayar K, Yakut E, et al. Reliability and validity of the Functional Rating Index in older people with low back pain: preliminary report. *Aging Clin Exp Res*. 2004;16(1):49–52.

362. Ceran F, Ozcan A. The relationship of the Functional Rating Index with disability, pain, and quality of life in patients with low back pain. *Med Sci Monit*. 2006;12(10):CR435–CR 439.

363. Hagg O, Fritzell P, Romberg K, et al. The General Function Score: a useful tool for measurement of physical disability. *Validity and Reliability Eur Spine J*. 2001;10(3):203–210.

364. Holm I, Friis A, Storheim K, et al. Measuring self-reported functional status and pain in patients with chronic low back pain by postal questionnaires: a reliability study. *Spine*. 2003;28(8):828–833.

365. Evans K, Refshauge KM, Adams R. Trunk muscle endurance tests: reliability and gender differences in athletes. *J Sci Med Sport*. 2007;10:447–455.

366. Del Pozo-Cruz B, Mocholi MH, Del Pozo-Cruz J, et al. Reliability and validity of lumbar and abdominal trunk muscle endurance tests in office workers with nonspecific subacute low back pain. *J Back Musculoskelet Rehabil*. 2014;27:399–408.

367. Hall GL, Hetzler RK, Perrin D, et al. Relationship of timed sit-up tests to isokinetic abdominal strength. *Res Q Exerc Sport*. 1992;63(1):80–84.

368. Holt AE, Shaw NJ, Shetty A, et al. The reliability of the low back outcome score for back pain. *Spine*. 2002;27(2):206–210.

369. Razmjou H, Kramer JF, Yamada R. Intertester reliability of the McKenzie evaluation in assessing patients with mechanical low-back pain. *J Orthop Sports Phys Ther*. 2000;30(7):368–389.

370. Kilpikoski S, Airaksinen O, Kankaanpaa M, et al. Interexaminer reliability of low back pain assessment using the McKenzie method. *Spine*. 2002;27(8):E207–E214.

371. Clare HA, Adams R, Maher CG. Reliability of McKenzie classification of patients with cervical or lumbar pain. *J Manip Physiol Ther*. 2005;28(2):122–127.

372. Werneke MW, Deutscher D, Hart DL, et al. McKenzie lumbar classification. *Spine*. 2014;39(3):E182–E190.

373. Donahue MS, Riddle DL, Sullivan MS. Intertester reliability of a modified version of McKenzie's lateral shift assessments obtained on patients with low back pain. *Phys Ther*. 1996;76(7):706–716.

374. John C, Piva SR, Fritz JM. Responsiveness of the numeric pain rating scale in patients with low back pain. *Spine*. 2005;30(11):1331–1334.

375. Wittink H, Turk DC, Carr DB, et al. Comparison of the redundancy, reliability, and responsiveness to change among SF-36, Oswestry Disability Index, and Multidimensional Pain Inventory. *Clin J Pain*. 2004;20(3):133–142.

376. Gronblad M, Hupli M, Wennerstrand P, et al. Intercorrelation and test-retest reliability of the Pain Disability Index (PDI) and the Oswestry Disability Questionnaire (ODQ) and their correlation with pain intensity in low back pain patients. *Clin J Pain*. 1993;9(3):189–195.

377. Copay AG, Glassman SD, Subach BR, et al. Minimum clinically important difference in lumbar spine surgery patients: a choice of methods using the Oswestry Disability Index, Medical Outcomes Study Questionnaire SF 36 and Pain Scales. *Spine J*. 2008;8:968–974.

378. Fritz JM, Piva SR. Physical Impairment Index: reliability, validity and responsiveness in patients with acute low back pain. *Spine*. 2003;28(11):1189–1194.

379. Hodges P, Richardson C, Jull G. Evaluation of the relationship between laboratory and clinical test of transversus abdominis function. *Physiother Res Int*. 1996;1(1):30–40.

380. Tong TK, Wu S, Nie J. Sport-specific endurance plank test for evaluation of global core muscle function. *Phys Ther Sport*. 2014;15(1):58–63.

381. Bruno PA, Millar DP, Goertzen DA. Inter-rater agreement, sensitivity, and specificity of the prone hip extension test and active straight leg raise test. *Chiropractic Man Ther*. 2014;22(1):1–16.

382. Demoulin C, Ostelo R, Knottnerus JA, Smeets RJEM. Quebec Back Pain Disability Scale was responsive and showed reasonable interpretability after a multidisciplinary treatment. *J Clin Epidemiol*. 2010;63:1249–1255.

383. Alaranta H, Hurri H, Heliovaara M, et al. Non-dynamometric trunk performance tests:

reliability and normative data. *Scand J Rehab Med*. 1994;26:211–215.

384. Stratford PW, Binkley JM, Riddle DL. Development and initial validation of the Back Pain Functional Scale. *Spine*. 2000;25(16):2095–2102.

385. Brouwer S, Kuijer W, Dijkstra PU, et al. Reliability and stability of the Roland Morris Disability Questionnaire: intra class correlation and limits of agreement. *Disabil Rehabil*. 2004;26(3):162–165.

386. Riddle DL, Stratford PW, Binkley JM. Sensitivity to change of the Roland-Morris Back Pain questionnaire: part 2. *Phys Ther*. 1998;78(11):1197–1207.

387. Jordan K, Dunn KM, Lewis M, Croft P. A minimal clinically important difference was derived for the Roland-Morris Disability Questionnaire for low back pain. *J Clin Epidemiol*. 2006;59:45–52.

388. Archenholtz B, Ahlmen M, Bengtsson C, et al. Reliability of articular indices and function tests in a population study of rheumatic disorders. *Clin Rheumatol*. 1989;8(2):215–224.

389. Williams R, Binkley J, Bloch R, et al. Reliability of the modified-modified Schober and double inclinometer methods for measuring lumbar flexion and extension. *Phys Ther*. 1993;73(1):33–44.

390. Perret C, Poiraudeau S, Fermanian J, et al. Validity, reliability, and responsiveness of the fingertip-to-floor test. *Arch Phys Med Rehabil*. 2001;82(11):1566–1570.

391. Potter BK, Freedman BZ, Andersen RC, et al. Correlation of Short Form-36 and disability status with outcomes of arthroscopic acetabular labral debridement. *Am J Sports Med*. 2005;33(6):864–870.

392. Taylor S, Frost H, Taylor A, et al. Reliability and responsiveness of the shuttle walking test in patients with chronic low back pain. *Physiother Res Int*. 2001;6(3):170–178.

393. Zwierska I, Nawaz S, Walker RD, et al. Treadmill versus shuttle walk tests of walking ability in intermittent claudication. *Med Sci Sports Exerc*. 2004;36(11):1835–1840.

394. Gabbe BJ, Bennell KL, Majswelner H, et al. Reliability of common lower extremity musculoskeletal screening tests. *Phys Ther Sports*. 2004;5:90–97.

395. Vincent-Smith B, Gibbons P. Inter-examiner and intra-examiner reliability of the standing flexion test. *Man Ther*. 1999;4(2):87–93.

396. van den Hoogen HJ, Koes BW, Deville W, et al. The inter-observer reproducibility of Lasègue's sign in patients with low back pain in general practice. *Br J Gen Pract*. 1996;46(413):727–730.

397. Kosteljanetz M, Bang F, Schmidt-Olsen S. The clinical significance of straight leg raising (Lasègue's sign) in the diagnosis of prolapsed lumbar disc: interobserver variation and correlation with surgical finding. *Spine*. 1988;13:393–395.

398. Majlesi J, Togay H, Unalan H, Toprak S. The sensitivity and specificity of the Slump and the Straight Leg Raising Tests in patients with lumbar disc herniation. *J Clin Rheumatol*. 2008;14(2):87–91.

399. Vanderwint DAWM, Simons E, Riphagen IL, et al. Physical examination for lumbar radiculopathy due to disc herniation in patients with low back pain. *Cochrane Database Sys Rev*. 2010;2:1–62.

400. Deen Jr HG, Zimmerman RS, Lyons MK, et al. Test-retest reproducibility of the exercise treadmill examination in lumbar spinal stenosis. *Mayo Clin Proc*. 2000;75(10):1002–1007.

401. Barz T, Melloh M, Staub L, et al. The diagnostic value of a treadmill test in predicting lumbar spinal stenosis. *Eur Spine J*. 2008;17:686–690.

402. Fritz JM, Erhard RE, Delitto A, et al. Preliminary results of the use of a two-stage treadmill test as a clinical diagnostic tool in the differential diagnosis of lumbar spinal stenosis. *J Spinal Disord*. 1997;10(5):410–416.

403. Heiss DG, Fitch DS, Fritz JM, et al. The interrater reliability among physical therapists newly training in a classification system for acute low back pain. *J Orthop Sports Phys Ther*. 2004;34:430–439.

404. Stanton TR, Fritz JM, Hancock MJ, et al. Evaluation of a treatment-based classification algorithm for low back pain: a cross-sectional study. *Phys Ther*. 2011;91(4):496–509.

CHAPTER 10

Pelvis

The sacroiliac joints form the "key" of the arch between the two pelvic bones; with the symphysis pubis, they help to transfer weight from the spine to the lower limbs and vice versa; they also provide elasticity to the pelvic ring (Fig. 10.1). Restriction (i.e., decreased range of motion [ROM]), loss of strength, or muscle imbalance in any of the lower limb joints can alter the kinetic chain, putting greater stress on the joints above the joint that is restricted, is weak, or has an imbalance of the controlling muscles. This, in turn, interferes with the efficient transmission of kinetic energy.[1] In addition, this triad of joints also acts as a buffer to decrease the force of jars and bumps to the spine and upper body caused by contact of the lower limbs with the ground. Because of this shock-absorbing function, the structure of the sacroiliac and symphysis pubis joints is different from that of most other joints. Assessment of the pelvic joints is often an assessment of exclusion. Because the symptoms that arise from the sacroiliac joints are similar to those arising in the lumbar spine and/or hip, because these symptoms occur in the same areas (i.e., back and leg [lateral thigh]), and because injury or degeneration are seen more commonly in the lumbar spine and hip, the examiner will commonly do an assessment of the lumbar spine and/or hip. If it is found that the problems are not coming from these areas (i.e., assessment has cleared these areas), the examiner will do an assessment of the pelvic joints. The only case where this might not occur is when there has been direct trauma to the pelvic joints.[2-4]

Applied Anatomy

The **sacroiliac joints** are part synovial (i.e., diarthrosis) joint and part syndesmosis; thus they are sometimes called amphiarthrosis (slightly movable) joints. A syndesmosis is a type of fibrous joint in which the intervening fibrous connective tissue forms an interosseous membrane or ligament. The synovial portion of the joint is C shaped, with the convex iliac surface of the C facing anteriorly and inferiorly. Kapandji[5] states that the greater or more acute the angle of the C, the more stable the joint and the less the likelihood of a lesion to the joint. The sacral surface is slightly concave. The sacroiliac joints act as shock absorbers to shear forces and provide a torsional load-attenuation mechanism for forces between the lower legs

and trunk that arise during daily activities.[6,7] The normal overall motion at the joints is about 7°.[4]

Sacroiliac Joint	
Resting position:	Neutral
Capsular pattern:	Pain when joints are stressed
Close pack:	Nutation
Loose pack:	Counternutation

The size, shape, and roughness of the articular surfaces of the sacrum vary greatly among individuals. In the child, these surfaces are smooth. In the adult, they become irregular depressions and elevations that fit into one another; by so doing, they restrict movement at the joint and add strength to it for transferring weight from the lower limb to the spine. The articular surface of the ilium is covered with fibrocartilage; the articular surface of the sacrum is covered with hyaline cartilage that is three times thicker than that of the ilium. In older persons, parts of the joint surfaces may be obliterated by adhesions.

Although the sacroiliac joints are relatively mobile in young people, they become progressively stiffer with age. In some cases, ankylosis results. The movements that occur in the sacroiliac and symphysis pubis joints are slight compared with the movements occurring in the spinal joints.

The sacroiliac joints are supported by several strong ligaments (Fig. 10.2)—the long posterior sacroiliac ligaments that limit anterior pelvic rotation[8] or sacral counternutation, the short posterior sacroiliac ligament that limits all pelvic and sacral movement, the posterior interosseous ligament that forms part of the sacroiliac articulation (the syndesmosis), and the anterior sacroiliac ligaments.[9] The sacrotuberous and sacrospinous ligaments limit nutation and posterior innominate rotation; they also provide vertical stability.[9] The iliolumbar ligament stabilizes L5 on the ilium.[9,10] These ligaments and the complex arrangement of dense connective tissue acting like a "ligamentous stocking" play a major role in stabilizing the sacroiliac joints.[11,12] The interosseous sacroiliac ligament is the major connection between the sacrum and the ilium and is one of the strongest ligaments in the body.[10,13]

The sacroiliac joints and symphysis pubis have no muscles that control their movements directly, although muscles do provide pelvic stability, so they are influenced by the action of the muscles moving the lumbar spine and hip because many of these muscles attach to the sacrum and pelvis (Table 10.1). The sacroiliac joints are stabilized through two mechanisms—form closure and force closure.[14,15] **Form closure** is due to specific anatomic features of the joint themselves (e.g., rough texture, ridges, depressions), which prevent shear. It refers to the close packed position of the joint where no outside forces are necessary to hold the joint stable. Thus intrinsic factors such as joint shape, coefficient of

friction of the joint surfaces, and the integrity of the ligaments contribute to form closure.[15-17] **Force closure** is the compression generated by the muscles and, through them, the tensing of the ligaments when they act to accommodate specific load situations. It is the effect of changing joint reaction forces generated by tissue tension, resulting in a self-bracing mechanism (Fig. 10.3).[10,15,17-21] Force closure would be similar to the loose packed position in that extrinsic factors, primarily the muscles and their neurological control as well as their ability to tension the ligaments, along with the capsule are needed to maintain functional stability of the joint as well as the forces applied to the joint.[15-17,20,21] These two forms of closure and neurological control enable the sacroiliac joints to self-lock as they go into close pack and to release slightly when the joints unlock. (See later discussion under "Observation" on nutation and counternutation and under "Active Movements").

The muscles that support the pelvic girdle as well as the lumbar spine and hips can be divided into groups.[16,22,23] The outer group consists of four groupings, which act primarily in crossing or oblique patterns of force couples to stabilize the pelvis. The **deep posterior longitudinal system** consists of the erector spinae, thoracolumbar fascia, and hamstring muscles along with the sacrotuberous ligament (Fig. 10.4). The **superficial posterior oblique system** includes the latissimus dorsi, gluteus maximus, and intervening thoracolumbar fascia (Fig. 10.5A). The **anterior oblique system** consists of the internal and external obliques, the contralateral adductors, and the abdominal fascia in between (Fig. 10.5B). The **lateral system** consists of the gluteus medius and minimus and the contralateral adductors (Fig. 10.6). The **innermost muscle group** consists of the multifidus, transverse abdominis, diaphragm (Fig. 10.7), and pelvic floor muscles (Fig. 10.8), which can play a role in stabilizing the pelvis and indirectly the lumbar spine. The **anterior-posterior superficial group** controls the anteroposterior rotation of the pelvis on the fixed femur. This group consists of the hamstrings and

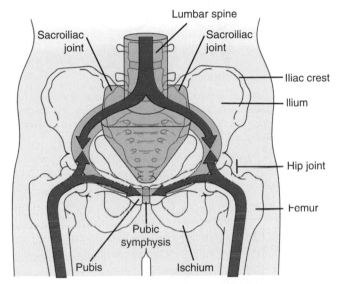

Fig. 10.1 The components of the pelvic ring. The *arrows* show the direction of body weight force as it is transferred between the pelvic ring, trunk, and femora. The keystone of the pelvic ring is the sacrum, which is wedged between the two ilia and secured bilaterally by the sacroiliac joints. (Redrawn from Neumann DA: *Kinesiology of the musculoskeletal system*, ed 2, St Louis, 2010, CV Mosby, p 360. Redrawn after Kapandji LA: *The physiology of joints*, vol 3, New York, 1974, Churchill Livingstone.)

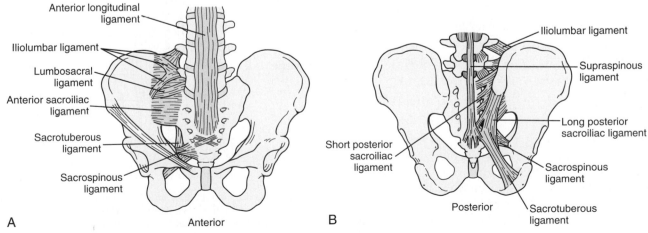

Fig. 10.2 Ligaments of the pelvis. (A) Anterior view. (B) Posterior view.

TABLE **10.1**

Muscles Attaching to the Pelvis

Muscles	Nerve Root Derivation
Latissimus dorsi	Thoracodorsal (C6–C8)
Erector spinae	L1–L3
Multifidus	L1–L5
External oblique	T7–TI2
Internal oblique	T7–T12, L1
Transverse abdominis	T7–T12, L1
Rectus abdominis	T6–T12
Pyramidalis	Subcostal (T12)
Quadratus lumborum	T12, L1–L4
Psoas minor	L1
Iliacus	Femoral (L2, L3)
Levator ani	S4, inferior rectal nerve/ pudendal nerve
Sphincter ani externus	S2–S4
Superficial transverse perineal ischiocavernous	S2–S4
Coccygeus	S4, S5
Gluteus maximus	Inferior gluteal (L5, S1,S2)
Gluteus medius	Superior gluteal (L5, S1)
Gluteus minimus	Superior gluteal (L5, S1)
Obturator internus	Nerve to obturator internus (L5, S1)
Obturator externus	Obturator (L3, L4)
Piriformis	L5, S1, S2
Interior gemellus	Nerve to quadratus femoris (L5, S1)
Superior gemellus	Nerve to obturator internus (L5, S1)
Pectineus	Femoral (L2, L3)
Semimembranosus	Sciatic (L5, S1, S2)
Semitendinosus	Sciatic (L5, S1, S2)
Biceps femoris	Sciatic (L5, S1, S2)
Tensor fascia lata	Superior gluteal (L4, L5)
Sartorius	Femoral (L2, L3)
Rectus femoris	Femoral (L2–L4)
Gracilis	Obturator (L2, L3)
Adductor magnus	Obturator/sciatic (L2–L4)
Adductor longus	Obturator (L2–L4)
Adductor brevis	Obturator (L2–L4)

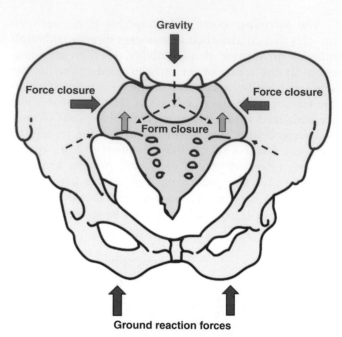

Fig. 10.3 Form closure stabilizes because of the shape of the sacroiliac joints. Force closure stabilizes because of the action of the muscles, ligaments, and fascia. The two closures act together to form a self-bracing mechanism *(dashed lines)*.

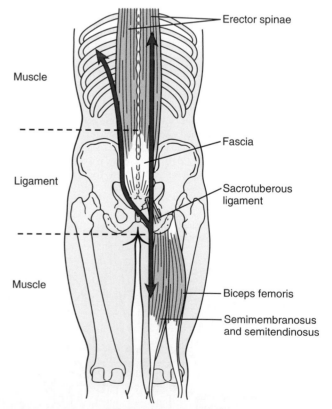

Fig. 10.4 The deep longitudinal muscle system of the outer group (includes the erector spinae, deep lamina of the thoracolumbar fascia, sacrotuberous ligament, and biceps femoris muscle).

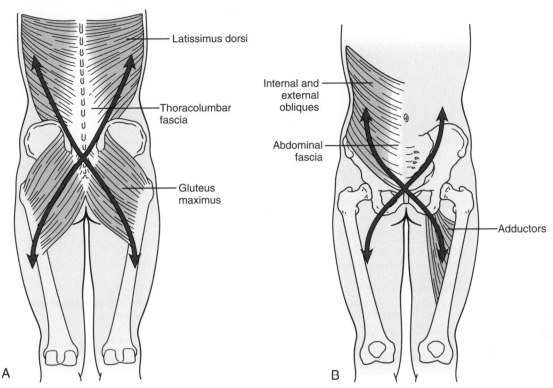

Fig. 10.5 (A) The posterior oblique muscle system of the outer group (includes the latissimus dorsi, gluteus maximus, and intervening thoracolumbar fascia). (B) The anterior oblique muscle system of the outer group (includes the external and internal obliques, contralateral adductors of the thigh, and intervening anterior abdominal fascia).

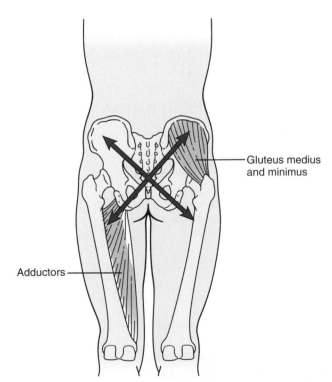

Fig. 10.6 The lateral muscle system of the outer group (includes the gluteus medius and minimus and contralateral adductors of the thigh).

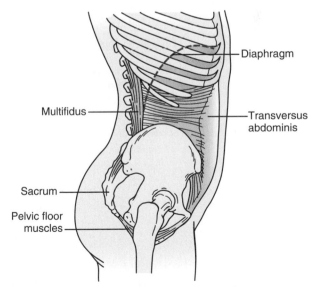

Fig. 10.7 The inner muscle unit including the multifidus, transverse abdominis, and pelvis floor muscles.

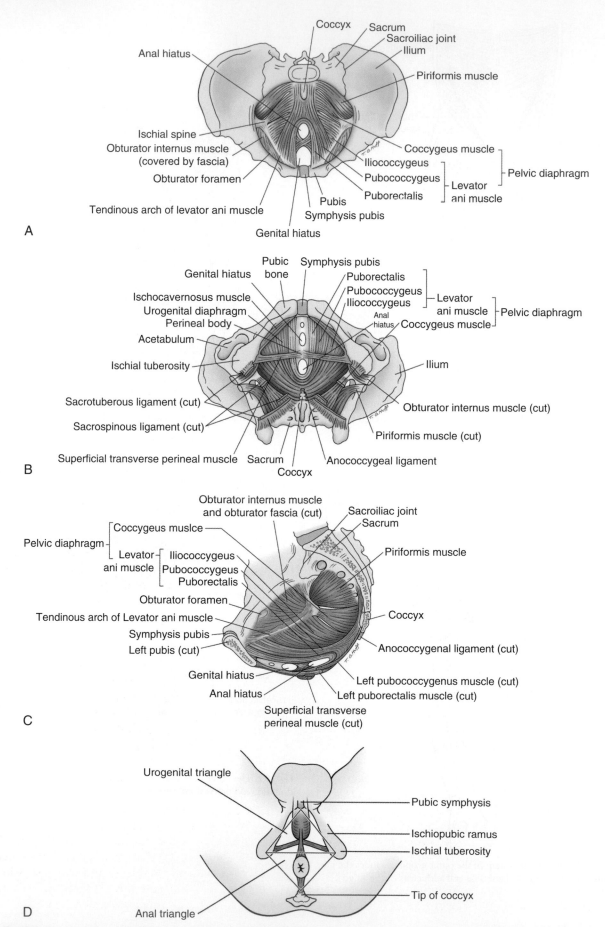

Fig. 10.8 Muscles of the pelvic floor. (A) Superior view. (B) Inferior view. (C) Medial view (female). (D) Subdivisions of the perineum.

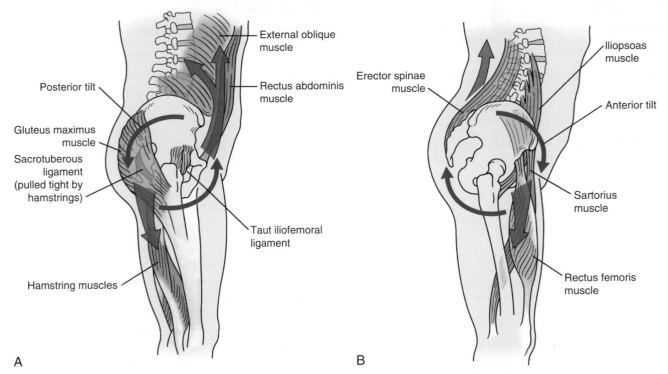

Fig. 10.9 The anterior-posterior superficial muscle group. (A) Muscles and ligaments involved in posterior tilt. (B) Muscles and ligaments involved in anterior tilt.

gluteus maximus, erector spinae, rectus abdominis, internal and external obliques, psoas, rectus femoris and sartorius, and iliofemoral and sacrotuberous ligaments (Fig. 10.9). These muscle systems help to actively stabilize the pelvic joints and contribute significantly to load transfer during gait and pelvic rotational activities.[16]

The **symphysis pubis** is a fibrocartilaginous joint held together by the pubic ligament. There is a disc of fibrocartilage between the two joint surfaces called the **interpubic disc.** This joint does allow limited movement.

The **sacrococcygeal joint** is usually a fused line (symphysis) united by a fibrocartilaginous disc. It is found between the apex of the sacrum and the base of the coccyx. Occasionally the joint is freely movable and synovial. With advanced age, the joint may fuse and be obliterated.

Patient History

In addition to the questions listed under "Patient History" in Chapter 1, the examiner should obtain the following information from the patient:

1. *Was there any known mechanism of injury? Has there been more than one episode?* For example, the sacroiliac joints are commonly injured by a sudden jar caused by inadvertently stepping off a curb, an overzealous kick (either missing the object or hitting the ground), a fall on the buttocks, or a lift and twist maneuver, thus commonly combining axial loading and rotation.[24,25] Has the patient experienced any recent falls, twists, or strains? These movements increase the chance of sacroiliac joint sprains.

2. *Where is the pain and does it radiate?* With a lesion of the sacroiliac joint, deep, diffuse, dull, undefined pain that is difficult to localize, tends to be unilateral and can be referred to the posterior thigh, iliac fossa, and buttock on the affected side.[7] Sacroiliac joint pain can spread to the abdominal area and sometimes to the groin, although groin pain is more commonly associated with hip problems.[6] The pain has been described as sclerotomal pain.[7] Sacroiliac pain does not commonly extend below the knee, although it can.[6] Both pain and numbness can originate from the sacroiliac joint and its ligaments, primarily the posterior sacroiliac ligaments.[11] Symptoms from sacroiliac problems do not usually follow a dermatomal pattern, which is common in the lumbar spine if the nerve roots are aggravated.[6] Most patients with sacroiliac joint pathology indicate pain around the posterior superior iliac spine (PSIS) or buttock. Thus the **point sign** (**Fortin finger test**), in which the patient points slightly inferior and medial to the PSIS as the source of pain, may help with diagnosis.[26] Pain arising from the posterior sacroiliac ligament is mainly on the lateral, posterolateral, and posteromedial thigh.[4,7,27] When doing movements, it is often better to ask whether the movement or test reproduces the pain of complaint rather than if it is just painful. If the pain of complaint is reproduced, it is likely that the tissue at fault is being stressed.[4]

TABLE **10.2**

Pelvic Motions With Lumbar Spine Movement

Lumbar Spine	Innominate	Sacrum
Flexion	Anterior rotation	Nutation followed by counternutation
Extension	Posterior rotation (slight)	Nutation
Rotation	Same side: posterior rotation Opposite side: anterior rotation	Nutation on same side
Side flexion	Same side: anterior rotation Opposite side: posterior rotation	Side bend

Adapted from Dutton M: *Orthopedic examination, evaluation and intervention*, ed 3, New York, 2012, McGraw-Hill.

3. *When does the pain occur? Does the pain keep the patient awake?* Pain that is caused by sacroiliac joint problems is usually felt when turning in bed, getting out of bed, or stepping up with the affected leg. Often, the pain is constant and unrelated to position. Symphysis pubis pain tends to be localized and increases with any movement involving the adductor or rectus abdominis muscles.
4. *What particular movements bother the patient?* Usually transitional-type movements (e.g., sit to stand, single-leg squat) cause pain in the sacroiliac joint if it is involved.
5. *What is the patient's habitual working stance? Is a great deal of sitting or twisting involved?* The examiner should look for postures that potentially increase the stress on the sacroiliac joints (e.g., standing, especially on one leg).
6. *Are there any risk factors that may be present?*[28] Risk factors include obesity, leg length discrepancy, gait abnormalities, low-grade/persistent trauma (e.g., jogging), vigorous prolonged exercise, scoliosis, pregnancy, surgery.[25,28]
7. *What is the patient's usual activity or pastime?* Again, would any of these activities stress the sacroiliac joints? Has endurance capacity for standing, walking, or sitting decreased? In the presence of sacroiliac joint pathology, endurance will decrease.[18,29]
8. *Is there any particular position or activity that aggravates the condition?* Climbing or descending stairs, walking, and standing from a sitting position all stress the sacroiliac joint (Tables 10.2 and 10.3).
9. *What is the patient's age?* Apophyseal injuries and avulsion fractures of the pelvis can occur in young athletes.[30] Ankylosing spondylitis is found primarily in men between the ages of 15 and 35 years.

TABLE **10.3**

Pelvic Motions With Hip Movement

Hip	Innominate
Flexion	Posterior rotation
Extension	Anterior rotation
Medial rotation	Inflare (medial rotation)
Lateral rotation	Outflare (lateral rotation)
Abduction	Superior glide
Adduction	Inferior glide

Adapted from Dutton M: *Orthopedic examination, evaluation and intervention*, ed 3, New York, 2012, McGraw-Hill.

Hypomobility is likely to be seen in men between 40 and 50 and in women after 50 years of age.[31]

10. *Does the patient have or feel any weakness in the lower limbs?* Neurological deficit in the limbs can be present if the sacroiliac joint is affected.
11. *Has the patient had any difficulty with micturition?* It has been reported that sacroiliac joint dysfunction can lead to urinary problems.[32]
12. *Has there been a recent pregnancy?* In females, sprain of the sacroiliac ligaments can be the result of increased laxity of the ligaments caused by hormonal changes. It may take 3 to 4 months or longer for the ligaments to return to their normal state after a pregnancy.
13. *Does the patient have a past history of rheumatoid arthritis, Reiter syndrome, or ankylosing spondylitis?* Each of these conditions can involve the sacroiliac joints.
14. *Are there any psychosocial issues that are relevant in the presence of pathology?* Questions about anxiety, depression, and other psychosocial issues should be addressed if considered important.[15]

Observation

The patient must be suitably undressed. For the sacroiliac joints to be observed properly, the patient is often required to be nude from the middle of the chest to the toes. If he or she wishes to wear shorts, they must be rolled down as far as possible so that the sacroiliac joints are visible. The posterior, superior, and inferior iliac spines must be visible. The patient stands and is viewed from the front, side, and back. The examiner should note the following:

1. Are the posture (see Chapter 15) and gait (see Chapter 14) normal? **Nutation**[16,33] (sacral locking) is the forward motion of the base of the sacrum into the pelvis; it could also be described as the backward rotation of the ilium on the sacrum (Fig. 10.10). It is the most stable position of the sacroiliac joint, increases the tension of the major ligaments of the sacroiliac joints including the short dorsal sacroiliac ligaments and interosseous ligament, and is an example of **form closure**.[12] When moving from supine

lying to standing, the sacrum normally moves bilaterally, just as it does in early movement of trunk flexion. The ilia move closer together and the ischial tuberosities move farther apart.[31] Unilaterally, the sacrum normally moves with hip flexion of the lower limb.[16] Pathologically, if nutation occurs only on one side (when it should occur bilaterally), the examiner will find that the anterior superior iliac spine (ASIS) is higher and the PSIS is lower on that side.[33] The result is an apparent or functional short leg on the same side.[34] Nutation is limited by the anterior sacroiliac ligaments, sacrospinous ligament, and sacrotuberous ligament and is more stable than counternutation. Nutation occurs when a person assumes a "pelvic tilt" position. During nutation, the sacrum will slide down its short part and then posteriorly along its long part (Fig. 10.11).[16]

Counternutation (sacral unlocking), or *contranutation* as it is sometimes called, is the opposite movement to nutation. It indicates an anterior rotation of the ilium on the sacrum or backward motion of the base of the sacrum out of the pelvis.[16] The iliac bones move farther apart and the ischial tuberosities approximate.[31] Pathologically, if counternutation occurs only on one side as it does during extension of the extremity on that side, the lower limb on that side will probably be medially rotated.[16] Pathological or abnormal counternutation on one side occurs when the ASIS is lower and the PSIS is higher on one side.[33] Counternutation is limited by the posterior sacroiliac ligaments. Counternutation occurs when a

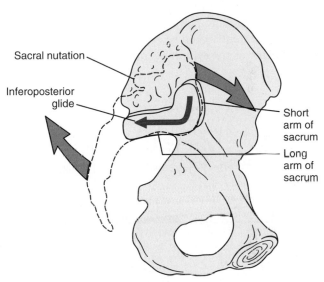

Fig. 10.11 When the sacrum nutates, its articular surface glides inferoposteriorly relative to the innominate bones. (Redrawn from Lee D: *The pelvic girdle*, ed 3, Edinburgh, 2004, Churchill Livingstone, p 60.)

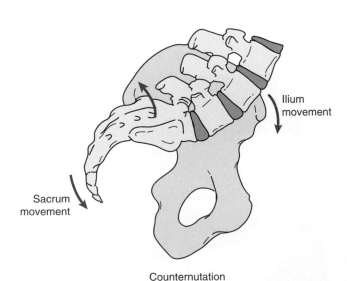

Fig. 10.10 Movements of nutation and counternutation occurring at the sacroiliac joint.

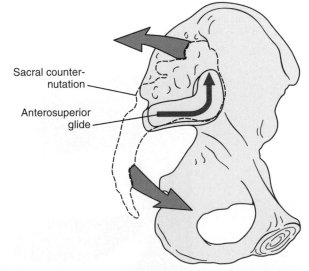

Fig. 10.12 When the sacrum counternutates, its articular surface glides anterosuperiorly relative to the innominate bones. (Redrawn from Lee D: *The pelvic girdle*, ed 3, Edinburgh, 2004, Churchill Livingstone, p 60.)

person assumes a "lordotic" or "anterior pelvic tilt" position. During counternutation, the sacrum will slide anteriorly along its long arm and then superiorly up its short arm (Fig. 10.12).[16] This motion is resisted by the long posterior sacroiliac ligament supported by the multifidus (contraction of multifidus causes nutation of the sacrum).[16]

Levine and Whittle[35] found that anterior and posterior pelvic tilt has an effect on lumbar lordosis with an average change of 20° being possible (9° posteriorly and 11° anteriorly). Thus looking for the **"neutral pelvis"** position becomes important, especially for later rehabilitation. Based on their data, a neutral pelvis would be somewhere between the two extremes. Pelvic tilt is the angle between a line joining the ASIS and PSIS and a horizontal line (Fig. 10.13). Average pelvic tilt is 11° ± 4°.[35,36] Ideal pelvic alignment would see the ASIS on the same vertical plane as the symphysis pubis.[37]

Three questions should be considered when one is looking for a neutral pelvis and whether the pelvis can be stabilized:

i. Can the patient get into the neutral pelvis position? If not, what is restricting the movement or what is weak so that the movement does not occur?
ii. Can the patient hold (i.e., stabilize) the neutral pelvis statically while moving distal joints dynamically? If not, what muscles need to be strengthened?
iii. Can the patient hold (i.e., stabilize) the neutral pelvis when moving it dynamically? If not, which muscles are weak and/or not functioning correctly (i.e., functioning isometrically, concentrically, eccentrically)?

These questions will help the examiner determine if the pelvis (and lumbar spine) can be stabilized during different movements or positions so that other muscles that originate from the pelvis can function properly. The ability to stabilize the pelvis statically or dynamically plays a significant role in proper functioning of the whole kinetic chain. For example, it should be possible to perform side-lying hip abduction with the lower limbs, pelvis, trunk, and shoulders aligned in the frontal plane (**active hip abduction test** ☑).[38] If the leg wobbles, the pelvis tips, the shoulders or trunk rotate, the hip flexes, or the abducted limb rotates medially, it is an indication of lack of movement control, lack of muscle balance, and inability to stabilize the pelvis while doing the movement so that the muscles have a firm base from which to function.

Gait is often affected if the pathology involves the pelvis. If the sacroiliac joints are not free to move, the stride length is decreased and a vertical limp may be present.[24] A painful sacroiliac joint may also cause reflex inhibition of the gluteus medius, leading to a Trendelenburg gait or lurch.

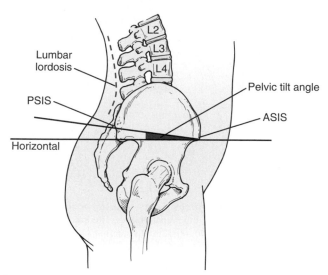

Lumbar lordosis
PSIS
Horizontal
Pelvic tilt angle
ASIS

Fig. 10.13 Pelvic tilt angle (7° to 15°). *ASIS,* anterior superior iliac spine; *PSIS,* posterior superior iliac spine.

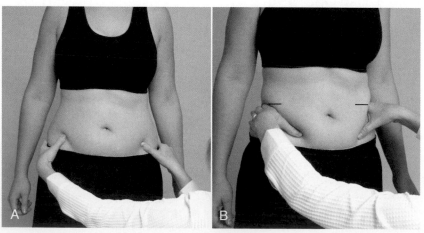

Fig. 10.14 Anterior observational view. (A) Level of the anterior superior iliac spines. (B) Level of the iliac crests.

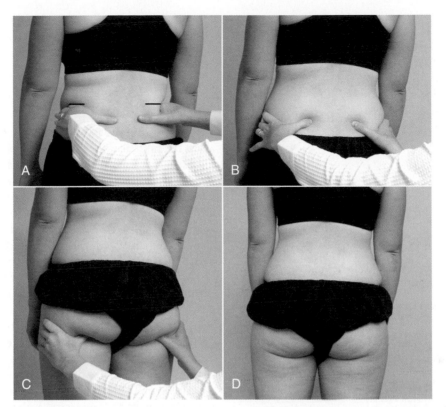

Fig. 10.15 Posterior observational view. (A) Level of the iliac crests. (B) Level of the posterior superior iliac spines. (C) Level of the ischial tuberosities. (D) Level of the gluteal folds.

2. Are the ASISs level when viewed anteriorly (Fig. 10.14)? On the affected side, the ASIS often tends to be higher and slightly forward. The examiner must remember this difference, if present, when the patient is viewed from behind (Fig. 10.15). If the ASIS and PSIS on one side are higher than the ASIS and PSIS on the other, this indicates an **upslip** of the ilium on the sacrum on the high side, a short leg on the opposite side, or muscle spasm caused by lumbar pathology (e.g., a disc lesion).[39–42] If the ASIS is higher on one side and the PSIS is lower at the same time, it indicates an **anterior torsion** of the sacrum (pathological nutation) on that side.[39] This torsion may result in a spinal scoliosis, an altered functional leg length, or both. Anterior rotational dysfunction is seen most frequently following a posterior horizontal thrust of the femur (dashboard injury), golf or baseball swing, or any forced anterior diagonal pattern.[40] The sacrum is lower on the side of the pelvis that has rotated backward. The most common rotation of the innominate bones is left posterior torsion or rotation (pathological counternutation). The posterior rotational dysfunctions are usually the result of falling on an ischial tuberosity, lifting when the body is forward flexed with the knees straight, repeated standing on one leg, vertical thrusting onto an extended leg, or sustaining hyperflexion and abduction of the hips.

3. Are both pubic bones level at the symphysis pubis? The examiner tests for level equality by placing one

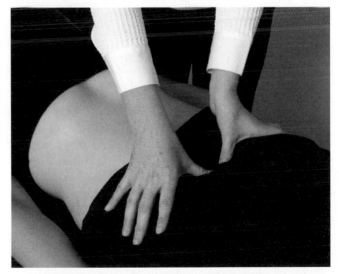

Fig. 10.16 Determining the level of the pubic bones.

finger or thumb on the superior aspect of each pubic bone and comparing the heights (Fig. 10.16). If the ASIS on one side is higher, the pubic bone on that side is suspected to be higher; this can be confirmed by this procedure, indicating a backward torsion problem of the ilium on that side. This procedure is usually done with the patient lying supine.

4. Does the patient, when standing, have equal weight on both feet, favor one leg, or have a lateral pelvic tilt? This finding may indicate pathology in the sacroiliac joints, the leg, the spine, or a short leg.

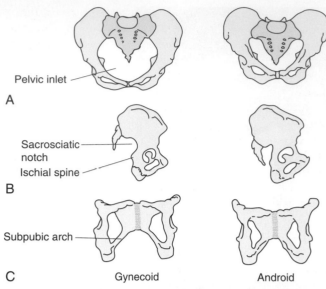

Fig. 10.17 Gynecoid (predominantly female) and android (primarily male) pelvises. (A) Superior view. (B) Lateral view. (C) Anterior view of the pubis and ischium.

TABLE **10.4**

A Comparison of the Two Most Common Types of Pelvis

Feature	Gynecoid	Android
Inlet	Round	Triangular
Sacrosciatic notch	Average size	Narrow
Sacrum	Average	Forward
Subpubic arch	Inclination curved	Inclination straight

5. Are the ASISs equidistant from the center line of the body?
6. What type of pelvis does the patient have?[43] Gynecoid and android types are the most common (as described in Fig. 10.17 and Table 10.4).
7. Are the iliac crests level? Altered leg length may alter their height.
8. Are the PSISs level?
9. Are the buttock contours or gluteal folds normal? The painful side is often flatter if there is loss of tone in the gluteus maximus muscle.
10. Is there any unilateral or bilateral spasm of the erector spinae muscles?
11. Are the ischial tuberosities level? If one tuberosity is higher, it may indicate an upslip of the ilium on the sacrum on that side.[39]
12. Is there excessive lumbar lordosis? Forward or backward sacral torsion may increase or decrease the lordosis.
13. Are the PSISs equidistant from the center line of the body?
14. Are the sacral sulci equal? If one is deeper, it may indicate a sacral torsion.

15. Do the feet face forward to the same degree? Often, the affected limb is medially rotated. With spasm of the piriformis muscle, the limb is laterally rotated more on the affected side.

Examination

Before assessing the pelvic joints, the examiner should first assess the lumbar spine and hip unless the history definitely indicates that one of the pelvic joints is at fault. The lumbar spine and hip can and frequently do refer pain to the sacroiliac joint area. Because the sacroiliac joints are in part a syndesmosis, movements at these joints are minimal compared with those of the other peripheral joints. It should also be remembered that any condition that alters the position of the sacrum relative to the ilium causes a corresponding change in the position of the symphysis pubis.

Although numerous tests and test movements have been described to help determine if there is sacroiliac dysfunction, many of them are imprecise and their reliability has been questioned.[44-56] However, at present they are the best tests available. It is important for the examiner to consider all aspects of the assessment, including the history and the patient's symptoms along with the various tests and movements before diagnosing sacroiliac joint problems.[9,16,44,57-59]

Active Movements

Unlike other peripheral joints, the sacroiliac joints do not have muscles that directly control their movement. However, because contraction of the muscles of the other joints may stress these joints or the symphysis pubis, the examiner must be careful during the active or resisted isometric movements of other joints and must be sure to ask the patient about the exact location of the pain on each movement. Table 10.1 outlines the muscles that attach to the pelvis. For example, if the joint is injured, resisted abduction of the hip can cause pain in the sacroiliac joint on the same side because the gluteus medius muscle pulls the ilium away from the sacrum when it contracts strongly. In addition, side flexion to the same side increases the shearing stress to the sacroiliac joint on that side. When the patient is doing active movements, the examiner is attempting to reproduce the patient's symptoms rather than just looking for pain.

The sacroiliac joints move in a "nodding" fashion of anteroposterior rotation. Normally the PSISs approximate when the patient stands and separate when the patient lies prone. When he or she stands on one leg, the pubic bone on the supported side moves forward in relation to the pubic bone on the opposite side as a result of rotation at the sacroiliac joint.

During the active movements of the pelvic joints, the examiner looks for unequal movement, loss of or increase in movement (hypomobility or hypermobility), tissue contracture, tenderness, or inflammation.

Active Movements That Stress the Sacroiliac Joints

- Forward flexion of the spine (40° to 60°)
- Extension of the spine (20° to 35°)
- Rotation of the spine, left and right (3° to 18°)
- Side flexion of the spine, left and right (15° to 20°)
- Flexion of the hip (100° to 120°)
- Abduction of the hip (30° to 50°)
- Adduction of the hip (30°)
- Extension of the hip (0° to 15°)
- Medial rotation of the hip (30° to 40°)
- Lateral rotation of the hip (40° to 60°)

The movements of the spine put stress on the sacroiliac joints as well as on the lumbar and lumbosacral joints. During forward flexion of the trunk, the innominate bones and pelvic girdle as a whole rotate anteriorly as a unit on the femoral heads bilaterally. The same thing occurs when one rises from supine lying to sitting. If one leg is actively extended at the hip, the innominate on that side will unilaterally rotate anteriorly.[16] During the anterior rotation of the innominate bones (counternutation), the innominate slides posteriorly along its long arm and inferiorly down its short arm (Fig. 10.18).[16] Initially, the sacrum nutates up to about 60° of forward flexion, but once the deep posterior structures (deep and posterior oblique muscle systems, thoracolumbar fascia, and the sacrotuberous ligament) become tight, the innominates continue to rotate anteriorly on the femoral heads but the sacrum begins to counternutate.[16] This counternutation causes the sacroiliac joint to be vulnerable to instability, as greater muscle action (force closure) is required to maintain stability with counternutation.[23] Thus the earlier counternutation occurs during forward flexion, the more vulnerable the sacroiliac joint will be to instability problems. Excessive counternutation is more likely to occur in patients who have tight hamstrings.[16]

To test forward flexion, the patient stands with weight equally distributed on both legs. The examiner sits behind the patient and palpates both PSISs (Fig. 10.19). The patient is asked to bend forward while keeping the knees straight (i.e., extended) (see Tables 10.2 and 10.3), and the symmetry of movement of the PSIS superiorly is noted. As long as both PSISs move equally and symmetrically, the movement is normal. If one PSIS moves upward less than the other, the hypomobile side is considered positive for limited movement of the ilium on the sacrum (called the **standing flexion test**).[60] At the same time, the examiner should note the amount of flexion that has occurred when sacral nutation begins. This can be done by having the patient repeat the forward bending motion while the examiner palpates the PSIS (inferior aspect) on one side with one thumb while the other thumb palpates the sacral base so that the thumbs are parallel. In the first 45° of forward flexion, the sacrum will move forward (nutation) (Fig. 10.20A), but near 60° (normally), the sacrum will begin to counternutate or move backward (Fig. 10.20B).[16] During the sacral counternutation, the two PSISs should move upward equally in relation to the sacrum and toward each other or approximate. At the same time, the ASIS will tend to flare out.

During extension, the opposite movements occur (see Tables 10.2 and 10.3).[16,24] During extension or backward bending of the trunk, the innominate bones

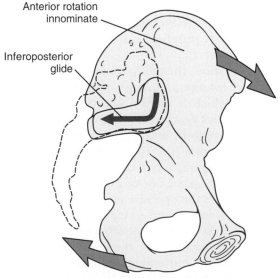

Fig. 10.18 When the innominate rotates anteriorly, its articular surface glides inferoposteriorly relative to the sacrum. (Redrawn from Lee D: *The pelvic girdle*, ed 2, Edinburgh, 1999, Churchill Livingstone, p 51.)

Anterior rotation innominate

Inferoposterior glide

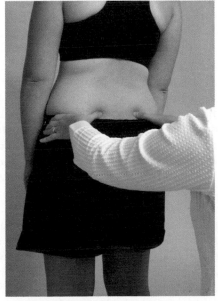

Fig. 10.19 Examiner palpating the posterior superior iliac spine prior to forward flexion.

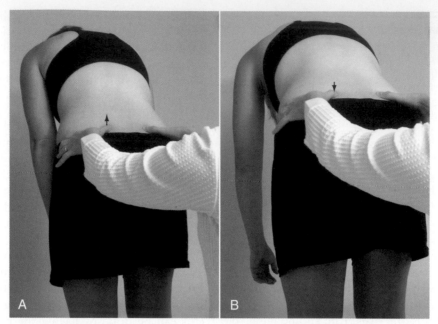

Fig. 10.20 Examiner palpating for sacral nutation. One thumb is on the posterior superior iliac spine; the other thumb is parallel to it on the sacrum. The examiner is feeling for forward movement (nutation) of the sacrum, which occurs early in movement (A), and backward movement (counternutation) of the sacrum, which normally occurs at around 60° of hip flexion (B).

(the pelvic girdle) as a whole unit rotate posteriorly (nutation) on the femoral heads bilaterally. If one leg is actively flexed at the hip, the innominate on that side unilaterally rotates posteriorly.[16] During the posterior rotation of the innominate bones, the innominate slides anteriorly along the long arm and superiorly up the short arm. This movement is the same as sacral nutation (Fig. 10.21). With backward bending, both PSISs move inferiorly an equal amount. Lee[16] advocates doing active hip extension (**active prone hip extension test**) with the leg straight under three conditions (also called **prone active straight leg raise test**). The first condition is hip extension (Fig. 10.22A). With sacroiliac pathology, there is a significant delay in gluteus maximus contraction. The second condition includes the same movement as the first with the examiner applying manual compression to the innominate bones (i.e., form closure) (Fig. 10.22B). This decreases the delay in the contraction of the gluteus maximus muscle. The third condition has the examiner resisting extension of the contralateral medially rotated leg or extended arm (i.e., force closure) as the patient extends the straight leg (Fig. 10.22C). If function improves when force closure stabilization is used, exercise will probably benefit the patient.[61]

To test backward bending, the patient stands with weight equally distributed on both legs. The examiner sits behind the patient and palpates both PSISs. The patient is asked to bend backward while the examiner notes any asymmetry (Fig. 10.23). Normally, the PSISs move inferiorly. During backward bending, the innominate bones and sacrum remain in the same

position, so there should be no change in their relationship.[16] The examiner palpates both sides of the sacrum at the level of S1. As the patient extends, the sacrum should normally move forward. This is called the **sacral flexion test.**

Side flexion normally produces a torsion movement between the ilia and the sacrum. As the patient side flexes, the innominate bones bend to the same side and the sacrum rotates slightly in the opposite direction; the thumb of the examiner on the same side (the thumbs are palpating on each side of the sacrum at the level of S1) moves forward. This is called the **sacral rotation test.**[16] If this torsion movement does not occur (e.g., in hypomobility), the patient finds that more effort is required to side flex and it is harder to maintain balance.[24]

During rotation, the pelvic girdle moves in the direction of the rotation, causing intrapelvic torsion. The innominate, which is on the side to which rotation is occurring, rotates posteriorly while the opposite innominate rotates anteriorly, pushing the sacrum into rotation in the same direction (i.e., right rotation of the trunk and pelvis causes right rotation of the sacrum). This causes the sacrum to nutate on the side to which rotation occurs and counternutate on the opposite side.[16]

The hip movements performed are also affected by sacroiliac lesions. As the patient flexes each hip maximally, the examiner should observe the ROM present, the pain produced, and the movement of the PSISs. The examiner first notes whether the PSISs are level before the patient flexes the hip. Normally, flexion of the hip with the knee flexed to 90° or more causes the sacroiliac joint

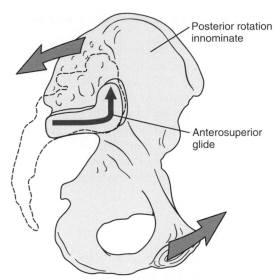

Posterior rotation
innominate

Anterosuperior
glide

Fig. 10.21 When the innominate rotates posteriorly, its articular surface glides anterosuperiorly relative to the sacrum. (Redrawn from Lee D: *The pelvic girdle*, ed 2, Edinburgh, 1999, Churchill Livingstone, p 51.)

on that side to drop or move caudally in relation to the other sacroiliac joint **(Gillet test).** If this drop does not occur, it may indicate hypomobility on the flexed side. The examiner can observe this movement by placing one thumb over the PSIS and the other thumb over the spinous process of S2 (Fig. 10.24A). In the patient with a normal sacroiliac joint, the thumb on the PSIS drops (Fig. 10.24B). If it is hypomobile, the thumb moves up on hip flexion. The two sides are compared. Sturesson and colleagues[62] have questioned whether much movement occurs at all because the stress of doing the test on one leg causes "force closure" of the sacroiliac joints, thus limiting movement.

The examiner then leaves the one thumb over the sacral spinous process and moves the other thumb over the ischial tuberosity (Fig. 10.24C). The patient is again asked to flex the hip as far as possible. Normally, the thumb over the ischial tuberosity moves laterally (Fig. 10.24D). With a fixed or hypomobile joint, the thumb moves superiorly or toward the head. Again, the two sides are compared.

The examiner then sits in front of the standing patient and palpates the ASIS. Testing one leg at a time, the patient pivots the leg on the heel into medial and lateral rotation. When doing these movements, the ASIS should move medially and laterally. Both sides are compared and the movement should be equal.[16] Depending on where the patient complains of pain, the affected joint may be hypomobile or hypermobile.

The position of the sacrum can then be determined. To do this, the examiner tests the patient in two positions—sitting and prone—doing three movements: flexion, staying in neutral, and extension. Before testing,

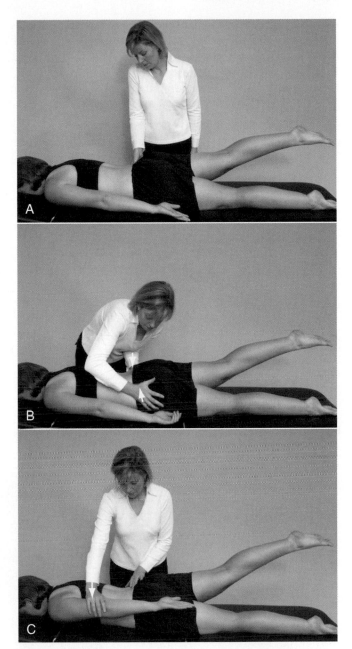

Fig. 10.22 Functional testing of prone active hip extension or prone straight leg raise. (A) Patient actively extends straight leg to provide comparison with ease of doing the test in other two positions. (B) Second part of the test with form closure augmented (compression of innominate bones). (C) Third part of the test with force closure augmented (resisted muscle action).

the examiner palpates the base of the sacrum and the inferior lateral angle (near the apex) of the sacrum on both sides (Fig. 10.25). Normally, the sacral bone and the inferior lateral angle of the sacrum are level (i.e., one is not more anterior or posterior than the other). The first test involves the patient sitting with the feet supported and the spine fully flexed. The examiner palpates the four points (Fig. 10.26) and determines their relationship to one another. The patient is then put in prone lying with the spine in neutral and the relationship of the four points determined. The examiner then asks the patient to fully extend the spine and then determines the relationship of the four points. In any of the positions tested, if the examiner found, for example, an anterior left sacral base along with a

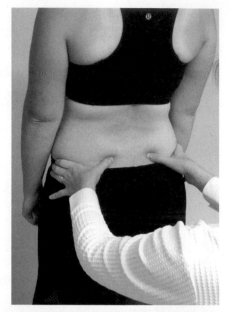

Fig. 10.23 Examiner palpating posterior superior iliac spine for asymmetric movement on backward bending.

posterior right inferior lateral angle, it would indicate a left rotated sacrum.[16]

The final active movements of the pelvis that the examiner may observe is the action of the pelvic floor muscles (Table 10.5; see Figs. 8.37 and 8.38). If the pelvis has been found to be unstable or the patient is suffering from incontinence, the examiner can ask the patient to contract the muscles by asking him or her to squeeze the muscles tight by trying to stop peeing and holding the contraction. With strong pelvic floor muscles, the patient should have little trouble holding the contraction for at least 30 seconds.

Passive Movements

The passive movements of the pelvic joints involve stressing of the ligaments and the joints themselves. They are not true passive movements, like those done at other joints, but are in reality stress or provocative tests. It should be noted, however, that the effectiveness of these tests in confirming sacroiliac joint problems has been questioned even when combined in a clinical prediction rule.[57,63,64] Lee[15] feels these passive movements or tests should be used to determine symmetry or asymmetry of stiffness rather than normal, hypermobile, or hypomobile. It is her contention that asymmetry at the two sacroiliac joints is the problem, not the amount of movement. Laslett et al.[56] and van der

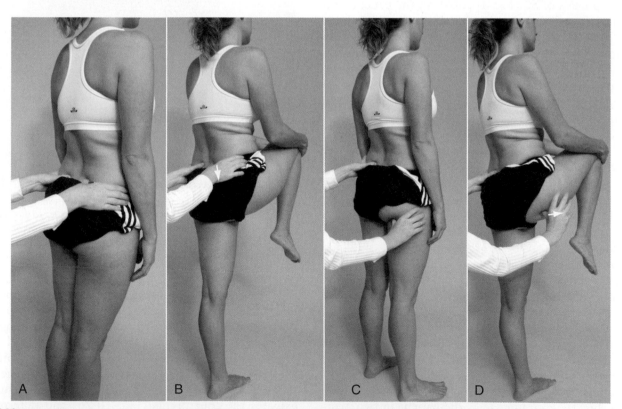

Fig. 10.24 Active movements demonstrating how to show hypomobility of the sacroiliac joints. (A) Starting position for sacral spine and posterior superior iliac spine. (B) Hip flexion; the ilium drops, as it normally should *(arrow)*. (C) Starting position for sacral spine and ischial tuberosity. (D) Hip flexion. Ischial tuberosity moves laterally *(arrow)*, as expected.

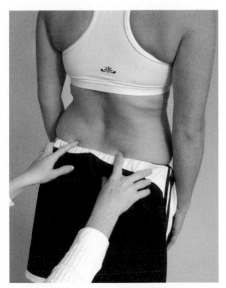

Fig. 10.25 Examiner palpating the base of the sacrum and inferior lateral angle of the sacrum for anteroposterior symmetry.

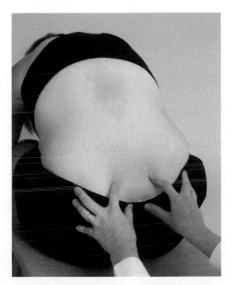

Fig. 10.26 Examiner palpating the position of the sacrum in flexed sitting.

Wurff et al.[48,54] felt that individually the sacroiliac provocative tests were not reliable enough to make a diagnosis but that a combination of the tests was. If two of four tests were positive, these tests were the best predictors of an intra-articular sacroiliac joint block. If all six tests were negative, sacroiliac joint pathology could be ruled out.[55] Doing the passive movement is more likely to eliminate muscle tension effects that cause compression and increased stiffness.[15] Because of their anatomic makeup, the pelvic joints do not move to the same degree or in the same fashion as other joints of the body. When doing these provocative passive movements/tests, the examiner is looking for the **reproduction of the patient's symptoms,** not just pain or discomfort.[59,65]

Key Stress Tests (Passive Movements) of the Sacroiliac Joints[a]

⚠ Approximation test

⚠ Femoral shear (POSH) test

✓ Gapping test

⚠ Hip abduction and external (lateral) rotation (HABER) test

❓ Ipsilateral prone kinetic test

✓ Knee-to-shoulder test

❓ Passive extension and medial rotation of ilium on sacrum

❓ Passive flexion and lateral rotation of ilium on sacrum

⚠ Prone gapping test

⚠ Sacral thrust test

✓ Thigh thrust test

[a]See Chapter 1, Key for Classifying Special Tests.

Laslett et al.'s Clinical Prediction Rule for Sacroiliac Joint Involvement[7,11,26,54,56]

SACROILIAC PROVOCATION TESTS (SIJ SPECIAL JOINT CLUSTER):
1. Approximation test (compression provocation test)
2. Gapping test (distraction provocation test)
3. Sacral thrust test
4. Thigh thrust test
5. Gaenslen's test (see "Special Tests")
6. Pain on palpation of the sacral sulcus medial to posterior superior iliac spine

Note: If two of the first four tests or three or more of the six tests are positive, then the sacroiliac joint pathology is present.

⚠ *Approximation (Transverse Posterior Stress) Test.*[16,56] The patient is in the side-lying position and the examiner's hands are placed over the upper part of the iliac crest, pressing toward the floor (Fig. 10.27). The movement causes forward pressure on the sacrum. An increased feeling of pressure in the sacroiliac joints indicates a possible sacroiliac lesion and/or a sprain of the posterior sacroiliac ligaments.

⚠ *Femoral Shear (Posterior Shear [POSH]) Test.* The patient lies in the supine position. The examiner slightly flexes, abducts, and laterally rotates the patient's thigh at approximately 45° from the midline. The examiner then applies a graded force through the long axis of the femur, which causes an anterior-to-posterior shear stress to the sacroiliac joint on the same side (Fig. 10.28).[66]

✓ *Gapping (Transverse Anterior Stress or Distraction Provocation) Test.*[16,56] The patient lies supine while the examiner applies crossed-arm pressure to the ASIS (Fig. 10.29A) (some examiners prefer not to cross arms; Fig. 10.29B). The examiner pushes down and out with the arms. The test is positive only if unilateral gluteal or posterior leg

TABLE **10.5**

Muscles of the Pelvic Floor, Their Actions, and Their Nerve Root Derivation

Muscles	Action	Nerve Root Derivation
Obturator internus	Rotates thigh laterally Abducts flexed thigh at hip	Nerve to obturator internus
Piriformis	Rotates thigh laterally Abducts flexed thigh Stabilizes hip	Ventral rami of S1, S2
Gluteus maximus	Extends thigh Rotates pelvis back on femur Rotates thigh laterally Abducts thigh	Inferior gluteal nerve, L5, S1, S2
Levator ani[a,b]	Supports pelvic viscera Raises pelvic floor	Ventral rami of S3, S4 Perineal nerve
Coccygeus[b] (also called *ischiococcygeus*)	Supports pelvic viscera Draws coccyx forward	Ventral rami of S4, S5
Superficial transverse perineal (transverse peroneal profundus)	Supports pelvic viscera	Pudendal nerve, S2, S3, S4

[a]Made up of three muscles: iliococcygeus, pubococcygeus and puborectalis depending on origin and insertion.
[b]These two muscles make up the pelvic or urogenital diaphragm.

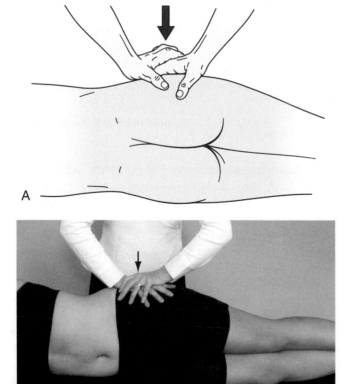

Fig. **10.27** Approximation test. (A) Diagram of posterior view. (B) Anterior view.

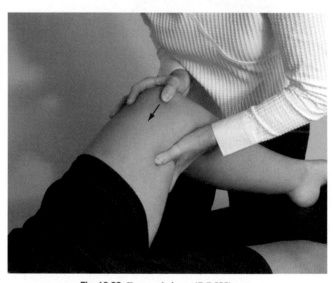

Fig. **10.28** Femoral shear (POSH) test.

pain is produced, indicating a sprain of the anterior sacroiliac ligaments. Care must be taken when performing this test. The examiner's hands pushing against the ASISs can elicit pain because the soft tissue is being compressed between the examiner's hands and the patient's pelvis.

⚠ *Hip Abduction and External (Lateral) Rotation (HABER) Test.*[29] The patient lies prone. Starting with the unaffected leg, the examiner flexes the patient's knee to 90° to facilitate lateral rotation of the hip. The examiner then abducts and laterally rotates the hip in 10° increments until the patient complains of pain or the end of the range is reached (Fig. 10.30). The result is compared with the

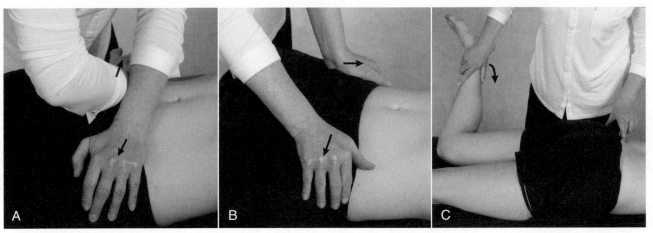

Fig. 10.29 Gapping test. (A) In supine with crossed arms. (B) In supine with arms not crossed. (C) In prone using hip medial rotation.

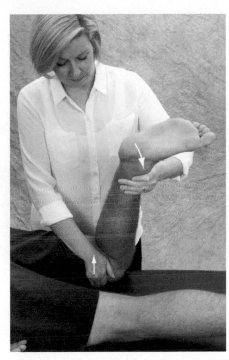

Fig. 10.30 Hip abduction and external (lateral) rotation (HABER) test.

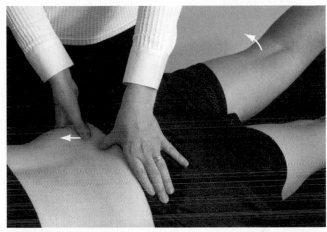

Fig. 10.31 Ipsilateral prone kinetic test. On extension, the posterior superior iliac spine and sacral crest move superiorly and laterally.

affected leg. The lateral rotation and abduction progressively increase the stress on the ipsilateral sacroiliac joint. Any difference between the two legs of greater than 30° is considered a positive test for sacroiliac joint involvement.

❓ *Ipsilateral Prone Kinetic Test.*[16,24] This test is designed to assess the ability of the ilium to flex and to rotate laterally or posteriorly. The patient lies prone while the examiner places one thumb on the PSIS and the other thumb parallel to it on the sacrum. The patient is then asked to actively extend the leg on the same side (Fig. 10.31). Normally, the PSIS should move superiorly and laterally. If it does not, it indicates hypomobility with a posterior rotated ilium, or **outflare.**

❓ *Passive Extension and Medial Rotation of Ilium on Sacrum.*[16,24] The patient is in side-lying position on the side that is not being tested. The examiner places one hand over the ASIS area of the anterior ilium. The other hand is placed over the PSIS in such a way that the fingers of the hand palpate the posterior ilium and sacrum. The examiner then pulls the ilium forward with the hand over the ASIS and pushes the posterior ilium forward with the other hand while feeling the relative movement of the ilium on the sacrum (Fig. 10.32). The unaffected side is then tested for comparison. If the affected side moves less, it indicates hypomobility and a posterior rotated ilium, or **outflare.**

❓ *Passive Flexion and Lateral Rotation of Ilium on Sacrum.* The patient is positioned as for the previously mentioned test. In this case, the examiner pushes the anterior ilium backward with the anterior hand, and the posterior hand and arm pull the ilium posteriorly while palpating the relative movement (Fig. 10.33). The unaffected side is then tested for comparison. If the affected side moves less, it is a sign of hypomobility and an anterior rotated ilium, or **inflare.**

If both this test and the previously mentioned one are positive, it means that an upslip has occurred to the ilium relative to the sacrum.

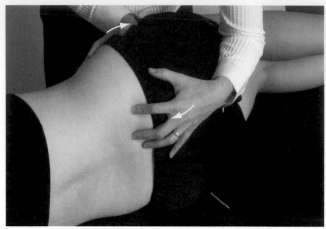

Fig. 10.32 Passive extension and medial rotation of the ilium on the sacrum. The innominate bone is held in extension and medial rotation. The examiner palpates the sacrum and ilium with the fingers while rotating the ilium forward. With hypomobility, the relative movement is less than on the unaffected side, indicating an outflare.

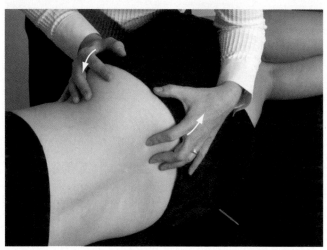

Fig. 10.33 Passive flexion and lateral rotation of the ilium on the sacrum. The innominate bone is held in flexion and lateral rotation. The examiner palpates the sacrum and ilium with the left fingers while rotating the ilium backward. With hypomobility, the relative movement is less than on the unaffected side, indicating an inflare.

❓ *Passive Lateral Rotation of the Hip.* The patient lies supine. The examiner flexes the hip and knee to 90° and then laterally rotates the hip to end range. This movement, provided that the hip is normal, stresses the sacroiliac joint on the test side.[31]

⚠ *Prone Gapping (Hibb's) Test.* The posterior sacroiliac ligaments may be stressed with the patient in the prone position (Fig. 10.29C). To perform the test, the patient's hips must have full ROM and be free of pathology. The patient lies prone and the examiner stabilizes the pelvis with his or her chest. The patient's knee is flexed to 90° or greater and the hip is rotated medially as far as possible. While pushing the hip into the very end of medial rotation, the examiner palpates the sacroiliac joint on the same side. The test is repeated on the other side, with

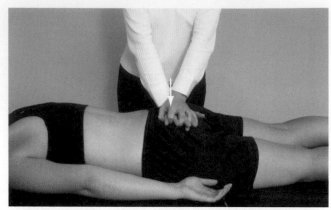

Fig. 10.34 Sacral apex pressure test. Patient is lying prone.

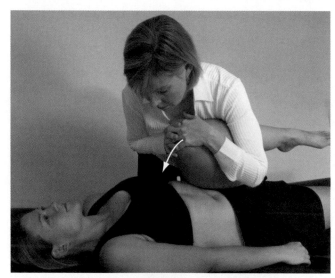

Fig. 10.35 Sacroiliac rocking (knee-to-shoulder) test.

the examiner comparing the degree of opening and the quality of the movement at each sacroiliac joint as well as stressing the posterior sacroiliac ligaments.

⚠ *Sacral Apex Pressure (Prone Springing, Cranial Shear, Midline Sacral Thrust, or Sacral Thrust) Test.*[28,56] The patient lies in a prone position on a firm surface while the examiner places the base of his or her hand at the apex of the patient's sacrum (Fig. 10.34). Pressure is then applied to the apex of the sacrum, directed cranially causing a shear of the sacrum on the ilium. The test may indicate a sacroiliac joint problem if pain is produced over the joint. If pressure is applied anteriorly instead of cranially, it causes a rotational stress to the sacroiliac joints.

✔ *Sacroiliac Rocking (Knee-to-Shoulder) Test.* This test is also called the sacrotuberous ligament stress test. The patient is in a supine position (Fig. 10.35). The examiner flexes the patient's knee and hip fully and then adducts the hip. To perform the test properly, both the hip and knee must demonstrate no pathology and have full ROM. The sacroiliac joint is "rocked" by flexion and adduction of the patient's hip. To do the test properly, the

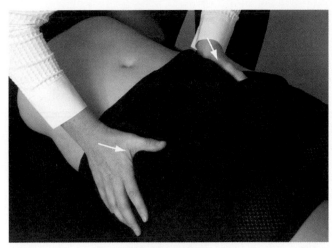

Fig. 10.36 "Squish" test.

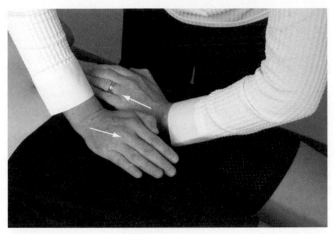

Fig. 10.37 Superoinferior symphysis pubis stress test. Patient is lying supine.

knee is moved toward the patient's opposite shoulder. Some authors[16,66] believe that the hip should be medially rotated as it is flexed and adducted to increase the stress on the sacroiliac joint. Simultaneously, the sacrotuberous ligament may be palpated (see Fig. 10.2 for location) for tenderness. Pain in the sacroiliac joints indicates a positive test. Care must be taken, because the test places a great deal of stress on the hip and sacroiliac joints. If a longitudinal force is applied through the hip in a slow, steady manner (for 15 to 20 seconds) in an oblique and lateral direction, further stress is applied to the sacrotuberous ligament.[16] While performing the test, the examiner may palpate the sacroiliac joint on the test side to feel for the slight amount of movement that normally is present.

❓ "Squish" Test. With the patient in the supine position, the examiner places both hands on the patient's ASISs and iliac crests and pushes down and in at a 45° angle (Fig. 10.36). This movement tests the posterior sacroiliac ligaments. A positive test is indicated by pain.

❓ Superoinferior Symphysis Pubis Stress Test.[16,24] The patient lies supine. The examiner places the heel of one hand over the superior pubic ramus of one pubic bone and the heel of the other hand over the inferior pubic ramus of the other pubic bone. The examiner then squeezes his or her hands together, applying a shearing force to the symphysis pubis (Fig. 10.37). Production of pain in the symphysis pubis is considered a positive test.

✓ Thigh Thrust Test (Oostagard, 4P, Sacrotuberous Stress, or Posterior Pelvic Pain Provocation Test).[12,56,60] The patient lies supine while the examiner passively flexes the hip on the test side to 90°. Using one hand to palpate the sacroiliac joint, the examiner thrusts down through the patient's knee and hip on the test side (Fig. 10.38). Pain in the sacroiliac joint on thrusting is a positive test.

❓ Torsion Stress Test.[16] The patient lies prone. The examiner palpates the spinous process of L5 with one

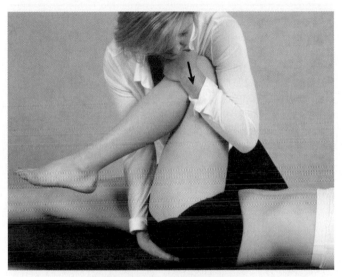

Fig. 10.38 Thigh thrust test.

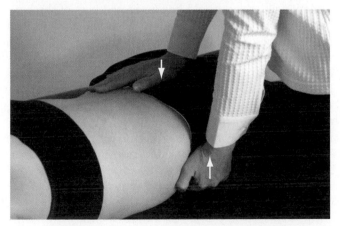

Fig. 10.39 Torsion stress test. Patient is lying prone.

thumb holding it stable. The examiner's other hand is placed around the anterior ilium on the opposite side and lifts the contralateral ilium up (Fig. 10.39). This rotational movement stresses the lumbosacral junction, the iliolumbar ligament, the anterior sacroiliac ligament, and the sacroiliac joint.

Resisted Isometric Movements

As previously stated, there are no specific muscles acting directly on the sacroiliac joints and symphysis pubis. However, contraction of adjacent muscles can stress these joints and cause force closure.[17] The examiner performs these movements with the patient supine and attempts to reproduce the patient's symptoms. It has been reported that if the leg is abducted to 30° with the patient in supine and with legs extended and the examiner resists further isometric abduction by the patient, pain in the area of the sacroiliac joint is considered a positive test.[60]

Resisted Isometric Movements Stressing the Sacroiliac Joints

- Forward flexion of spine (the abdominals stress the symphysis pubis)
- Flexion of hip (the iliacus stresses the sacroiliac joint)
- Abduction of hip (the gluteus medius stresses the sacroiliac joint)
- Adduction of the hip (the adductors stress the symphysis pubis)
- Extension of hip (the gluteus maximus and erector spinae cause force closure)
- Pelvic floor muscles—transverse abdominis/multifidus force couple causes force closure
- Abdominal obliques cause force closure
- Latissimus dorsi causes force closure

Functional Assessment

Functional assessment of the pelvic joints by themselves is very difficult because these joints do not work in isolation. Functionally, they should be considered part of the lumbar spine or part of the hip joint, depending on the area that the presenting pathology most affects. Individuals who have been diagnosed with sacroiliac joint dysfunction show a pattern similar to that seen in patients with low back pain or hip pain when completing the **sit-to-stand test**. When doing the movement from sit to stand, these patients put more load on the uninjured side, having a greater vertical reaction force on the unaffected side. This generates greater hip peak moments on the unaffected side having smaller ROM on the affected side, disrupting key muscle activity in the muscles providing force closure on the affected side.[67]

Special Tests

The examiner should use only those special tests that are considered necessary to confirm the diagnosis. Few special tests have been validated to accurately diagnose sacroiliac joint pathology.[17,48] In fact, a combination of tests appears to be needed to determine if the sacroiliac

joints are at fault[68] (see "Passive Movements," earlier). Dreyfuss et al.[57,69] showed that the sacral sulcus (the area of soft tissue just medial to the PSIS) was tender in 89% of sacroiliac joint patients. When these tests are performed, especially the stress or provocative tests, the examiner is attempting to reproduce the patient's symptoms.

Key Tests Performed on the Sacroiliac Joints Depending on Suspected Pathology[a,70,71]

- **For neurological involvement:**
  - ☑ Prone active straight leg raise test (three parts)
  - ☑ Straight leg raise test
  - ☑ Supine active straight leg raise test (three parts)
- **For joint involvement:**
  - ⚠ Drop test
  - ☑ Flamingo test
  - ☑ Gaenslen's test
  - ⚠ Gillet test
  - ☑ Patrick test
  - ⚠ Piedallu's sign
  - ⚠ Posterior superior iliac spine distraction test
  - ⚠ Supine-to-sit test
  - ☑ Yeoman's test
- **For limb length:**
  - ☑ Leg length measurement
- **For muscle dysfunction:**
  - ☑ 90–90 straight leg raise test
  - ☑ Trendelenburg test

[a]See Chapter 1, Key for Classifying Special Tests.

If muscle tightness is suspected as part of the problem, muscle should be tested for length.

For the reader who would like to review them, the reliability, validity, specificity, sensitivity, and odds ratios of some of the special tests used in the pelvis are available in eAppendix 10.1.

Tests for Neurological Involvement

❓ *Prone Knee Bending (Nachlas) Test.* Normally this is used to test for a tight rectus femoris, an upper lumbar joint lesion, an upper spine nerve root lesion, or a hypomobile sacroiliac joint. The patient lies prone and the examiner flexes the knee so that the heel is brought to the buttocks. If pain is felt in the front of the thigh before full range is reached, the problem is with the rectus femoris muscle flexibility. If the pain is in the lumbar spine, the problem is in the lumbar spine, usually the L3 nerve root, especially if these are radicular symptoms. If the problem is a hypomobile sacroiliac joint, the ipsilateral pelvic rim (ASIS) rotates forward, usually before the knee reaches 90° flexion.[66,72]

☑ *Straight Leg Raising (Lasègue's) Test.* Although the Lasègue sign is primarily considered a test of the neurological tissue around the lumbar spine, this test also places a stress on the sacroiliac joints. With the patient in the supine position (Fig. 10.40), the examiner passively flexes the patient's hip with the knee extended. Pain occurring after 70° is usually indicative of joint pain (i.e., hip, sacroiliac, or lumbar facet pain). In most people, the lumbar nerve roots are fully stretched by this point. However, in hypermobile persons, joint pain is often not experienced until after 120° of hip flexion. Therefore, it is more important to watch for the production of the patient's symptoms than for the actual ROM. In addition, the ROM obtained should be compared with the unaffected side. If the examiner then does a passive bilateral straight leg raising (SLR) test in a similar fashion, pain occurring before 70° is usually indicative of sacroiliac joint problems. DonTigny[73] has reported that the straight leg raise can be affected by sacroiliac problems. If, when doing SLR, the pain in the sacroiliac joint is unaltered or decreases, the examiner may suspect an anterior torsion. If the pain in the sacroiliac joint increases, a posterior torsion is possible. If pain increases on the opposite side, an anterior torsion on the opposite side should be suspected.

Lee[16] advocated several modifications to the straight leg test (Fig. 10.41A) if sacroiliac joint problems are suspected. These tests are called **active SLR tests** and were originally designed to test for postpartum pelvic problems.[74–76] In the first modification, Lee recommends

that the test be done actively by the patient in supine (**supine active straight leg raise test** ☑).[15,74–76] As the patient actively lifts the leg, the examiner asks whether the patient notes any "effort differences" between the two sides. The examiner then stabilizes and compresses the pelvis while the patient actively does the straight leg raise, providing form closure of the joints by squeezing the innominate bones together anteriorly (Fig. 10.41B). If the pain decreases or the SLR is easier to do with form closure (with no increased neurological signs), the test is

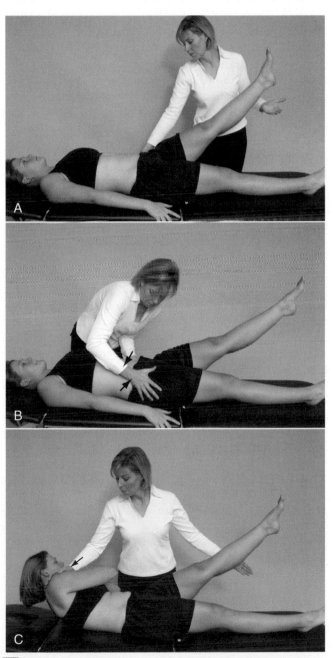

Fig. 10.41 Functional test of supine-active straight leg raise. (A) Patient actively does straight leg raise to provide comparison with ease of doing test in other two positions. (B) With form closure augmented (compression of innominate bones). (C) With force closure augmented (resisted muscle action).

Fig. 10.40 Straight leg raising test. (A) Unilateral (head may be flexed, ankle may be dorsiflexed, or both). (B) Bilateral.

considered positive for possible sacroiliac joint problems. At the same time, the examiner can check the contraction of the pelvic floor/transverse abdominis/multifidus force couple by palpating medial to the ASIS bilaterally. If the force couple functions properly, tension is felt symmetrically and the abdomen moves inward. If superficial tension is felt, it means that the internal obliques are contracting and there is a force-couple imbalance.[15] The multifidus may be palpated close to the spinous process, and it should contract when the pelvic floor muscles contract. Another modification tests force closure at the sacroiliac joints.[16] The patient is asked to flex and rotate the trunk toward the side on which the SLR is actively being performed. The trunk motion is resisted by the examiner (Fig. 10.41C). The two sides are compared for any difference. Force closure tests the ability of the muscles to stabilize the sacroiliac joints during movement.

A more detailed description of the SLR test is given in Chapter 9.

Tests for Sacroiliac Joint Involvement

Lee[15] has reported that active mobility tests should not be used to test the passive mobility of the sacroiliac joints. She felt that passive movements used to look for asymmetry were more effective.

Drop Test.[7] Starting with the good leg, the patient is asked to stand on one leg with the knee straight. The patient then stands "on the toes" of the foot by lifting the heel off the floor. The patient is then asked to allow the heel to suddenly drop, delivering an ipsilateral mechanical "jolt" to the pelvis. The test is then repeated on the affected side. The test mimics one of the possible mechanisms in which the sacroiliac joint is injured. A positive test would be reproduction of symptoms.

Flamingo Test or Maneuver. The patient is asked to stand on one leg (Fig. 10.42). When the patient is standing on one leg, the weight of the trunk causes the sacrum to shift forward and distally (caudally) with forward rotation. The ilium moves in the opposite direction.

On the non–weight-bearing side, the opposite occurs, but the stress is greatest on the stance side.[31] Pain in the symphysis pubis or sacroiliac joint indicates a positive test for lesions in whichever structure is painful. The stress may be increased by having the patient hop on one leg. This position is also used to take a stress x-ray of the symphysis pubis.

Gaenslen's Test. The patient lies on the side with the upper leg (test leg) hyperextended at the hip (Fig. 10.43A). The patient holds the lower leg flexed against the chest. The examiner stabilizes the pelvis while extending the hip of the uppermost leg. Pain indicates a positive test. The pain may be caused by an ipsilateral sacroiliac joint lesion, hip pathology, or an L4 nerve root lesion.

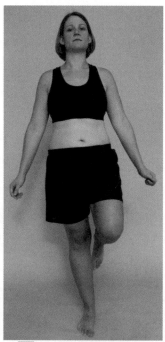

Fig. 10.42 Flamingo test.

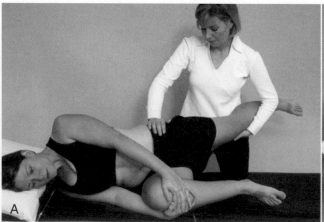
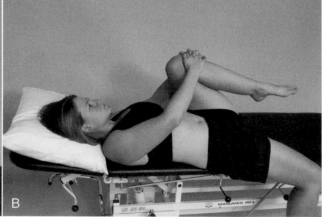

Fig. 10.43 Gaenslen's test. (A) With patient in side-lying position, the examiner extends the test leg. (B) With patient supine, the test leg is extended over the edge of the table.

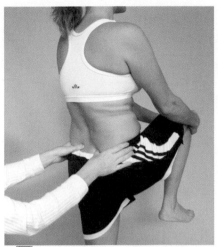

Fig. 10.44 Gillet (sacral fixation) test.

The Gaenslen's test is sometimes done with the patient supine (Fig. 10.43B), but this position may limit the amount of hyperextension available. The patient is positioned so that the test hip extends beyond the edge of the table. The patient draws both legs up onto the chest and then slowly lowers the test leg into extension. The other leg is tested in a similar fashion for comparison. Pain in the sacroiliac joints is indicative of a positive test.

⚠ *Gillet (Sacral Fixation, Stork Standing, Stork) Test.*[40] This test is also called the **ipsilateral posterior rotation test.** While the patient stands, the sitting examiner palpates the PSISs with one thumb and the other thumb parallel with the first thumb on the sacrum. The patient is then asked to stand on one leg while pulling the opposite knee up toward the chest. This causes the innominate bone on the same side to rotate posteriorly. The test is repeated with the other leg palpating the other PSIS. If the sacroiliac joint on the side on which the knee is flexed (i.e., the ipsilateral side) moves minimally or up, the joint is said to be hypomobile, or "blocked," indicating a positive test.[50] On the normal side, the test PSIS moves down or inferiorly (Fig. 10.44). This test is similar to the test performed during hip flexion in active movement; the only difference is the points of palpation during the movement. The test may also show altered muscle activation patterns with the weight transfer to one leg. With sacroiliac pathology, there is early activation of biceps femoris (i.e., lateral hamstrings) and delayed activation of the internal obliques and multifidus (in normal subjects, the opposite occurs).[12] It can also be used as the Trendelenburg test to test gluteus medius.[18]

Jackson[9] has suggested a modification to the test. After completing the Gillet test, he suggests that the examiner palpate the same PSIS and sacrum and ask the patient to do a repeat of the Gillet test using the other leg, which causes the opposite innominate bone to rotate posteriorly. As the patient flexes the hip and knee, the lumbar spine begins to flex, causing the sacrum to move inferiorly,

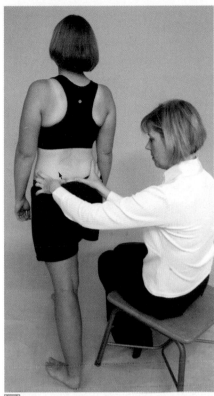

Fig. 10.45 Ipsilateral anterior rotation test.

resulting in the test innominate (side opposite to the leg being flexed) to rotate anteriorly.

❓ *Goldthwait Test.* The patient lies supine. The examiner places one hand under the lumbar spine so that each finger is in an interspinous space (i.e., L5–S1, L4–L5, L3–L4, and L2–L3 interspaces). The examiner uses the other hand to perform SLR. If pain is elicited before movement occurs at the interspaces, the problem is in the sacroiliac joint. Pain during interspace movement indicates a lumbar spine dysfunction. As with the SLR test, pain may be referred along the course of the sciatic nerve if there is neurological (e.g., nerve root) involvement.[72]

❓ *Ipsilateral Anterior Rotation Test.*[16] The patient stands with weight equally distributed on both feet. The examiner sits behind the patient and palpates one PSIS with one thumb and the sacrum on a parallel line with the other thumb. The patient is asked to extend the ipsilateral leg. Normally, the PSIS should move superiorly and laterally (Fig. 10.45). The other side is tested for comparison. This test determines the ability of the innominate on the test side to rotate anteriorly while the sacrum rotates to the opposite side.[16]

❓ *Laguere's Sign.* The patient lies supine (Fig. 10.46). To test the left sacroiliac joint, the examiner flexes, abducts, and laterally rotates the patient's left hip, applying an overpressure at the end of the ROM. The examiner must stabilize the pelvis on the opposite side by holding the opposite ASIS down. Pain in the left sacroiliac joint constitutes a positive test. The other side is tested

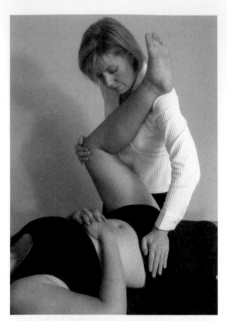

Fig. 10.46 Laguere's sign.

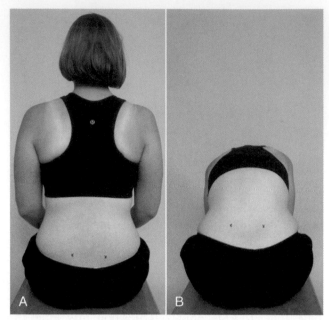

Fig. 10.47 Piedallu's sign. (A) Starting position. (B) Test position.

for comparison. This test should be performed with caution for patients with hip pathology because hip pain may ensue.

❓ *Mazion's Pelvic Maneuver (Standing Lunge Test).* [77] The patient stands in a straddle position with the limb on the unaffected side forward so that the feet are 0.5 to 1 m (2 to 3 feet) apart. The patient bends forward, trying to touch the floor, until the heel of the back leg lifts off the floor. If pain is produced in the lower trunk on the affected side, it is considered a positive test for unilateral forward displacement of the ilium relative to the sacrum.

✓ *Patrick Test.* See Chapter 11.

⚠ *Piedallu's Sign.* The patient is asked to sit on a hard flat surface (Fig. 10.47). This position keeps the muscles (e.g., hamstrings) from affecting the pelvic flexion symmetry and increases the stability of the ilia. In effect, it is a test of the sacrum on the ilia. The examiner palpates the PSISs and compares their heights. If one PSIS, usually the painful one, is lower than the other, the patient is asked to forward flex while remaining seated. If the lower PSIS becomes the higher one on forward flexion, the test is positive; it is that side that is affected. Because the affected joint does not move properly and is hypomobile, it goes from a low to a high position. This is believed to indicate an abnormality in the torsion movement at the sacroiliac joint.

⚠ *Posterior Superior Iliac Spine Distraction Test.* [78] The patient lies prone on the examining table with the arms by the side with the PSIS exposed. The examiner stands to one side of the patient at the level of the patient's hips and positions the thumbs on the inside of the PSIS (Fig. 10.48). The examiner then applies a quick forceful medial to lateral distraction force with the thumbs (or pisiform bones) to the insides of the PSIS. A positive test is indicated by pain or reproduction of the patient's symptoms.

⚠ *Supine-to-Sit (Long Sitting) Test.* The patient lies supine with the legs straight. The examiner ensures that the medial malleoli are level. The patient is asked to sit up, and the examiner observes whether one leg moves up (proximally) farther than the other (Figs. 10.49 and 10.50). If so, it is believed that there is a functional leg length difference resulting from a pelvic dysfunction caused by pelvic torsion or rotation. [66,79,80] It may also be caused by spasm of the lumbar muscles in the presence of lumbar pathology.

✓ *Yeoman's Test.* [3] The patient lies prone. The examiner flexes the patient's knee to 90° and extends the hip (Fig. 10.51). Pain localized to the sacroiliac joint indicates pathology in the anterior sacroiliac ligaments. Lumbar pain indicates lumbar involvement. [72] Anterior thigh paresthesia may indicate a femoral nerve stretch.

Tests for Limb Length

❓ *Functional Limb Length Test.* [81] The patient stands relaxed while the examiner palpates the ASISs and PSISs, noting any asymmetry. The patient is then placed in the "correct" stance (subtalar joints neutral, knees extended [not hyperextended], and toes facing straight ahead), and the ASISs and PSISs are palpated with the examiner noting whether the asymmetry has been corrected. If the asymmetry has been corrected by "correct" positioning of the limb, the leg is structurally normal (i.e., the bones have proper length), but abnormal joint mechanics (functional deficit) are producing a functional leg length difference. Therefore, if the asymmetry is corrected by proper positioning, the test is positive for a functional leg length difference. See Table 9.9 for lower limb joint changes that can affect functional leg length.

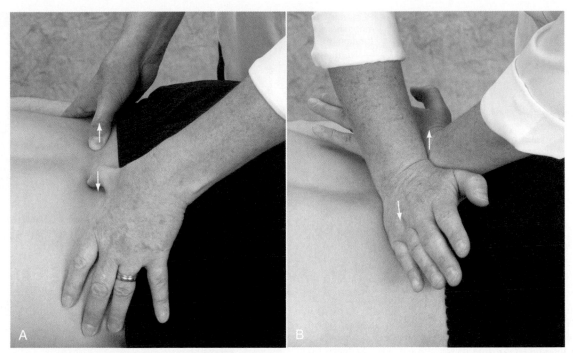

Fig. 10.48 Posterior superior iliac spine distraction test. (A) Using thumbs. (B) Using pisiform bones.

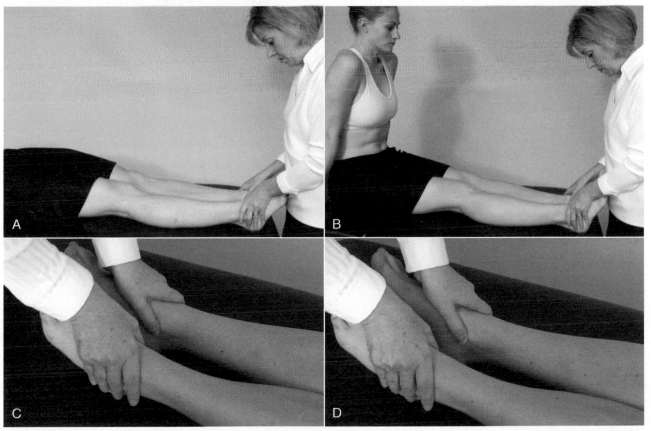

Fig. 10.49 Supine-to-sit test for functional leg length discrepancy. (A) Initial position. (B) Final position. (C) Symmetric leg lengths. (D) Asymmetric leg lengths.

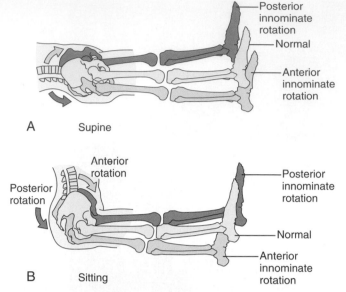

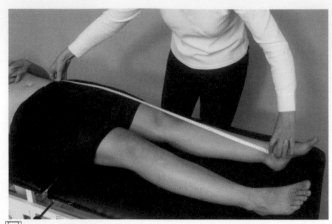

Fig. 10.52 Measuring leg length (anterior superior iliac spine to medial malleolus).

Fig. 10.50 Supine-to-sit test. Leg length reversal; supine (A) versus sitting (B). If the lower limb on the affected side appears longer when a patient lies supine but shorter when sitting, the test is positive, implicating anterior innominate rotation of the affected side. (Redrawn from Wadsworth CT, editor: *Manual examination and treatment of the spine and extremities*, Baltimore, MD, 1988, Williams & Wilkins, p 82.)

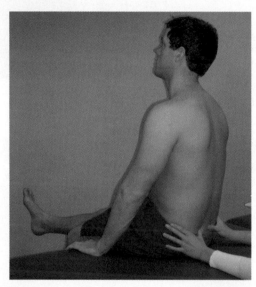

Fig. 10.53 Test of functional length of hamstrings and the sacrotuberous ligament.

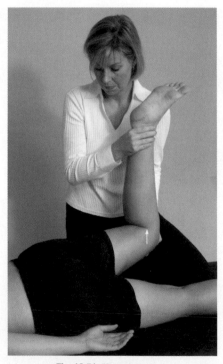

Fig. 10.51 Yeoman's test.

✓ **Leg Length Test.** The leg length test, described in detail in Chapter 11, should always be performed if the examiner suspects a sacroiliac joint lesion. Nutation (backward rotation) of the ilium on the sacrum results in a decrease in leg length—as does counternutation (anterior rotation) on the opposite side. If the iliac bone on one side is lower, the leg on that side is usually longer.[73] True

leg length is measured by placing the patient in a supine position with the ASISs level and the patient's lower limbs perpendicular to the line joining the ASISs (Fig. 10.52). Using a flexible tape measure, the examiner obtains the distance from the ASIS to the medial or lateral malleolus on the same side. The measurement is repeated on the other side and the results are compared. A difference of 1 to 1.3 cm (0.5 to 1 inch) is considered normal. It should be remembered, however, that leg length differences within this range may also be pathological if symptoms result.[82]

Other Tests

❓ **Functional Hamstring Length.**[16] The patient sits on the examining table with the knees flexed to 90°, no weight on the feet, and the spine in neutral. The examiner sits behind the patient and palpates the PSIS with one thumb while the other thumb rests parallel on the sacrum. The patient is asked to actively extend the knee (Fig. 10.53). Normally, full knee extension is possible

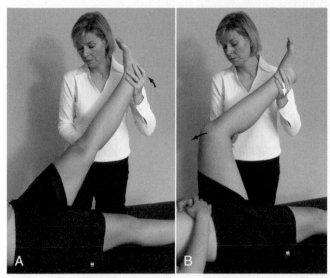

Fig. 10.54 Sign of the buttock test. (A) Hip is flexed with knee straight until resistance or pain is felt. (B) The knee is then flexed to see whether further hip flexion can be achieved. If further hip flexion can be achieved, the test is negative.

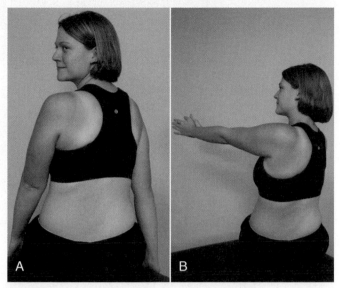

Fig. 10.55 Test of functional length of the thoracolumbar fascia and the latissimus dorsi muscle. (A) Test without stretch. (B) Test with muscle and fascia under stretch. Hands are rotated laterally so palms face upward.

without posterior rotation of the pelvis or flexion of the lumbar spine. Tight hamstrings would cause the pelvis to rotate posteriorly and/or the spine to flex.

☑ *90–90 Straight Leg Raising Test for Hamstring Tightness.* See Chapters 11 and 12.

❷ *Sign of the Buttock Test.* With the patient supine, the examiner performs a passive unilateral SLR test as done previously (Fig. 10.54). If restriction or pain is found on one side, the examiner flexes the patient's knee while holding the patient's thigh in the same position. Once the knee is flexed, the examiner tries to flex the hip further. If the problem is in the lumbar spine or hamstrings, hip flexion increases. This finding indicates a negative sign of the buttock test. If hip flexion does not increase when the knee is flexed, it is a positive sign of the buttock test and indicates pathology in the buttock, such as a bursitis, tumor, or abscess. The patient with this pathology would also exhibit a noncapsular pattern of the hip.

❷ *Thoracolumbar Fascial Length.*[16] The patient sits on the examining table with the knees bent to 90° and a neutral spine. The examiner stands behind the patient. The patient is asked to rotate left and right fully and the examiner notes the ROM available (Fig. 10.55A). The patient is then asked to forward flex the arms to 90° and laterally rotate and adduct the arms so the little fingers touch each other and palms face up (Fig. 10.55B). Holding this arm position, the patient is again asked to rotate left and right as far as possible. The motion will be restricted in the second set of rotations if the thoracolumbar fascia or latissimus dorsi is tight.

☑ *Trendelenburg Test or Sign.* The patient is asked to stand or balance first on one leg and then the other (Fig. 10.56). While the patient is balancing on one leg, the examiner watches the movement of the pelvis. If the

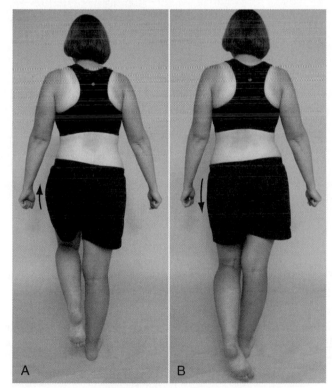

Fig. 10.56 Trendelenburg sign. (A) Negative test. (B) Positive test.

pelvis on the side of the nonstance leg rises, the test is considered negative, because the gluteus medius muscle on the opposite (stance) side lifts it up as it normally does in one-legged stance. If the pelvis on the side of the nonstance leg falls, the test is considered positive and is an indication of weakness or instability of the hip abductor muscles, primarily the gluteus medius on the stance leg

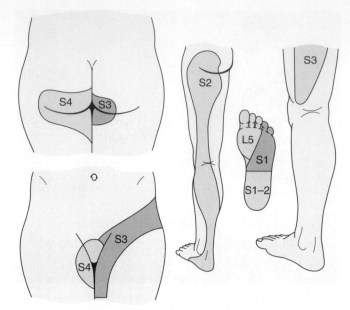

Fig. 10.57 Posterior sacral dermatomes. The representation at the lower left is an anterior view.

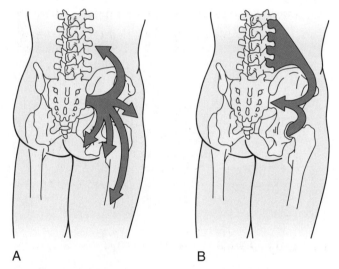

Fig. 10.58 Referred pain from the sacroiliac joint (A) and to the sacroiliac joint (B).

side. Therefore, although the examiner is watching what happens on the nonstance side, it is the stance side that is being tested.

Reflexes and Cutaneous Distribution

There are no reflexes to test for the pelvic joints. However, the examiner must be aware of the dermatomes from the sacral nerve roots (Fig. 10.57). Pain may be referred to the sacroiliac joints from the lumbar spine and the hip (Fig. 10.58). It has been reported that pain from the sacroiliac joints is localized to the gluteal region (94%) and referred to the lower lumbar area (72%), groin (14%), upper lumbar region (6%) or abdomen (2%), and lower

TABLE 10.6

Muscles and Referral of Pain to Pelvic Area

Muscle	Referral Pattern
Longissimus thoracis	From lower thoracic spine to posterior iliac crest and gluteal area
Iliocostalis lumborum	From area lateral to lumbar spine to sacral and gluteal area
Multifidus	Sacral area

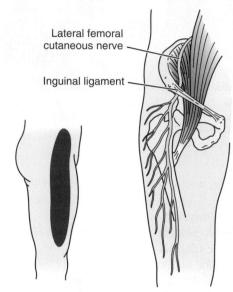

Fig. 10.59 Meralgia paresthetica. The lateral femoral cutaneous nerve supplies the skin of the lateral thigh. An area from the inguinal ligament to the knee may be affected.

limb (28%).[26] Typically the pain runs from the back/buttock outer thigh to the knee. In addition, the sacroiliac joint may refer pain to these same structures or along the courses of the superior gluteal and obturator nerves. The muscles of the spine may also refer pain to the sacral area (Table 10.6).

Peripheral Nerve Injuries About the Pelvis

Meralgia Paresthetica.[83,84] This condition is the result of pressure or entrapment of the lateral femoral cutaneous nerve near the ASIS because the nerve passes under the inguinal ligament. It may result from trauma such as that caused by a seat belt in a car accident, during delivery (in stirrups), by tight clothing, or as a complication of surgery (e.g., hernia). This nerve is sensory only, so the patient experiences sensory alteration and/or burning pain on the lateral aspect of the thigh (Fig. 10.59).

Ilioinguinal Nerve.[85] This nerve, which lies within the transverse abdominis muscle, may be compressed by spasm of the muscle (Fig. 10.60). The nerve is sensory only, and the sensory alteration and/or pain occurs in the superior aspect of the anterior thigh (in the L1 dermatome area) as well as in the scrotum or labia. There have

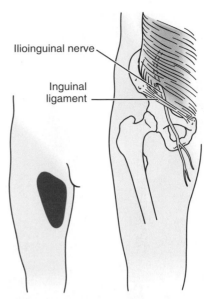

Fig. 10.60 Ilioinguinal syndrome. The ilioinguinal nerve lies within the transversus abdominis and emerges below the inguinal ligament. An area of skin on the medial thigh near the genitalia is affected.

been reports in the literature[86-89] that this nerve may be entrapped with injury to the external oblique muscle aponeurosis (hockey player's syndrome). The patient feels pain especially on ipsilateral hip extension and contralateral torso rotation. The pain may radiate to the groin, scrotum, hip, and back.

Joint Play Movements

The joint play movements (Fig. 10.61) are minimal for the sacroiliac joints and are similar to the passive movements in that they are stress or provocative tests.

Joint Play Movements of the Sacroiliac Joints

- Cephalad movement of the sacrum with caudal movement of the ilium (left and right)
- Cephalad movement of the ilium with caudal movement of the sacrum (left and right)
- Anterior movement of the sacrum on the ilium
- Anteroposterior translation of ilium on sacrum
- Superoinferior translation of ilium on sacrum
- Inferoposterior translation of ilium on sacrum
- Superoanterior translation of ilium on sacrum

To test each of these movements, the patient is in the prone position. For the first joint play movement, the examiner places the heel of one hand over the iliac crest and the heel of the other hand over the apex of the sacrum. The ilium is pushed down or caudally with one hand while the sacrum is pushed up or cephalad with the other hand. The test is repeated for the other ilium (see Fig. 10.61A). The examiner should feel only

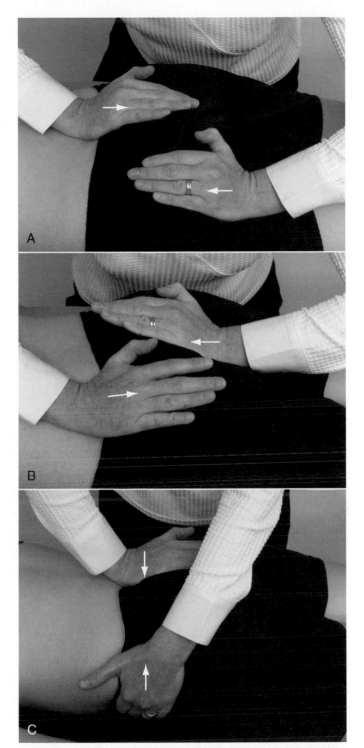

Fig. 10.61 Joint play movements of the sacroiliac joints. (A) Cephalad movement of sacrum with caudal movement of ilium. (B) Cephalad movement of the ilium with caudal movement of the sacrum. (C) Anterior movement of the sacrum on the ilium (left side demonstrated).

minimal movement, and there should be no pain in the joint if the joint is normal. In an affected sacroiliac joint, there is usually pain over the joint and little or no movement. This positioning tests for cephalad movement of the sacrum and caudal movement of the ilium.

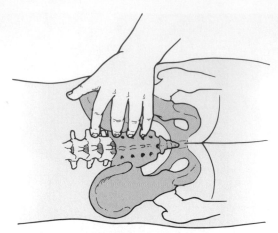

Fig. 10.62 Position of the posterior hand for palpation during mobility and stability testing of the sacroiliac joint.

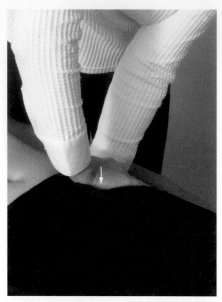

Fig. 10.63 Anteroposterior translation of the ilium on the sacrum.

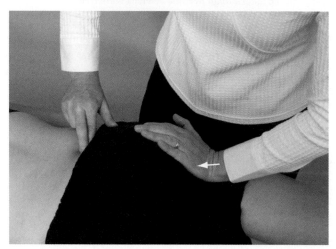

Fig. 10.64 Superoinferior translation of the ilium on the sacrum.

To test caudal movement of the sacrum and cephalad movement of the ilium, the examiner places the heel of one hand over the base of the sacrum and the heel of the other hand over the ischial tuberosity (see Fig. 10.61B). The examiner then pushes the pelvis cephalad and the sacrum caudally. The test is repeated with the other half of the pelvis being moved. The movement and amount of pain are compared.

The anterior movement of the sacrum on the ilium is tested with the patient lying prone (see Fig. 10.61C). The examiner places the heel of one hand over the sacrum and places the other hand under the iliac crest in the area of the ASIS on one side. The hand is then pushed down on the sacrum while the other hand lifts up. The process is repeated on the other side, and the results are compared. Similarly, with the patient supine, a wedge may be used against the sacrum with the patient's body weight acting to push the sacrum forward.

Lee[16,90] has advocated a way to test other translations at the sacroiliac joint. The patient lies supine with the hips and knees in the resting position. The examiner palpates the sacral sulcus just medial to the PSIS with the middle and ring fingers of one hand and the lumbosacral junction with the index finger of the same hand (Fig. 10.62). The middle and ring fingers monitor movement between the sacrum and innominate (ilium) bone while the index finger notes movement between the sacrum and L5.

To test anteroposterior translation of the ilium on the sacrum, the examiner, using the other hand, applies pressure through the iliac crest and ASIS. Posterior movement of the ilium should be noted and end range is achieved at the sacroiliac joint when the pelvis is felt to rotate or move at L5–S1 (Fig. 10.63). The motion is compared with the other side.

To test superoinferior translation of the innominate (ilium) bone on the sacrum, the examiner applies a superior force through the ischial tuberosity (Fig. 10.64). The end of motion is reached when the pelvic girdle is felt to laterally bend beneath L5–S1. The motion is compared with the opposite side.

To test inferoposterior translation of the innominate on the sacrum, the examiner, using the heel of the other hand, applies an anterior rotation force to the ipsilateral ASIS and iliac crest (Fig. 10.65). This produces an inferoposterior glide at the sacroiliac joint and is associated with nutation of the sacrum.

To test superoanterior translation of the innominate on the sacrum, the examiner, using the heel of the other hand, applies a posteriorly rotating force to the ipsilateral ASISs and iliac crest (Fig. 10.66). This produces a superoanterior glide at the sacroiliac joint and is associated with counternutation of the sacrum.

An unstable sacroiliac joint has a softer end feel, increased translation, and possible production of symptoms.[90]

Superoinferior Translation of the Symphysis Pubis.[16] The patient lies supine. The examiner places the heel of one hand on the superior aspect of the superior ramus of

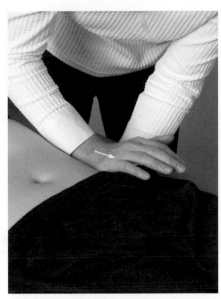

Fig. 10.65 Anterior rotation of the innominate requires an inferoposterior glide at the sacroiliac joint.

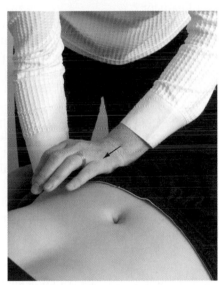

Fig. 10.66 Posterior rotation of the innominate requires a superoanterior glide at the sacroiliac joint.

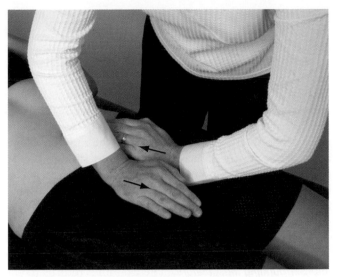

Fig. 10.67 Superoinferior translation of one pubic bone on the other.

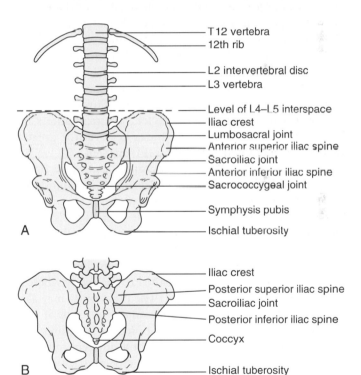

Fig. 10.68 Landmarks of the sacroiliac joints and symphysis pubis. (A) Anterior view. (B) Posterior view.

Palpation[91]

Because many structures are included in the assessment of the pelvic joints, palpation of this area may be extensive, beginning on the anterior aspect and concluding posteriorly. While palpating, the examiner should note any

one pubic bone and the heel of the other hand on the inferior aspect of the superior ramus of the opposite pelvic bone. A slow steady inferior force is applied with the uppermost hand while a superior force is applied with the lower hand (Fig. 10.67). The examiner is testing the end feel and looking for the production of symptoms.

tenderness, muscle spasm, or other signs that may indicate the source of pathology.

Anterior Aspect

The following structures should be carefully and thoroughly palpated (Fig. 10.68A).

Iliac Crest and Anterior Superior Iliac Spine. The palpating fingers are placed on the iliac crests on both sides and gently moved anteriorly until each ASIS is reached. **"Hip pointers"** (crushing or contusion of abdominal muscles that insert into iliac crest) may result in tenderness or pain on palpation of the iliac crest, as may undisplaced fractures. The inguinal ligament attaches to the ASIS and runs downward and medially to the symphysis pubis.

McBurney's Point and Baer's Point. The examiner may then draw an imaginary line from the right ASIS to the umbilicus. The **McBurney's point** lies along this line approximately one third of the distance from the ASIS and is especially tender in the presence of acute appendicitis. The **Baer's point** is located in the right iliac fossa anterior to the right sacroiliac joint and slightly medial to the McBurney's point. It is tender in the presence of infection or when there are sprains of the right sacroiliac ligament and indicates spasm and tenderness of the iliacus muscle.

Lymph Nodes, Symphysis Pubis (Pubic Tubercles), Greater Trochanter of the Femur, Trochanteric Bursa, Femoral Triangle, and Surrounding Musculature. The examiner returns to the ASIS and gently palpates the length of the inguinal ligament, feeling for any tenderness or swelling of the lymph nodes or possible inguinal hernia. At the distal end of the inguinal ligament, the examiner comes to the pubic tubercles and symphysis pubis,[92] which should be carefully palpated for tenderness or signs of pathology.

The examiner then places the thumbs over the pubic tubercles and moves the fingers laterally until the bony greater trochanter of the femur is felt. The trochanters are usually level. The trochanteric bursa lies over the greater trochanter and is palpable only if it is swollen.

Returning to the ASIS, the examiner can move on to palpate the **femoral triangle,** which has as its boundaries the inguinal ligament superiorly, the adductor longus muscle medially, and the sartorius muscle laterally. It is in the superior aspect of the triangle that the examiner palpates for swollen lymph nodes. The **femoral pulse** can be palpated deeper in the triangle. Although it is almost impossible to palpate, the femoral nerve lies lateral to the artery whereas the femoral vein lies medial to it. The psoas bursa may also be palpated within the femoral triangle, but only if it is swollen. Before moving on to the posterior structures, the examiner should determine whether the adjacent musculature—the abductor, flexor, and adductor muscles—shows any indication of pathology (e.g., muscle spasm, pain).

Posterior Aspect

To complete the posterior palpation, the patient lies in the prone position and the following structures are palpated (Fig. 10.68B).

Iliac Crest and Posterior Superior Iliac Spine. Again, the examiner places the fingers on the iliac crest and moves posteriorly until they rest on the PSIS, which is at the level of the S2 spinous process. On many patients, dimples indicate the position of the PSIS. The long dorsal sacroiliac ligament which has a close relationship with the erector spinae muscles (see Fig. 10.2) may be palpated distal to the PSIS and inner lip of the iliac crest as a thick band that attaches distally and medially to the lateral sacral crest

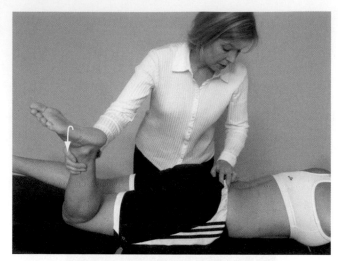

Fig. 10.69 Palpation of the right sacroiliac joint.

of S3 and S4.[12] The ligament becomes taut and painful to palpation when the pelvis is counternutated in the presence of sacroiliac pathology.[8,12] The reverse occurs for the sacrotuberous ligament.[8]

Ischial Tuberosity. If the examiner then moves distally from the PSIS and down to the level of the gluteal folds, the ischial tuberosities may be palpated. It is important that they be palpated because the hamstring muscles attach here and the bony prominences are what one "sits on."

Sacral Sulcus and Sacroiliac Joints. Returning to the PSIS as a starting point, the examiner should palpate slightly below it on the sacrum adjacent to the ilium. (This area is sometimes referred to as the **sacral sulcus.**) The depth on the right side should be compared with that on the left side. If one side is deeper or shallower than the other, sacral torsion or rotation on the ilium around the horizontal plane may be indicated.

If the examiner then moves slightly medially and distal to the PSIS, the fingers rest adjacent to the sacroiliac joints. To palpate these joints, the patient's knee is flexed to 90° or greater and the hip is passively medially rotated while the examiner palpates the sacroiliac joint on the same side (Fig. 10.69). This procedure is identical to the prone gapping test previously described under "Passive Movements." The procedure is repeated on the other side and the two results are compared.

Sacrum, Lumbosacral Joint, Coccyx, Sacral Hiatus, Sacral Cornua, and Sacrotuberous and Sacrospinous Ligaments. The examiner again returns to the PSIS and moves to the midline of the sacrum, where the S2 spinous process can be palpated.

Moving superiorly over two spinous processes, the fingers now rest on the spinous process of L5. As a check, the examiner may look to see if the fingers rest just below a horizontal line drawn from the high point of the iliac crests. This horizontal line normally passes through the interspace between L4 and L5. Having

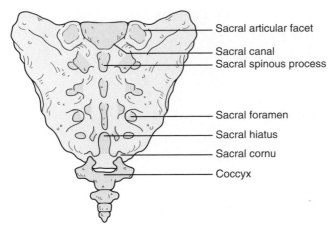

Fig. 10.70 Posterior view of the sacrum and coccyx.

Sacral articular facet
Sacral canal
Sacral spinous process
Sacral foramen
Sacral hiatus
Sacral cornu
Coccyx

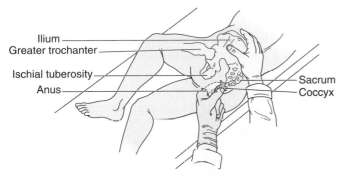

Fig. 10.71 Palpation of the coccyx.

Ilium
Greater trochanter
Ischial tuberosity
Anus
Sacrum
Coccyx

found the L5 spinous process, the examiner then palpates between the spinous processes of L5 and S1, feeling for signs of pathology at the lumbosacral joint. Moving laterally approximately 2 to 3 cm (0.8 to 1.2 inches), the fingers lie over the lumbosacral facet joints, which are not palpable. However, the overlying structures may be palpated for tenderness or spasm, which may indicate pathology of these joints or related structures. In a similar fashion, the spinous processes and facet joints of the other lumbar spines and intervening structures can be palpated.

The examiner then returns to the S2 spinous process or tubercle. Carefully palpating farther distally (just before the coccyx), the examiner may be able to palpate the sacral hiatus lying in the midline. If the fingers are moved slightly laterally, the sacral cornua, which constitute the distal aspect of the sacrum, may be palpated (Fig. 10.70).

To palpate the coccyx properly, the examiner performs a rectal examination (Fig. 10.71). A rubber glove is put on, and the index finger is lubricated. The index finger is then carefully pushed into the rectum as the patient relaxes the sphincter muscles. The index finger then palpates the anterior surface of the coccyx while the thumb of the same hand palpates its posterior aspect. While holding the coccyx between the finger and thumb, the examiner is able to move it back and forth, rocking it

at the sacrococcygeal joint. Normally this action should not cause pain.

The examiner then returns to the PSIS. Moving straight down or distally from the PSIS, the fingers follow the path of the **sacrotuberous ligament,** which should be palpated for tenderness. Conversely, the examiner may palpate the insertion of the long head of biceps femoris (i.e., lateral hamstrings) into the ischium and move superiorly to the superior aspect of the ischium where the ligament inserts just above the ischial tuberosity and follow it superiorly. Slightly more than halfway between the PSIS and ischial tuberosity and slightly medially, the fingers pass over the **sacrospinous ligament,** which is deep to the sacrotuberous ligament. Tenderness in this area may indicate pathology of this ligament.

Diagnostic Imaging[93]

Plain Film Radiography

X-rays that may be commonly taken in the pelvic area if pathology is suspected are shown in the following box.

Common X-Ray Views of the Pelvic Area

- Anteroposterior view (see Fig. 10.76)
- Judet view of the hip and pelvis (Fig. 10.79)
- Sacroiliac joints—Ferguson view (30° cephalad angulated anteroposterior) (Fig. 10.80)
- Pelvis—pelvic inlet/outlet views (for pelvic ring fracture) (Fig. 10.81)

On plain film radiography, anteroposterior views (bilateral and single stance) (Figs. 10.72 through 10.74), the examiner should look for or note the following:

1. Ankylosis of sacroiliac joints (e.g., ankylosing spondylitis; Fig. 10.75).
2. Displacement of one sacroiliac joint and/or the symphysis pubis (Fig. 10.76).[94]

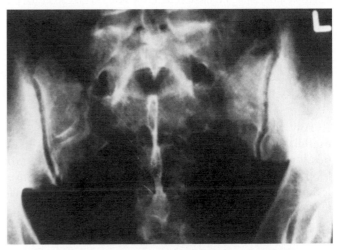

Fig. 10.72 Anteroposterior radiograph of the sacroiliac joint.

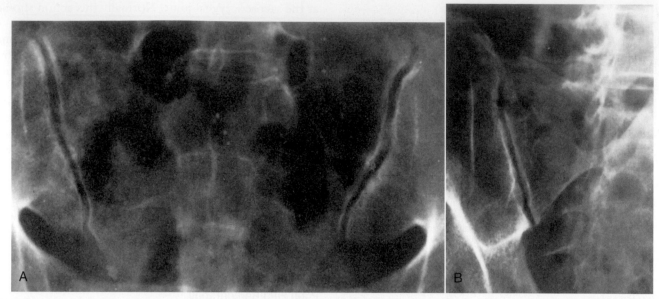

Fig. 10.73 Normal sacroiliac joints. Angled (A) and oblique (B) anteroposterior views show normally maintained cortices and cartilage spaces. (From Weissman BNW, Sledge CB: *Orthopedic radiology*, Philadelphia, 1986, WB Saunders, p 347.)

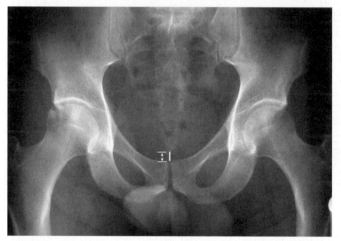

Fig. 10.74 A properly centered anteroposterior radiograph must be controlled for rotation and tilt. Proper rotation is confirmed by alignment of the coccyx over the symphysis pubis *(vertical line)*. Proper tilt is controlled by maintaining the distance between the tip of the coccyx and the superior border of the symphysis pubis at 1 to 2 cm. (From Byrd JWT: Arthroscopic management of femoroacetabular impingement, *Op Tech Sports Med* 19:81–94, 2011.)

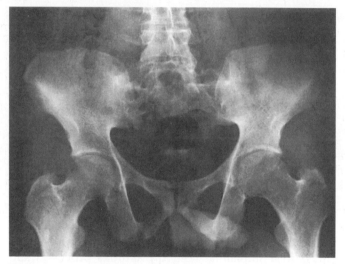

Fig. 10.75 Fusion of sacroiliac joint spaces in the late stage of sacroiliitis of ankylosing spondylitis (anteroposterior view). The sclerosis has resorbed, and there is slight narrowing of the left hip joint. (From Rothman RH, Simeone FA: *The spine*, Philadelphia, 1982, WB Saunders, p. 921.)

3. Demineralization, sclerosis, or periosteal reaction of one or both pubic bones at the symphysis pubis (e.g., osteitis pubis; Fig. 10.77).
4. Any fracture.
5. Relation of the sacrum to the ilium.
6. Single leg stance (Flamingo) x-rays can show up to 5 mm of movement at the symphysis pubis in asymptomatic subject comparing alternate leg views.[95,96]
7. Ferguson's angle (also called *lumbosacral angle, sacral base angle,* or *sacral slope*)[97] is formed by a line along the top of the sacral base and a horizontal line (normal: 41°) (Fig. 10.78).

Diagnostic Ultrasound Imaging

At present, there is minimal use for musculoskeletal diagnostic ultrasound imaging (DUSI) in the sacroiliac region. Le Goff et al.[98] have examined the posterior sacroiliac ligaments. There are several ligaments that maintain sacroiliac joint stability—the anterior ligament, the interosseous ligament, and the posterior sacroiliac ligaments. The posterior ligaments have been identified as a potential source of atypical back pain.[99] To find the posterior sacroiliac ligaments, the patient is positioned prone. The bony spinous process in the midline of the sacrum and the sacral wings are seen as regular echogenic lines on each side of the spinous process. The transducer is

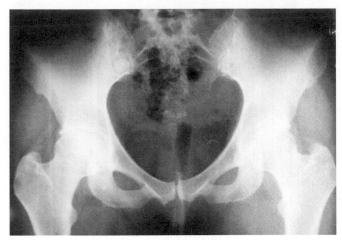

Fig. 10.76 Anteroposterior radiograph of the pelvis. Note the higher left pubic bone.

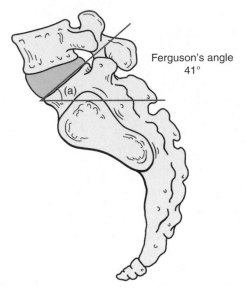

Ferguson's angle 41°

(a)

Fig. 10.78 Ferguson's angle (normal is approximately 41°).

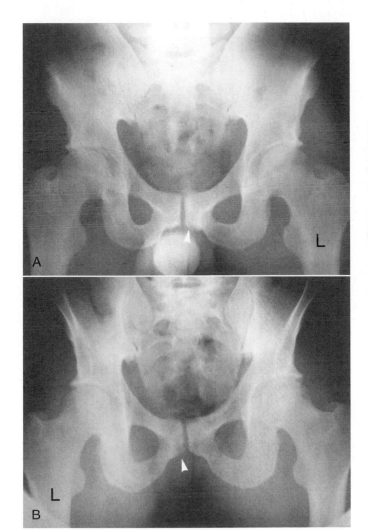

A

L

L

B

Fig. 10.77 Osteitis pubis. (A) Anteroposterior view of the pelvis showing a well-concealed bony lesion at the inferior corner of the left pubis at the symphysis *(arrowhead)*. (B) Posterior view of the same pelvis; the bone fragment is well delineated in this view. (From Wiley JJ: Traumatic osteitis pubis: the gracilis syndrome, *Am J Sports Med* 11:360–363, 1983.)

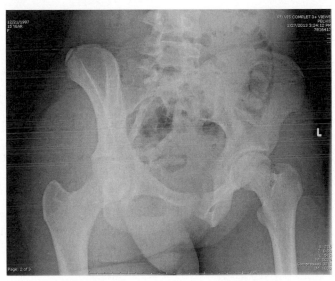

Fig. 10.79 Judet view of the left hip and pelvis.

then moved in the short axis laterally (Fig. 10.82) until the PSIS is visualized as a curved echogenic line (Fig. 10.83).[98] The short posterior sacroiliac ligament is the oblique ligament stretching from the posterior tuberosity of the ilium to the sacral wings. The transducer can then be rotated slightly obliquely (Fig. 10.84) where the long sacroiliac ligament appears as the structure attached superiorly to the PSIS and inferiorly to the third sacral transverse tubercle (Fig. 10.85).

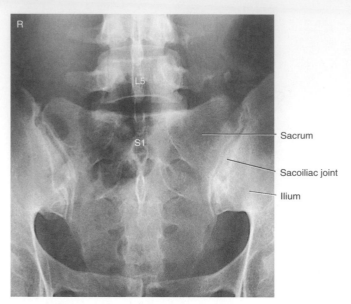

Fig. 10.80 Ferguson view (30° cephalad angulated anteroposterior) of the lumbosacral junction and sacroiliac joints. (From Frank ED, Long BW, Smith BJ: *Merrill's atlas of radiographic positioning and procedures: 3-volume set*, ed 12, St Louis, 2012, Mosby.)

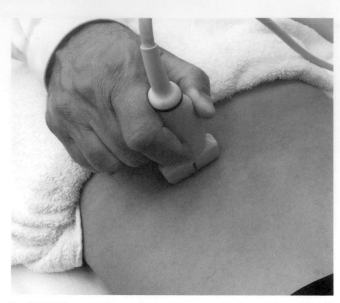

Fig. 10.82 Ultrasound transducer placement in short axis to identify the posterior inferior iliac spine, the ilium and short posterior sacral ligament.

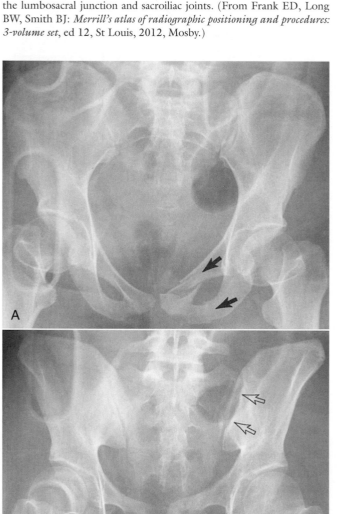

Fig. 10.81 (A) An anteroposterior inlet projection of a 22-year-old man who suffered a type III Malgaigne fracture-dislocation reveals minimally displaced vertical fractures *(arrows)* of both the left superior pubic ramus and the left ischiopubic ramus. On this view, the sacrum, ilium, and sacroiliac joints appear normal. (B) On the anteroposterior outlet view, the diastasis of the left sacroiliac joint becomes obvious *(open arrows)*. (From Taylor JA, et al: *Skeletal imaging*, ed 2, St Louis, 2010, WB Saunders.)

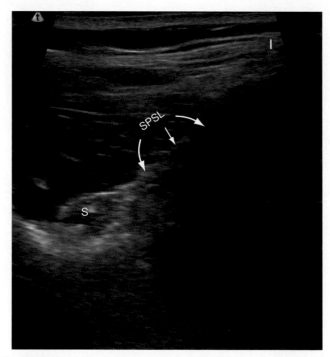

Fig. 10.83 Short-axis ultrasound scan of the short posterior sacroiliac ligament *(SPSL)*, the sacrum *(S)*, and the ilium *(I)*.

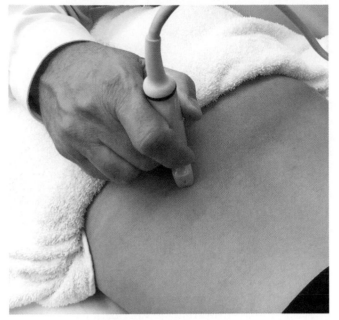

Fig. 10.84 Ultrasound transducer placement in long axis and slightly oblique to identify the long posterior sacroiliac ligament, the posterior inferior iliac spine, and the sacrum.

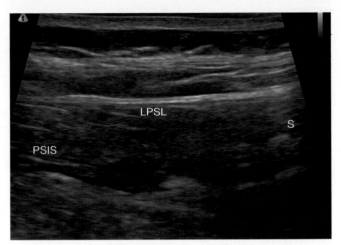

Fig. 10.85 Long-axis oblique ultrasound image of the long posterior sacroiliac ligament *(LPSL)*, the posterior superior iliac spine *(PSIS)*, and the sacrum *(S)*.

PRÉCIS OF THE PELVIS ASSESSMENT[a]

NOTE: Suspected pathology will determine which Special Tests are to be performed.

History (sitting)
Observation (standing)
Examination
  Active movements (standing)
    Flexion of the spine
    Extension of the spine
    Rotation of the spine (left and right)
    Side flexion of the spine (left and right)
    Flexion of the hip
    Abduction of the hip
    Adduction of the hip
    Extension of the hip
    Medial rotation of the hip
    Lateral rotation of the hip
  Special tests (standing)
    Drop test
    Flamingo test
    Gillet test
    Trendelenburg test
  Special tests (sitting)
    Piedallu's sign
  Passive movements (supine)
    Femoral shear test
    Gapping test
    Rocking (knee-to-shoulder) test
    Sacral apex pressure test
    Sacral thrust test
    Thigh thrust test
  Resisted isometric movements (supine)[b]
    Forward flexion of the spine
    Flexion of the hip
    Abduction of the hip
    Adduction of the hip
    Extension of the hip
  Special tests (supine)
    Leg length measurement
    90–90 straight leg raise
    Patrick test
    Straight leg raise test
    Supine active straight leg raise test
    Supine-to-sit (long sitting) test
  Passive movements (side lying)
    Approximation test
    Passive extension and medial rotation of ilium on sacrum
    Passive flexion and lateral rotation of ilium on sacrum
  Special tests (side lying)
    Gaenslen's test
  Reflexes and cutaneous distribution (supine, then prone)
  Passive movements (prone)
    Hip abduction and external (lateral) rotation (HABER) test
    Ipsilateral prone kinetic test
    Prone gapping (Hibb's) test
    Sacral apex pressure test
  Special tests (prone)
    Posterior superior iliac spine distraction test
    Prone active straight leg raise test
    Yeoman's test
  Joint play movements (prone)
    Cephalad movement of the sacrum with caudal movement of the ilium
    Cephalad movement of the ilium with caudal movement of the sacrum
  Palpation (prone, then supine)
  Diagnostic imaging

As previously stated, assessment of the sacroiliac joints and symphysis pubis is done only after an assessment of the lumbar spine and hips unless there has been specific trauma to the sacroiliac joints or symphysis pubis. Completion of the examination of the sacroiliac joints and symphysis pubis, therefore, may involve only passive movements, special tests, joint play movements, and palpation because the other tests would have been completed when the other joints were assessed.

After any examination, the patient should be warned of the possibility of exacerbation of symptoms as a result of the assessment.

[a]The précis is shown in an order that will limit the amount of moving or changing position that the patient has to do and yet ensure that all necessary structures are tested.
[b]If not done in standing.

CASE STUDIES

When doing these case studies, the examiner should list the appropriate questions to be asked and why they are being asked, what to look for and why, and what things should be tested and why. Depending on the patient's answers (and the examiner should consider different responses), several possible causes of the patient's problem may become evident (examples are given in parentheses). A differential diagnosis chart (Table 10.7) should be made up. The examiner can then decide how different diagnoses may affect the treatment plan.

1. A 20-year-old female softball player reports an insidious onset of bilateral lower back and hip pain that causes radiating pain along the lateral hip and into the anterior thigh; the pain is increased with running. She does not remember any traumatic event that caused these symptoms. They are usually worse after softball practice. Describe your assessment of this condition and how to differentiate (sacroiliac vs. neurological dysfunction).

2. A 54-year-old male professor fell on ice a week earlier and landed directly on his buttocks. He reports right-sided low back and sacroiliac pain. He reports feeling as though his hip and sacroiliac joint were "jammed up" on the right. He is walking with a limp on the right due to pain. His ASIS and PSIS are both higher on the right as compared with the left. He has significant lumbar paraspinal muscle tone on the right compared with the left. Describe your assessment of his condition and how to differentiate (sacroiliac dysfunction vs. leg length difference vs. up slip).

3. A 26-year-old male soccer player complains of lower abdominal pain that is referred into the right groin. Sit-ups are painful, and he experiences pain when he kicks the ball. Describe your assessment plan for this patient (abdominal strain vs. osteitis pubis).

4. A 35-year-old man complains of "back pain." He says that his back is stiff and sore when he gets up in the morning and that the stiffness remains for most of the day. Sclerosis of the sacroiliac is evident on x-ray. Describe your assessment plan for this patient (ankylosing spondylitis vs. osteoarthritis of the sacroiliac joints).

5. An 18-year-old female figure skater complains of back pain that increases when she is skating; the pain is prominent on one leg. The ASIS and PSIS are higher on the right side. Describe your assessment plan for this patient (sacroiliac dysfunction vs. short leg syndrome).

TABLE 10.7

Differential Diagnosis Between Ankylosing Spondylitis and Sacroiliac Arthritis

	Ankylosing Spondylitis	Sacroiliac Arthritis
History	Bilateral sacroiliac pain that may refer to posterior thigh Morning stiffness Male predominance	Bilateral sacroiliac pain referring to gluteal area (S1–S2 dermatomes) Morning stiffness (prolonged) Coughing painful
Observation	Stiff, controlled movement of pelvis	Controlled movement of pelvis
Active movement	Decreased	Side flexion and extension full Slight limitation of flexion
Passive movement	Decreased	Normal
Resisted isometric movement	Pain and weakness, especially if sacroiliac joints are stressed	Pain, especially if sacroiliac joints are stressed
Special tests	Sacral stress tests probably positive	Sacral stress tests probably positive
Sensation and reflexes	Normal	Normal
Palpation	Tender over sacroiliac joints	Tender over sacroiliac joints
Diagnostic imaging	X-rays diagnostic	X-rays diagnostic
Lab tests	Erythrocyte sedimentation rate increased human leukocyte antigen (HLA)—B27 HLA present in 80%	Normal

References

1. Kim SB, You JS, Kwon OY, Yi CH. Lumbopelvic kinematic characteristics of golfers with limited hip rotation. *Am J Sports Med*. 2014;43(1):113–120.

2. Schwarzer AC, Aprill CN, Bogduk N. The sacroiliac joint in chronic low back pain. *Spine*. 1995;20:31–37.

3. Ombregt L. *A System of Orthopedic Medicine*. 3rd ed. Edinburgh: Churchill Livingstone; 2013.

4. Polly DW. The sacroiliac joint. *Neurosurg Clin N Am*. 2017;28(3):301–312.

5. Kapandji LA. *The trunk and vertebral column. The Physiology of the Joints*. Vol. 3. New York: Churchill Livingstone; 1974.

6. Murakami E, Aizawa T, Kurosawa D, Noguchi K. Leg symptoms associated with sacroiliac joint disorder and related pain. *Clin Neurol Neurosurg*. 2017;157:55–58.

7. McGrath MC. Composite sacroiliac joint pain provocation tests: a question of clinical significance. *Int J Osteopath Med*. 2010;13(1):24–30.

8. Vleeming A, Pool-Goudzwaard AL, Hammudoghu D, et al. The function of the long dorsal sacroiliac ligament-its implication for understanding low back pain. *Spine*. 1996;21:556–562.

9. Jackson R. Diagnosis and treatment of pelvic girdle dysfunction. *Orthop Phys Ther Clin North Am*. 1998;7:413–445.

10. Vleeming A, Schuenke MD, Masi AT, et al. The sacroiliac joint: an overview of its anatomy, function and potential clinical implications. *J Anat*. 2012;221(6):537–567.

11. Soto Quijano DA, Otero Loperena E. Sacroiliac joint interventions. *Phys Med Rehabil Clin N Am*. 2018;29(1):171–183.

12. Cusi MF. Paradigm for assessment and treatment of SIJ mechanical dysfunction. *J Body Mov Thor*. 2010;14(2):152–161.

13. Rosatelli AL, Agur AM, Chhaya S. Anatomy of the interosseous region of the sacroiliac joint. *J Orthop Sports Phys Ther*. 2006;36(4):200–208.

14. Arumugam A, Milosavljevic S, Woodley S, et al. Effects of external pelvic compression on form closure, force closure and neuromotor control of the lumbopelvic spine—a systematic review. *Man Ther*. 2012;17:275–284.

15. Lee D. The pelvic girdle. In: Magee DJ, Zachazewski JE, Quillen WS, eds. *Musculoskeletal Rehabilitation—Pathology and Intervention*. Philadelphia: Elsevier; 2007.

16. Lee D. *The Pelvic Girdle*. 2nd ed. Edinburgh: Churchill Livingstone; 1999.

17. Pool-Goudzwaard AL, Vleeming A, Stoeckart R, et al. Insufficient lumbopelvic stability: a clinical, anatomical and biomechanical approach to "a-specific" low back pain. *Man Ther*. 1998;3(1):12–20.

18. Vleeming A, Albert HB, Ostgaard HC, et al. European guidelines for the diagnosis and treatment of pelvic girdle pain. *Eur Spine J*. 2008;17(6):794–819.

19. van Wingerden JP, Vleeming A, Buyruk HM, Raissadat K. Stabilization of the sacroiliac joint in vivo: verification of muscular contribution to force closure of the pelvis. *Eur Spine J*. 2004;13(3):199–205.

20. Vleeming A, Stoeckart R, Volkers AC, Snijders CJ. Relation between form and function in the sacroiliac joint. Part 1: clinical anatomical aspects. *Spine*. 1990;15(2):130–132.

21. Vleeming A, Stoeckart R, Volkers AC, Snijders CJ. Relation between form and function in the sacroiliac joint. Part 2: biomechanical aspects. *Spine*. 1990;15(2):133–136.

22. Vleeming A, Pool-Goudzwaard AL, Hammudoghu D, et al. The posterior layer of the thoracolumbar fascia: its function in load transfer from spine to legs. *Spine*. 1995;20:753–758.

23. Vleeming A, Snidjers CJ, Stoeckart R, et al. The role of the sacroiliac joints in coupling between spine, pelvis, legs and arms. In: Vleeming A, Mooney V, Dorman T, et al., eds. *Movement, Stability and Low Back Pain*. Edinburgh: Churchill Livingstone; 1997.

24. Lee DG. Clinical manifestations of pelvic girdle dysfunction. In: Boyling JD, Palastanga N, eds. *Grieve's Modern Manual Therapy: The Vertebral Column*. 2nd ed. Edinburgh: Churchill Livingstone; 1994.

25. Cohen SP. Sacroiliac joint pain: a comprehensive review of anatomy, diagnosis and treatment. *Anesth Analg*. 2005;101(5):1440–1453.

26. Vanelderen P, Szadek K, Cohen SP, et al. Sacroiliac joint syndrome. *Pain Pract*. 2010;10(5):470–478.

27. Liebenson C. The relationship of the sacroiliac joint, stabilization musculature, and lumbo-pelvic instability. *J Body Mov Ther*. 2004;8:43–45.

28. Cohen SP. Sacroiliac joint pain. In: Benzon H, Raja SN, Fishman SM, et al., eds. *Essentials of Pain Medicine*. 4th ed. Philadelphia: Elsevier; 2018.

29. Adhia DB, Tumilty S, Mani R, et al. Can hip abduction and external rotation discriminate sacroiliac joint pain? *Man Ther*. 2016;21:191–197.

30. Patella GA, Andrish JT. Injuries about the hip and pelvis in the young athlete. *Clin Sports Med*. 1995;14:591–628.

31. Ombregt L, Bisschop B, ter Veer HJ, et al. *A System of Orthopedic Medicine*. London: WB Saunders; 1995.

32. Dangaria TR. A case report of sacroiliac joint dysfunction with urinary symptoms. *Man Ther*. 1998;3:220–221.

33. Maigne R. *Orthopaedic Medicine: A New Approach to Vertebral Manipulation*. Springfield, IL: Charles C Thomas; 1972.

34. Maigne R. *Diagnosis and Treatment of Pain of Vertebral Origin*. Baltimore: Williams & Wilkins; 1996.

35. Levine D, Whittle MW. The effects of pelvic movement on lumbar lordosis in the standing position. *J Orthop Sports Phys Ther*. 1996;24:130–135.

36. Hagins M, Brown M, Cook C, et al. Intratester and intertester reliability of the palpation meter (PALM) in measuring the pelvic position. *J Man Manip Ther*. 1998;6:130–136.

37. Kendall FP, McCreary EK, Provance PG. *Muscles: Testing and Function*. Baltimore: Williams & Wilkins; 1993.

38. Nelson-Wong E, Flynn T, Callaghan JP. Development of acute hip abduction as a screening test for identifying occupational low back pain. *J Orthop Sports Phys Ther*. 2009;39:649–657.

39. Mitchell FL, Moran PS, Pruzzo NA. *An Evaluation and Treatment Manual of Osteopathic Muscle Energy Procedures*. Valley Park, MO: Mitchell, Moran & Pruzzo; 1979.

40. Woerman AL. Evaluation and treatment of dysfunction in the lumbar-pelvic-hip complex. In: Donatelli R, Wooden MJ, eds. *Orthopedic Physical Therapy*. Edinburgh: Churchill Livingstone; 1989.

41. Levangie PK. The association between static pelvic asymmetry and low back pain. *Spine*. 1999;24:1234–1242.

42. Greenman PE. Innominate shear dysfunction in the sacroiliac syndrome. *Man Med*. 1986;2:114–121.

43. Bookhout MM, Boissonnault JS. Musculoskeletal dysfunction in the female pelvis. *Orthop Phys Ther Clin North Am*. 1996;5:23–45.

44. Oldrieve WL. A critical review of the literature on tests of the sacroiliac joint. *J Man Manip Ther*. 1995;3:157–161.

45. Levangie PK. Four clinical tests of sacroiliac joint dysfunction: the association of test results with innominate torsion among patients with and without low back pain. *Phys Ther*. 1999;79:1043–1057.

46. Freburger JK, Riddle DL. Measurement of sacroiliac joint dysfunction: a multicenter intertester reliability study. *Phys Ther*. 1999;79:1135–1141.

47. van der Wurff P, Hagmeijer RH, Meijne W. Clinical tests of the sacroiliac joint—a systematic methodological review. Part 1—reliability. *Man Ther*. 2000;5:30–36.

48. van der Wurff P, Meijne W, Hagmeijer RH. Clinical tests of the sacroiliac joint—a systematic methodological review, Part 2—validity. *Man Ther*. 2000;5:89–96.

49. Cibulka MT, Koldehoff R. Clinical usefulness of a cluster of sacroiliac joint tests in patients with and without low back pain. *J Orthop Sports Phys Ther*. 1999;29:83–92.

50. Meijne W, van Neerbos K, Aufdemkampe G, et al. Intraexaminer and interexaminer reliability of the Gillet test. *J Manip Physiol Ther*. 1999;22:4–9.

51. Hancock MJ, Maher CG, Latimer J, et al. Systematic review of tests to identify the disc, SIJ or facet joint as a source of low back pain. *Eur Spine J*. 2007;16(10):1539–1550.

52. Laslett M, Young SB, Aprill CN, McDonald B. Diagnosing painful sacroiliac joints: a validity study of a McKenzie evaluation and sacroiliac provocation tests. *Aust J Physiother*. 2003;49(2):89–97.

53. Kokmeyer DJ, Van der Wurff P, Aufdemkampe G, et al. The reliability of multitest regimens with sacroiliac pain provocation tests. *J Manip Physiol Ther*. 2002;25(1):42–48.

54. van der Wurff P, Buijs EJ, Groen GJ. A multitest regimen of pain provocation tests as an aid to reducing unnecessary minimally invasive sacroiliac joint procedures. *Phys Med Rehabil*. 2006;87:10–14.

55. Szadek KM, van der Wurff P, Tulder MW, et al. Diagnostic validity of criteria for sacroiliac joint pain: a systematic review. *J Pain*. 2009;10:354–368.

56. Laslett M, Aprill CN, McDonald B, et al. Diagnosis of sacroiliac joint pain: validity of individual provocation tests and composites of tests. *Man Ther*. 2005;10:207–218.

57. Dreyfuss P, Michaelsen M, Pauza K, et al. The value of medical history and physical examination in diagnosing sacroiliac joint pain. *Spine*. 1996;21:2594–2602.

58. Dreyfuss P, Dreyer S, Griffin J, et al. Positive sacroiliac screening tests in asymptomatic adults. *Spine*. 1994;10:1138–1143.

59. Laslett M, Williams M. The reliability of selected pain provocation tests for sacroiliac joint pathology. *Spine*. 1994;19:1243–1249.

60. Soleimanifar M, Karimi N, Arab AM. Association between composites of selected motion palpation and pain provocation tests for sacroiliac joint disorders. *J Bodyw Mov Ther*. 2017;21(2):240–245.

61. Takasaki H, Iizawa T, Hall T, et al. The influence of increasing sacroiliac joint force closure of the hip and lumbar spine extensor muscle firing pattern. *Man Ther*. 2009;14(5):484–489.

62. Sturesson B, Udeu A, Vleeming A. A radiostereometric analysis of movements of the sacroiliac joints during the standing hip flexion test. *Spine*. 2000;25:364–368.

63. Ozgocmen S, Bozgeyik Z, Kalcik M, et al. The value of sacroiliac pain provocative tests in early active sacroiliitis. *Clin Rheum*. 2008;27:1275–1282.

64. Cattley P, Winyard J, Trevaskis J, Eaton S. Validity and reliability of clinical tests for the sacroiliac joint. A review of the literature. *Australas Chiropr Osteopathy*. 2002;10(2):73–80.

65. Dreyfus P, Dreyer S, Griffin J, et al. Positive sacroiliac screening tests in asymptomatic adults. *Spine*. 1994;19:1138–1143.

66. Porterfield JA, DeRosa C. *Mechanical Low Back Pain: Perspectives in Functional Anatomy*. Philadelphia: WB Saunders; 1991.

67. Capobianco RA, Feeney DF, Jeffers JR, et al. Patients with sacroiliac joint dysfunction exhibit altered movement strategies when performing a sit-to-stand task. *Spine J*. 2018;18(8):1434–1440.

68. Rubinstein SM, van Tulder M. A best evidence review of diagnostic procedures for neck and low back pain. *Best Pract Res Clin Rheumat*. 2008;22(3):471–482.

69. Dreyfuss P, Deyer SJ, Cole A, et al. Sacroiliac joint pain. *J Am Acad Ortho Surg*. 2004;12:255–265.

70. Cook CE, Hegedus EJ. *Orthopedic Physical Examination Tests—An Evidence Based Approach*. Upper Saddle River, NJ: Prentice Hall/Pearson; 2008.

71. Cleland JA, Koppenhaver S. In: *Netter's Orthopedic Clinical Examination—An Evidence Based Approach*. Philadelphia: Saunders; 2011.

72. Cipriano JJ. *Photographic Manual of Regional Orthopedic Tests*. Baltimore: Williams & Wilkins; 1985.

73. DonTigny RL. Dysfunction of the sacroiliac joint and its treatment. *J Orthop Sports Phys Ther*. 1979;1:23–35.

74. Mens JM, Vleeming A, Snijders CJ, et al. The active straight leg raising test and mobility of the pelvic joints. *Eur Spine*. 1999;8:468–473.

75. Mens JM, Vleeming A, Snijders CJ, et al. Reliability and validity of the active straight leg raise test in posterior pelvic pain since pregnancy. *Spine*. 2001;26:1167–1171.

76. Mens JM, Vleeming A, Snijders CJ, et al. Validity of the active straight leg raise test for measuring disease severity in patients with posterior pelvic pain after pregnancy. *Spine*. 2002;27:196–200.

77. Evans RC. *Illustrated Essentials in Orthopedic Physical Assessment*. St Louis: CV Mosby; 1994.

78. Werner CM, Hoch A, Gautier L, et al. Distraction test of the posterior superior iliac spine (PSIS) in the diagnosis of sacroiliac arthropathy. *BMC Surg*. 2013;13:52–57.

79. Palmer MC, Epler M. *Clinical Assessment Procedures in Physical Therapy*. Philadelphia: JB Lippincott; 1990.

80. Bemis T, Daniel M. Validation of the long sitting test on subjects with iliosacral dysfunction. *J Orthop Sports Phys Ther*. 1987;8:336–345.

81. Wallace LA. Limb length difference and back pain. In: Grieve GP, ed. *Modern Manual Therapy of the Vertebral Column*. Edinburgh: Churchill Livingstone; 1986.

82. Fischer P. Clinical measurement and significance of leg length and iliac crest height discrepancies. *J Man Manip Ther*. 1997;5:57–60.

83. Pecina MM, Krmpotic-Nemanic J, Markiewitz AD. *Tunnel Syndromes*. Boca Raton, FL: CRC Press; 1991.

84. Ivins GK. Meralgia paresthetica, the elusive diagnosis: clinical experience with 14 adult patients. *Ann Surg*. 2000;232(2):281–286.

85. Borenstein DG, Wiesel SW, Boden SD. *Low Back Pain: Medical Diagnosis and Comprehensive Management*. Philadelphia: WB Saunders; 1995.

86. Lacroix VJ. Lower abdominal pain syndrome in National Hockey League players: a report of 11 cases. *Clin J Sports Med*. 1998;8:5–9.

87. Lacroix VJ. A complete approach to groin pain. *Phys Sportsmed*. 2000;28(1):66–86.

88. Simonet WT, Saylor HL, Sim L. Abdominal wall muscle tears in hockey players. *Int J Sports Med*. 1995;16:126–128.

89. Taylor DC, Meyers WC, Moylan JA, et al. Abdominal musculature abnormalities as a cause of groin pain in athletes-inguinal hernias and pubalgia. *Am J Sports Med*. 1991;19:239–242.

90. Lee D. Instability of the sacroiliac joint and the consequences to gait. *J Man Manip Ther*. 1996;4:22–29.

91. O'Haire C, Gibbons P. Inter-examiner and intra-examiner agreement for assessing sacroiliac anatomical landmarks using palpation and observation: pilot study. *Man Ther*. 2000;5:13–20.

92. Williams PR, Thomas DP, Downes EM. Osteitis pubis and instability of the pubic symphysis—when nonoperative measures fail. *Am J Sports Med*. 2000;28:350–355.

93. Ebraheim NA, Mekhail AO, Wiley WF, et al. Yeasting: radiology of the sacroiliac joint. *Spine*. 1997;22:869–876.

94. Rodriguez C, Miguel A, Lima H, et al. Osteitis pubis syndrome in the professional soccer athlete: a case report. *J Athl Train*. 2001;36:437–440.

95. Garras DN, Carothers JT, Olson SA. Single-leg-stance (flamingo) radiographs to assess pelvic stability: how much motion is normal. *J Bone Joint Surg Am*. 2008;90:2114–2118.

96. Siegel J, Templeman DC, Tornetta P. Single-leg-stance radiographs in the diagnosis of pelvic instability. *J Bone Joint Surg Am*. 2008;90:2119–2125.

97. Hellems HK, Keats TE. Measurement of the normal lumbosacral angle. *Am J Radiol*. 1971;113:642–645.

98. Le Goff B, Berthelot JM, Maugars Y. Ultrasound assessment of the posterior sacroiliac ligaments. *Clin Exp Rheumatol*. 2011;29(6):1014–1017.

99. Berthelot JM, Labat JJ, Le Goff B, et al. Provocative sacroiliac joint maneuvers and sacroiliac joint block are unreliable for diagnosing sacroiliac joint pain. *Joint Bone Spine*. 2006;73(1):17–23.

100. Leboeuf C. The sensitivity and specificity of seven lumbo-pelvic orthopedic tests and the arm-fossa test. *J Manip Physiol Ther*. 1990;13(3):138–143.

101. Cooperstein R, Blum C, Cooperstein EC. Assessment of consistency between the arm-fossa test and Gillet test: a pilot study. *J Chiropr Med*. 2015;14:24–31.

102. Levin U, Stenstrom CH. Force and time recording for validating the sacroiliac distraction test. *Clin Biomech*. 2003;18:821–826.

103. Meijne W, van Neerbos K, Aufdemkampe G, et al. Intraexaminer and interexaminer reliability of the Gillet test. *J Manip Physiol Ther*. 1999;22(1):4–9.

104. Carmichael JP. Inter and intra examiner reliability of palpation for sacroiliac joint dysfunction. *J Manip Physiol Ther*. 1987;10(4):164–171.

105. O'Haire C, Gibbons P. Inter-examiner and intra-examiner agreement for assessing sacroiliac anatomical landmarks using palpation and observation: pilot study. *Man Ther*. 2000;5(1):13–20.

106. Cooperstein R, Hickey M. The reliability of palpating the posterior superior iliac spine: a systematic review. *J Can Chiropr Assoc*. 2016;60(1):36–46.

107. Riddle DL, Freburger JK. Evaluation of the presence of sacroiliac joint region dysfunction using a combination of tests: a multicenter intertester reliability study. *Phys Ther*. 2002;82(8):772–781.

108. Petersen T, Laslett M, Carsten J. Clinical classification in low back pain: best-evidence diagnostic rules based on systematic reviews. *BMC Musculoskelet Disord*. 2017;18(188):1–23.

109. Arnbak B, Jurik AG, Jensen RK, et al. The diagnostic accuracy of three sacroiliac joint pain provocation tests for sacroiliitis identified by magnetic resonance imaging. *Scand J Rheumatol*. 2017;46(2):130–137.

CHAPTER 11

Hip

The hip joint is one of the largest and most stable joints in the body. If it is injured or exhibits pathology, the lesion is usually immediately perceptible during walking, as any hip pathology will affect the patient's ability to ambulate.[1] Because pain from the hip can be referred to the sacroiliac joint, lumbar spine, or abdominal area (e.g., athletic pubalgia [i.e., involvement of the pubic bone], sports hernia, Gilmore's groin, osteitis pubis) or vice versa, it is imperative—unless there is evidence of direct trauma to the hip—that these joints be examined along with the hip.[2,3] In addition, in some cases, assessment of the gastrointestinal, urinary, or genital systems may have to be considered.[4] That being said, a limp, groin pain, or limited medial rotation is more likely to indicate a hip problem.[5,6] In the last two decades, issues of impingement and related dysplasias, ligamentum teres tears, and labral lesions have become major areas of focus in pathology of the hip.

Applied Anatomy

The hip joint is a multiaxial ball-and-socket joint that has maximal stability because of the deep insertion of the head of the femur into the acetabulum (Fig. 11.1). The femoral head is much more stable in the acetabulum for the hip than the humerus is in the glenoid for the shoulder. To allow sufficient movement and proper alignment to occur at the hip joint, the femur has a longer neck than the humerus and is anteverted (Fig. 11.2). The hip joint has a strong capsule and very strong muscles that control its actions (Fig. 11.3). The acetabulum is formed by fusion of parts of the ilium, ischium, and pubis, which—taken as a group—are sometimes called the *innominate bone* or *pelvis*. The normal acetabulum opens outward, forward, and downward. It is half of a sphere, and the femoral head is two-thirds of a sphere.

Hip Joint

Resting position:	30° flexion, 30° abduction, slight lateral rotation
Close packed position:	Full extension, medial rotation, abduction
Capsular pattern:	Flexion, abduction, medial rotation (but in some cases, medial rotation is limited)

In addition, the hip, like the shoulder, has a labrum, which helps to deepen and stabilize the joint.[7,8] The dense, horseshoe-shaped fibrocartilaginous **acetabular labrum** runs around the perimeter of the acetabulum and holds the femoral head in the acetabulum at extreme ranges of motion (ROM), stabilizing the hip. It increases the articular surface area and volume of the acetabulum and provides proprioceptive feedback for dynamic stability.[9–11] It creates a seal for the central compartment, which is part of the intra-articular hip joint. The seal resists distraction of the femoral head from the socket by maintaining a negative intra-articular pressure (i.e., a suction seal), allowing the femoral head to "float" on the surface of the cartilage and thus protecting the cartilage.[11–19] It also resists fluid flow by regulating synovial fluid, which enhances nutrition of the hip's articular cartilage, which in turn provides a smooth gliding surface. The labrum also acts as a shock absorber when assisting in force distribution during load bearing.[2,20,21] The acetabular labrum plays a secondary role in stabilizing the hip during lateral rotation while also preventing anterior translation.[22] Mechanisms of injury to the labrum include hip hyperabduction, twisting, falling, hyperextension, dislocation, a direct blow, or a motor vehicle accident.[23] Some 90% of patients with labral pathology have associated bony abnormalities (e.g., hip dysplasia).[24,25] The labrum is avascular except at its margins and therefore has poor healing potential.[17] Labral tears may be seen with **femoroacetabular impingement (FAI)**, hip dysplasia (e.g., Legg-Calvé-Perthes disease), slipped capital femoral epiphysis (SCFE), trauma, osteoarthritis, and iliopsoas impingement.[9,17] A tear to the labrum may occur as an activity-induced or positional pain that fails to improve (most common) or may occur with a sudden twisting or pivoting motion with a click, pop, or locking sensation.[17] These twisting and pivoting movements, especially at the end range of rotation and falling,[9] lead to labral fraying, chondral degeneration, or delamination and can ultimately lead to osteoarthritis.[9,16] Hip dysplasia causes abnormal loading on the acetabular rim, which can lead to labral tears, damage to the chondral surface, and capsular laxity.[9,14,26]

The hip, already a stable joint because of its bony configuration, is supported by three strong ligaments—the iliofemoral, ischiofemoral, and pubofemoral ligaments—which are thickenings of the capsule (Fig. 11.4).[27] The **iliofemoral ligament (Y ligament of Bigelow)** is considered to be one of the strongest ligaments in the body.[11] It is positioned to

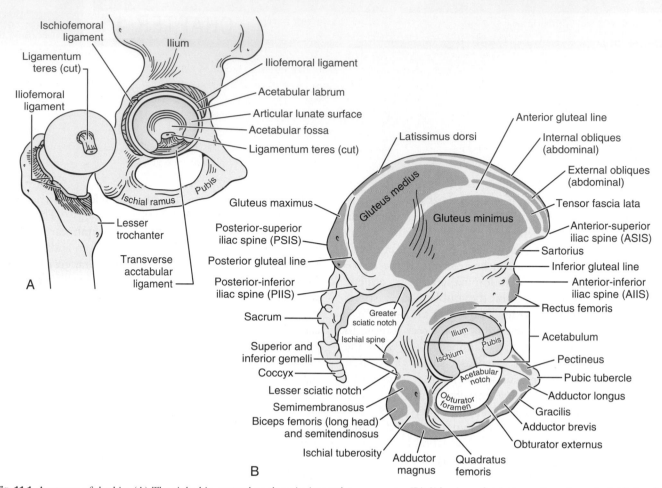

Fig. 11.1 Anatomy of the hip. (A) The right hip opened to show its internal components. (B) Side view of right innominate bone (pelvis) showing muscle attachments. (Modified from Neumann DA: *Kinesiology of the musculoskeletal system—foundations for physical rehabilitation*, St Louis, 2002, CV Mosby, pp 388, 397.)

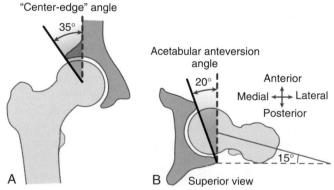

Fig. 11.2 (A) The center-edge angle measures the fixed orientation of the acetabulum within the frontal plane relative to the pelvis. This measurement defines the extent to which the acetabulum covers the top of the femoral head. The center-edge angle is measured as the intersection of a vertical fixed reference line *(stippled)* with the acetabular reference line *(bold solid line)* that connects the upper lateral edge of the acetabulum with the center of the femoral head. A more vertical acetabular reference line results in a smaller center-edge angle, providing less superior coverage of the femoral head. (B) The acetabular anteversion angle measures the fixed orientation of the acetabulum within the horizontal plane relative to the pelvis. This measurement indicates the extent to which the acetabulum covers the front of the femoral head. The angle is formed by the intersection of a fixed anteroposterior reference line *(stippled)* with an acetabular reference line *(bold solid line)* that connects the anterior and posterior rims of the acetabulum. A larger acetabular anteversion angle creates less acetabular containment of the anterior side of the femoral head. (A normal femoral anteversion of 15° is also shown.) (From Neumann DA: *Kinesiology of the musculoskeletal system—foundations for physical rehabilitation*, St Louis, 2010, Mosby, p 474.)

prevent excessive extension and plays a significant role in stabilizing the body and maintaining upright posture at the hip while also limiting anterior translation. The ligament tightens during lateral rotation and adduction.[9,11] Repeated forced lateral rotation of the hip can lead to iliofemoral insufficiency.[9] If this occurs, rotating (twisting) the hips (e.g., swinging a golf club) can lead to a feeling of instability.[9] The **ischiofemoral ligament**, the weakest of these three strong ligaments, winds tightly on extension, helping to stabilize the hip; it also tightens during medial rotation and abduction.[9] Repeated forced medial rotation of the hip can lead to ischiofemoral insufficiency.[9] The **pubofemoral ligament** prevents excessive abduction of the femur and limits lateral rotation, especially in extension, while tightening during lateral rotation and abduction.[9,11] All three ligaments also limit medial rotation of the femur. A fourth ligament of the hip that is sometimes injured is the **ligamentum teres,** or "ligament of the head," which

is intra-articular, strong, and acts as a hip stabilizer, especially in adduction, flexion, and lateral rotation when the hip is in its least stable position (see Fig. 11.1). The ligament supports the vascular system supplying the femoral head.[11,28,29] It is lax in abduction and medial rotation[11,27,30] and tight in adduction, flexion, and lateral rotation.[9] Interestingly, this position, in which the ligament is tightest, is the position in which the hip joint is most unstable.[28] The ligament provides a physical attachment of the head of the femur to the acetabulum.[31] It is only in the last two decades that the ligamentum teres has been investigated in depth, leading to a better understanding of its importance. Some feel that it may act similarly to the anterior cruciate ligament of the knee, serving as a strong intrinsic secondary stabilizer that resists subluxation forces,[28,30,32,33] while others have refuted this idea.[34] The ligamentum teres acts like a sling wrapping around and pulling the femoral head into the acetabulum during rotational

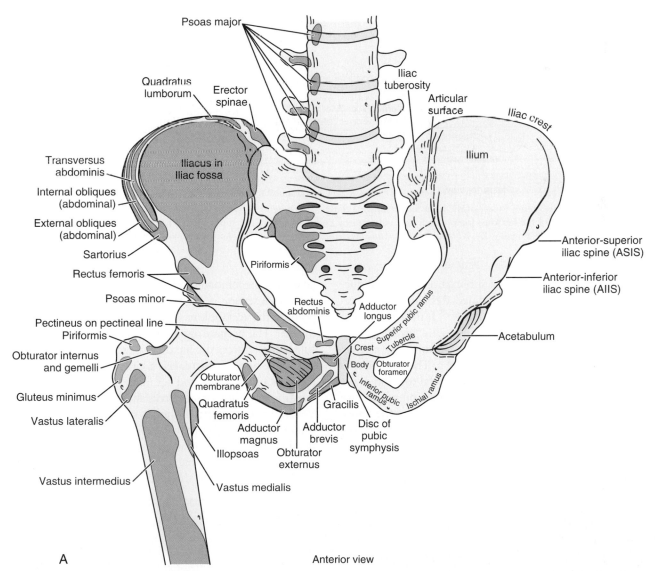

Fig. 11.3 (A) The anterior aspect of the pelvis, sacrum, and right proximal femur showing muscle attachments *(origins are shown in red and insertions are shown in blue)*. A section of the left side of the sacrum is removed to expose the articular surface of the sacroiliac joint. The pelvic attachments of the capsule around the sacroiliac joint are indicated by *dashed lines*.

Continued

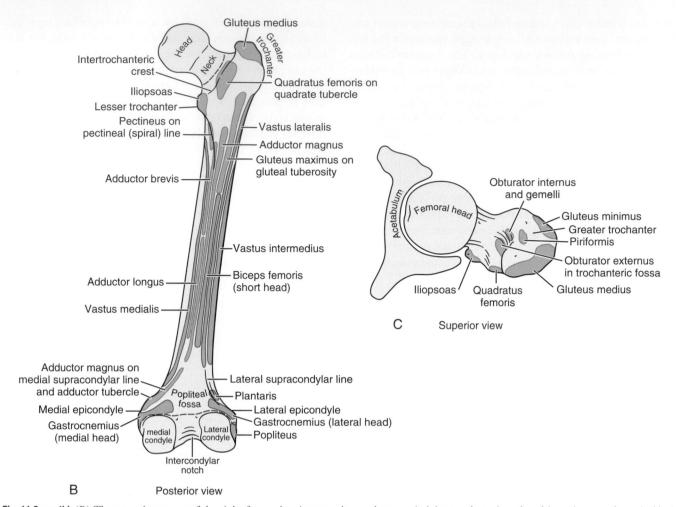

Fig. 11.3, cont'd (B) The posterior aspect of the right femur showing muscle attachments *(origins are shown in red and insertions are shown in blue).* The femoral attachments of the hip knee joint capsules are indicated by *dashed lines.* (C) The superior aspect of the right femur showing muscle attachments. (Redrawn from Neumann DA: *Kinesiology of the musculoskeletal system—foundations for physical rehabilitation,* St Louis, 2002, CV Mosby, pp 389, 393.)

movements, preventing inferior subluxation during abduction, posterior subluxation during medial rotation, and anterior dislocation during lateral rotation.[34,35] If the ligamentum teres is torn, **microinstability** of the hip (i.e., "giving way" of the hip) results, which can damage the labrum and cartilage, resulting in possible chondral lesions.[34,36] The instability is most evident in flexion, adduction, and lateral rotation of the hip.[36] Others feel that the ligament also has a proprioceptive role and may help to distribute synovial fluid over the femoral head via a "windshield-wiper effect."[27,28,34] Tears of the ligament are associated with dislocations, but partial tears can occur from flexion/adduction stresses, hyperabduction, a fall on the ipsilateral knee with the hip flexed, or a sudden twisting injury, such as those occurring in high-impact sports (e.g., football, hockey, tennis) and in activities requiring movement into extreme ROM (e.g., ballet, martial arts).[30,37,38] The ligament may also be affected by developmental disorders such as Legg-Calvé-Perthes disease and developmental dysplasia (i.e., congenital dislocation of the hip [CDH]) and connective tissue disorders (e.g., Marfan's and Ehler-Danlos syndromes), which put more stress on the ligament. The **fovea capitis** is

an area of the femoral head where there is no cartilage; it provides an insertion point for the ligamentum teres and is the point in the acetabulum where the ilium, ischium, and pubis meet.[11] The **arcuate ligament** is part of the posterior capsule and reinforces the hip during extreme flexion and extension. The **zona orbicularis,** a circular ligament, surrounds the neck of the femur and lies inferior to the femoral head; it resists inferior distraction forces and aids in stabilization.[11,27]

Under low loads, the joint surfaces are incongruous; under heavy loads, they become congruous, providing maximum surface contact, which brings the load per unit area down to a tolerable level. Depending on the activity, the forces exerted on the hip will vary.[39]

Forces on the Hip

Standing:	0.3 times body weight
Standing on one limb:	2.4–2.6 times body weight
Walking:	1.3–5.8 times body weight
Walking up stairs:	3 times body weight
Running:	4.5+ times body weight

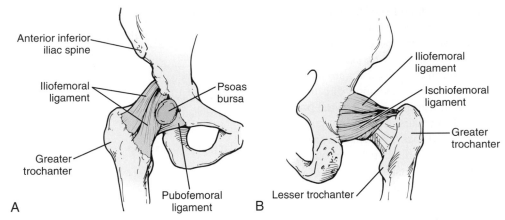

Fig. 11.4 Three of the main ligaments of the hip. (A) Anterior view. (B) Posterior view.

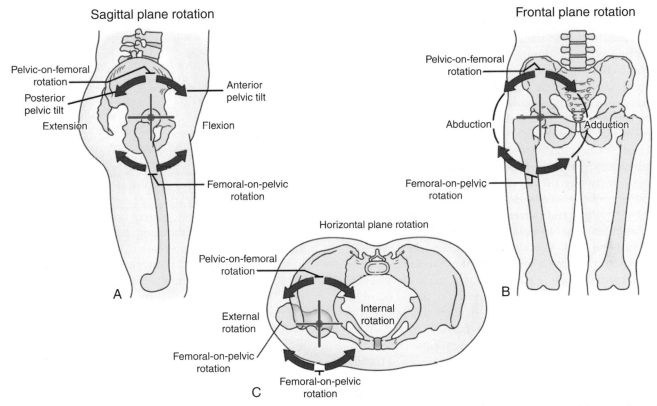

Fig. 11.5 The osteokinematics of the right hip joint. Femoral-on-pelvic and pelvic-on-femoral rotations occur in three planes. The axis of rotation for each plane of movement is shown as a *colored dot,* located at the center of the femoral head. (A) Side view shows sagittal plane rotations around a mediolateral axis of rotation. (B) Front view shows frontal plane rotations around an anteroposterior axis of rotation. (C) Top view shows horizontal plane rotations around a longitudinal, or vertical, axis of rotation. (Redrawn from Neumann DA: *Kinesiology of the musculoskeletal system—foundations for physical rehabilitation,* St Louis, 2010, Mosby, p 477.)

With regard to movement or kinematics at the hip joint, one must consider whether the pelvis is moving on a stationary femur (i.e., weight bearing) or the femur (i.e., non–weight bearing) is moving on the pelvis (Fig. 11.5).

Patient History

In addition to the questions listed under "Patient History" in Chapter 1, the examiner should obtain the following information from the patient:

1. *What is the patient's age?* Different conditions occur in different age groups, and ROM decreases with age. For example, congenital hip dysplasia is seen in infancy, primarily in girls, although its effect is often greater in adolescents and young adults; Legg-Calvé-Perthes disease is more common in boys 3 to 12 years old, and elderly women are more prone to osteoporotic femoral neck fractures. In young people, issues related to physeal injuries (e.g., avulsions/apophysitis, SCFE), state of skeletal maturity and morphological abnormalities (e.g., Legg-Calvé-Perthes

disease) must be considered, and the examiner must understand that these conditions have clinical features similar to or associated with labral tears and chondral injuries.[18]

2. *If trauma was involved, what was the mechanism of injury?* Typically, mechanical hip symptoms are worse with activities, especially twisting or changing directions; sitting with the hip flexed; rising from the seated position; ascending and descending stairs; getting into and out of a car; putting on shoes and socks. Patients may also complain of dyspareunia (i.e., painful sexual intercourse).[40–43] Did the patient land on the outside of the hip (e.g., trochanteric bursitis) or hit the knee, thus jarring the hip (e.g., subluxation, acetabular labral tear)? Is there any feeling of instability? The labrum may be injured with lateral rotation when the hip is hyperextended.[9] Such an injury may be an isolated event due to structural abnormalities, or it may arise from repetitive trauma. It can also be due to traction from the rectus femoris, occurring primarily during kicking or sprinting, or iliacus contraction, primarily occurring during a change of direction.[13,44,45] Hip injuries may cause mechanical symptoms such as intra-articular clicking, giving way, locking, or catching. An abnormal gait with a shortened stance phase may be observed.[46] Labral tears rarely occur in isolation.[46] Chondral lesions are commonly associated with labral tears.[13] Was the patient involved in repetitive loading activity (e.g., femoral neck stress fracture) or have osteoporotic problems developed (e.g., insufficiency injury)?[1,47] A careful determination of the mechanism of injury often leads to a diagnosis of the problem.

Femoral neck stress fractures occur when excessive or repetitive stress is applied to the trabecular bone in the femoral neck (e.g., running a marathon). These fractures, categorized as compression sided, occur at the inferomedial neck and are unlikely to displace. On the other hand, traction-sided fractures occur at the superolateral neck and, because any torque creates tension, are more likely to be displaced (see Fig. 11.135). The compression type is usually treated conservatively, whereas the traction type, which may displace, is a high-risk stress fracture that may require surgical stabilization.[48,49] Acute groin injuries are usually due to high running loads, changes in direction, or kicking.[44]

Traumatic instability occurs with a dislocation or subluxation involving a motor vehicle accident or sports injury. With a posterior dislocation (most common), the hip is slightly flexed, adducted, and medially rotated with the leg shortened.[11,50] An anterior dislocation results in the hip being extended, abducted, and laterally rotated.[11,50] If such an injury occurs, a neurological exam involving the sciatic and femoral nerves as well as examination of the knee should be performed. In the presence of a dislocation, reduction should be performed within 6 hours.[11,50] **Microinstability** or atraumatic instability occurs with repetitive microtrauma from axial loading and lateral rotation and is associated with FAI.[14,50–53] It

TABLE 11.1

Diagnostic Clues in Hip Pain

Type of Pain	Possible Causes
Dull, deep, aching	Arthritis, Paget disease
Sharp, intense, sudden, associated with weight bearing	Fracture
Tingling that radiates	Radiculopathy, spinal stenosis, meralgia paresthetica
Increased pain while sitting with the affected leg crossed	Trochanteric bursitis
Pain at sitting, legs not crossed	Ischiogluteal bursitis
Pain after standing, walking	Hip arthrosis
Pain on attempted weight bearing	Occult fracture, severe arthrosis
Unremitting, long duration	Paget disease, metastatic carcinoma, severe arthrosis (occasionally)

From Schon L, Zuckerman JD: Hip pain in the elderly: evaluation and diagnosis, *Geriatrics* 43:58, 1988.

is seen in activities that involve end-range stress to the joint, such as ice hockey (especially goal tending), ballet, figure skating, golf, martial arts, gymnastics, tennis, and football.[11,14,27] If the static stabilizers (i.e., ligaments, labrum, bone) are compromised, then the dynamic stabilizers (i.e., the muscles) must work harder to stabilize the joint; thus the biomechanics of joint movement are modified, leading to abnormal movement patterns (including muscle tightness).[14] For example, if a patient presents with an internally snapping hip (i.e., iliopsoas snapping), a labral tear, and a pincer-type FAI, it is called **triple impingement;** this may overlap or lead to microinstability.[27] With microinstability, the patient can complain of the leg "giving way" during activities or walking, apprehension, snapping, abnormal gait patterns (i.e., abductor lurch or Trendelenburg gait) with no defined injury.[14,27]

3. *What are the details of the present pain and other symptoms* (Tables 11.1 and 11.2)?[54,55] If the hip is at fault, the patient may demonstrate the **"C" sign** (Fig. 11.6); this means that if asked to show where the pain is, the patient will cup a hand above the greater trochanter with the fingers gripping the anterior groin, describing the pain as deep in the joint.[18,42,56–61] What brings the pain on? Does the pain occur with walking? Does it disappear when the patient stops? Is the pain static or dynamic? Do particular movements provoke pain? If so, what movements? Is the pain an ache or a sudden, sharp, unexpected pain?[18,62] Does the pain come on right away or does it take time during the activity for the pain to increase? This will give the clinician some idea of the patient's functional impairment. In

TABLE **11.2**

Classification System for Groin Pain in Athletes

Nomenclature	Symptoms	Definition	More Likely if Patient Presents With
Adductor-related groin pain[a]	Pain around the insertion of the adductor longus tendon at the pubic bone; pain may radiate distally along the medial thigh	Adductor tenderness and pain on resisted adduction testing	Pain on adductor stretching
Iliopsoas-related groin pain[a]	Pain in the anterior part of the proximal thigh, more laterally located than adductor-related groin pain	Iliopsoas tenderness (either suprainguinal or infrainguinal)	Pain reproduced with resisted hip flexion and/or pain with hip flexor stretching
Inguinal-related groin pain[a]	Pain in the inguinal region that worsens with activity. If pain is severe, inguinal pain often occurs when patient is coughing or sneezing or sitting up in bed.	Pain in the inguinal canal and inguinal canal tenderness, or pain with Valsalva maneuver, coughing, and/or sneezing. No palpable inguinal hernia found, including on invagination of the scrotum to palpate the inguinal canal.	Pain reproduced with resisted abdominal muscle testing
Pubic-related groin pain[a]	Pain in the region of the symphysis joint and the immediately adjacent bone	Local tenderness of the pubic symphysis and the immediately adjacent bone	No particular resistance test but more likely if pain is reproduced by resisted abdominal and hip adductor testing
Hip-related groin pain[a]		Clinical suspicion that the hip joint is the source of the pain, either through history or clinical examination	Mechanical symptoms present, such as catching, locking, clicking, or giving way
FAI syndrome[b]	Motion- or position-related pain in the hip or groin. Pain may also be felt in the back, buttock, or thigh. Patients may also describe clicking, catching, locking, stiffness, restricted range of motion, or giving way.	Motion-related clinical disorder of the hip with a triad of symptoms, clinical signs, and imaging findings. Cam and/or pincer morphology must be present on imaging.	Limited range of hip motion, typically restricted internal rotation, and evidence of labral and/or chondral damage on imaging
Other[a]	Clinical suspicion if symptoms cannot easily be classified into any of the commonly defined clinical entities	Any other orthopedic, neurological, rheumatological, urological, gastrointestinal, dermatological, oncological, or surgical condition causing pain in the groin region	

FAI, Femoroacetabular impingement.
[a]Doha agreement.
[b]Warwick agreement.
From Thorborg K, Reiman MP, Weir A, et al: Clinical examination, diagnostic imaging, and testing of athletes with groin pain: an evidence-based approach to effective management, *J Orthop Sports Phys Ther* 48(4):242, 2018.

older adults, osteoarthritis and fractures should be considered first.[60] Anterior or groin pain may be related to intra-articular hip problems, apophysitis in children (at the anterosuperior iliac spine [ASIS] or anterior inferior iliac spine [AIIS]), iliopsoas or adductor tendinitis, FAI, labral or chondral injuries, or athletic pubalgia.[18,58] Lateral hip pain may be related to extra-articular hip problems such as abductor injuries, **greater trochanteric pain syndrome**

(GTPS), and acetabular dysplasia.[63] Isolated posterior buttock pain is usually related to lumbar or sacroiliac pathology or issues with the sciatic nerve (e.g., **deep gluteal pain syndrome**).[18,58] Like pain in the shoulder, pain in the hip can be derived from several structures that produce the same signs and symptoms.[64] Pain that is not reproduced by high-level strenuous activity, does not have a predictable pattern, or involves only vague symptoms should lead the

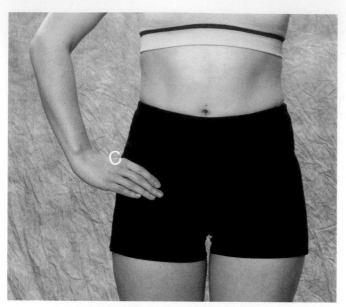

Fig. 11.6 "C" sign indicating hip pathology.

examiner to consider a systemic problem rather than a hip problem.[65] Hip intra-articular pain—including labral tears, FAI, and L4 nerve root pain—is felt mainly in the groin and along the front or medial side of the thigh to the knee. It is often described as a sharp, stabbing pain often accompanied by catching, locking, or clicking.[7,42,56,61] Buttock pain, on the other hand, is associated with posterior labral tears and lumbar spine problems.[7,66] Gradual onset of pain usually indicates osteoarthritis.[1] When did the pain start? What brought it on?[62] Adductor pain may be the result of overactive adductors caused by pelvic instability.[67] Pain when doing resisted sit-ups, hip flexion, or adduction may indicate **athletic pubalgia.** Pain may also be referred to the hip area from several structures (Fig. 11.7). Pain from the lumbar spine may commonly be referred to the back or lateral aspect of the hip.

A **sports hernia**—which is commonly caused by a deficient inguinal canal posterior wall, nerve entrapment, or adductor tendonopathies—may have an insidious

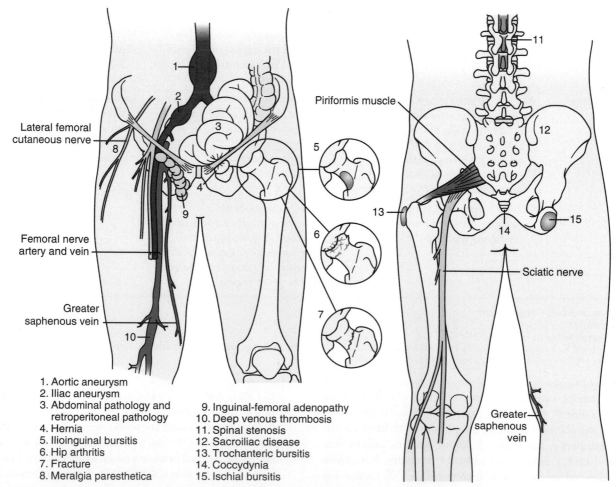

1. Aortic aneurysm
2. Iliac aneurysm
3. Abdominal pathology and retroperitoneal pathology
4. Hernia
5. Ilioinguinal bursitis
6. Hip arthritis
7. Fracture
8. Meralgia paresthetica
9. Inguinal-femoral adenopathy
10. Deep venous thrombosis
11. Spinal stenosis
12. Sacroiliac disease
13. Trochanteric bursitis
14. Coccydynia
15. Ischial bursitis

Fig. 11.7 Pain in the region of the hip can represent different musculoskeletal and nonmusculoskeletal problems. (Redrawn from Schon L, Zuckerman JD: Hip pain in the elderly: evaluation and diagnosis, *Geriatrics* 43:52, 1988.)

TABLE 11.3

Causes of Snapping Hip (Coxa Saltans) Symptoms

External	Internal	Intra-articular
• Posterior iliotibial band (over greater trochanter) • Anterior gluteus maximus • Trochanteric bursitis	• Iliopsoas tendon snapping (over anterior hip and pectineal eminence) • Iliofemoral ligament snapping • Hamstring syndrome • Iliopsoas bursal/capsular thickening	• Labral or ligamentum teres tears • Loose bodies • Synovial chondromatosis • Displaced fractures • Capsular instability

Modified from Wahl CJ, Warren RF, Adler RS, et al: Internal coxa saltans (snapping hip) as a result of overtraining, *Am J Sports Med* 32:1303, 2004.

onset of unilateral dull, aching pain in the groin that may be sharp or burning and may radiate into the proximal thigh, low back, lower abdominal muscles, perineum, and/or scrotum. The symptoms are aggravated by sudden acceleration, cutting, or kicking.[16,57,68–71]

Lateral hip pain may be due to a trochanteric bursitis (i.e., GTPS) or tear of the gluteus medius tendon, most commonly in older patients.[72] Lateral hip pain may also simulate L4 nerve root pain; therefore assessment of the lumbar spine should also be considered for lateral or posterior symptoms. Hip pain may also be referred to the knee or back and may increase on walking.

Clicking is common with labral tears when the hip moves into medial or lateral rotation.[73,74] **Snapping** in and around the hip (**coxa saltans**) has many causes and is an extra-articular sound (Table 11.3).[9,18,75,76] First and most commonly, it may be caused by slipping of the iliopsoas tendon over the osseous ridge of the lesser trochanter or anterior acetabulum, or the iliofemoral ligament may be riding over the femoral head.[1,60,77–79] Some call this **internal snapping.** If due to the iliopsoas tendon or iliofemoral ligament, the snapping often occurs at approximately 45° of flexion when the hip is moving from flexion to extension, especially with the hip abducted and laterally rotated (**snapping hip sign** or **extension test**) (Fig. 11.8).[80,81] The snap, which may be accompanied by pain or a jerk, is palpated anteriorly in the inguinal region and can also be the result of a labral tear or loose body if the patient complains of a sharp pain into the groin and anterior thigh, especially during pivoting movements.[21,80,82] Second, the snapping may be caused by a tight iliotibial band, snapping over the iliopectineal eminence, the femoral head, or the greater trochanter as the hip moves from flexion to extension,[9,83] or the gluteus maximus tendon riding over the greater trochanter of the femur.[77,78] This is sometimes called **external snapping** or **external coxa saltans.** This snapping or popping, which tends to be felt more laterally, occurs when the hip is brought from the flexed, abducted, and laterally rotated position into extension and medial rotation[42,84] during hip flexion and extension, especially if the hip is held in medial rotation; it may be made worse if the trochanteric bursa is inflamed.[82] The third cause of a snapping hip

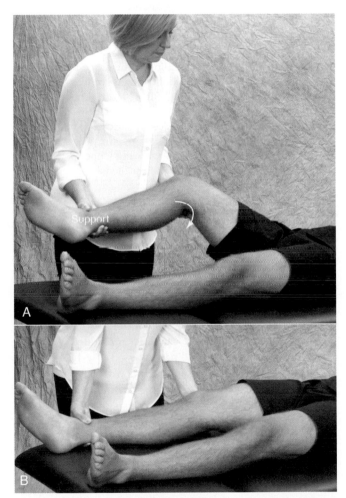

Fig. 11.8 Testing for snapping of the iliopsoas tendon (snapping hip sign). (A) Start position. Patient actively moves the hip from the start flexed position to the end extension position. (B) End position.

is acetabular labral tears (80%), loose bodies, cartilage defects, or ligamentum teres tears, which may be the result of trauma or degeneration.[57,78,85–87] This is sometimes referred to as **intra-articular snapping.** In this case, the patient (commonly between 20 and 40 years of age) complains of a sharp pain into the groin and anterior thigh, especially on pivoting movements. Passively, clicking may be felt and heard when the extended hip is adducted and laterally rotated.[78,82] Each of these conditions may be referred to as **snapping hip syndrome.**

TABLE **11.4**

Classification Criteria for Osteoarthritis of the Hip

Clinical (history, physical examination, laboratory) classification criteria for osteoarthritis of the hip, classification tree format[a]	1. Hip pain, and 2a. Hip internal rotation <15°, and 2b. ESR ≤45 mm/hour (if ESR not available, substitute hip flexion ≤115°), or 3a. Hip internal rotation ≥15°, and 3b. Pain on hip internal rotation, and 3c. Morning stiffness of the hip ≥60 min, and 3d. Age >50 years
Combined clinical (history, physical examination, laboratory) and radiographic classification criteria for osteoarthritis of the hip, traditional format[b]	Hip pain, and at least two of the following three features: • ESR <20 mm/h • Radiographic femoral or acetabular osteophytes • Radiographic joint space narrowing (superior, axial, and/or medial)

[a]This classification method yields a sensitivity of 86% and a specificity of 75%.

[b]This classification method yields a sensitivity of 89% and a specificity of 91%.

ESR, Erythrocyte sedimentation rate (Westergren).

Modified from Altman R, Alarcon G, Appelrouth D, et al: The American College of Rheumatology criteria for the classification and reporting of osteoarthritis of the hip, *Arth Rheum* 34:511–512, 1991.

4. *Is the condition improving? Worsening? Staying the same?* Such a question gives the examiner some idea of the present state of the joint and pathology. Table 11.4 outlines criteria for osteoarthritis in patients with hip pain.[88]

5. *Does any type of activity ease the pain or make it worse?* For example, trochanteric bursitis (i.e., GTPS) often results from abnormal running mechanics with the feet crossing over midline (increased hip adduction), a wide pelvis and genu valgum, or running on running tracks with no banking.[82] Pain on sitting may be due to pinching of an inflamed psoas bursa or an FAI.

6. *Are there any movements that the patient feels are weak or abnormal?* For example, in **piriformis syndrome** (also called **deep gluteal space syndrome**),[89] the sciatic nerve may be compressed, the piriformis muscle is tender, and hip abduction and lateral rotation are weak. Does the hip feel as though it "gives way"? FAI, trauma (e.g., lateral impact force to greater trochanter), labral lesions and avascular necrosis may lead to chondral lesions.[9,26] Cam-type FAI leads to damage to the labrum and articular surface to the anterosuperior acetabulum, and a pincer type of impingement causes more circumferential damage to the acetabular cartilage.[26] More information on FAI and other types of impingement can be found in the "Active Movements"

section. All of these conditions cause similar signs and symptoms, which makes a definitive diagnosis based on physical findings hard to achieve.[26]

7. *What is the patient's usual activity or pastime?* By listening to the patient, the examiner should be able to tell whether repetitive or sustained positions have contributed to the problem. Also, the examiner can develop some idea of the functional impairment felt by the patient.

8. *Is there any past medical and/or surgical history, such as developmental disorders (e.g., hip dysplasia, Legg-Calvé-Perthes disease), systemic illnesses, metabolic, or inflammatory disorders?*[61] A history of alcohol, corticosteroid, or tobacco use can increase the risk of osteonecrosis.[61] Depending on the history, it may also be necessary to clear the lumbar spine, abdominal (i.e., genitourinary and gastrointestinal systems), and neurovascular problems.[3,43]

Observation

As the patient comes into the assessment area, the gait should be observed. If the hip is affected, the weight is lowered carefully on the affected side and the knee bends slightly to absorb the shock. The length of the step on the affected side is shorter so that weight can be taken off the leg quickly. If the hip is stiff, the entire trunk and affected leg swing forward together. It is also important to watch for "balance" of the pelvis on the hip. In standing, the patient commonly has the hip slightly flexed if there is pain in the hip. When asked about pain, the patient may demonstrate the "C" sign (see Fig. 11.6), indicating where the pain is felt.

Pathology in the hip region can lead to tight adductors, iliopsoas, piriformis, tensor fasciae latae, rectus femoris, and hamstrings; at the same time, the gluteus maximus, medius, and minimus become weak.[90,91] Weak abductors can lead to a **Trendelenburg gait** or an "**abductor lurch,**" which is a lateral pelvic shift of more than 2 cm (0.8 inches) toward the weight-bearing side and may be accompanied by trunk inclination.[60,61,92,93] Internal hip pathology or a flexion contracture may lead to a "**pelvic wink**" or "**butt wink.**" This is excessive posterior pelvic rotation in the axial plane (more than 40°) (i.e., loss of lordosis) toward the affected hip as the patient flexes the hip and knee in an attempt to obtain terminal hip extension in the opposite leg.[43,92–94] It may be due to muscle tightness (i.e., iliopsoas) or structural change (e.g., anteversion angle of acetabulum or femoral neck, diameter of femoral neck, or depth of acetabulum). If there is an imbalance of the flexors or extensors in the sagittal plane, the forward–backward motion of the trunk is altered to help maintain balance. For example, a bilateral hip flexion contracture causes the lumbar spine to extend to a greater degree (i.e., increased lordosis) as a compensating mechanism. Weak extensors cause the patient to move the trunk backward to maintain balance and avoid falling as a result of the unopposed action of the flexors. If the lateral rotators are significantly stronger than the medial rotators, as is normally the case, excessive toe-out can result. In addition, the patellae may have a "frog eyes" appearance (i.e., they face or turn out). Contracture of either of the rotators may lead to a pivoting at the hip during gait.[95] The different types of gait are discussed in greater detail in Chapter 14.

If the patient uses a cane, it should be held in the hand opposite the affected side to negate some of the force of gravity on the affected hip.[96] The proper use of a cane can decrease the load on the hip by as much as 40%.[96,97]

The patient should be standing and suitably undressed for the examiner to perform a proper observation. The following aspects are noted from the front, side, and behind:

1. **Posture**: Can the patient stand with a correctly aligned posture? Is his or her stance comfortable and symmetrical? Is the weight taken equally in both legs? Is there any obvious muscle wasting? Excessive "toeing out" may be due to external hip neck retroversion or SCFE in adolescents, or pelvic torsion.[62] Posterior rotation of the innominate bone can cause lateral rotation of the leg.[62] "Toeing in" may be due to femoral neck anteversion.[62] See Table 13.3 for other causes of toeing in or toeing out in children. The examiner should watch for pelvic obliquity caused by, for example, unequal leg length, muscle contractures, or scoliosis (see Chapter 15 for more details). It must be remembered that injury to the iliopsoas may also affect the spine. Therefore, when patients are asked to do movements involving these muscles, the examiner must watch the effect on the spine and spinal movement (see the "Thomas Test" later in this chapter). Tightness of the iliopsoas can cause deviation of the spine to the same side.[98] The position of the pelvic tilt can affect the functional orientation of the acetabulum; therefore the examiner should observe whether the patient can achieve and hold the **neutral pelvis position,** which, in turn, can affect terminal hip ROM, which may affect the occurrence of FAI.[99]

   a. *Anterior View.* The examiner should note any abnormality of the bony and soft tissue contours. With many patients, differences in these contours are difficult to detect because of muscle bulk and other soft tissue deposition around the hips. Therefore the examiner must look closely. The same is true for swelling. Swelling in the hip joint itself is virtually impossible to detect by observation, and swelling resulting from a psoas or trochanteric bursitis can easily be missed if the examiner is not carefully observant.

   b. *Lateral View.* While the patient is being viewed from the side, the contour of the buttock should be observed for any abnormality (gluteus maximus atrophy or atonia). In addition, a hip flexion deformity is best observed from this position. The examiner should take the time to compare the two sides and note any subtle differences.

   c. *Posterior View.* The position of the hip and the effect, if any, of this position on the spine should be noted. For example, a hip flexion contracture may lead to an increased lumbar lordosis. Any differences in bony and soft tissue contours should again be noted.

2. Whether the patient can or will stand on both legs: Two bathroom scales may be used to check the symmetry of weight bearing. Asymmetrical skinfolds may indicate anatomical variations such as pelvic obliquity, leg-length discrepancy, developmental dysplasia of the hip (DDH) (i.e., CDH), or muscle atrophy.

3. **Balance**: It is important to check the patient's proprioceptive control in the joints being assessed. This control may be evaluated by asking the patient to balance first on one leg (the good one) and then the other—first with the eyes open and then with the eyes closed. Differences should be noted through comparison. Loss of proprioceptive control is especially obvious when the patient's eyes are closed. The use of the **stork standing test** (Fig. 11.9)[95] has also been advocated for testing proprioception. This test may also test stability at the sacroiliac joints, the knee, and the ankle and foot. With both methods, the examiner should watch for a positive Trendelenburg sign, which would negate the proprioceptive tests. It has been reported[100] that the star excursion balance test and the Y-balance test (see Chapter 2),[101,102] especially in the posteromedial and posterolateral directions, can be effective along with other measures in helping to diagnose FAI and susceptibility to injury.

4. Whether the limb positions are equal and symmetric: The position of the limb may indicate the type of injury. With traumatic posterior hip dislocation, the limb is shortened, adducted, and medially rotated, and the greater trochanter is prominent. If the piriformis (or other lateral rotators) is in spasm, then the affected leg will be laterally rotated when the patient is relaxed and lying supine (Fig. 11.10). With an anterior hip dislocation, the limb is abducted and laterally rotated; it may appear cyanotic or swollen owing to pressure in the femoral triangle. With intertrochanteric fractures, the limb is shortened and laterally rotated. As well, the examiner is looking for bilateral symmetry in the soft tissues (primarily muscle) and also bone symmetry. Certain sports or positions played or working postures may lead to asymmetric differences between the right and left sides, which may lead to problems. For example, tennis players or baseball players may show asymmetric differences in the upper limbs, which may or may not be present in the lower limbs.[103] Thus—especially if high-level, end-range activities are involved—it is imperative that the examiner consider the whole-body kinetic chain while doing the assessment.

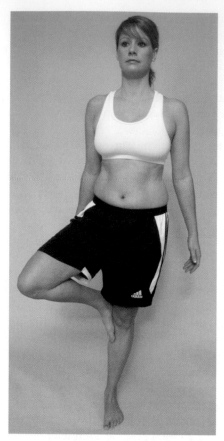

Fig. 11.9 Stork standing test.

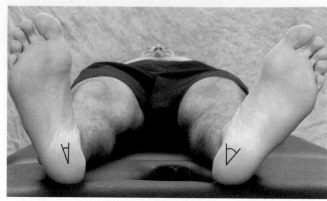

Fig. 11.10 Ipsilateral lateral rotation of the left hip in supine caused by spasm of the lateral rotators (primarily piriformis) of the hip.

5. Any obvious shortening of a leg: Shortening of the leg may be demonstrated by a spinal scoliosis if the shortening is present in only one lower limb. Shortening may be structural or functional. Structural changes at the hip that may lead to altered limb length include hip angulation deformity, congenital hypoplasia, femoral growth plate problems, or developmental disorders.[61] If the hips are unstable (e.g., bilateral unreduced CDH), an increased lumbar lordosis may be evident because the head of the femur usually rests above and behind the acetabulum, causing the patient to have an increased lordosis to maintain the center of gravity.

6. Color and texture of the skin

7. Any scars or sinuses

8. **Gait**: When the examiner has finished the static observation, time should be taken to review dynamic movement. This would involve the patient walking while the examiner looks for abnormal gait patterns, especially on the affected side (i.e., antalgic [i.e., painful] gait, Trendelenburg gait [i.e., abductor-deficient gait], pelvic [butt] wink, excessive rotation [either medial or lateral—at least 10° medial rotation is necessary at midstance of normal gait but less than 20° is abnormal[92]], contracture [especially flexion], leg-length limp, abnormal foot progression, arm swing, short stride length [on affected side], short stance phase [on affected side], heel strike, foot position, hip extension avoidance gait) or asking the patient to do the movement that causes the pain or discomfort.[1,3,18,42,58] The examiner should note the patient's willingness to move. If the hip is painful, the patient will have an antalgic gait (see Chapter 14) and will not want to move the hip. If the hip is unstable, the patient will have more difficulty in controlling its movement. Are any ambulatory aids used? What is their effect on gait and pain? Is the aid being used in the correct (i.e., opposite) hand?

9. During the observation and examination, as previously mentioned, the examiner must consider the whole kinetic chain. Abnormal kinematics in one joint can affect the mechanics in another joint, so the examiner must be prepared to look beyond the area of pain or weakness. For example, abnormal kinematics in the hip has been suggested to be one of the reasons for patellofemoral syndrome. Thus, although the pain may be in the knee, as in this case, weakness or abnormal mechanics in the hip may contribute to the problem and to provide a successful treatment, the examiner must consider the whole kinetic chain.[104]

Examination

During an examination of the hip, the examiner must keep in mind that pain may be referred to the hip from the sacroiliac joints or lumbar spine, and vice versa. Therefore the examination may be an extensive one. If there is any doubt as to the location of the lesion, an assessment of the lumbar spine and sacroiliac joints should be performed along with that of the hip. For example, lateral hip pain is often the result of lumbar pathology, but it may also be the result of GTPS.[105] It is only through a careful examination of the three areas, especially if there has been no history of trauma, that the examiner will be able to discern the location of the injury.

As with any examination, the examiner should compare one side of the body with the other, noting any differences. This comparison is necessary because of the individual differences among normal people.[106] It is also

TABLE **11.5**

Layered Approach to Clinical Assessment of the Hip Joint

Layer	Name	Structures	Purpose/Function	Pathology
Layer 1	Osteochondral layer	Femur Pelvis Acetabulum	Joint congruence and normal osteo-/ arthrokinematics	*Dynamic impingement* Cam, rim, femoral retroversion, femoral varus, acetabular overcoverage (focal or global), trochanteric impingement, subspine impingement *Static overload* Acetabular undercoverage, femoral anteversion, femoral valgus, acetabular version *Dynamic instability*
Layer 2	Inert layer	Labrum Joint capsule Ligamentous complex Ligamentum teres	Static stability of the hip joint	*Labral injury* *Ligamentum teres tear* *Ligament tears* *Capsular instability, adhesive capsulitis*
Layer 3	Contractile layer	Periarticular musculature Anterior structures Medial structures Posterior structures Lateral structures Lumbosacral and pelvic floor	Dynamic stability of the hip, pelvis, and trunk	*Anterior* Rectus femoris tendonopathy, psoas, subspine *Medial* Adductor strain, rectus abdominis strain, osteitis pubis *Posterior* Proximal hamstring, deep gluteal syndrome *Lateral* Abductor tears, iliotibial band syndrome, bursitis
Layer 4	Neuromechanical layer	Neural Femoral, lateral, femoral cutaneous, sciatic, ilioinguinal, genitofemoral, pudendal, and iliohypogastric nerves Regional mechanoreceptors Thoracolumbar mechanics Lower extremity mechanics	Properly sequenced kinetic linking and appropriate balance neuromuscular control presence or absence of neuromechanical shortcomings	*Neural* Pain syndrome Neuromuscular dysfunction Spinal referral patterns Nerve entrapments *Mechanical* Foot structure and mechanics Scoliosis Pelvic posture over femur Osteitis pubis, pubic symphysis pathology Sacroiliac dysfunction

From Poultsides LA, Bedi A, Kelly BT: An algorithmic approach to mechanical hip pain, *Hosp Special Surgery (HSSJ)* 8:219, 2012.

important to be sure that if the patient complains of pain during a test, that the pain is the same pain the patient experiences with activity.[56]

Table 11.5 provides a layered approach to assessment that enables the examiner to consider the various structures around the hip that may be injured.[107,108]

Active Movements

The active movements (Fig. 11.11) are done in such a way that the most painful ones are done last. To keep movement of the patient to a minimum, some movements are tested with the patient in the supine position and others in the prone position. For ease of description, the movements are described together. The examiner should follow the order as stated in the précis at the end of the chapter. If the history has indicated that repetitive movements, sustained postures, or combined movements have caused symptoms, the examiner should ensure that these movements are tested as well. For example, sustained extension of the hip may provoke gluteal pain in the presence of claudication in the common or internal iliac artery.[109] During the active movements, the examiner should always watch for the possibility of muscle or force-couple imbalances that lead to abnormal muscle recruitment patterns. For example, during extension, the

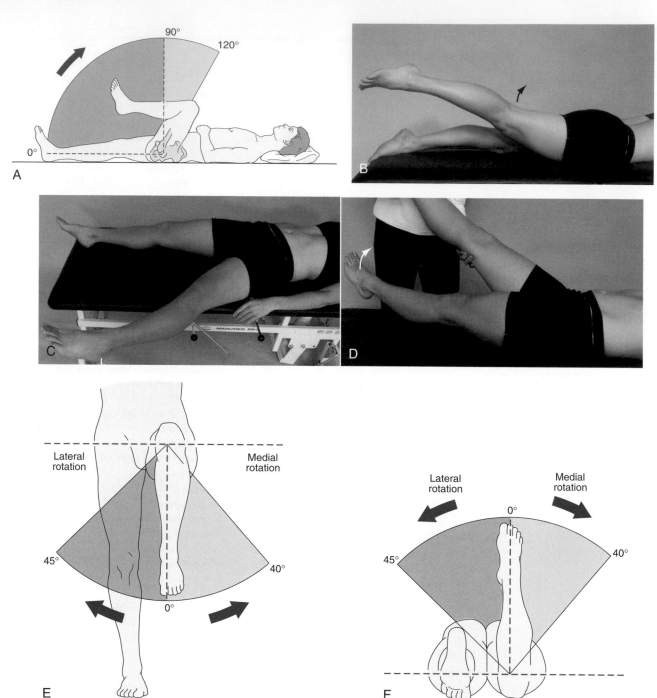

Fig. 11.11 Active movements of the hip. (A) Flexion. (B) Extension. (C) Abduction. (D) Adduction. (E) Rotation in the supine position. (F) Rotation in the prone position. (A, E, and F, Redrawn from Beetham WP, Polley HF, Slocumb CH, et al: *Physical examination of the joints*, Philadelphia, 1965, WB Saunders, pp 134, 137, and 138, respectively.)

normal pattern is contraction of the gluteus maximus followed by the erector spinae on the opposite side and the hamstrings (depending on the load being extended). If the erector spinae contract first, the pelvis rotates anteriorly and hyperextension of the lumbar spine occurs. During the active movements, the examiner should watch the pelvis and the anterosuperior (supine) and posterosuperior (prone) iliac spines. During hip movement, if the pelvic force couples are normal, the pelvis and ASIS/posterior superior iliac spine (PSIS) will not move. If they do, it may be an indication of muscle imbalance (Fig. 11.12).

Active Movements of the Hip

- Flexion (110°–120°)
- Extension (10°–15°)
- Abduction (30°–50°)
- Adduction (30°)
- Lateral rotation (40°–60°)
- Medial rotation (30°–40°)
- Sustained postures (if necessary)
- Repetitive movements (if necessary)
- Combined movements (if necessary)

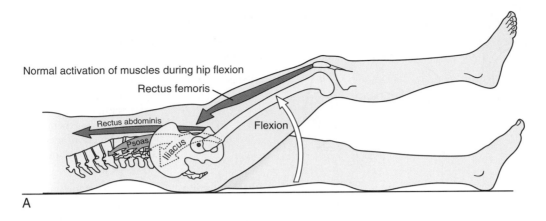

Normal activation of muscles during hip flexion
Rectus femoris
Rectus abdominis
Psoas
Iliacus
Flexion

A

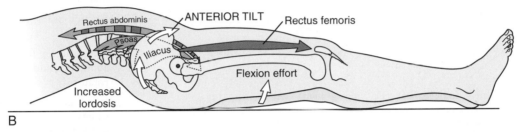

Muscle (force-couple) imbalance pattern (weak rectus abdominus)

Rectus abdominis
ANTERIOR TILT
Rectus femoris
Psoas
Iliacus
Flexion effort
Increased lordosis

B

Fig. 11.12 Force-couple action during a unilateral straight leg raise. (A) With normal activation of the rectus abdominis and the hip flexors (psoas and rectus femoris), the pelvis is stabilized and prevented from anterior tilting by the pull of the hip flexor muscles. (B) With reduced activation of the rectus abdominis, contraction of the hip flexor muscles causes a marked anterior tilt of the pelvis. Note the increase in lumbar lordosis accompanying the anterior tilt of the pelvis. (Modified from Neumann DA: *Kinesiology of the musculoskeletal system—foundations for physical rehabilitation*, St. Louis, 2002, CV Mosby, p 413.)

Flexion of the hip is tested in the supine position and normally ranges from 110° to 120° with the knee flexed. If the ASIS begins to move, the movement is stopped because pelvic rotation is occurring rather than hip flexion. The patient's knee is flexed during the test to prevent limitation of movement caused by hamstring tightness. Symptoms related to impingement worsen with higher degrees of flexion. If sharp anterior groin pain that may refer to the gluteal or trochanteric region is elicited on full flexion, adduction and medial rotation, the pain may be the result of anterolateral impingement of the femoral neck against the anterior acetabular rim (FAI), especially during end-range hip flexion and medial rotation, resulting in limited medial rotation of the flexed hip and pain at the extremes of flexion, medial rotation, and adduction.[110-117] Even in the asymptomatic patient, such findings may indicate future risk of pathological changes.[117] The pain is made worse by certain movements (e.g., pivoting, movement into extreme rotation) or long periods of sitting, standing, or walking.[118] This FAI (Fig. 11.13) is an abnormal relationship between the head of the femur and/or the femoral neck and the acetabulum. It may be the cam or pincer type and can lead to an early-onset osteoarthritis.[19,53,56] If medial rotation is limited relative to other movements, it is predictive of mild to moderate osteoarthritis.[9] Both types are usually associated with developmental dysplasia (e.g., Legg-Calvé-Perthes disease, SCFE) or acetabular dysplasia, which appears to have an ethnic component[119] and may be associated with high stresses that affect the hip during maturation. Both types can lead to joint damage and osteoarthritis.[19,56,120-134] The **cam-type impingement** (see Fig. 11.13B)—also called an inclusion-type injury as the bony deformity at the femoral head-neck junction enters the joint when the hip flexes—is commonly due to impingement of a large aspherical femoral head in a tight acetabulum (i.e., an abnormally shaped femoral head in a normal acetabulum).[15,16,18,56,76,132,135] The deformed (flattened) head (pistol-grip deformity or head-tilt deformity) leads to shearing of the labrum and acetabular cartilage and instability.[15,56,130,136,137] The cam-type impingement, more commonly seen in young adult males (20 to 30 years of age) and those who are physically active,[133,138,139] may also lead to increased stress at the symphysis pubis and may be a precursor to athletic pubalgia.[140] **Pincer type (rim) impingement** (see Fig. 11.13C), also called an impaction-type injury with an abnormal acetabulum, is more commonly seen in older females (40+ years of age)[138,139] and is due to overcoverage of the femoral head by a prominent acetabular rim (i.e., the anterolateral acetabulum overhangs the femoral head due to acetabular dysplasia, SCFE, acetabular retroversion, or coxa profunda), leading to pinching of the femoral neck against the labrum. The ultimate result

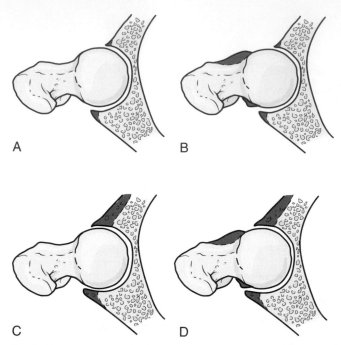

Fig. 11.13 Femoroacetabular impingement (hip impingement). (A) Normal hip. (B) Reduced femoral head-neck offset (cam-type impingement). (C) Excessive overcoverage of the femoral head (pincer-type impingement). (D) Combination of cam and pincer types of impingement.

TABLE 11.6

Clinical Characteristics of Patients with Femoroacetabular Impingement

Patient history	Patient reports "anterior groin related pain," demonstrates "C" sign, pain reported with different positions such as flexion and adduction; mechanical pain such a "clicking" or "giving way" may be present.
Pelvis position	Greater static standing anterior pelvic tilt or posterior pelvic tilt.
Soft tissue and joint restriction	Tight iliopsoas, hip joint, and lumbosacral mobility restrictions may be present.
Joint ROM	Decreased hip flexion and medial rotation.
Muscle weakness	Weakness in hip flexors, extensors, abductors, adductors, and external rotators.
Function	Limited motion with bilateral squats, stair ambulation, decreased motion with motion that causes hip flexion and adduction.
Gait	Slower cadence, kinematically less peak hip extension, adduction, and medial rotation during stance phase. Less peak hip flexion and lateral rotation moments may be present.
Special testing	Positive impingement tests.
Diagnostic imaging	Radiographs: Pincer-type FAIs include a lateral center edge angle >40° and acetabular index (Tönnis angle) of less than 0°. Cam-type FAI includes an alpha angle >50.5° and head-neck offset less than 8 mm.

FAI, femoroacetabular impingement; *ROM,* range of motion.
From Cheatham SW, Enseki KR, Kobler MJ: The clinical presentation of individuals with femoral acetabular impingement and labral tears: a narrative review of the evidence, *J Bodyw Mov Ther* 20(2):349, 2016.

is the same as as that of cam-type degeneration of the labrum and adjacent cartilage.[15,56,130,132,135,141–143] In the presence of acetabular retroversion or decreased femoral anteversion, hip flexion in the neutral line is limited to as little as 90° but full range is accomplished if the hip is allowed to rotate laterally and abduct. Lateral rotation may exceed 60°, with medial rotation limited.[122,144] Pincer and cam types of FAI may occur in isolation or more commonly together (see Fig. 11.13D).[13,84] If they are not combined, the cam type is more common.[13] Signs and symptoms of FAI include anterior groin pain—which can be referred to the buttock, greater trochanter, thigh, and medial knee—clicking, locking, catching, instability, stiffness, and giving way (Table 11.6).[13,137] ROM will be decreased and impingement tests (see "Special Tests" section) may be positive.

The examiner should palpate the ASIS when testing hip movements. In the presence of FAI, the ASIS moves early due to limited hip flexion as the lumbar spine flexes to allow more movement.[84,145] If medial rotation is measured at 90° of flexion, medial rotation in the FAI patient will be limited.[84] The amount of medial rotation occurring at 90° of hip flexion correlates with the amount of space between the femoral neck and the acetabular rim.[35] Excessive end-range repetitions into medial rotation (cam type—e.g., butterfly position in hockey goal tenders; hockey, basketball, and soccer players; or dancers) or lateral rotation (pincer type—e.g., dancers) or front-back or side splits (dancers) and other ballet maneuvers can lead to FAI.[35,146–148] During the movement, if the abdominals are weak, the pelvis rotates anteriorly (see Fig. 11.11). If the hip flexors are weak, the pelvis rotates posteriorly.

Iliopsoas impingement may also occur with flexion and has been linked to acetabular labral tears.[59,149–151] Likewise, **subspine impingement** between the AIIS and the femoral neck can occur with knee flexion and hip extension and can lead to avulsion of the AIIS (i.e., an osteochondral lesion) from overactivity of the rectus femoris in an adolescent patient (Table 11.7).[59,149]

Extension of the hip normally ranges from 0° to 15°. The patient is in the prone position, and the examiner must differentiate between hip extension and spinal

TABLE **11.7**

Common Types of Extra-articular Hip Impingement

	Patient Demographics	Clinical Presentation	Pathological Characteristics
Iliopsoas impingement	Average age: 25–35 years Gender: females more than males	Patients are typically active individuals with reports of "anterior hip pain." Clinical findings include a positive hip impingement test.	The pathology may be caused by: (1) a tight or inflamed iliopsoas tendon that causes impingement during hip extension, (2) a repetitive traction injury by the iliopsoas tendon that is scarred or adherent to the capsule-labrum complex of the hip.
Subspine (AIIS) impingements	Average age: 14–30 years Gender: males more than females	Patients are typically active individuals with reports of "anterior hip or groin pain." Clinical findings include limited hip flexion and palpable tenderness over the AIIS.	The pathology is caused by a prominent AIIS abnormally contacting the distal femoral neck during hip flexion. This may be due to an avulsion injury to the AIIS due to excessive muscular activity of the rectus femoris during repetitive knee flexion and hip extension.
Ischiofemoral impingement	Average age: 51–53 years Gender: females more than males	Patients typically report nonspecific pain in the hip, groin, buttock, or lower extremity. There are no specific clinical tests. Diagnosis is typically done with MRI.	The pathology is caused by a narrowed space between the ischial tuberosity and the lesser trochanter resulting in repetitive pinching of the quadratus femoris muscle.

AIIS, Anterior inferior iliac spine; *MRI*, magnetic resonance imaging.
From Cheatham SW, Enseki KR, Kobler MJ: The clinical presentation of individuals with femoral acetabular impingement and labral tears: a narrative review of the evidence, *J Bodyw Mov Ther* 20(2):348, 2016.

extension. Patients often have a tendency to extend the lumbar spine at the same time that they are extending the hip, giving the appearance of increased hip extension. Elevation of the pelvis or superior movement of the PSIS indicates that the patient has passed the end of hip extension.

Posteriorly, there are several places where extra-articular impingement of the hip can occur; most are rare and will result in symptoms at the end range of extension, adduction, and lateral rotation.[152–154] The most common are the **ischiofemoral impingement (IFI)** between the ischium and lesser trochanter of the femur; the **deep gluteal syndrome (DGS)** (Table 11.8), which includes the piriformis muscle (i.e., piriformis syndrome); the **greater trochanteric-pelvic impingement** seen with morphological abnormalities of the hip (e.g., Legg-Calvé-Perthes disease), where abduction is limited; and **psoas impingement** of the psoas tendon against the anterior aspect of the labrum. IFI occurs during extension in the narrow space between the ischial tuberosity and the lesser trochanter and may involve the quadratus femoris muscle.[149,152,154–158] This muscle assists lateral rotation and adduction of the hip.[155] Pinching of contractile or neurological tissue can also occur between the lateral aspect of the ischium and the lesser trochanter of the proximal femur by combined extension, adduction, and lateral rotation.[152,159,160] These patients have chronic groin or lower buttock pain with no history of injury. The pain may

radiate into the lower leg, as the sciatic nerve lies close by.[152,155] Limitation of hip extension can lead, over time, to increased load on L3-L4 and L4-L5 lumbar facets, leading to back pain (sometimes called **hip-spine syndrome** because of hyperlordosis and excessive pelvic rotation).[157] On examination, most end-range movements are painful and there may be a snapping sensation, crepitation, or locking.[155,161] The mean femoral anteversion is greater in patients with this problem.[159] In the posterior hip, the examiner must be able to differentiate between different extra-articular impingements—IFI, DGS, and **hamstring syndrome**—all of which involve the sciatic nerve.[159,162] If the sciatic nerve is trapped along its course through the hip area, the patient will demonstrate an inability to sit for more than 30 minutes, with radicular pain and paresthesia into the affected leg.[162] Activities that hold the hip in 30° hip flexion can produce sciatic symptoms when the hamstrings are activated (hamstring syndrome). Patients with IFI are comfortable sitting, while long-stride walking can exacerbate the pain.[157] Patients with IFI may also present with low back pain.[157,159,162] Short stride or hip abduction alleviates the pain.[163] With IFI there is deep gluteal pain and distal pain lateral to the ischium.[162,163] The condition is caused by narrowing between the ischium and the lesser trochanter, increased neck-shaft angle, or **coxa breva** (i.e., short femoral neck). If the foot is medially rotated and if the hip adducts during gait, the pelvic tilt associated with the rotary motion may contribute to lesser

TABLE **11.8**

Differential Diagnosis of Deep Gluteal Syndromes

Diagnosis	History	Physical Examination	Ancillary Tests
Pudendal nerve entrapment	Pain in the anatomical territory of the pudendal nerve, worsened by sitting, does not wake the patient at night Numbness	Tenderness at the medial ischium	Injection guided by imaging Intrapelvic tests
Ischiofemoral impingement	Sciatic nerve complaints Lower back pain Limping	Long stride walking reproduces the pain during terminal hip extension Tenderness at the lateral ischium Positive ischiofemoral impingement test	MRI showing decreased ischiofemoral and quadratus femoris space, and quadratus femoris muscle edema
Greater trochanter ischial impingement	Sciatic nerve complaints Laxity? Limping	Tenderness at the posterior aspect of the greater trochanter Pain in deep flexion, abduction, and external rotation	Injection guided by imaging
Ischial tunnel syndrome	Sciatic nerve complaints Limping Pain increased by flexion of the hip and extension of the knee	Tenderness at lateral ischium Positive hamstring active test	Injection guided by imaging MRI showing hamstring origin avulsion with edema around the sciatic nerve

MRI, Magnetic resonance imaging.
From Martin HD, Reddy M, Gomez-Hoyos J: Deep gluteal syndrome, *J Hip Preserv Surg* 2(2):103, 2015.

trochanteric impingement against the ischium.[162] The test for IFI is discussed under "Special Tests," later. The condition is more common in women.[83] The pain often begins without a precipitating event and is usually felt in adduction and lateral rotation.

The final, relatively rare impingement is **greater trochanteric-pelvic impingement,** in which a high greater trochanter (decreased neck-shaft angle—coxa vara) abuts against the ilium during hip abduction in extension.[59,149] This impingement is typically caused by Legg-Calvé-Perthes disease that has resulted in a morphological change in the femoral head and femoral neck, leading to contact between the ilium and greater trochanter when the hip is extended in abduction.[83,167] Patients may have a shortened involved leg (due to arrested growth of the proximal femoral physis) and a positive Trendelenburg gait. The "**gear-stick sign**" will be positive (see "Special Tests," later).

The examiner should also be aware that coxa valga (i.e., neck-shaft angle >135°) and femoral anteversion, which are associated with hip dysplasia, will also demonstrate limited extension, adduction, and lateral rotation.[149]

For the hamstring syndrome (or **ischial tunnel syndrome**), the pain is lateral to the ischium and pain occurs at heel strike (Fig. 11.14).[164,165] During the heel strike, the hamstrings act eccentrically, decelerating the forward leg. If pain is referred lateral to the ischium, there has probably been a proximal hamstring injury.[162] It is often associated with recurrent proximal hamstring

tears,[164,166] as posttraumatic scar tissue or congenital fibrotic bands may irritate the sciatic nerve.[160] If pain is felt in the extended hip, it is more likely due to hip pathology (e.g., arthritis). Pain is in the lower gluteal area and may spread to the popliteal space. Sitting is painful, as is forcefully driving the leg forward (e.g., sprinting, hurdling, or kicking a ball hard). There will be local tenderness around the ischial tuberosity.[166]

For DGS (including piriformis syndrome), the spinal, sacroiliac, and intrapelvic structures as well as the gluteal space must be examined and cleared. Pain is more proximal at the level of the piriformis, and is felt when the active and passive piriformis tests—the **Pace's** and **Freiberg's tests**—are positive (see "Special Tests," later).[162,165] Tenderness is usually felt over the piriformis muscle and retrotrochanteric area, and sitting for more than 20 to 30 minutes is painful.[165] In addition to piriformis syndrome, the DGS may include involvement of fibrous bands, obturator internus/gemellus syndrome, and quadratus femoris muscle. They all result in neurological signs due to involvement of the sciatic nerve.[63]

Hip abduction normally ranges from 30° to 50° and is tested with the patient in the supine position. Before asking the patient to do the abduction or adduction movement, the examiner should ensure that the patient's pelvis is "balanced," or level, with the ASISs being level and the legs being perpendicular to a line joining the two ASISs. The patient is then asked to abduct one leg at a time. Abduction is stopped when the pelvis begins

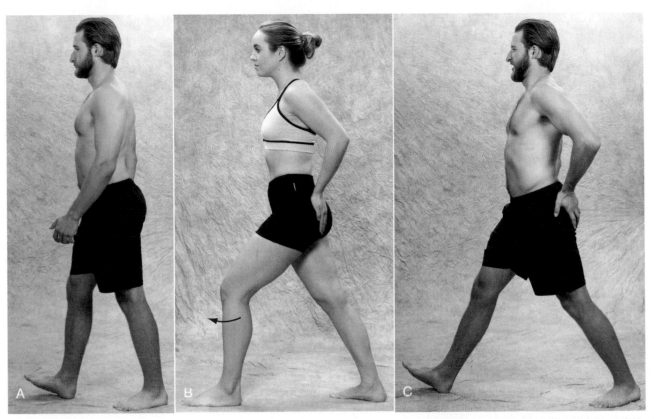

Fig. 11.14 Hamstring syndrome. (A) Short-stride walking—no pain in either leg. (B) Long-stride walking with right knee in extension—pain in the left hamstring, a positive sign. (C) If there is pain in the left hamstring on extension, the pain is probably due to hip pathology.

to move. Normally, the patient should be able to do hip abduction while the lower extremities, pelvis, trunk, and shoulders remain aligned in the frontal plane.[168] Pelvic motion is detected by palpation of the ASIS and by telling the patient to stop the movement as soon as the ASIS on either side starts to move. Normally, the ASIS on the movement side elevates while the opposite ASIS may drop or elevate. When the patient abducts the leg, the opposite ASIS tends to move first; with an **adduction contracture;** this occurs earlier in the ROM.

If, during abduction, lateral rotation and slight flexion occur early in the movement, the tensor fascia lata may be stronger and gluteus medius/minimus weak. If lateral rotation occurs later in the ROM, the iliopsoas or piriformis may be overactive. If the pelvis tilts up at the beginning of movement, the quadratus lumborum is overactive. All of these movements demonstrate imbalance patterns.

Hip adduction is normally 30° and is measured from the same starting position as abduction. The patient is asked to adduct one leg over the other while the examiner ensures that the pelvis does not move. An alternative method is for the patient to flex the opposite hip and knee and hold the limb in flexion with the arms; the patient then adducts the test leg under the other leg. This method is useful only for thin patients. When the patient adducts the leg, the ASIS on the same side moves first. This movement occurs earlier in the ROM if there is an **abduction**

contracture. Adduction can also be measured by asking the patient to abduct one leg and leave it abducted; the other leg is then tested for the amount of adduction present. The advantage of this method is that the test leg does not have to be flexed to clear the other leg before doing the adduction movement.

Rotational movements can be performed with the patient supine, prone, or sitting. The seated position ensures that the ischium is square to the table, but the testing is done in 90° of flexion; therefore, if the patient complains of symptoms while walking or running, supine or prone is the preferred test position.[3] In the flexed position, the iliofemoral ligament is relaxed. In flexion and extension, the ischiofemoral ligament is under tension.[3] Medial rotation normally ranges from 30° to 40° and lateral rotation from 40° to 60°. Asymmetric lateral rotation may indicate acetabular retroversion, femoral retrotorsion, or femoral head-neck abnormalities (e.g., FAI).[3] Loss of medial rotation is one of the first signs of internal hip pathology.[43] In the supine position, the patient simply rotates the straight leg on a balanced pelvis (i.e., leg rolling). Turning the foot or leg outward tests lateral rotation; turning the foot or leg inward tests medial rotation. If, in supine lying, the patient demonstrates enough lateral rotation that the lateral border of the foot touches the table, there is probably a lax anterior capsule or hip retroversion. Conversely, limited lateral rotation may indicate capsular hypomobility or hip anteversion.[6] In another supine test (see Fig. 11.11E), the patient is asked to flex both the hip and knee to 90° as the patient would do when being tested in sitting.[169] When this method is used, it must be recognized that having the patient rotate the leg outward tests medial rotation, whereas having the patient rotate the leg inward tests lateral rotation. With the patient prone, the pelvis is balanced by aligning the legs at right angles to a line joining the PSISs. The patient then flexes the knee to 90°. Again, medial rotation is being tested when the leg is rotated outward, and lateral rotation is being tested when the leg is rotated inward (see Fig. 11.11F). Usually one of these last two methods (i.e., sitting or prone) is used to measure hip rotation, because it is easier to measure the angle when the test is being performed. However, in prone, the measurement is done on a straight leg, whereas in sitting or supine, rotation is measured with the hip flexed to 90°. It has been found that there is a difference in the amount of lateral rotation between the flexed (less) and straight position, whereas medial rotation shows little difference when measured in the two positions.[169]

Flexibility can also be tested using the **Bent-Knee Fall-Out Test,** in which the patient is in the supine crook-lying position (i.e., hip at 45° flexion, knee at 90° flexion) with the knees together. The patient then allows the knees to fall outward while keeping the feet together (Fig. 11.15A). The examiner tests the end feel at the end of the ROM and then bilaterally measures from the head of the fibula to the table (Fig. 11.15B).[170]

Passive Movements

If the ROM was not full and the examiner was unable to test end feel during the active movements, passive movements should be performed to determine the end feel and passive range of motion (PROM). The passive movements performed are the same as the active movements. All the movements except extension can be tested with the patient in the supine position. Because of the many different structures around the hip, passive **end feel** becomes an important part of the examination to help differentiate the tissue that is causing problems.[3] It is also at this point that the examiner may check general laxity (see the **Carter and Wilkinson criteria** in Chapter 17) to determine whether the problem may have a systemic component.[3]

Passive Movements of the Hip and Normal End Feel

- Flexion (tissue approximation or tissue stretch)
- Extension (tissue stretch)
- Abduction (tissue stretch)
- Adduction (tissue approximation or tissue stretch)
- Medial rotation (tissue stretch)
- Lateral rotation (tissue stretch)

The capsular pattern of the hip is flexion, abduction, and medial rotation. These movements are always the ones most limited in a capsular pattern, although the order of restriction may vary. For example, medial rotation may be most limited, followed by flexion and abduction. The hip joint is the only joint to exhibit this altered pattern of the same movements.

Pain on passive flexion and medial rotation indicates there may be an intra-articular source of the problem.[56] Snapping of iliopsoas can be assessed by passively (or actively) moving the hip from a flexed, abducted, and laterally rotated position to one of extension and medial

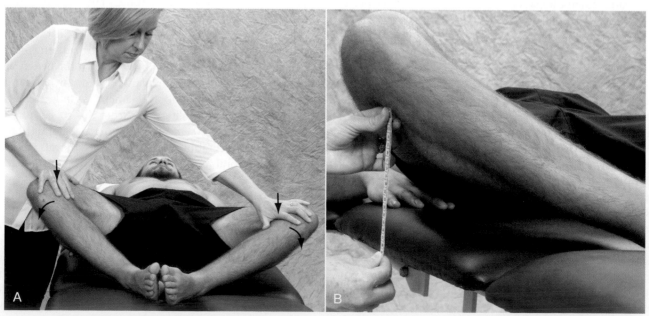

Fig. 11.15 Bent knee fall-out test. (A) Examiner is testing end feel. (B) Examiner measures from head of fibula to bed.

rotation (see Fig. 11.8).[56] Normally, if the contralateral hip is flexed to its normal end range (approximately 120°), the posterior aspect of the opposite leg should be able to touch the examining table. If it does not, a flexion contracture may be present in the straight leg.[61]

The pelvis should not move during passive hip movements. Groin discomfort and a limited ROM on medial rotation are good indications of hip problems. Passive hip flexion, adduction, and medial rotation, if painful, may indicate acetabular rim problems or labral tears, especially if clicking and pain into the groin is elicited.[171]

Intra-abdominal inflammation in the lower pelvis, as in the case of an abscess, may cause pain on passive medial and lateral rotation of the hip when the patient is supine with the hip and knee at 90°.

Resisted Isometric Movements

The resisted isometric movements are performed with the patient in the supine position (Fig. 11.16). The muscles of the hip play a very significant role in stabilizing the pelvis, so they must be included in any assessment dealing with issues of pelvic control. Manual muscle testing or a handheld dynamometer may be used.[172] The examiner should note whether the muscles are weak or strong and tight and whether the muscle force-couples are acting correctly.[173] When these muscles and the back and abdominal muscles are being dealt with, the examiner must be able to answer the following three questions in the affirmative to ensure that pelvic control is present:

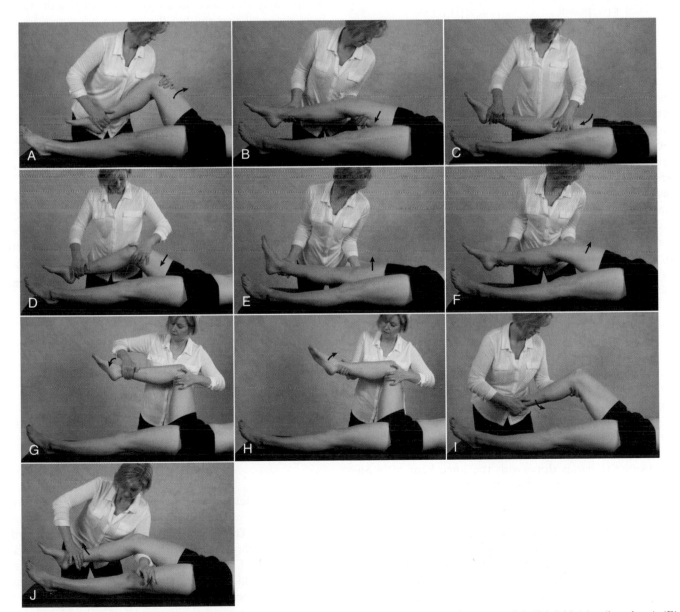

Fig. 11.16 Resisted isometric movements around the hip. (A) Flexion. (B) Extension. (C) Adduction (knee straight). (D) Adduction (knee bent). (E) Abduction (knee straight). (F) Abduction (knee bent). (G) Medial rotation. (H) Lateral rotation. (I) Knee flexion. (J) Knee extension.

1. Can the patient actively position the pelvis in neutral (especially while doing hip movements)?
2. Can the patient hold the neutral position statically while doing hip movements? (This may include distal movement.)
3. Can the patient control dynamic movement of the pelvis while doing hip movements?

Resisted Isometric Movements of the Hip

- Flexion of the hip
- Extension of the hip
- Abduction of the hip
- Adduction of the hip
- Medial rotation of the hip
- Lateral rotation of the hip
- Flexion of the knee
- Extension of the knee

Because the hip muscles are very strong and there are many of them (Table 11.9; Fig. 11.17), the examiner should position the patient's hip properly and say to the patient, "Don't let me move your hip," to ensure that the movement is isometric and that the patient does not initiate any compensatory movements (e.g., grasping the table, rotating the trunk).[89] Delahunt et al.[175–177] advocate testing the adductors with the hip flexed to 30° to 45° as the optimal test position (**thigh adductor squeeze test** or the **fist squeeze test**)[178] [also see "Special Tests," later]). Reiman et al.[89] reported that testing the adductors bilaterally with the knees extended (**bilateral adductor test**) was the most diagnostic of the adductor tests. By carefully noting which movements cause pain or show weakness when the tests are done isometrically, the examiner should be able to determine which muscle, if any, is at fault (see Table 11.9).[44,89] For example, the gluteus maximus is the only muscle that is involved in all of the following movements: extension, adduction, and lateral rotation. Therefore, if pain resulted from only these three movements, the examiner would expect the gluteus maximus muscle to be at fault. As with active movements, the most painful movements are performed last.

If the examiner does a resisted isometric test of abduction with the patient's knee straight, it is primarily gluteus maximus and tensor fascia lata that are being tested. If the isometric test is done with the knee bent, it is primarily gluteus medius and minimus being tested.[18] Boren et al.[179] showed that side plank abduction elicited the highest electromyography (EMG) value for gluteus medius, whereas front plank with hip extension (knee at 90°) elicited the highest EMG value for gluteus maximus. Almeida et al.[180] advocated using the hip stability isometric test (HipSIT) to test gluteal muscle strength.

Resisted isometric flexion and extension of the knee must also be performed, because there are two joint muscles (hamstrings and rectus femoris) that act over the knee as well as the hip. If the history has indicated that concentric, eccentric, or econcentric movement causes symptoms, these movements should also be tested, but only after the isometric tests have been completed. For example, strength of the hamstrings may be determined by doing a **supine plank test** in which the patient is in crook lying, resting on his or her elbows (Fig. 11.18).[181] The patient then lifts the buttocks off the table while maintaining the body weight on the elbows and heels. The patient then alternately lifts the injured leg and then the good leg. If pain occurs at the ischial origin or in the hamstrings musculature, or if pelvic "collapse" or rotation occurs, the test is positive for weak hamstrings.

The examiner must be aware that intra-abdominal inflammation in the area of the psoas muscle may cause pain on resisted hip flexion. Intra-abdominal inflammation may also result in a rigid abdominal wall. It has been reported that the hip flexors and hip extensors are almost equal in strength[182] and that the adductors are 2.5 times as strong as the abductors.[183] These ratios may vary depending on whether the movement is tested isometrically or isokinetically.

Functional Assessment

Hip motion is necessary for more activities than just ambulation. In fact, more hip ROM is required for activities of daily living (ADLs) than for gait; activities such as shoe tying, sitting, getting up from a chair, and picking up things from the floor all require a greater ROM. Table 11.10 illustrates the ROM necessary for various activities. Ideally, the patient should have functional ranges of 120° of flexion, 20° of abduction, and 20° of lateral rotation.

Functional Tests of the Hip

- Squatting
- Going up and down stairs one at a time
- Crossing the legs so that the ankle of one foot rests on the knee of the opposite leg
- Going up and down stairs two or more at a time
- Running straight ahead
- Running and decelerating
- Running and twisting
- One-legged hop (time, distance, crossover)
- Jumping

There are several numerical rating scales or patient-reported outcome measures with which to rate hip function.[59,184–192] These rating methods are based primarily on pain, mobility, and gait. Tables 11.11 through 11.13 and eTools 11.1 and 11.2 illustrate different rating scales. D'Aubigné and Postel[184] (see Tables 11.11 through 11.13) developed one of the first hip rating scales based on pain, mobility, and ability to walk.[185] The **Harris Hip Function Scale**[186] (see eTool 11.1) is one of the more

TABLE **11.9**

Muscles of the Hip: Their Actions, Innervation, and Nerve Root Derivation[174]

Action	Muscles Acting	Innervation	Nerve Root Derivation
Flexion of hip	1. Psoas	L1–L3	L1–L3
	2. Iliacus	Femoral	L2, L3
	3. Rectus femoris	Femoral	L2–L4
	4. Sartorius	Femoral	L2, L3
	5. Tensor fasciae latae	Superior gluteal	L5, S1, S2
	6. Pectineus	Femoral	L2, L3
	7. Adductor longus	Obturator	L2–L4
	8. Adductor brevis	Obturator	L2, L3
	9. Gracilis	Obturator	L2, L3
	10. Gluteus medius (anterior fibers)	Superior gluteal	L5, S1
Extension of hip	1. Biceps femoris (long head)	Sciatic	L5, S1, S2
	2. Semimembranosus	Sciatic	L5, S1, S2
	3. Semitendinosus	Sciatic	L5, S1, S2
	4. Gluteus maximus	Inferior gluteal	L5, S1, S2
	5. Gluteus medius (middle and posterior part)	Superior gluteal	L5, S1
	6. Adductor magnus (ischiocondylar part)	Sciatic	L2–L4
Abduction of hip	1. Tensor fasciae latae	Superior gluteal	L4, L5
	2. Gluteus minimus	Superior gluteal	L5, S1
	3. Gluteus medius	Superior gluteal	L5, S1
	4. Gluteus maximus	Inferior gluteal	L5, S1, S2
	5. Sartorius	Femoral	L2, L3
	6. Piriformis	L5, S1, S2	L5, S1, S2
	7. Rectus femoris	Femoral	L2–L4
Adduction of hip	1. Adductor longus	Obturator	L2–L4
	2. Adductor brevis	Obturator	L2–L4
	3. Adductor magnus (ischiofemoral part)	Obturator	L2–L4
	4. Gracilis	Obturator	L2, L3
	5. Pectineus	Femoral	L2, L3
	6. Biceps femoris (long head)	Sciatic	L5, S1, S2
	7. Gluteus maximus (posterior fibers)	Inferior gluteal	L5, S1, S2
	8. Quadratus femoris	N. to quadratus femoris	L5, S1
	9. Obturator externus	Obturator	L3–L4
Medial rotation of hip	1. Adductor longus	Obturator	L2–L4
	2. Adductor brevis	Obturator	L2–L4
	3. Adductor magnus (posterior head)	Obturator and sciatic	L2–L4
	4. Gluteus medius (anterior part)	Superior gluteal	L5, S1
	5. Gluteus minimus (anterior part)	Superior gluteal	L5, S1
	6. Tensor fasciae latae	Superior gluteal	L4, L5
	7. Pectineus	Femoral	L2, L3
	8. Gracilis	Obturator	L2, L3
Lateral rotation of hip	1. Gluteus maximus	Inferior gluteal	L5, S1, S2
	2. Obturator internus	N. to obturator internus	L5, S1
	3. Obturator externus	Obturator	L3, L4
	4. Quadratus femoris	N. to quadratus femoris	L5, S1
	5. Piriformis	L5, S1–S2	L5, S1, S2
	6. Gemellus superior	N. to obturator internus	L5, S1
	7. Gemellus inferior	N. to quadratus femoris	L5, S1
	8. Sartorius	Femoral	L2, L3
	9. Gluteus medius (posterior part)	Superior gluteal	L5, S1
	10. Gluteus minimus (posterior part)	Superior gluteal	L5, S1
	11. Biceps femoris (long head)	Sciatic	L5, S1, S2

N, Nerve.

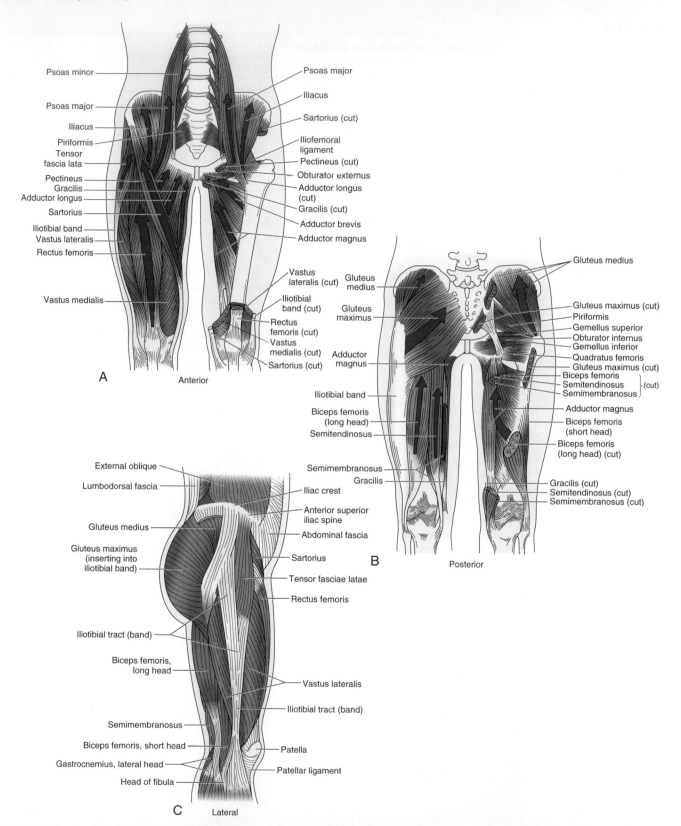

Fig. 11.17 Muscles of the hip and knee. (A) Anterior view. The right side shows the primary flexor and adductor muscles of the hip. Many muscles on the left side are cut to expose the adductor brevis and adductor magnus. (B) Posterior view. The left side highlights the gluteus maximus and hamstring muscles (long head of biceps femoris, semitendinosus, and semimembranosus). The right side shows the hamstring muscles cut to expose the adductor magnus and short head of the biceps femoris. The right side shows the gluteus medius and five of the six short external rotators (i.e., piriformis, gemellus superior and inferior, obturator internus, and quadratus femoris). (C) Lateral view showing extent of tensor fasciae latae and iliotibial band. (A and B, Redrawn from Neumann DA: *Kinesiology of the musculoskeletal system—foundations for physical rehabilitation*, St Louis, 2002, CV Mosby, pp 411, 419; C, From Paulsen F, Washcke: *Sobotta atlas of human anatomy*, ed 16, Munich, 2019, Urban & Fischer.)

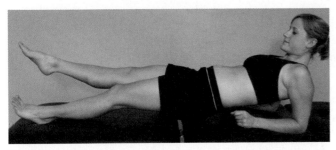

Fig. 11.18 The supine plank test is used to assess hamstring strength. The patient elevates the pelvis while keeping the body weight on the elbows and heels. The legs are alternately lifted, starting with lifting the injured leg. (This tests the good leg first.) Pelvic collapse or rotation or pain at the hamstring origin as the contralateral leg is lifted indicates hamstring weakness.

common questionnaires and is useful for rating hips before and after surgery.[92] This scale is most often used because it emphasizes pain and function. The Victorian Institute of Sport Australia developed the **VISA-G questionnaire** for GTPS (i.e., trochanteric bursitis) (eTool 11.3).[193] The **Western Ontario and McMaster Universities Osteoarthritis Index (WOMAC)**[194–199] and the **Lower Extremity Function Scale (LEFS)** (eTool 11.4)[200–203] were developed to evaluate clinically important and patient-relevant changes in health status primarily with arthroplasties of the hip and knee. The WOMAC scale is made up of three sections, with scores ranging from 1 (none) to 5 (extreme). The sum of three scores is called the *index* or *global score*. The higher the score, the greater the disability. The **SF-36 questionnaire** is also sometimes used as a functional assessment tool in arthroplasty cases.[199,204] The **Iowa Scale** (see eTool 11.2) provides

a single rating value. The **Oxford Hip Score,**[205] the **Mayo Hip Score,**[187] and the **Hip Outcome Score**[206,207] (eTool 11.5) for hip arthroplasty make use of greater patient (functional) and radiographic input (to predict long-term results). These scores correlate well with the Harris scale.[185,187] Johanson and colleagues[188] developed a numerical scale that is related to what patients are able to do functionally after total hip replacement. Its value

TABLE **11.10**

Range of Motion Necessary at the Hip for Selected Activities

Activity	Average Range of Motion Necessary
Shoe tying	120° of flexion
Sitting (average seat height)	112° of flexion
Stooping	125° of flexion
Squatting	115° of flexion/20° of abduction/20° of medial rotation
Ascending stairs (average stair height)	67° of flexion
Descending stairs (average stair height)	36° of flexion
Putting foot on opposite thigh (putting on socks)	120° of flexion/20° of abduction/20° of lateral rotation
Putting on trousers	90° of flexion
Walking on level surface	30°–44° of hip flexion

TABLE **11.11**

Method of Grading Functional Value of Hip[a]

Grade	Pain	Mobility	Ability to Walk
0	Pain is intense and permanent	Ankylosis with bad position of the hip	None
1	Pain is severe, even at night	No movement; pain or slight deformity	Only with crutches
2	Pain is severe when walking; prevents any activity	Flexion less than 40°	Only with canes
3	Pain is tolerable with limited activity	Flexion between 40° and 60°	With one cane, for less than 1 hour; very difficult without a cane
4	Pain is mild when walking; it disappears with rest	Flexion between 60° and 80°; patient can reach own foot	A long time with a cane; a short time without cane and with limp
5	Pain is mild and inconstant; normal activity	Flexion between 80° and 90°; abduction at least 15°	Without cane but with slight limp
6	No pain	Flexion more than 90°; abduction to 30°	Normal

[a]Values used in conjunction with Table 11.12.
From D'Aubigné RM, Postel M: Functional results of hip arthroplasty with acrylic prosthesis, *J Bone Joint Surg Am* 36:459, 1954.

TABLE **11.12**

D'Aubigné and Postel Scale for Functional Grading of the Hip

Pain (P)	Ability to Walk (W)	Mobility Normal or Nearly Normal	Grade
		Very Good	*P + W = 11 or 12*
6	6	Walk without cane, with no pain and no limp	
6	5	Walk without cane, with no pain but slight limp	
5	6	Walk without cane, with no limp but slight pain when starting	
		Good	*P + W = 10*
5	5	Walk without cane, with slight pain and slight limp	
4	6	Walk without cane, with pain but no limp	
6	4[a]	Walk without cane, without pain; a cane used to go outdoors	
		Medium	*P + W = 9*
5	4	Slight pain; a cane is used outdoors	
4	5	Pain after walking some minutes; no cane is used, but there is a slight limp	
6	3[b]	No pain; a cane used all the time	
		Fair	*P + W = 8*
5	3	Slight pain; a cane is used all the time	
4	4	Pain after walking; a cane is used outdoors	
≤3	≤3	*Poor*	*P + W = 7 or less*

[a]If the mobility is reduced to 4, the result is classified one grade lower.
[b]If the mobility is reduced to 3 or less, the result is classified two grades lower.
Adapted from D'Aubigné RM, Postel M: Functional results of hip arthroplasty with acrylic prosthesis, *J Bone Joint Surg Am* 36:460, 1954.

TABLE **11.13**

Method of Evaluating Improvement Brought About by Operation in Problems of the Hip (Relative Result)

	Preoperative Grading	Postoperative Grading	Difference	Improvement
Pain	3	5	$2 \times 2 = 4$	
Mobility	2	5	$3 = 3$	= 9
Ability to walk	3	4	$1 \times 2 = 2$	

Very great improvement = 12 or more, great improvement = 7–11, fair improvement = 3–7, failure = less than 3.
From D'Aubigné RM, Postel M: Functional results of hip arthroplasty with acrylic prosthesis, *J Bone Joint Surg Am* 36:461, 1954.

comes from its focus on the outcome from the patient's perspective (eTool 11.6). As Burton and coworkers[189] have pointed out, the notion of expectations is more important than the notion of success. Table 11.14 gives a testing scheme for functional strength and endurance of the hip.

Two of the newer outcome scales are the **International Hip Outcome Tool**[208–212] (in two versions, iHOT33 and iHOT12) [eTools 11.7 and 11.8]), which are geared toward hip problems in young people, and the **Copenhagen Hip and Groin Outcome Score (HAGOS),**[212,213] which has six subscales assessing pain, symptoms, physical function in ADLs, physical function in sport and recreation, participation in physical activities, and hip/groin-related quality of life.

Several **walking tests** have been developed, especially for the elderly, to give an indication of musculoskeletal functional impairment of the lower limb. These may be included in any assessment involving injury to the lower limb joints.[214] Testing dynamic stability, endurance, falls risk, and ability to step over low objects, they include the

TABLE **11.14**

Functional Testing of the Hip

Starting Position	Action	Functional Test
Standing	Lift foot onto 20-cm (8-inch) step and return (hip flexion-extension)	5–6 Repetitions: functional 3–4 Repetitions: functionally fair 1–2 Repetitions: functionally poor 0 Repetitions: nonfunctional
Standing	Sit in chair and return to standing (hip extension-flexion)	5–6 Repetitions: functional 3–4 Repetitions: functionally fair 1–2 Repetitions: functionally poor 0 Repetitions: nonfunctional
Standing	Lift leg to balance on one leg keeping pelvis straight (hip abduction)	Hold 1–1.5 minutes: functional Hold 30–59 seconds: functionally fair Hold 1–29 seconds: functionally poor Cannot hold: nonfunctional
Standing	Walk sideways 6 m (20 feet) (hip adduction/abduction)	6–8 m one way: functional 3–6 m one way: functionally fair 1–3 m one way: functionally poor 0 m: nonfunctional
Standing	Test leg off floor (patient may hold on to something for balance): medially rotate non–weight-bearing hip	10–12 Repetitions: functional 5–9 Repetitions: functionally fair 1–4 Repetitions: functionally poor 0 Repetitions: nonfunctional
Standing	Test leg off floor (patient may hold on to something for balance) laterally rotate non–weight-bearing hip	10–12 Repetitions: functional 5–9 Repetitions: functionally fair 1–4 Repetitions: functionally poor 0 Repetitions: nonfunctional

Data from Palmer ML, Epler M: *Clinical assessment procedures in physical therapy*, Philadelphia, 1990, JB Lippincott, pp 251–254.

Timed Up-and-Go test (TUG test) (see eTool 2.16), 13-minute walk test, 6-minute walk test (6-MWT), self-paced walk test, 2-minute walk test, 10-m walk test, 12-minute walk test, 4-square step test, step test, and sit to stand.[214–227]

Sutlive[228] developed the following clinical prediction rule for osteoarthritis of the hip: if four of the five tests are positive, the patient has osteoarthritis of the hip.

Clinical Prediction Rule for Hip Osteoarthritis[a,228]

- Limited active hip flexion with lateral hip pain
- Active hip extension causes pain
- Limited passive hip medial rotation (25° or less)
- Squatting limited and painful
- Scour test with adduction causes lateral hip or groin pain

[a]Four out of five variables must be positive.

The University of Delaware Physical Therapy Program has provided method, patient, and clinician instructions along with norms for the 6-minute walk test, the single-leg stance test,[226] stair-climbing test, and single-limb step test (eTool 11.9), which can be used to aid functional assessment.

In addition to the outcome measures directed specifically at the hip, the **EQ-5D Questionnaire** has been developed to determine a patient's present perceived health status and quality of life.[229–234] Other tools may be used to try to predict injuries to the lower extremity.[235]

If the patient is able to perform normal active movements with little difficulty, the examiner may use a series of functional tests to determine whether increased intensity of activity produces pain or other symptoms. These tests must be geared to the individual patient.[236] Older persons should not be expected to perform difficult activities unless they have been doing these movements or similar ones in the recent past. Wahoff and Ryan[237] recommended the **Functional Hip Sport Test** for athletes who want to return to sport following hip arthroscopy. The test includes single knee bends, side-to-side lateral movement, diagonal side-to-side movement, and forward box lunges. Patients must score 17/20 or higher to pass each of the four components. Thus the test could be used to determine a prearthroscopy score as well.[6,19]

Special Tests

Only those tests that the examiner believes are necessary should be performed when the hip is being assessed. Most tests are done primarily to confirm a diagnosis or to determine pathology; they should **not** be used as "stand-alone" tests when a diagnosis is being considered.[238] This is because many of the problems cause similar symptoms and the physical tests are seldom definitive.[19,59] In fact, for most of the physical tests, the best one can say is that the test increases suspicion for a certain condition. It is only through diagnostic imaging, primarily magnetic resonance imaging arthrography (MRI-A), that the examiner is able to be sure of the diagnosis, especially with impingement and labral problems.[130,139,239,240] As with all special tests, if the test is positive, it is highly likely that the problem exists; but if it is negative, it does not necessarily rule out the problem. Clustering of the tests may provide more promising findings.[238] Therefore special tests should not be taken in isolation but should be used to support the history, observation, and clinical examination.

For the reader who would like to review them, the reliability, validity, specificity, sensitivity, and odds ratios of some of the special tests used in the hip are available in eAppendix 11.1.

Tests for Hip Pathology

Hip pathology can cover a number of conditions, many of which demonstrate similar signs and symptoms. This can make diagnosing the problem difficult. Lesions such as FAI, labral lesions, microinstability (i.e., loss of dynamic muscle control of small movements of the hip), ligamentum teres tears, and osteochondral lesions often produce similar signs and symptoms. Some of the additional signs and symptoms that may be reported in the history include decreased extension and/or medial rotation, painful straight leg raising, and locking of the joint.[27] Tests that can be used to indicate intra-articular pathology include

Key Tests Performed on the Hip Depending on Suspected Pathology[a,241,242]

- **For hip pathology:**
  - Abduction, extension, and lateral rotation test
  - Anterior apprehension test
  - Drehmann sign
  - Flexion-adduction test
  - ✓ Hip scour test
  - Internal rotation overpressure test
  - Lateral FABER test
  - Ligamentum teres test
  - ✓ Log roll test
  - McCarthy hip extension sign
  - ✓ Patrick's test
  - Posterior apprehension test
  - Prone external rotation test
- **For impingement:**
  - Anteroposterior impingement test
  - "Gear stick" sign
  - Impingement provocation test
  - Ischiofemoral impingement test
  - Lateral FADDIR test
  - Lateral rim impingement test
  - Posteroinferior impingement test
  - ❓ Squat test
- **For labral lesions:**
  - ✓ Anterior labral tear test
  - External rotation test
  - Flexion-internal rotation test
  - Posterior labral tear test
  - THIRD test
- **For femoral neck stress fractures:**
  - Heel-strike test
  - Patellar-pubic percussion sign
- **For pediatric hip pathology:**
  - Abduction test

- ✓ Barlow's test
- Galleazzi sign
- ✓ Ortolani's sign
- Telescoping sign
- **For leg length:**
  - True leg length
  - Weber-Barstow maneuver
- **For muscle tightness or pathology:**
  - Abduction contracture test
  - Active piriformis stretch test
  - Adduction contracture test
  - Adductor squeeze (fist) test
  - Beatty's test
  - Bent-knee stretch test for proximal hamstrings
  - ❓ Eccentric hip flexion
  - Ely's test
  - External de-rotation test
  - Freiberg's maneuver
  - Hamstring syndrome test
  - Heel contralateral knee maneuver
  - ✓ Hip lag sign
  - Hip rotator tightness
  - Long stride heel-strike test
  - ✓ 90-90 straight leg raising test
  - Noble compression test
  - Ober's test
  - Pace's maneuver
  - Puranen-Orava test
  - Rectus femoris contracture test
  - Seated piriformis stretch test
  - Thomas test
  - ✓ Trendelenburg sign
- **Other tests:**
  - Femoral nerve tension (prone knee bending) test
  - Timed "up and go" test

[a]The authors recommend that these key tests be learned by the clinician to facilitate diagnosis. See Chapter 1: Key for Classifying Special Tests.

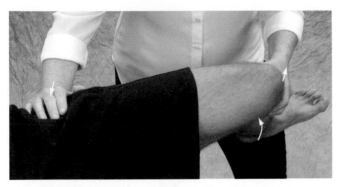

Fig. 11.19 Abduction, extension, and lateral rotation test.

the log roll test, resisted straight leg raising test, and McCarthy test.[28]

⚠ *Abduction, Extension, and Lateral Rotation Test.*[36,93,243] The patient is in the side-lying position with the test leg uppermost and laterally rotated. The examiner passively abducts the hip to 30° while pushing on the posterior aspect of the greater trochanter to push it forward while slowly extending the hip from 10° of flexion to full extension (Fig. 11.19). A positive test is reproduction of the patient's symptoms and indicates anterior instability. The test is purported to be similar to the apprehension test in the shoulder.[43]

⚠ *Anterior Apprehension Test (Hyperextension–Lateral Rotation Test).*[36,93,243] The patient is supine with the buttocks on the edge of the examining table (Fig. 11.20) and the test leg extended. The patient holds the contralateral extremity in flexion while the examiner rotates the test hip laterally. The maneuver reproduces anterior hip pain and/or apprehension for anterior instability or an anterior labral tear.

❓ *Bryant's Triangle.* With the patient lying supine, the examiner drops an imaginary perpendicular line from the ASIS of the pelvis to the examining table.[244] A second imaginary line is projected up from the tip of the greater trochanter of the femur to meet the first line at a right angle (Fig. 11.21). This line is measured and the two sides are compared. Differences may indicate conditions such as coxa vara or CDH. This measurement can be done with radiographs, in which case the lines may be drawn on the radiograph.

❓ *Craig's Test.* Craig's test measures **femoral anteversion** or forward torsion of the femoral neck (Fig. 11.22). Anteversion of the hip is measured primarily by the angle made by the femoral neck with the femoral condyles (Fig. 11.23), although some rotation also occurs in the femoral shaft.[245] It is the degree of forward projection of the femoral neck from the coronal plane of the shaft (Fig. 11.24), and it decreases during the growing period. At birth, the mean angle is approximately 30°; in the adult, the mean angle is 8° to 15° (Fig. 11.25). Increased anteversion leads to squinting patellae and toeing in (Fig. 11.26).[246] Excessive anteversion is twice as common in girls as in

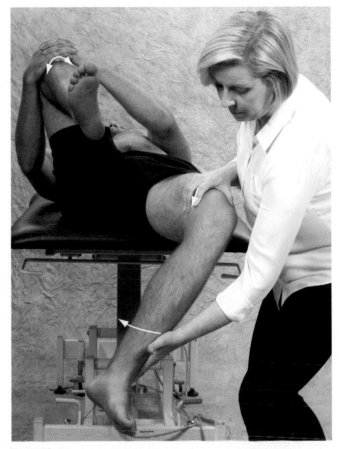

Fig. 11.20 Anterior apprehension test (hyperextension–lateral rotation test). Note: With the knee flexed, when the foot moves medially, the hip rotates laterally.

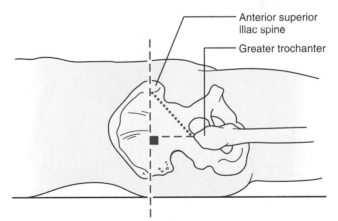

Fig. 11.21 Bryant's triangle.

boys. A common clinical finding of excessive anteversion is excessive medial hip rotation (more than 60°) and decreased lateral rotation in extension.[246] Gelberman et al.[247] pointed out, however, that rotation should be viewed both in neutral (as in the Craig's test) and with 90° of hip flexion, because rotation shows greater variability in flexion. They felt that greater medial rotation than lateral rotation in both positions was a better indicator of increased femoral anteversion. In retroversion, the plane of the femoral neck rotates backward in relation to

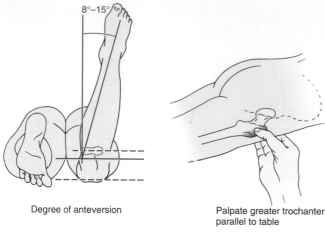

Degree of anteversion

Palpate greater trochanter parallel to table

Fig. 11.22 Craig's test to measure femoral anteversion.

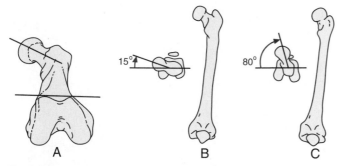

A   B   C

Fig. 11.23 Anteversion of the hip. (A) Femoral anteversion angle. (B) Normal angle. (C) Excessive angle. (A, Redrawn from the American Orthopaedic Association: *Manual of Orthopaedic Surgery*, Chicago, 1979, AOA, p 45.)

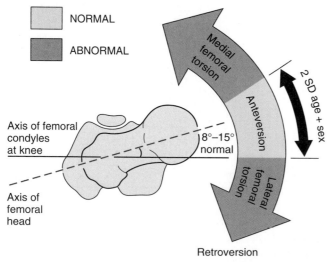

Fig. 11.24 Axial view of right femur showing approximately normal angle of anteversion and torsional deformity beyond. (Redrawn from Staheli LT: Medial femoral torsion, *Orthop Clin North Am* 11:40, 1980.)

the coronal condylar plane (see Fig. 11.26), or the acetabulum itself may be retroverted.[122,244,247–250]

For Craig's test, which has been found to correlate well with x-rays (within 4°) in children,[251] the patient lies prone with the knee flexed to 90°. The examiner

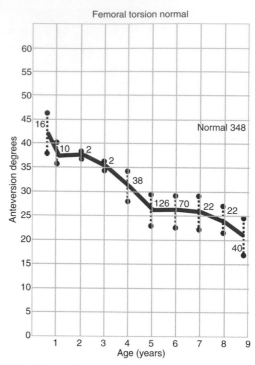

Femoral torsion normal

Fig. 11.25 The degree of normal femoral torsion in relation to age. *Solid lines* represent the mean; *vertical lines* represent the standard deviation. (Redrawn from Crane L: Femoral torsion and its relation to toeing-in and toeing-out, *J Bone Joint Surg Am* 41:423, 1959.)

palpates the posterior aspect of the greater trochanter of the femur. The hip is then passively rotated medially and laterally until the greater trochanter is parallel with the examining table or reaches its most lateral position. The degree of anteversion can then be estimated based on the angle of the lower leg with the vertical.[252] The test is also called the **Ryder method** for measuring anteversion or retroversion.

❓ *Dial Test of the Hip.*[18,253] The patient lies supine with the hips in neutral (i.e., no rotation). The examiner rotates the limb medially and then releases it, allowing the leg to go into lateral rotation. If the patient's leg rotates passively greater than 45° from vertical in the axial plane and if, on testing, there is no mechanical endpoint, the test is positive for hip instability (Fig. 11.27). Both limbs are compared, starting with the unaffected side.

⚠ *Drehmann Sign.*[254] This is a clinical feature of SCFE in adolescents and young adults showing excessive, unavoidable passive lateral rotation and abduction in hip flexion performed by the examiner (Fig. 11.28). It can also be used to help diagnose FAI because of SCFE. The diagnosis of SCFE is confirmed by diagnostic imaging.

⚠ *Flexion-Adduction Test.*[255] This test is used in older children and young adults in looking for hip disease. The patient lies supine while the examiner flexes the patient's hip to at least 90° with the knee flexed (Fig. 11.29). The examiner then adducts the flexed leg. Normally the knee will pass over the opposite hip without rolling the pelvis.

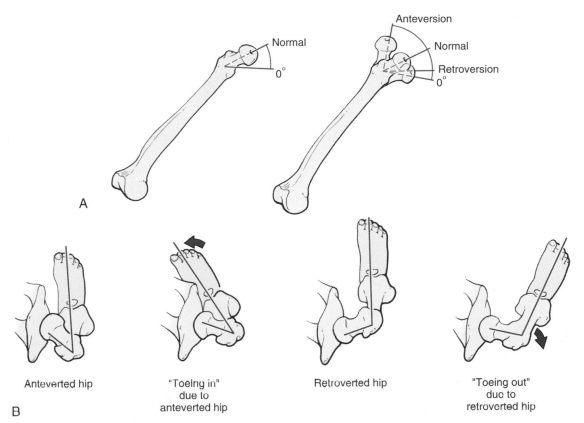

Fig. 11.26 Torsion angles of the hip. (A) Positions of femoral neck. (B) Different foot positions with anteversion and retroversion at the hip (coronal views). (Redrawn from Echternach J, editor: *Physical therapy of the hip*, New York, 1990, Churchill Livingstone, p 25.)

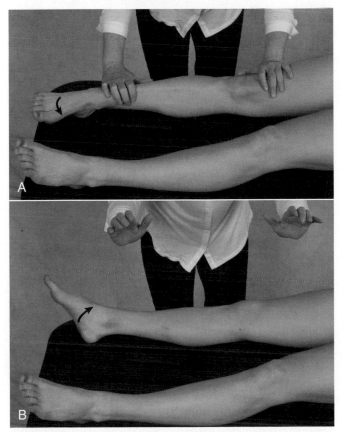

Fig. 11.27 Dial test of the hip. (A) The examiner rotates the hip medially. (B) The examiner releases the medial rotation and watches the hip roll into lateral rotation.

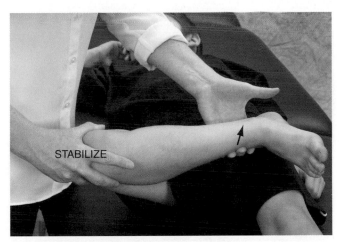

Fig. 11.28 Drehmann sign.

In pathological hips, adduction is limited and accompanied by pain or discomfort.

❓ *Foveal Distraction Test.*[61] The patient is in supine. The examiner abducts the hip to 30° and applies an axial traction to the leg, which reduces intra-articular pressure (Fig. 11.30). Relief of pain indicates that the pain is intra-articular.

✓ *Hip Scour (Grind) Test (Flexion-Adduction Test).* Maitland[256] called the flexion-adduction test the **quadrant** or **scouring test**. He felt that the test stressed or compressed the femoral neck against the acetabulum or pinched the adductor longus, pectineus, iliopsoas, sartorius, or tensor fascia lata. The patient lies supine. The

ZONES: 3   2   1

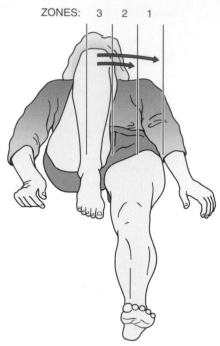

Fig. 11.29 The normal hip permits the ipsilateral knee to move convincingly across the midline of the body without rolling the pelvis. The knee should enter *zone 1* by overlapping the opposite hip and, in the youthful or supple patient, reaches a position lateral to the thigh. Progressive pathologic changes in the hip limit adduction to *zones 2* and *3*, producing pain with this maneuver. (Redrawn from Woods D, Macnicol M: The flexion-adduction test: an early sign of hip disease, *J Pediatr Orthop* 10:181, 2001.)

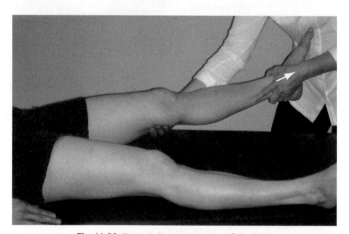

Fig. 11.30 Foveal distraction test of the hip.

examiner flexes and adducts the patient's hip so that the hip faces the patient's opposite shoulder and resistance to the movement is felt (Fig. 11.31). As slight resistance (i.e., a compressive force) is maintained, the patient's hip is taken into abduction while flexion is maintained in an arc of movement.[18,23] As the movement is performed, the examiner should look for any irregularity in the movement (e.g., "bumps"), pain, or patient apprehension, which may give an indication of where the pathology is occurring in the hip.[256] This motion also causes impingement of the femoral neck against

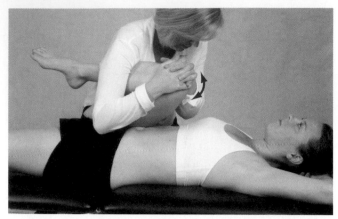

Fig. 11.31 Hip scour test.

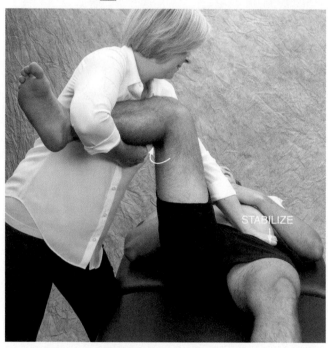

Fig. 11.32 Internal rotation overpressure (IROP) test.

the acetabular rim (i.e., FAI) and pinches the adductor longus, pectineus, iliopsoas, sartorius, and/or tensor fascia lata, depending on the position of the hip in the ROM. Therefore this maneuver should be performed with care.[110–112]

⚠ *Internal Rotation Overpressure (IROP) Test.*[130,257] The patient is in supine with the hip held in 90° flexion by the examiner with the patient's knee at 90°. The examiner rotates the hip medially by moving the leg/foot backwards while stabilizing the knee (Fig. 11.32). The examiner's other hand stabilizes the pelvis by applying a downward pressure on the contralateral ASIS. The examiner watches for resisted ROM, pain, and an abnormal end feel, which would indicate a positive test for hip pathology.

⚠ *Lateral FABER (Flexion, Abduction, and External Rotation) Test.*[3,107] The patient is in the side-lying position. The examiner holds the patient's upper leg with one hand while palpating over the hip joint with the other hand.

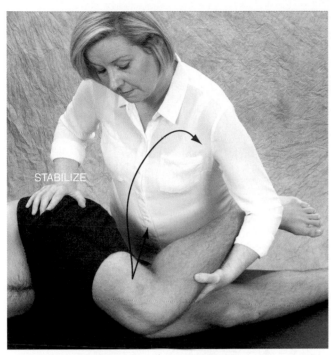

Fig. 11.33 Lateral FABER test.

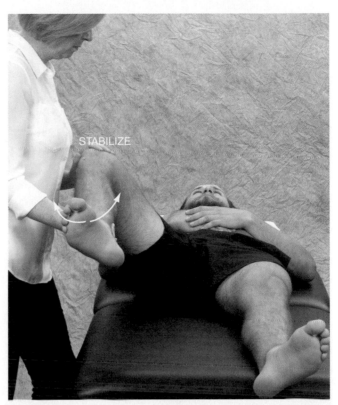

Fig. 11.34 Ligamentum teres test. Test leg is positioned as shown and then the hip is passively rotated medially and laterally to the end range of motion to stress the ligamentum teres.

The examiner passively takes the test hip through a wide abduction arc from flexion to extension (Fig. 11.33). Reproduction of pain indicates a positive test for intra-articular hip involvement.

⚠ *Ligamentum Teres Test.*[6,258] The patient is supine and the examiner stands beside the hip to be examined. The examiner then passively flexes the patient's knee to 90° and the hip to 70°, being sure that the pelvis has not moved or rotated. The patient's hip is then abducted as far as possible, followed by adduction until it is 30° short of the previous full abduction (Fig. 11.34). In this position, maximum tension is placed on the ligamentum teres while the femoral head and neck are positioned to avoid bony and soft tissue impingement. The hip is fully medially and laterally rotated to stress the ligamentum teres maximally. If pain results in either of these two rotations, the test is considered positive in the direction tested.

✓ *Log Roll (Passive Supine Rotation) Test.*[3,18,75] This test is often used if an intra-articular problem is suspected, as it does not stress extra-articular tissues, only intra-articular tissues.[38] The patient lies supine with both lower extremities extended (i.e., straight). The examiner passively rotates the femur medially and laterally to end range, comparing both hips (Fig. 11.35). Normally, the examiner rotates the leg medially and then lets the leg fall passively into lateral rotation.[36] The advantage of the test is that only rotation of the femoral head in the acetabulum occurs and only the capsule is stressed but not the surrounding tissues.[56,259] The maneuver also shows hip rotational mobility. If this is restricted or painful, it indicates intra-articular hip joint pathology.[9,11,41,260] A "click" during the test is suggestive of a labral tear, whereas increased lateral rotation may indicate a lax iliofemoral ligament.[9]

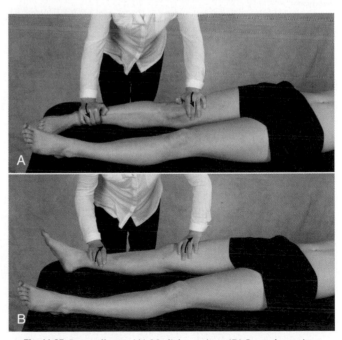

Fig. 11.35 Log roll test. (A) Medial rotation. (B) Lateral rotation.

⚠ *McCarthy Hip Extension Sign.*[23,41,43,261,262] The patient lies supine on the examining table with both hips flexed. The examiner then takes the good hip and extends it from the flexed position, first with the hip in lateral rotation and then with the hip in medial rotation.[23] The other leg is kept in flexion. The test is then repeated with

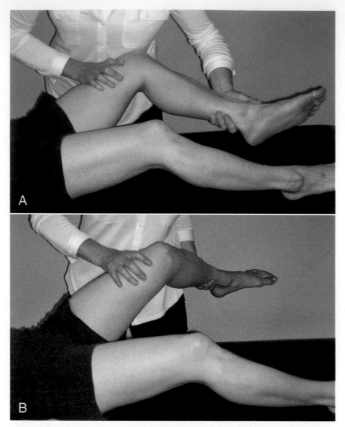

Fig. 11.36 McCarthy hip extension sign. (A) Lateral rotation. (B) Medial rotation.

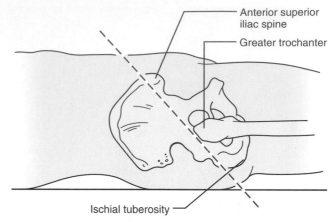

Fig. 11.37 Nélaton's line.

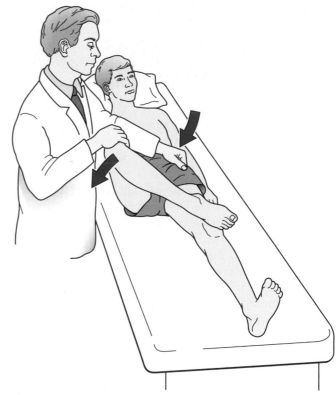

Fig. 11.38 Patrick's test (FABER or Figure 4 test) for the detection of limitation of motion in the hip. (Redrawn from Beetham WP, Polley HF, Slocumb CH, et al: *Physical examination of the joints*, Philadelphia, 1965, WB Saunders, p 139.)

the affected hip. Reproduction of the patient's pain and a "pop" would indicate a positive test.[3] The test is designed to simulate normal walking and creates a force double the patient's body weight across the hip.[23,61] McCarthy et al.[261] believed that there were three positive tests that would help to predict labral pathology: (1) pain with the McCarthy hip extension test (Fig. 11.36), (2) painful impingement with hip flexion abduction and lateral rotation (the anterior labial tear test), and (3) inguinal pain on resisted straight leg raising (Stinchfield resisted hip flexion test).

❓ Nélaton's Line. This is an imaginary line drawn from the ischial tuberosity of the pelvis to the ASIS of the pelvis on the same side (Fig. 11.37).[248] If the greater trochanter of the femur is palpated well above the line, it indicates a dislocated hip, or coxa vara. The two sides should be compared.

☑ Patrick's Test (FABER, "Figure-4" or Jansen's Test).[58,75,93,263,264] The patient lies supine, and the examiner places the foot of the patient's test leg on top of the knee of the opposite leg (the figure-4 position) (Fig. 11.38).[265] The examiner then slowly lowers the knee of the test leg toward the examining table. This position displaces the anterosuperior part of the femoral head-neck junction to the 12 o'clock position of the acetabular rim.[107] If the application of downward pressure on the knee produces lateral pain, superolateral and lateral FAI

are suggested; groin pain indicates iliopsoas pathology or psoas impingement against the femoral head or anterior capsule involvement; posterolateral pain is suggestive of ischiotrochanteric impingement, especially if femoral anteversion is increased; and posterior pain indicates sacroiliac involvement.[107] A negative test is indicated by the test leg's knee falling to the table or at least being parallel with the opposite leg. A positive test is indicated by pain provocation and by the test leg's knee remaining above the opposite straight leg.[9,11,130] If desired, the examiner can measure from the lateral knee joint line to

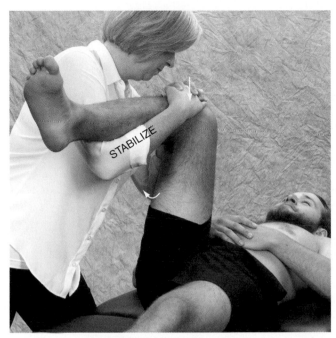

Fig. 11.39 Posterior apprehension test.

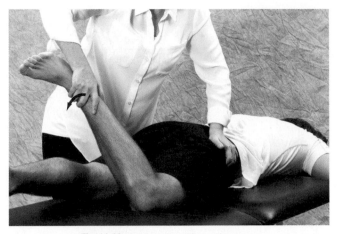

Fig. 11.40 Prone external rotation test.

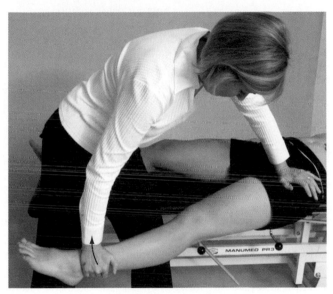

Fig. 11.41 Torque test.

the table and compare both sides. In FAI, the distance will be greater because ROM at the hip is decreased.[13] If positive, the test indicates that the posterior hip joint may be affected; that there may be iliopsoas spasm or weakness, or interarticular problems such as a psoas contraction stressing the labrum; or that the sacroiliac joint or lumbar spine may be affected. **Flexion, abduction, and external rotation (FABER)** is the position of the hip at which the patient begins the test.

⚠ *Posterior Apprehension Test.*[36] The patient is in supine with the test hip in 90° flexion, adduction, and medial rotation (Fig. 11.39). The examiner then applies a posteriorly directed force at the knee and a positive test results in pain and/or apprehension.

⚠ *Prone External Rotation Test.*[36] The patient is lying prone and the test hip is maximally laterally rotated by the examiner with one hand with an anteriorly directed pressure on the posterior greater trochanter with the other hand (Fig. 11.40) to translate the femoral head anteriorly. A positive test is reproduction of the patient's symptoms.

❓ *Stinchfield Resisted Hip Flexion (Straight-Leg Test Against Resistance) Test.*[3,43,75,266–268] The patient lies supine and then actively elevates the straight leg (i.e., flexes the hip) to about 20° to 30° while the examiner applies resistance proximal to the knee. The test is thought to load the hip joint anterosuperiorly, causing anterior groin pain if an intra-articular lesion is present.[23] If the test is repeated in lateral rotation, the iliopsoas is tightened and more tension is put on the labrum.[23] In a positive test, pain may be referred into the sensory distribution of the femoral, obturator, or sciatic nerves. A positive test indicates intra-articular pathology, which may include a labral tear, synovitis, arthritis, occult femoral neck fractures,

iliopsoas tendinitis/bursitis, or prosthetic failure or loosening.[9,265,269]

❓ *Torque Test.* The patient lies supine close to the edge of the examining table with the femur of the test leg extended over the edge of the table (Fig. 11.41). The test leg is extended until the pelvis (i.e., the ASIS) begins to move. The examiner uses one hand to medially rotate the femur to the end of range and the other to apply a slow posterolateral pressure along the line of the neck of the femur for 20 seconds to stress the capsular ligaments and test the stability of the hip joint.[270]

Rotational Deformities

Rotational deformities can occur anywhere between the hip and the foot (Table 11.15). Many of these deformities are hereditary or may be the result of cultural habit (e.g., kneeling). The patient lies supine with the lower limbs straight while the examiner looks at the patellae.[249] If the patellae face in (squinting patellae), it is a possible indication of medial rotation of the femur or the tibia.

TABLE **11.15**

Hip Malalignment

Malalignment	Related Posture	Possible Compensating Postures
Excessive anteversion	Toeing in Subtalar pronation Lateral patellar subluxation Medial tibial torsion Medial femoral torsion	Lateral tibial torsion Lateral rotation at knee Lateral rotation of tibia, femur, and/or pelvis Lumbar rotation on same side
Excessive retroversion	Toeing out Subtalar supination Lateral tibial torsion Lateral femoral torsion	Medial rotation at knee Medial rotation of tibia, femur, and/or pelvis Lumbar rotation on opposite side
Coxa vara	Pronated subtalar joint Medial rotation of leg Short ipsilateral leg Anterior pelvic rotation	Ipsilateral subtalar supination Contralateral subtalar pronation Ipsilateral plantar flexion Contralateral genu recurvatum Contralateral hip and/or knee flexion Ipsilateral posterior pelvic rotation and ipsilateral lumbar rotation
Coxa valga	Supinated subtalar joint Lateral rotation of leg Long ipsilateral leg Posterior pelvic tilt	Ipsilateral subtalar pronation Contralateral subtalar supination Contralateral plantar flexion Ipsilateral genu recurvatum Ipsilateral hip and/or knee flexion Ipsilateral anterior pelvic rotation and contralateral lumbar rotation

Adapted from Reigger-Krugh C, Keysor, JJ: Skeletal malalignments of the lower quarter: correlated and compensatory motions and postures, *J Orthop Sports Phys Ther* 23:166–167, 1996.

If the patellae face up, out, and away from each other ("frog eyes" or "grasshopper eyes"), it is a possible indication of lateral rotation of the femur or the tibia. If the tibia is affected, the feet face in ("pigeon toes") for medial rotation and face out more than 10° for excessive lateral rotation of the tibia (Fig. 11.42) while the patellae face straight ahead. Normally, the feet angle out 5° to 10° (**Fick angle**) for better balance.

Tests for Impingement

Impingement can lead to altered hip mechanics, which in turn lead to changes in dynamic (muscle) forces acting on the pelvis and hip. The muscles most commonly affected include the proximal hamstrings, adductors, abductors, and hip flexors.[24]

⚠ *Anteroposterior Impingement Test.*[9,18,75,120,124,271,272] This is a test for hip dysplasia (e.g., acetabular retroversion), SCFE, and FAI.[84] The patient lies supine with the hip flexed to 90°. The examiner then maximally medially rotates and adducts the hip, which leads to impingement of femoral neck against the acetabular rim (Fig. 11.43A).[17] Forced medial rotation can lead to a labral lesion, chondral lesion, or both. Pain is a positive sign. The hip is similarly tested in different degrees of flexion (45° to 120°), with pain increasing with increased flexion.[84]

⚠ *"Gear-Stick" Sign.*[83,149] This test is designed to test for greater trochanter-pelvic impingement. The patient

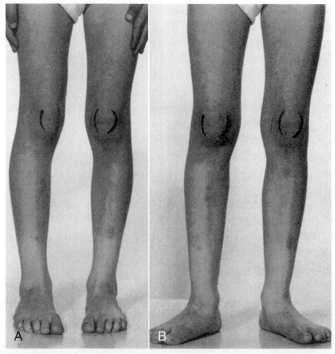

Fig. 11.42 Clinical appearance of excessive femoral torsion in a girl. (A) With the knees in full extension and the feet aligned (pointing straight forward), the legs appear bowed and the patellae face inward (squinting patella). (B) On lateral rotation of the hips so that the patellae are facing to the front, the feet and legs point outward and the bowleg appearance is corrected. (From Tachdjian MO: *Pediatric orthopedics*, Philadelphia, 1990, WB Saunders, p 2802.)

is in the side-lying position with the hip to be tested uppermost. The hip is passively abducted in extension by the examiner, who notes any limited ROM and whether symptoms are reproduced (Fig. 11.44A). The examiner then flexes and abducts the hip, noting whether abduction ROM has improved (Fig. 11.44B). Hip flexion allows the greater trochanter to move posteriorly, avoiding contact with the ilium.

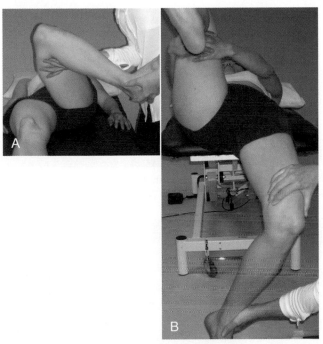

Fig. 11.43 (A) Anteroposterior impingement test. (B) Posteroinferior impingement test.

⚠ *Impingement Provocation Test.*[59] The patient lies supine at the end of the examining table with both legs extended. The examiner stands on the test-leg side of the table. The examiner lowers the test leg passively and slowly into hyperextension, abduction, and lateral rotation with overpressure (Fig. 11.45). Reproduction of the patient's symptoms (i.e., pain) indicates a positive test for a posterior labral tear.

⚠ *Ischiofemoral Impingement Test.*[52,162,273] The patient is in the side-lying position with the test leg uppermost. The examiner stands behind the patient and holds the patient's leg in slight flexion at the hip and flexion of the knee by holding the knee with one hand and the patient's foot/ankle supported between the examiner's side and elbow. With the other hand, the examiner stabilizes the pelvis (Fig. 11.46). The examiner passively extends, then adducts and laterally rotates the patient's hip. Reproduction of the patient's symptoms and a hard end feel indicate a positive test for IFI. If the test is repeated with hip abduction, the symptoms will be relieved.[162]

⚠ *Lateral FADDIR (Flexion, Adduction, and Internal Rotation) Test.*[93] The patient is in the side-lying position with the test leg uppermost. The examiner stands behind the patient with one hand supporting the patient's knee while the other palpates the hip with the fingers anteriorly (Fig. 11.47). The patient then flexes, adducts, and medially rotates the leg. Reproduction of the patient's symptoms indicates a positive test for FAI.

⚠ *Lateral Rim Impingement Test.*[3,107] The patient is supine with legs straight. The examiner stands beside the hip to be tested. While stabilizing the pelvis with one hand, the examiner abducts the neutral hip (i.e., not rotated) off the table as far as possible (Fig. 11.48). Lateral pain

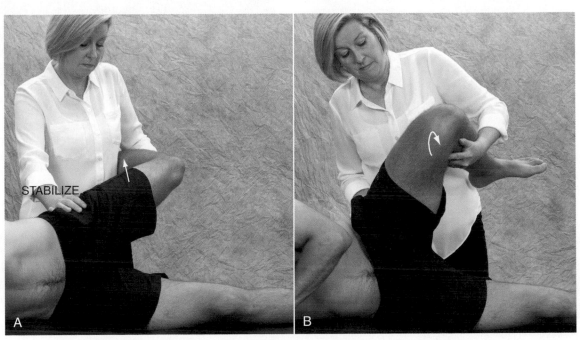

Fig. 11.44 "Gear-stick" sign. (A) Hip abducted in extension. (B) Hip abducted in flexion.

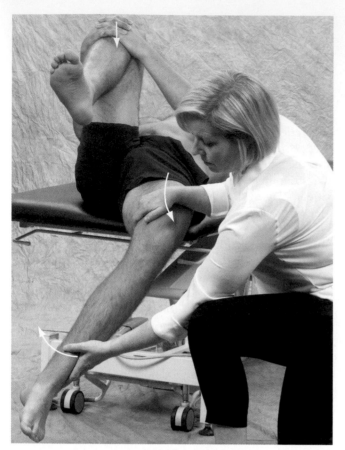

Fig. 11.45 Impingement provocation test.

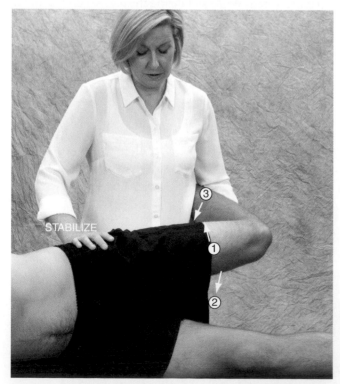

Fig. 11.46 Ischiofemoral impingement test. Extend *(1)*, adduct *(2)*, and laterally rotate the leg *(3)*.

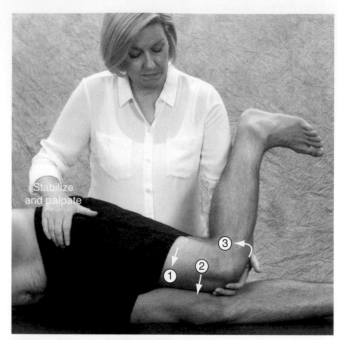

Fig. 11.47 Lateral FADDIR test actively done by patient (flexion *[1]*, adduction *[2]*, and internal rotation *[3]*).

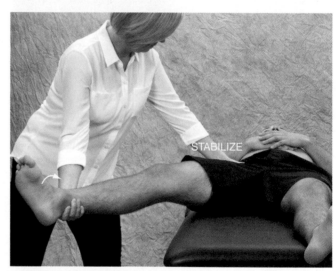

Fig. 11.48 Lateral rim impingement test. Note that no hip rotation should be allowed.

indicates impingement of the superolateral part of the femoral neck against the superoposterior acetabular rim.

⚠ ***Posteroinferior Impingement Test.***[75,84,120,124,253] This is a test for global acetabular overcoverage (e.g., coxa profunda [i.e., deep acetabular socket], coxa protrusion [i.e., the femoral head appears to be displaced into pelvic cavity]), global femoral neck offset abnormalities, and posterior acetabular cartilage damage. The test is also positive in people who place the hip in extremes of ROM (e.g., ballet dancers, martial artists, hockey goal tenders, mountain climbers, yoga practitioners, long-striding runners).[84] The patient lies supine with the legs hanging free over the edge of the bed to ensure maximal hip extension. The examiner then quickly rotates and abducts the hip laterally

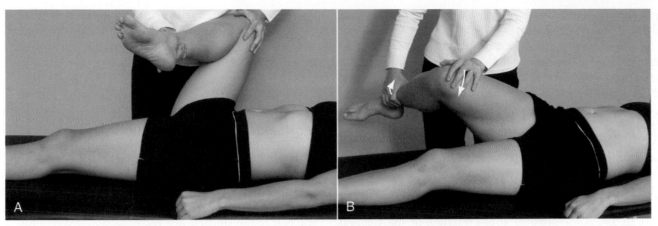

Fig. 11.49 Anterior labral tear test. (A) Starting position. (B) End position.

(Fig. 11.43B). Deep-seated posterior groin or buttock pain is an indication of posteroinferior impingement, but the examiner should be aware that the lateral rotation can lead to anterior translation of the femoral head, which could result in symptoms from anterior instability (i.e., microinstability) or an anterior labral tear.[56,84,120,124] The movement assesses the congruence of the posterolateral part of the femoral neck against the posterior rim of the acetabulum.[107] If pain arises anteriorly, it is more likely related to instability or a labral tear.[107]

The **dynamic internal (medial) rotation impingement (DIRI) test** and the **dynamic external (lateral) rotation impingement test (DEXRIT**) are modifications of the previous two tests, which are commonly used in arthroscopies of the hip.[3,61,107] In both cases, the patient is supine. The examiner takes the test hip into 90° of flexion. For the DIRI test, the hip is passively moved through a wide arc of adduction and medial rotation. If, when doing the DIRI test, a pop is heard, the test is referred to as the **McCarthy's test** (see tests under "Tests for Hip Pathology," earlier).[3] Some advocate stabilizing the pelvis by holding the contralateral leg in greater than 90° flexion as in the DEXRIT test.[3] For DEXRIT, the hip is passively moved through a wide arc of abduction and lateral rotation while the patient holds the contralateral leg in flexion beyond 90° to eliminate any lumbar lordosis.[3] Pain is a positive test.

Squat Test.[263,274] In the presence of an FAI, doing a full squat may cause groin pain and decreased ROM because of abnormal contact between the femoral head and the acetabulum. Most patients who have FAI will not be able to do a full squat.

Tests for Labral Lesions

Acetabular labral tears rarely occur without some structural osseous abnormality (e.g., FAI) often accompanied by a history of the patient repeatedly going into extreme ROMs, especially rotation.[118] These tears may be accompanied by damage to the acetabular cartilage.[118,275] Symptoms of a labral tear include anterior groin pain; feelings of catching, clicking, or locking; and activities

such as prolonged sitting, pivoting, kicking, walking, and running increase symptoms.[19,73,275,276]

Anterior Labral Tear Test (FADDIR, Fitzgerald's, FADER Test).[3,17,41,85,89,93,94,124,263,275,277] This test, also called the **anterior apprehension test,**[11,14] is used to test for anterosuperior impingement syndrome, anterior labral tears, and iliopsoas tendinitis. The patient is supine. The examiner takes the hip into full flexion, lateral rotation, and full abduction as a starting position. The examiner then extends the hip combined with medial rotation and adduction (Fig. 11.49). A positive test is indicated by the production of pain, the reproduction of the patient's symptoms with or without a click, or apprehension. The test places the greatest strain on the anterolateral labrum. The examiner should be careful to equate any findings with the patient's symptoms.[9,41]

External Rotation Test.[14] The patient is prone with hips extended (i.e., in neutral on the table) and test knee flexed. The examiner takes the test leg into lateral rotation while applying a posteroanterior force on the greater trochanter by progressively extending the hip (Fig. 11.50). Anterior pain or feeling of instability (i.e., apprehension) indicates a positive test for anterior labral lesion or anterior instability.

Flexion-Internal Rotation Test.[89,263] The patient lies supine with the legs extended (i.e., in neutral on the table). The examiner stands beside the hip to be tested and passively takes the hip to 90° flexion while medially rotating the hip (Fig. 11.51). Overpressure may be applied. A positive test is production of the patient's pain; locking, clicking, or catching indicate a labral tear.

Posterior Labral Tear Test.[85,124] The patient is supine. The examiner takes the hip into full flexion, adduction, and medial rotation as a starting position.[23] The examiner then takes the hip into extension combined with abduction and lateral rotation (Fig. 11.52). A positive test is indicated by the production of groin pain, patient apprehension, or the reproduction of the patient's symptoms, with or without a click. A positive test is an indication of a labral tear, anterior hip instability, or posteroinferior impingement. The test is sometimes called the **posterior**

apprehension test if apprehension occurs toward the end of ROM when doing the test.[14]

⚠ *THIRD (The Hip Internal Rotation with Distraction) Test.*[263,278,279] The patient lies supine with the hip flexed to 90° and adducted 10°. The hip is then medially rotated while a downward compressive force is applied by the examiner to the patient's hip (Fig. 11.53A). The test is repeated with traction to the hip (i.e., distraction) (Fig. 11.53B). The test is considered positive if pain is greater in the compression part of the test and less with distraction.

Tests for Femoral Neck Stress Fractures

❓ *Fulcrum Test of the Hip.* The fulcrum test[43,89,280] is used to assess for possible stress fracture of the femoral shaft. The patient sits with the knees bent over the end of the bed with feet dangling. The examiner places an arm under the patient's thigh to act as a fulcrum (Fig. 11.54). The fulcrum arm is moved from distal to proximal along the thigh as gentle pressure is applied to the

dorsum of the knee with the examiner's opposite hand. If a stress fracture is present, the patient complains of a sharp pain and expresses apprehension when the fulcrum arm is under the fracture site. A bone scan confirms the diagnosis.

⚠ *Heel-Strike Test.*[61] The patient is lying supine. The examiner firmly strikes the heel to stimulate heel strike during walking. Pain in the groin may be suggestive of a femoral neck stress fracture. A **single-leg hop** (see Chapter 12) would have the same effect, with a positive test showing pain in the groin.

⚠ *Patellar-Pubic Percussion Sign.*[89,238,281] The patient lies supine with the legs extended. The examiner places the bell of the stethoscope over the symphysis pubis. The examiner then percusses each patella with a finger, starting

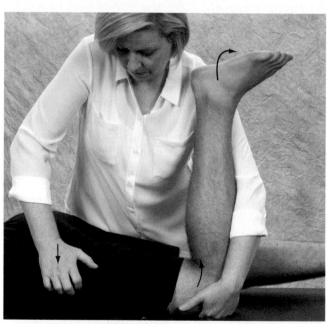

Fig. 11.50 External rotation test.

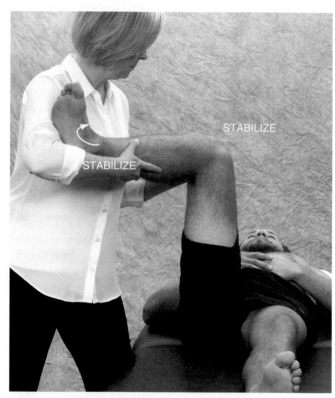

Fig. 11.51 Flexion–internal rotation test.

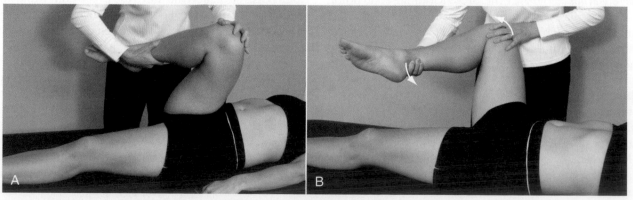

Fig. 11.52 Posterior labral tear test. (A) Starting position. (B) End position.

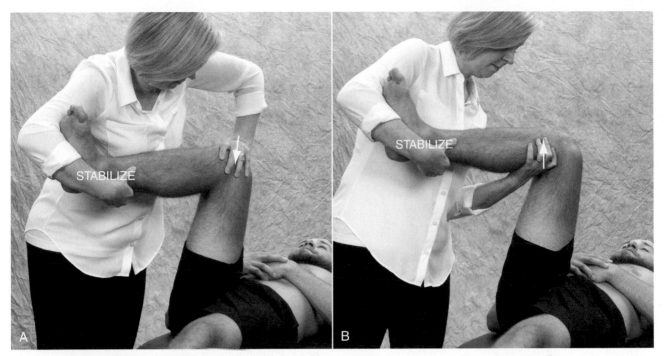

Fig. 11.53 THIRD (the hip internal rotation with distraction) test. (A) Compression. (B) Distraction.

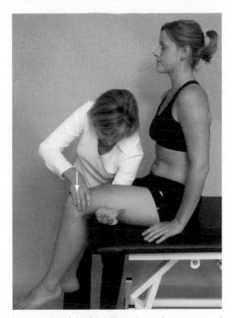

Fig. 11.54 Fulcrum test of the hip. Examiner places arm under femur and carefully applies a downward force at the knee.

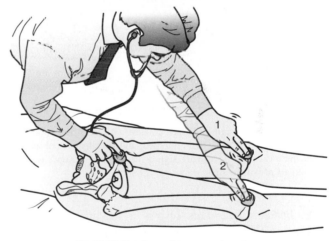

Fig. 11.55 Patellar-pubic percussion sign.

with the uninvolved side. Both sides are compared for differences in pitch and loudness. Normally the sounds are equal. If bone pathology is present (e.g., hip fracture) the affected side has a duller sound (Fig. 11.55). The test has been reported to be effective in identifying periacetabular, iliopubic, and ischiopubic ramus fractures as well as femoral fractures.[282]

Pediatric Tests for Hip Pathology

Orthopedic tests are commonly performed in newborns to detect problems, especially CDH (also called **DDH**)

that covers more than congenital problems, which may be amenable to conservative treatment if caught early.[156,283–285] Most of the tests are performed by pediatricians in the first 24 hours after birth.[286] Gooding and McClead[286] provide a good overview of the assessment of the newborn, including assessment for musculoskeletal issues.

⚠ ***Abduction Test (Hart's Sign).***[287] If CDH is not diagnosed early, parents often note that when they change the child's diapers, one leg does not abduct as far as the other.[284] That is the basis for this test. The child lies supine with the hips and knees flexed to 90°. The examiner then passively abducts both legs, noting any asymmetry or limitation of movement. In addition, if one hip is dislocated, the child often demonstrates asymmetry of fat folds in the gluteal and upper leg area because of the "riding up" of the femur on the affected side.

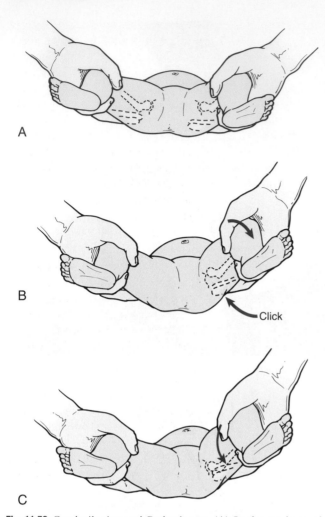

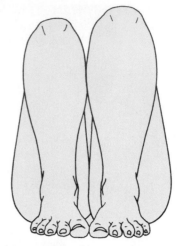

Fig. 11.57 Galeazzi sign (Allis test).

Fig. 11.56 Ortolani's sign and Barlow's test. (A) In the newborn, the two hips can be equally flexed, abducted, and laterally rotated without producing a click. (B) Ortolani's sign or first part of Barlow's test. (C) Second part of Barlow's test.

☑ **Barlow's Test.** This test is a modification of the Ortolani test[249] (Fig. 11.56) used for DDH.[284] The infant lies supine with the legs facing the examiner. The hips are flexed to 90°, with the knees fully flexed. Each hip is evaluated individually while the examiner's other hand steadies the opposite femur and the pelvis. The examiner's middle finger of each hand is placed over the greater trochanter, and the thumb is placed adjacent to the inner side of the knee and thigh opposite the lesser trochanter. The hip is taken into abduction while the examiner's middle finger applies forward pressure behind the greater trochanter. If the femoral head slips forward into the acetabulum with a click, clunk, or jerk, the test is positive, indicating that the hip was dislocated. This part of the test is identical to the Ortolani test. The examiner then uses the thumb to apply pressure backward and outward on the inner thigh. If the femoral head slips out over the posterior lip of the acetabulum and then reduces again when pressure is removed, the hip is classified as unstable. The hip is not dislocated but is dislocatable. The procedure is repeated for the other hip.

This test may be used for infants up to 6 months of age. It should not be repeated too often because it can result in a dislocated hip as well as articular damage to the head of the femur.[288]

⚠ *Galeazzi Sign (Allis or Galeazzi Test).* This test is good only for assessing unilateral DDH; it can be used in children from 3 to 18 months of age.[268] The child lies supine with the knees flexed and the hips flexed to 90°. A positive test is indicated if one knee is higher than the other (Fig. 11.57).

☑ *Ortolani's Sign.* This test can determine whether an infant has a DDH (see Fig. 11.56A and B).[247] With the infant supine, the examiner flexes the hips and grasps the legs so that the examiner's thumbs are against the insides of the knees and thighs; the examiner's fingers are then placed along the outsides of the thighs to the buttocks. With gentle traction, the thighs are abducted and pressure is applied against the greater trochanters of each femur. Resistance to abduction and lateral rotation begins to be felt at approximately 30° to 40°. The examiner may feel a click, clunk, or jerk, which indicates a positive test and that the hip has reduced; in addition, increased abduction of the hip is obtained. The femoral head has slipped over the acetabular ridge into the acetabulum, and normal abduction of 70° to 90° can be obtained.

This test is valid only for the first few weeks after birth and only for dislocated and lax hips, not for dislocations that are difficult to reduce. The examiner should take care to feel the quality of the click. Soft clicks may occur without dislocation and are thought to be caused by the iliofemoral ligament's clicking over the anterior surface of the head of the femur as it is laterally rotated. Soft clicking usually occurs without the prior resistance that is seen with dislocations. By repeated rotation of the hip, the exact location of the click can be palpated. However, this test should not be repeated too often because it can lead to damage of the articular cartilage of the femoral head. As with all clinical tests, if the test is positive, it is highly suggestive that the problem (i.e., CDH) exists; if it is negative, it does not necessarily rule out the problem.

▲ *Telescoping Sign (Piston or Dupuytren's Test).*[287] The telescoping sign is evident in a child with a dislocated hip. The child lies in the supine position. The examiner flexes the knee and hip to 90°. The femur is pushed down onto the examining table. The femur and leg are then lifted up and away from the table (Fig. 11.58). With the normal hip, little movement occurs with this action. With the dislocated hip, however, there is a lot of relative movement. This excessive movement is called **telescoping** or **pistoning**.

Tests for Leg Length

There are two types of leg-length discrepancy. The first, called **true leg-length discrepancy** or **true shortening,** is caused by an anatomic or structural change in the lower leg resulting from congenital maldevelopment (e.g., adolescent coxa vara, congenital hip dysplasia, bony abnormality) or trauma (e.g., fracture). Because an anatomic short leg results, the spine and pelvis are often affected, leading to lateral pelvic tilt and scoliosis.[61,289,290]

The second type of leg-length discrepancy is called **functional leg-length discrepancy** or **functional shortening;** it is the result of compensation for a change that may have occurred because of positioning rather than

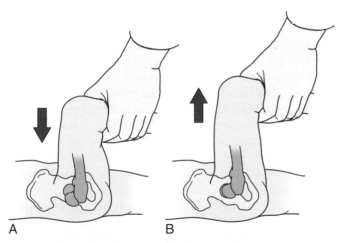

Fig. 11.58 Telescoping of the hip. Because the hip is not fixed in the acetabulum, it moves down (A) and up (B).

structure. For example, a functional leg-length discrepancy could occur because of unilateral foot pronation, spinal scoliosis, or pelvic obliquity[61,107] (e.g., measuring leg length from the umbilicus).[289,290] Scoliosis, hip contractures, pelvic deformities, and muscle spasm have been implicated as causes of functional leg-length discrepancy.[107]

▲*True Leg Length.* Before any measuring is done, the examiner must set the pelvis square, level, or in balance with the lower limbs.[291–293] The legs should be 15 to 20 cm (4 to 8 inches) apart and parallel to each other (Fig. 11.59). If the legs are not placed in proper relation to the pelvis, apparent shortening of the limb may occur. The lower limbs must be placed in comparable positions relative to the pelvis, because abduction of the hip brings the medial malleolus closer to the ASIS on the same side and adduction of the hip takes the medial malleolus farther from the ASIS on the same side. If one hip is fixed in abduction or adduction as a result of contracture or some other cause, the normal hip should be adducted or abducted an equal amount to ensure accurate leg-length measurement.

In North America, leg-length measurement is usually taken from the ASIS to the medial malleolus; however, these values may be altered by muscle wasting or obesity. Measuring to the lateral malleolus is less likely to be affected by the muscle bulk. To obtain the leg length, the examiner measures from the ASIS to the lateral or medial malleolus. The flat metal end of the tape measure is placed immediately distal to the ASIS and pushed up against it. The thumb then presses the tape end firmly against the bone, rigidly fixing the tape measure against the bone. The index finger of the other hand is placed immediately distal to the lateral or medial malleolus and pushed against it. The thumbnail is brought down against the tip of the index finger so that the tape measure is pinched between them. A slight difference (as much as 1 to 1.5 cm) in leg length is considered normal; however, this difference can still cause symptoms.

The **Weber-Barstow maneuver** (visual method) ▲ can also be used to measure leg length asymmetry. The patient lies supine with the hips and knees flexed (Fig. 11.60). The examiner stands at the patient's feet and palpates the distal aspect of the medial malleoli with the thumbs. The

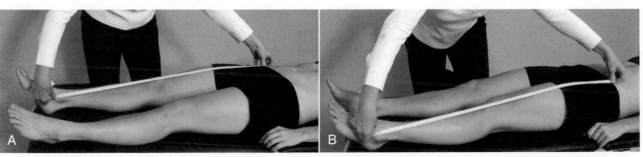

Fig. 11.59 Measuring true leg length. (A) Measuring to the medial malleolus. (B) Measuring to the lateral malleolus.

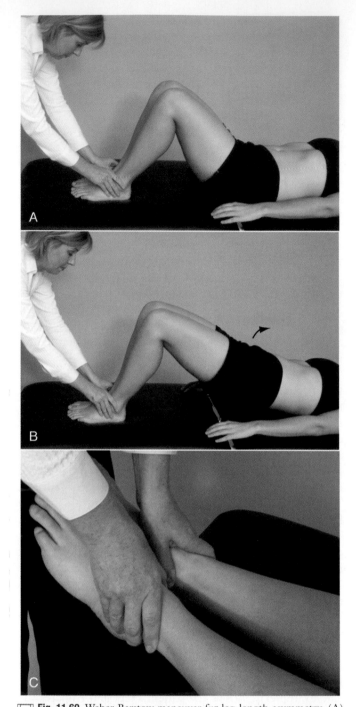

Fig. 11.60 Weber-Barstow maneuver for leg-length asymmetry. (A) Starting position. (B) Patient lifts hips off bed. (C) Comparing height of medial malleoli with the legs extended.

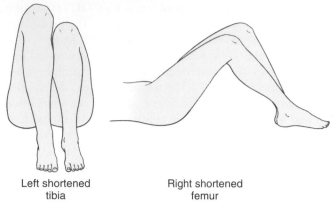

Left shortened tibia   Right shortened femur

Fig. 11.61 Leg-length discrepancy.

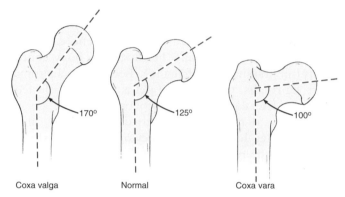

Coxa valga   170°   Normal   125°   Coxa vara   100°

Fig. 11.62 Neck shaft angles of the femur in adults.

patient then lifts the pelvis from the examining table and returns to the starting position. Next, the examiner passively extends the patient's legs and compares the positions of the malleoli using the borders of the thumbs. Different levels indicate asymmetry.[294]

If one leg is shorter than the other (Fig. 11.61), the examiner can determine where the difference is by measuring the following:

1. From the iliac crest to the greater trochanter of the femur (for coxa vara or coxa valga): The neck-shaft angle of the femur (Fig. 11.62) is normally 150° to 160° at birth and decreases to between 120° and 135° in the adult (Fig. 11.63). If this angle is less than 120° in an adult, it is known as **coxa vara;** if it is more than 135° in the adult, it is known as **coxa valga.**
2. From the greater trochanter of the femur to the knee joint line on the lateral aspect (for femoral shaft shortening).
3. From the knee joint line on the medial side to the medial malleolus (for tibial shaft shortening).

The relative length of the tibia may also be examined with the patient lying prone. The examiner places the thumbs transversely across the soles of the feet just in front of the heels. The knees are flexed 90°, and the relative heights of the thumbs are noted. Care must be taken to ensure that the legs are perpendicular to the examining table (Fig. 11.64).[294]

Similarly, the femoral lengths can be compared by having the patient lie supine with the hips and knees flexed to 90°. If one femur is longer than the other, its height will be higher (Fig. 11.65).[290]

Apparent shortening, or functional shortening (Fig. 11.66), of the leg is evident if the patient has a lateral pelvic tilt when the measurement is taken. Apparent or functional shortening of the limb is the result of adaptations the patient has made in response to pathology or contracture somewhere in the spine, pelvis, or lower

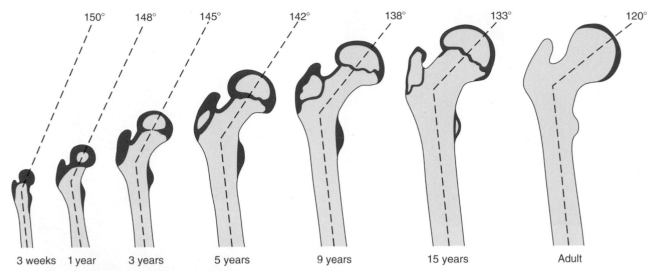

Fig. 11.63 Mean angle of the femoral neck shaft in different age groups. *Red area* indicates cartilage. (Modified from von Lanz T, Wachsmuth W: *Praktische anatomie*, Berlin, 1938, Julius Springer, p 143.)

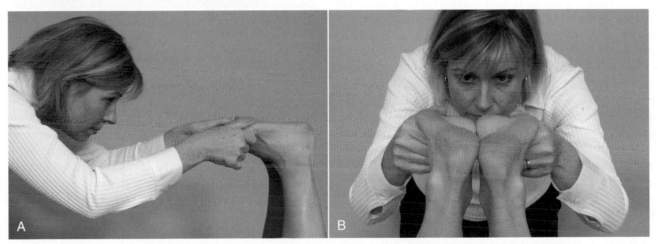

Fig. 11.64 Prone knee flexion test for tibial shortening. The prone knee flexion test is completed as the examiner (A) passively flexes the patient's knees to 90° and (B) sights through the plane of the heel pads to see whether a difference in height is noticeable.

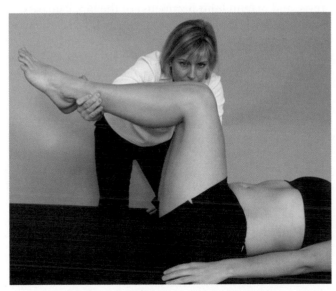

Fig. 11.65 Hip flexion test for femoral shortening.

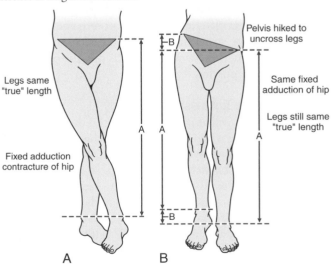

Fig. 11.66 Functional shortening due to adduction contracture. (A) Legs crossed. (B) Legs uncrossed. Note that uncrossing causes the pelvis to elevate on one side, but true leg length is equal on both sides. (Redrawn from the American Orthopaedic Association: *Manual of orthopaedic surgery*, Chicago, 1972, AOA, p 45.)

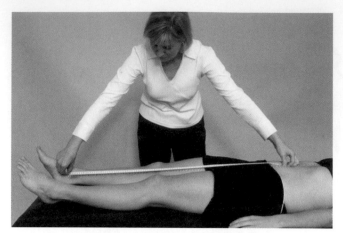

Fig. 11.67 Measuring functional leg length.

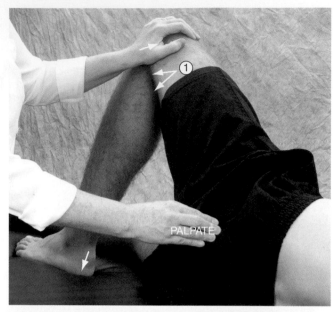

Fig. 11.68 Active piriformis stretch test or sign. Patient actively abducts and laterally rotates the hip *(1)* while the examiner resists.

limbs. In reality, there is no structural or anatomic difference in bone lengths. If there were, it would be called true shortening of the limb. When the apparent shortening of leg length is being measured, the examiner obtains the distance from the tip of the xiphisternum or umbilicus to the medial malleolus (Fig. 11.67). If true leg length is normal but the umbilicus-to-malleolus measurements are different, a functional leg-length discrepancy is present.[290] Values obtained by these measurements may be affected by muscle wasting, obesity, asymmetric position of the xiphisternum or umbilicus, or asymmetric positioning of the lower limbs.

⚠ **Standing (Functional) Leg Length.** The patient is first assessed in a relaxed stance, with the examiner palpating the ASIS and the PSIS, noting any asymmetry. The examiner then places the patient in a symmetric stance, ensuring that the subtalar joint is in neutral position (see Chapter 13), the toes are facing straight ahead, and the knees are extended. The ASIS and PSIS are again assessed for asymmetry. If differences are still noted, the examiner should check for structural leg-length differences, sacroiliac joint dysfunction, or weak gluteus medius or quadratus lumborum muscles.

Tests for Muscle Tightness or Pathology

Muscle function will also have been tested during resisted isometric testing, whereas ROM would have been tested during active and passive movement.

⚠ **Abduction Contracture Test.** This test is used to test the length of the abductor muscles (gluteus medius and minimus) of the hip. The patient lies supine with the ASISs level. If a contracture is present, the affected leg forms an angle of more than 90° with a line joining each ASIS. If the examiner then attempts to balance the lower limb with the pelvis, the pelvis (i.e., the ASIS) shifts down on the affected side or up on the unaffected side and balancing is not possible. Hip adduction should normally be about 30° before the ASIS moves. If the ASIS moves before this and there is a muscle-stretch end feel, the abductors will be tight. This type of contracture can

lead to **functional lengthening** of the limb rather than true lengthening.

⚠ **Active Piriformis Stretch Test or Sign.**[63,65,162,263,273] The patient is in the side-lying position with the hip flexed, so that the foot rests on the examining table (Fig. 11.68) with the patient pushing the heel into the table to stabilize the foot. The patient then actively abducts and laterally rotates the leg while the examiner offers resistance at the knee and, with the other hand, palpates the piriformis lateral to the ischium. A positive test is indicated by reproduction of the patient's neurological symptoms and indicates that the problem is at the piriformis muscle or obturator internus/gemelli complex.[65]

⚠ **Adduction Contracture Test.** This test is designed to test the length of the adductor muscles (adductor longus, brevis, and magnus and pectineus) of the hip. The patient lies supine with the ASISs level. Normally the examiner can easily "balance" the pelvis on the legs. This "balancing" implies that a line joining the ASIS is perpendicular to the two lines formed by the straight legs (Fig. 11.69). If a contracture is present, the affected leg forms an angle of less than 90° with the line joining the two ASISs. If the examiner then attempts to balance the lower limb with the pelvis, the pelvis (i.e., ASIS) shifts up on the affected side or down on the unaffected side and balancing is not possible. Normally hip abduction should be 30° to 50° before the ASIS moves. If the ASIS moves before this, the adductors are tight if there is a muscle-stretch end feel. This type of contracture can lead to functional shortening of the limb rather than true shortening (see Fig. 11.66).

Patients, especially children, with adductor spasticity may also be tested by abduction. With the patient supine, the examiner quickly abducts the leg. If there is a "grab" or "kicking in" of the stretch reflex at less than 30°, the test for adductor spasticity is considered positive. The

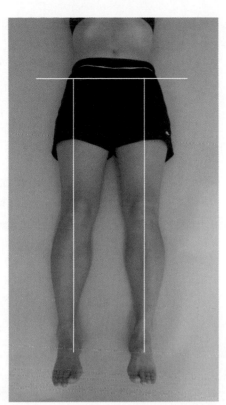

Fig. 11.69 Balancing the pelvis on the legs (femora).

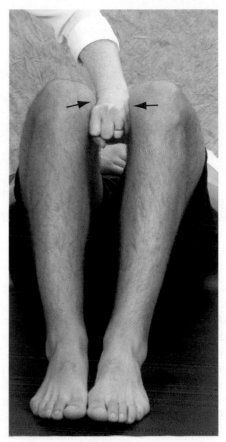

Fig. 11.70 Adductor squeeze (fist) test.

test should be repeated with the knee flexed to rule out a medial hamstring contracture.[295]

⚠ *Adductor Squeeze Test (Fist Squeeze Test).*[89,175–178] The patient is supine with the hips flexed to 45°, knees at 90°, and feet on the examining table. The examiner stands beside the patient's knees, placing a fist between them (a handheld dynamometer or sphygmomanometer may be used in place of the fist if a numerical value is desired) (Fig. 11.70).[6] The patient is asked to squeeze the fist by contracting the adductor muscles in both legs simultaneously. Reproduction of the patient's pain indicates a positive test for adductor pathology. The test may also be used to determine symmetry of the symphysis pubis (also see "Resisted Isometric Movements" earlier) and may result in a pop occurring at the symphysis pubis.

⚠ *Beatty's Test or Maneuver.*[52,63,263,296–298] The patient is in the side-lying position with the test leg uppermost and flexed and the knee resting on the examining table. The patient is asked to lift the flexed knee off the examining table several inches/centimeters and hold the position for 10 seconds (Fig. 11.71). Buttock pain when the knee is lifted off the examining table is a positive test for piriformis pathology.

⚠ *Bent-Knee Stretch Test for Proximal Hamstrings.*[181,299] The patient lies supine while the examiner flexes the hip and knee of the test leg maximally (Fig. 11.72A). The examiner then slowly extends the knee (Fig. 11.72B). It has also been suggested that the knee be extended quickly during the test.[263] Pain in the hamstrings at the ischial origin indicates a positive test. It should be noted that

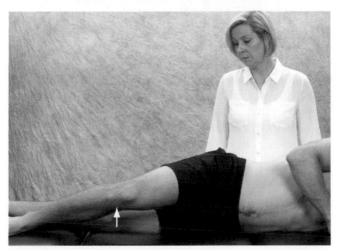

Fig. 11.71 Beatty's test or maneuver. Note examiner watching movement.

neurological tissues must also be cleared before the test can be considered positive.

❓ *Eccentric Hip Flexion.*[23] The patient lies supine and actively lifts the lower extremity into full hip flexion with full knee extension (i.e., the knee straight). The patient then eccentrically slowly lowers the leg to the examining table. Any reports of a click, clunk, or pain indicates a possible iliopsoas snapping and may be mistaken for a labral tear.[46]

⚠ *Ely's Test (Tight Rectus Femoris, Method 2).* The patient lies prone and the examiner passively flexes the patient's

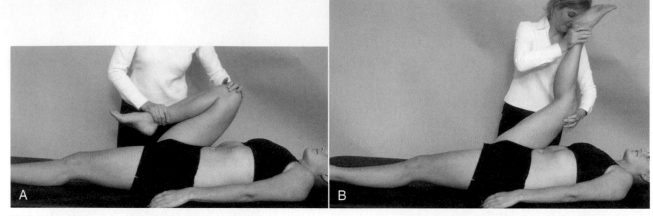

Fig. 11.72 The bent-knee stretch test for proximal hamstring tightness is performed with the patient supine. The hip and knee of the test leg are maximally flexed (A); then the examiner slowly straightens the knee (B).

knee (Fig. 11.73).[300] On flexion of the knee, the patient's hip on the same side spontaneously flexes, indicating that the rectus femoris muscle is tight on that side and that the test is positive. The two sides should be tested and compared.

⚠ *External De-rotation Test.*[52,89,263,297] The patient is supine. Starting with the good leg and the patient's hip and knee at 90°, the examiner asks the patient to resist lateral rotation of the hip (by isometrically medially rotating the leg) applied by the examiner (Fig. 11.74A). If lateral hip pain results, the diagnosis is GTPS. If passive ROM is greater than active ROM (i.e., 1.5x), then pain on passive medial rotation indicates osteoarthritis whereas no pain suggests GTPS.[259] If the first part of the test is negative, the test is repeated with the patient in prone, hip extended, and knee flexed to 90° (Fig. 11.74B). In either case, spontaneous reproduction of the patient's pain is a positive test, with lateral pain indicating GTPS, whereas groin pain indicates osteoarthritis.[89]

⚠ *Freiberg's Maneuver.*[52,63,263,296,297,298] The patient is lying prone. The examiner passively rotates the hip medially with the thigh extended. Buttock pain or tenderness in the sciatic notch indicates a positive test due to stretching of the piriformis muscle or a piriformis strain.

❓ *Hamstring Contracture Test.* The patient is instructed to sit with one knee flexed against the chest to stabilize the pelvis and the other knee extended (Fig. 11.75). The patient then attempts to flex the trunk and touch the toes of the extended lower limb (test leg) with the fingers. The test is repeated on the other side. A comparison is made between the two sides. Normally the patient should be able to at least touch the toes while keeping the knee extended. If he or she is unable to do so, it is an indication of tight hamstrings on the straight leg.

⚠ *Hamstring Syndrome (Active Hamstring) Test.*[160,162,164,166,301] The patient is sitting with the knee at 90°. The examiner isometrically resists as the patient tries to bend the knee further (Fig. 11.76A). For the second part of the test, the examiner holds the patient's leg in

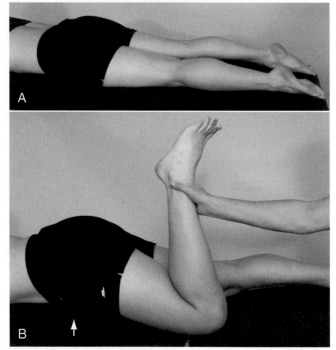

Fig. 11.73 Ely's test for a tight rectus femoris. (A) Position for the test. (B) Positive test shown by hip flexion when the knee is flexed.

30° of knee flexion and then isometrically resists as the patient tries to bend the knee (Fig. 11.76B). If ischial pain and weakness are less at 90° than at 30°, the test is considered positive for hamstring injury at the muscle's origin.

⚠ *Heel Contra-Lateral Knee (HCLK) Maneuver.*[298] When the hip is flexed beyond 90°, the piriformis muscle becomes a lateral rotator instead of a medial rotator. This maneuver can be used as a test or a stretching treatment for the piriformis. The patient is supine with both hips flexed and the knees at 90°, so that the feet rest on the examining table. The patient is then asked to put the test foot on the opposite knee (Fig. 11.77A). The examiner then lifts the unaffected leg, pushing the affected leg into

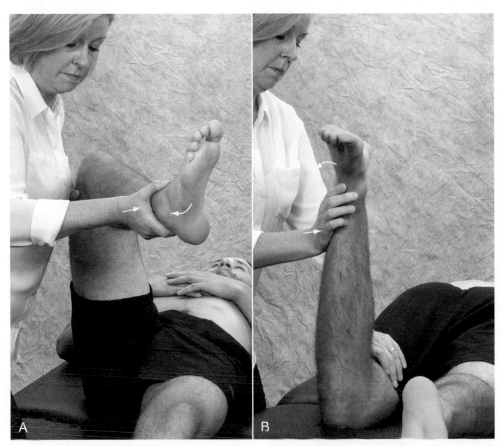

Fig. 11.74 External de-rotation test. (A) In supine. (B) In prone.

more lateral rotation, flexion, and abduction (see Fig. 11.77B) and holding the position for 10 seconds (if this maneuver were used for treatment, the stretch would be held longer). Buttock pain and/or sciatic neurological symptoms would be a positive sign of a tight piriformis.

☑ *Hip Lag Sign.* This is a test for the hip abductors. The patient is in the side-lying position. The examiner passively abducts and medially rotates the extended leg to about 45° and asks the patient to actively hold the position for 10 seconds (Fig. 11.78). If the patient cannot hold the position (i.e., if the leg drops more than 10 cm [4 inches]) or the medial rotation decreases, the test is considered positive for a gluteus medius tear.[259]

❓ *Lateral Step-Down Maneuver (Pelvis Drop Test).*[302] A 20-cm (8-inch) stool or step is placed in front of the patient. The patient is asked to place one foot on the stool and stand up straight on the stool on one foot. The patient then slowly lowers the non–weight-bearing leg to the floor. This should normally be accomplished with the arms by the side and the trunk relatively erect and no hip adduction or medial rotation (Fig. 11.79). If, however, on lowering, the arms abduct, the trunk inclines forward, the weight-bearing hip adducts or medially rotates, and/or the pelvis flexes forward or rotates backward, it is an indication of an unstable hip or weak lateral rotators.

⚠ *Long-Stride Heel-Strike Test.*[65,164,301] The patient is standing and is instructed to take a long stride forward

and to make sure that the heel strikes hard when the forward foot lands (Fig. 11.80). A positive test is ischial pain on heel strike.[164] It should be noted that if the examiner is asking the patient to stride forward with the good leg first, ischial pain may be felt in the back (i.e., bad) leg as it goes into hyperextension.[164]

☑ *90–90 Straight Leg Raising Test (Hamstring Contracture Test).* The supine patient flexes both hips to 90° while the knees are bent. The patient may grasp behind the knees with both hands to stabilize the hips at 90° of flexion. The patient actively extends each knee in turn as much as possible. For normal flexibility in the hamstrings, knee extension should be within 20° of full extension (Fig. 11.81).[95,303] Kuo et al.[304] called this angle the *popliteal angle* (the angle between two lines—one line along the shaft of femur and one line along the line of the tibia). They reported this angle to be 180° from birth to 2 years of age, which then decreases to about 155° by age 6 and remains fairly constant after that. If the angle is less than 125°, the hamstrings are considered to be tight. Normally or if the hamstrings are tight, the end feel is muscle stretch. Nerve root symptoms may also result, because this positioning is similar to the slump test done with the patient supine instead of sitting.

A modification of this test may also be used to test the length of gluteus maximus. The patient assumes the same starting position. While the examiner palpates the

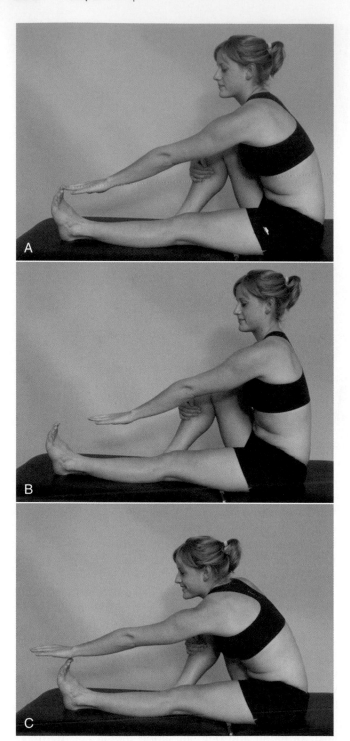

Fig. 11.75 Test for hamstring tightness. (A) Negative test. (B) Positive test. (C) Hypermobility of hamstrings.

ASIS on the same side, he or she also flexes the hip with the knee flexed (Fig. 11.82). If the thigh flexes 110° to 120° before the ASIS moves up, gluteus maximus length is normal. If the ASIS moves up before the thigh reaches the trunk, the gluteus maximus is tight. Both sides should be compared.

Janda[90,91] has reported that the gluteus maximus, medius, and minimus are more likely to be weak than

tight. To test gluteus maximus strength, the patient is placed prone with the hip straight and the knee flexed to 90°. The patient is asked to extend the hip, keeping the knee flexed, while the examiner applies an anterior force to the posterior thigh (Fig. 11.83A). Both legs are tested (good side first) and compared. If the patient attempts to further flex the knee while doing the test, it indicates that greater use of the hamstrings is occurring. To test the strength of the gluteus medius and minimus, the patient is placed in the side-lying position. The examiner stabilizes the pelvis and asks the patient to abduct the leg against the examiner's resistance, which is applied to the lateral aspect of the thigh (Fig. 11.83B). Both legs are tested (good side first) and compared.

▲ *Noble Compression Test.* This test is used to determine whether iliotibial band friction syndrome exists near the knee (Fig. 11.84).[305] This syndrome is a chronic inflammation of the iliotibial band near its insertion adjacent to the femoral condyle. The patient lies supine and the knee is flexed to 90°, accompanied by hip flexion. The examiner then applies pressure with the thumb to the lateral femoral epicondyle or 1 to 2 cm (0.4 to 0.8 inch) proximal to it. While the pressure is maintained, the patient slowly extends the knee. At approximately 30° of flexion (0° being a straight leg), if the patient complains of severe pain over the lateral femoral condyle, a positive test is indicated. The patient usually says it is the same pain that accompanies the patient's activity (e.g., running).

▲ *Ober's Test.* This test assesses the tensor fasciae latae (iliotibial band) for contracture (Fig. 11.85).[306–308] Tightness of the iliotibial band is the most common cause of lateral knee pain in runners. It has also been reported that it tests the gluteus medius and minimus muscles as well as the hip joint capsule. Thus if the test is found to be positive, these structures as well as the iliotibial band should be differentially diagnosed.[309] The patient is in the side-lying position with the lower leg flexed at the hip and knee for stability. The examiner then passively abducts and extends the patient's upper leg with the knee straight while the hip remains extended (see Fig. 11.85). It has been reported in the literature[3] that flexing the knee eliminates the iliotibial band, and the gluteus medius muscle is the main muscle tested. The examiner slowly lowers the upper limb; if a contracture is present, the leg remains abducted and does not fall to the table. When this test is being done, it is important to extend the hip slightly so that the iliotibial band passes over the greater trochanter of the femur. To do this, the examiner stabilizes the pelvis at the same time to stop the pelvis from "falling backward." Ober[306] originally described the test with the knee flexed. However, the iliotibial band has a greater stretch placed on it when the knee is extended. Additionally, when the knee is flexed during the test, greater stress is placed on the femoral nerve (Fig. 11.86A). If neurological signs (i.e., nerve pain, paresthesia) occur during the

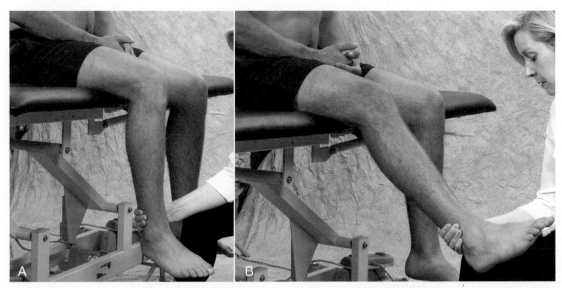

Fig. 11.76 Hamstring syndrome test. (A) Test at 90°. (B) Test at 30°.

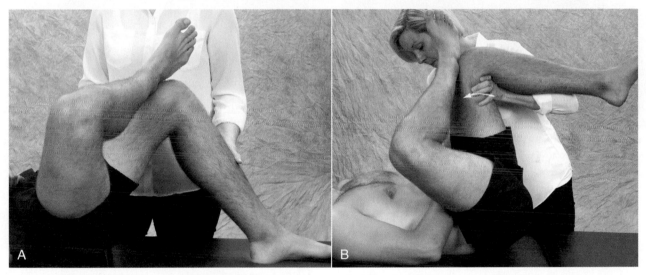

Fig. 11.77 Heel contra-lateral knee (HCLK) maneuver to stretch piriformis. (A) Start position. (B) Stretch position.

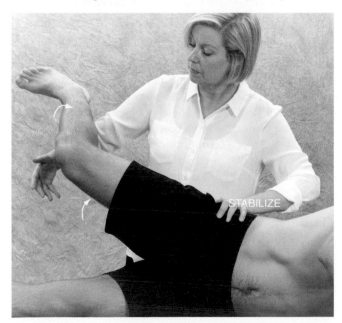

Fig. 11.78 Hip lag sign. Patient attempts to hold position isometrically.

test, the examiner should consider pathology affecting the femoral nerve. If the examiner then asks the patient to rotate the ipsilateral shoulder backward with the hip flexed and knee extended, tension will be placed on the gluteus maximus (Fig. 11.86B).[3] Likewise, tenderness over the greater trochanter should lead the examiner to consider trochanteric bursitis.

⚠ *Pace's (Pace and Nagle) Maneuver.*[52,63,263,296,297,298,310] The patient is seated and asked to abduct both legs as far as possible. Pain on contraction is a positive test for a piriformis strain. Neurogenic pain would indicate sciatic nerve involvement.

❓ *Phelps' Test.*[264] The patient lies prone with the knees extended. The examiner passively abducts both of the patient's legs as far as possible. The knees are then flexed to 90° (Fig. 11.87) and the examiner tries to abduct the hips further. If abduction increases, the test is considered positive for contracture of the gracilis muscle.

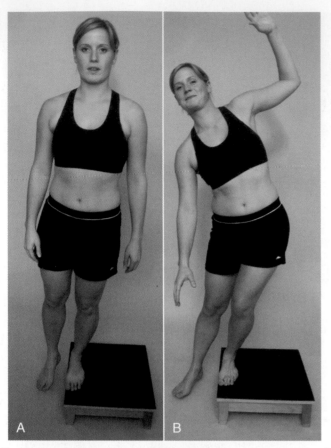

Fig. 11.79 Lateral step-down maneuver (pelvic drop test). (A) Normal (negative test). (B) Positive test.

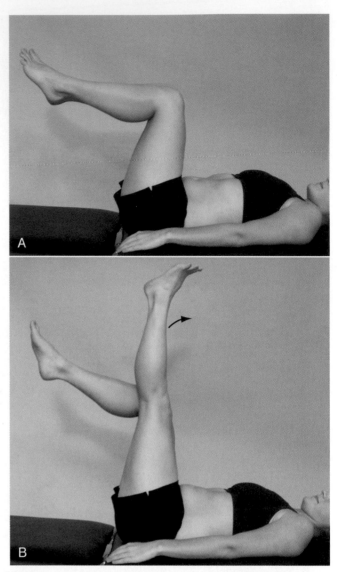

Fig. 11.81 The 90-90 straight leg raising test. (A) Start position. (B) End position. Knee angle is measured to show any limitation.

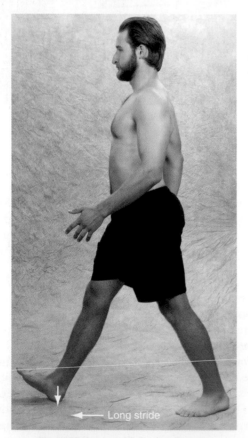

Fig. 11.80 Long-stride heel-strike test.

❓ *Piriformis (Flexion, Adduction, and Internal [Medial] Rotation [FAIR]; Fishman) Test.*[52,297,310–312] In about 15% of the population, the sciatic nerve, all or in part, passes through the piriformis muscle rather than below it (Figs. 11.88 and 11.89).[82,313] These people are more likely to suffer from piriformis syndrome, a relatively rare condition that is now more commonly called DGS.[314] The patient is in the side-lying position with the test leg uppermost. The patient flexes the test hip to 60° with the knee flexed. The leg is slightly rotated medially as it rests on the examining table. This is called the FAIR position (i.e., flexion, adduction, and internal [medial] rotation).[63] The examiner stabilizes the hip with one hand and applies a downward pressure to the knee (Fig. 11.90). If the piriformis muscle is tight, pain is elicited in the muscle. If the piriformis muscle is pinching the sciatic nerve, neurologic pain in the buttock and sciatica may be experienced by the patient.[95,270,273]

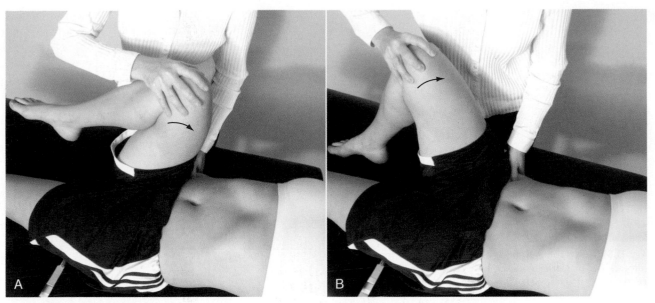

Fig. 11.82 Testing for length of gluteus maximus. (A) Negative test. (B) Positive test.

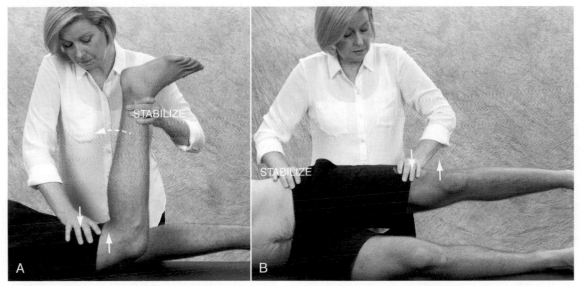

Fig. 11.83 (A) Testing strength of gluteus maximus. *Dashed arrow* indicates hamstring involvement. (B) Testing strength of gluteus medius and minimus. For both tests, the examiner watches/palpates the pelvis to ensure no movement.

Resisted lateral rotation with the muscle on stretch (i.e., hip medially rotated) can cause the same sciatica.[315]

❓ *Prone-Lying Test for Iliotibial Band Contracture.*[316] The patient lies prone while the examiner stands on the opposite side to the leg being tested. The examiner holds the ankle of the test leg and maximally abducts it at the hip while the other hand applies pressure to the buttock on the same side as the test leg to flatten the pelvis and correct any hip flexion deformity (Fig. 11.91). While maintaining the hip in neutral rotation and the knee flexed to 90°, the examiner then adducts the hip until there is a firm end feel. The angle is measured relative to the body's vertical axis and compared with the other side.[316] This test is more commonly done in children.

⚠ *Puranen-Orava Test.*[10,164,166,263,299] The patient stands about 2 to 3 feet (0.6 to 0.9 m) from an examining table (preferably one with electronic height adjustment). The patient flexes the hip to 90° so that the foot can rest on the table (Fig. 11.92). The patient then attempts to extend the knee. To stabilize the pelvis, the patient reaches one arm toward the toes. The angle at the knee between the two sides is compared. These maneuvers may also test whether the sciatic nerve is causing neurological symptoms.

⚠ *Rectus Femoris Contracture Test (Kendall Test).* The patient lies supine with the knees bent over the end or edge of the examining table. The patient flexes one knee onto the chest and holds it (Fig. 11.93). The angle of the test knee

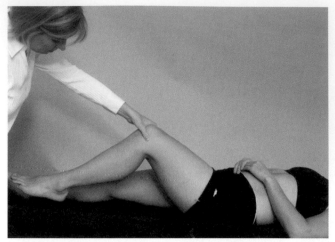

Fig. 11.84 Noble compression test for iliotibial band friction syndrome. The patient extends the knee. The examiner is indicating where pain is felt at about 30° of flexion.

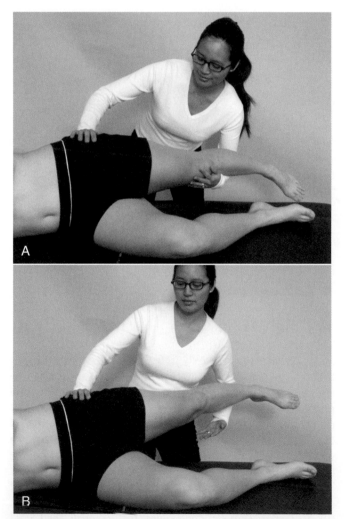

Fig. 11.85 Ober's test. (A) Knee straight. (B) The hip is passively extended by the examiner to ensure that the tensor fasciae latae runs over the greater trochanter. A positive test is indicated when the leg remains abducted while the patient's muscles are relaxed.

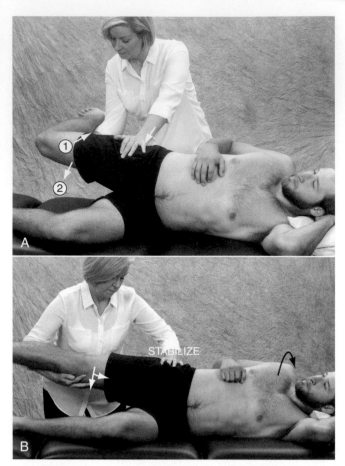

Fig. 11.86 (A) Test for gluteus medius contracture. Hip kept extended *(1)*. Leg allowed to fall into adduction *(2)*. (B) Test for gluteus maximus contracture. Patient rotates trunk posteriorly, then examiner adducts and flexes the hip while stabilizing the pelvis.

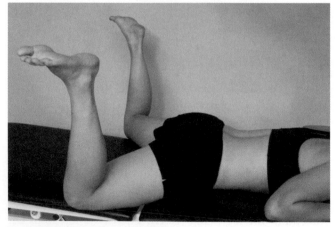

Fig. 11.87 Phelps' test. Hips are abducted and knees flexed to 90°. If abduction increases with knee flexion, the test is positive.

should remain at 90° when the opposite knee is flexed to the chest. If it does not (i.e., the test knee extends slightly), a contracture is probably present. The examiner may attempt to passively flex the knee to see whether it remains at 90° of its own volition. The examiner should always palpate for muscle tightness when any contracture test is being done. If

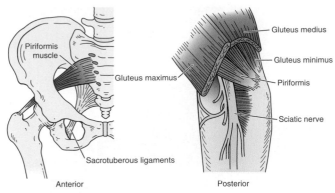

Fig. 11.88 Position of the piriformis muscle. (Redrawn from Norris C: *Sports injuries: diagnosis and management*, ed 3, London, 2004, Butterworth-Heinemann, p 205.)

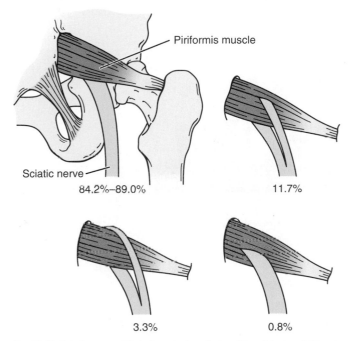

Fig. 11.89 Sciatic nerve: Variations in its relationship with the piriformis muscle. (Redrawn from Levin P: Hip dislocations. In Browner BD, et al., editors: *Skeletal trauma*, Philadelphia, 1992, WB Saunders, p 1333.)

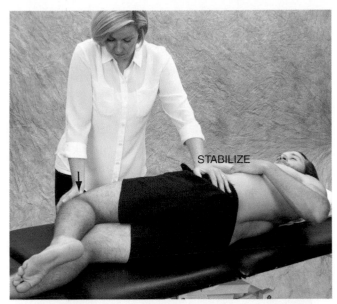

Fig. 11.90 Piriformis (flexion, adduction, and internal rotation—Fishman FAIR) test. FAIR position is illustrated.

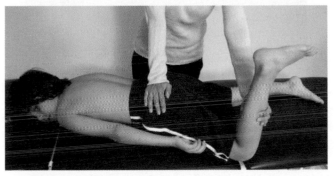

Fig. 11.91 Prone lying test for iliotibial band contracture.

there is no palpable tightness, the probable cause of restriction is tight joint structures (e.g., the capsule), and the end feel will be different (muscle stretch versus capsular). The two sides should be tested and compared.

⚠ *Seated Piriformis Stretch Test.*[63,65,162] With the patient seated, the examiner extends the knee (to stretch the sciatic nerve) and passively moves the hip, which is flexed, into adduction and medial rotation while palpating the piriformis lateral to the ischium or proximally at the sciatic notch (Fig. 11.94). A positive test is indicated by production of the patient's pain at the level of the piriformis. This position is thought to involve the deep rotators of the hip.[65]

❓ *Sign of the Buttock.* The patient lies supine and the examiner performs a straight leg raising test. If there is limitation on straight leg raising, the examiner flexes the patient's knee to see whether further hip flexion can be obtained. If hip flexion does not increase, the lesion is in the buttock or the hip, not the sciatic nerve or hamstring muscles. There may also be some limited trunk flexion. Causes of a positive test include ischial bursitis, a neoplasm, an abscess in the buttock, fracture, or hip pathology.

❓ *"Taking off the Shoe" Test.*[317] For the "taking off the shoe" test (TOST), the patient stands wearing shoes. The patient is asked to remove the shoe on the affected side with the help of the shoe on the opposite side (Fig. 11.95) by putting the heel of the affected side into the medial longitudinal arch of the stance (good) leg to pry the shoe off. In this position, the affected hip is laterally rotated about 90° with 20° to 25° flexion at the knee, leading to contraction of the biceps femoris on the affected side. If a sharp pain is felt in the biceps femoris, it indicates a 1° or 2° muscle strain. If the patient has no difficulty removing the shoe (or putting on a shoe) but has pain on palpating the greater trochanter, the problem is probably GTPS.[259]

⚠ *Thomas Test.* The Thomas test is used to assess a hip flexion contracture, the most common contracture of the hip. The patient lies supine while the examiner checks

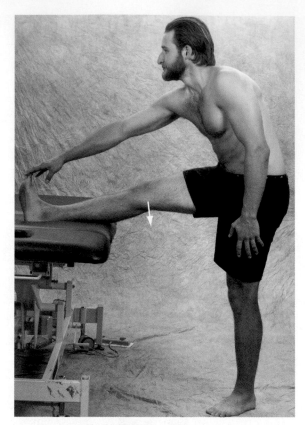

Fig. 11.92 Puranen-Orava test.

for excessive lordosis, which is usually present with tight hip flexors. The examiner flexes one of the patient's hips, bringing the knee to the chest to flatten out the lumbar spine and stabilize the pelvis. The patient holds the flexed hip against the chest. If there is no flexion contracture, the hip being tested (the straight leg) remains on the examining table. If a contracture is present, the patient's straight leg rises off the table, resulting in a muscle-stretch end feel (Fig. 11.96). The angle of contracture can be measured. If the lower limb is pushed down onto the table, the patient may exhibit an increased lordosis; again, this result indicates a positive test. If measurements are taken when the test is being done, the examiner must be sure that the restriction is in the hip and not the pelvis or lumbar spine.[318] If the leg does not lift off the table but abducts as the other leg is flexed to the chest, it is called the **"J" sign** or **stroke** and is indicative of a tight iliotibial band on the extended leg side.

⚠ *Tightness of Hip Rotators.* The medial and lateral hip rotators can be tested by placing the patient in the supine position with the hip and knee flexed to 90°. To test for tightness of the lateral rotators, the patient is asked to rotate the hip medially by rotating the leg outward (Fig. 11.97A). If the lateral rotators are tight, medial rotation will be less than 30° to 40° and the end feel is one of muscle stretch rather than tissue (capsular) stretch. To test for tightness of the medial rotators, the patient is asked to laterally rotate the hip by rotating the leg inward

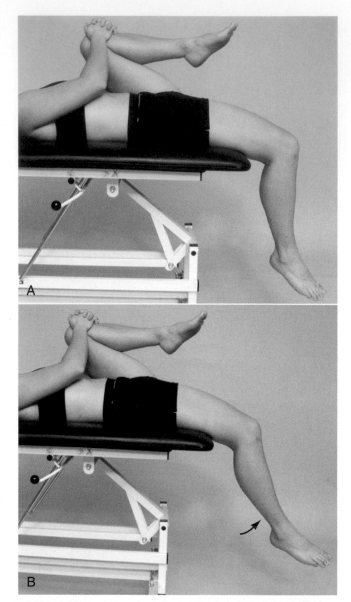

Fig. 11.93 Rectus femoris contracture test. (A) The movement leg is brought to the chest. The test leg remains bent over the end of the examining table, indicating a negative test. (B) The test knee extends, indicating a positive test.

(Fig. 11.97B). If the medial rotators are tight, lateral rotation will be less than 40° to 60° and the end feel will be muscle stretch rather than tissue (capsular) stretch.

✓ *Trendelenburg Sign.*[263,319] This test assesses the stability of the hip and the ability of the hip abductors to stabilize the pelvis on the femur. The patient is asked to stand on one leg and hold the position for 6 to 30 seconds.[3,53,107,320] Normally the pelvis on the opposite side should rise; this finding indicates a negative test (Figs. 11.98 and 11.99A). If the pelvis on the opposite side (non-stance side) drops and the drop is more than 2 cm when the patient stands on the affected leg, a positive test is indicated.[3,107] The test should always be performed on the normal side first so that the patient will understand

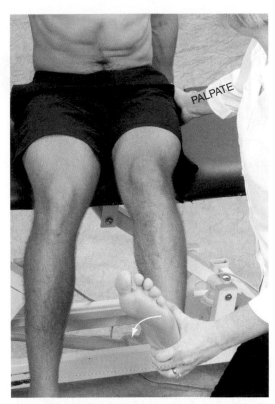

Fig. 11.94 Seated piriformis stretch test.

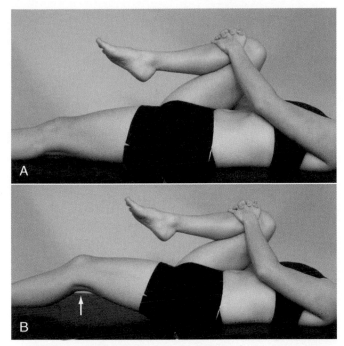

Fig. 11.96 Thomas test. (A) Negative test. (B) Positive test.

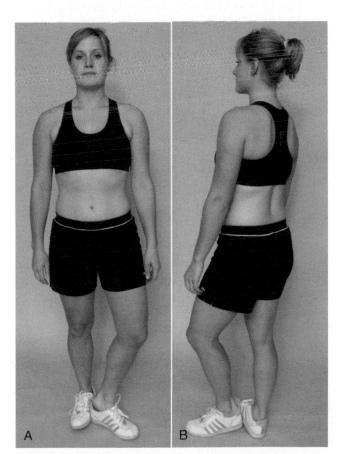

Fig. 11.95 "Taking off the shoe" test while standing. (A) Anterior view. (B) Posterior view.

what to do. If the pelvis drops on the opposite side, it indicates a weak gluteus medius or an unstable hip (e.g., as a result of hip dislocation) on the affected or stance side. To add difficulty to the test and to test overall stability of the hip and pelvis, the patient may be asked to do a **single-leg squat** (Fig. 11.99B) and the **corkscrew test,**[321] which involves rotating left and then right while doing a single-leg squat. During the squat and the corkscrew test, the examiner should watch for a positive Trendelenburg sign on the non–weight-bearing side as well as for hip, knee, and ankle movement control (i.e., alignment remains in a straight line). Abnormality could be **stance "leg collapse"** with medial hip rotation, valgus movement at the knee, and/or pronation of the foot (Fig. 11.99C). The normal result should be the same as that from a negative Trendelenburg test.[322] Grimaldi et al.[323] advocated doing a single-leg stance in which the test leg has the hip in neutral with the knee flexed to 90°. The patient can use a finger against a wall to help balance. If the patient cannot hold this non–weight-bearing position for 30 seconds and there is reproduction of the patient's pain or symptoms within the 30 seconds, the test is positive for GTPS.[323]

❓ *Tripod Sign (Hamstring Contracture Test).* The patient is seated with both knees flexed to 90° over the edge of the examining table (Fig. 11.100).[324] The examiner then passively extends one knee. If the hamstring muscles on that side are tight, the patient extends the trunk to relieve the tension in the hamstring muscles. The leg is returned to its starting position, and the other leg is tested and compared with the first side. Extension of the spine is indicative of a positive test. The examiner must be aware that

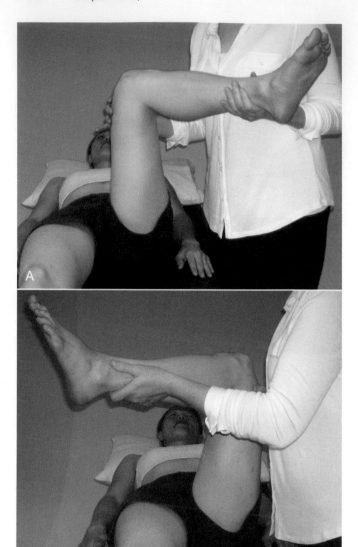

Fig. 11.97 (A) Testing for tightness of the lateral rotators. (B) Testing for tightness of the medial rotators.

nerve root problems (stretching of the sciatic nerve) can cause a similar positive sign, although the symptoms will be slightly different.

Other Tests

▲ *Femoral Nerve Tension (Prone Knee Bending) Test.*[296] See Chapter 9.

▲ *Timed "Up and Go" (TUG) Test.* For the TUG test, the patient sits in an armchair (seat height: 45 cm/17.7 inches). From this position, the patient is asked to rise on the command "ready, go!" and walks 3 m (9.8 feet) to a line on the floor, turns, and returns to the same seated position while the examiner times the movement with a stopwatch. If the patient takes more than 24 seconds to complete the task, the test is considered positive as a predictor for falls within 6 months of a hip fracture surgery.[325]

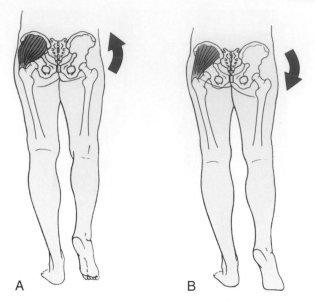

Fig. 11.98 Trendelenburg sign. (A) Negative test. (B) Positive test.

Reflexes and Cutaneous Distribution

There are no reflexes around the hip that can easily be evaluated. However, the examiner should assess the normal dermatomal patterns of the nerve roots (Fig. 11.101) as well as the sensory distribution of the peripheral nerves (Fig. 11.102). Because dermatomes vary from person to person, the accompanying diagrams are based on estimates only. Testing for altered sensation is performed as the examiner runs his or her relaxed hands and fingers over the pelvis and legs anteriorly, posteriorly, and laterally in a sensation-scanning assessment. Any difference in sensation should be noted and can be mapped out more precisely using a pinwheel, pin, cotton batten, and/or small brush.

True hip pain is usually referred to the groin, but it may also be referred to the ankle, knee, lumbar spine, and/or sacroiliac joints (Fig. 11.103). In children with hip problems (e.g., SCFE, Legg-Calvé-Perthes disease), sensory symptoms may be manifested only in the knee. Similarly, the knee, sacroiliac joints, and lumbar spine may refer pain to the hip. Table 11.16 illustrates muscles of the hip and their referral pattern if injured.

Peripheral Nerve Injuries About the Hip

There are several places where a peripheral nerve can become entrapped around the hip. Table 11.17 outlines anterior and posterior entrapments.

Pudendal Nerve (L2 to S4). The pudendal nerve is the main nerve of the perineum, providing sensation for the external genitalia and skin around anus and perineum and some pelvic muscles. Injury to the nerve causes numbness in the pelvic floor and genitals. Sitting may be painful. The nerve may be compressed as it leaves the pelvis between

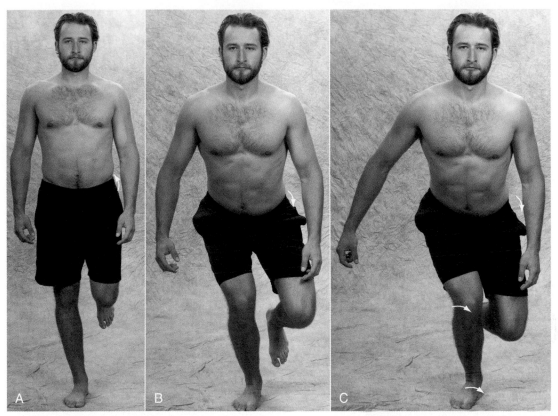

Fig. 11.99 (A) Trendelenburg sign—normal. (B) Trendelenburg squat—positive test. (C) Trendelenburg squat with stance leg collapse—positive test.

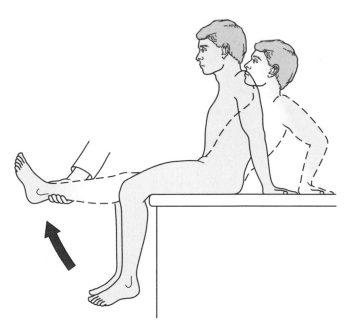

Fig. 11.100 Tripod sign.

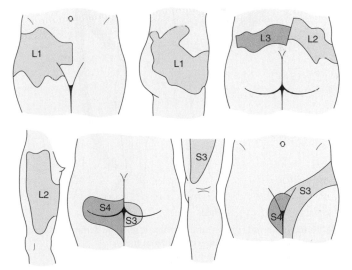

Fig. 11.101 Dermatomes around the hip. Only one side is illustrated.

the piriformis and coccygeus in the gluteal region near the ischial spine.

Sciatic Nerve (L4 to S3). The sciatic nerve (Fig. 11.104 and Table 11.18) may be injured anywhere along its path, from the lumbosacral spine down the back of the leg to the knee. It is the most commonly injured nerve in the hip region.[326–329] If it is injured in the pelvis or upper femoral area (e.g., posterior hip dislocation), the hamstrings and all muscles below the knee can be affected. The result is a high steppage gait with an inability to stand on the heel or toes. There is sensory alteration in the entire foot except the instep and medial malleolus as well as muscle atrophy. Usually the symptoms are primarily in the common peroneal branch of the sciatic nerve. In the hip region, the

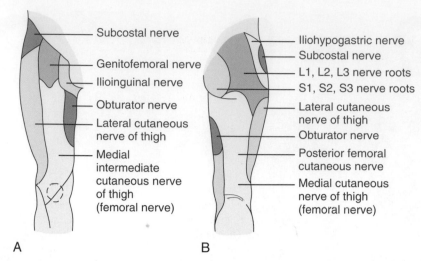

Fig. 11.102 Sensory distribution of peripheral nerves around the hip. (A) Anterior view. (B) Posterior view.

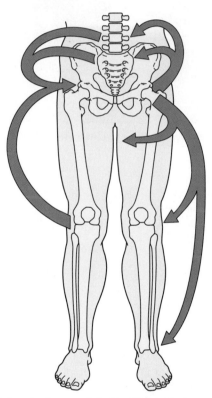

Fig. 11.103 Referred pain around the hip. Right side demonstrates referral to the hip. Left side shows referral from hip.

TABLE **11.16**

Hip Muscles and Referral of Pain

Muscle	Referral Pattern
Iliopsoas	Lateral to lumbar spine, anterior thigh
Gluteus maximus	Sacral and gluteal area to lateral aspect of pelvis and posterosuperior thigh
Gluteus medius	Lumbar and sacral gluteal area to lateral aspect of pelvis and upper thigh
Gluteus minimus	Gluteal area to area below iliac crest down lateral aspect of thigh and leg
Piriformis	Sacrum, gluteal area down posterior aspect of thigh
Tensor fasciae latae	Lateral thigh
Sartorius	Anteromedial thigh (along course of muscle)
Pectineus	Groin to upper medial thigh
Rectus femoris	Anterior thigh to knee
Adductor longus and brevis	Anterior thigh to medial thigh to anterior knee to anteromedial leg to ankle
Adductor magnus	Groin along medial thigh to above knee
Gracilis	Anteromedial thigh to knee
Hamstrings	Gluteal area along posterior thigh to knee and posteromedial calf

sciatic nerve may be compressed by the piriformis muscle (piriformis syndrome) (see Fig. 11.89).[330] If the piriformis is affected, there is pain and weakness on abduction and lateral rotation of the hip **(sign of Pace and Nagle).** The pain on passive medial rotation of the extended hip **(Freiberg sign)** is also elicited because this action stretches the piriformis.[331] Burning pain and hyperesthesia may be felt in the sacral and/or gluteal region as well as in the sciatic nerve distribution. Medial rotation with flexion of the hip accentuates the problem.

Superior Gluteal Nerve (L4 to S1). The superior gluteal nerve may be compressed as it passes between the piriformis and inferior border of the gluteus minimus muscle. It may also be injured during hip surgery.[327] The patient complains of acute gluteal pain that increases with ambulation. The hip is often medially rotated, and there is weakness of the hip abductors, resulting in a Trendelenburg

TABLE **11.17**

Sites of Entrapment, Key Signs and/or Symptoms with Nerves in the Anterior and Posterior Hip Region

Involved Nerve	Common Site of Entrapment	Key Signs and/or Symptoms
Posterior Nerve Entrapments		
Sciatic	Piriformis and obturator internus/ gemelli complex	Positive seated piriformis stretch and/or active piriformis tests
	Proximal hamstring	Ischial tenderness
		Pain in the posterior thigh to the popliteal fossa aggravated with running
	Lesser trochanter and ischium	Positive ischial femoral impingement test
Pudendal	Ischial spine, sacrospinous ligament, and lesser sciatic notch entrance	Pain medial to ischium
	Greater sciatic notch and piriformis	Sciatic notch tenderness and piriformis muscle spasm and tenderness
	Alcock's canal and obturator internus	Obturator internus spasm and tenderness
Anterior Nerve Entrapments		
Obturator	Obturator canal	Pain in medial thigh
	Adductor muscle fascia	Aggravation with movement into abduction
Femoral	Beneath iliopsoas tendon	Reproduction of symptoms with modified Thomas test position
	Inguinal ligament	Quadriceps muscle weakness
	Adductor canal	Pain in the anteromedial knee joint, medial leg, and foot
Lateral femoral cutaneous (meralgia paresthetica)	Inguinal ligament	Positive pelvic compression test

Used with permission of the *International Journal of Sports Physical Therapy* from Martin R, Nartin HD, Kivlan BR: Nerve entrapment in the hip region: current concepts review, *Int J Sports Phys Ther* 12(7):1169, 2017.

gait. Tenderness may be palpated just lateral to the greater sciatic notch.

Femoral Nerve (L2 to L4). The femoral nerve (Fig. 11.105), although not commonly injured, may be compressed during childbirth or with anterior dislocation of the femur, or it may be traumatized during hernia surgery, stripping of varicose veins, or adverse neural tension (i.e., inability of nerve to glide freely), which may be affected by muscle hypomobility and vice versa, hip surgery, or fractures.[327,332,333] The patient is not able to flex the thigh on the trunk or extend the knee. The deep tendon knee reflex is also lost. Wasting of the quadriceps is most evident. Sensory loss includes the medial aspect of the distal thigh (**anterior femoral cutaneous nerve**) and the medial aspect of the leg and foot (**saphenous nerve**). The nerve is tested using the prone knee bending test (see Chapter 9).

Obturator Nerve (L2 to L4). The obturator nerve (Fig. 11.106) may be compressed as it leaves the pelvis and enters the leg in the obturator tunnel or canal, the obturator externus tunnel, or the fascial plane deep to the pectineus and adductor brevis.[273,334] Injury to the nerve may be caused by pelvic or hip surgery, pregnancy (obstetric palsy), hemorrhaging, fascial entrapment, fractures, or tumors. It has been reported as a cause of groin pain in athletes.[16,327,330,335] Because the obturator nerve controls primarily the adductors, hip adduction is affected, as are knee flexion (gracilis) and hip lateral rotation (obturator externus). Sensory deficit is small but is often the most common symptom, involving a small area in the middle medial part of the thigh, although the patient may complain of pain from the symphysis pubis to the groin to the medial aspect of the knee.[336] Repetitive extension and lateral leg movement may aggravate the condition.[336] During ambulation, the hip will be abnormally laterally rotated and abducted relative to the other leg.[336] The neuropathy is usually diagnosed by EMG assessment.[336]

If the examiner feels that the vascular system may be involved, the popliteal (posterior knee), posterior tibial (below and behind medial malleolus), and dorsalis pedis (dorsum of foot distal to the navicular between the extensor hallucis longus and extensor digitorum longus tendons) pulses should be palpated for pulse rate and strength.[107]

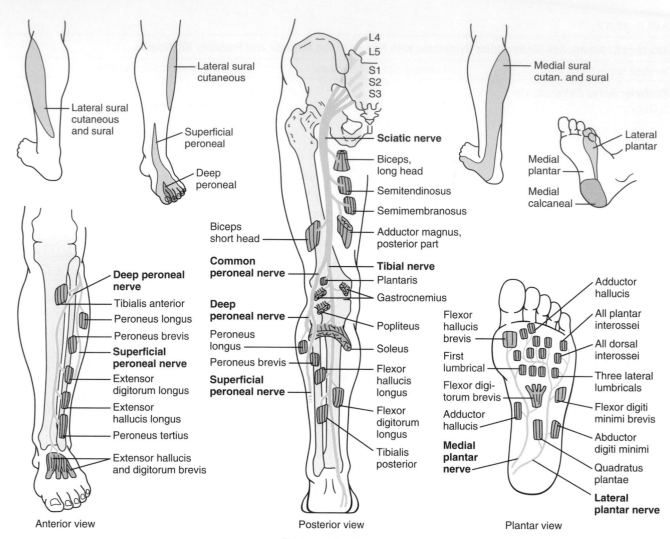

Fig. 11.104 Sciatic nerve.

Joint Play Movements

The joint play movements (Fig. 11.107) are completed with the patient in the supine position. The examiner should attempt to compare the amounts of available movement on the two sides. Small differences may be difficult to detect because of the large muscle bulk in the area.

Joint Play Movements of the Hip

- Caudal glide of the femur (long leg traction or long-axis extension)
- Compression
- Lateral distraction
- Quadrant test

Caudal Glide (Long Leg Traction). The examiner places both hands around the patient's leg slightly above the ankle. The examiner then leans back, applying a long-axis extension (traction) to the entire lower limb. Part of the movement occurs in the knee. If some pathology in the knee is suspected or the knee is stiff, both hands should be placed around the thigh just proximal to the knee, and traction force should again be applied (see

Fig. 11.107A). The first method enables the examiner to apply a greater force. During the movement, any telescoping or excessive movement occurring in the hip should be noted, since it may indicate an unstable joint or ligament laxity.[9] Martin et al.[9] advised doing the traction in 30° hip flexion, 30° hip abduction, and 10° plus 15° of hip lateral rotation. They found that if the patient had capsular laxity, then increased motion and a feeling of apprehension would occur in this position.[9]

Compression. The examiner places the patient's knee in the resting position and then applies a compressive force to the hip through the longitudinal axis of the femur by pushing through the femoral condyles (see Fig. 11.107B). Normally the end feel is hard, with no pain.

Lateral Distraction. The examiner applies a lateral distraction force to the hip by placing a wide strap around the leg as high up in the groin as possible. The strap is then wrapped around the examiner's buttocks. The examiner leans back, using the buttocks to apply the distraction force to the hip. The proximal hand is used to palpate the hip or greater trochanter movement while the distal hand prevents abduction of the leg and hence torque to the hip (see Fig. 11.107C).

TABLE **11.18**

Peripheral Nerve Injuries (Neuropathy) About the Hip

	Muscle Weakness	Sensory Alteration	Reflexes Affected
Sciatic nerve (L4 through S3)	Hamstrings Tibialis anterior Extensor digitorum longus Extensor digitorum brevis Extensor hallucis longus Peroneus tertius Peroneus longus Peroneus brevis Gastrocnemius Soleus Plantaris Tibialis posterior Flexor digitorum longus Flexor hallucis longus Flexor accessorious (quadratus plantae) Abductor digiti minimi Flexor digiti minimi Lumbricals Interossei Adductor hallucis Abductor hallucis Flexor digitorum brevis Flexor hallucis brevis	Posterior thigh and leg Whole foot except instep and medial malleolus	Medial hamstrings (L5–S1) Lateral hamstrings (S1–S2) Achilles (S1–S2) Tibialis posterior (L4–L5)
Superior gluteal nerve	Gluteus medius Gluteus minimus Tensor fasciae latae	None	None
Femoral nerve (L2–L4)	Iliacus Psoas Sartorius Pectineus Quadriceps	Medial side of thigh and leg	Patellar (L3–L4)
Obturator nerve (L2 through L4)	Adductor brevis Adductor magnus Adductor longus Obturator externus Gracilis	Middle thigh on anterior aspect	None

Palpation

During palpation of the hip and associated muscles, the examiner should note any tenderness, temperature, muscle spasm, or other signs and symptoms that may indicate the source of pathology. Intra-articular pain in the hip is rarely palpable.[337]

Anterior Aspect

The following structures should be palpated anteriorly, as shown in Fig. 11.108.

Iliac Crest, Greater Trochanter, and Anterosuperior Iliac Spine. The iliac crests are easily palpated and should be level. Each crest should be palpated for any tenderness because several muscles insert into this structure. In athletes, a condition called a **hip pointer** may be located on the iliac crest.[61] This occurs from a strain or contusion of the muscles that insert into the crest and can be very painful and debilitating as any trunk or pelvic movements can put stress on the muscles. The iliac tubercle is felt during palpation along the lateral aspect of the crest. The examiner then moves anteriorly to the ASIS. This is the insertion site of sartorius which may become avulsed (i.e., osteochondral fracture), especially in adolescents. Below this is the AIIS (the origin of the rectus femoris), which can be palpated for any tenderness.[107] The greater trochanter, located approximately 10 cm (4 inches) distal to the iliac tubercle of the iliac crest, is palpated next. If the examiner's thumbs are placed over each ASIS, the fingers will naturally lie along the lateral aspect of each thigh and the greater trochanter can be felt with the fingers on each side. If one or more of the trochanteric bursae (there are about 20 in the trochanteric area) are swollen (i.e., GTPS or trochanteric bursitis), lateral hip pain may

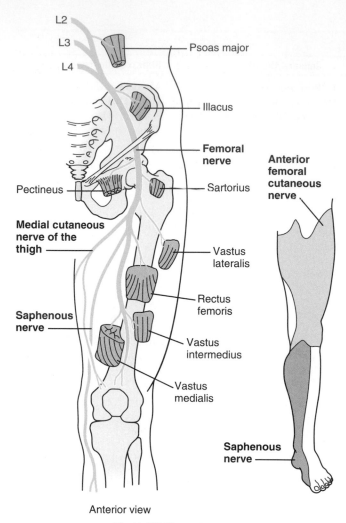

Fig. 11.105 Femoral nerve.

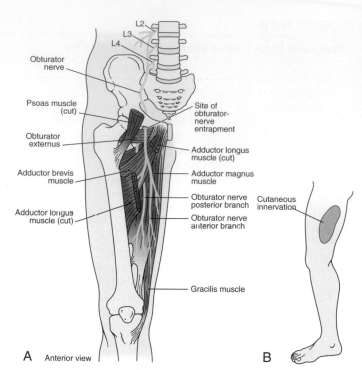

Fig. 11.106 Obturator nerve. (A) Anatomy of the obturator nerve. (B) Cutaneous sensory distribution of the anterior branch of the obturator nerve.

result.[105,259,338] The bursae may also be palpated in the area of the greater trochanter, although one would have difficulty in trying to determine which bursa is affected. Commonly the generic term *trochanteric bursa* is used.[339,340] If a bursa is pathologic, pain may extend down the thigh in a nondermatomal pattern and is often exacerbated by lying on the affected side, sitting with legs crossed, unilateral standing, stair climbing, walking, or running. Pain on resisted medial rotation with the hip in 90° flexion or maximum lateral rotation implicates gluteal tendinopathy.[263] At the same time, the examiner may palpate for tenderness/pain in the gluteus medius or minimus, tensor fascia lata tendinopathy or tear, or **external coxa saltans,** which is the anterior fibers of gluteus maximus or the iliotibial band snapping over the greater trochanter as the leg moves from hip extension to flexion.[259,339,341] If, with the clicking, external coxa saltans is suspected, the patient should be asked to do the movement with the leg laterally rotated, which would alleviate the problem.[259,338] If the greater trochanter is palpated carefully, the gluteus medius will be found to insert onto the lateral facet in two areas. The posterior fibers insert on the superoposterior portion of the lateral facet and the central and anterior portions insert more inferiorly on the lateral facet. The gluteus minimus inserts into the anteroinferior facet of the greater tuberosity, deep to gluteus medius.[259]

Inguinal Ligament, Femoral Triangle, Hip Joint, and Symphysis Pubis. The examiner's fingers are placed on the ASIS. Palpation gently continues along the inguinal ligament to the pelvic tubercles (symphysis pubis), with the examiner noting any signs of pathology. The psoas bursa, if swollen, is usually palpable under the inguinal ligament at its midpoint. Moving distal to the inguinal ligament, the examiner palpates the femoral triangle, the boundaries of which are the inguinal ligament superiorly, the sartorius muscle laterally, and the adductor longus muscle medially (Fig. 11.109). Within the femoral triangle, the examiner may palpate swollen lymph glands (Fig. 11.110) and the femoral artery. The femoral nerve lies lateral to the artery and the femoral vein lies medial to it, but neither of these structures is easily palpated. At this stage, the examiner may decide to palpate for an inguinal hernia in the male. The head of the femur is then palpated. Although the hip joint is deep and not easily palpable, the surrounding structures may show signs of pathology. The head of the femur is 1 to 2 cm (0.4 to 0.8 inch) below the middle third of the inguinal ligament and is found on a horizontal line running halfway between the pubic tubercle and the greater trochanter.

The examiner can palpate for muscle tenderness by palpating while the patient does a resisted contraction. Fig. 11.111A–D shows palpation of hip flexors, adductors, rectus abdominus, and gluteus medius.[342]

The examiner concludes the anterior palpation by palpating the hip flexor, adductor, and abductor muscles for signs of pathology.

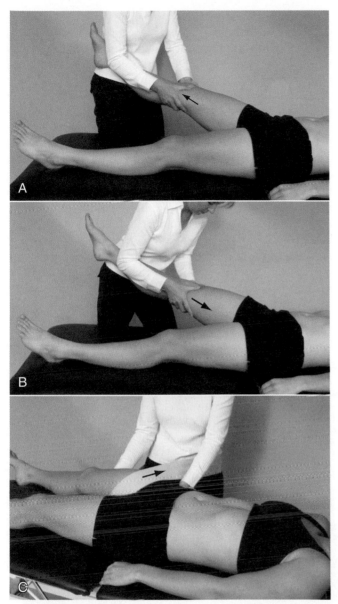

Fig. 11.107 Joint play movements of the hip. (A) Long leg traction (applied above the knee). (B) Compression. (C) Lateral distraction.

Posterior Aspect

The patient is then asked to lie in the prone position so that the following structures can be palpated posteriorly.

Iliac Crest, Posterosuperior Iliac Spine, Ischial Tuberosity, and Greater Trochanter. The examiner begins posterior palpation by following the iliac crests, which are easily palpable, posteriorly to the PSIS. Below the crest and lateral to the PSIS, the gluteals (i.e., gluteus maximus, medius, and minimus) may be palpated along with the sacroiliac joint, piriformis, tensor fascia lata, and iliotibial band.[107] On most patients, each PSIS is evident by the presence of overlying skin dimples. As the examiner moves caudally, the ischial tuberosities, which are approximately at the level of the gluteal folds, may be felt. If the ischial bursa is swollen, it is sometimes palpable over the ischial tuberosities.

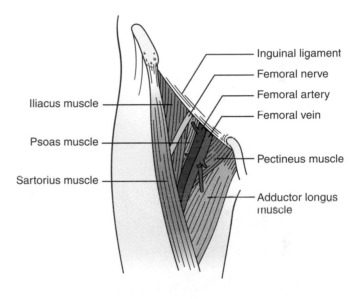

Fig. 11.109 Femoral triangle containing the femoral artery, vein, and nerve. Note the inguinal ligament above, iliacus and psoas laterally, and adductors medially. The sartorius attaches to the anterosuperior spine, whereas the adductor muscles attach along the pubic ramus. (Modified from Anson BJ: *Atlas of human anatomy*, Philadelphia, 1963, WB Saunders, p 583.)

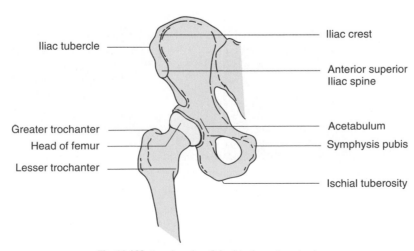

Fig. 11.108 Landmarks of the hip (anterior view).

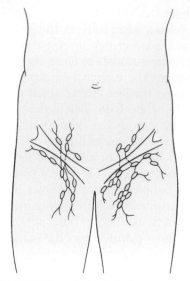

Fig. 11.110 Lymph glands in the groin area.

The tuberosities should also be palpated for possible tenderness of the hamstring muscle insertions. If one palpates the sciatic notch and piriformis and finds tenderness plus neurological symptoms, DGS may be suspected. If the tenderness is lateral to the ischium, hamstring syndrome or IFI may be suspected. Medial tenderness may indicate **pudendal nerve involvement**.[163] Laterally, the posterior aspect of the greater trochanter is felt. If the distance between the ischial tuberosity and greater trochanter is divided in half, the fingers lie over the sciatic nerve as it enters the lower limb. Normally the nerve is not palpable, but one can palpate the posterior muscles that insert into the greater trochanter (i.e., lateral rotators),[343] or they may be palpated about 1 to 1.5 inches (2.5 to 3.8 cm) below the PSIS and just lateral to the lateral edge of the sacrum.[344] The examiner then palpates upward from the midpoint to determine whether there is any tenderness of the hip lateral rotators, especially the piriformis muscle. In

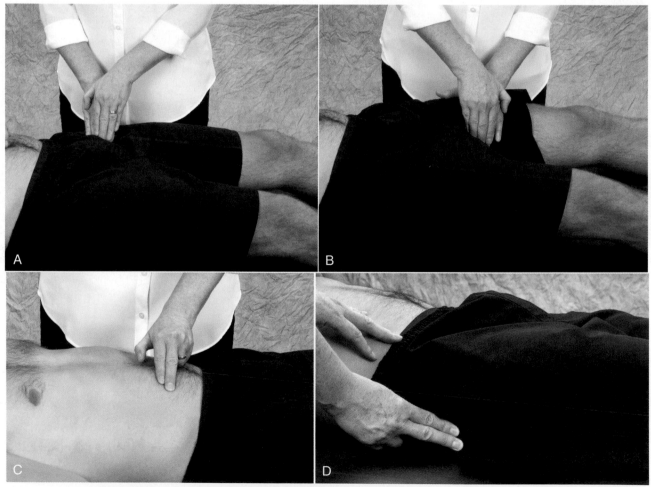

Fig. 11.111 Palpation of (A) hip flexors, (B) adductors, (C) rectus abdominis, and (D) gluteus medius.

addition, the gluteal and hamstring muscle bellies should be palpated for signs of pathology.

Sacroiliac, Lumbosacral, and Sacrococcygeal Joints. If the examiner suspects pathology in these joints, they should be palpated. Detailed descriptions of their palpation are given in Chapters 9 and 10.

Diagnostic Imaging

Plain Film Radiography[345]

Normally the standard views of the hip include anteroposterior views and axial or frog-leg views.[345] The following box shows common x-ray views used for the hip. Table 11.19 outlines what to look for in plain radiographs.[1]

Common X-Ray Views of the Hip Depending on Pathology

- Anteroposterior view of the hip (Fig. 11.112)
- Lateral view (cross table, only affected hip) (see Fig. 11.147)
- Lateral axial ("frog-leg") view (see Fig. 11.150)
- Anteroposterior view of both hips and pelvis (see Fig. 11.116)
- Anteroposterior oblique view (Fig. 11.113)
- Anteroposterior internal (medial) rotation view

Anteroposterior View.[99,346,347] The examiner should compare the two hips, noting the following features:

1. Neck-shaft angle, femoral head uncovering, and head–teardrop distance (Fig. 11.114): Abnormal head-neck offset (i.e., flattening of superior femoral head so that it is aspherical and flattening of the normal concave surface of the lateral femoral neck[348]) is called a **pistol-grip deformity** (Fig. 11.115; see Fig. 11.133), which may be seen in FAI, femoral head dysplasia, SCFE, and Legg-Calvé-Perthes disease.[123,348]
2. Joint spaces and pelvic lines and other landmarks (Figs. 11.116 and 11.117).
3. Is there any bone disease (i.e., Legg-Calvé-Perthes disease, bony cysts, or tumors; Fig. 11.118)? With Legg-Calvé-Perthes disease, prominence of the ischial spine indicates retroversion of the acetabulum.[349]

4. What is the neck-shaft angle?[350] The examiner should note whether the angle is normal or whether the patient exhibits a coxa vara or coxa valga (Figs. 11.119 and 11.120).
5. What is the shape of the femoral head?[351] The femoral head is normally spherical but can show changes with DDH, Legg-Calvé-Perthes disease, SCFE, and FAI.
6. The obturator foramen should be symmetrical.[345]
7. The distance from the symphysis pubis to the tip of the coccyx should be 1 to 3 cm (0.4 to 1.2 inches) (see Fig. 10.74).[345]

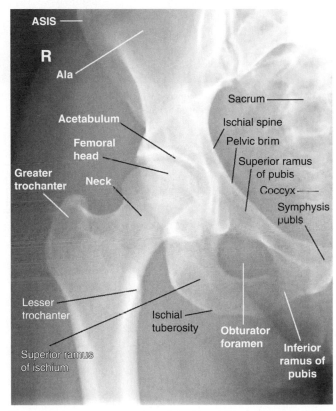

Fig. 11.112 Anteroposterior view of the hip. *ASIS,* Anterosuperior iliac spine. (From McQuillen Martensen K: *Radiographic image analysis,* ed 3, St Louis, 2011, Saunders/Elsevier, p 397.)

TABLE **11.19**

Interpreting Plain Radiographs of the Hip

	Alignment	Bone Mineralization	Articular Cartilage	Soft Tissue
What to look for	• Fracture • Dislocation • Angle of inclination • Acetabular index • Femoral offset and abductor lever arm • Inter-teardrop line • Teardrop sign • Bryant's triangle and Nelaton's line • Shenton's line	• Osteoporosis • Osteopenia • Avascular necrosis	• Joint-space narrowing • Osteophytes • Subchondral sclerosis • Subchondral cysts • Subluxation	• Signs of effusion

From Wang R, Bhandari M, Lachowski RJ: A systematic approach to adult hip pain. Part 1, *Can J Diagnosis* April:116, 2001.

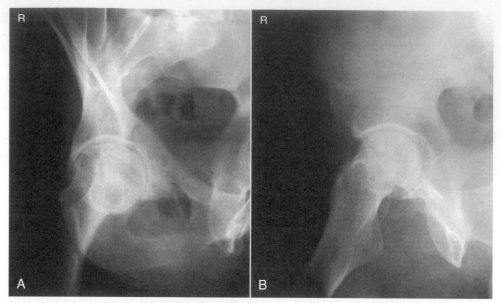

Fig. 11.113 Anteroposterior oblique view of the hip (Judet method). (A) Left posterior oblique. (B) Right posterior oblique. (From Long BW, Rafert JA: *Orthopedic radiography*, Philadelphia, 1995, Saunders.)

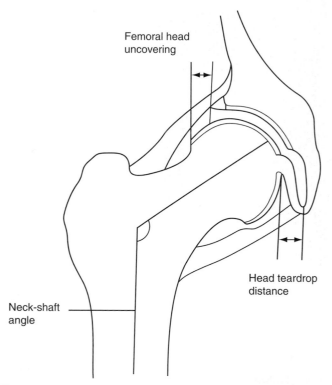

Fig. 11.114 Three radiologic measurements of the hip. (From Richardson JK, Iglarsh ZA: *Clinical orthopedic physical therapy*, Philadelphia, 1994, WB Saunders, p 358.)

8. Is coxa profunda (i.e., acetabular overcoverage) (Fig. 11.121) or coxa protrusion (i.e., the medial aspect of the femoral head being medial to the ischiofemoral line) present?[56]

9. Is protrusio acetabuli, which occurs if the medial aspect of the femoral head is medial to the ilioischial line, present (Fig. 11.122)?

10. Is the acetabulum anteverted (normal) or retroverted (see Fig. 11.2B)? A retroverted acetabulum is indicated by the **crossover sign** (Fig. 11.123).[56,352,353] Normally the anterior wall should cover less of the femoral head than the posterior wall, which should be at the level of the center of the femoral head or lateral to it (**posterior wall sign**).[84] The crossover sign or figure-eight sign occurs because the anterior aspect of the acetabular rim is more lateral than the posterior aspect of the acetabulum (Fig. 11.124).[142] The posterior wall sign occurs when the posterior aspect of the acetabular rim is more medial than the center of the hip joint, so there is less posterior coverage of the femoral head.[142]

11. Is the femoral head in the normal position? The distance from the femoral head to the ilioischial line should be less than 10 mm (Fig. 11.125).

12. Are the femoral head and acetabulum congruent (Fig. 11.126)?

13. Are the femoral head and acetabulum normal on both sides? In DDH, both structures may show dysplasia, and the **acetabular index** on the affected side may be more than the normal 30° in the newborn (20° in 2-year-olds). The acetabular index is determined by first drawing a horizontal line between the inferior aspects of the pelvic "teardrops." A second line is drawn between the lateral margin of the acetabular roof (i.e., lateral sourcil) and the teardrop on the same side. The intersection of the two lines is called the *acetabular index,* the **Hilgenreiner angle** or acetabular angle of Sharp (Table 11.20). Angles greater than 36° indicate acetabular dysplasia. The greater the slope angle, the less stable the femoral head in the acetabulum. Fig. 11.127 shows measurements that may be taken with DDH.

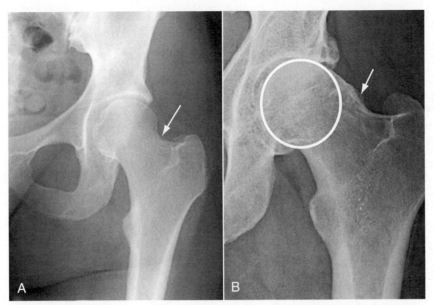

Fig. 11.115 (A) Normal frontal radiograph of hip shows concavity of femoral head and neck *(arrow)*. (B) Pistol-grip deformity with abnormal extension of epiphyseal scar in a patient with cam impingement. (From Patel K, Wallace R, Busconi BD: Radiology, *Clin Sports Med* 30:254, 2011.)

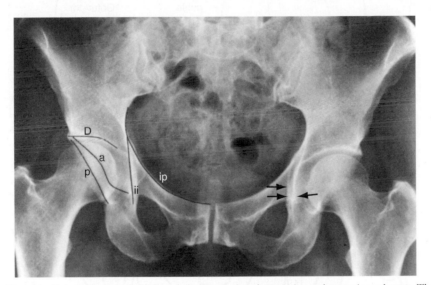

Fig. 11.116 Pelvic lines. The iliopubic *(ip)* and ilioischial *(ii)* lines help in assessing the anterior and posterior columns. The acetabular dome *(D)* and anterior *(a)* and posterior *(p)* lips *(rims)* of the acetabulum are seen. The teardrop figure *(arrows)* is a composite shadow made up laterally of the anterior aspect of the acetabular fossa and medially of the quadrilateral surface of the ilium. The more posterior aspect of the quadrilateral surface *(represented by the ilioischial line)* is superimposed on the teardrop in this nonrotated view. (From Weissman BNW, Sledge CB: *Orthopedic radiology*, Philadelphia, 1986, WB Saunders, p 343.)

14. What is the **femoral head extrusion index?** Normal is about 25% (Fig. 11.128).

15. Are there any osteophytes or is there arthritis (Fig. 11.129)? Kellgren and Lawrence[354] have developed a radiographic grading scale for hip osteoarthritis (Table 11.21). **Cardinal features of osteoarthritis** include narrowed or loss of joint space, presence of osteophytes, subchondral sclerosis, and subchondral bone cysts.[1]

16. Whether the **Shenton's line** is normal: Normally this line is curved, drawn along the medial curved edge of the femur and continuing upward in a smooth arc along the inferior edge of the pubis (Fig. 11.130). If the head of the femur is dislocated or fractured, two lines form two separate arcs, indicating a broken line. A broken Shenton's line is diagnostic of pathology.

17. The **acetabular (Tonnis) angle** or **index** should be between 0° and 10° in adults (Fig. 11.131). An angle greater than 10° is suggestive of acetabular dysplasia.[36]

18. The **lateral central edge angle** is normally less than 25° on an anteroposterior pelvic view (Fig. 11.132): If the angle is less than 25°, it could indicate insufficient coverage of the femoral head or dysplasia.[355]

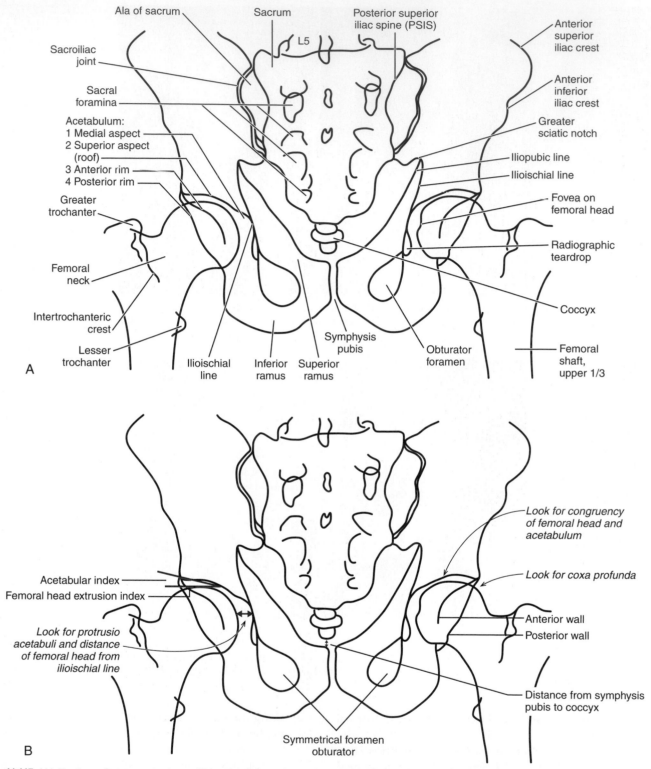

Fig. 11.117 (A) Tracing of anteroposterior radiograph of the pelvis. (B) Measurements and things to look for on an anteroposterior radiograph. (Redrawn and modified from McKinnis LN: *Fundamentals of musculoskeletal imaging*, Philadelphia, 2005, FA Davis, p 297.)

19. Is there evidence of FAI (Table 11.22; Fig. 11.133)?
20. Is there any evidence of fracture or dislocation (Figs. 11.134 and 11.135)? Is the pelvic ring intact, or has it been disrupted? Disruption of the pelvic ring indicates a severe injury.

21. Is there evidence of pelvic distortion (i.e., the ilia are counterrotated on the sacrum)?
22. Are the Hilgenreiner's and Perkins' lines within normal limits?[356] The **Hilgenreiner's line** is horizontal, drawn between the inferior parts of the ilium. The

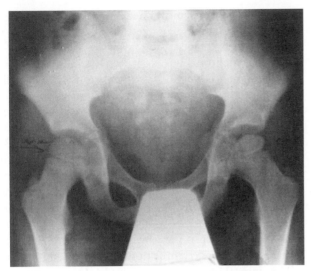

Fig. 11.118 Legg-Calvé-Perthes disease of the left hip.

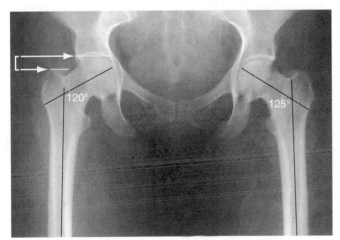

Fig. 11.119 Anteroposterior view of the pelvis in an adult patient with coxa vara of the hip joint shows a neck-shaft angle of less than 125° and a decreased trochanteric acetabular distance *(white arrows)*. This configuration contributes to the potential for abnormal joint reaction forces with an increased risk of a medial osteoarthritis developing at the hip joint. In this patient, loss of the medial joint space and/or early arthrokatadysis or medial migration of the femoral heads can be seen, as can early development of osteophytes at the acetabulum and femoral head. (From Johnson TR, Steinbach LS: *Essentials of musculoskeletal imaging*, Rosemont, IL, 2004, American Academy of Orthopedic Surgeons, p 458.)

Perkins' line is vertical, drawn through the upper outer point of the acetabulum (Fig. 11.136). Normally the developing femoral head or ossification center of the femoral head lies in the inner distal quadrant formed by the two lines. If the ossification center lies in the upper outer quadrant, the finding is indicative of a dislocation or DDH.[284] In the newborn, the ossification center is not visible (Fig. 11.137).

23. **"Sagging rope" sign:** With Legg-Calvé-Perthes disease, only the head of the femur is affected. If avascular necrosis of a developing femoral head occurs,

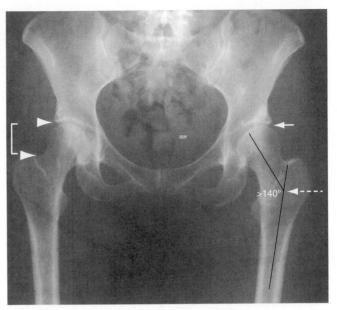

Fig. 11.120 Anteroposterior view of an adult patient with a valgus alignment at the hip joint shows a neck-shaft angle that exceeds 140° *(white dotted arrow)*. Note also the increased portion of the articular aspect of the femoral head that is uncovered *(white arrow)*. This attribute becomes even more important if the superior aspect of the weight-bearing surface of the acetabulum is smaller than normal. In this patient, the trochanteric acetabular distance (the distance from a line drawn parallel to the superior aspect of the weight-bearing surface of the dome to a line parallel to the superior aspect of the tip of the greater trochanter) exceeds 2.5 cm *(arrowheads)* Normally, the trochanteric acetabular distance in adults averages about 2.2 cm. (From Johnson TR, Steinbach LS: *Essentials of musculoskeletal imaging*, Rosemont, IL, 2004, American Academy of Orthopedic Surgeons, p 457)

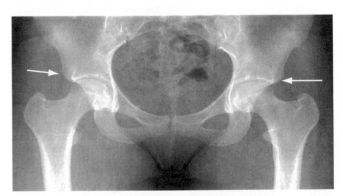

Fig. 11.121 Anteroposterior radiograph demonstrating global acetabular overcoverage (i.e., coxa profunda), which may lead to cam-type femoroacetabular impingement. (From Sierra RJ, Trousdale RT, Ganz R, et al: Hip disease in the young active patient: evaluation and nonarthroplasty surgical options, *J Am Acad Orthop Surg* 16:693, 2008.)

the "sagging rope" sign may be seen (Fig. 11.138). It indicates damage to the growth plate with marked metaphyseal reaction. Its presence indicates a severe disease process.

24. **"Teardrop" sign:** Migration of the femoral head upward in relation to the pelvis, caused by degeneration as seen in osteoarthritis, may be detected

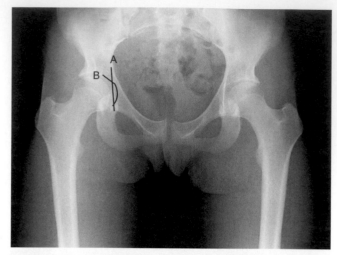

Fig. 11.122 The radiographic appearance of protrusio acetabuli on an anteroposterior pelvic view. *Line A* represents the ilioischial line and *line B* represents the floor of the acetabular fossa, which is medial to *line A*. A similar pathologic condition can also be seen on the radiograph of the patient's left hip. (From Clohisy JC, Carlisle JC, Beaulé PE, et al: A systematic approach to the plain radiographic evaluation of the young adult hip. *J Bone Joint Surg Am* 90:53, 2008.)

by the teardrop sign (Fig. 11.139). The teardrop is visible at the base of the pubic bone, extending vertically downward to terminate in a round teardrop, or head. The x-ray beam must be centered relative to the pelvis. A line is drawn between the two teardrops and extended to the femoral heads on both sides. The examiner can then measure from the teardrop to the femoral head. A difference of more than 10 mm between the two sides indicates significant migration of the head of the femur. Serial films or films taken over time often show a progression of the migration.

25. **"Head at risk" signs:** With Legg-Calvé-Perthes disease, the examiner should note the following radiologic head-at-risk signs on an anteroposterior film:
    a. The Cage sign, a small osteoporotic segment on the lateral side of the epiphysis that appears to be translucent (Fig. 11.140)
    b. Calcification lateral to the epiphysis (if collapse is occurring)
    c. Lateral subluxation of the head (an increase in the inferomedial joint space)
    d. Angle of the epiphyseal line (horizontal, in this case)
    e. Metaphyseal reaction
    Patients who exhibit three or more head-at-risk signs have a poor prognosis, and surgery is usually performed.

26. Signs of an SCFE[357]: With a SCFE (Fig. 11.141), the following x-ray signs may be noted:
    a. The epiphyseal line may widen.
    b. Lipping or stepping may be seen, as occurs on lateral films.
    c. The superior femoral neck line does not transect the overhanging ossified epiphysis as it does in the normal hip.
    d. The Shenton's line does not describe a continuous arc. (The line is also broken if the hip is dislocated or subluxed.)
    In addition to an SCFE causing a coxa vara, other causes such as fractures or congenital malformations can lead to the same deformity (Figs. 11.142 and 11.143).

27. Normally if, on each side of the body, a line (i.e., the **shoemaker's line**) is projected from the greater trochanter to the ASIS until the lines intersect, the lines will meet at midline at or above the umbilicus (Fig. 11.144). If the lines intersect below the umbilicus or are off center, it indicates a femoral neck fracture, dislocation of one femur upward, or malalignment.

28. The **lateral coverage index (LCI)** is a measure used to determine hip dysplasia and is defined as the center-edge (CE) angle minus the acetabular inclination (Fig. 11.145). Ligamentum teres tears are less frequent with higher LCI scores.[32,320]

29. Acetabular coverage of the femoral head may be determined by the **lateral center-edge (LCE)** angle, the **anterior LCE angle**, **acetabular inclination (Tönnis angle)**, and **acetabular index** (Fig. 11.146).[11,358] The normal LCE angle is 25° or greater. Less than 25° indicates acetabular dysplasia.

30. For FAI, the cam type is diagnosed from the **alpha angle** greater than 57°, pistol-grip deformity, acetabular index (Tönnis angle) less than 0°, femoral head-neck offset less than 8 mm, offset ratio, or triangular index, whereas the pincer type is diagnosed from the crossover sign, the posterior wall sign, anterior and LCE angle greater than 40°, the prominence of the ischial spine sign, or coxa profunda.[59,135,138,139,359–362]

31. The orientation of the acetabulum can affect hip stability. A retroverted acetabulum may lead to posterior instability and an anteverted acetabulum or an anteverted femoral neck may lead to anterior instability.[11,50,363] Acetabular retroversion is suggested by the posterior wall sign and/or ischial spine sign.[36]

32. It should be noted that osteopenia is not evident on plain films until there has been 40% loss in bone mineral density.[1]

33. Signs of joint effusion in the hip:
    a. Lateral subluxation of femoral head so that joint space is larger (common in juvenile rheumatoid arthritis)
    b. Absence of a vacuum effect—if traction (long leg) is applied as the x-ray is taken, normally the negative pressure is observed as a radiolucent crescent between the joint surfaces. This phenomenon does not appear in joints with even small amounts of extra fluid.

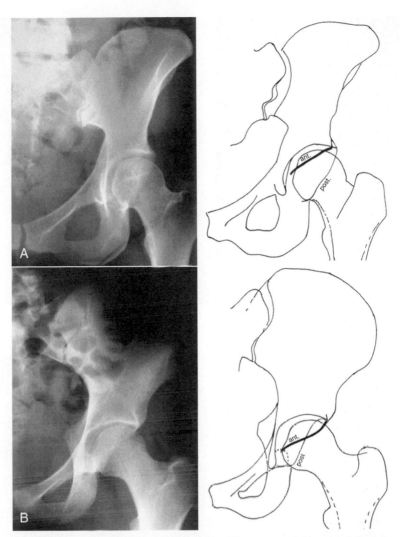

Fig. 11.123 (A) Radiograph and tracing of the normal (anteverted) acetabulum. The posture of this pelvis is flexed more at the lumbosacral junction than in the case described in (B). The outline of the obturator foramen is more circular and the ischial spine is obscured. In such a flexed pelvis, the anteverted attitude of the acetabulum is seen at a maximum. When an acetabulum is retroverted, adoption of a similar posture minimizes the appearance of retroversion. The line of the edge of the posterior wall is located at or even lateral to the center of the femoral head. (B) Radiograph and tracing showing acetabular retroversion and the "crossover" or figure-eight sign. Compare with (A). The line of the posterior wall appears thin whereas that of the anterior wall looks thick. The line of the edge of the posterior wall is located well medial to the center of the femoral head. (From Reynolds D: Retroversion of the acetabulum: a cause of hip pain, *J Bone Joint Surg Br* 81:285, 1999.)

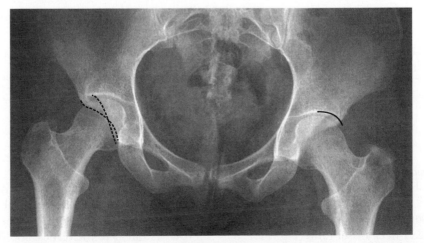

Fig. 11.124 Anteroposterior radiograph of the pelvis of a 22-year-old woman who presented with groin pain. Clinical examination strongly suggested femoroacetabular impingement. The radiograph demonstrates bilateral acetabular retroversion as determined by crossover of the anterior and posterior acetabular walls *(dotted lines)* (crossover sign) on the right hip. The left hip demonstrates a pistol-grip deformity. (From Parvizi J, Leunig M, Ganz R: Femoroacetabular impingement, *J Am Acad Orthop Surg* 15[9]:561–570, 2007.)

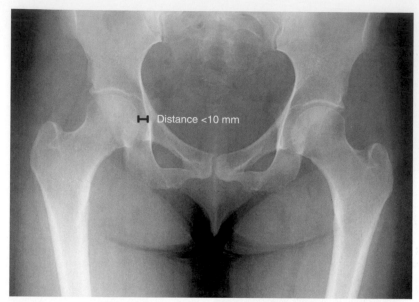

Fig. 11.125 Normal position of the femoral head in the acetabulum. (From Clohisy JC, Carlisle JC, Beaulé PE, et al: A systematic approach to the plain radiographic evaluation of the young adult hip, *J Bone Joint Surg Am* 90:59, 2008.)

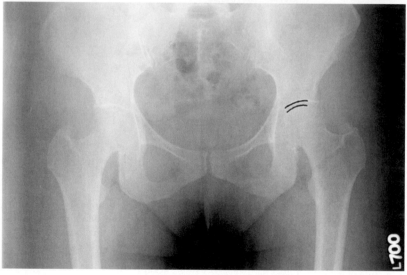

Fig. 11.126 Congruency of the femoral head and the acetabulum. (From Clohisy JC, Carlisle JC, Beaulé PE, et al: A systematic approach to the plain radiographic evaluation of the young adult hip, *J Bone Joint Surg Am* 90:62, 2008.)

TABLE 11.20

Average Values of Hilgenreiner's Angle (Acetabular Index)

	Newborn	6 Months Old	1 Year Old
Male	26°	20°	20°
Female	28°	22°	20°

c. Demineralization of subchondral bone is seen as fading of the sharp subchondral white line of the femoral head.[1]

Cross-Table Lateral View. This view (Fig. 11.147) can be used to measure the head-neck offset ratio (Fig. 11.148). This ratio is used when FAI (cam type) is suspected. If the ratio is less than 0.17, a cam deformity may be present.[345]

False-Profile Hip Radiograph.[345] This view is used to calculate the anterior CE angle. A vertical line is drawn through the center of the femoral head. A second line is drawn from the most anterior point of the acetabular "eyebrow" (sourcil) to the vertical line. The angle created is the anterior CE angle (Fig. 11.149; see Fig. 11.2A). Structural instability is indicated if the angle is less than 20°.

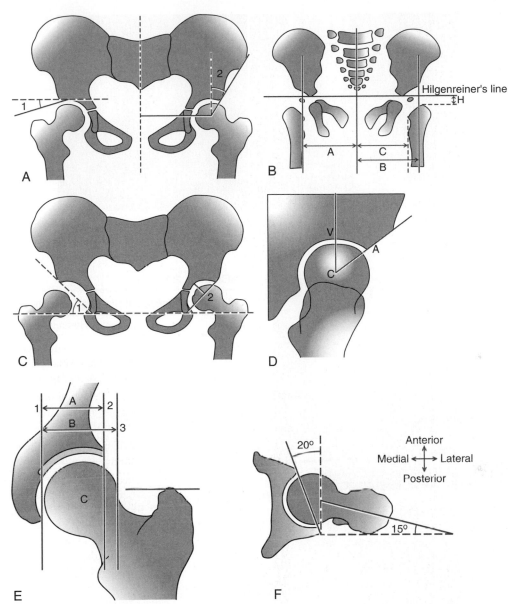

Fig. 11.127 Additional measurements performed on conventional radiographs in patients with developmental dysplasia of the hip. (A) *1:* Slope of the lateral edge of the acetabulum. The angle formed between a line that is parallel to the Hilgenreiner line and tangent to the roof of the acetabulum; a line that is parallel to the lateral edge of the acetabulum is termed *the slope.* The normal acetabulum has a slope of the lateral edge that is defined as positive. *2:* Center-edge *(CE)* angle. This angle lies between a line drawn from the center of the femoral head, perpendicular to the line connecting the centers of each femoral head, and a line drawn from the center of the head to the superolateral ossified edge of the acetabulum. The CE angle has a negative value. (B) *Right hip:* The pelvic midline is drawn vertically through the centers of the sacrum and the symphysis pubis. The lateral displacement of each femoral head is indicated by the length of a line *(A)* drawn horizontally from the pelvic midline to the center of the femoral head. *Left hip:* The *C/B* ratio compared *C,* the distance from the pelvic midline to the medial beak of the femoral metaphysis, and *B,* the distance from the pelvic midline to the lateral acetabular edge. (C) *1:* The angle that lies between a line connecting the teardrops on the inferior margin of the acetabula and a line drawn from the most superolateral ossified edge of the acetabulum to the teardrop constitutes the adult acetabular index or angle. *2:* The greatest perpendicular distance between the medial articular surface of the acetabulum and a line drawn from the teardrop to the superolateral ossified edge of the acetabulum is the acetabular depth. (D) Vertical center-edge angle, drawn on a false profile view. It is defined as the angle subtended by a line *(V–C)* drawn from the center of the femoral head extending vertically upward and a line *(C–A)* drawn from the center of the femoral head obliquely to the anterior edge of the acetabulum. The angle lies between the two lines. (E) Percentage of the femoral head covered by the acetabulum. This represents the relative width of the weight-bearing surface of the acetabulum *(A),* represented by line *1–2,* and that of the femoral head, represented by line *1–3.* Normal acetabular coverage is 75% or above when the ratio of *1–2:1–3* is determined. (F) The acetabular anteversion angle describes the extent to which the acetabulum surrounds the femoral head within the horizontal plane. Measured from above, this angle is normally about 20°. As shown, the angle is formed by the intersection of an anterior-posterior reference line *(stippled)* and a line across the rim of the acetabulum. The 15° of normal anteversion of the proximal femur is also indicated. (A–D, Redrawn from Restrick D, Kransdorf MJ: *Bone and joint imaging,* Philadelphia, 2005, Elsevier, p 1286; Courtesy N. Lektakul, MD, Bangkok, Thailand. E, Redrawn from Delaunay S, Dussault RG, Kaplan PA, et al: Radiographic measurements of dysplastic adult hips, *Skeletal Radiol* 26:75, 1997. F, Redrawn from Neumann DA: *Kinesiology of the musculoskeletal system—foundations for physical rehabilitation,* St Louis, 2002, CV Mosby, p 398.)

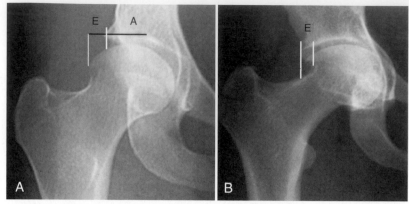

Fig. 11.128 Femoral head extrusion index [E/A + E]. Normal extrusion index (A) is about 25%. In coxa profunda and protrusio acetabuli (B), more femoral head is covered and the index is zero, or negative. (From Patel K, Wallace R, Busconi BD: Radiology, *Clin Sports Med* 30:257, 2011.)

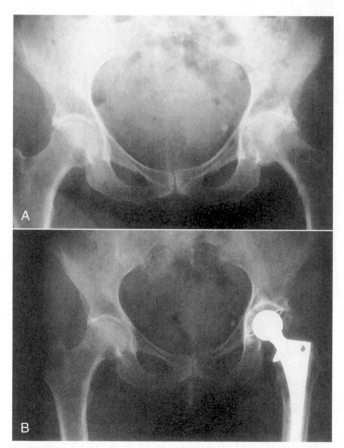

Fig. 11.129 Arthritis of the left hip. (A) Before surgery. Note decreased joint space and unevenness of femoral head. (B) After total hip surgery.

Lateral (Axial "Frog-Leg") View. For this view, the patient is supine with the hips in flexion, abduction, and lateral rotation. This view provides a true lateral view of the femoral head and neck (Fig. 11.150).[364] This view is useful if a vascular necrosis is suspected.[1] The examiner looks for any pelvic distortion or any slipping of the femoral head, as may be seen in SCFE. The lateral view is the first in which slipping may be seen. This view will also show head-neck offset deformity.[345]

TABLE 11.21

Kellgren and Lawrence Grading Scale for Hip Osteoarthritis

Grade	Radiographic Findings
0	No evidence of joint space narrowing, osteophyte formation, or sclerosis (normal radiograph)
1	Possible narrowing of the joint space medially and possible osteophytes around the femoral head
2	Definite narrowing of the joint space, definite osteophytes, and slight sclerosis
3	Marked narrowing of the joint space, slight osteophytes, some sclerosis, and cyst formation, and deformity of the femoral head and acetabulum
4	Gross loss of joint space with sclerosis and cysts, marked deformity of femoral head and acetabulum, large osteophytes

Modified from Kellgren JH, Lawrence JS: Radiological assessment of osteo-arthrosis, *Ann Rheum Dis* 16:494–502, 1957.

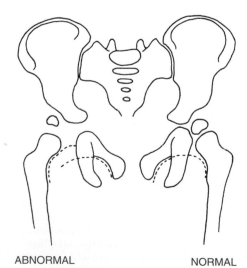

ABNORMAL   NORMAL

Fig. 11.130 Shenton's line.

Text continued on p. 849.

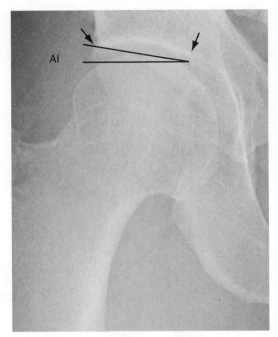

Fig. 11.131 The acetabular index *(AI)* is an angle formed by a horizontal line and a line connecting the medial point of the sclerotic zone *(small black arrow)* with the lateral center of the acetabulum. Normal acetabular index is positive while in coxa profunda and in protrusio acetabula, the acetabular index is zero, or negative. (From Patel K, Wallace R, Busconi BD: Radiology, *Clin Sports Med* 30:256, 2011.)

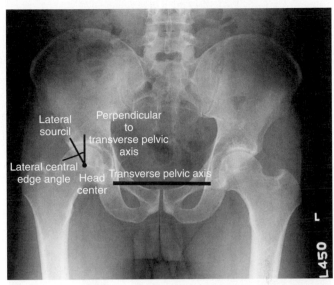

Fig. 11.132 Lateral central edge angle. (Modified from Clohisy JC, Carlisle JC, Beaulé PE, et al: A systematic approach to the plain radiographic evaluation of the young adult hip, *J Bone Joint Surg Am* 90:55, 2008.)

TABLE 11.22

Key Radiographic Features of Dysplasia and Femoroacetabular Impingement

	Dysplasia	FEMOROACETABULAR IMPINGEMENT	
		Pincer Type	Cam Type
Anteroposterior pelvic/ hip radiograph	Center-edge angle <25°, Tonnis angle >10°	Crossover and/or posterior wall sign, ischial sign, coxa profunda	Pistol-grip deformity
Lateral radiograph	—	—	Alpha angle >50.5°, offset ratio <0.15
False-profile radiograph	Anterior center-edge angle <25°	Narrowing of posterior articular surface	—

From Beaulé PE, O'Neill M, Rakhra K: Acetabular labral tears, *J Bone Joint Surg Am* 91:705, 2009.

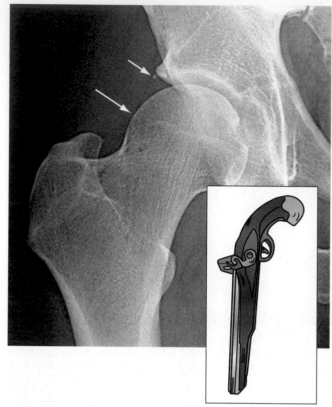

Fig. 11.133 A 36-year-old male with cam-type femoroacetabular impingement (FAI). Anteroposterior view of the right hip demonstrates the pistol-grip deformity of the lateral femoral head-neck junction *(long arrow)*. Note the calcifications of the labrum *(short arrow)*. (Modified from Zaragoza EJ, Beaulé PE: Imaging of the painful non-arthritic hip: a practical approach to surgical relevancy. *Oper Tech Orthop* 14:44, 2004.)

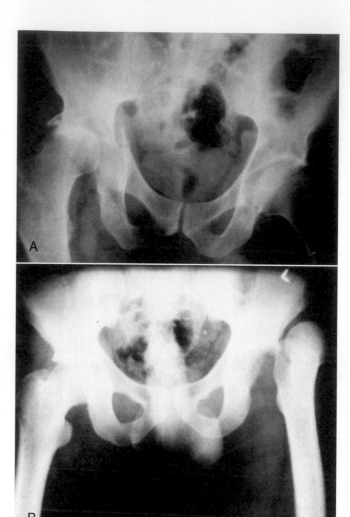

Fig. 11.134 Trauma to the hip. (A) Fractured right acetabulum. (B) Dislocated left femur.

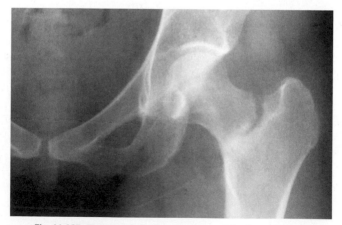

Fig. 11.135 Traction-type stress fracture of the femoral neck.

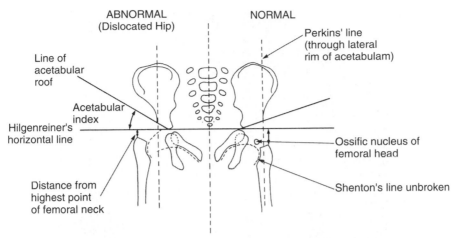

Fig. 11.136 Radiological findings in congenital dislocation of the hip compared with normal findings in a 12- to 15-month-old child. Acetabular index: normal = 30°, in newborn = 27.5°. If the ossific nucleus of the femoral head is present, it should sit in the inner lower quadrant.

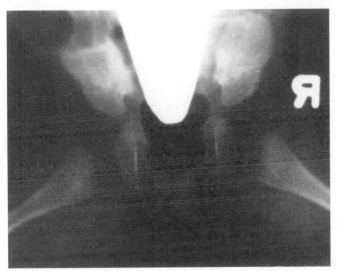

Fig. 11.137 Radiograph of the hip in the newborn. Ossification of the femoral head has not yet developed.

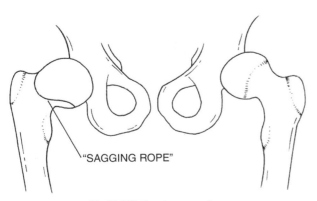

Fig. 11.138 Sagging rope sign.

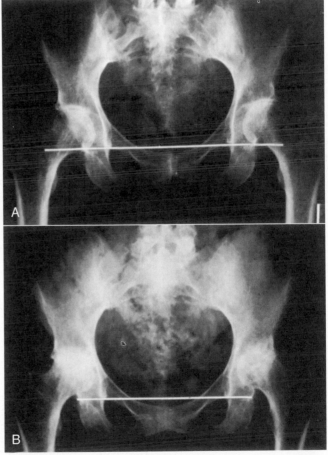

Fig. 11.139 Teardrop sign. (A) A line has been drawn between the tips of the two "teardrops" and extended into the femoral neck. Osteoarthritis of both hip joints appears to be equal, with equivalent narrowing of the joint space, but the left hip is already at a slightly higher level than the right in relation to the line. (B) Later, both hips have gradually moved upward as a result of loss of the bone at the apex of each femoral head. The left hip is now at a higher level than the right, confirming the original observation that the process of destruction in the left hip was more advanced. (From Greubel-Lee DM: *Disorders of the hip*, Philadelphia, 1983, JB Lippincott, pp 61, 146.)

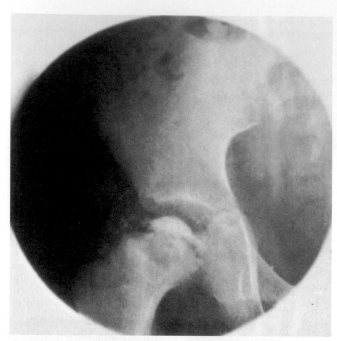

Fig. 11.140 All of the signs of the "head at risk" are present: lateral sub-luxation, abnormal direction of the growth plates, Cage sign, lateral calcification, and irregularity of the epiphysis. (From Greubel-Lee DM: *Disorders of the hip*, Philadelphia, 1983, JB Lippincott, p 146.)

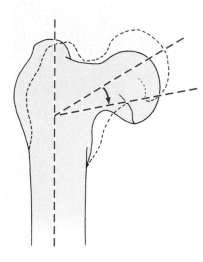

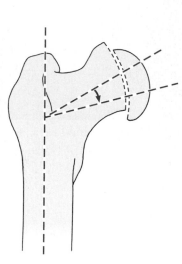

Congenital

Fracture

Slipped capital
femoral epiphysis

Fig. 11.141 Some causes of coxa vara.

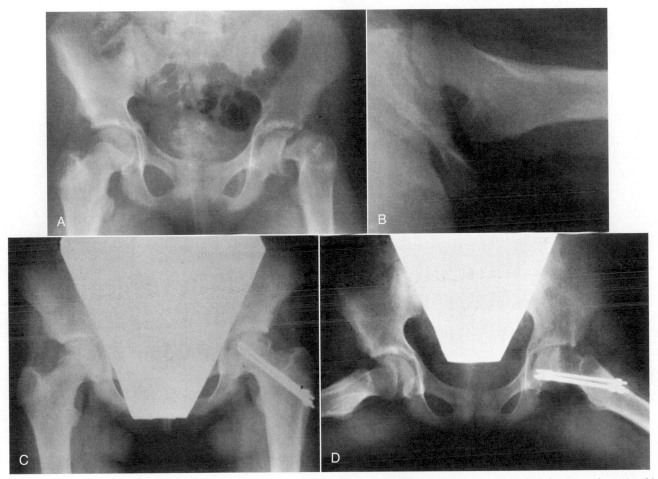

Fig. 11.142 Acute slipped femoral epiphysis in a 14-year-old boy. After a fall, the patient complained of severe pain in the left groin and anterior thigh and was unable to bear weight on the left lower limb. (A and B) Preoperative radiographs show the severe slip on the left. The patient was placed in bilateral split Russell traction with medial rotation straps on the left thigh and leg. Gradually, within a period of 3 to 4 days, the slip was reduced. (C and D) Postoperative radiographs approximately 6 months later show closure of epiphyseal plate and normal position of femoral head. The hip had full range of motion. (From Tachdjian MO: *Pediatric orthopedics*, Philadelphia, 1972, WB Saunders, p 470.)

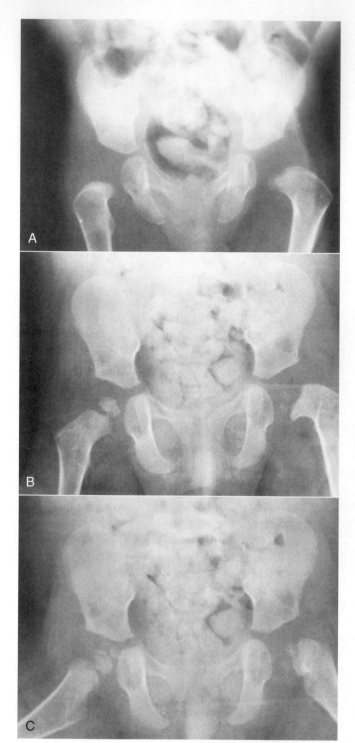

Fig. 11.143 Congenital coxa vara of the left hip in an infant. (A) Anteroposterior radiographs of both hips at 3 months of age, taken because of limited abduction of left hip and suspicion of congenital hip dislocation. It was interpreted to be normal. (B and C) Radiographs of the hips of same patient at 1 year of age when he started walking with a painless gluteus medius lurch on the left. Varus deformity of the left hip is evident. (From Tachdjian MO: *Pediatric orthopedics*, Philadelphia, 1972, WB Saunders, p 587.)

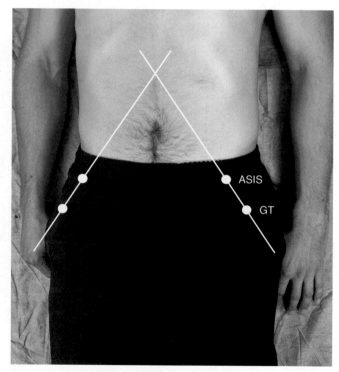

Fig. 11.144 Shoemaker's line. *ASIS,* Anterior superior iliac spine; *GT,* greater trochanter.

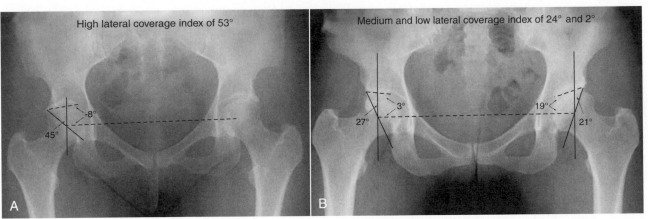

Fig. 11.145 Radiographic measurement examples for the lateral coverage index (LCI). (A) Example of high LCI (53°) composed of center-edge (CE) angle of 45° and acetabular inclination of –8°. (B) Example of medium and low LCI on the right and left hip, respectively. On the right hip, CE angle of 27° and acetabular inclination of 3° yield an LCI of 24°, whereas on the left hip, a CE angle of 21° and acetabular inclination of 19° yield a low LCI of 2°. (From Domb BG, Martin DE, Botser IB: Risk factors for ligamentum teres tears, *Arthroscopy* 29[1]:65, 2013.)

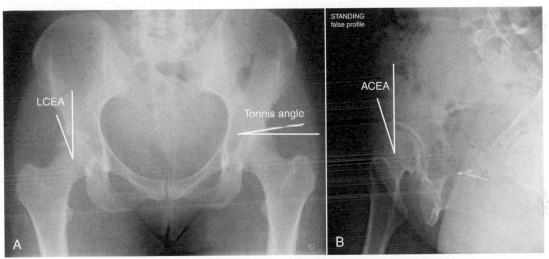

Fig. 11.146 (A) Evaluation of acetabular coverage starts with a well-rotated and tilted anteroposterior pelvic radiograph on which the lateral central edge angle *(LCEA)* and Tonnis angle are measured. (B) The anterior center edge angle *(ACEA)* is measured on a false profile radiograph. (From Dumont GD: Hip instability—current concepts and treatment options, *Clin Sport Med* 35[3]:435–447, 2016.)

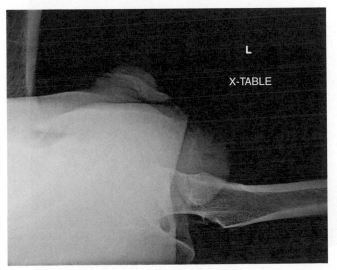

Fig. 11.147 Cross-table lateral view of the hip used to measure the head-neck offset ratio.

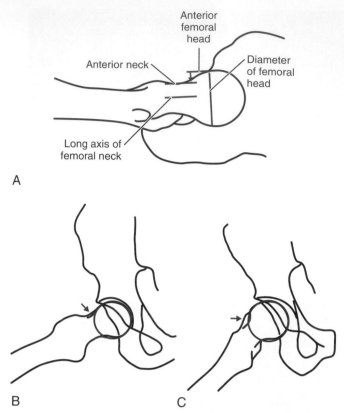

A

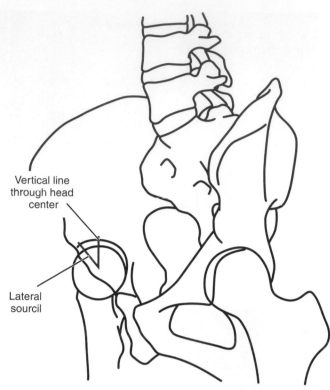

B   C

Fig. 11.148 (A) Tracing to show technique for calculating the head-neck offset ratio. Three parallel lines are drawn, with *line 1* passing through the center of the long axis of the femoral neck, *line 2* passing through the anteriormost aspect of the femoral neck, and *line 3* passing through the anteriormost aspect of the femoral head. The head-neck offset ratio is calculated by measuring the distance between *lines 2* and *3* and dividing by the diameter of the femoral head. (B) Moderate head-neck offset and/or mild cam impingement. (C) Anterolateral head-neck offset reduced.[345] (From Clohisy JC, Carlisle JC, Beaulé PE, et al: A systematic approach to the plain radiographic evaluation of the young adult hip, *J Bone Joint Surg Am* 90:47–66, 2008.)

Fig. 11.149 Tracing to show technique for calculating the anterior center-edge angle on a false-profile radiograph. A vertical line is drawn through the center of the femoral head. A second line is drawn through the center of the femoral head, passing through the most anterior point of the acetabular sourcil. The angle created by the intersection of these two lines is the anterior center-edge angle. Values of less than 20° can be indicative of structural instability.[345] (Clohisy JC, Carlisle JC, Beaulé PE, et al: A systematic approach to the plain radiographic evaluation of the young adult hip, *J Bone Joint Surg Am* 90:47–66, 2008.)

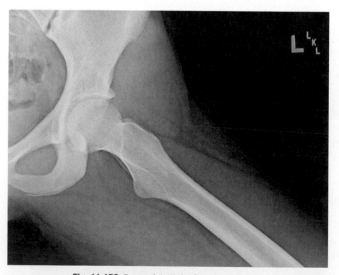

Fig. 11.150 Lateral (axial "frog-leg") view.

Arthrography

Although arthrograms are not routinely done on the hip, they may be done if the hip cannot be reduced following a dislocation (Fig. 11.151). The arthrogram may indicate a possible inverted limbus (infolding of a meniscus-like structure) or an hourglass configuration from a contracted capsule. It is also useful in CDH to show where the unossified femoral head lies relative to the labrum. A normal hip arthrogram is shown in Fig. 11.152.

Diagnostic Ultrasound Imaging

The hip is a large synovial joint that can have multiple pathologies, both intra- and extraarticular, that could be the cause of symptoms. A large and thick articular capsule and associated ligaments including the iliofemoral, ishiofemoral and pubofemoral that help provide joint stability. The femoral head is covered with hyaline articular cartilage, whereas the acetabulum is lined with the same cartilage and has a fibrocartilagenous labrum attached to the edge. Many of these structures can be visualized via ultrasonography.

Anterior Hip. The ultrasound examination of the hip begins anteriorly. An initial view can be performed with the patient supine. The transducer is placed in the long axis with the probe in line with the femoral neck. This position is slightly oblique to follow the neck (Fig. 11.153). The outline of the femoral head, neck, and acetabulum will be clearly seen. Just inferior to the head and anterior to the neck is the anterior joint recess, which may show swelling due to fluid or excessive synovial fluid due to synovitis and/ or inflammation of the joint capsule (Fig. 11.154). The joint space here should be symmetrical and not excessively large in any area along the anterior femur. Proximally, the labrum should appear hyperechoic and triangular. Turning the transducer to the transverse plane in the short axis (Fig. 11.155) allows the examiner to visualize the iliopsoas

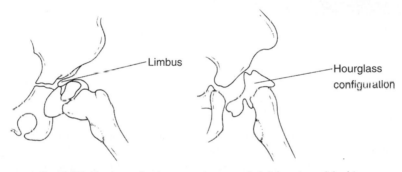

Fig. 11.151 Tracings of arthrograms in congenital dislocation of the hip.

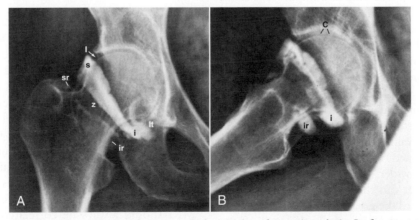

Fig. 11.152 Normal hip arthrogram. Normal examination after intra-articular injection of approximately 6 mL of contrast medium. (A) Anteroposterior view. (B) Frog-leg lateral views. *c*, Contrast agent outlining articular cartilage (recess capitis); *i*, inferior articular recess; *ir*, recess colli inferior; *1*, acetabular labrum; *lt*, defect on contrast from transverse ligament; *s*, superior articular recess; *sr*, recess colli superior; *z*, zona orbicularis (impression on the intra-articular contrast by the iliofemoral ischiofemoral ligaments of the hip joint capsule). (From Weissman BNW, Sledge CB: *Orthopedic radiology*, Philadelphia, 1986, WB Saunders, p 396.)

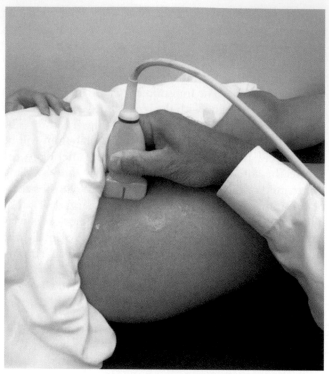

Fig. 11.153 Anterior hip long-axis transducer placement.

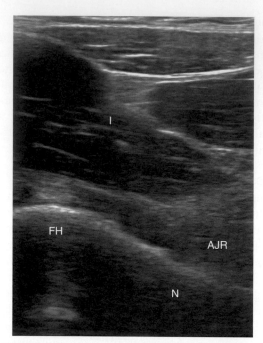

Fig. 11.154 Anterior hip long-axis view demonstrating hypoechoic hyaline cartilage over the femoral head *(FH)*, the femoral neck *(N)*, the anterior joint recess *(AJR)*, and the iliopsoas *(I)*.

superficially and the rounded femoral head underneath. Moving proximal to this in the inguinal region, the iliopsoas tendon, rectus femoris tendon, and femoral artery and nerve can be seen as well as the AIIS (Fig. 11.156).

Lateral Hip. To start the lateral hip ultrasound examination, the patient rolls onto the contralateral hip. The transducer is placed directly over the lateral hip to locate the lateral greater trochanter while in the short axis (Fig. 11.157). The apex of the greater trochanter is found to visualize the anterior and lateral facets (Fig. 11.158). The gluteus minimus rests above the anterior facet while the gluteus medius sits over the lateral facet. The transducer can be turned 90° to view these structures in the long axis. The transducer can then be placed over each of the facets—anterior and lateral. The gluteus minimus may be seen over the anterior facet and the gluteus medius over the lateral facet. Each should appear as a hyperechoic tendon as they run toward the greater trochanter.

Posterior Hip. The posterior hip ultrasound examination begins in the short axis evaluating the sacral foramen and the sacroiliac joint (see Chapter 10). The more superior portion of the sacroiliac joint is wider, whereas the inferior joint is narrower. The transducer can then be moved obliquely in the lateral direction toward the greater trochanter, where the piriformis can be viewed in the long axis. In this position, the tendon of the piriformis will be just above the bony outline of the ilium. The hip can be rotated to see passive movement of the piriformis tendon at this location.

Computed Tomography

CT scanning is useful in assessing abnormalities of the hip, especially bony ones.[251] In fact, CT and MR

arthrography (CT-A and MR-A) are the primary means of assessing intra-articular lesions of the hip.[30,275] For example, either one can be used to measure anteversion and retroversion, also showing the size and shape of the acetabulum and femoral head as well as the congruity and position of the femoral head relative to the acetabulum (Figs. 11.159 and 11.160). This technique can be used to assess FAI.[365] In newborns, however, the lack of ossification limits its use.

Magnetic Resonance Imaging[366]

MRI (Figs. 11.161 and 11.162) is a useful technique to study the hip because it is able to show soft tissue (e.g., labral lesions [Fig. 11.163], cartilage lesions, bursitis, ligamentous teres lesions, tendon lesions) as well as osseous tissue (e.g., osteonecrosis, femoral neck stress fractures) (Fig. 11.164).[47,275,367–370] This ability makes it an excellent technique to use for the study of congenital abnormalities. It is also the examination of choice for the evaluation of unexplained hip pain.[337] When combined with MR-A, it is often more sensitive to hip lesions but also produces more false positives.[371,372] Signs seen on MRI should always be correlated with clinical findings, as abnormal hip findings are common in asymptomatic patients.[373]

Scintigraphy (Bone Scan)

Bone scans may be used in the hip to help diagnose stress fractures (especially of femoral neck), necrosis, and tumors (Figs. 11.165 and 11.166).

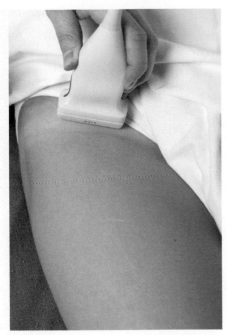

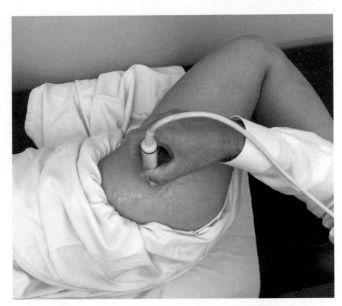

Fig. 11.157 Lateral hip view in short-axis transducer placement.

Fig. 11.155 Iliopsoas evaluation in short-axis transducer placement. (From Jacobson A: *Fundamentals of musculoskeletal ultrasound*, ed 2, Philadelphia, 2013, Elsevier, p 169.)

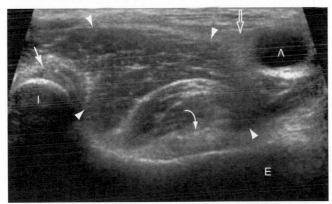

Fig. 11.156 Transverse image of iliopsoas demonstrating the iliopsoas tendon *(curved arrow)* and muscle *(arrowheads)*, rectus femoris direct head *(arrow)*, femoral artery *(A)*, and femoral nerve *(open arrow)*, iliopecineal eminence *(E)*, and anteroinferior iliac spine *(I)*. (From Jacobson A: *Fundamentals of musculoskeletal ultrasound*, ed 2, Philadelphia, 2013, Elsevier, p 169.)

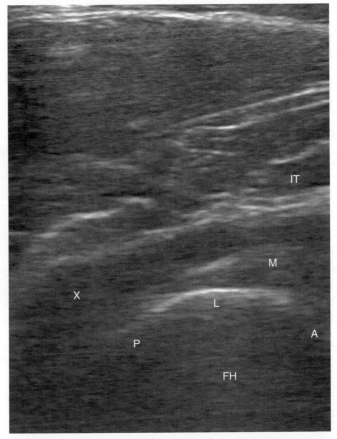

Fig. 11.158 Lateral view demonstrating the femoral head *(FH)*, posterior facet of greater trochanter *(P)*, lateral facet of greater trochanter *(L)*, anterior facet of greater trochanter *(A)*, gluteus medius *(M)*, gluteus maximus *(X)*, and iliotibial band *(IT)*.

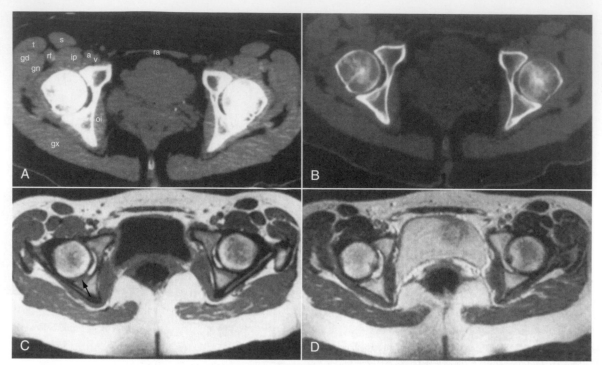

Fig. 11.159 (A) Normal computed tomography (CT) image at the level of the midacetabulum obtained with soft tissue window settings, showing the homogenous intermediate signal of musculature. *a,* Common femoral artery; *gd,* gluteus medius; *gn,* gluteus minimus; *gx,* gluteus maximus; *ip,* iliopsoas; *oi,* obturator internus; *ra,* rectus abdominis; *rf,* rectus femoris; *s,* sartorius; *t,* tensor fasciae latae; *v,* common femoral vein. (B) Axial CT at bone window settings reveals improved delineation of cortical and medullary osseous details. Note anterior and posterior semilunar acetabular articular surfaces and the central nonarticular acetabular fossa. (C) Normal midacetabular T1-weighted axial 0.4-T magnetic resonance image (MRI) (TR, 600 ms; TE, 20 ms) of a different patient shows a normal high-signal-intensity image of muscle and absence of signal in the cortical bone. The thin articular hyaline cartilage is of intermediate signal intensity *(arrow).* (D) T2-weighted MRI (TR, 2000 ms; TE, 80 ms) shows decreasing high-signal intensity in fatty marrow and subcutaneous tissue with increased signal intensity in the fluid-filled urinary bladder. (From Pitt MJ, Lund PJ, Speer DP: Imaging of the pelvis and hip, *Orthop Clin North Am* 21:553, 1990.)

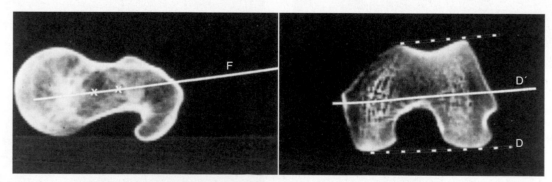

Fig. 11.160 Computed tomography for determining femoral anteversion (using a femoral specimen). The diacondylar line *(D)* is drawn along the condyles, although Hernandez and coworkers construct it *(D')* midway between the anterior and posterior femoral surfaces *(dashed lines).* The axis of the femoral neck *(F)* is shown. The angle between the femoral neck axis *(F)* and the diacondylar line is the angle of anteversion. In this case, there are 2° of retroversion. (From Weissman BNW, Sledge CB: *Orthopedic radiology,* Philadelphia, 1986, WB Saunders, p 399.)

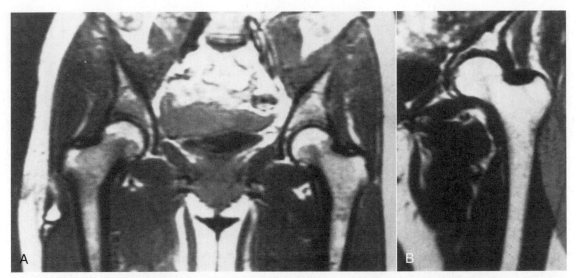

Fig. 11.161 (A) Normal magnetic resonance imaging scan of a young adult. Spin-echo T1-weighted image (600/25). Note the bright signal of fat in the region of the femoral epiphysis and the greater trochanter. The intermediate signal intensity in the femoral neck represents hemopoietic marrow. (B) Normal elderly woman with same imaging sequence shows replacement of hemopoietic marrow in the femoral neck by fatty marrow. (From Dalinka MK, Neustadter LM: Radiology of the hip. In Steinberg ME, editor: *The hip and its disorders*, Philadelphia, 1991, WB Saunders, p 68.)

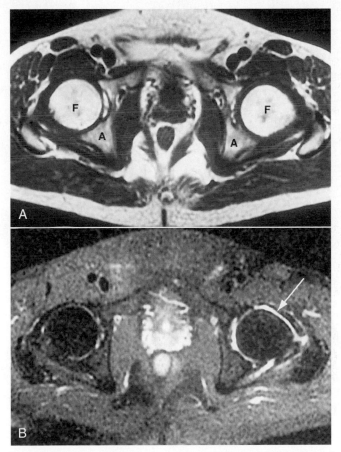

Fig. 11.162 Normal adult bone marrow. (A) Transaxial T1-weighted (TR/TE, 600/8) spin-echo magnetic resonance image (MRI) of the pelvis. Yellow marrow within the femoral heads *(F)* is isointense to subcutaneous fat. Red marrow within the acetabulae *(A)* has signal intensity between that of muscle and fat. (B) Transaxial fat-suppressed T2-weighted (TR/TEeff, 4000/60) fast spin-echo MRI. The signal intensity of both yellow and red marrow decreases. A small effusion is seen in the left hip *(arrow)*. (From Resnick D, Kransdorf MJ: *Bone and joint imaging*, Philadelphia, 2005, Elsevier, p 119.)

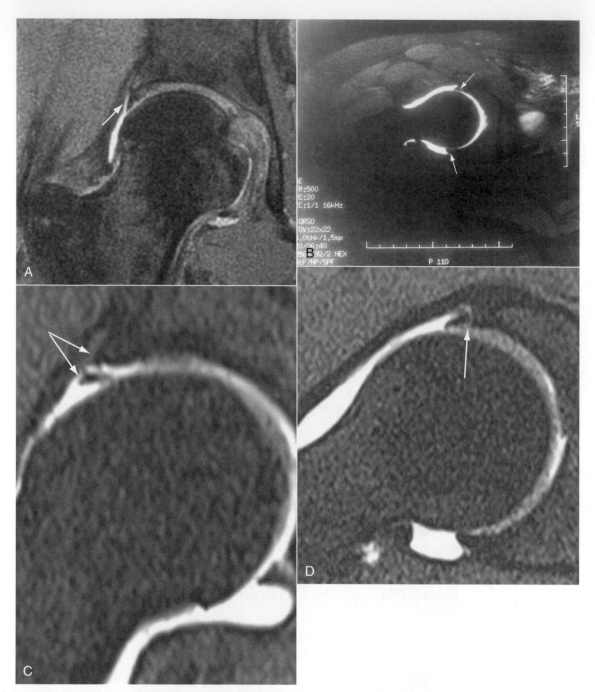

Fig. 11.163 Acetabular labral tears. (A) Normal hip. *Arrow* indicates the normal space (perilabral sulcus) between the capsule, lateral acetabular rim, and labrum. (B) Acetabular labral tear *(arrows)*. (C) Corneal T1 F5-weighted magnetic resonance image (MRI) shows longitudinal bucket handle–type tear with labral fragments *(arrows)*. (D) Oblique axial T1 F5-weighted MRI showing detachment *(arrow)* of the anterior labrum. (A, C, and D, From Patel K, Wallace R, Busconi BD, et al: Radiology, *Clin Sports Med* 30:241, 247, 2011. B, From DeLee J, Drez D, Miller MD: *DeLee and Drez's orthopaedic sports medicine*, ed 2, Philadelphia, 2003, WB Saunders.)

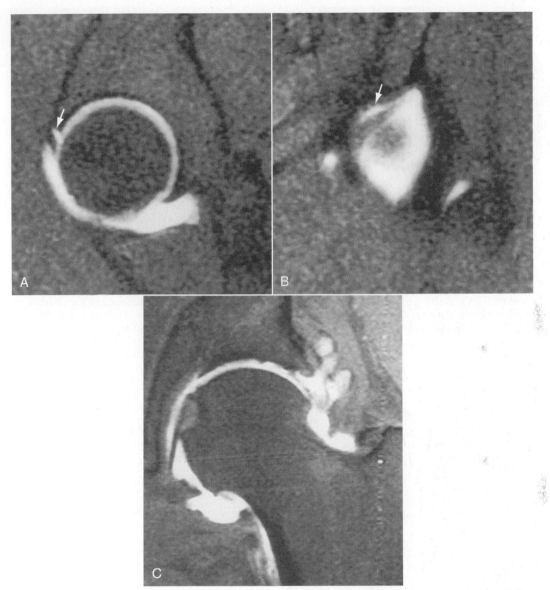

Fig. 11.164 Acetabular labrum: tear and cystic degeneration. (A and B) Partial detachment of the anterosuperior portion of the labrum *(arrows)* is seen on fat-suppressed sagittal (A) and coronal (B) T1-weighted (TR/TE, 600/16) spin-echo magnetic resonance (MR) arthrographic images. (C) In a different patient, a fat-suppressed coronal T1-weighted (TR/TE, 700/12) spin-echo MR arthrographic image demonstrates a massive superior labral tear with a perilabral ganglion cyst. (From Resnick D, Kransdorf MJ: *Bone and joint imaging*, Philadelphia, 2005, Elsevier. A and B, Courtesy J. Tomanek, MD, Johnson City, TN.)

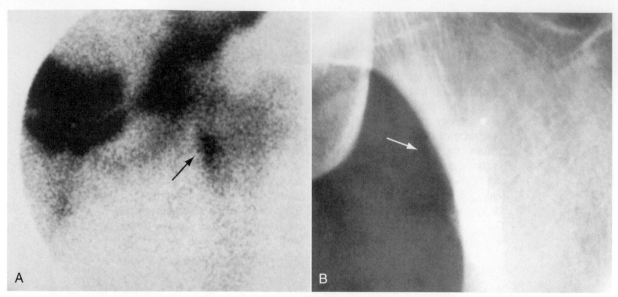

Fig. 11.165 Stress fracture. This athletic young woman complained of persistent hip pain aggravated by activity. (A) Radionuclide examination reveals a focal, sharply marginated area of increased activity in the femoral neck *(arrow)*. (B) Radiograph of the hip delineates a minimal amount of indistinct new bone formation along the medial aspect of the femoral neck *(arrow)*. (From Resnick D, Kransdorf MJ: *Bone and joint imaging*, Philadelphia, 2005, Elsevier, p 797.)

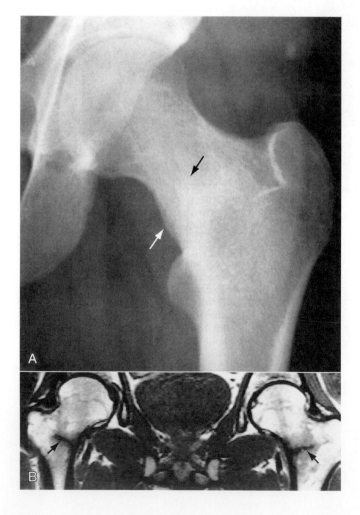

Fig. 11.166 Femoral neck stress fracture (compression type). (A) In the medial portion of the femoral neck, observe the presence of buttressing and sclerosis *(arrows)*. (B) Coronal intermediate-weighted (TR/TE, 2000/20) spin echo magnetic resonance image reveals bilateral fatigue fractures *(arrows)* in the medial portion of the femoral neck. The fracture itself and the surrounding marrow edema are of low signal intensity. (From Resnick D, Kransdorf MJ: *Bone and joint imaging*, Philadelphia, 2005, Elsevier, p 800.)

PRÉCIS OF THE HIP ASSESSMENT[a]

NOTE: Suspected pathology will determine which special tests are to be performed.

History

Observation

Examination

Functional assessment

Special tests (sitting)
  Hamstring syndrome test
  Pace's maneuver
  Seated piriformis stretch test
  Timed up-and-go (TUG) test

Special tests (standing)
  Long-stride heel-strike test
  Puranen-Orava test
  Trendelenburg test

Active movements (supine)
  Hip flexion
  Hip abduction
  Hip adduction
  Hip lateral rotation
  Hip medial rotation

Passive movements (supine), as in active movements (if necessary)

Resisted isometric movements (supine)
  Hip flexion
  Hip extension
  Hip adduction
  Hip abduction
  Hip medial rotation
  Hip lateral rotation
  Knee flexion
  Knee extension

Special tests (supine)
  Abduction/adduction contracture tests
  Adductor squeeze (fist) test
  Anterior apprehension test
  Anterior labral tear test
  Anteroposterior impingement test
  Bent-knee stretch test for proximal hamstrings
  Drehmann sign
  External de-rotation test
  Flexion-adduction test
  Flexion-internal rotation test
  Heel contra-lateral knee maneuver
  Heel-strike test
  Hip rotator tightness
  Hip scour test
  Impingement provocation test
  Internal rotation overpressure test
  Lateral rim impingement test
  Leg-length tests
  Ligamentum teres test
  Log roll test
  McCarthy hip extension sign

90-90 straight leg raising test
Noble compression test
Patellar-pubic percussion sign
Patrick's test
Posterior apprehension test
Posterior labral tear test
Posteroinferior impingement test
Rectus femoris test
THIRD test
Thomas test

Reflexes and cutaneous distribution (supine)
  Reflexes
  Sensory scan
  Peripheral nerves

Joint play movements (supine)
  Caudal glide
  Compression
  Lateral distraction
  Quadrant test

Palpation (supine)

Special tests (side lying)
  Abduction, extension and lateral rotation test
  Active piriformis stretch test
  Beatty's test
  "Gear stick" sign
  Hip lag sign
  Ischiofemoral impingement test
  Lateral FABER test
  Lateral FADDIR test
  Ober's test

Active movement (prone)
  Hip extension

Passive movement (prone)
  Hip extension

Resisted isometric movements (prone)
  Hip medial rotation (if not previously done)
  Hip lateral rotation (if not previously done)
  Knee flexion (if not previously done)
  Knee extension (if not previously done)

Special tests (prone)
  Ely's test
  External rotation test
  Femoral nerve tension test
  Freiberg's maneuver
  Prone external rotation test

Reflexes and cutaneous distribution (prone)

Palpation (prone)

Diagnostic imaging

After the rest of the examination is completed, the examiner can ask the patient to perform any appropriate additional functional tests.

After any examination, the patient should be warned of the possibility of exacerbation of symptoms as a result of the assessment.

[a]The précis is shown in an order that limits the amount of moving that the patient must do but ensures that all necessary structures are tested.

CASE STUDIES

When doing these case studies, the examiner should list the appropriate questions to be asked and why they are being asked, what to look for and why, and what things should be tested and why. Depending on the patient's answers (and the examiner should consider different responses), several possible causes of the patient's problem may become evident (examples are given in parentheses). A differential diagnosis chart (Table 11.23) should be made up. The examiner can then decide how different diagnoses may affect the treatment plan.

1. A 20-year-old female collegiate dancer comes to see you reporting onset of pain in the right hip 2 years earlier. She has continued to dance for the university dance team despite pain with activities such as walking, climbing and descending stairs, and squatting. She has clicking in her right hip, which is painful, or sometimes actually relieved of pain after it happens. She is unable to run because her pain becomes severe. Her pain is rated at 2/10 at rest and sometimes increases to 8/10 with activity. She is extremely flexible throughout her body. Hip strength is rated at 5/5 for most hip muscles except for hip flexion and extension, which are 4/5 and painful. Describe special tests that you would use to differentiate a labral tear from FAI.

2. A 64-year-old male is being seen 3 weeks following a left total hip replacement. During the first few weeks, he did really well with his recovery. His strength had improved. He was able to start ambulating without an assistive device. He reported that over the weekend, his hip started hurting more despite no real increase in activity. He feels as though it were swelling although there is no observable swelling. In the back of your mind, there is concern about infection. Describe some signs and symptoms that you would see in a patient following a total hip arthroplasty if a postsurgical infection had developed.

3. A 14-year-old boy was well until he fell from a chair onto his buttocks. He did not appear hurt, but 1 week later his parents brought him in for assessment because of a limp and pain in his right thigh and knee. The teenager is a tall, thin boy who prefers to walk with the right foot laterally rotated. Design your assessment plan for this patient (SCFE vs. ischial bursitis).

4. A 71-year-old woman had an Austin Moore prosthesis inserted into her left hip a day earlier, which has relieved the pain she had had in her hip. X-rays reveal that the prosthesis is solid. The surgeon has asked you to get the patient up and moving. Before doing this, however, you must do a bedside assessment. Outline how you would do the assessment.

5. His parents bring a 7-year-old boy in for assessment. He walks with a limp and has done so during the past 5 weeks at irregular times, the limp becoming more pronounced when the boy becomes tired. The boy also complains of a painful left knee. Describe your assessment plan for this patient (Legg-Calvé-Perthes disease vs. SCFE).

6. A 3-week-old girl is referred to you to be fitted with a Pavlik harness for CDH (i.e., DDH). Before you can fit the harness, you must do an assessment. Design your assessment plan for this patient.

7. A 55-year-old man complains of hip and back pain. There is some sciatica with pain into the groin, which is especially bad when he walks. He has a desk job but has been very active throughout his life. Describe your assessment plan for this patient (piriformis syndrome vs. lumbar spondylosis).

8. A 35-year-old woman complains of lateral hip pain. She states that she was in a motor vehicle accident 2 weeks earlier in which she was hit from the passenger side (she was driving) and her car was pushed against a telephone pole. She was wearing a seat belt. Describe your assessment plan for this patient (trochanteric bursitis vs. muscle contusion).

9. An 18-year-old man was surfing when he was thrown by a wave and hurt his hip. The hip is medially rotated and shortened. He has some sciatic pain. Describe your assessment plan for this patient (posterior hip dislocation vs. trochanteric fracture).

10. A 23-year-old female diver comes to you complaining of hip pain. She says it bothers her when she does any quick flexion of the hip. Describe your assessment plan for this patient (psoas bursitis vs. psoas strain).

TABLE **11.23**

Differential Diagnosis of Hip Pain

Diagnosis	Pain Characteristics	History/Risk Factors	Examination Findings	Additional Testing
Anterior Thigh Pain				
Meralgia paresthetica	Paresthesia, hypesthesia	Obesity, pregnancy, tight pants or belt, conditions with increased intra-abdominal pressure	Anterior thigh hypesthesia, dysesthesia	None
Anterior Groin Pain				
Athletic pubalgia (sports hernia)	Dull, diffuse pain radiating to inner thigh; pain with direct pressure, sneezing, sit-ups, kicking, Valsalva maneuver	Soccer, rugby, football, hockey players	No hernia, tenderness of the inguinal canal or pubic tubercle, adductor origin, pain with resisted sit-up or hip flexion	Radiography: no bony involvement MRI: can show tear or detachment of the rectus abdominis or adductor longus
Anterolateral Hip and Groin Pain ("C" Sign)				
Femoral neck fracture/stress fracture	Deep, referred pain; pain with weight bearing	Females (especially with female athlete triad), endurance athletes, low aerobic fitness, steroid use, smokers	Painful ROM, pain on palpation of greater trochanter	Radiography: cortical disruption MRI: early bony edema
Femoroacetabular impingement	Deep, referred pain; pain with standing after prolonged sitting	Pain with getting in and out of a car	FADDIR and FABER tests are sensitive	Radiography: cam or pincer deformity, acetabular retroversion, coxa profunda
Hip labral tear	Dull or sharp, referred pain; pain with weight bearing	Mechanical symptoms, such as catching or painful clicking; history of hip dislocation	Trendelenburg or antalgic gait, loss of internal rotation, positive FADDIR and FABER tests	MRI: can show a labral tear Magnetic resonance arthrography: offers added sensitivity and specificity
Iliopsoas bursitis (internal snapping hip)	Deep, referred pain; intermittent catching, snapping, or popping	Ballet dancers, runners	Snap with FABER to extension, adduction, and internal rotation; reproduction of snapping with extension of hip from flexed position	Radiography: no bony involvement MRI: bursitis and edema of the iliotibial band Ultrasonography: tendinopathy, bursitis, fluid around tendon Dynamic ultrasonography: snapping of iliopsoas or iliotibial band over greater trochanter
Legg-Calvé-Perthes disease	Deep, referred pain; pain with weight bearing	2–12 years of age, male predominance	Antalgic gait, limited ROM or stiffness	Radiography: early small femoral epiphysis, sclerosis and flattening of the femoral head
Loose bodies and chondral lesions	Deep, referred pain; painful clicking	Mechanical symptoms, history of hip dislocation or low-energy trauma, history of Legg-Calvé-Perthes disease	Limited ROM, catching and grinding with provocative maneuvers, positive FADDIR and FABER tests	Radiography: can show ossified or osteochondral loose bodies MRI: can detect chondral and fibrous loose bodies

TABLE **11.23**

Differential Diagnosis of Hip Pain—cont'd

Diagnosis	Pain Characteristics	History/Risk Factors	Examination Findings	Additional Testing
Osteoarthritis of the hip	Deep, aching pain and stiffness; pain with weight bearing	Older than 50 years, pain with activity that is relieved with rest	Medial rotation <15°, flexion <115°	Radiography: presence of osteophytes at the acetabular joint margin, asymmetrical joint-space narrowing, subchondral sclerosis and cyst formation
Osteonecrosis of the hip	Deep, referred pain; pain with weight bearing	Adults: Lupus, sickle cell disease, human immunodeficiency virus infection, corticosteroid use, smoking, and alcohol use; insidious onset, but can be acute with history of trauma	Pain on ambulation, positive log roll test, gradual limitation of ROM	Radiography: femoral head lucency and subchondral sclerosis, subchondral collapse (i.e., crescent sign), flattening of the femoral head MRI: bony edema, subchondral collapse
Slipped capital femoral epiphysis	Deep, referred pain; pain with weight bearing	11–14 years of age, overweight (80th–100th percentile)	Antalgic gait with foot externally rotated on occasion, positive log roll and straight leg raise against resistance tests, pain with hip internal rotation relieved with external rotation	Radiography: widened epiphysis early, slippage of femur under epiphysis later
Septic arthritis	Refusal to bear weight, pain with leg movement	Children: 3–8 years of age, fever, ill appearance Adults: Older than 80 years, diabetes mellitus, rheumatoid arthritis, recent joint surgery, hip or knee prostheses	Guarding against any ROM; pain with passive ROM	Hip aspiration guided by fluoroscopy, computed tomography, or ultrasonography; Gram stain and culture of joint aspirate MRI: useful for differentiating septic arthritis from transient synovitis
Transient synovitis	Refusal to bear weight	Children: 3–8 years of age, sometimes fever and ill appearance	Pain with extremes of ROM	
Lateral Pain				
External snapping hip[a]	Pain with direct pressure, radiation down lateral thigh, snapping or popping	All age groups, audible snap with ambulation	Positive Ober test, snap with Ober test, pain over greater trochanter	Radiography: no bony involvement MRI: bursitis and edema of the iliotibial band Ultrasonography: tendinopathy, bursitis, fluid around tendon
Greater trochanteric bursitis[a]	Pain with direct pressure, radiation down lateral thigh	Runners, middle-aged women	Pain over greater trochanter	Dynamic ultrasonography: snapping of iliopsoas or iliotibial band over greater trochanter
Greater trochanteric pain syndrome (GTPS)	Pain with direct pressure, radiation down lateral thigh	Associated with knee osteoarthritis, increased body mass index, low back pain; female predominance	Proximal iliotibial band tenderness, Trendelenburg gait is sensitive and specific	

TABLE **11.23**

Differential Diagnosis of Hip Pain—cont'd

Diagnosis	Pain Characteristics	History/Risk Factors	Examination Findings	Additional Testing
Posterolateral Pain				
Gluteal muscle tear or avulsion[a]	Pain with direct pressure, radiation down lateral thigh and buttock	Middle-aged women	Weak hip abduction, pain with resisted external rotation, Trendelenburg gait is sensitive and specific	MRI: gluteal muscle edema or tears
Iliac crest apophysis avulsion	Tenderness to direct palpation	History of direct trauma, skeletal immaturity (younger than 25 years)	Iliac crest tenderness and/or ecchymosis	Radiography: apophysis widening, soft tissue swelling around iliac crest
Posterior pain				
Hamstring muscle strain or avulsion	Buttock pain, pain with direct pressure	Eccentric muscle contraction while hip flexed and leg extended	Ischial tuberosity tenderness, ecchymosis, weakness to leg flexion, palpable gap in hamstring	Radiography: avulsion or strain of hamstring attachment to ischium
Ischial apophysis avulsion	Buttock pain, pain with direct pressure	Skeletal immaturity, eccentric muscle contraction (cutting, kicking, jumping)		MRI: hamstring edema and retraction
Ischiofemoral impingement	Buttock or back pain with posterior thigh radiation, sciatica symptoms	Groin and/or buttock pain that may radiate distally	None established	MRI: soft tissue edema around quadratus femoris muscle
Piriformis syndrome	Buttock pain with posterior thigh radiation, sciatica symptoms	History of direct trauma to buttock or pain with sitting, weakness and numbness are rare compared with lumbar radicular symptoms	Positive log roll test, tenderness over the sciatic notch	MRI: lumbar spine has no disc herniation, piriformis muscle atrophy or hypertrophy, edema surrounding the sciatic nerve
Sacroiliac joint dysfunction	Pain radiates to lumbar back, buttock, and groin	Female predominance, common in pregnancy, history of minor trauma	FABER test elicits posterior pain localized to the sacroiliac joint, sacroiliac joint line tenderness	Radiography: possibly no findings, narrowing and sclerotic changes of the sacroiliac joint space

From Wilson JJ, Furukawa M: Evaluation of the patient with hip pain, *Am Fam Physician* 89(1):27–34, 2014.
FABER, Flexion, abduction, external rotation; *FADDIR,* flexion, adduction, internal rotation; *MRI,* magnetic resonance imaging; *ROM,* range of motion.
[a]Conditions associated with greater trochanteric pain syndrome (GTPS).

References

1. Wang R, Bhandari M, Lachowski RJ. A systematic approach to adult hip pain. *Can J Diagnosis April.* 2001:109–120.
2. Uchida S, Utsunomiya H, Mori T, et al. Clinical and radiographic predictors for worsened clinical outcomes after hip arthroscopic labral preservation and capsular closure in developmental dysplasia of the hip. *Am J Sports Med.* 2015;44(1):28–38.
3. Martin HD, Kelly BT, Leunig M, et al. The pattern and technique in the clinical evaluation of the adult hip: the common physical examination tests of hip specialists. *Arthroscopy.* 2010;26(2):161–172.
4. Poulsen E, Overgaard S, Vestergaard JT, et al. Pain distribution in primary care patients with hip osteoarthritis. *Fam Pract.* 2016;33(6):601–606.
5. Brown MD, Gomez-Marin O, Brookfield KF, Stokes P. Differential diagnosis of hip disease versus spine disease. *Clin Orthop Relat Res.* 2004;419:280–284.
6. Reiman MP, Thorborg K. Clinical examination and physical assessment of hip joint-related pain in athletes. *Int J Sports Phys Ther.* 2014;9(6):737–755.
7. Lewis CL, Sahrmann SA. Acetabular labral tears. *Phys Ther.* 2006;86:110–121.
8. Huffman GR, Safran M. Tears of the acetabular labrum in athletes: diagnosis and treatment. *Sports Med Arthro Rev.* 2002;10:141–150.
9. Martin RL, Enseki KR, Draovitch P, et al. Acetabular labral tears of the hip: examination and diagnostic challenges. *J Orthop Sports Phys Ther.* 2006;36:503–515.
10. Cacchio A, Borra F, Severini G, et al. Reliability and validity of three pain provocation tests used for the diagnosis of chronic proximal hamstring tendinopathy. *Br J Sports Med.* 2012;46(12):883–887.
11. Shu B, Safran MR. Hip instability: anatomic and clinical considerations of traumatic and atraumatic instability. *Clin Sports Med.* 2011;30:349–367.
12. Wolff AB, Grossman J. Management of the acetabular labrum. *Clin Sports Med.* 2016;35(3):345–360.
13. Ejnisman L, Philippon MJ, Lertwanich P. Acetabular labral tears: diagnosis, repair, and a method for labral reconstruction. *Clin Sports Med.* 2011;30(2):317–329.
14. Dangin A, Tardy N, Wettstein M, et al. Microinstability of the hip: a review. *Orthop Traumatol Surg Res.* 2016;102(8S):S301–S309.
15. Lischuk AW, Dorantes TM, Wong W, Haims AH. Imaging of sports-related hip and groin injuries. *Sports Health.* 2010;2(3):252–261.
16. Tammareddi K, Morelli V, Reyes M. The athlete's hip and groin. *Prim Care.* 2013;40(2):313–333.
17. Blankenbaker DG, Tuite MJ. Acetabular labrum. *Magn Reson Imaging Clin N Am.* 2013;21(1):21–33.
18. Giordano BD. Assessment and treatment of hip pain in the adolescent athlete. *Pediatr Clin North Am.* 2014;61(6):1137–1154.
19. Reiman MP, Mather RC, Hash TW, Cook CE. Examination of acetabular labral tear: a continued diagnostic challenge. *Br J Sports Med.* 2014;48(4):311–319.
20. Safran MR. The acetabular labrum: anatomic and functional characteristics and rationale for surgical intervention. *J Am Acad Orthop Surg.* 2010;18:338–345.
21. Frechill MT, Safran MR. The labrum of the hip: diagnosis and rationale for surgical correction. *Clin Sports Med.* 2011;30(2):293–315.
22. Myers CA, Register BC, Lertwanich P, et al. Role of the acetabular labrum and the iliofemoral ligament in hip stability. *Am J Sports Med.* 2011;39(suppl 1):S85–S91.

23. Springer BA, Gill NW, Freedman BA, et al. Acetabular labral tears: diagnostic accuracy of clinical examination by a physical therapist, orthopaedic surgeon, and orthopaedic residents. *N Am J Sports Phys Ther.* 2009;4(1):38–45.
24. Bedi A, Dolan M, Leunig M, Kelly BT. Static and dynamic mechanical causes of hip pain. *Arthroscopy.* 2011;27(2):235–251.
25. Wenger DE, Kendall KR, Miner MR, Trousdale RT. Acetabular labral tears rarely occur in the absence of bony abnormalities. *Clin Orthop Relat Res.* 2004;426:145–150.
26. Logan ZS, Redmond JM, Spelsberg SC, et al. Chondral lesions of the hip. *Clin Sports Med.* 2016;35(3):361–372.
27. Cerezal L, Arnaiz J, Canga A. Emerging topics on the hip: ligamentum teres and hip microinstability. *Eur J Radiol.* 2012;81(12):3745–3754.
28. Bardakos NV, Villar RN. The ligamentum teres of the adult hip. *J Bone Joint Surg Br.* 2009;91(1):8–15.
29. Rao J, Zhou YZ, Villar RN. Injury to the ligamentum teres. Mechanism, findings, and results of treatment. *Clin Sports Med.* 2001;20(4):791–799.
30. Cerezal L, Kassarjian A, Canga A, et al. Anatomy, biomechanics, imaging and management of ligamentum teres injuries. *Radiographics.* 2010;30(6):1637–1651.
31. Botser IB, Martin DE, Stout CE, et al. Tears of the ligamentum teres—prevalence in hip arthroscopy using two classification systems. *Am J Sports Med.* 2011;39(suppl 1):S117–S125.
32. Domb BG, Martin DE, Botser IB. Risk factors for ligamentum teres tears. *Arthroscopy.* 2013;29(1):64–73.
33. de Sa D, Phillips M, Philippon MJ, et al. Ligamentum teres injuries at the hip: a systematic review examining surgical indications, treatment options, and outcomes. *Arthroscopy.* 2014;30(12):1634–1641.
34. O'Donnell JM, Devitt BM, Arora M. The role of the ligamentum teres in the adult hip: redundant or relevant? A Review. *J Hip Preservation Surg.* 2018;5(1):15–22.
35. Martin RL, McGovern RP, Martin HD, Kivlan BR. A mechanism for ligamentum teres injuries in femoroacetabular impingement: an anatomical study. *Int J Sports Phys Ther.* 2018;13(2):208–213.
36. Kalisvaart MM, Safran MR. Microinstability of the hip – it does exist: etiology, diagnosis and treatment. *J Hip Preserv Surg.* 2015;2(2):123–135.
37. Economopoulos K, O'Donnell J. Posterior bony impingement – potential mechanism of ligamentum teres tears. *Arthroscopy.* 2018;34(7):2123–2128.
38. Byrd JW, Jones KS. Traumatic rupture of the ligamentum teres as a source of hip pain. *Arthroscopy.* 2004;20(4):385–391.
39. Van Den Bogert AJ, Read L, Nigg BM. An analysis of hip joint loading during walking, running and skiing. *Med Sci Sports Exer.* 1999;31:131–142.
40. Byrd JW. Physical examination. In: Byrd JW, ed. *Operative Hip Arthroscopy.* 2nd ed. New York: Springer; 2005.
41. Domb BG, Brooks AG, Byrd JW. Clinical examination of the hip joint in athletes. *J Sports Rehabil.* 2009;18:3–23.
42. Byrd JW. Evaluation of the hip: history and physical examination. *N Am J Sports Phys Ther.* 2007;2(4):231–240.
43. Martin HD. Clinical examination of the hip. *Oper Techniques Orthop.* 2005;15(3):177–181.
44. Serner A, Tol JL, Jomaah N, et al. Diagnosis of acute groin injuries: a prospective study of 110 athletes. *Am J Sports Med.* 2015;43(8):1857–1864.

45. Serner A, Weir A, Tol JT, et al. Characteristics of acute groin injuries in the hip flexor muscles – a detailed MRI study in athletes. *Scand J Med Sci Sports.* 2018;28(2):677–685.
46. Bharam S. Labral tears, extra-articular injuries, and hip arthroscopy in the athlete. *Clin Sports Med.* 2006;25(2):279–292.
47. Gurney B, Boissonault WG, Andrews R. Differential diagnosis of a femoral neck/head stress fracture. *J Orthop Sports Phys Ther.* 2006;36:80–88.
48. Ramey LN, McInnis KC, Palmer WE. Femoral neck stress fracture: can MRI grade help predict return-to-running time? *Am J Sports Med.* 2016;44(8):2122–2129.
49. Boden BP, Osbahr DC. High-risk stress fractures: evaluation and treatment. *J Am Acad Orthop Surg.* 2000;8(6):344–353.
50. Dumont GD. Hip instability: current concepts and treatment options. *Clin Sport Med.* 2016;35(3):435–447.
51. Abrams GD, Luria A, Sampson J, et al. Decreased synovial inflammation in atraumatic hip microinstability compared with femoroactetabular impingement. *Arthroscopy.* 2017;33(3):553–558.
52. Battaglia PJ, D'Angelo K, Kettner NW. Posterior, lateral, and anterior hip pain due to musculoskeletal origin: a narrative literature review of history, physical examination, and diagnostic imaging. *J Chiropr Med.* 2016;15(4):281–293.
53. Tibor LM, Sekiya JK. Differential diagnosis of pain around the hip joint. *Arthroscopy.* 2008;24(12):1407–1421.
54. Schon L, Zuckerman JD. Hip pain in the elderly: evaluation and diagnosis. *Geriatrics.* 1988;43:48–62.
55. Thorborg K, Reiman MP, Weir A, et al. Clinical examination, diagnostic imaging, and testing of athletes with groin pain: an evidence-based approach to effective management. *J Orthop Sports Phys Ther.* 2018;48(4):239–249.
56. Byrd JW. Femoroacetabular impingement in athletes: current concepts. *Am J Sports Med.* 2013;42(3):737–751.
57. Fernandez E, Gastaldi P. Hip pain from the orthopedic point of view. *Eur J Radiol.* 2012;81(12):3737–3739.
58. Ward D, Parvizi J. Management of hip pain in young adults. *Orthop Clin North Am.* 2016;47(3):485–496.
59. Cheatham SW, Enseki KR, Kobler MJ. The clinical presentation of individuals with femoral acetabular impingement and labral tears: a narrative review of the evidence. *J Body Mov Ther.* 2016;20(2):346–355.
60. Wilson JJ, Furukawa M. Evaluation of the patient with hip pain. *Am Fam Physician.* 2014;89(1):27–34.
61. Plante M, Wallace R, Busconi BD. Clinical diagnosis of hip pain. *Clin Sports Med.* 2011;30:225–238.
62. Ombregt L: Clinical examination of the hip and buttock. In: Ombregt L, ed. *A System of Orthopaedic Medicine.* 3d ed. Elsevier; 2013. Available at www.orthopaedicmedicineonline.com.
63. Carro LP, Hernando MF, Cerezal L, et al. Deep gluteal space problems: piriformis syndrome, ischiofemoral impingement and sciatic nerve release. *Muscles Ligaments Tendons J.* 2016;6(3):384–396.
64. Rankin AT, Bleakly CM, Cullen M. Hip joint pathology as a leading cause of groin pain in the sporting population: a 6 year review of 894 cases. *Am J Sports Med.* 2015;43(7):1698–1703.
65. Martin HD, Kivlan BR, Palmer IJ, Martin RL. Diagnostic accuracy of clinical tests for sciatic nerve entrapment in the gluteal region. *Knee Surg Sports Traumatol Arthrosc.* 2014;22(4):882–888.
66. Hase T, Ueo T. Acetabular labral tear: arthroscopic diagnosis and treatment. *Arthroscopy.* 1999;15:138–141.

67. Mens J, Inklaar H, Koes BW, et al. A new view on adduction-related groin pain. *Clin J Sports Med.* 2006;16:15–19.

68. Minnich JM, Hanks JB, Muschaweck U, et al. Sports hernia—diagnosis and treatment highlighting a minimal repair surgical technique. *Am J Sports Med.* 2011;39:1341–1349.

69. Morales-Conde S, Socas M, Barranco A. Sportsman hernia: what do we know? *Hernia.* 2010;14:5–15.

70. Garvey JF, Read JW, Turner A. Sportsman hernia: what can we do? *Hernia.* 2010;14:17–25.

71. Litwin DE, Sneider EB, McEnaney PM, et al. Athletic pubalgia (sports hernia). *Clin Sports Med.* 2011;30:417–434.

72. Kagan A. Rotator cuff tears of the hip. *Clin Orthop Relat Res.* 1999;368:135–140.

73. Narvani AA, Tsiridis E, Kendall S, et al. A preliminary report on prevalence of acetabular labrum tears in sports patients with groin pain. *Knee Surg Sports Traumatol Arthrosc.* 2003;11:403–408.

74. Safran MR, Giordano G, Lindsey DP, et al. Strains across the acetabular labrum during hip motion—a cadaveric model. *Am J Sports Med.* 2011;39(suppl 1):S92–S102.

75. Prather H, Colorado B, Hunt D. Managing hip pain in the athlete. *Phys Med Rehabil Clin N Am.* 2014;25(4):789–812.

76. Hasan BA. The presenting symptoms, differential diagnosis, and physical examination of patients presenting with hip pain. *Dis Mon.* 2012;58(9):477–491.

77. Reid DC. *Sports Injury Assessment and Rehabilitation.* New York: Churchill Livingstone; 1992.

78. Allen WC. Coxa saltans: the snapping hip revisited. *J Am Acad Orthop Surg.* 1995;3:303–308.

79. Wahl CJ, Warren RF, Adler RS, et al. Internal coxa saltans (snapping hip) as a result of overtraining. *Am J Sports Med.* 2004;32:1302–1309.

80. Johnston CA, Wiley JP, Lindsay DM, et al. Iliopsoas bursitis and tendinitis: a review. *Sports Med.* 1998;25:271–283.

81. Philippon MJ, Devitt BM, Campbell KJ, et al. Anatomic variance of the iliopsoas tendon. *Am J Sports Med.* 2014;42(4):807–811.

82. Mellman MR, McPherson EJ, Dorr LD, et al. Differential diagnosis of back and lower extremity problems. In: Watkins RG, ed. *The Spine in Sport.* St Louis: CV Mosby; 1996.

83. Beckmann JT, Safran MR, Abrams GD. Extra-articular impingement: ischiofemoral impingement and trochanteric-pelvic. *Oper Techniques Sports Med.* 2015;23(3):184–189.

84. Sierra RJ, Trousdale RT, Ganz R, et al. Hip disease in the young active patient: evaluation and nonarthroplasty surgical options. *J Am Acad Orthop Surg.* 2008;16:689–703.

85. Fitzgerald RH. Acetabular labrum tears—diagnosis and treatment. *Clin Orthop Relat Res.* 1995;311:60–68.

86. Dorrell JH, Catterall A. The torn acetabular labrum. *J Bone Joint Surg Br.* 1986;68:400–403.

87. Rashleigh-Belcher HJ, Cannon SR. Recurrent dislocation of the hip with a "Bankart type" lesion. *J Bone Joint Surg Br.* 1986;68:398–399.

88. Altman R, Alarcon G, Appelrouth D, et al. The American College of Rheumatology criteria for the classification and reporting of osteoarthritis of the hip. *Arth Rheum.* 1991;34:505–514.

89. Reiman MP, Mather RC, Cook CE. Physical examination tests for hip dysfunction and injury. *Br J Sports Med.* 2015;49(6):357–361.

90. Janda V. On the concept of postural muscles and posture in man. *Aust J Physiother.* 1983;29:83–85.

91. Jull JA, Janda V. Muscles and motor control in low back pain: Assessment and management. In: Twomey LT, Taylor JR, eds. *Physical Therapy of the Low Back.* New York: Churchill Livingstone; 1987.

92. Martin HD, Palmer IJ. History and physical examination of the hip: the basics. *Curr Rev Musculoskelet Med.* 2013;6(3):219–225.

93. Domb BG, Brooks AG, Guanche CA. Physical examination of the hip. In: Guanche CA, ed. *Hip and Pelvis Injuries in Sports Medicine.* Philadelphia: Lippincott Williams & Wilkins; 2010.

94. Braly BA, Beall DP, Martin HD. Clinical examination of the athletic hip. *Clin Sports Med.* 2006;25:199–210.

95. Saudek CE. The hip. In: Gould JA, ed. *Orthopedic and Sports Physical Therapy.* St Louis: CV Mosby; 1990.

96. Krebs DE, Robbins CE, Lavine L, et al. Hip biomechanics during gait. *J Orthop Sports Phys Ther.* 1998;28:51–59.

97. Brand RA, Crowninshield RD. The effect of cane use on hip contact force. *Clin Orthop.* 1980;147:181–184.

98. Aspinall W. Clinical implications of iliopsoas dysfunction. *J Man Manip Ther.* 1993;1:41–46.

99. Ross JR, Nepple JJ, Philippon MJ, et al. Effect of changes in pelvic tilt on range of motion to impingement and radiographic parameters of acetabular morphologic characteristics. *Am J Sports Med.* 2014;42(10):2402–2409.

100. Johansson AC, Karlsson H. The Star Excursion Balance Test: criterion and divergent validity on patients with femoral acetabular impingement. *Man Ther.* 2016;26:104–109.

101. Gonell AC, Romero JA, Soler LM. Relationship between the Y balance test scores and soft tissue injury incidence in a soccer team. *Int J Sports Phys Ther.* 2015;10(7):955–966.

102. Smith CA, Chimera NJ, Warren M. Association of Y balance test reach asymmetry and injury in Division 1 athletes. *Med Sci Sports Exerc.* 2015;47(1):136–141.

103. Sauers EL, Huxel Bliven KC, Johnson MP, et al. Hip and glenohumeral rotational range of motion in healthy professional baseball pitchers and position players. *Am J Sports Med.* 2013;42(2):430–436.

104. Thomson C, Krouwel O, Kuisma R, Hebron C. The outcome of hip exercise in patellofemoral pain: a systematic review. *Man Ther.* 2016;26:1–30.

105. Tan LA, Benkli B, Tuchman A, et al. High prevalence of greater trochanteric pain syndrome among patients presenting to a spine clinic for evaluation of degenerative lumbar pathologies. *J Clin Neurosci.* 2018;53:89–91.

106. Kemp JL, Schache AG, Makdissi M, et al. Greater understanding of normal hip physical function may guide clinicians in providing targeted rehabilitation programmes. *J Sci Med Sport.* 2013;16(4):292–296.

107. Poultsides LA, Bedi A, Kelly BT. An algorithmic approach to mechanical hip pain. *HSS J.* 2012;8(3):213–224.

108. Draovitch P, Edelstein J, Kelly BT. The layer concept: utilization in determining the pain generators, pathology and how structure determines treatment. *Curr Rev Musculoskelet Med.* 2012;5(1):1–8.

109. Ombregt L, Bissehop P, ter Veer HJ, et al. *A System of Orthopedic Medicine.* London: WB Saunders; 1995.

110. Ito K, Minka MA, Leunig M, et al. Femoroacetabular impingement and the cam-effect—a MRI-based quantitative anatomical study of the femoral head-neck offset. *J Bone Joint Surg Br.* 2001;83:171–176.

111. Leunig M, Werlen S, Ungersbock A, et al. Evaluation of the acetabular labrum by MR arthrography. *J Bone Joint Surg Br.* 1997;79:230–234.

112. Klaue K, Durnin CW, Ganz R. The acetabular rim syndrome-a clinical presentation of dysplasia of the hip. *J Bone Joint Surg Br.* 1991;73:423–429.

113. Crawford JR, Villar RN. Current concepts in the management of femoroacetabular impingement. *J Bone Joint Surg Br.* 2005;87:1459–1462.

114. Ferguson TA, Matta J. Anterior femoroacetabular impingement: a clinical presentation. *Sports Med Arthro Rev.* 2002;10:134–140.

115. Santori N, Villar RN. Acetabular labral tears: result of arthroscopic partial limbectomy. *Arthroscopy.* 2000;16:11–15.

116. Philippon MJ, Maxwell RB, Johnson TL, et al. Clinical presentation of femoroacetabular impingement. *Knee Surg Sports Traumatol Arthrosc.* 2007;15:1041–1047.

117. Yuan BJ, Bartelt RB, Levy BA, et al. Decreased range of motion is associated with structural hip deformity in asymptomatic adolescent athletes. *Am J Sports Med.* 2013;41(7):1519–1525.

118. Reaulé PE, O'Neill M, Rakhra K. Acetabular labral tears. *J Bone Joint Surg Am.* 2009;91:701–710.

119. Mosler AB, Crossley KM, Waarsing JH, et al. Ethnic differences in bony hip morphology in a cohort of 445 professional male soccer players. *Am J Sports Med.* 2016;44(11):2967–2974.

120. Ganz R, Parvizi J, Beck M, et al. Femoroacetabular impingement—a case for osteoarthritis of the hip. *Clin Orthop Relat Res.* 2003;417:112–120.

121. Zaragoza EJ, Beaulé PE. Imaging of the painful nonarthritic hip: a practical approach to surgical relevancy. *Oper Tech Orthop.* 2004;14:42–48.

122. Reynolds D, Lucas J, Klaue K. Retroversion of the acetabulum. *J Bone Joint Surg Br.* 1999;81:281–288.

123. Beck M, Kalhor M, Leung M, et al. Hip morphology influences the pattern of damage to the acetabular cartilage—femoroacetabular impingement as a cause of early osteoarthritis of the hip. *J Bone Joint Surg Br.* 2005;87:1012–1018.

124. Parvizi J, Leung M, Ganz R. Femoroacetabular impingement. *J Am Acad Orthop Surg.* 2007;15:561–570.

125. Ejnisman L, Philippon MJ, Lertwanich P. Femoroacetabular impingement: the femoral side. *Clin Sports Med.* 2011;30:369–377.

126. Byrd JW, Jones KS, Gwathmey FW. Femoroacetabular impingement in adolescent athletes: outcomes of arthroscopic management. *Am J Sports Med.* 2016; 44(8):2106–2111.

127. Khanna V, Caragianis A, Diprimio G, et al. Incidence of hip pain in a prospective cohort of asymptomatic volunteers: is the cam deformity a risk factor for hip pain? *Am J Sports Med.* 2014;42(4):793–797.

128. Agricola R, Heijboer MP, Ginai AZ, et al. A cam deformity is gradually acquired during skeletal maturation in adolescent and young male soccer players: a prospective study with minimum 2-year follow-up. *Am J Sports Med.* 2014;42(4):798–806.

129. Nepple JJ, Vigdorchik JM, Clohisy JC. What is the association between sports participation and the development of proximal femoral cam deformity? A systematic review and meta-analysis. *Am J Sports Med.* 2015;43(11):2833–2840.

130. Pacheco-Carrillo A, Medina-Porqueres I. Physical examination tests for the diagnosis of femoroacetabular impingement. A systematic review. *Phys Ther Sport.* 2016;21:87–93.

131. Wright AA, Naze GS, Kavchak AE, et al. Radiological variables associated with progression of femoroacetabular impingement of the hip: a systematic review. *J Sci Med Sport.* 2015;18(2):122–127.

132. Cross MB, Fabricant PD, Maak TG, Kelly BT. Impingement (acetabular side). *Clin Sports Med.* 2011;30(2):379–390.

133. Byrd JW, Jones KS. Arthroscopic femoroplasty in the management of cam-type femoroacetabular impingement. *Clin Orthop Relat Res.* 2009;467(3):739–746.

134. van Klij P, Heerey J, Waarsing JH, Agricola R. The prevalence of Cam and Pincer morphology and its association with development of hip osteoarthritis. *J Orthop Sports Phys Ther.* 2018;48(4):230–238.

135. Tibor LM, Leung M. The pathoanatomy and arthroscopic management of femoroacetabular impingement. *Bone Joint Res.* 2012;1(10):245–257.

136. Allen D, Beaulé PE, Ramadan D, et al. Prevalence of associated deformities and hip pain with cam-type femoroacetabular impingement. *J Bone Joint Surg Br.* 2009;91:589–594.

137. Canham CD, Yen YM, Giordano BD. Does femoroacetabular impingement cause hip instability? A systematic review. *Arthroscopy.* 2016; 32(1):203–208.

138. Anderson SE, Siebenrock KA, Tannast M. Femoroacetabular impingement. *Eur J Radiol.* 2012;81 (12):3740–3744.

139. Hendry D, England E, Kenter K, Wissman RD. Femoral acetabular impingement. *Semin Roentgenol.* 2013;48(2):158–166.

140. Birmingham PM, Kelly BT, Jacobs R, et al. The effect of dynamic femoroacetabular impingement on pubic symphysis motion—a cadaveric study. *Am J Sports Med.* 2012;40:1113–1118.

141. Beaulé PE, Allen DJ, Clohisy JC, et al. The young adult with hip impingement: deciding on the optimal intervention. *J Bone Joint Surg Am.* 2009;91:210–221.

142. Siebenrock KA, Schoeniger R, Ganz R. Anterior femoro-acetabular impingement due to acetabular retroversion—treatment with periacetabular osteotomy. *J Bone Joint Surg Am.* 2003;85:278–286.

143. Byrd JW, Jones KS. Arthroscopic management of femoroacetabular impingement in athletes. *Am J Sports Med.* 2011;39(suppl 1):S7–S13.

144. Audenaert EA, Peeters I, Vigneron L, et al. Hip morphology characteristics and range of internal rotation in femoroacetabular impingement. *Am J Sports Med.* 2012;40:1329–1336.

145. Matsuda DK, Schnieder CP, Sehgal B. The critical corner of cam femoroacetabular impingement: clinical support of an emerging concept. *Arthroscopy.* 2014;30(5):575–580.

146. Whiteside D, Deneweth JM, Bedi A, et al. Femoroacetabular impingement in elite ice hockey goaltenders: etiological implications of on-ice hip mechanics. *Am J Sports Med.* 2015;43(7):1689–1697.

147. Harris JD, Gerrie BJ, Varner KE, et al. Radiographic prevalence of dysplasia, cam and pincer deformities in elite ballet. *Am J Sports Med.* 2016;44(1):20–27.

148. Lerebours F, Robertson W, Neri B, et al. Prevalence of cam-type morphology in elite ice hockey players. *Am J Sports Med.* 2016;44(4):1024–1030.

149. Bardakosa NV. Hip impingement: beyond femoroacetabular. *J Hip Preserv Surg.* 2015;2(3):206–223.

150. Domb BG, Shindle MK, McArthur B, et al. Iliopsoas impingement: a newly identified cause of labral pathology in the hip. *Hosp Special Surg J.* 2011;7: 145–150.

151. Tey M, Alvarez S, Rios JL. Hip labral cyst caused by psoas impingement. *Arthroscopy.* 2012;28(8):1184–1186.

152. Gollwitzer H, Banke IJ, Schauwecker J, et al. How to address ischiofemoral impingement? Treatment algorithm and review of the literature. *J Hip Preserv Surg.* 2017;4(4):289–298.

153. Safran M, Ryu J. Ischiofemoral impingement of the hip: a novel approach to treatment. *Knee Surg Sports Traumatol Arthrosc.* 2014;22(4):781–785.

154. Kivlan BR, Martin RL, Martin HD. Ischiofemoral impingement: defining the lesser trochanter-ischial space. *Knee Surg Sports Traumatol Arthrosc.* 2017;25(1):72–76.

155. Taneja AK, Bredella MA, Torriani M. Ischiofemoral impingement. *Magn reson imaging. Clin N Am.* 2013;21(1):65–73.

156. Singer AD, Subhawong TK, Jose J, et al. Ischiofemoral impingement syndrome: a meta-analysis. *Skeletal Radiol.* 2015;44(6):831–837.

157. Gomez-Hoyos J, Khoury A, Schroder R, et al. The hip-spine effect: a biomechanical study of ischiofemoral impingement effect on lumbar facet joints. *Arthroscopy.* 2017;33(1):101–107.

158. Lee S, Kim I, Lee SM, Lee J. Ischiofemoral impingement syndrome. *Ann Rehabil Med.* 2013;37(1):143–146.

159. Gomes-Hoyos J, Schroder R, Reddy M, et al. Femoral neck anteversion and lesser trochanteric retroversion in patients with ischiofemoral impingement: a case-control magnetic resonance imaging study. *Arthroscopy.* 2016;32(1):13–18.

160. Migliorini S, Merlo M. The hamstring syndrome in endurance athletes. *Br J Sports Med.* 2011;45(4):363.

161. Mittal G, Parry J, Saifuddin A. Atypical hip pain: is it ischiofemoral impingement? *Rheumatology.* 2015;54(suppl 1):i182.

162. Martin HD, Khoury A, Schroder R, Palmer IJ. Ischiofemoral impingement and hamstring syndrome as causes of posterior hip pain: where do we go next? *Clin Sports Med.* 2016;35(3):469–486.

163. Hatem MA, Palmer IJ, Martin HD. Diagnosis and 2-year outcomes of endoscopic treatment for ischiofemoral impingement. *Arthroscopy.* 2015;31(2):239–246.

164. Matsuda DK. Editorial commentary: proximal hamstring syndrome: another pain in the buttock. *Arthroscopy.* 2018;34(1):122–125.

165. Martin HD, Reddy M, Gomez-Hoyos J. Deep gluteal syndrome. *J Hip Preserv Surg.* 2015;2(2):99–107.

166. Puranen J, Orava S. The hamstring syndrome. A new diagnosis of gluteal sciatic pain. *Am J Sports Med.* 1988;16(5):517–521.

167. Comez-Hoyos J, Martin RL, Martin HD. Current concepts review: evaluation and management of posterior hip pain. *J Am Acad Orthop Surg.* 2018;26(17):597–609.

168. Davis AM, Bridge P, Miller J, et al. Interrater and intrarater reliability of the active hip abduction test. *J Orthop Sports Phys Ther.* 2011;41:953–960.

169. Simoneau GG, Hoenig KJ, Lepley JE, et al. Influence of hip position and gender on active hip internal and external rotation. *J Orthop Sports Phys Ther.* 1998;28:158–164.

170. Malliaras P, Hogan A, Nowrocki A, et al. Hip flexibility and strength measures: reliability and association with athletic groin pain. *Br J Sports Med.* 2009;43(10):739–744.

171. Klaue K, Durnin CW, Ganz R. The acetabular rim syndrome: a clinical presentation of dysplasia of the hip. *J Bone Joint Surg Br.* 1991;73:423–429.

172. Jackson SM, Cheng MS, Smith AR, Kolber MJ. Intrarater reliability of hand held dynamometer in measuring lower extremity isometric strength using a portable stabilization device. *Musculoskelet Sci Pract.* 2017;27:137–141.

173. Ward SR, Winters TM, Blemken SS. The architectural design of the gluteal muscle group: implications for movement and rehabilitation. *J Orthop Sports Phys Ther.* 2010;40:95–102.

174. Neuman DA. Kinesiology of the hip: a focus on muscular actions. *J Orthop Sports Phys Ther.* 2010;40:83–94.

175. Delahunt E, Kennelly C, McEntee BL, et al. The high adductor squeeze test: 45° of hip flexion as the optimal test position for eliciting adductor muscle activity and maximum pressure values. *Manual Therapy.* 2011;16:476–480.

176. Delahunt E, McEntee BL, Kennelly C, et al. Intrarater reliability of the adductor squeeze test in Gaelic Games athletes. *J Athl Train.* 2011;46(3):241–245.

177. Nevin F, Delahunt E. Adductor squeeze test values and hip joint range of motion in Gaelic football athletes with longstanding groin pain. *J Sci Med Sport.* 2014;17(2):155–159.

178. Hodgson L, Hignett T, Edwards K. Normative adductor squeeze test scores in rugby. *Phys Ther Sport.* 2015;16(2):93–97.

179. Boren K, Conrey C, Le Coguic J, et al. Electromyographic analysis of gluteus medius and gluteus maximus during rehabilitation exercises. *Int J Sports Phys Ther.* 2011;6(3):206–223.

180. Almeida GP, das Neves Rodrigues HL, de Freitas BW, de Paula Lima PO. Reliability and validity of the hip stability isometric test (HipSIT): a new method to assess hip posterolateral muscle strength. *J Orthop Sports Phys Ther.* 2017;47(12):906–913.

181. Fredericson M, Moore W, Guillet M, et al. High hamstring tendinopathy in runners. *Phys Sportsmed.* 2005;33:32–43.

182. Tis LL, Perrin DH, Snead DB, et al. Isokinetic strength of the trunk and hip in female runners. *Isok Exerc Sci.* 1991;1:22–25.

183. Donatelli R, Catlin PA, Backer GS, et al. Isokinetic hip abductor to adductor torque ratio in normals. *Isok Exerc Sci.* 1991;1:103–111.

184. D'Aubigné RM, Postel M. Functional results of hip arthroplasty with acrylic prosthesis. *J Bone Joint Surg Am.* 1954;36:451–475.

185. Murray D. The hip. In: Pynsent P, Fairbank J, Carr A, eds. *Outcome Measures in Orthopedics.* Oxford: Butterworth Heinemann; 1994.

186. Harris WH. Traumatic arthritis of the hip after dislocation and acetabular fractures: treatment by mold arthroplasty. An end result study using a new method of result evaluation. *J Bone Joint Surg Am.* 1969;51:737–755.

187. Kavanagh BF, Fitzgerald RH. Clinical and roentgenographic assessment of total hip arthroplasty: a new hip score. *Clin Orthop.* 1985;193:133–140.

188. Johanson NA, Charlson ME, Szatrowski TP, et al. A self-administered hip-rating questionnaire for the assessment of outcome after total hip replacement. *J Bone Joint Surg Am.* 1992;74:587–597.

189. Burton KE, Wright V, Richards J. Patients' expectations in relation to outcome of total hip replacement surgery. *Ann Rheum Dis.* 1979;38:471–474.

190. Jaglal S, Lakhani Z, Schatzker J. Reliability, validity, and responsiveness of the lower extremity measure for patients with a hip fracture. *J Bone Joint Surg Am.* 2000;82:955–962.

191. Tijssen M, van Cingel R, van Melick N, de Visser E. Patient-reported outcome questionnaires for hip arthroscopy: a systematic review of psychometric evidence. *BMC Musculoskelet Disord.* 2011;12:117–125.

192. Lodhia P, Slobogean GP, Noonan VK, Gilbart MK. Patient-reported outcome instruments for femoroacetabular impingement and hip labral pathology: a systematic review of the clinimetric evidence. *Arthroscopy.* 2011;27(2):279–286.

193. Fearon AM, Ganderton C, Scarvell JM, et al. Development and validation of a VISA tendinopathy questionnaire for greater trochanteric pain syndrome, the VISA–G. *Man Ther.* 2015;20(6):805–813.

194. Jogi P, Spaulding SJ, Zecevic AA, et al. Comparison of the original and reduced versions of the Berg Balance Scale and the Western Ontario and McMaster Universities Osteoarthritis Index in patients following hip or knee arthroplasty. *Physiother Can.* 2011;63:107–114.

195. McConnell S, Kolopack P, Park AM. The Western Ontario and McMaster Universities Osteoarthritis Index (WOMAC): a review of its utility and measurement properties. *Arth Rheum.* 2001;45:453–461.

196. Jogi P, Kraemer JF, Birmingham T. Comparison of the Western Ontario and McMaster Universities Osteoarthritis Index (WOMAC) and the Lower Extremity Functional Scale (LEFS) questionnaires in patients awaiting or having undergone total knee arthroplasty. *Physiother Can.* 2005;57:208–216.

197. Jones CA, Voaklander DC, Johnston DW, et al. The effect of age on pain, function, and quality of life after total hip and knee arthroplasty. *Arch Intern Med.* 2001;161(3):454–460.

198. Bellamy N, Buchanan WW, Goldsmith CH, et al. Validation study of WOMAC: a health status instrument for measuring clinically important patient relevant outcomes to antirheumatic drug therapy in patients with osteoarthritis of the hip or knee. *J Rheumatol.* 1988;15(12):1833–1840.

199. Jones CA, Voaklander DC, Johnston DW, et al. Health related quality of life outcomes after total hip and knee arthroplasties in a community based population. *J Rheumatol.* 2000;27:1745–1752.

200. Stratford PW, Binkley JM, Watson J, et al. Validation of the LEFS on patients with total joint arthroplasty. *Physiother Can.* 2000;52:97–105.

201. Binkley JM, Stratford PW, Lott SA, et al. The lower extremity functional scale (LEFS): scale development, measurement properties, and clinical application. *Physical Therapy.* 1999;79:371–383.

202. Yeung TS, Wessel J, Stratford P, et al. Reliability, validity and responsiveness of the lower extremity functional scale for inpatients of an orthopedic rehabilitation ward. *J Orthop Sports Phys Ther.* 2009;39:468–477.

203. Lin CW, Moseley AM, Refshauge KM, et al. The lower extremity functional scale has good clinimetric properties in people with ankle fracture. *Physical Therapy.* 2009;89:580–588.

204. Ritter MA, Albohm MJ, Keating M, et al. Comparative outcomes of total joint arthroplasty. *J Arthroplasty.* 1995;10:737–741.

205. Impellizzeri FM, Mannion AF, Naal FD, Leunig M. Validity, reproducibility, and responsiveness of the Oxford Hip Score in patients undergoing surgery for femoroacetabular impingement. *Arthroscopy.* 2015;31(1):42–50.

206. Martin RL, Philippon MJ. Evidence of validity for the hip outcome score in hip arthroplasty. *Arthroscopy.* 2007;23(8):822–826.

207. Nwachukwu BU, Fields K, Chang B, et al. Preoperative outcome scores are predictive of achieving the minimally clinically important difference after arthroscopic treatment of femoroacetabular impingement. *Am J Sports Med.* 2016;45(3):612–619.

208. Ruiz-Iban MA, Seijas R, Sallant A, et al. The international Hip Outcome Tool-33 (iHOT-33): multicenter validation and translation to Spanish. *Health Qual Life Outcomes.* 2015;13:62–69.

209. Thorborg K, Roos EM, Christensen R, et al. The iHOT-33: how valid is it? *Arthroscopy.* 2012;28(9):1194–1195.

210. Griffin DR, Parsons N, Mohtadi NG, et al. A short version of the International Hip Outcome Tool (iHOT-12) for use in routine clinical practice. *Arthroscopy.* 2012;28(5):611–618.

211. Mohtadi NG, Griffin DR, Pedersen ME, et al. The development and validation of a self-administered quality-of-life outcome measure for young, active patients with symptomatic hip disease: the International Hip Outcome Tool (iHOT-33). *Arthroscopy.* 2012;28(5):595–610.

212. Weir A, Brukner P, Delahunt E, et al. Doha agreement meeting on terminology and definitions in groin pain athletes. *Br J Sports Med.* 2015;49(12):768–774.

213. Thorborg K, Holmich P, Christensen R, et al. The Copenhagen Hip and Groin Outcome Score (HAGOS): development and validation according to the COSMIN checklist. *Br J Sports Med.* 2011;45(6):478–491.

214. Mori B, Lundon K, Kreder HJ. 13-metre walk test applied to the elderly with musculoskeletal impairment: validity study. *Physiother Can.* 2005;57:217–224.

215. Nordin E, Rosendahl E, Lundin-Olsson L. Time "up and go" test: reliability in older people dependent in activities of daily living—focus on cognitive state. *Phys Ther.* 2006;86:646–655.

216. Yeung TS, Wessel J, Stratford P, et al. The timed up and go test for use on an inpatient orthopedic rehabilitation ward. *J Orthop Sports Phys Ther.* 2008;38:410–417.

217. Wright AA, Cook CE, Baxter GD, et al. A comparison of 3 methodological approaches to defining major clinically important improvement of 4 performance measures in patients with hip osteoarthritis. *J Orthop Sports Phys Ther.* 2011;41(5):319–327.

218. Butland RJ, Pang J, Gross ER, et al. Two-, six- and 12-minutes walking tests in respiratory disease. *Br Med J.* 1982;284:1607–1608.

219. Peel C, Ballard D. Reproducibility of the 6-minute walk test in older women. *J Aging Phys Act.* 2001;9:184–193.

220. Rikli RE, Jones CJ. The reliability of validity of a 6-minute walk test as a measure of physical endurance in older adults. *J Aging Phys Act.* 1998;6:363–375.

221. Harada ND, Chin V, Stewart AL. Mobility-related function in older adults: assessment with a 6-minute walk test. *Arch Phys Med Rehabil.* 1999;80:837–841.

222. Segura-Orti F, Martinez Olmos FJ. Test-retest reliability and minimal detectable change scores for sit to stand to sit tests, the six minute walk test, the one leg heel rise test and handgrip strength in people undergoing hemodialysis. *Physical Therapy.* 2011;91(8):1244–1252.

223. Ekblom B, Day WC, Hartley LH, et al. Reproducibility of exercise prescribed by pace description. *Scand J Sports Sci.* 1979;1:16–19.

224. Cunningham DA, Rechnitzer PA, Pearce ME, et al. Determinates of self-selected walking pace across ages 19 to 66. *J Gerontol.* 1982;37:560–564.

225. Bassey J, Fentem PH, MacDonald IC, et al. Self-paced walking as a method for exercise testing in elderly and young men. *Clin Sci Mol Med.* 1976;51:609–612.

226. Cibulka MT, Bloom NJ, Enseki KR, et al. Hip pain and mobility deficits – hip osteoarthritis: revision 2017 – clinical practice guidelines. *J Orthop Sports Phys Ther.* 2017;47(6):A1–A37.

227. Moore M, Barker K. The validity and reliability of the four square step test in different adult populations: a systematic review. *Syst Rev.* 2017;6:187–196.

228. Sutlive TG, Lopez HP, Schnitker DE, et al. Development of a clinical prediction rule for diagnosing hip osteoarthritis in individuals with unilateral hip pain. *J Orthop Sports Phys Ther.* 2008;38:542–550.

229. Bansback N, Tsuchiya A, Brazier J, Anis A. Canadian valuation of EQ-5D health states: preliminary value set and considerations for future valuation studies. *PLoS One.* 2012;7(2):e31115.

230. Granja C, Teixeira-Pinto A, Costo-Pereira A. Quality of life after intensive care – evaluation with EQ-5D questionnaire. *Intensive Care Med.* 2002;28(7):898–907.

231. Konig HH, Bernert S, Angermeyer MC, et al. Comparison of population health status in six European countries: results of a representative survey using the EQ-5D questionnaire. *Med Care.* 2009;47(2):255–261.

232. van Hout B, Janssen MF, Feng YS, et al. Interim scoring for the EQ-5D-5L: mapping the EQ-5D-5L to EQ-5D-3L value sets. *Value Health.* 2012;15(5):708–715.

233. McClure NS, Sayah FA, Xie F, et al. Instrument-defined estimates of the minimally important difference for EQ-5D-5L index scores. *Value Health.* 2017;20(4):644–650.

234. Balestroni G, Bertolotti G. EuroQuol-5D (EQ-5D): an instrument for measuring quality of life. *Monaldi Arch Chest Dis.* 2012;78(3):155–159.

235. Dallinga JM, Benjaminse A, Lemmink KA. Which screening tools can predict injury to the lower extremities in team sports?: a systematic review. *Sports Med.* 2012;42(9):791–815.

236. Tinetti ME. Performance-oriented assessment of mobility problems in elderly patients. *J Am Geriatr Soc.* 1986;34:119–126.

237. Wahoff M, Ryan M. Rehabilitation after hip femoroacetabular impingement arthroscopy. *Clin Sports Med.* 2011;30(2):463–482.

238. Reiman MP, Goode AP, Hegedus EJ, et al. Diagnostic accuracy of clinical tests of the hip: a systematic review with meta-analysis. *Br J Sports Med.* 2013;47(14):893–902.

239. Reiman MP, Goode AP, Cook CE, et al. Diagnostic accuracy of clinical tests for the diagnosis of hip femoroacetabular impingement/labral tear: a systematic review with meta- analysis. *Br J Sports Med.* 2015;49(12):811–824.

240. Tijssen M, van Cingel R, Willemsen L, de Visser E. Diagnostics of femoroacetabular impingement and labral pathology of the hip: a systematic review of the accuracy and validity of physical tests. *Arthroscopy.* 2012;28(6):860–871.

241. Cook CE, Hegedus EJ. *Orthopedic Physical Examination Tests—An Evidence Based Approach.* Upper Saddle River, NJ: Prentice Hall/Pearson; 2008.

242. Cleland JA, Koppenhaver S. *Netter's orthopedic Clinical Examination—An Evidence Based Approach.* 2nd ed. Philadelphia. Saunders/Elsevier; 2011.

243. Domb BG, Stake CE, Lindner D, et al. Arthroscopic capsular plication and labral preservation in borderline hip dysplasia: two-year clinical outcomes of a surgical approach to a challenging problem. *Am J Sports Med.* 2013;41(11):2591–2598.

244. Crane L. Femoral torsion and its relation to toeing-in and toeing-out. *J Bone Joint Surg Am.* 1959;41:421–428.

245. Seitlinger G, Moroder P, Scheurecker G, et al. The contribution of different femur segments to overall femoral torsion. *Am J Sports Med.* 2016;44(7):1796–1800.

246. Tonnis D, Heinecke A. Acetabular and femoral anteversion: relationship with osteoarthritis of the hip. *J Bone Joint Surg Am.* 1999;81:1747–1770.

247. Gelberman RH, Cohen MS, Desai SS, et al. Femoral anteversion: a clinical assessment of idiopathic intoeing gait in children. *J Bone Joint Surg Br.* 1987;69(1):75–79.

248. Adams MC. *Outline of Orthopaedics.* London: E & S Livingstone; 1968.

249. Tachdjian MO. *Pediatric Orthopedics.* Philadelphia: W.B. Saunders; 1972.

250. Staheli LT. Medial femoral torsion. *Orthop Clin North Am.* 1980;11:39–50.

251. Ruwe PA, Gage JR, Ozonoff MB, DeLuca PA. Clinical determination of femoral anteversion. *J Bone Joint Surg Am.* 1992;74:820–830.

252. Souza RB, Powers CM. Concurrent criterion-related validity and reliability of a clinical test to measure femoral anteversion. *J Orthop Sports Phys Ther.* 2009;39:586–592.

253. Boykin RE, Anz AW, Bushnell BD, et al. Hip instability. *J Am Acad Orthop Surg.* 2011;19(6):340–348.

254. Kamegaya M, Saisu T, Nakamura J, et al. Drehmann sign and femoro-acetabular impingement in SCFE. *J Pediatr Orthop.* 2011;31(8):853–857.

255. Woods D, Macnicol M. The flexion-adduction test: an early sign of hip disease. *J Pediatr Orthop.* 2001;10:180–185.

256. Maitland GD. *The Peripheral Joints: Examination and Recording Guide.* Adelaide, Australia: Virgo Press; 1973.

257. Maslowski E, Sullivan W, Forster Harwood J, et al. The diagnostic validity of hip provocation maneuvers to detect intra-articular hip pathology. *Am Acad Phys Med Rehabil.* 2010;2(3):174–181.

258. O'Donnell J, Economopoulos K, Singh P, et al. The ligamentum teres test: a novel and effective test in diagnosing tears of the ligamentum tercs. *Am J Sports Med.* 2014;42(1):138–143.

259. Mulligan EP, Middleton EF, Brunette M. Evaluation and management of greater trochanter pain syndrome. *Phys Ther Sport.* 2015;16(3):205–214.

260. Austin AB, Souza RB, Meyer JL, et al. Identification of abnormal hip motion associated with acetabular labral pathology. *J Orthop Sports Phys Ther.* 2008;38:558–565.

261. McCarthy JC, Lee J-O. Hip arthroscopy: indications, outcomes, and complications. *J Bone Joint Surg Am.* 2005;87:1138–1145.

262. Fagerson T. Hip and thigh. In: Magee DJ, Zachazewski JE, Quillen WS, eds. *Pathology and Intervention in Musculoskeletal Rehabilitation.* Philadelphia: Elsevier; 2009.

263. Heiderscheit B, McClinton S. Evaluation and management of hip and pelvis injuries. *Phys Med Rehabil Clin N Am.* 2016;27(1):1–29.

264. Evans RC. *Illustrated Essentials in Orthopedic Physical Assessment.* St Louis: CV Mosby; 1994.

265. Troelsen A, Mechlenburg I, Gelineck J, et al. What is the role of clinical tests and ultrasound in acetabular labral tear diagnostics? *Acta Orthop.* 2009;80(3):314–318.

266. McGrory BJ. Stinchfield resisted hip flexion test. *Hosp Physician.* 1999;35:41–42.

267. McCarthy JC, Noble PC, Schuck MR, et al. The role of labral lesions to development of early degenerative hip disease. *Clin Orthop Relat Res.* 2001;393:25–37.

268. McGrory BJ. Stinchfield resisted inflection test. *Hosp Phys.* 1999;35:41–42.

269. Callaghan JJ. Examination of the hip. In: Clarke CR, Bonfiglio M, eds. *Orthopedics: Essentials of Diagnosis and Treatment.* New York: Churchill Livingstone; 1994.

270. Lee D. *The Pelvic Girdle.* Edinburgh: Churchill Livingstone; 1989.

271. Hananouchi T, Yaui Y, Yamamoto K, et al. Anterior impingement test for labral lesions has high positive predictive value. *Clin Orthop Relat Res.* 2012;470(12):3524–3529.

272. Casartelli NC, Brunner R, Maffiuletti NA, et al. The FADIR test accuracy for screening cam and pincer morphology in youth elite ice hockey players. *J Sci Med Sport.* 2018;21(2):134–138.

273. Martin R, Nartin HD, Kivlan BR. Nerve entrapment in the hip region: current concepts review. *Int J Sports Phys Ther.* 2017;12(7):1163–1173.

274. Ayeni O, Chu R, Hetaimish B, et al. A painful squat test provides limited diagnostic utility in CAM-type femoroacetabular impingement. *Knee Surg Sports Traumatol Arthrosc.* 2014;22(4):806–811.

275. Burgess RM, Rushton A, Wright C, et al. The validity and accuracy of clinical diagnostic tests used to detect labral pathology of the hip: a systematic review. *Manual Therapy.* 2011;16:318–326.

276. Khoo-Summers L, Bloom NJ. Examination and treatment of a professional ballet dancer with a suspected acetabular labral tear: a case report. *Man Ther.* 2015;20(4):623–629.

277. Suenaga E, Noguchi Y, Jingushi S, et al. Relationship between the maximum flexion-internal rotation test and the torn acetabulum labrum of a dysplastic hip. *J Orthop Sci.* 2002;7:26–32.

278. Myrick KM, Nissen CW. THIRD test: diagnosing hip labral tears with a new physical examination technique. *J Nurse Practitioners.* 2013;9(8):501–505.

279. Myrick KM, Feinn R. Internal and external validity of THIRD test for hip labral tears. *J Nurse Practitioners.* 2014;10(8):540–544.

280. Johnson AW, Weiss CB, Wheeler DL. Stress fractures of the femoral shaft in athletes—more common than expected: a new clinical test. *Am J Sports Med.* 1994;22:248–256.

281. Adams SL, Yarnold PR. Clinical use of the patellar-pubic percussion sign in hip trauma. *Am J Emerg Med.* 1997;15:173–175.

282. Segat M, Casonato O, Margelli M, Pillon S. Is the Patellar Pubic Percussion Test useful to diagnose only femur fractures or something else? Two case reports. *Man Ther.* 2016;21:292–296.

283. Darmonov AV. Clinical screening for congenital dislocation of the hip. *J Bone Joint Surg Am.* 1996;78:383–388.

284. Guille JT, Pizzutillo PD, MacEwan GD. Developmental dysplasia of the hip from birth to six months. *J Am Acad Orthop Surg.* 2000;8:232–242.

285. Mahan ST, Katz JN, Kim YJ. To screen or not to screen? A decision analysis of utility of screening for developmental dysplasia of the hip. *J Bone Joint Surg Am.* 2009;91:1705–1719.

286. Gooding JR, McClead RE. Initial assessment and management of the newborn. *Pediatr Clin North Am.* 2015;62(2):345–365.

287. LeVeau B. Hip. In: Richardson JK, Iglarsh ZA, eds. *Clinical Orthopedic Physical Therapy.* Philadelphia: WB Saunders; 1994.

288. Moore FH. Examining infants' hips: can it do harm? *J Bone Joint Surg Br.* 1989;71:4–5.

289. Bolz S, Davies GJ. Leg length differences and correlation with total leg strength. *J Orthop Sports Phys Ther.* 1984;6:123–129.

290. Reider B. *The Orthopedic Physical Examination.* Philadelphia: WB Saunders; 1999.

291. Clarke GR. Unequal leg length: an accurate method of detection and some clinical results. *Rheumatol Phys Med.* 1972;11:385–390.

292. Fisk JW, Balgent ML. Clinical and radiological assessment of leg length. *N Z Med J.* 1975;81:477–480.

293. Woerman AL, Binder-Macleod SA. Leg-length discrepancy assessment: accuracy and precision in five clinical methods of evaluation. *J Orthop Sports Phys Ther.* 1984;5:230–239.

294. Woerman AL. Evaluation and treatment of dysfunction in the lumbar-pelvic-hip complex. In: Donatelli R, Wooden MJ, eds. *Orthopedic Physical Therapy.* Edinburgh: Churchill Livingstone; 1989.

295. Crawford AH. Neurologic disorders. In: Steinberg ME, ed. *The Hip and Its Disorders.* Philadelphia: WB Saunders; 1991.

296. Beatty RA. The piriformis muscle syndrome: a simple diagnostic maneuver. *Neurosurgery.* 1994;34(3):512–514.

297. Hopayian K, Song F, Riera R, Sandbandan S. The clinical features of the piriformis syndrome: a systematic review. *Eur Spine J.* 2010;19(12):2095–2109.

298. Michel F, Decavel P, Toussirot E, et al. The piriformis muscle syndrome: an exploration of anatomical context, pathophysiological hypotheses and diagnostic criteria. *Ann Phys Rehabil Med.* 2013;56(4):300–311.

299. Ahmad CS, Redler LH, Ciccotti MG, et al. Evaluation and management of hamstring injuries. *Am J Sports Med.* 2003;41(12):2933–2947.

300. Gruebel-Lee DM. *Disorders of the Hip.* Philadelphia: JB Lippincott; 1983.

301. Martin RL, Schroder RG, Gomez-Hoyos J, et al. Accuracy of 3 clinical tests to diagnose proximal hamstrings tears with and without sciatic nerve involvement in patients with posterior hip pain. *Arthroscopy.* 2018;34(1):114–121.

302. Zimney NJ. Clinical reasoning in the evaluation and management of undiagnosed chronic hip pain in a young adult. *Phys Ther.* 1998;78:62–73.

303. Palmar ML, Epler M. *Clinical Assessment Procedures in Physical Therapy.* Philadelphia: JB Lippincott; 1990.

304. Kuo L, Chung W, Bates E, et al. The hamstring index. *J Pediatr Ortho.* 1997;17:78–88.

305. Noble HB, Hajek MR, Porter M. Diagnosis and treatment of iliotibial band tightness in runners. *Phys Sportsmed.* 1982;10:67–68. 71–72, 74.

306. Ober FB. The role of the iliotibial and fascia lata as a factor in the causation of low-back disabilities and sciatica. *J Bone Joint Surg.* 1936;18:105–110.

307. Strauss EJ, Kim S, Calcei JG, et al. Iliotibial band syndrome: evaluation and management. *J Am Acad Orthop Surg.* 2011;19:728–736.

308. Baker RL, Fredericson M. Iliotibial band syndrome in runners: biomechanical implications and exercise interventions. *Phys Med Rehabil Clin N Am.* 2016;27(1):53–77.

309. Willett GM, Kleim SA, Shostrom VK, Lomneth CS. An anatomic investigation of the Ober test. *Am J Sports Med.* 2016;44(3):696–701.

310. Pace JB, Nagle D. Piriform syndrome. *West J Med.* 1976;124(6):435–439.

311. Fishman LM, Dombi GW, Michaelson C, et al. Piriformis syndrome: diagnosis, treatment, and outcome – a 10-year study. *Arch Phys Med Rehabil.* 2002;83(3):295–301.

312. Boyajian-O'Neill LA, McClain RL, Coleman MK, Thomas PP. Diagnosis and management of piriformis syndrome: an osteopathic approach. *J Am Osteopath Assoc.* 2008;108(11):657–664.

313. Lewis S, Jurak J, Lee C, et al. Anatomical variations of the sciatic nerve, in relation to the piriformis muscle. *Trans Res Anatomy.* 2016;5:15–19.

314. Tonley JC, Yun SM, Kochevar RJ, et al. Treatment of an individual with piriformis syndrome focusing on hip muscle strengthening and movement re-education: a case report. *J Orthop Sports Phys Ther.* 2010;40:103–111.

315. Garrick JG, Webb DR. *Sports Injuries: Diagnosis and Treatment.* Philadelphia: WB Saunders; 1990.

316. Gautam VK, Anand S. A new test for estimating iliotibial band contracture. *J Bone Joint Surg Br.* 1998;80:474–475.

317. Zeren B, Oztekin HH. A new self-diagnostic test for biceps femoris muscle strains. *Clin J Sports Med.* 2006;16:166–169.

318. Thurston A. Assessment of fixed flexion deformity of the hip. *Clin Orthop.* 1982;169:186–189.

319. Trendelenburg F. Trendelenburg's test (1895). *Clin Orthop Relat Res.* 1998;355:3–7.

320. Kuhns BD, Giordano BD, Perets I, et al. The lateral coverage index: a clinically relevant marker for acetabular coverage. *Arthroscopy.* 2018;34(12):e16.

321. Bailey R, Richards J, Selfe J. A biomechanical investigation of selected lumbo-pelvic hip tests: implications for the examination of running. *Phys Med Rehabil Int.* 2016;3(5):1096–1113.

322. Crossley KM, Zhang W-J, Schache AG, et al. Performance on the single-leg squat task indicates hip abductor muscle function. Am J Sports Med. 2011;39:866–873.

323. Grimaldi A, Mellor R, Nicolson P, et al. Utility of clinical tests to diagnose MRI-confirmed gluteal tendinopathy in patients presenting with lateral hip pain. Br J Sports Med. 2017;51:524–591.

324. American Orthopaedic Association. Manual of Orthopaedic Surgery. Chicago: AOA; 1972.

325. Kristensen MT, Foss NB, Kehlet H. Timed "up and go" test as a predictor of falls within 6 months after hip fracture surgery. Physical Therapy. 2007;87:24–30.

326. Cornwall R, Radomisli TE. Nerve injury in traumatic dislocation of the hip. Clin Orthop Relat Res. 2000;377:84–91.

327. Dettart MM, Riley LH. Nerve injuries in total hip arthroplasty. J Am Acad Orthop Surg. 1999;7:101–111.

328. Giannoudis PV, DaCosta AA, Raman R, et al. Double-crush syndrome after acetabular fractures—a sign of poor prognosis. J Bone Joint Surg Br. 2005;87:401–407.

329. Su EP. Post-surgical neuropathy after total hip arthroplasty: causality and avoidance. Sem Arthroplasty. 2016;27(1):70–73.

330. Pecina MM, Krmpotic-Nemanic J, Markiewitz AD. Tunnel Syndromes. Boca Raton, Florida: CRC Press; 1991.

331. Vandertop WP, Bosman NJ. The piriformis syndrome—a case report. J Bone Joint Surg Am. 1991;73:1095–1096.

332. Fleischman AN, Rothman RH, Parvizi J. Femoral nerve palsy following total hip arthroplasty: incidence and course of recovery. J Arthroplasty. 2018;33(4):1194–1199.

333. Anloague PA, Somers-Chorny W, Childs KE, et al. The relationship between femoral nerve tension and hip flexor muscle length. J Nov Physiothor. 2015;5:244–248.

334. Kumka M. Critical sites of entrapment of the posterior division of the obturator nerve: anatomical considerations. J Can Chiropr Assoc. 2010;54(1):33–42.

335. Bradshaw C, Bell S, Brukner P. Obturator nerve entrapment—a cause of groin pain in athletes. Am J Sports Med. 1997;25:402–408.

336. Tipton JS. Obturator neuropathy. Curr Rev Musculoskelet Med. 2008;1:234–237.

337. Kelly BT, Williams RJ, Philippon MJ. Hip arthroscopy: current indications, treatment options, and management issues. Am J Sports Med. 2003;31:1020–1037.

338. Mallow M, Nazarian LN. Greater trochanteric pain syndrome diagnosis and treatment. Phys Med Rehabil Clin N Am. 2014;25(2):279–289.

339. Reid D. The management of greater trochanteric pain syndrome: a systematic literature review. J Orthop. 2016;13(1):15–28.

340. Ganderton C, Pizzari T, Harle T, et al. A comparison of gluteus medius, gluteus minimus and tensor facia latae muscle activation during gait in post-menopausal women with and without greater trochanteric pain syndrome. J Electromyogr Kinesiol. 2017;33:39–47.

341. Klontzas ME, Karantanas AH. Greater trochanter pain syndrome: a descriptive MR imaging study. Eur J Radiol. 2014;83(10):1850–1855.

342. Holmich P, Holmich LR, Bjerg AM. Clinical examination of athletes with groin pain: an intraobserver and interobserver reliability study. Br J Sports Med. 2004;38(4):446–451.

343. Michel F, Decavel P, Toussirot E, et al. Piriformis muscle syndrome: diagnostic criteria and treatment of a monocentric series of 250 patients. Ann Phys Rehabil Med. 2013;56(5):371–383.

344. Khan D, Nelson A. Piriformis syndrome. In: Benzon H, Raja SN, Fishman SM, et al., eds. Essentials of Pain Management. 4th ed. Philadelphia: Elsevier; 2018.

345. Clohisy JC, Carlisle JC, Beaulé PE, et al. A systematic approach to the plain radiographic evaluation of the young adult hip. J Bone Joint Surg Am. 2008;90:47–66.

346. Lee WA, Saroki AJ, Loken S, et al. Radiographic identification of arthroscopically relevant proximal femoral structures. Am J Sports Med. 2015;44(1):60–66.

347. Lee WA, Saroki AJ, Loken S, et al. Radiographic identification of arthroscopically relevant acetabular structures. Am J Sports Med. 2015;44(1):67–73.

348. Harris WH. Etiology of osteoarthritis of the hip. Clin Orthop Relat Res. 1986;213:20–33.

349. Larson AN, Stans AA, Sierra RJ. Ischial spine sign reveals acetabular retroversion in Legg-Calvé-Perthes Disease. Clin Orthop Relat Res. 2011;469(7):2012–2018.

350. Oh CW, Thacker MM, Mackenzie WG, et al. Cox vara—a novel measurement technique in skeletal dysplasias. Clin Orthop Relat Res. 2006;147:125–131.

351. Sugano N, Kubo T, Takaoka K, et al. Diagnostic criteria for non-traumatic osteonecrosis of the femoral head. J Bone Joint Surg Br. 1999;81:590–599.

352. Zaltz I, Kelly BT, Hetsroni I, Bedi A. The crossover sign overestimates acetabular retroversion. Clin Orthop Relat Res. 2013;471(8):2463–2470.

353. Kappe T, Kocak T, Neuerburg C, et al. Reliability of radiographic signs for acetabular retroversion. Int Orthop. 2011;35(6):817–821.

354. Kellgren JH, Lawrence JS. Radiological assessment of osteo-arthrosis. Ann Rheum Dis. 1957;16:494–502.

355. Wylie JD, Kapron AL, Peters CL, et al. Relationship between the lateral center-edge angle and 3-dimensional acetabular coverage. Orthop J Sports Med. 2017;5(4):2325967117700589.

356. Perkins G. Signs by which to diagnose congenital dislocation of the hip. Clin Orthop. 1992;274:3–5.

357. Loder RT, Aronsson DD, Dobbs MB, et al. Slipped capital femoral epiphysis. J Bone Joint Surg Am. 2000;82:1170–1188.

358. Llopis E, Higueras V, Vano M, Altonaga JR. Anatomic and radiographic evaluation of the hip. Eur J Radiol. 2012;81(12):3727–3736.

359. Yamasaki T, Yasunaga Y, Shoji T, et al. Inclusion and exclusion criteria in the diagnosis of femoroacetabular impingement. Arthroscopy. 2015;31(7):1403–1410.

360. Hadeed MM, Cancienne JM, Gwathmey FW. Pincer impingement. Clin Sports Med. 2016;35(3):405–418.

361. Barrientos C, Barahona M, Diaz J, et al. Is there a pathological alpha angle for hip impingement? A diagnostic test study. J Hip Preserv Surg. 2016;3(3):223–228.

362. Sutter R, Dietrich TJ, Zingg PO, Pfirrmann CW. How useful is the alpha angle for discriminating between symptomatic patients with cam-type femoroacetabular impingement and asymptomatic volunteers? Radiology. 2012;264(2):514–521.

363. Wong TY, Jesse MK, Jensen A, et al. Upsloping lateral sourcil: a radiographic finding of hip instability. J Hip Preserv Surg. 2018;5(4):435–442.

364. Bigg-Wither G, Kelly P. Diagnostic imaging in musculoskeletal physiotherapy. In: Refshauge K, Gass E, eds. Musculoskeletal Physiotherapy. Oxford: Butterworth Heinemann; 1995.

365. Kang AC, Gooding AJ, Coates MH, et al. Computed tomography assessment of hip joints in asymptomatic individuals in relation to femoroacetabular impingement. Am J Sports Med. 2010;38:1160–1165.

366. Edwards DJ, Lomas D, Villar RN. Diagnosis of the painful hip by magnetic resonance imaging and arthroscopy. J Bone Joint Surg Br. 1995;77:374–376.

367. Guanch CA. MR imaging of the hip. Sports Med Arthrosc Rev. 2009;17:49–55.

368. Mitchell B, McCrory P, Brukner P, et al. Hip joint pathology: clinical presentation and correlation between magnetic resonance arthrography, ultrasound and arthroscopic findings in 25 consecutive cases. Clin J Sports Med. 2003;13:152–156.

369. McMahon PJ, Hodnett PA, Koulouris GC, et al. Hip and groin pain: radiological assessment. Open Sports Med J. 2010;4:108–120.

370. Byrne CA, Bowden DJ, Alkhayat A, et al. Sports-related groin pain secondary to symphysis pubis disorders: correlation between MRI findings and outcome after fluoroscopy-guided injection of steroid and local anesthetic. Am J Roentgenol. 2017;209(2):380–388.

371. Byrd JW, Jones KS. Diagnostic accuracy of clinical assessment, magnetic resonance imaging, magnetic resonance arthrography, and intra-articular injection in hip arthroscopy patients. Am J Sports Med. 2004;32(7):1668–1674.

372. Blankenbaker DG, Tuite MJ, Keene JS, del Rio AM. Labral injuries due to iliopsoas impingement: can they be diagnosed on MR arthrography? Am J Roentgenol. 2012;199(4):894–900.

373. Register B, Pennock AT, Ho CP, et al. Prevalence of abnormal hip findings in asymptomatic participants—a prospective, blended study. Am J Sports Med. 2012;40:2720–2724.

374. Jonson SR, Gross MT. Intraexaminer reliability, interexaminer reliability, and mean values for nine lower extremity skeletal measures in healthy naval midshipmen. J Orthop Sports Phys Ther. 1997;25:253–263.

375. Salen BA, Spangfort EV, Nygren AL, et al. The Disability Rating Index: an instrument for the assessment of disability in clinical settings. J Clin Epidemiol. 1994;47:1423–1434.

376. Parsons H, Bruce J, Achten J, et al. Measurement properties of the Disability Rating Index in patients undergoing hip replacement. Rheumatology (Oxford). 2015;54(1):64–71.

377. Lequesne M, Mathieu P, Vuillemin-Bodaghi V, et al. Gluteal tendinopathy in refractory greater trochanter pain syndrome: diagnostic value of two clinical tests. Arthritis Rheum. 2008;59(2):241–246.

378. Cliborne AV, Waineer RS, Rhon DI, et al. Clinical hip tests and a functional squat test in patients with knee osteoarthritis: reliability, prevalence of positive test findings, and short-term response to hip mobilization. J Orthop Sports Phys Ther. 2004;34:676–685.

379. Kaltenborn A, Bourg CM, Gutzeit A, Kalberer F. The Hip Lag Sign - prospective blinded trial of a new clinical sign to predict hip abductor damage. PLoS One. 2014;9(3):e91560.

380. Cibulka MT, White DM, Woehrle J, et al. Hip pain and mobility deficits—hip osteoarthritis: clinical practice guidelines. J Orthop Sports Phys Ther. 2009;39(4):A1–A25.

381. Burnett RS, Della Rocca GJ, Prather H, et al. Clinical presentation of patients with tears of the acetabular labrum. J Bone Joint Surg Am. 2006;88(7):1448–1457.

382. Philippon MJ, Briggs KK, Yen YM, Kuppersmith DA. Outcomes following hip arthroscopy for femoroacetabular impingement with associated chondrolabral dysfunction: minimum two-year follow-up. J Bone Joint Surg Br. 2009;91(1):16–23.

383. Hasler RM, Gal I, Biedert RM. Landmarks of the normal adult human trochlea based on axial MRI measurements: a cross-sectional study. Knee Surg Sports Traumatol Arthrosc. 2014;22(10):2372–2376.

384. Stepanovich M, Bomar JD, Pennock AT. Are the current classifications and radiographic measurements for trochlear dysplasia appropriate in the skeletally immature patient?. *Orthop J Sports Med*. 2016;4(10):232596711666949.

385. Bache JB, Cross AB. The Barford test. A useful diagnostic sign in fractures of the femoral neck. *Practitioner*. 1984;228(1389):305–308.

386. Tiru M, Goh SH. Low BY: Use of percussion as a screening tool in the diagnosis of occult hip fractures. *Singapore Med J*. 2002;43(9):467–469.

387. Ross MD, Nordeen MH, Barido M. Test-retest reliability of Patrick's hip range of motion test in healthy college-aged men. *J Strength Cond Res*. 2003;17(1):156–161.

388. Martin RL, Sekiya JK. The interrater reliability of 4 clinical tests used to assess individuals with musculoskeletal hip pain. *J Orthop Sports Phys Ther*. 2008;38(2):71–77.

389. Martin RL, Irrgang JJ, Sekiya JK. The diagnostic accuracy of a clinical examination in determining intra-articular hip pain for potential hip arthroscopy candidates. *Arthroscopy*. 2008;24(9):1013–1018.

390. Kapron AL, Anderson AE, Peters CL, et al. Hip internal rotation is correlated to radiographic findings of cam femoroacetabular impingement in collegiate football players. *Arthroscopy*. 2012;28(11):1661–1670.

391. Remy F, Chantelot C, Fontaine C, et al. Inter- and intra-observer reproducibility in radiographics diagnosis and classification of femoral trochlear dysplasia. *Surg Radiol Anat*. 1998;20:285–289.

392. Hinson R, Brown SH. Supine leg length differential estimation: an inter- and intra-examiner reliability study. *Chiropr Res J*. 1998;5(1):17–22.

CHAPTER 12

Knee

The knee joint is particularly susceptible to traumatic injury because it is located at the ends of two long lever arms, the tibia and the femur. In addition, because the joint connects one long bone "sitting" on another long bone, it depends on the ligaments and muscles that surround it for its strength and stability, not on its bony configuration.[1]

Because the knee joint depends on its ligaments to such a great extent, it is imperative that the ligaments be tested during the examination of the knee. Therefore, the ligamentous tests are not included under the "Special Tests" section but instead are listed in a separate section to ensure that they are always included in the examination of the knee.

Because of its anatomical arrangement, the knee is a complicated area to assess, and the examiner must take time to ensure that all relevant structures are tested. It must also be remembered that the lumbar spine, hip, and ankle may refer pain to the knee, and these joints must be assessed if it appears that joints other than the knee may be involved. For example, a slipped capital femoral epiphysis at the hip commonly refers pain to the knee, and this referred knee pain may predominate.

Applied Anatomy

The **tibiofemoral joint** is the largest joint in the body. It is a modified hinge joint having 2° of freedom. The synovium around the joint is extensive; it communicates with many of the bursae and pouches around the knee joint. Although the synovial membrane "encapsulates" the entire knee joint, its distribution within the knee is such that the cruciate ligaments, which run from the middle of the tibial plateau to the intercondylar area of the femur, are extrasynovial. (*Cruciate* means that the ligaments cross each other.)

The articular surfaces of the tibia and femur are not congruent, which enables the two bones to move different amounts, guided by the muscles and ligaments. The two bones approach congruency in full extension, which is the close packed position. Kaltenborn[2] has stated that the close packed position includes full lateral rotation of the tibia. The lateral femoral condyle projects anteriorly more than the medial femoral condyle to help prevent lateral dislocation of the patella. In females, this enlargement is important because of the female's broader pelvis and increased inward angle of the femur, which allow the femoral condyles to be parallel with the ground (Fig. 12.1). The resting position of the joint is approximately 25° of flexion, and the capsular pattern is flexion more limited than extension.

Tibiofemoral Joint	
Resting position:	25° flexion
Close packed position:	Full extension, lateral rotation of tibia
Capsular pattern:	Flexion, extension

The space between the tibia and femur is partially filled by two menisci that are attached to the tibia to add congruency. The **medial meniscus** is a small part of a large circle (i.e., C shaped) and is thicker posteriorly than anteriorly. The **lateral meniscus** is a large part of a small circle (i.e., O shaped) and is generally of equal thickness throughout. Both menisci are thicker along the periphery and thinner along the inner margin.

During the movement from extension to flexion, both menisci move posteriorly, the lateral meniscus being displaced more than the medial meniscus. The lateral meniscus has an excursion of 10 mm, and the medial meniscus has an excursion of 2 mm. In fact, evidence using healthy live adults with an open magnetic resonance imaging (MRI) system has shown that different parts of the lateral meniscus move different amounts. Backward excursion of the anterior horn is significantly more than the posterior horn, while excursion of the posterior horn of the lateral meniscus is significantly greater than that of the posterior horn of the medial meniscus.[3,4] The menisci are avascular in their cartilaginous inner two-thirds and are partly vascular and fibrous in their outer one-third.[5] They are held in place by the coronary ligaments attaching to the tibia.

The menisci serve several functions in the knee. They aid in lubrication and nutrition of the joint and act as shock absorbers (a meniscectomy can reduce shock absorption capacity at the knee by 20%),[6] spreading the stress over the articular cartilage and decreasing cartilage wear. They make the joint surfaces more congruent and improve weight distribution by increasing the area of

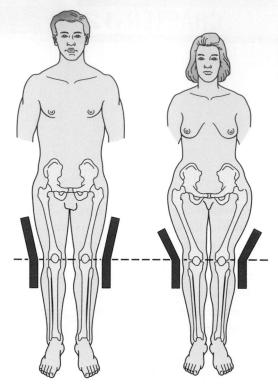

Fig. 12.1 Q-angle differences in males and females. Because of the broader pelvis in the female, it is necessary for the femur to come inward at an increased angle to make the distal end of the condyles parallel with the ground. The quadriceps, patella, and patellar tendon form an angle centered at the patella. As the quadriceps contracts, the angle tends to straighten, which forces the patella laterally. (Redrawn from O'Donoghue D: *Treatment of injuries to athletes*, ed 4, Philadelphia, 1984, WB Saunders, p 522.)

contact between the condyles. The menisci reduce friction during movement and aid the ligaments and capsule in preventing hyperextension. The menisci prevent the joint capsule from entering the joint and participate in the "locking" mechanism of the joint into close pack by directing the movement of the femoral articular condyles. Because more recent literature indicates that removal of the entire meniscus can lead to early degeneration of the joint,[7,8] most surgeons nowadays remove only the torn portion of the meniscus, or, if the tear is in the outer one-third where there is sufficient circulation to aid healing, the surgeon may attempt to surgically repair (suture) the meniscus.

It is generally believed that the meniscus possesses minimal innervation so there is minimal or no pain when it is damaged unless the coronary ligaments have been damaged as well. However, Gray[9] has reported that the menisci possess innervation in their outer two-thirds, with the anterior and posterior horns being well innervated. Because the menisci are primarily avascular, especially in the inner two-thirds, there is seldom bloody effusion in injury; however, there may be synovial effusion. Their poor blood supply, especially in the inner two-thirds, gives the menisci a low regeneration potential.

The lateral meniscus is not as firmly attached to the tibia as the medial meniscus and therefore is less prone to injury. The coronary ligaments, also referred to as the *meniscotibial ligaments,* tend to be longer on the lateral aspect, and the horns of the lateral meniscus are closer together.

The **patellofemoral joint** is a modified plane joint, the lateral articular surface of the patella being wider. The patella contains the thickest layer of cartilage in the body and, in reality, is a sesamoid bone found within the patellar tendon. It has five facets, or ridges: superior, inferior, lateral, medial, and odd. The odd facet is most frequently the first part of the patella to be affected in chondromalacia patellae (i.e., premature degeneration of the patellar cartilage) or patellofemoral syndrome.

During the movement from flexion to extension, different parts of the patella articulate with the femoral condyles (Fig. 12.2).[10,11] The odd facet does not come into contact with the femoral condyles until at least 135° of flexion is reached. Incorrect alignment or malalignment of the patellar movement over the femoral condyles can lead to patellofemoral arthralgia. The capsule of this joint is continuous with the capsule of the tibiofemoral joint.

The **patella** improves the efficiency of extension during the last 30° of extension (i.e., 30° to 0° of extension with the straight leg being 0°), because it holds the quadriceps tendon away from the axis of movement. The patella also functions as a guide for the quadriceps or patellar tendon, decreases friction of the quadriceps mechanism, controls capsular tension in the knee, acts as a bony shield for the cartilage of the femoral condyles, and improves the aesthetic appearance of the knee (Fig. 12.3). Loading on the articular surface of the patella also varies with activity.

Patellar Loading with Activity

Walking:	0.3 times the body weight
Climbing stairs:	2.5 times the body weight
Descending stairs:	3.5 times the body weight
Squatting:	7 times the body weight

Patellar stability is achieved through the bony structure of the trochlea and soft tissues consisting of the retinacular tissue, the medial and lateral patellofemoral ligaments (MPFL and LPFL), and the medial and lateral meniscopatellar ligaments.

The patellar retinaculum is a fibrous tissue covering the anterior knee that helps to bind structures and fill space between the patella, the patellar ligament, and the medial and lateral collateral ligaments. The lateral retinaculum has been shown to provide up to 19% of the resistance against lateral patellar displacement,[12] whereas the medial retinaculum provides only approximately 11% of the resistance to a lateral patellar displacement.[13] Recent

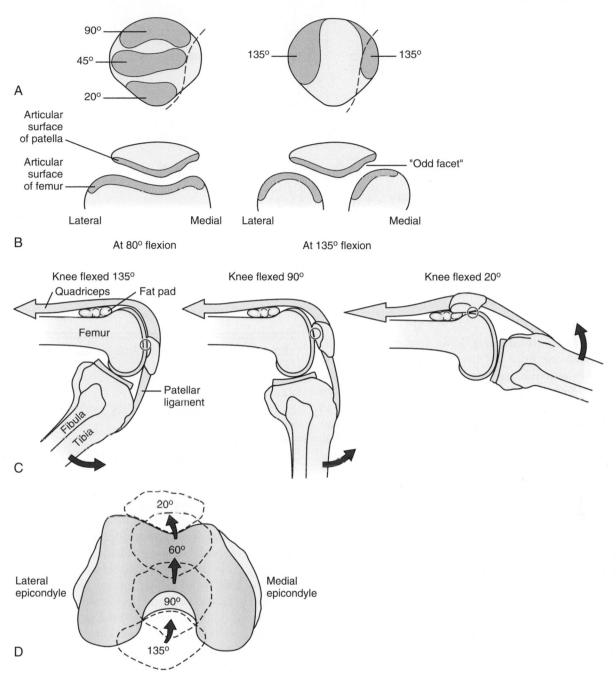

Fig. 12.2 (A) Area of contact of the patella during different degrees of flexion. (B) Articulation between patella and femur. (C) The *circles* depicted on the patella indicate the point of maximal contact between the patella and the femur. As the knee is extended, the contact point on the patella migrates from superior to inferior pole. Note the suprapatellar fat pad deep to the quadriceps. (D) The path and contact areas of the patella on the intercondylar groove of the femur. The degree values 135, 90, 60, and 20 indicate flexed positions of the knee. (C and D, Redrawn from Neumann DA: *Kinesiology of the musculoskeletal system—foundations for physical rehabilitation*, St Louis, 2002, Mosby, p 448.)

attention has been given to the importance of the MPFL. The MPFL is thought to provide a checkrein to lateral patellar displacement.[14] The MPFL runs from the medial femoral condyle to its attachment onto the medial border of the patella.[15–17] The MPFL is able to provide this stabilization function as it is the primary static restraint to lateral patellar displacement at 20° of knee flexion, contributing 60% of the total restraining force.[13] The medial meniscopatellar ligament is a thickening of the capsule that runs from the anterior horn of the medial meniscus to the inferior portion of the medial border of the patella.[18] The lateral meniscopatellar ligament runs between the anterior horn of the lateral meniscus and to the inferior aspect of the capsule. Both of these structures create a thickening of the joint capsule on their respective sides of the knee.

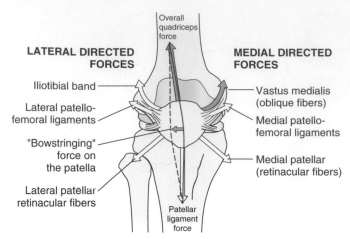

Fig. 12.3 The major guiding forces acting on the patella are shown as it moves through the intercondylar groove of the femur. Each structure has a natural tendency to pull the patella laterally or medially. In most cases the opposing forces counteract one another so that the patella moves optimally during flexion and extension. (Modified from Neumann DA: *Kinesiology of the musculoskeletal system—foundations for physical rehabilitation*, St Louis, 2002, Mosby, p 463.)

The **superior tibiofibular joint** is a plane synovial joint between the tibia and the head of the fibula. It is supported by anterior and posterior ligaments of the same name. Movement occurs in this joint with any activity involving the ankle. Hypomobility at this joint can lead to pain in the knee area on activity, because the fibula can bear up to one-sixth of the body weight. In approximately 10% of the population, the capsule of this joint is continuous with that of the tibiofemoral joint.

Patient History

In addition to the questions listed under the "Patient History" section in Chapter 1, the examiner should obtain the following information from the patient:

1. *How did the accident occur, or what was the mechanism of injury?*[19,20] The primary mechanisms of injury in the knee are a valgus force (with or without rotation or twisting), hyperextension, flexion with posterior translation, and a varus force.[21] The first often results in injury to the medial collateral ligament, frequently accompanied by injury to the posteromedial capsule, medial meniscus, and anterior cruciate ("terrible triad"). The second leads to anterior cruciate injuries, often associated with meniscus tears. The third mechanism of injury often involves the posterior cruciate ligament, and the fourth mechanism involves the lateral collateral ligament, the posterolateral capsule, and the posterior cruciate ligament. Was the injury the result of trauma, such as a direct or an indirect blow? Bauer et al.[22] developed a clinical prediction rule for determining whether a fracture was present in an acute knee injury. Was the patient bearing weight at the time of injury? From which direction did the injuring force come? For example, meniscal injuries, especially those on the medial side, occur as a result of a torsion injury that

> ### Bauer's Clinical Prediction Rule for Acute Knee Fracture[a,22]
>
> - Severe joint line tenderness
> - Severe localized swelling with effusion and ecchymosis
> - Flexion less than 90°
> - Inability to bear weight
>
> [a]The presence of these signs would indicate that an x-ray assessment is warranted.

combines compression and rotation. Slowly developing forces tend to cause bony avulsions, whereas rapidly developing forces tend to tear ligaments. If two or more ligaments have been torn, the knee may have been dislocated which, if it has occurred, may lead to a vascular injury. Thus, it is important to check the popliteal and dorsalis pedis pulse.[23] In young children, injuries to the growth plate or physis may occur instead of injury to the ligaments, especially during a rapid growth spurt when the physis is weaker than the ligaments. Injuries may occur to the distal femoral physis, the proximal tibial physis, and the tibial tubercle apophysis (traction epiphysis).[24,25] Injury to this last structure is called *Osgood-Schlatter disease*. Table 12.1 lists typical mechanisms of injury to the knee and the structures injured. The lower limb may be viewed as an open (foot off the ground) or a closed (foot on the ground) kinetic chain (Fig. 12.4). There is less chance of injury when the lower limb is an open kinetic chain. That being said, the hamstrings are often injured near the end of the swing phase when the muscles are at their maximum length and undergoing an eccentric contraction just before heel strike.[26] In some cases, hamstring injuries may occur following insidious onset of progressive hamstring tightness.[26] As a closed kinetic chain, the lower limb is an encapsulated system in which all

TABLE **12.1**

Mechanisms of Injury to the Knee and Possible Structures Injured

Mechanism of Injury	Structure Possibly Injured
Varus or valgus contact without rotation	1. Collateral ligament 2. Epiphyseal fracture 3. Patellar dislocation or subluxation
Varus or valgus contact with rotation	1. Collateral and cruciate ligaments 2. Collateral ligaments and patellar dislocation or subluxation 3. Meniscus tear
Blow to patellofemoral joint, or fall on flexed knee, foot dorsiflexed	1. Patellar articular injury or osteochondral fracture
Blow to tibial tubercle, or fall on flexed knee, foot plantar flexed	1. Posterior cruciate ligament
Anterior blow to tibia, resulting in knee hyperextension (contact hypertension)	1. Anterior cruciate ligament 2. Anterior and posterior cruciate ligament
Noncontact hyperextension	1. Anterior cruciate ligament 2. Posterior capsule
Noncontact deceleration	1. Anterior cruciate ligament
Noncontact deceleration, with tibial medial rotation or femoral lateral rotation on fixed tibia	1. Anterior cruciate ligament
Noncontact, quickly turning one way with tibia rotated in opposite direction	1. Patellar dislocation or subluxation
Noncontact, rotation with varus or valgus loading	1. Meniscus injury 2. Medial collateral ligament
Noncontact, compressive rotation	1. Meniscus injury 2. Osteochondral fracture
Hyperflexion	1. Meniscus (posterior horn) 2. Anterior cruciate ligament
Forced medial rotation	1. Meniscus injury (lateral meniscus)
Forced lateral rotation	1. Meniscus injury (medial meniscus) 2. Medial collateral ligament and possibly anterior cruciate ligament 3. Patellar dislocation
Flexion-varus-medial rotation	1. Anterolateral instability
Flexion-valgus-lateral rotation	1. Anteromedial instability
Dashboard injury	1. Isolated posterior cruciate ligament 2. Posterior cruciate ligament and posterior capsule 3. Posterolateral instability 4. Posteromedial instability 5. Patellar fracture 6. Tibial fracture (proximal) 7. Tibial plateau fracture 8. Acetabular and pelvic fracture

Adapted from Clancy W: Evaluation of acute knee injuries. In American Association of Orthopaedic Surgeons, *Symposium on sports medicine: the knee*, St Louis, 1985, Mosby; Strobel M, Stedtfeld HW: *Diagnostic evaluation of the knee*, Berlin, 1990, Springer-Verlag.

parts work in concert. Forces applied to one part of the chain must be absorbed by that part as well as by other parts of the closed chain. If the forces are too great, injury results. Bone tumors have a more insidious onset with swelling, unexplained deep pain, and a palpable mass as the first signs often combined with night pain, constant ache, and difficulty using the limb (i.e., limp)—all of which get progressively worse.[27]

2. *What type of playing surface was the patient playing on (if an athlete!) when the injury occurred?* Artificial playing surfaces increase the risk of anterior cruciate ligament injuries.[28] What type of shoe does the patient wear during the day and with different activities? Were the shoes designed for the surface they were competing on (if an athlete)? What is the "wear pattern" of the shoes? This will give the examiner an idea of stress put on the lower leg, ankle, and foot.

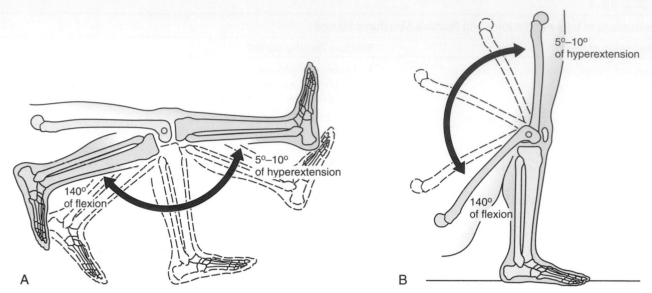

Fig. 12.4 Sagittal plane motion at the knee. (A) Tibial-on-femoral perspective (open kinetic chain). (B) Femoral-on-tibial perspective (closed kinetic chain). (Modified from Neumann DA: *Kinesiology of the musculoskeletal system—foundations for physical rehabilitation*, St Louis, 2002, Mosby, p 444.)

3. *Has the knee been injured before, or does it have any feeling of weakness?* The examiner should be aware of potential neuromuscular risk factors and altered neuromuscular activation patterns that may increase the risk of injury especially when the individual is fatigued (e.g., quadriceps/hamstrings strength imbalance, structural and functional deformities, bilateral strength and range-of-motion [ROM] differences, hypomobility/hypermobility laxity differences, dynamic balance alterations, mobility versus stability of different body segments).[29–31] These injuries can lead to arthritic changes.[32]

4. *Does the patient wear a brace?* If so, what type (e.g., neoprene, neoprene with metal/fiberglass stays, custom made)? The type of brace may indicate the type of injury. In addition, if the patient wears a brace, does it make him or her more functional?[33]

5. *What is the patient able or unable to do functionally? Is there disability on running, cutting, pivoting, twisting, climbing, or descending stairs?* Positive responses to these questions should alert the examiner to instability caused by injured ligaments, muscle dysfunction, joint articular problems, or meniscus problems.[34]

6. *Is there any "clicking," or was there a "pop" when the injury occurred?* A distinct pop may indicate an anterior cruciate ligament or medial collateral ligament tear or osteochondral fracture. Popping on the lateral aspect of the knee may be due to the popliteus tendon snapping over the lateral femoral inferoposterior tubercle within 2 cm of the muscle's attachment into the femur.[35] Posterior cruciate ligament injuries typically have more vague symptoms of unsteadiness or discomfort.[36] Patients with an acute posterior cruciate ligament injury have moderate effusion, posterior knee pain, or pain with kneeling.[37]

7. *Did the injury occur during acceleration, during deceleration, or when the patient was moving at a constant speed?* Acceleration and twisting and cutting injuries may involve the meniscus and ligaments. Deceleration injuries often involve the cruciate ligaments. Constant speed with cutting may involve the anterior cruciate ligament.[37]

8. *Is there any pain? If so, where? What type is it? Retropatellar? Does the patient point to one spot with one finger or a more general area indicating the problem is more diffuse, aching?*[38] Aching pain may indicate degenerative changes, whereas sharp, "catching" pain usually indicates a mechanical problem. Arthritic pain is more likely to be associated with stiffness in the morning and eases with activity. Anterior knee pain may be due to patellofemoral problems, bursa (prepatellar, infrapatellar) pathology, fat pad pathology, tendinosis, or Osgood-Schlatter disease.[39,40] Patellofemoral pain tends to be insidious and occurs spontaneously, often from overuse, which makes establishing the source of the problem important.[41,42] Pain at rest is not usually mechanical in origin. Pain during activity is usually seen in structural abnormalities, such as subluxation or patellar tracking disorders. Pain after activity or with overuse is characteristic of inflammatory disorders, such as synovial plica irritation or early tendinosis or paratenonitis leading to jumper's knee or Sinding-Larsen-Johansson syndrome.[43–48] Generalized pain in the area of the knee is usually characteristic of contusions or partial tears of muscles or ligaments. Instability rather than pain tends to be the major presenting factor in complex ligament disruptions or muscle dysfunction (e.g., quadriceps rupture). Pain in the knee on ankle movements may implicate the superior tibiofibular joint.

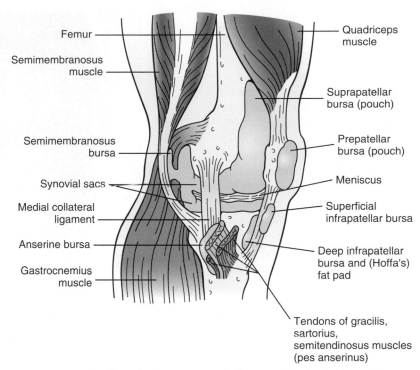

Fig. 12.5 The bursae around the knee (medial aspect).

9. *Do certain positions or activities have an increased or decreased effect on the pain? Which activities produce pain? How much activity is needed to produce pain? Which positions or activities ease the pain? Does the pain go away when activity ceases?* The examiner must take note of constant pain that is unrelated to activity, time, or posture, because it usually indicates serious pathology, such as a tumor. Does the patient have confidence in the knee? Such a question gives the examiner some idea of the functional impairment from the patient's perspective.[49]

10. *Does the knee "give way?"*[49] This finding usually indicates instability in the knee, meniscus pathology, patellar subluxation (if present when rotation or stopping is involved), undisplaced osteochondritis dissecans (OCD), patellofemoral syndrome, plica, or loose body. Giving way when walking uphill or downhill is more likely the result of a retropatellar lesion.[34,50,51] If the patient complains that the patella "slips out of place," it may be because of patellar subluxation or a pathological plica.[52]

11. *Has the knee ever locked?* True locking of the knee is rare. Loose bodies may cause recurrent locking. Locking must be differentiated from catching, which is momentary locking or giving way as a result of reflex inhibition or pain.[52] **Locking** in the knee usually means that the knee cannot fully extend with flexion often being normal, and it is related to meniscus pathology. Hamstring muscle spasm may also limit extension and is sometimes referred to as **spasm locking.**

12. *On movement, is there any grating or clicking in the knee?* Grating or clicking may be caused by degeneration or by one structure's snapping over another.

13. *Is the joint swollen? Does the swelling occur with activity or several hours after activity, or does the joint feel tight at rest?* Swelling with activity may be caused by instability, and tightness at rest may be caused by arthritic changes or patellofemoral dysfunction. Is the swelling recurrent? If so, what activity causes it? Swelling with pivoting or twisting may be a result of meniscus problems or instability at the tibiofemoral joint. Recurrent swelling caused by climbing or descending slopes or stairs may be related to patellofemoral dysfunction.[52] Often there is no swelling in the knee after severe injury, because the fluid extravasates into the soft tissues surrounding the joint and because a number of structures around the knee joint are avascular and can be injured without bloody swelling occurring. Synovial swelling may occur 8 to 24 hours after the injury; swelling caused by blood begins to occur almost immediately. Localized swelling may be caused by an inflamed bursa (Fig. 12.5).[53] The deep infrapatellar bursa has been noted as a source of anterior knee pain and could be misdiagnosed as patellofemoral arthralgia or Osgood-Schlatter disease.[54,55]

14. *Is the gait normal? Does the patient put weight on the limb? Can the patient extend the knee while walking? Is the stride length altered on the affected limb?* All these questions give an indication of the patient's functional disability and how much the knee is bothering the patient.

Observation

For a proper observation, the patient must be suitably undressed so that the examiner can observe the posture of the spine as well as the alignment of the hips, knees, and ankles. The alignment contributes to lower limb load distribution across each joint articular surface. In the neutrally aligned knee, the medial compartment bears 60% to 70% of the load across the knee.[56] Knee alignment is determined by tibiofemoral congruence, ligament integrity, meniscus degeneration and position, articular cartilage loss, bone attrition, and osteophytes.[56,57] Initially, the examiner should note whether the patient puts weight on the affected limb or stands with only a slight amount of weight on the affected side. In addition to the common observational items mentioned in Chapter 1, the examiner should look for the following alterations around the knee.

Anterior View, Standing

From the anterior aspect (Fig. 12.6), the examiner should note any malalignment, including **genu varum** (bowleg) or **genu valgum** (knock-knee) deformity (Fig. 12.7). Any observable malalignment may lead to or be the result of malalignment elsewhere (Table 12.2).[58] These deformities may be unilateral or bilateral. Although in adults the legs should be relatively straight, in the child, the normal development of the knee is from genu varum to straight, to genu valgum, and then to straight. Initially, a child's lower limbs are in genu varum until 18 or 19 months, when they straighten. The knee then goes into genu valgum until approximately 3 to 4 years of age (Fig. 12.8). The limbs should be almost straight by age 6 years and should remain that way. In the adult, the knee is normally in approximately 6° of valgus.

To observe genu varum and genu valgum, the patient is positioned so that the patellae face forward and the medial aspects of the knees and medial malleoli of both limbs are as close together as possible. If the knees touch and the ankles do not, the patient has a genu valgum. A distance of 9 to 10 cm (3.5 to 4 inches) between the ankles is considered excessive. If two or more fingers (4 cm [1.6 inches]) fit between the knees when the ankles are together, the patient has a varus deformity or genu varum.[59] On x-ray studies, the normal **tibiofemoral shaft angle** is approximately 6° (Fig. 12.9).

Alignment is often different between males and females.[60] Some of these misalignments, if excessive, can lead to patellofemoral symptoms or instability.[61] These excessive differences are sometimes referred to as **miserable malalignment syndrome** and can include anterior pelvic tilt, increased hip/femoral anteversion, tibial torsion, decreased tibiofemoral angle, genu recurvatum, navicular drop, and increased foot pronation (Figs. 12.10 and 12.11).[62] Similarly, excessive hip adduction and

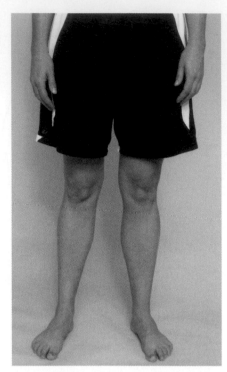

Fig. 12.6 Anterior view of the lower limbs. Note the wider than normal base width.

medial rotation along with relative medial deviation of the knee and tibial abduction can result in **dynamic knee valgus** which is the result of medial collapse during loading (e.g., when doing a squat) (Fig. 12.12).[63] This movement may also be accompanied by lateral rotation of the tibia, anterior translation of the knee, rear foot eversion or navicular drop, and decreased dorsiflexion.[63]

The patient is asked to extend the knees to see whether the movement can be performed and what effect it has on the knee. Both knees should extend equally. If not, something must be limiting the movement (swelling, loose body, or meniscus). Normally, a person does not stand with the knees fully extended. If, however, the patient has an excessive lordosis, the knees are often hyperextended to maintain the center of gravity. This change can lead to posterior knee pain.

Is there any apparent swelling or ecchymosis in or around the knees (see Fig. 1.6)? If there is intracapsular swelling, or at least sufficient swelling, the knee assumes a position of 15° to 25° of flexion, which provides the synovial cavity with the maximum capacity to hold fluid. This position is also called the **resting position** of the knee. Early signs of effusion include the loss of the peripatellar groove on each side of the patella (see Fig. 12.124).[38] Is the swelling intracapsular or extracapsular? Intracapsular swelling is evident over the entire joint; extracapsular swelling tends to be more localized. An example of extracapsular swelling is shown in Fig. 12.13, which illustrates **prepatellar bursitis**.

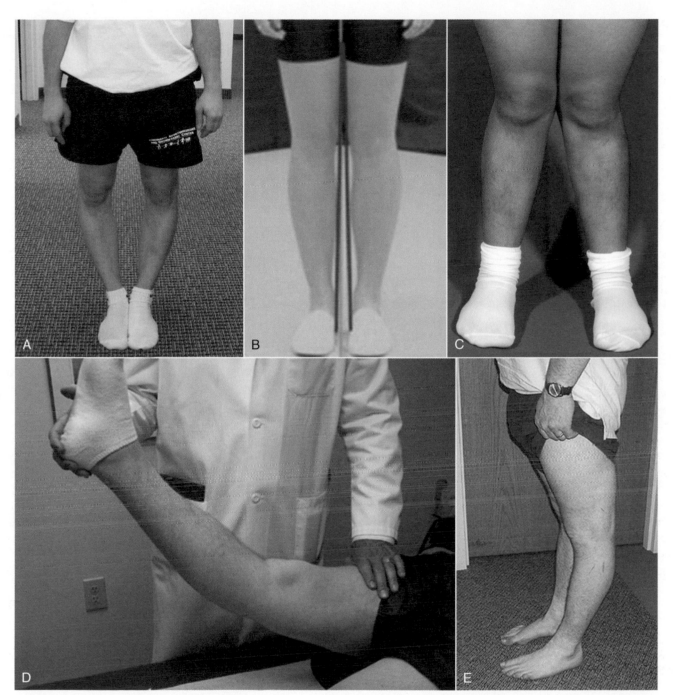

Fig. 12.7 Genu varum and genu valgum. (A) Bilateral genu varum. (B) Straight. (C) Bilateral genu valgum. (D) Hyperextension in supine. (E) Genu recurvatum. (A, From Noyes FR, Barber-Westin SD: Tibial and femoral osteotomy for varus and valgus knee syndromes: diagnosis, osteotomy techniques, and clinical outcomes. In Noyes FR, Barber-Westin SD, editors: *Noyes' knee disorders: surgery, rehabilitation, clinical outcomes*, ed 2, Philadelphia, 2017, Elsevier; B, From Seckiner D, Mallett X, Maynard P, et al: Forensic gait analysis—morphometric assessment from surveillance footage, *Forensic Sci Int* 296:57–66, 2019; C, From Johnston CE, Young M: Disorders of the leg. In Herring JA, editors: *Tachdjian's pediatric orthopaedics*, ed 5, Philadelphia, 2014, Elsevier; D and E, From Noyes FR, Barber-Westin SD: Medial and posteromedial ligament injuries: diagnosis, operative techniques and clinical outcomes. In Noyes FR, Barber-Westin SD, editors: *Noyes' knee disorders: surgery, rehabilitation, clinical outcomes*, ed 2, Philadelphia, 2017, Elsevier.)

The examiner should ask the patient to contract the quadriceps muscles to see whether there is any visible wasting of the muscles, especially of the vastus medialis obliquus (VMO). The prominence of the vastus medialis results from the obliquity of the distal fibers, the inferior position of its insertion, and the thinness of the fascial covering compared with the other quadriceps muscles. Quadriceps muscle defects (i.e., third-degree strain or rupture) should also be watched for when the patient contracts the muscles. Third-degree strains may be indicated by muscle "bunching," abnormal mechanics (e.g., unilateral patella alta with patella tendon rupture), a palpable

TABLE **12.2**

Malalignment About the Knee and Possible Correlated and Compensatory Motions or Postures

Malalignment	Possible Correlated Motions or Postures	Possible Compensatory Motions or Postures
Genu valgum	Pes planus Excessive subtalar pronation Lateral tibial torsion Lateral patellar subluxation Excessive hip adduction Ipsilateral hip excessive medial rotation Lumbar spine contralateral rotation	Forefoot varus Excessive subtalar supination to allow the lateral heel to contact the ground In-toeing to decrease lateral pelvic sway during gait Ipsilateral pelvic lateral rotation
Genu varum	Excessive lateral angulation of the tibia in the frontal plane; tibial varum Medial tibial torsion Ipsilateral hip lateral rotation Excessive hip abduction	Forefoot valgus Excessive subtalar pronation to allow the medial heel to contact the ground Ipsilateral pelvic medial rotation
Genu recurvatum	Ankle plantar flexion Excessive anterior pelvic tilt	Posterior pelvic tilt Flexed trunk posture Excessive thoracic kyphosis
Lateral tibial torsion	Out-toeing Excessive subtalar supination with related rotation along the lower quarter	Functional forefoot varus Excessive subtalar pronation with relaxed rotation along the lower quarter
Medial tibial torsion	In-toeing Metatarsus adductus Excessive subtalar pronation with related rotation along the lower quarter	Functional forefoot valgus Excessive subtalar supination with relaxed rotation along the lower quarter
Excessive tibial retroversion (posterior slant of tibial plateaus)	Genu recurvatum	
Inadequate tibial retrotorsion (posterior deflection of proximal tibia due to hamstrings pull)	Flexed knee posture	
Inadequate tibial retroflexion (bowing of the tibia)	Altered alignment of Achilles tendon causing altered associated joint motion	
Bowleg deformity of the tibia (tibial varum)	Medial tibial torsion	Forefoot valgus Excessive subtalar pronation

From Riegger-Krugh C, Keysor JJ: Skeletal malalignments of the lower quarter: correlated and compensatory motions and postures, *J Orthop Sports Phys Ther* 23:166–167, 1996.

defect, the knee not extending fully, and the knee only stable in full extension when standing as the position is held (i.e., full extension) by the iliotibial band.[52]

The position of the patella should be noted. When viewing the patellae, the examiner should note whether they face straight ahead, tilt outward ("grasshopper eyes" patellae), tilt inward ("squinting" patellae), or are rotated ("spin") in or out (Fig. 12.14).[64] Rotation and tilt may be caused by tight structures that alter the position of the patella. These tight structures may include muscles (e.g., rectus femoris, iliotibial band, gastrocnemius) or fascia (e.g., lateral retinaculum). Normally, the patellae should face straight ahead with no lateral tilt or rotation. If these deviations are seen in the observation phase, they are considered static problems, and the examiner should test patellar movement passively and watch the patellae during active movements to see whether it is a dynamic problem as well.[65] A squinting or rotated patella may indicate

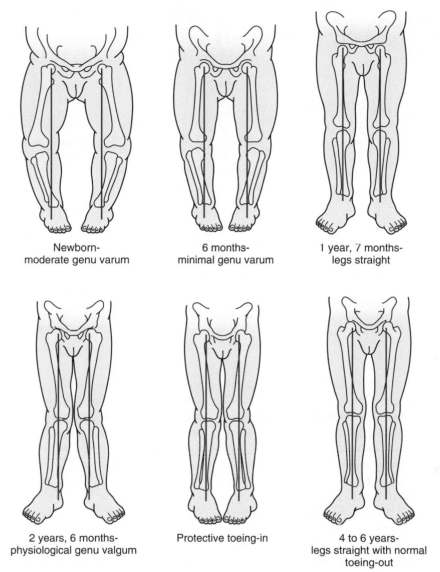

Fig. 12.8 Physiological evolution of lower limb alignment at various ages in infancy and childhood. (Redrawn from Tachdjian MO: *Pediatric orthopedics*, Philadelphia, 1972, WB Saunders, p 1463.)

Newborn-
moderate genu varum

6 months-
minimal genu varum

1 year, 7 months-
legs straight

2 years, 6 months-
physiological genu valgum

Protective toeing-in

4 to 6 years-
legs straight with normal
toeing-out

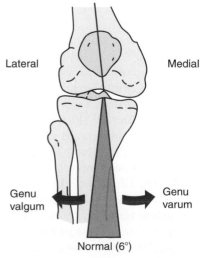

Fig. 12.9 Normal tibiofemoral shaft angle.

medial femoral or lateral tibial torsion (Fig. 12.15). Patients with abnormal torsion are prone to patellofemoral instability.

Any bruising or discoloration around the knee should also be noted, as well as any scars or signs indicating recent injury or surgery.

Lateral View, Standing

The examiner then views the patient from both sides for comparison. It should be noted whether **genu recurvatum** (hyperextended knee) (see Fig. 12.7E)[66] or a fixed flexion deformity (Fig. 12.16) is present and whether one or both patellae are higher **(patella alta)** or lower **(patella baja** or **patella infera)**[67] than normal (Fig. 12.17). For example, patella alta can increase the patellofemoral contact force during flexion, which may contribute to

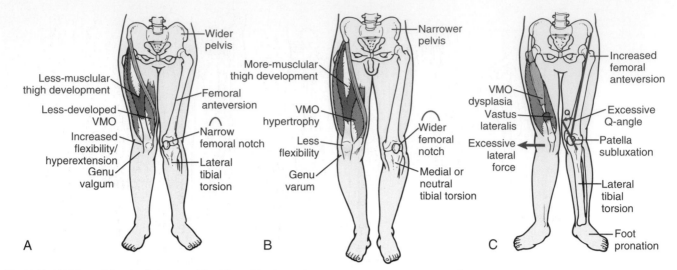

Fig. 12.10 (A) Normal female alignment with wider pelvis, femoral anteversion, genu valgum, hyperflexibility, lateral tibial torsion, and narrow notch. (B) Normal male alignment demonstrates a narrower pelvis, more developed musculature, genu varum, medial or neutral tibial torsion, and wider notch. (C) Miserable malalignment syndrome is a term coined to describe patients who have increased femoral anteversion, genu valgum, vastus medialis obliquus *(VMO)* dysplasia, lateral tibial torsion, and forefoot pronation. These factors create excessive lateral forces and contribute to patellofemoral dysfunction. (From Griffin LY, editor: *Rehabilitation of the injured knee*, St Louis, 1995, Mosby, pp 298–299.)

anterior knee pain.[68] With an abnormally high patella, a **"camel sign"** may be present (Fig. 12.18); because of the high patella (one "hump"), the infrapatellar fat pad (second hump) or an inflamed infrapatellar bursa (just anterior to the fat pad) becomes more prominent. This finding is especially noticeable in females. In this position, the examiner should also note (Fig. 12.19) whether the inferior pole of the patella is tilted in (inferior tilt). Ideally, the plane of the patella and that of the femoral condyles should be the same. If the inferior pole tilts in, fat pad irritation may occur.[69] Habitual genu recurvatum may make a patient prone to posterior cruciate tears because of the stretching of the posterior oblique ligament.[52] If one knee (normal) hyperextends and the other one (injured) does not, it may indicate meniscus pathology that is limiting extension. Osteoarthritic lipping (Fig. 12.20) or synovial hypertrophy (rheumatoid arthritis) may also limit movement.

Posterior View, Standing

Next, the examiner views the patient from behind, looking for findings similar to those from the anterior aspect. In addition, the examiner looks for abnormal swellings, such as a popliteal (Baker's) cyst, which is caused by herniation of synovial tissue through a weakening in the posterior capsule wall (Fig. 12.21).[70]

Anterior and Lateral Views, Sitting

For the final part of the observation, the patient sits with the knee flexed to 90° and the feet either partially bearing weight (on a stool) or dangling free. The patient is observed from the front and from the side. In this position, the patella should face forward and should rest on the distal end of the femur. With patella alta, the patella becomes more aligned with the anterior surface of the femur (angled upward). If the patella is laterally displaced or laterally displaced with a patella alta, the patellae take on the appearance of "frog eyes" or "grasshopper eyes" (Fig. 12.22), meaning that the patellae face upward and outward, away from each other. Patella alta sometimes causes a concavity proximal to the patella in thin patients.[52] Any bony enlargements, such as those seen in Osgood-Schlatter disease (i.e., an enlarged tibial tubercle), should be noted (Fig. 12.23), as should abnormal swelling. Swelling of the pes anserine bursa and a meniscal cyst (Fig. 12.24) are best visualized in the seated position.[52,71] Meniscal cysts may also present as isolated medial or lateral swelling.[50]

In the same position or in standing, any **tibial torsion** should be noted.[69,72] If there is tibial torsion, it is medial torsion that is associated with genu varum; genu valgum is associated with lateral tibial torsion (Fig. 12.25). Normally, the patella faces straight ahead while the foot faces slightly laterally (Fick angle). With medial tibial torsion, the feet point toward each other, resulting in a "pigeon-toed" foot deformity. These deformities can be exacerbated by habitual postures. The positions illustrated in Figs. 12.26, 12.27, and 12.28 cause problems only if they are used habitually. Excessive tibial torsion can contribute to conditions such as chondromalacia patellae, patellofemoral instability, and fat pad entrapment. When standing, most people exhibit a lateral tibial torsion, the

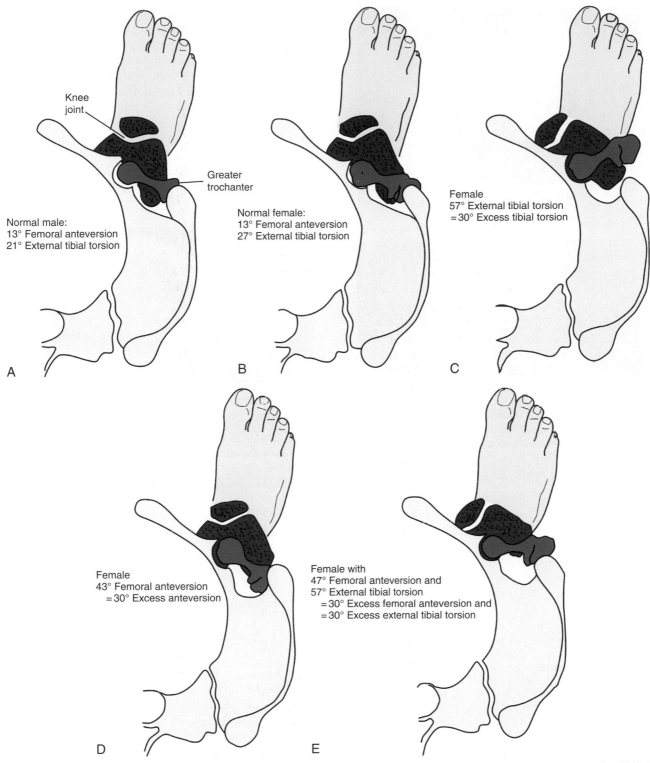

Fig. 12.11 (A) Normal male with femoral anteversion of 13° and external tibial torsion of 21°. Note that with a foot progression angle of 13° (Fick angle) the knee joint faces slightly outward. (B) Normal female with femoral anteversion of 13° and external tibial torsion of 27°. Note that the knee joint is pointing slightly more inward and the greater trochanter is slightly more anterior than the normal side. (C) Female with 30° of increase in tibial torsion to keep the foot progression angle normal; the knee joint axis points inward nearly 30° causing increased strain on the knee. The hip appears markedly medially rotated with the greater trochanter pointing somewhat anteriorly. (D) Female with 30° of increase in femoral anteversion. The knee joint points in the same direction, slightly inward, as in the normal female, but the greater trochanter points posteriorly, giving a poor mechanical advantage. At some point, the hip cannot laterally rotate enough to keep the knee joint pointed forward. With fatigue of the hip abductors, the knee points more inward to compensate for hip collapse, placing greater stress on the knee. (E) Female with 30° of increase in both femoral anteversion and external tibial torsion. Note the trochanter is pointed more anterior than normal, and with the foot progression angle normal, the knee joint axis points markedly inward. (From Teitge RA: Patellofemoral disorders: correction of rotational malalignment of the lower extremity. In Noyes FR, Barber-Westin SD, editors: *Noyes' knee disorders: surgery, rehabilitation, clinical outcomes*, ed 2, Philadelphia, 2017, Elsevier.)

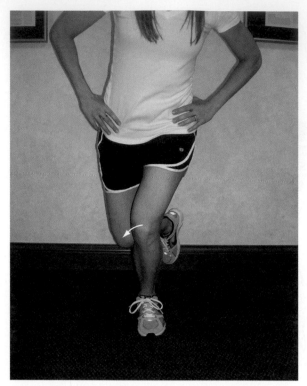

Fig. 12.12 Dynamic knee valgus. Note how the knee moves medially during squat and alters the alignment of the leg. (From Heckmann TP, Noyes FR, Barber-Westin SD: Correction of hyperextension gait abnormalities: preoperative and postoperative techniques. In Noyes FR, Barber-Westin SD, editors: *Noyes' knee disorders: surgery, rehabilitation, clinical outcomes*, ed 2, Philadelphia, 2017, Elsevier.)

Fick angle (see Fig. 13.13), which increases as the child grows. This angle is approximately 5° in babies and as much as 18° in adults. To test for tibial torsion, the examiner aligns the patient's straight legs (knees extended) so that the patellae face straight ahead. The examiner then looks at the feet to determine their angle relative to the shaft of the tibia.

Femoral torsion, or anteversion (discussed in Chapter 11), can also affect the position of the patella relative to the femur and tibia.

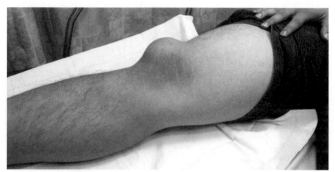

Fig. 12.13 Prepatellar bursitis. Swelling is confined to the bursa between the skin and the patella. (From Gupta N: Treatment of bursitis, tendinitis, and trigger points. In Roberts JR, Custalow CB, Thomsen TW, editors: *Roberts and Hedges' clinical procedures in emergency medicine and acute care*, ed 7, Philadelphia, 2019, Elsevier.)

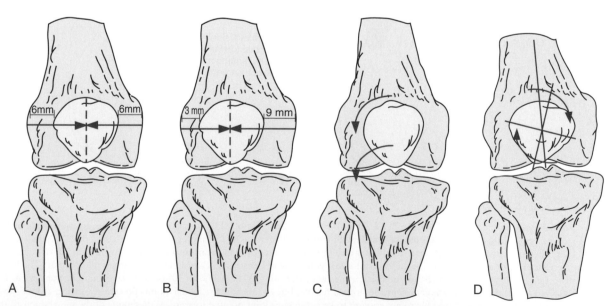

Fig. 12.14 Assessment of the patellar glide component. Ideally, the patella should be centered on the superior portion of the femoral articular surface at 20° flexion. (A) Ideal alignment. (B) Lateral glide of the patella. (C) Lateral tilt of the patella. (D) Lateral rotation ("spin") of inferior pole of patella. (From McConnell J, Fulkerson J: The knee: patellofemoral and soft tissue injuries. In Zachazewski JE, et al., editors: *Athletic injuries and rehabilitation*, Philadelphia, 1996, WB Saunders, pp 711–712.)

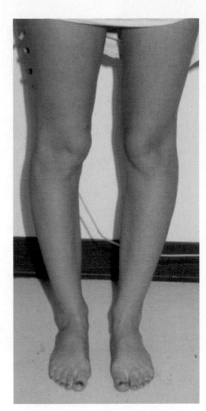

Fig. 12.15 Standing rotational malalignment shows "squinting patella" and miserable alignment syndrome. Both patellae point inward in a medial fashion, a sign of excessive femoral anteversion or increased medial femoral torsion. (From Teitge RA: Patellofemoral disorders: correction of rotational malalignment of the lower extremity. In Noyes FR, Barber-Westin SD, editors: *Noyes' knee disorders: surgery, rehabilitation, clinical outcomes*, ed 2, Philadelphia, 2017, Elsevier.)

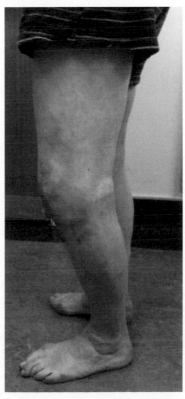

Fig. 12.16 Fixed flexion deformity of the knee. (From Ali F: Clinical examination of the knee, *Orthop Trauma* 27[1]:51, 2013.)

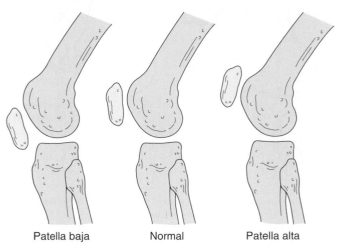

Patella baja   Normal   Patella alta

Fig. 12.17 The normal patellar posture for exerting deceleration forces in the functional position of 45° of knee flexion places the patellar articular surface squarely against the anterior femur. A lower posture represents patella baja. A higher posture represents patella alta. Patella alta makes the patella less efficient in exerting normal forces. (Redrawn from Hughston JC, Walsh WM, Puddu G: *Patellar subluxation and dislocation*, Philadelphia, 1984, WB Saunders, p 8.)

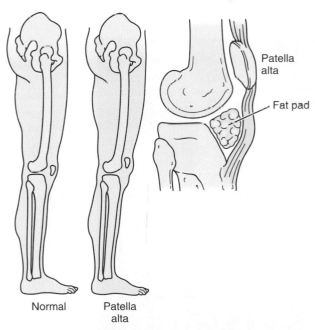

Normal   Patella alta

Fig. 12.18 Camel sign. Double hump seen from side caused by high-riding patella and uncovered infrapatellar fat pad. (Modified from Hughston JC, Walsh WM, Puddu G: *Patellar subluxation and dislocation*, Philadelphia, 1984, WB Saunders, p 22.)

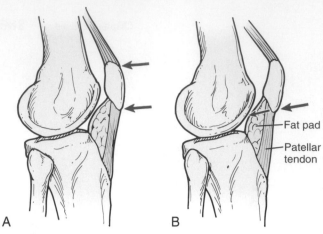

Fig. 12.19 Assessment of the anteroposterior component of the patella. Ideally, the superior and inferior poles of the patella should be parallel in the sagittal plane of the knee. (A) Commonly, in individuals with patellar malalignment, the inferior patellar pole pushes posteriorly into the infrapatellar fat pad. (B) This may irritate the fat pad. (Redrawn from McConnell J, Fulkerson J: The knee: patellofemoral and soft tissue injuries. In Zachazewski JE, et al., editors: *Athletic injuries and rehabilitation*, Philadelphia, 1996, WB Saunders, p 712.)

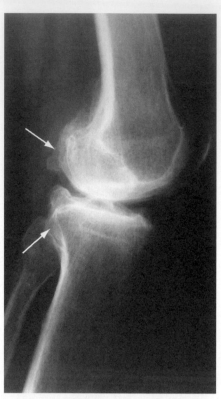

Fig. 12.20 Osteophytic lipping *(arrows)* in posterior knee limits flexion and produces a bone-to-bone end feel.

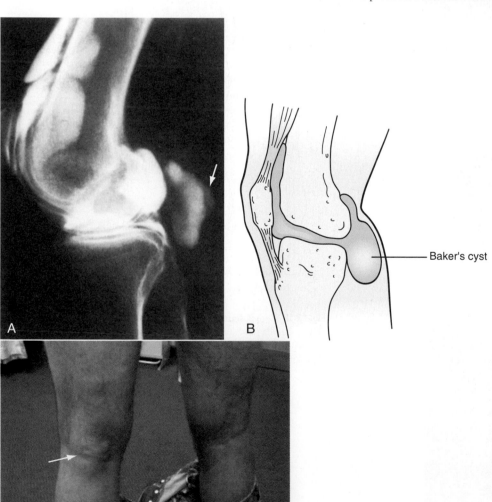

Fig. 12.21 Popliteal (Baker's) cysts. (A) This 74-year-old man presented with the acute onset of calf pain and swelling without knee pain. The initial suspected diagnosis was popliteal thrombosis. A venogram was normal. The arthrogram revealed a collection of dye posterior to the joint space—a popliteal cyst *(arrow)*. (B) Schematic diagram of Baker's cyst. (C) Popliteal cyst viewed from behind (posterior view). (A, From Reilly BM: *Practical strategies in outpatient medicine*, Philadelphia, 1991, WB Saunders, p 1179; C, From Ali F: Clinical examination of the knee, *Orthop Trauma* 27[1]:51, 2013.)

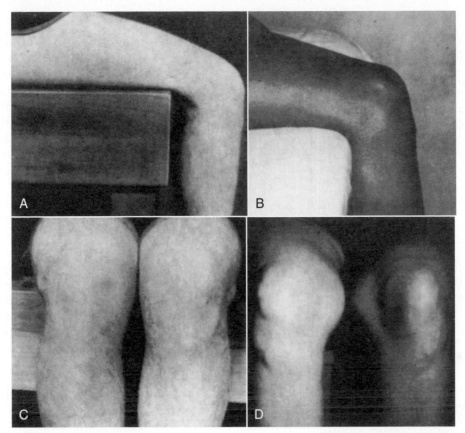

Fig. 12.22 (A) Normal knee seen from side; patella faces straight ahead in line with femur. (B) Patella alta seen from side; patella points toward ceiling. (C) Normal patellae seen from front; patellae centered in outline of knees. (D) High and lateral posturing of patellae seen from front, giving "grasshopper eyes" or "frog eyes" appearance. (From Hughston JC, Walsh WM, Puddu G: *Patellar subluxation and dislocation*, Philadelphia, 1984, WB Saunders, p 23.)

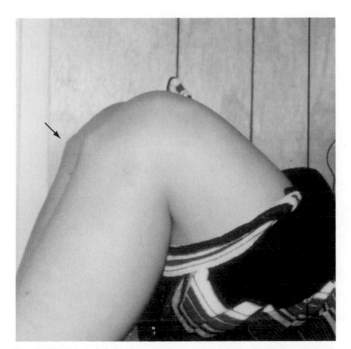

Fig. 12.23 Osgood-Schlatter disease with enlarged tibial tuberosity *(arrow)*.

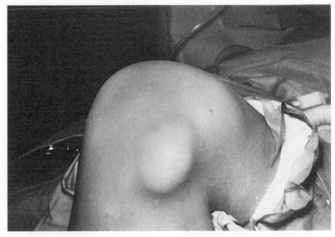

Fig. 12.24 Lateral meniscus cyst. (From Reider B: *The orthopedic physical examination*, Philadelphia, 1999, WB Saunders, p 209.)

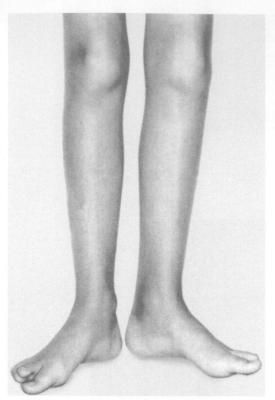

Fig. 12.25 Exaggerated lateral tibial torsion. In stance, with the patellae facing straight forward, the feet point outward. (From Tachdjian MO: *Pediatric orthopedics*, Philadelphia, 1990, WB Saunders, p 2816.)

Gait

The examiner should also observe the patient's gait (see Chapter 14), noting any differences in stride length, walking speed, cadence, or linear and angular displacement. In addition, the examiner should watch for abnormal patellar movement, indicating possible patellar tracking problems, and abnormal motion of the tibia relative to the femur, indicating possible instability problems. In patients with osteoarthritis, the examiner watches for a **varus thrust,** which is a dynamic alignment change and instability on loading the knee, that is most obvious in single leg midstance in which the knee, on weight bearing, is thrust laterally and is an indication of progressive medial tibiofemoral pathology.[73–77]

Movement at the pelvis, hip, and ankle should also be observed. For example, weak hip abductors (positive Trendelenburg sign) may lead to increased stress on the knee. If this is combined with medial tibial torsion, patellofemoral syndromes may result.[52,78] Tight heel cords may result in gait with the knee flexed, which can put extra pressure on the patellofemoral joint. Similarly, pronation of the foot and lateral tibial torsion may lead to patellofemoral pathology or anteromedial joint pain.[52] Tight hamstrings result in increased knee flexion, which can lead to the need for more ankle dorsiflexion. If no further dorsiflexion is possible, the foot pronates to compensate, thus increasing the **dynamic Q-angle.**[79]

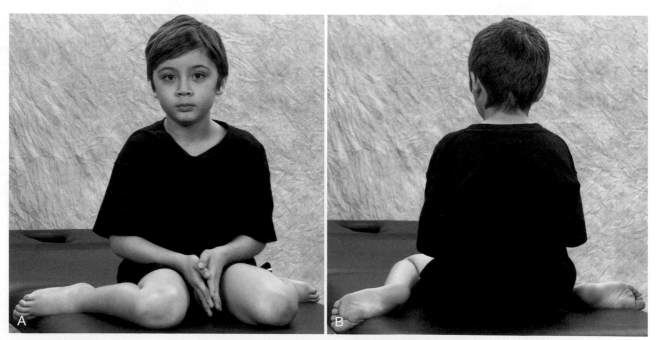

Fig. 12.26 "Television" or "W" sitting position may lead to excessive lateral tibial torsion. (A) Anterior view. (B) Posterior view.

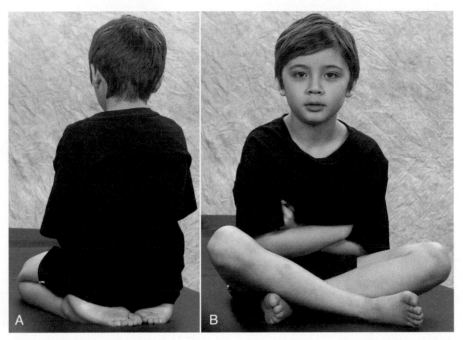

Fig. 12.27 Medial tibial torsion. (A) Position to be avoided to prevent excessive medial tibial torsion. (B) Tailor position maintains normal medial tibial torsion.

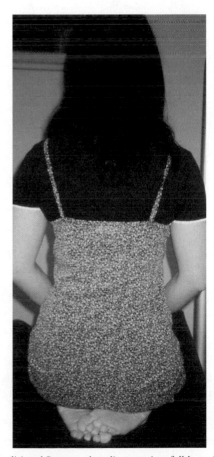

Fig. 12.28 Traditional Japanese kneeling requires full knee flexion, often accompanied by medial tibial rotation.

Examination

Although the examination focuses primarily on the knee, the examiner must keep in mind that knee pathology may be the result of biomechanical (e.g., alignment, asymmetry) and pathological (e.g., hypomobility, hypermobility, muscle weakness, instability) issues in other joints in the kinetic chain, including the lumbar spine, pelvis, hips, ankles, and feet. Thus the examination, like the history and observation, may be extensive to rule out other kinetic chain contributors.[80–85] For example, Dutton[86] believed the gracilis and adductor longus and magnus play a significant role along with the iliotibial band in knee stability. In addition, several muscles that are two-joint muscles acting over the hip and knee (e.g., rectus femoris, hamstrings, sartorius, gracilis) and knee and ankle (gastrocnemius) should be tested for functional mobility because their action at one joint can affect the other joint (Fig. 12.29). The examination should always start with the healthy knee to create trust between the patient and examiner and to allow the patient to relax.[38]

Active Movements

The examination is performed initially with the patient sitting and then with the patient in lying position. During the active movements, the examiner should observe (1) the excursion of the patella to ensure that it tracks freely and smoothly; (2) the ROM available; (3) whether pain occurs during the movement, and if so, where; and (4) what appears to be limiting the movement. The active

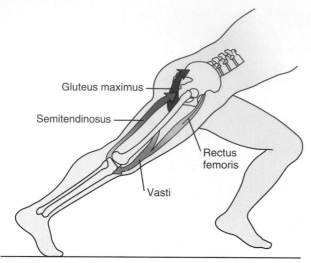

Fig. 12.29 The action of several one-joint and two-joint muscles is depicted during the hip-and-knee extension phase of running. Observe that the vasti extend the knee, which then stretches the distal end of the semitendinosus. The gluteus maximus extends the hip, which then stretches the proximal end of the rectus femoris. The stretch placed on the active biarticular muscles reduces the rate and amount of their overall contraction. (Redrawn from Neumann D: *Kinesiology of the musculoskeletal system—foundations for physical rehabilitation*, St Louis, 2002, Mosby, p 468.)

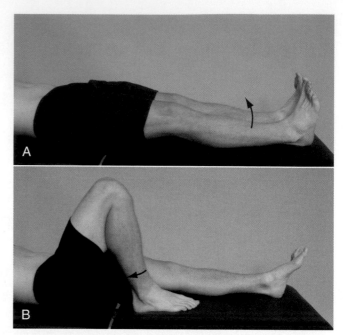

Fig. 12.30 Active movements of the knee. (A) Extension. (B) Flexion.

movements may be done in the sitting or supine position, and, as always, the most painful movements should be done last (Fig. 12.30).

Active Movements of the Knee Complex

- Flexion (0°–135°)
- Extension (0°–15°)
- Medial rotation of the tibia on the femur (20°–30°)
- Lateral rotation of the tibia on the femur (30°–40°)
- Repetitive movements (if necessary)
- Sustained postures (if necessary)
- Combined movements (if necessary)

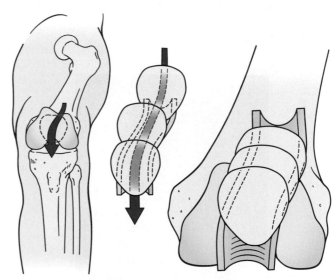

Fig. 12.31 Multiplanar patellar path during knee flexion. (Redrawn from Stanitski CL, DeLee JC, Drez D, editors: *Pediatric and adolescent sports medicine*, Philadelphia, 1994, WB Saunders, p 307.)

Full knee flexion is 135° (0° being straight knee). As the patient moves the knee through flexion and extension, the examiner should watch the movement of the patella as it "tracks" along the femoral trochlea. The examiner should note whether the movement is smooth from beginning to end or whether there is a lag or abrupt jump of the patella as it attempts to center in the groove.[87] The patella does not follow a straight path as the knee moves from extension to flexion. Normally, it follows a curved pattern moving medially in early flexion and then laterally engaging the femoral condyles at approximately 20° to 30° of knee flexion (Fig. 12.31).[88,89] In the presence of pathological patellar tracking and patellar instability, an inverted **"J" sign** (Fig. 12.32) may be noted.[89–92] During the initiation of flexion (e.g., going in to a squat), the laterally located patella moves suddenly medially to enter the trochlea. The key to the J sign is the sudden movement medially instead of the normal smooth movement pattern. It is indicative of excessive lateral patellar shift, patellar maltracking, or VMO insufficiency in terminal extension.[92] As in the observation phase, the examiner should note whether dynamic movement causes lateral tilt, anteroposterior tilt, or rotation of the patella during movement.[79,88]

Active knee extension is approximately 0° but may be –15°, especially in women, who are more likely to have hyperextended knees (genu recurvatum). The knee extensor muscles develop the greatest force near 60°,

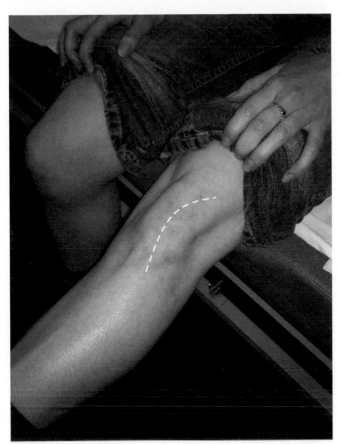

Fig. 12.32 The J sign can be demonstrated only with a patient sitting and hanging the leg over the side of the table and taking the leg from flexion to full extension. (From Ali F: Clinical examination of the knee, *Orthop Trauma* 27[1]:52, 2013.)

TABLE 12.3

Selected Factors That Contribute to the Inability to Completely Extend the Knee

Factor	Clinical Examples
Reduced force production from the quadriceps	Disuse atrophy of quadriceps following trauma and/or prolonged immobilization Lacerated femoral nerve Herniated disc compressing L3 or L4 nerve roots Severe pain Excessive swelling in the knee
Excessive resistance from connective tissues	Excessive tightness in hamstring or other knee flexor muscles Excessive stiffness in the anterior cruciate ligament, posterior capsule, or collateral ligaments Scarring of the skin in the popliteal fossa Excessive swelling in the knee
Faulty arthrokinematics	Lack of "screw-home" rotation mechanics Lack of anterior slide of the tibia[a] Meniscal block or other derangement Lack of superior slide of the patella[a]

[a]Assume tibial-on-femoral knee extension.
From Neumann DA: *Kinesiology of the musculoskeletal system—foundations for physical rehabilitation*, St Louis, 2002, Mosby, p 460.

and the knee flexor muscles develop their greatest force at 45° to 10°. To complete the last 15° of knee extension, a 60% increase in force of the quadriceps muscles is required. The examiner should also watch for evidence of **quadriceps lag,** which means the quadriceps muscles are not strong enough to fully extend the knee. The lag results from loss of mechanical advantage, muscle atrophy, decreasing power of the muscle as it shortens, adhesion formation, effusion, or reflex inhibition (Table 12.3). In non–weight bearing, active medial rotation of the tibia on the femur should be 20° to 30°, whereas active lateral rotation should be 30° to 40° at 90° flexion in non–weight bearing (Fig. 12.33A). In weight bearing (closed kinetic chain), the femur rotates on the tibia (Fig. 12.33B).

If, during the history, the patient has complained that repetitive or combined movements or sustained postures have resulted in symptoms, these movements should also be tested.

Passive Movements

If, on active movements, the ROM is full, overpressure may gently be applied to test the end feel of the various movements in the tibiofemoral joint. This action would

preclude the need to do passive movements to the tibiofemoral joint. However, the examiner must do movements of the patella passively (Fig. 12.34).

Passive Movements of the Knee Complex and Normal End Feel

- Flexion (tissue approximation)
- Extension (tissue stretch)
- Medial rotation of tibia on femur (tissue stretch)
- Lateral rotation of tibia on femur (tissue stretch)
- Patellar movement (tissue stretch—all directions)

At the tibiofemoral joint, the end feel of flexion is tissue approximation; the end feel of extension and of medial and lateral rotation of the tibia on the femur is tissue stretch. During passive movement, the examiner is also looking for a capsular pattern of the tibiofemoral joint.[93] This pattern is more limitation of flexion than of extension. Passive medial rotation of the tibia on the femur should be approximately 30° when the knee is flexed to 90°. Passive lateral rotation of the tibia on the femur at 90° of knee flexion should be 40°.

Although full knee extension is usually preferable for everyday activities (e.g., standing, walking), full flexion (135°) is often not necessary except where people kneel

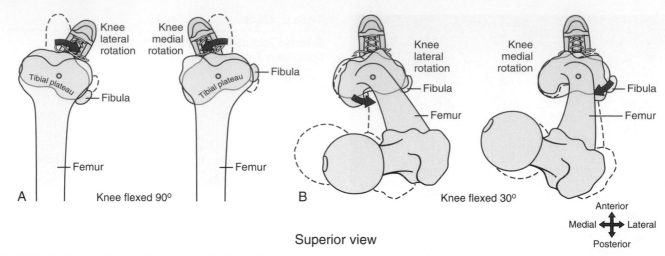

Fig. 12.33 Horizontal plane (axial) rotation at the knee. (A) Tibial-on-femoral rotation at 90° flexion (open kinetic chain—non–weight bearing). (B) Femoral-on-tibial rotation (closed kinetic chain—weight bearing). (Redrawn from Neumann DA: *Kinesiology of the musculoskeletal system—foundations for physical rehabilitation*, St Louis, 2002, Mosby, p 445.)

back on their heels. However, approximately 117° of flexion is necessary for activities, such as squatting to tie a shoelace or to pull on a sock. Sitting in a chair requires approximately 90° of flexion, and climbing stairs (average height) requires approximately 80° of flexion.

Lancaster et al.[94] advocated doing a **motion palpation test** when assessing the knee for articular damage when the damage is severe. The patient sits on the edge of the examining table with the knees flexed to approximately 90°. The examiner passively moves the patient's knee between 100° and 0° flexion three to four times at approximately 30°/s. While doing this movement with one hand, the examiner applies approximately 2.3 kg (5 lbs) compression over the patellofemoral joint while the index finger of the same hand palpates immediately distal to the inferior pole of the patella (Fig. 12.35). The examiner is palpating for joint crepitus and location, and severity of any discomfort that would indicate positive signs or possible articular damage (Table 12.4).

Passive medial and lateral movement of the patella is also carried out to determine its mobility and to compare it with the unaffected side. Normally, the patella should move up to half its width medially and laterally in extension (Fig. 12.36). Lateral glide greater than 75% of patellar width indicates MPFL insufficiency.[89] If the test is done with the knee flexed 30° and if the patella glides more than 75% of its width, the medial restraints are lax. If it glides less than 25%, then the lateral restraints are tight.[89] When the patella is pushed medially or laterally, the examiner should note whether it stays parallel to the femoral condyles or whether it tilts or rotates.[65] For example, if pushed medially when the medial structures are tight, the lateral border of the patella tilts up. Likewise, tight lateral structures cause the medial border to tilt up. If the lateral structures are tight superiorly, the inferior pole of the patella medially rotates. These are examples of dynamic tilt and rotation problems of the patella. The side to side

passive motion of the patella should also be tested in 45° of flexion, which is a more functional position and gives a better indication of functional instability of the patella.[95] The end feel of these movements is tissue stretch. Lateral displacement must be performed with care, especially in patients who have experienced a dislocated patella.

Objective measurements of patellar mobility can be made by describing the amount of movement based on quadrants or fourths of patellar movement (i.e., quadrants of mobility) (see Fig. 12.36). For example, if the patella has a normal passive medial translation of one-half of the width of the patella, a grade of two quadrants would be objectively described. A patella that has been dislocated laterally would have been objectively passively translated four quadrants or more. Kolowich et al.[96] reported that three quadrants of lateral glide suggest incompetent medial restraints, whereas a medial glide of less than one quadrant suggests a tight lateral retinaculum, and a medial glide of greater than three quadrants suggests patellar hypermobility.

The examiner must also ensure full and normal flexibility of the quadriceps, hamstring, iliotibial band, and abductor and adductor muscles of the thigh, as well as the gastrocnemius muscles (Fig. 12.37). Tightness of any of these structures or of the lateral retinaculum can alter gait and postural mechanics, which may lead to pathology. For example, tight hamstrings can contribute to patellofemoral pathology because of increased knee flexion at heel strike and during stance phase.[79] Limitation of hip rotation in extension can lead to patellofemoral pathology as well.[52] If the rectus femoris is tight, full excursion of the patella in the trochlea is not possible, especially if the hip is extended. A tight iliotibial band can lead to lateral tracking of the patella.[79,97] Tests for the hamstring, abductor, adductor, and rectus femoris muscles have been described in Chapter 11. A functional test for the quadriceps (described under the "Special Tests" section in this

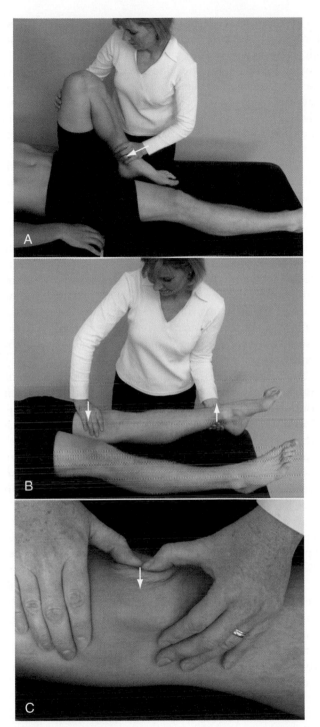

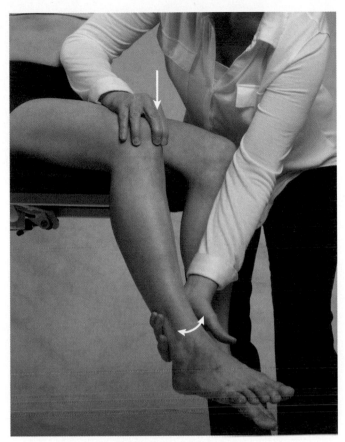

Fig. 12.35 Morton palpation test of the patellofemoral joint.

Fig. 12.34 Passive movements of the knee. (A) Flexion. (B) Extension. (C) Medial glide of patella.

TABLE **12.4**

Grades of Articular Cartilage Damage of Patella Seen with Arthritic Changes

Grade	Pathology
0	Normal cartilage
I	Softening and swelling of articular cartilage
II	Fragmentation and fissuring of articular cartilage affecting an area of less than 0.5 inch (1.3 cm)
III	Fragmentation and fissuring of articular cartilage affecting an area greater than 0.5 inch (1.3 cm)
IV	Cartilage erosion to bone

Modified from Park JY, Duong CT, Sharma AR, et al: Effects of hyaluronic acid and γ–globulin concentrations on the frictional response of human osteoarthritic articular cartilage, *PLoS One* 9(11):e112684, 2014.

chapter) is also a passive movement test (heel to buttock) for the femoral nerve. To test the gastrocnemius muscle, the examiner extends the patient's knee and, while holding it straight, dorsiflexes the patient's ankle. The examiner should be able to reach at least 90° (plantigrade), although 10° to 15° of dorsiflexion is more common.

During the examination, the examiner should also check the ROM available at the hip and ankle because restricted motion at these joints may increase the stress on the ligaments about the knee. For example, limited hip medial rotation can increase strain on the anterior cruciate ligament during cutting and pivoting activities.[98]

Resisted Isometric Movements

For a proper test of the muscles, resisted isometric movements must be performed (Fig. 12.38). In some cases (e.g., patellofemoral pain syndrome [PFPS]), hip strength

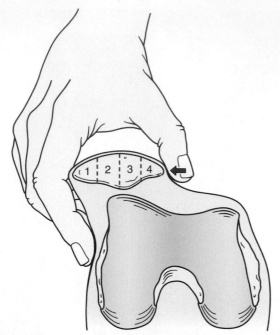

Fig. 12.36 Passive lateral glide test demonstrating a patella being subluxated laterally to its second quadrant. Decreased patellar mobility (hypomobile) is manifested by less than one quadrant of medial and lateral glide; movement of more than two quadrants (one-half of patellar width) is considered hypermobile. (Redrawn from Jackson DW, editor: *The anterior cruciate ligament: current and future concepts*, New York, 1993, Raven Press, p 358.)

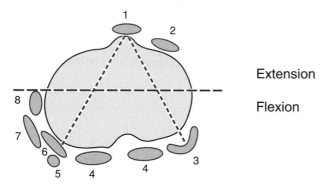

Extension

Flexion

Fig. 12.37 Movement diagram of the knee showing quadriceps-hamstrings tripod. *1*, Patellar tendon (quadriceps); *2*, iliotibial band; *3*, biceps femoris; *4*, gastrocnemius; *5*, semitendinosus; *6*, semimembranosus; *7*, gracilis; *8*, sartorius.

should also be tested because hip abductors, extensors, and lateral rotators have been found to be weak in PFPS patients and anterior cruciate ligament patients.[99,100] The patient should be tested in the supine position.

Resisted Isometric Movements of the Knee Complex

- Flexion of the knee
- Extension of the knee
- Ankle plantar flexion
- Ankle dorsiflexion
- Hip abductors (in alignment cases)
- Hip lateral rotators (in alignment cases)

Ideally, these resisted isometric movements are performed with the joint in its resting position. Segal and Jacob[101] suggest testing the quadriceps muscle at 0°, 30°, 60°, and 90° while observing any abnormal tibial movement (e.g., ligament instability) or excessive pain from patellar compression (e.g., patellofemoral syndrome). Fig. 12.39 shows the quadriceps complex components and their angle of pull. Table 12.5 lists the muscles acting at the knee (see Figs. 11.17 and 13.62).

Although these movements are tested with the patient in the supine position, the hamstrings are often tested with the patient prone or sitting. In prone, if the knee is flexed to 90° and the heel is turned out (i.e., lengthening the lateral hamstrings), the greatest tension is placed on the lateral hamstring muscle (biceps femoris). If the heel is turned in, the greatest tension is placed on the medial hamstring (semimembranosus and semitendinosus) muscles.[26,102] It has also been shown that testing the hamstrings at 30° flexion while in sitting is more likely to be positive (pain and weakness) than if tested at 90° for a proximal hamstring strain (**hamstring syndrome**).[103–106]

Ankle movements are tested because the gastrocnemius muscle crosses the posterior knee and both plantar and dorsiflexion movements cause movement of the fibula. Dorsiflexion causes the fibula to move up and increases the stress being applied to the ligaments supporting the superior tibiofibular joint. Plantar flexion decreases the stress on these ligaments and also brings the gastrocnemius into play, supporting the posterior knee and assisting knee flexion.

If the history has indicated concentric, eccentric, or econcentric movements have caused symptoms, these types of contractions should be tested as well but only after isometric testing has been performed.

Kannus and colleagues[107] developed a scoring scale for measuring isokinetic and isometric strength (eTool 12.1). The scale can be used to show improvement in strength over time.[108] When using isokinetic values, different test parameters may be used. However, it is important to realize that most knee isokinetic tests are not done with the knee in a functional position

---

Isokinetic Test Parameters Commonly Used for the Knee

- Left/right peak torque ratio
- Left/right average (mean) torque ratio
- Ratio of peak torque to body weight
- Torque curve analysis
- Bilateral total work comparison
- Hamstrings/quadriceps ratio (left and right)
- Ratio of average power to body weight
- Time ratio to torque development
- Time to 50% peak torque
- Endurance (fatigue) ratio (first to last repetition)

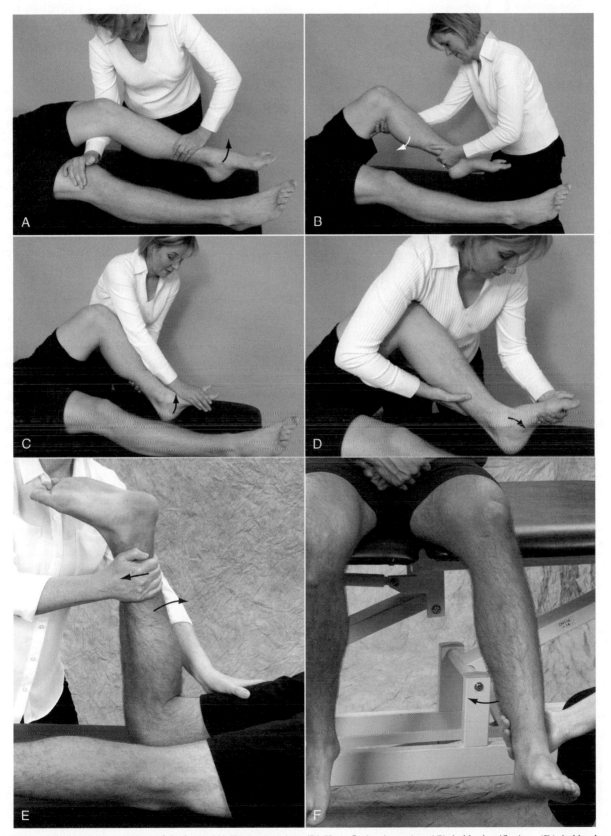

Fig. 12.38 Resisted isometric movements of the knee. (A) Knee extension. (B) Knee flexion in supine. (C) Ankle dorsiflexion. (D) Ankle plantar flexion. (E) Knee flexion in prone. (F) Knee flexion at 30° in sitting.

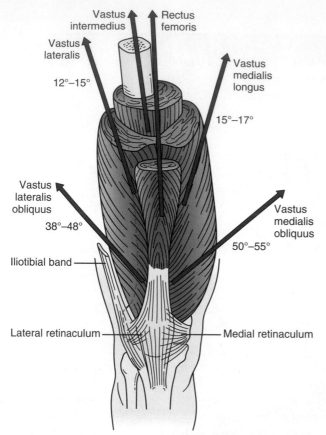

Fig. 12.39 Components of the quadriceps femoris complex. Note the angle of insertion of the various components of the complex. The orientation of the muscle fibers dictates the line of action and pull on the patella. (Redrawn from McConnell J, Fulkerson J: The knee: patellofemoral and soft tissue injuries. In Zachazewski JE, et al., editors: *Athletic injuries and rehabilitation*, Philadelphia, 1996, WB Saunders, p 697.)

Depending on the speed, the hamstring/quadriceps ratio is normally between 50% and 60%.[109] However, as the speed of isokinetic testing increases, the ratio approaches 1:1, or 100%.[110,111]

Functional Assessment

Physical function is the ability to perform daily activities and is important to determine as an outcome measure as it relates to the patient's daily function and quality of life.[112] Instabilities produced on the examining table are easily produced functionally, especially in athletes who participate in activities, such as vigorous cutting and jumping or rapid deceleration, which produce high physiological joint loads. In the knee, patients, especially those who have had surgery, are often grouped as copers (i.e., able to cope with the disability) or noncopers (i.e., cannot function close to their preinjury or presurgical level). The noncopers often show fear of reinjury, abnormal and asymmetrical gait patterns, and other functional shortcomings that are evident with functional testing.[113–115] The examiner should consider the necessary criteria (see following box) before doing functional testing. Functional tests and numerous numerical knee rating systems have been developed for the knee, many of them for specific populations (e.g., athletes) or to assess outcomes after surgery or for specific conditions. The examiner must pick the appropriate test or scale, realizing that each has advantages and disadvantages.[116–119]

TABLE 12.5

Muscles of the Knee: Their Actions, Nerve Supply, and Nerve Root Derivation

Action	Muscles Acting	Nerve Supply	Nerve Root Derivation
Flexion of knee	1. Biceps femoris	Sciatic	L5, S1, S2
	2. Semimembranosus	Sciatic	L5, S1, S2
	3. Semitendinosus	Sciatic	L5, S1, S2
	4. Gracilis	Obturator	L2, L3
	5. Sartorius	Femoral	L2, L3
	6. Popliteus	Tibial	L4, L5, S1
	7. Gastrocnemius	Tibial	S1, S2
	8. Tensor fasciae latae (in 45°–145° of flexion)	Superior gluteal	L4, L5
	9. Plantaris	Tibial	S1, S2
Extension of knee	1. Rectus femoris	Femoral	L2–L4
	2. Vastus medialis	Femoral	L2–L4
	3. Vastus intermedius	Femoral	L2–L4
	4. Vastus lateralis	Femoral	L2–L4
	5. Tensor fasciae latae (in 0°–30° of flexion)	Superior gluteal	L4, L5
Medial rotation of flexed leg (non–weight bearing)	1. Popliteus	Tibial	L4, L5
	2. Semimembranosus	Sciatic	L5, S1, S2
	3. Semitendinosus	Sciatic	L5, S1, S2
	4. Sartorius	Femoral	L2, L3
	5. Gracilis	Obturator	L2, L3
Lateral rotation of flexed leg (non–weight bearing)	1. Biceps femoris	Sciatic	L5, S1, S2

If the active, passive, and resisted isometric movements are performed with little difficulty, the examiner may put the patient through a series of **functional tests** or **physical performance tests (PPTs)** to see whether these sequential activities produce pain or other symptoms and whether there is near symmetry between the normal knee values and the injured knee values.[120] Lawrence et al.[121] reported that passive ROM, dynamic balance, single-leg hop, and the International Knee Documentation Committee (IKDC) subjective form were good measures for limb symmetry but that strength was not a good symmetrical measurement, especially when looking at injury risk potential. Sadeghi et al.,[122] in looking at limb differences, stated that the foot used for an activity (e.g., kicking a ball) is classed as the preferred foot while the nonpreferred foot provides stabilizing and postural support, demonstrating that both limbs play an important though different role during activity. These tests may be scored by the time taken to do the test or by the distance or height attained when doing the test. If the results are so measured, three measurements should be taken and averaged. In some cases the results of different tests may be combined. Fonseca and coworkers[123] found that the time ratio of figure-eight running to straight running was one of the most effective ways of differentiating patients with anterior cruciate ligament deficiencies from normal patients (Fig. 12.40). Some of these tests may involve walking (e.g., Timed "Up and Go" test

[TUG test], sit-to-stand test). These walking tests may be used when any lower limb joint is affected but are primarily designed for elderly people.[124] Boonstra et al.[124] believed the TUG test could be used as a global functional test following total knee arthroplasty, whereas the sit-to-stand was a more biomechanical function test.

These functional activities, which are provided as examples, must be geared to the individual patient, and in some cases, to specific pathology.[125] Paxton et al.[126] recommended doing knee-specific, activity-specific, and general health questionnaires to provide a more accurate assessment of outcomes. Squatting reveals limitations of flexion and may cause impingement with meniscal lesions. Duck waddle, if attempted, can demonstrate increased symptoms in meniscal and ligamentous lesions. Older patients should not be expected to accomplish the last five or six (see earlier) movements unless they have been doing these or similar activities in the recent past. Daniel and coworkers[127] outlined different functional and intensity levels that are useful, especially for getting an indication of functional activities from a patient's perspective (Table 12.6). Functional strength tests for sedentary individuals are shown in Table 12.7.

Strobel and Stedtfeld[128] put forward the **one-leg hop test.** The patient stands and does a "long jump" hop on one leg while landing on the same leg. This is a **single-leg hop for distance (hop and stop test)** (Fig. 12.41A).[129–132] Noyes and associates[129] considered symmetry of less than 85% between the legs to be abnormal. The test is repeated three times alternately with each leg. If instability is evident, the distance for the affected leg is less than that for the normal leg. Any functional deficit between the two limbs has been called the **limb symmetry index (LSI).**[133,134] When comparing limbs using PPTs or the LSI, the examiner should err on the side of caution because the index may overestimate or underestimate the performance deficits and may not identify residual deficits.[134–137] Likewise, PPTs are widely used to determine whether an individual is ready to return to different levels of activity and to determine the risk of injury. However, further research is necessary to determine whether their results are meaningful (e.g., when using PPTs, is the minimally important change or minimally detected change

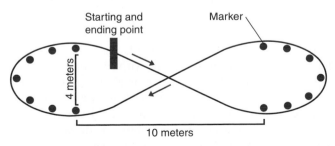

Fig. 12.40 Figure-eight running track. (Redrawn from Fonseca ST, Magee DJ, Wessel J, et al: Validation of a performance test for outcome evaluation of knee function. *Clin J Sport Med* 2:253, 1992.)

TABLE 12.6

Patient Activity Scale

Functional Levels

Level I:	Activities of daily living
Level II:	Straight running; sports that do not involve lower-limb agility activities; occupations involving heavy lifting
Level III:	Activities that require lower-limb agility but not involving jumping, hard cutting, or pivoting
Level IV:	Activities involving jumping, hard cutting, or pivoting

Intensity

W:	Work related or occupational
LR:	Light recreational
VR:	Vigorous recreational
C:	Competitive

Exposure

Number of hours per year of participation at any given functional level and intensity

From Daniel D, et al., editors: *Knee ligaments: structure, injury and repair*, New York, 1990, Raven Press, p 522.

TABLE 12.7

Functional Testing of the Knee

Starting Position	Action	Functional Test
Standing	1. Walking backward 2. Running forward 20° (knee flexion)	6–8 m (19.7–26.2 feet): Functional 3–6 m (9.8–19.7 feet): Functionally fair 1–3 m (3.3–9.8 feet): Functionally poor 0 m: Nonfunctional
Standing	1. Squat 20°–30° 2. Jump, lifting body off floor	5–6 Repetitions: Functional 3–4 Repetitions: Functionally fair 1–2 Repetitions: Functionally poor 0 Repetitions: Nonfunctional

Data from Palmar ML, Epler M: *Clinical assessment procedures in physical therapy*, Philadelphia, 1990, JB Lippincott, pp 275–276.

known?).[138–140] Thus it becomes another "tool in the toolbox" to help the examiner make decisions about return to activity following injury. Juris et al.[141] advocated doing a **maximal controlled leap** in addition to the one-leg hop test. For this test, which is said to test force absorption, the patient stands on one foot and "leaps forward" to land on the opposite foot. Patients should

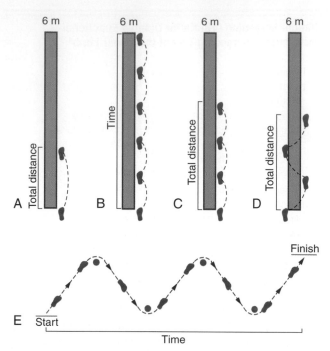

Fig. 12.41 Hop tests. (A) Single hop for distance. (B) Timed hop. (C) Triple hop for distance. (D) Crossover hop for distance. (E) A 30-m agility hop test.

be instructed to maintain the flexed hip/knee position during takeoff and extend the leg for landing. Patients must "stick" on landing with no movement of the landing foot and must be upright with hands on hips within 1 second. The distance is measured and the test repeated with the opposite start leg. Augustsson et al.[142] advocated doing the hop test after the legs have been fatigued. They believed the fatiguing was more likely to show functional deficits between limbs during the hop test.

Another concept that has become prevalent in the treatment of knee injuries is the idea of coactivation of the quadriceps and hamstrings during exercise. Begalle et al.[143] believed the most balanced coactivation activities were the single-leg dead lift, the lateral hop, the transverse hop, and lateral band–walk exercise (see later for description). Jang et al.[144] believed carioca tests and cocontraction tests showed a significant difference between those able to return to sport and those who could not. Lee et al.[145] found a strong correlation between knee numerical scoring scales and a single-leg vertical jump.

Since the advent of the single-leg hop, modifications and different iterations have been developed (e.g., single-leg vertical jump, medial hop, figure-eight hop, up-down hop).[146,147] Davies[137] recommends that the hop tests be modified so they are done with the hands clasped behind the back. They stated that allowing the patient to swing the arms, head, and trunk increased the jump distance approximately 20%. Thus, if the desire is to measure functional leg power, it is better to do so with the arm, head, and trunk movements eliminated. Each test is usually repeated three times, with the good limb tested first, followed by the injured limb, and the average of the three attempts attained with each leg are compared.[148] Practice trials may be used if desired.[149] Performance can be affected by gender and level of competition.[150] These modifications include the following:

1. **Single-leg hop for time:** With this test, the patient is assessed for the time taken to hop 6 m (20 ft) on one leg (Fig. 12.41B). The good leg is tested first, followed by the injured leg.[129,130,148]

2. **Triple hop:** With this test, the patient is asked to hop as far as possible, taking three hops. The distance for the good leg is compared with that for the injured leg (Fig. 12.41C).[129,130,148]

3. **Crossover hop:** A straight line is marked on the floor. The patient is asked to take three consecutive hops on one foot, crossing over the straight line each time (Fig. 12.41D). The good limb is tested, followed by the injured limb, and the average distances attained with each leg are compared.[129] Risberg and Ekeland[151] modified this test and called it the **side jump test.**[152] For this test, two 6-m parallel lines are placed 30 cm (12 inches) apart on the floor. Outside one line, 10 marks are made at 60-cm (24-inch) intervals. Outside the other line, marks are made at 60-cm (24-inch) intervals but starting at 30 cm (12 inches) so that the marks are staggered from one side to the other. The patient is asked to hop from marker to marker on each line. The good leg is timed, followed by the injured leg.

4. **Agility hop:** This hop test requires a space of 30 m (100 ft). Cones are placed 6 m (20 ft) apart (Fig. 12.41E). The patient is then timed as he or she hops through the cones (e.g., a figure-eight pattern could be used[153]).

5. **Stair hop test (stairs hopple test)[151]:** The patient is timed as he or she hops up and down several steps (20 to 25 steps recommended), first on the good leg and then on the injured leg. Hopper et al.[133] recommended a different stair hop test. For this test, patients are asked to hop up and then down a three-step platform, then turn about a marker fixed 1 m from the platform, and then hop back up and down the step (Fig. 12.42).

These functional tests are for active persons and can be quite demanding; however, they have been shown to have high test-retest reliability.[133] Losee[154] mentioned several additional tests. For example, in the **deceleration test,** the patient is asked to run at full speed and to stop suddenly on command.[49] The test is positive for rotary instability if the patient stops without using the quadriceps or decelerates in a crouched position (more than 30° flexion of the knee). The effect of the test can be accentuated by having the patient turn away from the affected leg just as he or she is about to stop.[155] As the patient does the test, the examiner should watch to ensure that the patient uses the affected leg to help stop. With instability problems, the patient uses only the good leg to stop, "hopping through" with the injured leg.

For the **"disco test,"** the patient stands on one leg with the knee flexed 10° to 20°. The patient is asked to rotate or twist left and right while holding the flexed position (Fig. 12.43).[49] Apprehension during the test or refusal to do the

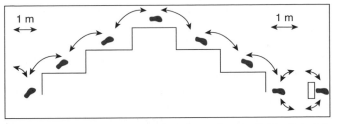

Fig. 12.42 Stair hop test. (Modified from Hopper DM, Goh SC, Wentworth LA, et al: Test-retest reliability of knee rating scales and functional hop tests one year following anterior cruciate ligament reconstruction, *Phys Ther Sport* 3:10–18, 2002.)

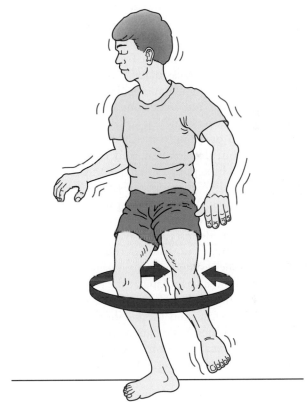

Fig. 12.43 Losee disco test. Flexion, compression, and rotation may lead to shift of femur on tibia, causing rotary instability.

test is a positive sign for rotary instability. If pain is felt on the joint line, it may indicate meniscus pathology, in which case it is called **Merke's sign.**[128] Pain on medial rotation along the joint line implies medial meniscus pathology, and pain on lateral rotation implies lateral meniscus pathology.

Larson[156] advocated the **leaning hop test.** For this test, the patient hops up and down on one leg while abducting the opposite leg. A positive test is apprehension during the test or refusal to do the test and is a positive sign for rotary instability.

Onate et al.[157] advocated using a **drop box screening test** as part of a landing error scoring system. To do the test, the patient jumps down from a 30-cm (12-inch) height onto both feet 30 cm (12 inches) from the box while the examiner watches to see whether there is any valgus movement of the knee on landing, noting the initial knee flexion angle and amount of flexion during the landing; whether there is any knee valgus throughout the movement; foot-ground symmetry; trunk flexion angle; ankle flexion angle; and foot stance width. The action of both limbs is compared. The system was developed to identify individuals with poor jump landing technique.

Tests that involve landing (single leg), cutting, and pivoting also play a role as screening tests that may identify at-risk individuals for noncontact anterior cruciate ligament injuries.[158] In some cases, scales that measure fear of injury/lack of confidence (e.g., Tampa Scale of Kinesiophobia [see eTool 1.5]) may be of benefit in directing a more appropriate rehabilitation program and improving quality of life.[114,159–166]

The **Vail Sport Test**[167] is a functional test to measure patients attempting to return to sport following anterior cruciate ligament injury (eTool 12.2). Similarly, the **Functional Sports Assessment**[168] measures postsurgical anterior cruciate ligament patients. Included in the test are ROM for the knee and ankle, single-leg hop, triple hop, crossover triple hop, single-leg squatting, lateral jumping (bounding) and pivoting, 6-m (20-feet) straight line run with acceleration, deceleration, and change in direction, and plyometric box jump 30-cm (12-inch) box height. Hildebrandt et al.[169] developed a seven-item test battery including a two-leg stability test, a one-leg stability test, a two-leg countermove jump (CMJ), a one-leg CMJ, plyometric jumps, speedy test, and quick feet test. During the tests, the examiner is not only determining whether the patient can do the test and measuring the time or distance, but the examiner is also looking at the position of the knee relative to the hip and ankle/foot, the patient's balance and balance recovery, and the position of the hip, knee, and ankle/foot joints as the patient completes the task.[170]

To assess physical function of older patients with hip or knee osteoarthritis, Lin et al.[171] recommended the following tests:

1. Walk a distance of 2.4 m (8 feet)
2. Ascend/descend four stairs
3. Rise from/sit down from a chair five times

In addition, they measured hip/knee flexion ROM and isometric quadriceps strength and had the patient complete the **Western Ontario and McMaster University Osteoarthritis Index (WOMAC)**. For other PPTs, see different sections of the Primary Care Assessment chapter (Chapter 17).

Numerical rating systems are commonly done to determine the state of the knee. Most of these measures combine clinical (e.g., ROM) and functional (e.g., stair climbing) measures. Many of these scoring systems have not been tested on normal subjects and show possible interviewer bias, nor are the values given to each measure explained. In addition, there may be male and female differences.[172–175]

Noyes and colleagues[176–180] developed the **Cincinnati Knee Rating System** (eTool 12.3), which deals with pain, swelling, stability, and activity level and is a good functional rating system for active persons. Irrgang and associates[181] use two scales, an **Activities of Daily Living Scale**[182]

and a **Sports Activity Scale** (eTools 12.4 and 12.5), to detect clinically significant changes over time. The Knee Society[183] also has a rating scale. The Knee Society advocates keeping knee rating and functional assessment separate. This knee-rating scale deals first with pain, ROM, and stability, giving positive points up to 100 and grouping deductions that can take away from the overall value. Function is dealt with separately on the scale.

Lysholm and Gillquist[184] developed a frequently used scale primarily designed to score clinical instability that may also be used for chondral lesions of the knee (eTool 12.6).[185–189] The **International Knee Documentation Committee (IKDC)** has also developed a number of assessment forms, three of which are included here (eTools 12.7 to 12.9).[180,190–201] The **Tegner Activity Scale**[185,189,202,203] is useful in determining the patient's current level of activity relative to his or her previous level and can also be used as a guide for rehabilitation and the level of activity the patient hopes to achieve.[204] The 12-item **ACL-Return to Sports After Injury (ACL-RSI) Scale** was developed to measure psychological responses to return to sport involving emotions, confidence in performance, and risk appraisal (eTool 12.10).[205] The **Knee Self-Efficacy Scale (K-SES)** was developed to measure self-sufficiency during daily activities (eTool 12.11).[206] The **Marx Activity Scale** (eTool 12.12) was designed to measure activity level rather than knee function on health status.[207–210] The **Patellofemoral Joint Evaluation Scale** (eTool 12.13), the **Kujala Score Questionnaire (Anterior Knee Pain Scale)** (eTool 12.14), and the **Banff Patella Instability Instrument**[211–213] (eTool 12.15) are examples of patellofemoral joint evaluation scales that can be used to assess functional levels in non-surgical patients with patellofemoral syndrome or after surgery.[214–218] Similar scales used to measure patellofemoral

---

Tegner Activity Levels for the Knee

- Level 0: Unable to work or on disability because of knee problems
- Level 1: Sedentary work
- Level 2: Light labour, walk on uneven ground, cannot hike or backpack
- Level 3: Light labour, some lifting
- Level 4: Moderately heavy labour (e.g., truck driving)
- Level 5: Heavy labour (e.g., construction), cycling, cross-country skiing, jogging on uneven ground 1 to 2 times per week
- Level 6: Racquet sports, downhill skiing, jogging 5 times per week
- Level 7: Competitive sports (e.g., handball, tennis, running); recreational sports (e.g., soccer, football, ice hockey, basketball, racquetball)
- Level 8: Competitive sports (e.g., racquet sports, downhill skiing, track and field sports)
- Level 9: Competitive sports (e.g., soccer, football, rugby, ice hockey, gymnastics, basketball, wrestling)
- Level 10: Competitive sports (national/elite level)

Data from Tegner Y, Lysholm J, Odensten M, et al: Evaluation of cruciate ligament injuries, *Acta Orthop Scand* 59:336–341, 1988; and, Tegner Y, Lysholm J: Rating systems in the evaluation of knee ligament injuries, *Clin Orthop Relat Res* 198:43-49, 1985.

TABLE **12.8**

Primary and Secondary Restraints of the Knee

Tibial Motion	Primary Restraints	Secondary Restraints
Anterior translation	ACL	MCL, LCL; middle third of mediolateral capsule; popliteus corner, semimembranosus corner, iliotibial band
Posterior translation	PCL	MCL, LCL; posterior third of mediolateral capsule; popliteus tendon; anterior and posterior meniscofemoral ligaments
Valgus rotation (medial gapping)	MCL	ACL, PCL; posterior capsule when knee fully extended, semimembranosus corner
Varus rotation (lateral gapping)	LCL	ACL, PCL; posterior capsule when knee fully extended, popliteus corner
Lateral rotation	MCL, LCL	Popliteus corner
Medial rotation	ACL, PCL	Anteroposterior meniscofemoral ligaments, semimembranosus corner Anterolateral ligament, anterolateral capsule

ACL, Anterior cruciate ligament; *LCL,* lateral collateral ligament; *MCL,* medial collateral ligament; *PCL,* posterior cruciate ligament.
Modified from Zachazewski JE, et al., editors: *Athletic injuries and rehabilitation,* Philadelphia, 1996, WB Saunders, p 627.

dysfunction also exist.[219–222] The Oslo Sports Trauma Research Centre has developed the **OSTRC Overuse Injury Questionnaire** for patients suffering from overuse injuries about the knee.[223–225] Other scales, such as the WOMAC, **Knee Injury and Osteoarthritis Outcome Score (KOOS),**[186,195,197,226–231] **Lequesne Index,** and the **Knee Quality of Life (KQol-26) Questionnaire,**[232] have been developed to determine the outcome of arthroplasties in osteoarthritis and for patients with suspected ligamentous or meniscus injuries[232]) (see Chapter 11).[229,233–242] Each of these knee-rating scales is slightly different. The scale that works best for the examiner and the examiner's clientele should be used. Other knee-rating scales are also available.[126,184,232,243–247]

Ligament Stability

Because the knee, more than any other joint in the body, depends on its ligaments to maintain its integrity, it is imperative that the ligaments be tested. The ligaments of the knee joint act as primary stabilizers and guide the movement of the bones in proper relation to one another. Depending on the motion being tested, the ligaments act as primary or secondary restraints (Table 12.8).[248] For example, the anterior cruciate ligament is the primary restraint to anterior tibial displacement and a secondary restraint to varus-valgus motion in full extension and rotation.[181,249] If the primary restraint is injured, pathological motion occurs. If the secondary restraint is injured but the primary restraint is not, pathological motion in that direction does not occur. If both primary and secondary restraints are injured, the pathological motion is greater.[181] Thus an understanding of the ligamentous structures around the knee is imperative, and the reader is referred to the appropriate papers for review.[250–255] There are several ligaments around the knee, but four deserve special mention (Fig. 12.44).

Collateral and Cruciate Ligaments

Collateral Ligaments. The **medial (tibial) collateral ligament** lies more posteriorly than anteriorly on the medial aspect of the tibiofemoral joint. It is made up of two layers, one superficial and one deep. The deep layer is a thickening of the joint capsule that blends with the medial meniscus; it is sometimes called the *medial capsular ligament.* The superficial layer is a strong, broad triangular strap. It starts distal to the adductor tubercle and extends to the medial surface of the tibia, approximately 6 cm (2.4 inches) below the joint line. It blends with the posterior capsule and is separated from the capsule and the medial meniscus by a bursa.

The entire medial collateral ligament is tight throughout the full ROM, although there is varying stress placed on different parts of the ligament as it moves through the full range because of the shape of the femoral condyles. All of its fibers are taut on full extension. In flexion, the anterior fibers are the most taut; in midrange, the posterior fibers are the most taut.[256]

The **lateral (fibular) collateral ligament** is round and lies under the tendon of the biceps femoris muscle. It runs from the lateral epicondyle of the femur to the fibular head. It also lies more posteriorly than anteriorly. This ligament is tight in extension and loosens in flexion, especially after 30° flexion. As the knee flexes, it provides protection to the lateral aspect of the knee. It is not attached to the lateral meniscus but rather is separated from it by a small fat pad.[256]

Cruciate Ligaments. The cruciate ligaments cross each other and are the primary rotary stabilizers of the knee.[257] These strong ligaments are named in relation to their attachment to the tibia and are intracapsular but extrasynovial. Each ligament has an anteromedial and a posterolateral portion. The anterior cruciate ligament has, in addition, an intermediate portion.

The **anterior cruciate ligament** extends superiorly, posteriorly, and laterally, twisting on itself as it extends from the tibia to the femur. Its main functions are to

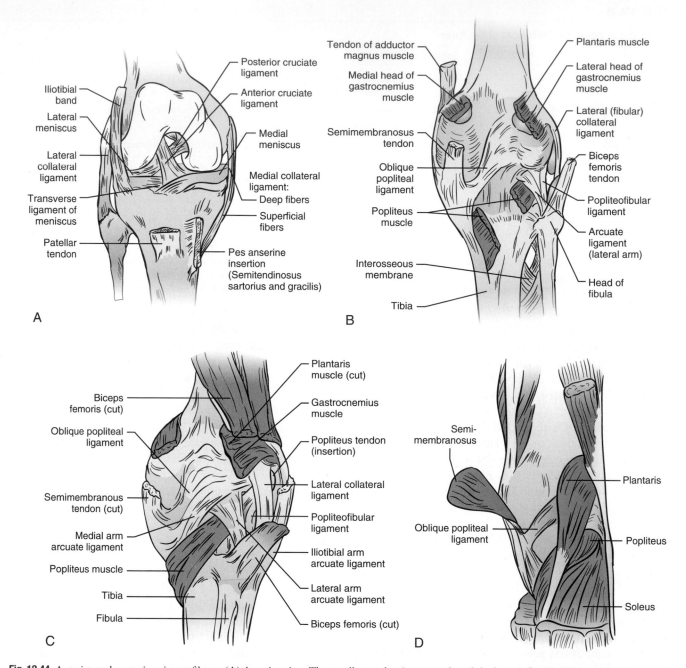

Fig. 12.44 Anterior and posterior views of knee. (A) Anterior view. The patellar tendon is removed, and the knee is flexed. Note that the cruciate ligament rises in front of the anterior tibial spine, not from it. Note also that the medial meniscus is firmly attached to the medial collateral ligament. (B) Posterior view with the knee extended and the posterior ligament removed. The two layers of the medial collateral ligament are shown, as is the tibial portion of the lateral collateral ligament. The posterior cruciate ligament rises behind the tibia, not on its upper surface. Note the femoral attachment of the anterior cruciate ligament on the back of the notch. (C) Posterior oblique view showing superficial structures of posterolateral corner. (D) Posterior oblique view showing deeper structures including popliteus.

prevent anterior movement of the tibia on the femur, to check lateral rotation of the tibia in flexion, and, to less extent, to check extension and hyperextension at the knee. It also helps to control the normal rolling and gliding movement of the knee. The anteromedial bundle is tight in both flexion and extension, limits anterior translation, and helps to stabilize medial and lateral rotation,[258,259] whereas the posterolateral bundle is tight in low flexion angles (closer to extension) and medial rotation. It limits anterior translation, hyperextension, and rotation.[258] As

a whole, the ligament has the least amount of stress on it between 30° and 60° flexion.[256,257,260,261]

The **posterior cruciate ligament** extends superiorly, anteriorly, and medially from the tibia to the femur. This strong, fan-shaped ligament, the stoutest ligament in the knee, is a primary stabilizer of the knee against posterior movement of the tibia on the femur, and it checks extension and hyperextension. In addition, the ligament helps to maintain rotary stability and functions as the knee's central axis of rotation. Along with the anterior cruciate

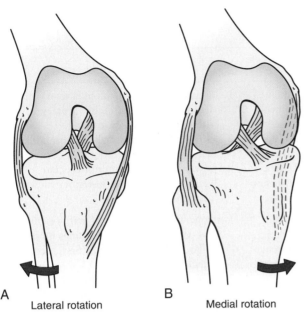

A   Lateral rotation   **B**   Medial rotation

Fig. 12.45 Effect of tibial rotation on cruciate and collateral ligaments. (A) The collateral ligament is taut; the cruciate ligament is lax. (B) The collateral ligament is lax; the cruciate ligament is taut.

ligament, it acts as a rotary guide to the "screwing home" mechanism of the knee.[256,261] For the posterior cruciate ligament, the bulk of the fibers are tight at 30° flexion, but the posterolateral fibers are loose in early flexion.

With lateral rotation of the tibia, both collateral ligaments become more taut and the cruciate ligaments become relaxed (Fig. 12.45). With medial rotation of the tibia, the reverse action occurs: the collateral ligaments become more relaxed and the cruciate ligaments become tighter.[256,262]

LaPrade et al.[263] have stressed the importance of the popliteus in controlling rotation of the tibia on the femur by contributing to lateral rotation stability. They believed the muscle, in fact, acts like a dynamic ligament to help stabilize the knee (see Fig. 12.44). Morgan et al.[264] reported that the oblique popliteal ligament, which is an expansion of the semimembranosus tendon (see Fig. 12.44), was the primary structure preventing hyperextension of the knee.

Testing of Ligaments

When testing the ligaments of the knee, the examiner must watch for four one-plane instabilities and four rotational instabilities (Table 12.9 and Fig. 12.46).

Instabilities About the Knee

- One-plane medial instability
- One-plane lateral instability
- One-plane anterior instability
- One-plane posterior instability
- Anteromedial rotary instability
- Anterolateral rotary instability
- Posteromedial rotary instability
- Posterolateral rotary instability

There are a number of tests for each type of instability. The examiner should use the one or two tests that he or she believes gives the best results. It is not essential to do all of the tests discussed. The techniques chosen must be practiced diligently so that the examiner becomes proficient at doing them; only with practice will the examiner be able to determine which structures are injured.[265] It is also important to understand that the direction of instability does not imply that only structures in that direction are injured. For example, with anterolateral rotary instability (ALRI), it is not necessarily structures on the anterolateral side of the knee that are injured. In fact, posterior structures are often commonly injured as well. With ALRI, the posterolateral capsule and the arcuate-popliteus complex may also be injured.[49]

Key Ligamentous Tests Performed on the Knee[a,b,271]

- **For one-plane medial instability:**
  - ✓ Hughston's valgus stress at 0° and 30°
  - ✓ Valgus stress at 0° and 30°
- **For one-plane lateral instability:**
  - ✓ Hughston's varus stress at 0° and 30°
  - ✓ Varus stress at 0° and 30°
- **For one-plane anterior instability:**
  - ⚠ Active drawer test
  - ✓ Drawer test
  - ✓ Lachman test or its modifications
  - ✓ Lelli test (lever sign)
- **For one-plane posterior instability:**
  - ✓ Active drawer test
  - ✓ Drawer test
  - ⚠ Godfrey test
  - ✓ Posterior sag
- **For anteromedial rotary instability:**
  - ⚠ Slocum test
- **For anterolateral rotary instability (ALRI):**
  - ⚠ Crossover test
  - ✓ Jerk test of Hughston
  - ✓ Losee test
  - ⚠ Noyes flexion-rotation drawer test
  - ✓ Pivot shift test
  - ⚠ Slocum ARLI test
  - ⚠ Supine internal rotation test
- **For posteromedial rotary instability:**
  - ⚠ Hughston's posteromedial drawer test
  - ⚠ Posteromedial pivot shift test
- **For posterolateral rotary instability:**
  - ⚠ External rotation recurvatum
  - ⚠ Hughston's posterolateral drawer test
  - ⚠ Jakob test
  - ⚠ Loomer's posterolateral rotary instability test
  - ⚠ Tibial external rotation (dial) test

[a]See Chapter 1, Key for Classifying Special Tests.
[b]If the pathology indicates a ligamentous problem, the clinician should have the ability to do at least one test well from each type of instability.

TABLE **12.9**

Tests tor Ligamentous Instability around the Knee

Instability	Tests Used to Determine Instability	Structures Injured to Some Degree If Test Positive[a]	Notes
One-plane medial (straight medial)	1. Abduction (valgus) stress with knee in **full extension**	1. Medial collateral ligament (superficial and deep fibers) 2. Posterior oblique ligament 3. Posteromedial capsule 4. Anterior cruciate ligament 5. Posterior cruciate ligament 6. Medial quadriceps expansion 7. Semimembranosus muscle	1. If either cruciate ligament is torn (third-degree sprain) or stretched, rotary instability will also be evident 2. Order of injury is usually medial collateral ligament, then posteromedial corner, posterior capsule, anterior cruciate ligament, and finally posterior cruciate ligament
	2. Abduction (valgus) stress with knee **slightly flexed (20°–30°)**	1. Medial collateral ligament (superficial and deep fibers) 2. Posterior oblique ligament 3. Posterior cruciate ligament	1. Depending on degree of pain, opening and end feel, primarily signifies medial collateral ligament sprain (first, second, or third degree) 2. If posterior cruciate ligament is torn (third-degree sprain), rotary instability will also be evident 3. Opening of 12°–15° signifies injury to posterior cruciate ligament 4. If tibia is laterally rotated, stress is taken off posterior cruciate ligament 5. If tibia is medially rotated, stress is increased on cruciate ligaments while medial collateral ligament relaxes
One-plane lateral (straight lateral)	1. Adduction (varus) stress with knee in **full extension**	1. Lateral collateral ligament 2. Posterolateral capsule 3. Arcuate-popliteus complex 4. Biceps femoris tendon 5. Anterior cruciate ligament 6. Posterior cruciate ligament 7. Lateral gastrocnemius muscle	1. If either cruciate ligament is torn (third-degree sprain) or stretched, rotary instability will also be evident 2. Order of injury is lateral collateral ligament, arcuate-popliteus complex, anterior cruciate ligament, posterior cruciate ligament 3. With severe injury (third degree), common peroneal nerve and circulation may be affected
	2. Adduction (varus) stress with knee **slightly flexed (20°–30°)** and tibia laterally rotated	1. Lateral collateral ligament 2. Posterolateral capsule 3. Arcuate-popliteus complex 4. Iliotibial band 5. Biceps femoris tendon	1. Depending on degree of pain, opening, and end feel, primarily signifies lateral collateral ligament sprain (first, second, or third degree) 2. If tibia is not laterally rotated, maximum stress will not be placed on lateral collateral ligament 3. Lateral rotation of tibia results in relaxation of both cruciate ligaments 4. With flexion, the iliotibial band lies over the center of the lateral joint line 5. If tibia is medially rotated, stress is increased on both cruciate ligaments while lateral collateral ligament relaxes 6. Order of injury is lateral collateral ligament, arcuate-popliteus complex, and iliotibial band and/or biceps femoris

TABLE **12.9**

Tests tor Ligamentous Instability around the Knee—cont'd

Instability	Tests Used to Determine Instability	Structures Injured to Some Degree If Test Positive[a]	Notes
One-plane anterior	1. Lachman test (**20°–30° knee flexion**) or its modifications 2. Lelli (Lever) test	1. Anterior cruciate ligament 2. Posterior oblique ligament 3. Arcuate-popliteus complex	1. Medial collateral ligament and iliotibial band lax in this position 2. Tests primarily posterolateral bundle of anterior cruciate ligament 3. Primarily tests anterior cruciate ligament but with severe injury (third degree); structures in posteromedial and posterolateral corners may also be injured
	3. Anterior drawer sign (**90° knee flexion**) 4. Active drawer test (**90° knee flexion**)	1. Anterior cruciate ligament 2. Posterolateral capsule 3. Posteromedial capsule 4. Medial collateral ligament 5. Iliotibial band 6. Posterior oblique ligament 7. Arcuate popliteus complex	1. Tests primarily anteromedial bundle of anterior cruciate ligament 2. If anterior cruciate ligament and medial or lateral structures are torn (third-degree sprain) or stretched, rotary instability will also be evident 3. Be sure posterior cruciate has not been injured, giving possible false-positive test
One-plane posterior	1. Posterior drawer sign (**90° knee flexion**) 2. Posterior sag sign 3. Active drawer test 4. Godfrey test 5. Reverse Lachman test (**20°–30° knee flexion**)	1. Posterior cruciate ligament 2. Arcuate-popliteus complex 3. Posterior oblique ligament 4. Anterior cruciate ligament	1. If posterior cruciate ligament and medial or lateral structures are torn (third-degree sprain) or stretched, rotary instability will also be evident 2. With severe injury (third degree), collateral ligaments may also be injured
Anteromedial rotary	1. Slocum test (foot laterally rotated 15°) 2. Lemaire's anteromedial jolt test 3. Dejour test	1. Medial collateral ligament (superficial and deep fibers) 2. Posterior oblique ligament 3. Posteromedial capsule 4. Anterior cruciate ligament	1. Test must not be done in extreme lateral rotation of tibia because passive stabilizing will result from "coiling" to maximum rotation
Anterolateral rotary	1. Slocum test (foot medially rotated 30°) 2. Losee test 3. Jerk test of Hughston 4. Active pivot shift 5. Nakajima test	1. Anterior cruciate ligament 2. Posterolateral capsule 3. Arcuate-popliteus complex 4. Lateral collateral ligament 5. Iliotibial band	1. **Tests go from flexion to extension** 2. Tests bring about anterior subluxation of the tibia on femur, causing patient to experience "giving way" sensation 3. Slocum test must not be done in extreme medial rotation of tibia because passive stabilization will result from "coiling" to maximum rotation 4. Shift may be "slip" (second degree) or "jerk" (third degree), depending on degree of sprain or injury
	1. Lateral pivot shift test of Macintosh 2. Slocum ALRI test 3. Crossover test 4. Flexion-rotation drawer test 5. Flexion-extension valgus test 6. Martens test	1. Anterior cruciate ligament 2. Posterolateral capsule 3. Arcuate popliteus complex 4. Iliotibial band	1. **Tests go from extension to flexion** 2. Tests cause reduction of anterior subluxed tibia on femur 3. Shift may be "slip" (second degree) or "jerk" (third degree), depending on degree of sprain or injury

Continued

TABLE **12.9**

Tests tor Ligamentous Instability around the Knee—cont'd

Instability	Tests Used to Determine Instability	Structures Injured to Some Degree If Test Positive[a]	Notes
Posteromedial rotary	1. Hughston's posteromedial drawer sign 2. Posteromedial pivot shift test	1. Posterior cruciate ligament 2. Posterior oblique ligament 3. Medial collateral ligament (superficial and deep fibers) 4. Semimembranosus muscle 5. Posteromedial capsule 6. Anterior cruciate ligament	1. Watch for changing position of tibial tubercle relative to femoral condyles
Posterolateral rotary	1. Hughston's posterolateral drawer sign 2. Jakob test (reverse pivot shift maneuver) 3. External rotational recurvatum test 4. Dynamic posterior shift test 5. Loomer's test 6. Active posterolateral drawer sign	1. Posterior cruciate ligament 2. Arcuate-popliteus ligament 3. Lateral collateral ligament 4. Biceps femoris tendon 5. Posterolateral capsule 6. Anterior cruciate ligament	1. Watch for changing position of tibial tubercle relative to femoral condyles

[a]The amount of displacement gives an indication of how badly and how much of the structure is injured (i.e., first-, second-, or third-degree sprain). *ALRI,* Anterolateral rotary instability.

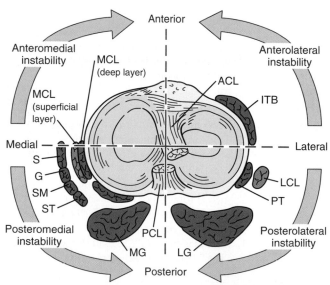

Fig. 12.46 Instabilities about the knee. *ACL,* Anterior cruciate ligament; *G,* gracilis; *ITB,* iliotibial band; *LCL,* lateral collateral ligament; *LG,* lateral gastrocnemius; *MCL,* medial collateral ligament; *MG,* medial gastrocnemius; *PCL,* posterior cruciate ligament; *PT,* popliteal tendon; *S,* sartorius; *SM,* semimembranosus; *ST,* semitendinosus.

When testing for ligament stability of the knee, the examiner should keep the following points in mind:

1. The normal knee is tested first to establish a baseline and to show the patient what to expect. This action helps to gain the patient's confidence by showing what the test involves.

2. When one is comparing the normal and injured limbs, the test must be the same for both limbs. The examiner must use the same initial starting position and the same amount of force, apply the same force at the same point or throughout the range, and note the position at which the displacement occurs.[266]

3. The muscles must be relaxed if the tests are to be valid. Muscle guarding by the hamstrings will adversely affect the outcome.[267] Maximum laxity would be demonstrated with the patient under anesthesia.[267,268]

4. The appropriate stress should be applied gently.

5. The stress is repeated several times and increased to the point of pain to demonstrate maximum laxity without causing muscle spasm.

6. It is not only the degree of opening but also the quality of the opening (i.e., the end feel) that is of concern. Left-right differences of 3 mm or more arc classified as pathological.[266]

7. If the ligament is intact, there should be an abrupt stop or end feel when the ligament is stressed. A soft or indistinct end feel usually signifies ligamentous injury.[269]

8. Ligaments of the knee tend to act in concert to maintain stability, and individual ligaments are difficult to isolate in terms of their function. Therefore more than one test may be found to be positive when assessing for the different instabilities. For example, a patient may exhibit a one-plane medial and one-plane anterior instability as well as an anteromedial rotary instability

(AMRI) and/or ALRI, depending on the severity of the injury to the various ligamentous structures.

9. Tests for ligament instability are more accurate for assessment of a chronic injury than for assessment of an acute injury in the unanesthetized knee because of the presence of muscle spasm and swelling in the acutely injured knee.

10. For the tests involving rotary instability in which the tibia is moved in relation to the femur, if the movement is into extension, subluxation of the tibia relative to the femur occurs in a positive test. If the movement is into flexion, reduction of the tibia relative to the femur occurs in a positive test.

11. Positive rotational tests should not be repeated too frequently because they may lead to articular cartilage damage, further meniscal tearing, or further damage to injured ligaments.

12. Because the ligamentous tests are subjective tests, the more experience the examiner has in doing them, the more accurate will be the interpretation of the test. The examiner should select only one or two from each group of tests and learn to do them well rather than learn all of the tests and risk doing them poorly.

13. It is common for examiners to use two or three tests in combination for each ligament to improve their diagnostic accuracy.[270]

Tests for One-Plane Medial Instability

The **abduction (valgus stress) test** ☑ is an assessment for one-plane (straight) medial instability, which means that the tibia moves away from the femur (i.e., gaps) on the medial side (Fig. 12.47). The examiner applies a valgus stress (pushes the knee medially) at the knee while the ankle is stabilized in slight lateral rotation either with the hand or with the leg held between the examiner's arm and trunk. The knee is first in full extension, and then it is slightly flexed (20° to 30°) so that it is "unlocked."[146]

It has been advocated that resting the test thigh on the examining table enables the patient to relax more and is easier for the examiner. The knee rests on the edge of the table; the lower leg is controlled by the examiner's stabilizing the thigh on the table, and the lower leg is abducted, applying a valgus stress to the knee (Fig. 12.48).[52] Similarly, a varus stress may be applied to stress the lateral structures.

Hughston[52] advocates a third way to do this test (**Hughston's valgus stress test** ☑). The patient is positioned as described earlier, and the examiner faces the patient's foot, placing his or her body against the patient's thigh to help stabilize the upper leg in combination with one hand, which can also palpate the joint line. With the other hand, the examiner grasps the patient's big toe and applies a valgus stress, allowing any natural rotation of the tibia (Fig. 12.49).

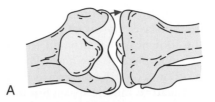

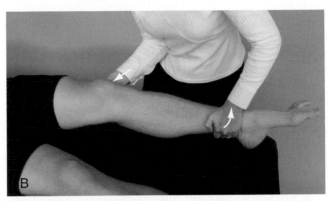

Fig. 12.47 Abduction (valgus stress) test. (A) "Gapping" on the medial aspect of the knee. (B) Positioning for testing the medial collateral ligament (extended knee).

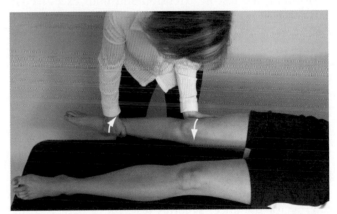

Fig. 12.48 Applying a valgus stress with thigh supported on examining table.

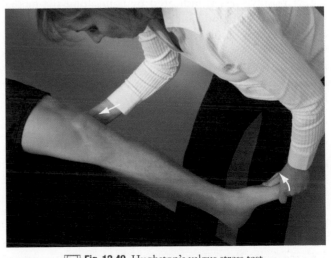

Fig. 12.49 Hughston's valgus stress test.

Similarly, a varus stress may be applied to test the lateral structures, but in this case, the examiner grasps the lateral aspect of the foot near the fifth and fourth toes. A varus stress is then applied to the knee. Doing the test in this fashion often allows the patient to relax more and is less likely to lead to muscle spasm limiting movement.

If the test is positive (i.e., the tibia moves away from the femur an excessive amount when a valgus stress is applied) when the knee is *in extension*, the following structures may have been injured to some degree:

1. Medial collateral ligament (superficial and deep fibers)
2. Posterior oblique ligament
3. Posteromedial capsule
4. Anterior cruciate ligament
5. Posterior cruciate ligament
6. Medial quadriceps expansion
7. Semimembranosus muscle

A positive finding on full extension is classified as a major disruption of the knee. The examiner usually finds that one or more of the rotary tests are also positive. If the examiner applies lateral rotation to the foot when performing the test in extension and finds excessive lateral rotation on the affected side, it is a sign of possible AMRI.

If the test is positive when the knee is *flexed* to 20° to 30°, the following structures may have been injured to some degree:

1. Medial collateral ligament
2. Posterior oblique ligament
3. Posterior cruciate ligament
4. Posteromedial capsule

This flexed part of the valgus stress test would be classified as the true test for one-plane medial instability.

Lonergan and Taylor[272] advocated doing the **Swain test** ⚠ for the knee. For this test, the patient is seated with the knees flexed to 90° over the edge of the examining table. The examiner then passively laterally rotates the tibia on the femur of the good leg followed by the injured leg. A positive test is indicated by pain along the medial side of the joint, indicating injury to the medial collateral ligament complex, because with the knee flexed to 90° the cruciates are lax, whereas the collateral ligaments are tight. Post surgery, pain on the medial joint line may indicate inadequate healing, or, in the chronic medial side laxity, joint line pain may be medial or posteromedial (Fig. 12.50).[273]

If a stress radiograph is taken when the test is performed in full extension, a 5-mm opening indicates a grade 1 injury; up to 10 mm, a grade 2 injury; and more than 10 mm, a grade 3 injury.[256,274] Both limbs should be viewed for differences.[275]

Tests for One-Plane Lateral Instability

The **adduction (varus stress) test** ✓ is an assessment for one-plane lateral instability (i.e., the tibia moves

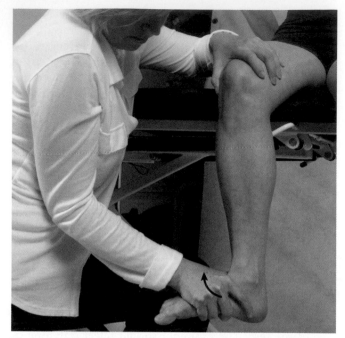

Fig. 12.50 Swain test. Pain along the medial side of the knee indicates medial collateral ligament complex injury.

away from the femur an excessive amount on the lateral aspect of the leg). The examiner applies a varus stress (pushes the knee laterally) at the knee while the ankle is stabilized (Fig. 12.51). The test is first done with the knee in full extension and then with the knee in 20° to 30° of flexion. If the tibia is laterally rotated in full extension before the test, the cruciate ligaments are uncoiled, and maximum stress is placed on the collateral ligaments.

As previously mentioned (see the "Tests for One-Plane Medial Instability" section), **Hughston's varus stress test** ✓ may be used. In this case, the examiner grasps the fifth and fourth toes and applies a varus stress to the knee in extension and slightly (20° to 30°) flexed.

If the test is positive (i.e., the tibia moves away from the femur when a varus stress is applied) *in extension*, the following structures may have been injured to some degree:

1. Fibular or lateral collateral ligament
2. Posterolateral capsule
3. Arcuate-popliteus complex
4. Biceps femoris tendon
5. Posterior cruciate ligament
6. Anterior cruciate ligament
7. Lateral gastrocnemius muscle
8. Iliotibial band

The examiner usually finds that one or more rotary instability tests are also positive. A positive test indicates major instability of the knee.

If the test is positive when the knee is *flexed* 20° to 30° with lateral rotation of the tibia, the following structures may have been injured to some degree:

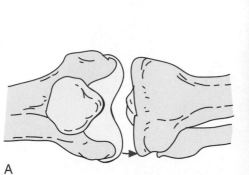

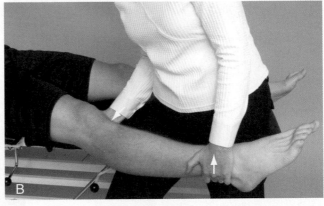

Fig. 12.51 Adduction (varus stress) test. (A) One-plane lateral instability "gapping" on the lateral aspect. (B) Positioning for testing lateral collateral ligament in extension.

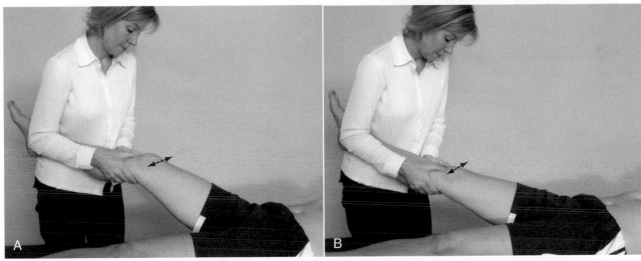

Fig. 12.52 Varus-valgus test. (A) Knee flexed. (B) Knee extended.

1. Lateral collateral ligament
2. Posterolateral capsule
3. Arcuate-popliteus complex
4. Iliotibial band
5. Biceps femoris tendon

This flexed part of the varus stress test is classified as the true test for one-plane lateral instability.

If a stress radiograph is taken when the test is performed in full extension, a 5-mm opening indicates a grade 1 injury; up to 8 mm, a grade 2 injury; and more than 8 mm, a grade 3 injury to the lateral ligaments of the knee.[256,274]

Both varus and valgus stress testing (**varus-valgus test**) can be performed at the same time while the examiner palpates the joint line. The examiner holds the ankle between the examiner's waist and forearm while the patient lies supine with the knee extended and then flexed. At the same time, the examiner palpates the medial and lateral joint lines with the fingers. Varus and valgus stresses are applied with the heels of the examiner's hands (Fig. 12.52).[128]

Tests for One-Plane Anterior Instability

Tests for one-plane anterior instability are designed to primarily test the anterior cruciate ligament.[276,277] Some clinicians[49,52] believe that the posterior cruciate ligament should be tested (see the "Tests for One-Plane Posterior Instability" section) or observed for a posterior sag before the anterior cruciate ligament is tested, to rule out false-positive tests for anterior translation. In either case the examiner should be aware that a torn posterior cruciate can lead to a false-positive anterior translation test if the patient is tested in supine position with the knee flexed, because gravity causes the tibia to sag posteriorly.

Active Drawer Test. For the active drawer test (also called the **quadriceps active test**), the patient is positioned as for the normal drawer test. The examiner holds the patient's foot down. The patient is asked to try to straighten the leg, and the examiner prevents the patient from doing so (isometric test). Muller[256] advocated allowing the foot to be free and noting when the foot is lifted off the table, which occurs only after the tibia has shifted forward and stabilized. If the anterior cruciate ligament or

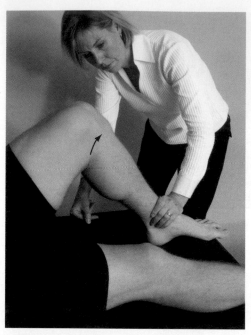

Fig. 12.53 Active anterior drawer test. Examiner watches for excessive anterior shift.

posterior cruciate ligament is torn, the anterior contour of the knee changes as the tibia is drawn forward. If the posterior cruciate ligament is torn, a posterior sag is evident before the patient contracts the quadriceps. Contraction of the quadriceps causes the tibia to shift forward to its normal position, indicating a positive test for a torn posterior cruciate ligament.[278,279] If there is no posterior sag present and if the tibia shifts forward more on the injured side than the noninjured side, it is a positive test for anterior cruciate ligament disruption (Fig. 12.53).[278] A second part of the test may be instituted by having the patient contract the hamstrings isometrically so that the tibial plateau moves posteriorly. This part of the test accentuates the posterior sag for posterior cruciate insufficiency, if present, and ensures maximum movement for anterior cruciate insufficiency if a quadriceps contraction is tried a second time.[128] The active drawer test is a better expression of posterior cruciate insufficiency than of anterior cruciate insufficiency.[280]

With the drawer sign or test, if the anterior or posterior cruciate ligament is torn (third-degree sprain), some rotary instability is evident when the appropriate ligamentous tests are performed.

☑ *Drawer Sign.* The drawer sign is a test for one-plane anterior and one-plane posterior instabilities.[281] The difficulty with this test is in determining the neutral starting position if the ligaments have been injured. The patient's knee is flexed to 90°, and the hip is flexed to 45°. In this position, the anterior cruciate ligament is almost parallel with the tibial plateau. The patient's foot is held on the table by the examiner's body with the examiner sitting on the patient's forefoot and the foot in neutral rotation. The examiner's hands are placed around the tibia to ensure that the hamstring muscles are relaxed (Figs.

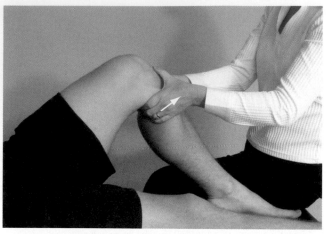

Fig. 12.54 Position for drawer sign.

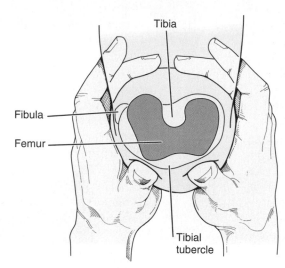

Fig. 12.55 This view of the knee from above shows the inside of the knee joint during performance of the anterior drawer test in flexion. The hands are in place, and the overlay of the femur on the tibia demonstrates that the anterior and posterior motions are normal. The index fingers are ensuring that the hamstrings are relaxed. If, on pulling or pushing tibia, rotation of tibial plateau occurs, the examiner should check for rotary instabilities. (Redrawn from Hughston JC: *Knee ligaments: injury and repair*, St Louis, 1993, Mosby, p 111.)

12.54 and 12.55). The tibia is then drawn forward on the femur (**anterior drawer test**). The normal amount of movement that should be present is approximately 6 mm. This part of the test assesses one-plane anterior instability. If the test is positive (i.e., the tibia moves forward more than 6 mm on the femur), the following structures may have been injured to some degree:

1. Anterior cruciate ligament (especially the anteromedial bundle)
2. Posterolateral capsule
3. Posteromedial capsule
4. Medial collateral ligament (deep fibers)
5. Iliotibial band
6. Posterior oblique ligament
7. Arcuate-popliteus complex

If only the anterior cruciate ligament is torn, the test is negative, because other structures (posterior capsule and posterolateral and posteromedial structures) limit movement. In addition, hemarthrosis, a torn medial meniscus (posterior horn) wedged against the medial femoral condyle, or hamstring spasm may result in a false-negative test. Hughston[52] points out that tearing of the coronary or meniscotibial ligament can allow the tibia to translate forward more than normal, even in the presence of an intact anterior cruciate ligament. In this case, when the anterior drawer test is performed, anteromedial rotation (subluxation) of the tibia occurs.

When performing this test, the examiner must ensure that the posterior cruciate ligament is not torn or injured. If it has been torn, it allows the tibia to drop or slide back on the femur, and when the examiner pulls the tibia forward, a large amount of movement occurs, giving a false-positive sign (see the "Posterior Sag Sign" section). Therefore, the test should be considered positive only if it is shown that the posterior sag is not present.

Weatherwax[282] described a modified way of testing the anterior drawer (**90–90 anterior drawer**). The patient lies supine. The examiner flexes the patient's hip and knee to 90° and supports the lower leg between the examiner's trunk and forearm. The examiner places the hands around the tibia, as with the standard test, and applies sufficient force to slowly lift the patient's buttock off the table (Fig. 12.56). A positive test is excessive anterior tibial translation.

If, when doing the anterior drawer test, there is an audible snap or palpable jerk (**Finochietto jumping sign**) when the tibia is pulled forward and the tibia moves forward excessively, a meniscus lesion is probably accompanying the torn anterior cruciate ligament.[128]

After the anterior movement of the tibia on the femur, the posterior movement of the tibia on the femur should be completed (**posterior drawer test**). In this part of the test, the tibia is pushed back on the femur. This phase is a test for one-plane posterior instability. If the test is positive or a posterior sag is evident, the following structures may have been injured to some degree:

1. Posterior cruciate ligament
2. Arcuate-popliteus complex
3. Posterior oblique ligament
4. Anterior cruciate ligament

If the arcuate-popliteus complex remains intact, a positive posterior drawer sign may not be elicited.[283] If, when the tibia is pushed backward, the examiner forcefully rotates the tibia laterally and excessive movement occurs, the test is positive for posterolateral instability. Warren[284] calls this maneuver the **arcuate spin test.**

Feagin[285] advocated doing the drawer test with the patient sitting with the leg hanging relaxed over the end of the examining table (**sitting anterior drawer test**). The examiner places the hands as with the standardized test and slowly draws the tibia first forward and then backward to test the anterior and posterior drawer (Fig. 12.57). The examiner uses the thumbs to palpate the

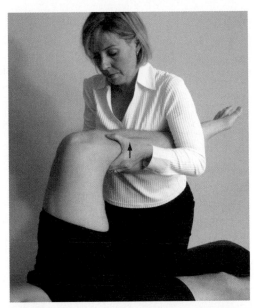

Fig. 12.56 Anterior drawer test in 90° flexion with the hip flexed 90°.

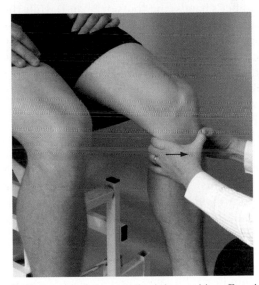

Fig. 12.57 Anterior drawer test in sitting position. Examiner feels anterior shift with thumbs.

tibial plateau movement relative to the femur. The examiner may also note any rotational deformity. The advantage of doing the test this way is that the posterior sag is eliminated because the effect of gravity is eliminated.

✓ *Lachman Test.* The Lachman test, which may also be referred to as the **Ritchie, Trillat,** or **Lachman-Trillat test,** is the best indicator of injury to the anterior cruciate ligament, especially the posterolateral band,[286–291] although this has been questioned.[292] It is a test for one-plane anterior instability and for many is considered the "gold standard" for a clinical diagnosis of an anterior cruciate ligament injury.[146,267,293–296] The patient lies supine with the involved leg beside the examiner. The examiner holds the patient's knee between full extension and 30° of flexion. This position is close to the functional position of the knee, in which the anterior cruciate ligament plays a major role. The patient's femur is stabilized with one of

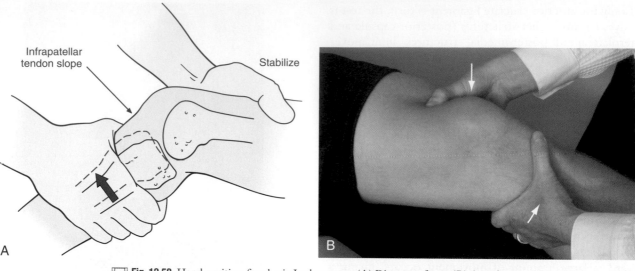

Infrapatellar
tendon slope

Stabilize

A

B

Fig. 12.58 Hand position for classic Lachman test (A) Diagram of test. (B) Actual test.

the examiner's hands (the "outside" hand) while the proximal aspect of the tibia is moved forward with the other ("inside") hand (Fig. 12.58). Frank[297] reported that to achieve the best results, the tibia should be slightly laterally rotated and the anterior tibial translation force should be applied from the posteromedial aspect. Therefore, the hand on the tibia should apply the translation force. A positive sign is indicated by a "mushy" or soft end feel when the tibia is moved forward on the femur (increased anterior translation with medial rotation of the tibia) and disappearance of the infrapatellar tendon slope.[291] A false-negative test may occur if the femur is not properly stabilized, if a meniscus lesion blocks translation, or if the tibia is medially rotated.[297] A positive sign indicates that the following structures may have been injured to some degree:

1. Anterior cruciate ligament (especially the posterolateral bundle)
2. Posterior oblique ligament
3. Arcuate-popliteus complex

Other ways of doing the Lachman test have also been advocated. The method that works for the examiner and that the examiner can use competently should be selected. Another method **(modification 1)** has the patient sitting with the leg over the edge of the examining table. The examiner sits facing the patient and supports the foot of the test leg on the examiner's thigh so that the patient's knee is flexed 30°. The examiner stabilizes the thigh with one hand and pulls the tibia forward with the other hand (Fig. 12.59). Excessive forward motion is considered to be a positive test.[298]

For examiners with small hands, the **stable Lachman test (modification 2)** is recommended. The patient lies supine with the knee resting on the examiner's knee (Fig. 12.60). One of the examiner's hands stabilizes the femur against the examiner's thigh, and the other hand applies

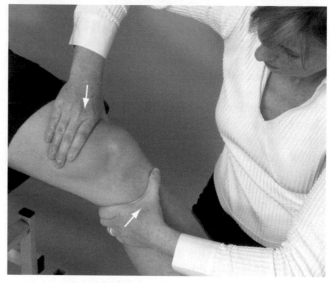

Fig. 12.59 Lachman test (modification 1).

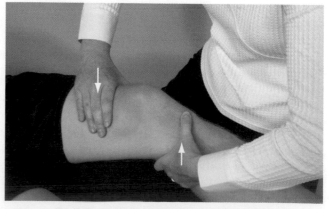

Fig. 12.60 Stable Lachman test (modification 2).

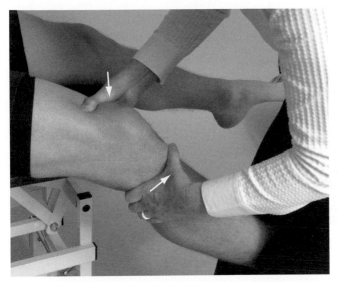

Fig. 12.61 Drop leg Lachman test (modification 3).

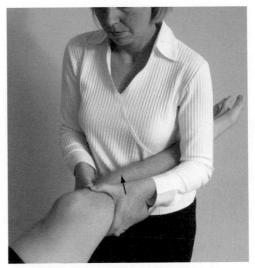

Fig. 12.62 Lachman test (modification 4).

an anterior stress.[128,299] Adler and associates[300] described a modification of this method, which they called the **drop leg Lachman test (modification 3).** The patient lies supine, and the leg to be examined is abducted off the side of the examining table and the knee is flexed to 25°. One of the examiner's hands stabilizes the femur against the table while the patient's foot is held between the examiner's knees. The examiner's other hand is then free to apply the anterior translation force (Fig. 12.61). They found there was greater anterior laxity demonstrated when doing the test this way than when doing it the classical way.[300]

Modification 4 has the patient lying supine while the examiner stabilizes the foot between the examiner's thorax and arm. Both hands are placed around the tibia, the knee is flexed 20° to 30°, and an anterior drawer movement is performed.[128] This technique allows gravity to control movement of the femur, which may not be sufficient to show a good positive test (Fig. 12.62).

Another way of doing the test **(modification 5)** is for the patient to lie supine while the examiner stands beside the leg to be tested with the eyes level with the knee. The examiner grasps the femur with one hand and the tibia with the other hand.[128] The tibia is pulled forward, and any abnormal motion is noted (Fig. 12.63). As with the regular Lachman test, the examiner may have difficulty stabilizing the femur if the examiner has small hands.

To perform the **prone Lachman test (modification 6),**[285,301,302] the patient lies prone, and the examiner stabilizes the foot between the examiner's thorax and arm and places one hand around the tibia. The other hand stabilizes the femur (Fig. 12.64). Gravity assists anterior movement with this method, but it is more difficult to determine the quality of the end feel.

For the **active (no touch) Lachman test (modification 7),**[128,303,304] the patient lies supine with the knee over the examiner's forearm so that the knee is flexed

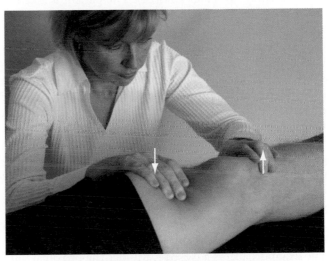

Fig. 12.63 Lachman test (modification 5).

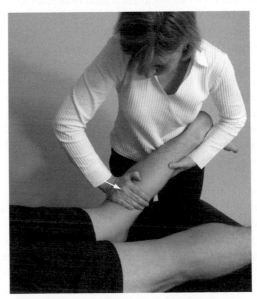

Fig. 12.64 Prone Lachman test (modification 6).

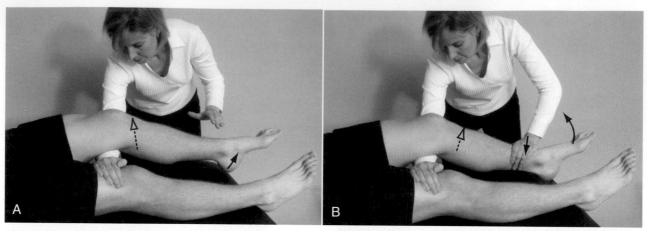

Fig. 12.65 (A) No-touch Lachman test (modification 7). *Open arrow* shows where the examiner watches for shift. (B) Active Lachman (maximum quadriceps) test (modification 8).

approximately 30° (Fig. 12.65A). The patient is asked to actively extend the knee, and the examiner watches for anterior displacement of the tibia relative to the unaffected side. The test may also be carried out with the foot held down on the table to increase the pull of the quadriceps. In this case the test has been called the **maximum quadriceps test (modification 8)** (Fig. 12.65B).[128] The examiner must be certain that there is no posterior sag before performing the test.

The Lachman test may be graded with a stress radiograph: a 3- to 6-mm anterior movement of the tibia relative to the femur is classified as a grade 1 injury; 6 to 9 mm, grade 2; 10 to 16 mm, grade 3; and 16 to 20 mm, grade 4.[128]

✓ *Lelli Test (Lever Sign).*[267,295,305–309] The patient is in supine with the knee fully extended on the examining table. The examiner places a closed fist under the proximal third of the patient's calf which causes the knee to flex slightly. The examiner's other hand then slowly applies a moderate downward force to the distal third of the quadriceps (i.e., the femur) while watching the relation of the tibial plateau to the femoral condyles. If the anterior cruciate ligament is intact, the patient's heel will lift off the examining table (Fig. 12.66A). If the anterior cruciate ligament is partially or completely torn (i.e., a positive test), the heel will not raise off the examining table and the tibial plateau will slide forward relative to the femoral condyles (Fig. 12.66B). The test should not be used in isolation when making an anterior cruciate ligament tear diagnosis.[295]

Tests for One-Plane Posterior Instability[310,311]

One-plane posterior instability implies injury to the posterior cruciate ligament.[36] However, it has been pointed out that isolated posterior cruciate injuries are rare, and if a posterior cruciate ligament injury is suspected, it is important to complete a full knee examination looking at all the ligaments, especially those involving the posterolateral corner.[36,312]

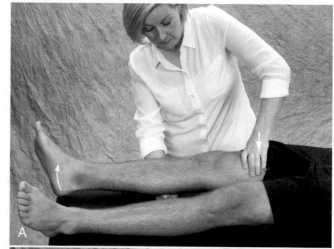

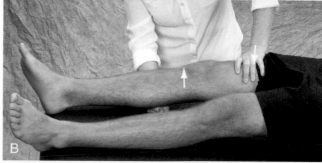

Fig. 12.66 Lelli test (Lever sign). (A) Note the examiner watching what happens at the knee. (B) Positive test. Heel does not lift off the bed, and the tibia shifts forward relative to the femur.

⚠ *Active Drawer Test.* This test has been described previously.

✓ *Drawer Sign or Test.* This test has been described previously. Veltri and Warren[279] report that the posterior drawer test is one of the most effective means of clinically diagnosing posterior cruciate and posterolateral (popliteus) corner injuries.

⚠ *Godfrey (Gravity) Test.*[128] The patient lies supine, and the examiner holds both legs while flexing the patient's

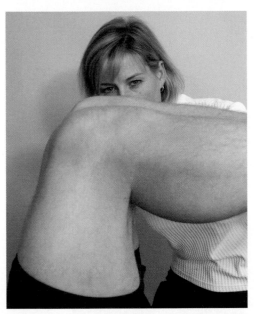

Fig. 12.67 Godfrey test. Examiner watches for posterior shift, which is not evident in this case.

hips and knees to 90° (Fig. 12.67). If there is posterior instability, a posterior sag of the tibia is seen. If manual posterior pressure is applied to the tibia, posterior displacement may increase.

Posterior Sag Sign (Gravity Drawer Test).[146] The patient lies supine with the hip flexed to 45° and the knee flexed to 90°. In this position the tibia "drops back," or sags back, on the femur because of gravity if the posterior cruciate ligament is torn (Fig. 12.68). Posterior tibial displacement is more noticeable when the knee is flexed 90° to 110° than when the knee is only slightly flexed. It is a test for one-plane posterior instability. Normally, the medial tibial plateau extends 1 cm anteriorly beyond the femoral condyle when the knee is flexed 90°. If this "step" is lost, which is what occurs with a positive posterior sag caused by a torn posterior cruciate ligament, this **step-off test** or **thumb sign** is considered positive.[59,78,280,310] The examiner must be careful because the position could result in a false-positive anterior drawer test for the anterior cruciate ligament if the sag remains unnoticed. If there is minimal or no swelling, the sag is evident because of an obvious concavity distal to the patella. If the posterior sag sign is present, the following structures may have been injured to some degree:

1. Posterior cruciate ligament
2. Arcuate-popliteus complex
3. Posterior oblique ligament
4. Anterior cruciate ligament

If it appears that the patient has a positive posterior sag sign, the patient should carefully extend the knee while the examiner holds the hip in 90° to 100° of flexion. This action is sometimes called the **voluntary anterior drawer sign,** and the results are similar to those of the active anterior drawer test. As the patient does this slowly, the tibial plateau moves or shifts forward to its normal position,

indicating that the tibia was previously posteriorly subluxated (posterior cruciate tear) on the femur.

Reverse Lachman Test.[128] The patient lies prone with the knee flexed to 30°, and the examiner grasps the tibia with one hand while fixing the femur with the other hand (Fig. 12.69). The examiner ensures that the hamstring muscles are relaxed. The examiner then pulls the tibia up (posteriorly), noting the amount of movement and the quality of the end feel. It is a test for the posterior cruciate ligament. The examiner should be wary of a false-positive test if the anterior cruciate ligament has been torn, because gravity may cause an anterior shift. This test is not as accurate for the posterior cruciate ligament as the posterior drawer test because, when the posterior cruciate ligament is torn, the greatest posterior displacement is at 90°.

Tests for Anteromedial Rotary Instability

For these rotary tests, the examiner is watching for abnormal tibial motion. In this case the examiner watches the medial side of the tibia to see if it rotates anteriorly more than the uninjured side.

Dejour Test.[49] The patient lies supine. The examiner holds the patient's leg with one arm against the body and the hand under the calf to lift the tibia while applying a valgus stress. The other hand pushes the femur down (Fig. 12.70). In extension, this action causes anteromedial subluxation in the pathological knee. If the knee is then flexed, the tibial plateau reduces suddenly, indicating a positive test. If the jolt is painful, it indicates that the medial meniscus has been injured. If it is not painful, the posteromedial corner has been injured.

Slocum Test. The Slocum test assesses both anterior rotary instabilities.[313] The patient's knee is flexed to 80° or 90°, and the hip is flexed to 45°. The foot is first placed in 30° medial rotation (Fig. 12.71). The examiner then sits on the patient's forefoot to hold the foot in position and draws the tibia forward; if the test is positive, movement occurs primarily on the lateral side of the knee. This movement is excessive relative to the unaffected side and indicates ALRI. It also indicates that the following structures may have been injured to some degree:

1. Anterior cruciate ligament
2. Posterolateral capsule
3. Arcuate-popliteus complex
4. Lateral collateral ligament
5. Posterior cruciate ligament
6. Iliotibial band

If the examiner finds ALRI during this first position of the Slocum test, the second part of the test, which assesses AMRI in this position, is of less value.[314]

In the second part of the test, the foot is placed in 15° of lateral rotation, and the tibia is drawn forward by the examiner. This part of the test is sometimes referred to as **Lemaire's T drawer test.** If the test is positive, the movement occurs primarily on the medial side of the knee. This movement is excessive relative to the unaffected side and

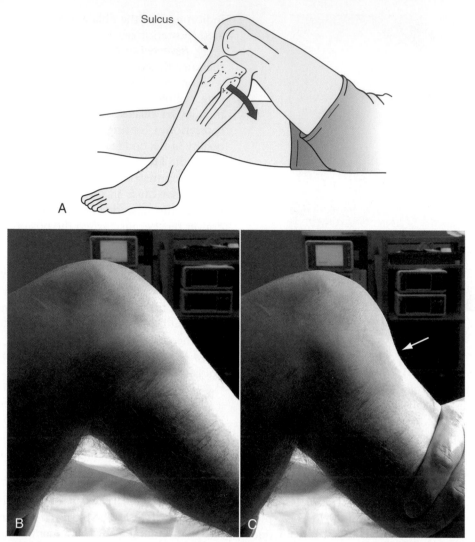

Sulcus

Fig. 12.68 (A) Illustration of posterior sag sign. (B and C) These surgical images are from a dislocated knee. Bruising can be seen in the thigh and calf areas. (B) shows the tibia reduced under the femur at 90°. (C) shows a minimal posterior force applied to the knee revealing a grade III posterior drawer (positive sag) test and the sulcus sign *(arrow)*. (A, Redrawn from O'Donoghue DH: *Treatment of injuries to athletes*, ed 4, Philadelphia, 1984, WB Saunders, p 450; B and C, From Lamb JN, Guy SP: Soft tissue knee injuries, *Surgery* 34[9]:456, 2016.)

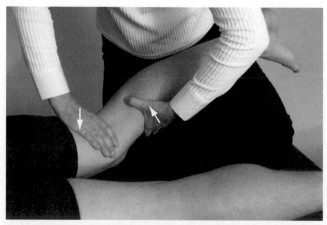

Fig. 12.69 Reverse Lachman test.

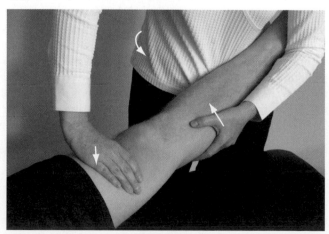

Fig. 12.70 Dejour test.

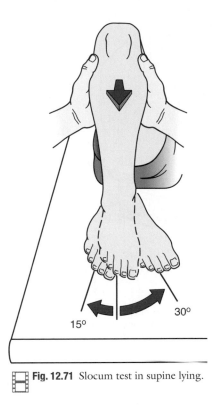

Fig. 12.71 Slocum test in supine lying.

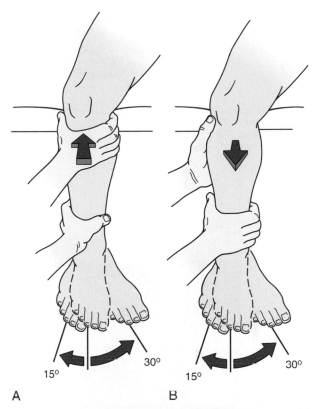

A   B

Fig. 12.72 Slocum test with the patient in the sitting position. Examiner rotates foot one way (i.e., medially or laterally) and then pushes the tibia backwards (A) or pulls it forward (B), comparing the amount of rotation and anterior and posterior movement in each knee.

indicates AMRI. It also indicates that the following structures may have been injured to some degree:

1. Medial collateral ligament (especially the superficial fibers, although the deep fibers may also be affected)
2. Posterior oblique ligament
3. Posteromedial capsule
4. Anterior cruciate ligament

For the Slocum test, it is imperative that the examiner medially or laterally rotate the foot to the degrees shown. If the examiner rotates the tibia as far as it will go, the test will be negative for movement because this action tightens all of the remaining structures.

If a stress radiograph is taken during the test, minimal or no movement indicates a negative test; 1 mm or less, a grade 1 injury; 1 to 2 mm, a grade 2 injury; and more than 2 mm, a grade 3 injury.[274]

The test may also be performed with the patient sitting with the knees flexed over the edge of the examining table (Fig. 12.72).[256] The examiner applies an anterior or a posterior force while holding the foot medially or laterally rotated. If this procedure is used, the examiner must remember that use of the anterior force tests for anterior rotary instability, whereas use of the posterior force tests for posterior rotary instability (see "Hughston Posteromedial and Posterolateral Drawer Sign" in later sections). The examiner should note whether the movement is excessive on the medial or on the lateral side of the knee relative to the normal knee. Excessive movement indicates a positive test.

Tests for Anterolateral Rotary Instability

When performing these tests, the examiner is looking for abnormal (excessive) anterior rotation of the tibia on the lateral side relative to the femur. The iliotibial band plays a major role in restraining anterior subluxation of the lateral tibial plateau and tibial medial rotation. If excessive motion is found on testing, the examiner should be aware of possible iliotibial band injury, especially if the laxity is found between 30° and 90° flexion.[248] The superficial medial collateral ligament resists the valgus component of the tests while the posterior oblique ligament helps the anterior cruciate ligament near extension.[315] During the rotation that occurs with the tests, the anterolateral ligament plays a role in stabilization through the changing degrees of knee flexion.[316]

? *Active Pivot Shift Test.*[267,294,295,317,318] The patient sits with the foot on the floor in neutral rotation and the knee flexed 80° to 90°. The patient is asked to isometrically contract the quadriceps while the examiner stabilizes the foot. A positive test is indicated by anterolateral subluxation of the lateral tibial plateau and is indicative of ALRI (Fig. 12.73).

⚠ *Crossover Test of Arnold.* The patient is asked to cross the uninvolved leg in front of the involved leg (Fig. 12.74). The examiner then carefully steps on the patient's involved foot to stabilize it and instructs the patient to rotate the upper torso away from the injured leg approximately 90° from the fixed foot. When this position is achieved, the patient contracts the quadriceps muscles,

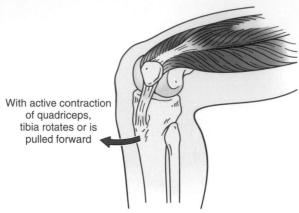

With active contraction of quadriceps, tibia rotates or is pulled forward

Fig. 12.73 Active pivot shift test.

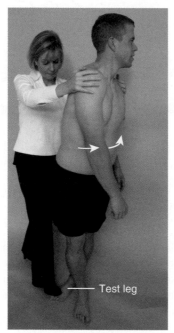

Test leg

Fig. 12.74 Crossover test.

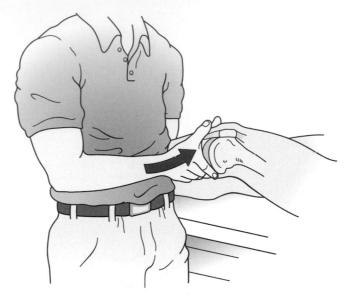

Fig. 12.75 Flexion-extension valgus test. *Arrow* shows compression. (Redrawn from Hanks GA, Joyner DM, Kalenak A: Anterolateral instability of the knee, *J Sports Med* 9:226, 1981.)

producing the same symptoms and testing the same structures as in the lateral pivot shift test.

Flexion-Extension Valgus Test. The patient lies supine, and the examiner holds the patient's leg as in the Noyes test. The examiner palpates the joint line with the thumb and fingers of both hands, and a valgus stress and axial compression are applied while the knee is flexed and extended (Fig. 12.75). If the anterior cruciate ligament is torn, the examiner feels the reduction and subluxation. The tibia is not rotated, so the subluxation is easily felt.[319]

Jerk Test of Hughston.[320] This test is similar to the pivot shift maneuver. The positioning of the patient and the examiner is the same, except that the patient's hip is flexed to 45°. With this test, the knee is first flexed to 90°. The leg is then extended, maintaining medial rotation and a valgus stress (Fig. 12.76). At approximately 20° to 30° of flexion, the tibia shifts forward, causing a

subluxation of the lateral tibial plateau with a jerk if the test is positive. If the leg is carried into further extension, it spontaneously reduces. A positive jerk test indicates that the same structures are injured as indicated by a positive pivot shift maneuver and assesses ALRI. According to the literature,[256] this test is not as sensitive as the pivot shift test.

Lateral Pivot Shift Maneuver (Test of MacIntosh). This is the primary test used to assess ALRI of the knee and is an excellent test for ruptures (third-degree sprains) of the anterior cruciate ligament.[321–324] However, like most provocative tests, it does have a disadvantage. In the apprehensive patient, because of the forces applied during the test, protective muscle contraction may lead to a false-negative test.[49] Lane et al.[325] stated that the pivot shift test closely correlates with patient outcomes. The presence of a pivot shift post surgery often precludes return to sports, is associated with continuation of symptoms, correlates with decreased patient satisfaction, and increases the likelihood of osteoarthrosis. During this test, the tibia moves away from the femur on the lateral side (but rotates medially) and moves anteriorly in relation to the femur (Fig. 12.77). Table 12.10 outlines the effect of some soft-tissue changes that can affect the pivot shift test.

Normally, the knee's center of rotation changes constantly through its ROM as a result of the shape of the femoral condyles, ligamentous restraint, and muscle tension. The path of movement of the tibia on the femur is described as a combination of rolling and sliding, with rolling predominating when the instant center is near the joint line and sliding predominating when the instant center shifts distally from the contact area. The MacIntosh test is a duplication of the anterior subluxation-reduction phenomenon that occurs during the normal gait cycle

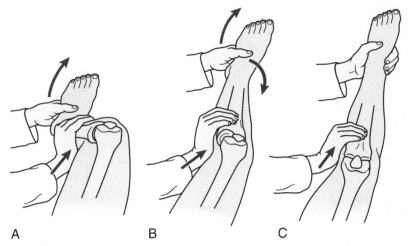

Fig. 12.76 Jerk test of Hughston. (A) The knee is flexed to 90°, and the heel of one hand is placed behind the fibular head to produce medial rotation of the tibia. (B) At 20°–30°, the lateral tibial plateau subluxates anteriorly. (C) At full extension, the lateral tibial plateau is reduced. (Redrawn from Irrgang JJ, et al: The knee: ligamentous and meniscal injuries. In Zachazewski JE, et al., editors: *Athletic injuries and rehabilitation*, Philadelphia, 1996, WB Saunders, pp 683–644.)

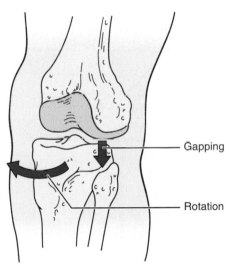

Fig. 12.77 Anterolateral rotary instability (ALRI).

TABLE 12.10

Effect of Soft-Tissue Characteristics on Pivot Shift Examination in the Anterior Cruciate Ligament–Deficient Knee

Soft-Tissue Factors	Effect on Pivot Shift	Mechanism
ITB tightness	Decreases	Restricts subluxation
ITB tightness	Decreases	Allows internal rotation throughout ROM so that there is no shift
MCL laxity	Decreases	Limits compression of lateral compartment with valgus stress
PLC	Increases	Increases external rotation
Medial meniscectomy	Increases	Increases anterior translation
Bucket-handle meniscus tear	Decreases	Blocks extension
Flexion contracture	Decreases	Prevents extension

ITB, Iliotibial band; *MCL*, medial collateral ligament; *PLC*, posterolateral corner; *ROM*, range of motion.
From Lane CG, Warren R, Pearle AD: The pivot shift, *J Am Acad Orthop Surg* 16:686, 2008.

when the anterior cruciate ligament is torn. Therefore, it illustrates a **dynamic subluxation.** This shift occurs between 20° and 40° of flexion (0° being full extension). It is this phenomenon that gives the patient the clinical description of feeling the knee "give way" (Fig. 12.78).

The patient lies supine with the hip both flexed and abducted 30° and relaxed in slight medial rotation (20°). The examiner holds the patient's foot with one hand while the other hand is placed at the knee, holding the leg in slight medial rotation. This is done by placing the heel of the hand behind the fibula and over the lateral head of the gastrocnemius muscle with the tibia medially rotated, causing the tibia to subluxate anteriorly as the knee is taken into extension (Fig. 12.79). Bach and colleagues[326] modified the position to slight lateral rotation because they believed that lateral tibial rotation gives a more pronounced pivot shift when the test is positive. In slight

flexion, the secondary restraints (i.e., hamstrings, lateral femoral condyle, lateral meniscus) are less efficient than in full flexion. It is important to realize that in full extension subluxation does not occur, because of the "locking home" of the tibia on the femur.[49] However, with slight flexion, the secondary restraints are less restrictive, and subluxation occurs. The examiner then applies a valgus stress to the knee while maintaining a medial rotation

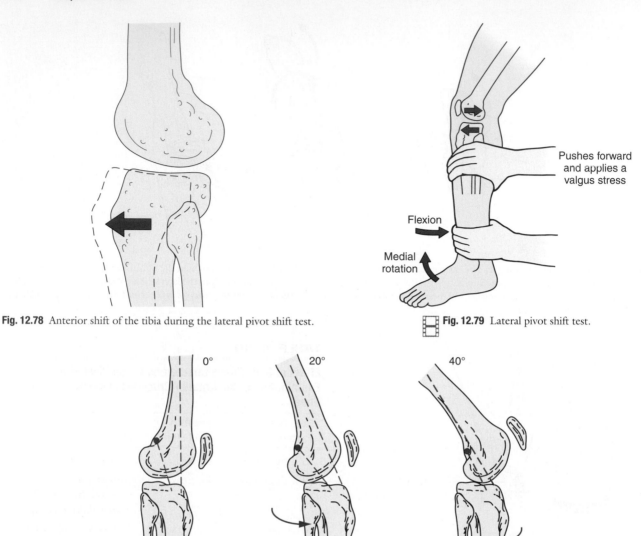

Fig. 12.78 Anterior shift of the tibia during the lateral pivot shift test.

Fig. 12.79 Lateral pivot shift test.

Fig. 12.80 Biomechanics of the pivot shift. Three phases occur during the pivot shift maneuver. Under load transmission in the lateral compartment, the tibia rolls from a reduced position in neutral rotation to anterior subluxation and some medial rotation. Under increasing flexion to 20°, the condyle becomes jammed behind the posterior slope of the lateral plateau. The iliotibial band, especially the femorotibial portion, becomes tight until, at 30°–40°, it is gliding behind the flexion axis, initiating reduction in more flexion and some lateral rotation.

torque on the tibia at the ankle. Kurosaka et al.[327] recommend applying an axial (compression) load to the knee while doing the test. If a click occurred during the test, they related the click to meniscus pathology. The leg is then flexed, and at approximately 30° to 40°, the tibia reduces or "jogs" backward. The patient says that that is what the "giving way" feels like, indicating a positive test. The reduction of the tibia on the femur is caused by the change in position of the iliotibial band when it switches from an extensor function to a flexor function, pulling the tibia back into its normal position (Fig. 12.80). The test involves two phases: first subluxation and then reduction. The iliotibial band must be intact for the test to work. In cases of ALRI in which the iliotibial band has also been torn, the test does not work (the subluxation will be evident, but the "jog" will not occur). In addition, if either

meniscus has been torn, it may limit or prevent the subluxation reduction motion seen in the test.

If the patient is tense or apprehensive, the test can be modified; this is called the **soft pivot shift test** (Fig. 12.81). The patient lies supine, and the examiner supports the test foot with one hand while placing the other hand over the calf muscle 10 to 20 cm (4 to 8 inches) distal to the knee joint. The examiner flexes and extends the knee slowly and gently to relax the patient. After three to five cycles, the examiner applies axial compression while the other hand over the calf exerts an anterior pressure. In a positive test, the tibia subluxates and reduces but not with the same apprehensive, jerky feeling.[128] Kennedy[274] advocated pushing on the fibular head with the thumb when performing this maneuver. Because hip abduction and adduction have an effect on the iliotibial band, hip

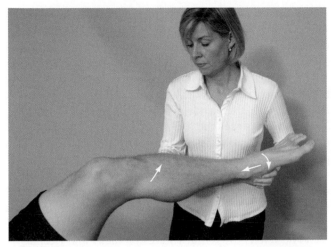

Fig. 12.81 Soft pivot shift test. Examiner watches for anterior shift.

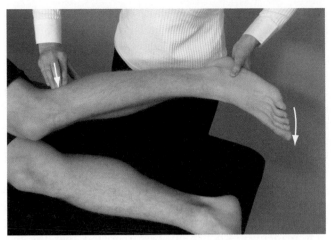

Fig. 12.82 Lemaire's jolt test for anterolateral rotary instability.

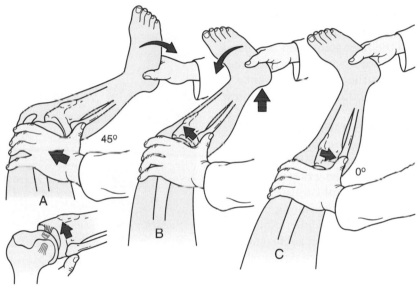

Fig. 12.83 The Losee test begins with the knee in flexion and the tibia in lateral rotation and valgus stress (A). As the knee is extended (B), the foot is allowed to medially rotate, and the previously reduced (A) tibia subluxes as the knee approaches full extension (C). A palpable "clunk" correlates with anterior cruciate ligament tear. (Redrawn from Scott WN, editor: *Ligament and extensor mechanism injuries of the knee: diagnosis and treatment*, St Louis, 1991, Mosby, p 96.)

position plays an important role in the test. Subluxation is most obvious when the hip is abducted and least obvious when it is adducted. In addition, lateral rotation of the tibia allows greater subluxation because, like abduction, it decreases the stress on the iliotibial band.[128] If the test is positive, the following structures have probably been injured to some degree:

1. Anterior cruciate ligament
2. Posterolateral capsule
3. Arcuate-popliteus complex
4. Lateral collateral ligament
5. Iliotibial band

Lemaire's Jolt Test.[49] The patient is in side-lying position with the test leg uppermost. For the test to work, the patient must be relaxed. With one hand, the examiner medially rotates the tibia by grasping the foot and medially rotating it with the knee in extension. The back of

the other hand pushes lightly against the biceps tendon and head of the fibula while the hand on the foot flexes and extends the knee (Fig. 12.82). In a positive test, at approximately 15° to 20° of flexion, a "jolt" occurs with displacement of the tibia, indicating a positive test for anterolateral instability.

Losee Test. This test is a clinical duplication of the ALRI mechanism of injury. The patient lies supine while relaxed.[328] The examiner holds the patient's ankle and foot so that the leg is laterally rotated. The knee is then flexed to 30°, and the examiner ensures that the hamstring muscles are relaxed (Fig. 12.83). The lateral rotation ensures that the subluxation of the knee is reduced at the beginning of the test. With the examiner's other hand positioned so that the fingers lie over the patella and the thumb is hooked behind the fibular head, a valgus force is applied to the knee; the examiner can use the abdomen as a fulcrum while extending the patient's knee and applying forward pressure behind the fibular head with the thumb. The valgus stress compresses the structures in the lateral compartment and makes the anterior subluxation, if present, more noticeable. At the same time, the foot and ankle are allowed to drift into medial rotation. If the foot and ankle are not allowed to rotate medially, the anterior subluxation of the lateral tibial plateau may be prevented. Just before full extension of the knee, there is a "clunk" forward if the test is positive, and the patient must recognize the movement as the instability that was previously experienced. This clunk means that the tibia has subluxated anteriorly and indicates injury to the same structures as those indicated by a positive pivot shift maneuver. Kocher et al.[329] reported that the test could be used as a good check of functional instability after surgical reconstruction.

❓ Martens Test.[128] The patient and examiner are positioned as for the Noyes test. The examiner grips the patient's leg distal to the knee joint with one hand and pushes the femur posteriorly with the other hand. A valgus stress is applied to the knee as the knee is flexed until the tibia reduces, indicating a positive test (Fig. 12.84).

❓ Nakajima Test.[128] The patient lies supine, and the examiner stands on the side of the test leg. The patient's foot is held with one hand, which medially rotates the tibia. The knee is flexed to 90°. The examiner's other hand is placed over the lateral femoral condyle with the thumb behind the head of the fibula, pushing it forward. The examiner slowly extends the knee while pushing the head of the fibula forward, noting whether subluxation of the fibula occurs, which indicates a positive test.

⚠ Noyes Flexion-Rotation Drawer Test. Described by Noyes et al,[330] this test is a modification of the pivot shift maneuver. It can be used in the acutely injured knee and is believed by some[21] to be more sensitive than the other ALRI tests. The patient lies supine, and the examiner holds the patient's ankle between the examiner's trunk and arm with the hands around the tibia (Fig. 12.85). The examiner flexes the patient's knee to 20° to 30° while maintaining the tibia in neutral rotation. The tibia is then pushed posteriorly, as in a posterior drawer test. This posterior movement reduces the subluxation of the tibia, indicating a positive test for ALRI. If the tibia is alternately pushed posteriorly and released and the femur is allowed to rotate freely, the reduction and subluxation are seen and felt as the femur rotates medially and laterally.

⚠ Slocum Test. This test has been described previously.

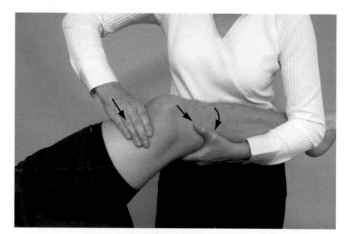

Fig. 12.84 Martens test.

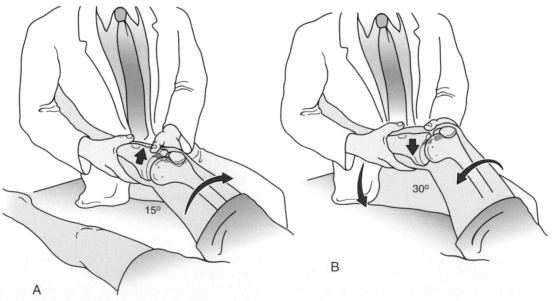

Fig. 12.85 Flexion-rotation drawer test combines elements of Lachman test and lateral pivot shift. Flexion from (A B) results in posterior reduction of subluxated tibia and medial rotation of femur. Positive test results correlate with anterior cruciate ligament disruption. (Redrawn from Scott WN, editor: *Ligament and extensor mechanism injuries of the knee: diagnosis and treatment*, St Louis, 1991, Mosby, p 94.)

▲ *Slocum Anterolateral Rotary Instability Test.* ALRI is also assessed by the Slocum ALRI test.[256,314] The patient is in the side-lying position (approximately 30° from supine). The bottom leg is the uninvolved leg. The knee of the uninvolved leg is flexed to add stability (Fig. 12.86). The foot of the involved leg rests and is stabilized on the examining table, with the patient's foot in medial rotation and the knee in extension and valgus. This position helps to eliminate hip rotation during the test. The examiner applies a valgus stress to the knee while flexing the knee. The subluxation of the knee reduces at between 25° and 45° of flexion if the test is positive. A positive test indicates injury to the same structures as indicated in the pivot shift maneuver. The main advantage of this test is that it aids in relaxation of the patient's hamstring muscles and is easier to perform on heavy or tense patients.

Tests for Posteromedial Rotary Instability[331–334]

When performing these tests, the examiner is looking for abnormal (excessive) posterior rotation of the medial side of the tibia relative to the femur. A note of caution: If the leg is positioned so that gravity may affect the relation of the tibia to the femur (e.g., supine-lying position, hip at 45°, knee at 90°), the medial side of the tibia may "drop back" into excessive posterior rotation just by positioning and the effect of gravity. In this case,

if the examiner is not aware of this abnormal position, a false-positive test for AMRI may occur if testing for AMRI when in fact the real problem is posteromedial rotary instability (PMRI).

▲ *Hughston's Posteromedial and Posterolateral Drawer Sign.* The patient lies supine with the knee flexed to 80° to 90° and the hip flexed to 45° (Fig. 12.87).[335] The examiner medially rotates the patient's foot slightly and sits on the foot to stabilize it. The examiner then pushes the tibia posteriorly. If the tibia moves or rotates posteriorly on the medial aspect an excessive amount relative to the normal knee, the test is positive and indicates PMRI. A positive test indicates that the following structures have probably been injured to some degree:

1. Posterior cruciate ligament
2. Posterior oblique ligament
3. Medial collateral ligament (superficial and deep fibers)
4. Semimembranosus tendon
5. Posteromedial capsule
6. Anterior cruciate ligament
7. Medial meniscus

The medial tubercle rotates posteriorly around the posterior cruciate ligament when the tibia is in mild medial rotation. If the posterior cruciate ligament is also torn, the posteromedial movement is greater, and the tibia subluxates posteriorly (Fig. 12.88).

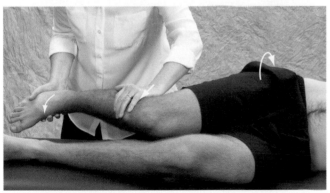

Fig. 12.86 Slocum anterolateral rotary instability test.

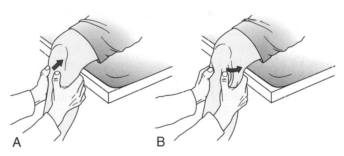

Fig. 12.87 Posteromedial and posterolateral drawer test, anterior view. (A) Starting position for posterolateral drawer test. (B) Positive posterolateral drawer test with posterior and lateral rotation of the lateral tibial condyle.

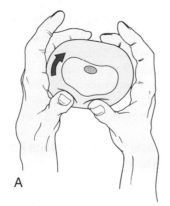
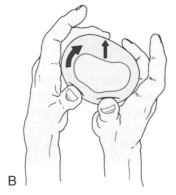

Fig. 12.88 Posterolateral drawer test. (A) If the posterior cruciate ligament is intact, the tibia rotates posterolaterally. (B) If the posterior cruciate ligament is torn, the tibia rotates posterolaterally and subluxates posteriorly.

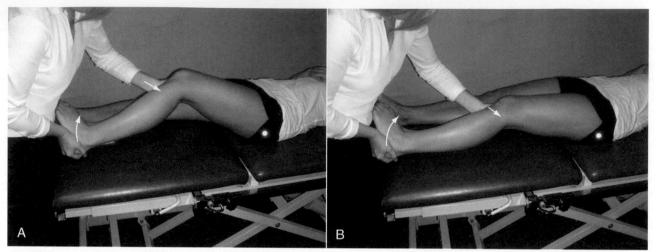

Fig. 12.89 Posteromedial pivot shift test. (A) Starting position. (B) In a positive test, the tibia will jog into reduction at between 20° and 40° of flexion as the knee is extended.

The test may also be done with the patient sitting with the knee flexed over the edge of the examining table. The examiner pushes posteriorly while holding the patient's leg in medial rotation, watching for the same excessive movement.

Posterolateral rotary instability (PLRI) may be tested in a similar fashion.[335] The patient and examiner are in the same position, but the patient's foot is slightly laterally rotated. If the tibia rotates posteriorly on the lateral side an excessive amount relative to the uninvolved leg when the examiner pushes the tibia posteriorly, the test is positive for PLRI. The test is positive only if the posterior cruciate ligament and lateral collateral ligaments are torn.[336] The examiner may palpate the fibula while doing the movement to feel for excessive movement.

? *Posteromedial Pivot Shift Test.*[337] The patient lies relaxed in the supine position. The examiner passively flexes the knee more than 45° while applying a varus stress, compression, and medial rotation of the tibia; in a "positive" knee, these movements cause subluxation of the medial tibial plateau posteriorly (Fig. 12.89A). The examiner then takes the knee into extension. At approximately 20° to 40° of flexion, the tibia shifts into the reduced position (Fig. 12.89B). A positive test indicates that the following structures are injured:
1. Posterior cruciate ligament
2. Medial collateral ligament
3. Posterior oblique ligament

⚠ *Supine Internal (Medial) Rotation Test.*[338] The patient lies supine with the examiner standing beside the knee to be tested. The examiner flexes the patient's knee with one hand while the other hand holds the patient's ankle and rotates the tibia. The examiner flexes the knee to 60° flexion (and hip to 80°) and applies a medial rotation torque to the patient's foot (Fig. 12.90). The amount of rotation is graded by the location of the tibial tubercle relative to its neutral position in millimeters. The test is repeated at 75°, 90°, 105°, and 120° of knee flexion. Both knees are

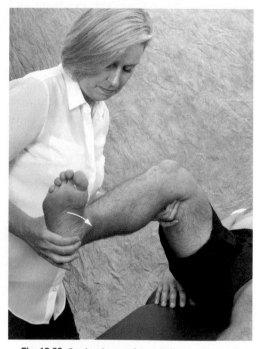

Fig. 12.90 Supine internal (medial) rotation test.

compared. Grade 0 is 0 mm excursion; grade 1 is between 0 and less than 3 mm excursion; grade 2 is between 3 mm and less than 6 mm excursion; grade 3 is between 6 mm and less than 9 mm excursion; and grade 4 is greater than or equal to 9 mm excursion. The test is designed to test the integrity of the posterior cruciate ligament. If the ligament is injured, the excursion should increase at all the angles tested.

Tests for Posterolateral Rotary Instability[336,339–344]
The examiner is looking for abnormal (excessive) posterior rotation of the lateral side of the tibia when performing these tests. As with the posteromedial rotation, the examiner must always be aware that positioning the leg (gravity may cause the lateral tibia to "drop back") may

lead to a false-positive ALRI when, in fact, the problem is actually a PLRI problem.

❓ *Active Posterolateral Drawer Sign.* [345] The patient sits with the foot on the floor in neutral rotation. The knee is flexed to 80° to 90°. The patient is asked to isometrically contract the hamstrings, primarily the lateral one (biceps femoris), while the examiner stabilizes the foot. A positive test for PLRI is posterior subluxation of the lateral tibial plateau (Fig. 12.91).

❓ *Dynamic Posterior Shift Test.* [346] The patient lies supine, and the examiner flexes the hip and knee of the

test leg to 90° with the femur in neutral rotation. One hand of the examiner stabilizes the anterior thigh while the other hand extends the knee. If the test is positive, the tibia reduces anteriorly with a clunk as extension is reached. The test is positive for posterior and posterolateral instabilities. If the knee is painful before extension is accomplished, the hip flexion may be decreased, but the hamstrings must be kept tight (Fig. 12.92).

⚠ *External Rotation Recurvatum Test.* There are three methods for performing this test. In the first method, the patient lies in the supine position with the lower limbs relaxed. The examiner gently grasps the big toe of each foot and lifts both feet off the examining table (Fig. 12.93A).[335,339,347] The patient is told to keep the quadriceps muscles relaxed (i.e., it is a passive test). While elevating the legs, the examiner watches the tibial tuberosities. LaPrade et al.[348] suggest one of the examiner's hands should hold the toes while the other hand gently holds the distal thigh near the knee to prevent the thigh lifting off the table (method 2). In this case, the tibia will sublux anteriorly (Fig. 12.93B) and the affected leg will show a higher heel height indicating injury to the posterolateral structures. With a positive test, the affected knee goes into relative hyperextension on the lateral aspect because of the force of gravity with the tibia and tibial tuberosity rotating laterally. The affected knee has the appearance of a relative genu varum. It is a test for PLRI in extension and injury to the anterior cruciate ligament.[348]

In the third method, the patient lies supine, and the examiner's hand holds the patient's heel or foot and flexes the knee to 30° to 40° (Fig. 12.94).[335] The examiner's other hand holds the posterolateral aspect of the patient's knee and slowly extends it. With the hand on the knee, the examiner feels the relative hyperextension and lateral rotation occurring in the injured limb compared with the uninjured limb.

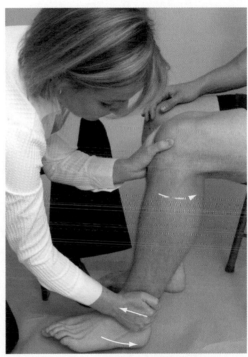

Fig. 12.91 Active posterolateral drawer sign or test. Examiner watches for posterolateral shift of tibia.

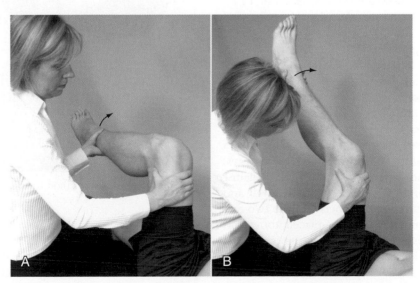

Fig. 12.92 Dynamic posterior shift test. (A) Starting position in flexion. (B) Extended position in which posterior shift occurs.

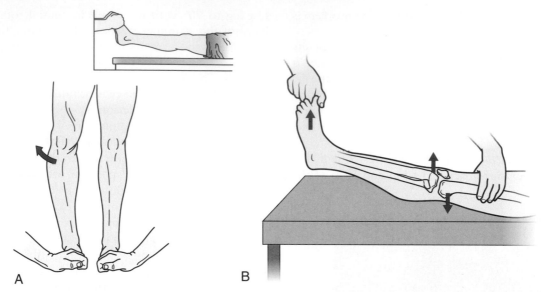

Fig. 12.93 External rotational recurvatum test. (A) Method 1, the examiner grasps the big toe of each foot. (B) Method 2, the examiner grasps the big toe with one hand while the other gently holds the distal thigh near the knee to prevent the thigh from lifting off the table. In a positive test, differences in heel height from the table are demonstrated.

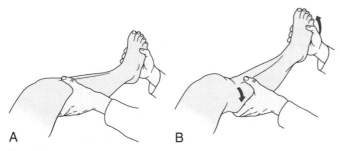

Fig. 12.94 External rotation recurvatum test (method 3). (A) The test is begun by holding the knee in flexion. (B) As the knee is slowly extended, the hand at the knee feels the lateral rotation and recurvatum at the posterolateral aspect of the knee.

⚠️ *Hughston's Posteromedial and Posterolateral Drawer Sign.* This test has been described previously. For PLRI to occur, the following structures must have been injured to some degree:

1. Posterior cruciate ligament
2. Arcuate-popliteus complex
3. Lateral collateral ligament
4. Biceps femoris tendon
5. Posterolateral capsule
6. Anterior cruciate ligament

⚠️ *Jakob Test (Reverse Pivot Shift Maneuver).* This is a test for PLRI,[256,349] and it can be performed in two ways. In the first method, the patient stands and leans against a wall with the uninjured side adjacent to the wall and the body weight distributed equally between the two feet (Fig. 12.95). The examiner's hands are placed above and below the involved knee, and a valgus stress is exerted while flexion of the patient's knee is initiated. If there is a jerk in the knee or the tibia shifts posteriorly and the "giving way" phenomenon occurs during this maneuver, it

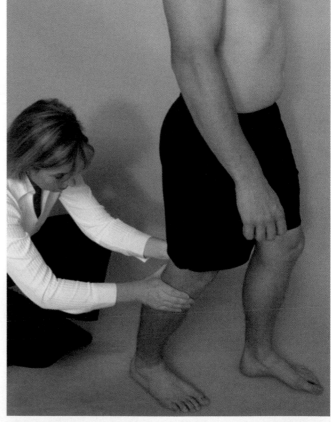

Fig. 12.95 Jakob test (method 1, showing valgus stress and flexion).

indicates injury to the lateral collateral ligament, arcuate-popliteus complex, and mid-third of the lateral capsule.[336]

In the second method, the patient lies in the supine position with the hamstring muscles relaxed. The examiner faces the patient, lifts the patient's leg, and supports

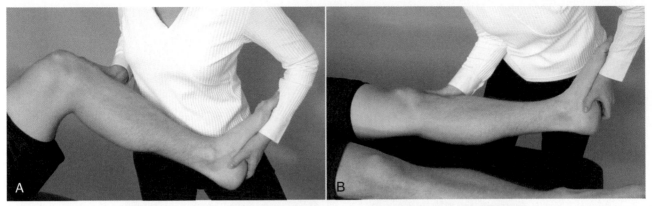

Fig. 12.96 Reverse pivot shift test, method 2. (A) Flexed position with lateral rotation causes lateral tibial tubercle to subluxate. (B) As the extended position is approached, the lateral tibial tubercle reduces.

the leg against the examiner's pelvis. The examiner's other hand supports the lateral side of the calf with the palm on the proximal fibula. The knee is flexed to 70° to 80° of flexion, and the foot is laterally rotated, causing the lateral tibial plateau to subluxate posteriorly (Fig. 12.96A). The knee is taken into extension by its own weight while the examiner leans on the foot to impart a valgus stress to the knee through the leg. As the knee approaches 20° of flexion, the lateral tibial tubercle shifts forward or anteriorly into the neutral rotation and reduces the subluxation, indicating a positive test (Fig. 12.96B). The leg is then flexed again, and the foot falls back into lateral rotation and posterior subluxation.

⚠ *Loomer's Posterolateral Rotary Instability Test.*[347,350] The patient lies supine and flexes both hips and both knees to 90°. The examiner then grasps the feet and maximally laterally rotates both tibias (Fig. 12.97). The test is considered positive if the injured tibia laterally rotates excessively and there is a posterior sag of the affected tibial tubercle; both signs must be present for a positive test. This test is similar to the **Bousquet external hypermobility test.**[49]

Veltri and associates[351–354] describe a modification of the Loomer test that is called the **tibial lateral rotation test** or **dial test of the knee** ⚠ (Fig. 12.98). This test is designed to show loss of the posterolateral support structures of the knee. Griffith et al. reported that this test could also test medial knee joint structures.[355] The patient may be placed supine or prone. The examiner places one hand behind the posterior proximal tibia to support the tibia and maintain it in the reduced (normal) position.[354] The examiner then flexes the knee to 30°, extends the foot over the side of the examining table, and stabilizes the femur on the table.[356] The examiner then laterally rotates the tibia on the femur and compares the amount of rotation with that on the good side. If the test is done in supine position, the examiner can observe the amount of tibial tubercle movement and compare. The test is then repeated with the knee flexed to 90° and the thigh still on the examining table. If the tibia rotates less at 90° than at

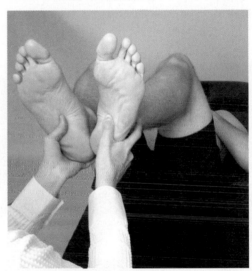

▣ **Fig. 12.97** Loomer's test for posterolateral rotary instability.

30°, an isolated posterolateral (popliteus corner) injury is more likely. If the knee rotates more at 90°, injury to both the popliteus corner and posterior cruciate injury are more likely.[279,336,339–341] If the pain is on the medial joint line, a positive test may indicate injury to the medial ligament complex (see Swain test).[272,273]

❓ *Standing Apprehension Test.*[357] The patient stands on the affected knee. The examiner then pushes anteriorly and medially on the anterolateral part of the lateral femoral condyle crossing the joint line. The patient is then asked to slightly flex the knee while the examiner pushes with the thumb (Fig. 12.99). Condylar movement and a "giving way" sensation are considered positive signs for PLRI.

Ligament Testing Devices

Ligament testing devices for the knee have been developed to help quantify the displacement occurring in the knee and how this displacement is modified when ligaments are injured. Most commonly, these devices test anteroposterior displacement, although more expensive

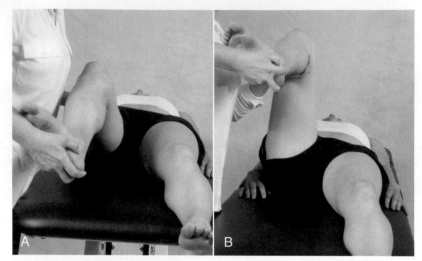

Fig. 12.98 Tibial lateral rotation test or dial test in supine position. (A) At 30° flexion. (B) At 90° flexion. The examiner watches for increased lateral rotation on the affected side, which may occur at 30° or 90° (see text).

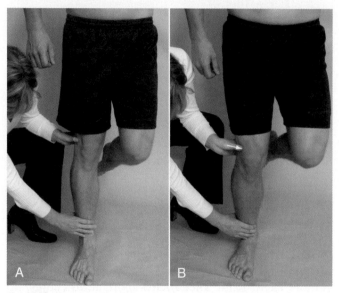

Fig. 12.99 Standing apprehension test for posterolateral instability. (A) Starting position. (B) With knee flexed.

ones may test other displacements. These devices are used primarily to assist in diagnosing ligament injuries (third-degree sprains) by detecting abnormal (pathological) motion, to provide a quantified measurement of motion, and to measure the amount of motion after surgery (e.g., whether normal motion limits were reestablished).[358–361]

The most commonly used ligament testing devices are the KT-1000 arthrometer (most common), the Genucom, the Stryker knee laxity tester, the Rolimeter, and the Telos device. The KT-1000 and Rolimeter are reported to be best for anterior laxity, whereas the Telos device is best for posterior laxity.[362] Other units have been developed but are not commonly used.[49,363–366] These devices should be considered adjuncts to clinical assessment and should be used primarily to confirm a clinical diagnosis.[52]

Each of these devices works on the principle of positioning the limb in a specific manner, applying a force that causes displacement, and subsequently measuring the amount of displacement or translation caused by the applied force.[358,367,368] The measurements obtained depend on the experience and ability of the examiner, the joint position, muscle activity or inactivity, the constraints present in the joint and those imposed by the testing systems, the amount of displacing force, and the measurement system used.[358] The greatest sources of error when using the arthrometer are the inability to stabilize the patellar sensor pad and lack of muscle relaxation.[369]

Because the KT-1000 arthrometer is the most commonly used testing device for anteroposterior displacement, it is briefly described here. More detailed descriptions of its use are found elsewhere[181,367–369] and should be consulted if the examiner plans to use this device. The arthrometer is placed on the anterior aspect of the tibia and is held in place with two Velcro straps (Figs. 12.100 and 12.101). A thigh support and foot support help to hold the leg in proper alignment with straps if necessary. There are two sensor pads, one on the tibial tubercle and one on the patella. Because the patella is one of the sensor points, knees that are swollen and demonstrate a ballotable patella should not be tested unless the knee is aspirated to minimize false-positive readings.[370] These pads detect relative movement. Forces to translate the tibia are applied through a force-sensing handle.

After the device is properly positioned and the leg is properly relaxed, several tests may be performed, first on the good knee and then on the injured knee.

Quadriceps Neutral Test. The patient's knee is flexed to 90°, and the arthrometer is positioned on the leg. A 9-kg (20-lb) posterior force is applied through the apparatus to establish a reference position. The patient is then asked to perform an isolated quadriceps contraction. If the tibia shifts forward, the knee angle is altered until there is no

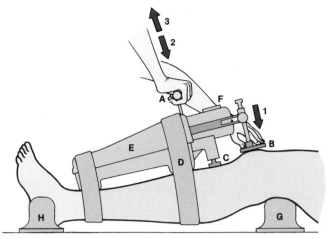

Fig. 12.100 KT-1000 arthrometer. A posterior *(2)* or anterior *(3)* force is applied. A constant force *(1)* is applied to stabilize the patellar sensor pad. *A,* Force handle; *B,* patellar sensor pad; *C,* tibial sensor pad; *D,* Velcro straps; *E,* arthrometer body; *F,* displacement dial; *G,* thigh support; *H,* foot support. (From Daniel D, Akeson W, O'Conner J, editors: *Knee ligaments: structure, injury and repair,* New York, 1990, Raven Press, p 428.)

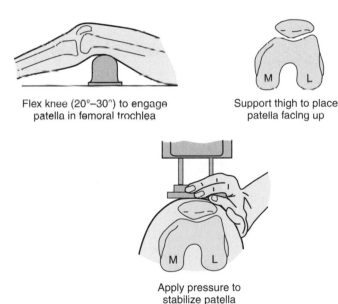

Flex knee (20°–30°) to engage patella in femoral trochlea

Support thigh to place patella facing up

Apply pressure to stabilize patella

Fig. 12.101 The knee is supported in a flexed position to engage the patella in the femoral trochlea. In some patients, the thigh support must be raised an additional 3–6 cm (1.2–2.4 inches) to provide sufficient knee flexion to engage the patella in the femoral trochlea. This may be done by placing a board under the thigh support. The thigh should be supported so that the patella is facing up. Occasionally, a thigh strap is used to accomplish this task. The examiner stabilizes the patellar sensor with manual pressure. The stabilizing hand should rest against the lateral thigh and should apply 1–2.25 kg (2–5 lbs) of pressure on the patellar sensor pad. The hand position, patellar sensor position, and patellar sensor pressure must remain constant throughout the test. Variation of the pressure on the patellar sensor pad and rotation of the pad is a common cause of measurement error. (From Daniel D, et al., editors: *Knee ligaments: structure, injury and repair,* New York, 1990, Raven Press, p 428.)

movement of the tibia when the quadriceps contracts. This position is called the **quadriceps neutral angle** or **quadriceps active position,** and it usually occurs at approximately 70° flexion (see Fig. 12.135). This position

is found on the good knee and is used as a reference or starting position for the injured knee. If, when the injured knee is tested in this position, the anterior displacement is greater than 1 mm, the translation is abnormal and probably indicates a posterior cruciate ligament sprain.[358,369]

Test in Quadriceps Active Position. With the patient's leg positioned at the quadriceps neutral angle, the examiner applies a 9-kg (20-lb) anterior force, followed by a 9-kg (20-lb) posterior force. The results for the good and injured knee are compared.[358,369]

Test in 30° Flexion. With the patient's leg positioned as shown in Fig. 12.100, five tests are performed:

1. 9-kg (20-lb) posterior displacement
2. 7-kg (15-lb) anterior (Lachman) displacement
3. 9-kg (20-lb) anterior (Lachman) displacement
4. Maximum anterior (Lachman) displacement, usually 14 to 18 kg (30 to 40 lb)
5. Quadriceps active anterior displacement

The difference between the 7- and the 9-kg anterior displacement tests is called the **compliance index.** For the maximum anterior displacement test, the examiner manually pulls or translates the tibia forward on the femur, using a pull of approximately 14 to 18 kg (30 to 40 lb). For the quadriceps active test, the patient is asked to lift the heel slowly off the table; displacement as the heel leaves the table is noted. Differences of more than 3 mm between the good and injured legs are considered diagnostic for injury to the anterior cruciate or posterior cruciate.[358,369] Force displacement curves (Fig. 12.102) and frequency-distribution curves (Fig. 12.103) demonstrate differences between the normal and pathological knees. Tests involving larger translation forces have been found to be more responsive to translation differences.[371]

It is important to realize that the accuracy of the readings for these devices depends very much on positioning, muscle relaxation, and the experience of the operator. Reliability of any of these measuring devices may be greatly affected if these factors are not controlled.[358,363,364,368,372–379]

Special Tests

Although most special tests on the knee are done only if the examiner suspects certain pathologies and wants to do a confirming test, tests for swelling should always be performed. The findings or outcomes of special tests depend on many factors and when individually performed only rarely rule in or out a particular pathology.[200,380] Only those special tests that are relevant to being used to confirm a diagnosis from information gleaned from the history, observation, and the remainder of the examination would be used in an assessment.

For the reader who would like to review them, the reliability, validity, specificity, sensitivity, and odds ratios of some of the special tests used on the knee are available in eAppendix 12.1.

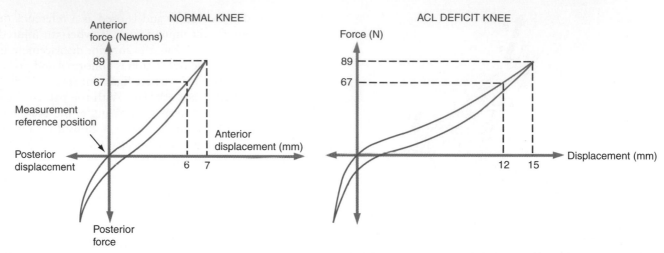

Fig. 12.102 Force-displacement curves for normal knees and for knees with anterior cruciate ligament *(ACL)* deficit. The compliance index is obtained by measuring the displacement between the 67- and 89-N anterior-force levels. On this curve, the compliance index for the normal knee is 1 mm; for the knee with an ACL deficit, it is 3 mm. (From Daniel D, et al., editors: *Knee ligaments: structure, injury and repair*, New York, 1990, Raven Press, p. 433.)

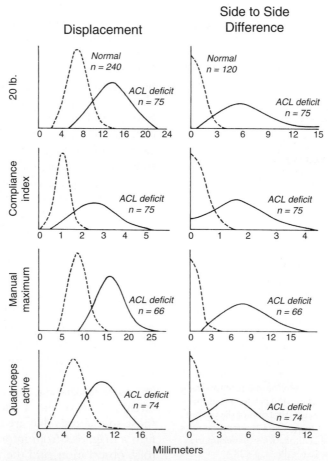

Fig. 12.103 Frequency distribution curves of anterior laxity in normal knee in 30° of flexion and in knees with unilateral chronic anterior cruciate ligament disruption. *ACL,* Anterior cruciate ligament. (From Daniel DM, Stone ML: Diagnosis of knee ligament injury: test and measurements of joint laxity. In Feagin JA, editor: *The crucial ligaments*, New York, 1988, Churchill Livingstone, p 298.)

Key Tests Performed on the Knee Depending on Suspected Pathology[a,271]

- **For meniscus lesions:**
  - ☑ Apley's test
  - ⚠ "Bounce home" test
  - ⚠ Childress' sign (squat and duck walk test)
  - ⚠ Dynamic knee test
  - ⚠ Ege's test
  - ❓ Figure-of-four meniscal stress maneuver
  - ☑ McMurray test
  - ⚠ O'Donohue's test
  - ⚠ Thessaly test
- **For plica lesions:**
  - ⚠ Hughston's plica test
  - ⚠ Mediopatellar plica test
  - ⚠ Patellar bowstring test
  - ⚠ Plica "stutter" test
- **For swelling:**
  - ☑ Brush, stroke or bulge test (minimal swelling)
  - ⚠ Fluctuation test (moderate swelling)
  - ⚠ Indentation test
  - ☑ Patellar tap test (moderate swelling)
- **For patellofemoral syndrome:**
  - ⚠ Clarke's sign
  - ⚠ Eccentric step (lateral step down) test
  - ⚠ McConnell test
  - ⚠ Motion palpation test
  - ⚠ Step up test
- **For quadriceps:**
  - ⚠ Q-angle
  - ⚠ Tubercle sulcus test
- **Coactivation tests for quadriceps and hamstrings:**
  - ⚠ Single-limb dead-lift
  - ⚠ Lateral hop
  - ⚠ Transverse hop
  - ⚠ Lateral band walks
- **For patellar instability:**
  - ☑ Fairbank's apprehension test
  - ⚠ Moving patellar apprehension test
- **For iliotibial band friction syndrome:**
  - ⚠ Noble compression test

[a]The authors recommend these key tests be learned by the clinician to facilitate a diagnosis. See Chapter 1, Key for Classifying Special Tests.

Tests for Meniscus Injury

Although there are several tests for a meniscus injury, none can be considered definitive without considerable experience on the part of the examiner.[381–383] Even with experience, the examiner must do a thorough history and examination, because a positive test is more likely to be found if one suspects the condition is present.[384–386] Because the menisci are avascular and have no nerve supply on their inner two-thirds, an injury to the meniscus can result in little or no pain or swelling, making diagnosis even more difficult. Often, a combination of tests and clinical signs is needed to have a high level of suspicion of meniscus injury.[386–388] However, in some cases, joint line pain or tenderness, if the ligaments have been ruled out as causes of the pain, is the result of meniscus pathology.[389] However, it has been found that only approximately 50% of meniscus injuries have joint line pain or tenderness, especially with anterior cruciate tears, so this finding should not be used in isolation for diagnosis.[390–392] Antunes et al.[267] recommended combining three clinical tests for meniscus injury (Steinman test, joint line tenderness, and McMurray test) to improve diagnostic accuracy for meniscus injuries.

Signs and Symptoms of Meniscus Injury

- Joint line pain
- Loss of flexion (more than 10°)
- Loss of extension (more than 5°)
- Swelling (synovial)
- Crepitus
- Positive special test

❓ **Anderson Medial-Lateral Grind Test.**[393] The patient lies supine. The examiner holds the test leg between the trunk and the arm while the index finger and thumb of the opposite hand are placed over the anterior joint line (Fig. 12.104). A valgus stress is applied to the knee as it is passively flexed to 45°; then a varus stress is applied to the knee as it is passively extended, producing a circular motion to the knee. The motion is repeated, increasing the varus and valgus stresses with each rotation. A distinct grinding is felt on the joint line if there is meniscus pathology. The test may also show a pivot shift if the anterior cruciate ligament has been torn.

☑ **Apley's Test.**[394] The patient lies in the prone position with the knee flexed to 90°. The patient's thigh is then anchored to the examining table with the examiner's knee (Fig. 12.105). The examiner medially and laterally rotates the tibia, combined first with distraction, while noting any restriction, excessive movement, or discomfort. Then the process is repeated using compression instead of distraction. If rotation plus distraction is more painful or shows increased rotation relative to the normal side, the lesion is probably ligamentous. If the rotation plus compression is more painful or shows decreased rotation relative to the normal side, the lesion is probably a meniscus injury.

❓ **Bohler's Sign.** The patient lies in the supine position, and the examiner applies varus and valgus stresses to the knee. Pain in the opposite joint line (valgus stress for lateral meniscus) on stress testing is a positive sign for meniscus pathology.[128]

⚠ **"Bounce Home" Test.** The patient lies in the supine position, and the heel of the patient's foot is cupped in the examiner's hand (Fig. 12.106). The patient's knee is completely flexed, and the knee is passively allowed to extend. If extension is not complete or has a rubbery end feel ("springy block"), there is something blocking full extension. The most likely cause of a block is a torn meniscus.

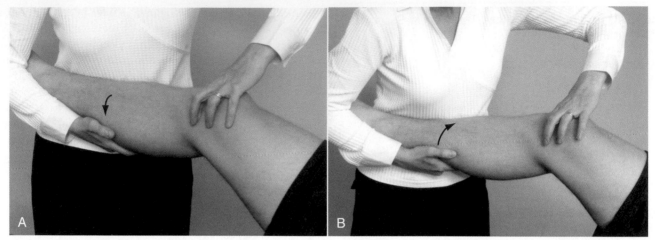

Fig. 12.104 Anderson medial-lateral grind test. (A) Flexion and valgus stress. (B) Extension and varus stress.

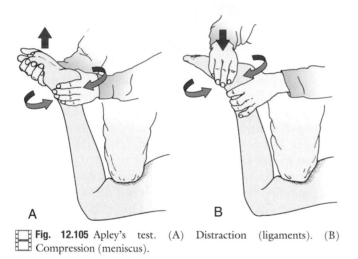

A   B

Fig. 12.105 Apley's test. (A) Distraction (ligaments). (B) Compression (meniscus).

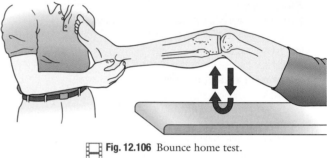

Fig. 12.106 Bounce home test.

Oni[395] reported that if the knee is allowed to quickly extend in one movement or jerk and the patient experiences a sharp pain on the joint line, which may radiate up or down the leg, the test is positive for a meniscus lesion.

Bragard's Sign. The patient lies supine, and the examiner flexes the patient's knee. The examiner then laterally rotates the tibia and extends the knee (Fig. 12.107). Pain and tenderness on the medial joint line indicate medial meniscus pathology. If the examiner then medially rotates the tibia and flexes the knee, the pain and tenderness decrease.[128] Both of these symptoms indicate medial meniscus pathology.

Cabot's Popliteal Sign.[128] The patient lies supine, and the examiner positions the test leg in the figure-four position. The examiner palpates the joint line with the thumb and forefinger of one hand and places the other hand proximal to the ankle of the test leg. The patient is asked to isometrically straighten the knee while the examiner resists the movement. A positive test, signifying a meniscus lesion, is indicated by pain on the joint (Fig. 12.108).

Childress' Sign (Squat and Duck Walk Test).[396] The patient is asked to squat and then is asked to "walk" or "waddle"

forward in the squatted position (i.e., duck walking) (Fig. 12.109). If, when doing the test, the patient complains of joint line pain or painful clicking, the test is considered positive for a posterior horn lesion of the meniscus.

Dynamic Knee Test. The patient lies supine with the hip flexed, abducted to 60° and laterally rotated 45° with the knee in 90° flexion so that the lateral border of the foot of the test leg rests on the examining table (Fig. 12.110A). The examiner palpates the lateral joint line while adducting the hip (knee still in 90° flexion) (Fig. 12.110B). If there is increased pain on joint line or a sharp pain at end of adduction, the test is considered positive for a lateral meniscus tear.

Ege's Test. This test has been described as a weight-bearing McMurray test.[397] The patient stands with the knees in extension and the feet 30 to 40 cm (11 to 15 inches) away from each other. To test the medial meniscus, the patient laterally rotates each tibia maximally and squats causing the distance between the knees and lateral rotation to increase. The patient then stands slowly while leaving the feet laterally rotated (Fig. 12.111A and B). To test the lateral meniscus, both tibias are medially rotated maximally while the patient squats and then stands up (Fig. 12.111C and D). A full squat in medial rotation is very difficult even in healthy individuals. Both tests are considered positive if pain and/or a click is felt by the patient along the joint line or heard by the examiner. The pain or click may be heard when squatting or

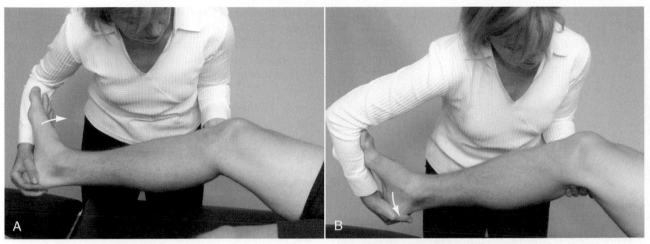

Fig. 12.107 Bragard's sign for a meniscus lesion. (A) Medial meniscus test. (B) Lateral meniscus test.

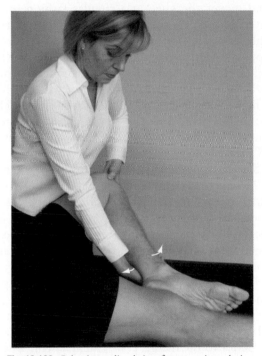

Fig. 12.108 Cabot's popliteal sign for a meniscus lesion.

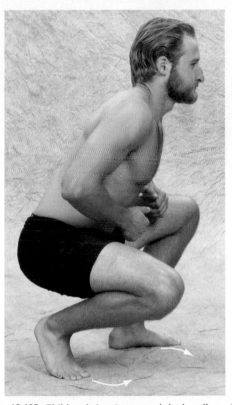

Fig. 12.109 Childress' sign (squat and duck walk test).

coming out of the squat. It was reported that anterior tears are more likely to occur in earlier knee flexion while posterior horn tears cause the click or pain in more flexion. The test may not be as useful in acute cases (<6 weeks). It is purported to be as or more accurate than joint line pain.

❓ *Figure-of-Four Meniscal Stress Maneuver.*[89] The patient lies supine. The examiner puts the test leg in the figure-four position (i.e., test foot on the knee of the opposite leg) and then lifts the foot of the test leg and swings the leg rapidly from a varus to valgus stress using one hand while pushing a finger of the other hand in the joint line (Fig. 12.112). The varus-valgus stress is reported to bring the meniscus toward the joint periphery while the finger pushes it away from the periphery.

The combined action causes a sharp pain in a positive case indicating a meniscal tear.

❓ *Kromer's Sign.* This test is similar to Bohler sign except that the knee is flexed and extended while the varus and valgus stresses are applied.[128] A positive test is indicated by the same pain on the opposite joint line.

✓ *McMurray Test.* The McMurray test is the grandfather of meniscus tests of the knee. However, the reliability and sensitivity of the test has been found to be low.[381,383,398] The patient lies in the supine position with the knee completely flexed (the heel to the buttock).[399,400] The examiner then medially rotates

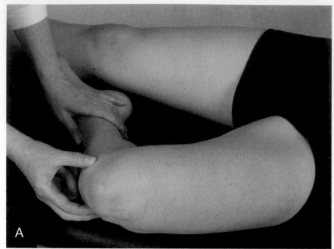

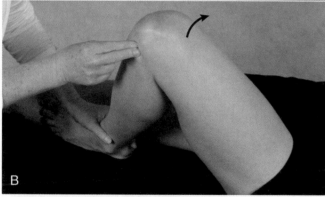

Fig. 12.110 Dynamic knee test. (A) Starting position. Hip flexed and abducted, knee at 90°. (B) The examiner then adducts the flexed hip while palpating the lateral joint line.

the tibia and extends the knee (Fig. 12.113). If there is a loose fragment of the lateral meniscus, this action causes a snap or click that is often accompanied by pain. By repeatedly changing the amount of flexion and then applying the medial rotation to the tibia followed by extension, the examiner can test the entire posterior aspect of the meniscus from the posterior horn to the middle segment. The anterior half of the meniscus is not as easily tested because the pressure on the meniscus is not as great. To test the medial meniscus, the examiner performs the same procedure with the knee laterally rotated. Kim and colleagues[401] reported that meniscus lesions may be found on the medial side with medial rotation and on the lateral side with lateral rotation.

The test may be modified by medially rotating the tibia, extending the knee, and moving through the full ROM to test the lateral meniscus. The process is repeated several times. The tibia is then laterally rotated, and the process is repeated to test the medial meniscus. Both methods are described by McMurray.[383,399]

? *Modified Helfet Test.*[402] In the normal knee, the tibial tuberosity is in line with the midline of the patella when the knee is flexed to 90°. However, when the knee is extended, the tibial tubercle is in line with the

lateral border of the patella (Fig. 12.114). If this change does not occur with the change in movement, rotation is blocked, indicating that there is injury to the meniscus, there is a possible cruciate injury, or the quadriceps muscles have insufficient strength to "screw home" the knee.

⚠ *O'Donohue's Test.* If a patient experiences pain along the joint line, the patient is asked to lie in the supine position. The examiner flexes the knee to 90°, rotates it medially and laterally twice, and then fully flexes and rotates it both ways again. A positive sign is indicated by increased pain on rotation in either or both positions and is indicative of capsular irritation or a meniscus tear.

? *Passler Rotational Grind Test.*[128] The patient sits with the test knee extended and held at the ankle between the examiner's legs proximal to the examiner's knees. The examiner places both thumbs over the medial joint line and moves the knee in a circular fashion, medially and laterally rotating the tibia while the knee is rotated through various flexion angles. Simultaneously, the examiner applies a varus or a valgus stress (Fig. 12.115). Pain elicited on the joint line indicates a meniscus lesion.

? *Payr's Test.* The patient lies supine with the test leg in the figure-four position (Fig. 12.116). If pain is elicited on the medial joint line, the test is considered positive for a meniscus lesion, primarily in the middle or posterior part of the meniscus.[128]

? *Steinman's Tenderness Displacement Test.* Steinman's sign is indicated by point tenderness and pain on the joint line that appears to move anteriorly when the knee is extended and moves posteriorly when the knee is flexed. It indicates a possible meniscus tear. Medial pain is elicited on lateral rotation, and lateral pain is elicited on medial rotation.

⚠ *Test for Retreating or Retracting Meniscus.* The patient sits on the edge of the examining table or lies in the supine position with the knee flexed to 90°.[402] The examiner places one finger over the joint line of the patient's knee anterior to the medial collateral ligament, where the curved margin of the medial femoral condyle approaches the tibial tuberosity (Fig. 12.117). The patient's leg and foot are then passively laterally rotated, and the meniscus normally disappears. The leg is medially and laterally rotated several times with the meniscus appearing and disappearing. The knee must be flexed and the muscles relaxed to do the test. If the meniscus does not appear, a torn meniscus is indicated because rotation of the tibia is not occurring. The examiner must palpate carefully because a distinct structure is difficult to palpate. If the examiner medially and laterally rotates the unaffected leg several times first, the meniscus can be felt pushing against the finger on medial rotation, and it disappears on lateral rotation.

Seil et al.[403] reported a test for an avulsion of the posterior horn of the medial meniscus. When the examiner applies a valgus stress to the knee, in the presence of an avulsion, the medial meniscus is extruded (i.e., forced) anteromedially

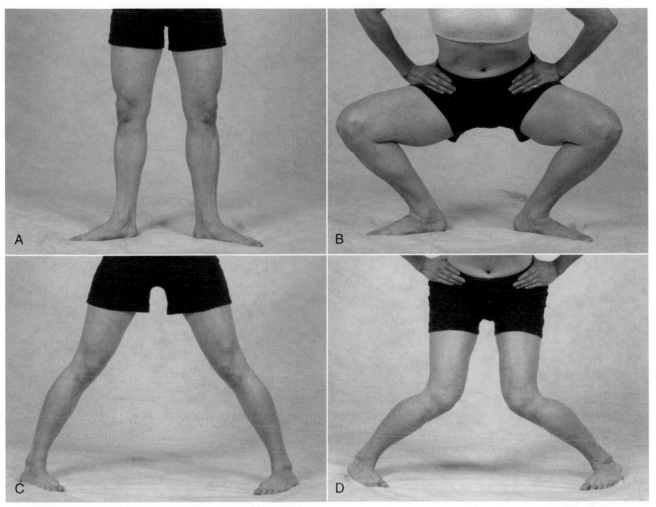

Fig. 12.111 Ege's test. The patient is weight bearing. To detect a medial meniscal tear, both lower extremities are first held in maximum lateral rotation (A). The patient then squats while maintaining the lateral rotation (B). For lateral meniscal tears, both lower extremities are held in maximum medial rotation (C). Maximum medial rotations of both lower extremities are preserved during squatting (D).

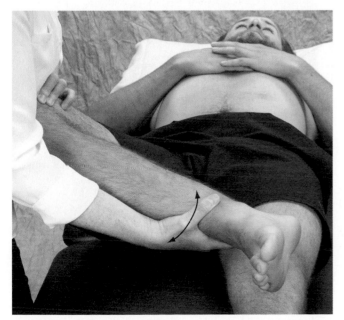

Fig. 12.112 Figure-of-four meniscal stress maneuver. Examiner's left hand is palpating the patient's knee joint line while the right hand applies varus-valgus stress to the knee.

and becomes more apparent on the anteromedial joint line. By palpating the anteromedial joint line while doing the test, the examiner will feel the meniscus extrude.

⚠ ***Thessaly Test.***[200,404,405] The patient stands flat footed on one leg while the examiner provides his or her hands for balance. The patient then flexes the knee to 5° and rotates the femur on the tibia medially and laterally three times while maintaining the 5° flexion (Fig. 12.118A). The good leg is tested first, and then the injured leg. The test is then repeated at 20° flexion (Fig. 12.118B). The test is considered positive for a meniscus tear if the patient experiences medial or lateral joint line discomfort. The patient may also have a sense of locking or catching in the knee. The test should not be used if an anterior cruciate ligament injury is also suspected.[406]

Tests for Plica Lesions

In the knee, plica are embryological remnants that have remained in some people after birth.[407–410] Normally, they are reabsorbed by the time of birth, although remnants may be present in 20% to 50% of knees.[411–413] Because an abnormal plica can mimic meniscus pathology, it is

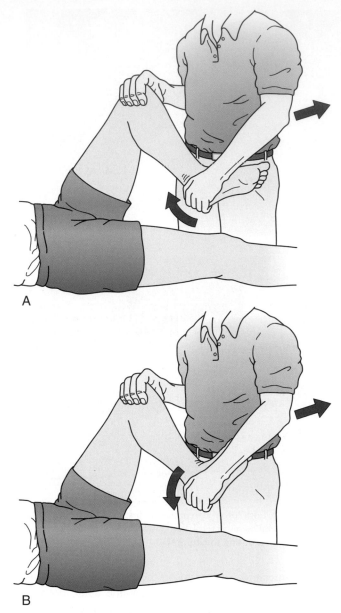

A

B

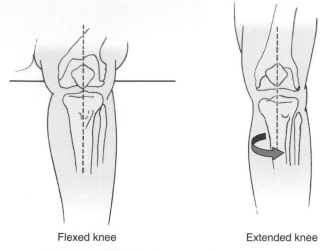

Flexed knee Extended knee

Fig. 12.114 Modified Helfet test (negative test shown).

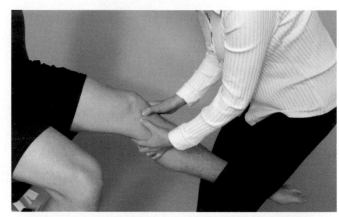

Fig. 12.115 Passler rotational grind test for meniscus pathology.

Fig. 12.113 McMurray test. (A) For medial meniscus test. (B) For lateral meniscus test.

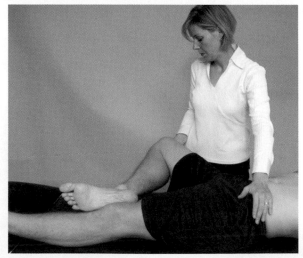

Fig. 12.116 Payr's sign for a meniscus lesion.

essential that the plica tests be performed as well as the meniscus tests if a meniscus or plica injury is suspected.[414]

⚠ *Hughston's Plica Test.* The patient lies in the supine position, and the examiner flexes the knee and medially rotates the tibia with one arm and hand while pressing the patella medially with the heel of the other hand and palpating the medial femoral condyle with the fingers of the same hand (Fig. 12.119). The patient's knee is passively flexed and extended while the examiner feels for "popping" of the plica band under the fingers. The popping indicates a positive test.[320]

⚠ *Mediopatellar Plica Test (Mital-Hayden Test or Medial Plica Shelf Test).* The patient lies in the supine position with the affected knee flexed to 30° resting on a support or the examiner's arm (Fig. 12.120). The examiner then

pushes the patella medially with the thumb. If the patient complains of pain or a click, it indicates a positive test caused by pinching of the edge of the plica between the medial femoral condyle and the patella. The pain may indicate a mediopatellar plica.[415]

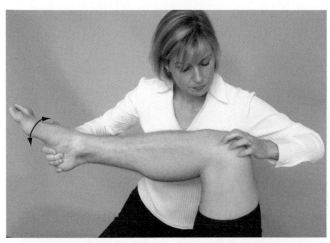

Fig. 12.117 Test for a retreating meniscus.

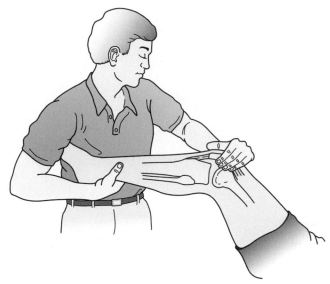

Fig. 12.119 Examination for suprapatellar plica. The foot and tibia are held in medial rotation. The patella is displaced slightly medially with the fingers over the course of the plica. The knee is passively flexed and extended, eliciting a "pop" of the plica and associated tenderness. (Redrawn from Hughston JC, Walsh WM, Puddu G: *Patellar subluxation and dislocation*, Philadelphia, 1984, WB Saunders, p 29.)

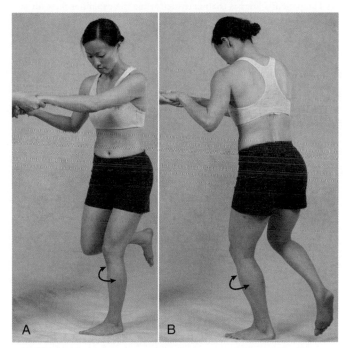

Fig. 12.118 Thessaly test. Patient stands on test leg. (A) In 5° flexion with rotation. (B) In 20° flexion with rotation.

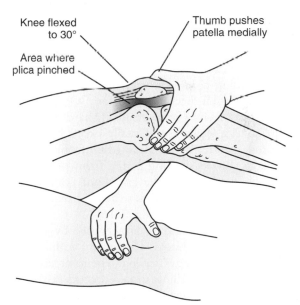

Knee flexed to 30°

Area where plica pinched

Thumb pushes patella medially

Fig. 12.120 Positioning for mediopatellar plica test.

⚠ *Patellar Bowstring Test.*[86] The patient lies on his or her side with the test leg uppermost. Using the heel of one hand, the examiner pushes the patella medially and holds it there. The examiner then flexes the patient's knee and medially rotates the tibia with the other hand. The patient's knee is then extended (Fig. 12.121) while the examiner listens for any sounds or feels for any grinding.

⚠ *Plica "Stutter" Test.* The patient is seated on the edge of the examining table with both knees flexed to 90°. The examiner places a finger over one patella to palpate during movement. The patient is then instructed to slowly extend the knee. If the test is positive, the patella stutters or jumps somewhere between 60° and 45° of flexion (0° being straight leg) during an otherwise smooth movement. The test is effective only if there is no joint swelling.

Tests for Swelling

When assessing swelling, the examiner must determine the type and amount of swelling that are present. Although the tests for swelling are listed under the "Special Tests" section, the examiner should always be testing for swelling when examining the knee. In addition, the examiner must differentiate between swelling and synovial thickening. With swelling, the knee assumes its resting position of 15° to 25° of flexion, which allows the synovial cavity

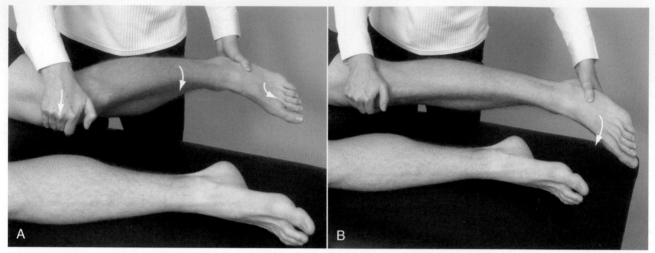

Fig. 12.121 Bowstring test for plica. (A) Using the heel of one hand, the examiner pushes the patella medially and holds it there. The examiner then flexes the patient's knee and medially rotates the tibia with the other hand. (B) The patient's knee is then extended while the examiner feels for any sounds.

the maximum capacity for holding fluid. If the injury is sufficiently severe, the fluid extravasates into the soft tissue surrounding the joint as a result of torn structures (i.e., ligaments, capsule, synovium). Therefore, lack of effusion should not lull the examiner into thinking the injury is a minor one.

If the swelling consists of blood that results in a hemarthrosis (within the joint), it may be caused by a ligament tear, osteochondral fracture, or peripheral meniscus tear. "Blood" swelling comes on very quickly (within 1 to 2 hours), and the skin becomes very taut. On palpation, it has a "doughy" feeling and is relatively hard to the touch. The joint surface feels warm. Usually, excess blood should be aspirated, or osteoarthritis may result from irritation of the cartilage. Blood swelling in the form of ecchymosis may also be seen around the knee, but commonly this blood will begin to "track" down the leg because of gravity as it becomes visible (see Fig. 1.16).

Normally, synovial fluid swelling caused by joint irritation occurs in 8 to 24 hours. The feeling within the joint is a fluctuating or "boggy" feeling. The joint surface feels warm and tender. Swelling usually occurs with activity and disappears after a few days of inactivity.

The third type of joint swelling is purulent or pus swelling, in which the joint surface is hot to the touch. Often it is red, and the patient has general signs of infection or pyrexia.

Signs and Symptoms of Knee Joint Infection

- Intra-articular effusion
- Pain
- Redness
- Warmth
- Gray or brownish liquid draining/drained from knee
- Fever
- Night chills or sweats

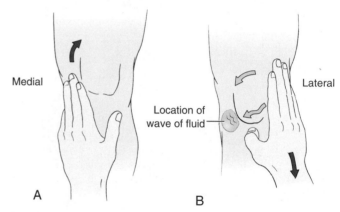

Fig. 12.122 Brush test for swelling. (A) Hand strokes up. (B) Hand strokes down.

✔ **Brush, Stroke, or Bulge Test.** Also called the *wipe test,* this test assesses minimal effusion. The examiner commences just below the joint line on the medial side of the patella, stroking proximally toward the patient's hip as far as the suprapatellar pouch two or three times with the palm and fingers (Fig. 12.122). With the opposite hand, the examiner strokes down the lateral side of the patella. A wave of fluid passes to the medial side of the joint and bulges just below the medial distal portion or border of the patella. The wave of fluid may take up to 2 seconds to appear. Normally, the knee contains 1 to 7 mL of synovial fluid. This test shows as little as 4 to 8 mL of extra fluid within the knee. Sturgill et al.[416] developed an effusion grading scale based on the stroke test (Table 12.11).[146]

⚠ **Fluctuation Test.** The examiner places the palm of one hand over the suprapatellar pouch and the palm of the other hand anterior to the joint with the thumb and index finger just beyond the margins of the patella (Fig. 12.123). By pressing down with one hand and then the other, the examiner may feel the synovial fluid fluctuate

TABLE **12.11**

Effusion Grading Scale of the Knee Joint Based on the Stroke Test

Grade	Test Result
Zero	No wave produced on downstroke
Trace	Small wave on medial side with downstroke
1+	Larger bulge on medial side with downstroke
2+	Effusion spontaneously returns to medial side after upstroke (no downstroke necessary)
3+	So much fluid that it is not possible to move the effusion out of the medial aspect of the knee

From Sturgill LP, Snyder-Mackler L, Manal TJ, et al: Interrater reliability of a clinical scale to assess knee joint effusion, *J Orthop Sports Phys Ther* 39:846, 2009.

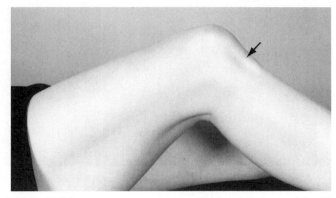

Fig. 12.124 Indentation test. *Arrow* indicates where to watch for filling of indentation.

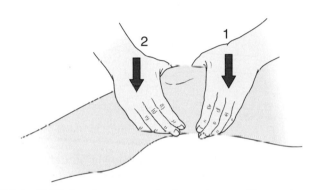

Fig. 12.123 Hand positioning for fluctuation test. First one hand is pushed down *(arrow 1);* then the other hand is pushed down *(arrow 2).* The examiner will feel fluid shifting back and forth under one hand and then the other.

under the hands and move from one hand to the other, indicating significant effusion.

⚠ *Indentation Test.*[417] The patient lies supine. The examiner passively flexes the good leg, noting an indentation on the lateral side of the patellar tendon (Fig. 12.124). The good knee is fully flexed, and the indentation remains. The injured knee is then slowly flexed while the examiner watches for the disappearance of the indentation. At that point, knee flexion is stopped. The disappearance of the indentation is caused by swelling and indicates a positive test. The angle at which the indentation disappears depends on the amount of swelling. The greater the swelling, the sooner the indentation disappears. If the thumb and finger are placed on each side of the patellar tendon, the fluid can be made to fluctuate back and forth. This method, like the brush test, can detect minimal levels of swelling.

✓ *Patellar Tap Test ("Ballotable Patella").* With the patient's knee extended or flexed to discomfort, the examiner applies a slight tap or pressure over the patella (Fig. 12.125). When this is done, a floating of the patella should be felt. This is sometimes called the **"dancing patella"** sign. A modification of this test calls for the examiner to apply the thumb and forefinger of one hand lightly on both sides of the patella. The examiner then strokes down on the suprapatellar pouch with the other hand.[128] A positive test is indicated by separation of the thumb and forefinger. This test can detect a large amount of swelling (40 to 50 mL) in the knee, which can also be noted by observation.

❓ *Peripatellar Swelling Test.*[418] The patient lies supine with the knee extended. The examiner carefully milks fluid from the suprapatellar pouch distally. With the opposite hand, the examiner palpates adjacent to the patellar tendon (usually on the medial side) for fluid accumulation or a wave of fluid passing under the fingers. Reider[71] calls this a **palpable fluid wave.** If less swelling is evident, Reider[71] suggests the **visible fluid wave.** The examiner strokes the fluid into the suprapatellar pouch. With one hand, the examiner then squeezes or pushes down on the suprapatellar pouch while watching the hollows on each side of the patella for a wave of fluid to pass. This test is similar to the brush test.

Tests for Patellofemoral Dysfunction

Patellofemoral dysfunction, or patellofemoral pain syndrome (PFPS), implies there is some pathology affecting the patellofemoral joint.[90,200,419,420] This pathology may be the result of biomechanical factors, pathophysiological processes, trochlear dysplasia, or loss of tissue homeostasis resulting in synovitis and an inflamed fat pad.[51,421,422] Commonly, patients with patellofemoral problems experience pain when climbing or descending stairs, when stepping up or down, with prolonged sitting (movie sign), when squatting, or when getting up from a chair. The reliability of most PFPS tests is low, and thus multiple tests are often recommended.[196] Nunes et al.[423] reported that the patellar tilt and squatting test showed evidence of supporting a diagnosis of PFPS. Piva et al.[424] reported that there are several measures of impairment for PFPS that are reliable (e.g., hamstrings, quadriceps, plantar flexors, and iliotibial band length, hip abductor strength, and foot pronation). The examiner should consider assessing the whole lower kinetic chain and its effect on the

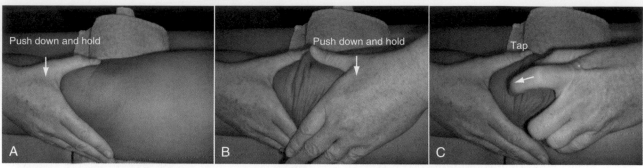

Fig. 12.125 Patellar tap test ("ballotable patella"). (A) Step 1. (B) Step 2. (C) Step 3.

patellofemoral joint when PFPS is suspected.[80–85,425–428] For example, it has been found that hip abductors and lateral rotators are weak and the iliotibial band is tight in PFPS patients.[99,429–432] In some cases the pain may cause reflex inhibition, resulting in buckling or giving way of the knee.[433] Cook et al.[434] believed the diagnosis of PFPS was a diagnosis of exclusion, meaning that other conditions (e.g., plica syndrome, tibiofemoral arthritis) had to be ruled out before a diagnosis of PFPS could be considered.

Risk Factors That May Contribute to Patellofemoral Pain Syndrome[a]

- Patellar dysplasia (e.g., patella alta or baja)
- Tight patellar retinaculum (especially lateral)
- Abnormal patellar tracking
- Abnormal patellar tilt or rotation
- Abnormal patellar alignment relative to the femur (e.g., Q-angle outside the normal 13°–18°)
- Crossover gait
- Excessive genu valgum/varum
- Muscle weakness (e.g., vastus medialis obliquus, hip abductor and lateral rotators, ankle dorsiflexors)
- Muscle imbalance (e.g., quadriceps/hamstrings ratio)
- Excessive tibial torsion (especially medial)
- Foot malalignment (e.g., rearfoot varus or valgus, excessive pronation/supination of the foot)
- Muscle hypomobility (e.g., quadriceps, hamstrings, gastrocnemius, iliotibial band, hip adductors)
- Trauma to patella (e.g., dislocation, direct blow)
- Abnormal repetitive stress to patella (e.g., running on the same side of road or sidewalk continually [camber of road or sidewalk affects foot-knee mechanics])
- Training shoes worn (e.g., control shoe versus cushioning shoe, shoes "broken down")
- Excessive pelvic tilt (anterior/posterior, medial/lateral)

[a]Patellofemoral pain syndrome may be the result of any or all of the above. In reality, the definitive cause of patellofemoral pain syndrome is unknown.

Nijs et al.[435] reported that the vastus medialis coordination test, the patellar apprehension test, and the eccentric step test had the most positive likelihood ratio in patients with PFPS.

Active Patellar Grind Test.[71] The patient sits on the examining table with the knee flexed 90° over the edge

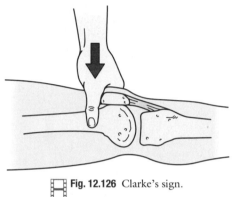

Fig. 12.126 Clarke's sign.

of the table. While the patient slowly straightens the knee, the examiner places a hand over the patella to feel for crepitus. Where in the ROM that pain occurs gives an indication of what part of the patella is demonstrating pathology (see Fig. 12.2). Greater force can be applied through the patella by asking the patient to step up and step down on a small stool while the examiner gently palpates the patella for crepitus and pain (**step up–step down test**).[71]

Clarke's Sign (Patellar Grind Test). This test assesses the presence of a problem with the articulation between the articular surface of the patella and the articular surfaces of the femoral condyles, but it is not specific to one pathology, and the validity of the test has been questioned.[436] The examiner presses down slightly proximal to the upper pole or base of the patella with the web of the hand as the patient lies relaxed with the knee extended (Fig. 12.126). Reider[71] recommends pushing down on the patella directly. The patient is then asked to contract the quadriceps muscles while the examiner pushes down. If the patient can complete and maintain the contraction without pain, the test is considered negative. If the test causes retropatellar pain and the patient cannot hold a contraction, the test is considered positive. Because the examiner can achieve a positive test on anyone if sufficient pressure is applied to the patella, the amount of pressure that is applied must be carefully controlled. The best way to do this is to repeat the procedure several times, increasing the pressure each time and comparing the results with those of the unaffected side. To test different parts of the

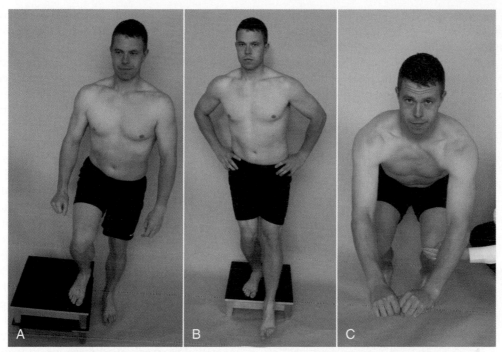

Fig. 12.127 Step tests. (A) Step up test. (B) Eccentric step down test. (C) Waldron test.

patella, the knee should be tested in 30°, 60°, and 90° of flexion and in full extension.

⚠ *Eccentric Step (Lateral Step Down) Test.*[246,247,424,435] The patient stands on a 15-cm (6-inch)-high step or stool while keeping the hands on the hips. The patient steps down, first leading with the injured leg (this tests the good leg first) as slowly and smoothly as he or she can while the examiner watches the quality of movement (Fig. 12.127B).[424] The test is considered positive if pain is felt by the patient during the test. Table 12.12 outlines the scoring criteria for the test.[424]

❓ *Frund's Sign.* The patient is in the sitting position. The examiner percusses the patella in various positions of knee flexion. Pain indicates a positive test and may signify chondromalacia patellae.

❓ *Lateral Pull Test.* The patient lies supine with the leg extended. The patient contracts the quadriceps while the examiner watches the movement of the patella.[96] Normally, the patella moves superiorly, or superiorly and laterally in equal proportions (Fig. 12.128). If lateral movement is excessive, the test is positive for lateral overpull of the quadriceps, resulting in a patellofemoral arthralgia. Watson et al.[437] have questioned the reliability of this test, especially when performed by inexperienced examiners.

⚠ *McConnell Test for Chondromalacia Patellae.* The patient is sitting with the femur laterally rotated. The patient performs isometric quadriceps contractions at 120°, 90°, 60°, 30°, and 0°, with each contraction held for 10 seconds (Fig. 12.129). If pain is produced during any of the contractions, the patient's leg is passively returned to full extension by the examiner. The patient's

TABLE 12.12

Scoring the Eccentric Step (Lateral Step Down) Test

Criteria	Points
Use of arms to maintain balance	1
Trunk lean (medial or lateral)	1
Pelvis rotation and/or elevation	1
Genu Valgum	
Tibial tubercle medial to second toe	1
Tibial tubercle medial to foot	2
Unsteady unilateral stance	1

Score: 0–1 good quality of movement; 2–3 medium quality of movement; 4+ poor movement.
Adapted from Piva SR, Fitzgerald K, Irrgang JJ, et al: Reliability of measures of impairments associated with patellofemoral pain syndrome, *BMC Muscloskelet Disord* 7:33, 2006.

leg is then fully supported on the examiner's knee, and the examiner pushes the patella medially. The medial glide is maintained while the knee is returned to the painful angle, and the patient performs an isometric contraction, again with the patella held medially. If the pain is decreased, the pain is patellofemoral in origin. Each angle is tested in a similar fashion.[438]

⚠ *Motion Palpation Test.*[94] The patient is seated with the knees flexed to approximately 90° over the end of the examining table so the feet do not touch the floor. The examiner sits beside the knee to be examined with one hand resting over the patella and one hand holding the ankle (Fig. 12.130). Using the hand at the ankle, the examiner passively moves the patient's knee between full extension (0°) and 100° flexion while applying approximately 2.3 kg (5 lb) of compression over the patellofemoral joint, with the index finger positioned immediately distal to the inferior patellar pole. During the passive motion, the examiner is palpating for crepitus and discomfort severity and location. The passive motion is repeated three or four times. The crepitus grade is determined using the criteria in Table 12.13.

❓ *Passive Patellar Tilt Test.*[424] The patient lies supine with the knee extended and the quadriceps relaxed. The examiner stands at the end of the examining table and lifts the lateral edge of the patella away from the lateral femoral condyle. The patella should not be pushed medially or laterally but rather should remain in the femoral trochlea.[96] The normal angle is 15°, although males may have an angle 5° less than that of females (Fig. 12.131). Patients with angles less than this are prone to patellofemoral syndrome, specifically excessive lateral pressure syndrome. Watson et al.[437] have questioned the reliability of this test, especially when performed by inexperienced examiners.

⚠ *Step Up Test.*[433] The patient stands beside a stool that is 25 cm (10 inches) high. The examiner asks the patient to step up sideways onto the stool using the good leg. The test is repeated with the other leg. Normally, the patient should have no difficulty doing the test and have no pain. Inability to do the test may indicate patellofemoral arthralgia, weak quadriceps, or an inability to stabilize the pelvis (Fig. 12.127A).

❓ *Vastus Medialis Coordination Test.*[435,439] The patient lies supine while the examiner places a fist under the patient's knee (Fig. 12.132). The patient is asked to slowly extend the knee without pressing into the examiner's fist or lifting the leg away from the fist while trying to achieve full extension. The test is considered positive if the patient cannot fully extend the knee or has difficulty achieving full extension smoothly or tries to use the hip flexors or extensors to accomplish the task.

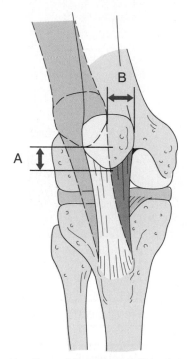

Fig. 12.128 Lateral pull test. Normally, A > B or A = B; with lateral overpull of the quadriceps, B > A. (From Kolowich PA, Paulos LE, Rosenberg TD, et al: Lateral release of the patella: indications and contraindications, *Am J Sports Med* 18:361, 1990.)

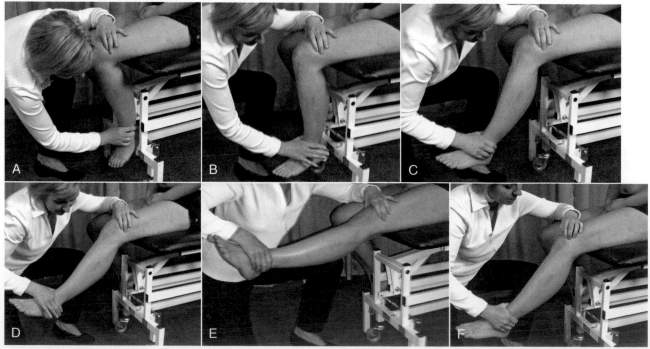

Fig. 12.129 McConnell test for chondromalacia patellae. (A) 120°. (B) 90°. (C) 60°. (D) 30°. (E) 0°. (F) Testing at 60°, holding patella medially.

? *Waldron Test.* This test also assesses the presence of patellofemoral syndrome and functions in a similar fashion to the step up test and the eccentric step test.[72] The examiner palpates the patella while the patient performs several slow deep knee bends (these may be unilateral squats or bilateral for easier comparison) (Fig. 12.127C). As the patient goes through the ROM, the examiner should note the amount of crepitus (significant only if accompanied by pain), where it occurs in the ROM, the amount of pain, and whether there is "catching" or poor tracking of the patella (see Fig. 12.31) throughout the movement. If pain and crepitus occur together during the movement, it is considered a positive sign.[72]

? *Zohler's Sign.*[128] The patient lies supine with the knees extended. The examiner pulls the patella distally and holds it in this position. The patient is asked to contract the quadriceps (Fig. 12.133). Pain indicates a positive test for chondromalacia patellae. However, the test may be positive (false-positive) in a large proportion of the normal population.

Other Tests

⚠ *Coactivation Tests for Quadriceps and Hamstrings.*[143]

1. **Single-Limb Dead-Lift**: The patient balances on one leg (the uninjured one to begin) with the knees and hips flexed approximately 30°. The patient slowly flexes the hip and trunk so as to touch the contralateral finger to the foot or ground beside the support foot and returns to starting position (Fig. 12.134 A and B). Ideally, the knee is kept at

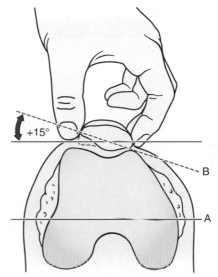

Fig. 12.131 Passive patellar tilt test. (Redrawn from Kolowich PA, Paulos LE, Rosenberg TD, et al: Lateral release of the patella: indications and contraindications, *Am J Sports Med* 18:361, 1990.)

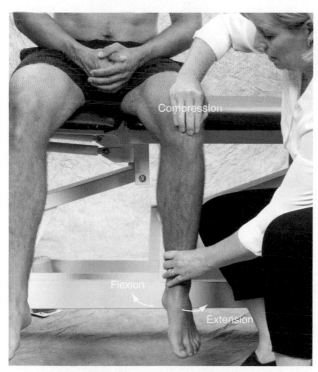

Fig. 12.130 Motion palpation test.

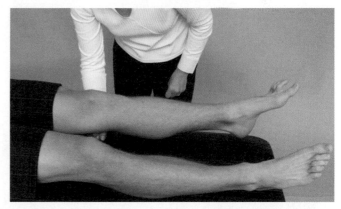

Fig. 12.132 Vastus medialis coordination test.

TABLE **12.13**

Crepitation Grading Scale for Patella with Cartilage Damage

	None	Mild	Moderate	Severe
Tactile Friction	Smooth motion	Fine-grade sandpaper	Medium-grade sandpaper	Bone-on-bone grinding
Sound	No sound	No sound	Squeaky floorboard	Popping-cracking-crunching

Modified from Lancaster AR, Nyland J, Roberts CS: The validity of the motion palpation test for determining patellofemoral joint articular cartilage damage, *Phys Ther Sport* 8(2):59–65, 2007.

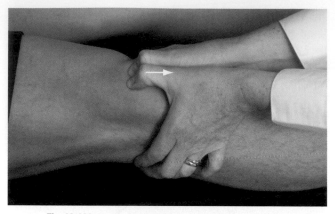

Fig. 12.133 Zohler's sign for chondromalacia patellae.

30° throughout the movement so the knee is over the toes of the same foot. Both legs are compared for form and timing.

2. **Lateral Hop**: The patient stands with the feet close together. The patient (starting with the uninjured leg) hops laterally one-half of his or her body height, being instructed to "land as softly as possible" with the knee flexed and over the toes (Fig. 12.134C and D). The patient is instructed to balance on the "hopped" leg for 3 seconds. Both legs are compared for form and timing.

3. **Transverse/Diagonal Hop**: The patient stands with the feet close together. The patient (starting with the uninjured leg) hops in a transverse plane one-half of

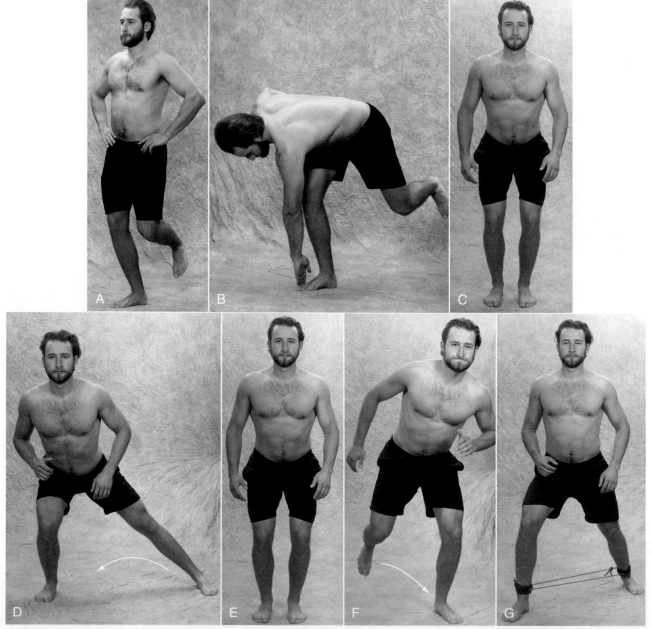

Fig. 12.134 Coactivation tests for quadriceps and hamstrings. (A) Single-limb dead-lift—start position. (B) Single-limb dead-lift—end position. (C) Lateral hop—start position. (D) Lateral hop—end position. (E) Transverse/diagonal hop—start position. (F) Transverse/diagonal hop—end position. (G) Rubber bands ("ankle tubes") may be used to offer resistance in different directions and during walking.

his or her body height, being instructed to "land as softly as possible" with the knee flexed and over the toes (Fig. 12.134, E and F). The patient is instructed to balance on the "hopped" leg for 3 seconds. Both legs are compared for form and timing.

4. **Lateral Band Walks:** The patient stands with an elastic band tied around the ankles while standing upright and feet together (approximately 30 cm [11.8 inches] expansion should be allowed in the band). While keeping the hips and knees flexed to 30°, the patient (starting with the uninjured leg) side steps a distance of 130% of his or her shoulder width (marked on the floor) to assume a single limb stance on the side-stepped foot while keeping the toes pointing straight ahead and the knee over the toes (Fig. 12.134G). The patient may also move in an oblique direction. Both legs are compared for form and timing.

❓ *Daniel's Quadriceps Neutral Angle Test.*[440] The patient lies supine, and the unaffected leg is tested first. The patient's hip is flexed to 45°, and the knee is flexed to 90° with the foot flat on the examining table. The patient is asked to extend the knee isometrically while the examiner holds down the foot. If tibial displacement is noted, knee flexion is decreased (posterior tibial displacement) or increased (anterior tibial displacement). The process is repeated until the angle at which there is no tibial displacement is reached (Fig. 12.135). This angle, the quadriceps neutral angle, averages 70° (range, 60° to 90°). The injured knee is placed in the same neutral angle position, and the patient is asked to contract the quadriceps. Any anterior displacement indicates posterior cruciate ligament insufficiency. The quadriceps neutral angle is primarily used for machine testing of laxity (e.g., KT-1000 arthrometer, Stryker knee laxity test apparatus).

✓ *Fairbank's Apprehension Test.* This is a test for **dislocation of the patella.**[320,441] The patient lies in the supine position with the quadriceps muscles relaxed and the knee flexed to 30° while the examiner carefully and slowly pushes the patella laterally (Fig. 12.136). Tanner et al.[442] believed the patella should be pushed laterally and distally to make the test more sensitive. If the patient feels the patella is going to dislocate, the patient contracts the quadriceps muscles to bring the patella back "into line." This action indicates a positive test. The patient will also have an apprehensive look.

Functional Leg Length. The patient stands in the normal relaxed stance. The examiner palpates the anterior superior iliac spines (ASISs) and then the posterior superior iliac spines (PSISs) and notes any differences. The examiner then positions the patient so that the patient's subtalar joints are in neutral while bearing weight (see Chapter 13). While the patient holds this position with the toes straight ahead and the knee straight, the examiner repalpates the ASISs and the PSISs. If the previously noted differences remain, the pelvis and sacroiliac joints should be evaluated further. If the previously noted differences

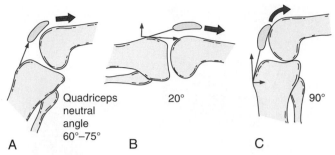

Fig. 12.135 During open chain knee extension, tibial translation is a function of the shear force produced by the patellar tendon. (A) Quadriceps neutral position. The patellar tendon force is perpendicular to the tibial plateaus and results in compression of the joint surfaces without shear force. (B) At flexion angles less than the angle of the quadriceps neutral position, orientation of the patellar tendon produces anterior shear of the tibia. (C) At angles greater than the angle of the quadriceps neutral position, patellar tendon force causes a posterior shear of the tibia. (From Daniel DM, Stone ML, Barnett P, et al: Use of the quadriceps active test to diagnose posterior cruciate ligament disruption and measure posterior laxity of the knee, *J Bone Joint Surg Am* 70:386–391, 1988.)

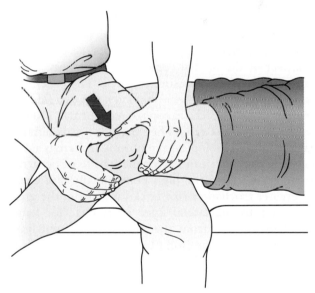

Fig. 12.136 Apprehension test. (Redrawn from Hughston JC, Walsh WM, Puddu G: *Patellar subluxation and dislocation,* Philadelphia, 1984, WB Saunders, p 29.)

disappear, the examiner should suspect a functional leg length difference caused by hip, knee, ankle, or foot problems—primarily ankle or foot problems.

❓ *Functional Test for Quadriceps Contusion.* The patient lies in the prone position while the examiner passively flexes the knee as much as possible. If passive knee flexion is 90° or more, it is only a mild contusion. If passive knee flexion is less than 90°, the contusion is moderate to severe, and the patient should not be allowed to bear weight. Normally, the heel-to-buttock distance should not exceed 10 cm (4 inches) in men and 5 cm (2 inches) in women. This test may also be used to test tightness of the quadriceps (vasti) muscles. If the range is limited and the end feel is muscle stretch, the vastus medialis,

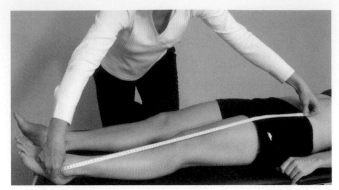

Fig. 12.137 Measuring leg length (to the lateral malleolus).

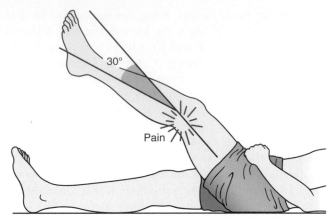

Fig. 12.138 Noble compression test for iliotibial band friction syndrome.

lateralis, and/or intermedius is tight. Testing for a tight rectus femoris is described in Chapter 11.

☑ *Measurement of Leg Length.* The patient lies in the supine position with the legs at a right angle to a line joining the two ASISs. With a tape measure, the examiner obtains the distance from one ASIS to the lateral or medial malleolus on that side, placing the metal end of the tape measure immediately distal to and up against the ASIS (Fig. 12.137). The tape is stretched so that the other hand pushes the tape against the distal aspect of the medial (or lateral) malleolus, and the reading on the tape measure is noted. The other side is tested similarly. A difference between the two sides of as much as 1.0 to 1.5 cm is considered normal. However, the examiner must remember that even this difference may result in pathological symptoms. If there is a difference, the examiner can determine its site of occurrence by measuring from the high point on the iliac crest to the greater trochanter (for coxa vara), from the greater trochanter to the lateral knee joint line (for femoral shaft length), and from the medial knee joint line to the medial malleolus (for tibial length). The two legs are then compared. The examiner must also remember that torsion deformities to the femur or tibia can alter leg length.

❓ *Measurement of Muscle Bulk (Anthropometric Measurements for Effusion and Atrophy).* The examiner selects areas where muscle bulk or swelling is greatest and measures the circumference of the leg. It is important to note on the patient's chart how far above or below the apex or base of the patella one is measuring and whether the tape measure is placed above or below that mark. The following are common measurement points:
1. 15 cm (6 inches) below the apex of the patella
2. Apex of the patella or joint line
3. 5 cm (2 inches) above the base of the patella
4. 10 cm (4 inches) above the base of the patella
5. 15 cm (6 inches) above the base of the patella
6. 23 cm (9 inches) above the base of the patella

Hughston[78] advocated using the lateral joint line rather than the patella for the beginning point of measurement; he believed that the joint line was more constant. The examiner must also note, if possible, whether swelling or muscle bulk is being measured and remember that there is no correlation between muscle bulk and strength.

It is important to understand that circumferential measurements are useful for swelling and noting atrophy; however, the values do not give a good indication of muscle strength, power, or function. The values can show change but are not correlated with torque output.[443]

▲ *Moving Patellar Apprehension Test (MPAT) for Lateral Patellar Instability.*[444] For the moving patellar apprehension test, the patient lies supine with the thigh on the examining table and the examiner holding the leg in full extension off the table. The examiner then translates the patella laterally using the examiner's thumb, and the patella is held laterally while the examiner passively flexes the knee to 90° and then returns the leg to full extension (step 1). If there is patient apprehension or contraction of the quadriceps, the test is considered positive. If the patella is then translated medially and the knee flexed, there will be no apprehension or protective quadriceps contraction (step 2) because the patella most commonly subluxes or dislocates laterally. For the test to be positive, both step 1 (apprehension) and step 2 (no apprehension) must occur.

▲ *Noble Compression Test.* This is a test for **iliotibial band friction syndrome.**[445] The patient lies in the supine position, and the examiner flexes the patient's knee to 90°, accompanied by hip flexion (Fig. 12.138). Pressure is then applied to the lateral femoral epicondyle, or 1 to 2 cm (0.4 to 0.8 inch) proximal to it, with the thumb. While the pressure is maintained, the patient's knee is passively extended. At approximately 30° of flexion (0° being straight leg), the patient experiences severe pain over the lateral femoral condyle. Pain indicates a positive test. The patient states that it is the same pain that occurs with activity.

▲ *Quadriceps Angle (Q-Angle) or Patellofemoral Angle.* The Q-angle is defined as the angle between the quadriceps muscles (primarily the rectus femoris) and the patellar tendon and represents the angle of quadriceps muscle force (Fig. 12.139).[446–449] The angle is obtained by first ensuring that the lower limbs are at a right angle to the line joining the two ASISs with the patient usually in supine

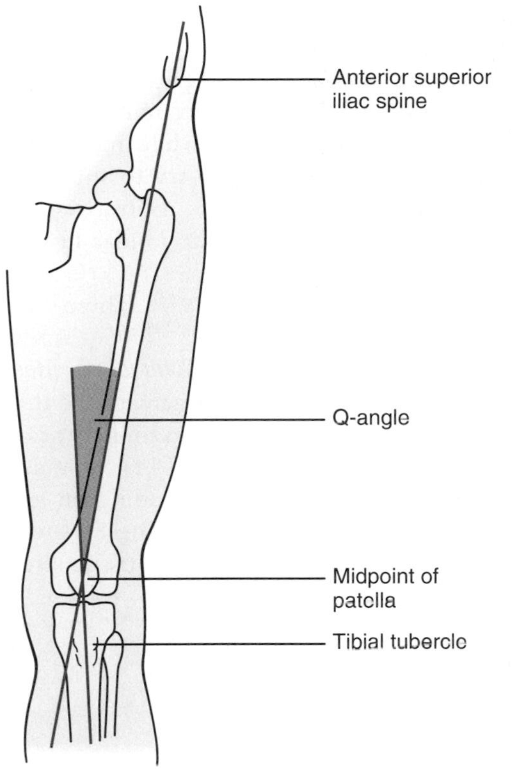

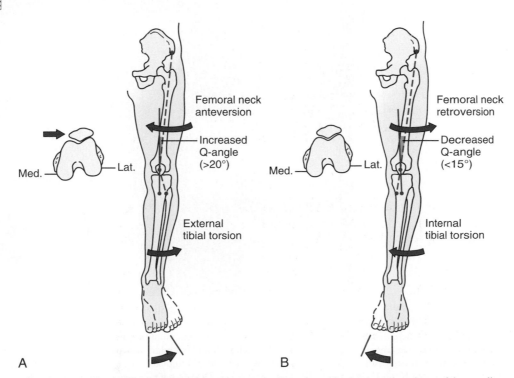

Fig. 12.139 Quadriceps angle (Q-angle).

- Anterior superior iliac spine
- Q-angle
- Midpoint of patella
- Tibial tubercle

(standing may also be used), legs straight, and quadriceps relaxed.[450] Some feel the knee should be in 20° to 30° flexion because the patella is more centralized in this position and may represent the gait stance phase better.[447,450] A line is then drawn from the ASIS to the midpoint of the patella on the same side and from the tibial tubercle to the midpoint of the patella. The angle formed by the crossing of these two lines is called the *Q-angle*. The foot should be placed in a neutral position in regard to supination and pronation and the hip in a neutral position in regard to medial and lateral rotation, because it has been found that different foot and hip positions alter the Q-angle.[451]

Normally, the Q-angle is 13° for males and 18° for females when the knee is straight (Fig. 12.140), although Grelsamer et al.[452] reported male and female values are similar when patient height is considered. Any angle less than 13° may be associated with chondromalacia patellae, patella alta, or patellar instability.[450] An angle greater than 18° is often associated with PFPS, chondromalacia patellae, subluxing patella, increased femoral anteversion, genu valgum, lateral displacement of tibial tubercle, or increased lateral tibial torsion. During the test, which may be done either with radiographs or physically on the patient, the quadriceps should be relaxed. If measured with the patient in the sitting position, the Q-angle should be 0° (Fig. 12.141). While the patient is in a sitting position, the presence of the "**bayonet sign,**" which indicates an abnormal alignment of the quadriceps musculature, patellar tendon, or tibial shaft, should be noted (Fig. 12.142).

Fig. 12.140 (A) Femoral neck anteversion and lateral tibial torsion increase the Q-angle and lead to lateral tracking of the patella on the femoral sulcus. (B) Femoral neck retroversion and medial tibial torsion decrease the Q-angle and tend to centralize the tracking of the patella. (Redrawn from Tria AJ, Palumbo RC: Conservative treatment of patellofemoral pain, *Semin Orthop* 5:116–117, 1990.)

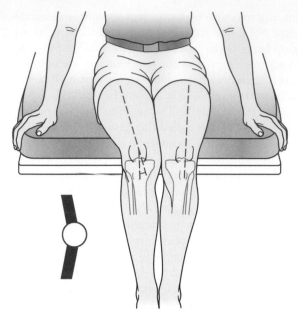

Fig. 12.141 Q-angle in flexed position. Exaggerated Q-angle in the patient's right knee is seen as residual positive Q-angle with the knee flexed. Normally, the Q-angle in flexion should be 0°. (Redrawn from Hughston JC, Walsh WM, Puddu G: *Patellar subluxation and dislocation*, Philadelphia, 1984, WB Saunders, p 24.)

Hughston et al.[320] advocate doing the test with the quadriceps contracted. If measured with the quadriceps contracted and the knee fully extended, the Q-angle should be 8° to 10°. Any angle greater than 10° is considered abnormal. The examiner must ensure that a standardized measurement procedure is used to ensure consistent values.[453]

❓ *Radulescu Sign.*[454,455] The patient lies prone with the knee flexed to 90°. The examiner stabilizes the patient's thigh with one hand while medially rotating the tibia with the other hand to try to sublux the fibular head anteriorly (Fig. 12.143). A positive test is indicated by pain, subluxation of the fibular head, and/or apprehension.

***Tests for Hamstring Tightness.*[456]** These tests are described in Chapter 11.

⚠ *Test for Knee Extension Contracture (Heel Height Difference).*[457] The patient lies prone with the thighs supported and the legs relaxed. The examiner measures the difference in heel height (Fig. 12.144). One centimeter of difference approximates 1°, depending on leg length. The test, along with the accompanying end feel, would be used to test for joint contracture (tissue stretch) and

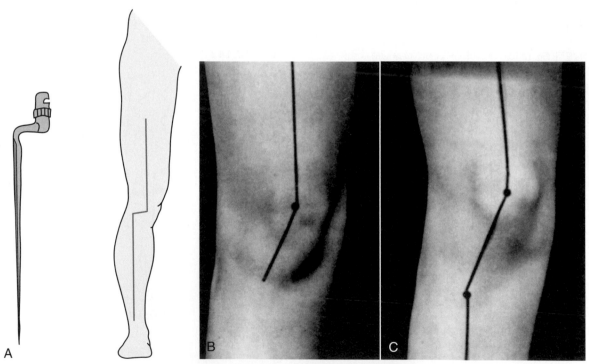

Fig. 12.142 Increased Q-angle. (A) Bayonet sign. Tibia vara of proximal third causes a markedly increased Q-angle. Alignment of the quadriceps, patellar tendon, and tibial shaft resembles a French bayonet. (B) Q-angle with the knee in full extension is only slightly increased over normal. (C) However, with the knee flexed at 30°, there is failure of the tibia to derotate normally and failure of the patellar tendon to line up with the anterior crest of the tibia. This is not an infrequent finding in patients with patellofemoral arthralgia. Increased medial femoral torsion (anteversion) combined with increased lateral tibial torsion causes the same bayonet sign. (A, From Hughston JC, et al: *Patellar subluxation and dislocation*, Philadelphia, 1984, WB Saunders, p 26; B and C, From Ficat RP, Hungerford DS: *Disorders of the patello-femoral joint*, Baltimore, 1977, Williams & Wilkins, p 117.)

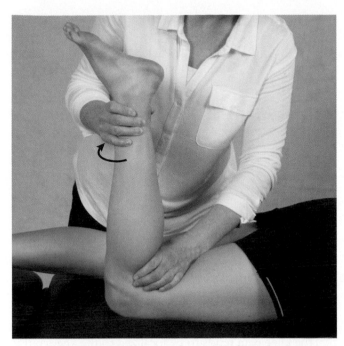

Fig. 12.143 Radulescu test for unstable fibular head.

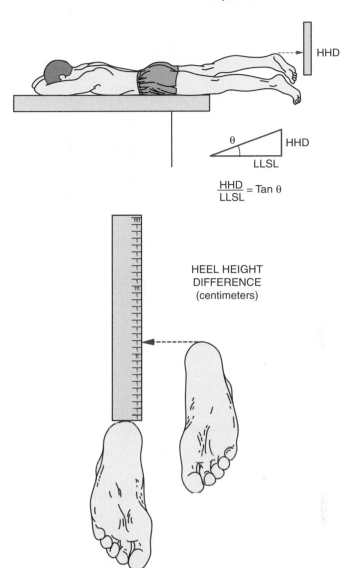

possibly tight hamstrings (muscle stretch). Swelling may also cause a positive test.

⚠ *Tubercle Sulcus Angle (Q-Angle at 90°).*[52,438] This measurement is also used to measure the angle of quadriceps pull. A vertical line is drawn from the center of the patella to the center of the tibial tubercle. A second horizontal line is drawn through the femoral epicondyle (Fig. 12.145). Normally the lines are perpendicular. Angles greater than 10° from the perpendicular are considered abnormal. Lateral patellar subluxation may affect the results.

Another measurement, which is similar to the Q-angle, is the **A-angle,** which measures the relation of the patella to the tibial tubercle. This measurement, which is not as commonly used as the Q-angle, consists of a vertical line that divides the patella into two halves and a line drawn from the tibial tubercle to the apex of the inferior pole of the patella. The resulting angle is called the *A-angle* (Fig. 12.146).[458,459] Some have questioned the reliability of this measurement because of the difficulty in consistently finding appropriate landmarks.[460]

❓ *Wilson Test.* This is a test for **OCD**.[461] The patient sits with the knee flexed over the examining table. The knee is then actively extended with the tibia medially rotated. At approximately 30° of flexion (0° being straight leg), the pain in the knee increases, and the patient is asked to stop the flexion movement. The patient is then asked to rotate the tibia laterally, and the pain disappears. This finding means a positive test, which is indicative of OCD of the femoral condyle. The

Fig. 12.144 Heel height difference *(HHD)*. The patient lies prone on the examining table with the lower limbs supported by the thighs. The difference in heel height is measured. The conversion of HHD to degrees of extension lost depends on the leg length. The tangent of angle q is the HHD divided by the lower-leg segment length *(LLSL)*. The LLSL is proportional to patient height. (From Daniel D, Akeson W, O'Conner J, editors: *Knee ligaments: structure, injury and repair,* New York, 1990, Raven Press, p 32.)

test is positive only if the lesion is at the classic site for OCD of the knee, namely, the lateral side of the medial femoral condyle near the intercondylar notch (Fig. 12.147).

Reflexes and Cutaneous Distribution

Having completed the ligamentous and other tests of the knee, if a scanning examination has not been carried out, the examiner next determines whether the reflexes around the knee joint are normal, especially if

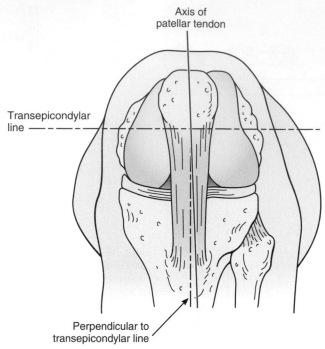

Fig. 12.145 Tubercle sulcus angle of 90°. With the knee flexed to 90°, the transepicondylar line is assessed. The axis of the patellar tendon is compared with a perpendicular to the transepicondylar line. (Modified from Kolowich PA, Paulos LE, Rosenberg TD, et al: Lateral release of the patella: indications and contraindications, *Am J Sports Med* 18:361, 1990.)

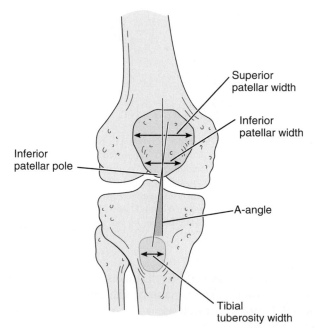

Fig. 12.146 Location of landmarks of the A-angle. (Redrawn from Ehrat M, Edwards J, Hastings D, et al: Reliability of assessing patellar alignment: the A-angle, *J Orthop Sports Phys Ther* 19:23, 1994.)

neurological involvement is suspected (Fig. 12.148). The patellar (L3–L4) and medial hamstring (L5–S1) reflexes should be checked for differences between the two sides.

The examiner must keep in mind the dermatome patterns of the various nerve roots (Fig. 12.149) as well as the cutaneous distribution of the peripheral nerves (Fig. 12.150). To test for altered sensation, a sensation

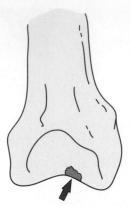

Fig. 12.147 Classic site of osteochondritis dissecans.

scanning examination should be performed using relaxed hands and fingers to cover all aspects of the thigh, knee, and leg. Any differences in sensation should be noted and can be mapped out further with the use of a pinwheel, pin, cotton batting, or soft brush.

True knee pain tends to be localized to the knee, but it may also be referred to the hip or ankle (Fig. 12.151). In a similar fashion, pain may be referred to the knee from the lumbar spine, hip (e.g., slipped capital femoral epiphysis in children), and ankle. Sometimes a lesion of the medial meniscus leads to irritation of the infrapatellar branch of the saphenous nerve. The result is a hyperaesthetic area the size of a quarter on the medial side of the knee. This finding is called **Turner's sign.**[128] Muscles about the knee and their pain referral pattern are shown in Table 12.14.

Peripheral Nerve Injuries About the Knee

Peripheral nerve injuries about the knee occur primarily from trauma (e.g., fracture, dislocation, direct blow, compression).[23,462]

Common Peroneal Nerve (L4–S2). This nerve is vulnerable to injury in the posterolateral knee and as it winds around the head of the fibula. It has also been reported that the nerve may be stretched as a result of pulling on the peroneus longus muscle in a lateral ankle sprain,[457,463,464] direct trauma, injury to the posterolateral corner, or a varus stress to the knee.[52,342] The result is weakness or paralysis of muscles supplied by the deep and superficial peroneal nerves, the two branches of the common peroneal nerve (Table 12.15). This causes an inability to dorsiflex the foot (drop foot), resulting in a steppage gait and an inability to evert the foot. Sensory loss is as shown in Fig. 12.152.

Saphenous Nerve (L2–L4). The saphenous nerve is a sensory branch of the femoral nerve that arises near the inguinal ligament and passes down the leg to supply the skin on the medial side of the knee and calf. The nerve is sometimes injured during surgery or trauma, or it may be entrapped as it passes between the vastus medialis and adductor magnus muscles. Entrapment may lead to medial knee pain (burning) that is aggravated by walking, standing, and quadriceps exercises.[465–467] Depending on the peripheral nerve that is injured, sensory loss after surgery or trauma is shown in Fig. 12.150.

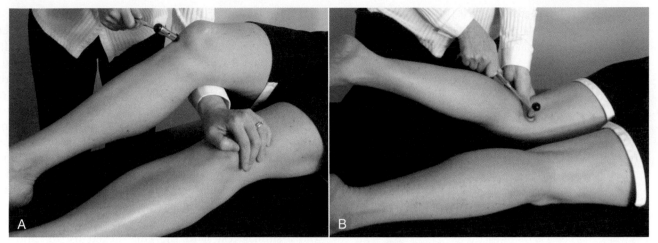

Fig. 12.148 Reflexes of the knee. (A) Patellar (L3). (B) Medial hamstrings (L5).

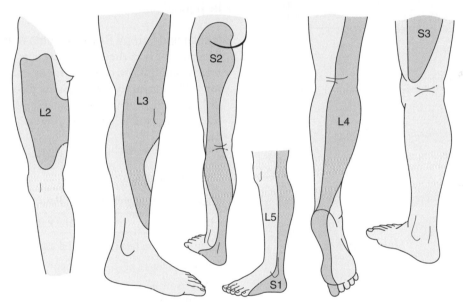

Fig. 12.149 Dermatomes about the knee.

Joint Play Movements

For joint play movements on the knee, the patient is placed in the supine position (Fig. 12.153). The movement on the affected side is compared with that on the normal side.

Joint Play Movements of the Knee Complex

- Backward glide of tibia on femur
- Forward glide of tibia on femur
- Medial translation of tibia on femur
- Lateral translation of tibia on femur
- Medial displacement of patella
- Lateral displacement of patella
- Distal movement of patella
- Proximal movement of patella
- Anteroposterior movement of the head of the fibula on the tibia

Backward and Forward Movements of Tibia on Femur

The patient is asked to lie in the supine position with the test knee flexed to 25° to 30° (loose packed position) and the hip flexed to 45°. The examiner then places the heel of the hand over the tibial tuberosity while stabilizing the patient's limb with the other hand and pushing backward with the heel of the hand. The end feel of the movement is normally tissue stretch. To perform the forward movement, the examiner places both hands around the posterior aspect of the tibia. Before performing the joint play movement, the examiner must ensure that the hamstrings and gastrocnemius muscles are relaxed. The tibia is then drawn forward on the femur. The examiner feels the quality of the movement, which normally is tissue stretch. These joint play movements are similar to those used in the anterior and posterior drawer tests for ligamentous stability.

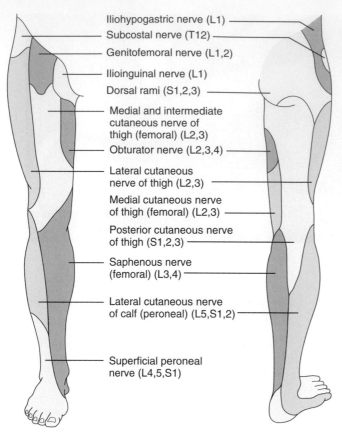

Iliohypogastric nerve (L1)

Subcostal nerve (T12)

Genitofemoral nerve (L1,2)

Ilioinguinal nerve (L1)

Dorsal rami (S1,2,3)

Medial and intermediate
cutaneous nerve of
thigh (femoral) (L2,3)

Obturator nerve (L2,3,4)

Lateral cutaneous
nerve of thigh (L2,3)

Medial cutaneous nerve
of thigh (femoral) (L2,3)

Posterior cutaneous nerve
of thigh (S1,2,3)

Saphenous nerve
(femoral) (L3,4)

Lateral cutaneous nerve
of calf (peroneal) (L5,S1,2)

Superficial peroneal
nerve (L4,5,S1)

Fig. 12.150 Peripheral nerve sensory distribution about the knee.

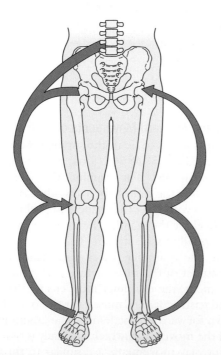

Fig. 12.151 Patterns of referred pain to and from the knee.

Medial and Lateral Translation of Tibia on Femur

The patient lies supine, and the patient's leg is held between the examiner's trunk and arm. To test medial translation, the examiner puts one hand on the lateral side of the tibia and one hand on the medial side of the femur. The tibia is then pushed or translated medially on the femur. Excessive movement may indicate a torn anterior cruciate ligament (Fig. 12.154). To test lateral translation, the examiner puts one hand on the medial side of the tibia and one hand on the lateral side of the femur. The tibia is then pushed or translated laterally on the femur. Excessive movement may indicate a torn posterior cruciate ligament. The normal end feel of each movement is tissue stretch.[128] Liorzou[49] reports that Galway did a similar test with the knee flexed to 90° and the foot on the examining table. If the tibial plateau bulges laterally, Wrisberg ligament or the lateral meniscus may be injured.

Medial and Lateral Displacements of Patella

The patient is in the supine position with the knee slightly flexed on a pillow or over the examiner's knee (30° flexion). The examiner's thumbs are placed against the medial or lateral edge of the patella, and a force is applied to the side of the patella with the fingers used for stabilization.

TABLE **12.14**

Knee Muscles and Referral of Pain

Muscle	Referral Pattern
Tensor fasciae latae	Lateral aspect of thigh
Sartorius	Over course of muscle (anterior thigh)
Quadriceps	Anterior thigh, patella, lateral thigh, and knee (vastus lateralis)
Adductor longus and brevis	Superior anteromedial thigh, anterior thigh, proximal to patella and sometimes down anteromedial leg
Adductor magnus	Medial thigh from groin to adductor tubercle
Gracilis	Medial thigh (primarily the midportion)
Semimembranosus and semitendinosus	Ischial tuberosity, posterior thigh, and posteromedial calf
Biceps femoris	Posterior knee up posterior thigh
Popliteus	Posterior knee
Gastrocnemius	Posterior knee, posterolateral calf, and posteromedial calf to foot instep
Plantaris	Posterior knee and calf

TABLE **12.15**

Peripheral Nerve Injuries (Neuropathy) About the Knee

Nerve	Muscle Weakness	Sensory Alteration	Reflexes Affected
Common peroneal nerve	Tibialis anterior (DP) Extensor digitorum brevis (DP) Extensor digitorum longus (DP) Extensor hallucis longus (DP) Peroneus tertius (DP) Peroneus longus (SP) Peroneus brevis (SP)	Area around head of fibula Web space between first and second toes (DP) Lateral aspect of leg and dorsum of foot (SP)	None
Saphenous nerve	None	Medial side of knee, may extend down medial side of leg to medial malleolus	None

DP, Deep peroneal branch; *SP,* superficial peroneal branch.

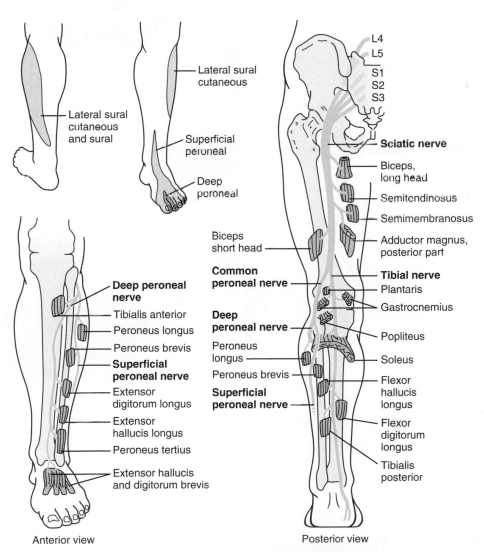

Fig. 12.152 Common peroneal nerve.

The process is then repeated with pressure applied to the other side of the patella. The other knee is tested as a comparison.

This joint play is similar to the passive movements of the patella; as in the passive test, the patella can be displaced by approximately half of its width medially and laterally with the knee in extension. The examiner must do the movements slowly and carefully to ensure that the patella is not prone to dislocation, especially laterally.

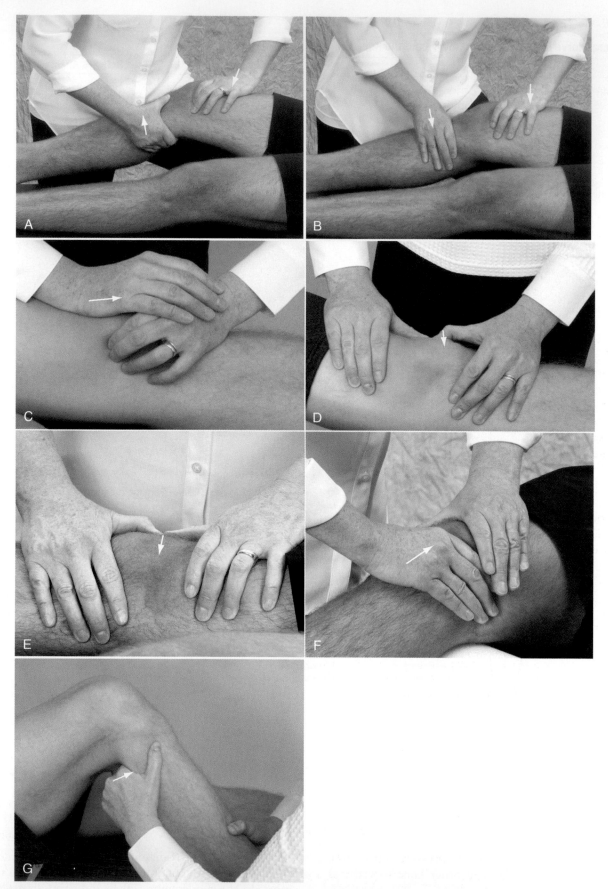

Fig. 12.153 Joint play movements of the knee. (A) Anterior movement of the tibia on the femur (similar to the Lachman test). (B) Posterior movement of the tibia on the femur (similar to the posterior drawer test). (C) Patellar movement, distally. (D) Patellar movement, medially. (E) Patellar movement laterally. (F) Patellar movement proximally (*C to F*, similar to passive movements of the patella). (G) Anterior movement of the superior tibiofibular joint.

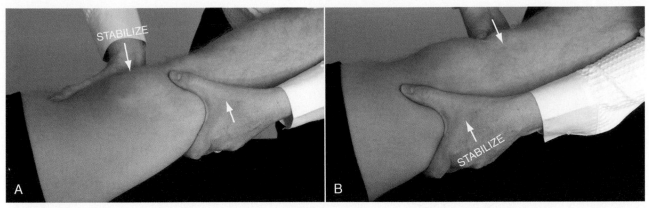

Fig. 12.154 Medial and lateral shift of tibia on femur. (A) Medial translation for anterior cruciate pathology. (B) Lateral translation for posterior cruciate pathology.

Depression (Distal Movement) of Patella

The patient is in a supine position with the knee slightly flexed. The examiner then places one hand over the patient's patella so that the pisiform bone rests over the base of the patella. The other hand is placed so that the finger and thumb can grasp the medial and lateral edges of the patella to direct its movement. The examiner then rests the first hand over the second hand and applies a caudal force to the base of the patella, directing the caudal movement with the second hand so that the patella does not grind against the femoral condyles.

Anteroposterior Movement of the Head of the Fibula on the Tibia

The patient is supine with the knee flexed to 90° and the hip to 45°. The examiner then sits on the patient's foot and places one hand around the patient's knee to stabilize the knee and leg. The mobilizing hand is placed around the head of the fibula. The fibula is drawn forward on the tibia, and the movement and end feel are tested. The fibula then slides back to its resting position of its own accord. The movement is tested several times and compared with that of the other side. Care must be taken when performing this test because the common peroneal nerve, which winds around the head of the fibula, may be easily compressed, causing pain. If the superior tibiofibular joint is stiff or hypomobile, the test itself will cause discomfort. In most cases, foot dorsiflexion will cause lateral knee pain if the superior tibiofibular joint is hypomobile.

Palpation

The patient lies supine with the knee slightly flexed. It is wise to put the knee in several positions during palpation. For example, meniscal cysts are best palpated at 45°, whereas the joint line is easiest to palpate at 90°. When palpating, the examiner looks for abnormal tenderness, swelling, nodules, or abnormal temperature. The following structures should be palpated (Fig. 12.155).

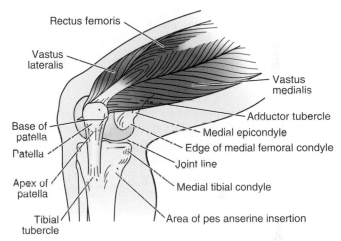

Fig. 12.155 Palpation landmarks of the knee.

Anterior Palpation with Knee Extended

Patella, Patellar Tendon, Patellar Retinaculum, Associated Bursa, Cartilaginous Surface of the Patella, and Plica. The patella can easily be palpated over the anterior aspect of the knee. The base of the patella lies superiorly, and the apex lies distally. After palpating the apex of the patella (for possible jumper's knee), the examiner moves distally, palpating the patellar tendon (for paratenonitis or tendinosis) and the overlying infrapatellar bursa (for Parson's knee), as well as the fat pad that lies behind the tendon (**Hoffa's sign**). When the knee is extended, the fat pad often extends beyond the sides of the tendon. Moving distally, the examiner comes to the tibial tuberosity, which should be palpated for enlargement (possible Osgood-Schlatter disease).

Returning to the patella, the examiner can palpate the skin lying over the patella for pathology (prepatellar bursitis or housemaid's knee) and then extend medially and laterally to palpate the patellar retinaculum on both sides of the patella. With the examiner pushing down on the lateral aspect of the patella, the medial retinaculum can be brought under tension and then palpated for tender areas.

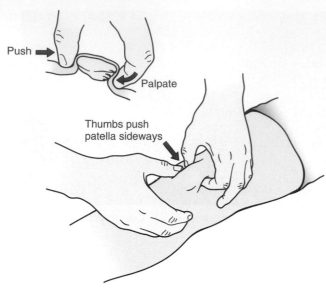

Fig. 12.156 Checking for patellar medial and lateral facet tenderness. Note that tenderness may be related to structures other than patellar surfaces beneath the examining finger. (Redrawn from Hughston JC, Walsh WM, Puddu G: *Patellar subluxation and dislocation*, Philadelphia, 1984, WB Saunders, p 28.)

The lateral retinaculum can be palpated in a similar fashion with the examiner pushing down on the medial aspect of the patella. By stressing the retinaculum, the examiner is separating the retinaculum from the underlying tissue.

With the quadriceps muscles relaxed, the articular facets of the patella are palpated for tenderness (possible chondromalacia patellae), as shown in Fig. 12.156. This palpation is often facilitated by carefully pushing the patella medially to palpate the medial facets and laterally to palpate the lateral facet.

As the medial edge of the patella is palpated, the examiner should carefully feel for the presence of a mediopatellar plica. The plica, if pathological, may be palpated as a thickened ridge medial to the patella. To help confirm the presence of the plica, the examiner flexes the patient's knee to 30° and pushes the patella medially. If the plica is present and pathological, this maneuver often causes pain.

Suprapatellar Pouch. Returning to the anterior surface of the patella and moving proximally beyond the base of the patella, the examiner's fingers lie over the suprapatellar pouch. The examiner then lifts the skin and underlying tissue between the thumb and fingers (Fig. 12.157). In this way, the synovial membrane of the suprapatellar pouch, which is continuous with that of the knee joint, can be palpated as a very slippery surface normally. The examiner should feel for any thickness, tenderness, or nodules, the presence of which may indicate pathology.

Quadriceps Muscles (Vastus Medialis, Vastus Intermedius, Vastus Lateralis, Rectus Femoris) and Sartorius. After palpating the suprapatellar pouch, the examiner palpates the quadriceps for tenderness (possible first- or second-degree strain), defects (third-degree strain), atonia, or hard masses (myositis ossificans).

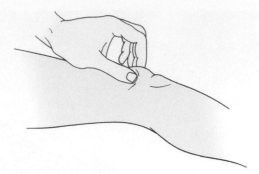

Fig. 12.157 Palpation of the suprapatellar pouch.

Medial Collateral Ligament. If the examiner moves medially from the patella so that the fingers lie over the medial aspect of the tibiofemoral joint, the fingers will lie over the medial collateral ligament, which should be palpated along its entire length for tenderness (possible sprain) or other pathology (e.g., Pellegrini-Stieda syndrome—bone development in the medial collateral ligament).

Pes Anserinus. Medial and slightly distal to the tibial tuberosity, the examiner may palpate the pes anserinus (the common aponeurosis of the tendons of gracilis, semitendinosus, and sartorius muscles) for tenderness. Any associated swelling may indicate either pes anserine bursitis or tendinitis.

Tensor Fascia Lata (Iliotibial Band and Head of Fibula). As the examiner moves laterally from the tibial tuberosity, the head of the fibula can be palpated. Medial and slightly superior to the fibula, the examiner palpates the insertion of the iliotibial band into the lateral condyle of the tibia. When the knee is extended, it stands out as a strong, visible ridge anterolateral to the knee joint. As the examiner moves proximally, the iliotibial band is palpated along its entire length distally to its attachment at the Gerdy's tubercle on the lateral side of the tibial plateau.

Anterior Palpation with Knee Flexed

Tibiofemoral Joint Line and Meniscus. The patient's knee is flexed at 45°, and the examiner palpates the joint line for tenderness, especially the anterior half of each meniscus. Medial rotation of the tibia makes the medial edge of the medial meniscus easier to palpate, whereas lateral rotation allows easier palpation of the lateral meniscus. The meniscus is palpated for tenderness (possible meniscal tear), swelling (possible meniscal cyst), or other pathology.[265,468] Joint line tenderness for lateral meniscus tears is more accurate (96%), sensitive (89%), and specific (97%) than for medial meniscus tears (accuracy 74%; sensitivity 86%; and, specificity 67%).[469]

Tibiofemoral Joint Line, Tibial Plateau, Femoral Condyles, and Adductor Muscles. The patient's knee is flexed to 90°. If the examiner returns to the patella, palpates the apex of the patella, and moves medially or laterally, the fingers lie on the tibiofemoral joint line, which should be palpated along its entire length. As the joint line is palpated, the

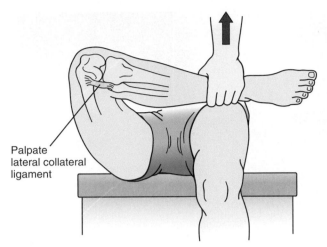

Palpate
lateral collateral
ligament

Fig. 12.158 Palpation of the lateral (fibular) collateral ligament.

examiner should also palpate the tibial plateau (for possible coronary ligament sprain) medially and laterally which are commonly injured with meniscus tears.

Both condyles should be palpated carefully for any tenderness (e.g., OCD).[470] OCD of the knee is four times more likely to be seen in males than females, and patients aged 12 to 19 years are three times more likely to risk OCD than children aged 6 to 11 years.[470] Beginning at the superior aspect of the femoral condyles, the examiner should note that the lateral condyle extends farther anteriorly (i.e., higher) than the medial condyle. The trochlear groove between the two condyles can then be palpated. As the medial condyle is palpated, a sharp edge appears on the condyle medially. If the edge is followed posteriorly, the adductor tubercle can be palpated on the posteromedial portion of the medial femoral condyle. The area around the adductor tubercle may be tender following patellar dislocation as it is a common location for attachment of the MPFL. After palpating the adductor tubercle, the examiner moves proximally, palpating the adductor muscles of the hip for tenderness or other signs of pathology.

Anterior Palpation with Foot of Test Leg Resting on Opposite Knee

Kennedy[274] has advocated palpation of the lateral collateral ligament by having the patient in the sitting or lying position (Fig. 12.158). The patient's knee is flexed to 90°, and the hip is laterally rotated so that the ankle of the test leg rests on the knee of the other leg (figure-four position) (**Cabot's maneuver**[89]). The examiner then places the knee into a varus position, and the ropelike ligament stands out if the ligament is intact.

Posterior Palpation with the Knee Slightly Flexed

Posterior Aspect of Knee Joint. The soft tissue on the posterior aspect of the knee should be palpated for tenderness or swelling (e.g., Baker's cyst). In some patients,

the popliteal artery (pulse) may be palpated by running the hand down the center of the posterior knee.

Posterolateral Aspect of Knee Joint. The posterolateral corner of the knee is sometimes called the *popliteus corner*. The examiner should attempt to palpate the arcuate-popliteus complex, the lateral gastrocnemius muscle, the biceps femoris muscle, and possibly the lateral meniscus in this area. A sesamoid bone is sometimes found inserted in the tendon of the lateral head of the gastrocnemius muscle. This bone, referred to as the **fabella,** may be interpreted as a loose body in the posterolateral aspect of the knee by an unwary examiner (see Fig. 12.174).

Posteromedial Aspect of Knee Joint. The posteromedial corner of the knee joint is sometimes referred to as the **semimembranosus corner.** The examiner should attempt to palpate the posterior oblique ligament, the semimembranosus muscle, the medial gastrocnemius muscle, and possibly the medial meniscus in this area for tenderness or pathology.

Hamstring and Gastrocnemius Muscles. After the various parts of the posterior aspect of the knee have been palpated, the tendons and muscle bellies of the hamstring muscle group (biceps femoris, semitendinosus, semimembranosus) proximally and of the gastrocnemius muscle distally should be palpated for tenderness, swelling, or other signs of pathology.

Diagnostic Imaging

Plain Film Radiography

For evaluation of knee injuries, anteroposterior and lateral views are most commonly obtained. Depending on the suspected pathology, other views may be taken as well. Usually, the anteroposterior view is taken with the patient bearing weight. Imaging should not be used indiscriminately but should be considered an adjunct to examination; it is used primarily to confirm a diagnosis obtained by careful assessment.[22,471–474] Stiell and associates[475] have developed the **Ottawa knee rules** for the use of radiography in acute knee injuries.[311,476,477] They believed knee radiography was only necessary in acute knee injuries if the patient is 55 years of age or older or had isolated tenderness of the patella, tenderness at the head of the fibula, inability to flex the knee to 90°, or an inability to walk four steps (bearing weight). The use of the Ottawa knee rules in children is supported by some[478,479] and questioned by others.[480] Seaberg and Jackson[481] developed the **Pittsburgh Knee Rules**. They believed patients should undergo radiography if there was blunt trauma or a fall as a mechanism of injury, plus either the patient was younger than 12 or older than 50, or the patient had an inability to walk four weight-bearing steps. Many clinicians combine both knee rules when making a decision about radiographs of the knee.[482] The American College of Rheumatology has three sets of criteria for osteoarthritis.[477,483]

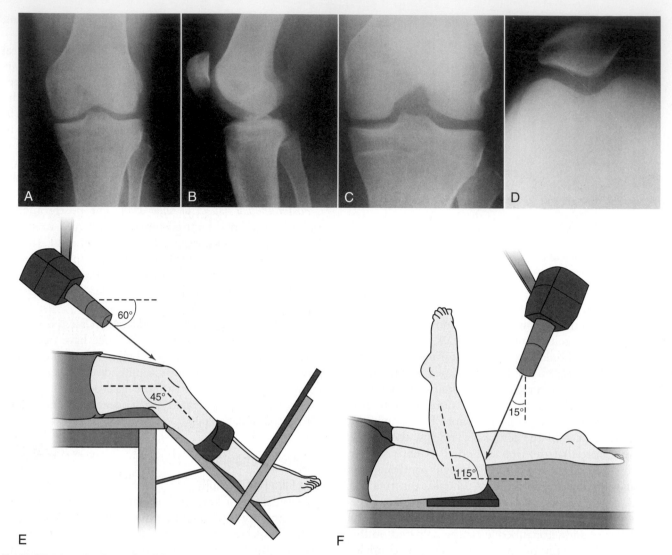

Fig. 12.159 Normal radiographs of the knee. (A) Anteroposterior view. (B) Lateral view. (C) Tunnel view. (D) Patellofemoral joint skyline (merchant) view. (E) Positioning for merchant view of patellofemoral joint (supine). (F) Positioning for prone view of patellofemoral joint. (A–D, From Reilly BM: *Practical strategies in outpatient medicine*, Philadelphia, 1991, WB Saunders, p 1188.)

Common X-Ray Views of the Knee Depending on Pathology

- AP view[a] (see Fig. 12.159A)
- Lateral view—90° flexion (note if fabella present posteriorly) (see Fig. 12.169)
- Lateral view—30° flexion[a] (see Fig. 12.159B)
- Intercondylar notch (tunnel) view (AP 45° flexion) (see Fig. 12.159C)
- Axial (skyline/sunrise) view of patellofemoral joint (see Fig. 12.159D)
- Standing AP (both knees) (see Fig. 12.188)
- Standing PA—30° flexion (Fig. 12.189)
- Merchant view (patient supine, knee flexed 45°, x-ray beam directed caudally through patella at 60° from vertical) (patellar subluxation, patellofemoral arthritis) (Fig. 12.190)
- Tunnel view (see Fig. 12.161)

[a]Should be weight bearing for arthritis.[324]
AP, Anteroposterior; *PA*, posteroanterior.

Ottawa Knee Rules for Radiographs of Acute Knee Injuries[471]

- Patient age younger than 55 or older than 18 years
- Fibular head tenderness
- Patellar tenderness
- Inability to flex knee to 90°
- Inability to bear weight and walk four steps when examined and at time of injury

Pittsburgh Knee Rules[478]

- Blunt trauma or fall
- Patient age younger than 12 years or older than 50 years
- Inability to walk four weight-bearing steps on affected leg

Criteria for Diagnosis of Osteoarthritis Based on Three Sets of Criteria[477,483,484]

SET ONE (CLINICAL AND RADIOLOGICAL FINDINGS):

- Osteophytes
- At least 1 of 3 of the following:
  - >50 years of age
  - Crepitus
  - Morning stiffness ≤30 min
  - Female
  - Overweight

SET TWO (CLINICAL FINDINGS):

- At least 3 of the following:
  - >50 years of age
  - Stiffness <30 min
  - Crepitus
  - Bony tenderness
  - Bony enlargement
  - No palpable warmth
  - Female
  - Overweight

SET THREE (CLINICAL AND LABORATORY FINDINGS):

- At least 5 of 9 of the following:
  - >50 years of age
  - Stiffness <30 min
  - Crepitus
  - Bony tenderness
  - Bony enlargement
  - No palpable warmth
  - Female
  - Overweight
  - ESR <40 mm/h
  - Rheumatoid factor titer <1:40
  - Synovial fluid clear, viscous with leukocyte count <2 × 10^9 cells/L

ESR, Erythrocyte sedimentation rate.
Modified from Jackson JL, O'Malley FG, Kroenke K: Evaluation of acute knee pain in primary care, *Ann Intern Med* 139:575–588, 2003; Altman R, Asch E, Bloch D, et al: Development of criteria for the classification and reporting of osteoarthritis—classification of osteoarthritis of the knee, *Arthr Rheum* 29(8):1039–1049, 1986; and, Zhang W, Doherty M, Peat G, et al: EULAR evidence-based recommendations for the diagnosis of knee osteoarthritis, *Ann Rheum Dis* 69(3):483–489, 2010.

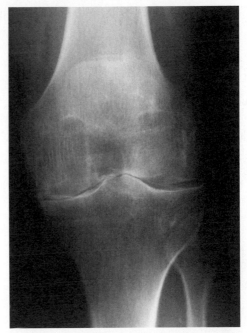

Fig. 12.160 Anteroposterior x-ray showing degenerative arthritis of the knee. Note the loss of joint space caused by loss of cartilage (both sides) and meniscus (on medial side).

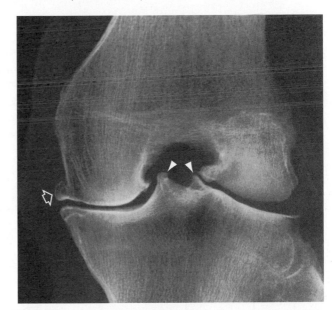

Fig. 12.161 Tunnel view: osteoarthritis of the knee—femorotibial compartment abnormalities. Radiograph of a coronal section of a cadaveric knee indicates osteoarthritis changes that are more prominent in the medial femorotibial compartment. Findings include joint space narrowing related to cartilage erosion, subchondral bony sclerosis, osteophytosis *(open arrow),* and sharpening of the tibial spines *(arrowheads).* Degeneration of both the medial meniscus and the lateral meniscus is evident. View may also be used to look for osteochondritis dissecans. (From Resnick D, Kransdorf MJ: *Bone and joint imaging,* Philadelphia, 2005, WB Saunders, p 386.)

Anteroposterior View. When looking at radiographs of the knee (Fig. 12.159), the examiner should note any possible fractures (e.g., osteochondral, fibular head), diminished joint space (possible osteoarthritis; Figs. 12.160 and 12.161), epiphyseal damage, lipping (see Fig. 12.161), loose bodies, alterations in bone texture, abnormal calcification, ossification (e.g., Pellegrini-Stieda syndrome; Fig. 12.162) or tumors, accessory ossification centers, varus or valgus deformity, patellar position, patella alta (Figs. 12.163 and 12.164) or baja, and asymmetry of femoral condyles.[485,486] Weight-bearing radiographs of knees in 30° flexion are recommended for cases of suspected arthritis or degeneration.[487] Stress, non–weight-bearing radiographs of this view illustrate excessive gapping medially or laterally, indicating ligamentous instability (Fig. 12.165). The examiner should also remember the possible presence of the fabella (see Fig. 12.174), which is seen in 20% of the population. Epiphyseal fractures (Fig. 12.166) and OCD (Fig. 12.167) may also be seen in this

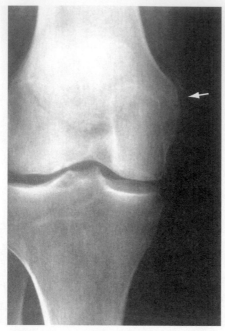

Fig. 12.162 Pellegrini-Stieda syndrome. Note calcium formation within the substance of the medial collateral ligament *(arrow)*.

view.[488–490] The presence of the **Segund sign** or **lateral capsular sign,** which is an avulsion fracture, often indicates severe lateral capsular injury and probably anterior cruciate ligament disruption (Fig. 12.168).[21,491–493]

Lateral View. With this view,[320,485,494] the examiner should note the same structures as seen with the anteroposterior view (Figs. 12.169 to 12.171). This view is usually done in side-lying position with the knee flexed to 45°.[495] To determine the normal positioning of the patella, the standing, weight-bearing lateral view is used to determine the ratio of patellar length to patellar tendon length (Fig. 12.172); several methods are possible.[496–499] Berg and associates[500] reported that the Blackburne-Peel method was the most consistent. This view also illustrates Osgood-Schlatter disease (Fig. 12.173), the presence of the fabella (Fig. 12.174), the arcuate sign (avulsion fracture of the arcuate complex leading to posterolateral instability; Fig. 12.175),[342,501] myositis ossificans (Figs. 12.176 and 12.177), and avulsion of the anterior cruciate insertion (Fig. 12.178). Stress radiographs of this view in kneeling can be used to show complete tears (8 mm or more) of the posterior cruciate ligament.[502,503]

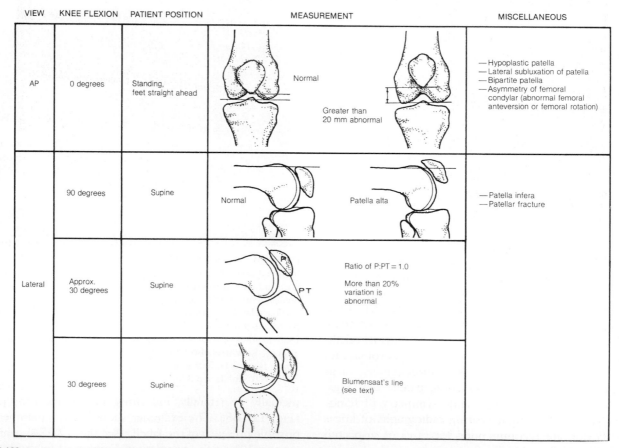

Fig. 12.163 Summary of radiographic findings in patella alta. (From Carson WG Jr, James SL, Larson RL, et al: Patellofemoral disorders: physical and radiographic evaluation. I. Physical examination, *Clin Orthop* 185:179, 1984.)

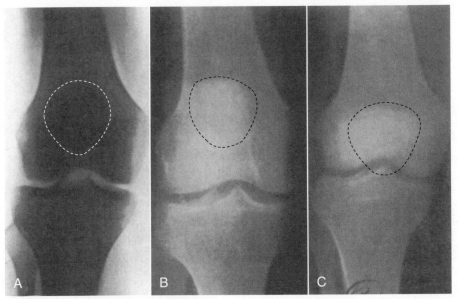

Fig. 12.164 Anteroposterior view of the knee. (A) Normal patellar position. (B) Patella alta. (C) Patella baja. (From Hughston JC, et al: *Patellar subluxation and dislocation*, Philadelphia, 1984, WB Saunders, p 50.)

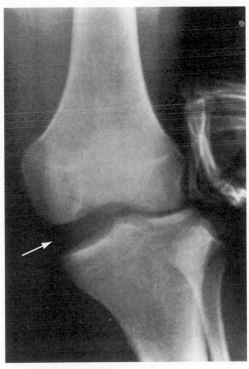

Fig. 12.165 This valgus stress radiograph shows the patient's knee in full extension. Note the gapping on the medial side *(arrow)* caused by the stress applied by the examiner's hand (bones to right of knee). (From Mital MA, Karlin LI: Diagnostic arthroscopy in sports injuries. *Orthop Clin North Am* 11:775, 1980.)

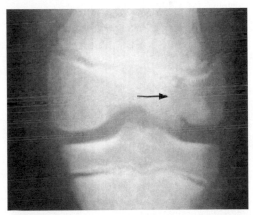

Fig. 12.166 A Salter-Harris type III injury *(arrow)* of the growth plate and epiphysis. Main attention should be directed toward restitution of the joint surface. (From Ehrlich MG, Strain RE: Epiphyseal injuries about the knee, *Orthop Clin North Am* 10:93, 1979.)

Intercondylar Notch (Tunnel View X-Ray). With this view (patient prone, knee flexed from 45° to 90°) (Fig. 12.179), the tibia and intercondylar attachments of the cruciate ligaments can be examined as well as the width of the intercondylar notch, which is less in women.[504] This narrower notch can put the anterior cruciate at

greater risk of tearing.[504] In addition, any loose bodies or possibility of OCD, subluxation, trochlear dysplasia, patellar tilt (lateral or medial), or dislocation should be noted.[490,505]

Axial (Skyline) View. This 30° tangential view (Fig. 12.180) is primarily used for suspected patellar problems, such as patellar subluxation and dysplasia (Fig. 12.181).[82,486,494,506–510] It may be taken at different angles, as shown in Figs. 12.182 to 12.184, or it may be used to determine the type of patella present, as shown in Fig. 12.185.[511] Fig. 12.186 illustrates abnormal patellar forms. Other patellofemoral measurements include lateral patellar displacement (see Fig. 12.183) and the lateral/medial trochlear ratio or sulcus angle (see Fig. 12.184).[494,511]

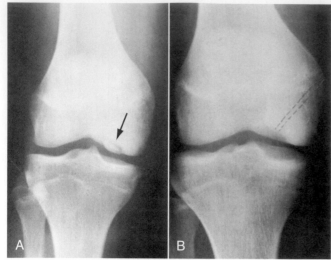

Fig. 12.167 (A) Osteochondritis dissecans—actually an osteochondral fracture *(arrow)* of the femoral condyle—with almost the entire femoral attachment of the posterior cruciate ligament remaining attached to the fragment. (B) Three months after repair of posterior cruciate to femur. Excellent function is restored. Complete filling in of this defect is unlikely at this age. (From O'Donoghue DH: *Treatment of injuries to athletes,* ed 4, Philadelphia, 1984, WB Saunders, p 575.)

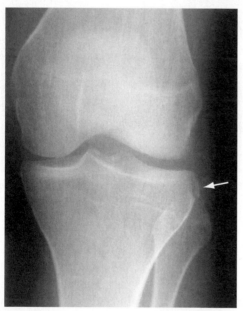

Fig. 12.168 Segund sign. Note avulsion fracture adjacent to lateral tibial plateau *(arrow)*. This lateral capsular injury often signifies an anterior cruciate ligament tear.

Fixed Flexion Posteroanterior View (10° to 30° Knee Flexion). This view is best for determining narrowing of the joint space (Fig. 12.187).

Standing Anteroposterior View. This view is best for knee alignment (Fig. 12.188).

Arthrography

Arthrograms of the knee are used primarily to diagnose tears in the menisci (Fig. 12.191) and plica (Fig. 12.192), although their use is being replaced by arthroscopy. Double-contrast

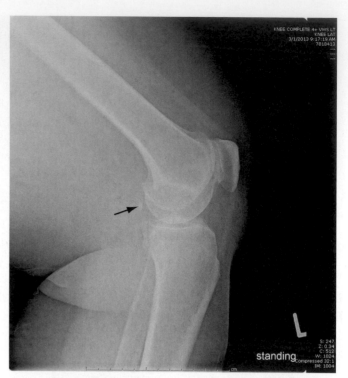

Fig. 12.169 Lateral view of the knee—90° flexion. Note fabella (sesamoid bone) posteriorly *(arrow)*.

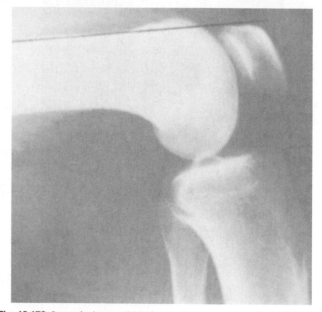

Fig. 12.170 Lateral view at 90° shows the normal position of the patella. (From Hughston JC, et al: *Patellar subluxation and dislocation,* Philadelphia, 1984, WB Saunders, p 52.)

arthrograms are also used (Fig. 12.193). Arthrograms combined with computed tomography (CT) scans (CT arthrograms) are useful for assessing meniscus tears, articular cartilage, meniscal and popliteal cysts, and synovial plica.[512]

Arthroscopy

The arthroscope is being used increasingly to diagnose lesions of the knee and to repair many of them surgically.[513–515] By using various approaches (portals) to the

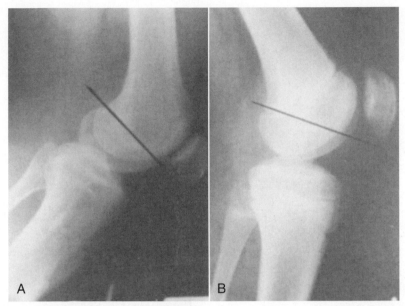

Fig. 12.171 Lateral view of the patella at 45°. (A) Normal patellar position in relation to the intercondylar notch. (B) Patella alta. (From Hughston JC, et al: *Patellar subluxation and dislocation*, Philadelphia, 1984, WB Saunders, p 52.)

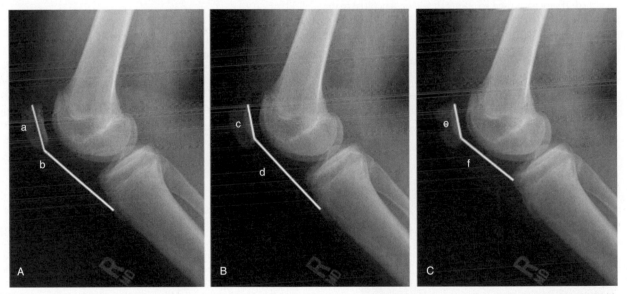

Fig. 12.172 Measurement of patellar height indices. (A) The Insall-Salvati Ratio is measured as the ratio of patellar tendon length *(b)* divided by patellar length *(a)*. (B) The Modified Insall-Salvati Ratio is measured as the ratio of patellar tendon length *(d)* divided by patellar articular surface length *(c)*. (C) The Caton-Deschamps Index is measured as the ratio of the length from the tibial plateau to the inferior pole of the patella *(f)* divided by patellar articular surface length *(e)*. (From Fabricant PD, Ladenhauf HN, Salvati EA, Green DW: Medial patellofemoral ligament (MPFL) reconstruction improves radiographic measures of patella alta in children, *The Knee* 21[6]:1180-1184, 2014.)

knee, the surgeon is able to view all of the structures to determine whether they have been injured (Fig. 12.194).

Diagnostic Ultrasound Imaging

The knee is a large synovial joint that has many isolated, specific, and localized superficial structures that could cause pathology. Internal structures such as meniscus, articular cartilage, and cruciate ligaments, and even some patellofemoral conditions, will cause more diffuse patterns of pain. The knee will generally be examined in all

four quadrants with the lateral portion being examined both anteriorly and posteriorly.

Anterior Knee. The patellar tendon along the anterior knee is one of the most commonly examined and accessible tendons in the body. To decrease the anisotropy effect, the anterior knee may be better seen with some slight tension on the soft tissues. This can be done by placing a towel roll under the knee putting it in slight flexion. The normal tendon is easily seen as striated fibrillary structure. When viewed in the short axis, the tendon proper will

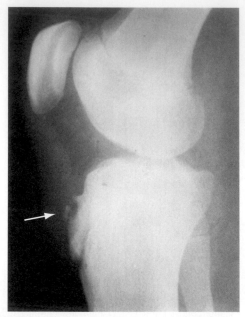

Fig. 12.173 Osgood-Schlatter disease, showing epiphysitis of the entire epiphysis *(arrow)*, with irregularity of the epiphyseal line. Because this epiphyseal cartilage is continuous with that of the upper tibia, it should not be disturbed. If surgery is used, exposure should be superficial to the epiphyseal cartilage. (From O'Donoghue DH: *Treatment of injuries to athletes*, ed 4, Philadelphia, 1984, WB Saunders, p 574.)

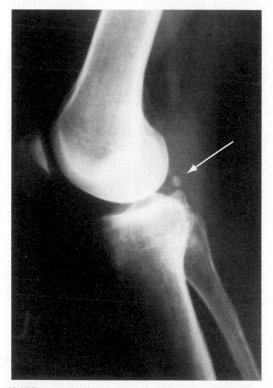

Fig. 12.174 Sesamoid bone (fabella) in the gastrocnemius muscle.

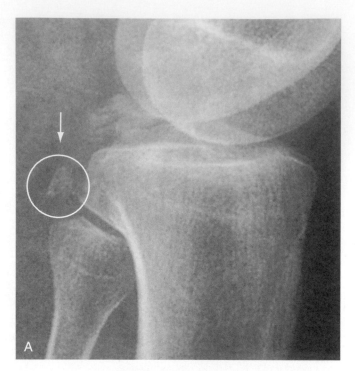

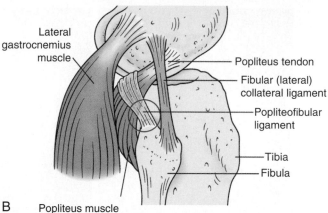

Fig. 12.175 Arcuate sign or fibular styloid fracture on lateral radiograph, (A) with comparative diagram (B). The arcuate sign is pathognomonic of posterolateral corner injuries. It is an avulsion fracture of the arcuate complex. The fracture *(denoted by arrow)* is small and posteriorly located with minimal displacement. *Circles* denote the insertions of the arcuate complex. (A, From Bahk MS, Cosgarea AJ: Physical examination and imaging of the lateral collateral ligament and posterolateral corner of the knee, *Sports Med Arthrosc Rev* 14:16, 2006.)

be seen in a transverse cross section with the Hoffa fat pad directly below it (Fig. 12.195). The tendon can be followed from the distal pole of the patella to the tibial tubercle. The normal appearance at the proximal pole is variable. The attachment can be similar dimensions as the tendon itself, whereas in others, it may be triangular in shape (Fig. 12.196).[516] While still in the short axis view, the medial and lateral gutter or recess can be visualized. In this plane, the thin hyperechoic retinaculum will be seen both medially and laterally. More specifically on the medial side, the MPFL may be seen as a thickening of the medial retinaculum. Moving the transducer 90° into long axis (Fig. 12.197), the tendon is a hyperechoic, fibrillary, and uniform structure. Because there is some degree of asymmetry in this plane between the patella and tibial tubercle, the transducer may need to be floated in gel. With this image, the patella, tendon, and tibial tubercle

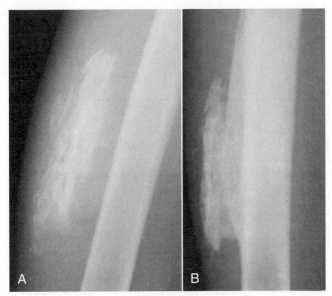

Fig. 12.176 Myositis ossificans traumatica: maturing ossification. In this 11-year-old boy who fell from the steps of a swimming pool, lateral radiographs of the femur 1 month (A) and 5 months (B) after the injury show maturation of the ossifying process. Initially separated from the bone, the process subsequently merged with the anterior femoral surface. (From Resnick D, Kransdorf MJ: *Bone and joint imaging*, Philadelphia, 2005, WB Saunders. Courtesy G Greenway, MD, Dallas, TX, p 1361.)

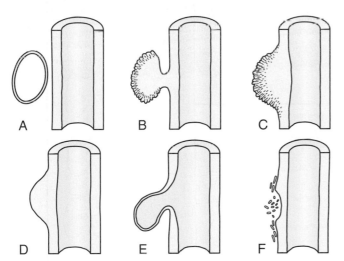

Fig. 12.177 Myositis ossificans traumatica: differential diagnosis. (A) Myositis ossificans traumatica. The shell-like configuration of the ossification, with a clear zone between it and the underlying bone, is typical of this condition. In some cases, there may be a cortical bridge. (B) Parosteal osteosarcoma. These lesions appear as central ossifying foci with irregular outlines and may be connected to the underlying bone by a stalk. (C) Periosteal osteosarcoma. These tumors arise in the cortex of the diaphysis of a tubular bone and produce cortical thickening and speculated osteoid matrix. (D) Osteoma. Characteristic of this lesion is a localized excrescence that produces bulging of the cortical contour. (E) Osteochondroma. An exostosis protrudes from the cortical surface. Its medullary and cortical bone is continuous with that of the underlying osseous structure. (F) Juxtacortical (periosteal) chondroma. These periosteal lesions produce localized excavation of the cortex, with periostitis. They may contain calcification. (Redrawn from Resnick D, Kransdorf MJ: *Bone and joint imaging*, Philadelphia, 2005, WB Saunders, p 1361.)

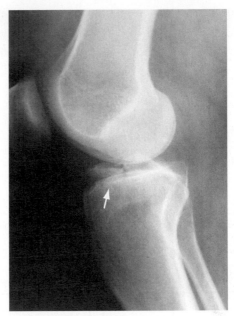

Fig. 12.178 Avulsion fracture of the tibial insertion of the anterior cruciate ligament.

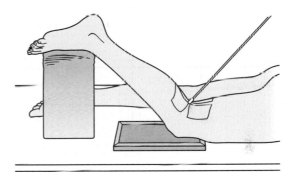

Fig. 12.179 Position for intercondylar notch view. (Redrawn from Larson RL, Grana WA, editors: *The knee: form, function, pathology and treatment*, Philadelphia, 1993, WB Saunders, p 106.)

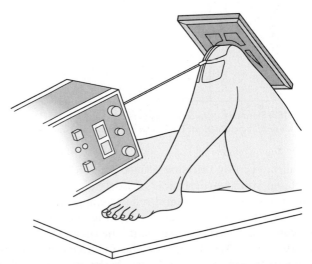

Fig. 12.180 Positioning for the patellofemoral (skyline) view. (Redrawn from Larson RL, Grana WA, editors: *The knee: form, function, pathology and treatment*, Philadelphia, 1993, WB Saunders, p 107.)

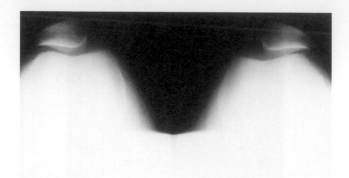

Fig. 12.181 Skyline (sunrise) view of patellofemoral joints. Note the lateral displacement of both patellae and shallow trochlea (trochlear dysplasia), especially the one on the right. Note also the Alpine hunter's cap shape of patella.

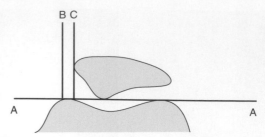

Fig. 12.183 Lateral patellar displacement. A line is drawn through the highest points of the medial and lateral femoral condyles *(AA)*. A perpendicular to that line, at the medial edge of the medial femoral condyle *(B)*, normally lies 1 mm or less medial to the patella *(line C)*. (Redrawn from Laurin CA, Dussault R, Levesque HP: The tangential x-ray investigation of the patellofemoral joint, *Clin Orthop* 144:22, 1979.)

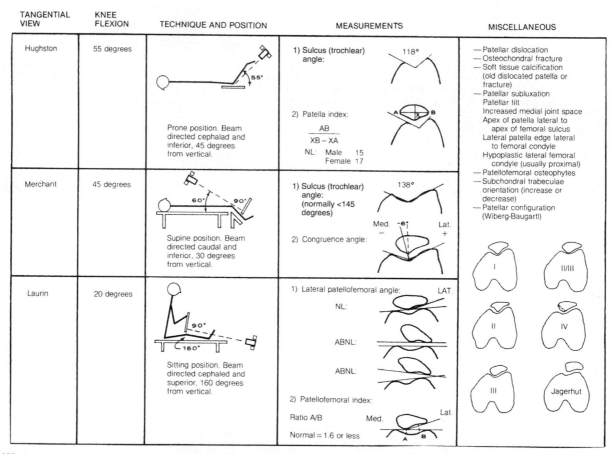

Fig. 12.182 Summary of radiographic findings, tangential view. (From Carson WG Jr, James SL, Larson RL, et al: Patellofemoral disorders: physical and radiographic evaluation. I. Physical examination, *Clin Orthop* 185:182, 1984.)

can all be seen on one single view. This view will also see Hoffa fat pad as hyperechoic or isoechoic (Fig. 12.198). The fat pad has a bright and reflective appearance typical of fat and has very few vessels. Moving superiorly above the patella in the transverse plane, the quadriceps tendon can be viewed. At this position, the quadriceps tendon will appear hyperechoic and fibrillary. If the transducer is set for deep enough viewing, the quadriceps tendon, patella, and femur underneath can all be clearly delineated. In the short axis, the quadriceps tendon cross section can be seen transversely.

Moving the transducer proximally above the patella, the clinician can view the quadriceps tendon in the long axis (Fig. 12.199). Again, it may be helpful to have a towel roll under the knee to place the quadriceps tendon in slight flexion to decrease the effect of anisotropy. The quadriceps tendon has several portions that can be seen individually. If centrally located, one might be able

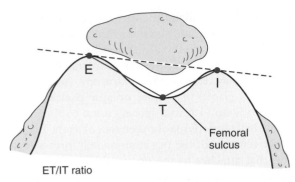

Fig. 12.184 The lateral/medial trochlear ratio is the ratio between the external and internal segments (*ET* and *IT*) joining the highest points of the femoral condyles to the deepest point of the trochlear groove (sulcus angle). It measures the dysplasia of the medial aspect of the trochlea. (Redrawn from Beaconsfield T, Pintore E, Maffulli N, et al: Radiographic measurements in patellofemoral disorders, *Clin Orthop* 308:22, 1994.)

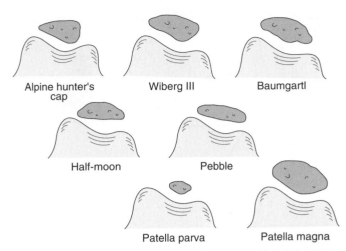

Fig. 12.186 Variations in patellar form that are considered dysplastic. (Redrawn from Ficat RP, Hungerford DS: *Disorders of the patellofemoral joint*, Baltimore, 1977, Williams & Wilkins, p 55.)

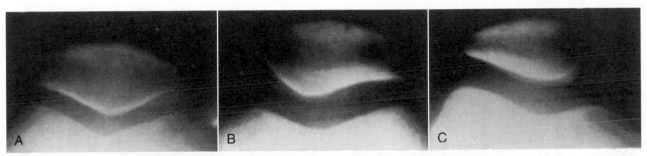

Fig. 12.185 Examples of patellar variations. (A) Wilberg type I. (B) Wilberg type II. (C) Wilberg type III. Trochlea of femur also show variations. (From Ficat RP, Hungerford DS: *Disorders of the patello-femoral joint*, Baltimore, 1977, Williams & Wilkins, p 53.)

to see distinct upper and lower bands separated by fascia. In the central position, the upper band would be the rectus femoris, while the lower band would be the vastus intermedius. Moving the probe slightly laterally will visualize the vastus lateralis, while moving medially will allow viewing of the vastus medialis. By rotating the transducer 90° to the short axis, the quadriceps tendon can be clearly seen in the transverse view to see a hyperechoic, fibrillary pattern of tendon tissue.

Moving the transducer over the medial and lateral knee longitudinally anterior to posterior will view the MPFL and LPFL. They can generally be followed by their posterior attachments near the medial collateral ligament and the iliotibial band and as they run anterior to their insertions on the medial and lateral border of the patella.

Lastly, in deeper knee flexion, the transducer can be placed transversely in the short axis just superior to the patella to view the hypoechoic hyaline cartilage covering the anterior and central aspects of the femoral condyles (Fig. 12.200). Spannow et al.[517] have provided normal cartilage measurements in the knee as a function of age and sex based on axial measurements obtained in this position. Spannow found that the rates of decrease in

cartilage thickness in boys and girls were shown to differ, likely related to sex differences in the rate of skeletal maturation.[517]

Medial Knee. An important structure on the medial side of the knee is the medial collateral ligament. It runs proximally from the medial femoral condyle and extends distally to the anterior proximal tibia. It can be viewed by rotating the patient's leg slightly laterally, exposing the medial side of the knee. With the transducer placed in the long axis in the sagittal plane, the bony contours of the femur and tibia can be clearly seen (Fig. 12.201). The medial collateral ligament can be seen as a thick hyperechoic and fibrillary structure. In this same view, the meniscus will be situated between the tibia and femur as will its attachments to the medial collateral ligament and the meniscofemoral and meniscotibial connections, named in reference to their attachment sites on their respective bones (Fig. 12.202). The meniscus itself is seen as a hyperechoic triangular-shaped structure directly between and slightly protruding from the medial edges of the tibia and femur. If the transducer is rotated 90° into the short transverse axis (Fig. 12.203), the medial collateral ligament can be seen as a more hyperechoic structure distinguishable clearly from the other surrounding tissues.

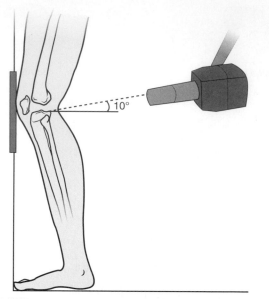

Fig. 12.187 Patient positioning for fixed flexion posteroanterior view.

The transducer, still in the short axis, can be moved further distally and anteriorly to follow the tendons of the pes anserine muscle group (i.e., sartorious, gracillis, and semitendinosus). With the transducer in a straight short axis, the tendons may demonstrate anisotropy; however, if the transducer is placed in a more oblique position approximately 4 to 5 cm (1.6 to 2 inches) distal to the joint line, the individual tendons may be seen more clearly. Eventually, the three tendons of the pes anserine will form a cojoined tendon that attaches to the proximal tibia. Lastly, if continued distally, the semimembranosus tendon can be seen at its attachment to the small recess in the tibia. This view is seen with the transducer in the long axis as the tendon appears as a normal hyperechoic fibrillary structure seen clearly demarcated from the tibial cortex.

Lateral Knee. To image the lateral side of the knee, the patient's leg is medially rotated slightly or the patient can lay on his or her contralateral side. To view the iliotibial tract, the transducer is placed in the long axis along

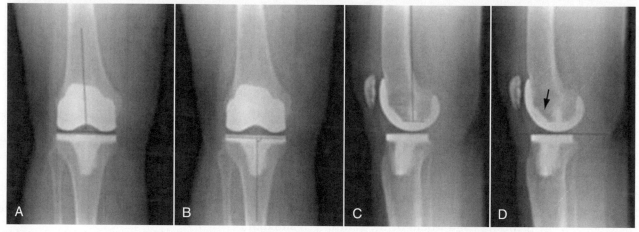

Fig. 12.188 Normal component positioning on standing knee radiographs. (A) Anteroposterior view of the knee demonstrates the method of measuring femoral component alignment. (B) The tibial tray should be 90° to the long axis of the tibial shaft. (C) Lateral radiographs show the femoral component parallel to the femoral shaft. (D) The tibial tray is at approximately 90° to the tibial shaft. Osteopenia *(arrow)* is seen about the femoral component, consistent with stress shielding. (From Scott WN: *Insall & Scott Surgery of the knee*, ed 5, Philadelphia, 2011, Churchill Livingstone.)

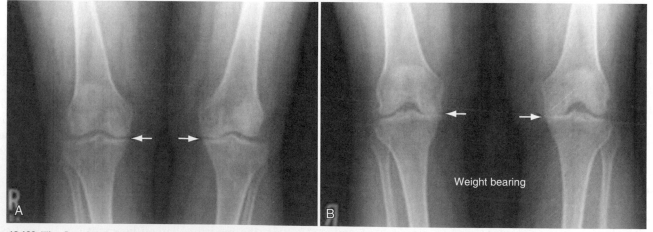

Fig. 12.189 The flexed weight-bearing posteroanterior *(PA)* view. (A) Routine standing anteroposterior (AP) film demonstrates moderate bilateral medial compartment joint space narrowing with proliferative changes *(arrows)*. (B) PA flexion view demonstrates the findings to be more severe with marked narrowing of bilateral medial joint compartments, complete loss of the joint space, and bone-on-bone apposition *(arrows)*. (From Scott WN: *Insall & Scott Surgery of the knee*, ed 5, Philadelphia, 2011, Churchill Livingstone.)

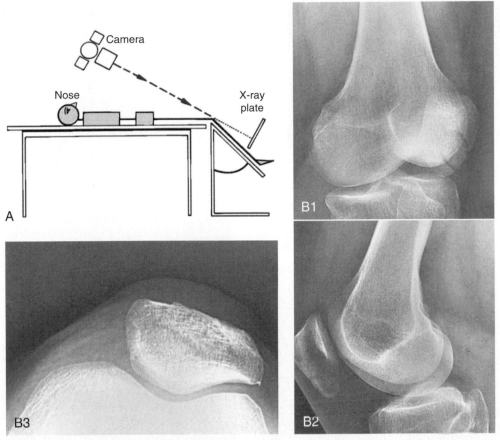

Fig. 12.190 (A) Merchant tangential view of the patella is made with the knee flexed 45° and the radiograph exposed as shown. (B) Patellar fracture of the middle and inferior pole is best seen on the oblique view *(B1)*. *B2*, Lateral view. *B3*, Merchant (sunrise) view. (From Johnson GA, et al: *Atlas of emergency radiology*, St Louis, 2001, WB Saunders; and, Resnick D, Niwayama G: *Diagnosis of bone and joint disorders*, ed 2, Philadelphia, 1988, WB Saunders.)

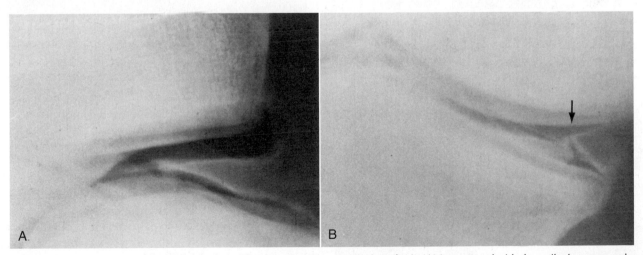

Fig. 12.191 Arthrogram demonstrating a torn meniscus. The normal meniscus on the lateral side (A) is compared with the easily demonstrated tear in the medial meniscus *(arrow)* in the same patient (B). (From Reilly BM: *Practical strategies in outpatient medicine*, Philadelphia, 1991, WB Saunders, p 1198.)

the anterolateral knee and moved posteriorly or laterally (Fig. 12.204). The first structure that is encountered is the iliotibial band, which inserts onto the proximal lateral tibia at the Gerdy's tubercle (Fig. 12.205). As the transducer continues laterally and is rotated slightly oblique, the lateral collateral ligament will come into view. This is seen as a long hyperechoic fibular structure that extends from the fibular head to the lateral femoral condyle. As the transducer is moved further posteriorly, the biceps femoris tendon will come into view. This muscle tendon

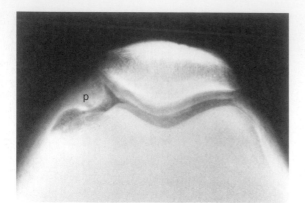

Fig. 12.192 Tangential patellar view after arthrography, showing thinning and slight roughening of the patellar cartilage, especially medially. The mediopatellar plica *(p)* is markedly thickened. (From Weissman BNW, Sledge CB: *Orthopedic radiology*, Philadelphia, 1986, WB Saunders, p 536.)

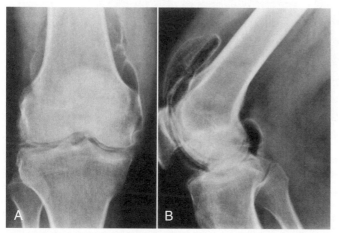

Fig. 12.193 Double-contrast arthrogram. (A) The anteroposterior view demonstrates the menisci and articular cartilage. (B) The lateral projection illustrates the extent of the joint space. (From Forrester DM, Brown JC: *The radiology of joint disease*, ed 3, Philadelphia, 1987, WB Saunders, p 200.)

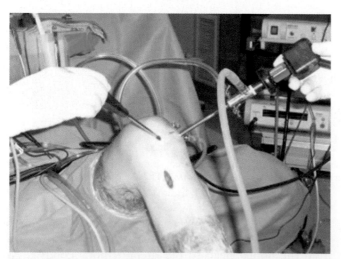

Fig. 12.194 Arthroscopy of the left knee. (From Harner CD, Honkamp NJ, Ranawat AS: Anteromedial portal technique for creating the anterior cruciate ligament femoral tunnel, *Arthroscopy* 24[1]:113–115, 2008.)

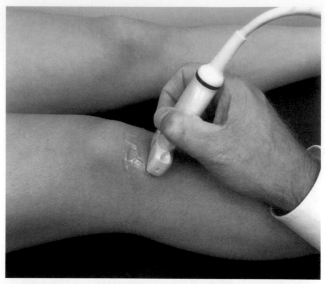

Fig. 12.195 Transducer placement for patellar tendon short axis.

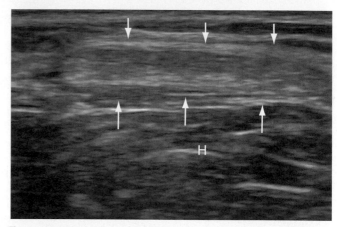

Fig. 12.196 Patellar tendon in short-axis view. Normal tendon seen as fibrillar structure *(arrows)*. *H*, Hoffa fat pad under patellar tendon.

will be clearly differentiated from the lateral collateral ligament by its muscular structure proximally from the tendon. The distal tendinous portion will appear hyperechoic and fibular, while the more muscular portion of muscle will appear more hypoechoic than ligament and tendon. Slightly posterior to the biceps femoris tendon will be the common peroneal nerve, which will appear as a hyperechoic linear structure seen in this view, the long axis.

Posterior Knee. The posterior knee is full of contents that are best seen with the patient lying prone. Beginning with the transducer in the short axis, the examination can commence at midcalf, where multiple muscle groups including the gastrocnemius and soleus can be visualized (Fig. 12.206). The transducer can be moved superiorly, still in the short axis, to follow the medial gastrocnemius tendon, at which point a Baker's cyst (if present) may be seen in the popliteal fossa. A Baker's cyst can be swelling that is seen as a distension of the semimembranosus and semitendinosus bursae. The transducer can be moved medially on the posterior knee to view the posterior portion of the medial meniscus.

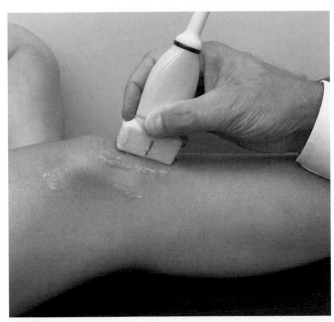

Fig. 12.197 Transducer placement for patellar tendon long-axis view.

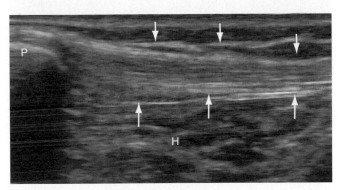

Fig. 12.198 Patellar tendon in sagittal long-axis view. Normal tendon is seen as hyperechoic, fibrillar structure in appearance *(arrows)*. *H*, Hoffa fat pad; *P*, patella.

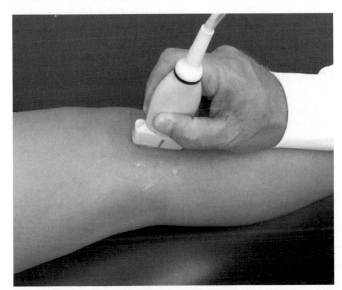

Fig. 12.199 Transducer placement for quadriceps tendon long-axis view.

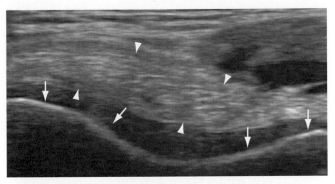

Fig. 12.200 View of proximal tendon just off patella in short-axis view with hypoechoic articular cartilage from underlying trochlea *(arrows)*; outline of quadriceps tendon *(arrowheads)*.

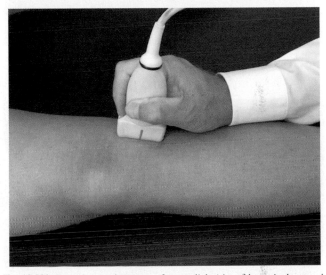

Fig. 12.201 Transducer placement for medial side of knee in long-axis view.

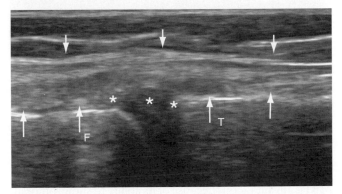

Fig. 12.202 View of medial collateral ligament in long-axis view along medial joint line. Superficial *(arrows)*; deep portion of ligament *(*)*; *F*, femur; *T*, tibia.

As the transducer is moved midline, the posterior cruciate ligament can be visualized as a hyperechoic structure. Due to anisotropy, the viewer may need to use the heel-toe technique to better visualize the ligament. Multiple studies have determined that an injured posterior cruciate ligament is thicker than an uninjured ligament.[518–522] Cho et al.[518] have recommended a posterior cruciate thickness of greater than 10 mm as a diagnostic criterion for an MRI-confirmed acutely torn posterior cruciate ligament.

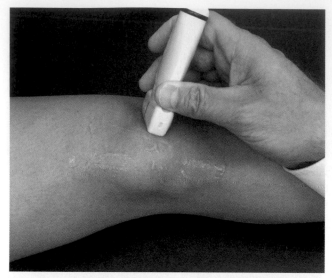

Fig. 12.203 Transducer placement for medial knee in short-axis view.

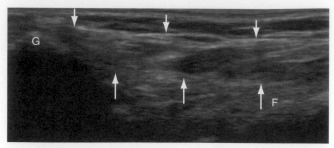

Fig. 12.205 Lateral knee long-axis view. Illiotibial tract *(arrows)*; *F*, femur; *G*, Gerdy tubercle of tibia.

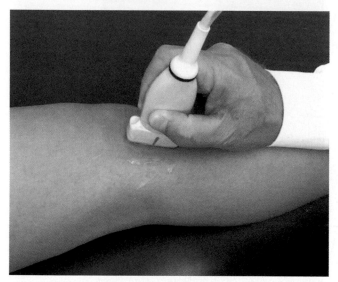

Fig. 12.204 Transducer placement for lateral knee in long-axis view.

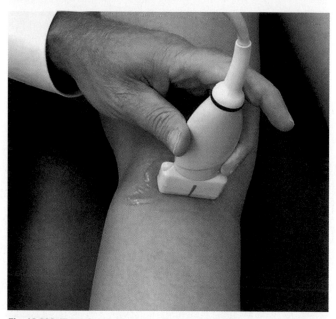

Fig. 12.206 Transducer placement for posterior knee in short-axis view.

Computed Tomography

CT scans are often used to view soft tissue as well as bone (Fig. 12.207).

Magnetic Resonance Imaging

MRI is advantageous because of its ability to show soft tissue as well as bone tissue while providing no exposure to ionizing radiation.[523] It has largely replaced CT scans for evaluation of the knee, and its use should not be indiscriminate but based on history and clinical findings indicating a need for MRI imaging.[524–527] MRI has been found to be useful in diagnosing lesions of the tendon (Fig. 12.208), bone bruises (Fig. 12.209), menisci (Figs. 12.210 and 12.211), plica (Fig. 12.212), collateral ligaments (Fig. 12.213), cruciate ligaments (Fig. 12.214), Baker's cyst (Fig. 12.215), muscle strains (Fig. 12.216), chondromalacia patellae (Fig. 12.217), osteochondral defects, patellar tendon tears, and fractures, but it should be used only to confirm or clarify a clinical diagnosis.[155,493,528–543] Camp et al.[544] provided methods of determining different patellar instability ratios using MRI images to predict recurrent patellar instability. Sagittal proton density MRI and other MRI techniques for cartilage (e.g., 3T imaging, T2 mapping, T1-delayed gadolinium-enhanced MRI) are also becoming more common.[540,545] Sanders and Miller[530] provide a good overview of the use of MRI about the knee.

Xeroradiography

Xeroradiography may be used to delineate the edge of bone (Fig. 12.218).

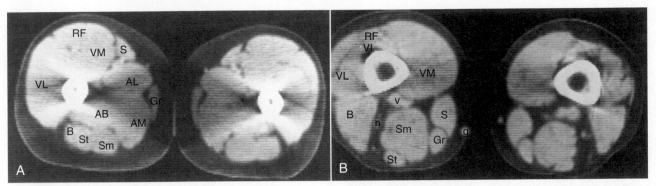

Fig. 12.207 Muscular anatomy as shown on computed tomography scan; images through the upper femur (A) and lower third of femur (B) are shown. *AB,* Adductor brevis; *AL,* adductor longus; *AM,* adductor magnus; *B,* biceps femoris; *g, Gr,* gracilis; *n,* tibial and common peroneal nerves; *RF,* rectus femoris; *S,* sartorius; *Sm,* semimembranosus; *St,* semitendinosus; *V,* deep femoral vein and artery; *VI,* vastus intermedius; *VL,* vastus lateralis; *VM,* vastus medialis. (From Weissman BNW, Sledge CB: *Orthopedic radiology,* Philadelphia, 1986, WB Saunders, p 504.)

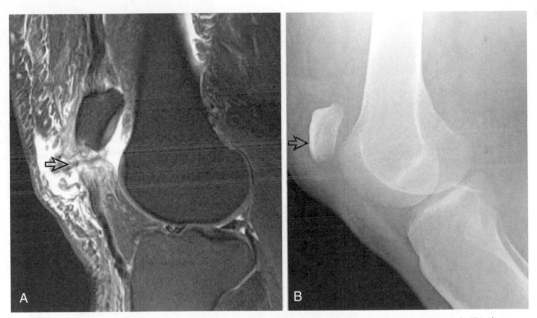

Fig. 12.208 Patellar tendon rupture. Sagittal fat suppressed proton density MR image (A) and lateral knee radiograph (B) show complete rupture of the patellar tendon at its patellar origin (*open black arrow,* A). The patella is proximally retracted (*arrow,* B). (From Petchprapa CN: Imaging of the extensor mechanism. In Scott WN, ed: *Insall & Scott surgery of the knee,* ed 6, Philadelphia, 2018, Elsevier.)

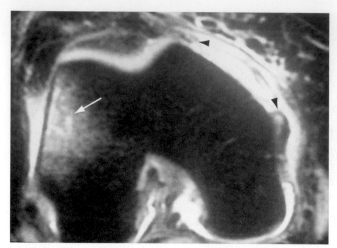

Fig. 12.209 Bone bruise from patellar dislocation-relocation injury. Transverse fat-suppressed intermediate-weighted (TR/TEeff, 3500/12) fast spin-echo magnetic resonance (MR) image. A high-signal-intensity contusion *(arrow)* is apparent in the lateral femoral condyle. Also note the torn medial patellofemoral ligament *(arrowheads)*. (From Resnick D, Kransdorf MJ: *Bone and joint imaging*, Philadelphia, 2005, WB Saunders, p 121.)

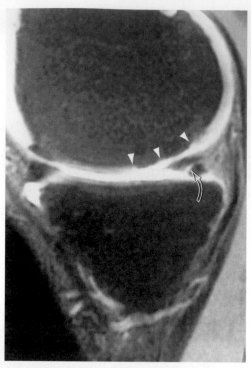

Fig. 12.210 Recurrent meniscal tear after partial medial meniscectomy. Sagittal fat-suppressed T1-weighted (TR/TE, 800/15) spin-echo magnetic resonance image after a knee arthrogram performed with a dilute gadolinium mixture. Injected contrast enters the substance of a new meniscal tear *(arrow)* in the remnant of the posterior horn. Also note the degenerative cartilage loss along the medial femoral surface *(arrowheads)*. (From Resnick D, Kransdorf MJ: *Bone and joint imaging*, Philadelphia, 2005, WB Saunders, p 126.)

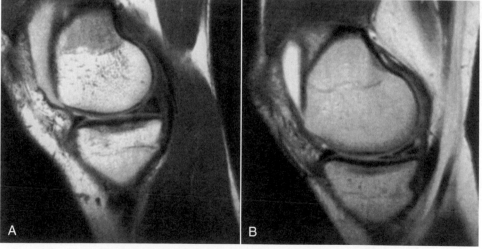

Fig. 12.211 Magnetic resonance image showing lesion of the posterior horn of the medial meniscus. (A) In some cases, contrast can be enhanced by the intra-articular injection of gadolinium diethylenetriamine pentaacetic acid. (B) Inferior longitudinal tear with an associated horizontal tear. (From Strobel M, Stedtfeld HW: *Diagnostic evaluation of the knee*, Berlin, 1990, Springer-Verlag, p 240.)

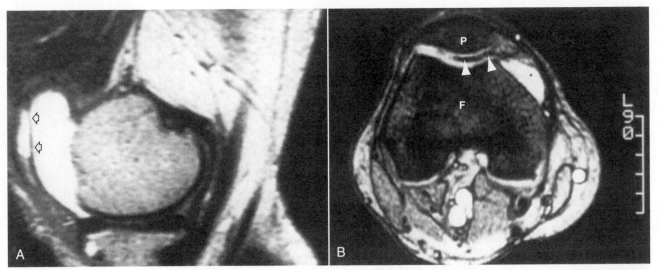

Fig. 12.212 Magnetic resonance image of mediopatellar plica. (A) Sagittal, T2-weighted image located medial to the patella demonstrates an effusion present within the knee joint that appears white. The vertical linear band seen within the joint *(open arrows)* represents the medial plica. (B) Transaxial STIR (Short-TI Inversion Recovery) image through the patellofemoral joint again demonstrates the effusion *(arrowheads)*, which appears bright and surrounds a tonguelike extension of tissue arising from the medial joint line and located between the patella *(P)* and the femur *(F)*. This tissue represents a medial plica. In this location, plicae can become hypertrophied and lead to symptoms and signs of internal derangement. (From Kursunoglu-Brahme S, Resnick D: Magnetic resonance imaging of the knee, *Orthop Clin North Am* 21:571, 1990.)

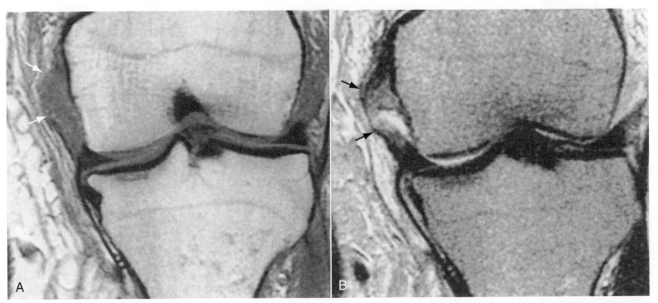

Fig. 12.213 Injuries of the medial collateral ligament: complete tear. Coronal intermediate-weighted (TR/TE, 1500/12) (A) and T2-weighted (TR/TE, 1500/80) (B) spin-echo magnetic resonance (MR) images show complete disruption *(arrows)* of the fibers of the medial collateral ligament. Note the increase in signal intensity in the ligament and soft tissues in (B). A joint effusion is present. Additional injuries in this patient included tears of the lateral meniscus and anterior cruciate ligament. (From Resnick D, Kransdorf MJ: *Bone and joint imaging*, Philadelphia, 2005, WB Saunders, p 959. Courtesy V. Chandnani, MD, Pittsburgh.)

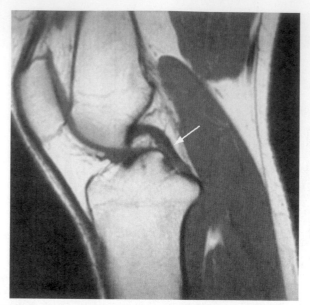

Fig. 12.214 Magnetic resonance image showing intact posterior cruciate ligament *(arrow).* (From Strobel M, Stedtfeld HW: *Diagnostic evaluation of the knee,* Berlin, 1990, Springer-Verlag, p 243.)

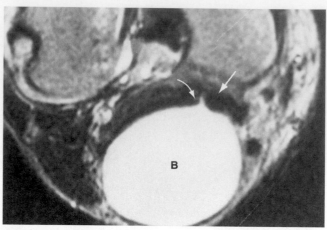

Fig. 12.215 Baker's cyst. Transverse T2-weighted (TR/TE, 2500/80) spin-echo magnetic resonance image of the knee. Fluid distends the semimembranosus-gastrocnemius recess *(B).* The neck of the popliteal cyst is located between the tendons of the medial gastrocnemius *(curved arrow)* and semimembranosus *(straight arrow)* tendons. (From Resnick D, Kransdorf MJ: *Bone and joint imaging,* Philadelphia, 2005, WB Saunders, p 124.)

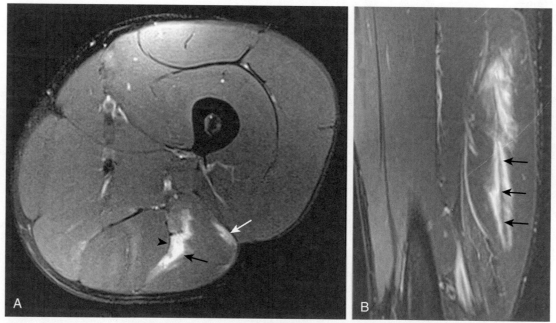

Fig. 12.216 (A) Axial, fat-suppressed, fast spin-echo, T2-weighted MR image of a grade 2 myotendinous tear of biceps femoris. Hematoma *(black arrow)* is demonstrated, and there is muscle fiber retraction from the myotendinous junction *(arrowhead).* Further intramuscular hematoma is seen peripherally close to the epimysium *(white arrow).* (B) Sagittal, fast spin-echo, T2-weighted MR image in the same patient shows the irregular and thickened myotendinous junction *(arrows).* (From Johnson MB, Grainger AJ: Muscle injury and sequelae. In Pope TL, Bloem HL, Beltran J, et al, eds: *Musculoskeletal imaging,* ed 2, Philadelphia, 2015, Saunders.)

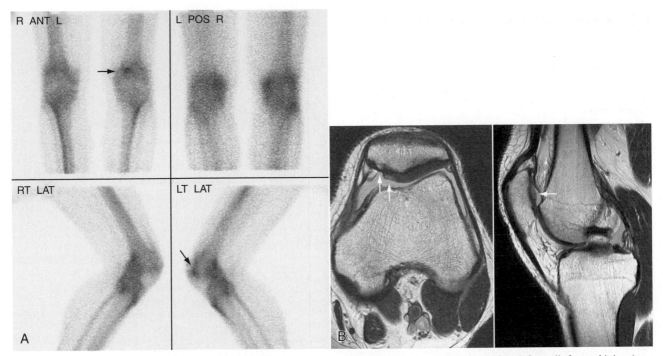

Fig. 12.217 Chondromalacia patellae. (A) Bone scan shows a focal area of increased uptake in the medial aspect of the left patellofemoral joint *(arrows)*. (B) Intermediate-weighted spin-echo magnetic resonance image shows abnormal signal and erosion in the medial aspect of the patellar cartilage *(arrows)*. (From Resnick D, Kransdorf MJ: *Bone and joint imaging*, Philadelphia, 2005, WB Saunders, p 112.)

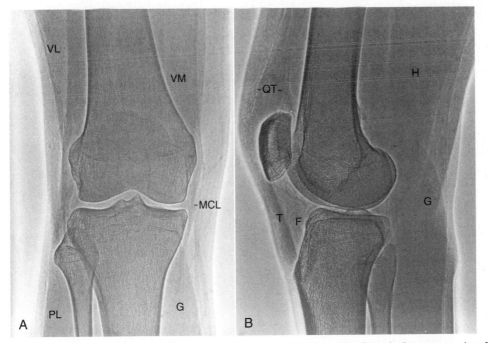

Fig. 12.218 Xeroradiography of the knee. (A) Anteroposterior view. (B) Lateral view. *F*, Infrapatellar fat pad; *G*, gastrocnemius; *H*, hamstrings; *MCL*, medial collateral ligament; *PL*, peroneus longus; *QT*, quadriceps tendon; *T*, patellar tendon; *VL*, vastus lateralis; *VM*, vastus medialis. (From Weissman BNW, Sledge CB: *Orthopedic radiology*, Philadelphia, 1986, WB Saunders, p.504.)

PRÉCIS OF THE KNEE ASSESSMENT[a]

NOTE: Suspected pathology will determine which *Special Tests* are to be performed.

History

Observation

Examination

Active movements (sitting or supine lying)
Knee flexion
Knee extension
Medial rotation of the tibia on the femur
Lateral rotation of the tibia on the femur

Passive movements (as in active movements) (sitting or supine lying)

Resisted isometric movements (sitting or supine lying)
Knee flexion
Knee extension
Ankle plantar flexion
Ankle dorsiflexion

Tests for ligament stability (sitting or supine lying)
For one-plane medial instability:
Hughston's valgus stress at 0° and 30°
Valgus stress at 0° and 30°
For one-plane lateral instability:
Hughston's varus stress at 0° and 30°
Varus stress at 0° and 30°
For one-plane anterior instability:
Active drawer test
Drawer test
Lachman test or its modifications
Lelli test
For one-plane posterior instability:
Active drawer test
Drawer test
Godfrey test
Posterior sag
For anteromedial rotary instability:
Slocum test
For anterolateral rotary instability:
Jerk test of Hughston
Losee test
Noyes flexion-rotation drawer test
Pivot shift test
Slocum anterolateral rotary instability test
For posteromedial rotary instability:
Hughston's posteromedial drawer test
Posteromedial pivot shift test
Supine internal rotation test
For posterolateral rotary instability:
External rotation recurvatum
Hughston's posterolateral drawer test
Loomer's posterolateral rotary instability test
Tibial external rotation (Dial) test

Functional assessment

Special tests (sitting or supine lying)
For meniscus lesions:
Figure-of-four meniscal stress maneuver
McMurray test

For plica lesions:
Hughston plica test
Mediopatellar plica test
Plica "stutter" test
For swelling:
Brush test (minimal swelling)
Fluctuation test (moderate swelling)
Indentation test
Patellar tap test (moderate swelling)
For patellofemoral syndrome:
Clarke sign
McConnell test
Motion palpation test
For quadriceps pull:
Q-angle
Tubercle sulcus test
For patellar instability:
Fairbank apprehension test
Moving patellar apprehension test
For iliotibial band friction syndrome:
Noble compression test

Reflexes and cutaneous distribution

Joint play movements (supine)
Backward and forward movements of the tibia on the femur
Medial and lateral translation of the tibia on the femur
Medial and lateral displacements of the patella
Depression of the patella
Elevation of the patella
Anteroposterior movement of the head of the fibula on the tibia

Palpation (supine)

Tests for ligament stability (prone lying)
For one-plane anterior instability:
Lachman test modification 6

Special tests (prone lying)
For meniscus lesions:
Apley's test

Tests for ligament stability (standing)
For anterolateral rotary instability:
Crossover test
For posterolateral rotary instability:
Jakob test

Special tests (standing)
For meniscus lesions:
Childress' sign (squat and duck walk test)
Ege's test
Thessaly test
For patellofemoral syndrome:
Eccentric step (lateral step down) test
Step up test
Coactivation tests for quadriceps and hamstrings

Diagnostic imaging

After any examination, the patient should be warned of the possibility of exacerbation of symptoms as a result of the assessment.

[a]Although examination of the knee may be carried out with the patient in the supine position, some of the tests may require the patient to move to other positions (e.g., standing, lying, prone, sitting). When these tests are used, the examination should be planned in such a way that the movement and therefore the discomfort experienced by the patient are kept to a minimum. The sequence should be from standing to sitting, to supine lying, to side lying, and, finally, to prone lying.

CASE STUDIES

When doing these case studies, the examiner should list the appropriate questions to be asked and why they are being asked, what to look for and why, and what things should be tested and why. Depending on the answers of the patient (and the examiner should consider different responses), several possible causes of the patient's problem may become evident (examples are given in parentheses). A differential diagnosis chart should be made. The examiner can then decide how different diagnoses may affect the treatment plan. For example, a 16-year-old female volleyball player comes to you with knee pain (Table 12.16). Her knee is painful when she plays, and she sometimes feels a clicking when going up and down stairs. Describe your assessment plan for this patient (meniscus pathology versus plica syndrome).

1. A 14-year-old male wrestler comes to see you for medial knee pain that is thought to be from an injury at his very first wrestling match where he was taken down by his opponent and landed awkwardly on his leg twisting his knee. His diagnosis is medial knee sprain. However, he complains of pain with weight bearing and twisting while the knee is loaded and popping with pain along medial joint line. Your differential diagnosis is between medial collateral ligament or medial meniscus tear. Describe your assessment and which tests you would use to determine what his pathology actually is.

2. A 22-year-old collegiate female basketball player comes to see you for a complaint of medial knee pain that has come about with insidious onset over the past 4 weeks. She cannot describe any trauma that may have caused her problem but does report she plays fairly aggressively and has taken several falls diving for basketballs and getting knocked down during game situations. She has had radiographs to rule out any potential fractures. Describe every bony, ligamentous or soft-tissue structure that could be a source of medial knee pain that may be contributing to her symptoms.

3. A 59-year-old man presents to you with moderate pain and swelling of 4 months' duration in his right knee. There is no history of trauma. The pain and swelling have become worse during the past month. Describe your assessment plan for this patient (osteoarthritis vs. meniscus pathology).

4. A 24-year-old male football player is referred to you for treatment after a surgical repair to the anterior cruciate and medial collateral ligaments of the right knee. He is still in a splint, but the surgeon says the splint can be removed for treatment. Describe your assessment plan for this patient.

5. A 54-year-old man comes to you for treatment. He has difficulty walking and pain in the left hamstrings that is referred into the area of the gluteal fold. There is ecchymosis evident in the posterior knee and a small amount in the superior calf area. Describe your assessment plan for this patient (hamstring strain vs. sciatica).

6. An 18-year-old woman presents to your clinic with anterior knee pain. Design your assessment plan for this patient (chondromalacia patellae vs. plica syndrome).

7. A 17-year-old male soccer player comes to you saying that his knee feels unstable. He says he was playing soccer, twisted to challenge a player, and felt a pop in his knee. Describe your assessment plan for this patient (osteochondral fracture vs. anterior cruciate sprain).

8. A 10-year-old boy is brought to you by his parents. He is experiencing anterior knee pain. Describe your assessment plan for this patient (Osgood-Schlatter syndrome vs. chondromalacia patellae).

9. A 20-year-old female rugby player comes to you with lateral knee pain that is sometimes referred down the leg. The knee hurts when she walks. She vaguely remembers being kicked in the knee while playing rugby 10 days earlier. Describe your assessment plan for this patient (superior tibiofibular joint subluxation vs. common peroneal nerve neuropraxia).

10. An 18-year-old female swimmer presents to you with medial knee pain. She has just increased her training to 10,000 m per day. Describe your assessment plan for this patient (medial collateral ligament sprain vs. chondromalacia patellae).

TABLE **12.16**

Differential Diagnosis of Meniscus and Medial Patellar Plica Syndrome

	Medial Meniscus	Medial Patellar Plica Syndrome
History	Mechanism of injury: rotation, flexion, and valgus stress (may be acute or insidious) while weight bearing	Mechanism of injury: flexion, rotation (usually insidious onset)
Pain	Joint line	May be joint line but also superomedial to joint line
Swelling	May be present	May be present
Locking or giving way	Locking more likely	Giving way more likely
Active movement	May be limited	Usually full but extremes of motion may be painful, catching may occur on movement
Passive movement	Pain at extremes	Pain possible at extreme of flexion
Resisted isometric movement	Normal	Normal unless pinching causes pain and reflex inhibition
Ligament tests	Negative	Negative
Special tests	McMurray test may be positive; Apley's test may be positive	Mediopatellar plica test positive, plica "stutter" test positive, Hughston's plica test positive
Palpation	Joint line tenderness	Plica may demonstrate thickening and be bandlike

References

1. Muller W. Form and function of the knee—its relation to high performance and to sports. *Am J Sports Med.* 1996;24:S104–S106.
2. Kaltenborn F. *Mobilization of the Extremity Joints.* Oslo: Olaf Norles Bokhandel; 1980.
3. Thompson WO, Thaete FL, Fu FH, et al. Tibial meniscal dynamics using three-dimensional reconstruction of magnetic resonance images. *Am J Sports Med.* 1991;19:210–215.
4. Hamamoto K, Tobimatsu Y, Zabinska-Uroda K. Magnetic resonance imaging evaluation of the movement and morphological changes of the meniscus during deep knee flexion. *J Phys Ther Sci.* 2004;16(2):143–149.
5. Arnoczsky S. The blood supply of the meniscus and its role in healing and repair. In: *American Association of Orthopaedic Surgeons, Symposium on Sports Medicine: The Knee.* St Louis: Mosby; 1985.
6. Volashin AS, Wosk J. Shock absorption of meniscectomized and painful knees: a comparative in vivo study. *J Biomech Eng.* 1983;5:157–193.
7. Radin EL, de Lamotte R, Maquet P. Role of the menisci in the distribution of stress in the knee. *Clin Orthop.* 1984;185:290–294.
8. Seedhom BB. Loadbearing function of the menisci. *Physiotherapy.* 1976;62:223–226.
9. Gray JC. Neural and vascular anatomy of the menisci of the human knee. *J Orthop Sports Phys Ther.* 1999;29:23–30.
10. Ficat RP, Hungerford DS. *The Patello-Femoral Joint.* Baltimore: Williams & Wilkins; 1977.
11. Goodfellow J, Hungerford DS, Zindel M. Patellofemoral joint mechanics and pathology: functional anatomy of the patellofemoral joint. *J Bone Joint Surg Br.* 1976;58:287–290.
12. Christoforakis J, Bull AM, Strachan RK, et al. Effects of lateral retinacular release on the lateral stability of the patella. *Knee Surg Sports Traumatol Arthrosc.* 2006;14(3):273–277.
13. Desio SM, Burks RT, Bachus KN. Soft tissue restraints to lateral patellar translation in the human knee. *Am J Sports Med.* 1998;26(1):59–65.

14. Steensen RN, Dopirak RM, McDonald WG. The anatomy and isometry of the medial patellofemoral ligament: implications for reconstruction. *Am J Sports Med.* 2004;32(6):1509–1513.
15. Baldwin JL. The anatomy of the medial patellofemoral ligament. *Am J Sports Med.* 2009;37(12):2355–2361.
16. Nomura E, Inoue M, Osada N. Anatomical analysis of the medial patellofemoral ligament of the knee, especially the femoral attachment. *Knee Surg Sports Traumatol Arthrosc.* 2005;13(7):510–555.
17. Stephen JM, Lumpaopong P, Deehan DJ, et al. The medial patellofemoral ligament: location of the femoral attachment and length change patterns resulting from anatomic and nonanatomic attachments. *Am J Sports Med.* 2012;40(8):1871–1879.
18. Conlan T, Garth WP, Lemons JE. Evaluation of the medial soft-tissue restraints of the extensor mechanism of the knee. *J Bone Joint Surg Am.* 1993;75(5):682–693.
19. Delfico AJ, Garrett WE. Mechanisms of injury of the anterior cruciate ligament in soccer players. *Clin Sports Med.* 1998;17:779–785.
20. Levine JW, Kiapour AM, Quatman CE, et al. Clinically relevant injury patterns after an anterior cruciate ligament injury provide insight into injury mechanisms. *Am J Sports Med.* 2013;41:385–395.
21. Tria AJ, Hosea TM. Diagnosis of knee ligament injuries: clinical. In: Scott WN, ed. *Ligament and Extensor Mechanism Injuries of the Knee: Diagnosis and Treatment.* St Louis: Mosby; 1991.
22. Bauer SJ, Hollander JE, Fuchs SH, et al. A clinical decision rule in the evaluation of acute knee injuries. *J Emerg Med.* 1995;13:611–615.
23. Welton KL, Bernas GA, Wojtys EM. Management of acute knee dislocation before surgical intervention. In: Noyes FR, Barber-Westin SD, eds. *Noyes' Knee Disorders: Surgery Rehabilitation, Clinical Outcomes.* 2nd ed. Philadelphia: Elsevier; 2017.
24. Edwards PH, Grana WA. Physeal fractures about the knee. *J Am Acad Orthop Surg.* 1995;3:63–69.
25. Veenema KR. Valgus knee instability in an adolescent-ligament sprain or physeal injury. *Phys Sportsmed.* 1999;27:62–75.

26. Ahmad CS, Redler LH, Ciccotti MG, et al. Evaluation and management of hamstring injuries. *Am J Sports Med.* 2013;41(12):2933–2947.
27. Gosling LC, Rushton AB. Identification of adult knee primary bone tumor symptom presentation: a qualitative study. *Man Ther.* 2016;26:54–61.
28. Balazs GC, Pavey GJ, Brelin AM, et al. Risk of anterior cruciate ligament injury in athletes on synthetic playing surfaces: a systematic review. *Am J Sports Med.* 2014;43(7):1798–1804.
29. Read PJ, Oliver JL, De Ste Croix MB, et al. Neuromuscular risk factors for knee and ankle ligament injuries in male youth soccer players. *Sports Med.* 2016;46(8):1059–1066.
30. Alentorn-Geli E, Alvarez-Diaz P, Ramon S, et al. Assessment of neuromuscular risk factors for anterior cruciate ligament injury through tensiomyography in male soccer players. *Knee Surg Sports Traumatol Arthrosc.* 2015;23(9):2508–2513.
31. Smeets A, Marfait B, Dingenen B, et al. Is knee neuromuscular activity related to anterior cruciate ligament injury risk? A pilot study. *Knee.* 2019;26(1):40–51.
32. Driban JB, Eaton CB, Lo GH, et al. Knee injuries are associated with accelerated knee osteoarthritis progression: data from the osteoarthritis initiative. *Arthritis Care Res.* 2014;66(11):1673–1679.
33. Ewing KA, Begg RK, Galea MO, Lee PV. Effects of prophylactic knee bracing on lower limb kinematics, kinetics, and energetics during double-leg drop landing at 2 heights. *Am J Sports Med.* 2016;44(7):1753–1761.
34. Levy M, Smith AD. Diagnosing meniscus injuries: focus on the office exam. *Phys Sportsmed.* 1994;22:47–54.
35. Cooper DE. Snapping popliteus syndrome—a cause of mechanical knee popping in athletes. *Am J Sports Med.* 1999;27:671–674.
36. LaPrade CM, Civitarese DM, Rasmussen MT, LaPrade RF. Emerging updates on the posterior cruciate ligament: a review of current literature. *Am J Sports Med.* 2015;43(12):3077–3092.
37. Marshall BM, Franklyn-Miller AD, King EA, et al. Biomechanical factors associated with time to

complete a change of direction cutting maneuver. *J Strength Cond Res.* 2014;28(10):2845–2851.

38. Solomon DH, Simel DL, Bates DW, et al. Does this patient have a torn meniscus or ligament of the knee? Value of the physical examination. *JAMA.* 2001;286(13):1610–1620.

39. Cutbill JW, Ladly KO, Bray RC, et al. Anterior knee pain: a review. *Clin J Sports Med.* 1997;7:40–45.

40. Biedert RM, Sanchis-Alfonso V. Sources of anterior knee pain. *Clin Sports Med.* 2002;21:335–347.

41. Fulkerson JP. Diagnosis and treatment of patients with patellofemoral pain. *Am J Sports Med.* 2002;30:447–456.

42. Post WR, Fulkerson J. Knee pain diagrams: correlation with physical examination findings in patients with anterior knee pain. *Arthroscopy.* 1994;10:618–623.

43. Khan KM, Cook JL, Bonar F, et al. Histopathology of common tendinopathies—update and implications for clinical management. *Sports Med.* 1999;27:393–408.

44. Bassett FH, Soucacous PN, Carr WA. Jumper's knee: patellar tendinitis and patellar tendon rupture. In: *American Academy of Orthopedic Surgeons: Symposium on the Athlete's Knee.* St Louis: Mosby; 1980.

45. Medlar RC, Lyne ED. Sinding-Larsen-Johansson disease. *J Bone Joint Surg Am.* 1978;60:1113–1116.

46. Khan KM, Maffulli N, Coleman BD, et al. Patellar tendinopathy: some aspects of basic science and clinical management. *Br J Sports Med.* 1998;32:346–355.

47. DePalma MJ, Perkins RH. Patellar tendinosis—acute patellar tendon rupture and jumper's knee. *Phys Sportsmed.* 2004;32(5):41–45.

48. Hale SA. Etiology of patellar tendinopathy in athletes. *J Sports Rehab.* 2005;14:258–272.

49. Liorzou G. *Knee Ligaments: Clinical Examination.* Berlin: Springer-Verlag; 1991.

50. Grelsamer RP. Patellar malalignment. *J Bone Joint Surg Am.* 2000;82:1639–1650.

51. Nissen CW, Cullen MC, Hewitt TE, Noyes FR. Physical and arthroscopic examination techniques of the patellofemoral joint. *J Orthop Sports Phys Ther.* 1998;28(5):277–285.

52. Hughston JC. *Knee Ligaments: Injury and Repair.* St Louis: Mosby; 1993.

53. McFarland EG, Mamanee P, Queale WS, et al. Olecranon and prepatellar bursitis. *Phys Sportsmed.* 2000;28(3):40–52.

54. LaPrade RF. The anatomy of the deep infrapatellar bursa of the knee. *Am J Sports Med.* 1998;26:129–132.

55. Fulkerson RP, Hungerford DS. Evaluation and rehabilitation of nonarthritic anterior knee pain. In: Fulkerson JP, Hungerford DS, eds. *Disorders of the Patellofemoral Joint.* Baltimore: Williams & Wilkins; 1990.

56. Hunter DJ, Sharma L, Skaife T. Alignment and osteoarthritis of the knee. *J Bone Joint Surg Am.* 2009;91:85–89.

57. Khan FA, Koff MF, Noiseux NO, et al. Effect of local alignment on compartment patterns of knee osteoarthritis. *J Bone Joint Surg Am.* 2008;90(9):1961–1969.

58. Riegger-Krugh C, Keysor JJ. Skeletal malalignments of the lower quarter: correlated and compensatory motions and postures. *J Orthop Sports Phys Ther.* 1996;23:164–170.

59. Hawkins RJ. *Musculoskeletal Examination.* St Louis: Mosby; 1995.

60. Fulkerson JP, Arendt EA. Anterior knee pain in females. *Clin Orthop Relat Res.* 2000;372:69–73.

61. Boden BP, Pearsall AW, Garrett WE, et al. Patellofemoral instability: evaluation and management. *J Am Acad Orthop Surg.* 1997;5:47–57.

62. Shultz SJ, Nguyen AD, Levine BJ. The relationship between lower extremity alignment characteristics and anterior knee joint laxity. *Sports Health.* 2009;1:54–60.

63. Bell-Jenje T, Olivier B, Wood W, et al. The association between loss of ankle dorsiflexion range of movement, and hip adduction and internal rotation during a step down test. *Man Ther.* 2016;21:256–261.

64. Post WR, Teitge R, Amis A. Patellofemoral malalignment: looking beyond the view box. *Clin Sports Med.* 2002;21:521–546.

65. McConnell J. Management of patellofemoral problems. *Man Ther.* 1996;1:60–66.

66. Loudon JK, Goist HL, Loudon KL. Genu recurvatum syndrome. *J Orthop Sports Phys Ther.* 1998;27:361–367.

67. Grelsamer RP. Patellar nomenclature—the Tower of Babel revisited. *Clin Orthop Relat Res.* 2005;436:60–65.

68. Luyckx T, Didden K, Vandenneucker H, et al. Is there a biomechanical explanation for anterior knee pain in patients with patella alta? *J Bone Joint Surg Br.* 2009;91:344–350.

69. Staheli LT, Engel GM. Tibial torsion: a method of assessment and a survey of normal children. *Clin Orthop.* 1972;86:183–186.

70. Fritschy D, Fasel J, Imbert JC, et al. The popliteal cyst. *Knee Surg Sports Traumatol Arthrosc.* 2006;14(7):623–628.

71. Reider B. *The Orthopedic Physical Examination.* Philadelphia: WB Saunders; 1999.

72. Waldron VD. A test for chondromalacia patellae. *Orthop Rev.* 1983;12:103.

73. Sharma L, Chang AH, Jackson RD, et al. Varus thrust and incident and progressive knee osteoarthritis. *Arthritis Rheumatol.* 2017;69(11):2136–2143.

74. Fukutani N, Iijima H, Fukumoto T, et al. Association of varus thrust with pain and stiffness and activities of daily living in patients with medial knee osteoarthritis. *Phys Ther.* 2016;96(2):167–175.

75. Lo GH, Harvey WF, McAlindon TE. Associations of varus thrust and alignment with pain in knee osteoarthritis. *Arthritis Rheumatol.* 2012;64(7):2252–2259.

76. Sosdian L, Hinman RS, Wrigley TV, et al. Quantifying varus and valgus thrust in individuals with severe knee osteoarthritis. *Clin Biomech.* 2016;39:44–51.

77. Kuroyanagi Y, Nagura T, Kiriyama Y, et al. A quantitative assessment of varus thrust in patients with medial knee osteoarthritis. *Knee.* 2012;19(2):130–134.

78. Hughston JC. Extensor mechanism examination. In: Fox JM, Del Pizzo W, eds. *The Patellofemoral Joint.* New York: McGraw-Hill; 1993.

79. McConnell J, Fulkerson J. The knee: patellofemoral and soft tissue injuries. In: Zachazewski JE, Magee DJ, Quillen WS, eds. *Athletic Injuries and Rehabilitation.* Philadelphia: WB Saunders; 1996.

80. Earl JE, Hertel J, Denegar CR. Patterns of dynamic malalignment, muscle activation, joint motion, and patellofemoral pain syndrome. *J Sports Rehab.* 2005;14:215–233.

81. Arendt E. Anatomy and malalignment of the patellofemoral joint: its relation to patellofemoral arthrosis. *Clin Orthop Relat Res.* 2005;436:71–75.

82. Shibanuma N, Sheehan FT, Stanhope SJ. Limb positioning is critical for defining patellofemoral alignment and femoral shape. *Clin Orthop Relat Res.* 2005;434:198–206.

83. Post WR. Anterior knee pain: diagnosis and treatment. *J Am Acad Orthop Surg.* 2005;13:534–543.

84. Tyler TF, Nicholas SJ, Mullaney MJ, et al. The role of hip muscle function in the treatment of patellofemoral pain syndrome. *Am J Sports Med.* 2006;34:630–636.

85. Gibulka MT, Threlkeld-Watkins J. Patellofemoral pain and asymmetrical hip rotation. *Phys Ther.* 2005;85:1201–1207.

86. Dutton M. *Orthopedic Examination, Evaluation and Intervention.* New York: McGraw Hill; 2004.

87. Fulkerson JP. Patellofemoral pain disorders: evaluation and management. *J Am Acad Orthop Surg.* 1994;2:124–132.

88. Katchburian MV, Ball AM, Shih YF, et al. Measurement of patellar tracking: assessment and analysis of the literature. *Clin Orthop Relat Res.* 2003;412:241–259.

89. Rossi R, Dettoni F, Bruzzone M, et al. Clinical examination of the knee: know your tools for diagnosis of knee injuries. *Sports Med Arthrosc Rehabil Ther Technol.* 2011;3:25–35.

90. Post WR. Clinical evaluation of patients with patellofemoral disorders. *Arthroscopy.* 1999;15:841–851.

91. Nissen CW, Cullen MC, Hewett TE, et al. Physical and arthroscopic examination techniques of the patellofemoral joint. *J Orthop Sports Phys Ther.* 1998;26:277–285.

92. Sheehan FT, Derasari A, Fine KM, et al. Q-angle and J-sign: indicative of maltracking subgroups in patellofemoral pain. *Clin Orthop Relat Res.* 2010;468(1):266–275.

93. Fritz JM, Delitto A, Erhard RE, et al. An examination of the selective tissue tension scheme, with evidence for the concept of a capsular pattern of the knee. *Phys Ther.* 1998;78:1046–1061.

94. Lancaster AR, Nyland J, Roberts CS. The validity of the motion palpation test for determining patellofemoral joint articular cartilage damage. *Phys Ther Sport.* 2007;8:59–65.

95. Jacobson KE, Flandry FC. Diagnosis of anterior knee pain. *Clin Sports Med.* 1989;8:179–195.

96. Kolowich PA, Paulos LE, Rosenberg TD, et al. Lateral release of the patella: indications and contraindications. *Am J Sports Med.* 1990;18:359–365.

97. Rouse SJ. The role of the iliotibial tract in patellofemoral pain and iliotibial band friction syndromes. *Physiotherapy.* 1996;82:199–202.

98. Beaulieu ML, Oh YK, Bedi A, et al. Does limited internal femoral rotation increase peak anterior cruciate ligament strain during a simulated pivot landing? *Am J Sports Med.* 2014;42(12):2955–2963.

99. Cichanowski HR, Schmitt JS, Johnson RJ, et al. Hip strength in collegiate female athletes with patellofemoral pain. *Med Sci Sports Exerc.* 2007;39:1227–1232.

100. Khayambashi K, Ghoddosi N, Staub RK, Powers CM. Hip muscle strength predicts noncontact anterior cruciate ligament injury in male and female athletes: a prospective study. *Am J Sports Med.* 2015;44(2):355–361.

101. Segal P, Jacob M. *The Knee.* Chicago: Year Book Medical; 1983.

102. Liu H, Garrett WE, Moorman CT, Yu B. Injury rate, mechanism, and risk factors of hamstring strain injuries in sports: a review of the literature. *J Sport Health Sci.* 2012;1(2):92–101.

103. Martin HD, Khoury A, Schröder R, Palmer IJ. Ischiofemoral impingement and hamstring syndrome as causes of posterior hip pain: where do we go next? *Clin Sports Med.* 2016;35(3):469–486.

104. Matsuda DK. Editorial commentary: Proximal hamstring syndrome: another pain in the buttock. *Arthroscopy.* 2018;34(1):122–125.

105. Migliorini S, Merlo M. The hamstring syndrome in endurance athletes. *Br J Sports Med.* 2011;45(4):363.

106. Martin RL, Schroder RG, Gomez-Hoyos J, et al. Accuracy of 3 clinical tests to diagnose proximal hamstrings tears with and without sciatic nerve involvement in patients with posterior hip pain. *Arthroscopy.* 2018;34(1):114–121.

107. Kannus P, Jarvineaa M, Latvala K. Knee strength evaluation. *Scand J Sport Sci.* 1987;9(9).

108. Sole G, Hamren J, Milosavljevic S, et al. Test-retest reliability of isokinetic knee extension and flexion. *Arch Phys Med Rehabil.* 2007;88(5):626–631.

109. Goslin BR, Charteris J. Isokinetic dynamometry: normative data for clinical use in lower extremity (knee) cases. *Scand J Rehab Med.* 1979;11:105–109.

110. Stafford MG, Grana WA. Hamstring/quadriceps ratios in college football players: a high velocity evaluation. *Am J Sports Med.* 1984;12:209–211.

111. Aagaard P, Simonsen EB, Magnusson SP, et al. A new concept for isokinetic hamstring: quadriceps muscle strength ratio. *Am J Sports Med.* 1998;26:231–237.

112. Terwee CB, Mokkink LB, Steultjens MPM, et al. Performance-based methods for measuring the physical function of patients with osteoarthritis of the hip or knee: a systematic review of measurement properties. *Rheumatol.* 2006;45:890–902.

113. Di Stasi SL, Logerstedt D, Gardinier ES, Snyder-Mackler L. Gait patterns differ between ACL-reconstructed athletes who pass return-to-sport criteria and those who fail. *Am J Sports Med.* 2013;41(6):1310–1318.

114. Flanigan DC, Everhart JS, Pedroza A, et al. Fear of reinjury (kinesiophobia) and persistent knee symptoms are common factors for lack of return to sport after anterior cruciate ligament reconstruction. *Arthroscopy.* 2013;29(8):1322–1329.

115. Eitzen I, Moksnes H, Snyder-Mackler L, et al. Functional tests should be accentuated more in the decision for ACL reconstruction. *Knee Surg Sports Traumatol Arthrosc.* 2010;18(11):1517–1525.

116. Sgaglione NA, Del Pizzo W, Fox JM, et al. Critical analysis of knee ligament rating systems. *Am J Sports Med.* 1995;23:660–667.

117. Borsa PA, Lephart SM, Irrgang JJ. Sport-specificity of knee scoring systems to assess disability in anterior cruciate ligament-deficient athletes. *J Sports Rehab.* 1998;7:44–60.

118. Wright RW. Knee injury outcomes measures. *J Am Acad Orthop Surg.* 2009;17:31–39.

119. Clark NC. Functional performance testing following knee ligament injury. *Phys Ther Sport.* 2001;2:91–105.

120. Rohman E, Steubs JT, Tompkins M. Changes in involved and uninvolved limb function during rehabilitation after anterior cruciate ligament reconstruction: implications for limb symmetry index measures. *Am J Sports Med.* 2015;43(6):1391–1398.

121. Lawrence S, Killian C, Rundquist P, Jenkins W. Measures of limb symmetry used for injury risk identification: what is normal? *Br J Sports Med.* 2017;51(4):347.

122. Sadeghi H, Allard P, Prince F, Labelle H. Symmetry and limb dominance in able-bodied gait: a review. *Gait Posture.* 2000;12(1):34–45.

123. Fonseca ST, Magee DJ, Wessel J, et al. Validation of a performance test for outcome evaluation of knee function. *Clin J Sport Med.* 1992;2:251–256.

124. Boonstra MC, deWaal Malefijt MC, Verdonschot N. How to quantify knee function after total knee arthroplasty? *The Knee.* 2008;15:390–395.

125. Garratt AM, Brealey S, Gillespie WJ. Patient-assessed health instruments of the knee: a structured review. *Rheumatology.* 2003;43:1414–1423.

126. Paxton EW, Fithian DC, Stone ML, et al. The reliability and validity of knee specific: general health instruments in assessing acute patellar dislocation outcomes. *Am J Sports Med.* 2003;31:487–492.

127. Daniel DM, Stone ML, Riehl B. Ligament surgery: the evaluation of results. In: Daniel D, Akeson W, O'Conner J, eds. *Knee Ligaments: Structure, Injury and Repair.* New York: Raven Press; 1990.

128. Strobel M, Stedtfeld HW. *Diagnostic Evaluation of the Knee.* Berlin: Springer-Verlag; 1990.

129. Noyes FR, Barber SD, Mangine RE. Abnormal lower limb symmetry determined by functional hop tests after anterior cruciate rupture. *Am J Sports Med.* 1991;19:513–518.

130. Barber SD, Noyes FR, Mangine RE, et al. Quantitative assessment of functional limitations in normal and anterior cruciate ligament-deficient knees. *Clin Orthop.* 1990;255:204–214.

131. Grindem H, Logerstedt D, Eitzen I, et al. Single-legged hip tests as predictors of self-reported knee function in nonoperatively treated individuals with anterior cruciate ligament injury. *Am J Sports Med.* 2011;39:2347–2354.

132. O'Donnell SO, Thomas SG, Marks P. Improving the sensitivity of the hop index in patients with an ACL deficient knee by transforming the hop distance scores. *BMC Musculoskelet Disord.* 2006;7:9–14.

133. Hopper DM, Goh SC, Wentworth LA, et al. Test-retest reliability of knee rating scales and functional hop tests one year following anterior cruciate ligament reconstruction. *Phys Ther Sport.* 2002;3:10–18.

134. Gokeler A, Welling W, Benjaminse A, et al. A critical analysis of limb symmetry indices of hop tests in athletes after anterior cruciate reconstruction: a case control study. *Orthop Traumatol Surg Res.* 2017;103(6):947–951.

135. Zwolski C, Schmitt LC, Thomas S, et al. The utility of limb symmetry indices in return-to-sport assessment in patients with bilateral anterior cruciate ligament reconstruction. *Am J Sports Med.* 2016;44(8):2030–2038.

136. Fitzgerald GK, Axe MJ, Snyder-Mackler L. A decision-making scheme for returning patients to high-level activity with nonoperative treatment after anterior cruciate ligament rupture. *Knee Surg Sports Traumatol Arthrosc.* 2000;8(2):76–82.

137. Davies GJ. Individualizing the return to sports after anterior cruciate ligament reconstruction. *Oper Tech Orthop.* 2017;27(1):70–78.

138. Hegedus EJ, McDonough S, Bleakly C, et al. Clinician-friendly lower extremity physical performance measures in athletes: a systematic review of measurement properties and correlation with injury, part 1. The tests for knee function including the hop tests. *Br J Sports Med.* 2015;49(10):642–648.

139. Hegedus EJ, McDonough S, Bleakly C, et al. Clinician-friendly lower extremity physical performance measures in athletes: a systematic review of measurement properties and correlation with injury, part 2. The tests for the hip, thigh, foot and ankle including the star excursion balance test. *Br J Sports Med.* 2015;49(10):649–656.

140. Wellsandt E, Failla MJ, Synder-Mackler L. Limb symmetry indexes can overestimate knee function after anterior cruciate ligament injury. *J Orthop Sports Phys Ther.* 2017;47(5):334–338.

141. Juris PM, Phillips EM, Dalpe C, et al. A dynamic test of lower extremity function following anterior cruciate ligament reconstruction and rehabilitation. *J Orthop Sports Phys Ther.* 1997;26:184–191.

142. Augustsson J, Thomeé R, Karlsson J. Ability of a new hop test to determine functional deficits after anterior cruciate ligament reconstruction. *Knee Surg Sports Traumatol Arthrosc.* 2004;12:350–356.

143. Begalle RL, Distefano LJ, Blackburn T, Padua DA. Quadriceps and hamstrings coactivation during common therapeutic exercises. *J Athl Train.* 2012;47(4):396–405.

144. Jang SH, Kim JG, Ha JK, et al. Functional performance tests as indicators of returning to sports after anterior cruciate ligament construction. *Knee.* 2014;21(1):95–101.

145. Lee DW, Yang SJ, Cho SI, et al. Single-leg vertical jump test as a functional test after anterior cruciate ligament reconstruction. *Knee.* 2018;25(6):1016–1026.

146. Logerstedt DS, Snyder-Mackler L, Ritter RC, et al. Knee stability and movement coordination impairments: knee ligament sprain. *J Orthop Sports Phys Ther.* 2010;40:A1–A37.

147. Penna A, Bullock G, Ubben C, et al. Single limb hop tests, Rehabilitation Measures Database; 2015. Available at https://www.sralab.org/rehabilitation-measures.

148. Booher LD, Hench KM, Worrell TW, et al. Reliability of three single-leg hop tests. *J Sports Rehab.* 1993;2:165–170.

149. Krishnan C. Are practice trials required for hop tests? *Gait Posture.* 2015;41(4):960–963.

150. Myers BA, Jenkins WL, Killian C, Rundquist P. Normative data for hop tests in high school and collegiate basketball and soccer players. *Int J Sports Physical Ther.* 2014;9(5):596–603.

151. Risberg MA, Ekeland A. Assessment of functional tests after anterior cruciate ligament surgery. *J Orthop Sports Phys Ther.* 1994;19:212–217.

152. Gustavsson A, Neeter C, Thomeé P, et al. A test battery for evaluating hop performance in patients with an ACL injury and patients who have undergone ACL reconstruction. *Knee Surg Sports Traumatol Arthrosc.* 2006;14(8):778–788.

153. Itoh H, Kurosaka M, Yoshiya S, et al. Evaluation of functional deficits determined by four different hop tests in patients with anterior cruciate ligament deficiency. *Knee Surg Sports Traumatol Arthrosc.* 1998;6(4):241–245.

154. Losee RE. Diagnosis of chronic injury to the anterior cruciate ligament. *Orthop Clin North Am.* 1985;16:83–97.

155. Jackson DW, Jennings LD, Maywoods RM, et al. Magnetic resonance imaging of the knee. *Am J Sports Med.* 1988;16:29–37.

156. Larson RL. Physical examination in the diagnosis of rotary instability. *Clin Orthop.* 1983;172:38–44.

157. Onate J, Cortes N, Welch C, Van Lunen B. Expert versus novice interrater reliability and criterion validity of the landing error scoring system. *J Sport Rehabil.* 2010;19(1):41–56.

158. Jones PA, Herrington LC, Munro AG, Graham-Smith P. Is there a relationship between landing, cutting, and pivoting tasks in terms of the characteristics of dynamic valgus? *Am J Sports Med.* 2015;42(9):2095–2102.

159. Lentz TA, Zeppieri G, George SZ, et al. Comparison of physical impairment, functional, and psychosocial measures based on fear of reinjury/lack of confidence and return-to-sport status after ACL reconstruction. *Am J Sports Med.* 2015;43(2):345–353.

160. Filbay SR, Crossley KM, Ackerman IN. Activity preferences, lifestyle modifications and re-injury fears influence longer-term quality of life in people with knee symptoms following anterior cruciate ligament reconstruction: a qualitative study. *J Physiother.* 2016;62:103–110.

161. Ardern CL, Taylor NF, Feller JA, Webster KE. Fear of re-injury in people who have returned to sport following anterior cruciate ligament reconstruction surgery. *J Sci Med Sport.* 2012;15(6):488–495.

162. Harput G, Ulusoy B, Ozer H, et al. External supports improve knee performance in anterior cruciate ligament reconstructed individuals with higher kinesiophobia levels. *Knee.* 2016;23(5):807–813.

163. Panken AM, Heymans MW, van Oort L, Verhagen AP. Clinical prognostic factors for patients with anterior knee pain in physical therapy; a systematic review. *Int J Sports Phys Ther.* 2015;10(7):929–945.

164. Ardern CL, Webster KE, Taylor NF, Feller JA. Return to sport following anterior cruciate ligament reconstruction surgery: a systematic review and meta-analysis of the state of play. *Br J Sports Med*. 2011;45(7):596–606.

165. Podlog L, Dimmock J, Miller J. A review of return to sport concerns following injury rehabilitation: practitioner strategies for enhancing recovery outcomes. *Phys Ther Sport*. 2011;12(1):36–42.

166. Tjong VK, Murnaghan ML, Nyhof-Young JM, Ogilvie-Harris DJ. A qualitative investigation of the decision to return to sport after anterior cruciate ligament construction: to play or not to play. *Am J Sports Med*. 2014;42(2):336–342.

167. Garrison JC, Shanley E, Thigpen C, et al. The reliability of the Vail Sport Test™ as a measure of physical performance following anterior cruciate ligament reconstruction. *Int J Sports Phys Ther*. 2012;7(1):20–30.

168. Williams D, Heidloff D, Haglage E, et al. Anterior cruciate ligament functional sports assessment. *Oper Tech Sports Med*. 2015;24:59–64.

169. Hildebrandt C, Müller L, Zisch B, et al. Functional assessments for decision-making regarding return to sports following ACL reconstruction. Part 1: development of a new test battery. *Knee Surg Sports Traumatol Arthrosc*. 2015;23:1273–1281.

170. Myer GD, Schmitt LS, Brent JL, et al. Utilization of modified NFL combine testing to identify functional deficits in athletes following ACL reconstruction. *J Orthop Sports Phys Ther*. 2011;41(6):377–387.

171. Lin YC, Davey RC, Cochrane T. Tests for physical function of the elderly with hip and knee osteoarthritis. *Scand J Med Sci Sports*. 2001;11(5):280–286.

172. Demirdjian AM, Petrie SG, Guanche CA, et al. The outcomes of two knee scoring questionnaires in a normal population. *Am J Sports Med*. 1998;26:46–51.

173. Hoher J, Bach T, Munster A, et al. Does the mode of data collection change result in a subjective knee score? Self administration vs. interview. *Am J Sports Med*. 1997;25:642–647.

174. Marx RG. Knee rating scales. *Arthroscopy*. 2003;19(10):1103–1108.

175. Barber-Westin SD, Noyes FR. Rating of athletic and daily functional activities: knee specific scales and global outcome instruments. In: Noyes FR, Barber-Westin SD, eds. *Noyes' Knee Disorders: Surgery Rehabilitation, Clinical Outcomes*. 2nd ed. Philadelphia: Elsevier; 2017.

176. Noyes FR, Barber-Westin SD. Cincinnati knee rating system. In: Noyes FR, Barber-Westin SD, eds. *Noyes' Knee Disorders: Surgery Rehabilitation, Clinical Outcomes*. 2nd ed. Philadelphia: Elsevier; 2017.

177. Noyes FR, McGinniss GH, Mooar LA. Functional disability in the anterior cruciate insufficient knee syndrome: review of knee rating systems and projected risk factors in determining treatment. *Sports Med*. 1984;1:278–302.

178. Noyes FR, Barber SD, Mooar LA. A rationale for assessing sports activity levels and limitations in knee disorders. *Clin Orthop*. 1989;246:238–249.

179. Barber-Westin SD, Noyes FR, McCloskey JW. Rigorous statistical reliability, validity and responsiveness testing on the Cincinnati knee rating system in 350 subjects with uninjured, injured, or anterior cruciate ligament-reconstructed knees. *Am J Sports Med*. 1999;27:402–416.

180. Agel J, LaPrade RF. Assessment of differences between the modified Cincinnati and International Knee Documentation Committee patient outcome scores—a prospective study. *Am J Sports Med*. 2009;37:2151–2157.

181. Irrgang JC, Safran MC, Fu FH. The knee: ligamentous and meniscal injuries. In: Zachazewski JE, Magee DJ, Quillen WS, eds. *Athletic Injuries and Rehabilitation*. Philadelphia: WB Saunders; 1996.

182. Irrgang JJ, Snyder-Mackler L, Wainner RS, et al. Development of a patient-reported measure of function of the knee. *J Bone Joint Surg Am*. 1998;80:1132–1145.

183. Insall JN, Dorr LD, Scott RD, et al. Rationale of the Knee Society clinical rating system. *Clin Orthop*. 1989;248:13–14.

184. Lysholm J, Gillquist J. Evaluation of knee ligament surgery results with special emphasis on use of a scoring scale. *Am J Sports Med*. 1982;10:150–154.

185. Briggs KK, Lysholm J, Tegner Y, et al. The reliability, validity and responsiveness of the Lysholm Score and Tegner Activity Scale for anterior cruciate injuries of the knee. *Am J Sports Med*. 2009;37:890–897.

186. Heintjes EM, Bierma-Zeinstra SM, Berger MY, et al. Lysholm scale and WOMAC index were responsive in prospective cohort of young general practice patients. *J Clin Epidemiol*. 2008;61:481–488.

187. Smith HJ, Richardson JB, Tennant A. Modification and validation of the Lysholm knee scale to assess articular cartilage damage. *Osteoarthritis Cartilage*. 2009;17:53–58.

188. Kocher MS, Steadman JR, Briggs KK, et al. Reliability, validity and responsiveness of the Lysholm knee scale for various chondral disorders of the knee. *J Bone Joint Surg Am*. 2004;86:1139–1145.

189. Briggs KK, Steadman JR, Hay CJ, et al. Lysholm Score and Tegner Activity Level in individuals with normal knees. *Am J Sports Med*. 2009;37:898–901.

190. Ilefti F, Mullen W, Jakob RP, et al. Evaluation of knee ligament injuries with the IKDC form. *Knee Surg Sports Traumatol Arthrosc*. 1993;1:226–234.

191. Anderson AF, Irrgang JJ, Kocher MS, et al. The international knee documentation committee subjective knee evaluation form—normative data. *Am J Sports Med*. 2006;34:128–135.

192. Kocher MS, Smith JT, Iverson MD, et al. Reliability, validity and responsiveness of a modified international knee documentation committee subjective knee form (Pedi-IKDC) in children with knee disorders. *Am J Sports Med*. 2011;39:933–939.

193. Schmitt LC, Paterno MV, Huang S. Validity and internal consistency of the International Knee Documentation Committee subjective knee evaluation form in children and adolescents. *Am J Sports Med*. 2010;38:2443–2447.

194. Greco NJ, Anderson AF, Mann BJ, et al. Responsiveness of the International Knee Documentation Committee subjective knee form in comparison to the Western Ontario and McMaster Universities Osteoarthritis Index, Modified Cincinnati knee rating system and short form 36 in patients with focal articular cartilage defects. *Am J Sports Med*. 2010;38:891–902.

195. Hambly K, Griva K. IKDC or KOOS—which one captures symptoms and disabilities most important to patients who have undergone initial anterior cruciate ligament reconstruction. *Am J Sports Med*. 2010;38:1395–1404.

196. Oak SR, O'Rourke C, Strnad G, et al. Statistical comparison of the pediatric versus adult IKDC subjective knee evaluation form in adolescents. *Am J Sports Med*. 2015;43(9):2216–2221.

197. van de Graaf VA, Wolterbeek N, Scholtes VA, et al. Reliability and validity of the IKDC, KOOS, and WOMAC for patients with meniscus injuries. *Am J Sports Med*. 2014;42(6):1408–1416.

198. Collins NJ, Misra D, Felson DT, et al. Measures of knee function: International Knee Documentation Committee (IKDC) Subjective Knee Evaluation Form, Knee Injury and Osteoarthritis Outcome Score (KOOS), Knee Injury and Osteoarthritis Outcome Score Physical Function Short Form (KOOS-PS), Knee Outcome Survey Activities of Daily Living Scale (KOS-ADL), Lysholm Knee Scoring Scale, Oxford Knee Score (OKS), Western Ontario and McMaster Universities Osteoarthritis Index (WOMAC), Activity Rating Scale (ARS), and Tegner Activity Score (TAS). *Arthritis Care Res*. 2011;63:S208–S228.

199. Nasreddine AY, Connell PL, Kalish LA, et al. The Pediatric International Knee Documentation Committee (Pedi-IKDC) subjective knee evaluation form: normative data. *Am J Sports Med*. 2017;45(3):527–534.

200. Décary S, Ouellet P, Vendittoli PA, Desmeules F. Reliability of physical examination tests for the diagnosis of knee disorders: evidence from a systematic review. *Man Ther*. 2016;26:172–182.

201. Barber-Westin SD, Noyes FR. International knee documentation committee rating system. In: Noyes FR, Barber-Westin SD, eds. *Noyes' Knee Disorders: Surgery Rehabilitation, Clinical Outcomes*. 2nd ed. Philadelphia: Elsevier; 2017.

202. Tegner Y, Lysholm J, Odensten M, et al. Evaluation of cruciate ligament injuries. *Acta Orthop Scand*. 1988;59:336–341.

203. Letchford R, Button K, Sparkes V, van Deursen R. Assessing activity participation in the ACL injured population: a systematic review of activity rating scale measurement properties. *Phys Ther Rev*. 2012;17(2):99–109.

204. Bell DR, Pfeiffer KA, Cadmus-Bertram LA, et al. Objectively measured physical activity in patients after anterior cruciate ligament reconstruction. *Am J Sports Med*. 2017;45(8):1893–1900.

205. Webster KE, Feller JA, Lambros C. Development and preliminary validation of a scale to measure the psychological impact of returning to sport following anterior cruciate ligament reconstruction surgery. *Phys Ther Sport*. 2008;9(1):9–15.

206. Thomeé P, Wahrborg P, Borjesson M, et al. A new instrument for measuring self-efficacy in patients with anterior cruciate ligament injury. *Scand J Med Sci Sports*. 2006;16(3):181–187.

207. Marx RG, Stump TJ, Jones EC, et al. Development and evaluation of an activity rating scale for disorders of the knee. *Am J Sports Med*. 2001;29(2):213–218.

208. Cox CL, Huston LJ, Dunn WR, et al. Are articular cartilage lesions and meniscus tears predictive of IKDC, KOOS, and Marx Activity level outcomes after ACL reconstruction? A 6-year multicentre cohort study. *Am J Sports Med*. 2014;42(5):1058–1067.

209. Shirazi CP, Israel HA, Kaar SG. Is the Marx Activity Scale reliable in patients younger than 18 years? *Sports Health*. 2015;8(2):145–148.

210. Cameron KL, Peck KY, Thompson BS, et al. Reference values for the Marx Activity Rating Scale in a young athletic population: history of knee ligament injury is associated with higher scores. *Sports Health*. 2015;7(5):403–408.

211. Hiemstra LA, Kerslake S, Lefaave MR, et al. Initial validity and reliability of the Banff Patella Instability Instrument. *Am J Sports Med*. 2013;41(7):1629–1635.

212. Hiemstra LA, Kerslake S, Lefaave MR, et al. Concurrent validation of the Banff Patella Instability Instrument to the Norwich Patellar Instability Score and the Kujala Score in Patients with patellofemoral instability. *Orthop J Sports Med*. 2016;4(5):2325967116646085.

213. Barber-Westin SD, Noyes FR. Knee arthroplasty and patellofemoral rating systems. In: Noyes FR, Barber-Westin SD, eds. *Noyes' Knee Disorders: Surgery Rehabilitation, Clinical Outcomes*. 2nd ed. Philadelphia: Elsevier; 2017.

214. Shea KP, Fulkerson JP. Preoperative computed tomography scanning and arthroscopy in predicting outcome after lateral retinacular release. *Arthroscopy.* 1992;8:327–334.

215. Karlsson J, Thomeé R, Sward L. Eleven year follow up of patellofemoral pain syndromes. *Clin J Sport Med.* 1996;6:22–26.

216. Ittenbach RF, Huang G, Berber Foss KD, et al. Reliability and validity of the anterior knee pain scale: applications for use as an epidemiologic screener. *PLoS One.* 2016;11(7):e159204.

217. Crossley KM, Bennell KL, Cowan SM, et al. Analysis of outcome measurement for persons with patellofemoral pain: which are reliable and valid? *Arch Phys Med Rehabil.* 2004;85:815–822.

218. Green A, Liles C, Rushton A, Kyte DG. Measurement properties of patient-reported outcome measures (PROMS) in patellofemoral pain syndrome: a systematic review. *Man Ther.* 2014;19:517–526.

219. Kujala UM, Jaakkola LH, Koskinen SK, et al. Scoring of patellofemoral disorders. *Arthroscopy.* 1993;9:159–163.

220. Bennell K, Bartam S, Crossley K, et al. Outcome measures in patellofemoral pain syndrome: test retest reliability and inter-relationships. *Phys Ther Sport.* 2000;1:31–41.

221. Eng J, Pierrynowski MR. Evaluation of soft shoe orthotics in the treatment of patellofemoral pain syndrome. *Phys Ther.* 1993;73:62–68.

222. Flandry F, Hunt J, Terry G, et al. Analysis of subjective knee complaints using visual analog scales. *Am J Sports Med.* 1991;19:112–118.

223. Clarsen B, Myklebust G, Bahr R. Development and validation of a new method for the registration of overuse injuries in sports injury epidemiology: the Oslo Sports Trauma Research Centre (OSTROC) Overuse Injury Questionnaire. *Br J Sports Med.* 2013;47:495–502.

224. Andersen CA, Clarsen B, Johansen TV, Engebretsen L. High prevalence of overuse injury among iron–distance triathletes. *Br J Sports Med.* 2013;47(13):857–861.

225. Clarsen B, Ronsen O, Myklebust G, et al. The Oslo Sports Trauma Research Center Questionnaire on health problems: a new approach to prospective monitoring of illness and injury in elite athletes. *Br J Sports Med.* 2014;48:754–760.

226. Jinks C, Jordan K, Croft P. Measuring the population impact of knee pain and disability with the Western Ontario and McMaster Universities Osteoarthritis Index (WOMAC). *Pain.* 2002;100:55–64.

227. Samuelsson K, Magnussen RA, Alentorn-Geli E, et al. Equivalent knee injury and osteoarthritis outcome scores 12 and 24 months after anterior cruciate ligament reconstruction: results from the Swedish National Knee Ligament Register. *Am J Sports Med.* 2017;45(9):2085–2091.

228. Williamson T, Sikka R, Tompkins M, Nelson BJ. Use of the knee injury and osteoarthritis outcome score in a healthy United States population. *Am J Sports Med.* 2015;44(2):440–446.

229. Roos EM, Roos HP, Lohmander LS, et al. Knee injury and osteoarthritis outcome score (KOOS) development of a self-administered outcome measure. *J Orthop Sports Phys Ther.* 1998;78:88–96.

230. Roos EM, Lohmander LS. The Knee Injury and Osteoarthritis Outcome Score (KOOS): from joint injury to osteoarthritis. *Health Qual Life Outcomes.* 2003;1:64–72.

231. Muller B, Yabroudi MA, Lynch A, et al. Defining thresholds for the patient acceptable symptom state for the IKDC subjective knee form and KOOS for patients who underwent ACL reconstruction. *Am J Sports Med.* 2016;41(11):2820–2826.

232. Garratt AM, Brealey S, Robling M, et al. Development of the knee quality of life (KQual-26) 26-item questionnaire: data quality, reliability, validity and responsiveness. *Health Quality Life Outcomes.* 2008;6:48–59.

233. Brazier JE, Harper R, Munro J, et al. Generic and condition-specific outcome measures for people with osteoarthritis of the knee. *Rheumatology.* 1999;38:870–877.

234. Anderson JG, Wixson RL, Tsai D, et al. Functional outcome and patient satisfaction in total knee patients over the age of 75. *J Arthroplasty.* 1996;11:831–840.

235. Kreibich DN, Vaz M, Bourne RB, et al. What is the best way of assessing outcome after total knee replacement? *Clin Orthop Relat Res.* 1996;331:221–225.

236. Kantz ME, Harris WJ, Levitsky K, et al. Methods for assessing condition-specific and generic functional status outcomes after total knee replacement. *Med Care.* 1992;30(5):MS240–MS252.

237. Bombardier C, Melfi CA, Paul J, et al. Comparison of a generic and a disease-specific measure of pain and physical function after knee replacement surgery. *Med Care.* 1995;33:AS131–AS144.

238. Hartley RC, Barton-Hanson NG, Finley R, et al. Early patient outcomes after primary and revision total knee arthroplasty—a prospective study. *J Bone Joint Surg Br.* 2002;84:994–999.

239. Faucher M, Poiraudeau S, Lefevre-Colan MM, et al. Assessment of the test-retest reliability and construct validity of a modified Lequesne Index in knee osteoarthritis. *Joint Bone Spine.* 2003;70:520–525.

240. Faucher M, Poiraudeau S, Lefevre-Colan MM, et al. Algo-functional assessment of knee osteoarthritis: comparison of the test-retest reliability and construct validity of the WOMAN and Lequesne Indexes. *Osteoarthritis Cartilage.* 2002;10:602–610.

241. Roos EM, Toksvig-Larsen S. Knee Injury and Osteoarthritis Outcome Score (KOOS)—validation and comparison to the WOMAN in total knee replacements. *Health Qual Life Outcomes.* 2003;1:17–27.

242. Rejeski WJ, Ettinger WH, Schumaker S, et al. Assessing performance-related disability in patients with knee osteoarthritis. *Osteoarthritis Cartilage.* 1995;3:157–167.

243. Kettlekamp DB, Thompson C. Development of a knee scoring scale. *Clin Orthop.* 1975;107:93–99.

244. Aichroth P, Freeman MA, Smillie IS, et al. A knee function assessment chart. *J Bone Joint Surg Br.* 1978;60:308–309.

245. Larson R. Rating sheet for knee function. In: Smillie I, ed. *Diseases of the Knee Joint.* Edinburgh: Churchill Livingstone; 1974.

246. Selfe J, Harper L, Pederson I, et al. Four outcome measures for patellofemoral joint problems. 1. development and validity. *Physiotherapy.* 2001;87:507–515.

247. Selfe J, Harper L, Pederson I, et al. Four outcome measures for patellofemoral joint problems. 2. reliability and clinical sensitivity. *Physiotherapy.* 2001;87:516–522.

248. Kittl C, El-Daou H, Athwal KK, et al. The role of the anterolateral structures and the ACL in controlling laxity of the intact and ACL-deficient knee. *Am J Sports Med.* 2015;44(2):345–354.

249. Shoemaker SC, Daniel DM. The limits of knee motion: in vitro studies. In: Daniel D, Akeson W, O'Conner J, eds. *Knee Ligaments: Structure, Injury and Repair.* New York: Raven Press; 1990.

250. LaPrade RF, Engebretsen AH, Ly TV, et al. The anatomy of the medial part of the knee. *J Bone Joint Surg Am.* 2007;89(9):2000–2010.

251. James EW, LaPrade CM, LaPrade RF. Anatomy and biomechanics of the lateral side of the knee and surgical implications. *Sports Med Arthrosc Rev.* 2015;23(1):2–9.

252. Recondo JA, Salvador E, Villanúa JA, et al. Lateral stabilizing structures of the knee: functional anatomy and injuries assessed with MR imaging. *Radiographics.* 2000;20:S91–S102.

253. LaPrade RF, Morgan PM, Wentorf FA, et al. The anatomy of the posterior aspect of the knee. An anatomic study. *J Bone Joint Surg Am.* 2007;89(4):758–764.

254. LaPrade RF, Johansen S, Wentorf FA, et al. An analysis of an anatomical posterolateral knee reconstruction: an in vitro biomechanical study and development of a surgical technique. *Am J Sports Med.* 2004;32(6):1405–1414.

255. LaPrade RF, Ly TV, Wentorf FA, Engebretsen L. The posterolateral attachments of the knee: a qualitative and quantitative morphologic analysis of the fibular collateral ligament, popliteus tendon, popliteofibular ligament, and lateral gastrocnemius tendon. *Am J Sports Med.* 2003;31(6):854–860.

256. Muller W. *The Knee: Form, Function and Ligament Reconstruction.* New York: Springer-Verlag; 1983.

257. Detenbeck LC. Function of the cruciate ligaments in knee stability. *Am J Sports Med.* 1974;2:217–221.

258. DeFranco MJ, Bach BR. A comprehensive review of partial anterior cruciate ligament tears. *J Bone Joint Surg Am.* 2009;91:198–208.

259. Wu JL, Seon JK, Gadikota HR, et al. In situ forces in the anteromedial and posterolateral bundles of the anterior cruciate ligament under simulated functional loading conditions. *Am J Sports Med.* 2010;38:558–563.

260. Furman W, Marshall JL, Girgis FG. The anterior cruciate ligament: a functional analysis based on postmortem studies. *J Bone Joint Surg Am.* 1976;58:179–185.

261. Girgis FG, Marshall JL, Al Monajem ARS. The cruciate ligaments of the knee joint: anatomical, functional and experimental analysis. *Clin Orthop.* 1975;106:216–231.

262. Baker CL, Norwood LA, Hughston JC. Acute combined posterior and posterolateral instability of the knee. *Am J Sports Med.* 1984;12:204–208.

263. LaPrade RF, Wozniczka JK, Stellmaker MP, et al. Analysis of the static function of the popliteus tendon and evaluation of an anatomic reconstruction—the "fifth ligament" of the knee. *Am J Sports Med.* 2010;38:543–549.

264. Morgan PM, LaPrade RF, Wentorf FA, et al. The role of the oblique popliteal ligament and other structures in preventing knee hyperextension. *Am J Sports Med.* 2010;38:550–557.

265. Malanga GA, Andrus S, Nadler SF, et al. Physical examination of the knee: a review of common orthopaedic tests. *Arch Phys Med Rehabil.* 2003;84:592–603.

266. Daniel DM. Diagnosis of a ligament injury. In: Daniel D, Akeson W, O'Conner J, eds. *Knee Ligaments: Structure, Injury and Repair.* New York: Raven Press; 1990.

267. Antunes LC, de Souza JM, Cerqueira NB, et al. Evaluation of clinical tests and magnetic resonance imaging for knee meniscal injuries: correlation with video arthroscopy. *Rev Bras Ortop.* 2017;52(5):582–588.

268. Deveci A, Cankaya D, Yilmaz S, et al. The arthroscopical and radiological correlation of lever sign test for the diagnosis of anterior cruciate ligament rupture. *Springerplus.* 2015;4:830–835.

269. Marshall JL, Baugher WH. Stability examination of the knee: a single anatomic approach. *Clin Orthop.* 1980;146:78–83.

270. Swain MS, Henschke N, Kamper SJ, et al. Accuracy of clinical tests in the diagnosis of anterior cruciate ligament injury: a systematic review. *Chiropr Man Therap.* 2014;22:25–35.

271. Cleland JA, Koppenhaver S. *Netter's Orthopedic Clinical Examination—An Evidence Based Approach.* 2nd ed. Philadelphia: Saunders/Elsevier; 2011.

272. Lonergan KT, Taylor DC. Medial collateral ligament injuries of the knee: an evolution of surgical reconstruction. *Tech Knee Surg.* 2002;1(2):137–145.

273. Marchant MH, Tibor LM, Sekiya JK, et al. Management of medial-sided knee injuries, part 1: medial collateral ligament. *Am J Sports Med.* 2011;39:1102–1113.

274. Kennedy JC. *The Injured Adolescent Knee.* Baltimore: Williams & Wilkins; 1979.

275. LaPrade RF, Bernhardson AS, Griffith CJ, et al. Correlation of valgus stress radiographs with medial knee ligament injuries—an in vitro biomechanical study. *Am J Sports Med.* 2010;38:330–338.

276. Lange T, Freiberg A, Dröge P, et al. The reliability of physical examination tests for the diagnosis of anterior cruciate ligament rupture – a systematic review. *Man Ther.* 2015;20(3):402–411.

277. Wagemakers HP, Luijsterburg PA, Boks SS, et al. Diagnostic accuracy of history taking and physical examination for assessing anterior cruciate ligament lesions of the knee in primary care. *Arch Phys Med Rehabil.* 2010;91(9):1452–1459.

278. Daniel DM, Stone ML, Barnett P, et al. Use of the quadriceps active test to diagnose posterior cruciate ligament disruption and measure posterior laxity of the knee. *J Bone Joint Surg Am.* 1988;70:386–391.

279. Veltri DM, Warren RF. Isolated and combined posterior cruciate ligament injuries. *J Am Acad Orthop Surg.* 1993;1:67–75.

280. De Lee JC. Ligamentous injury of the knee. In: Stanitski CL, DeLee JC, Drez D, eds. *Pediatric and Adolescent Sports Medicine.* Philadelphia: WB Saunders; 1994.

281. Butler DL, Noyes FR, Grood ES. Ligamentous restraints to anterior-posterior drawer in the human knee. *J Bone Joint Surg Am.* 1980;62:259–270.

282. Weatherwax RJ. Anterior drawer sign. *Clin Orthop.* 1981;154:318–319.

283. Hughston JC. The absent posterior drawer test in some acute posterior cruciate ligament tears of the knee. *Am J Sports Med.* 1988;16:39–43.

284. Warren RF. Physical diagnosis of the knee. In: Post M, ed. *Physical Examination of the Musculoskeletal System.* Chicago: Year Book Medical; 1987.

285. Feagin JA. *The Crucial Ligaments.* Edinburgh: Churchill Livingstone; 1988.

286. Jonsson T, Althoff B, Peterson L, et al. Clinical diagnosis of ruptures of the anterior cruciate ligament: a comparative study of the Lachman test and the anterior drawer sign. *Am J Sports Med.* 1982;10:100–102.

287. Paessler HH, Michel D. How new is the Lachman test? *Am J Sports Med.* 1992;20:95–98.

288. Torg JS, Conrad W, Allen V. Clinical diagnosis of anterior cruciate ligament instability in the athlete. *Am J Sports Med.* 1976;4:84–93.

289. Jackson R. The torn ACL: natural history of untreated lesions and rationale for selective treatment. In: Feagin JA, ed. *The Crucial Ligaments.* Edinburgh: Churchill Livingstone; 1988.

290. Rosenberg TD, Rasmussen GL. The function of the anterior cruciate ligament during anterior drawer and Lachman's testing. *Am J Sports Med.* 1984;12:318–322.

291. Logan MC, Williams A, Lavelle J, et al. What really happens during the Lachman test—a dynamic MRI analysis of tibiofemoral motion. *Am J Sports Med.* 2004;32:369–375.

292. Cooperman JM, Riddle DL, Rothstein JM. Reliability and validity of judgments of the integrity of the anterior cruciate ligament of the knee using the Lachman's test. *Phys Ther.* 1990;70:225–233.

293. Johnson DS, Ryan WG, Smith RB. Does the Lachman testing method affect the reliability of the International Knee Documentation Committee (IKDC) Form? *Knee Surg Sports Traumatol Arthrosc.* 2004;12(3):225–228.

294. Kuroda R, Hoshino Y, Kubo S, et al. Similarities and differences of diagnostic manual tests for anterior cruciate ligament insufficiency: a global survey and kinematics assessment. *Am J Sports Med.* 2012;40(1):91–99.

295. Mulligan EP, Anderson A, Watson S, Dimeff RJ. The diagnostic accuracy of the lever sign for detecting anterior cruciate ligament injury. *Int J Sports Phys Ther.* 2017;12(7):1057–1067.

296. Scholten RJ, Opstelten W, Van der Plas CG, et al. Accuracy of physical diagnostic tests for assessing ruptures of the anterior cruciate ligament: a meta-analysis. *J Fam Pract.* 2003;52(9):689–694.

297. Frank C. Accurate interpretation of the Lachman test. *Clin Orthop.* 1986;213:163–166.

298. Bechtel SL. Ellman BR, Jordon JL. Skier's knee: the cruciate connection. *Phys Sports Med.* 1984;12:50–54.

299. Wroble RR, Lindenfeld TN. The stabilized Lachman test. *Clin Orthop.* 1988;237:209–212.

300. Adler GG, Hockman RA, Beach DM. Drop leg Lachman test—a new test of anterior knee laxity. *Am J Sports Med.* 1995;23:320–323.

301. Rebman LW. Lachman's test: an alternative method. *J Orthop Sports Phys Ther.* 1988;9:381–382.

302. Mulligan EP, Harwell JL, Robertson WJ. Reliability and diagnostic accuracy of the Lachman test performed in the prone position. *J Orthop Sports Phys Ther.* 2011;41:749–757.

303. Cross MJ, Crichton KJ. *Clinical Examination of the Injured Knee.* Baltimore: Williams & Wilkins; 1987.

304. Cross MJ, Schmidt DR, Mackie IG. A no-touch test for the anterior cruciate ligament. *J Bone Joint Surg Br.* 1987;69:300.

305. Chong AC, Whitetree C, Priddy MC, et al. Evaluating different clinical diagnosis of anterior cruciate ligament ruptures in providers with different training backgrounds. *Iowa Ortho J.* 2017;37:71–79.

306. Jarbo KA, Hartigan DE, Scott KL, et al. Accuracy of the lever sign test in the diagnosis of anterior cruciate ligament injuries. *Orthop J Sports Med.* 2017;5(10):1–7.

307. Lelli A, Di Turi RP, Spenciner DB, Domini M. The "lever sign": a new clinical test for the diagnosis of anterior cruciate ligament rupture. *Knee Surg Sports Traumatol Arthrosc.* 2014;24(9):2794–2797.

308. Lichtenberg MC, Koster CH, Teunissen LP, et al. Does the lever sign test have added value for diagnosing anterior cruciate ligament ruptures? *Orthop J Sports Med.* 2018;6(3):1–7.

309. Thapa SS, Lamichhane AP, Mahara DP. Accuracy of Lelli test for anterior cruciate ligament tear. *J Institute Med.* 2015;37(2):91–94.

310. Wind WM, Bergfeld JA, Parker RD. Evaluation and treatment of posterior cruciate ligament injuries revisited. *Am J Sports Med.* 2004;32:1765–1775.

311. Emparanza JI, Aginaga JR. Validation of the Ottawa knee rules. *Ann Emerg Med.* 2001;38:364–368.

312. Voos JE, Mauro CS, Wente T, et al. Posterior cruciate ligament—anatomy, biomechanics and outcomes. *Am J Sports Med.* 2012;40:222–231.

313. Slocum DB, Larson RL. Rotary instability of the knee. *J Bone Joint Surg Am.* 1968;50:211–225.

314. Slocum DB, James SL, Larson RL, et al. A clinical test for anterolateral rotary instability of the knee. *Clin Orthop.* 1976;118:63–69.

315. Schafer KA, Tucker S, Griffith T, et al. Distribution of force in the medial collateral ligament complex during simulated clinical tests of knee stability. *Am J Sports Med.* 2015;44(5):1203–1208.

316. Sonnery-Cottet B, Lutz C, Daggett M, et al. The involvement of the anterolateral ligament in rotational control of the knee. *Am J Sports Med.* 2015;44(5):1209–1214.

317. Peterson L, Pitman MI, Gold J. The active pivot shift: the role of the popliteus muscle. *Am J Sports Med.* 1984;12:313–317.

318. Huang W, Zhang Y, Yao Z, Ma L. Clinical examination of anterior cruciate ligament rupture: a systematic review and meta-analysis. *Acta Orthop Traumatol Turc.* 2016;50(1):22–31.

319. Hanks GA, Joyner DM, Kalenak A. Anterolateral instability of the knee. *Am J Sports Med.* 1981;9:225–231.

320. Hughston JC, Walsh WM, Puddu G. *Patellar Subluxation and Dislocation.* Philadelphia: WB Saunders; 1984.

321. Fetto JF, Marshall JL. Injury to the anterior cruciate ligament producing the pivot shift sign: an experimental study on cadaver specimens. *J Bone Joint Surg Am.* 1979;61:710–714.

322. Galway HR, MacIntosh DL. The lateral pivot shift: a symptom and sign of anterior cruciate ligament insufficiency. *Clin Orthop.* 1980;147:45–50.

323. Tamea CD, Henning CE. Pathomechanics of the pivot shift maneuver. *Am J Sports Med.* 1981;9:31–37.

324. Katz JW, Fingeroth RF. The diagnostic accuracy of ruptures of the anterior cruciate ligament comparing the Lachman test, the anterior drawer sign and the pivot shift test in acute and chronic knee injuries. *Am J Sports Med.* 1986;14:88–91.

325. Lane CG, Warren R, Pearle AD. The pivot shift. *J Am Acad Orthop Surg.* 2008;16:679–688.

326. Bach BR, Warren RF, Wickiewitz TL. The pivot shift phenomenon: results and description of a modified clinical test for anterior cruciate ligament insufficiency. *Am J Sports Med.* 1988;16:571–576.

327. Kurosaka M, Yagi M, Yoshiya S, et al. Efficacy of the axially loaded pivot shift test for the diagnosis of a meniscal tear. *Int Orthop.* 1999;23:271–274.

328. Losee RE, Ennis TRJ, Southwick WO. Anterior subluxation of the lateral tibial plateau: a diagnostic test and operative review. *J Bone Joint Surg Am.* 1978;60:1015–1030.

329. Kocher MS, Steadman JR, Briggs KK, et al. Relationships between objective assessment of ligament stability and subjective assessment of symptoms and function after anterior cruciate ligament reconstruction. *Am J Sports Med.* 2004;32:629–634.

330. Noyes FR, Butler DL, Grood ES, et al. Clinical paradoxes of anterior cruciate ligament and a new test to detect its instability. *Orthop Trans.* 1978;2(36).

331. Sims WF, Jacobson KE. The posterolateral corner of the knee—medial-sided injury patterns revisited. *Am J Sports Med.* 2004;32:337–345.

332. Jacobson KE, Chi FS. Evaluation and treatment of medial collateral ligament and medial-sided injuries of the knee. *Sports Med Arthrosc Rev.* 2006;14:58–66.

333. Kurzweil PR, Kelley ST. Physical examination and imaging of the medial collateral ligament and posteromedial corner of the knee. *Sports Med Arthrosc Rev.* 2006;14:67–73.

334. Tibor LM, Marchant MH, Taylor DC, et al. Management of medial-sided knee injuries, part 2. *Am J Sports Med.* 2011;39:1332–1340.

335. Hughston JC, Norwood LA. The posterolateral drawer test and external rotational recurvatum test for posterolateral rotary instability of the knee. *Clin Orthop.* 1980;147:82–87.

336. LaPrade RF, Terry GC. Injuries to the posterolateral aspect of the knee—association of anatomic injury patterns with clinical instability. *Am J Sports Med.* 1997;25:433–438.

337. Owens TC. Posteromedial pivot shift of the knee: a new test for rupture of the posterior cruciate ligament. *J Bone Joint Surg Am.* 1994;76:532–539.

338. Moulton SG, Cram TR, James EW, et al. The supine internal rotation test: a pilot study evaluating tibial internal rotation in grade III posterior cruciate ligament tears. *Orthop J Sports Med.* 2015;3(2):1–7.

339. Chen FS, Rokito AS, Pitman MI. Acute and chronic posterolateral rotary instability of the knee. *J Am Acad Orthop Surg.* 2000;8:97–110.

340. Ferrari JD, Bach BR. Posterolateral instability of the knee: diagnosis and treatment of acute and chronic instability. *Sports Med Arthrosc Rev.* 1999;7:273–288.

341. Covey DC. Injuries of the posterolateral corner of the knee. *J Bone Joint Surg Am.* 2001;83:106–117.

342. Bahk MS, Cosgarea AJ. Physical examination and imaging of the lateral collateral ligament and posterolateral corner of the knee. *Sports Med Arthrosc Rev.* 2006;14:12–19.

343. Lunden JB, Bzdusek PJ, Monson JK, et al. Current concepts in the recognition and treatment of the posterolateral corner injuries of the knee. *J Orthop Sports Phys Ther.* 2010;40(8):502–515.

344. Fanelli GC, Larson RV. Practical management of posterolateral instability of the knee. *Arthroscopy.* 2002;18(2 suppl 1):1–8.

345. Shino K, Horibe S, Ono K. The voluntary evoked posterolateral drawer sign in the knee with posterolateral instability. *Clin Orthop.* 1987;215:179–186.

346. Shelbourne KD, Benedict F, McCarroll JR, et al. Dynamic posterior shift test: an adjuvant in evaluation of posterior tibial subluxation. *Am J Sports Med.* 1989;17:275–277.

347. Swain RA, Wilson FD. Diagnosing posterolateral rotary knee instability: two clinical tests hold key. *Phys Sportsmed.* 1993;21:95–102.

348. LaPrade RF, Ly TV, Griffith C. The external rotation recurvatum test revisited—reevaluation of the sagittal plane tibiofemoral relationship. *Am J Sports Med.* 2008:709–712.

349. Jakob RP, Hassler H, Staeubli HU. Observations on rotary instability of the lateral compartment of the knee. *Acta Orthop Scand.* 1981;52(suppl 191):1–32.

350. Loomer RL. A test for knee posterolateral rotary instability. *Clin Orthop.* 1991;264:235–238.

351. Veltri DM, Warren RF. Posterolateral instability of the knee. *J Bone Joint Surg Am.* 1994;76:460–472.

352. Veltri DM, Warren RF. Anatomy, biomechanics and physical findings in posterolateral knee instability. *Clin Sports Med.* 1994;13:599–614.

353. Veltri DM, Deng XH, Torzelli PA, et al. The role of the cruciate and posterolateral ligaments instability of the knee—a biomechanical study. *Am J Sports Med.* 1995;23:436–443.

354. Ranawat A, Baker CL, Henry S, et al. Posterolateral corner injury of the knee: evaluation and management. *J Am Acad Orthop Surg.* 2008;16:506–518.

355. Griffith CJ, LaPrade RF, Johansen S, et al. Part 1: static function of the individual components of the main medial knee structures. *Am J Sports Med.* 2009;37:1762–1770.

356. LaPrade RF, Wentorf F. Acute knee injuries—on the field and sideline evaluation. *Phys Sportsmed.* 1999;27:55–61.

357. Ferrari DA, Ferrari JD, Coumas J. Posterolateral instability of the knee. *J Bone Joint Surg Am.* 1994;76:187–192.

358. Daniel DM, Stone ML. Instrumented measurement of knee motion. In: Daniel D, Akeson W, O'Conner J, eds. *Knee Ligaments: Structure, Function, Injury and Repair.* New York: Raven Press; 1990.

359. Harter RA, Osternig LR, Singer KM. Instrumented Lachman tests for the evaluation of anterior laxity after reconstruction of the anterior cruciate ligament. *J Bone Joint Surg Am.* 1989;71:975–983.

360. Daniel DM, Malcolm LL, Losse G, et al. Instrumented measurement of anterior laxity of the knee. *J Bone Joint Surg Am.* 1985;67:720–726.

361. Tyler TF, McHugh MP, Gleim GW, et al. Association of KT-1000 measurements with clinical tests of the knee stability 1 year following anterior cruciate ligament reconstruction. *J Orthop Sports Phys Ther.* 1999;29:540–545.

362. Pugh L, Mascarenhas R, Arneja S, et al. Current concepts in instrumented knee laxity testing. *Am J Sports Med.* 2009;37:199–210.

363. Edixhoven P, Huiskes R, De Graff R, et al. Accuracy and reproducibility of instrumented knee drawer tests. *J Orthop Res.* 1987;5:378–387.

364. Andersson C, Gillquist J. Instrumented testing for evaluation of sagittal knee laxity. *Clin Orthop.* 1990;256:178–184.

365. Markolf KL, Amstutz HC. The clinical relevance of instrumented testing for ACL insufficiency: experience with the UCLA clinical knee testing apparatus. *Clin Orthop.* 1987;223:198–207.

366. Anderson AF, Snyder RB, Federspiel CF, et al. Instrumented evaluation of knee laxity: a comparison of five arthrometers. *Am J Sports Med.* 1992;20:135–140.

367. Daniel DM, Stone ML. Diagnosis of knee ligament injury: tests and measurements of joint laxity. In: Feagin JA, ed. *The Crucial Ligaments.* Edinburgh: Churchill Livingstone; 1988.

368. Bach BR, Johnson JC. Ligament testing devices. In: Scott WN, ed. *Ligament and Extensor Mechanism Injuries of the Knee: Diagnosis and Treatment.* St Louis: Mosby Year Book; 1991.

369. Daniel DM, Stone ML. KT-1000 anterior-posterior displacement measurements. In: Daniel D, Akeson W, O'Conner J, eds. *Knee Ligaments: Structure, Function, Injury and Repair.* New York: Raven Press; 1990.

370. Wright RW, Luhmann SJ. The effect of knee effusions on KT-1000 arthrometry—a cadaver study. *Am J Sports Med.* 1998;26:571–574.

371. Stratford PW, Miseferi D, Ogilvie R, et al. Assessing the responsiveness of five KT 1000 knee arthrometer measures used to evaluate anterior laxity at the knee joint. *Clin J Sport Med.* 1991;1:225–228.

372. Wroble RR, Grood ES, Noyes FR, et al. Reproducibility of genucom knee analysis system testing. *Am J Sports Med.* 1990;18:387–395.

373. Wroble RR, Van Ginkel LA, Grood ES, et al. Repeatability of the KT-1000 arthrometer in a normal population. *Am J Sports Med.* 1990;18:396–399.

374. Highgenboten CL, Jackson A, Meske NB. Genucom, KT-1000 and Stryker knee laxity measuring device comparisons: device reproducibility and interdevice comparison in asymptomatic subjects. *Am J Sports Med.* 1989;17:743–746.

375. McQuade KJ, Sidles JA, Larson KV. Reliability of the genucom knee analysis system. *Clin Orthop.* 1989;245:216–219.

376. Highgenboten CL, Jackson AW, Jansson KA, et al. KT-1000 arthrometer: conscious and unconscious test results using 15, 20 and 30 pounds of force. *Am J Sports Med.* 1992;20:450–454.

377. Kowalk DL, Wojtys EM, Disher J, et al. Quantitative analysis of the measuring capabilities of the KT-1000 knee ligament arthrometer. *Am J Sports Med.* 1993;21:744–747.

378. Forster IW, Warren-Smith CD, Tew M. Is the KT-1000 knee ligament arthrometer reliable? *J Bone Joint Surg Br.* 1989;71:843–847.

379. Huber FE, Irgang JJ, Harner C, et al. Intratester and intertester reliability of the KT-1000 arthrometer in the assessment of posterior laxity of the knee. *Am J Sports Med.* 1997;25:479–485.

380. Decary S, Ouellet P, Vendittoli PA, et al. Diagnostic validity of physical examination tests for common knee disorders: an overview of systematic reviews and meta-analysis. *Phys Ther Sport.* 2017;23:143–155.

381. Galli M, Ciriello V, Menghi A, et al. Joint line tenderness and McMurray tests for the detection of meniscal lesions: what is their real diagnostic values? *Arch Phys Med Rehabil.* 2013;94(6):1126–1131.

382. Scholten RJ, Devilli WL, Opsteuten W, et al. The accuracy of physical diagnostic tests for assessing meniscal lesions of the knee: a meta-analysis. *J Fam Pract.* 2001;50(11):938–944.

383. Hing W, White S, Reid D, et al. Validity of the McMurray's test and modified versions of the test: a systematic literature review. *J Man Manip Ther.* 2009;17:22–35.

384. Stratford PW, Binkley J. A review of the McMurray test: definition, interpretation and clinical usefulness. *J Orthop Sports Phys Ther.* 1995;22:116–120.

385. Bernstein J. Meniscal tears of the knee—diagnosis and individualized treatment. *Phys Sportsmed.* 2000;28:83–90.

386. Smith BE, Thacker D, Crewesmith A, Hall M. Special tests for assessing meniscal tears within the knee: a systematic review and meta-analysis. *Evid Based Med.* 2015;20(3):88–97.

387. Metcalf MH, Barrett GR. Prospective evaluation of 1485 meniscal tear patterns in patients with stable knees. *Am J Sports Med.* 2004;32:675–680.

388. Hegedus EJ, Cook C, Hasselbald V, et al. Physical examination tests for assessing a torn meniscus in the knee: a systematic review with meta-analysis. *J Orthop Sports Phys Ther.* 2007;37:541–550.

389. Haviv B, Bronak S, Kosashvili Y, Thein R. Gender differences in the accuracy of joint line tenderness for arthroscopically confirmed meniscal tears. *Arch Orthop Trauma Surg.* 2015;135:1567–1570.

390. Shelbourne KD, Martini DJ, McCarrell JR, et al. Correlation of joint line tenderness and meniscal lesions in patients with acute anterior cruciate ligament tears. *Am J Sports Med.* 1995;23:166–169.

391. Rose RE. The accuracy of joint line tenderness in the diagnosis of meniscal tears. *West Indian Med J.* 2006;55(5):323–326.

392. Meserve BB, Cleland JA, Boucher TR. A meta-analysis examining clinical test utilities for assessing meniscal injury. *Clin Rehabil.* 2008;22:143–161.

393. Anderson AF, Lipscomb AB. Clinical diagnosis of meniscal tears: description of a new manipulative test. *Am J Sports Med.* 1988;14:291–293.

394. Apley AG. The diagnosis of meniscus injuries: some new clinical methods. *J Bone Joint Surg Br.* 1947;29:78–84.

395. Oni O. The knee jerk test for diagnosis of torn meniscus. *Clin Orthop.* 1985;193:309.

396. Van der Post A, Noorduyn JC, Scholtes VA, Mutsaerts EL. What is the diagnostic accuracy of the duck walk test in detecting meniscal tears? *Clin Orthop Relat Res.* 2017;475(12):2963–2969.

397. Akseki D, Ozcan O, Boya H, et al. A new weight bearing meniscal test and a comparison with McMurray's test and joint line tenderness. *Arthroscopy.* 2004;20:951–958.

398. Galli M, Marzetti E. Accuracy of McMurray and joint line tenderness tests in the diagnosis of chronic meniscal tears: an ad hoc receiver operator characteristic analysis approach. *Arch Phys Med Rehabil.* 2017;98(9):1897–1899.

399. McMurray TP. The semilunar cartilages. *Br J Surg.* 1942;29:407–414.

400. Evans PJ, Bell GD, Frank C. Prospective evaluation of the McMurray test. *Am J Sports Med.* 1993;21:604–608.

401. Kim SJ, Min BH, Han DY. Paradoxical phenomena of the McMurray test: an arthroscopic examination. *Am J Sports Med.* 1996;24:83–87.

402. Helfet A. *Disorders of the Knee.* Philadelphia: JB Lippincott; 1974.

403. Seil R, Dück K, Pape D. A clinical sign to detect root avulsions of the posterior horn of the medial meniscus. *Knee Surg Sports Traumatol Arthrosc.* 2011;19(12):2072–2075.

404. Karachalios T, Hantes M, Zibis AH, et al. Diagnostic accuracy of a new clinical test (the Thessaly Test) for early detection of meniscal tears. *J Bone Joint Surg Am.* 2005;87:955–962.

405. Hegedus EJ. Thessaly test is no more accurate than standard clinical tests for meniscal tears. *Evid Based Med.* 2016;21(1):39.

406. Mirzatolooei F, Yekta Z, Bayazidchi M, et al. Validation of the Thessaly test for detecting meniscal tears in anterior cruciate deficient knees. *Knee.* 2010;17(3):221–223.

407. Kent M, Khanduja V. Synovial plicae around the knee. *Knee.* 2010;17(2):97–102.

408. Johnson DP, Eastwood DM, Witherow PJ. Symptomatic synovial plica of the knee. *J Bone Joint Surg Am.* 1993;75:1485–1496.

409. Gray DJ, Gardner E. Prenatal development of the human knee and superior tibiofibular joints. *Am J Anat.* 1950;56:235–287.

410. Ogata S, Uhthoff HK. The development of synovial plica in human knee joints: an embryologic study. *Arthroscopy.* 1990;6:315–321.

411. Hardaker WG, Shipple TL, Bassett FH. Diagnosis and treatment of the plica syndrome of the knee. *J Bone Joint Surg Am.* 1980;62:221–225.

412. Zanoli S, Piazzai E. The synovial plica syndrome of the knee—pathology, differential diagnosis and treatment. *Ital J Orthop Traumatol.* 1983;9:241–250.

413. Jackson RW, Marshall DJ, Fujisawa Y. The pathologic medial shelf. *Orthop Clin North Am.* 1982;13:307–312.

414. Stubbings N, Smith T. Diagnostic test accuracy of clinical and radiological assessments for medial patella plica syndrome: a systematic review and meta-analysis. *Knee.* 2014;21(2):486–490.

415. Mital MA, Hayden J. Pain in the knee in children: the medial plica shelf syndrome. *Orthop Clin North Am.* 1979;10:713–722.

416. Sturgill LP, Snyder-Mackler L, Manal TJ, et al. Interrater reliability of a clinical scale to assess knee joint effusion. *J Orthop Sports Phys Ther.* 2009;39:845–849.

417. Mann G, Finsterbush A, Frankel U, et al. A method of diagnosing small amounts of fluid in the knee. *J Bone Joint Surg Br.* 1991;73:346–347.

418. Sibley MB, Fu FH. Knee injuries. In: Fu FH, Stone DA, eds. *Sports Injuries: Mechanisms, Prevention, Treatment.* Baltimore: Williams & Wilkins; 1994.

419. Haim A, Yaniv M, Dekel S, et al. Patellofemoral pain syndrome: validity of clinical and radiological features. *Clin Orthop Relat Res.* 2006;451:223–228.

420. Boling MC, Padua DA, Marshall SW, et al. A prospective investigation of biomechanical risk factors for patellofemoral pain syndrome. *Am J Sports Med.* 2009;37:2108–2116.

421. Dye SF. The pathophysiology of patellofemoral pain. *Clin Orthop Relat Res.* 2005;436:100–110.

422. Van Haver A, De Roo K, De Beule M, et al. The effect of trochlear dysplasia on patellofemoral biomechanics: a cadaveric study with simulated trochlear deformities. *Am J Sports Med.* 2015;43(6):1354–1361.

423. Nunes GS, Stapait EL, Kirsten MH, et al. Clinical test for diagnosis of patellofemoral pain syndrome: systematic review with meta-analysis. *Phys Ther Sport.* 2013;14(1):54–59.

424. Piva SR, Fitzgerald K, Irrgang JJ, et al. Reliability of measures of impairments associated with patellofemoral pain syndrome. *BMC Muscloskelet Disord.* 2006;7:33–46.

425. LaBotz M. Patellofemoral syndrome—diagnostic pointers and individualized treatment. *Phys Sportsmed.* 2004;32:22–31.

426. Witvroux E, Lysons R, Bellemans J, et al. Intrinsic risk factors for the development of anterior knee pain in an athletic population—a 2 year prospective study. *Am J Sports Med.* 2000;28:480–489.

427. Witvrouw E, Werner C, Mikkelsen C, et al. Clinical classification of patellofemoral pain syndrome: guidelines for non-operative treatment. *Knee Surg Sports Traumatol Arthrosc.* 2005;13(2):122–130.

428. Barton CJ, Levinger P, Crossley KM, et al. The relationship between rearfoot, tibial and hip kinematics in individuals with patellofemoral pain syndrome. *Clin Biomech.* 2012;27:702–705.

429. Souza RB, Powers CM. Predictors of hip internal rotation during running—an evaluation of hip strength and femoral structure in women with and without patellofemoral pain. *Am J Sports Med.* 2009;37:579–587.

430. Hudson Z, Darthuy E. Iliotibial band tightness and patellofemoral pain syndrome: a case control study. *Manual Therapy.* 2009;14:147–151.

431. Souza RB, Powers CM. Differences in hip kinematics, muscle strength, and muscle activation between subjects with and without patellofemoral pain. *J Orthop Sports Phys Ther.* 2009;39(1):121–129.

432. Thomson C, Krouwel O, Kuisma R, Hebron C. The outcome of hip exercise in patellofemoral pain: a systematic review. *Man Ther.* 2016;26:1–30.

433. Muller K, Snyder-Mackler L. Diagnosis of patellofemoral pain after arthroscopic meniscectomy. *J Orthop Sports Phys Ther.* 2000;30:138–142.

434. Cook C, Mabry L, Reiman MP, Hegedus EJ. Best tests/clinical findings for screening and diagnosis of patellofemoral pain syndrome: a systematic review. *Physiotherapy.* 2012;98(2):93–100.

435. Nijs J, VanGeel C, Vanderauwera C, et al. Diagnostic value of five clinical tests in patellofemoral syndrome. *Man Ther.* 2006;11:69–77.

436. Doberstein ST, Romeyn RL, Reinke DM. The diagnostic value of the Clarke sign in assessing chondromalacia patella. *J Athl Train.* 2008;43:190–196.

437. Watson CJ, Leddy HM, Dynjan TD, et al. Reliability of the lateral pull test and tilt test to assess patellar alignment in subjects with symptomatic knees: student raters. *J Orthop Sports Phys Ther.* 2001;3:368–374.

438. McConnell J. The management of chondromalacia patellae: a long term solution. *Aust J Physiother.* 1986;32:215–223.

439. Souza TA. The knee. In: Hyde TE, Gengenbach MS, eds. *Conservative Management of Sport Injuries.* Baltimore: Williams & Wilkins; 1997.

440. Daniel DM, Stone ML, Barnett P, et al. Use of the quadriceps active test to diagnose posterior cruciate ligament disruption and measure posterior laxity of the knee. *J Bone Joint Surg Am.* 1988;70:386–391.

441. Fairbank HAT. Internal derangement of the knee in children and adolescents. *Proc R Soc Med.* 1937;30:427–432.

442. Tanner SM, Garth WP, Soileau R, et al. A modified test for patellar instability—the biomechanical basis. *Clin J Sports Med.* 2003;13:327–338.

443. Cooper H, Dobbs WN, Adams ID, et al. Use and misuse of the tape-measure as a means of assessing muscle strength and power. *Rheumatol Rehabil.* 1981;20(4):211–218.

444. Ahmad CS, McCarthy M, Gomez JA, et al. The moving patellar apprehension test for lateral patellar instability. *Am J Sports Med.* 2009;37:791–796.

445. Noble HB, Hajek MR, Porter M. Diagnosis and treatment of iliotibial band tightness in runners. *Phys Sportsmed.* 1982;10:67–74.

446. Schulthies SS, Francis RS, Fisher AG, et al. Does the Q-angle reflect the force on the patella in the frontal plane. *Phys Ther.* 1995;75:24–30.

447. Herrington L, Nester C. Q-angle undervalued? The relationship between Q-angle and medio-lateral position of the patella. *Clin Biomech.* 2004;19:1070–1073.

448. Smith TO, Hunt NJ, Donell ST. The reliability and validity of the Q-angle: a systematic review. *Knee Surg Sports Traumatol Arthrosc.* 2008;16:1068–1079.

449. Insall J, Falvo KA, Wise DW. Chondromalacia patellae: a prospective study. *J Bone Joint Surg Am.* 1976;58(1–8).

450. Smith TO, Hunt NJ, Donell ST. The reliability and validity of the Q-angle: a systematic review. *Knee Surg Sports Traumatol Arthrosc.* 2008;16(12):1068–1079.

451. Olerud C, Berg P. The variation of the Q angle with different positions of the foot. *Clin Orthop.* 1984;191:162–165.

452. Grelsamer RP, Dubey A, Weinstein CH. Men and women have similar Q-angles—a clinical and trigonometric evaluation. *J Bone Joint Surg Br.* 2005;87:1498–1501.

453. Guerra JP, Arnold MJ, Gajdosik RL. Q-angle: effects of isometric quadriceps contraction and body position. *J Orthop Sports Phys Ther.* 1994;19:200–204.

454. Cook CE, Hegedus EJ. *Orthopedic Physical Examination Tests—An Evidence Based Approach.* Upper Saddle River, NJ: Prentice-Hall/Pearson; 2008.

455. Baciu CC, Tudor A, Olaru I. Recurrent luxation of the superior tibio-fibular joint in the adult. *Acta Orthop Scand.* 1974;45:772–777.

456. Fournier-Farley C, Lamontagne M, Gendron P, Gagnon DH. Determinants of return to play after the nonoperative management of hamstring injuries in athletes: a systematic review. *Am J Sports Med.* 2016;44(8):2166–2172.

457. Daniel DM, Stone ML. Case studies. In: Daniel D, Akeson W, O'Conner J, eds. *Knee Ligaments: Structure, Injury and Repair.* New York: Raven Press; 1990.

458. Arno S. The A-angle: a quantitative measurement of patella alignment and realignment. *J Orthop Sports Phys Ther.* 1990;12:237–242.

459. DiVeta JA, Vogelbach WD. The clinical efficacy of the A-angle in measuring patellar alignment. *J Orthop Sports Phys Ther.* 1992;16:136–139.

460. Ehrat M, Edwards J, Hastings D, et al. Reliability of assessing patellar alignment: the A-angle. *J Orthop Sports Phys Ther.* 1994;19:22–27.

461. Crawford DC, Safran MR. Osteochondritis dissecans of the knee. *J Am Acad Orthop Surg.* 2006;14:90–100.

462. Dellon AL. Knee pain of neural origin. In: Noyes FR, Barber-Westin SD, eds. *Noyes' Knee Disorders: Surgery Rehabilitation, Clinical Outcomes.* 2nd ed. Philadelphia: Elsevier; 2017.

463. Hyslop GH. Injuries of the deep and superficial peroneal nerves complicating ankle sprain. *Am J Surg.* 1941;51:436–438.

464. Sidey J. Weak ankles: a study of common peroneal entrapment neuropathy. *Br Med J.* 1969;56:623–626.

465. Pecina MM, Krmpotic-Nemanic J, Markiewitz AD. *Tunnel Syndromes.* Boca Raton, FL: CRC Press; 1991.

466. Worth RM, Kettlekamp DB, Defalque RJ, et al. Saphenous nerve entrapment: a cause of medial nerve pain. *Am J Sports Med.* 1984;12:80–81.

467. Cox JS, Blanda JB. Periarticular pathologies. In: DeLee JC, Drez D, eds. *Orthopedic Sports Medicine.* Philadelphia: WB Saunders; 1994.

468. Lin J, Chang C. A medial soft tissue mass of the knee. *Phys Sportsmed.* 1999;27:87–90.

469. Eren OT. The accuracy of joint line tenderness by physical examination in the diagnosis of meniscal tears. *Arthroscopy.* 2003;19(8):850–854.

470. Kessler JI, Nikizad H, Shea KG, et al. The demographics and epidemiology of osteochondritis dissecans of the knee in children and adolescents. *Am J Sports Med.* 2014;42(2):320–326.

471. O'Shea KJ, Murphy KP, Heekin D, et al. The diagnostic accuracy of history, physical examination and radiographs in the evaluation of traumatic knee disorders. *Am J Sports Med.* 1996;24:164–167.

472. Gelb HJ, Glasgow SG, Sapega AA, et al. Magnetic resonance imaging of knee disorders: clinical value and cost-effectiveness in a sports medicine practice. *Am J Sports Med.* 1996;24:99–103.

473. Luhmann SJ, Schootman M, Gordon JE, et al. Magnetic resonance imaging of the knee in children and adolescents. *J Bone Joint Surg Am.* 2005;87:497–502.

474. Bedson J, Croft PR. The discordance between clinical and radiographic knee osteoarthritis: a systematic search and summary of the literature. *BMC Musculoskelet Disord.* 2008;9:116–127.

475. Stiell IG, Wells GA, Hoag RH. Implementation of the Ottawa knee rules for the use of radiography in acute knee injuries. *JAMA.* 1997;278:2075–2079.

476. Nugent P. The Ottawa knee rule—avoiding unnecessary radiographs in sports. *Phys Sportsmed.* 2004;32(5):26–32.

477. Jackson JL, O'Malley FG, Kroenke K. Evaluation of acute knee pain in primary care. *Ann Intern Med.* 2003;139:575–588.

478. Cohen DM, Jasser JW, Kean JR, et al. Clinical criteria for using radiography for children with acute knee injuries. *Ped Emerg Care.* 1998;14:185–187.

479. Bulloch B, Neto G, Plint A, et al. Validation of the Ottawa knee rule in children: a multicentre study. *Ann Emerg Med.* 2003;42:48–55.

480. Khine H, Dorfman DH, Avner JR. Applicability of Ottawa knee rule for knee injury in children. *Ped Emerg Care.* 2001;17:401–404.

481. Seaberg DC, Jackson R. Clinical decision rule for knee radiographs. *Am J Emerg Med.* 1994;12(5):541–543.

482. Tandeter HB, Shvartzman P, Stevens MA. Acute knee injuries: use of decision rules for radiograph ordering. *Am Fam Physician.* 1999;60(9):2599–2608.

483. Altman R, Asch E, Bloch D, et al. Development of criteria for the classification and reporting of osteoarthritis – classification of osteoarthritis of the knee. *Arthritis Rheumatism.* 1986;29(8):1039–1049.

484. Zhang W, Doherty M, Peat G, et al. EULAR evidence-based recommendations for the diagnosis of knee osteoarthritis. *Ann Rheum Dis.* 2010;69(3):483–489.

485. Carson Jr WG, James SL, Larson RL, et al. Patellofemoral disorders: physical and radiographic evaluation. I. Physical examination. *Clin Orthop.* 1984;185:178–186.

486. Merchant AC. Extensor mechanism injuries: classification and diagnosis. In: Scott WN, ed. *Ligament and Extensor Mechanism Injuries of the Knee: Diagnosis and Treatment.* St Louis: Mosby; 1991.

487. Davies AP, Calder DA, Marshall T, et al. Plain radiography in the degenerate knee. *J Bone Joint Surg Br.* 1999;81:632–635.

488. Tatum R. Osteochondritis dissecans of the knee: a radiology case report. *J Manip Physiol Ther.* 2000;23:347–351.

489. Schenck RC, Goodnight JM. Osteochondritis dissecans—current concepts review. *J Bone Joint Surg Am.* 1996;78:439–456.

490. Wall EJ, Polousky JD, Shea KG, et al. Novel radiographic feature classification of knee osteochondritis dissecans: a multicenter reliability study. *Am J Sports Med.* 2015;43(2):303–309.

491. Woods GW, Stanley RF, Tullos HS. Lateral capsular sign: x-ray clue to a significant knee instability. *Am J Sports Med.* 1979;7:27–33.

492. Altchek DW. Diagnosing acute knee injuries: the office exam. *Phys Sportsmed.* 1993;21:85–96.

493. Schils JP, Resnick D, Sartoris DJ. Diagnostic imaging of ligamentous injuries of the knee. In: Daniel D, Akeson W, O'Conner J, eds. *Knee Ligaments: Structure, Injury and Repair.* New York: Raven Press; 1990.

494. Beaconsfield T, Pintore E, Maffulli N, et al. Radiographic measurements in patellofemoral disorders. *Clin Orthop.* 1994;308:18–28.

495. Grana WA. Diagnostic evaluation. In: Larson RL, Grana WA, eds. *The Knee: Form, Function, Pathology and Treatment.* Philadelphia: WB Saunders; 1993.

496. Grelsamer RP, Meadows S. The modified Insall-Salvati ratio for assessment of patellar height. *Clin Orthop.* 1992;282:170–176.

497. Haas SB, Scuderi GR. Examination and radiographic assessment of the patellofemoral joint. *Semin Orthop.* 1990;5:108–114.

498. Grelsamer RP, Proctor CS, Brazos AN. Evaluation of patellar shape in the sagittal plane: a clinical analysis. *Am J Sports Med.* 1994;22:61–66.

499. Phillips CL, Silver DA, Schranz PJ, et al. The measurement of patellar height—a review of the methods of imaging. *J Bone Joint Surg Br.* 2010;92:1045–1053.

500. Berg EE, Mason SL, Zucas MJ. Patellar height ratios: a comparison of four measurement methods. *Am J Sports Med.* 1996;24:218–221.

501. LaPrade RF, Ly TV, Wentorf FA, et al. The posterolateral attachments of the knee: a qualitative and quantitative morphologic analysis of the fibular collateral ligament, popliteus tendon, popliteofibular ligament and lateral gastrocnemius tendon. *Am J Sports Med.* 2003;31:854–860.

502. Hewett TE, Noyes FR, Lee MD. Diagnosis of complete and partial posterior cruciate ligament ruptures—stress radiography compared with KT-1000 and posterior drawer testing. *Am J Sports Med.* 1997;25:648–655.

503. Jackman T, LaPrade RF, Pontinen T, et al. Intraobserver and interobserver reliability of the kneeling technique of stress radiography for the evaluation of posterior knee laxity. *Am J Sports Med.* 2008;36:1571–1576.

504. Shelbourne KD, Davis TJ, Klootwyk TE. The relationship between intercondylar notch width of the femur and the incidence of anterior cruciate ligament tears—a prospective study. *Am J Sports Med.* 1998;26:402–408.

505. Bollier M, Fulkerson JP. The role of trochlear dysplasia in patellofemoral instability. *J Am Acad Orthop Surg.* 2011;19:8–16.

506. Speakman HB, Weisberg J. The vastus medialis controversy. *Physiotherapy.* 1977;63:249–254.

507. Murray TF, Dupont JY, Fulkerson JP. Axial and lateral radiographs in evaluating patellofemoral malalignment. *Am J Sports Med.* 1999;27:580–584.

508. Tscholl PM, Wanivenhaus F, Fucentese SF. Conventional radiographs and magnetic resonance imaging for the analysis of trochlear dysplasia: the influence of selected levels on magnetic resonance imaging. *Am J Sports Med.* 2017;45(5):1059–1065.

509. Carlson VR, Boden BP, Sheehan FT. Patellofemoral kinematics and tibial tuberosity-trochlear groove distances in female adolescents with patellofemoral pain. *Am J Sports Med.* 2017;45(5):1102–1109.

510. Carlson VR, Boden BP, Shen A, et al. The tibial tubercle-trochlear groove distance is greater in patients with patellofemoral pain: implications for the origin of pain and clinical interventions. *Am J Sports Med.* 2017;45(5):1110–1116.

511. Davies AP, Costa ML, Donnell ST, et al. The sulcus angle and malalignment of the extensor mechanisms of the knee. *J Bone Joint Surg Br.* 2000;82:1162–1166.

512. Ghelman B, Schraft S. Arthrography of the knee. In: Scott WN, ed. *Ligament and Extensor Mechanism Injuries of the Knee: Diagnosis and Treatment.* St Louis: Mosby; 1991.

513. Mital MA, Karlin LI. Diagnostic arthroscopy in sports injuries. *Orthop Clin North Am.* 1980;11:771–785.

514. McClelland CJ. Arthroscopy and arthroscopic surgery of the knee. *Physiotherapy.* 1984;70:154–156.

515. Noyes FR, Bassett RW, Grood ES, et al. Arthroscopy in acute traumatic hemarthrosis of the knee. *J Bone Joint Surg Am.* 1980;62:687–695, 757.

516. McNally E. Knee joint and calf: Anatomy and techniques. In: McNally E, ed. *Practical Musculoskeletal Ultrasound.* 2nd ed. London: Churchill Livingstone; 2014.

517. Spannow AH, Pheiffer-Jensen M, Andersen NT, et al. Ultrasonographic measurements of joint cartilage thickness in healthy children: age- and sex-related standard reference values. *J Rheumatol.* 2010;37:2595–2601.

518. Cho KH, Lee DC, Chhem RK, et al. Normal and acutely torn posterior cruciate ligament of the knee at US evaluation: preliminary experience. *Radiology.* 2001;219(2):375–380.

519. Hsu CC, Tsai WC, Chen CP, et al. Ultrasonographic examination of the normal and injured posterior cruciate ligament. *J Clin Ultrasound.* 2005;33(6):277–282.

520. Miller TT. Sonography of injury of the posterior cruciate ligament of the knee. *Skeletal Radiol.* 2002;31(3):149–154.

521. Sorrentino F, Iovane A, Nicosia A, et al. Role of high-resolution ultrasonography without and with real-time spatial compound imaging in evaluating the injured posterior cruciate ligament: preliminary study. *Radiol Med.* 2009;114(2):312–320.

522. Wang LY, Yang TH, Huang YC, et al. Evaluating posterior cruciate ligament injury by using two-dimensional ultrasonography and sonoelastography. *Knee Surg Sports Traumatol Arthrosc.* 2017;25(10):3108–3115.

523. LaPrade RF, Gilbert TJ, Bollom TS, et al. The magnetic resonance imaging appearance of individual structures of the posterolateral knee—a prospective study of normal knees and knees with surgically verified grade III injuries. *Am J Sports Med.* 2000;28:191–199.

524. Potter HG. Imaging of the multiple-ligament-injured knee. *Clin Sports Med.* 2000;19:425–441.

525. Thomas S, Pullagura M, Robinson E, et al. The value of magnetic resonance imaging in our current management of ACL and meniscal injuries. *Knee Surg Sports Traumatol Arthrosc.* 2007;15:533–536.

526. Rose NE, Gold SM. A comparison of accuracy between clinical examination and magnetic resonance imaging in the diagnosis of meniscal and anterior cruciate ligament tears. *Arthroscopy.* 1996;12(4):398–405.

527. Kocabey Y, Tetik O, Isbell WM, et al. The value of clinical examination versus magnetic resonance imaging in the diagnosis of meniscal tears and anterior cruciate ligament rupture. *Arthroscopy.* 2004;20(7):696–700.

528. Cross TM, Gibbs N, Houang MT, et al. Acute quadriceps muscle strains—magnetic resonance imaging features and prognosis. *Am J Sports Med.* 2004;32:710–719.

529. Chin KR, Sodl JF. Infrapatellar fat pad disruption—a radiographic sign of patellar tendon rupture. *Clin Orthop Relat Res.* 2005;440:222–225.

530. Sanders TG, Miller MD. A systematic approach to magnetic resonance imaging interpretation of sports medicine injuries of the knee. *Am J Sports Med.* 2005;33:131–148.

531. Glashow JL, Friedman MJ. Diagnosis of knee ligament injuries: magnetic resonance imaging. In: Scott WN, ed. *Ligament and Extensor Mechanism Injuries of the Knee: Diagnosis and Treatment.* St Louis: Mosby; 1991.

532. Arendt EA. Assessment of the athlete with an acutely injured knee. In: Griffin LY, ed. *Rehabilitation of the Injured Knee.* St Louis: Mosby; 1995.

533. Gelb HJ, Glasgow SG, Sapega AA, et al. Magnetic resonance imaging of knee disorders: clinical value and cost effectiveness in a sports medicine practice. *Am J Sports Med.* 1996;24:99–103.

534. Adalberth T, Roos H, Lauren M, et al. Magnetic resonance imaging, scintigraphy and arthroscopic evaluation of traumatic hemarthrosis of the knee. *Am J Sports Med.* 1997;25:231–237.

535. Munshi M, Davidson M, MacDonald PB, et al. The efficacy of magnetic resonance imaging in acute knee injuries. *Clin J Sports Med.* 2000;10:34–39.

536. Potter HG, Linklater JM, Allen AA, et al. Magnetic resonance imaging of articular cartilage of the knee. *J Bone Joint Surg Am.* 1998;80:1276–1284.

537. Ross G, Chapman AW, Newberg AR, et al. Magnetic resonance imaging for the evaluation of acute posterolateral complex injuries of the knee. *Am J Sports Med.* 1997;25:444–448.

538. Schneider-Kolsky ME, Hoving JL, Warren P, et al. A comparison between clinical assessment and magnetic resonance imaging of acute hamstring injuries. *Am J Sports Med.* 2006;34:1008–1015.

539. Ben-Galim P, Steinberg EL, Amir H, et al. Accuracy of magnetic resonance imaging of the knee and justified surgery. *Clin Orthop Relat Res.* 2006;447:100–104.

540. Miller TT. Imaging of the knee. *Sports Med Arthrosc Rev.* 2008;17:56–67.

541. Quatman CE, Hettrich CM, Schmitt LC, et al. The clinical utility and diagnostic performance of magnetic resonance imaging for identification of early and advanced knee osteoarthritis—a systematic review. *Am J Sports Med.* 2011;39:1557–1568.

542. Krampla W, Roesel M, Svoboda K, et al. MRI of the knee: how do field strength and radiologist's experience influence diagnostic accuracy and interobserver correlation in assessing chondral and meniscal lesions and the integrity of the anterior cruciate ligament. *Eur Radiol.* 2009;19:1519–1528.

543. van der Heijden RA, de Kanter JL, Bierma-Zeinstra SM, et al. Structural abnormalities on magnetic resonance imaging in patients with patellofemoral pain: a cross-sectional case-control study. *Am J Sports Med.* 2016;44(9):2339–2346.

544. Camp CL, Heidenreich MJ, Dahm DL, et al. Individualizing the tibial tubercle-trochlear groove distance: patellar instability ratios that predict recurrent instability. *Am J Sports Med.* 2015;44(2):393–399.

545. Black BR, Chong LR, Potter HG. Cartilage imaging in sports medicine. *Sports Med Arthrosc Rev.* 2008;17:68–80.

546. Jakobsen TL, Kehlet H, Bandholm T. Reliability of the 6-min walk test after total knee arthroplasty. *Knee Surg Sports Traumatol Arthrosc.* 2013;21(11):2625–2628.

547. McCarthy CJ, Oldham JA. The reliability, validity and responsiveness of an aggregated locomotor function (ALF) score in patients with osteoarthritis of the knee. *Rheumatology.* 2004;43:514–517.

548. Irrgang JJ, Anderson AF, Boland AL, et al. International Knee Documentation Committee: Responsiveness of the International Knee Documentation Committee subjective knee form. *Am J Sports Med.* 2006;34(10):1567–1573.

549. Liow RYL, Walker K, Wajid MA, et al. The reliability of the American Knee Society Score. *Acta Orthop Scand.* 2000;71(6):603–608.

550. Kim S, Lee D, Kim T. The relationship between the MPP test and arthroscopically found medial patellar plica pathology. *J Arthrosc Relat Surg.* 2007;23(12):1303–1308.

551. Peeler J, Leiter J, Macdonald P. Accuracy and reliability of anterior cruciate ligament clinical examination in a multidisciplinary sports medicine setting. *Clin J Sport Med.* 2010;20(2):80–85.

552. Boeree NR, Ackroyd CE. Assessment of the menisci and cruciate ligaments: an audit of clinical practice. *Injury.* 1991;22:291–294.

553. Bomberg BC, McGinty JB. Acute hemarthrosis of the knee: indications for diagnostic arthroscopy. *Arthroscopy.* 1990;6:221–225.

554. Braunstein EM. Anterior cruciate ligament injuries: a comparison of arthrographic and physical diagnosis. *Am J Roentgenol.* 1982;138:423–425.

555. Hughston JC, Andrews JR, Cross MJ, et al. Classification of knee ligament instabilities. I. The medial compartment and cruciate ligaments. *J Bone Joint Surg Am.* 1976;58:159–172.

556. Lee LK, Yao L, Phelps CT, et al. Anterior cruciate ligament tears: MR imaging compared with arthroscopy and clinical tests. *Radiology.* 1988;166:861–864.

557. Noyes FR, Paulos L, Mooar LA, et al. Knee sprains and acute knee hemarthrosis: misdiagnosis of anterior cruciate ligament tears. *Phys Ther.* 1980;60:1596–1601.

558. Rubinstein RA, Shelbourne KD, McCarroll JR, et al. The accuracy of the clinical examination in the setting of posterior cruciate ligament injuries. *Am J Sports Med.* 1994;22:550–557.

559. Sandberg R, Balkfors B, Henricson A, et al. Stability tests in knee ligament injuries. *Arch Orthop Trauma Surg.* 1986;106:5–7.

560. Warren RF, Marshall JL. Injuries of the anterior cruciate and medial collateral ligaments of the knee: a retrospective analysis of clinical records. I. *Clin Orthop Relat Res.* 1978;136:191–197.

561. Jonsson T, Althoff B, Peterson L, et al. Clinical diagnosis of ruptures of the anterior cruciate ligament: a comparative study of the Lachman test and the anterior drawer sign. *Am J Sports Med.* 1982;10:100–102.

562. Benjaminse A, Gokeler A, van der Schans CP. Clinical diagnosis of an anterior cruciate ligament rupture: a meta-analysis. *J Orthop Sports Phys Ther.* 2006;36:267–288.

563. Davis E. Clinical examination of the knee following trauma: an evidence-based perspective. *Trauma.* 2002;4:135–145.

564. Smith C. Evaluating the painful knee: a hands-on approach to acute ligamentous and meniscal injuries. *Sports Med.* 2004;4(7):362–370.

565. Steinbruck K, Wiehmann JC. Examination of the knee joint. The value of clinical findings in arthroscopic control. *Z Orthop Ihre Grenzgeb.* 1988;126:289–295.

566. Tonino AJ, Huy J, Schaafsma J. The diagnostic accuracy of knee testing in the acutely injured knee. Initial examination versus examination under anaesthesia with arthroscopy. *Acta Orthop Belg.* 1986;52:479–487.

567. Anderson AF, Lipscomb AB. Preoperative instrumented testing of anterior and posterior knee laxity. *Am J Sports Med.* 1986;17:1299–1306.

568. DeHaven KE. Diagnosis of acute knee injuries with hemarthrosis. *Am J Sports Med.* 1980;8:9–14.

569. Donaldson WF, Warren RF, Wickiewicz T. A comparison of acute anterior cruciate ligament examinations: initial vs examination under anesthesia. *Am J Sports Med.* 1985;13:5–9.

570. Hardaker WT, Garrett WE, Bassett FH. Evaluation of acute traumatic hemarthrosis of the knee joint. *South Med J.* 1990;83:640–644.

571. Liu SH, Osti L, Henry M, et al. The diagnosis of acute complete tears of the anterior cruciate ligament: comparison of MRI, arthrometry and clinical examination. *J Bone Joint Surg Br.* 1995;77:586–588.

572. Kim SJ, Kim HK. Reliability of the anterior drawer test, the pivot shift test, and the Lachman test. *Clin Orthop Relat Res.* 1995;317:237–242.

573. Harilainen A. Evaluation of knee instability in acute ligamentous injuries. *Am Chir Gynaecol.* 1987;76:269–273.

574. Mitsou A, Vallianatos P. Clinical diagnosis of ruptures of the anterior cruciate ligament: a comparison between the Lachman test and the anterior drawer sign. *Injury.* 1988;19:427–428.

575. Makhmalbaf H, Moradi A, Ganji S, Omidi-kashani F. Accuracy of Lachman and anterior drawer tests for anterior cruciate ligament injuries. *Arch Bone Joint Surg.* 2013;1(2):94–97.

576. Watson CJ, Propps M, Ratner J, et al. Reliability and responsiveness of the lower extremity functional scale and the anterior knee pain scale in patients with anterior knee pain. *J Orthop Sports Phys Ther.* 2005;35:136–146.

577. Fowler PJ, Lubliner JA. The predictive value of five clinical signs in the evaluation of meniscal pathology. *Arthroscopy.* 1989;5:1846.

578. Muellner T, Weinstabl R, Schabus R, et al. The diagnosis of meniscal tears in athletes: a comparison of clinical and magnetic resonance imaging investigations. *Am J Sports Med.* 1997;25(1):7–12.

579. Niskanen RO, Paavilainen PJ, Jaakkola M, Korkala OL. Poor correlation of clinical signs with patellar cartilaginous changes. *Arthroscopy.* 2001;17:307–310.

580. Clark NC, Gumbrell CJ, Rana S, et al. Intratester reliability and measurement error of the adapted crossover hop for distance. *Phys Ther Sport.* 2002;3:143–151.

581. Bolgla LA, Keskula DR. Reliability of lower extremity functional performance test. *J Orthop Sports Phys Ther.* 1997;26:138–142.

582. Ross MD, Langford B, Wheland PJ. Test-retest reliability of 4 single leg horizontal hop tests. *J Strength Cond Res.* 2002;16:617–622.

583. Bandy WD, Rusche KR, Tekulve FY. Reliability and limb symmetry for five unilateral functional tests for the lower extremities. *Isokinetics Exerc Sci.* 1994;4:108–111.

584. Reid A, Birmingham TB, Stratford PW, et al. Hop testing provides a reliable and valid outcome measure during rehabilitation after anterior cruciate ligament reconstruction. *Physical Therapy.* 2007;87(3):337–349.

585. Haitz K, Shultz R, Hodgins M, Matheson GO. Test-retest and interrater reliability of the functional lower extremity evaluation. *J Orthop Sports Phys Ther.* 2014;44(12):947–954.

586. Logerstedt D, Grindem H, Lynch A, et al. Single-legged hop tests as predictors of self-reported knee function after anterior cruciate ligament reconstruction: the Delaware-Oslo ACL cohort study. *Am J Sports Med.* 2012;40(10):2348–2356.

587. Impellizzeri FM, Bizzini M, Rampinini E, et al. Reliability of isokinetic strength imbalance ratios measured using Cybex NORM dynamometer. *Clin Physiol Funct Imaging.* 2008;28:113–119.

588. Mokkink LB, Terwee CB, Van Lummel RC, et al. Construct validity of the Dynaport knee test: a comparison with observations of physical therapists. *Osteoarthr Cartilage.* 2005;13:738–743.

589. Arjun RH, Kishan R, Dhillon MS, Chouhan D. Reliability of clinical methods in evaluating patellofemoral pain syndrome with malalignment. *Int J Res Orthop.* 2017;3:334–338.

590. Hayes KW, Petersen CM. Reliability of assessing end-feel and pain and resistance sequence in subjects

with painful shoulders and knees. *J Orthop Sports Phys Ther*. 2001;31:432–445.

591. Harrison E, Quinney H, Magee DJ, et al. Analysis of outcome measured used in the study of patellofemoral pain syndrome. *Physiother Can*. 1995;47:264–272.

592. Anderson AF, Rennirt GW, Standeffer WC. Clinical analysis of the pivot shift tests: description of the pivot drawer test. *Am J Knee Surg*. 2000;13:19–23.

593. Ikjaer T, Henriksen M, Dyhre-Poulsen P, et al. Forward lunge as a functional performance test in ACL deficient subjects: test-retest reliability. *The Knee*. 2009;16(3):176–182.

594. Smith TO, Davies L, O'Driscoll M, et al. An evaluation of the clinical tests and outcome measures used to assess patellar instability. *The Knee*. 2008;15:255–262.

595. Loudon JK, Wiesner D, Goist-Foley HL, et al. Intrarater reliability of functional performance tests for subjects with patellofemoral pain syndrome. *J Athl Train*. 2003;37:256–261.

596. Bremander AB, Dahl LL, Roos EM. Validity and reliability of functional performance tests in meniscotomized patients with or without knee osteoarthritis. *Scand J Med Sci Sports*. 2007;17:120–127.

597. Piva SR, Fitzgerald GK, Irrgang JJ, et al. Get up and go test in patients with knee osteoarthritis. *Arch Phys Med Rehabil*. 2004;85:284–289.

598. Johanson NA, Liang MH, Daltroy L, et al. American Academy of Orthopaedic Surgeons lower limb outcomes assessment instruments: reliability, validity, and sensitivity to change. *J Bone Joint Surg Am*. 2004;86:902–909.

599. Bennell KL, Hinman RS, Crossley KM, et al. Is the human activity profile a useful measure in people with knee osteoarthritis? *J Rehabil Res Dev*. 2004;41(4):621–630.

600. Mehta VM, Paxton LW, Fornalski SX, et al. Reliability of the International Knee Documentation Committee radiographic grading system. *Am J Sports Med*. 2007;35:933–935.

601. Munich H, Cipriani D, Hall C, et al. The test-retest reliability of an inclined squat strength test protocol. *J Orthop Sports Phys Ther*. 1997;26:209–213.

602. Sanfridson J, Ryd L, Svahn S. Radiographic measurement of femoral rotation in weight-bearing. *Acta Radiol*. 2001;42:207–217.

603. Hartmann A, Knols R, Murer K, et al. Reproducibility of an isokinetic strength-testing protocol of the knee and ankle in older adults. *Gerontology*. 2009;55:259–268.

604. Wadley V, Mohtadi N, Bray R, Frank C. Positive predictive value of maximal posterior joint-line tenderness in diagnosing meniscal pathology: a pilot study. *Can J Surg*. 2007;50:96–100.

605. Konan S, Rayan F, Haddad FS. Do physical diagnostic tests accurately detect meniscal tears? *Knee Surg Sports Traumatol Arthrosc*. 2009;17:806–811.

606. Salavati M, Akhbari B, Mohammadi F, et al. Knee Injury and Osteoarthritis Outcome Score (KOOS): reliability and validity in competitive athletes after anterior cruciate ligament reconstruction. *Osteoarthr Cartil*. 2011;19(4):406–410.

607. Stillman BC, McMeeken JM. The role of weightbearing in the clinical assessment of knee joint position sense. *Austr J Phyiother*. 2001;47:247–253.

608. Lingard EA, Katz JN, Wright J, et al. Kinemax Outcomes Group: Validity and responsiveness of the knee society clinical rating system in comparison with the SF-36 and WOMAC. *J Bone Joint Surg*. 2001;83:1856–1864.

609. Kessler S, Käfer W. Comparative assessment of outcome in osteoarthritis: the utility of the knee. *Acta Chir Orthop Traumatol Cech*. 2007;74(5):332–335.

610. Berry J, Kramer K, Binkley J, et al. Error estimates in novice and expert raters for the KT-1000 arthrometer. *J Orthop Sports Phys Ther*. 1999;29:49–55.

611. Denti M, Monteleone M, Trevisan C, et al. Instrumental lachman test: comparison between two arthrometers. Intraoperator and interoperator reproducibility in

subjects asymptomatic and subjects operated for reconstruction of the anterior cruciate ligament. *J Sports Traumatol Rel Res*. 1993;15(1):29–36.

612. Robnett NJ, Riddle DL, Kues JM. Intertester reliability of measurements obtained with the KT-1000 on patients with reconstructed anterior cruciate ligaments. *J Orthop Sports Phys Ther*. 1995;21(2):113–119.

613. Ballantyne BT, French AK, Heimsoth SL, et al. Influence of examiner experience and gender on interrater reliability of KT-1000 arthrometer measurements. *Phys Ther*. 1995;75(10):898–906.

614. Brosky JA, Nitz AJ, Malone TR, et al. Intrarater reliability of selected clinical outcome measures following anterior cruciate ligament reconstruction. *J Orthop Sports Phys Ther*. 1999;29(1):39–48.

615. Sernet N, Kartus J, Kohler K, et al. Evaluation of the reproducibility of the KT-1000 arthrometer. *Scand J Med Sci Sports*. 2001;11:120–125.

616. Wiertsema SH, van Hooff HJA, Migchelsen LAA, et al. Reliability of the KT1000 arthrometer and the Lachman test in patients with an ACL rupture. *The Knee*. 2008;15:107–110.

617. Mulligan EP, Mcguffie DQ, Coyner K, Khazzam M. The reliability and diagnostic accuracy of assessing the translation endpoint during the Lachman test. *Int J Sports Phys Ther*. 2015;10(1):52–61.

618. Steiner ME, Brown C, Zarins B, et al. Measurement of anterior-posterior displacement of the knee. *J Bone Joint Surg Am*. 1990;72(9):1307–1315.

619. Leamouth DJ. Incidence and diagnosis of anterior cruciate injuries in the accident and emergency department. *Injury*. 1991;22:287–290.

620. Katz JW, Fingeroth RJ. The diagnostic accuracy of ruptures of the anterior cruciate ligament comparing the Lachman test, the anterior drawer sign, and the pivot shift test in acute and chronic knee injuries. *Am J Sports Med*. 1986;14:88–91.

621. Schwarz W, Hagelstein J, Minholz R, et al. Manual ultrasound of the knee joint: a general practice method for diagnosis of fresh rupture of the anterior cruciate ligament. *Unfallchirurg*. 1997;100(4):280–285.

622. Dahlstedt LJ, Dalen N. Knee laxity in cruciate ligament injury: value of examination under anesthesia. *Acta Orthop Scand*. 1989;60:181–184.

623. Cook JL, Khan KM, Kiss ZS, et al. Reproducibility and clinical utility of tendon palpation to detect patellar tendinopathy in young basketball players. *Br J Sports Med*. 2001;35(1):65.

624. Stratford PW, Binkley JM, Watson J, et al. Validation of the LEFS on patient with total joint arthroplasty. *Physiother Can*. 2000;52:97–105.

625. Yeung TS, Wessel J, Stratford P, Macdermid J. Reliability, validity, and responsiveness of the lower extremity functional scale for inpatients of an orthopaedic rehabilitation ward. *J Orthop Sports Phys Ther*. 2009;39(6):468–477.

626. Bengtsson J, Mollborg J, Werner S. A study for testing the sensitivity and reliability of the Lysholm knee scoring scale. *Knee Surg Sports Traumatol Arthrosc*. 1996;4:27–31.

627. Briggs KK, Kocher MS, Rodkey WG, et al. Reliability, validity, and responsiveness of the Lysholm knee score and Tegner activity scale for patients with meniscal injury of the knee. *J Bone Joint Surg Am*. 2006;88(4):698–705.

628. Marx RG, Jones EC, Allen AA, et al. Reliability, validity, and responsiveness of four knee outcome scales for athletic patients. *J Bone Joint Surg Am*. 2001;83:1459–1469.

629. Risberg MA, Holm I, Steen H, et al. Sensitivity to changes over time for the IKDC form, the Lysholm score, and the Cincinnati knee score: a prospective study of 120 CL reconstructed patients with a 2-year follow-up. *Knee Surg Sports Traumatol Arthrosc*. 1999;7:152–159.

630. Lee SY, Jee W, Kim J. Radial tear of the medial meniscal root: reliability and accuracy of MRI for diagnosis. *Am J Roentgenol*. 2008;7:81–85.

631. Raynauld JP, Kauffmann C, Beaudoin G, et al. Reliability of a quantification imaging system using magnetic resonance images to measure cartilage thickness and volume in human normal and osteoarthritic knees. *Osteoarthritis Cartilage*. 2003;11(5):351–360.

632. Winters K, Tregonning R. Reliability of magnetic resonance imaging for traumatic injury of the knee. *NZ Med J*. 2005;118(1209):U1301.

633. Watson CJ, Prepps M, Galt W, et al. Reliability of McConnell's classification of patellar orientation in symptomatic and asymptomatic subjects. *J Orthop Sports Phys Ther*. 1999;29:378–385.

634. Herrington LC. The inter tester reliability of a clinical measurement used to determine the medial/lateral orientation of the patella. *Man Ther*. 2000;7(3):163–167.

635. Corea JR, Moussa M, Othman AA. McMurray's test tested. *Knee Surg Sports Traumatol Arthrosc*. 1994;2:70–72.

636. Lowery D, Farley T, Wing D, et al. A clinical composite score accurately detects meniscal pathology. *Arthroscopy*. 2006;22(11):1174–1179.

637. Laoruengthana A, Jarusriwanna A. Sensitivity and specificity of magnetic resonance imaging for knee injury and clinical application for the Naresuan University Hospital. *J Med Assoc Thai*. 2012;95(suppl 10):S151–S157.

638. Esmaili Jah AA, Keyhani S, Zarei R, Moghaddam AK. Accuracy of MRI in comparison with clinical and arthroscopic findings in ligamentous and meniscal injuries of the knee. *Acta Orthop Belg*. 2005;71(2):189–196.

639. Yaqoob J, Alam MS, Khalid N. Diagnostic accuracy of magnetic resonance imaging in assessment of meniscal and ACL tear: correlation with arthroscopy. *Pak J Med Sci*. 2015;31(2):263–268.

640. Lundberg M, Odensten M, Thuomas KA, Messner K. The diagnostic validity of magnetic resonance imaging in acute knee injuries with hemarthrosis. a single-blinded evaluation in 69 patients using high-field MRI before arthroscopy. *Int J Sports Med*. 1996;17(3):218–222.

641. Ercin E, Kaya I, Sungur I, et al. History, clinical findings, magnetic resonance imaging, and arthroscopic correlation in meniscal lesions. *Knee Surg Sports Traumatol Arthrosc*. 2012;20(5):851–856.

642. Ramos LA, Carvalho RT, Garms E, et al. Prevalence of pain on palpation of the inferior pole of the patella among patients with complaints of knee pain. *Clinics (Sao Paulo)*. 2009;64:199–202.

643. Muellner T, Funovics M, Nikolic A, et al. Patellar alignment evaluated by MRI. *Acta Orthop Scand*. 1998;69(5):489–492.

644. Sallay PI, Poggi J, Speer KP, et al. Acute dislocation of the patella. A correlative pathoanatomic study. *Am J Sports Med*. 1996;24:52–60.

645. Chatman AB, Hyams SP, Neel JM, et al. The patient-specific functional scale: measurement properties in patients with knee dysfunction. *Physical Therapy*. 1997;77:820–829.

646. Lucie RS, Wiedel JD, Messner DG. The acute pivot shift: clinical correlation. *Am J Sports Med*. 1984;12:189–191.

647. Rubinstein Jr RA, Shelbourne KD, McCarroll JR, et al. The accuracy of the clinical examination in the setting of posterior cruciate ligament injuries. *Am J Sports Med*. 1994;22:550–557.

648. Loos WC, Fox JM, Blazina ME, et al. Acute posterior cruciate ligament injuries. *Am J Sports Med*. 1981;9:86–92.

649. Moore HA, Larson RL. Posterior cruciate ligament injuries. Results of early surgical repair. *Am J Sports Med*. 1980;8:68–78.

650. Hughston JC, Andrews JR, Cross MJ, et al. Classification of knee ligament instabilities. Part II The lateral compartment. *J Bone Joint Surg Am*. 1976;58:173–179.

651. Clendenin MB, DeLee JC, Heckman JD. Interstitial tears of the posterior cruciate ligament of the knee. *Orthopedics*. 1980;3:764–772.

652. Fowler PJ, Messieh SS. Isolated posterior cruciate ligament injuries in athletes. *Am J Sports Med*. 1987;15:553–557.

653. Staubli JU, Jakob RP. Posterior instability of the knee near extension. A clinical and stress radiographic analysis of acute injuries of the posterior cruciate ligament. *J Bone Joint Surg Br*. 1990;72:225–230.

654. Greene CC, Edwards TB, Wade MR, et al. Reliability of the quadriceps angle measurement. *Am J Knee Surg*. 2001;14:97–103.

655. Fredericson M, Yoon K. Physical examination and patellofemoral pain syndrome. *Am J Phys Med Rehabil*. 2006;85:234–243.

656. Caylor D, Fites R, Worrell TW. The relationship between quadriceps angle and anterior knee pain syndrome. *J Orthop Sport Phys Ther*. 1993;17:11–16.

657. Bremander AB, Peterson IF, Ross EM. Validation of the rheumatoid and arthritis outcome scores (RAOS) for the lower extremity. *Health and Quality of Life Outcomes*. 2003;1:1–11.

658. Gill S, McBurney H. Reliability of performance-based measures in people awaiting joint replacement surgery of the hip or knee. *Physiother Res Int*. 2008;13:141–152.

659. Kennedy DM, Stratford PW, Wessel J, et al. Assessing stability and change of four performance measures: a longitudinal study evaluating outcome following total hip and knee arthroplasty. *BMC Musculoskelet Disord*. 2005;6(3).

660. Fransen M, Crosbie J, Edmonds J. Reliability of gait measurements in people with osteoarthritis of the knee. *Phys Ther*. 1997;77:944–953.

661. Augustsson J, Thomeé R, Linden C, et al. Single-leg hop testing following fatiguing exercise: reliabilty and biomechanical analysis. *Scand J Med Sci Sports*. 2006;16:111–120.

662. Kea J, Kramer J, Forwell L, et al. Hip abduction-adduction stretch and one-leg hop test: test-retest reliability and relationship to function in elite ice hockey players. *J Orthop Sports Phys Ther*. 2001;31(8):446–455.

663. Paterno MV, Greenberger HB. The test-retest reliability of a one legged hop for distance in young adults with and without ACL reconstruction. *Isokinetics Exerc Sci*. 1996;6:1–6.

664. Kramer JF, Nusca D, Fowler P, et al. Test-retest reliability of the one-leg hop test following ACL reconstruction. *Clin J Sport Med*. 1992;2:240–243.

665. Ageberg E, Zatterstrom R, Mortiz U. Stabiliometry and one leg hop test have high test-retest reliability. *Scand J Med Sci Sports*. 1998;8:198–202.

666. Birmingham TB. Test-retest reliability of lower extremity functional instability measures. *Clin J Sports Med*. 2000;10:264–268.

667. DiMattia MA, Livengood AL, Uhl TL, et al. What are the validity of the single-leg squat test and its relationship to hip-abduction strength? *Sport Rehabil*. 2005;14:108–123.

668. Shields RK, Enloe LJ, Evans RF, et al. Reliability, validity, and responsiveness of functional tests in patients with total joint replacement. *Phys Ther*. 1995;75:169–179.

669. Björklund K, Sköld C, Andersson L, et al. Reliability of a criterion-based test of athletes with knee injuries: where the physiotherapist and the patient independently and simultaneously assess the patient's performance. *Knee Surg Sports Traumatol Arthrosc*. 2006;14:165–175.

670. Björklund K, Andersson L, Dalén N. Validity and responsiveness of the test of athletes with knee injuries: the new criterion based functional performance test instrument. *Knee Surg Sports Traumatol Arthrosc*. 2009;17:435–445.

671. Harrison B, Abell B, Gibson T. The Thessaly test for detection of meniscal tears: validation of a new physical examination technique for primary care medicine. *Clin J Sport Med*. 2009;19(1):9–12.

672. Hamilton RT, Shultz SJ, Schmitz RJ, Perrin DH. Triple-hop distance as a valid predictor of lower limb strength and power. *J Athl Train*. 2008;43(2):144–151.

673. Gebhard F, Authenrieth M, Strecker W, et al. Ultrasound evaluation of gravity induced anterior drawer following anterior cruciate ligament lesion. *Knee Surg Sports Traumatol Arthrosc*. 1999;7(3):166–172.

674. McClure PW, Rothstein JM, Riddle DL. Intertester reliability of clinical judgements of medial knee ligament integrity. *Phys Ther*. 1989;69(4):268–275.

675. Garvin GJ, Munk PL, Vellet AD. Tears of the medial collateral ligament: magnetic resonance imaging findings and associated injuries. *Can Assoc Radiol J*. 1993;44:199–204.

676. Salaffi F, Leardini G, Canesi B, et al. Reliability and validity of the Western Ontario and McMaster Universities (WOMAC) Osteoarthritis Index in Italian patients with osteoarthritis of the knee. *Osteoarthr Cartil*. 2003;11(8):551–560.

CHAPTER 13

Lower Leg, Ankle, and Foot

At least 80% of the general population has foot problems, but these problems can often be corrected by proper assessment, treatment, and, above all, care of the feet. Lesions of the ankle and foot can alter the mechanics of gait resulting in movement impairments and, as a result, cause stress on other lower limb joints, which in turn may lead to pathology in these joints.[1]

The foot and ankle combine flexibility with stability because of the many bones, their shapes, and their attachments. The lower leg, ankle, and foot have three principal functions: impact absorption and adaptation to uneven surfaces, propulsion, and support.[2] For impact absorption and adaptation to uneven surfaces and propulsion, they act like a flexible lever; for support, they act like a rigid structure that holds up the entire body.[2]

Functions of the Foot

- Acts as a support base that provides the necessary stability for upright posture with minimal muscle effort
- Provides a mechanism for rotation of the tibia and fibula during the stance phase of gait
- Provides flexibility to adapt to uneven terrain
- Provides flexibility for absorption of shock
- Acts as a lever during push-off

Although the joints of the lower leg, ankle, and foot are discussed separately, they act as functional groups, not as isolated joints. As the terminal part of the lower kinetic chain, the lower leg, ankle, and foot have the ability to distribute and dissipate the different forces (e.g., compressive, shearing, rotary, tensile) acting on the body through contact with the ground.[3] The ankle joint sustains the greatest load per surface area of any joint in the body.[4] This is especially evident during gait. In the foot, the movement occurring at each individual joint is minimal. However, when combined, there normally is sufficient range of motion (ROM) in all of the joints to allow functional mobility as well as functional stability. For ease of understanding, the joints of the foot are divided into three sections: hindfoot (rearfoot), midfoot, and forefoot.

Because the foot is distally located, there is very little referred pain from lesions of the foot but injuries in the spine, sacroiliac joints, hips, and knees may refer pain to the foot.[5] The foot is difficult to examine because of the strong structures with limited individual mobility.[5]

Applied Anatomy

Hindfoot (Rearfoot)

Tibiofibular Joint. The inferior (distal) tibiofibular joint is a fibrous or syndesmosis type of joint. It is supported by the anterior tibiofibular, posterior tibiofibular, and inferior transverse ligaments as well as the interosseous ligaments (Fig. 13.1). The movements at this joint are minimal but allow a small amount of spread (1 to 2 mm) at the ankle joint during dorsiflexion. This same action allows the fibula to move up and down during dorsiflexion and plantar flexion. Dorsiflexion at the ankle joint causes the fibula to move superiorly, putting stress on both the inferior tibiofibular joint at the ankle and the superior tibiofibular joint at the knee. The fibula carries more of the axial load when it is dorsiflexed. On average, the fibula carries about 17% of the axial loading.[6] The joint is supplied by the deep peroneal and tibial nerves.

Talocrural (Ankle) Joint. The talocrural joint is a uniaxial, modified hinge, synovial joint located between the **talus,** the **tibial plafond,** the **medial malleolus** of the tibia, and the **lateral malleolus** of the fibula.[7] The talus is shaped so that in dorsiflexion it is wedged between the malleoli,

---

Joints of the Hindfoot

Tibiofibular Joint

Resting position:	Plantar flexion
Close packed position:	Maximum dorsiflexion
Capsular pattern:	Pain when joint is stressed

Talocrural (Ankle) Joint

Resting position:	10° plantar flexion, midway between inversion and eversion
Close packed position:	Maximum dorsiflexion
Capsular pattern:	Plantar flexion, dorsiflexion

Subtalar Joint

Resting position:	Midway between extremes of range of motion (ROM)
Close packed position:	Supination
Capsular pattern:	Limited ROM (varus, valgus)

allowing little or no inversion or eversion at the ankle joint. It is this shape that provides a major source of natural stability to the ankle.[8,9] The talus is approximately 2.4 mm (0.1 inch) wider anteriorly than posteriorly. The talocrural joint is lined with about 3 mm of articular cartilage and is compressed about 30% to 40% in response to peak physiologic loads.[10] The medial malleolus is shorter, extending halfway down the talus, whereas the lateral malleolus extends almost to the level of the subtalar joint. The joint is supplied by branches of the tibial and deep peroneal nerves.

The talocrural joint is designed for stability, especially in dorsiflexion. In plantar flexion, it is much more mobile. This joint is responsible for the anterior-posterior (dorsiflexion-plantar flexion) movement that occurs in the ankle-foot complex. Its close packed position is maximum dorsiflexion, and its capsular pattern is more a limitation of plantar flexion than of dorsiflexion. This joint is most stable in the dorsiflexed position due to joint congruency and ligamentous tension. The resting position is 10° of plantar flexion, midway between maximum inversion and

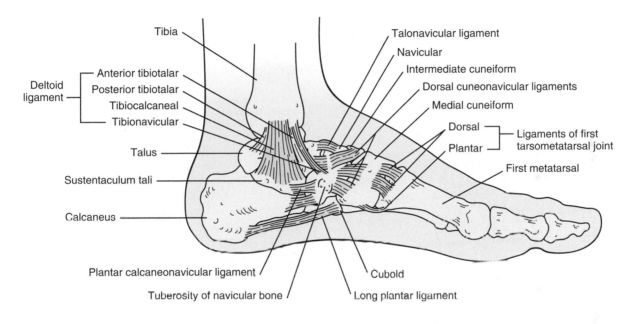

A

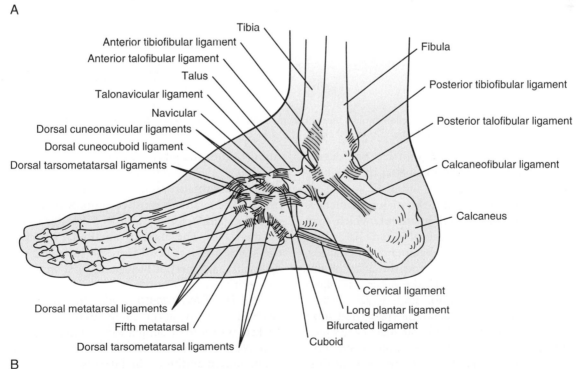

B

Fig. 13.1 Ligaments of the hindfoot and midfoot. (A) Medial view. (B) Lateral view.

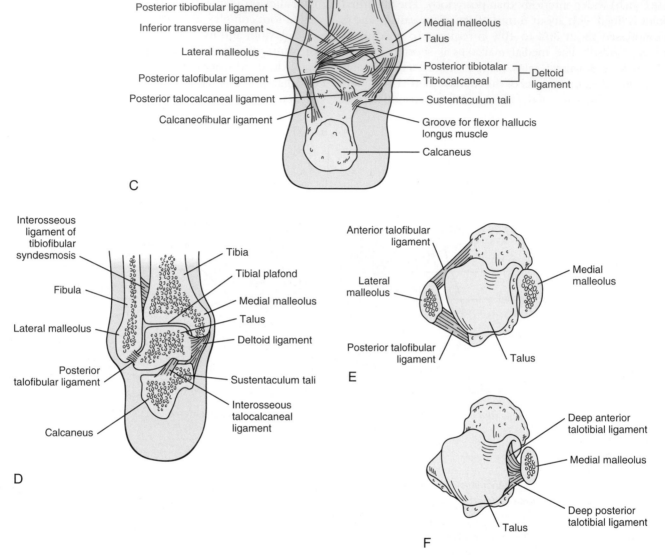

Fig. 13.1, cont'd (C) Posterior view. (D) Coronal section through the left talocrural and talocalcaneal joints. (E) Superior view of ligaments on the lateral aspect. (F) Superior view of deep deltoid ligament on the medial aspect.

maximum eversion. The talocrural joint has one degree of freedom, and the movements possible at this joint are dorsiflexion and plantar flexion.

On the medial side of the joint, the major ligament is the **deltoid** or **medial collateral ligament,** which consists of four separate ligaments: the tibionavicular, tibiocalcaneal, and posterior tibiotalar ligaments superficially, all of which resist talar abduction, and the anterior tibiotalar ligament, which lies deep to the other three ligaments and resists lateral translation and lateral rotation of the talus. On the lateral aspect, the talocrural joint is supported by the anterior talofibular ligament, which provides stability against excessive inversion of the talus; the posterior talofibular ligament, which resists ankle dorsiflexion, adduction ("tilt"), medial rotation, and medial

translation of the talus; and the calcaneofibular ligament, which provides stability against maximum inversion at the ankle and subtalar joints. The anterior talofibular ligament is the ligament most commonly injured by a lateral inversion ankle sprain, followed by the calcaneofibular ligament.[11,12] The anterior talofibular ligament requires the lowest maximal load to result in failure of the lateral ligaments, although it has the highest strain to failure of the entire lateral group.[13]

Subtalar (Talocalcaneal) Joint. The subtalar joint is a synovial joint having three degrees of freedom and a close packed position of supination. Supporting the subtalar joint are the lateral talocalcaneal and medial talocalcaneal ligaments. In addition, the interosseous talocalcaneal and cervical ligaments limit eversion.

The movements possible at the subtalar joint are gliding and rotation. With injury to the area (e.g., sprain, fracture), this joint and the talocrural joint often become hypomobile, partially because the talus has no muscles attaching to it. Medial rotation of the leg causes a valgus (outward) movement of the calcaneus, whereas lateral rotation of the leg produces a varus (inward) movement of the calcaneus. The normal varus-valgus ROM is between 20° and 45°.[5] The axis of the joint is at an angle of 41° inclined vertically from the transverse plane and 23° medially from the longitudinal reference of the foot (see Fig. 13.157).

Midfoot (Midtarsal Joints)

In isolation, the midtarsal joints allow only a minimal amount of movement. Taken together, however, they allow significant movement to enable the foot to adapt to many positions without putting undue stress on the joints. **Chopart joint** refers collectively to the midtarsal joints between the talus-calcaneus and the navicular-cuboid.

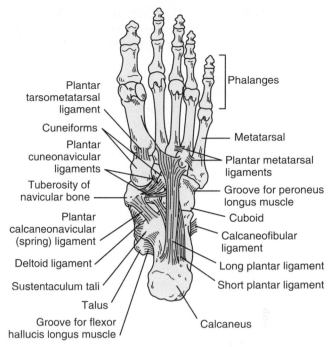

Fig. 13.2 Ligaments on plantar aspect of foot.

Joints of the Midfoot (Midtarsal Joints)

Resting position:	Midway between extremes of range of motion (ROM)
Close packed position:	Supination
Capsular pattern:	Dorsiflexion, plantar flexion, adduction, medial rotation

---

Talocalcaneonavicular Joint. The talocalcaneonavicular joint is a ball-and-socket synovial joint with 3° of freedom. Its close packed position is supination, and the dorsal talonavicular ligament, bifurcated ligament, and plantar calcaneonavicular (spring) ligament support the joint (Fig. 13.2). Movements possible at this joint are gliding and rotation.

Cuneonavicular Joint. The cuneonavicular joint is a plane synovial joint with a close packed position of supination. The movements possible at this joint are slight gliding and rotation.

Cuboideonavicular Joint. The cuboideonavicular joint is fibrous, its close packed position being supination. The movements possible at this joint are slight gliding and rotation.

Intercuneiform Joints. The intercuneiform joints are plane synovial joints with a close packed position of supination. The movements possible at these joints are slight gliding and rotation.

Cuneocuboid Joint. The cuneocuboid joint is a plane synovial joint with a close packed position of supination. The movements of slight gliding and rotation are possible at this joint.

Calcaneocuboid Joint. The calcaneocuboid joint is saddle shaped with a close packed position of supination. Supporting this joint are the bifurcated ligament, the calcaneocuboid ligament, and the long plantar ligaments. The movement possible at this joint is gliding with conjunct rotation.

Forefoot

Tarsometatarsal Joints. The tarsometatarsal joints are plane synovial joints with a close packed position of supination. The movement possible at these joints is gliding. Taken together, these joints are referred to as **Lisfranc joint.**[14]

Joints of the Forefoot

Tarsometatarsal Joints

Resting position:	Midway between extremes of range of motion (ROM)
Close packed position:	Supination
Capsular pattern:	None

Metatarsophalangeal Joints

Resting position:	10° extension
Close packed position:	Full extension
Capsular pattern:	Hallux (big toe): extension, flexion
	Second to fifth toe: variable

Interphalangeal Joints

Resting position:	Slight flexion
Close packed position:	Full extension
Capsular pattern:	Flexion, extension

Intermetatarsal Joints. The four intermetatarsal joints are plane synovial joints with a close packed position of supination. The movement possible at these joints is gliding.

Metatarsophalangeal Joints. The five metatarsophalangeal joints are condyloid synovial joints with 2° of freedom. Their close packed position is full extension. Their capsular pattern is variable for the lateral four joints and more limitation of extension than flexion for the hallux (big toe); their resting position is 10° of extension. The movements possible at these joints are flexion, extension, abduction, and adduction.

Interphalangeal Joints. The interphalangeal joints are synovial hinge joints with 1° of freedom. The close packed position is full extension, and the capsular pattern is more limitation of flexion than of extension. The resting position of the distal and proximal interphalangeal joints is slight flexion. The movements possible at these joints are flexion and extension.

Patient History

It is important to take a detailed and complete history when assessing the lower leg, ankle, and foot.[15] In addition to the questions listed under the "Patient History" section in Chapter 1 the examiner should obtain the following information from the patient:

1. *What is the patient's occupation?* Whether the patient stands a great deal and the types of surfaces on which the patient usually stands may have bearing on what is causing the problem.
2. *What was the mechanism of injury?* What was the position of the foot at the time of the injury? Ankle sprains occur most often when the foot is plantar flexed, inverted, and adducted, with injury to the anterior talofibular ligament, anterolateral capsule, and possibly the distal tibiofibular ligament.[16–18] This same mechanism can lead to peroneal tendon injury, tibialis posterior tendon injury, common peroneal nerve injury, a malleolar or talar dome fracture, or sinus tarsi syndrome.[19–21] Fig. 13.3 outlines some of the common mechanisms of injury to the ankle. Table 13.1 outlines the **West Point Sprain Grading System** that can be used to determine the severity of ankle sprains.[22] With injury to the lateral ligaments, the structures (articular surfaces) may be damaged on the medial side owing to compression leading to medial as well as lateral pain.[23] In fact, if the lateral ligaments are completely torn and the capsule disrupted, medial pain may predominate. Anterolateral pain without a history of trauma may be the result of anterior impingement especially after injury to the

anterior talofibular ligament. Syndesmosis injuries ("high ankle sprains") are usually the result of forced lateral rotation of the tibia and/or hyperdorsiflexion. Fig. 13.4 illustrates the most common mechanisms for syndesmosis sprains.[24] Liu et al.[25] developed a clinical prediction rule for ankle impingement that would preclude the need for magnetic resonance imaging (MRI). The impingement may be due to thickening of the joint capsule and/or bone spurs adjacent to the anterior talocrural joint.[26] Achilles tendinosis or paratenonitis often arises as the result of overuse, increased activity, or change in a high-stress training program. Achilles tendon ruptures are reported as a pop or snap as though the patient had been hit or kicked in the area of the rupture although, in most cases, there was no one near them.[27–29] The pain is sudden and quickly dissipates with weakness of plantar flexion. Osteochondral lesions most commonly occur with trauma and may accompany ankle sprains and fractures with symptoms being exacerbated by prolonged weight bearing or high-impact activities.[30] A dorsiflexion injury, accompanied by a snapping and pain on the lateral aspect that rapidly diminishes, may indicate a tear of the peroneal retinaculum.[31] Individuals such as dancers, soccer players, and track and field athletes may have **posterior ankle impingement** because of excessive repetitive plantar flexion of the foot which may be accompanied by or result in an **os trigonum** (separate ossicle), a **Stieda's process** (protruding lateral tubercle of the talus), or **Shepherd's fracture** (fracture of the lateral tubercle).[32,33] The flexor hallucis longus tendon pathology may also result in similar pain.[33] Anteriorly, synovial impingement may lead to chronic pain following an anterolateral talocrural sprain.[34] Taunton et al.[35] list some causes of overuse injuries in the lower limb.

Clinical Prediction Rule for Anterolateral Ankle Impingement

Note: Five of six symptoms must be positive.
- Anterolateral ankle joint tenderness
- Anterolateral ankle joint swelling
- Pain on forced dorsiflexion
- Pain on affected side with single leg squat
- Pain with activities
- Absence of ankle instability

From Liu SH, Nuccion SL, Finerman G: Diagnosis of anterolateral ankle impingement: comparison between magnetic resonance imaging and clinical examination, *Am J Sports Med* 25:389–393, 1997.

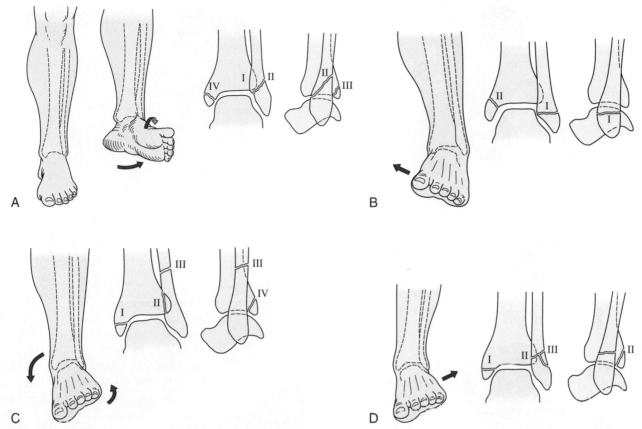

Fig. 13.3 Ankle fracture injury mechanisms. (A) Supination-lateral rotation injury. Lateral rotation forces applied to a supinated foot initially result in rupture of the anterior tibiofibular ligament (stage I). As the forces continue, a short oblique fracture of the distal portion of the fibula occurs (stage II). Stage III involves a fracture of the posterior aspect of the tibia. Stage IV is a fracture of the medial malleolus. (B) Supination-adduction injury. Adduction forces applied to a supinated foot initially result in a traction or avulsion fracture of the distal portion of the fibula or rupture of the lateral ligaments (stage I). As forces continue, fracture of the medial malleolus or rupture of the deltoid ligament occurs (stage II). The fibular fracture is typically transverse, and that of the medial malleolus is oblique or nearly vertical. (C) Pronation-lateral rotation injury. Forces of lateral rotation applied to a pronated foot initially result in rupture of the deltoid ligament or fracture of the medial malleolus (stage I). As forces continue, the anterior tibiofibular ligament is ruptured (stage II). A high fibular fracture (stage III) and fracture of the posterior tibial margin (stage IV) are the final stages in this mechanism of injury. (D) Pronation-abduction injury. The first two stages of this injury are identical to those of the pronation-external rotation fracture complex. Stage III is a transverse supramalleolar fibular fracture that may be comminuted laterally. (Redrawn from Resnick D, Kransdorf MJ: *Bone and joint imaging*, Philadelphia, 2005, WB Saunders, pp 867–868.)

TABLE **13.1**

The West Point Ankle Sprain Grading System

Criterion	Grade I	Grade II	Grade III
Location of tenderness	Anterior talofibular ligament	Anterior talofibular ligament and calcaneofibular ligament	Anterior talofibular ligament, calcaneofibular ligament, and posterior talofibular ligament
Edema and ecchymosis	Slight and local	Moderate and local	Significant and diffuse
Weight-bearing ability	Full or partial	Difficult without crutches	Impossible without significant pain
Ligament damage	Stretched	Partial tear	Complete tear
Instability	None	None or slight	Definite

From Dutton M: *Dutton's orthopedic examination, evaluation and intervention*, ed 3, New York, 2012, McGraw Hill. Data from Gerber JP, Williams GN, Scoville CR, et al: Persistent disability associated with ankle sprains: a prospective examination of an athletic population, *Foot Ankle Int* 19:653-660, 1998.

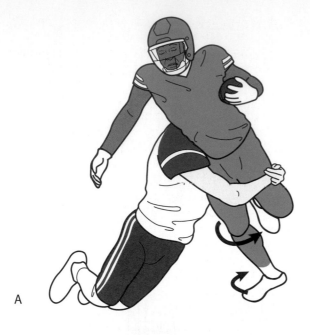

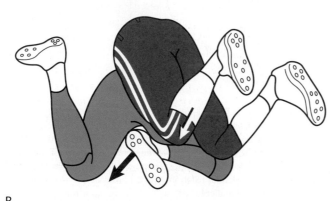

Fig. 13.4 Typical mechanisms of injury for syndesmotic sprains/fractures. (A) The foot is fixed in a position of lateral rotation with the ankle dorsiflexing while a lateral force at the trunk or hip causes a medial rotation of the lower limb. (B) The athlete is in a prone position and receives a direct blow to the lateral leg forcing the dorsiflexed ankle into excessive lateral rotation. (Redrawn from Mulligan EP: Evaluation and management of ankle syndesmosis injuries, *Phys Ther Sport* 12(2):59, 2011.)

Causes of Overuse Injuries to the Lower Limb

- Prolonged training season
- Impact force of activity
- Training or competing on hard surfaces
- Change of training surface
- Downhill running
- Lack of flexibility
- Individual muscle weakness or poor reciprocal muscle strength
- Overstriding
- Poor posture
- High mileage or sudden change in mileage
- Too much, too soon
- Overtraining
- Anatomical factors (e.g., malalignment)
- Wrong type of footwear
- Road or sidewalk camber

From Taunton J, Smith C, Magee DJ: Leg, foot and ankle injuries. In Zachazewski JE, Magee DJ, Quillen WS, editors: *Athletic injuries and rehabilitation*, Philadelphia, 1996, WB Saunders.

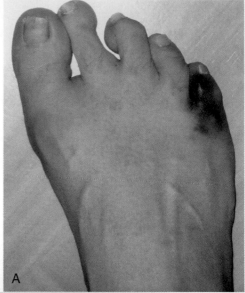

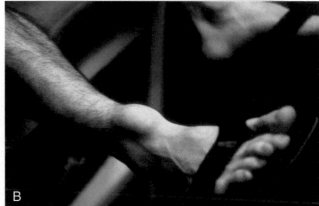

Fig. 13.5 (A) Ecchymosis following fracture of small toe. (B) "Skate or lace bite." Swelling over extensor tendons.

3. *Did the patient notice a transient or fixed deformity of the foot or ankle at the time of injury?* Was there any transitory locking (e.g., loose body, muscle spasm)? An affirmative answer may indicate a fracture causing immediate swelling that decreased as it spread into the surrounding tissue.

4. *Was the patient able to continue the activity after the injury?* If so, the injury is probably not too severe, provided there is no loss of stability. Inability to bear weight, severe pain, and rapid swelling indicate a severe injury.[31] Walking is compatible with a second-degree sprain; pain with running usually indicates a first-degree injury.[36]

5. *Was there any swelling or bruising (ecchymosis)* (Fig. 13.5A)? *How quickly and where did it develop?* This question can elicit some idea of the type of swelling (e.g., blood, synovial, purulent) and whether it is intracapsular or extracapsular. Fig. 13.5B shows "skate bite" in which there is swelling over the extensor tendons of the foot caused by irritation from doing up (i.e., lacing up) stiff ice skates too tight.

6. *Are symptoms improving, becoming worse, or staying the same?* It is important to know the type of onset (macrotrauma, microtrauma) and the duration and intensity of symptoms (acute, subacute, chronic). Edwards et al.[37] outlined some of the chronic causes of leg pain in athletes. Chronic recurrent ankle instability will be indicated by one or more significant lateral ankle sprains involving functional and mechanical instability, increased subtalar laxity and greater anterior laxity, or history of giving way usually during initial contact when walking, running, cutting, or rapidly decelerating in the last 6 months. Outcome score cutoffs on functional ankle instruments are: **Ankle Instability Instrument** (answer "yes" to at least 5 yes/no questions); **Cumberland Ankle Instability Tool** (<24); **Identification of Functional Ankle Instability (IdFAI)** (>11); **Foot and Ankle Ability Measure** (ADL scale <90%; sport scale <80%); and **Foot and Ankle Outcome Score** (<75% on 3 or more categories).[38–43] Mechanical instability is due to disruption of one or more ligaments while functional instability is loss of neuromuscular or proprioceptive movement control.[44]

Differential Diagnosis of Chronic Leg Pain in the Athlete

Bone Periosteum
- Medial tibial stress syndrome ("shin splints")[a]
- Stress fracture[a]

Vascular
- Popliteal artery entrapment syndrome
- Intermittent claudication

Referred Pain
- Nerve entrapment
  - Peripheral
  - Spinal/radiculopathy
- Referred pain
  - Knee abnormality
  - Hip abnormality (especially in young patients)

Muscle/Tendon
- Chronic exertional compartment syndrome
- Muscle strains
- Tendinitis/tendinosis

Neoplasm

Infection

[a]These two conditions are commonly different stages of the same pathological continuum.
Modified from Edwards PH, Wright ML, Hartman JF: A practical approach for the differential diagnosis of chronic leg pain in the athlete. *Am J Sports Med* 33:1244, 2005.

---

7. *What are the sites and boundaries of pain or abnormal sensation?* The examiner should note whether the pattern is one of a dermatome, a peripheral nerve, or another painful structure. If pain and other physical findings are "out of proportion" to what would normally be expected with injury especially in the rearfoot/talar region, a more diligent examination including extra radiographic images of the talus and calcaneus may be necessary.[45]

8. *What is the patient's usual activity or pastime?* Answers to this question should give some idea of the stresses placed on the lower leg, ankle, and foot; how frequently they are applied; and whether the patient is suffering from a repetitive stress injury. For example, tarsal navicular stress fractures may be seen in runners resulting in dorsal midfoot pain radiating into the medial arch with little swelling.[46]

9. *Does activity make a difference?* Pain after activity suggests overuse.[47] For example, with overuse injuries, pain initially comes on after the activity. As the injury progresses, pain or soreness is present at the beginning of the activity, and then it goes away during the activity only to return afterward. In later stages of the problem, the pain is constantly present. Pain during the activity suggests stress on the injured structure.

10. *Where is the pain? Does the patient indicate a specific location or area?* For example, with shin splints **(medial tibial stress syndrome [MTSS])** or a compartment syndrome (acute or chronic exertional type), the patient usually indicates a diffuse area.[48–52] With a stress fracture, the area of pain tends to be more specific. Anterolateral ankle impingement demonstrates anterolateral ankle joint tenderness, anterolateral ankle joint swelling (extracapsular), pain with force dorsiflexion and eversion, pain with single leg squat, pain with activities, and possible absence of ankle instability.[25] Peroneal tendon problems show posterolateral pain and may be associated with lateral ankle instability.[53] Plantar fasciitis is the most common cause of heel pain on the antero-medial aspect of the heel.[54] It may be accompanied by a heel spur (see Fig. 13.144C), which is the result of the plantar fasciitis.

    Systemic problems may also lead to problems in the leg and foot. **Deep venous thrombosis (DVT)** in the leg can lead to pulmonary embolism especially in sedentary people due to venous stasis and can have devastating consequences. Diabetes may also lead to foot problems (Table 13.2).[15,55,56]

11. *Does walking on various terrains make a difference in regard to the foot problem?* If so, which terrains cause the most obvious problem? For example, walking on grass (an uneven surface) may bother the patient more than walking on a sidewalk (a relatively even surface), or the patient may find walking on a relatively soft surface (e.g., grass) easier than walking on a hard surface (e.g., cement). Prepared surfaces, such as sidewalks, roads, and playing fields, often have a camber to allow water runoff. This camber can cause problems in some cases of overuse.

12. *What types of shoes does the patient wear? What kind of heel do the shoes have? Are the shoes in good condition? Does the patient make use of orthoses? If so, are they still functional?*[57] When an appointment is being made for an assessment, the patient should be

TABLE 13.2

Diabetic Foot Screening Guidelines

Ulcer Risk Factors	Historical Features	Essential Physical Examination
• Peripheral neuropathy • Foot deformity • Foot trauma • Previous amputation • Past foot ulcer history • Peripheral vascular disease • Visual impairment • Diabetic nephropathy • Poor glycemic control • Cigarette smoking	• Past medical history: ◦ Ulceration, amputation, Charcot joint, vascular surgery, angioplasty, cigarette smoking • Neuropathic symptoms: ◦ Burning, shooting, pain, electrical, or sharp sensations ◦ Numbness, dead feet • Vascular symptoms: ◦ Claudication, rest pain, nonhealing ulcer • Other complications: ◦ Renal, retina	• Skin assessment ◦ Color, thickness, dryness, cracking; sweating; infection (check between toes for fungal); ulceration; calluses/blistering (hemorrhage into callus?) • Musculoskeletal assessment ◦ Deformity, such as claw toes, prominent metatarsal heads, Charcot joint, hallux valgus; muscle wasting (guttering between metatarsals) • Neurologic assessment ◦ 10-g monofilament + 1 of the following 4: Vibration using 128-Hz tuning fork; pinprick sensation; ankle reflexes; vibration perception threshold testing • Vascular assessment ◦ Foot pulses (ankle-brachial index[a] if indicated)

[a]Ankle-brachial index: comparison of systolic blood pressure in arm and leg.
From Papaliodis DN, Vanushkina MA, Richardson NG, DiPreta JA: The foot and ankle examination, *Med Clin North Am* 98(2):184, 2014. Data from Rogers LC, Frykberg RG, Armstrong DG, et al: The Charcot foot in diabetes, *Diabetes Care* 34(9):2123–2129, 2011.

Signs, Symptoms and Risk Factors for Deep Venous Thrombosis (DVT)[52]

Signs and Symptoms[a]
• Unilateral leg pain (tenderness, cramping, throbbing)
• Shortness of breath
• Dizziness/confusion
• Visible swelling (possible painful lump)
• Red, patchy skin/color change
• Chest pain
• Legs feel tired
• Warm skin (body temperature increase)
• Visible or bulging veins
• Bloody cough

Risk Factors
• Overweight
• Smoker
• Sedentary lifestyle
• Over age 60
• Stationary while travelling long distances
• Genetics
• Heart disease history
• Pregnancy
• Hormonal changes
• Cancer

[a]In some cases, there may be no visible signs or symptoms.

---

told not to wear new shoes so that the examiner can use the shoes to determine the patient's usual shoe wear pattern. Over pronators show more medial shoe wear while over supinators show more lateral wear. Bulging of the medial shoe wall indicates an everted foot while a lateral bulge indicates an inverted foot. The toe box crease should occur at the metatarsal heads and the end of the toe box should be about one thumb's width from the longest toe.[2] The examiner should also note whether the shoes offer proper support. The patient should bring any orthoses he or she is using to the assessment. Poor footwear may contribute to patient pain and subsequent impairment.[58–60] There are several footwear assessment tools to evaluate the fit and function of footwear.[61–64]

13. *Is there a history of previous injury, affliction, or surgery?* For example, poliomyelitis may lead to a pes cavus. Systemic conditions, such as diabetes, gout, psoriasis, and collagen diseases, may manifest themselves first in the foot. If there was previous surgery, did the pain resolve following surgery? Is the pain the same as before surgery? Is it new pain?

14. For active people, especially runners or joggers, the following questions should also be considered[65]:
   a. *How long has the patient been running or jogging?*
   b. *On what type of terrain and surface does the patient train?*
   c. *In what types of workouts does the patient participate? Have the workouts changed lately? How many workouts are done per week? How far does the patient run per week?* (Joggers run approximately 2 to 30 km [1.2 to 18.6 miles] per week at a pace of 5 to 10 minutes/km, and sports runners run 30 to 65 km [18.6 to 40 miles] per week at a pace of 5 to 6 minutes/km. Long-distance runners run 60 to 180 km [37 to 112 miles] per week at a pace of 4 to 5 minutes/km. Elite runners run 100 to 270 km [62 to 168 miles] per week at a pace of 3.3 to 4 minutes/km.)
   d. *What types of warmup, stretching, and postexercise routines does the patient do?* The answers give

the examiner some idea of whether the warmup and stretching activities are static or ballistic and whether these activities could be detrimental.

e. *What types and styles of athletic shoes does the patient wear?* (The patient should have the shoes at the examination.) Are they "control" or "cushioning" shoes? People with a cavus foot are more likely to need a cushioning shoe, whereas those with a planus foot are more likely to need a control shoe. The examiner should be able to tell if the shoes fit properly. Is there any evidence of a subungual hematoma (i.e., blood under the nail) which, in runners, is due to microtrauma from the nail (especially of the hallux) rubbing on the end of the shoe?[66]

f. *Does the patient wear socks while training?* If so, what kind (e.g., cotton, wool, nylon), and how many pairs?

g. *When was the patient's last race? How long was it? When is the patient's next race?* The answers give the examiner some idea of how long the problem has been present and how long it will be until maximum stress is again placed on the joints.

15. *What impact has the injury/deformity had on the patient's quality of life?*

Observation

Observation of the foot is extensive. Because of the stresses the foot is subjected to and because it, like the hand, can project signs of systemic problems and disease, the examiner should carefully and meticulously inspect the foot.

When performing the observation, the examiner should remember to compare the weight-bearing (closed-chain) with the non–weight-bearing (open-chain) posture of the foot.[67] During open-chain motion, the talus is considered fixed; during closed-chain motion, the talus moves to help the foot and leg adapt to the terrain and to the stresses that are applied to the foot. Even though the calcaneus is touching a surface in closed-chain movement, for descriptive purposes, it is still considered to be moving. The weight-bearing stance of the foot shows how the body compensates for structural abnormalities (Fig. 13.6). The non–weight-bearing posture shows functional and structural abilities without compensation (Fig. 13.7). The observation includes looking at the patient from the front, from the side, and from behind in the weight-bearing (standing) position and from the front, from the side, and from behind in the sitting position with the legs and feet not bearing weight. The examiner should note the patient's willingness and ability to use the feet. The bony and soft-tissue contours of the foot should be normal, foot type should be determined (see Fig. 13.15), and any deviation should be noted.[68] Often, painful callosities (hyperkeratosis) may be found over abnormal bony prominences due to increased friction or loading.[2] The examiner should also note any scars or sinuses.

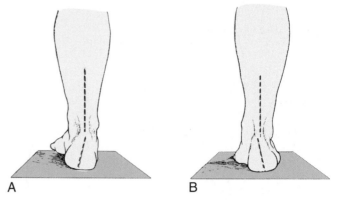

Fig. 13.6 (A) Closed-chain (weight-bearing) supination of the subtalar joint (right foot). Supination of the subtalar joint in the weight-bearing foot results in motion of both the calcaneus and the talus. The calcaneus moves in the frontal plane, and the talus moves in the transverse and sagittal planes. The calcaneus inverts, and the talus simultaneously abducts and dorsiflexes relative to the calcaneus. The leg follows the motion of the talus in the transverse plane and laterally rotates. The leg also follows the sagittal plane motion of the talus to some degree. The dorsiflexion motion of the talus on the calcaneus, therefore, tends to impart a slight extension motion to the knee. (B) Closed-chain (weight-bearing) pronation of the subtalar joint (right foot). Pronation of the subtalar joint in the weight-bearing foot results in eversion of the calcaneus; the talus adducts and plantar flexes relative to the calcaneus. The leg follows the talus in a transverse plane and medially rotates. In a sagittal plane, the leg also moves to some extent with the talus. As the talus plantar flexes, the proximal aspect of the tibia moves forward to flex the knee slightly. (Redrawn from Root ML, Orien WP, Weed JH: *Normal and abnormal function of the foot*, Los Angeles, 1977, Clinical Biomechanics, p 30.)

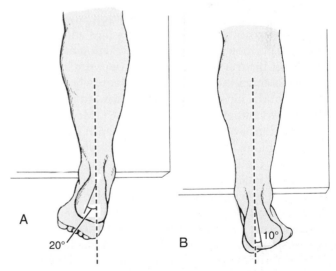

Fig. 13.7 (A) Open-chain (non–weight-bearing) supination of the subtalar joint (right foot). When the non–weight-bearing foot is moved at the subtalar joint in the direction of supination, the talus is stable, and the calcaneus and foot move around the talus. The calcaneus and foot invert, plantar flex, and adduct. These positional changes, associated with subtalar joint supination, are readily visible when compared with the pronated position of the subtalar joint. (B) Open-chain (non–weight-bearing) pronation of the subtalar joint (right foot). When the subtalar joint is moved into a pronated position in the non–weight-bearing foot, the foot abducts, everts, and dorsiflexes around the stable talus. The positional variances can best be appreciated by comparing this illustration with the supinated position of the subtalar joint. (Redrawn from Root ML, Orien WP, Weed JH: *Normal and abnormal function of the foot*, Los Angeles, 1977, Clinical Biomechanics, p 29.)

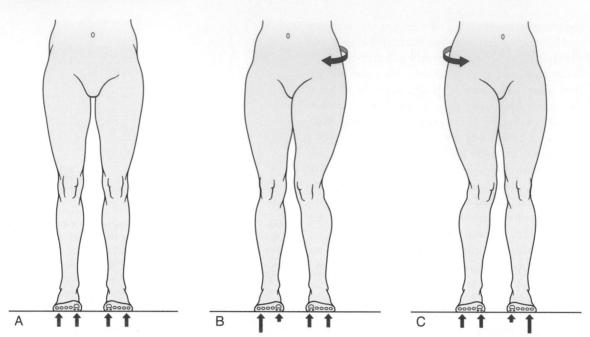

Fig. 13.8 (A) During static stance, ground reaction forces *(arrows)* directed upward against the plantar aspects of both feet maintain the transverse plane equilibrium and stability of the lower extremities and pelvis. Equal ground reaction forces are exerted on the lateral and medial plantar surfaces of both feet. (B) When the trunk is rotated to the right, the right foot supinates and the left pronates. The right forefoot inverts from the ground; vertical ground reaction forces are greater against the lateral side of the forefoot *(large arrow)* and less against the medial side of the forefoot *(small arrow)*. The left forefoot remains flat on the ground, and vertical ground reaction forces are distributed evenly against the forefoot *(equal arrows)*. (C) When the trunk is rotated to the left, ground reaction exerts unequal forces against the left forefoot and equal forces against the right forefoot. (Redrawn from Root ML, Orien WP, Weed JH: *Normal and abnormal function of the foot*, Los Angeles, 1977, Clinical Biomechanics, p 102.)

Weight-Bearing Position, Anterior View

With the patient in a standing position, the examiner should observe whether the patient's hips and trunk are in normal position. Excessive lateral rotation of the hip or rotation of the trunk away from the opposite hip elevates the medial longitudinal arch of the foot, whereas medial rotation of the hip or trunk rotation toward the opposite hip tends to flatten the arch (Fig. 13.8). Medial rotation of the hip can also cause pigeon toes, which is a condition more commonly associated with medial tibial torsion or rotation. If the iliotibial band is tight, the tightness may cause eversion and lateral rotation of the foot.

The examiner should also look at the tibia to note any local or general bone swelling (Fig. 13.9). Does the tibia have a normal shape, or is it bowed? Is there any torsional deformity? The medial malleolus usually lies anterior to the lateral malleolus. Pigeon toes, or toe-in deformity, result from a medial tibial torsion deformity; it does not constitute a foot deformity (Table 13.3).

Fig. 13.10 shows the anterosuperior view of the feet in the weight-bearing stance. The examiner should note whether there is any asymmetry, malalignment (Table 13.4), or excessive supination or pronation of the foot.[69] **Supination** of the foot involves inversion and outward rotation of the heel, adduction of the forefoot with inward rotation at the tarsometatarsal joints to maintain contact with the ground and outward rotation at the midtarsal joints, and plantar flexion at the subtalar joint and midtarsal joints so that the medial

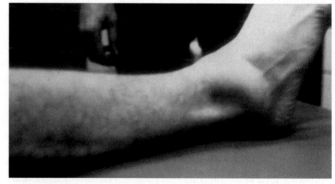

Fig. 13.9 Swelling within the talocrural and subtalar joint capsule.

longitudinal arch is accentuated (see Fig. 13.57). In addition, along with lateral rotation of the talus, there is lateral rotation of the leg in relation to the foot (Fig. 13.11). Supination of the foot causes the proximal aspect of the tibia to move posteriorly. It is required during propulsion to give rigidity to the foot and requires less muscle work than pronation.

Pronation of the foot involves eversion and inward rotation of the heel, abduction of the forefoot with outward rotation at the tarsometatarsal joints and inward rotation at the midtarsal joints, and medial rotation of the talus causing medial rotation of the leg in relation to the foot, and dorsiflexion of the subtalar and midtarsal joints (Fig. 13.12), resulting in a decrease in the medial longitudinal arch (see Fig. 13.57). This movement causes the proximal aspect of the tibia to move anteriorly. The pronated foot has greater subtalar motion than the supinated

TABLE **13.3**

Causes of Toeing-In and Toeing-Out in Children

Level of Affection	Toe In	Toe Out
Feet-ankles	Pronated feet (protective toeing-in) Metatarsus varus Talipes varus and equinovarus	Pes valgus due to contracture of triceps surae muscle Talipes calcaneovalgus Congenital convex pes planovalgus
Leg-knee	Tibia vara (Blount disease) and developmental genu varum Abnormal medial tibial torsion Genu valgum—developmental (protective toeing-in to shift body center of gravity medially)	Lateral tibial torsion Congenital absence of hypoplasia of the fibula
Femur-hip	Abnormal femoral antetorsion Spasticity of medial rotators of hip (cerebral palsy)	Abnormal femoral retroversion Flaccid paralysis of medial rotators of hip
Acetabulum	Maldirected—facing anteriorly	Maldirected—facing posteriorly

From Tachdjian MO: *Pediatric orthopedics*, Philadelphia, 1990, WB Saunders, p 2817.

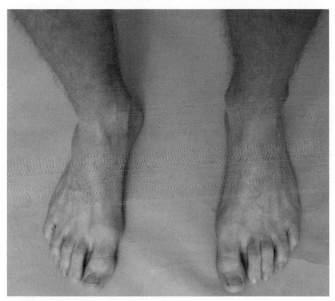

Fig. 13.10 Anterosuperior view of the feet (weight-bearing position) showing an index plus or Egyptian-type foot.

foot and requires more muscle work to maintain stance stability than the supinated foot. The foot is much more mobile in this pronated position.

The definitions used in this chapter are the ones preferred by orthopedists and podiatrists. Anatomists and kinesiologists, such as Kapandji, refer to inversion as a combination of adduction and supination and to eversion as a combination of abduction and pronation.[70] Lipscomb and Ibrahim[71] and Williams and Warwick[72] have defined supination and pronation as opposite the terms just mentioned. Because of the confusion in terminology concerning the terms supination and pronation, readers of books and articles on the foot must be careful to discern exactly what each author means.

In the infant, the foot is normally pronated. As the child matures, the foot begins to supinate, accompanied by development of the medial longitudinal arch. The foot

also appears to be more pronated in the infant because of the fat pad in the medial longitudinal arch.

The examiner should note how the patient stands and walks. Normally, in standing, 50% to 60% of the weight is taken on the heel and 40% to 50% is taken by the metatarsal heads. The foot assumes a slight toe-out position. This angle (the **Fick angle**) is approximately 12° to 18° from the sagittal axis of the body, developing from 5° in children (Fig. 13.13).[73] Asymmetrical or excessive lateral rotation of the foot may be due to acetabular retroversion, femoral retrotorsion, or femoral head neck abnormalities (see Chapter 11).[74] During movement, the foot is subjected to high loading, and pathology may cause the gait to be altered. The cumulative force to which each foot is subjected during the day is the equivalent of 639 metric tons in a person who weighs approximately 90 kg, or the equivalent of walking 13 km/day.

Foot Loading During Gait

Walking:	1.2 times the body weight
Running:	2 times the body weight
Jumping (from height of 60 cm [2 feet]):	5 times the body weight

---

When weight-bearing, if the relation of the foot to the ankle is normal, all of the metatarsal bones bear weight, and all of the metatarsal heads lie in the same transverse plane. The forefoot and hindfoot should be parallel to each other and to the floor. The midtarsal joints are in maximum pronation, and the subtalar joint is in neutral position. The subtalar and talocrural joints should be parallel to the floor. Finally, the posterior bisection of the calcaneus and distal one third of the leg should form two vertical, parallel lines.[75]

If the examiner has noted any asymmetry in standing, the examiner should place the talus (or foot) in neutral (see the "Special Tests" section) to see if the asymmetry disappears. If the asymmetry is present in normal standing, it is a **functional asymmetry.** If it is

TABLE **13.4**

Malalignment About the Foot and Ankle

Malalignment	Possible Correlated Motions or Postures	Possible Compensatory Motions or Postures
Ankle equinus		Hypermobile first ray Subtalar or midtarsal excessive pronation Hip or knee flexion Genu recurvation
Rearfoot varus Excessive subtalar supination (calcaneal varus)	Tibial; tibial and femoral; or tibial, femoral, and pelvic lateral rotation	Excessive medial rotation along the lower quarter chain Hallux valgus Plantar flexed first ray Functional forefoot valgus Excessive or prolonged midtarsal pronation
Rearfoot valgus Excessive subtalar pronation (calcaneal valgus)	Tibial; tibial and femoral; or tibial, femoral, and pelvic medial rotation Hallux valgus	Excessive lateral rotation along the lower quarter chain Functional forefoot varus
Forefoot varus	Subtalar supination and related rotation along the lower quarter	Plantar flexed first ray Hallux valgus Excessive midtarsal or subtalar pronation or prolonged pronation Excessive tibial; tibial and femoral; or tibial, femoral, and pelvic medial rotation, or all with contralateral lumbar spine rotation
Forefoot valgus	Hallux valgus Subtalar pronation and related rotation along the lower quarter	Excessive midtarsal or subtalar supination Excessive tibial; tibial and femoral; or tibial, femoral, and pelvic lateral rotation, or all with ipsilateral lumbar spine rotation
Metatarsus adductus	Hallux valgus Medial tibial torsion Flatfoot Toeing-in	
Hallux valgus	Forefoot valgus Subtalar pronation and related rotation along the lower quarter	Excessive tibial; tibial and femoral; or tibial, femoral, and pelvic lateral rotation, or all with ipsilateral lumbar spine rotation

From Riegger-Krugh C, Keysor JJ: Skeletal malalignment of the lower quarter: correlated and compensatory motions and postures, *J Orthop Sports Phys Ther* 23:166, 1996.

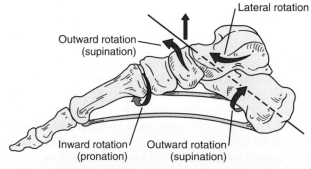

Fig. 13.11 Supination of the foot produced by lateral rotation of the tibia. The rearfoot and midfoot outwardly rotate (supinate) and the forefoot inwardly rotates (pronates) on the midfoot. As foot is plantar flexed, plantar fascia becomes tight along with ligaments to provide stable foot for push-off. (Modified from Richardson JK, Iglarsh ZA, editors: *Clinical orthopedic physical therapy*, Philadelphia, 1994, WB Saunders, p 513.)

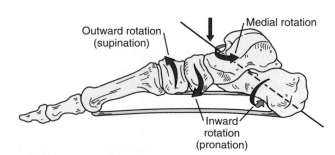

Fig. 13.12 Pronation of the foot produced by medial rotation of the tibia. The rearfoot and midfoot inwardly rotate (pronate) and the forefoot outwardly rotate (supinates) on the midfoot. Plantar fascia and plantar ligaments become taut as they absorb the ground reaction forces. (Modified from Richardson JK, Iglarsh ZA, editors: *Clinical orthopedic physical therapy*, Philadelphia, 1994, WB Saunders, p 513.)

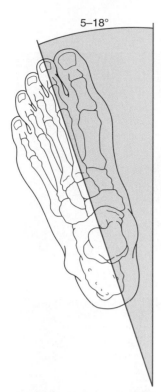

Fig. 13.13 Fick angle.

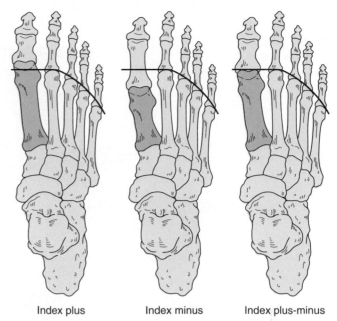

Index plus   Index minus   Index plus-minus

Fig. 13.14 Metatarsal classification.

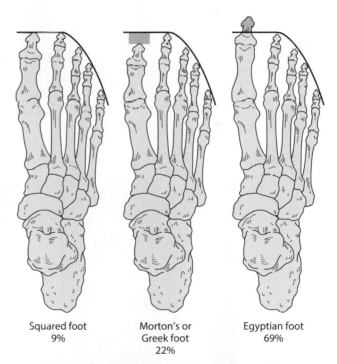

Squared foot   Morton's or   Egyptian foot
9%   Greek foot   69%
                    22%

Fig. 13.15 Types of feet seen in the general population.

still present when the foot is in neutral, it is also an **anatomical** or **structural asymmetry,** in which case a structural deformity is probably causing the asymmetry. Leg-heel and forefoot-heel alignment (see the "Special Tests" section) may also be checked, especially if asymmetry is present.

The examiner should note whether the patient uses a cane or other walking aid. Use of a cane in the opposite hand diminishes the stress on the ankle joint and foot by approximately one third.

Any prominent bumps or exostoses should be noted, as should any splaying (widening) of the forefoot. Splaying of the forefoot and metatarsus primus varus is more evident in weight bearing. There are three types of forefoot,[76] based on the length of the metatarsal bones (Fig. 13.14):

1. **Index plus type:** The first metatarsal (1) is longer than the second (2), with the others (3, 4, and 5) of progressively decreasing lengths, so that 1 > 2 > 3 > 4 > 5. This can result in an Egyptian-type foot (Fig. 13.15).
2. **Index plus-minus type:** The first metatarsal is equal in length to the second metatarsal, with the others progressively diminishing in length, so that 1 = 2 > 3 > 4 > 5. This results in a squared-type foot (see Fig. 13.15).
3. **Index minus type:** The second metatarsal is longer than the first and third metatarsals. The fourth and fifth metatarsals are progressively shorter than the third, so that 1 < 2 > 3 > 4 > 5. This results in a Morton's or Greek type foot (see Fig. 13.15).

The examiner should note whether the toenails appear normal. Older individuals have more brittle nails. The examiner should look for warts, calluses, and corns. Warts

are especially tender to the pinch (but not to direct pressure), but calluses are not. Plantar warts also tend to separate from the surrounding tissues, but calluses do not. Corns are similar to calluses but have a central nidus. They may be hard (on outside or upper aspect of toes) or soft (between toes) because of moisture.

Any swelling or pitting edema within the Achilles tendon, ankle, and foot should be noted (Fig. 13.16). If there is any swelling, the examiner should note whether it is intracapsular or extracapsular. Swelling above the lateral malleolus may be related to a fibular fracture or disruption of the syndesmosis ("high" ankle sprain).[77,78] This injury takes

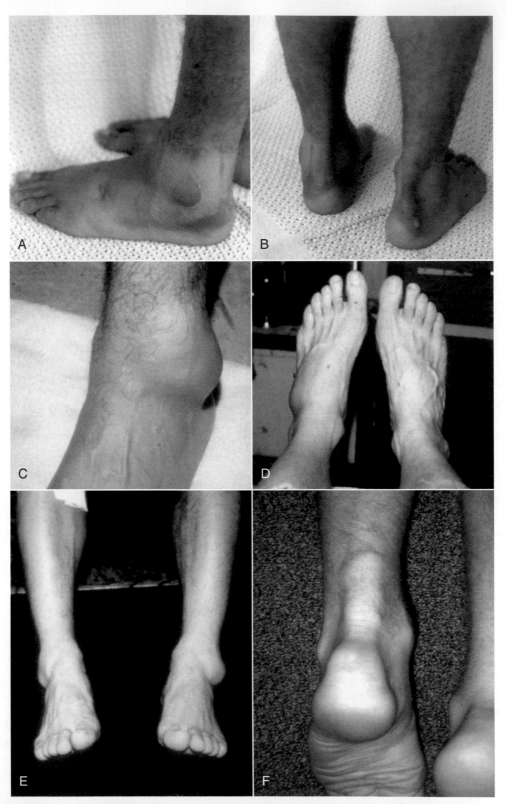

Fig. 13.16 Ankle sprain. (A) Note pattern of pitting edema on top of the left foot. (B) The swelling is intracapsular, as indicated by swelling on both sides of the left Achilles tendon. (C) Extracapsular swelling. (D) Midtarsal swelling of left foot. (E) Bilateral synovial thickening (not swelling) because of repeated ankle sprains. (F) Achilles swelling.

TABLE **13.5**

Classification of Ankle Sprains

Severity	Pathology	Signs and Symptoms	Disability
Grade I (mild) stable	Mild stretch No instability Single ligament involved (usually anterior talofibular ligament)	No hemorrhage Minimal swelling Point tenderness No anterior drawer sign No varus laxity	No or little limp Minimal functional loss Difficulty hopping Recovery 8 days (range, 2–10)
Grade II (moderate) stable	Large spectrum of injury Mild to moderate instability Complete tearing of anterior talofibular ligament, or partial tearing of anterior talofibular plus calcaneofibular ligaments	Some hemorrhage Localized swelling (margins of Achilles tendon less defined) Anterior drawer sign may be present No varus laxity	Walking with limp Unable to toe raise Unable to hop Unable to run Recovery 20 days (range, 10–30)
Grade III (severe) two-ligament, unstable	Significant instability Complete tear of anterior capsule, anterior talofibular and calcaneofibular ligaments	Diffuse swelling on both sides of Achilles tendon, early hemorrhage Possible tenderness medially and laterally Positive anterior drawer sign Positive varus laxity	Unable to bear weight fully Significant pain inhibition Initially almost complete loss of ROM Recovery 40 days (range, 30–90)

ROM, Range of motion.
From Reid DC: *Sports injury assessment and rehabilitation*, New York, 1992, Churchill Livingstone, p 226.

a long time to heal and may involve the anterior and/or posterior tibiofibular ligament as well as the ligaments of the talocrural joint. Swelling posterior to the lateral malleolus may indicate peroneal retinacular injury. Lateral ankle sprains initially swell distal to the lateral malleolus, but swelling may spread into the foot if the capsule has been torn (Table 13.5).[31] The examiner should also check the patient's gait for the position of the foot at heel strike, at foot flat, and at toe off. The gait cycle is described in greater detail in Chapter 14.

Any vasomotor changes should be recorded, including loss of hair on the foot, toenail changes, osteoporosis as seen on radiographs, and possible differences in temperature between the limbs. Systemic diseases such as diabetes can also lead to foot problems as a result of altered sensation, which facilitates injury.

The examiner should look for any circulatory impairment or presence of varicose veins. Brick-red color or cyanosis when the limb is dependent is an indication of impairment. Does this condition change to rapid blanching, or does it stay normal on elevation of the limbs? Change indicates circulatory impairment.

Weight-Bearing Position, Posterior View

From behind, the examiner compares the bulk of the calf muscles and notes any differences. Variation may be caused by peripheral nerve lesions, nerve root problems, or atrophy resulting from disuse after injury. The Achilles tendons on each side should be compared (see Fig. 13.16F). If a tendon appears to curve out (Fig. 13.17), it

may indicate a fallen medial longitudinal arch, resulting in a pes planus (flatfoot) condition **(Helbing sign).**[79]

The examiner observes the calcaneus for normality of shape and position. Runners often build up bone and a callus on the heel, producing a "pump bump" (**Haglund disease or deformity**) as a result of pressure on the heel (Fig. 13.18).[80-83]

The malleoli are compared for positioning. Normally, the lateral malleolus extends farther distally than the medial malleolus; however, the medial malleolus extends farther anteriorly.

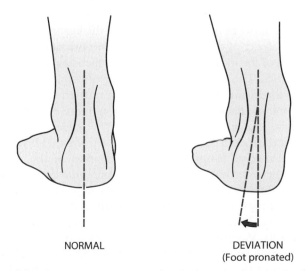

NORMAL   DEVIATION
                (Foot pronated)

Fig. 13.17 Normal and deviated Achilles tendon. The deviation is often seen with pes planus (flatfoot) and when the medial longitudinal arch is lower or has "dropped."

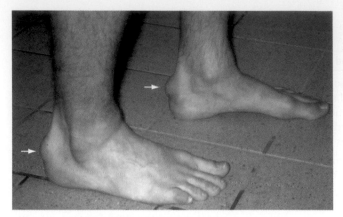

Fig. 13.18 "Pump bumps" from tight ice skates.

Weight-Bearing Position, Lateral View

With the side view, the examiner is primarily observing the longitudinal arches of the foot (Fig. 13.19). The structure of the foot and the arches allows the foot to act as a shock attenuator during early and midstance, and as a rigid lever during push off.[84] As long as the foot does these things during gait, it is usually "functionally normal" regardless of the arch height.[85] However, rigidity or instability can alter the interplay of the bones of the foot and weaken the whole lower-extremity kinetic chain.[85] High-arch feet (i.e., pes cavus) tend to be stiffer while low-arched (i.e., pes planus) feet tend to be more flexible.[84] **Pes rectus** is a normal arch.[86] Pronating the foot lowers the arch; thus functionally shortening the leg while supinating the foot raises the arch functionally lengthening the leg.[84] The examiner should note whether the medial arch is higher than the lateral arch (as would be expected). Differences in the arches may often be determined by looking at the footprint patterns (Fig. 13.20). The footprint pattern can be established by putting a light film of baby oil and then powder on the patient's foot and asking the patient to step down on a piece of colored paper.

The arches of the feet (Fig. 13.21) are maintained by three mechanisms[87]: (1) wedging of the interlocking tarsal and metatarsal bones; (2) tightening of the ligaments on the plantar aspect of the foot; and (3) the intrinsic and extrinsic muscles of the foot and their tendons, which help to support the arches. The longitudinal arches form a cone as a result of the angle of the metatarsal bones in relation to the floor. With the medial longitudinal arch being more evident, this angle is greater on the medial side. The angle formed by each of the metatarsals with the floor is shown in Fig. 13.22.

The **medial longitudinal arch** consists of the calcaneal tuberosity, the talus, the navicular, three cuneiforms, and the first, second, and third metatarsal bones with the navicular representing the highest point of the medial arch (Figs. 13.23 and 13.24).[86,88] The best measurement for the medial longitudinal arch is the navicular height-to-foot length ratio (ratio = 0.8 to 0.9).[89] Normally, the height of the apex of the medial arch is about 1 cm (0.4 inch) when weight bearing.[2] This arch is maintained by the tibialis

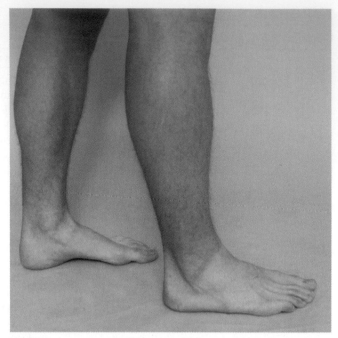

Fig. 13.19 Lateral and medial views of the feet showing longitudinal arches.

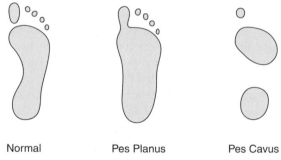

Normal   Pes Planus   Pes Cavus

Fig. 13.20 Footprint patterns.

anterior, tibialis posterior, flexor digitorum longus, flexor hallucis longus, abductor hallucis, and flexor digitorum brevis muscles; the plantar fascia or aponeurosis; and the plantar calcaneonavicular ligament. The plantar aponeurosis plays a major role during the stance and push-off phases of gait and helps maintain the longitudinal arches of the foot to help distribute Achilles tendon forces under the forefoot to the metatarsal heads and phalanges (see Fig. 13.63A).[90,91]

The calcaneus, cuboid, and fourth and fifth metatarsal bones make up the **lateral longitudinal arch** (Fig. 13.25). This arch is more stable and less adjustable than the medial longitudinal arch. The arch is maintained by the peroneus longus, peroneus brevis, peroneus tertius, abductor digiti minimi, and flexor digitorum brevis muscles; the plantar fascia; the long plantar ligament; and the short plantar ligament.[87]

The **transverse arch** is maintained by the tibialis posterior, tibialis anterior, and peroneus longus muscles and the

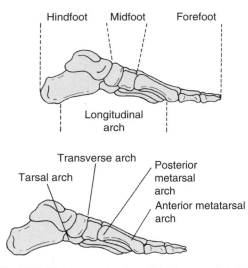

Fig. 13.21 Divisions and arches of the foot (medial view).

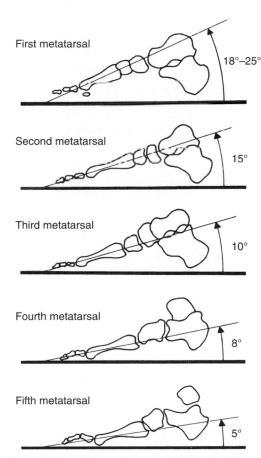

Fig. 13.22 Angle formed by each metatarsal with the floor. (Modified from Jahss MH: *Disorders of the foot*, Philadelphia, 1991, WB Saunders, p 1231.)

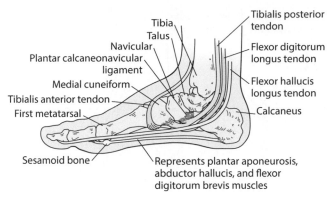

Fig. 13.23 Supports of the medial longitudinal arch of the foot.

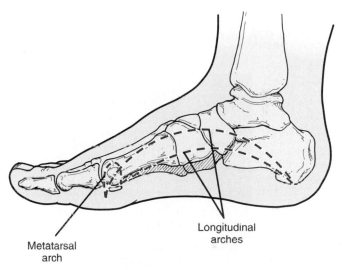

Fig. 13.24 Arches of the foot (medial view).

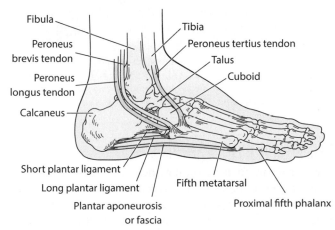

Fig. 13.25 Supports of the lateral longitudinal arch of the foot: plantar aponeurosis (including the abductor digiti minimi and the flexor digitorum brevis IV and V); long plantar ligament; short plantar ligament.

plantar fascia (Fig. 13.26). This arch consists of the navicular, cuneiforms, cuboid, and metatarsal bones. The arch is sometimes divided into three parts: tarsal, posterior metatarsal, and anterior metatarsal. A loss of the anterior metatarsal arch results in callus formation under the heads of the metatarsal bones (especially the second and third metatarsal heads). The metatarsophalangeal joints are slightly extended when the patient is in the normal standing position because the longitudinal arches of the foot curve down toward the toes.[87]

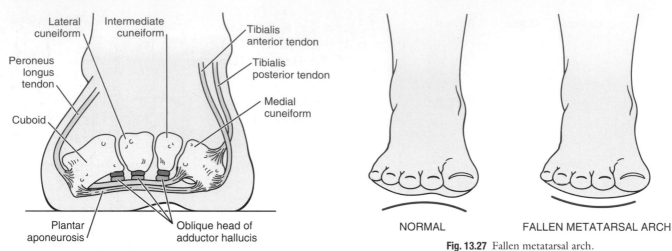

Fig. 13.26 Supports of the transverse arch of the foot.

Fig. 13.27 Fallen metatarsal arch.

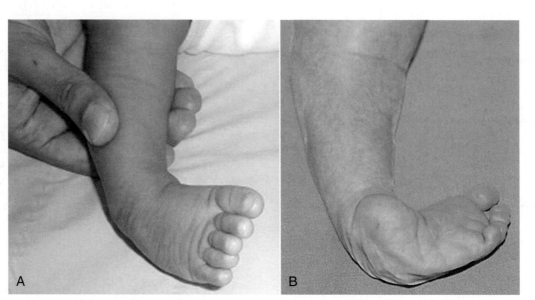

Fig. 13.28 Talipes equinovarus (clubfoot) in a child. (A) Anterior view. (B) Posterior view. (A, From Foster A, Davis N: Congenital talipes equino-varus [clubfoot], *Surgery* 25(4), 171–175, 2007; B, From Moore KL, Persaud TV, Torchia MG: Musculoskeletal system. In Moore KL, Persaud TV, Torchia MG, eds: *Before we are born: essentials of embryology and birth defects*, ed 9, Philadelphia, 2016, Elsevier. Courtesy AE Chudley, MD, Section of Genetics and Metabolism, Department of Pediatrics and Child Health, University of Manitoba, Children's Hospital, Winnipeg, Manitoba, Canada.)

Non–Weight-Bearing Position

With the patient in a supine, non–weight-bearing posi-tion, the examiner should look for abnormalities, such as callosities, plantar warts, scars, and sinuses or pressure sores on the soles of the feet, as well as swelling, which is more prominent on the dorsum of the foot. In addi-tion, by looking at the foot from anterior to posterior, as shown in Fig. 13.27, the examiner can observe whether the patient has a "fallen" metatarsal arch. Normally, in the non–weight-bearing position, the arch is visible. If the arch falls, callosities are often found over the metatarsal heads. The arch may be reversed, or it may fall because of an equinus forefoot, pes cavus, rheumatoid arthritis, short heel cord, or hammer toes. Abnormal width of one ankle in relation to the other (**Keen sign**) may be caused by swelling, loss of integrity of the syndesmosis, or a mal-leolar fracture.

Young children should be assessed for clubfoot defor-mities, the most common of which is talipes equinovarus (Figs. 13.28 and 13.29; Table 13.6). These types of deformities are often associated with other anomalies, such as spina bifida.

Common Deformities, Deviations, and Injuries

Bunionette (Tailor's Bunion). This deformity is character-ized by prominence of the lateral aspect of the fifth toe metatarsal head (Fig. 13.30).[92] If associated with hallux valgus, it results in a splayed foot. It is often associated with a pronated foot.

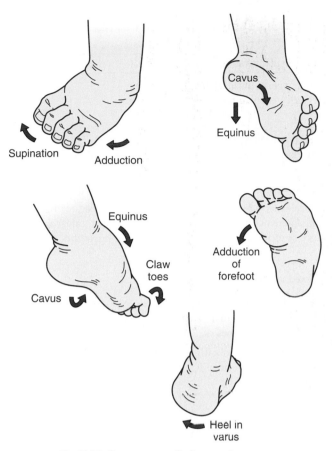

Fig. 13.29 Components of talipes equinovarus.

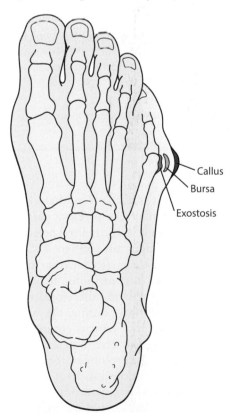

Fig. 13.30 A bunionette or tailor's bunion.

Claw Toes. A claw-toe deformity results in hyperextension of the metatarsophalangeal joints and flexion of the proximal and distal interphalangeal joints (Fig. 13.31A). Claw toes usually result from the defective actions of lumbrical and interosseus muscles that cause the toes to become functionless. This condition may be unilateral or bilateral and may be associated with pes cavus, fallen metatarsal arch, spina bifida, or other neurological problems.

Clubfoot. This congenital deformity is relatively common and can take many forms, the most common of which is **talipes equinovarus.** Its cause is unknown, but there are probably multifactorial genetic causes modified by environmental factors.[93] It sometimes coexists with other congenital deformities, such as spina bifida and cleft palate. The flexible form is easily treated, but the resistant type often requires surgery. On assessment, the ROM is limited and the foot has abnormal form (see Fig. 13.29).

Crossover Toe. Crossover toe is the result of weakening of the lateral collateral ligament of the metatarsophalangeal joint and insufficiency of the plantar plate along with the pull of the extrinsic muscles resulting in medial deviation of the toe, most commonly in the second or third toe. It is often associated with hallux valgus.[94]

Curly Toe. A curly toe deformity involves a flexion deformity of both the proximal and distal interphalangeal joints with the metatarsophalangeal joint in neutral or flexion, often combined with rotation. It is the result of contracture of flexor digitorum brevis and longus tendons and is most commonly seen in the fifth toe in children.[94]

Equinus Deformity (Talipes Equinus). This deformity is characterized by limited dorsiflexion (less than 10°) at the talocrural joint, usually as a result of contracture of the gastrocnemius or soleus muscles or Achilles tendon. It may also be caused by structural bone deformity (primarily in the talus), trauma, or inflammatory disease. The deformity causes increased stress to the forefoot, which may lead to a rocker-bottom foot and excessive pronation at the subtalar joint. This deviation can contribute to conditions such as plantar fasciitis, metatarsalgia, heel spurs, and talonavicular pain.[65]

Exostosis (Bony Spur). Exostosis is an abnormal bony outgrowth extending from the surface of the bone (Fig. 13.32). It is actually an increase in the bone mass at the site of an irritative lesion in response to overuse, trauma, or excessive pressure. The common areas of occurrence in the foot are on the dorsal aspect of the tarsometatarsal joint, the head of the fifth metatarsal bone, the calcaneus (where it is often called a pump bump or runner's bump), the insertion of the plantar fascia, and the superior aspect of the navicular bone. Most often these exostoses are the result of poorly fitting footwear that leads to undue pressure on the bone.

TABLE **13.6**

Differential Diagnosis of Postural Clubfoot and Talipes Equinovarus

	Postural Clubfoot	Talipes Equinovarus
Etiology	Intrauterine malposture	Primary germ plasm defect
		Defective cartilaginous anlage of the talus
Pathologic Anatomy		
Head and neck of talus	Normal	Medial and plantar tilt
	Declination angle of talus normal (150°–155°)	Declination angle of talus decreased (115°–135°)
Talocalcaneonavicular joint	Normal	Subluxed or dislocated medially and plantarward
Effect of manipulation in fetal specimens	Normal alignment of foot can be restored	Talocalcaneonavicular subluxation cannot be reduced unless ligaments connecting navicular to calcaneus, talus, and tibia are sectioned and posterior capsule and ligaments divided
Clinical Features		
Severity of deformity	Mild and flexible	Marked and rigid
Heel	Normal size	Small, drawn up
Relation between navicular and medial malleolus	Normal space between two bones; can insert finger	Navicular abuts medial malleolus; finger cannot be inserted between two bones
Lateral malleolus	Normal position	Posteriorly displaced with anterior part of talus very prominent in front of it
Skin creases on:		
Dorsolateral aspect of foot	Present; normal	Thin or absent
Medial and plantar aspects of foot	No furrowed skin	Furrowed skin
Posterior aspect of ankle	Normal	Deep crease
Calf and leg atrophy	None or very minimal	Moderate to marked
Treatment	Passive manipulation followed by retention by adhesive strapping, splint, or cast	Primary open reduction of talocalcaneonavicular joint often required; surgery is conservative
		Closed methods of reduction often unsuccessful
		Prolonged retentive apparatus essential
Prognosis	Excellent; result is normal foot	Poor with closed methods
		Prolonged cast immobilization results in smaller foot and atrophied leg

From Tachdjian MO: *The child's foot*, Philadelphia, 1985, WB Saunders, p 163.

Forefoot Valgus. This structural midtarsal deviation involves eversion of the forefoot on the hindfoot when the subtalar joint is in the neutral position because the normal valgus tilt (35° to 45°) of the head and neck of the talus to its trochlea has been exceeded. With this deformity, during the weight-bearing phase of gait, the midtarsal joint is supinated so that the lateral aspect of the foot is brought into contact with the ground. Like hindfoot valgus, it contributes to decreasing the medial longitudinal arch and, therefore, clinically resembles a planus foot. The prolonged supination can contribute to conditions such as lateral ankle sprains, iliotibial band syndrome, plantar fasciitis, anterior tarsal tunnel syndrome, toe deformities, sesamoiditis, and leg and thigh pain (Fig. 13.33B).[65,95]

Forefoot Varus. This structural midtarsal joint deviation involves inversion of the forefoot on the hindfoot when the subtalar joint is in the neutral position. It occurs because the normal valgus tilt (35° to 45°) of the head and neck of the talus to its trochlea has not been achieved.[65,95,96] Clinically, it contributes to decreasing the medial longitudinal arch and, therefore, resembles pes planus. With this deformity, during the weight-bearing phase of gait, the midtarsal joint is completely pronated in an attempt to bring the first metatarsal head in contact with the ground. The prolonged rotation that results can contribute to conditions, such as tibialis posterior paratenonitis, patellofemoral syndrome, toe deformities, ligamentous stress (medially), shin splints, plantar fasciitis, postural fatigue, and Morton's neuroma (Fig. 13.33A).

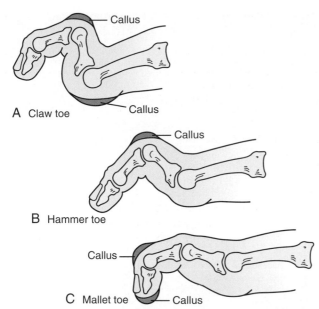

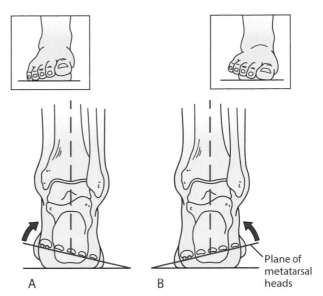

Fig. 13.33 Forefoot deformities (right foot). (A) Forefoot varus (metatarsal heads raised on medial side). (B) Forefoot valgus (metatarsal heads raised on lateral side).

Fig. 13.31 Toe deformities. (A) Claw toe. Note that the proximal and distal interphalangeal joints are hyperflexed and the metatarsophalangeal joint is dorsally subluxated. (B) Hammer toe. Note the flexion deformity of the proximal interphalangeal joints. The distal interphalangeal joint is in neutral position or slight flexion. (C) Mallet toe. There is flexion contracture of the distal interphalangeal joint. The proximal interphalangeal and metatarsophalangeal joints are in neutral position.

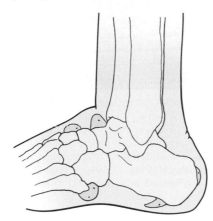

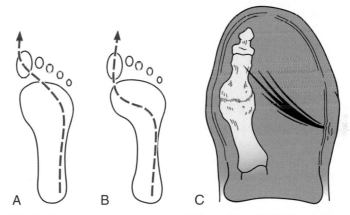

Fig. 13.34 Weight-bearing patterns in hallux rigidus. (A) Hallux rigidus gait pattern. (B) Normal gait pattern. (C) Shoe develops oblique creases with hallux rigidus. (C, Redrawn from Jahss MH: *Disorders of the foot*, Philadelphia, 1991, WB Saunders, p 60.)

Fig. 13.32 Common areas of exostosis formation in the foot.

Hallux Rigidus. Hallux rigidus is a condition in which dorsiflexion or extension of the big toe is limited because of osteoarthritis of the first metatarsophalangeal joint.[97] Hallux rigidus may also be caused by an anatomical abnormality of the foot, an abnormally long first metatarsal bone (index plus type forefoot; see Fig. 13.14), pronation of the forefoot, or trauma. There are two types: acute and chronic.

The acute, or adolescent, type occurs primarily in young people with long, narrow, pronated feet and occurs more frequently in boys than in girls. Pain and stiffness in the big toe come on quickly; the pain is described as constant, burning, throbbing, or aching. Tenderness may be palpated over the metatarsophalangeal joint, and

the toe is initially held stiff because of muscle spasm. The first metatarsal head may be elevated, large, and tender. The weight distribution pattern in the gait is shown in Fig. 13.34.

The second (chronic) type of hallux rigidus is much more common and occurs primarily in adults—again, in men more frequently than in women. It is frequently bilateral and is usually the result of repeated minor trauma resulting in osteoarthritic changes to the metatarsophalangeal joint of the big toe. The toe stiffens gradually, and the pain, once established, persists. The patient complains primarily of pain at the base of the big toe on walking.

Hallux Valgus. Hallux valgus is a relatively common condition in which there is medial deviation of the head of the first metatarsal bone in relation to the center of the body and lateral deviation of the head in relation to the center of the foot (Fig. 13.35). Although, upon visual inspection, it seems that the condition only surrounds the metatarsophalangeal joint, it is actually a problem with the entire first ray. In most instances, there is an associated adduction of the first metatarsal at the tarsometatarsal joint.[98–100] The cause of hallux valgus is varied. It may result from a hereditary factor and is often familial. Women tend to be affected more than men. Trying to keep up with fashion may be a contributing factor if the patient wears tight or pointed shoes, tight stockings, or high-heeled shoes.[101]

As the metatarsal bones move medially, the base of the proximal phalanx is carried with it, and the phalanx pivots around the adductor hallucis muscle that inserts into it, causing the distal end as well as the distal phalanx to deviate laterally in relation to the center of the body. The long flexor and extensor muscles then have a bow-string effect as they are displaced to the lateral side of the joint, which can lead to increased stress on the proximal phalanx.[102]

A callus develops over the medial side of the head of the metatarsal bone, and the bursa becomes thickened and inflamed; excessive bone (exostosis) forms, resulting in a **bunion** (Fig. 13.36).[35,103] These three changes—callus, thickened bursa, and exostosis—make up the bunion, a condition separate from hallux valgus, although it is the result of hallux valgus.

In normal persons, the **metatarsophalangeal angle** (the angle between the longitudinal axis of the metatarsal bone and the proximal phalanx) is 8° to 20° (Fig. 13.37). This angle is increased to varying degrees in hallux valgus.

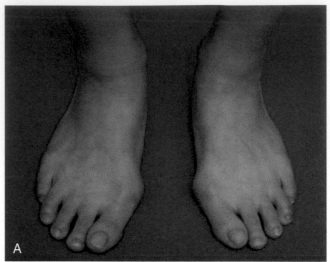
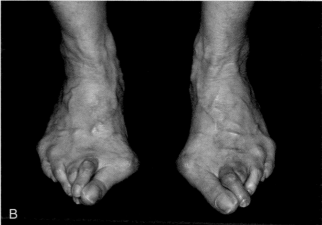

Fig. 13.35 (A) An example of congruent (i.e., no lateral subluxation) hallux valgus. (B) Pathological (incongruent) hallux valgus with bilateral bunions and overlapped toes. Note how the deviating big toe (hallux) rotates and pushes over the second toe (crossover toe). (A, From Makhdom AM, Sinno H, Aldebeyan S, et al: Bilateral hallux valgus: a utility outcome score assessment, *J Foot Ankle Surg* 55(5):944–47, 2016. B, From Davies MB: Common disorders of the adult foot and ankle, *Surgery* 31(9):488–494, 2013.)

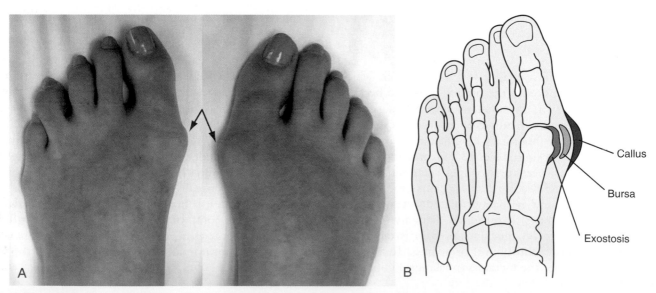

Fig. 13.36 (A) Bunions on both feet. (B) Schematic line drawing of a bunion. (A, From Khosroabadi A, Lamm BM: Modified percutaneous hallux abductovalgus correction, *J Foot Ankle Surg* 55(6):1336–42, 2016.)

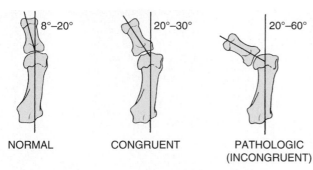

Fig. 13.37 Metatarsophalangeal (hallux valgus) angle.

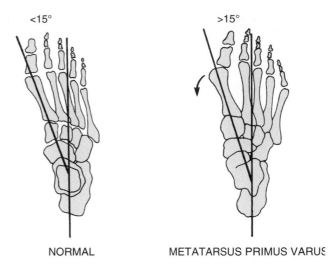

Fig. 13.38 Normal foot and metatarsus primus varus. (Note increased intermetatarsal angle.)

The first type (**congruous hallux valgus**) is a simple exaggeration of the normal relation of the metatarsal to the phalanx of the big toe. The deformity does not progress, and the valgus deformity is between 20° and 30°. The opposing joint surfaces are congruent. It requires little treatment, and often the biggest problem is cosmetic.

The second type (**pathological hallux valgus**) is a potentially progressive deformity, increasing from 20° to 60°. The joint surfaces are no longer congruent, and some may even go to subluxation. This type may occur in deviated (early) and subluxed (later) stages.

When looking at the foot, the examiner may find that there is a widening gap between the first and second metatarsal bones (increased **intermetatarsal angle**) and a lateral deflection of the phalanx at the metatarsophalangeal joint. The joint capsule lengthens on the medial aspect and is contracted on the lateral aspect. The toes rotate on the long axis so that the toenail faces medially because of the pull of the adductor hallucis muscle. Sometimes, the big toe deviates so far that it lies over or under the second toe.

Of all hallux valgus cases, 80% are caused by **metatarsus primus varus,** in which the intermetatarsal or metatarsal angle is increased to more than 15° (Fig. 13.38).[104,105] Metatarsus primus varus is an abduction deformity of the first metatarsal bone in relation to the tarsal and other metatarsal bones so that the medial border of the forefoot is curved. Normally, this angle is between 0° and 15°.

Hammer Toe. A hammer toe deformity consists of an extension contracture at the metatarsophalangeal joint and flexion contracture at the proximal interphalangeal joint; the distal interphalangeal joint may be flexed, straight, or hyperextended (Fig. 13.31B).[103,106] The interosseus muscles are unable to hold the proximal phalanx in the neutral position and, therefore, lose their flexion effect. This results in clawing of the toe by the long flexors and extensors leading to and accentuating the deformity. The causes of hammer toe include an imbalance of the synergic muscles, hereditary factors, and mechanical factors, such as poorly fitting shoes or hallux valgus. It is usually seen only in one toe— the second toe. Often, there is a callus or corn over the dorsum of the flexed joint. The condition is often asymptomatic, especially if the hammer toe is flexible or semiflexible. The rigid type of hammer toe is likely to cause the greatest problems.

Hindfoot Valgus (Subtalar or Rearfoot Valgus). This structural position involves eversion of the calcaneus when the subtalar joint is in the neutral position. Normally, individuals have a rearfoot valgus that is about 4°.[107] The hindfoot is mobile, which may lead to excessive pronation and limited supination. It may result from genu valgum (knock knees) and may contribute to the appearance of a pes planus foot with the medial longitudinal arch appearing flattened.[108] Because of the increased mobility, it is less likely to cause problems than hindfoot varus. It is often associated with tibia valgus (Fig. 13.39B) and has been associated with posterior tibial tendon insufficiency.[109]

Hindfoot Varus (Subtalar or Rearfoot Varus). This structural deviation involves inversion of the calcaneus when the subtalar joint is in the neutral position. The hindfoot is mildly rigid with calcaneal eversion; therefore, pronation is limited. It may contribute to the appearance of a pes cavus foot, making the medial longitudinal arch appear accentuated. It may be the result of tibia varus (genu varum), and, because of the extra subtalar pronation necessary at the beginning of stance, normal supination during early propulsion may be prevented. This deviation can contribute to conditions, such as retrocalcaneal exostosis (pump bumps), shin splints, plantar fasciitis, hamstring strains, and knee and ankle pathology (Fig. 13.39A).[65]

Mallet Toe. Mallet toe is associated with a flexion deformity of the distal interphalangeal joint (Fig. 13.31C).[103,106] It can occur on any of the four lateral toes. Often, a corn or callus is present over the dorsum of the affected joint. The condition is usually asymptomatic. It is commonly seen with ill-fitting or poorly designed footwear.[92]

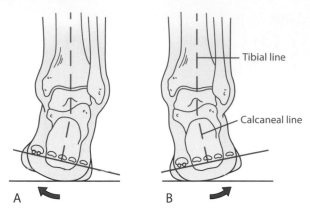

Fig. 13.39 Hindfoot (rearfoot) deformities (right foot). (A) Hindfoot varus (heel appears inverted). (B) Hindfoot valgus (heel appears everted).

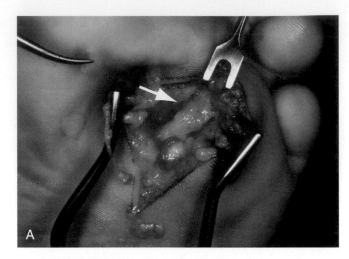

Metatarsus Adductus (Hooked Forefoot). This deformity is the most common foot deviation in children. It may be seen at birth but often is not noticed until the child begins to stand. The foot appears to be adducted and supinated (kidney shaped with medial deviation), and the hindfoot may or may not be in valgus.[110] It may be associated with hip dysplasia. Eighty-five to 90% of cases resolve spontaneously.[93]

Morton's (Atavistic or Grecian) Foot. With a Morton's foot, the second toe is longer than the first.[2] The length difference may be due to different lengths of the metatarsals (see Fig. 13.14). Increased stress is put on this longer toe, and the hallux (i.e., big toe) tends to be hypomobile. There is often hypertrophy of the second metatarsal bone because more stress is put through the second toe. In fact, the second metatarsal can become as large as the first metatarsal. People with this deformity often have difficulty putting on tight-fitting footwear (e.g., skates, ski boots) or dancing (e.g., en pointe in ballet). The different types of feet and their proportional representations in the population are shown in Fig. 13.15.

Morton's Metatarsalgia (Interdigital Neuroma).[111–113] Morton's metatarsalgia (Morton's neuroma) refers to the formation of an interdigital neuroma as a result of injury to one of the digital nerves (Fig. 13.40). Usually, it is the digital nerve between the third and fourth toes, so the examiner must take care to differentially diagnose the condition from a stress fracture of one of the metatarsals in the same area **(march fracture).** (A stress fracture will be more painful when the bone is palpated and a bone scan would be positive.) Title et al.[114] point out that if a Morton's neuroma is suspected, pressure palpation should be applied on the plantar aspect avoiding counterpressure on the dorsal aspect. Dorsal palpation pain is more likely to be associated with a stress fracture, metatarsophalangeal synovitis, or dorsal neuralgia. While walking or running, the patient is suddenly seized with an agonizing pain on the outer border of the forefoot. The pain is often intermittent, like a cramp, shooting up the side and to the tip of the affected toe or the

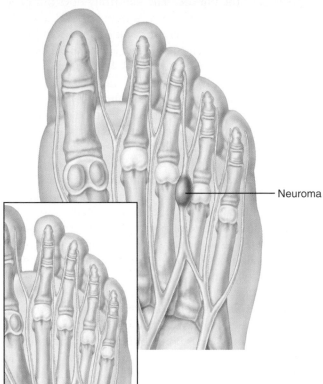

Fig. 13.40 (A) The applied anatomy of Morton's metatarsalgia. The interdigital nerve to the space between the third and fourth digits has been divided 2 cm above the neuroma and is reflected. The communicating nerve is shown entering the neuroma *(arrow).* (B) Schematic line drawing of interdigital neuroma. (A, From Grear BJ: Neurogenic disorders. In Azar FM, Beaty JH, Canale ST, eds: *Campbell's operative orthopaedics,* ed 13, Philadelphia, 2017, Elsevier. B, From Powell BD: Morton neuroma (plantar interdigital neuroma). In Miller MD, Hart JA, MacKnight JM, eds: *Essential orthopaedics,* ed 2, Philadelphia, 2020, Elsevier.)

adjacent two toes. Squeezing the metatarsal bones together elicits pain because of the pressure on the digital nerve. On palpation, pain is more likely to be between the bones rather than on the bone. The condition tends to occur more frequently in women than in men.

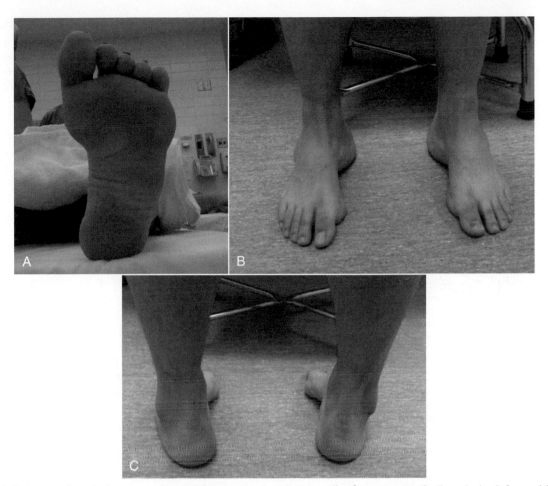

Fig. 13.41 Clinical pictures of a typical cavovarus foot. (A) Plantar view demonstrates callus formation specifically at the heel, first and fifth metatarsal heads. (B) Anterior view demonstrates accentuation of the medial arch ("hollow foot") and "peek-a-boo" heel. (C) Hindfoot alignment view shows calcaneal varus and fat pad hypertrophy of the first metatarsal head. (From DeVries JG, McAlister JE: Corrective osteotomies used in cavus reconstruction, *Clin Pod Med Surg* 32[3]:375–387, 2015.)

Pes Cavus ("Hollow Foot" or Rigid Foot). A pes cavus may be caused by a congenital problem; a neurological problem, such as spina bifida, poliomyelitis, or Charcot-Marie-Tooth disease; talipes equinovarus; or muscle imbalance. There may also be a genetic factor because it tends to run in families.

The longitudinal arches are accentuated (Fig. 13.41), and the metatarsal heads are lower in relation to the hindfoot so that there is a dropping of the forefoot on the hindfoot at the tarsometatarsal joints (Fig. 13.42). The soft tissues of the sole of the foot are abnormally short, which gives the foot a shortened appearance. If the deformity persists, the bones eventually alter their shape, perpetuating the deformity. The heel is normal, at least initially. Claw toes are often associated with the condition because of the dropping of the forefoot combined with the pull of the extensor tendons. The examiner often finds painful callosities beneath the metatarsal heads that are caused by the loss of the metatarsal arch and tenderness along the deformed toes. There is pain in the tarsal region after time because of osteoarthritic changes in these joints.

The longitudinal arches are high on both the medial and lateral aspects so that a lateral longitudinal arch occurs in some severe cases, and the forefoot is thickened and splayed (Table 13.7). The metatarsal heads are prominent on the sole of the foot, and the toes do not touch the ground, even on active or passive movement. This type of deformity leads to a rigid foot with little ability to absorb shock and adapt to stress. People with this deformity have difficulty doing repetitive stress activity (e.g., long-distance running, ballet) and require a cushioning shoe. In severe cases, the cavus foot is often associated with neurological disorders.[93]

Pes Planus (Flatfoot or Mobile Foot).[115–117] Flatfoot may be congenital, or it may result from trauma, muscle weakness, ligament laxity, dropping of the talar head, paralysis, or a pronated foot. For example, a traumatic flatfoot may follow fracture of the calcaneus. It may also be caused by a postural deformity, such as medial rotation of the hips or medial tibial torsion. A patient with a flexible pes planus has a near normal arch when non-weight bearing but the height of the arch decreases significantly when weight bearing.[2] It is a relatively common foot deformity

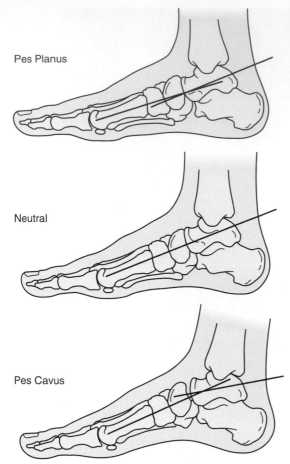

Pes Planus

Neutral

Pes Cavus

Fig. 13.42 Talometatarsal angle used to define pes planus, neutral, and pes cavus foot types. (Redrawn from Jahss MH, editor: *Disorders of the foot and ankle: medical and surgical management*, ed 2, vol 1, Philadelphia, 1991, WB Saunders.)

TABLE 13.7

Pes Cavus Classification

Classification	Features
1. Mild	Longitudinal arch appears high NWB
	Longitudinal arch almost normal WB
	Toes clawed NWB
	Toes may be normal WB
	May have hindfoot varus
2. Moderate	Longitudinal arch high NWB and WB
	Claw toes evident NWB and WB
	Calluses under prominent metatarsal heads
	Dorsiflexion may be limited
	Forefoot plantar flexed on hindfoot
3. Severe	Calcaneus cannot evert past 5° varus
	Heel in varus, foot in valgus
	Decreased ROM in foot

NWB, Non–weight-bearing; *ROM,* range of motion; *WB,* weight-bearing.

that often causes little or no problem. Therefore, the examiner should not necessarily assume that a flat, mobile foot needs to be treated.[118] Because the foot is mobile, patients with flatfoot function well without treatment and often need only a control shoe to avoid problems in prolonged stress situations which can lead to alteration in the lower-extremity kinetic chain.[85]

It must be remembered that all infants have flatfeet up to approximately 2 years of age. This appearance in part results from the fat pad in the longitudinal arch and in part from the incomplete formation of the arches. With pes planus, the medial longitudinal arch is reduced, the rearfoot is in valgus, the talonavicular joint is everted, the talocalcaneal joint is dorsiflexed, and the forefoot is abducted so that on standing its borders are close to or in contact with the ground.[119] This results from the hindfoot dropping in relation to the forefoot (see Fig. 13.42). If the condition persists into adulthood, it may become a permanent structural deformity, leading to a defect or alteration of the tarsal bones and the talonavicular joints.

There are two types of flatfoot deformities. The first type (**rigid** or **congenital flatfoot**) is relatively rare. The calcaneus is found in a valgus position, whereas the midtarsal region is in pronation. The talus faces medially and downward, and the navicular is displaced dorsally and laterally on the talus. There are accompanying soft-tissue contractures and bony changes. The second type is **acquired** or **flexible flatfoot** (Fig. 13.43). In this case, the deformity is similar to the rigid flatfoot, but the foot is mobile (Table 13.8); and there are few, if any, soft-tissue contractures and bony changes. It is usually caused by hereditary factors and is sometimes called a **hypermobile flatfoot.** Flexible flatfoot may result from tibial or femoral torsion, coxa vara, a defect in the subtalar joint, or injury to the posterior tibial tendon.[120] If the arch appears when the patient stands on tiptoes, the patient may have a mobile flatfoot. This type of flatfoot seldom needs treatment.

Plantar Flexed First Ray. This structural deformity occurs when the first ray (big toe) lies lower than the other four metatarsal bones so that the forefoot is everted when the metatarsal bones are aligned. If present congenitally, it is indicative of a cavus foot. In its acquired form, it occurs as compensation for tibia varum (genu varum) with limited calcaneal eversion. This deformity can contribute to the same conditions seen with forefoot valgus.[65] The neutral position of the first ray is the position in which the first metatarsal head lies in the same transverse plane as the second through fourth metatarsal heads when they are maximally dorsiflexed.[121]

Polydactyly. This developmental anomaly is characterized by the presence of an extra digit or toe (Fig. 13.44). It may be seen in isolation or with other anomalies, such as polydactyly of the hands and syndactyly (webbing) of the

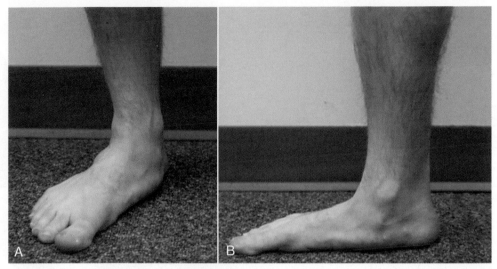

Fig. 13.43 (A) Anterior and (B) side views of the weight-bearing flatfoot demonstrate the absence of the medial arch and the forefoot hyperabduction. (From Sheikh Taha AM, Feldman DS: Painful flexible flatfoot, *Foot Ankle Clin* 20(4):693–704, 2015.)

TABLE **13.8**

Pes Planus Classification

Classification	Features
1. Mild	4°–6° hindfoot valgus 4°–6° forefoot valgus
2. Moderate	6°–10° hindfoot valgus 6°–10° forefoot varus Poor shock absorption at heel strike
3. Severe	10°–15° hindfoot valgus 8°–10° forefoot varus Equinus deformity may be present

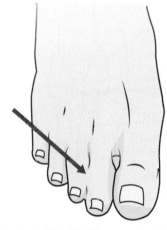

Fig. 13.45 Syndactyly (webbing) of the second and third toe *(arrow)*.

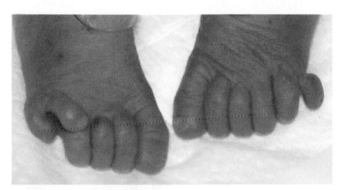

Fig. 13.44 Polydactyly (extra digit). (From Balest AL, Riley MM, Bogen DL: Neonatology. In Zitelli BJ, McIntire SC, Nowalk AJ, eds: *Zitelli and Davis' atlas of pediatric physical diagnosis*, ed 7, Philadelphia, 2018, Elsevier.)

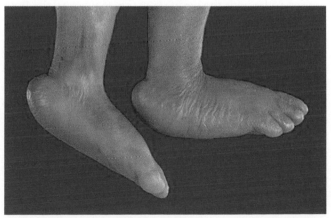

Fig. 13.46 Rigid flat foot with a rocker bottom caused by a congenital vertical talus with dorsal dislocation of the navicular on the talus associated with myelodysplasia and arthrogryposis. (From Miller MA: History and examination of the pediatric patient. In Cifu DX, Kaelin DL, Kowalske KJ, et al, eds: *Braddom's physical medicine and rehabilitation*, ed 5, Philadelphia, 2016, Elsevier.)

toes or hands (Fig. 13.45). The primary concern with this anomaly is cosmesis.[122] These digits are commonly amputated early in life.

Rocker-Bottom Foot. In the rocker-bottom foot deformity, the forefoot is dorsiflexed on the hindfoot (Fig. 13.46). This results in a "broken midfoot," so that the medial and longitudinal arches are absent and the foot

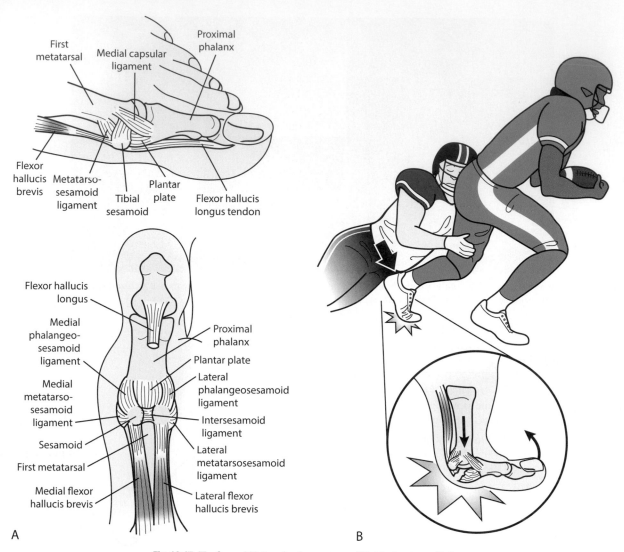

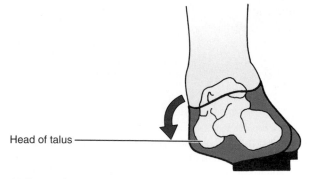

Fig. 13.47 Turf toe. (A) Involved structures. (B) Mechanism of injury.

appears to be bent the wrong way (i.e., convex to the floor instead of the normal concave).

Splay Foot. This deformity, which is broadening of the forefoot, is often caused by weakness of the intrinsic muscles and associated weakness of the intermetatarsal ligament and dropping of the anterior metatarsal arch.

Turf Toe. Turf toe is a hyperextension injury (sprain) combined with compressive loading to the metatarsophalangeal joint of the hallux (Fig. 13.47). It can cause a significant functional disability, especially in sports, where the hallux is put under high loads. It is often related to the use of flexible footwear and artificial turf.[64,123–125]

Shoes

The examiner looks at the patient's shoes, both inside and outside, for weight-bearing and wear patterns

Fig. 13.48 Pes planus (flatfoot) or calcaneus in valgus can lead to misshapen shoes. Note the prominence of the talar head.

(Figs. 13.48 and 13.49). With the normal foot, the greatest wear on the shoe is beneath the ball of the foot and slightly to the lateral side and the posterolateral aspect of the heel. If shoes are too small or too narrow,

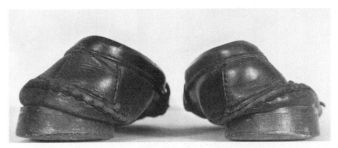

Fig. 13.49 Misshapen shoes caused by severely pronated feet. (From Gartland JJ: *Fundamentals of orthopedics*, Philadelphia, 1987, WB Saunders, p 398.)

they may pinch the feet, causing deformities and affecting normal growth. If shoes are worn out, they offer little support. If shoes are stiff, they limit proper movement of the foot.

Platform-type or high-heeled shoes often cause painful knees because the patient wearing these shoes usually walks with the knees flexed, which may increase the stress on the patella. Continuous wearing of high-heeled shoes may cause the calf muscles to contract and may lead to sore knees and a painful back, because the lumbar spine goes into increased lordotic posture to maintain the center of gravity in its normal position. In addition, these shoes increase the potential for ankle sprains and fractures because a raised center of gravity puts the wearer off balance.

High-heeled and pointed shoes often contribute to hallux valgus, bunions, march fractures, and Morton's metatarsalgia that may result because the toes are being pushed together. Shoes with a negative heel may lead to hyperextension of the knees and patellofemoral syndrome. High-cut or high-top shoes that cover the medial and lateral malleoli offer more support than low-cut shoes or those that do not cover the malleoli.

Excessive bulging on the medial side of the shoe suggests a valgus or everted foot, whereas excessive bulging on the lateral side suggests an inverted foot. Drop foot resulting from musculature weakness or peroneal nerve injury scuffs the toe of the shoe. Oblique forefoot creases in the shoe indicate possible hallux rigidus; absence of forefoot creases indicates no toe-off action during gait.

Examination

As with any assessment, the examiner must compare one side with the other and note any asymmetry. This comparison is necessary because of individual differences among normal people.

Active Movements

The first movements tested during the examination are active, with painful movements being tested last. These movements should be done in both weight-bearing (Figs. 13.50 and 13.51) and non–weight-bearing (long leg sitting or supine lying; Fig. 13.52) positions, and the examiner should note any differences because foot deformities and deviations in addition to decreased ROM can lead to injury.[126] Lindsjo and colleagues advocated testing weight-bearing ROM by putting the test foot on a 30-cm (12-inch) stool for ease of measurement and flexing the knee.[127]

Weight-Bearing Active Movements of the Lower Leg, Ankle, and Foot

- Plantar flexion (flexion), standing on the toes
- Dorsiflexion (extension), standing on the heels
- Supination, standing on the lateral edge of the foot
- Pronation, standing on the medial edge of the foot
- Toe extension
- Toe flexion
- Combined movements (if necessary)
- Sustained positions (if necessary)
- Repetitive movements (if necessary)

Non–Weight-Bearing Active Movements of the Lower Leg, Ankle, and Foot

- Plantar flexion (flexion), 50°
- Dorsiflexion (extension), 20°
- Supination, 45°–60°
- Pronation, 15°–30°
- Toe extension, lateral four toes (MTP, 40°; PIP, 0°; DIP, 30°) and great toe (MTP, 70°;IP, 0°)
- Toe flexion, lateral four toes (MTP, 40°; PIP, 35°; DIP, 60°) and great toe (MTP, 45°; IP, 90°)
- Toe abduction
- Toe adduction
- Combined movements (if necessary)
- Sustained positions (if necessary)
- Repetitive movements (if necessary)

DIP, Distal interphalangeal joint; *IP,* interphalangeal joint; *MTP,* metatarsophalangeal joint; *PIP,* proximal interphalangeal joint.

Plantar Flexion

Plantar flexion of the ankle is approximately 50° (see Fig. 13.52A), and the patient's heel normally inverts when the movement is performed in weight bearing (Fig. 13.53). If heel inversion does not occur, the foot is unstable, or there is tibialis posterior weakness or tightness.[80,128,129] The tibialis posterior muscle and tendon balance the pull of the peroneal muscles, protect the spring ligament, and

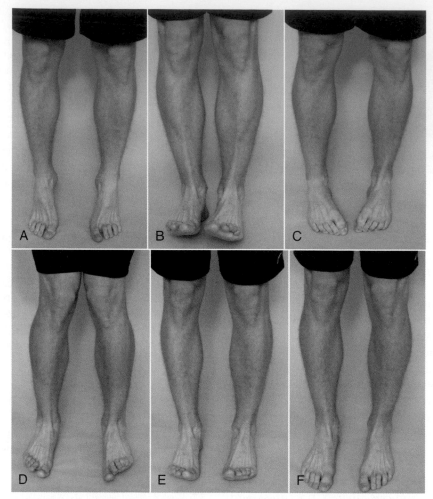

Fig. 13.50 Active movements (weight-bearing posture). (A) Plantar flexion. (B) Dorsiflexion. (C) Supination. (D) Pronation. (E) Toe extension. (F) Toe flexion.

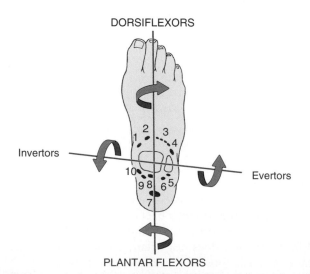

Fig. 13.51 Motion diagram of the ankle. *1,* Tibialis anterior; *2,* extensor hallucis longus; *3,* extensor digitorum longus; *4,* peroneus tertius; *5,* peroneus brevis; *6,* peroneus longus; *7,* Achilles tendon (soleus and gastrocnemius); *8,* flexor hallucis longus; *9,* flexor digitorum longus; *10,* tibialis posterior.

invert and stabilize the hindfoot during toe off.[130] Pain in the spring ligament as well as the medial midfoot and hindfoot ligaments, hindfoot valgus, plantar flexed talar head, and forefoot abduction should lead the examiner to assessing the tibialis posterior for proper function.[80]

Dorsiflexion

Dorsiflexion of the ankle is usually 20° past the anatomical position (plantigrade), which is with the foot at 90° to the bones of the leg (see Fig. 13.52B). For normal locomotion, 10° of dorsiflexion and 20° to 25° of plantar flexion at the ankle are required. Functional dorsiflexion may be measured by the **ankle lunge test** ☑.[131–134] For this weight-bearing test, the patient is asked to place one foot perpendicular to a wall and lunge the same knee toward the wall (Fig. 13.54A). The foot is progressively moved away from the wall until the knee barely touches the wall and the foot remains flat on the floor. The distance from the wall to the big toe is measured (Fig. 13.54B). Both sides are compared. If desired, the angle of the tibial shaft to a vertical line can also be measured (Fig. 13.55).[135]

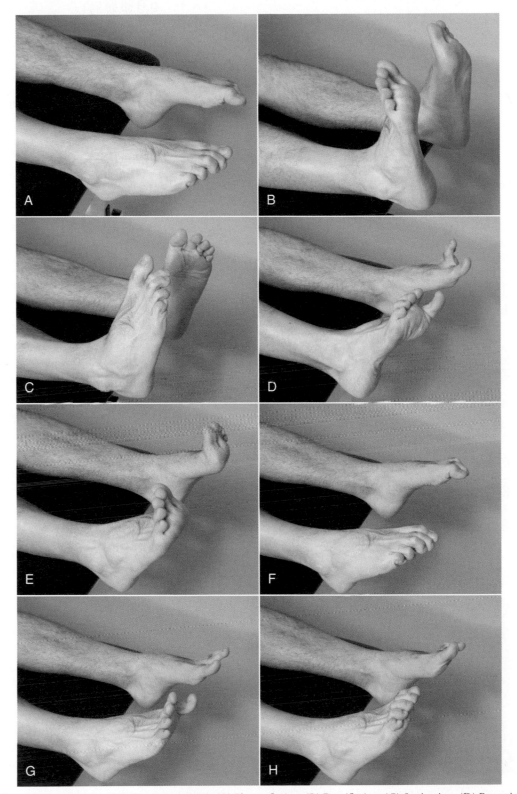

Fig. 13.52 Active movements (non-weight-bearing posture). (A) Plantar flexion. (B) Dorsiflexion. (C) Supination. (D) Pronation. (E) Toe extension. (F) Toe flexion. (G) Toe abduction. (H) Toe adduction.

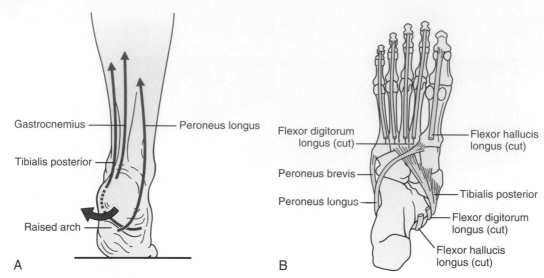

Fig. 13.53 (A) Inversion of heel while standing on toes (plantar flexion of ankle). Note that peroneus longus and tibialis posterior support the medial longitudinal and transverse arches. This motion is sometimes called "sickling" of the foot. (B) Plantar view of the right foot shows the distal course of the tendons of the peroneus longus, peroneus brevis, and tibialis posterior. The tendons of the flexor digitorum longus and flexor hallucis longus are cut. Note the force couple relationship between the two peroneal muscles and tibialis posterior to control inversion and eversion along with the long flexors and extensors. (B, Redrawn from Neumann DA: *Kinesiology of the musculoskeletal system: foundations for physical rehabilitation*, St Louis, 2002, Mosby, p 511.)

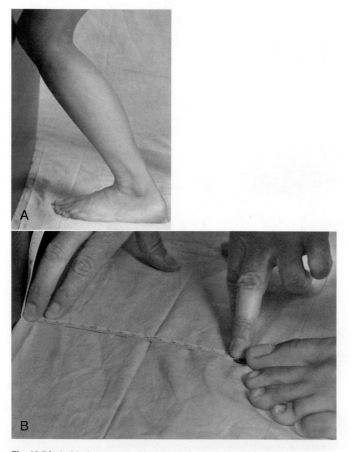

Fig. 13.54 Ankle lunge test. (A) Normal position: ankle fully dorsiflexed and knee against the wall. Note heel is firmly on floor. (B) Measurement of the distance of the toes from the wall.

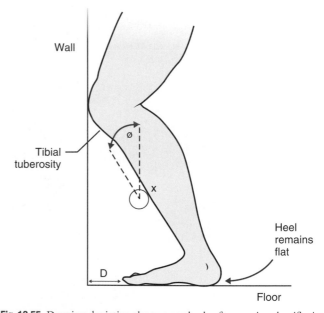

Fig. 13.55 Drawing depicting the two methods of measuring dorsiflexion lunge—distance from wall to big toe *(D)* and angle *(φ)* between line along anterior tibia *(x)* and vertical line.

Differences between sides may be due to a tight Achilles tendon or talocrural dorsiflexion restriction or stiffness.[136]

Supination and Pronation

Supination and pronation are the two primary movements that enable the foot to adapt to uneven ground, aid in shock absorption, and transition to a rigid lever for forward propulsion.[137] Supination is 45° to 60° and pronation is 15° to 30°, although individuals vary (see Fig. 13.52C and D). It is more important to compare the movement with that of the patient's normal side (Figs. 13.56 and 13.57). Supination combines the movements of inversion, adduction, and plantar flexion moving the foot into close packed making the foot more rigid while pronation makes the foot more mobile and flexible to absorb shock and allow adaptation to terrain.[2] Pronation combines the movements of eversion, abduction, and dorsiflexion of the foot and ankle. As the foot accepts weight, the foot moves into pronation, achieving maximum pronation in midstance and the midtarsal joint unlocks. As the foot moves into supination, the midtarsal joint locks (close pack), providing a rigid lever for push off.[137] As the patient does the movement, the examiner should watch for the possibility of subluxation of various tendons. The peroneal tendons are especially prone to subluxation, and their subluxation is evident on eversion (Fig. 13.58). If tibialis anterior is weak, supination is affected. If the peronei are weak or the tendons sublux, pronation is affected.

Walking on the lateral side of the foot tests inversion strength (primarily tibialis posterior and the tibial nerve), while walking on the medial side of the foot tests eversion strength (primarily peroneal muscles and superficial peroneal nerve).[2]

Toe Extension and Flexion

Movement of the toes occurs at the metatarsophalangeal and proximal and distal interphalangeal joints (see Fig. 13.52E and F). Extension of the great toe occurs primarily at the metatarsophalangeal joint (70°); there is minimal or no extension at the interphalangeal joint. For the great toe, 45° flexion occurs at the metatarsophalangeal joint, and 90° occurs at the interphalangeal joint.

For the lateral four toes, extension occurs primarily at the metatarsophalangeal (40°) and distal interphalangeal joints (30°). Extension at the proximal interphalangeal joints is negligible. For the lateral four toes, 40° flexion occurs at the metatarsophalangeal joints, 35° occurs at

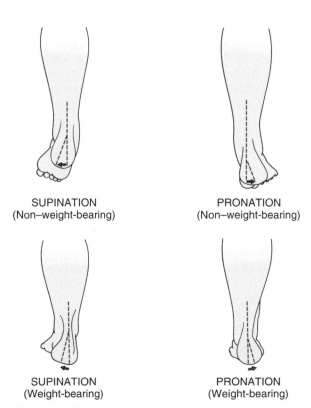

SUPINATION
(Non–weight-bearing)

PRONATION
(Non–weight-bearing)

SUPINATION
(Weight-bearing)

PRONATION
(Weight-bearing)

Fig. 13.56 Posterior view of the foot in supination and pronation (weight-bearing and non-weight-bearing stances).

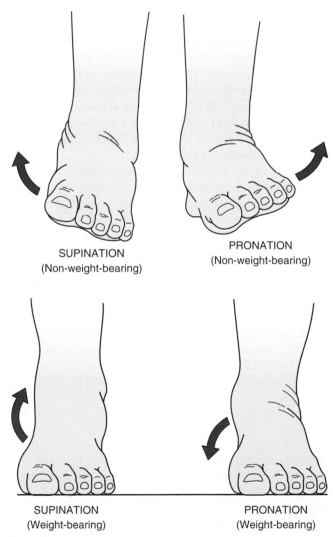

SUPINATION
(Non-weight-bearing)

PRONATION
(Non-weight-bearing)

SUPINATION
(Weight-bearing)

PRONATION
(Weight-bearing)

Fig. 13.57 Anterior view of the foot in supination and pronation (weight-bearing and non–weight-bearing stances).

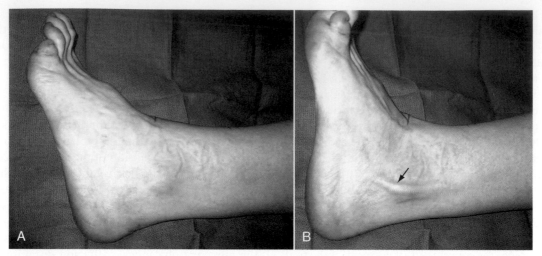

Fig. 13.58 Subluxation of the peroneal tendons. (A) With plantar-flexion and inversion, the tendons are reduced in the fibular groove. (B) With dorsi-flexion and eversion, tendon instability is reproduced. Note the subluxed position of the peroneal tendon *(arrow)*. (From Perumal V, Wilkinson GL: Peroneal tendon disorders. In Miller MD, Hart JA, MacKnight JM, eds: *Essential orthopaedics*, ed 2, Philadelphia, 2020, Elsevier.)

the proximal interphalangeal joints, and 60° occurs at the distal interphalangeal joints.

Toe Abduction and Adduction

Abduction and adduction of the toes are measured with the second toe as midline. Although the ROM of abduction can be measured, this is not usually done. The common practice is to ask the patient to spread the toes and then bring them back together (see Fig. 13.52G and H). The amount and quality of movement are compared with those of the unaffected side.

If the history has indicated that weight-bearing or non–weight-bearing combined or repetitive movements or sustained postures result in symptoms, these movements should also be tested. The examiner should ask the patient to walk on the toes, heels, and outer and inner borders of the feet. These actions indicate the patient's muscle power and control and the functional ROM. With a third-degree strain (rupture) of the Achilles tendon, the patient is not able to walk on the toes. Lack of dorsiflexion makes it difficult for the patient to walk on the heels. When the patient walks on the inner or outer borders of the feet, pain and difficulty are experienced in the presence of a subtalar lesion.

The examiner should also check the efficiency of the toes. Are the toes straight and parallel? Is the patient able to flex, extend, adduct, and abduct the toes? The toes have a primarily ambulatory function, although, with training, they can develop a prehensile function. The toes extend the weight-bearing area forward and, by so doing, reduce the load on the metatarsal heads. The great toe also has a primary function of pushing off during gait.

When assessing the active movements, the examiner must remember that peripheral nerve injuries may alter the pattern of movement. For example, the common peroneal

nerve may be injured, because it winds around the head of the fibula, resulting in altered nerve conduction to the peroneus longus and brevis muscles (superficial peroneal nerve) or the tibialis anterior, extensor digitorum longus, and extensor hallucis longus (deep peroneal nerve).[138] In such cases, the movements controlled by these muscles are altered. In addition, there are sensory changes that must be noted.

Passive Movements

The passive movements of the lower leg, ankle, and foot are performed with the patient in a non–weight-bearing position (Fig. 13.59). As with other joints, if the active ROM is full, overpressure can be applied to test end feel during the active, non–weight-bearing movements to negate the need to do passive movements. Each movement should be carefully checked, especially if deformities or asymmetries have been noticed during the observation. These deformities or asymmetries may cause problems in other areas of the lower kinetic chain. For example, limited dorsiflexion or tight heel cords may lead to anterior knee pain or ankle injuries.[139] Because the gastrocnemius is a two-joint muscle, dorsiflexion should be tested with the knee straight to test this muscle for tightness. Testing with the knee bent to 90° isolates the soleus. Stovitz and Coetzee recommended testing the Achilles tendon and its associated muscles with the subtalar joint in neutral with a lateral force applied to the talar neck to lock the foot during testing.[129] This eliminates calcaneal eversion or forefoot dorsiflexion from contributing to an apparent normal Achilles tendon. There is greater mobility and flexibility in the Achilles tendon in a baby or young child than there is in an adult. For example, in the newborn, the foot can readily be

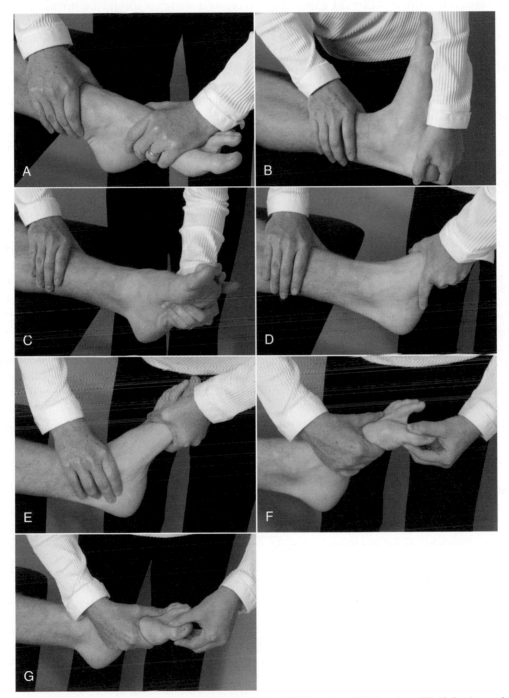

Fig. 13.59 Passive movements of the ankle. (A) Plantar flexion. (B) Dorsiflexion. (C) Inversion. (D) Eversion. (E) Abduction and adduction. (F) Toe flexion and extension. (G) Toe abduction.

dorsiflexed passively so that the toes and dorsum of the foot touch the skin over the tibia. In the adult, however, dorsiflexion is limited to 20° more than plantigrade. If the patient can only attain plantigrade (90°), then the gastrocnemius or soleus is tight or there is loss of talocrural joint mobility. If gastrocnemius is tight, the ankle ROM is limited with the knee extended. If the soleus is tight, the ankle ROM is limited with the knee flexed. Conversely, increased ankle dorsiflexion (**Matles test** ⚠), compared to the other side, may indicate a torn Achilles tendon, especially if combined with decreased plantar flexion strength.[140] If tibialis posterior is tight, pronation of the foot is limited.

Passive Movements of the Lower Leg, Ankle, and Foot and Normal End Feel

- Plantar flexion at the talocrural joint (tissue stretch)
- Dorsiflexion at the talocrural joint (tissue stretch)
- Inversion at the subtalar joint (tissue stretch)
- Eversion of the subtalar joint (tissue stretch)
- Adduction at the midtarsal joints (tissue stretch)
- Abduction at the midtarsal joints (tissue stretch)
- Flexion of the toes (tissue stretch)
- Extension of the toes (tissue stretch)
- Adduction of the toes (tissue stretch)
- Abduction of the toes (tissue stretch)

Some movements may be tested in combination to more closely approximate what occurs functionally. For example, instead of testing plantar flexion, adduction, and inversion separately, supination, as a combined movement, may be tested. Similarly, pronation may be tested as a combined movement, instead of dorsiflexion, abduction, and eversion.

During passive movements of the ankle and foot, any capsular patterns should be noted. The capsular pattern of the talocrural joint is more limitation of plantar flexion than of dorsiflexion; the subtalar joint capsular pattern shows more limitation of varus range than of valgus ROM. The midtarsal joint capsular pattern is dorsiflexion most limited, followed by plantar flexion, adduction, and medial rotation. The first metatarsophalangeal joint has a capsular pattern in which extension is most limited, followed by flexion. The pattern for the second through fifth metatarsophalangeal joints is variable. The capsular pattern of the interphalangeal joints is flexion most limited, followed by extension.

The **Foot Posture Index (FPI-6)**[141–147] may be used to rate foot posture and to quantify the amount of supination or pronation, or neutral position when standing. The patient stands relaxed with the arms by the side and looking straight ahead. The patient may be asked to "march in place" and to then settle into a comfortable stance. The patient will need to stand for about 2 minutes in place while the assessment is performed. If an observation cannot be made, it is left blank. The data sheet (Fig. 13.60) is used based on the observed criteria in Table 13.9. Features of a neutral foot posture are graded as 0 while pronated postures are graded positively and supinated postures are graded negatively. The scores are combined to give an aggregate score of overall foot posture.

Foot Posture Index (6-item) Datasheet

Patient name   *ID number*

	COMPONENT	PLANE	SCORE 1 Date_____ Comment_____		SCORE 2 Date_____ Comment_____		SCORE 3 Date_____ Comment_____	
			Left (-2 to +2)	Right (-2 to +2)	Left (-2 to +2)	Right (-2 to +2)	Left (-2 to +2)	Right (-2 to +2)
Rearfoot	Talar head palpation	Transverse						
	Curves above and below lateral malleoli	Frontal/trans						
	Inversion/eversion of the calcaneus	Frontal						
Forefoot	Bulge in the region of the TNJ	Transverse						
	Congruence of the medial longitudinal arch	Sagittal						
	Abduction/adduction of the forefoot on the rearfoot (too many toes).	Transverse						
	TOTAL							

Fig. 13.60 Foot Posture Index (6-Item) (FPI-6) Datasheet. (©Anthony Redmond 1998. From Redmond AC, Crosbie J, Ouvrier RA: Development and validation of a novel rating system for scoring standing foot posture: the Foot Posture Index. *Clin Biomech* 21[1]:89–98, 2006.)

TABLE **13.9**

Observation Criteria for Foot Posture Index

Criteria	-2	-1	0	+1	+2
Talar head palpation	Talar head palpable on lateral side but not on medial side	Talar head palpable on lateral/slightly palpable on medial side	Talar head equally palpable on lateral and medial side	Talar head slightly palpable on lateral side/palpable on medial side	Talar head not palpable on lateral side but palpable on medial side
Supra- and infra-lateral malleoli curvature (viewed from behind)	Curve below the malleolus either straight or convex	Curve below the malleolus concave, but flatter/more than the curve above the malleolus	Both infra- and supramalleolar curves roughly equal	Curve below the malleolus more concave than curve above malleolus	Curve below the malleolus markedly more concave than curve above malleolus
Calcaneal frontal plane position (viewed from behind)	More than an estimated 5° inverted (varus)	Between vertical and an estimated 5° inverted (varus)	Vertical	Between vertical and an estimated 5° everted (valgus)	More than an estimated 5° everted (valgus)
Prominence in region of the talonavicular joint (viewed at an angle from inside)	Area of talonavicular joint markedly concave	Area of talonavicular joint slightly, but definitely concave	Area of talonavicular joint flat	Area of talonavicular joint bulging slightly	Area of talonavicular joint bulging markedly
Congruence of medial longitudinal arch (viewed from inside)	Arch high and acutely angled toward the posterior end of the medial arch	Arch moderately high and slightly acute posteriorly	Arch height normal and concentrically curved	Arch lowered with some flattening in the central position	Arch very low with severe flattening in the central portion—arch making ground contact
Abduction/adduction of forefoot on rearfoot (view from behind)	No lateral toes visible. Medial toes clearly visible	Medial toes clearly more visible than lateral	Medial and lateral toes equally visible	Lateral toes clearly more visible than medial	No medial toes visible. Lateral toes clearly visible

From Lee JS, Kim KB, Jeong JO, et al: Correlation of Foot Posture Index with plantar pressure and radiographic measurements in pediatric flatfoot. *Ann Rehab Med* 39[1]:13, 2015.

Resisted Isometric Movements

The resisted isometric movements are performed to test the strength of contractile tissue around the foot, ankle, and lower leg. The patient is in the sitting or supine lying position, and the patient's foot is placed in the anatomical position (plantigrade or 90°; Fig. 13.61). Table 13.10 shows the muscles acting over the foot and ankle (Figs. 13.62 to 13.64). Strength results may vary depending on age and sex.[148]

Resisted Isometric Movements of the Lower Leg, Ankle, and Foot

- Knee flexion
- Plantar flexion
- Dorsiflexion
- Supination
- Pronation
- Toe extension
- Toe flexion

Dorsiflexion is sometimes tested with the patient's hip flexed to 45° and the knee flexed to 90°, as illustrated in Fig. 13.61B. Testing with the patient in this position enables the examiner to exert a greater isometric force. Resisted isometric knee flexion must be performed, because the triceps surae (gastrocnemius and soleus muscles together) act on the knee as well as on the ankle and foot.

If the history has indicated that eccentric, concentric, or econcentric muscle action has caused symptoms, these movements should also be tested, but only after the isometric tests have been completed. It has also been shown that hip strength (i.e., hip extension) can be a risk factor in lateral ankle sprains so the examiner should consider testing the muscle strength of the muscles in the lower kinetic chain if imbalances are suspected or if chronic injuries have occurred.[149]

Functional Assessment

If the patient is able to do the movements already described with little difficulty, functional tests may be performed to

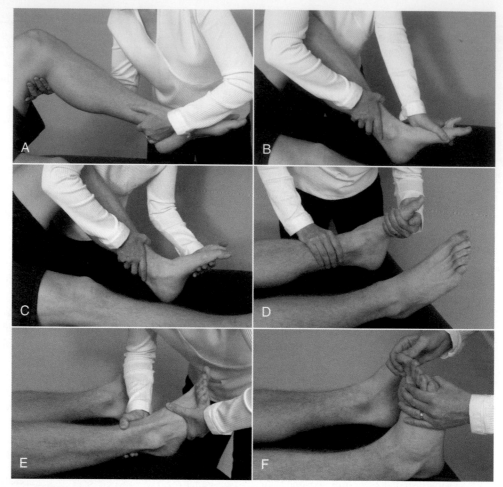

Fig. 13.61 Resisted isometric movements of the lower leg, ankle, and foot. (A) Knee flexion. (B) Dorsiflexion. (C) Plantar flexion. (D) Supination. (E) Pronation. (F) Toe extension.

TABLE 13.10

Muscles of the Lower Limb, Ankle, and Foot: Their Actions, Nerve Supply, and Nerve Root Derivation (Peripheral Nerves)

Action	Muscles Acting	Nerve Supply	Nerve Root Derivation
Plantar flexion (flexion) of ankle	1. Gastrocnemius[a]	Tibial	S1, S2
	2. Soleus[a]	Tibial	S1, S2
	3. Plantaris	Tibial	S1, S2
	4. Flexor digitorum longus	Tibial	S2, S3
	5. Peroneus longus	Superficial peroneal	L5, S1, S2
	6. Peroneus brevis	Superficial peroneal	L5, S1, S2
	7. Flexor hallucis longus	Tibial	S2, S3
	8. Tibialis posterior	Tibial	L4, L5
Dorsiflexion (extension) of ankle	1. Tibialis anterior	Deep peroneal	L4, L5
	2. Extensor digitorum longus	Deep peroneal	L5, S1
	3. Extensor hallucis longus	Deep peroneal	L5, S1
	4. Peroneus tertius	Deep peroneal	L5, S1
Inversion	1. Tibialis posterior	Tibial	L4, L5
	2. Flexor digitorum longus	Tibial	S2, S3
	3. Flexor hallucis longus	Tibial	S2, S3
	4. Tibialis anterior	Deep peroneal	L4, L5
	5. Extensor hallucis longus	Deep peroneal	L5, S1
Eversion	1. Peroneus longus	Superficial peroneal	L5, S1, S2
	2. Peroneus brevis	Superficial peroneal	L5, S1, S2
	3. Peroneus tertius	Deep peroneal	L5, S1
	4. Extensor digitorum longus	Deep peroneal	L5, S1

TABLE **13.10**

Muscles of the Lower Limb, Ankle, and Foot: Their Actions, Nerve Supply, and Nerve Root Derivation (Peripheral Nerves)—cont'd

Action	Muscles Acting	Nerve Supply	Nerve Root Derivation
Flexion of toes	1. Flexor digitorum longus	Tibial	S2, S3
	2. Flexor hallucis longus	Tibial	S2, S3
	3. Flexor digitorum brevis	Tibial (medial plantar branch)	S2, S3
	4. Flexor hallucis brevis	Tibial (medial plantar branch)	S2, S3
	5. Flexor accessorius (Quadratus plantae)	Tibial (lateral plantar branch)	S2, S3
	6. Interossei	Tibial (lateral plantar branch)	S2, S3
	7. Flexor digiti minimi brevis	Tibial (lateral plantar branch)	S2, S3
	8. Lumbricals (metatarsophalangeal joints)	Tibial (first by medial plantar branch; second through fourth by lateral plantar branch)	S2, S3
Extension of toes	1. Extensor digitorum longus	Deep peroneal	L5, S1
	2. Extensor hallucis longus	Deep peroneal	L5, S1
	3. Extensor digitorum brevis	Deep peroneal (lateral terminal branch)	S1, S2
	4. Lumbricals (interphalangeal joints)	Tibial (first by medial plantar branch; second through fourth by lateral plantar branch)	S2, S3
Abduction of toes	1. Abductor hallucis	Tibial (medial plantar branch)	S2, S3
	2. Abductor digiti minimi	Tibial (lateral plantar branch)	S2, S3
	3. Dorsal interossei	Tibial (lateral plantar branch)	S2, S3
Adduction of toes	1. Adductor hallucis	Tibial (lateral plantar branch)	S2, S3
	2. Plantar interossei	Tibial (lateral plantar branch)	S2, S3

[a]The gastrocnemius and soleus muscles are sometimes grouped together as the triceps surae muscles.

see whether these sequential activities produce pain or other symptoms. Full ROM is often not necessary for the patient to lead a functional life.

Functional Activities of the Lower Leg, Ankle, and Foot (in Sequential Order)

- Squatting (both ankles should dorsiflex symmetrically)
- Standing on toes (both ankles should plantar flex symmetrically)
- Squatting and bouncing at the end of a squat
- Standing on one foot at a time
- Standing on the toes, one foot at a time
- Going up and down stairs
- Walking on the toes
- Running straight ahead
- Running, twisting, and cutting
- Jumping
- Jumping and going into a full squat

Range of Motion Necessary at the Foot and Ankle for Selected Locomotion Activities

Descending stairs: Full dorsiflexion (20°)
Walking: Dorsiflexion (10°); plantar flexion (20°–25°)

These activities, which are examples only, must be geared to the individual patient. Older patients should

not be expected to do some of the activities unless they have been doing these or similar ones in the recent past (Table 13.11). More active individuals may be tested using the **Functional Movement Screen** (see Chapter 17) or the **Star Excursion Balance Test** (see Chapter 2).[150–154] The most commonly used measures of these two tests are the anterior posteromedial and posterolateral reach in centimeters. Because the functional tests place a stress on the other lower limb joints (e.g., knee, hip, sacroiliac, lumbar joints), the examiner must ensure that these joints exhibit no pathology before all of the tests are completed. Wikstrom et al.,[155] Buchanan et al.,[156] Linens et al.,[157] and Sharma et al.[158] felt a modified hop test (jump test), the side hop test, figure-of-8 hop test, the square hop test, and the **single limb hurdle test**[156,158,159] (Fig. 13.65) were an effective way to determine functional ankle instability. Eechaute et al.[160,161] likewise, found a **multiple hop test** (Fig. 13.66) to be a reliable functional test. The test involves standing on two feet, jumping forward half the height of the patient's vertical jump, and landing on one leg (good leg first).

Conditions, such as vascular intermittent claudication and anterior compartment syndrome, that occur within a specific time frame must also be considered in an assessment and when considering function.[162,163]

Balance and proprioception are tested by asking the patient to stand on the unaffected leg and then on

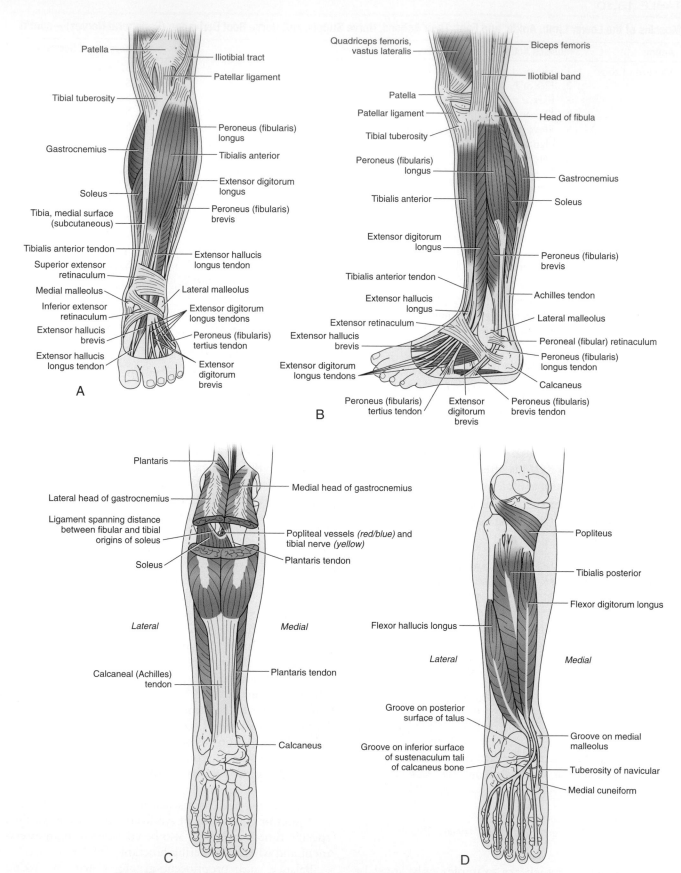

Fig. 13.62 Muscles of the leg. (A) Anterior. (B) Lateral. (C) Posterior superficial. (D) Posterior deep.

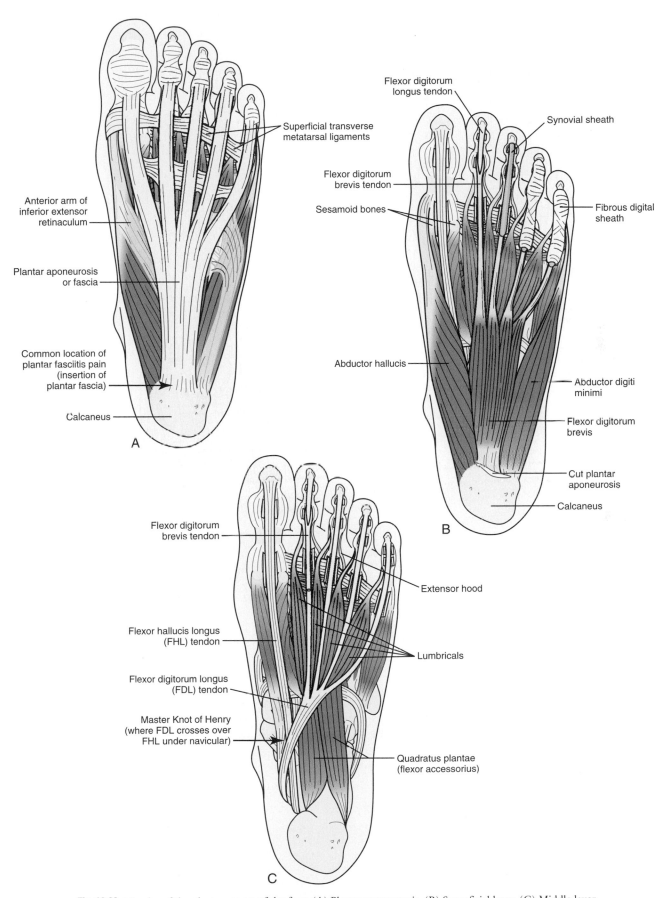

Superficial transverse metatarsal ligaments

Anterior arm of inferior extensor retinaculum

Plantar aponeurosis or fascia

Common location of plantar fasciitis pain (insertion of plantar fascia)

Calcaneus

A

Flexor digitorum longus tendon

Synovial sheath

Flexor digitorum brevis tendon

Sesamoid bones

Fibrous digital sheath

Abductor hallucis

Abductor digiti minimi

Flexor digitorum brevis

Cut plantar aponeurosis

Calcaneus

B

Flexor digitorum brevis tendon

Extensor hood

Flexor hallucis longus (FHL) tendon

Lumbricals

Flexor digitorum longus (FDL) tendon

Master Knot of Henry (where FDL crosses over FHL under navicular)

Quadratus plantae (flexor accessorius)

C

Fig. 13.63 Muscles of the plantar aspect of the foot. (A) Plantar aponeurosis. (B) Superficial layer. (C) Middle layer.

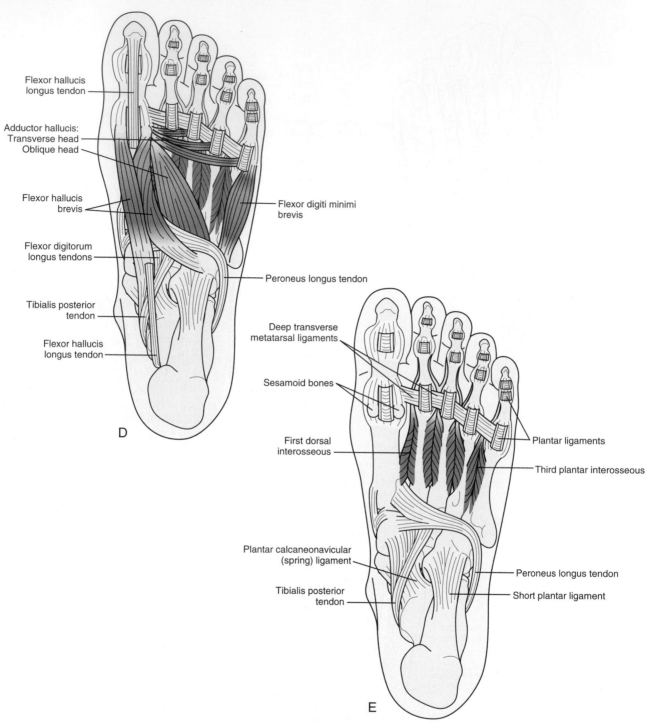

Flexor hallucis
longus tendon

Adductor hallucis:
Transverse head
Oblique head

Flexor hallucis
brevis

Flexor digitorum
longus tendons

Tibialis posterior
tendon

Flexor hallucis
longus tendon

Flexor digiti minimi
brevis

Peroneus longus tendon

D

Deep transverse
metatarsal ligaments

Sesamoid bones

First dorsal
interosseous

Plantar calcaneonavicular
(spring) ligament

Tibialis posterior
tendon

Plantar ligaments

Third plantar interosseous

Peroneus longus tendon

Short plantar ligament

E

Fig. 13.63, cont'd (D) Deep layer. (E) Interossei.

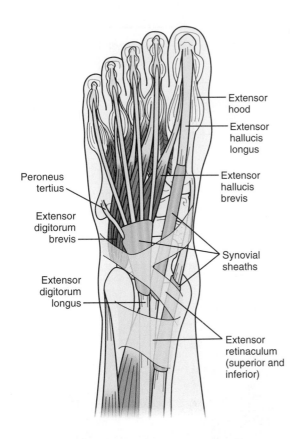

Extensor hood

Extensor hallucis longus

Extensor hallucis brevis

Peroneus tertius

Extensor digitorum brevis

Synovial sheaths

Extensor digitorum longus

Extensor retinaculum (superior and inferior)

Fig. 13.64 Muscles of the dorsum of the foot.

the affected leg, first with the eyes open and then with the eyes closed. Any differences in balance time or difficulty in balancing give an idea of proprioceptive ability, especially differences that occurred when the patient's eyes were closed (Fig. 13.67).[164] It has been reported that the **Balance Error Scoring System (BESS)** can be used to screen individuals for postural deficits following lower limb injuries.[165]

Kaikkonen and colleagues[166] developed a numerical scoring system to evaluate functional outcome after ankle injury (eTool 13.1). The **Ankle Joint Functional Assessment Tool (AJFAT)** (eTool 13.2); the **Foot and Ankle Ability Measure (FAAM)**[167–170] (eTool 13.3); the **Foot and Ankle Outcome Score (FAOS)**[167,171] (eTool 13.4); the **Foot Function Index (FFI)**[2,26,167,168,172–180] (eTool 13.5), which was developed for an elderly outpatient population; and the **Foot and Disability Index (FADI)**[169,181] (eTool 13.6), which has two modules—Activities of Daily Living and Sports—are other functional tests. The **Foot Health Status Questionnaire (FHSQ)**[177] (eTool 13.7), the **Bristol Foot Score,**[182] the **Manchester-Oxford Foot Questionnaire (MOxFQ),**[183–185] and the **Podiatry Health Questionnaire** measure foot health relative to quality of life.[176,177,186–188] Other scales such as the **Ankle Arthritis Scale,**[189] the American Orthopedic Foot and Ankle Society's **Ankle**

TABLE 13.11

Functional Testing of the Foot and Ankle

Starting Position	Action	Functional Test
Standing on one leg[a]	Lift toes and forefeet off ground (dorsiflexion)	10–15 Repetitions: Functional 5–9 Repetitions: Functionally fair 1–4 Repetitions: Functionally poor 0 Repetitions: Nonfunctional
Standing on one leg[a]	Lift heels off ground (plantar flexion)	10–15 Repetitions: Functional 5–9 Repetitions: Functionally fair 1–4 Repetitions: Functionally poor 0 Repetitions: Nonfunctional
Standing on one leg[a]	Lift lateral aspect of foot off ground (ankle eversion)	5–6 Repetitions: Functional 3–4 Repetitions: Functionally fair 1–2 Repetitions: Functionally poor 0 Repetitions: Nonfunctional
Standing on one leg[a]	Lift medial aspect of foot off ground (ankle inversion)	5–6 Repetitions: Functional 3–4 Repetitions: Functionally fair 1–2 Repetitions: Functionally poor 0 Repetitions: Nonfunctional
Seated	Pull small towel up under toes or pick up and release small object (i.e., pencil, marble, cotton ball) (toe flexion)	10–15 Repetitions: Functional 5–9 Repetitions: Functionally fair 1–4 Repetitions: Functionally poor 0 Repetitions: Nonfunctional
Seated	Lift toes off ground (toe extension)	10–15 Repetitions: Functional 5–9 Repetitions: Functionally fair 1–4 Repetitions: Functionally poor 0 Repetitions: Nonfunctional

[a]Hand may hold something for balance only.
Data from Palmer ML, Epler M: *Clinical assessment procedures in physical therapy*, Philadelphia, 1990, JB Lippincott, pp 308–310.

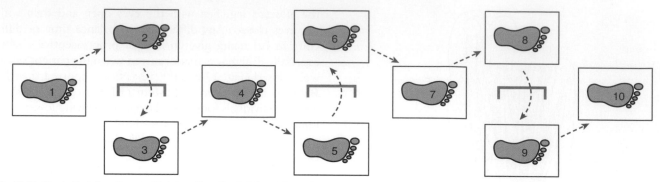

Fig. 13.65 Single limb hurdle test. Height of hurdles is 10 to 15 cm (4 to 6 inches). The test involves two lateral jumps and one medial jump over hurdles. Right leg test is shown.

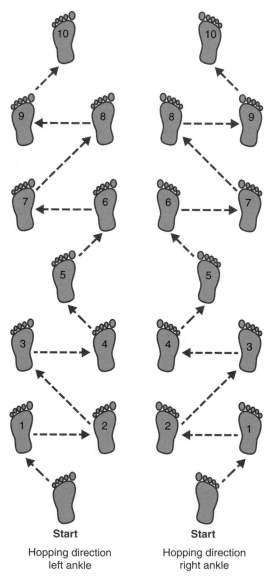

Start   **Start**

Hopping direction   Hopping direction
left ankle   right ankle

Fig. 13.66 Multiple hop test. (Modified from Eechaute C, Vaes P, Duquet W: Functional performance deficits in patients with chronic ankle instability: validity of the multiple hop test, *Clin J Sports Med* 18:124–129, 2008.)

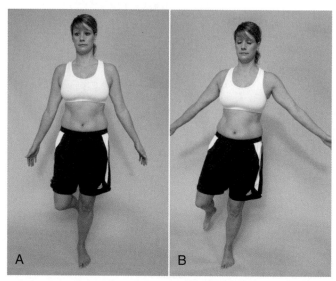

Fig. 13.67 Balance and proprioception. (A) One leg, with eyes open. (B) One leg, with eyes closed.

Hindfoot Scale[190–192] which is one of four scales for the foot,[190,191,193–196] the **Ankle Joint Functional Assessment Tool,**[197] the **Identification of Functional Ankle Instability** form[198–200] (eTool 13.8), the **Sports Ankle Rating System,**[201] the **Cumberland Ankle Instability Tool (CAIT),**[202–204] the **Ankle Instability Instrument,**[203,204] the **Foot and Ankle Outcome Score,**[205] and the **VISA-A Questionnaire** (for Achilles tendinopathy)[206] have been developed to evaluate function in specific conditions, specific activities, or specific parts of the lower leg, ankle, and foot.[183,207] Other scales have been developed for specific pathologies (e.g., fractures, osteoarthritis) about the ankle or can be applied to injuries in any part of the lower limb (e.g., Lower Extremity Function [LEF] Scale; see Chapter 11).[201,208–218]

Special Tests

When assessing the lower leg, ankle, and foot, it is important to always assess the neutral position of the talus in both weight-bearing and non–weight-bearing situations. This will help the examiner to differentiate functional from structural deformities. Other tests that should be carried out include alignment, functional leg length, and tibial torsion tests. Of the other tests, only those that the examiner wishes to use as confirming tests need be performed. Special tests should never be used in isolation but can be used to confirm clinical findings.

It has been found that functional movement screens that may be used to assess risk of potential ankle and foot injuries have, to date, not been recommended because of low predictive value and injury risk miscalculation.[219,220] That being said however, programs such as the FIFA 11+ Injury Prevention Program have been shown to prevent or reduce injuries.[221]

For the reader who would like to review them, the reliability, validity, specificity, sensitivity, and odds ratios of some of the special tests used in the lower leg, ankle, and foot are available in eAppendix 13.1.

Tests for Neutral Position of the Talus

The neutral position of the talus is often referred to as the *neutral* or *balanced position* of the foot. This so-called neutral position is an ideal position that, in reality, is not commonly found in people in normal weight bearing.[67,222,223] For most patients, the subtalar joint is normally in slight valgus with the forefoot in slight varus and the calcaneus in slight valgus. The tibia is in slight varus,[224] so each joint slightly compensates for the adjacent one. The neutral position is used as a starting position to determine foot and leg deviations. When the subtalar joint is in neutral, calcaneal inversion is twice (2×) calcaneal eversion.[26,225] Functional asymmetry may occur in the lower limb in normal standing; the examiner should then put the talus in the neutral position to see whether the asymmetry remains. If it does, there is anatomical or structural asymmetry as well as functional asymmetry. If the asymmetry disappears, there is only functional asymmetry, which is often easier to treat.

⚠ *Neutral Position of the Talus (Prone—Non–Weight-Bearing Position).* The patient lies prone with the foot extended over the end of the examining table (Fig. 13.68). The examiner grasps the patient's foot over the fourth and fifth metatarsal heads with the index finger and thumb of one hand. The examiner palpates both sides of the talus on the dorsum of the foot, using the thumb and index finger of the other hand. The examiner then passively and gently dorsiflexes the foot until resistance is felt (Fig. 13.69). While maintaining the dorsiflexed position, the examiner moves the foot back and forth through an arc of supination (talar head bulges laterally) and pronation (talar head bulges medially). As the arc of movement is performed, there is a point in the arc at which the foot appears to fall off to one side or the other more easily. This point is the neutral, non–weight-bearing position of the subtalar joint.[75,96,121,226] This prone test position is best for determining the relation of the hindfoot to the leg.

Key Tests Performed on the Lower Leg, Ankle, and Foot Depending on Suspected Pathology[a]

- *For determining the position of the talus:*
  - ❓ Navicular drop test
  - ⚠ Talar neutral position (non–weight-bearing) (supine and prone)
  - ⚠ Talar neutral position (weight-bearing)
- *For alignment:*
  - ⚠ Forefoot-heel alignment
  - ⚠ Leg-heel alignment
  - ⚠ Tibial torsion (prone)
  - ⚠ Tibial torsion (sitting)
  - ⚠ Tibial torsion (supine)
  - ⚠ "Too many toes" sign
- *For ligamentous instability:*
  - ✔ Anterior drawer test (supine and prone)
  - ⚠ Talar tilt
- *For joint instability (syndesmosis):*
  - ⚠ Cotton test
  - ✔ External rotation stress test
  - ⚠ Fibular translation test
  - ✔ Medial subtalar glide test

- *For medial tibial stress syndrome:*
  - ⚠ Shin oedema test (SOT)
  - ⚠ Shin palpation test (SPT)
- *For third-degree strain (rupture):*
  - ⚠ Matles (knee flexion) test
  - ⚠ Thompson's (Simmonds') test
- *For swelling:*
  - ⚠ Figure-eight measurement
- *Other tests:*
  - ⚠ Dorsiflexion-eversion test for tarsal tunnel syndrome
  - ⚠ Functional hallux limitus test
  - ⚠ Leg length discrepancy/functional leg length
  - ⚠ Morton's (squeeze) test
  - ⚠ Synovial impingement test
  - ⚠ Tests for peroneal tendon dislocation
  - ✔ Tinel's sign (3 positions)
  - ⚠ Triple compression test
  - ⚠ Windlass test (great toe extension)

[a]The authors recommend these key tests be learned by the clinician to facilitate a diagnosis. See Chapter 1, Key for Classifying Special Tests.

⚠ *Neutral Position of the Talus (Supine—Non–Weight-Bearing Position).* The patient lies supine with the feet extending over the end of the examining table. The examiner grasps the patient's foot over the fourth and fifth metatarsal heads, using the thumb and index finger of one hand. The examiner palpates both sides of the head of the talus on the dorsum of the foot with the thumb and index finger of the other hand (Fig. 13.70). The examiner then gently, passively dorsiflexes the foot until resistance is felt. While the examiner maintains the

dorsiflexion, the foot is passively moved through an arc of supination (talar head bulges laterally) and pronation (talar head bulges medially). If the foot is positioned so that the talar head does not appear to bulge to either side, the subtalar joint will be in its neutral non–weight-bearing position.[75,96,121,226] This supine test position is best for determining the relation of the forefoot to the hindfoot.

⚠ *Neutral Position of the Talus (Weight-Bearing Position).* The patient stands with the feet in a relaxed standing position so that the base width and Fick angle are normal for the patient. Usually, only one foot is tested at a time. The examiner palpates the head of the talus on the dorsal aspect of the foot with the thumb and forefinger of one hand (Fig. 13.71). The patient slowly rotates the trunk to the right and then to the left, which causes the tibia to medially and laterally rotate so that the talus supinates and pronates. If the foot is positioned so that the talar head does not appear to bulge to either side, then the subtalar joint will be in its neutral position in weight bearing.[96] Mueller et al.[227] described a progression of the neutral talus position in standing called the **navicular drop test ❓** to quantify midfoot mobility and its effect on other parts of the kinetic chain.[86,228] Using a small rigid ruler, the examiner first measures the height of the navicular from the floor in the neutral talus position using the most prominent part of the navicular tuberosity and then measures the height of the navicular in normal relaxed standing (Fig. 13.72A and B). The difference is called the *navicular drop* and indicates the amount of foot pronation or flattening of the medial longitudinal arch during standing (Fig. 13.72C).[228,229] Any measurement greater than 10 mm is considered abnormal. Experience in measuring is necessary to ensure reliable measures.[230] The test does not measure the amount of deformation that occurs

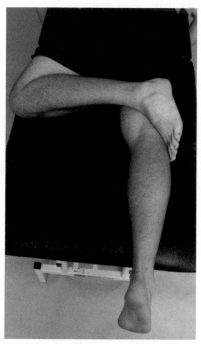

Fig. 13.68 Prone lying with leg, which is not being assessed, in figure-4 position to allow easier assessment of the neutral position of the right subtalar joint.

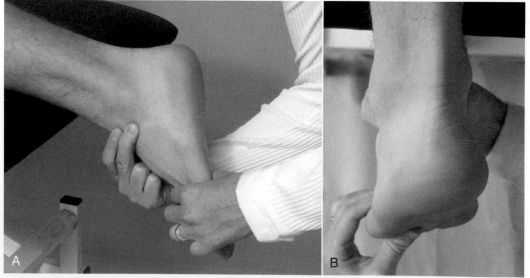

Fig. 13.69 Determining the neutral position of the subtalar joints in the prone position. (A) Side view. (B) Superior view.

with functional activities, such as walking or running.[231] McPoil et al.[232] advocated measuring the change in navicular height by doing a sit-to-stand test measuring navicular height in sitting (i.e., non-weight-bearing) and then in standing (i.e., weight-bearing) to measure navicular drop.

Tests for Alignment

Alignment tests are used to determine the relation of the leg to the hindfoot and the relation of the hindfoot to the forefoot.[233,234] These tests are used to differentiate functional from anatomical (structural) deformities or asymmetries.

🛇 *Coleman Block Test.*[235] This test differentiates a hindfoot varus resulting from a forefoot valgus from a hindfoot varus resulting from a tight tibialis posterior. If the patient is found to have a hindfoot varus in standing, the examiner places a lift or block under the lateral side of the forefoot. If the hindfoot varus is corrected, it indicates the hindfoot is flexible and the hindfoot varus is due to a plantar flexed first ray or a valgus forefoot (Fig. 13.73). If it does not correct, the tibialis posterior is tight.

⚠ *Forefoot-Heel Alignment.* The patient lies supine with the feet extending over the end of the examining table. The examiner positions the subtalar joint in supine neutral position. While maintaining this position, the examiner pronates the midtarsal joints maximally and then observes the relation between the vertical axis of the heel

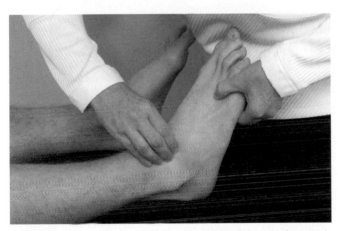

Fig. 13.70 Determining the neutral position of the subtalar joint in supine position.

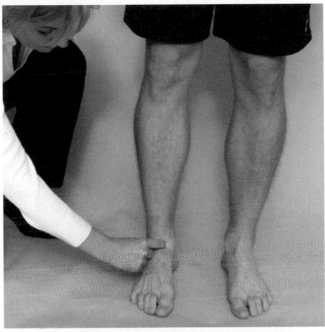

Fig. 13.71 Determining the neutral position of the subtalar joint in standing (weight bearing).

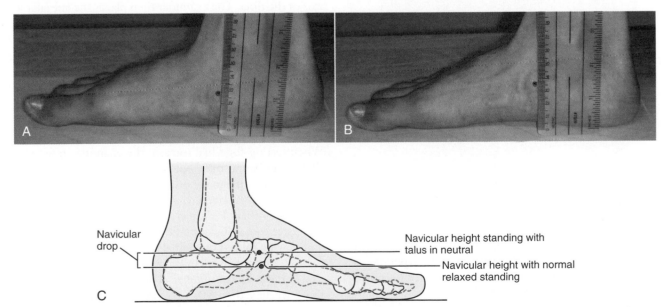

Fig. 13.72 Navicular drop test. "Drop" is the difference in height between the navicular height in standing relaxed (A) and standing with talus in neutral (B). (C) Illustration of two different foot positions required for navicular drop measurement.

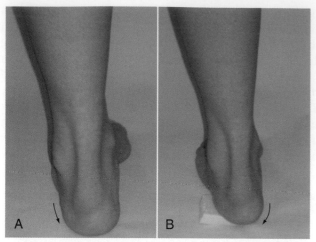

Fig. 13.73 Coleman block test. (A) On initial examination, the hindfoot is in varus. (B) The patient stands with a book or block under the lateral side of the forefoot, and the hindfoot is reexamined. Heel varus correction indicates that the hindfoot deformity is flexible and that the varus position is secondary to the plantar flexed first ray, or valgus position of the forefoot.

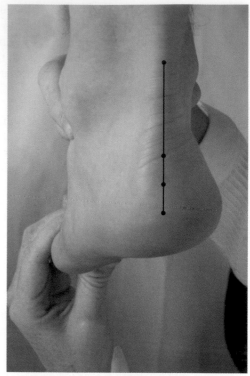

Fig. 13.75 Alignment of leg and heel.

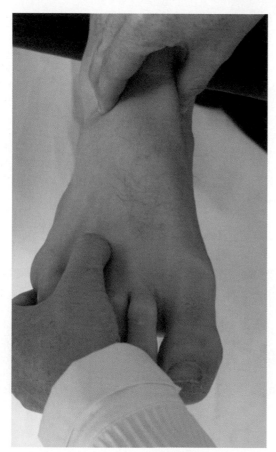

Fig. 13.74 Alignment of forefoot and heel (superior view).

and the plane of the second through fourth metatarsal heads (Fig. 13.74). Normally, the plane is perpendicular to the vertical axis. If the medial side of the foot is raised, the patient has a forefoot varus; if the lateral side of the foot is raised, the patient has a forefoot valgus.[75,226]

▲ *Leg-Heel Alignment.* The patient lies in the prone position with the foot extending over the end of the examining table. The examiner places a mark over the midline of the calcaneus at the insertion of the Achilles tendon. The examiner makes a second mark approximately 1 cm distal to the first mark and as close to the midline of the calcaneus as possible. A **calcaneal line** is then made to join the two marks. Next, the examiner makes two marks on the lower third of the leg in the midline. These two marks are joined, forming the **tibial line,** which represents the longitudinal axis of the tibia. The examiner then places the subtalar joint in the prone neutral position. While the subtalar joint is held in neutral, the examiner looks at the two lines. If the lines are parallel or in slight varus (2° to 8°), the leg-to-heel alignment is considered normal.[226] If the heel is inverted, the patient has hindfoot varus; if the heel is everted, the patient has hindfoot valgus (Fig. 13.75).

Tests for Tibial Torsion

When testing for tibial torsion, the examiner must realize that some lateral tibial torsion (13° to 18° in adults, less in children) is normally present.[236] If tibial torsion is more than 18°, it is referred to as a *toe-out position*. If tibial torsion is less than 13°, it is referred to as a *toe-in position*. Excessive toeing-in is sometimes referred to as pigeon toes and may be caused by medial tibial torsion, medial femoral torsion, or excessive femoral anteversion (see Table 13.3).

▲ *Tibial Torsion (Prone).* The patient lies prone with the knee flexed to 90°. The examiner views from above the angle formed by the foot and thigh (Fig. 13.76) after

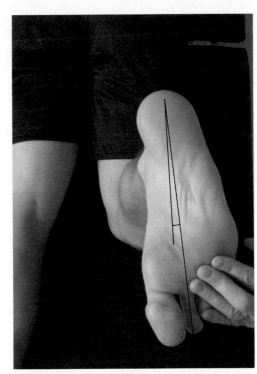

Fig. 13.76 Measurement of tibial torsion in the prone position.

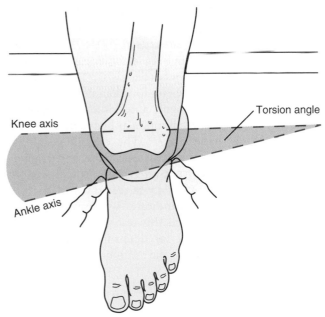

Knee axis

Torsion angle

Ankle axis

Fig. 13.77 Determination of tibial torsion in sitting (superior view). The torsion angle (normal: 12° to 18°) determined by the intersection of the knee axis and the ankle axis. (Modified from Hunt GC, editor: *Physical therapy of the foot and ankle, clinics in physical therapy*, New York, 1988, Churchill Livingstone, p 80.)

the subtalar joint has been placed in the neutral position, noting the angle the foot makes with the tibia.[237] This method is most often used in children, because it is easier to observe the feet from above.

⚠ *Tibial Torsion (Sitting).* Tibial torsion is measured by having the patient sit with the knees flexed to 90° over the edge of the examining table (Fig. 13.77). The

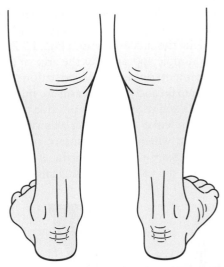

Fig. 13.78 "Too many toes" sign signifying lateral foot or tibial rotation. Two-and-one-half toes shown on the left foot, four toes on the abnormal right foot. (Redrawn from Baxter DE, editor: *The foot and ankle in sport*, St Louis, 1995, Mosby, p 45.)

examiner places the index finger of one hand over the apex of one malleolus and the index finger of the other hand over the apex of the other malleolus. Next, the examiner visualizes the axes of the knee and of the ankle. The lines are not normally parallel but instead form an angle of 12° to 18° owing to lateral rotation of the tibia.[65]

⚠ *Tibial Torsion (Supine).* The patient lies supine. The examiner ensures that the femoral condyle lies in the frontal plane (patella facing straight up). The examiner palpates the apex of both malleoli with one hand and draws a line on the heel representing a line joining the two apices. A second line is drawn on the heel parallel to the floor. The angle formed by the intersection of the two lines indicates the amount of lateral tibial torsion.

⚠ *"Too Many Toes" Sign.* The patient stands in a normal relaxed position while the examiner views the patient from behind. If the heel is in valgus, the forefoot abducted, or the tibia laterally rotated more than normal (tibial torsion), the examiner can see more toes on the affected side than on the normal side (Fig. 13.78).[238] Similarly, lateral femoral torsion could cause the "too many toes" test to be positive. If the talus is positioned in neutral and the calcaneus is in neutral, the "too many toes" sign means the forefoot is adducted on the rearfoot and may be seen with excessive pronation (hyperpronation).[129,239] Hyperpronation is often associated with metatarsalgia, plantar fasciitis, hallux valgus, and posterior tibial tendon pathology.[129]

Tests for Ligamentous (Joint) Instability

✓ *Anterior Drawer Test of the Ankle.* This test is designed primarily to test for injuries to the anterior talofibular ligament, the most frequently injured ligament in the ankle.[240–242] The patient lies supine with the foot relaxed.

The examiner stabilizes the tibia and fibula, holds the patient's foot in 20° of plantar flexion, and draws the talus forward in the ankle mortise (Fig. 13.79A).[243–246] Sometimes, a dimple appears over the area of the anterior talofibular ligament on anterior translation (**dimple** or **suction sign**) if pain and muscle spasm are minimal.[247–249] In the plantar-flexed position, the anterior talofibular ligament is perpendicular to the long axis of the tibia. By adding inversion, which gives an anterolateral stress, the examiner can increase the stress on the anterior talofibular ligament and the calcaneofibular ligament. A positive

anterior drawer test may be obtained with a tear of only the anterior talofibular ligament, but anterior translation is greater if both ligaments are torn, especially if the foot is tested in dorsiflexion.[250] If straight anterior movement or translation occurs (Fig. 13.80B), the test indicates both medial and lateral ligament insufficiencies. This bilateral finding, which is often more evident in dorsiflexion, means that the superficial and deep deltoid ligaments, as well as the anterior talofibular ligament and anterolateral capsule, have been torn. If the tear is on only one side, only that side would translate forward. For example, with a lateral tear, the lateral side would translate forward, causing medial rotation of the talus and resulting in anterolateral rotary instability (Fig. 13.80C), which is increasingly evident with plantar flexion of the foot.[73,76,251–253] Miller et al.[254] found that doing an anterolateral drawer movement rather than doing a straight anterior drawer test caused twice the lateral talar displacement.

Ideally, the knee should be placed in 90° of flexion to alleviate tension on the Achilles tendon. The test should be performed in plantar flexion and in dorsiflexion to test for straight and rotational instabilities.

The test may also be performed by stabilizing the foot and talus and pushing the tibia and fibula posteriorly on the talus (Fig. 13.79B). In this case, excessive posterior movement of the tibia and fibula on the talus indicates a positive test.

▲ *Cotton Test (Lateral Stress Test).*[26,255–259] This test is used to assess for syndesmosis instability caused by separation of the tibia and fibula (diastasis). The two bones are normally held together by four ligaments (the tibiofibular interosseous ligament, anteroinferior tibiofibular ligament, posteroinferior tibiofibular ligament, and transverse tibiofibular ligament).[259] The examiner stabilizes the distal tibia and fibula with one hand and applies a lateral translation force (not an eversion force) with the other hand to the foot.[26] Any lateral translation (more than 3 to 5 mm) or clunk indicates syndesmotic instability.[26,260] Stoffel et al.[261] felt this test was better than the lateral rotation stress test for determining syndesmotic instability on stress x-ray. If the examiner applies a medial

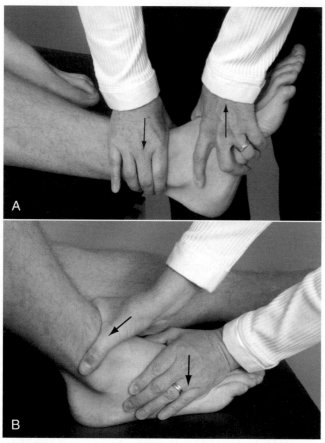

Fig. 13.79 Anterior drawer test. (A) Method 1—drawing the foot forward. (B) Method 2—pushing the leg back.

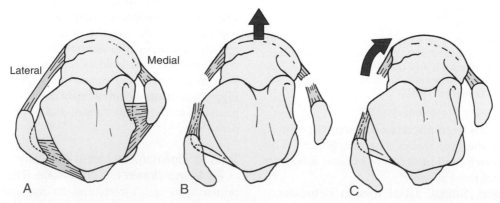

Fig. 13.80 Anterior drawer test. (A) Normal relation between talus and malleoli. (B) Straight anterior translation (one-plane anterior instability). (C) Anterolateral rotary translation (anterolateral rotary instability).

translation force, the test is called the **medial subtalar glide test** ✓.

? *Crossed Leg Test.*[24,262,263] The patient sits in a chair with the affected leg crossed over the opposite knee so the midpoint of the fibula is resting on the opposite knee (Fig. 13.81). The examiner then applies a gentle force to the medial aspect of the knee of the injured leg. If the patient experiences pain in the area of the distal syndesmosis, it indicates a positive test.

? *Dorsiflexion Compression Test.*[24,262,264] While in bilateral weight bearing, the patient is asked to move

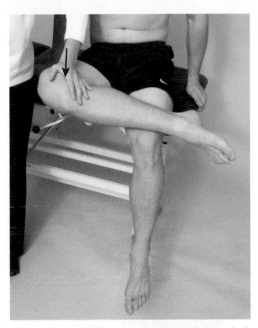

Fig. 13.81 Crossed-leg test. The patient sits in a chair, with the injured leg resting across the knee of the uninjured leg. The examiner applies a gentle force on the medial knee of the injured leg.

his or her ankle into extreme dorsiflexion (Fig. 13.82A). The patient is asked to note whether this maneuver is painful while the examiner notes the end ROM. The patient then assumes a normal standing position again. The examiner applies a compression force using two hands surrounding the malleoli of the injured leg. While this compression is maintained, the patient is asked to move into dorsiflexion again (Fig. 13.82B). A decrease in pain on dorsiflexion or an increase in dorsiflexion range indicates a positive test.

? *Dorsiflexion Maneuver.*[24,262,265,266] The patient sits on the edge of the table. The examiner stabilizes the patient's leg with one hand and with the other hand passively and forcefully dorsiflexes the foot by holding on to the heel and using the forearm to dorsiflex the foot (Fig. 13.83). Pain on forced dorsiflexion indicates a positive test for a syndesmosis problem.

✓ *External (Lateral) Rotation Stress Test (Kleiger Test).*[24,242,249,255,262,264,267–269] The patient is seated with the leg hanging over the examining table with the knee at 90°. The examiner stabilizes the leg with one hand. With the other hand, the examiner holds the foot in plantigrade (90°) and applies a passive lateral rotation stress to the foot and ankle. The test is positive for a **syndesmosis ("high ankle") injury** if pain is produced over the anterior or posterior tibiofibular ligaments and the interosseous membrane (Fig. 13.84).[24,270,271] It is important to note that syndesmosis sprains are associated with prolonged recovery with chronic ankle dysfunction and take longer to heal than medial or lateral ankle sprains.[22] If the patient has pain medially and the examiner feels the talus displace from the medial malleolus, it may indicate a tear of the deltoid ligament. On a stress radiograph, if the medial clear space is increased (see Fig. 13.138), it suggests rupture of the

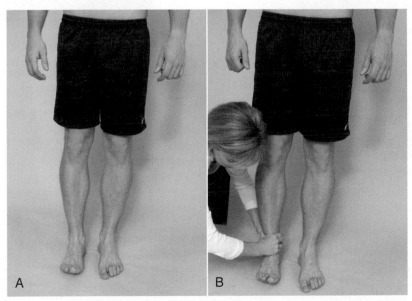

Fig. 13.82 Dorsiflexion compression test. (A) Step 1: Patient dorsiflexes feet while standing. (B) Step 2: Patient dorsiflexes feet while examiner squeezes malleoli together.

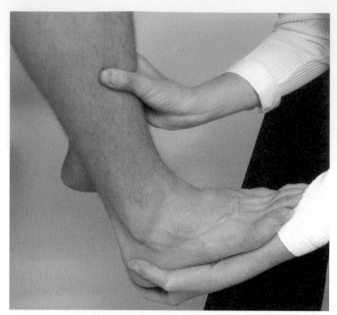

Fig. 13.83 Dorsiflexion maneuver. The examiner stabilizes the leg with one hand and passively moves the foot toward dorsiflexion with the other hand using the forearm.

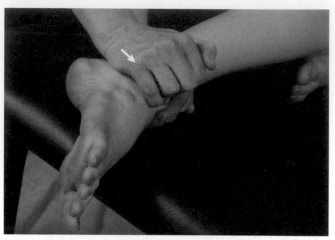

Fig. 13.85 Fibular translation test showing anterior translation.

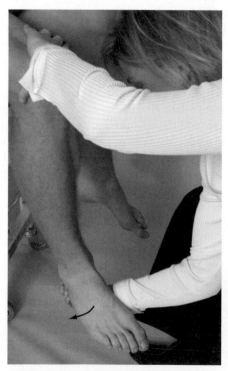

Fig. 13.84 External rotation stress test.

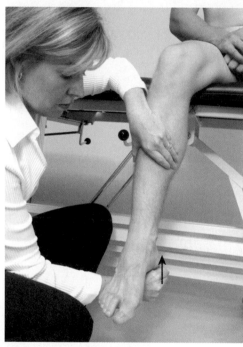

Fig. 13.86 Heel thump test. The examiner holds the patient's leg with one hand and with the other hand applies a gentle but firm thump on the heel with the fist.

ligament (see the discussion in the Diagnostic Imaging section) if the lateral malleolus is intact.

⚠ *Fibular Translation Test.*[257,258,272] The patient is side lying. The examiner faces the foot to be examined from behind and stabilizes the tibia with one hand and translates the fibular malleolus anteriorly and posteriorly with the other hand (Fig. 13.85). If pain occurs during the translation or if the movement is greater on the affected

side, the test is considered positive for a syndesmosis injury.

❓ *Heel Thump Test.*[24,262,273] The patient is sitting or lying. The examiner uses one hand to stabilize the leg. With the other hand, the examiner applies a firm thump on the heel with the fist so that the force is applied to the center of the heel and in line with the long axis of the tibia (Fig. 13.86). A positive test (i.e., pain) in the area of the ankle indicates a syndesmosis injury. Pain along the shaft of the tibia may indicate a stress fracture.

❓ *Point (Palpation) Test.*[78,262,264] The patient is positioned in sitting or supine. The examiner then applies a gradual pressure over the anteroinferior tibiofibular ligament (anterior aspect of the distal tibia fibular syndesmosis) using the thumb or index finger (Fig. 13.87). Pain in the syndesmosis area indicates a positive test.

✓ *Prone Anterior Drawer Test.*[274] The patient lies prone with the feet extending over the end of the examining table. With one hand, the examiner pushes the heel steadily forward (Fig. 13.88). Excessive anterior movement and a sucking in of the skin on both sides of the Achilles tendon indicate a positive sign. The test, like the previous one, indicates ligamentous instability, primarily the anterior talofibular ligament.

❓ *Single Leg Balance Test.*[275] The patient is asked to stand on one foot without shoes with the contralateral knee bent and not touching the floor or the test leg (i.e., weight-bearing leg). The patient starts with the eyes open fixing on a spot on a wall. The patient is then asked to close the eyes for 10 seconds. If the patient loses balance, the legs touch each other, the contralateral leg touches down, or the arms move from their start position, the test is considered positive for a potential ankle sprain.

❓ *Squeeze Test of the Leg.* The patient lies supine. The examiner grasps the lower leg at midcalf and squeezes the tibia and fibula together (Fig. 13.89).[24] The examiner then applies the same load at more distal locations moving toward the ankle. Pain in the lower leg may indicate a syndesmosis injury, provided that fracture, contusion, and compartment syndrome have been ruled out.[24,31,242,255,264,276,277] Brosky and associates called this test the **distal tibiofibular compression test** and applied the compression over the malleoli rather than the shaft of the tibia and fibula (Fig. 13.90).[266] Nussbaum et al.[267] reported that the "length of tenderness" above the lateral malleolus indicates severity.

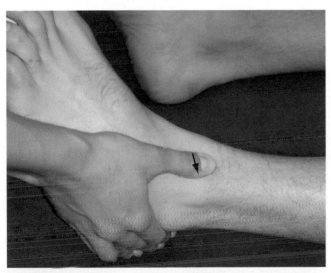

Fig. 13.87 Point (palpation) test. The examiner applies pressure over the anterior aspect of the distal tibiofibular syndesmosis.

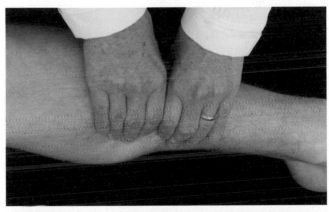

Fig. 13.89 Squeeze test for stress fracture or ankle syndesmosis pathology.

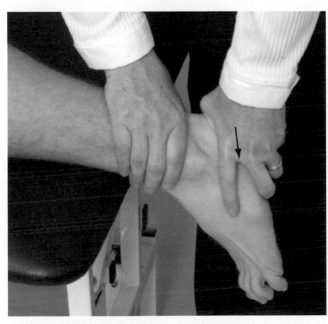

Fig. 13.88 Prone anterior drawer test.

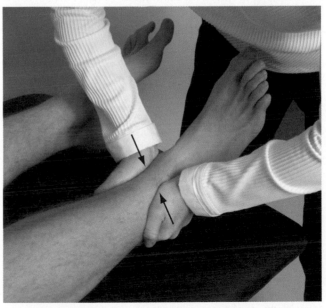

Fig. 13.90 Distal tibiofibular compression test.

⚠ *Talar Tilt.* The patient lies in the supine or side-lying position with the foot relaxed (Fig. 13.91).[73,278] The patient's gastrocnemius muscle may be relaxed by flexion of the knee. This test is to determine whether the calcaneofibular ligament is torn.[241,250] The normal side is tested first for comparison. The foot is held in the anatomical (90°) position, which brings the calcaneofibular ligament perpendicular to the long axis of the talus. If the foot is plantar flexed, the anterior talofibular ligament is more likely to be tested (**inversion stress test**).[249] The talus is then tilted from side to side into inversion and eversion. Inversion tests the calcaneofibular ligament and, to some degree, the anterior talofibular ligament by increasing the stress on the ligament.[36] Eversion stresses the deltoid ligament, primarily the tibionavicular, tibiocalcaneal, and posterior tibiotalar ligaments. On a radiograph, the talar tilt may be measured by obtaining the angle between the distal aspect of the tibia and the proximal surface of the talus (see the discussion of stress radiographs in the Diagnostic Imaging section).

Tests for Medial Tibial Stress Syndrome

⚠ *Shin Oedema Test (SOT).*[279] The patient is lying supine on the examining table with the test leg flexed to 45° at the hip and 90° at the knee. The examiner applies sustained palpation/pressure (for 5 seconds) to the distal two-thirds of the medial surface of the tibia (Fig. 13.92). Both legs are compared. Pitting edema indicates a positive test.

⚠ *Shin Palpation Test (SPT).*[279] The patient is lying supine on the examining table with the test leg flexed to 45° at the hip and 90° at the knee. The examiner palpates along the distal two-thirds of the posteromedial leg including the posteromedial border of the tibia and associated musculature (Fig. 13.93). Both legs are compared. Diffuse pain indicates a positive test. Localized point-specific pain may indicate a stress fracture if history indicates previous overload activity.

Other Tests

❓ *Buerger's Test.* This test is designed to test the arterial blood supply to the lower limb.[79] The patient lies supine while the examiner elevates the patient's leg to 45° for at least 3 minutes. If the foot blanches or the prominent veins collapse shortly after elevation, the test is positive for poor arterial blood circulation. The examiner then asks the patient to sit with the legs dangling over the edge of the bed. If it takes 1 to 2 minutes for the limb color to be restored and the veins to fill and become prominent, the test is confirmed positive.

⚠ *Dorsiflexion-Eversion Test for Tarsal Tunnel Syndrome.*[280] The patient sits on the examining table with the legs bent over the end of the table. The examiner takes the foot into full dorsiflexion with the heel everted and all the toes fully extended (Fig. 13.94). If neurological symptoms (i.e., pain, numbness) related to the tibial nerve and its branches result (i.e., medial aspect of sole, heel), the test is positive.

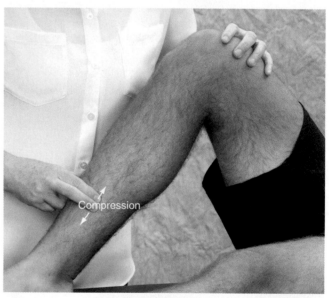

Fig. 13.92 Shin oedema test (SOT).

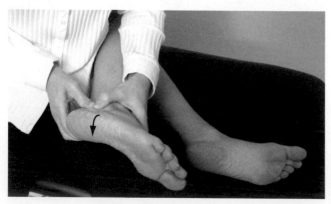

Fig. 13.91 Talar tilt test.

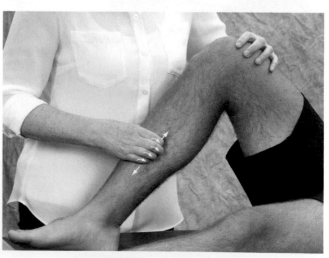

Fig. 13.93 Shin palpation test (SPT).

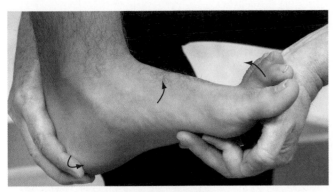

Fig. 13.94 Dorsiflexion-eversion test for tarsal tunnel syndrome.

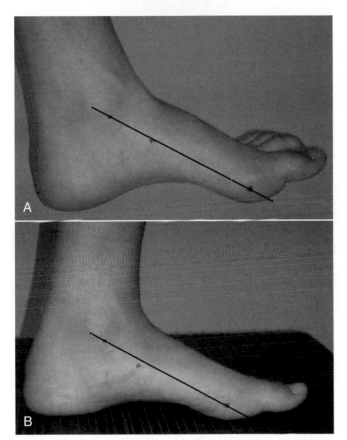

Fig. 13.95 (A) Feiss line in non–weight-bearing. Navicular is in normal position. (B) Feiss line in weight-bearing. Navicular is slightly below line (within normal limits).

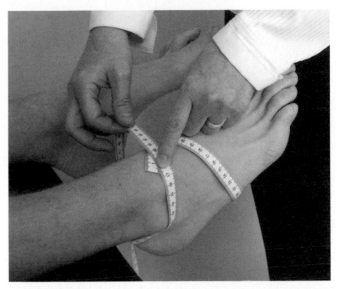

Fig. 13.96 Figure-eight ankle measurement for swelling.

❓ *Duchenne Test.*[79] The patient lies supine with the legs straight. The examiner pushes up on the head of the first metatarsal through the sole, pushing the foot into dorsiflexion. The test is positive for a lesion of the superficial peroneal nerve or a lesion of L4, L5, or S1 nerve root if, when the patient is asked to plantar flex the foot, the medial border dorsiflexes and offers no resistance while the lateral border plantar flexes.

❓ *Feiss Line.*[75,86] The examiner marks the apex of the medial malleolus and the plantar aspect of the first metatarsophalangeal joint while the patient is not bearing weight (Fig. 13.95A). The examiner then palpates the navicular tuberosity on the medial aspect of the foot, noting where it lies relative to a line joining the two previously made points. The patient then stands with the feet 8 to 15 cm (3 to 6 inches) apart. The two points are checked to ensure that they still represent the apex of the medial malleolus and the plantar aspect of the metatarsophalangeal joint. The navicular tubercle is again palpated. The navicular tubercle normally lies on or close to the line joining the two points (Fig. 13.95B). If the tubercle falls one third of the distance to the floor, it represents a first-degree flatfoot; if it falls two thirds of the distance, it represents a second-degree flatfoot; if it rests on the floor, it represents a third-degree flatfoot (see Fig. 13.42A).

⚠ *Figure-Eight Ankle Measurement for Swelling.*[281–284] The patient is positioned in long sitting with the ankle and lower leg beyond the end of the examining table with the ankle in plantigrade (90°). Rohner-Spengler et al.[285] recommend placing the ankle in 20° plantar flexion (called **figure-of-eight-20**). Using a 6-mm (¼ inch) wide plastic tape measure, the examiner places the end of the tape measure on the tibialis anterior tendon, drawing the tape medially across the instep just distal to the navicular tuberosity. The tape is then pulled across the arch of the foot just proximal to the base of the fifth metatarsal, across the tibialis anterior tendon, and then around the ankle joint just distal to the tip of the medial malleolus, across the Achilles tendon, and just distal to the lateral malleolus, returning to the starting position (Fig. 13.96). The measurement is repeated three times and an average taken.

⚠ *Functional Hallux Limitus Test.*[286,287] The patient lies supine with the leg supported on the bed. The examiner uses one hand to keep the subtalar joint in neutral while using the same hand to keep the first metatarsal in dorsiflexion. The examiner's other hand dorsiflexes the

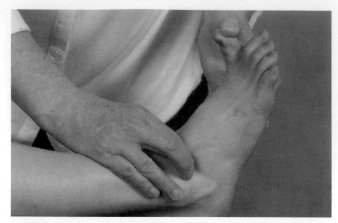

Fig. 13.97 Functional hallux limitus test. Note the right hand of the examiner ensuring the foot is in the neutral position while the hallux is dorsiflexed or extended.

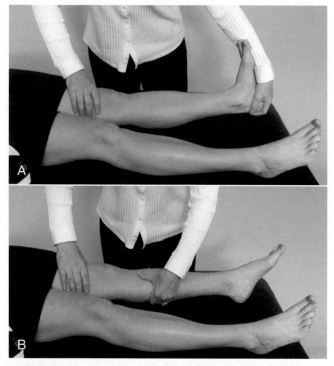

Fig. 13.98 Homans sign for thrombophlebitis. (A) Test. (B) Palpation for tenderness in thrombophlebitis.

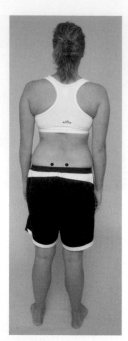

Fig. 13.99 Functional leg length in standing position (subtalar joint in neutral). *Dots on back* indicate posterior superior iliac spines.

proximal phalanx of the hallux. If the first metatarsal plantar flexes when the toe is dorsiflexed, the test is considered positive for abnormal midtarsal joint function leading to abnormal midtarsal joint pronation during late midstance (Fig. 13.97).

❓ *Hoffa's Test.* The patient lies prone with the feet extended over the edge of the examining table. The examiner palpates the Achilles tendon while the patient plantar flexes and dorsiflexes the foot. If one Achilles tendon (the injured one) feels less taut than the other one, the test is considered positive for a calcaneal fracture. Passive dorsiflexion on the affected side is also greater.

❓ *Homans Sign.* The patient's foot is passively dorsiflexed with the knee extended. Pain in the calf indicates a positive Homans sign for deep vein thrombophlebitis (Fig. 13.98). Tenderness is also elicited on palpation of the calf. In addition to these findings, the examiner may find pallor and swelling in the leg and a loss of the dorsalis pedis pulse.

⚠ *Leg Length Discrepancy (Anisomelia) and Functional Leg Length (see Chapter 11).*[288,289] The patient stands in the normal relaxed stance (Fig. 13.99). The examiner palpates the anterior superior iliac spines and then the posterior superior iliac spines and notes any differences. The examiner then positions the patient so that the patient's subtalar joints are in neutral position while weight bearing. The patient maintains this position with the toes straight ahead and the knees straight, and the examiner re-palpates the anterior and the posterior superior iliac spines. If the previously noted differences remain, the pelvis and sacroiliac joints should be evaluated further. If the previously noted differences disappear, the examiner should suspect a functional leg length difference resulting from hip, knee, or ankle and foot problems—primarily, ankle and foot problems (Table 13.12; see Table 9.9). The examiner must then determine what is causing the difference. For example, foot pronation is often seen with forefoot or hindfoot varus, tibial varus, tight muscles (e.g., calf, hamstrings, hip flexors), or weak muscles (e.g., ankle invertors, piriformis).

Leg length discrepancy may be structural (bony difference) or functional (altered mechanics), and can affect loading on the foot.[290] Structural leg length

TABLE **13.12**

Dynamic Limb Length Evaluation

Asymmetric Shoe Wear	Asymmetric Callus	Asymmetric Posture	Asymmetric Alignment or Movement
Shoe upper	Medial first distal interphalangeal	Foot	Toe-out
Heel counter	Medial first metatarsal	Ankle	Toe-grasp
Varus or valgus	Second and third metatarsal heads	Knee	Patellar alignment over foot
		Hip	Knee flexion
Shoe sole	Fourth and fifth metatarsal heads	Pelvis	Hip drop
Posterior lateral heel	Calcaneus		Propulsion
Posterior central heel	Lateral		
Posterior medial heel	Central		
	Medial		

Modified from Wallace LA. Limb length difference and back pain. In Grieve GP, editor: *Modern manual therapy of the vertebral column*, Edinburgh, 1986, Churchill Livingstone, p 469.

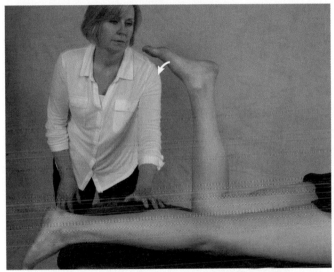

Fig. 13.100 Matles test. Negative test is demonstrated. If the Achilles tendon is ruptured, the foot would move into more dorsiflexion *(arrow)*.

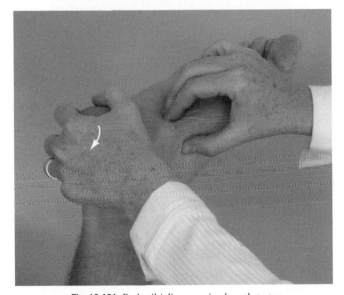

Fig. 13.101 Patla tibialis posterior length test.

deformity is sometimes called true leg length discrepancy. Compensation patterns may include pronation; hip or knee flexion on the longer leg; and/or supination, hip, or knee extension on the shorter leg. If there is no compensation, the anterior superior iliac spine and/or posterior superior iliac spine will be lower on the short leg resulting in postural or functional scoliosis. On the shorter side, stance time is decreased, walking velocity is decreased, cadence is increased, and step length is decreased.

⚠ *Matles Test (Knee Flexion Test).*[27,291] The patient lies prone with the foot over the end of the examining table while the clinician stands near the end of the table. The patient is asked to actively flex the knee to 90° (Fig. 13.100). During the motion, the examiner watches the foot. Normally, it will be slightly plantar flexed in knee flexion. If the foot falls into neutral or slight dorsiflexion, the test is positive for a 3° strain (rupture) of the Achilles tendon.

⚠ *Morton's (Squeeze) Test.*[79] The patient lies supine. The examiner uses the thumb and index finger of one hand to squeeze on the dorsal and plantar aspect of each intermetatarsal space. The examiner then grasps the foot around the metatarsal heads with the other hand and squeezes the heads together. Pain is a positive sign for stress fracture or neuroma. Sometimes a palpable click (**Mulder's click**) is felt during the test.[2]

❓ *Patla Tibialis Posterior Length Test.*[128] The patient is in prone lying with the knee flexed to 90° and the calcaneus held in eversion and the ankle in dorsiflexion with one hand (Fig. 13.101). With the other hand, the examiner's thumb contacts the plantar surface of the bases of the second, third, and fourth metatarsals while the index and middle fingers contact the plantar surface of the navicular.

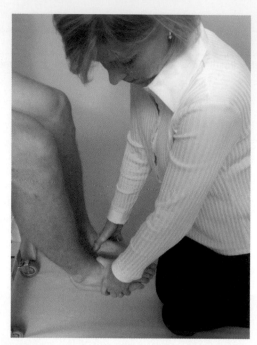

Fig. 13.102 Swing test for posterior tibiotalar subluxation.

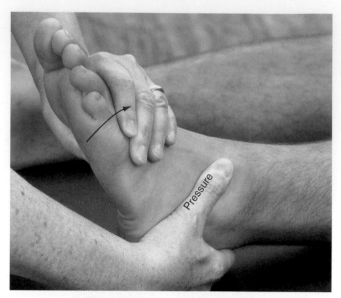

Fig. 13.103 Synovial impingement test.

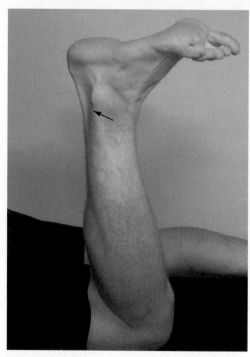

Fig. 13.104 Test for peroneal tendon dislocation. *Arrow* indicates where to look for subluxing tendon (also see Fig. 13.58).

The examiner then determines the end feel by pushing dorsally on the navicular and metatarsal heads. The end feel is compared with the normal side. A reproduction of the patient's symptoms indicates a positive test.

❓ *Swing Test for Posterior Tibiotalar Subluxation.*[292] The patient sits with feet dangling over the edge of the examining table (Fig. 13.102). The examiner places the hands around the dorsum of the foot using the fingers to keep the feet parallel to the floor. With the thumbs, the examiner palpates the anterior portion of the talus. The examiner then passively plantar flexes and dorsiflexes the foot and compares the quality and degree of movement between feet, especially into dorsiflexion. Resistance to normal dorsiflexion in the injured ankle indicates a positive test for posterior tibiotalar subluxation.

⚠ *Synovial Impingement Test.*[34] The patient is in long sitting on the examining table. The examiner stands at the end of the table and grasps the calcaneus so the thumb of one hand rests in the anterolateral gutter of the ankle joint. The other hand grasps the forefoot. The examiner first takes the foot into plantar flexion, then applies pressure in the lateral gutter. While maintaining the pressure in the lateral gutter, the examiner passively takes the patient's foot into dorsiflexion (Fig. 13.103). If hypertrophic synovium is present, it is forced into the joint by the examiner's thumb and is impinged between the neck of the talus and the distal tibia causing pain (or increasing pain caused by thumb pressure), indicating a positive test.

⚠ *Test for Peroneal Tendon Dislocation.*[293] The patient is placed in prone on the examining table with the knee flexed to 90°. The posterolateral region of the ankle is

inspected for swelling. The patient is then asked to actively dorsiflex and plantar flex the ankle along with eversion against the examiner's resistance (Fig. 13.104). If the tendon subluxes from behind the lateral malleolus, the test is positive.

⚠ *Thompson's (Simmonds') Test (Sign for Achilles Tendon Rupture).* The patient lies prone or kneels on a chair with the feet over the edge of the table or chair (Fig. 13.105). While the patient is relaxed, the examiner squeezes the calf muscles. The absence of plantar flexion when the

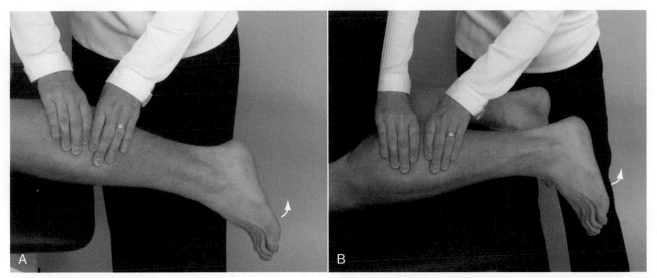

Fig. 13.105 Thompson's test for Achilles tendon rupture. (A) Prone lying position. (B) Kneeling position. In each case, foot plantar flexes *(arrow)* if the test result is negative.

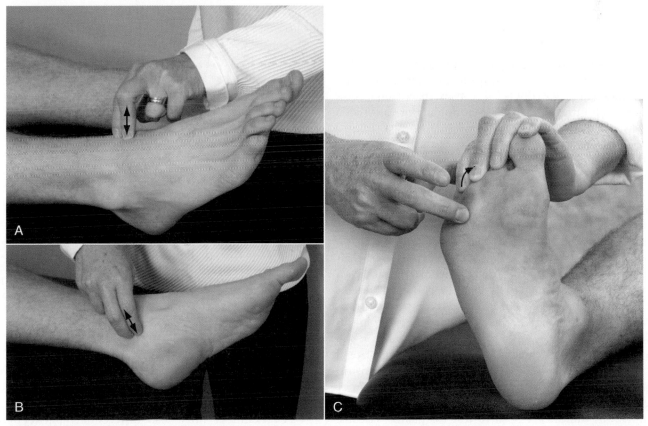

Fig. 13.106 Tinel's sign. (A) Anterior tibial branch of deep peroneal nerve. (B) Posterior tibial nerve. (C) Morton's neuroma. Tapping between third and fourth metatarsals.

muscle is squeezed indicates a positive test and a ruptured Achilles tendon (third-degree strain).[294–297] One should be careful not to assume that the Achilles tendon is not ruptured if the patient is able to plantar flex the foot while not bearing weight. The long flexor muscles can perform this function in the non–weight-bearing stance even with a rupture of the Achilles tendon.

✓ **Tinel's Sign at the Ankle (Percussion Sign).** Tinel sign may be elicited in three places around the ankle. The anterior tibial branch of the deep peroneal nerve may be percussed in front of the ankle (Fig. 13.106A). The posterior tibial nerve may be percussed as it passes behind the medial malleolus (Fig. 13.106B). The third place is for **Morton's neuroma.** With one hand, the examiner

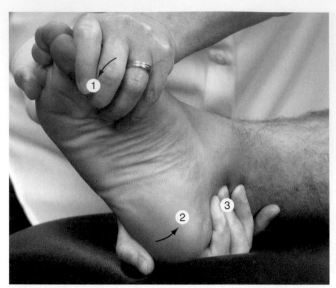

Fig. 13.107 Triple compression test for tibial nerve and tarsal tunnel syndrome involves three steps: *(1)* full plantar flexion, *(2)* heel inversion, and *(3)* compression over nerve.

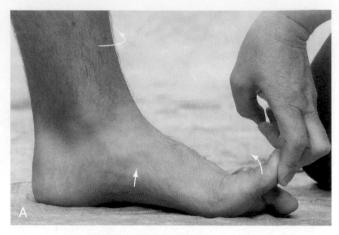

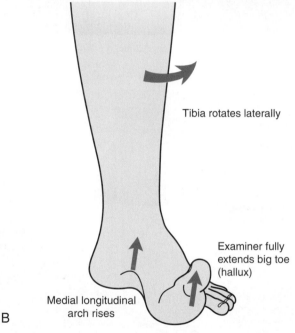

Tibia rotates laterally

Examiner fully extends big toe (hallux)

Medial longitudinal arch rises

B

Fig. 13.108 Windlass (great toe extension, first metatarsal rise) test. (A) The test. Examiner passively dorsiflexes the big toe. (B) Schematic diagram showing what should happen normally while doing the test. The medial longitudinal arch rises and the tibia laterally rotates. (B, Redrawn from Rose GK, Welton EA, Marshall T: The diagnosis of flat foot in the child, *J Bone Joint Surg Br* 67(1):71–78, 1985.)

passively extends the toes and while holding this position, uses the middle finger of the dominant hand to tap between the metatarsals proximal to the metatarsal heads five times (Fig. 13.106C).[15,111] Web space tenderness indicates a positive test. In all cases, tingling or paresthesia felt distally is a positive sign.

⚠ *Triple Compression Test.*[298] The test is used to assess for tarsal tunnel syndrome. The examiner takes the ankle into full plantar flexion and foot and heel inversion, and then applies an even constant pressure over the posterior tibial nerve for 30 seconds (Fig. 13.107). A positive test is reproduction of neurological symptoms.

⚠ *Windlass Test (Great Toe Extension Test, First Metatarsal Rise Test).*[2,55,287,299] The patient stands on a stool or chair with the foot positioned so that the metatarsal heads rest on the edge of the stool while the patient maintains weight through the leg. The examiner then passively dorsiflexes the big toe at the metatarsophalangeal going as far as it will go (Fig. 13.108A). Normally, this action will cause elevation of the medial longitudinal arch and lateral rotation of the tibia (Fig. 13.108B). If both actions do not occur, the foot cannot function normally.[300] Pain or increased pain at the insertion of the plantar fascia (see Fig. 13.25) indicates a positive test for plantar fasciitis. Lack of extension may indicate hallux rigidus.

The test may also be used to test for a flexible flatfoot. In this case, the test is performed the same way but is called the **Hubscher's maneuver** or **Jack's test**.[115]

Reflexes and Cutaneous Distribution

The examiner must be aware of the sensory distribution of the various peripheral nerves in the foot, especially the superficial peroneal, deep peroneal, and saphenous nerves, and the branches of the tibial nerve (sural, medial calcaneal, medial plantar, and lateral plantar; Fig. 13.109).

The examiner must also differentiate between the peripheral nerve sensory distribution and the sensory nerve root distribution or dermatomes (Fig. 13.110). Although dermatomes vary among individuals, their pattern is never identical to the peripheral nerve distribution, which tends to be more consistent among patients.

The examiner should test the patient's sensation by running his or her hands over the anterior, lateral, medial, and posterior surfaces of the patient's leg below the knee, foot, and toes (sensation scanning examination). Any difference in sensation should be noted and can be mapped out in more detail with a pinwheel, pin, cotton batten, or brush.

The examiner must test the patient's reflexes. Commonly checked in this region are the Achilles reflex[301]

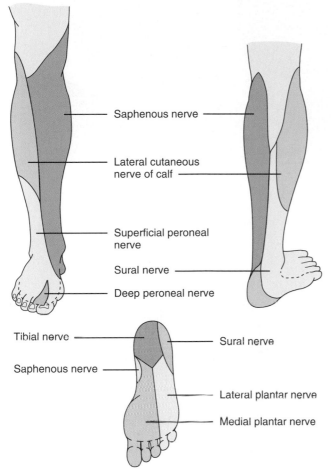

Fig. 13.109 Peripheral nerve distribution in the lower leg, ankle, and foot.

(S1–S2; Fig. 13.111) and the posterior tibial reflex (L4–L5; Fig. 13.112). These reflexes may be affected by age and may be absent in older normal individuals.[301] The examiner may also wish to test for pyramidal tract (upper motor neuron) disease. There are various methods for testing the pathological reflexes, including the Babinski, Chaddock, Oppenheim, and Gordon reflexes (Fig. 13.113). A positive sign in all of these tests is extension of the big toe. The Babinski reflex also causes fanning of the second through fifth toes. The most common and reliable test is the Babinski test.[302]

The examiner must remember that pain may be referred to the lower leg, ankle, or foot from the lumbar spine, sacrum, hip, or knee (Fig. 13.114). Conversely, pain from a lesion in the lower leg, ankle, or foot may be transmitted to the hip or knee. Table 13.13 shows the muscles of the lower leg, ankle, and foot, and their patterns of pain referral.

Peripheral Nerve Injuries of the Lower Leg, Ankle, and Foot

When assessing the patient, and depending on the history, the examiner should be able to differentiate between peripheral nerve injuries in the lower limb, peripheral neuropathy, referral of symptoms from lumbosacral or other lower limb peripheral joint pathologies, upper motor neuron disease, and central nervous system pathology based on the symptoms and where they occur.[303]

Deep Peroneal Nerve (L4 to S2). The deep peroneal nerve, a branch of the common peroneal nerve, which is itself a branch of the sciatic nerve (Figs. 13.115 and 13.116), is most commonly injured (compressed) in **anterior compartment syndrome** in the leg, and where it passes under the extensor retinaculum (**anterior tarsal tunnel syndrome**).[237,304–310] Compression may be caused by trauma, tight shoelaces, a ganglion, or pes

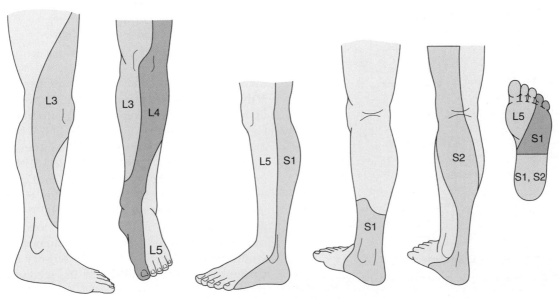

Fig. 13.110 Dermatomes of the lower leg, ankle, and foot.

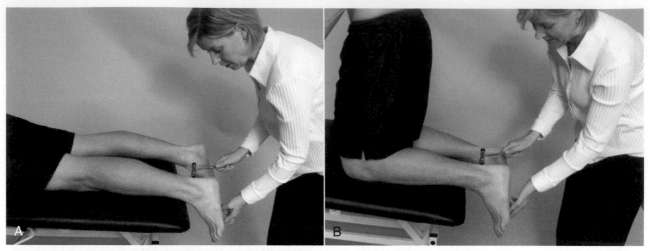

Fig. 13.111 Test of Achilles reflex (S1–S2). (A) Prone lying. (B) Kneeling.

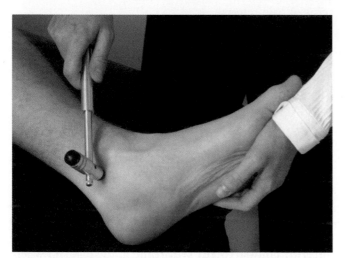

Fig. 13.112 Tibialis posterior reflex (L4–L5).

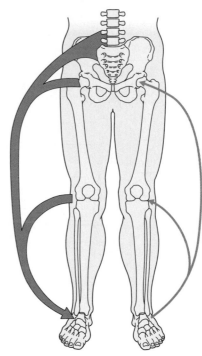

Fig. 13.114 Pattern of referred pain to and from the ankle.

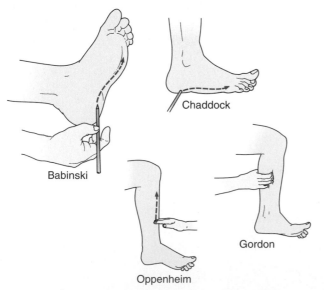

Fig. 13.113 Pathological reflexes for pyramidal tract disease.

cavus, or it may be due to intramuscular swelling with activity (**chronic exertional compartment syndrome**) in which there is increase in the intramuscular compartment pressure.[306] Roscoe et al.[311] have outlined diagnostic criteria for measuring the intramuscular compartment pressure. Motor loss (Table 13.14) includes an inability to dorsiflex the foot (**drop foot),** which results in a high steppage gait and an inability to control ankle movement. Because the deep peroneal nerve is primarily motor, there is minimal sensory loss, but this loss can be aggravating, especially in anterior tarsal tunnel syndrome (see Fig. 13.116). The sensory loss is a small triangular area between the first and second toes. Pain is

TABLE 13.13

Muscles of the Lower Leg, Ankle, and Foot and Referral of Pain

Muscle	Referral Pattern
Tibialis anterior	Anterior lower leg, medial dorsum of foot to hallux
Peroneus longus	Superolateral aspect of lower leg
Peroneus brevis	Lower lateral leg, over lateral malleolus and lateral aspect of foot
Peroneus tertius	Lower lateral leg, anterior to lateral malleolus and onto dorsum of foot, or behind lateral malleolus to lateral heel
Gastrocnemius	Behind knee, posterior leg to instep of foot
Soleus	Posterior leg to heel and sometimes to sole of foot
Plantaris	Posterior knee to upper half of posterior leg
Tibialis posterior	Posterior leg, Achilles tendon, heel, and sole of foot
Extensor digitorum longus	Anterolateral leg to dorsum of foot
Extensor hallucis longus	Anterior leg to dorsomedial foot
Flexor digitorum longus	Posteromedial leg, over medial malleolus, distal sole of foot
Flexor hallucis longus	Plantar aspect of hallux
Extensor digitorum brevis and extensor hallucis brevis	Dorsum of foot
Abductor hallucis	Medial heel and instep
Abductor digiti minimi	Sole of foot over fifth metatarsal
Flexor digitorum brevis	Over metatarsal head
Quadratus plantae (flexor accessorius)	Plantar aspect of heel
Adductor hallucis	Sole of foot over metatarsals
Flexor hallucis brevis	Dorsal and plantar aspect of first metatarsal and hallux
Interossei	Dorsum and plantar aspect of equivalent metatarsal and toe

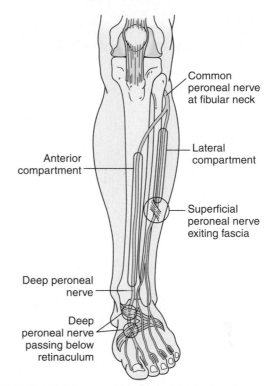

Fig. 13.115 Superficial peroneal nerve travels in the lateral compartment of the leg and can be entrapped as it pierces the fascia 8 to 12 cm proximal to the tip of the lateral malleolus. The deep peroneal nerve can be compressed as it pierces the intermuscular septum to travel in the anterior compartment and under the retinaculum.

often accentuated by plantar flexion.[306] With the tunnel syndrome, muscle weakness is minimal (extensor digitorum brevis); there is burning pain between the first and second toes that is sometimes referred to the dorsum of the foot.

Superficial Peroneal Nerve (L4 to S2). Injuries to the superficial peroneal nerve, a branch of the common peroneal nerve (Fig. 13.117; and see Fig. 13.115), are rare but they have been reported to be associated with lateral ankle (inversion) sprains causing stretching of the nerve, or the nerve may be entrapped as it pierces the deep fascia to become subcutaneous about 10 to 13 cm (4 to 5 inches) above the lateral malleolus (Fig. 13.118).[25,239,305,308,309,312–315] Motor loss with the high lesion near the head of the fibula is primarily loss of foot eversion and loss of ankle stability. With both lesions, the sensory loss is the same. The superficial peroneal nerve has a greater sensory role than the deep branch; it supplies the lateral side of the leg and dorsum of the foot (see Fig. 13.117). This sensory alteration is often greater with activity. If the examiner plantar flexes and inverts the foot while applying pressure over the distal site, symptoms usually result.[316]

Pahor and Toppenberg reported that the slump test (see Chapter 9) combined with plantar flexion and inversion of the foot can be performed to rule out neurological injury to the nerve following lateral ankle sprains.[317]

Tibial Nerve (L4 to S3). The tibial nerve, a branch of the sciatic nerve (Fig. 13.119), has a major role to play in the lower leg, ankle, and foot because it supplies all the muscles in the posterior leg and on the sole of the foot. The nerve may be injured in the popliteal area at the knee from trauma (e.g., dislocation, blow) or from entrapment as it passes over the popliteus and under the soleus. **Popliteal entrapment** syndrome or injury may accompany an ankle sprain.[313] In the odd case, the tibial nerve and/or popliteal artery may be compressed in the deep posterior compartment from chronic exertional activity (**deep posterior chronic**

TABLE **13.14**

Peripheral Nerve Injuries (Neuropathy) of the Lower Leg, Ankle, and Foot

Nerve	Muscle Weakness	Sensory Alteration	Reflexes Affected
Deep peroneal nerve (L4 through S2)	Tibialis anterior Extensor digitorum longus Extensor digitorum brevis Extensor hallucis longus Peroneus tertius	Triangular area between the first and second toes	None
Superficial peroneal nerve (L4 through S2)	Peroneus longus Peroneus brevis	Lateral aspect of leg and dorsum of foot	None
Tibial nerve (L4 through S3)	Gastrocnemius Soleus Plantaris Tibialis posterior Flexor digitorum longus Flexor hallucis longus Flexor accessorius (quadratus plantae) Abductor digiti minimi Flexor digiti minimi Lumbricals Interossei Adductor hallucis Abductor hallucis Flexor digitorum brevis Flexor hallucis brevis	Sole of foot except medial border, plantar surface of toes	Achilles (S1–S2) Tibialis posterior (L4–L5)

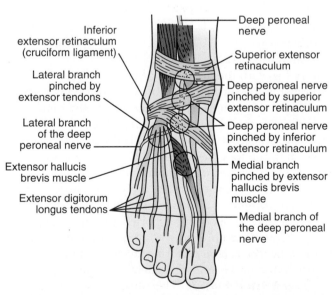

Fig. 13.116 Compression of deep peroneal nerve by the extensor retinaculum or other structures.

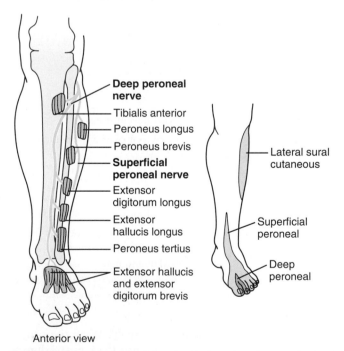

Fig. 13.117 Common peroneal nerve and its branches, the superficial and deep peroneal nerves.

exertional compartment syndrome) with the patient reporting pain and tightness in the calf within half an hour of starting activity (e.g., running) along with weakness of muscles supplied by the tibial nerve (see Table 13.10) and diminished sensation in the tibial nerve distribution.[52,318] At the ankle, the nerve may be compressed as it passes through the tarsal tunnel, which is formed by the medial malleolus, calcaneus,

and talus on one side and the deltoid ligament (primarily the tibiocalcaneal ligament) on the other. This compression is referred to as **tarsal tunnel syndrome** (Fig. 13.120).[120,305,310,319–321]

Injury to the nerve at the knee causes a major functional disability. Functionally, the patient is unable to plantar flex

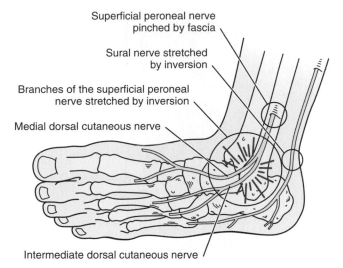

Superficial peroneal nerve pinched by fascia

Sural nerve stretched by inversion

Branches of the superficial peroneal nerve stretched by inversion

Medial dorsal cutaneous nerve

Intermediate dorsal cutaneous nerve

Fig. 13.118 Stretching of the superficial peroneal nerve as a result of inversion of ankle.

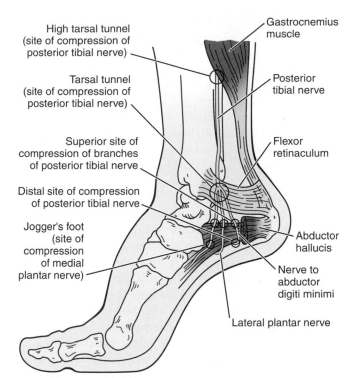

High tarsal tunnel (site of compression of posterior tibial nerve)

Tarsal tunnel (site of compression of posterior tibial nerve)

Superior site of compression of branches of posterior tibial nerve

Distal site of compression of posterior tibial nerve

Jogger's foot (site of compression of medial plantar nerve)

Gastrocnemius muscle

Posterior tibial nerve

Flexor retinaculum

Abductor hallucis

Nerve to abductor digiti minimi

Lateral plantar nerve

Fig. 13.120 Tarsal tunnel syndrome.

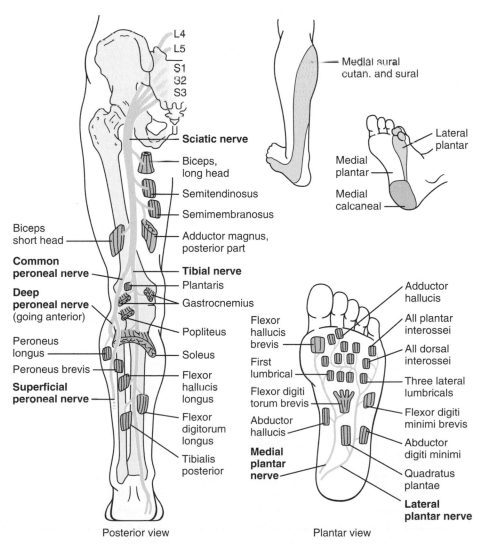

L4
L5
S1
S2
S3

Sciatic nerve

Biceps, long head

Semitendinosus

Semimembranosus

Adductor magnus, posterior part

Biceps short head

Common peroneal nerve

Deep peroneal nerve (going anterior)

Peroneus longus

Peroneus brevis

Superficial peroneal nerve

Tibial nerve

Plantaris

Gastrocnemius

Popliteus

Soleus

Flexor hallucis longus

Flexor digitorum longus

Tibialis posterior

Medial sural cutan. and sural

Lateral plantar

Medial plantar

Medial calcaneal

Flexor hallucis brevis

First lumbrical

Flexor digitorum brevis

Abductor hallucis

Medial plantar nerve

Adductor hallucis

All plantar interossei

All dorsal interossei

Three lateral lumbricals

Flexor digiti minimi brevis

Abductor digiti minimi

Quadratus plantae

Lateral plantar nerve

Posterior view

Plantar view

Fig. 13.119 Distribution of the sciatic nerve and its branches (tibial and common peroneal nerves).

and invert the foot, which has a major effect on gait. In addition, the patient is unable to flex, abduct, or adduct the toes. Sensory loss involves primarily the sole of the foot, lateral surface of the heel, and plantar surfaces of the toes. With popliteal entrapment syndrome, the popliteal artery is often compressed with the nerve, leading to vascular symptoms (e.g., numbness, tingling, intermittent cramping, weakened dorsalis pedis pulse) and neurological signs.

Compression in the tarsal tunnel may be caused by swelling after trauma, a space-occupying lesion (e.g., ganglion), inflammation (e.g., paratenonitis), valgus deformity, or chronic inversion.[122,307–309,322–329] Sammarco and associates reported the possibility of **double crush injury** in the lower limb involving the sciatic nerve (L4 to S3) and one of its branches.[330] The examiner must always keep this possibility in mind when assessing for nerve pathology in the lower limb, especially in patients who do not appear to be recovering. Pain and paresthesia into the sole of the foot are often present and are worse after long periods of standing or walking or at night.[305] The pain may be localized or may radiate over the medial side of the ankle distal to the medial malleolus. The condition is sometimes misdiagnosed as plantar fasciitis (Table 13.15).[331] In long-standing cases, motor weakness may become evident in the muscles of the sole of the foot that are supplied by the terminal branches of the tibial nerve (i.e., the medial and lateral plantar nerves).

The **sural nerve** (L5 to S2) is a sensory branch of the tibial nerve supplying the skin on the posterolateral aspect of the lower one third of the leg and the lateral aspect of the foot (Fig. 13.121). Injury can result from a blow, trauma (e.g., fracture), or stretching (e.g., accompanying an ankle sprain).[122,239,308,329] Shooting pain and paresthesia in its sensory distribution are diagnostic signs.[305]

The **medial plantar nerve** (Fig. 13.122), another branch of the tibial nerve that is found in the foot, may be entrapped in the longitudinal arch, causing aching in the arch, burning pain in the heel, and altered sensation

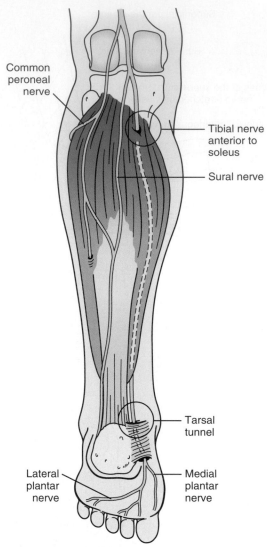

Fig. 13.121 Sural nerve travels between the two heads of the gastrocnemius muscle and then becomes superficial in the distal third of the leg. The common peroneal nerve may become entrapped as it courses anteriorly between the fibular head and the peroneus longus. The tibial nerve may be entrapped as it passes through soleus and in the tarsal tunnel.

TABLE 13.15

Differential Diagnosis of Plantar Fasciitis and Tarsal Tunnel Syndrome

	Plantar Fasciitis	Tarsal Tunnel Syndrome
Cause	Overuse	Trauma, space occupying lesion, inflammation, inversion, pronation, valgus deformity
Pain	Plantar aspect of foot, anterior calcaneus Worse with walking, running, and in the morning (sometimes improves with activity)	Medial heel and medial longitudinal arch Worse with standing, walking, and at night
Electrodiagnosis	Normal	Prolonged motor and sensory latencies
Active movements	Full ROM	Full ROM
Passive movements	Full ROM	May have pain on pronation
Resisted isometric movements	Normal	Weakness of foot intrinsics may be present
Sensory deficits	No	Possible
Reflexes	Normal	Normal

ROM, Range of motion.

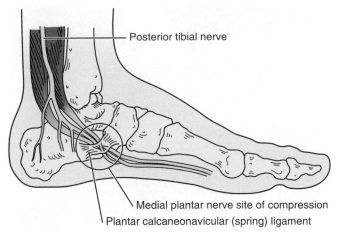

Fig. 13.122 Jogger's foot (entrapment of the medial plantar nerve).

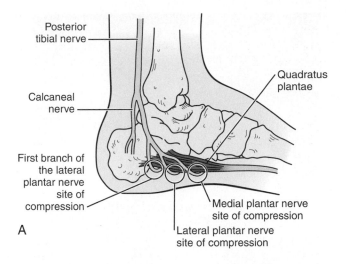

A

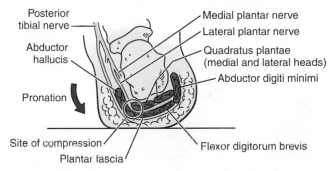

B

Fig. 13.123 Entrapment of the lateral plantar nerve as it changes direction. (A) Medial view. (B) Posterior view.

in the sole of the foot behind the hallux. This condition is associated with hindfoot valgus and may be referred to as **jogger's foot**.[305,310,332,333]

Similarly, the **lateral plantar nerve** (**Baxter's nerve**) may be entrapped between the deep fascia of the abductor hallucis and the quadratus plantae (flexor accessorius) muscles (Fig. 13.123).[305,334] The patient complains of chronic, dull, aching heel pain that is accentuated by walking and running. There is no complaint of numbness. The condition is accentuated by excessive foot pronation.[334]

The plantar digital nerves are branches of the tibial nerve. Injury to these nerves can result in a Morton's or interdigital neuroma[114] (see the earlier "Morton's Metatarsalgia [Interdigital Neuroma]" section).

Saphenous Nerve. This nerve is a sensory branch of the femoral nerve. If it is injured, sensation on the medial side of the leg and foot is affected.[335] More details are given in Chapter 12.

Joint Play Movements

The joint play movements (Figs. 13.124 to 13.127) are performed with the patient in the supine or side-lying position, depending on which movement is being performed. A comparison of movement between the normal or unaffected side and the injured side should be made.

Joint Play Movements of the Lower Leg, Ankle, and Foot

Talocrural (ankle joint)	Long-axis extension (traction)
	Anteroposterior glide
Subtalar joint	Talar rock
	Side tilt medially and laterally
Midtarsal joints	Anteroposterior glide
	Rotation
Tarsometatarsal joints	Anteroposterior glide
	Rotation
Metatarsophalangeal and	Long-axis extension (traction)
interphalangeal joints	Anteroposterior glide
	Lateral or side glide
	Rotation

Long-Axis Extension

Long-axis extension is performed by stabilizing the proximal segment and applying traction to the distal segment. For example, at the ankle, the examiner stabilizes the tibia and fibula by using a strap or just allowing the leg to relax. Both hands are then placed around the ankle, distal to the malleoli, and a longitudinal distractive force is applied. At the metatarsophalangeal and interphalangeal joints, the examiner stabilizes the metatarsal bone or proximal phalanx and applies a longitudinal distractive force to the proximal or distal phalanx, respectively.

Anteroposterior Glide

Anteroposterior glide at the ankle joint is performed by stabilizing the tibia and fibula and drawing the talus and foot forward. To test the posterior movement, the examiner pushes the talus and foot back on the tibia and fibula. There is a difference in the arc of movement between the two actions in tests of joint play. During the anterior movement, the foot should move in an arc into plantar flexion; during the posterior movement, the foot should move in an arc into dorsiflexion. Although similar to the anterior drawer test, the movements are not the same.

Anteroposterior glide at the midtarsal and tarsometatarsal joints is performed in a fashion similar to that used to

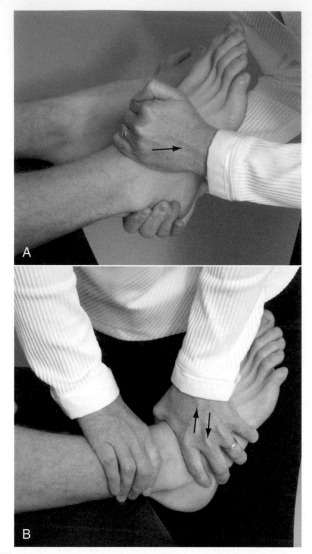

Fig. 13.124 Joint play movements at the talocrural joint. (A) Long-axis extension. (B) Anteroposterior glide at the talocrural joint.

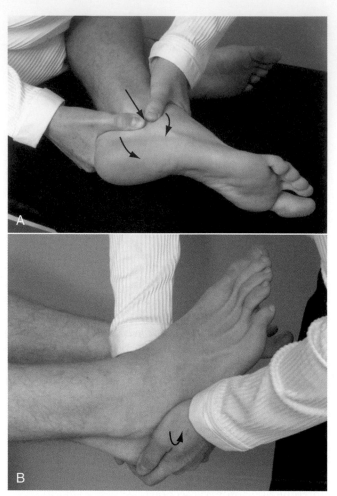

Fig. 13.125 Joint play movements at the subtalar joint. (A) Talar rock with slight traction applied. Talus is rocked anteriorly and posteriorly. (B) Side tilt.

test the carpal bones at the wrist. For the midtarsal joints, the examiner stabilizes the navicular, talus, and calcaneus with one hand by grasping the bones in the web space, thumb, and fingers. The other hand is placed around the distal row of tarsal bones (cuneiforms and cuboid). If the hands are positioned properly, they should touch each other, as in Fig. 13.126. An anteroposterior gliding movement of the distal row of tarsal bones is applied while the proximal row of tarsal bones is stabilized. The examiner's hands are then moved distally so that the stabilizing hand rests over the distal row of tarsal bones and the mobilizing hand rests over the proximal aspect of the metatarsal bones. Again, the hands should be positioned so that they touch each other. An anteroposterior gliding movement of the metatarsal bones is applied while the distal row of tarsal bones is stabilized.

Anteroposterior glide of the metatarsophalangeal and interphalangeal joints is performed by stabilizing the proximal bone (metatarsal or phalanx) and moving the distal bone (phalanx) in an anteroposterior gliding motion in relation to the stabilized bone.

Talar Rock

Talar rock is the only joint play movement performed with the patient in the side-lying position.[278] Both the hip and knee are flexed. The examiner sits with his or her back to the patient, as illustrated in Fig. 13.125A, and places both hands around the ankle just distal to the malleoli. A slight distractive force is applied to the ankle, and a rocking movement forward and backward (plantar flexion-dorsiflexion) is applied to the foot. Normally, the examiner should feel a clunk at the extreme of each movement. As with all joint play movements, the movement is compared with that of the unaffected side.

Side Tilt

Side tilt at the subtalar joint is performed by placing both hands around the calcaneus (see Fig. 13.125B). The wrists are flexed and extended, tilting the calcaneus medially and laterally on the talus. The examiner keeps the patient's foot in the anatomical position while performing

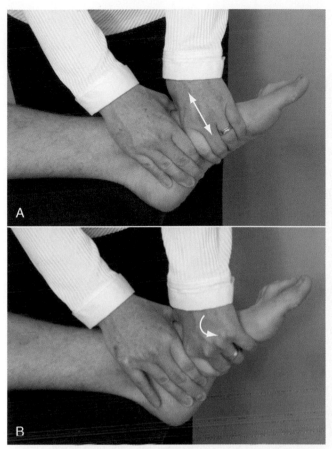

Fig. 13.126 Joint play movements in the midtarsal and tarsometatarsal joints. (A) Anteroposterior glide. (B) Rotation.

the movement. The movement is identical to that used to test the calcaneofibular ligament in the talar tilt test.

Rotation

Rotation at the midtarsal joints is performed in a similar fashion to the anteroposterior glide at these joints. The proximal row of tarsal bones (navicular, calcaneus, and talus) is stabilized, and the mobilizing hand is placed around the distal tarsal bones (cuneiforms and cuboid). The distal row of bones is then rotated on the proximal row of bones. Rotation at the tarsometatarsal joints is performed in a similar fashion. Rotation at the metatarsophalangeal and interphalangeal joints is performed by stabilizing the proximal bone with one hand, applying slight traction, and rotating the distal bone with the other hand.

Side Glide

Side glide at the metatarsophalangeal and interphalangeal joints is performed by stabilizing the proximal bone with one hand. The examiner then uses the other hand to apply slight traction to the distal bone and moves the distal bone sideways (right and left) in relation to the stabilized bone without causing torsion motion at the joint.

Tests for Tarsal Bone Mobility

In addition to testing of the tarsal bones as a group, the bones should be tested individually, especially if symptoms resulted from group testing. The examiner may test these individual bones using whatever method is desired realizing that the amount of movement normally is minimal. An example of individual tarsal bone testing was put forward by Kaltenborn,[336] who advocates 10 tests to determine the mobility of the tarsal bones.

Kaltenborn's Ten Tests for Tarsal Mobility

1. Fixate the second and third cuneiforms, and mobilize the second metatarsal bone.
2. Fixate the second and third cuneiform bones, and mobilize the third metatarsal bone.
3. Fixate the first cuneiform bone, and mobilize the first metatarsal bone.
4. Fixate the navicular bone, and mobilize the first, second, and third cuneiform bones.
5. Fixate the talus, and mobilize the navicular bone.
6. Fixate the cuboid bone, and mobilize the fourth and fifth metatarsal bones.
7. Fixate the navicular and third cuneiform bones, and mobilize the cuboid bone.
8. Fixate the calcaneus, and mobilize the cuboid bone.
9. Fixate the talus, and mobilize the calcaneus.
10. Fixate the talus, and mobilize the tibia and fibula.

Palpation

The examiner palpates for any swelling, noting whether it is intracapsular or extracapsular. Extracapsular swelling around the ankle is indicated by swelling on only one side of the Achilles tendon, whereas intracapsular swelling is indicated by swelling on both sides (see Fig. 13.16). Pitting edema, if present, should be noted. If swelling is present at the end of the day and absent after a night of recumbency, venous insufficiency, caused by a weakening or insufficiency of the action of the muscle pump of the lower leg muscles, may be implied. Swelling in the ankle may persist for many weeks after injury as a result of this insufficiency.

The examiner should also notice the texture of the skin and nails. The skin of an ischemic foot shows a loss of hair and becomes thin and inelastic. In addition, the nails become coarse, thickened, and irregular. Many of the nail changes seen in the hand (see Chapter 7) in the presence of systemic disease are also seen in the foot. With poor circulation, the foot will also feel colder. The foot is palpated in the non–weight-bearing and long leg sitting or supine positions. The following structures, including the joints between them, should be palpated.

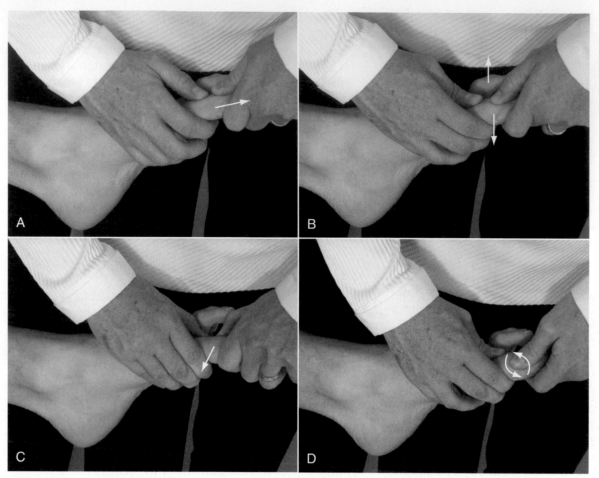

Fig. 13.127 Joint play movements at the metatarsophalangeal and interphalangeal joints. (A) Long-axis extension. (B) Anteroposterior glide. (C) Side glide. (D) Rotation.

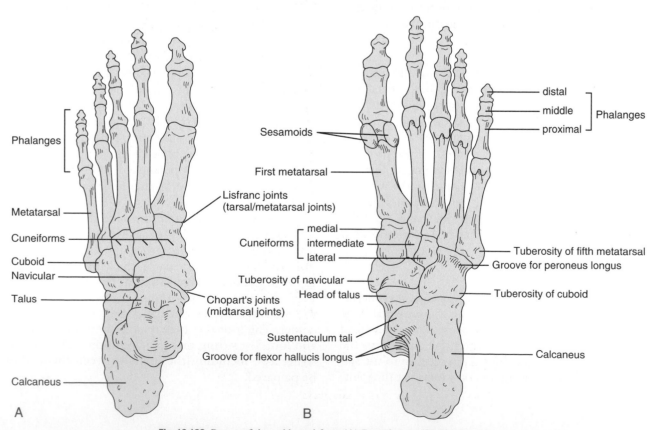

Fig. 13.128 Bones of the ankle and foot. (A) Dorsal view. (B) Plantar view.

Palpation Anteriorly and Anteromedially

Toes and Metatarsal, Cuneiform, and Navicular Bones.
Starting on the medial side, the great toe and its two phalanges are easily palpated. Moving proximally, the examiner comes to the first metatarsal bone (Fig. 13.128). The head of the first metatarsal should be palpated carefully. On the medial aspect of the foot, the examiner palpates for any evidence of a bunion (exostosis, callus, and inflamed bursa), which is often associated with hallux valgus. On the plantar aspect, the two sesamoid bones just proximal to the head of the first metatarsal may be palpated.[337] The examiner then palpates the first metatarsal bone along its length to the first cuneiform bone and notes any tenderness, swelling, or signs of pathology. While moving proximally past the first cuneiform on its medial aspect, the examiner will feel a bony prominence, the tubercle of the navicular bone. The examiner then returns to the first cuneiform bone and moves laterally on the dorsal and plantar surface, palpating the second and third cuneiforms (Fig. 13.129). Like the first cuneiform, the navicular and second and third cuneiform bones should be palpated on their dorsal and plantar aspects for signs of pathology such as fracture, exostosis, or **Köhler's bone disease** (osteochondritis of the navicular bone).

Moving laterally, the examiner palpates the three phalanges of each of the lateral four toes. Each of the lateral four metatarsals is palpated proximally to check for conditions, such as **Freiberg disease** (osteochondrosis of the second metatarsal head). Under the heads of the second and third metatarsals on the plantar aspect, the examiner should feel for any evidence of a callus, which may indicate a fallen metatarsal arch. Care must be taken to palpate the base of the fifth metatarsal (styloid process) and adjacent cuboid bone for signs of pathology such as a fracture or positional faults or **Morton's neuroma** which is usually found in the interspace between the third and fourth metatarsal bones. Also, the lateral aspect of the head of the fifth metatarsal may demonstrate a bunion similar to that seen on the first toe. This is called a **tailor's bunion** (see Fig. 13.30).

In addition to palpating the metatarsal bones, the examiner palpates between the bones for evidence of pathology (e.g., interdigital neuroma) as well as the intrinsic muscles of the foot.

Medial Malleolus, Medial Tarsal Bones, and Posterior Tibial Artery. The examiner stabilizes the patient's heel by holding the calcaneus with one hand and palpates the distal edges of the medial malleolus for tenderness or swelling with the other hand. Moving from the distal extent of the medial malleolus along a line joining the navicular tubercle, the examiner moves along the talus until the head of the talus is reached. As the head of the talus is palpated, the examiner may evert and invert the foot, feeling the movement between the talar head and navicular bone. Eversion causes the talar head to become more prominent, as does pes planus. At the same time, the tibialis posterior tendon may be palpated where it inserts into the navicular and cuneiform bones. Rupture (third-degree strain) of this

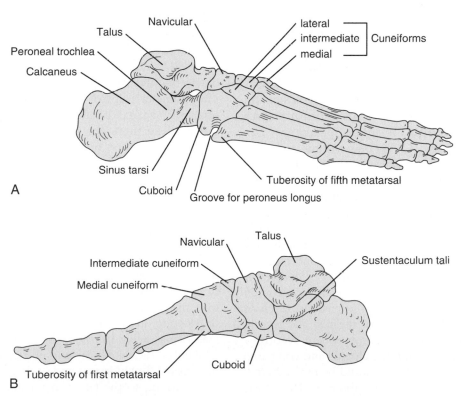

Fig. 13.129 Bones of the foot from the lateral (A) and medial (B) sides.

tendon leads to a valgus foot and a decreased arch. The four ligaments that make up the deltoid ligament may also be palpated for signs of pathology.

Returning to the medial malleolus at its distal extent, the examiner moves further distally (approximately one finger width) until he or she feels another bony prominence, the sustentaculum tali of the calcaneus. This bony prominence is often small and difficult to palpate. Moving further posteriorly, the examiner palpates the medial aspect of the calcaneus for signs of pathology (e.g., sprain, fracture, tarsal tunnel syndrome). As the examiner moves to the plantar aspect of the calcaneus, the heel fat pad, intrinsic foot muscles, and plantar fascia are palpated for signs of pathology (e.g., heel bruise, plantar fasciitis, bone spur).

The examiner then returns to the medial malleolus and palpates along its posterior surface, noting the movement of the tibialis posterior and long flexor tendons (and checking for paratenonitis) during plantar flexion and dorsiflexion and noting any swelling or crepitus. At the same time, the posterior tibial artery, which supplies blood to 75% of the foot, may be palpated as it runs posterior to the medial malleolus. This pulse is often difficult to palpate in individuals with "plump" ankles and in the presence of edema or synovial thickening.

As the examiner moves proximally along the shaft of the tibia, he or she should feel for any tenderness or swelling (i.e., pitted edema) which may indicate the development of a **medial tibial stress syndrome** (see **shin palpation test** and **shin oedema test** in Special Tests).[279]

Anterior Tibia, Neck of Talus, and Dorsalis Pedis Artery. The examiner moves to the anterior aspect of the medial malleolus and follows its course laterally onto the distal end of the tibia. As the examiner moves distally, the fingers rest on the talus. If the ankle is then plantar flexed and dorsiflexed, the anterior aspect of the articular surface of the talus can be palpated for signs of pathology (e.g., osteochondritis dissecans [OCD], talar dome fracture). As the examiner moves further distally, the fingers can follow the course of the neck of the talus to the talar head. Moving distally from the tibia, the examiner should be able to palpate the long extensor tendons, the tibialis anterior tendon, and, with care, the extensor retinaculum (Fig. 13.130). If the examiner moves further distally over the cuneiforms or between the first and second metatarsal bones, the dorsalis pedis pulse (branch of the anterior tibial artery) may be palpated. It may be found between the tendons of extensor digitorum longus and extensor hallucis longus over the junction of the first and second cuneiform bones. If an anterior compartment syndrome is suspected, this pulse should be palpated and compared with that of the opposite side. It should be remembered, however, that this pulse is normally absent in 10% of the population.

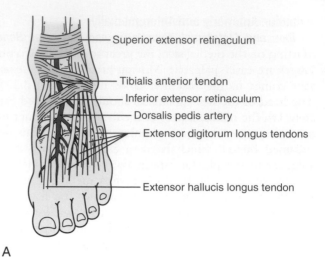

A

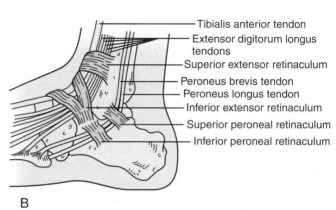

B

Fig. 13.130 Retinaculum of the ankle. (A) Anterior view. (B) Lateral view.

Palpation Anteriorly and Anterolaterally

Lateral Malleolus, Calcaneus, Sinus Tarsi, and Cuboid Bone. The lateral malleolus is palpated at the distal extent of the fibula. It should be noted that the lateral malleolus extends further distally and lies more posterior than the medial malleolus. The examiner palpates the calcaneus (**calcaneal squeeze test**), paying particular attention to the sides of the calcaneus (calcaneal fracture), the posterior calcaneus or tuberosity (retrocalcaneal bursa or fracture), and the medial calcaneal tubercle on the plantar aspect of the foot (plantar fasciitis). At the same time, the peroneal tendons can be palpated as they angle around the lateral malleolus to their insertion in the foot and up to their origin in the peroneal muscles of the leg. The peroneal retinaculum, which holds the peroneal tendons in place as they angle around the lateral malleolus, is also palpated for tenderness (see Fig. 13.130). While palpating the retinaculum, the examiner should ask the patient to invert and evert the foot. If the peroneal retinaculum is torn, the peroneal tendons will often slip out of their groove or dislocate on eversion (see Fig. 13.58). While the lateral malleolus is being palpated, the lateral ligaments (anterior talofibular, calcaneofibular, and posterior talofibular) should be palpated for tenderness and swelling (see Fig. 13.1).

Returning to the lateral malleolus, the examiner palpates its anterior surface and then moves anteriorly to the extensor digitorum brevis muscle, the only muscle on the dorsum of the foot. By palpating carefully and deeply through the muscle, the examiner can feel a depression (the sinus tarsi) which lies between the lateral talus and the calcaneus, usually under a fat pad (Fig. 13.131).[2] If the fingers are left in the depression and the foot is inverted, the examiner will feel the neck of the talus, and the fingers will be pushed deeper into the depression. Tenderness in this area may indicate a sprain to the anterior talofibular ligament (see Fig. 13.131), the most frequently injured ligament in the lower leg, ankle, and foot.

The cuboid bone may be palpated in two ways. The examiner may move further distally from the sinus tarsi (approximately one finger width) so that the fingers lie over the cuboid bone. Or the styloid process at the base of the fifth metatarsal bone may be palpated, and, as the examiner moves slightly proximally, the fingers lie over the cuboid bone. In either case, the cuboid should be palpated on its dorsal, lateral, and plantar surfaces for signs of pathology.

Inferior Tibiofibular Joint, Tibia, and Muscles of the Leg. Starting at the lateral malleolus and following its anterior border, the examiner should note any signs of pathology. The inferior tibiofibular joint is almost impossible to feel; however, it lies between the tibia and fibula and just superior to the talus. The examiner then follows the shin, or crest, of the tibia superiorly, observing for signs of pathology (e.g., shin splints, anterior compartment syndrome, stress fracture). At the same time, the muscles of the lateral compartment (peronei) and anterior compartment (tibialis anterior and long extensors) should be carefully palpated for tenderness or swelling.

Palpation Posteriorly

The patient is then asked to lie in the prone position with the feet over the end of the examining table. The examiner palpates the following structures.

Calcaneus and Achilles Tendon. The examiner palpates the calcaneus and surrounding soft tissue for swelling (i.e., retrocalcaneal bursitis), exostosis (e.g., pump bump—Haglund deformity), or other signs of pathology. In children, care should be taken in palpating the calcaneal epiphysis for evidence of **Sever's disease** (calcaneal apophysitis; Fig. 13.132). Moving proximally, the examiner palpates the Achilles tendon where it inserts into the calcaneus, 2 to 6 cm (0.8 to 2.4 inches) above the insertion where vascularity of the tendon is decreased, and the musculotendinous junction for pathology,[91] noting any swelling or thickening (e.g., paratenonitis, retro-Achilles bursitis) or crepitation on movement. A palpable gap in the Achilles tendon may indicate a rupture of the tendon.[140] Any swelling caused by an intracapsular sprain of the ankle would also be evident posteriorly. Proximal to the Achilles tendon, the dome or superior surface of the calcaneus may also be palpated.

Posterior Compartment Muscles of the Leg. Moving further proximally, the examiner palpates the superficial (triceps surae) and deep posterior compartment muscles (tibialis posterior and long flexors) of the leg

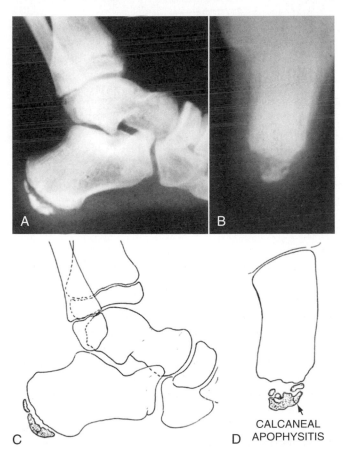

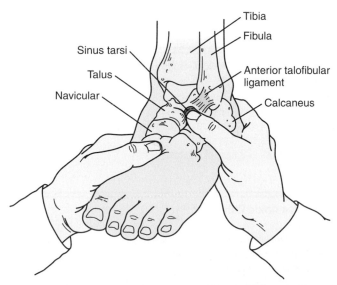

Fig. 13.131 Palpation of the sinus tarsi and the anterior talofibular ligament.

Fig. 13.132 In Sever's disease (calcaneal apophysitis), there is fragmentation of the posterior apophysis off the calcaneus, causing achillodynia. (A) Lateral roentgenogram of a 10-year-old boy with pain around the insertion of the Achilles tendon. (B) Axial view of the calcaneus. (C and D) Representations of films A and B, respectively. (From Kelikian H, Kelikian AS: *Disorders of the ankle*, Philadelphia, 1985, WB Saunders, p 121.)

along their lengths for signs of pathology (e.g., strain, thrombosis).

Diagnostic Imaging

Plain Film Radiography[338]

When viewing any radiograph, the examiner should look for changes and differences between the right and left lower legs, ankles, and feet, such as osteoporosis or alterations in soft tissue, joint space, fracture, and alignment.[339] Both weight-bearing and non–weight-bearing views should be taken.[340] Routinely, anteroposterior, lateral, and mortise views are taken.[31,341,342] However, x-rays should not be used indiscriminately and findings should be considered in conjunction with other clinical signs and symptoms.[343]

Common X-Ray Views of the Lower Leg, Ankle, and Foot Depending on Pathology

- Anteroposterior view of the leg and ankle (weight-bearing or non–weight-bearing) (Fig. 13.140)
- Anteroposterior view of the foot/toes (routine) (Fig. 13.141)
- Lateral view of the leg and ankle (see Fig. 13.142)
- Mortise view (anteroposterior oblique) (routine—ankle) (see Fig. 13.136B)
- Anteroposterior view of the ankle (routine) (see Fig. 13.136A)
- Dorsoplanar view of the foot (see Fig. 13.147)
- Medial 45° oblique view of the foot (non–weight-bearing) (see Fig. 13.148)
- Stress (inversion) oblique view (see Fig. 13.153)
- Anteroposterior lateral stress view (see Fig. 13.155)
- Lateral view of foot/toes (see Fig. 13.143)
- Medial oblique view of the ankle
- Lateral oblique view of the ankle
- Posterior tangential (subtalar)

Stiell and others have developed rules (**Ottawa ankle rules [OAR]** ☑) for the proper use of x-rays after ankle or foot injuries (Fig. 13.133).[344–351] Leddy and associates modified these rules with the Buffalo modification.[352] In addition to the Ottawa rules, the Buffalo modification includes the crest (midportion) of the malleolus, proximal to the ligament attachments (see Fig. 13.133). OAR do not apply to people under the age of 18, in the presence of multiple painful injury, head injury, intoxication, pregnancy, or neurological deficit.[249] The **Bernese Ankle Rules (BAR)** were developed to improve upon the OAR and can be used in conjunction with OAR. The BAR includes three steps: 1) direct pressure 10 cm (4 inches) proximal to fibular malleolus (Fig. 13.134A), 2) direct stress or pressure on the medial malleolus (Fig. 13.134B), and 3) simultaneous compression of the midfoot and hindfoot (Fig. 13.134C).[353–356] A third ankle rule was developed for

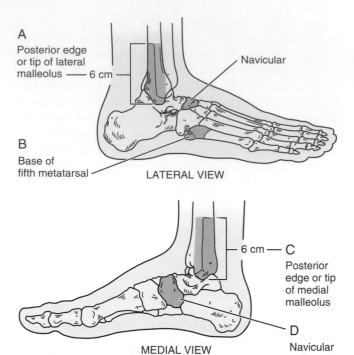

Fig. 13.133 Ottawa rules for ankle and foot radiographic series in ankle injury patients. Radiographic series are needed only if there is bone tenderness at *A, B, C,* or *D*; inability to bear weight, and malleolar or midfoot pain. *Gray shaded areas* show Buffalo modification.

fractures called the **Leiden Ankle Rule** in which 7 items are weighted. If the sum of the scores exceeds 7, radiography is recommended.[257,357] Concern must also be given for the mechanism of injury.[358] For example, snowboarders commonly fracture the lateral process of the talus. Thus, a history of falling while snowboarding with tenderness below the lateral malleolus indicates the need for an x-ray.[130] To be viewed properly, individual radiographs must be made of the ankle, lower leg, or foot, and in some cases, all three to rule out injury proximal or distal to where the patient is complaining of pain.[31,75,359–362]

Ottawa Rules for Ankle X-Rays (with Buffalo Modifications)

- Tenderness over lateral malleolus to 6 cm (2.4 inches) proximally
- Tenderness over medial malleolus to 6 cm (2.4 inches) proximally
- Tenderness over navicular
- Tenderness over base of fifth metatarsal

Bernese Ankle Rules[353–356]

- Pressure bilaterally 10 cm (4 inches) proximal to fibular malleolus
- Direct pressure on medial malleolus
- Compression of hindfoot
- Compression of midfoot

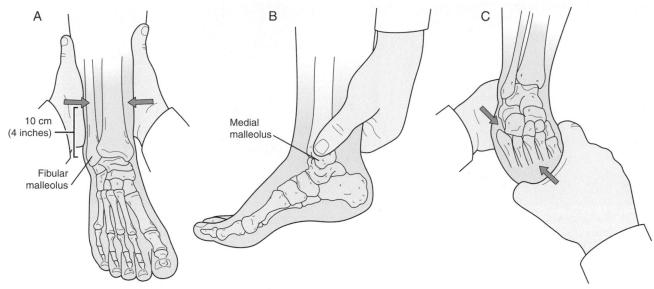

Fig. 13.134 Bernese ankle rules. (A) Pressure 10 cm (4 inches) proximal to fibular malleolus. (B) Direct pressure on medial malleolus. (C) Compression of midfoot and hindfoot.

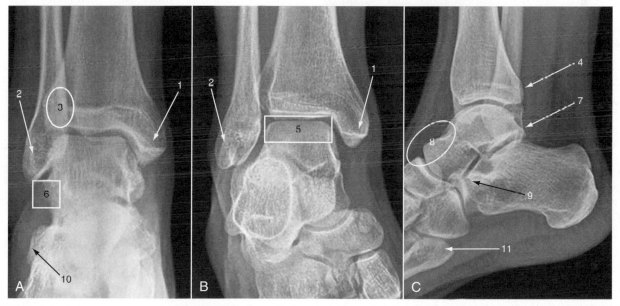

Fig. 13.135 Radiological assessment template for the ankle. A standard radiographic series of the ankle has a minimum of three views including an anterior-posterior view (A), a mortise view (B), and a lateral view (C). There are 11 target sites that represent vulnerable areas where fractures occur including the medial (1) and lateral (2) malleoli, anterior tibial tubercle (3) and posterior tibial malleolus (4), talar dome (5), lateral talar process (6), tubercles of the posterior talus process (7), dorsal to the talonavicular joint (8), anterior calcaneus process (9), calcaneal insertion of the extensor digitorum brevis (10), and the base of the fifth metatarsal bone (11). (From Yu JS, Cody ME: A template approach for detecting fractures in adults sustaining low-energy ankle trauma, *Emerg Radiol* 16[4]:309–318, 2009.)

Leiden Ankle Rules

Clinical Feature	Score[a]
• Deformity, instability, crepitation	5
• Inability to bear weight	3
• Pulseless or weakened posterior tibial artery	2
• Pain on palpation of malleoli or fifth metatarsal	2
• Swelling of the malleoli or fifth metatarsal	2
• Swelling or pain of the Achilles tendon	1
• Age divided by 10	Variable

[a]If the sum of the individual scores exceeds 7, radiography is recommended.
From Glas AS, Pijnenburg BA, Lijmer JG, et al: Comparison of diagnostic decision rules and structured data collection in assessment of acute ankle injury, *Can Med Assoc J* 166(6):728, 2002.

Yu and Cody[363] have suggested three views are necessary for detecting fractures in the ankle area (Fig. 13.135). Radiographs may also be used to identify and classify fractures and osteoarthritis.[364–367]

Anteroposterior View of the Ankle. The examiner notes the shape, position (whether the medial clear space is normal), and texture of the bones and determines whether there is any fractured or new subperiosteal bone (Fig. 13.136). Fig. 13.137 outlines the radiographic parameters of the ankle. The **medial clear space** is the space

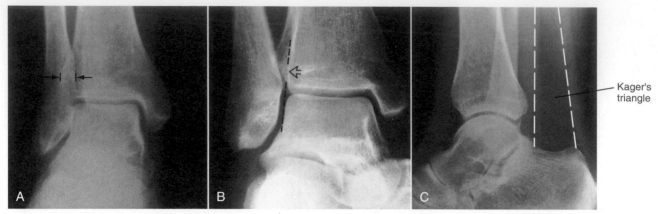

Fig. 13.136 Radiographs of normal ankle. (A) Anteroposterior view. Note tibiofibular overlap *(between arrows)*. (B) Internal oblique (mortise) view. *Arrow* demonstrates alignment of lateral talus with posterior cortex of tibia. (C) Lateral view. Note the presence of Kager's triangle with an intact Achilles tendon. (From Weissman BNW, Sledge CB: *Orthopedic radiology*, Philadelphia, 1986, WB Saunders, pp. 590–591.)

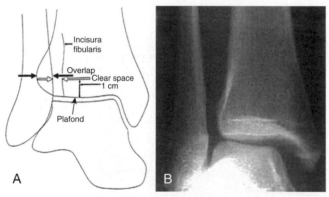

Fig. 13.137 Ankle radiographic parameters. (A) Normal syndesmotic relationships include a tibiofibular clear space *(open arrows)*, 6 mm in both the anteroposterior (AP) and mortise views, as well as a tibiofibular overlap *(solid arrows)* greater than 6 mm or greater than 42% of the width of the fibula on the AP view, or greater than 1 mm on the mortise view. The overlap is measured 1 cm proximal to the plafond (ceiling of ankle joint or the articular surface of the distal end of the tibia). (B) AP radiograph demonstrating a widened syndesmosis and increased medial clear space and no overlap. (A and B, From Stephen D: Ankle and foot injuries. In Kellam JF et al, editors: *Orthopaedic knowledge update: trauma 2*, Rosemont, IL, 2000, American Academy of Orthopaedic Surgeons, p 210.)

between the talus and medial malleolus (Fig. 13.138). It is normally ≤ 4 mm wide, and values greater than this indicate a lateral talar shift with disruption of the ankle mortise (e.g., fibular fracture)[259,343,368] with disruption of the deltoid and tibiofibular ligaments[369] and, therefore, of the tibiofibular syndesmosis.[31,255,262,370] The **tibiofibular overlap** or **tibiofibular clear space** (see Fig. 13.136A) should be at least 6 mm, and greater than 1 mm in the mortise view, although any alteration and related injury has been questioned.[259,369,371] In addition, the configuration, congruity, and inclination of the talar dome in relation to the tibial vault above it should be noted, because it may indicate an osteochondral lesion

or OCD (Fig. 13.139).[73] OCD is more likely to be seen in females (1.5 times more likely than males), and teenagers have 7 times the risk compared to children 6 to 11 years of age.[367,372,373] If epiphyseal plates are present, the examiner should note whether they appear normal. Any increase or decrease in joint space, greater reduction of the tibial overlap, widening of the interosseus space, and greater visibility of the digital fossa should also be noted.

Criteria for Syndesmosis Injury[75,374]

Medial clear space	>4 mm
Tibiofibular overlap	<2.1 mm ♀
	<5.7 mm ♂
Clear space between fibula and peroneal incisura of tibia	<5.2 mm ♀
	<6.5 mm ♂
Medial clear space	>Superior clear space

Mortise View of the Ankle. With this view, the ankle mortise and distal tibiofibular joint can be visualized (see Fig. 13.136B).[375] To obtain this view, which is a modification of the anteroposterior view, the foot and leg are medially rotated 15° to 30°.

Lateral View of Leg, Ankle, and Foot. With this view, the examiner notes the shape, position, and texture of bones, including the tibial tubercle (Figs. 13.142 and 13.143). Any fracture, new subperiosteal bone, or bone spurs should be noted (Fig. 13.144). The examiner must note whether the epiphyseal lines are normal and whether there is any increase or decrease in joint space. Although this view clearly shows the talus and calcaneus, there is overlap of the midtarsal, metatarsal, and phalangeal structures. On the lateral x-ray, the presence or

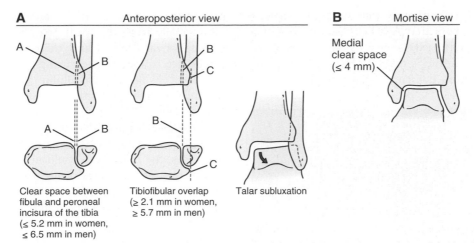

Fig. 13.138 Syndesmotic radiographic criteria. A finding outside any of these criteria indicates a syndesmosis injury. (A) Anteroposterior view. (B) Mortise view. *A,* Lateral border of posterior tibial malleolus; *B,* medial border of fibula; *C,* lateral border of anterior tibial tubercle.

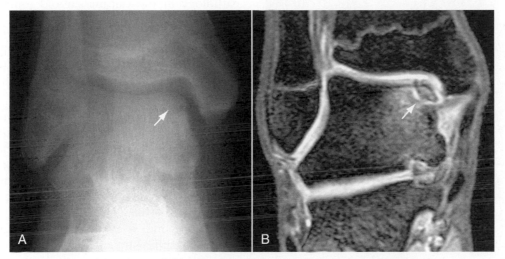

Fig. 13.139 Osteochondritis dissecans of the talus: medial lesion. (A) Note the lucent lesion of the medial talar dome *(arrow),* the site of an osteochondral fragment. (B) Corresponding coronal, volume gradient (TR/TE, 28/7; flip angle, 25°) magnetic resonance image shows the nondisplaced fragment. (From Resnick D, Kransdorf MJ: *Bone and joint imaging,* Philadelphia, 2005, WB Saunders, p 808.)

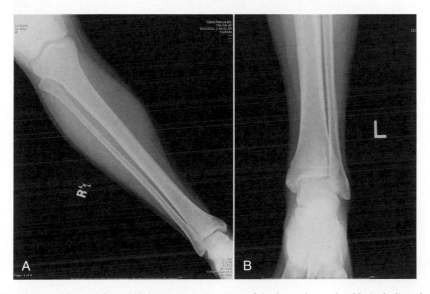

Fig. 13.140 Radiographs of lower leg, ankle, and foot. (A) Anteroposterior view of the lower leg and ankle including the knee. (B) Anteroposterior view of the lower leg, ankle, and foot.

absence of **Kager's triangle** (see Fig. 13.136C) may be used to diagnose a ruptured Achilles tendon.[376] When viewing lateral films, the examiner must also be aware of Sever's disease and Köhler's disease (Fig. 13.145). The presence of a Haglund deformity (abnormally enlarged

posterosuperior aspect of calcaneus) or "pump bump" (abnormally large calcaneal protuberance as a result of retrocalcaneal bursitis and thickened Achilles tendon) can be determined by measuring parallel pitch lines (Fig. 13.146).[80,81] Fowler and Phillip also used the posterior calcaneal angle to determine the same measurement (see Fig. 13.146B).[80,81,377]

Dorsoplanar View of the Foot. The dorsoplanar view is used primarily to project the forefoot. As with the previous views, the examiner should note the position, shape, and texture of the bones of the foot (Fig. 13.147). The presence of a metatarsus primus varus or a condition, such as Köhler disease, should be noted.

Medial Oblique View of the Foot. This view is often taken because it gives the clearest picture of the tarsal bones and joints and the metatarsal shafts and bases (Figs. 13.148 to 13.150). The medial oblique view shows any pathology in the calcaneocuboid joint as well as the presence of a calcaneonavicular bar (Figs. 13.151 and 13.152).

Stress Oblique View. The examiner should note whether there is a calcaneonavicular bar or abnormality of the calcaneus or navicular bones with this view (see Fig. 13.152; Fig. 13.153).

Stress Film. The stress radiograph is used to compare the two ankles for integrity of the ligaments (Figs. 13.154 and 13.155).[251,322,378–382] Anteroposterior views are most commonly used. With the application of an eversion or abduction stress, tilting of the talus by more than 10° is considered pathological.[383] An increase in the medial clear space (space between medial malleolus and talus) of more than 2 to 3 mm is considered pathological and usually indicates insufficiency of the deltoid ligament, especially

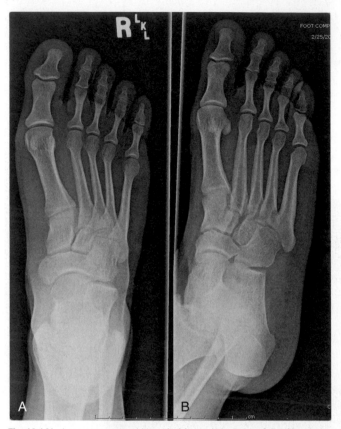

Fig. 13.141 Anteroposterior (A) and oblique (B) views of the foot/toes.

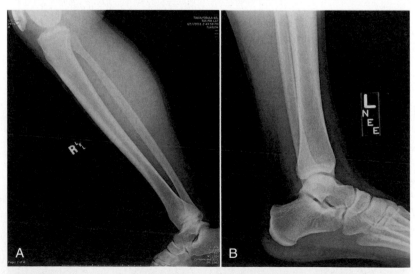

Fig. 13.142 (A) Lateral view of the right leg and ankle including the knee. (B) Lateral view of the left leg and ankle including the foot.

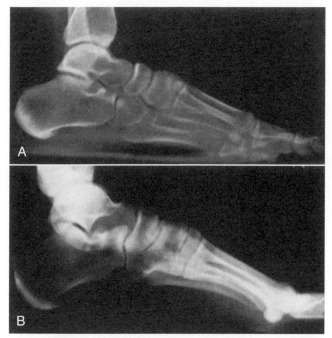

Fig. 13.143 Lateral view of the foot. (A) Weight-bearing posture. The soft-tissue pads are flattened beneath the heel and in the forepart of the foot, and the first metatarsal head is elevated by the sesamoids beneath it. (B) Non–weight-bearing posture. The bony alignment and configuration are satisfactory, but the lack of resistance from the floor to the body weight permits variations, which make such views unsatisfactory for determining foot contours. (From Jahss MH: *Disorders of the foot*, Philadelphia, 1991, WB Saunders, pp 68, 72.)

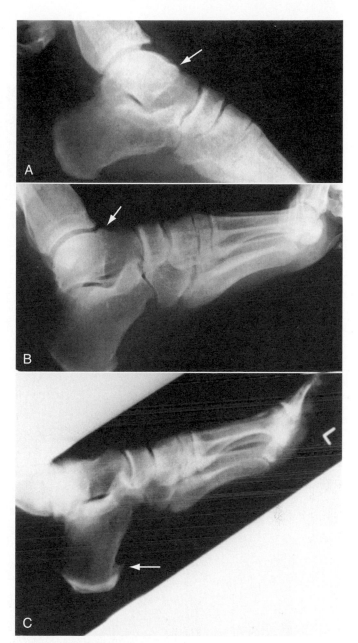

Fig. 13.144 (A) Talotibial spurs. (B) Impingement occurs when foot is dorsiflexed. (C) Heel spur. (A and B, From O'Donoghue DH: *Treatment of injuries to athletes*, ed 4, Philadelphia, 1984, WB Saunders, p 627.)

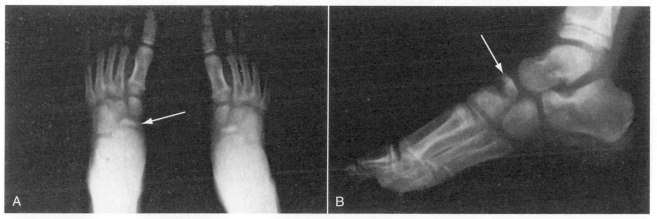

Fig. 13.145 Radiographs of the foot. (A) Bilateral involvement with condensation in the early stage of Köhler disease. (B) Same foot 2 years later shows restoration of contour on the way to completion. (From Jahss MH: *Disorders of the foot*, Philadelphia, 1991, WB Saunders, p 608.)

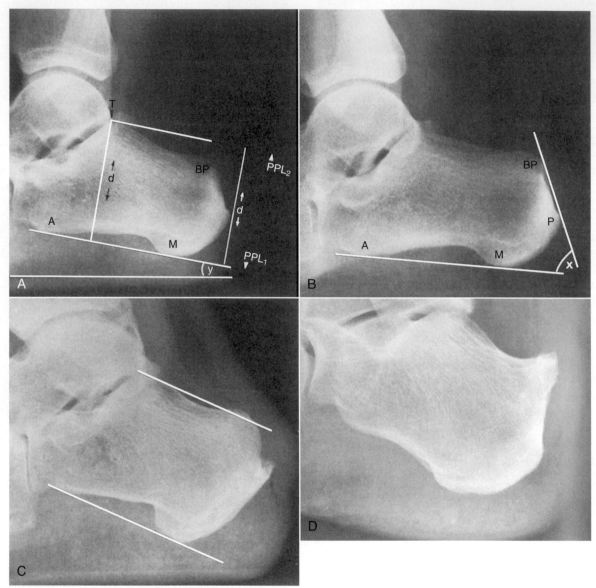

Fig. 13.146 Quantitative evaluation of the shape and pitch of the os calcis (calcaneus). (A) The parallel pitch lines *(PPL)* determine the prominence of the bursal projection *(BP)*. The lower PPL *(PPL$_1$)* is the base line, constructed as for the posterior calcaneal angle. A perpendicular *(d)* is constructed between the posterior lip of the talar articular facet *(T)* and the base line. The upper PPL *(PPL$_2$)* is drawn parallel to the base line at distance *d*. A bursal projection touching or below the PPL$_2$ is normal, not prominent, a –PPL. The pitch angle *(y)* is formed by the intersection of the base line *(PPL$_1$)* with the horizontal. (B) The posterior calcaneal angle *(x)* of Fowler and Philip is that angle formed by the intersection of the base line tangent to the anterior tubercle A,[377] and the medial tuberosity *(M)* with the line tangent to the posterior surface of the bursal project *(BP)* and the posterior tuberosity *(P)*. (C) Haglund syndrome is diagnosed on the lateral view of the heel by a +PPL; a cortically intact bursal projection; loss of the retrocalcaneal recess, indicating retrocalcaneal bursitis; thickening of the Achilles tendon, measuring over 9 mm at 2 cm above the bursal projection; loss of the sharp interface between the Achilles tendon and the pre-Achilles fat pad, indicating Achilles tendinitis; and convexity of the posterior soft tissues at the level of the Achilles tendon insertion, indicating superficial tendo Achilles bursitis. Clinically, this latter finding presents as a pump-bump. (D) Patient with hypertrophic osteoarthritic spurring of the bursal projection. This bony projection displaces the Achilles tendon and adjacent soft tissues posteriorly and creates a pump-bump, which is prone to trauma if improper shoes are worn. Although this patient clinically had a pump-bump, it was produced by the posterior displacement of normal tissues at the level of a prominent bursal projection. (From Pavlov H, Heneghan MA, Hersh A, et al: The Haglund deformity: initial and differential diagnosis. *Radiology* 144:85–86, 1982.)

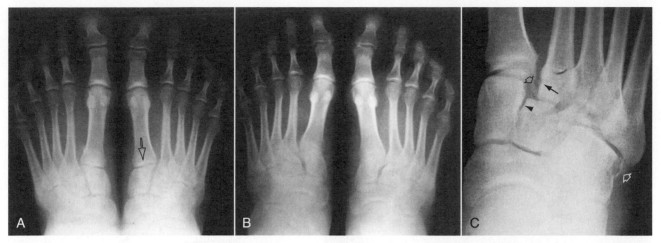

Fig. 13.147 Dorsoplanar view of the foot. (A) Weight-bearing posture. The cuneiform-first metatarsal joint is clearly shown *(arrow)*, as are the transverse intertarsal joints, in contrast to the non–weight-bearing radiographs. (B) Non–weight-bearing posture. The joint between the medial and middle cuneiforms is clearly shown; the other midtarsal joints are obscure. (C) In this patient, note the subtle displacement of the second through fifth metatarsal bases. The medial edge of the second metatarsal base *(solid arrow)* is not aligned with the medial edge of the second cuneiform *(arrowhead)*. Fractures of the base of the second metatarsal bone and cuboid are evident *(open arrows)*. (A and B, From Jahss MH: *Disorders of the foot*, Philadelphia, 1991, WB Saunders, pp 69, 71. C, From Resnick D, Kransdorf MJ: *Bone and joint imaging*, Philadelphia, 2005, WB Saunders, p 873.)

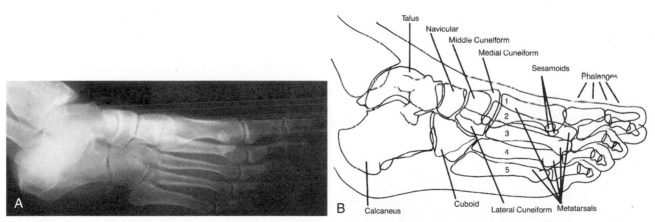

Fig. 13.148 Medial oblique projection of the foot. (A) Radiograph demonstrates the normal medial border alignment of the third and fourth metatarsophalangeal joints. It also allows evaluation of the talonavicular and calcaneocuboid relationships. (B) Anatomic drawing for correlation. (From Brotzman SB, Manske RC: *Clinical orthopaedic rehabilitation: an evidence-based approach*, ed 2, Philadelphia, 2003, Mosby.)

the tibiotalar ligament. Instability may also be demonstrated by widening of the **syndesmosis** (the mortise between the tibia and fibula). An inversion or adduction stress causing 8° to 10° more movement on one ankle than the other is considered pathological and is indicative of torn lateral ligaments. If the talus has not moved, or if it is fixed but its distal end is unduly prominent, subtalar instability is suggested.

Measurements on Plain Radiographs. Plain radiographs may be used to measure different angles and axes.[86] For example, Fig. 13.156 shows the ankle joint axis, and Fig. 13.157 shows the subtalar joint axis. Figs. 13.158 to 13.160 show various angles measured in the ankle and foot. These angles may change during development, so in some cases, serial radiographs may be of benefit.[384–386]

Abnormal Ossicles or Accessory Bones. The foot often exhibits abnormal ossicles, and their presence may lead to incorrect interpretation of radiographic films (Fig. 13.161). These bones are pieces of the prominences of various tarsal bones that for some reason (e.g., fracture, secondary ossification center) are separated from the normal bone (e.g., os trigonum; Fig. 13.162).[79,387] A sesamoid bone, on the other hand, is incorporated into the substance of a tendon with one surface articulating with the adjacent bones. A sesamoid bone moves with the tendon and is found over bony prominences or where the tendon makes a change in direction. In addition to the normal sesamoid bones under the big toe, sesamoid bones may also be found in the tendons of peroneus longus and tibialis posterior. Abnormal ossicles are more likely to occur in the foot than anywhere else in the body.

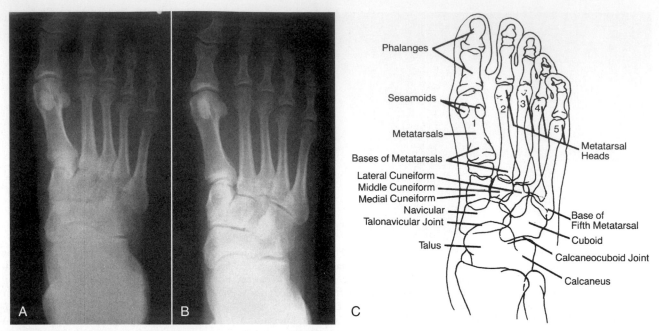

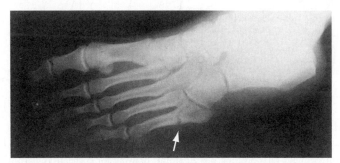

Fig. 13.149 Anteroposterior projection of the foot. (A) Perpendicular x-ray beam demonstrates the forefoot anatomy, particularly the phalanges and metatarsophalangeal (MTP) joints. Note the distal third and fourth metatarsal fractures. (B) Angled x-ray beam provides improved detail of the midfoot anatomy, particularly illustrating the normal alignment of the lateral border of the first MTP joint and the medial border of the second MTP joint. (C) Anatomic drawing for correlation. (From Brotzman SB, Manske RC: *Clinical orthopaedic rehabilitation: an evidence-based approach*, ed 2, Philadelphia, 2003, Mosby.)

Fig. 13.150 Fracture of the base of the fifth metatarsal. All fractures in this region have generally been referred to as "Jones fractures" after the original description put forth in 1902 by Sir Robert Jones, who personally sustained this fracture while dancing. Unfortunately, the persistence of this eponym has resulted in significant confusion in the management of these fractures, because at least two distinct fracture patterns occur at the base of the fifth metatarsal: avulsion fracture of the tuberosity at the attachment of the peroneus brevis, and transverse fracture of the proximal diaphysis, as shown here *(arrow)*. The management of these two types of fractures is distinctly different, because of the healing potential of the diaphyseal fracture is diminished and the rate of fibrous union or subsequent refracture is high. Inadequate initial treatment may contribute to nonunion or delayed union of the diaphyseal fracture, and thus this fracture must be distinguished from the less complicated, more proximal avulsion fracture. (From McKinnis LN: *Fundamentals of musculoskeletal imaging*, Philadelphia, 2005, FA Davis, p 397.)

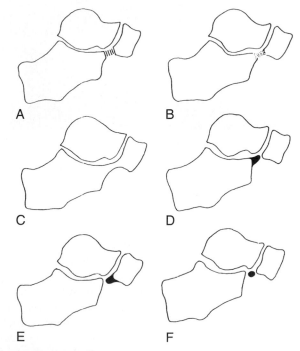

Fig. 13.151 Diagrammatic representation of the types of union. (A) Fibrous. (B) Cartilaginous. (C) Osseous. (D) Prominent process on the calcaneus. (E) Prominent process on the navicular. (F) Separate calcaneonavicular ossicle (calcaneum secondarium). (From Klenerman L: *The foot and its disorders*, Boston, 1982, Blackwell Scientific, p 336.)

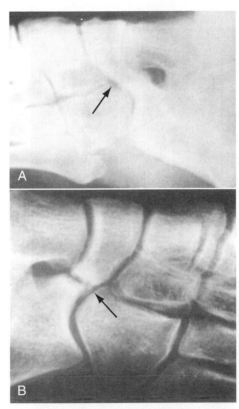

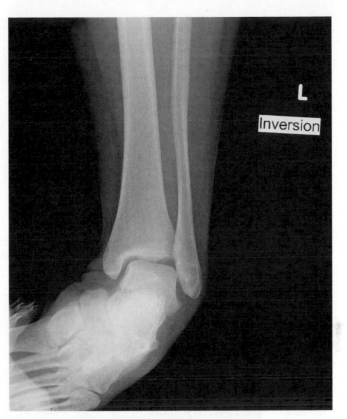

Fig. 13.152 Calcaneonavicular coalition or bar. (A) Total bony union, as well as bony breaks on the upper surfaces of the navicular and talus. The head of the talus may well be small. (B) Fibrous or cartilaginous, rather than osseous, union between the bones is shown with osteoarthritic changes of the opposing bone surfaces and an enlarged navicular. (From Klenerman L: *The foot and its disorders*, Boston, 1982, Blackwell Scientific, p 340.)

Fig. 13.153 Ankle stress (inversion) view.

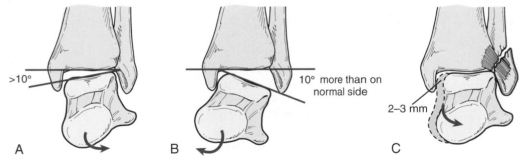

Fig. 13.154 Positive findings on diagrammatic stress radiographs. (A) Abduction stress. (B) Adduction stress. (C) Increased (2 to 3 mm) medial clear space (lateral rotary stress).

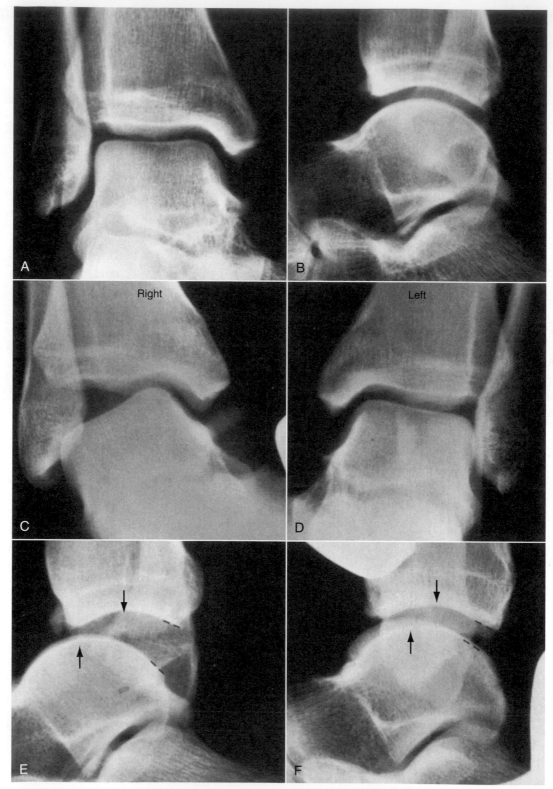

Fig. 13.155 Abnormal stress views: anterior talofibular and calcaneofibular ligament tears. Anteroposterior (A) and lateral (B) views of the right ankle showing hypertrophic lipping from the anterior tibia and talus. The syndesmosis is slightly wide. Comparison varus stress views of the right (C) and left (D) ankles show abnormal talar tilt on the right, particularly when compared with the normal left side. This is diagnostic of an anterior talofibular ligament tear on the right, with or without a calcaneofibular ligament tear. The anterior drawer test is abnormal on the right (E) compared with the left (F). Comparison can be made by noting the anterior shift of the midtalus in relation to the midtibia *(arrows)* on each side, the loss of parallelism of the subchondral cortices on the right, or the marked widening of the posterior joint space *(lines)* on the abnormal as compared with the normal side. This is consistent with an anterior talofibular ligament tear on the right. (From Weissman BNW, Sledge CB: *Orthopedic radiology*, Philadelphia, 1986, WB Saunders, p 600.)

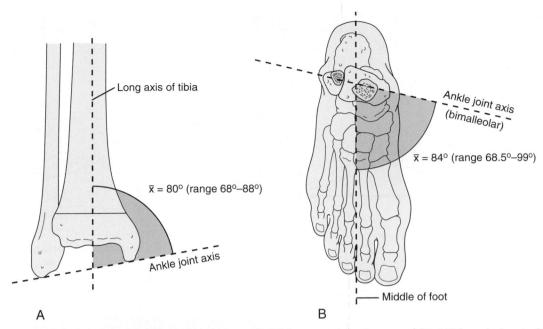

Fig. 13.156 Orientation of the ankle joint axis. Mean values measure (A) 80° from a vertical reference and (B) 84° from the longitudinal reference of the foot. (Adapted from Hunt GC, editor: *Physical therapy of the foot and ankle*, New York, 1988, Churchill Livingstone; and Isman RE, Inman VT: *Anthropometric studies of the human foot and ankle: technical report No. 58*, San Francisco, 1968, University of California.)

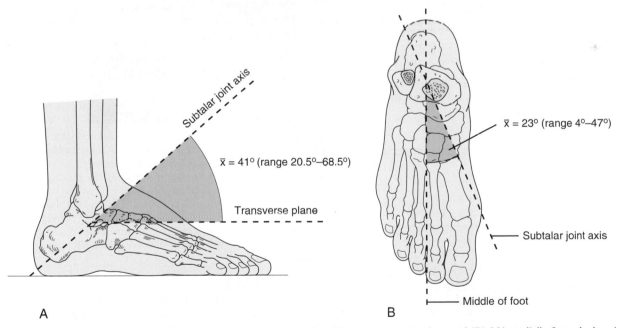

Fig. 13.157 Orientation of the subtalar joint axis. Mean values measure (A) 41° from the transverse plane and (B) 23° medially from the longitudinal reference of the foot. (Adapted from GC Hunt, editor: *Physical therapy of the foot and ankle*, New York, 1988, Churchill Livingstone; and Isman RE, Inman VT: *Anthropometric studies of the human foot and ankle: technical report no. 58*, San Francisco, 1968, University of California.)

Normal Alignment

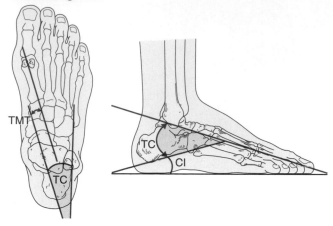

Flatfoot Deformity

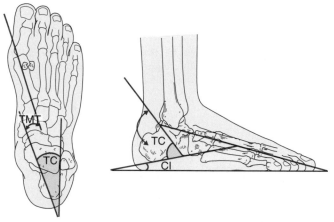

Fig. 13.158 Drawing of normal and pathologic alignment of a pes planus in anteroposterior and lateral views. *CI,* Calcaneal inclination; *TC,* talocalcaneal angle; *TMT,* talometatarsal angle.

Common Ossicles in the Foot

- Os trigonum (separate posterior talar tubercle)
- Os tibiale externum (separate navicular tuberosity)
- Bipartite medial cuneiform (separated into upper and lower halves)
- Os vesalianum (separate tuberosity of the base of the fifth metatarsal)
- Os sustentaculi (separate part of the sustentaculum tali)
- Os supranaviculare (dorsum of the talonavicular joint)

Films Showing Bone Development. Like the bones of the hand, the bones of the foot form within a certain time period (Fig. 13.163). However, because the foot is subjected to greater forces and environmental effects than the hand, it is not usually used to determine skeletal age. X-rays of the foot often show the developing bone deformities seen in clubfoot (Fig. 13.164). Although not all of the bones are present at birth, a series of films will show differences when compared with films of normal feet.

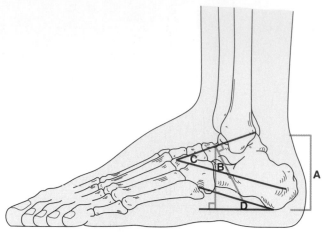

Fig. 13.159 Drawing of normal alignment of a healthy foot in lateral weight-bearing view. *A,* Hindfoot height; *B,* talar declination angle; *C,* lateral talocalcaneal angle (method 2); *D,* calcaneal pitch.

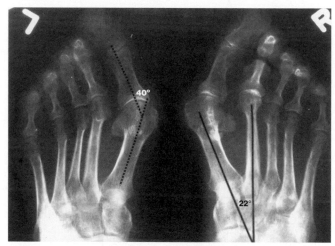

Fig. 13.160 Measurement of hallux valgus deformity. On the left, the angle of intersection of the long axes of the proximal phalangeal and the first metatarsal shafts *(dotted lines)* is 40°. Normally, this angle is no greater than 10°. On the right, there is rotation of the great toe and lateral subluxation of the proximal phalanx, leaving about one half of the articular surface of the metacarpal uncovered. The angle of the first and second metatarsal shafts *(solid lines)* is 22°. On standing views, angles of greater than 10° indicate metatarsus primus varus. (From Weissman BNW, Sledge CB: *Orthopedic radiology,* Philadelphia, 1986, WB Saunders, p 657.)

Arthrography

Arthrograms of the ankle are indicated whenever there is acute ligament injury, chronic ligament laxity, or indications of loose body or OCD (Figs. 13.165 and 13.166).[31,73,388,389] Leakage of the contrast medium indicates tearing of the joint capsule or capsular ligaments. Normally, the talocrural joint admits only about 6 mL of contrast medium.

Diagnostic Ultrasound Imaging

This technique makes use of the ultrasonic waves to determine possible tissue injury. With an experienced operator, it may show injury to growth plates in the presence of a

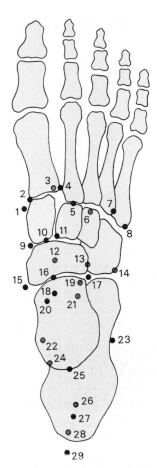

Fig. 13.161 Accessory tarsal bones. *1,* Os sesamoideum tibialis anterior; *2,* os cuneometatarsale I tibiale; *3,* os cuneometatarsale I plantare; *4,* os intermetatarsale I; *5,* os cuneometatarsale II dorsale; *6,* os unci; *7,* os intermetatarsale IV; *8,* os vesalianum; *9,* os paracuneiforme; *10,* os naviculo-cuneiforme I dorsale; *11,* os intercuneiforme; *12,* os sesamoideum tibialis posterior (according to Trolle, this may be the same as *15*); *13,* os cuboideum secundarium; *14,* os peroneum; *15,* os tibiale (externum); *16,* os talonaviculare dorsale; *17,* os calcaneus secundarius; *18,* os supertalare; *19,* os trochleae; *20,* os talotibiale dorsale; *21,* os in sinu tarsi; *22,* os sustentaculi proprium; *23,* calcaneus accessorius; *24,* os talocalcaneare posterior; *25,* os trigonum; *26,* os aponeurosis plantaris; *27,* os supracalcaneum; *28,* os subcalcaneum; *29,* os tendinis Achilles. (Redrawn from Klenerman L: *The foot and its disorders,* Boston, 1982, Blackwell Scientific, p 361.)

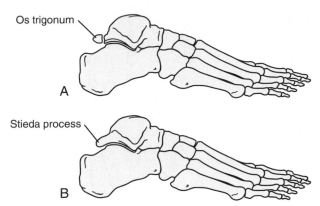

Fig. 13.162 Lateral view of the ankle, showing the os trigonum (A) and Stieda process (B). (Redrawn from Brodsky AE, Khalil MA: Talar compression syndrome. *Foot Ankle* 7:338–344, 1987.)

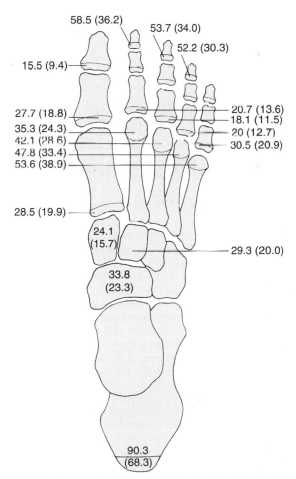

Fig. 13.163 Anteroposterior diagram of the foot showing the times of appearance (in months) of the centers of ossification for boys (and for girls, in parentheses). (Redrawn from Hoerr NL, Pyle SI, Francis CC: *Radiographic atlas of skeletal development of the foot and ankle,* Springfield, IL, 1962, Charles C Thomas, with kind permission of Charles C Thomas, Springfield, IL.)

normal radiograph or prenatal pathology.[390,391] It has been proposed that diagnostic ultrasound imaging (DUSI) may be used to diagnose ligament injuries in "real time," for example, using the ultrasound when doing the Thompson test to diagnose Achilles tendon ruptures.[392,393]

Ankle injuries account for nearly 15% of sports-related orthopedic emergency room visits.[394] Due to the superficial nature of structures surrounding the ankle, ultrasound imaging can be very beneficial during an evaluation. Examination should include ligaments and tendons around the ankle, as well as a more specific detailed examination around the lower leg and foot.

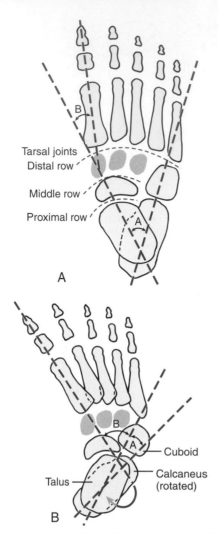

Fig. 13.164 Representations of the foot as seen on radiographs. (A) Representation of the normal foot. The cuboid blocks medial movement of the foot at the middle row of tarsal joints because of its unique location. It alone occupies a position in both rows of tarsal joints. The talocalcaneal angle *(angle A)* is measured by drawing lines through the long axes of the talus and calcaneus. One should attempt to be as accurate as possible in making these measurements. The normal range for this measurement is 20° to 40° in the young child. The talus-first metatarsal angle *(angle B)* is measured by drawing lines through the long axis of the talus and along the long axis of the first metatarsal. The normal range is 0° to –20°. (B) Hindfoot varus, as manifested by a decreased talocalcaneal angle *(angle A)*, and talonavicular subluxation, as manifested by a talocalcaneal angle of less than 15° and a talus-first metatarsal angle *(angle B)* of more than 15°. Talonavicular subluxation occurs through the medial movement of three bones, which move as a unit. The navicular, cuboid, and calcaneus move medially through the combined movements of medial translation and supination of the proximal tarsal bones, whereas the calcaneus inverts beneath the talus. (Redrawn from Simons GW: Analytical radiography and the progressive approach in talipes equinovarus. *Orthop Clin North Am* 9:189, 1978.)

Anterior. One of the first areas to be examined in the evaluation of the anterior ankle is the anterior joint recess. This is seen with the patient in supine with the foot relaxed. The distal tibia and the proximal talus are landmarks that guide the examiner to the anterior joint recess. The transducer is placed longitudinally along the tibia and talus (Fig. 13.167). The bony contours of the tibia and talus will appear

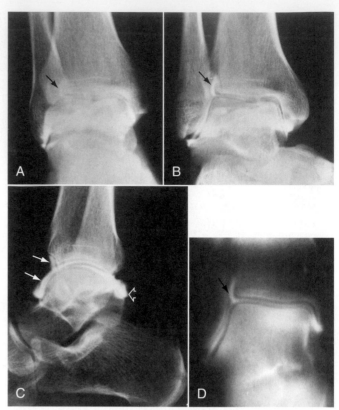

Fig. 13.165 Normal positive-contrast ankle arthrogram. (A) Anteroposterior view; (B) internal oblique or mortise view; (C) lateral view; and (D) a tomogram in the internal oblique projection show contrast agent coating the articular surfaces and filling normally present anterior *(white arrows)*, posterior *(open arrow)*, and syndesmotic *(black arrows)* recesses. There is no extension of contrast medium into the soft tissue medially or laterally. (From Weissman BNW, Sledge CB: *Orthopedic radiology*, Philadelphia, 1986, WB Saunders, p 596.)

hyperechoic. A thick line of hypoechoic articular cartilage can also be seen along the margins of the bone. Normally, a fat pad will sit between the tibia and the talus, and can be seen (Fig. 13.168). The transducer can then be moved into the short axis near the joint line to view the tendons of the anterior ankle including the tibialis anterior, extensor hallucis longus, and extensor digitorum. The tibialis anterior will be most medial and larger than all the other tendons. In its cross section, it will appear hyperechoic and fibrillar. The extensor hallucis longus tendon will run parallel and lateral to the tibialis anterior tendon, while the extensor digitorum longus will be most lateral. It is generally unmistakable due to its multiple tendons that run distally to the digits.

The dorsalis pedal artery lies near the extensor hallucis longus and will be seen in cross section. The deep peroneal nerve and the tibial artery can be seen in short axis at the level of the distal tibia.

Posterior. To best view the posterior ankle, the patient should lie comfortably in the prone position. The posterior evaluation can begin with the transducer placed on the posterior Achilles in the long axis (Fig. 13.169). The tendon should be thick and uniform in shape. The tendon can be viewed from the intermuscular attachment all the way distal to the calcaneus (Fig. 13.170). The transducer

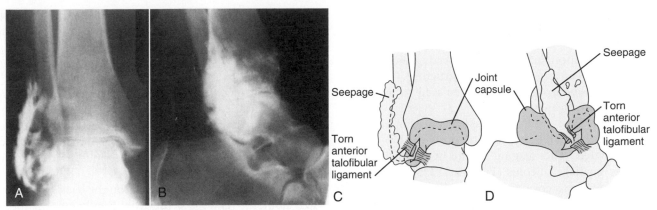

Fig. 13.166 Contrast arthrography showing acute tear of the anterior tibiofibular ligament. (A) Anteroposterior arthrogram of the right ankle 14 hours after the injury showing extravasation of contrast medium in front and around the lateral aspect of the fibula. (B) Lateral view of the same. (C and D) Illustrations of arthrograms A and B, respectively. (Modified from Kelikian H, Kelikian AS: *Disorders of the ankle*, Philadelphia, 1985, WB Saunders, p 143.)

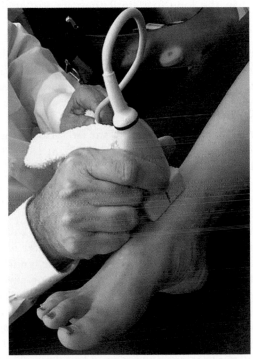

Fig. 13.167 Transducer placement for anterior joint recess long-axis view.

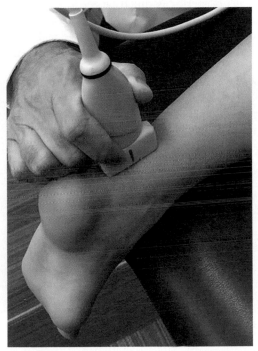

Fig. 13.169 Transducer placement for posterior ankle and Achilles tendon.

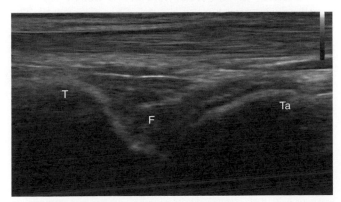

Fig. 13.168 Longitudinal image over anterior joint recess showing fat pad *(F)*, tibia *(T)*, and talus *(Ta)*.

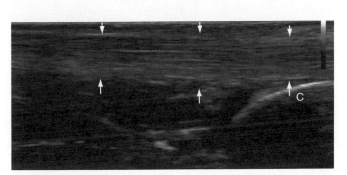

Fig. 13.170 Longitudinal image of Achilles tendon in long axis *(arrows)* and calcaneus *(C)*.

can then be rotated to the short axis. In this view, the tendon should be uniform and hyperechoic and relatively flat and broad.

The plantar aponeurosis can be viewed in the long axis which will appear as a hyperechoic structure. The insertion of the aponeurosis can clearly be seen to its attachment onto the calcaneus.

Medial. For best results, the medial ankle can be visualized with the foot relaxed and the proximal hip slightly laterally rotated. The imaging should begin in short axis above the medial malleolus (Fig. 13.171). As the transducer is moved posterior to the tibia, the tibialis posterior tendon, the flexor digitorum longus and the flexor hallucis longus are seen as hyperechoic fibrillary structures (Fig. 13.172). Because of the contour of the surrounding bone and soft tissues, anisotropy may occur requiring the examiner to toggle the transducer to get a clearer image. The tibialis posterior is much larger in size than that of the flexor hallucis and flexor digitorum longus.

In this same area, the tibial nerve will be situated between the flexor digitorum longus and flexor hallucis

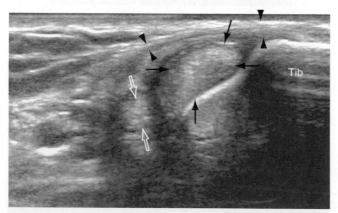

Fig. 13.171 Transducer placement for medial ankle short-axis view.

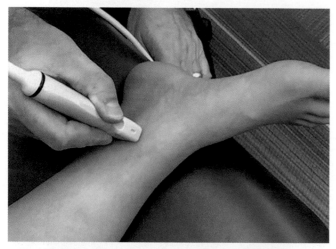

Fig. 13.172 Short-axis image superior and posterior to medial malleolus showing tibialis posterior *(arrows)*, and the flexor digitorum longus *(open arrows)* tendons, and flexor retinaculum *(arrowheads)*. *Tib*, Tibia. (From Jacobson JA: *Fundamentals of musculoskeletal ultrasound*, ed 3, Philadelphia, 2018, Elsevier.)

longus tendons. In the short axis view, the fascicles of the nerve can be seen surrounded by hyperechoic connective tissue.

The transducer can then be brought to the frontal or coronal plane as the tendons change direction under the medial malleolus. In this area, the sustentaculum tali protrudes from the medial calcaneus. At the sustentaculum tali, the tibialis posterior is more superficial and dorsal, while the flexor digitorum longus lies immediately superficial. The flexor hallucis longus tendon is inferior and lies in the bony groove of the calcaneus.[395]

The transducer can then be brought back to the long axis along the tendons as they run distally into the medial foot. The distal tibialis posterior will be able to be traced as it runs distally to insert onto the navicular, cuneiforms, and then the metatarsals on the sole of the foot. The flexor digitorum longus and flexor hallucis longus can be followed in the long axis until they are lost under the foot.

The deltoid ligament is the large broad ligament that provides a primary restraint to eversion of the ankle. The transducer can be placed in the coronal plane initially at the medial malleolus. The deltoid ligament can be seen running from the tibia to the calcaneus as a think superficial hyperechoic ligament.

Lateral. Because of injuries to the lateral ankle ligamentous structures, this is the area that DUSI is most often used. The patient can lay supine with the hip in slight medial rotation (Fig. 13.173). Starting with the transducer in the short axis posterior to the fibula, the peroneus brevis and longus tendons can be viewed (Fig. 13.174). If a muscle is seen by the peroneus longus, it will be the belly of the peroneus brevis. As the transducer is moved distally, the muscle belly should taper to the tendon.

As the transducer is rotated in an oblique axis under the tip of the lateral malleolus, the calcaneofibular ligament can be seen deep to the peroneal tendons. As the examiner continues distally, the peroneal tubercle will be seen. The peroneal tubercle is the site where the two peroneal tendons run in different locations. The peroneus brevis runs above the tubercle while the longus runs distal to the tubercle. The brevis can be followed distally to its attachment on the fifth metatarsal. The longus runs distally to dive under the peroneal or cuboid groove proximal to the fifth metatarsal to insert underneath the foot at the medial cuneiform and the base of the first metatarsal.

The peroneal tendons can also be viewed in the long axis. Starting above the malleolus, the transducer is moved posteriorly to the fibula in the recess behind the malleolus. With the transducer in an oblique plane, the brevis and longus can usually be seen in one isolated image. As they are followed distally, just like with the short axis, they can be followed distally to the fifth metatarsal or to the peroneal or cuboid groove.

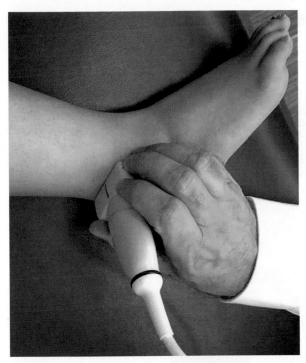

Fig. 13.173 Transducer placement for lateral ankle short axis slightly posterior to lateral malleolus.

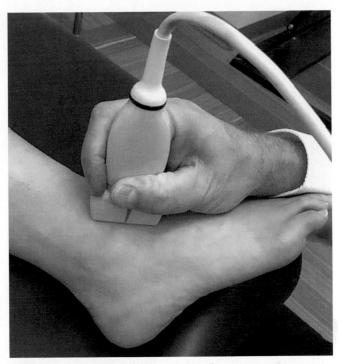

Fig. 13.175 Transducer placement longitudinally along the anterior talofibular ligament on the lateral ankle.

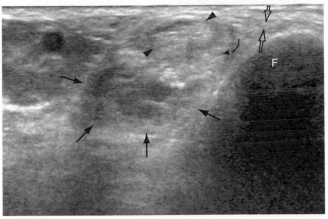

Fig. 13.174 Short-axis image superior and posterior to the lateral malleolus showing peroneal tendons including the peroneus longus tendon *(arrowheads)*, and the peroneus brevis muscle *(arrows)* and tendon *(curved arrow)*. *F*, Fibula. (From Jacobson JA: *Fundamentals of musculoskeletal ultrasound*, ed 3, Philadelphia, 2018, Elsevier.)

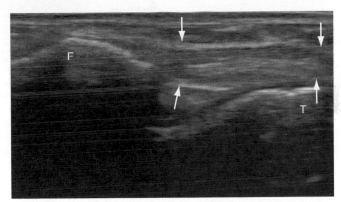

Fig. 13.176 Axial image of the anterior talofibular ligament in long axis *(arrows)*, as well as the fibula *(F)* and tibia *(T)*.

To assess the anterior talofibular ligament the transducer is placed along the ligament's long axis (Fig. 13.175). The ligament will appear as either a hyper- or a hypoechoic structure due to anisotropy and the oblique course of the ligament as it runs from the fibula to the talus (Fig. 13.176). To better view the ligament, the transducer may need to be toggled slightly. A normal ligament has full continuity.

The calcaneofibular ligament can be seen by placing the transducer at the tip of the fibula and slightly posterior toward the calcaneus. This ligament is also seen as a hyperechoic fibrillary structure. However, in the short axis, it may appear hypoechoic again due to anisotropy.

Lastly, the anterior inferior tibiofibular ligament should be examined as it is crucial if a high ankle sprain is suspected. In the short axis, the transducer is moved distally to the level of the distal tibia and fibula. At this level, the cortical outline of the tibia and fibula can be seen. As the transducer is moved inferiorly, there comes a location where the tibia ends and the fibula continues. The transducer should angle toward the continuing fibula and at this point, the hyperechoic fibrillary anterior inferior tibiofibular ligament can be found.

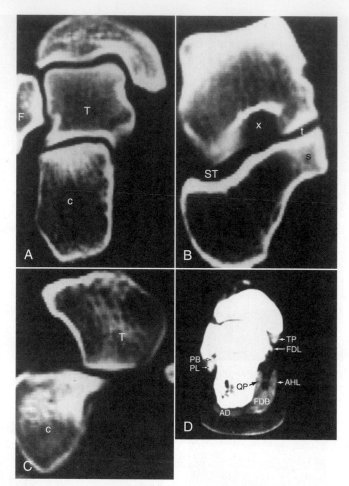

Fig. 13.177 Normal anatomy of the ankle and foot as seen on computed tomography scans. (A) Coronal section through the ankle and subtalar joint. *T,* Talus, *C,* calcaneus, *F,* fibula. (B) Farther anteriorly, the sustentaculum tali *(S),* the site of insertion of the talocalcaneal ligament *(X),* the subtalar joint *(ST),* and the mid-talocalcaneonavicular joint *(t)* are shown. (C) Anterior to the sustentaculum tali, the talus *(T)* and the calcaneus *(C),* are shown. (D) The peroneus brevis *(PB),* peroneus longus *(PL),* posterior tibial *(TP),* and flexor digitorum longus *(FDL)* muscles are shown. *AD,* Abductor digiti quinti pedis; *AHL,* abductor hallucis longus, *FDB,* flexor digitorum brevis, *QP,* quadratus plantae. This scan is at the level of the posterior aspect of the sustentaculum tali. (From Weissman BNW, Sledge CB: *Orthopedic radiology,* Philadelphia, 1986, WB Saunders, p. 632.)

Computed Tomography

Computed tomography scans are useful for determining the relation among the bones and for giving a view of the relation between bony and soft tissues (Figs. 13.177 and 13.178).

Magnetic Resonance Imaging

MRI is an especially useful, although sometimes overused, technique for delineating bony and soft tissues around the ankle and foot (Figs. 13.179 to 13.182).[25] MRI may be used to diagnose ruptured tendons (e.g., Achilles, peroneal), ligament tears (Fig. 13.183), and fractures (e.g., stress fractures, osteochondral fractures, osteonecrosis).[375,396–409]

Bone Scans

Bone scans are used in the lower limb, ankle, and foot to diagnose stress fractures. Areas of high risk for stress fractures include the tibia (anterior diaphysis) (Figs. 13.184 and 13.185), navicular, and proximal fifth metatarsal.[410]

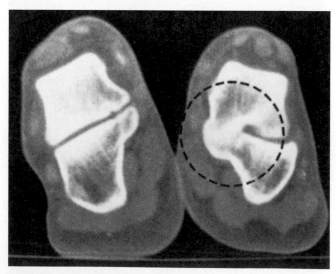

Fig. 13.178 Coronal computed tomographic view showing talocalcaneal coalition on the right. (From Rettig AC, Shelbourne KD, Beltz HF, et al: Radiographic evaluation of foot and ankle injuries in the athlete, *Clin Sports Med* 6:914, 1987.)

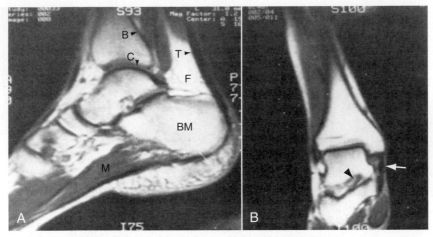

Fig. 13.179 Sagittal and coronal magnetic resonance images of the ankle. (A) Sagittal projection. Note the white bone marrow *(BM)* and subcutaneous fat *(F)*, black tendons *(T)* and ligaments, gray muscles *(M)* and articular cartilage *(C)*, and black cortical bone *(B)*. (B) Coronal projection. Note the black appearance of the deltoid ligament *(white arrow)* and interosseous ligament *(black arrowhead)* between the talus and calcaneus. (From Kingston S: Magnetic resonance imaging of the ankle and foot, *Clin Sports Med* 7:19, 1988.)

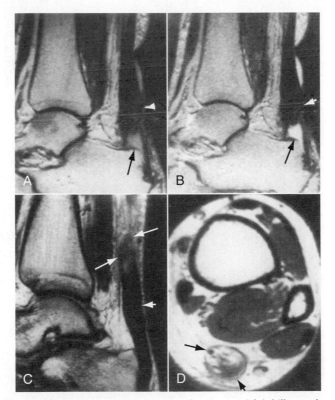

Fig. 13.180 Magnetic resonance images showing partial Achilles tendon tear. Sagittal, proton-density (A) and T2-weighted magnetic resonance images (B) reveal a large tear at the Achilles insertion with intratendinous fluid *(long arrow)* and fraying and thickening of the distal tendon *(short arrow)*. (C) Complete Achilles tendon tear. Sagittal, proton-density magnetic resonance (MR) image reveals disruption of the Achilles tendon *(long arrows)* and thickening of its distal portion *(short arrow)*. (D) On an axial, T1-weighted MR image, only gray granulation tissue is shown within the paratenon *(short arrow)*. The intact plantaris tendon passes along the medial border of the paratenon *(long arrow)*. (From Kerr R, Forrester DM, Kingston S: Magnetic resonance imaging of foot and ankle trauma, *Orthop Clin North Am* 21:593, 1990.)

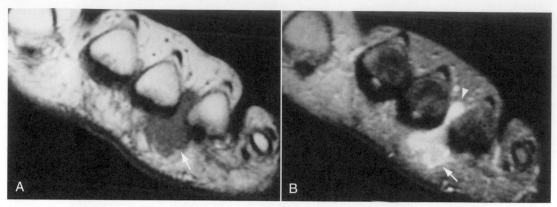

Fig. 13.181 Morton's neuroma. (A) Coronal T1-weighted (TR/TE, 600/20) spin-echo magnetic resonance (MR) image shows a mass *(arrow)* of low signal intensity between the third and fourth metatarsal heads. (B) This mass *(arrow)* has high signal intensity on a coronal fat-suppressed fast spin echo (TR/TE, 3500/50) MR image. A small amount of fluid may be present in the intermetatarsal bursa *(arrowhead)*. (From Resnick D, Kransdorf MJ: *Bone and joint imaging,* Philadelphia, 2005, WB Saunders, p 1051.)

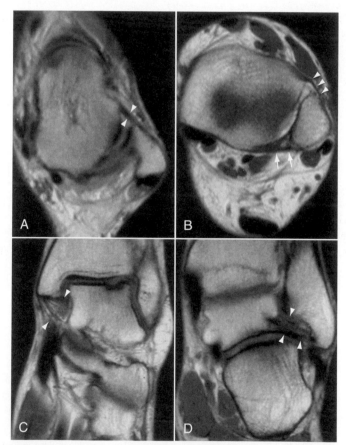

Fig. 13.182 Appearance of normal ankle ligaments. (A) The intact anterior talofibular ligament *(arrowheads)* is of low signal intensity on this T1-weighted transaxial image. Note the elliptical shape of the talus and the presence of the lateral malleolar fossa. (B) Intact anterior *(arrowheads)* and posterior *(arrows)* tibiofibular ligaments are of uniform low-signal intensity. The medial border of the lateral malleolus is flattened, indicating that this is the level of the tibiofibular ligaments. (C) Intact tibiotalar component of the deltoid *(arrowheads)*. Note the osteochondral defect of the lateral talar dome. (D) Posterior talofibular ligaments *(arrowheads)* on T1-weighted coronal image. The deltoid and posterior talofibular ligaments have a striated appearance rather than a homogeneous low-signal-intensity appearance like the anterior talofibular ligament. (© 2001 American Academy of Orthopaedic Surgeons. Reprinted from the Journal of the American Academy of Orthopaedic Surgeons, vol 9[3], pp. 187–199, with permission.)

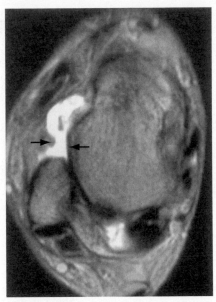

Fig. 13.183 Chronic tear of the anterior talofibular ligament. This transaxial T2-weighted image demonstrates the absence of the anterior talofibular ligament, with high-signal-intensity fluid *(arrows)* filling the expected location of the ligament. (© 2001 American Academy of Orthopaedic Surgeons. Reprinted from the Journal of the American Academy of Orthopaedic Surgeons, vol 9[3], pp. 187–199, with permission.)

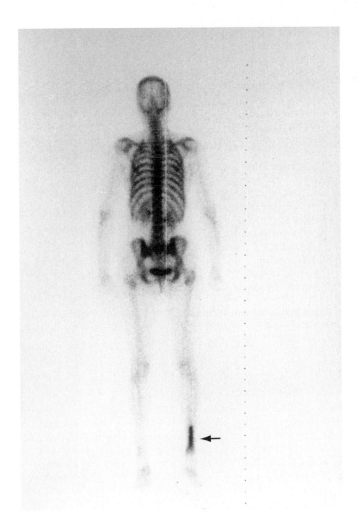

Fig. 13.184 Bone scan of whole body. *Arrow* indicates area of increased isotope uptake ("hot spot") in the right tibia, which is consistent with a stress-related lesion.

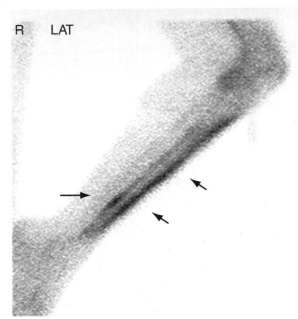

Fig. 13.185 Stress fracture of the tibia and anterior shin splint. A short fusiform area of increased uptake in the posterior aspect of the distal shaft of the tibia represents a stress fracture *(large arrow)*. A long longitudinal area of increased uptake in the anterior aspect of the tibial shaft is consistent with a shin splint *(small arrows)*. (From Resnick D, Kransdorf MJ: *Bone and joint imaging*, Philadelphia, 2005, WB Saunders, p 103.)

PRÉCIS OF THE LOWER LEG, ANKLE, AND FOOT ASSESSMENT[a]

NOTE: Suspected pathology will determine which *Special Tests* are to be performed.

History

Observation

Examination

Active movements, weight-bearing (standing)
Plantar flexion
Dorsiflexion
Supination
Pronation
Toe extension
Toe flexion

Functional assessment (standing)

Special tests (standing)
Neutral position of talus
"Too many toes" sign
Windlass test (great toe extension)

Active movements, non–weight-bearing (sitting or supine lying)
Plantar flexion
Dorsiflexion
Supination
Pronation
Toe extension
Toe flexion
Toe abduction
Toe adduction

Special tests (sitting)
Dorsiflexion-eversion test for tarsal tunnel syndrome
External rotation stress test
Navicular drop test
Synovial impingement test
Tibial torsion

Passive movements (supine lying)
Plantar flexion at the talocrural (ankle) joint
Dorsiflexion at the talocrural joint
Inversion at the subtalar joint
Eversion at the subtalar joint
Adduction at the midtarsal joints
Abduction at the midtarsal joints
Flexion of the toes
Extension of the toes
Adduction of the toes
Abduction of the toes

Resisted isometric movements (supine lying)
Knee flexion
Plantar flexion
Dorsiflexion
Supination
Pronation
Toe extension
Toe flexion

Special tests (supine lying)
Anterior drawer sign
Cotton test
Figure-eight measurement of ankle
Forefoot-heel alignment
Functional hallux limitus test
Leg length
Medial subtalar glide test
Morton's (squeeze) test
Neutral position of talus
Shin oedema test
Shin palpation test
Talar tilt
Tibial torsion
Tinel's sign at the ankle
Triple compression test

Reflexes and cutaneous distribution (supine lying)

Special tests (side lying)
Fibular translation test

Joint play movements (supine and side lying)
Long-axis extension
Anteroposterior glide
Talar rock
Side tilt
Rotation
Side glide
Tarsal bone mobility

Palpation (supine lying and prone lying)

Special tests (prone lying)
Leg-heel alignment
Matles test
Neutral position of talus
Prone anterior drawer test
Tibial torsion
Thompson test

Diagnostic imaging

[a]The précis is shown in an order that limits the amount of moving that the patient has to do but ensures that all necessary structures are tested. It does not follow the order of the text. After any examination, the patient should be warned of the possibility that symptoms will exacerbate as a result of the assessment.

CASE STUDIES

When doing these case studies, the examiner should list the appropriate questions to be asked and why they are being asked, identify what to look for and why, and specify what things should be tested and why. Depending on the patient's answers (and the examiner should consider different responses), several possible causes of the patient's problem may become evident (examples are given in parentheses). A differential diagnosis chart should be made (see Table 13.16 as an example). The examiner can then decide how different diagnoses may affect the treatment plan.

1. A 26-year-old male firefighter is being seen following a fascial release in the lower leg due to increased inter-compartmental pressures while running. He is a recreational athlete who enjoys ultra-marathon running. Describe your assessment plan for him following this surgical procedure. In particular, describe how you would assess entire neurological function of lower extremity and ROM specific to a high-level recreational runner.

2. A 36-year-old emergency room physician comes to see you as a direct access patient following a basketball injury. He reports that, while playing basketball over the weekend, he was kicked in the back of his right heel. He has swelling in the posterior heel but no discoloration at this time. He has enough weakness such that he is having trouble walking normally. He feels as though he has no control to stop dorsiflexion during gait, and has little strength during the push-off phase of gait in terminal stance. Describe your assessment plan for this patient (Achilles tendon rupture vs. Achilles tendinopathy).

3. A 38-year-old man ruptured his Achilles tendon 4 weeks earlier and had it surgically repaired. The cast has been removed. Describe your assessment plan for this patient.

4. A 24-year-old woman presents at your clinic with a painful left foot. There is no history of trauma; however, the pain has been present for approximately 6 years and has become worse in the past year. Describe your assessment plan for this patient (Morton's neuroma vs. plantar fasciitis).

5. A 59-year-old man comes to you complaining of pain in his right calf and some numbness in his right foot. He also complains of some stiffness in his back. Describe your assessment plan for this patient (lumbar spondylosis vs. tibial nerve palsy).

6. A 10-year-old boy recently had a triple arthrodesis for talipes equinovarus. The cast has now been removed. Describe your assessment plan for this patient.

7. A 16-year-old female volleyball player comes to you complaining of left ankle pain and difficulty walking after she stepped on another player's foot and went over on her ankle. The injury occurred 30 minutes earlier, and her ankle is swollen. Describe your assessment plan for this patient (malleolar fracture versus ligament sprain).

8. A 25-year-old woman tells you that she is training for a marathon but that every time she increases her mileage, her right foot hurts. Some time ago, someone told her she had a cavus foot. Describe your assessment plan for this patient.

9. Parents bring a 2-year-old boy to you and express concern that the child appears to have flat feet and "pigeon toes." Describe your assessment plan for this patient.

10. A 32-year-old woman comes to you complaining of ankle pain. She states that she sprained it 9 months earlier and thought it was better. However, she has now returned to training, and the ankle is bothering her. Describe your assessment plan for this patient (proprioceptive loss vs. instability).

TABLE **13.16**

Differential Diagnosis of Lower Leg Compartment Syndrome

	Compartment Syndrome	Shin Splints[a]	Stress Fracture[a]	Tumor
Pain (type)	Severe cramping, diffuse pain, and tightness	Diffuse along medial two-thirds of tibial border	Deep, nagging localized with minimal radiation	Deep, nagging (bone) with some radiation
Pain with rest	Decreases or disappears	Decreases or disappears	Present, especially night pain	Present, often night pain
Pain with activity	Increases	Increases	Present (may increase)	Present
Pain with warm-up	May increase or become present	May disappear	Unilateral	Unaltered
Range of motion	Limited in acute phase	Limited	Normal	Normal
Onset	Gradual to sudden	Gradual	Gradual	?
Altered sensation	Sometimes	No	No	Sometimes
Muscle weakness or paralysis	Maybe	No	No	Not usually
Stretching	Increases pain	Increases pain	Minimal pain alteration	No increase in pain
Radiography	Normal	Normal	Early, negative; late, positive (?)	Usually positive
Bone scan	Negative	Periosteal uptake	Positive	Positive
Pulse	Affected sometimes	Normal	Normal	Normal
Palpation	Tender, tight compartment	Diffuse tenderness	Point tenderness	Point or diffuse tenderness
Cause	Muscle expansion	Overuse	Overuse	?
Duration and recovery	None without surgery	None without rest	Up to 3 months	None without treatment

[a]These two conditions are different stages of tibial stress syndrome.
From Magee DJ: *Sports physiotherapy manual,* Edmonton, 1988, University of Alberta Bookstore.

References

1. Kangas J, Dankaerts W, Staes F. New approach to the diagnosis and classification of chronic foot and ankle disorders: identifying motor control and movement impairments. *Man Ther.* 2011;16:522–530.
2. Young CC, Niedfeldt MW, Morris GA, Eerkes KJ. Clinical examination of the foot and ankle. *Prim Care.* 2005;32(1):105–132.
3. Donatelli R. Abnormal biomechanics of the foot and ankle. *J Orthop Sports Phys Ther.* 1987;9:11–16.
4. Sartoris DJ. Diagnosis of ankle injuries: the essentials. *J Foot Ankle Surg.* 1994;33(1):102–107.
5. Ombregt L. *A System of Orthopedic Medicine.* 3rd ed. Philadelphia: Elsevier; 2013.
6. Wang Q, Whittle M, Cunningham J, et al. Fibula and its ligaments in load transmission and ankle joint stability. *Clin Orthop Relat Res.* 1996;330:261–270.
7. Hertel J. Functional anatomy, pathomechanics and pathophysiology of lateral ankle instability. *J Athl Train.* 2002;37(4):364–375.
8. Tochigi Y, Rudert MJ, Saltzman CL, et al. Contribution of articular surface geometry to ankle stabilization. *J Bone Joint Surg Am.* 2006;88(12):2704–2713.
9. Tome J, Nawoczenski DA, Flemister A, Houck J. Comparison of foot kinematics between subjects with posterior tibialis tendon dysfunction and healthy controls. *J Orthop Sports Phys Ther.* 2006;36(9):635–644.
10. Wan L, de Asla RJ, Rubash HE, Li G. In vivo cartilage contact deformation of human ankle joints under full body weight. *J Orthop Res.* 2008;26(8):1081–1089.
11. Gribble PA, Bleakley CM, Caulfield BM, et al. Evidence review for the 2016 International Ankle Consortium consensus statement on the prevalence, impact and long-term consequences of lateral ankle sprains. *Br J Sports Med.* 2016;50(24):1496–1505.
12. Gribble PA, Bleakley CM, Caulfield BM, et al. 2016 consensus statement in the International Ankle Consortium: prevalence, impact and long-term consequences of lateral ankle sprains. *Br J Sports Med.* 2016;50(24):1493–1495.
13. Attarian DE, McCrackin HJ, Devito DP, et al. A biomechanical study of human lateral ankle ligaments and autogenous reconstructive grafts. *Am J Sports Med.* 1985;13(6):377–381.
14. Mantas JP. Lisfranc injuries in the athlete. *Clin Sports Med.* 1994;13:719–730.
15. Papaliodis DN, Vanushkina MA, Richardson NG, DiPreta JA. The foot and ankle examination. *Med Clin North Am.* 2014;98(2):181–204.
16. Kleiger B. Mechanisms of ankle injury. *Orthop Clin North Am.* 1974;5:127–146.
17. Safran MR, Benedetti RS, Bartolozzi AR, et al. Lateral ankle sprains: a comprehensive review. Part 1: Etiology, pathoanatomy, histopathogenesis, and diagnosis. *Med Sci Sports Exerc.* 1999;31:S429–S437.
18. Czajka CM, Tran E, Cai AN, DiPreta JA. Ankle sprains and instability. *Med Clin North Am.* 2014;98(2):313–329.
19. Klausner VB, McKeigue ME. The sinus tarsi syndrome: a cause of chronic ankle pain. *Phys Sportsmed.* 2000;28:75–80.
20. Heckman DS, Gluck GS, Pavekh SG. Tendon disorders of the foot and ankle. Part 1—peroneal tendon disorders. *Am J Sports Med.* 2009;37:614–625.
21. Jackson LT, Dunaway LJ, Lundeen GA. Acute tears of the tibialis posterior tendon following ankle sprain. *Foot Ankle Int.* 2017;38(7):752–759.
22. Gerber JP, Williams GN, Scoville CR, et al. Persistent disability associated with ankle sprains: a prospective examination of an athletic populations. *Foot Ankle Int.* 1998;19:653–660.
23. van Dijk CN, Bossuyt PM, Marti RK. Medial ankle pain after lateral ligament rupture. *J Bone Joint Surg Br.* 1996;78:562–567.
24. Mulligan EP. Evaluation and management of ankle syndesmosis injuries. *Phys Ther Sport.* 2011;12(2):57–69.
25. Liu SH, Nuccion SL, Finerman G. Diagnosis of anterolateral ankle impingement: comparison between magnetic resonance imaging and clinical examination. *Am J Sports Med.* 1997;25:389–393.
26. Dutton M. *Dutton's Orthopedic Examination, Evaluation and Intervention.* 3rd ed. New York: McGraw-Hill; 2012.
27. Kauve M. Acute Achilles tendon rupture: clinical evaluation, conservative management, and early active rehabilitation. *Clin Podiatr Med Surg.* 2017;34(2):229–243.
28. Kraeutler MJ, Purchell JM, Hunt KJ. Chronic Achilles tendon ruptures. *Foot Ankle Int.* 2017;38(8):921–929.
29. Gravlee JR, Hatch RL, Galea AM. Achilles tendon rupture: a challenging diagnosis. *J Am Board Fam Pract.* 2000;13(5):371–373.
30. O'Loughlin PF, Heyworth BE, Kennedy JG. Current concepts in the diagnosis and treatment of osteochondral lesions of the ankle. *Am J Sports Med.* 2010;38:392–404.

31. Marder RA. Current methods for the evaluation of ankle ligament injuries. *J Bone Joint Surg Am.* 1994;76:1103–1111.

32. Russell JA, Kruse DW, Koutedakis Y, et al. Pathoanatomy of posterior ankle impingement in ballet dancers. *Clin Anat.* 2010;23(6):613–621.

33. Ribbans WJ, Ribbans HA, Cruikshank JA, Wood EV. The management of posterior ankle impingement syndrome in sport: a review. *Foot Ankle Surg.* 2015;21(1):1–10.

34. Molloy S, Solan MC, Bendall SP. Synovial impingement in the ankle. A new physical sign. *J Bone Joint Surg Br.* 2003;85(3):330–333.

35. Taunton J, Smith C, Magee DJ. Leg, foot and ankle injuries. In: Zachazewski JE, Magee DJ, Quillen WS, eds. *Athletic Injuries and Rehabilitation.* Philadelphia: WB Saunders; 1996.

36. Reid DC. *Sports Injury Assessment and Rehabilitation.* New York: Churchill Livingstone; 1992.

37. Edwards PH, Wright ML, Hartman JF. A practical approach for the differential diagnosis of chronic leg pain in the athlete. *Am J Sports Med.* 2005;33:1241–1249.

38. Gribble PA, Delahunt E, Bleakley CM, et al. Selection criteria for patients with chronic ankle instability in controlled research: a position statement of the International Ankle Consortium. *J Athl Train.* 2014;49(1):121–127.

39. Munn J, Sullivan SJ, Schneiders AG. Evidence of sensorimotor deficits in functional ankle instability: a systematic review with meta-analysis. *J Sci Med Sport.* 2010;13(1):2–12.

40. Wright CJ, Arnold BL, Ross SE, et al. Clinical examination results in individuals with functional ankle instability and ankle sprain copers. *J Athl Train.* 2013;48(5):581–589.

41. Hubbard TJ. Ligament laxity following inversion injury with and without chronic ankle instability. *Foot Ankle Int.* 2008;29(3):305–311.

42. Brown C, Padua D, Marshall SW, Guskiewicz K. Individuals with mechanical ankle instability exhibit different motion patterns than those with functional ankle instability and ankle sprain copers. *Clin Biomech.* 2008;23(6):822–831.

43. Hiller CE, Kilbreath SL, Refshauge KM. Chronic ankle instability: evolution of the model. *J Athl Train.* 2011;46(2):133–141.

44. Ritchie DH. Functional instability of the ankle and the role of neuromuscular control: a comprehensive review. *J Foot Ankle Surg.* 2001;40(4):240–251.

45. Kou JX, Fortin PT. Commonly missed peritalar injuries. *J Am Acad Orthop Surg.* 2009;17:775–786.

46. Coris EE, Lombardo JA. Tarsal navicular stress fractures. *Am Fam Physician.* 2003;67(1):85–90.

47. Fullem BW. Overuse lower extremity injuries in sport. *Clin Podiatr Med Surg.* 2015;32(2):239–251.

48. Yates B, White S. The incidence and risk factors in the development of medial tibial stress syndrome among naval recruits. *Am J Sports Med.* 2004;32:772–780.

49. Gabisan GG, Gentile DR. Acute peroneal compartment syndrome following ankle inversion injury: a case report. *Am J Sports Med.* 2004;32:1059–1061.

50. van den Brand JG, Nelson T, Verleisdonk EJ, et al. The diagnostic value of intracompartmental pressure management, magnetic resonance imaging, and near-infrared spectroscopy in chronic exertional compartment syndrome: a prospective study of 50 patients. *Am J Sports Med.* 2005;33:699–704.

51. Gabisan GG, Gentile DR. Acute peroneal compartment syndrome following ankle inversion injury: a case report. *Am J Sports Med.* 2004;32:1059–1061.

52. Burrus MT, Werner BC, Starman JS, et al. Chronic leg pain in athletes. *Am J Sports Med.* 2015;43(6):1538–1547.

53. Bonnin M, Tavernier T, Bouysset M. Split lesions of the peroneus brevis tendon in chronic ankle laxity. *Am J Sports Med.* 1997;25:699–703.

54. Neufeld SK, Cerrato R. Plantar fasciitis: evaluation and treatment. *J Am Acad Orthop Surg.* 2008;16:338–346.

55. Reilly K, Barker K, Shamley D, et al. The role of foot and ankle assessment of patients with lower limb osteoarthritis. *Physiotherapy.* 2009;95(3):164–169.

56. Golightly YM, Hannan MT, Shi XA, et al. Foot symptoms are independently associated with poor self-reported and performance-based physical function: The Johnston County Osteoarthritis Project. *Arthritis Care Res.* 2011;63(5):654–659.

57. Rao S, Riskowski J, Hannan MT. Musculoskeletal conditions of the foot and ankle: assessments and treatment options. *Best Pract Res Clin Rheumatol.* 2012;26(3):345–368.

58. Dufour AB, Broe KE, Nguyen US, et al. Foot pain: is current or past shoewear a factor? *Arthritis Rheum.* 2009;61(10):1352–1358.

59. Menz HB, Lord SR. Gait instability in older people with hallux valgus. *Foot Ankle Int.* 2005;26(6):483–489.

60. Riskowski J, Dufour AB, Hannan MT. Arthritis, foot pain and shoe wear: current musculoskeletal research on feet. *Curr Opin Rheumatol.* 2011;23(2):148–155.

61. Byrne M, Curran MJ. The development and use of a footwear assessment score in comparing the fit of children's shoes. *The Foot.* 1998;8(4):215–218.

62. Menz HB, Sherrington C. The Footwear Assessment Form: a reliable clinical tool to assess footwear characteristics of relevance to postural stability in older adults. *Clin Rehabil.* 2000;14(6):657–664.

63. Williams A. Footwear assessment and management – understanding shoe construction and materials aids in properly fitting patients. *Podiatry Management* October. 2007:165–177.

64. Barton CJ, Bonanno D, Menz HB. Development and evaluation of a tool for the assessment of footwear characteristics. *J Foot Ankle Res.* 2009;2:10–22.

65. Hunt GC, Brocato RS. Gait and foot pathomechanics. In: Hunt GC, ed. *Physical Therapy of the Foot and Ankle: Clinics in Physical Therapy.* Edinburgh: Churchill Livingstone; 1988.

66. Laird RC. Acute forefoot and midfoot injuries. *Clin Podiatr Med Surg.* 2015;32(2):231–238.

67. Lang LM, Volpe RG, Wernick J. Static biomechanical evaluation of the foot and lower limb: the podiatrist's perspective. *Man Ther.* 1997;2:58–66.

68. Chuckpaiwong B, Nunley JA, Queen RM. Correlation between static foot type measurements and clinical assessments. *Foot Ankle Int.* 2009;30(3):205–212.

69. Gulchet JM, Javed A, Russell J, Saleh M. Effect of the foot on the mechanical alignment of the lower limbs. *Clin Orthop Relat Res.* 2003;415:193–201.

70. Kapandji IA. *The Physiology of the Joints.* Lower limb. Vol 2. New York: Churchill Livingstone; 1970.

71. Lipscomb AB, Ibrahim AA. Acute peroneal compartment syndrome in a well conditioned athlete: report of a case. *Am J Sports Med.* 1977;5:154–157.

72. Williams PL, Warwick R, eds. *Gray's Anatomy.* 36th ed. British, Philadelphia: WB Saunders; 1980.

73. Kelikian H, Kelikian AS. *Disorders of the Ankle.* Philadelphia: WB Saunders; 1985.

74. Sierra RJ, Trousdale RT, Ganz R, et al. Hip disease in the young active patient: evaluation and nonarthroplasty surgical options. *J Am Acad Orthop Surg.* 2008;16:689–703.

75. Palmer ML, Epler M. *Clinical Assessment Procedures in Physical Therapy.* Philadelphia: JB Lippincott; 1990.

76. Jahss MH. *Disorders of the Foot.* Philadelphia: WB Saunders; 1982.

77. Smith AH, Bach BR. High ankle sprains: minimizing the frustration of a prolonged recovery. *Phys Sportsmed.* 2004;32(12):39–43.

78. Scranton PE. Isolated syndesmotic injuries: diastasis of the ankle in the athlete. *Tech Foot Ankle Surg.* 2002;1:88–90.

79. Evans RC. *Illustrated Essentials in Orthopedic Physical Assessment.* St Louis: Mosby; 1994.

80. Mizel MS, Hecht PJ, Marymount JV, et al. Evaluation and treatment of chronic ankle pain. *J Bone Joint Surg Am.* 2004;86:622–632.

81. Pavlov H, Heneghan MA, Hersh A, et al. The Haglund deformity: initial and differential diagnosis. *Radiology.* 1982;144:83–88.

82. Meininger AK, Koh JL. Evaluation of the injured runner. *Clin Sports Med.* 2012;31:203–215.

83. Myerson CL, Shimozono Y, Kennedy JG. Haglund's deformity and chronic Achilles tendonitis. *Oper Tech Orthop.* 2018;28(2):104–109.

84. Zifchock RA, Davis I, Hillstrom H, Song J. The effect of gender, age, and lateral dominance on arch height and arch stiffness. *Foot Ankle Int.* 2006;27(5):367–372.

85. Pedowitz WJ, Kovatis P. Flatfoot in the adult. *J Am Acad Orthop Surg.* 1995;3(5):293–302.

86. Razeghi M, Batt ME. Foot type classification: a critical review of current methods. *Gait Posture.* 2002;15(3):282–291.

87. Hamilton JJ, Ziemer LK. *Functional Anatomy of the Human Ankle and Foot, American Association of Orthopaedic Surgeons, Symposium on the Foot and Ankle.* St Louis: Mosby; 1983.

88. Williams DS, McClay IS. Measurements used to characterize the foot and the medial longitudinal arch: reliability and validity. *Physical Ther.* 2000;80(9):864–871.

89. Saltzman CL, Nawoczenski DA, Talbot KD. Measurement of the medial longitudinal arch. *Arch Phys Med Rehabil.* 1995;76(1):45–49.

90. Erdemir A, Hamel AJ, Fauth AR, et al. Dynamic loading of the plantar aponeurosis in walking. *J Bone Joint Surg Am.* 2004;86:546–552.

91. Tenforde AS, Yin A, Hunt KJ. Foot and ankle injuries in runners. *Phys Med Rehabil Clin N Am.* 2016;27(1):121–137.

92. Romash M. Deformities of the lesser toes and bunionette. In: Lutter LD, Mizel MS, Pfeffer GB, eds. *Orthopedic Knowledge Update: Foot and Ankle.* Rosemont, IL: American Academy of Orthopaedic Surgeons; 1994.

93. Bowe JA. The pediatric foot. In: Lutter LD, Mizel MS, Pfeffer GB, eds. *Orthopedic Knowledge Update: Foot and Ankle.* Rosemont, IL: American Academy of Orthopaedic Surgeons; 1994.

94. Shirzad K, Kiesau CD, deOrio JK, et al. Lesser toe deformities. *J Am Acad Orthop Surg.* 2011;19(8):505–514.

95. Brown LP, Yavorsky P. Locomotor biomechanics and pathomechanics: a review. *J Orthop Sports Phys Ther.* 1987;9:3–10.

96. McPoil TG, Brocato RS. The foot and ankle: biomechanical evaluation and treatment. In: Gould JA, ed. *Orthopedic and Sports Physical Therapy.* St Louis: Mosby; 1990.

97. McMaster MJ. The pathogenesis of the hallux rigidus. *J Bone Joint Surg Br.* 1978;60:82–87.

98. Dietze A, Bahlke U, Martin H, Mittlmeier T. First ray instability in hallux valgus deformity: a radiokinematic and pedobarographic analysis. *Foot Ankle Int.* 2013;34(1):124–130.

99. Glasoe WM, Phadke V, Pena FA, et al. An image-based gait simulation study of tarsal kinematics in women with hallux valgus. *Phys Ther.* 2013;93(11):1551–1562.

100. Koller U, Willegger M, Windhager R, et al. Plantar pressure characteristics in hallux valgus feet. *J Orthop Res.* 2014;32(12):1688–1693.

101. Pedowitz WJ. Deformities of the first ray. In: Lutter LD, Mizel MS, Pfeffer GB, eds. *Orthopedic Knowledge Update: Foot and Ankle.* Rosemont, IL: American Academy of Orthopaedic Surgeons; 1994.

102. Yokoe K, Kameyama Y. Relationship between stress fractures of the proximal phalanx of the great toe and hallux valgus. *Am J Sports Med.* 2004;32:1032–1034.

103. Thompson GH. Bunions and deformities of the toes in children and adolescents. *J Bone Joint Surg Am.* 1995;77:1924–1936.

104. Durman DC. Metatarsus primus varus and hallux valgus. *Arch Surg.* 1957;74:128–135.

105. Price GFW. Metatarsus primus varus, including various clinicoradiologic features of the female foot. *Clin Orthop.* 1979;145:217–223.

106. Coughlin MJ. Conditions of the forefoot. In: DeLee JC, Drez D, eds. *Orthopedic Sports Medicine: Principles and Practice.* Philadelphia: WB Saunders; 1994.

107. Sobel E, Levitz S, Caselli M, et al. Natural history of the rearfoot angle: preliminary values in 150 children. *Foot Ankle Int.* 1999;20(2):119–125.

108. Kanatli U, Gozil R, Besli K, et al. The relationship between the hindfoot angle and the medial longitudinal arch of the foot. *Foot Ankle Int.* 2006;27(8):623–627.

109. Beals TC, Pomeroy GC, Manoli A. Posterior tibial tendon insufficiency: diagnosis and treatment. *J Am Acad Orthop Surg.* 1999;7:112–118.

110. Churgay A. Diagnosis and treatment of pediatric foot deformities. *Am Fam Physician.* 1993;47:883–887.

111. Owens R, Gougoulias N, Guthrie H, Sakellariou A. Morton's neuroma: clinical testing and imaging in 76 feet, compared to a control group. *Foot Ankle Surg.* 2011;17(3):197–2009.

112. Mahadevan D, Venkatesan M, Bhatt R, Bhatia M. Diagnostic accuracy of clinical tests for Morton's neuroma compared with ultrasonography. *J Foot Ankle Surg.* 2015;54(4):549–553.

113. Pastides P, El-Sallakh S, Charalambides C. Morton's neuroma: a clinical versus radiological diagnosis. *Foot Ankle Surg.* 2012;18(1):22–24.

114. Title CI, Schon LC. Morton's neuroma: primary and secondary neurectomy. *J Am Acad Orthop Surg.* 2008;16:550–557.

115. Lee MS, Vanore JV, Thomas JL, et al. Diagnosis and treatment of adult flatfoot. *J Foot Ankle Surg.* 2005;44(2):78–113.

116. Harris EJ, Vanore JV, Thomas JL, et al. Diagnosis and treatment of pediatric flatfoot. *J Foot and Ankle Surg.* 2004;43(6):341–373.

117. Arangio GA, Wasser T, Rogman A. Radiographic comparison of standing medial cuneiform arch height in adults with and without acquired flatfoot deformity. *Foot Ankle Int.* 2006;27(8):636–638.

118. Buldt AK, Murley GS, Butterworth P, et al. The relationship between foot posture and lower limb kinematics during walking: a systematic review. *Gait Posture.* 2013;38(3):363–372.

119. Kido M, Ikoma K, Imai K, et al. Load response of the tarsal bones in patients with flatfoot deformity: in vivo 3D study. *Foot Ankle Int.* 2011;32(11):1017–1022.

120. Wukich DK, Tuason DA. Diagnosis and treatment of chronic ankle pain. *J Bone Joint Surg Am.* 2010;92:2002–2016.

121. Root ML, Orien WP, Weed JH. *Normal and Abnormal Function of the Foot.* Los Angeles: Clinical Biomechanics; 1977.

122. Lian G. Nerve problems in the foot. In: Lutter LD, Mizel MS, Pfeffer GB, eds. *Orthopedic Knowledge Update: Foot and Ankle.* Rosemont, IL: American Academy of Orthopaedic Surgeons; 1994.

123. Bowers KD, Martin RB. Turf toe: a shoe related football injury. *Med Sci Sports Exerc.* 1976;8:81–83.

124. Clanton TO, Ford JJ. Turf toe injury. *Clin Sports Med.* 1994;13:731–741.

125. Anderson RB, Hunt KJ, McCormick JJ. Management of common sports-related injuries about the foot and ankle. *J Am Acad Orthop Surg.* 2010;18:546–556.

126. Kaufman KR, Brodine SK, Schaffer RA, et al. The effect of foot structure and range of motion on musculoskeletal overuse injuries. *Am J Sports Med.* 1999;27:585–593.

127. Lindsjo U, Danckwardt-Lilliestrom G, Sahlstedt B. Measurement of the motion range in the loaded ankle. *Clin Orthop.* 1985;199:68–71.

128. Patla CE, Abbott JH. Tibialis posterior myofascial tightness as a source of heel pain: diagnosis and treatment. *J Orthop Sports Phys Ther.* 2000;30:624–632.

129. Stovitz SD, Coetzee JC. Hyperpronation and foot pain—steps toward pain-free feet. *Phys Sportsmed.* 2004;32(8):19–26.

130. McCrory P, Bladin C. Fractures of the lateral process of the talus: a clinical review: "snowboarder's ankle". *Clin J Sports Med.* 1996;6:124–128.

131. Bennell K, Talbot R, Wajswelner H, et al. Intra-rater and inter-rater reliability of a weight bearing lunge measure of ankle dorsiflexion. *Austr J Physio.* 1998;44:175–180.

132. Simondson D, Brock K, Cotton S. Reliability and smallest real difference of the ankle lunge test post ankle fracture. *Manual Therapy.* 2012;17:34–38.

133. Rabin A, Kozol Z, Spitzer E, Finestone AS. Weight-bearing ankle dorsiflexion range of motion – can side-to-side symmetry be assumed? *J Athl Train.* 2015;50(1):30–35.

134. Chisholm MD, Birmingham TB, Brown J, et al. Reliability and validity of a weight-bearing measure of ankle dorsiflexion range of motion. *Physiother Can.* 2012;64(4):347–355.

135. Konor MM, Morton S, Eckerson JM, Grindstaff TL. Reliability of three measures of ankle dorsiflexion range of motion. *Int J Sports Phys Ther.* 2012;7(3):279–287.

136. Hoch MC, McKeon PO. Normative range of weight bearing lunge test performance asymmetry in healthy adults. *Manual Therapy.* 2011;16:516–519.

137. Cote KP, Brunet ME, Gansneder BM, Shultz SJ. Effects of pronated and supinated foot postures on static and dynamic postural stability. *J Athl Train.* 2005;40(1):41–46.

138. Hyslop GH. Injuries of the deep and superficial peroneal nerves complicating ankle sprain. *Am J Surg.* 1941;51:436–438.

139. Tabrizi P, McIntyre WM, Quesnel MB, et al. Limited dorsiflexion predisposes to injuries of the ankle in children. *J Bone Joint Surg Br.* 2000;82:1103–1106.

140. Chiodo CP, Glazebrook M, Bluman EM, et al. Diagnosis and treatment of acute achilles tendon rupture. *J Am Acad Orthop Surg.* 2010;18:503–510.

141. Menz HB. Clinical hindfoot measurement: a critical review of the literature. *The Foot.* 1995;5(2):57–64.

142. Redmond AC, Crosbie J, Ouvrier RA. Development and validation of a novel rating system for scoring standing foot posture: the foot posture index. *Clin Biomech.* 2006;21:89–98.

143. Redmond AC, Crane YZ, Menz HB. Normative values for the foot posture index. *J Foot Ankle Res.* 2008;1(1):6–15.

144. Lowe R, Hashem M, Thomas E, Ager A. *Foot Posture Index (FPI – 6).* Physiopedia; 2018. Accessed at www.physio-pedia.com/index.php?title=Foot_Posture_Index_(FP1-6)andoldid=199552".

145. Redmond AL. *The Foot Posture Index (FPI – 6) – User Guide and Manual;* 2005. Available at https://www.leeds.ac.uk/medicine/FASTER/z/pdf/FPI-manual-form atted-August-2005v2.pdf.

146. Rokkedal-Lausch T, Lykke M, Hansen MS, Nielsen RO. Normative values for the foot posture index between right and left foot: a descriptive study. *Gait Posture.* 2013;38(4):843–846.

147. Nielsen RG, Rathleff MS, Moelgaard CM, et al. Video based analysis of dynamic midfoot function and its relationship with foot posture index scores. *Gait Posture.* 2010;31(1):126–130.

148. Jan MH, Chai AM, Lin YF, et al. Effects of age and sex on the results of an ankle plantar-flexor manual muscle test. *Phys Ther.* 2005;85:1078–1084.

149. De Ridder R, Witvrouw E, Dolphens M, et al. Hip strength as an intrinsic risk factor for lateral ankle sprains in youth soccer players: a 3-season prospective study. *Am J Sports Med.* 2017;45(2):410–416.

150. Richie DH, Izadi FE. Return to play after an ankle sprain: guidelines for the podiatric physician. *Clin Podiatr Med Surg.* 2015;32(2):195–215.

151. Plisky PJ, Rauh MJ, Kaminski TW, Underwood FB. Star excursion balance test as a predictor of lower extremity injury in high school basketball players. *J Orthop Sports Phys Ther.* 2006;36(12):911–919.

152. Gribble PA, Hertel J. Considerations for normalizing measures of the star excursion balance test. *Measure Phys Educ Exerc Sci.* 2003;7(2):89–100.

153. Hertel J, Braham RA, Hale SA, Olmsted-Kramer LC. Simplifying the Star Excursion Balance Test: analyses of subjects with and without chronic ankle instability. *J Orthop Sports Phys Ther.* 2006;36(3):131–137.

154. Gribble PA, Hertel J, Plisky P. Using the Star Excursion Balance Test to assess dynamic postural-control deficits and outcomes in lower extremity injury: a literature and systematic review. *J Athl Train.* 2012;47(3):339–357.

155. Wikstrom EA, Tillman MD, Borsa PA. Detection of dynamic stability deficits in subjects with functional ankle instability. *Med Sci Sports Exerc.* 2005;37(2):169–175.

156. Buchanan AS, Docherty CL, Schrader J. Functional performance testing in participants with functional ankle instability and in a healthy control group. *J Athl Train.* 2008;43(4):342–346.

157. Linens SW, Ross SE, Arnold BL, et al. Postural-stability tests that identify individuals with chronic ankle instability. *J Athl Train.* 2014;49(1):15–23.

158. Sharma N, Sharma A, Sandu JS. Functional performance testing in athletes with functional ankle instability. *Asian J Sports Med.* 2011;2(4):249–258.

159. Docherty CL, Arnold BL, Gansneder BM, et al. Functional-performance deficits in volunteers with functional ankle instability. *J Athl Train.* 2005;40(1):30–34.

160. Eechaute C, Vaes P, Duquet W. Functional performance deficits in patients with chronic ankle instability: validity of the multiple hop test. *Clin J Sports Med.* 2008;18:124–129.

161. Eechaute C, Vaes P, Duquet W. The dynamic postural control is impaired in patients with chronic ankle instability: reliability and validity of the multiple hop test. *Clin J Sports Med.* 2009;19(2):107–114.

162. Mubarak S, Hargens A. *Exertional Compartment Syndromes, American Association of Orthopaedic Surgeons, Symposium on the Foot and Leg in Running Sports.* St Louis: CV Mosby; 1982.

163. Reneman RS. The anterior and the lateral compartmental syndrome of the leg due to intensive use of muscles. *Clin Orthop.* 1975;113:69–80.

164. Freeman MAR, Dean MRE, Hanham IWF. The etiology and prevention of functional instability of the foot. *J Bone Joint Surg Br.* 1965;47:678–685.

165. Docherty CL, Valovich McLeod TC, Schultz SJ. Postural control deficits in participants with functional ankle instability as measured by the balance error scoring system. *Clin J Sports Med.* 2006;16(3):203–208.

166. Kaikkonen A, Kannus P, Jarvinen M. A performance test protocol and scoring scale for the evaluation of ankle injuries. *Am J Sports Med.* 1994;22:462–469.

167. Sierevelt IN, Zwiers R, Schats W, et al. Measurement properties of the most commonly used foot- and ankle-specific questionnaires: the FFI, FAOS and FAAM. A systematic review. *Knee Surg Sports Traumatol Arthrosc.* 2018;26(7):2059–2073.

168. Martin RL, Irrgang JJ, Burdett RG, et al. Evidence of validity for the foot and ankle ability measure (FAAM). *Foot Ankle Int.* 2005;26:968–983.

169. Eechaute C, Vaes P, van Aerschot L, et al. The clinimetric qualities of patient-assessed instruments for measuring chronic ankle instability: a systematic review. *BMC Musculoskel Disord.* 2007;8(6–17).

170. Houston MN, Hoch JM, Gabriner ML, et al. Clinical and laboratory measures associated with health-related quality of life in individuals with chronic ankle instability. *Physical Therapy in Sport.* 2015;16:169–175.

171. *FAOS (Foot and Ankle Outcome Score) User's Guide.* 2003. Access at: http://www.koos.nu/FAOSGuide2003.pdf.

172. Rozzi SL, Lephart SM, Scott M, et al. Balance training for persons with functionally unstable ankles. *J Orthop Sports Phys Ther.* 1999;29:478–486.

173. Roos EM, Brandsson S, Karlsson J. Validation of the foot and ankle outcome score for ankle ligament reconstruction. *Foot Ankle Int.* 2001;22:788–794.

174. Budiman-Mak E, Conrad KJ, Roach KE. The foot function index: a measure of foot pain and disability. *J Clin Epidemiol.* 1991;44:561–570.

175. Martin RL, Irrgang JJ. A survey of self-reported outcome instruments for the foot and ankle. *J Orthop Sports Phys Ther.* 2007;37(2):72–84.

176. Bennett PJ, Patterson C, Wearing S, Baglioni T. Development and validation of a questionnaire designed to measure foot-health status. *J Am Podiatr Med Assoc.* 1998;88(9):419–428.

177. Landorf KB, Radford JA. Minimal important difference: values for the Foot Health Status Questionnaire, Foot Function Index and Visual Analogue Scale. *The Foot.* 2008;18(1):15–19.

178. Budiman-Mak E, Conrad KJ, Mazza J, Stuck RM. A review of the Foot Function Index and the Foot Function Index – Revised. *J Foot Ankle Res.* 2013;6:5–42.

179. Budiman-Mak E, Conrad K, Stuck R, Matters M. Theoretical model and Rasch analysis to develop a revised Foot Function Index. *Foot Ankle Int.* 2006;27(7):519–527.

180. Agel J, Beskin JL, Brage M, et al. Reliability of the Foot Function Index: a report of the AOFAS Outcomes Committee. *Foot Ankle Int.* 2005;26(11):962–967.

181. Hale SA, Hertel J. Reliability and sensitivity of the Foot and Ankle Disability Index in subjects with chronic ankle instability. *J Athl Train.* 2004;40:35–40.

182. Barnett S, Campbell R, Harvey I. The Bristol Foot Score: developing a patient-based foot-health measure. *J Am Podiatr Med Assoc.* 2005;95(3):264–272.

183. Jia Y, Huang H, Gagnier JJ. A systematic review of measurement properties of patient-reported outcome measures for use in patients with foot or ankle diseases. *Qual Life Res.* 2017;26(8):1969–2010.

184. Morley D, Jenkinson C, Doll H, et al. The Manchester-Oxford Questionnaire (MOXFQ): development and validation of a summary index score. *Bone J Res.* 2013;2(4):66–69.

185. Schrier JC, Palmen LN, Verheyen CC, et al. Patient-reported outcome measures in hallux valgus surgery. A review of the literature. *Foot Ankle Surg.* 2015;21(1):11–15.

186. Riskowski JL, Hagedorn TJ, Hannan MT. Measures of foot function, foot health and foot pain. *Arthritis Care Res.* 2011;63(11):S229–S239.

187. Farndon L, Barnes A, Littlewood K, et al. Clinical audit of core podiatry treatment in the NHS. *J Foot Ankle Res.* 2009;2:7–13.

188. Macran S, Kind P, Collingwood J, et al. Evaluating podiatry services: testing a treatment specific measure of health status. *Qual Life Res.* 2003;12(2):177–188.

189. Croft S, Wing KJ, Daniels TR, et al. Association of ankle arthritis score with need for revision surgery. *Foot Ankle Int.* 2017;38(9):939–943.

190. Rodrigues RC, Masiero D, Mizusaki JM, et al. Translation, cultural adaptation and validation of the "American Orthopedic Foot and Ankle Society's (AOFAS) Ankle-Hindfoot Scale". *Acta Ortop Bras.* 2008;16(2):107–111.

191. Cook JJ, Cook EA, Rosenblum BI, et al. Validation of the American College of Foot and Ankle Surgeons Scoring Scales. *J Foot Ankle Surg.* 2011;50(4):420–429.

192. Schepers T, Heetveld MJ, Mulder PG, Patka P. Clinical outcome scoring of intra-articular calcaneal fractures. *J Foot Ankle Surg.* 2008;47(3):213–218.

193. Baumhauer JF, Nawoczenski DA, DiGiovanni BF, Wilding GE. Reliability and validity of the American Orthopedic Foot and Ankle Society Clinical Rating Scale: a pilot study for the hallux and lesser toes. *Foot Ankle Int.* 2006;27(12):1014–1019.

194. Kitaoka HB, Alexander IJ, Adelaar RS, et al. Clinical rating systems for the ankle-hindfoot, midfoot, hallux and lesser toes. *Foot Ankle Int.* 1994;15(7):349–353.

195. Hunt KJ, Hurwit D. Use of patient-reported outcome measures in foot and ankle research. *J Bone Joint Surg Am.* 2013;95(16):e118 (1–9).

196. Chan HY, Chen JY, Zainul-Abidin S, et al. Minimal clinically important differences for American Orthopedic Foot and Ankle Society Score in Hallux Valgus Surgery. *Foot Ankle Int.* 2017;38(5):551–557.

197. Ross SE, Guskiewicz KM, Gross MT, Yu B. Assessment tools for identifying functional limitations associated with functional ankle instability. *J Athl Train.* 2008;43(1):44–50.

198. Simon J, Donahue M, Docherty C. Development of the Identification of Functional Ankle Instability (IdFAI). *Foot Ankle Int.* 2012;33(9):755–763.

199. Gurav RS, Ganu SS, Panhale VP. Reliability of the Identification of Functional Ankle Instability (IdFAI) Scale across different age groups in adults. *N Am J Med Sci.* 2014;6(10):516–518.

200. Donahue M, Simon J, Docherty CL. Reliability and validity of a new questionnaire created to establish the presence of functional ankle instability: the IdFAI. *Athl Train Sports Health Care.* 2013;5(1):38–43.

201. Williams GN, Molloy JM, DeBerardino TM, et al. Evaluation of the sports ankle-rating system in young, athletic individuals with acute lateral ankle sprains. *Foot Ankle Int.* 2003;24:274–282.

202. Docherty CL, Gansneder BM, Arnold BL, Hurwitz SR. Development and reliability of the Ankle Instability Instrument. *J Athl Train.* 2006;41(2):154–158.

203. Hiller CE, Refshauge KM, Bundy AC, et al. The Cumberland ankle instability tool: a report of validity and reliability testing. *Arch Phys Med Rehabil.* 2006;87:1235–1241.

204. Donahue M, Simon J, Docherty CL. Critical review of self-reported functional ankle instability measures. *Foot Ankle Int.* 2011;32(12):1140–1146.

205. Koltsov JC, Greenfield ST, Soukup D, et al. Validation of patient-reported outcomes measurement information system computerized adaptive tests against the Foot and Ankle Outcome Score for 6 common foot and ankle pathologies. *Foot Ankle Int.* 2017;38(8):870–878.

206. Robinson JM, Cook JL, Purdam C, et al. The VISA-A questionnaire: a valid and reliable index of the clinical severity of Achilles tendinopathy. *Br J Sports Med.* 2001;35(5):335–341.

207. Pinsker E, Inrig T, Daniels TR, et al. Reliability and validity of 6 measures of pain, function, and disability for ankle arthroplasty and arthrodesis. *Foot Ankle Int.* 2015;36(6):617–625.

208. Shultz S, Olszewski A, Ramsey O, et al. A systematic review of outcome tools used to measure lower leg conditions. *Int J Sports Phys Ther.* 2013;8(6):838–848.

209. Seligson D, Gassman J, Pope M. Ankle instability: evaluation of the lateral ligaments. *Am J Sports Med.* 1980;8:39–42.

210. Hildebrand KA, Buckley RE, Mohtadi NG, et al. Functional outcome measures after displaced intra-articular calcaneal fractures. *J Bone Joint Surg Br.* 1996;75:119–123.

211. Merchant TC, Dietz FR. Long-term follow up after fractures of the tibial and fibular shafts. *J Bone Joint Surg Am.* 1989;71:599–606.

212. Olerud C, Molander H. A scoring scale for symptom evaluation after ankle fracture. *Arch Orthop Trauma Surg.* 1984;103:190–194.

213. Stafford PW, Hart DL, Binkley JM, et al. Interpreting lower extremity functional status scores. *Physiother Can.* 2005;57:154–162.

214. Halasi T, Kynsburg A, Tallay A, et al. Development of a new activity score for the evaluation of ankle instability. *Am J Sports Med.* 2004;32:899–908.

215. Domsic RT, Saltzman CL. Ankle arthritis scale. *Foot Ankle Int.* 1998;19:466–471.

216. Andre M, Hagelberg S, Stenstrom CH. The juvenile arthritis foot disability index: development and evaluation of measurement properties. *J Rheum.* 2004;31:2488–2493.

217. Heffernan G, Knan F, Awan N, et al. A comparison of outcome scores in os calcis fractures. *Irish J Med Sci.* 2000;169:127–128.

218. Rowan K. The development and validation of a multidimensional measure of chronic foot pain: the Rowan foot pain assessment questionnaire. *Foot Ankle Int.* 2001;22:795–809.

219. Bushman TT, Grier TL, Canham-Chervak M, et al. The Functional Movement Screen and Injury Risk: association and predictive value in active men. *Am J Sports Med.* 2016;44(2):297–303.

220. Gribble PA, Terada m, Beard MQ, et al. Prediction of lateral ankle sprains in football players based on clinical tests and body mass index. *Am J Sports Med.* 2016;44(2):460–467.

221. Silvers-Granelli H, Mandelbaum B, Adeniji O, et al. Efficacy of the FIFA 11+ Injury Prevention Program in the collegiate male soccer player. *Am J Sports Med.* 2015;43(11):2628–2637.

222. Jarvis HL, Nester CJ, Bowden PD, Jones RK. Challenging the foundations of the clinical model of foot function: further evidence that the root model assessments fail to appropriately classify foot function. *J Foot Ankle Res.* 2017;10:7–18.

223. Harradine P, Gates L, Bowen C. If it doesn't work, why do we still do it? The continuing use of subtalar joint neutral theory in the face of overpowering critical research. *J Orthop Sports Phys Ther.* 2018;48(3):130–132.

224. Astrom M, Arvidson T. Alignment and joint motion in the normal foot. *J Orthop Sports Phys Ther.* 1995;22:216–222.

225. Vaes PH, Duquet W, Casteleyn PP, et al. Static and dynamic roentgenographic analysis of ankle stability in braced and non-braced stable and functionally unstable ankle. *Am J Sports Med.* 1998;26:692–702.

226. Roy S, Irvin R. *Sports Medicine: Prevention, Evaluation, Management and Rehabilitation.* Englewood Cliffs, NJ: Prentice-Hall; 1983.

227. Mueller MJ, Host JV, Norton BJ. Navicular drop as a composite measure of excessive pronation. *J Am Pod Med Assoc.* 1993;83:198–202.

228. Shrader JA, Poporich JM, Gracey GC, et al. Navicular drop measurement in people with rheumatoid arthritis: interrater and intrarater reliability. *Phys Ther.* 2005;85:656–664.

229. Loudon JK, Jenkins W, Loudon KL. The relationships between static posture and ACL injury in female athletes. *J Orthop Sports Phys Ther.* 1996;24:91–97.

230. Picciano AM, Rowlando MS, Worrell T. Reliability of open and closed kinetic chain subtalar joint neutral positions and navicular drop test. *J Orthop Sports Phys Ther.* 1993;18:553–558.

231. Dicharry JM, Franz JR, Croce UD, et al. Differences in static and dynamic movements in evaluation of talonavicular mobility in gait. *J Orthop Sports Phys Ther.* 2009;39:628–634.

232. McPoil TG, Cornwall MW, Medoff L, et al. Arch height change during sit-to-stand: an alternative for the navicular drop test. *J Foot Ankle Res.* 2009;2:17–24.

233. Buchanan KR, Davis I. The relationship between the forefoot, midfoot, and rearfoot static alignment in pain-free individuals. *J Orthop Sports Phys Ther.* 2005;35:559–566.

234. Keenan AM, Redmond AC, Horton M, et al. The Foot Posture Index: Rasch analysis of a novel, foot-specific outcome measure. *Arch Phys Med Rehabil.* 2007;88(1):88–93.

235. Younger AS, Hansen ST. Adult cavovarus foot. *J Am Acad Orthop Surg.* 2005;13:302–315.

236. Staheli LT, Corbett M, Wyss C, et al. Lower extremity rotational problems in children: normal values to guide management. *J Bone Joint Surg Am.* 1985;67:39–47.

237. Staheli LT. Rotational problems of the lower extremities. *Orthop Clin North Am.* 1987;18:503–512.

238. Johnson KA. Posterior tibial tendon. In: Baxter DE, ed. *The Foot and Ankle in Sport.* St Louis: Mosby; 1995.

239. Pell RF, Khanuja HS, Cooley GR. Leg pain in the running athlete. *J Am Acad Orthop Surg.* 2004;12:396–404.

240. Lindstrand A. New aspects in the diagnosis of lateral ankle sprains. *Orthop Clin North Am.* 1976;7:247–249.

241. Hollis JM, Blasier RD, Flahiff CM. Simulated ankle ligamentous injury: change in ankle stability. *Am J Sports Med.* 1995;23:672–677.

242. Trojian TH, McKeag DB. Ankle sprains: expedient assessment and management. *Phys Sportsmed.* 1998;26(10):29–40.

243. Frost HM, Hanson CA. Technique for testing the drawer sign in the ankle. *Clin Orthop.* 1977;123:49–51.

244. Birrer RB, Cartwright TJ, Denton JR. Immediate diagnosis of ankle trauma. *Phys Sportmed.* 1994;22:95–102.

245. Tohyama H, Yasuda K, Ohkoshi Y, et al. Anterior drawer test for acute anterior talofibular ligament injuries of the ankle: how much load should be applied during the test? *Am J Sports Med.* 2003;31:226–232.

246. Parasher RK, Nagy DR, Em AL, et al. Clinical measurement of mechanical ankle instability. *Manual Therapy.* 2012;17:470–473.

247. Aradi AJ, Wong J, Walsh M. The dimple sign of a ruptured lateral ligament of the ankle: brief report. *J Bone Joint Surg Br.* 1988;70:327–328.

248. Davis PF, Trevino SG. Ankle injuries. In: Baxter DE, ed. *The Foot and Ankle in Sport.* St Louis: Mosby; 1995.

249. Hockenbury RT, Sammarco GJ. Evaluation and treatment of ankle sprains: clinical recommendations for a positive outcome. *Phys Sportsmed.* 2001;24(2):57–64.

250. Kjaersgaard-Andersen P, Frich LH, Madsen F, et al. Instability of the hindfoot after lesion of the lateral ankle ligaments: investigations of the anterior drawer and adduction maneuvers in autopsy specimens. *Clin Orthop.* 1991;266:170–179.

251. Colter JM. Lateral ligamentous injuries of the ankle. In: Hamilton WC, ed. *Traumatic Disorders of the Ankle.* New York: Springer-Verlag; 1984.

252. Hamilton WC. Anatomy. In: Hamilton WC, ed. *Traumatic Disorders of the Ankle.* New York: Springer-Verlag; 1984.

253. Rasmussen O, Tovberg-Jensen I. Anterolateral rotational instability in the ankle joint. *Acta Orthop Scand.* 1981;52:99–102.

254. Miller AG, Myers SH, Parks BG, Guyton GP. Anterolateral drawer versus anterior drawer test for ankle instability: a biomechanical model. *Foot Ankle Int.* 2016;37(4):407–410.

255. Peng JR. Solving the dilemma of the high ankle sprain in the athlete. *Sports Med Arthro Rev.* 2000;8:316–325.

256. Cotton FJ. *Fractures and Fracture-Dislocations.* Philadelphia: WB Saunders; 1910.

257. Kor A. Dynamic techniques for clinical assessment of the athlete. *Clin Podiatr Med Surg.* 2015;32(2):217–229.

258. Beumer A, Swierstra BA, Mulder PG. Clinical diagnosis of syndesmotic ankle instability: evaluation of stress tests behind the curtain. *Acta Orthop Scand.* 2002;73:667–669.

259. Stiehl JB. Complex ankle fracture dislocations with syndesmotic diastasis. *Ortho Rev.* 1990;19:499–507.

260. Adamson C, Cymet T. Ankle sprains: evaluation, treatment, rehabilitation. *Maryland Med J.* 1997;46:530–537.

261. Stoffel K, Wysocki D, Baddour E, et al. Comparison of two intraoperative assessment methods for injuries to the ankle syndesmosis. *J Bone Joint Surg Am.* 2009;91:2646–2652.

262. Lin CF, Gross MT, Weinfeld P. Ankle syndesmosis injuries: anatomy, biomechanics, mechanism of injury, and clinical guidelines for diagnosis and intervention. *J Orthop Sports Phys Ther.* 2006;36:372–384.

263. Kiter E, Bukurt M. The crossed-leg test for examination of ankle syndesmosis injuries. *Foot Ankle Int.* 2005;26:187–188.

264. Alonso A, Khoury L, Adams R. Clinical tests for ankle syndesmosis injury: reliability and prediction of return to function. *J Orthop Sports Phys Ther.* 1998;27:276–284.

265. Taylor DC, Engelhardt DL, Bassett FH. Syndesmosis sprains of the ankle. The influence of heterotopic ossification. *Am J Sports Med.* 1992;20:146–150.

266. Brosky T, Nyland J, Nitz A, et al. The ankle ligaments: consideration of syndesmotic injury and implications for rehabilitation. *J Orthop Sports Phys Ther.* 1995;21:197–205.

267. Nussbaum ED, Hosea TM, Sieler SD, et al. Prospective evaluation of syndesmotic ankle sprains without diastasis. *Am J Sports Med.* 2001;29:31–35.

268. Boytim MJ, Fischer DA, Neuman L. Syndesmotic ankle sprains. *Am J Sports Med.* 1991;19:294–298.

269. Wright RW, Barile RJ, Surprenant DA, et al. Ankle syndesmosis sprains in national hockey league players. *Am J Sports Med.* 2004;32:1941–1945.

270. Sman AD, Hiller CE, Refshauge KM. Diagnostic accuracy of clinical tests for diagnosis of ankle syndesmosis injury: a systematic review. *Br J Sports Med.* 2013;47(10):620–628.

271. D'Hooghe P, Alkhelaifi K, Abdelatif N, Kaux JF. From "low" to "high" athletic ankle sprains: a comprehensive review. *Oper Tech Orthop.* 2018;28(2):54–60.

272. Cook CE, Hegedus EJ. *Orthopedic Physical Examination Tests—An Evidence Based Approach.* Upper Saddle River, NJ: Prentice Hall/Pearson; 2008.

273. Lindenfeld T, Parikh S. Clinical tip: heel-thump test for syndesmotic ankle sprain. *Foot Ankle Int.* 2005;26:406–408.

274. Gungor T. A test for ankle instability: brief report. *J Bone Joint Surg Br.* 1988;70:487.

275. Trojian TH, McKeag DB. Single leg balance test to identify risk of ankle sprains. *Br J Sports Med.* 2006;40(7):610–613.

276. Hopkinson WJ, St Pierre P, Ryan JB, et al. Syndesmosis sprains of the ankle. *Foot Ankle.* 1990;10:325–330.

277. Norkus SA, Floyd RT. The anatomy and mechanisms of syndesmotic ankle sprains. *J Athletic Train.* 2001;36:68–73.

278. Mennell JM. *Foot Pain.* Boston: Little, Brown; 1969.

279. Newman P, Adams R, Waddington G. Two simple clinical tests for predicting onset of medial tibial stress syndrome: shin palpation test and shin oedema test. *Br J Sports Med.* 2012;46(12):861–864.

280. Kinoshita M, Okuda R, Morikawa J, et al. The dorsiflexion-eversion test for diagnosis of tarsal tunnel syndrome. *J Bone Joint Surg Am.* 2001;83(12):1835–1839.

281. Tatro-Adams D, McGann S, Carbone W. Reliability of the figure-of-eight method of ankle measurement. *J Orthop Sports Phys Ther.* 1995;22:161–163.

282. Petersen EJ, Irish SM, Lyons CL, et al. Reliability of water volumetry and the figure of eight method on subjects with ankle joint swelling. *J Orthop Sports Phys Ther.* 1999;29:609–615.

283. Mawdsley RH, Hoy DK, Erwin PM. Criterion-related validity of the figure of eight method of measuring ankle edema. *J Orthop Sports Phys Ther.* 2000;30:149–153.

284. Pugia ML, Middel CJ, Seward SW, et al. Comparison of acute swelling and function in subjects with lateral ankle injury. *J Orthop Sports Phys Ther.* 2001;31:384–388.

285. Rohner-Spengler M, Mannion AF, Babst R. Reliability and minimal detectable change for the figure-of-eight-20 method of measurement of ankle edema. *J Orthop Sports Phys Ther.* 2007;37:199–205.

286. Payne C, Chuter V, Miller K. Sensitivity and specificity of the functional hallux limitus test to predict foot function. *J Am Podiatr Med Assoc.* 2002;92:269–271.

287. Cleland JA, Koppenhaver S. *Netter's Orthopedic Clinical Examination—An Evidence-Based Approach.* 2nd ed. Philadelphia: Saunders/Elsevier; 2011.

288. Wallace LA. Limb length difference and back pain. In: Grieve GP, ed. *Modern Manual Therapy of the Vertebral Column.* Edinburgh: Churchill Livingstone; 1986.

289. Gurney B. Leg length discrepancy. *Gait Posture.* 2002;15(2):195–206.

290. O'Toole GC, Makwana NK, Lunn J, et al. The effect of leg length discrepancy on foot loading patterns and contact times. *Foot Ankle Int.* 2003;24(3):256–259.

291. Maffulli N. The clinical diagnosis of subcutaneous tear of the achilles tendon. *Am J Sports Med.* 1998;26:266–270.

292. Blood SD. Treatment of the sprained ankle. *J Am Osteopathic Assoc.* 1980;79:680–692.

293. Safran MR, O'Malley D, Fu FH. Peroneal tendon subluxation in athletes: new exam technique, case reports and review. *Med Sci Sports Exerc.* 1999;31:S487–S496.

294. Thompson T, Doherty J. Spontaneous rupture of the tendon of Achilles: a new clinical diagnostic test. *Anat Res.* 1967;158:126–129.

295. Scott BW, Al-Chalabi A. How the Simmonds-Thompson test works. *J Bone Joint Surg Br.* 1992;74:314–315.

296. Simmonds FA. The diagnosis of a ruptured Achilles tendon. *Practitioner.* 1957;179:56–58.

297. Thompson TC. A test for rupture of the tendoachilles. *Acta Orthop Scand.* 1962;32:461–465.

298. Abouelela AA, Zohiery AK. The triple compression stress test for diagnosis of tarsal tunnel syndrome. *Foot (Edinb).* 2012;22(3):146–149.

299. Garceau DD, Bean D, Requejo SM, et al. The association between diagnosis of plantar fasciitis and Windlass test results. *Foot Ankle Int.* 2003;24:251–255.

300. Rose GK, Welton EA, Marshall T. The diagnosis of flat foot in the child. *J Bone Joint Surg Br.* 1985;67(1):71–78.

301. Bowditch MG, Sanderson P, Livesey JP. The significance of an absent ankle reflex. *J Bone Joint Surg Br.* 1996;78:276–279.

302. Bassetti C. Babinski and Babinski's sign. *Spine.* 1995;20:2591–2594.

303. Wilton JP. Lower extremity focused neurologic examination. *Clin Podiatr Med Surg.* 2016;33(2):191–202.

304. Chusid JG, McDonald JJ. *Correlative Neuroanatomy and Functional Neurology.* Los Altos, CA: Lange Medical Publications; 1967.

305. Schon LC, Baxter DE. Neuropathies of the foot and ankle in athletes. *Clin Sports Med.* 1990;9:489–509.

306. Zengzhao L, Jiansheng Z, Li Z. Anterior tarsal tunnel syndrome. *J Bone Joint Surg Br.* 1991;73:470–473.

307. Pecina MM, Krmpotic-Nemanic J, Markiewitz AD. *Tunnel Syndromes.* Boca Raton, FL: CRC Press; 1991.

308. Wechsler LR, Busis NA. Sports neurology. In: Fu FH, Stone DA, eds. *Sports Injuries: Mechanisms, Prevention, Treatment.* Baltimore: Williams & Wilkins; 1994.

309. Baxter DE. Functional nerve disorders. In: Baxter DE, ed. *The Foot and Ankle in Sport.* St Louis: Mosby; 1995.

310. Beskin JL. Nerve entrapment syndromes of the foot and ankle. *J Am Acad Orthop Surg.* 1997;5:261–269.

311. Roscoe D, Roberts AJ, Hulse D. Intramuscular compartment pressure measurement in chronic exertional compartment syndrome: new and improved diagnostic criteria. *Am J Sports Med.* 2015;43(2):392–398.

312. Sidey JD. Weak ankles: a study of common peroneal entrapment neuropathy. *Br Med J.* 1969;3:623–626.

313. Nitz AJ, Dobner JJ, Kersey D. Nerve injury and grades II and III ankle sprains. *Am J Sports Med.* 1985;13:177–182.

314. Kleinrensink GJ, Stoeckart R, Meulstee J, et al. Lowered motor conduction velocity of the peroneal nerve after inversion trauma. *Med Sci Sports Exerc.* 1994;26:877–883.

315. Schon LC, Clanton TO. Chronic leg pain. In: Baxter DE, ed. *The Foot and Ankle in Sport.* St Louis: Mosby; 1995.

316. Styf J. Entrapment of the superficial peroneal nerve: diagnosis and results of decompression. *J Bone Joint Surg Br.* 1989;71:131–135.

317. Pahor S, Toppenberg R. An investigation of neural tissue involvement in ankle inversion sprains. *Man Ther.* 1996;1:192–197.

318. Winkes MB, van Zantvoort AP, de Bruijn JA, et al. Fasciotomy for deep posterior compartment syndrome in the lower leg: a prospective study. *Am J Sports Med.* 2016;44(5):1309–1316.

319. Romani W, Perrin DH, Whiteley T. Tarsal tunnel syndrome: case study of a male collegiate athlete. *J Sports Rehab.* 1997;6:364–370.

320. Kinoshita M, Okuda R, Abe M. Tarsal tunnel syndrome and athletes. *Am J Sports Med.* 2006;34:1307–1312.

321. Gould JS. Recurrent tarsal tunnel syndrome. *Foot Ankle Clin.* 2014;19(3):451–467.

322. Kaplan PE, Kernahan WT. Tarsal tunnel syndrome: an electrodiagnostic and surgical correlation. *J Bone Joint Surg Am.* 1981;63:96–99.

323. Massey EW, Plett AB. Neuropathy in joggers. *Am J Sports Med.* 1978;6:209–211.

324. Murphy PC, Baxter DE. Nerve entrapment of the foot and ankle in runners. *Clin Sports Med.* 1985;4:753–763.

325. Takakura Y, Kitada C, Sugimoto K, et al. Tarsal tunnel syndrome: causes and results of operative treatment. *J Bone Joint Surg Br.* 1991;73:125–128.

326. Stefko RM, Lauerman WC, Heckman JD. Tarsal tunnel syndrome caused by an unrecognized fracture of the posterior process of the talus (Cedell fracture). *J Bone Joint Surg Am.* 1994;76:116–118.

327. Trepman E. Tarsal tunnel syndrome following Achilles tendon injury in dancers: two cases. *Clin J Sports Med.* 1993;3:192–194.

328. Jackson DL, Haglund BL. Tarsal tunnel syndrome in runners. *Sports Med.* 1992;13:146–149.

329. Mann RA. Entrapment neuropathies of the foot. In: DeLee JC, Drez D, eds. *Orthopedic Sports Medicine: Principles and Practice.* Philadelphia: WB Saunders; 1994.

330. Sammarco GJ, Chalk DE, Feibel JH. Tarsal tunnel syndrome and additional nerve lesions in the same limb. *Foot Ankle.* 1993;14:71–77.

331. Jackson DL, Haglund B. Tarsal tunnel syndrome in athletes: case reports and literature review. *Am J Sports Med.* 1991;19:61–65.

332. Rask MR. Medial plantar neuropraxia (jogger's foot): report of three cases. *Clin Orthop.* 1978;134:193–195.

333. Pfeffer GB. Plantar heel pain. In: Baxter DE, ed. *The Foot and Ankle in Sport.* St Louis: Mosby; 1995.

334. Johnson ER, Kirby K, Lieberman JS. Lateral plantar nerve entrapment: foot pain in the power lifter. *Am J Sports Med.* 1992;20:619–620.

335. House JA, Ahmed K. Entrapment neuropathy of the infrapatellar branch of the saphenous nerve. *Am J Sports Med.* 1977;5:217–224.

336. Kaltenborn FM. *Mobilization of the Extremity Joints.* Oslo: Olaf Norlis Bokhandel; 1980.

337. Richardson EG. Hallucal sesamoid pain: causes and surgical treatment. *J Am Acad Orthop Surg.* 1999;7:270–278.

338. Koulouris G, Morrison WB. Foot and ankle disorders: radiographic signs. *Semin Roentgenol.* 2005;40(4):358–379.

339. Arunakul M, Amendola A, Gao Y, et al. Tripod index: a new radiologic parameter assessing foot alignment. *Foot Ankle Int.* 2013;34(10):1411–1420.

340. Miller CP, Ghorbanhoseini M, Ehrlichman LK, et al. High variability of observed weight bearing during standing foot and ankle radiographs. *Foot Ankle Int.* 2017;38(6):690–693.

341. Thordarson DB. Detecting and treating common foot and ankle fractures. Part 1: the ankle and hindfoot. *Phys Sportsmed.* 1996;24(9):29–38.

342. Thordarson DB. Detecting and treating common foot and ankle fractures. Part 2: the midfoot and forefoot. *Phys Sportsmed.* 1996;24(10):58–64.

343. Egol KA, Amirtharage M, Tejwani NC, et al. Ankle stress test for predicting the need for surgical fixation of isolated fibular fractures. *J Bone Joint Surg Am.* 2004;86:2393–2398.

344. Springer BA, Arceiro RA, Tenuta JJ, et al. A prospective study of modified Ottawa rules in a military population—interobserver agreement between physical therapists and orthopedic surgeons. *Am J Sports Med.* 2000;28:864–868.

345. Stiell IG, Greenberg GH, McKnight RD, et al. Decision rules for the use of radiography in acute ankle injuries: refinement and prospective validation. *JAMA.* 1993;269:1127–1132.

346. Stiell IG, McKnight RD, Greenberg GH, et al. Implementation of the Ottawa ankle rules. *JAMA.* 1994;271:827–832.

347. Stiell IG, Greenberg GH, McKnight RD, et al. A study to develop clinical decision rules for the use of radiography in acute ankle injuries. *Ann Emerg Med.* 1992;21:384–390.

348. Bachman LM, Kolb E, Koller MT, et al. Accuracy of Ottawa ankle rules to exclude fractures of the ankle and midfoot: systematic review. *Br Med J.* 2003;326:417–424.

349. Heyworth J. Ottawa ankle rules for the injured ankle. *Br Med J.* 2003;326:405–406.

350. Myers A, Canty K, Nelson T. Are the Ottawa ankle rules helpful in ruling out the need for x-ray examination in children? *Arch Dis Child.* 2005;90(12):1309–1311.

351. Beckenkamp PR, Lin CC, Macaskill P, et al. Diagnostic accuracy of the Ottawa Ankle and Midfoot Rules: a systematic review with meta-analysis. *Br J Sports Med.* 2017;51(6):504–510.

352. Leddy JJ, Smolinski RJ, Lawrence J, et al. Prospective evaluation of the Ottawa ankle rules in a university sports medicine centre—with a modification to increase specificity for identifying malleolar fractures. *Am J Sports Med.* 1998;26:158–165.

353. Derksen RJ, Knijnenberg LM, Fransen G, et al. Diagnostic performance of the Bernese versus Ottawa ankle rules: results of a randomized controlled trial. *Injury.* 2015;46(8):1645–1649.

354. Kose O, Gokhan S, Ozhasenekler A, et al. Comparison of Ottawa Ankle Rules and Bernese Ankle Rules in acute ankle and midfoot injuries. *Turk J Emerg Med.* 2010;10(3):101–105.

355. Jonckheer P, Willems T, De Riddler R, et al. Evaluating fracture risk in acute ankle sprains: Any news since the Ottawa Ankle Rules? A systematic review. *Eur J Gen Pract.* 2016;22(1):31–41.

356. Eggli S, Sclabas GM, Eggli S, et al. The Bernese ankle rules: a fast, reliable test after low-energy, supination-type malleolar and midfoot trauma. *J Trauma.* 2005;59(5):1268–1271.

357. Glas AS, Pijnenburg BA, Lijmer JG, et al. Comparison of diagnostic decision rules and structured data collection in assessment of acute ankle injury. *Can Med Assoc J.* 2002;166(6):727–733.

358. Alluri RK, Hill JR, Donohoe S, et al. Radiographic detection of marginal impaction of supination-adduction ankle fractures. *Foot Ankle Int.* 2017;38(9):1005–1010.

359. Black H. Roentgenographic considerations. *Am J Sports Med.* 1977;5:238–240.

360. Hoffman JD. Radiography of the ankle. In: Hamilton WC, ed. *Traumatic Disorders of the Ankle.* New York: Springer-Verlag; 1984.

361. Renton P, Stripp WJ. The radiology and radiography of the foot. In: Klenerman L, ed. *The Foot and Its Disorders.* 2nd ed. Boston: Blackwell Scientific; 1982.

362. Rettig AC, Shelbourne KD, Beltz HF, et al. Radiographic evaluation of foot and ankle injuries in the athlete. *Clin Sports Med.* 1987;6:905–919.

363. Yu JS, Cody ME. A template approach for detecting fractures in adults sustaining low-energy ankle trauma. *Emerg Radiol.* 2009;16(4):309–318.

364. Zammit GV, Munteanu SF, Menz HB. Development of a diagnostic rule for identifying radiographic osteoarthritis in people with first metatarsophalangeal joint pain. *Osteoarthritis Cartilage.* 2011;19(8):939–945.

365. Menz HB, Munteanu SE, Landorf KB, et al. Radiographic classification of osteoarthritis in commonly affected joints of the foot. *Osteoarthritis Cartilage.* 2007;15(11):1333–1338.

366. Howells NR, Hughes AW, Jackson M, et al. Interobserver and intraobserver reliability assessment of calcaneal fracture classification systems. *J Foot Ankle Surg.* 2014;53(1):47–51.

367. Schepers T, van Lieshout EM, Ginai AZ, et al. Calcaneal fracture classification: a comparative study. *J Foot Ankle Surg.* 2009;48(2):156–162.

368. Koulouris G, Morrison WB. Foot and ankle disorders: radiographic signs. *Semin Roentgenol.* 2005;40(4):358–379.

369. Nielson JH, Gardner MJ, Peterson MG, et al. Radiographic measurements do not predict syndesmotic injury in ankle fractures: an MRI study. *Clin Orthop Relat Res.* 2005;436:216–221.

370. Wuest TK. Injuries to the distal lower extremity syndesmosis. *J Am Acad Orthop Surg.* 1997;5:172–181.

371. Katcherian D. Soft-tissue injuries of the ankle. In: Lutter LD, Mizel MS, Pfeffer GB, eds. *Orthopedic Knowledge Update: Foot and Ankle.* Rosemont, IL: American Academy of Orthopaedic Surgeons; 1994.

372. Kessler JI, Weiss JM, Nikizad H, et al. Osteochondritis dissecans of the ankle in children and adolescents: demographics and epidemiology. *Am J Sports Med.* 2014;42(9):2165–2171.

373. Kraeutler MJ, Chahla J, Dean CS, et al. Current concepts review update: osteochondral lesions of the talus. *Foot Ankle Int.* 2016;38(3):331–342.

374. Beumer A, van Hemert WL, Niesing R, et al. Radiographic measurement of the distal tibiofibular syndesmosis has limited use. *Clin Orthop Relat Res.* 2004;423:227–234.

375. de Cesar PC, Avila EM, de Abreu MR. Comparison of magnetic resonance imaging to physical examination for syndesmotic injury after lateral ankle sprain. *Foot Ankle Int.* 2011;32(12):1110–1114.

376. Cetti R, Andersen I. Roentgenographic diagnosis of ruptured Achilles tendon. *Clin Orthop.* 1993;286:215–221.

377. Fowler A, Philip JF. Abnormality of calcaneus as a cause of painful heel: its diagnosis and operative treatment. *Br J Surg.* 1945;32:494–498.

378. Rubin G, Witten M. The talar-tilt angle and the fibular collateral ligaments: a method for the determination of talar-tilt. *J Bone Joint Surg Am.* 1960;42:311–326.

379. Rijke AM, Jones B, Vierhout PA. Stress examination of traumatized lateral ligaments of the ankle. *Clin Orthop.* 1986;210:143–161.

380. Grace DL. Lateral ankle ligament injuries: inversion and anterior stress radiography. *Clin Orthop.* 1984;183:153–159.

381. Rijke AM. Lateral ankle sprains: graded stress radiography for accurate diagnosis. *Phys Sportsmed.* 1991;19:107–118.

382. Karlsson J, Bergsten T, Peterson L, et al. Radiographic evaluation of ankle joint stability. *Clin J Sports Med.* 1991;1:166–175.

383. Cox JS, Hewes TF. "Normal" talar tilt angle. *Clin Orthop.* 1979;140:37–41.

384. Vanderwilde R, Staheli LT, Chew DE, et al. Measurements on radiographs of the foot in normal infants and children. *J Bone Joint Surg Am.* 1988;70:407–415.

385. Banerjee R, Saltzman C, Anderson RB, et al. Management of calcaneal malunion. *J Am Acad Orthop Surg.* 2011;19:27–36.

386. Gluck GS, Heckman DS, Parekh SG. Tendon disorders of the foot and ankle. Part 3—the posterior tibial tendon. *Am J Sports Med.* 2010;38:2133–2144.

387. Klenerman L. Examination of the foot. In: Klenerman L, ed. *The Foot and Its Disorders.* 2nd ed. Boston: Blackwell Scientific; 1982.

388. Pavlov H. Ankle and subtalar arthrography. *Clin Sports Med.* 1982;1:47–49.

389. Raatikainen T, Putkanen M, Puranen J. Arthrography, clinical examination and stress radiograph in the diagnosis of acute injury to the lateral ligaments of the ankle. *Am J Sports Med.* 1992;20:2–6.

390. Gleeson AP, Stuart MJ, Wilson B, et al. Ultrasound assessment and conservative management of inversion injuries of the ankle in children. *J Bone Joint Surg Br.* 1996;78:484–487.

391. Bar-On E, Mashiach R, Inbar O, et al. Prenatal ultrasound diagnosis of club foot: outcome and recommendations for counseling and followup. *J Bone Joint Surg Br.* 2005;87:990–993.

392. Griffin MJ, Olson K, Heckmann N, Charlton TP. Realtime Achilles Ultrasound Thompson (RAUT) Test for the evaluation and diagnosis of acute Achilles tendon ruptures. *Foot Ankle Int.* 2017;38(1):36–40.

393. Wiebking U, Pacha TO, Jagodzinski M. An accuracy evaluation of clinical, arthrometric and stress-sonographic acute ankle instability examinations. *Foot Ankle Surg.* 2015;21(1):42–48.

394. Fong DT, Man CY, Yung PS, et al. Sport-related ankle injuries attending an accident and emergency department. *Injury.* 2008;39(10):1222–1227.

395. Jacobson JA. Ankle, foot, and lower leg ultrasound. In: Jacobson JA, ed. *Fundamentals of Musculoskeletal Ultrasound.* 2nd ed. Philadelphia: Elsevier; 2013.

396. Kerr R, Forrester DM, Kingston S. Magnetic resonance imaging of foot and ankle trauma. *Orthop Clin North Am.* 1990;21:591–601.

397. Terk MR, Kwong PK. Magnetic resonance imaging of the foot and ankle. *Clin Sports Med.* 1994;13:883–908.

398. Rijke AM, Gietz HT, McCue FC, et al. Magnetic resonance imaging of injury to the lateral ankle ligaments. *Am J Sports Med.* 1993;21:528–534.

399. Verhaven EF, Shahabpour M, Handelberg FW, et al. The accuracy of three-dimensional magnetic resonance imaging in the diagnosis of ruptures of the lateral ligaments of the ligament. *Am J Sports Med.* 1991;19:583–587.

400. Haygood TM. Magnetic resonance imaging of the musculoskeletal system—the ankle. *Clin Orthop Relat Res.* 1997;336:318–336.

401. Patterson MJ, Cox WK. Peroneus longus tendon rupture as a cause of chronic lateral ankle pain. *Clin Orthop Relat Res.* 1999;365:163–166.

402. Stone JW. Osteochondral lesions of the talar dome. *J Am Acad Orthop Surg.* 1996;4:63–73.

403. Lazarus ML. Imaging of the foot and ankle in the injured athlete. *Med Sci Sports Exerc.* 1999;31:S412–S420.

404. Recht MP, Donley BG. Magnetic resonance imaging of the foot and ankle. *J Am Acad Orthop Surg.* 2001;9:187–199.

405. Bresler M, Mar W, Toman J. Diagnostic imaging in the evaluation of leg pain in athletes. *Clin Sports Med.* 2012;31:217–245.

406. Baker JC, Hoover EG, Hillen TJ. Subradiographic foot and ankle fractures and bone contusions detected by MRI in elite ice hockey players. *Am J Sports Med.* 2016;44(5):1317–1323.

407. Wright AA, Hegedus EJ, Lenchik L, et al. Diagnostic accuracy of various imaging modalities for suspected lower extremity stress fractures: a systematic review with evidence-based recommendations for clinical practice. *Am J Sports Med.* 2016;44(1):255–263.

408. Jolman S, Robbins J, Lewis L, et al. Comparison of magnetic resonance imaging and stress radiographs in the evaluation of chronic lateral ankle instability. *Foot Ankle Int.* 2017;38(4):397–404.

409. Donovan A, Rosenberg ZS, Bencardino JT, et al. Plantar tendons of the foot: MR imaging and US. *RadioGraphics.* 2013;33(7):2065–2085.

410. Shindle MK, Endo Y, Warren RF, et al. Stress fractures about the tibia, foot and ankle. *J Am Acad Orthop Surg.* 2012;20(3):167–176.

411. Brodovicz KG, McNaughton K, Uemura N, et al. Reliability and feasibility of methods to quantitatively assess peripheral edema. *Clin Med Res.* 2009;7:21–31.

412. Dennis RJ, Finch CF, Elliott BC, et al. The reliability of musculoskeletal screening tests used in cricket. *Phys Ther Sport.* 2008;9:25–33.

413. Menz HB, Tiedemann A, Kwan MM, et al. Reliability of clinical tests of foot and ankle characteristics in older people. *J Am Podiatr Med Assoc.* 2003;93(5):380–387.

414. Martin RL, McPoil TG. Reliability of ankle goniometric measurements: a literature review. *J Am Podiatr Med Assoc.* 2005;95(6):564–572.

415. Greninger LO, Kark LA. The reliability of active ankle plantar flexion assessment. *Clin Kinesiol.* 2000;54(1):19–24.

416. Yildiz Y, Sekir U, Hazneci B, et al. Reliability of a functional test battery evaluating functionality, proprioception and strength of the ankle joint. *Turk J Med Sci.* 2009;1:115–123.

417. Spahn G. The ankle meter: an instrument for evaluation of anterior talar drawer in ankle sprain. *Knee Surg Sports Traumatol Arthrosc.* 2004;12:338–342.

418. Lohrer H, Nauck T, Arentz S, et al. Observer reliability in ankle and calcaneocuboid stress radiography. *Am J Sports Med.* 2008;36(6):1143–1149.

419. Phisitkul P, Chaichankul C, Sripongsai R, et al. Accuracy of anterolateral drawer test in lateral ankle instability: a cadaveric study. *Foot Ankle Int.* 2009;30(7):690–695.

420. Wilkin EG, Hunt A, Nightingale EJ, et al. Manual testing for ankle instability. *Manual Therapy.* 2012;17:593–596.

421. Docpherty CL, Rybak-Webb K. Reliability of the anterior drawer and talar tilt tests using the ligmaster joint arthrometer. *J Sport Rehabil.* 2009;18:389–397.

422. Vela L, Tourville TW, Hertel J. Physical examination of acutely injured ankles: an evidence-based approach. *Athletic Ther Today.* 2003;8(5):13–19.

423. Schwieterman B, Haas D, Columber K, et al. Diagnostic accuracy of physical examination tests of the ankle/foot complex: a systematic review. *Int J Sports Phys Ther.* 2013;8(4):416–426.

424. Croy T, Koppenhaver S, Saliba S, Hertel J. Anterior talocrural joint laxity: diagnostic accuracy of the anterior drawer test of the ankle. *J Orthop Sports Phys Ther.* 2013;43(12):911–919.

425. Menz HB, Munteanu SE. Validity of 3 clinical techniques for the measurement of static foot posture in older people. *J Orthop Sports Phys Ther.* 2005;35:479–486.

426. Friends J, Augustine E, Danoff J. A comparison of different assessment techniques for measuring foot and ankle volume in healthy adults. *J Am Podiatr Med Assoc.* 2008;98(2):85–94.

427. Eechaute C, Vaes P, Duquet W. The chronic ankle instability scale: clinimetric properties of a multidimensional, patient-assessed instrument. *Phys Ther Sport.* 2008;9:57–66.

428. Shambaugh P, Sclafani L, Fanselow AD. Reliability of the Derifeild-Thompson test for leg length inequality, and use of the test to demonstrate cervical adjusting efficacy. *J Manip Physiol Ther.* 1988;11(5):396–399.

429. Kerkhoffs GM, Blankevoort L, Sierevelt LN, et al. Two ankle joint laxity testers: reliability and validity. *Knee Surg Sports Traumatol Arthrosc.* 2005;13:699–705.

430. Kim J, Hwang SK, Lee KT, et al. A simpler device for measuring the mobility of the first ray of the foot. *Foot Ankle Int.* 2008;29(2):213–218.

431. Weaver K, Price R, Czerniecki J, et al. Design and validation of an instrument package designed to increase the reliability of ankle range of motion measurements. *J Rehabil Res Dev.* 2001;38(5):471–475.

432. Meyer DC, Werner CM, Wyss T, et al. A mechanical equinometer to measure the range of motion of the ankle joint: interobserver and intraobserver reliability. *Foot Ankle Int.* 2006;27(3):202–205.

433. Evans AM, Copper AW, Scharfbillig RW, et al. Reliability of the foot posture index and traditional measures of foot position. *J Am Podiatr Med Assoc.* 2003;93(3):203–213.

434. Jonson SR, Gross MT. Intraexaminer reliability, interexaminer reliability, and mean values for nine lower extremity skeletal measures in healthy naval midshipmen. *J Orthop Sports Phys Ther.* 1997;25(4):253–263.

435. Hubbard TJ, Kaminski TW, Vander Griend RA, et al. Quantitative assessment of mechanical laxity in the functional unstable ankle. *Med Sci Sports Exerc.* 2004;36(5):760–766.

436. Neelly K, Wallmann HW, Backus CJ. Validity of measuring leg length with a tape measure compared to a computed tomography scan. *Physiother Theory Pract.* 2013;29(6):487–492.

437. Rose KJ, Burns J, Ryan MM, et al. Reliability of quantifying foot and ankle muscle strength in very young children. *Muscle Nerve.* 2008;37:626–631.

438. Kelln BM, McKeon PO, Gontkof LM, et al. Hand-held dynamometry: reliability of lower extremity muscle testing in healthy, physically active, young adults. *J Sport Rehab.* 2008;17:160–170.

439. Möller M, Lind K, Styf J, et al. The reliability of isokinetic testing of the ankle joint and a heel-raise test for endurance. *Knee Surg Sports Traumatol Arthrosc.* 2005;13:60–71.

440. Power CM, Maffucci R, Hampton S. Rearfoot posture in subjects with patellofemoral pain. *J Orthop Sports Phys Ther.* 1995;22(4):155–160.

441. Erichsen N, Lund H, Moller JO, et al. Inter-rater and intra-rater reliability of tests of translatoric movements and range of movements in the subtalar and talocrural joints. *Adv Physiother.* 2006;8:161–167.

442. Kwon OY, Tuttle LJ, Commean PK, et al. Reliability and validity of measures of hammer toe deformity angle and tibial torsion. *The Foot.* 2009;19:149–155.

443. Rosen AB, Do J, Brown CN. Diagnostic accuracy of instrumented and manual talar tilt tests in chronic ankle instability populations. *Scand J Med Sci Sports.* 2015;25:214–221.

444. Van den Bekerom MPJ, Mutsaerts EL, Niek van Dijk C. Evaluation of the integrity of the deltoid ligament in supination external rotation ankle fractures: a systematic review. *Arch Orthop Trauma Surg.* 2009;129:227–235.

445. Cornwall MW, McPoil TG, Lebec M, et al. Reliability of the modified foot posture index. *J Am Podiatr Med Assoc.* 2008;98(1):7–13.

446. Glasoe WM, Getsoian S, Myers M, et al. Criterion-related validity of a clinical measure of dorsal first ray mobility. *J Orthop Sports Phys Ther.* 2005; 35:589–593.

447. Gaebler C, Kukla C, Breitenseher MJ, et al. Diagnosis of lateral ankle ligament injuries: comparison between talar tilt, MRI and operative findings in 112 athletes. *Acta Orthop Scand.* 1997;68(3):286–290.

448. Picciano AM, Rowlands MS, Worrel T. Reliability of open and closed kinetic chain subtalar joint neutral positions and navicular drop test. *J Orthop Sports Phys Ther.* 1993;18(4):553–558.

449. Shultz SJ, Nguyen A, Windley TC, et al. Intratester and intertester reliability of clinical measures of lower extremity anatomic characteristics: implications for multicenter studies. *Clin Sport Med.* 2006;16(2): 155–161.

450. Torbum L, Perry J, Gronley JK. Assessment of rearfoot motion: passive positioning, one-legged standing gait. *Foot Ankle Int.* 1998;19(10):688–693.

451. Smith-Oricchio K, Harris BA. Interrater reliability of subtalar neutral, calcaneal inversion and eversion. *J Orthop Sports Phys Ther.* 1990;12(1):10–15.

452. Elveru RA, Rothstein JM, Lamb RL. Goniometric reliability in a clinical setting: subtalar and ankle joint measurements. *Phys Ther.* 1988;68(5): 672–677.

453. Sell KE, Verity TM, Worrell TW, et al. Two measurement techniques for assessing subtalar joint position: a reliability study. *J Orthop Sports Phys Ther.* 1994;19:162–167.

454. Yamamoto K, Miyata T, Onozuka A, et al. Plantar flexion as an alternative to treadmill exercise for evaluating patients with intermittent claudication. *Eur J Vasc Endovasc Surg.* 2007;33:325–329.

455. Troester JC, Jasmin JG, Duffield R. Reliability of single-leg balance and landing tests in rugby union; prospect of using postural control to monitor fatigue. *J Sports Sci Med.* 2018;17(2):174–180.

456. Pieper B, Templin TN, Birk TJ, et al. The standing heel-rise test: relation to chronic venous disorders and balance, gait, and walk time injection drug users. *Ostomy Wound Manage.* 2008;54(9):18–22, 24, 26–30.

457. Burns J, Redmond A, Ouvrier R, et al. Quantification of muscle strength and imbalance in neurogenic pes cavus, compared to health controls, using hand-held dynamometry. *Foot Ankle Int.* 2005;26 (7):540–544.

CHAPTER 14

Assessment of Gait

Walking is the simple act of falling forward and catching oneself. One foot is always in contact with the ground, and within a cycle, there are two periods of single-leg support and two periods of double-leg support. With running, there is a period of time during which neither foot is in contact with the ground, a period called "double float."

Winter[1] felt that walking gait performs five main functions. First, it helps to support the head, arms, and trunk by maintaining a semirigid lower limb. Second, it helps to maintain upright posture and balance. Third, it controls the foot to allow it to clear obstacles and enables gentle heel or toe landing through eccentric muscle action. Fourth, it generates mechanical energy by concentric muscle contraction to initiate, maintain, and, if desired, increase forward velocity. Finally, through eccentric action of the muscles, it provides shock absorption and stability and decreases the forward velocity of the body.

The locomotion pattern tends to be variable and irregular until about the age of 7 years.[2] Several functional tasks are involved in gait, including forward progression, which is executed in a stepping movement in a wide range of rapid and comfortable walking speeds. Second, the body must be balanced alternately on one limb and then the other; this is accompanied by repeated adjustments of limb length. Finally, there is support of the upright body.

Gait assessment or analysis takes a great deal of time, practice, and technical skill combined with standardization for the clinician to develop the necessary skills.[3–5] Most gait analysis today is performed with force platforms to measure ground reaction forces, electromyography to measure muscle activity, and high-speed video motion analysis systems to measure movement. Discussion of these techniques, however, is beyond the scope of this book. This chapter gives only a brief overview of a complex task, which is the assessment of normal and pathological gait; detailed assessment of gait is left to other authors.[6–15] The various terms commonly used to describe gait, the normal pattern of gait, the assessment of gait, and common abnormal gaits are reviewed.

Definitions[5–10]

Gait Cycle

The **gait cycle** is the time interval or sequence of motions occurring between two consecutive initial contacts of the same foot (Fig. 14.1). It is synonymous with the stride length. For example, if heel strike is the initial contact, the gait cycle for the right leg is from one heel strike to the next heel strike on the same foot. The gait cycle is a description of what happens in one leg. The same sequence of events is repeated with the other leg, but it is 180° out of phase.[8] There are spatial descriptors of gait, such as stride length, step length, and step width; time or temporal descriptors, such as cadence, stride time, and step time; and also descriptors that involve time and space, such as walking speed.[16] Another spatial descriptor that is sometimes discussed with gait is foot angle (Fick angle; see Fig. 14.14). Each of these descriptors can and should be very similar for both limbs. For example, osteoarthritis in one hip can change many of the descriptors, and the examiner should watch for these changes. Simoneau[17] clearly described the terminology that applies to the gait cycle events (Fig. 14.2). Table 14.1 demonstrates the periods or phases of the gait cycle, the function of each phase, and what is happening in the opposite limb.[8] The gait cycle consists of two phases for each foot: **stance phase,** which makes up 60% to 65% of the walking cycle, and **swing phase,** which makes up 35% to 40% of the walking cycle. In addition, there are two periods of double support and one period of single-leg stance during the gait cycle.

As the velocity of the cycle increases, the cycle length or stride length decreases. For example, in jogging, the gait cycle is 70% of the walking cycle, and in running, the gait cycle is 60% that of walking.[18] In addition, as the speed of movement increases, the function of the muscles changes somewhat, and their electromyographic activity may increase or decrease. Generally, gait velocity decreases with age.[19,20] Montero-Odasso et al.[21] found that the gait velocity (<0.8 m/s) could be used to determine mobility impairment in the elderly.

Stance Phase

The stance phase of gait occurs when the foot is on the ground and bearing weight (Fig. 14.3). It allows the lower leg to support the weight of the body and, by so doing, acts as a shock absorber while allowing the body to advance over the supporting limb.[18] Normally, this phase

The **load response** and **midstance** instants consist of the **single-leg support** or **single-leg stance**, which accounts for the next 40% of the gait cycle. During this period, one leg alone carries the body weight while the other leg goes through its swing phase. The stance leg must be able to hold the weight of the body, and the body must be able to balance on the one leg. In addition, lateral hip stability must be exhibited to maintain balance, and the tibia of the stance leg must advance over the stationary foot.

The **terminal stance** and **preswing** instants make up the **weight-unloading period**, which accounts for the next 10% of the gait cycle. During this period, the stance leg is unloading the body weight to the contralateral limb and preparing the leg for the swing phase. As with the first two instants, both feet are in contact, so double support occurs for the second time during the gait cycle.

Swing Phase

The swing phase of gait occurs when the foot is not bearing weight and is moving forward (Fig. 14.4). The swing phase allows the toes of the swing leg to clear the floor and also allows for leg length adjustments. In addition, it allows the swing leg to advance forward. It makes up approximately 40% of the gait cycle and consists of three subphases.

Stages (Instants) of Stance Phase

- Initial contact (heel strike)
- Load response (foot flat)
- Midstance (single-leg stance)
- Terminal stance (heel off)
- Preswing (toe off)

---

makes up 60% of the gait cycle and consists of five subphases, or instants.

The **initial contact** instant is the **weight-loading** or **weight-acceptance period** of the stance leg, which accounts for the first 10% of the gait cycle. During this period, one foot is coming off the floor while the other foot is accepting body weight and absorbing the shock of initial contact. Because both feet are in contact with the floor, it is a period of **double support** or **double-leg stance**.

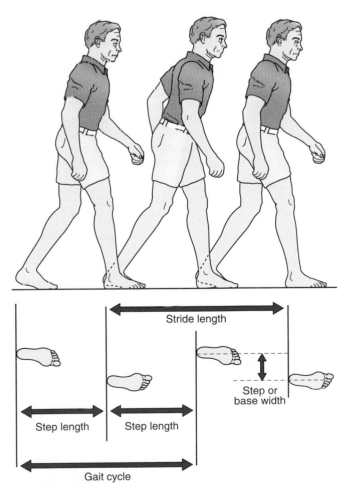

Fig. 14.1 Gait cycle, stride length, and step length and width.

Subphases (Instants) of Swing Phase

- Initial swing (acceleration)
- Midswing
- Terminal swing (deceleration)

Acceleration occurs when the foot is lifted off the floor. During normal gait, rapid knee flexion and ankle dorsiflexion occur to allow the swing limb to accelerate forward. In some pathological conditions, loss or alteration of knee flexion and ankle dorsiflexion leads to alterations in gait.

The **midswing** instant occurs when the swing leg is adjacent to the weight-bearing leg, which is in midstance.

During the final instant (**terminal swing** or **deceleration**), the swinging leg slows down in preparation for initial contact with the floor. With normal gait, active quadriceps and hamstring muscle actions are required. The quadriceps muscles control knee extension, and the hamstrings control the amount of hip flexion.

During running or with increased velocity, the stance phase decreases and a **float phase** or **double unsupported phase** occurs while the double support phase

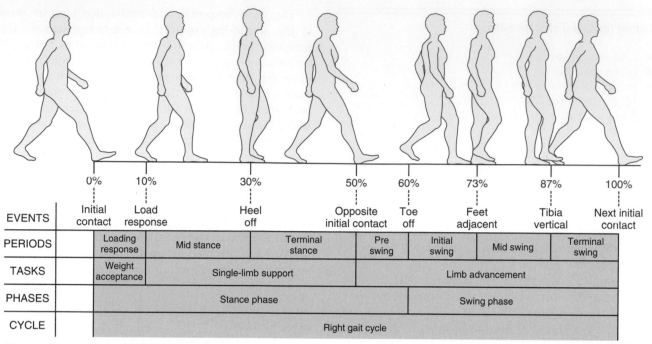

Fig. 14.2 Terminology to describe the events of the gait cycle. *Initial contact* corresponds to the beginning of stance when the foot first contacts the ground at 0% of gait cycle. *Load response* occurs when the contralateral foot leaves the ground at 10% of gait cycle. *Heel off* corresponds to the heel lifting from the ground and occurs at approximately 30% of gait cycle. *Opposite initial contact* corresponds to the foot contact of the opposite limb, typically at 50% of gait cycle. *Toe off* occurs when the foot leaves the ground at 60% of gait cycle. *Feet adjacent* takes place when the foot of the swing leg is next to the foot of the stance leg at 73% of gait cycle. *Tibia vertical* corresponds to the tibia of the swing leg being oriented in the vertical direction at 87% of gait cycle. The final event is, again, initial contact, which in fact is the start of the next gait cycle. These eight events divide the gait cycle into seven periods. *Loading response*, between initial contact and opposite toe off, corresponds to the time when the weight is accepted by the lower extremity, initiating contact with the ground. *Midstance* is from opposite toe off to heel rise (10% to 30% of gait cycle). *Terminal stance* begins when the heel rises and ends when the contralateral lower extremity touches the ground, from 30% to 50% of gait cycle. *Preswing* takes place from foot contact of the contralateral limb to toe off of the ipsilateral foot, which is the time corresponding to the second double-limb support period of gait cycle (50% to 60% of gait cycle). *Initial swing* is from toe off to feet adjacent, when the foot of the swing leg is next to the foot of the stance leg (60% to 73% of gait cycle). *Midswing* is from feet adjacent to when the tibia of the swing leg is vertical (73% to 87% of gait cycle). *Terminal swing* is from a vertical position of the tibia to immediately before heel contact (87% to 100% of gait cycle). The first 10% of the gait cycle corresponds to a task of weight acceptance—when body mass is transferred from one lower extremity to the other. Single-limb support, from 10% to 50% of gait cycle, bears the weight of the body as the opposite limb swings forward. The last 10% of stance phase and the entire swing phase advance the limb forward to a new location. (Modified from Simoneau GG: Kinesiology of walking. In Neumann DA, editor: *Kinesiology of the musculoskeletal system: foundations of physical rehabilitation*, ed 2, St Louis, 2010, Mosby, p 636.)

TABLE **14.1**

Gait Cycle: Periods and Functions

Period	Percentage of Cycle	Function	Contralateral Limb
Initial double-limb support	0–12	Loading, weight transfer	Unloading and preparing for swing (preswing)
Single-limb support	12–50	Support of entire body weight: center of mass moving forward	Swing
Second double-limb support	50–62	Unloading and preparing for swing (preswing)	Loading, weight transfer
Initial swing	62–75	Foot clearance	Single-limb support
Midswing	75–85	Limb advances in front of body	Single-limb support
Terminal swing	85–100	Limb deceleration, preparation for weight transfer	Single-limb support

From Sutherland DH, Kaufman KR, Moitoza JR: Kinematic of normal human walking. In Rose J, Gamble JG, editors: *Human locomotion*, Baltimore, 1994, Williams & Wilkins, p 27.

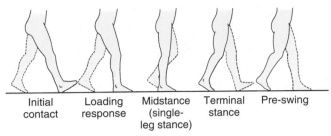

Fig. 14.3 Stance phase of gait.

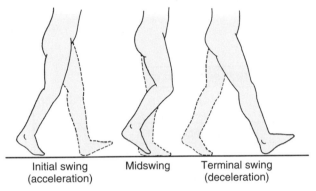

Fig. 14.4 Swing phase of gait.

disappears (Fig. 14.5).[18,22] Although the single-leg stance phase decreases, the load increases two or three times.[23] The motion occurring at each of the joints (pelvis, hip, knee, ankle) is similar for walking and for running, but the required range of motion (ROM) increases with the speed of the activity. For example, hip flexion in walking is about 40° to 45°, whereas in running it is 60° to 75°.[24]

Double-Leg Stance

Double-leg stance is that phase of gait in which parts of both feet are on the ground. In normal gait, it occurs twice during the gait cycle and represents about 25% of the cycle. This percentage increases the more slowly one walks; it becomes shorter as walking speed increases (Fig. 14.6) and disappears in running.

Single-Leg Stance

The single-leg stance is that phase of gait in which only one leg is on the ground; this occurs twice during the normal gait cycle and takes up approximately 30% of the cycle.

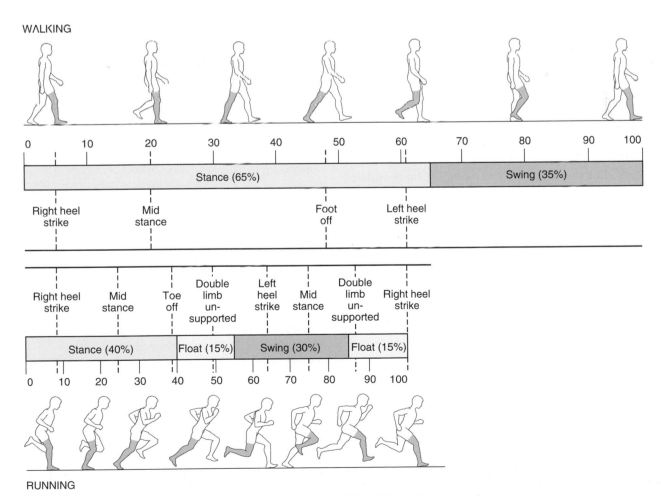

Fig. 14.5 Comparison of the phases of the walking and running cycles.

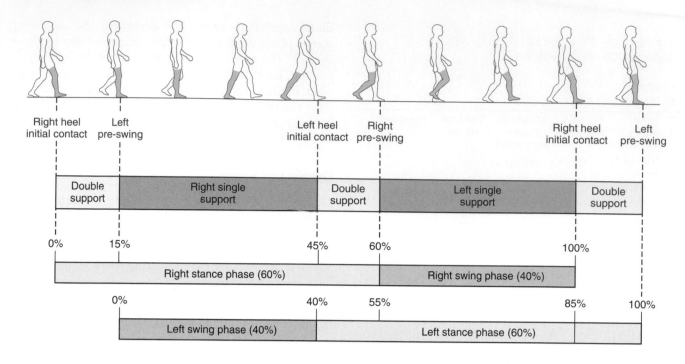

Fig. 14.6 Time dimensions of the walking cycle. (Adapted from Inman VT, Ralston HJ, Todd F: *Human walking*, Baltimore, 1981, Williams & Wilkins, p 26.)

Normal Parameters of Gait[7–11,25]

The parameters that follow and their values are considered normal for a population between the ages of 8 and 45 years. It should be pointed out, however, that a relatively normal gait pattern is seen in persons as young as 3 years of age,[2] although there are differences between individuals of the same gender and between men and women.[26] For the majority of the population outside of these ages, there are alterations caused by neurological development, balance control, aging, changes in limb length, and maturation.[2] For example, with maturity, walking velocity and step length increase and cadence decreases.[27] It is also important to evaluate gait on the basis of normal gait for someone the same age. This is especially true for children.

Base (Step) Width

The normal base width, which is the distance between the two feet, is 8 to 10 cm (3 to 4 inches) (Fig. 14.7).[28–30] If the base is wider, the examiner may suspect some pathology (e.g., cerebellar or inner ear problems) that results in poor balance, or a condition such as diabetes or peripheral neuropathy, which may indicate a loss of sensation or a musculoskeletal problem (e.g., tight hip abductors). In the first two cases, the patient tends to have a wider base to maintain balance. With

Gait Descriptors or Parameters for Which the Examiner Should Watch While Observing Gait[16]

Stride:	The sequence of events between successive heel strikes of the same foot
Step:	The sequence of events between successive heel strikes of the opposite feet
Stride length:	The distance between two successive heel strikes of the same foot (average: 144 cm or 57 inches)
Step length:	The distance between successive heel strikes of two different feet (average: 72 cm or 28 inches)
Step or base width:	The lateral distance between the heel centers of two consecutive foot contacts (average: 8–10 cm or 3–4 inches)
Cadence (step rate):	Number of steps per minute (average: 90–120/min)
Stride time:	Time for a full gait cycle
Step time:	Time for completion of heel strike of right foot to heel strike of left foot
Walking or gait speed:[a]	Distance covered in a given amount of time (average: 1.4 m/second or 3 mph)

[a]All other values will vary depending on walking speed.

increased speed, the base width normally decreases to zero, and in some cases, crossover occurs, in which one foot lands where the other should and vice versa. Such **crossover** can lead to gait alterations and other problems.[31]

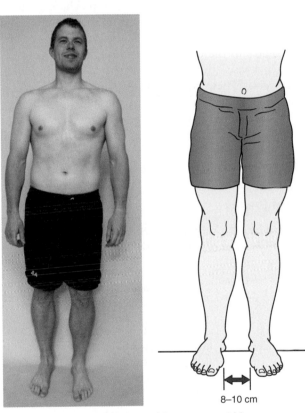

8–10 cm

Fig. 14.7 Normal base or step width.

Step Length

Step length, or gait length, is the distance between successive contact points on opposite feet (see Fig. 14.1). Normally, this distance is about 72 cm (28 inches), being relatively constant for each individual (i.e., step length is commonly related to preferred walking speed)[32] and equal for both legs. It varies with age and gender, with children taking smaller steps than adults and females taking smaller steps than males.[23] Height also has an effect: a taller person takes larger steps. Step length tends to decrease with age, fatigue, pain, and disease. If step length is normal for both legs, the **rhythm of walking** is smooth. If there is pain in one limb, the patient attempts to take weight off that limb as quickly as possible, thus altering the rhythm.

Stride Length

Stride length is the linear distance in the plane of progression between successive points of foot-to-floor contact of the same foot. The stride length is normally about 144 cm (56 inches) and in reality is one gait cycle.[17] Stride length, like step length, decreases with age, pain, disease, and fatigue.[19,33] The age changes are often the result of decreased walking pace or speed.[33,34]

Lateral Pelvic Shift (Pelvic List)

Lateral pelvic shift, or pelvic list, is the side-to-side movement of the pelvis during walking. It is necessary to center the weight of the body over the stance leg for balance (Fig. 14.8). The lateral pelvic shift is normally 2.5 to 5 cm (1 to 2 inches). It increases if the feet are farther apart. The pelvic list causes relative adduction of the weight-bearing limb, facilitating the action of the hip adductors. If the abductor muscles are weak, a **Trendelenburg gait** results (see Fig. 14.18).

Vertical Pelvic Shift

Vertical pelvic shift keeps the center of gravity from moving up and down more than 5 cm (2 inches) during normal gait. By means of a vertical pelvic shift, the high point occurs during midstance and the low point during initial

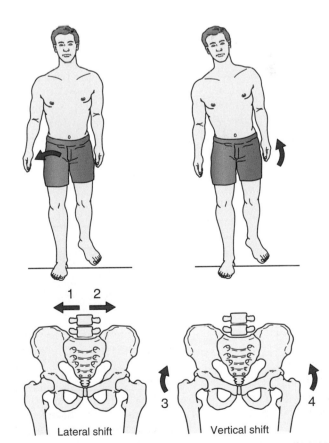

1 2

Lateral shift   Vertical shift

3   4

Fig. 14.8 Pelvic shift. Numbers indicate that one lateral or vertical shift occurs and then the other; they do not occur at the same time. *1,* Right lateral shift; *2,* left lateral shift; *3,* right vertical shift; *4,* left vertical shift.

contact; the height of these points may increase during the swing phase if the knee is fused or does not bend because of protective spasm or swelling. The head is never higher during normal gait than it is when the person is

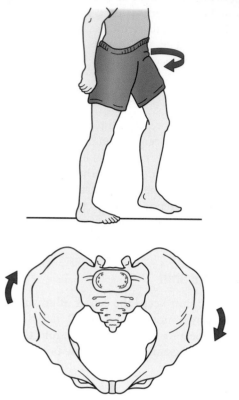

Fig. 14.9 Pelvic rotation. Left forward pelvic rotation is illustrated.

standing on both feet. Therefore, if a person can stand in an opening, he or she should be able to move through the opening without hitting the head.[7] On the swing phase, the hip is lower on the swing side, and the patient must flex the knee and dorsiflex the foot to clear the toe. This action shortens the extremity length at midstance and decreases the rise of the center of gravity.

Pelvic Rotation

Pelvic rotation is necessary to lessen the angle of the femur with the floor; in so doing, it lengthens the femur (Fig. 14.9). The rotation decreases the amplitude of displacement along the path traveled by the center of gravity and thereby decreases the center-of-gravity dip. There is a total of 8° pelvic rotation with 4° forward on the swing leg and 4° posteriorly on the stance leg. To maintain balance, the thorax rotates in the opposite direction. When the pelvis rotates clockwise, the thorax rotates counterclockwise, and vice versa. These concurrent rotations provide counterrotation forces and help regulate the speed of walking.

In the lower limb, rotation is evident at each joint (Fig. 14.10). The farther the joint is from the trunk, the greater the amount of rotation. For example, rotation in the tibia is three times greater than rotation in the pelvis.[7]

Center of Gravity

In the standing position, the center of gravity is normally 5 cm (2 inches) anterior to the second sacral vertebra; it

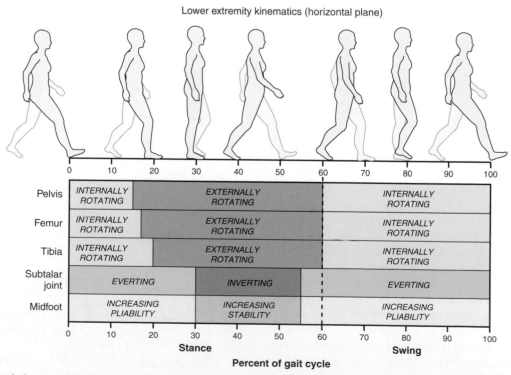

Fig. 14.10 Horizontal plane rotation of the major bones of the lower extremity and subtalar joint during walking. The graph shows the direction of rotation, which is not necessarily the same as the absolute joint position. (From Simoneau GG: Kinesiology of walking. In Neumann DA: *Kinesiology of the musculoskeletal system: foundations of physical rehabilitation*, ed 2, St Louis, 2010, Mosby, p 647.)

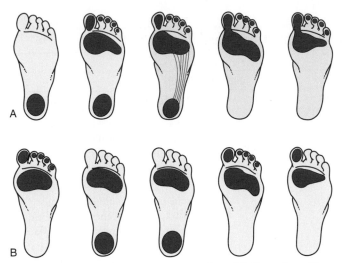

Fig. 14.11 The cadence of gait. (A) Normal foot. (B) Cavus foot. (From Viladot A: *Patologia del Antepié*, Barcelona, 1975, Ediciones Toray, SA.)

tends to be slightly higher in men than in women because men tend to have a greater body mass in the shoulder area. The vertical and horizontal displacements of the center of gravity describe a figure eight, occupying a 5-cm (2-inch) square within the pelvis during walking. The vertical displacement, which describes a smooth sinusoidal curve during walking, can be observed from the side. The patient's head descends during weight-loading and weight-unloading periods and rises during single-leg stance.

Normal Cadence

The normal cadence is between 90 and 120 steps per minute, which varies in part because of the height of the individual.[35–38] The cadence of women is usually six to nine steps per minute higher than that of men.[37] Even with anthropometrically matched men and women, women still have a higher cadence and shorter step length than men when they are ambulating at the same speed.[39–41] With age, the cadence decreases. Fig. 14.11A illustrates the cadence of normal gait from heel strike to toe off, showing the changing weight distribution. With pathology or deformity (e.g., a cavus foot [Fig. 14.11B]), this weight-bearing pattern may be altered. As the pace of walking increases, the stride width increases and the toeing-out angle decreases. Gait speed is about 1.4 m/s (3 mph).[17] Cadence is also affected by age, decreasing from age 4 to 7 and then again in advancing years.[42]

Normal Pattern of Gait[6–11,17,35,43,44]

Stance Phase

As previously mentioned, five instants are involved during the stance phase of gait. These are now described in order of occurrence. This phase is the **closed kinetic chain** phase of gait. The action occurring at the various joints causes a chain reaction because of the stresses put on the joints and supporting structures with weight bearing. The foot becomes the fixed stable segment, and alterations occur from the foot up, with the joints of the foot adapting first, followed by those of the ankle, knee, hip, pelvis, spine, and finally the upper limb, which acts as a counterbalance to movement in the lower limb.[45] The relations between the joints are constantly changing. Table 14.2 summarizes the movement at the hip, knee, ankle, and foot during the stance phase.[46]

Initial Contact (Heel Strike)

Initial contact occurs when the limb first strikes the ground. Normally, this occurs when the heel strikes and the limb is being prepared to take weight. During the initial contact, the pelvis is level and medially rotated on the side of initial contact, whereas the trunk is aligned between the two lower limbs. The hip is flexed 30° to 49° and is medially rotated; the knee is slightly flexed or extended; the tibia is laterally rotated; the ankle is at 90° with the foot supinated; and the hindfoot is everted. At this instant, there is little force going through the limb.

If pain occurs in the heel at this time, it may be caused by a heel spur, bone bruise, heel fat-pad bruise, or bursitis. This pain may cause increased flexion of the knee, with early plantar flexion to relieve the stress or pressure on the painful tissues. If the knee is weak, the patient may extend the knee by using a hand or may hit the heel hard on the ground to whip the knee into extension. A patient may do this because of weakness of the muscles (e.g., reflex inhibition, poliomyelitis, an internal derangement of the knee, a nerve root lesion [L2, L3, or L4], femoral neuropathy). In the past, this instant was referred to as "heel strike"; however, with some pathological gaits, heel strike may not be the first instant. Instead, the toes, the forefoot, or the entire foot may initially contact the ground. If the dorsiflexor muscles are weak, the foot drops, slaps, or flops down. The weakness may be caused by a peroneal neuropathy or nerve root lesion (L4). A knee flexion contracture or spasticity may cause the same alteration.

Load Response (Weight Acceptance or Foot Flat)

Load response is a critical event in that the person subconsciously decides whether the limb is able to bear the weight of the body. The trunk is aligned with the stance leg. The pelvis drops slightly on the swing leg side and rotates medially on the same side. The flexed and laterally rotated hip moves into extension, and the knee flexes 15° to 25°. The tibia is medially rotated and begins to move forward over the fixed foot as the body swings over the foot. The ankle is plantar flexed and the hindfoot is inverted. The foot moves into pronation because this position unlocks the foot and enables it to adapt to different terrains and postures. The forefoot is pronated, unlocking the subtalar and metatarsal joints to enable them to absorb the shock more effectively, and the plantar aspect is in contact with the floor.

Abnormal responses include excessive or no knee motion as a result of weak quadriceps, plantar flexor contractures, or spasticity.[9]

TABLE **14.2**

Summary of Joint Motions at the Hip, Knee, Tibia, Foot, and Ankle During the Stance Phase of Normal Gait

Hip

Phase	KINEMATIC MOTION	KINETIC MOTION	
	Hip	External Forces	Internal Forces
Heel strike	20° to 40° hip flexion moving toward extension; slight adduction and lateral rotation	Reaction force in front of joint; flexion moment moving toward extension; forward pelvic rotation	Gluteus maximus and hamstrings working eccentrically to resist flexion moment; erector spinae working eccentrically to resist forward bend
Foot flat	Hip moving into extension, adduction, medial rotation	Flexion moment	Gluteus maximus and hamstrings contracting concentrically to bring hip into extension; erector spinae resisting trunk flexion
Midstance	Moving through neutral position; pelvis rotating posteriorly	Reaction force posterior to hip joint; extension moment	Iliopsoas working eccentrically to resist extension; gluteus medius contracting in reverse action to stabilize opposite pelvis; iliopsoas activity continuing
Heel off	10° to 15° extension of hip abduction, lateral rotation	Extension moment decreasing after double-limb support begins	
Toe off	Moving toward 10° extension, abduction, lateral rotation	Decrease of extension moment	Adductor magnus working eccentrically to control or stabilize pelvis; iliopsoas activity continuing

Knee and Tibia

Phase	KINEMATIC MOTION		KINETIC MOTION	
	Knee	Tibia	External Forces	Internal Forces
Heel strike	In full extension before heel contact; flexing as heel strikes floor	Slight lateral rotation	Rapidly increasing reaction forces behind knee joint causing flexion moment	Quadriceps femoris contracting eccentrically to control rapid knee flexion and to prevent buckling
Foot flat	In 20° flexion moving toward extension	Medial rotation	Flexion moment	After foot is flat, quadriceps femoris activity becoming concentric to bring femur over tibia
Midstance	In 15° flexion moving toward extension	Neutral	Maximum flexion moment	Quadriceps femoris activity decreasing; gastrocnemius working eccentrically to control excessive knee extension
Heel off	In 4° flexion moving toward extension	Lateral rotation	Reaction forces moving anterior to joint; extension moment	Gastrocnemius beginning to work concentrically to start knee flexion
Toe off	Moving from near full extension to 40° flexion	Lateral rotation	Reaction forces moving posterior to joint as knee flexes; flexion moment	Quadriceps femoris contracting eccentrically

Foot and Ankle

Phase	KINEMATIC MOTION		KINETIC MOTION	
	Foot	Ankle	External Forces	Internal Forces
Heel strike	Supination (rigid) at heel contact	Moving into plantar flexion	Reaction forces behind joint axis; plantar flexion moment at heel strike	Dorsiflexors (tibialis anterior, extensor digitorum longus, and extensor hallucis longus) contracting eccentrically to slow plantar flexion

TABLE **14.2**

Summary of Joint Motions at the Hip, Knee, Tibia, Foot, and Ankle During the Stance Phase of Normal Gait—cont'd

Foot and Ankle

	KINEMATIC MOTION		KINETIC MOTION	
Phase	**Foot**	**Ankle**	**External Forces**	**Internal Forces**
Foot flat	Pronation, adapting to support surface	Plantar flexion to dorsiflexion over a fixed foot	Maximum plantar flexion moment; reaction forces beginning to shift anterior, producing a dorsiflexion moment	Dorsiflexion activity decreasing; tibialis posterior, flexor hallucis longus, and flexor digitorum longus working eccentrically to control pronation
Midstance	Neutral	3° of dorsiflexion	Slight dorsiflexion moment	Plantar flexor muscles (gastrocsoleus and peroneal muscles), activated to control dorsiflexion of the tibia and fibula over a fixed foot, contracting eccentrically
Heel off	Supination as foot becomes rigid for push off	15° dorsiflexion toward plantar flexion	Maximal dorsiflexion moment	Plantar flexor muscles beginning to contract concentrically to prepare for push off
Toe off	Supination	20° plantar flexion	Dorsiflexion moment	Plantar flexor muscles at peak activity but becoming inactive as foot leaves ground

Modified from Giallonardo LM: Gait. In Myers RS, editor: *Saunders manual of physical therapy practice*, Philadelphia, 1995, WB Saunders, pp 1108–1109.

Midstance (Single-Leg Support)

The midstance instant is a period of stationary foot support. Normally, the weight of the foot is evenly distributed over the entire foot. The trunk is aligned over the stance leg, and the pelvis shows a slight drop to the swing leg side.

During this stage, there is maximum extension of the hip (10° to 15°) with lateral rotation, and the greatest force is on the hip. Painful hip, knee, or ankle conditions cause this phase to be shortened as the patient hurries through the phase to decrease the pain. If the gluteus medius (L5 nerve root) is weak, the Trendelenburg sign will be present. The knee flexes, and the ankle is locked at 5° to 8° of dorsiflexion, rolling forward on the forefoot (roll off). The foot is in contact with the floor, the forefoot is pronated, and the hindfoot is inverted. This instant is a critical event for the ankle. If pain is elicited during this period, the phase is shortened and the heel may lift off early. This pain is commonly caused by conditions such as arthritis, rigid pes planus, fallen metatarsal or longitudinal arches, plantar fasciitis, or Morton metatarsalgia. Therefore pathology at the hip, ankle, or knee can modify the gait in this phase.

Terminal Stance (Heel Off)

In the final stages, the trunk is initially aligned over the lower limbs and moves toward the stance leg. The pelvis is initially level and posteriorly rotated and then dips to the swing leg side, remaining posteriorly rotated. The heel is in neutral and slight medial rotation; the knee is extended with the tibia laterally rotated. At the ankle, plantar flexion occurs as the critical event. This action helps to smooth the pathway of the center of gravity. The

forefoot is initially in contact with the floor, and then the weight on the foot moves forward with plantar flexion so that only the big toe is in contact with the floor. At the same time, the forefoot moves from inversion to eversion.

Preswing (Toe Off)

The preswing phase is the acceleration phase as the toe pushes the leg forward. The trunk remains erect, the pelvis remains posteriorly rotated, and the hip is extended and slightly medially rotated. The knee flexes to 30° to 35° (critical event), and the ankle is plantar flexed. Because the center of gravity is anterior to the hip, the hip can be accelerated forward in initial swing.

If pain is elicited during this instant, it may be caused by a hallux rigidus, turf toe, or any other pathology involving the great toe (hallux), especially the metatarsophalangeal joint of the hallux. With injury to the joint, the patient is unable to push off on the medial aspect of the foot; instead, the patient pushes off on the lateral aspect of the foot to compensate for the painful metatarsophalangeal joint or, in some cases, a painful metatarsal arch resulting from increased pressure on the metatarsal heads. If the plantar flexors are weak (e.g., S1–S2 nerve root pathology), push off may be absent. During this phase, the foot pronates so that there is a rigid base for better push off.

During walking, a cane can be used to decrease the load on the limb. Lyu and associates[47] have shown that when a cane is used in the contralateral upper limb and the cane tip touches the ground at the same time as the heel, the force at heel strike can be reduced by 34%, at midstance by 25%, and at toe off by about 30%.

TABLE **14.3**

Summary of Joint Motion and Forces During Swing Phase: Acceleration to Midswing and Midswing to Deceleration

Joint	ACCELERATION TO MIDSWING		MIDSWING TO DECELERATION	
	Kinematic Motion	Kinetic Motion	Kinematic Motion	Kinetic Motion
Hip	Slight flexion (0° to 15°) moving to 30° flexion and lateral rotation to neutral	Hip flexors working concentrically to bring limb through; contralateral gluteus medius contracting concentrically to maintain position of pelvis	Continued flexion at about 30° to 40°	Gluteus maximus contracting eccentrically to slow hip flexion
Knee	30° to 60° knee flexion and lateral rotation of tibia moving toward neutral	Hamstrings contracting concentrically	Moving to near full extension and slight lateral tibial rotation	Quadriceps femoris contracting concentrically and hamstrings contracting eccentrically
Ankle and foot	20° dorsiflexion and slight pronation	Dorsiflexors contracting concentrically	Ankle in neutral; foot in slight supination	Dorsiflexors contracting isometrically

From Giallonardo LM: Gait. In Myers RS, editor: *Saunders manual of physical therapy practice*, Philadelphia, 1995, WB Saunders, p 1110.

Swing Phase

The swing phase of gait involves the lower limb in an **open kinetic chain;** the foot is not fixed on the ground, and the stresses on the limb are therefore less and easier to dissipate. During this phase, alterations occur from the spine down through the pelvis, hip, ankle, and foot. The pelvis and hip provide the most stability in the lower limb during the non–weight-bearing phase. Table 14.3 summarizes the motions occurring in the lower limb during the swing phase.

The three instants composing the swing phase of gait are now described in order of occurrence.

Initial Swing

During the first subphase of acceleration (Fig. 14.12), flexion and medial rotation of the hip and flexion of the knee occur. The pelvis rotates medially and dips to the swing leg side. The trunk is aligned with the stance leg. In addition, the ankle continues to plantar flex. The foot is not in contact with the floor. The forefoot continues supinating, and the hindfoot continues everting. The dorsiflexor muscles of the ankle contract to allow the foot to clear the ground, and the knee exhibits its maximum flexion of about 60° during gait. If the quadriceps muscles are weak, the trunk muscles thrust the pelvis forward to provide forward momentum to the leg.

Midswing

During the midswing instant, the hip continues to flex and rotate medially, and the knee continues to flex. The ankle is in the anatomic or plantigrade position (90°) for the first 25% of the stance phase to permit the foot and midtarsal joints to unlock so that the foot can adapt to uneven terrain when it begins to bear weight, The forefoot is supinated and

the hindfoot is everted. The pelvis and trunk are in the same position as in the previous stage. If the ankle dorsiflexor muscles are weak (e.g., drop foot), the patient demonstrates a **steppage gait** (see Fig. 14.24). In such a gait, the hip flexes excessively so that the toes will clear the ground.

Terminal Swing (Deceleration)

During the final subphase, the hip continues to flex and rotate medially and the knee reaches its maximum extension. At the ankle, dorsiflexion has occurred. The forefoot is supinated and the hindfoot is everted. The trunk and pelvis maintain the same position as before. The hamstring muscles contract during the terminal phase to slow the swing; if the hamstrings are weak (e.g., S1–S2 nerve root lesion), heel strike may be excessively harsh to lock the knee in extension.

Joint Motion During Normal Gait

Although there is a tendency to talk about gait as action around joints, the examiner must not forget that muscles play a significant role in what happens at the joints. Table 14.4 illustrates the actions of some of the muscles used during gait.[48]

Hip. The function of the hip is to extend the leg during the stance phase and flex the leg during the swing phase. The ligaments of the hip help to stabilize it in extension. The hip extensors help to initiate movement, as do the hip flexors; both groups of muscles work phasically.[49] Deficits in the gluteus maximus strength may be seen as functional deficits during stair climbing, sit to stand, and step ups.[50] The gluteals—maximus, medius, and minimus—all play a role in gait; disease and running can alter the activity of these muscles.[51–55] The hip flexors (primarily the iliopsoas muscle) contract to slow extension; the hip extensors (primarily the

RANGE OF MOTION SUMMARY

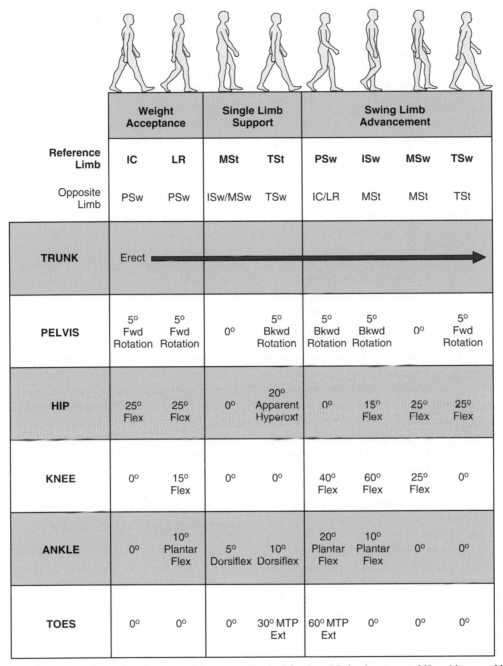

	Weight Acceptance		Single Limb Support		Swing Limb Advancement			
Reference Limb	IC	LR	MSt	TSt	PSw	ISw	MSw	TSw
Opposite Limb	PSw	PSw	ISw/MSw	TSw	IC/LR	MSt	MSt	TSt
TRUNK	Erect ──▶							
PELVIS	5° Fwd Rotation	5° Fwd Rotation	0°	5° Bkwd Rotation	5° Bkwd Rotation	5° Bkwd Rotation	0°	5° Fwd Rotation
HIP	25° Flex	25° Flex	0°	20° Apparent Hyperext	0°	15° Flex	25° Flex	25° Flex
KNEE	0°	15° Flex	0°	0°	40° Flex	60° Flex	25° Flex	0°
ANKLE	0°	10° Plantar Flex	5° Dorsiflex	10° Dorsiflex	20° Plantar Flex	10° Plantar Flex	0°	0°
TOES	0°	0°	0°	30° MTP Ext	60° MTP Ext	0°	0°	0°

Fig. 14.12 Normal range of motion during gait cycle. *IC,* Initial contact; *ISw,* initial swing; *LR,* load response; *MSt,* midstance; *MSw,* midswing; *PSw,* preswing; *TSt,* terminal stance; *TSw,* terminal swing. (Copyright 1991 LAREI, Rancho Los Amigos Medical Center, Downey, CA 90242; From The Pathokinesiology Service and The Physical Therapy Department, Rancho Los Amigos Medical Center: Observational Gait Analysis. Downey, CA, Los Amigos Research and Educational Institute, Inc., 1996, p 30.)

hamstring muscles) contract to slow flexion. In this way they work eccentrically. The abductor muscles provide stability during single-leg support, a critical event for the hip.[49]

If there is loss of movement of the hip, the compensatory mechanisms are increased mobility of the knee on the same side and increased mobility of the contralateral hip. In addition, the lumbar spine will show increased mobility.

Knee. When the knee is in flexion during the first three instants of the stance phase of gait, it acts as a shock absorber. Painful knees are not able to do this. One of the critical events of the knee is extension. The functions of the knee during gait are to bear weight, absorb shock, extend the stride length, and allow the foot to move through its swing. The quadriceps muscles use only 4% to 5% of their maximum voluntary contraction to extend the knee, but in so doing they help to control weight acceptance. The hamstring muscles flex the knee and slow the leg in the swing phase, working eccentrically.

TABLE **14.4**

Muscle Actions During the Gait Cycle

Phase of Gait	Mechanical Goals	Active Muscle Groups	Examples
Stance Phase			
Initial contact	Position foot, begin deceleration	Ankle dorsiflexors, hip extensors, knee flexors	Anterior tibialis, gluteus maximus, hamstrings
Loading response	Accept weight, stabilize pelvis, decelerate mass	Knee extensors, hip abductors, ankle plantar flexors	Vasti, gluteus medius, gastrocnemius, soleus
Midstance	Stabilize knee, preserve momentum	Ankle plantar flexors (isometric)	Gastrocnemius, soleus
Terminal stance	Accelerate mass	Ankle plantar flexors (concentric)	Gastrocnemius, soleus
Swing Phase			
Preswing	Prepare for swing	Hip flexors	Iliopsoas, rectus femoris
Initial swing	Clear foot, vary cadence	Ankle dorsiflexors, hip flexors	Tibialis anterior, iliopsoas, rectus femoris
Midswing	Clear foot	Ankle dorsiflexors	Tibialis anterior
Terminal swing	Decelerate shank, decelerate leg, position foot, prepare for contact	Knee flexors, hip extensors, ankle dorsiflexors, knee extensors	Hamstrings, gluteus maximus, tibialis anterior, vasti

From Rab GT: Muscle. In Rose J, Gamble JG, editors: *Human locomotion*, Baltimore, 1994, Williams & Wilkins, p 113.

If the knee has a flexion deformity, the hip will be flexed and therefore will lose its extension power, which is a critical event for the hip. Pathological conditions such as patellofemoral syndrome also cause deviations from normal gait. For example, patients with patellofemoral syndrome show less knee flexion during the single-leg stance phase combined with lateral femoral rotation during the swing phase.[56] On heel strike to foot flat, the femur then rotates medially, and if this compensating medial rotation is too great, it will cause excessive pronation, which then stresses the medial aspect of the patellofemoral joint.

Gastrocnemius and Soleus. The gastrocnemius and soleus muscles are important in gait. They use 85% of their maximum voluntary contraction during normal walking. These muscles help to restrain the body's momentum during forward movement. They also contribute to knee and ankle stability, restrain forward rotation of the tibia on the talus during the stance phase, and minimize the vertical pelvic shift, thereby conserving energy.[57] To accomplish these functions during gait, the triceps surae work eccentrically and concentrically.

Foot and Ankle. The foot and ankle play major roles in gait in that the various joints allow the foot to accommodate to the ground. The joints of the foot and ankle work interdependently during normal gait. When the heel contacts the ground, the lower limb becomes a closed kinetic chain and movements and stresses must be absorbed by the structures of the lower limb.

When the examiner looks at the ankle, he or she should observe immediate plantar flexion at initial contact. Loss of this plantar flexion (e.g., tibial nerve neuropathy) results in an inability to transfer weight to the anterior foot, increased ankle dorsiflexion, and increased knee flexion. In addition,

the duration of single-leg stance on the affected side decreases and the step length on the opposite side decreases. Furthermore, quadriceps action at the knee increases because of the lack of knee stability caused by the loss of the triceps surae, with the end result being that walking velocity decreases.[57] The foot then dorsiflexes through midstance or single-leg stance, with maximum dorsiflexion being reached just before heel off. The examiner should note whether there is sufficient plantar flexion during push off.

Overview and Patient History

The assessment of a patient's gait should be included in any assessment of the lower limb. The examiner must keep in mind that the posture of the head, neck, thorax, and lumbar spine can affect gait even if no pathology is evident in the lower limb. The examiner must be able to identify the action of each body segment and note any deviation from normal during the individual phases of gait. For this reason it is important to understand the normal parameters of gait and the mechanism of gait as it occurs. With this knowledge, the ways in which the gait is altered under pathological conditions can be better understood.

Musculoskeletal pathology tends to modify gait because of muscle weakness, pain, or altered ROM, so the examiner should watch closely for these factors in observing gait. Many patients can adapt automatically to these changes provided that they have normal sensation and can develop selective control.[9] In fact, a recent study has shown that an individual can tolerate up to a 40% overall muscle weakness while still maintaining a relatively normal gait.[58] Patients with upper motor neuron lesions have greater alterations and cannot easily adapt because, in addition to the musculoskeletal problems, they also present with spasticity, control problems, and sensory disturbances.[9] It is important that the examiner read the patient's chart and take a history from the patient regarding any disease or injury, past or present, that may be causing gait problems.

Observation

The examiner should first perform a general overview of the patient's posture, looking for any asymmetry, and then observe the patient's gait, looking at stride length, step frequency, time of swing, speed of walking, and duration of the complete walking cycle. This is normally done with the patient in shorts, wearing no shoes or socks. If gait is observed while the patient is wearing shoes, the same shoes should be used for each test.[59] A steady gait pattern is usually established **within three steps**; it is initiated by the body's becoming unbalanced, so that the patient can lift one foot off the ground to take the first step.[60] After this overview is completed, the examiner can look at specific parts of the gait in terms of phases and what happens at each joint during these phases.

Because gait constantly changes as one stops and starts, hurries, dawdles, and walks with others, it is important to remember whether the movements the patient is capable of are normal and whether the speeds, phases, strides, and durations of the cycles occur in normal combinations. In addition to observing walking at a normal speed, the patient's slow and fast gait speeds should be examined to see whether these changes affect the gait. The examiner must watch the upper limbs and trunk as well as the lumbar spine, pelvis, hips, knees, feet, and ankles during these changes. Female patients should be in a bra and briefs, and male patients should be in shorts. The patient should walk barefoot. In this way, the motions of the toes, feet, legs, pelvis, trunk, and upper limbs can properly be observed.

The examiner should ask the patient to walk in the usual manner, using any aids necessary (e.g., parallel bars, crutches, walker, canes). While the patient is walking, the examiner makes an initial general observation of any obvious limp or deformity.

The examiner should observe the gait from the front, from behind, and from the side, in each instance observing from proximal to distal and watching the pelvis and lumbar spine down to the ankle and foot as well as from the foot up. For example, in the swing phase (open kinetic chain), movement starts proximally and moves distally. In the stance phase (closed kinetic chain), movement is reversed, starting in the foot and moving proximally. The examiner should observe the movements in the trunk and upper limbs, which normally are in the opposite direction to those of the lower limbs. This method provides a sequential and thorough manner of assessment. Rancho Los Amigos Medical Center has developed a useful gait analysis chart (Fig. 14.13). By using the chart during observation, the examiner can determine deviations and their effect on gait in an easily used and retained method of recording. The dark-blue boxes indicate what normally should occur; the light-blue and white boxes indicate minor and major deviations from the normal, respectively. Minor deviations imply that the functional task of walking is not affected. Major deviations imply that the mechanics of walking are affected adversely.[61]

Anterior View

While observing from the front as the patient walks, the examiner should note whether the head moves only slightly up and down. Additionally, the head should not move much at all in the lateral direction during gait. A bouncing gait would be seen with excessive superior and inferior head movement during walking. The examiner should observe whether any lateral tilt of the pelvis occurs, whether there is any sideways swaying of the trunk, whether the pelvis rotates on a horizontal plane, whether the trunk and upper extremity rotate in the opposite direction to the pelvis, and whether reciprocal arm swing is present. Usually, the rotation of the trunk and upper extremity is approximately 180° out of phase with the pelvis—that is, as the pelvis and lower limb rotate one way, the trunk and upper limb rotate in the opposite direction. This action helps provide a balancing effect and smooths the forward progression of the body. The examiner may also note movements at the hip (rotation and abduction/adduction), knee (rotation and abduction/adduction), and ankle and foot (amount of toe out and toe in, dorsiflexion/plantar flexion and supination/pronation). Excessive varus or valgus at the knee can indicate a **varus extension thrust**, which is characteristic of injuries to the posterolateral corner of the knee and may also lead to an increased Fick angle.[62,63] The examiner should note any bowing of the femur or the tibia; any medial or lateral rotation of the hips, femur, or tibia; and the position of the feet as the patient goes through the gait cycle (Fig. 14.14).[30,64] This view is best used to examine the weight-loading period of the gait cycle. The examiner should also note whether there is any abduction or circumduction of the swing leg, whether there is atrophy of the musculature of the anterior thigh and leg, and whether the base width is normal.

Lateral View

From the side, the examiner should observe rotation of the shoulder and thorax during the gait cycle as well as reciprocal arm swing. Spinal posture (e.g., lordosis), pelvic rotation, and movements in the joints of the lower limbs should be noted. The trunk should remain erect and level. The trunk may compensate for lost motor control at the hip. Excessive trunk extension may be due to weak hip extensors or loss of hip flexion ROM. A forward trunk lean may be due to many factors including but not limited to pathology of the hip, knee or ankle; abdominal weakness; decreased spinal mobility; and/or hip flexor contractures. These movements include flexion/

GAIT ANALYSIS: FULL BODY

RANCHO LOS AMIGOS MEDICAL CENTER
PHYSICAL THERAPY DEPARTMENT

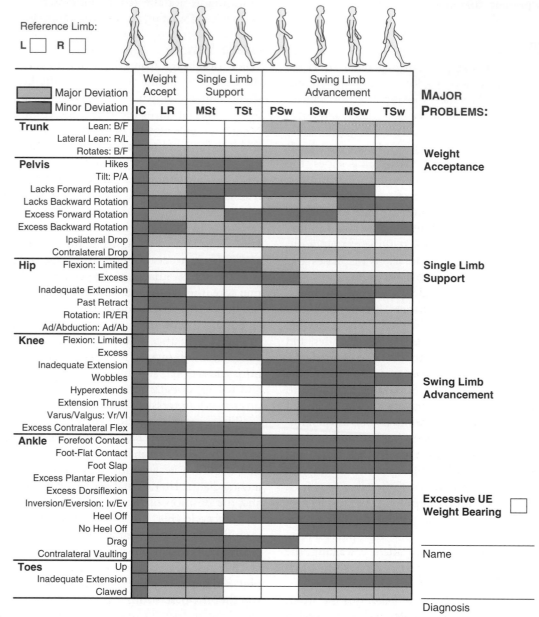

Fig. 14.13 Gait analysis of the full body. (Copyright 1996 LAREI, Rancho Los Amigos Medical Center, Downey, CA 90242; From the Pathokinesiology Service and the Physical Therapy Department, Rancho Los Amigos Medical Center: Observational Gait Analysis. Downey, CA, Los Amigos Research and Educational Institute, Inc., 1996, p 64.)

extension at the hip, flexion/extension at the knee, and dorsiflexion/plantar flexion at the ankle. From the lateral aspect, the examiner may also observe step length, stride length, cadence, and the other time dimensions of gait (see Fig. 14.6).[44] This view enables observation of the interactions between the walking surface and the various body parts.

The examiner must remember that there may be some compensation by the lumbar spine for limitation of movement in the hip. For example, a swayback posture may increase stress on the anterior structures of the hip.[65] The patient should be observed to determine whether there is sufficient knee extension at initial contact, followed almost immediately by slight flexion until the foot makes contact with the floor; whether there is control of the slightly flexed knee during load response and midstance; and whether there is sufficient flexion during preswing and initial swing. Also, any hyperextension of the knee during the gait cycle should be noted. Finally, the examiner should note whether there is coordination

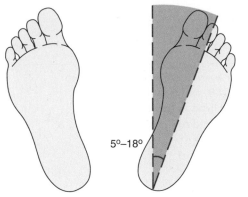

Fig. 14.14 During stance and gait, the toes angle out 5° to 18° in adults (Fick angle).

of movement between the hip, knee, and ankle; even or uneven gait length; and even or uneven duration of steps.

As the patient moves from initial contact to loading response, the foot flexes immediately and the knee flexes until the foot is flat on the floor. During this period the hip is also flexed. During midstance the ankle dorsiflexes as the body pivots in an arc over the stationary foot. At the same time, the hip and knee extend, lengthening the leg. As the patient moves from terminal stance to preswing, the ankle plantar flexes to raise the heel and the hip and knee flex as the weight is transferred to the opposite leg.

During the initial swing, the ankle plantar flexes and the hip and knee are maximally flexed. As the leg progresses to midswing, the ankle dorsiflexes and the hip and knee begin to extend. As the patient moves from midswing to terminal swing, the ankle remains in the neutral position while the hip and knee continue extending. As the leg moves from terminal swing to initial contact, the knee reaches maximum extension; the ankle remains in neutral, and no further hip extension occurs at this stage.

Posterior View

While observing the gait cycle from behind, the examiner should notice the same structures that were viewed from the front. Rotation of the shoulders and thorax, reciprocal arm swing, and pelvic list and rotation may be noted posteriorly, as well as hip, knee, ankle, and subtalar joint movement. Heel rise and base of support (base width) are easier to view posteriorly. Any abnormal abduction or adduction movements or lateral displacement of the body segments should be noted. This view is best to examine the weight-unloading period of the gait cycle. The examiner can note whether heel rise is equal for both feet and whether the heels turn in or out. The observation should also include lateral movement of the spine and the musculature of the back, buttocks, posterior thigh, and calf.

Footwear

The patient should be asked to walk in normal footwear as well as in bare feet. The examiner should take time to observe the patient's footwear and any wearing down of the heels or socks, the condition of the shoe uppers, creases, and so on. The feet should also be examined for callus formations, blisters, corns, and bunions. Different shoes can modify a patient's gait and the amount of energy necessary to perform gait. For example, high-heeled shoes alter movement, especially at the knee and ankle, which in turn increases the vertical loading.[66]

Examination

Most gait assessment involves observation. However, the examiner should take time, especially if he or she notices altered gait, to measure muscle strength (active and resisted movement) and range of movement (active and passive movement) at each joint involved in the gait cycle.

The parameters of gait (see "Normal Parameters of Gait," earlier) may also be measured to see if there are differences between the left and right gait cycles.[67,68] Leg length discrepancies (see Chapter 11 for leg length measurement) may also affect gait. Children tend to have better compensation mechanisms for leg length discrepancies than do adults.[69] Table 9.9 gives functional causes of leg length differences. Tables 11.15, 12.2, and 13.4 outline malalignments that may also affect gait.

Locomotion Scores

In addition to the detailed assessment of gait, locomotion scales or grading systems have been developed that include subjective and objective scores, which are combined for a total score. eTool 14.1 is a locomotion scoring scale that was developed for rheumatoid arthritis.[70] eTool 14.2 shows the modified **Gait Abnormality Scale (GARS-M)** for elderly people who may be at high risk for falling.[71–73] In addition to including all aspects of locomotion, it gives an overall estimation of functional disability for patients with rheumatoid arthritis. Wolf and associates reported on the Emory Functional Ambulation Profile and established its reliability and validity.[74,75] The profile measures different tasks and surfaces for stroke patients and can differentiate between those suffering from a stroke and normals. The profile does time trials and measures such things as a 5 m (16.4-feet) walk on bare floor and carpeted floor, an "up and go" task, negotiating an obstacle course, and stair climbing. The **Walking Safety Scale** (Grille d'évaluation de la sécurité à la marche [GEM]) is a scale developed to measure walking ability and safety.[16,76] It is a functional scale divided into basic level (walking short distances in different directions), advanced level (walking and doing other activities or walking on different surfaces), and outdoor activities; it can also test patients with walking aids. It has both patient input (perception and safety)

TABLE **14.5**

Walking Items for Each Subscale of the Walking Safety Scale

Sub-scale	Items
Sub-scale A: Basic level	A1: Stand up from a chair (or wheelchair) and walk 10 m
	A2: Walk 1 m, then turn 180° and walk 1 m
	A3: Walk 2 m and turn the head to the right
	A4: Walk 2 m and turn the head to the left
	A5: Walk 2 m and stop abruptly
	A6: Walk backward 1 m
	A7: Walk sideways 1 m to the right
	A8: Walk sideways 1 m to the left
	A9: Walk 1 m, make an S around two chairs, and walk 1 m
	A10: Walk 1 m and sit down on the chair (or wheelchair)
Sub-scale B: Advanced level	B1: Walk 1 m and then sit on a chair without armrests
	B2: Get up from a chair without armrests and walk 1 m
	B3: Walk 1 m, go over a doorsill, and then walk 1 m
	B4: Walk 1 m, pick up a shoe, and walk 1 m
	B5: Walk 1 m and open then close a door
	B6: On carpet, walk 5 m
	B7: On carpet, walk 1 m, then turn 180° and walk 1 m
	B8: On carpet, walk backward 1 m
	B9: On carpet, walk 1 m sideways to the right
	B10: On carpet, walk 1 m sideways to the left
	B11: On carpet, walk 1 m, make an S around two chairs, and walk 1 m
	B12: Walk 1 m, climb stairs, and walk 1 m
	B13: Walk 1 m, descend stairs, and walk 1 m
Sub-scale C: Pretest for outdoor walking	C1: Walk 1 m and step up onto a platform 15 cm high
	C2: Step down from a platform 15 cm high and walk 1 m
	C3: On mat, walk 2 m
	C4: On mat, walk 1 m then turn 180° and walk 1 m
	C5: On mat, walk 1 m and stop abruptly
	C6: On mat, walk backward 1 m
	C7: Walk 3 m up an incline
	C8: Walk 3 m down an incline
	C9: Walk 1 m, climb stairs, and walk 1 m
	C10: Walk 1 m, descend stairs, and walk 1 m

From Kaegi C, Boudreau R, Rousseau J, et al: Development of a walking safety scale for older adults. Part 1: content validity of the GEM scale, *Physiother Can* 60:264–273, 2008.

and examiner (rater) input. Table 14.5 shows the walking items for each subscale. The **modified Gait Efficacy Scale (mGES)** (eTool 14.3) was designed to measure walking confidence in older adults during everyday activities.[77] Other functional tests include the **Get Up and Go Test,**[78] the **Functional Ambulatory Classification Scale,**[79,80] **Figure-of-8 Walk Test,**[81] **Functional Gait Assessment** (for assessing postural stability during gait in adults over 60 years of age),[82–85] **Dynamic Gait Index,**[86–88] and the **Performance Oriented Balance and Mobility Assessment (POMA).**[89]

Compensatory Mechanisms

The examiner must try to determine the primary cause of gait faults and the compensatory factors used to maintain an energy-saving gait. The patient tries to use the most energy-saving gait possible.[90] Speed of walking can also modify many of the normal parameters of gait.[91] Therefore not only the gait pattern but also the speed of the activity and its effects must be noted. This type of assessment allows the examiner to set appropriate goals and plan a logical approach to treatment.

Abnormal Gait

Gait deviations can occur for three reasons. First, they may occur because of pathology or injury in the specific joint (Table 14.6). Second, they may occur as compensations for injury or pathology in other joints on the same or ipsilateral side. Finally, they may occur as compensations for injury or pathology on the opposite limb (Table 14.7).[17] Some of the more common gait abnormalities are discussed next, but this list is by no means all inclusive.

TABLE **14.6**

Gait Deviations Secondary to Specific Impairments[a,b]

Gait Deviations at the Hip/Pelvis/Trunk Secondary to Specific Hip/Pelvis/Trunk Impairments

Observed Gait Deviation at the Hip/Pelvis/Trunk	Likely Impairment	Selected Pathologic Precursors	Mechanical Rationale and/or Associated Compensations
Backward trunk lean during **loading response**	Weak hip extensors	Paralysis of poliomyelitis	This action moves the line of gravity of the trunk behind the hip and reduces the need for hip extension torque
Lateral trunk lean toward the **stance** leg; since this movement compensates for a weakness, it is often called "compensated" Trendelenburg gait and is referred to as a waddling gait if bilateral	Marked weakness of the hip abductors	Guillain-Barré syndrome or poliomyelitis	Shifting the trunk over the supporting limb reduces the demand on the hip abductors
	Hip pain	Arthritis	Shifting the trunk over the supporting lower extremity reduces compressive joint forces associated with the action of hip abductors
Excessive downward drop of the contralateral pelvis during **stance** (referred to as positive Trendelenburg sign if present during single-limb standing)	Mild weakness of the gluteus medius of the stance leg	Guillain-Barré syndrome or poliomyelitis	Although the Trendelenburg sign may be seen in single-limb standing, a compensated Trendelenburg gait is often seen when there is severe weakness of the hip abductors
Forward bending of the trunk during **mid- and terminal stance** as the hip is moved over the foot	Hip flexion contracture	Hip osteoarthritis	Forward trunk leaning is used to compensate for lack of hip extension; an alternate adaptation could be excessive lumbar lordosis
	Hip pain	Hip osteoarthritis	Keeping the hip at 30° of flexion minimizes intra-articular pressure
Excessive lumbar lordosis in **terminal stance**	Hip flexion contracture	Arthritis	Lack of hip extension in terminal stance is compensated for by increased lordosis
Trunk lurches backward and toward the unaffected stance leg from **heel off to midswing**	Hip flexor weakness	L2–L3 nerve compression	Hip flexion is passively generated by a backward movement of the trunk
Posterior tilt of the pelvis during **initial swing**	Hip flexor weakness	L2–L3 nerve compression	Abdominals are used during initial swing to advance the swing leg
Hip circumduction: semicircular movement of the hip during **swing**—combining hip flexion, hip abduction and forward rotation of the pelvis	Hip flexor weakness	L2–L3 nerve compression	Semicircular movement combining hip flexion, hip abduction, and forward rotation of the pelvis

Gait Deviations at the Knee Secondary to Specific Knee Impairments

Observed Gait Deviation at the Knee	Likely Impairment	Selected Pathologic Precursors	Mechanical Rationale and/or Associated Compensations
Rapid extension of the knee (knee extensor thrust) immediately altering **initial contact**	Spasticity of the quadriceps	Upper motor neuron lesion	Depending on the status of the posterior structures of the knee, may occur with or without knee hyperextension

TABLE **14.6**

Gait Deviations Secondary to Specific Impairments—cont'd

Gait Deviations at the Knee Secondary to Specific Knee Impairments

Observed Gait Deviation at the Knee	Likely Impairment	Selected Pathologic Precursors	Mechanical Rationale and/or Associated Compensations
Knee remains extended during the **loading response** but without extensor thrust	Weak quadriceps	Femoral nerve palsy, L3–L4 compression neuropathy	Knee remains fully extended throughout stance; an associated anterior trunk lean in the early part of stance moves the line of gravity of the trunk slightly anterior to the axis of rotation of the knee; this keeps the knee extended without action of the knee extensors; this gait deviation may lead to an excessive stretching of the posterior capsule of the knee and eventual knee hyperextension (genu recurvatum) during stance
	Knee pain	Arthritis	Knee is kept in extension to reduce the need for quadriceps activity and associated compressive forces; it may be accompanied by an antalgic gait pattern characterized by a reduced stance time and shorter step length
Genu recurvatum (hyperextension) during **stance**	Knee extensor weakness (see the two previously described gait deviations)	Poliomyelitis	Secondary to progressive stretching of the posterior capsule of the knee
Varus thrust during **stance**	Laxity of the posterior and lateral ligamentous joint structures of the knee	Traumatic injury or progressive laxity	Rapid varus deviation of the knee during midstance, typically accompanied by knee hyperextension
Flexed position of the knee during **stance** and lack of knee extension in **terminal swing**	Knee flexion contracture >10° (genu flexum); hamstring overactivity (spasticity)	Upper motor neuron lesion	Associated increase in hip flexion and ankle dorsiflexion during stance
	Knee pain and joint effusion	Trauma or arthritis	Knee is kept in flexion since this is the position of lowest intra-articular pressure
Reduced or absent knee flexion during **swing**	Spasticity of knee extensors; knee extension contracture	Upper motor neuron lesion; immobilization (cast, brace) or surgical fusion	Compensatory hip hiking and/or hip circumduction could be noted

Gait Deviations at the Ankle/Foot Secondary to Specific Ankle/Foot Impairments

Observed Gait Deviation at the Ankle/Foot	Likely Impairment	Selected Pathologic Precursors	Mechanical Rationale and/or Associated Compensations
"Foot slap": rapid ankle plantar flexion occurs following **heel contact**; the name *foot slap* is derived from the characteristic noise made by the forefoot hitting the ground	Mild weakness of ankle dorsiflexors	Common peroneal nerve palsy and distal peripheral neuropathy	Ankle dorsiflexors have sufficient strength to dorsiflex the ankle during swing but not enough to control ankle plantar flexion after heel contact; no other gait deviations
"Foot flat": Entire plantar aspect of the foot touches the ground at **initial contact**,[c] followed by normal, passive ankle dorsiflexion during the rest of stance	Marked weakness of ankle dorsiflexors	Common peroneal nerve palsy and distal peripheral neuropathy	Sufficient strength of the dorsiflexors to partially but not completely dorsiflex the ankle during swing; normal dorsiflexion occurs during stance as long as the ankle has normal ROM; no other gait deviations

TABLE **14.6**

Gait Deviations Secondary to Specific Impairments—cont'd

Gait Deviations at the Ankle/Foot Secondary to Specific Ankle/Foot Impairments

Observed Gait Deviation at the Ankle/Foot	Likely Impairment	Selected Pathologic Precursors	Mechanical Rationale and/or Associated Compensations
Initial contact with the ground is made by the forefoot, followed by the heel region; normal passive ankle dorsiflexion occurs during stance	Severe weakness of ankle dorsiflexors	Common peroneal nerve palsy and distal peripheral neuropathy	No active ankle dorsiflexion is possible during swing; normal dorsiflexion occurs during stance as long as the ankle has normal ROM; likely requires excessive knee and hip flexion during swing to avoid catching toes on the ground
Initial contact is made with the forefoot, but the heel never makes contact with the ground during stance	Heel pain Plantar flexion contracture (pes equinus deformity) or spasticity of ankle plantar flexors	Calcaneal fracture, plantar fasciitis Upper motor neuron lesion (cerebral palsy, CVA)	Purposeful strategy to avoid weight bearing on the heel To maintain the weight over the foot, the knee and hip are kept in flexion throughout stance, leading to a "crouched gait"; requires short steps
Initial contact is made with the forefoot, and the heel is brought to the ground by a posterior displacement of the tibia **at midstance**	Plantar flexion contracture (pes equinus deformity) or spasticity of ankle plantar flexors	Upper motor neuron lesion (cerebral palsy, CVA) Ankle fusion in a plantar flexed position	Knee hyperextension occurs during stance owing to the inability of the tibia to move forward over the foot; hip flexion and excessive forward trunk lean during terminal stance occur to shift the weight of the body over the foot
Premature elevation of the heel in **midstance or terminal stance**	Lack of ankle dorsiflexion	Congenital or acquired muscular tightness of ankle plantar flexors	Characteristic bouncing gait pattern
Heel remains in contact with the ground late in **terminal stance**	Weakness or flaccid paralysis of plantar flexors with or without a fixed dorsiflexed position of the ankle (pes calcaneus deformity)	Peripheral or central nervous system disorders; excessive surgical lengthening of the Achilles tendon	Excessive ankle dorsiflexion results in prolonged heel contact, reduced push off, and a shorter step length
Supinated foot position and weight bearing on the lateral aspect of the foot during **stance**	Pes cavus deformity	Congenital structural deformity	A high medial longitudinal arch is noted with reduced midfoot mobility throughout swing and stance
Excessive foot pronation occurs during **stance,** with failure of the foot to supinate in midstance; normal medial longitudinal arch noted during swing	Rearfoot varus and/or forefoot varus	Congenital or acquired structural deformity	Excessive foot pronation and associated flattening of the medial longitudinal arch may be accompanied by a general medial rotation of the lower extremity during stance
Excessive foot pronation with weight bearing on the medial portion of the foot during **stance;** the medial longitudinal arch remains absent during **swing**	Weakness (paralysis) of ankle invertors Pes planus deformity	Upper motor neuron lesion Congenital structural deformity	An overall excessive medial rotation of the lower extremity during stance is possible

Continued

TABLE **14.6**

Gait Deviations Secondary to Specific Impairments—cont'd

Gait Deviations at the Ankle/Foot Secondary to Specific Ankle/Foot Impairments

Observed Gait Deviation at the Ankle/Foot	Likely Impairment	Selected Pathologic Precursors	Mechanical Rationale and/or Associated Compensations
Excessive inversion and plantar flexion of the foot and ankle occur during swing and at **initial contact**	Pes equinovarus due to spasticity of the plantar flexors and inverters	Upper motor neuron lesion (cerebral palsy, CVA)	Contact with the ground is made with the lateral border of the forefoot; weight bearing on the lateral border of the foot during stance
Ankle remains plantar flexed during **swing** and can be associated with dragging of the toes, typically called *drop foot*	Weakness of dorsiflexors and/or pes equinus deformity	Common peroneal nerve palsy	Hip hiking, hip circumduction, or excessive hip and knee flexion of the swing leg or vaulting of the stance leg may be noted to lift the toes off the ground and prevent the toes from dragging during swing

[a]An impairment is a loss or an abnormality in physiologic, psychologic, or anatomic structure or function.
[b]Note: Terms in **boldface** indicate when in the gait cycle the gait deviation is expressed.
[c]Initial contact is often used instead of heel contact to reflect the fact that with many gait deviations the heel is not the part of the foot that makes initial contact with the ground.
CVA, Cerebrovascular accident; *ROM*, range of motion.
From Simoneau GG: Kinesiology of walking. In Neumann DA, editor: *Kinesiology of the musculoskeletal system: foundations of physical rehabilitation*, ed 2, St Louis, 2010, Mosby, pp 665, 666, 668.

TABLE **14.7**

Gait Deviations as a Compensation for a Lower Extremity Impairment[a]

Gait Deviations Seen at the Hip/Pelvis/Trunk as a Compensation for an Impairment of the Ipsilateral Ankle, Ipsilateral Knee, or Contralateral Lower Extremity

Observed Gait Deviation at the Hip/Pelvis/Trunk	Likely Impairment	Mechanical Rationale
Forward bending of the trunk during the **loading response**	Weak quadriceps	Trunk is brought forward to move the line of gravity anterior to the axis of rotation of the knee, thereby reducing the need for knee extensors
Forward bending of the trunk during **mid- and terminal stance**	Pes equinus deformity	Lack of ankle dorsiflexion during stance results in knee hyperextension and forward trunk lean to move the weight of the body over the stance foot
Excessive hip and knee flexion during **swing**	Often due to lack of dorsiflexion of the swing leg; may also be due to a functionally or anatomically short contralateral stance leg	Used to clear the toes of the swing leg
Hip circumduction during **swing**	Lack of shortening of the swing leg secondary to reduced hip flexion, reduced knee flexion, and/or lack of ankle dorsiflexion	Used to lift the foot of the swing leg off the ground and provide toe clearance
Hip hiking (elevation of the ipsilateral pelvis during **swing**)	Lack of shortening of the swing leg secondary to reduced hip flexion, reduced knee flexion, and/or lack of ankle dorsiflexion / Functionally or anatomically short stance leg	Used to lift the foot of the swing leg off the ground and provide toe clearance
Excessive backward horizontal rotation of the pelvis on the side of the stance leg in **terminal stance**	Ankle plantar flexor weakness	Ankle plantar flexor weakness leads to prolonged heel contact and lack of push off; an increased pelvic horizontal rotation is used to lengthen the limb and maintain adequate step length

TABLE **14.7**

Gait Deviations as a Compensation for a Lower Extremity Impairment—cont'd

Gait Deviations Seen at the Knee as a Compensation for an Impairment of the Ipsilateral Ankle, Ipsilateral Hip, or Contralateral Lower Extremity

Observed Gait Deviation at the Knee	Likely Impairment	Mechanical Rationale
Knee is kept in flexion during **stance** despite the knee having normal ROM on examination	Impairments at the ankle or the hip, including a pes calcaneus deformity, plantar flexor weakness, and hip flexion contracture	Exaggerated ankle dorsiflexion or hip flexion during stance forces the knee in a flexed position; the contralateral (healthy) swing leg shows exaggerated hip and knee flexion to clear the toes owing to the functionally shorter stance leg
Hyperextension of the knee (genu recurvatum) from **initial contact to preswing**	Ankle plantar flexion contracture (pes equinus deformity) or spasticity of ankle plantar flexors	Knee must hyperextend to compensate for the lack of forward displacement of the tibia during midstance
Antalgic gait	Painful stance leg	This is characterized by a shorter step length and stance time on the side of the painful lower extremity; it may be accompanied by ipsilateral trunk lean; if hip pain, contralateral trunk lean occurs with knee and foot pain
Excessive knee flexion in **swing**	Lack of ankle dorsiflexion of the swing leg or a short stance leg	Strategy to increase toe clearance of the swing leg, typically accompanied by increased hip flexion

Gait Deviations Seen at the Ankle and Foot as a Compensation for an Impairment of the Ipsilateral Ankle, Ipsilateral Hip, or Contralateral Lower Extremity

Observed Gait Deviation at the Ankle/Foot	Likely Impairment	Mechanical Rationale
Vaulting: compensatory mechanism demonstrated by exaggerated ankle plantar flexion during **midstance**; leads to excessive vertical movement of the body	Any impairment of the contralateral lower extremity that reduces hip flexion, knee flexion, or ankle dorsiflexion during swing	Strategy used to allow the foot of a functionally long, contralateral lower extremity to clear the ground during swing
Excessive foot angle during **stance**, called *toeing out*	Retroversion of the neck of the femur or tight hip lateral rotators	Foot is in excessive toeing out due to excessive lateral rotation of the lower extremity
Reduction of the normal foot ankle during **stance**, called *toeing in*	Excessive femoral anteversion or spasticity of the hip adductors and/or hip medial rotators	General medial rotation of the lower extremity

[a]Note: Terms in **boldface** indicate when in the gait cycle the gait deviation is expressed.
ROM, Range of motion.
From Simoneau GG: Kinesiology of walking. In Neumann DA: *Kinesiology of the musculoskeletal system: foundations of physical rehabilitation*, ed 2, St Louis, 2010, Mosby, pp 665–670.

Antalgic (Painful) Gait

The antalgic or painful gait is self-protective and is the result of injury to the pelvis, hip, knee, ankle, or foot. The stance phase on the affected leg is shorter than that on the nonaffected leg because the patient attempts to remove weight from the affected leg as quickly as possible; therefore the amount of time on each leg should be noted. The swing phase of the uninvolved leg is decreased. The result is a shorter step length on the uninvolved side, decreased walking velocity, and decreased cadence.[44] In addition, the painful region is often supported by one hand if it is within reach of a supporting structure, and the other arm, acting as a counterbalance, is outstretched. If a painful hip is causing the problem, the patient also shifts the body weight over the painful hip. This shift decreases the pull of the abductor muscles, which decreases the pressure on the femoral head from more than two times the body weight to approximately body weight owing to vertical instead of angular placement of the load over the hip. Flynn and Widmann have outlined some of the causes of a painful limp in children[92] (Table 14.8). In those with ankle osteoarthritis, both genders minimize limb loading on the affected side by increasing swing time and reducing stance time on the affected side.[93]

TABLE **14.8**

Differential Diagnosis of Antalgic Gait

Less Than 4 Years	4–10 Years	More Than 10 Years
• Toddler's fracture (tibia or foot) • Osteomyelitis, septic arthritis, discitis • Arthritis (juvenile rheumatoid arthritis, Lyme disease) • Discoid lateral meniscus • Foreign body in the foot • Benign or malignant tumor	• Fracture (especially physeal) • Osteomyelitis, septic arthritis, discitis • Legg-Calvé-Perthes disease • Transient synovitis • Osteochondritis dissecans (knee or ankle) • Discoid lateral meniscus • Sever's apophysitis (calcaneus) • Accessory tarsal navicular • Foreign body in the foot • Arthritis (juvenile rheumatoid arthritis, Lyme disease) • Benign or malignant tumor	• Stress fracture (femur, tibia, foot, pars interarticularis) • Osteomyelitis, septic arthritis, discitis • Slipped capital femoral epiphysis • Osgood-Schlatter disease or Sinding-Larsen-Johanssen syndrome • Osteochondritis dissecans (knee or ankle) • Chondromalacia patellae • Arthritis (Lyme disease, gonococcal) • Accessory tarsal navicular • Tarsal coalition • Benign or malignant tumor

© 2001 American Academy of Orthopaedic Surgeons. Reprinted from the Journal of the American Academy of Orthopaedic Surgeons, vol 9(2), pp. 89–98.

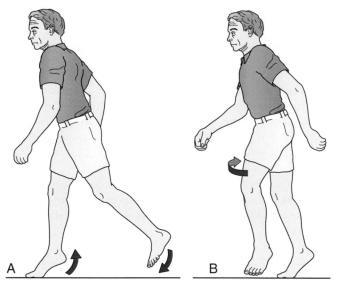

Fig. 14.15 Arthrogenic (stiff knee or hip) gait. (A) Excessive plantar flexion. (B) Circumduction.

Arthrogenic (Stiff Hip or Knee) Gait

The arthrogenic gait results from stiffness, laxity, or deformity; it may be painful or pain free. If the knee or hip is fused or the knee has recently been removed from a cylinder cast, the pelvis must be elevated by exaggerated plantar flexion of the opposite ankle and circumduction of the stiff leg (**circumducted gait**) to provide toe clearance. The patient with this gait lifts the entire leg higher than normal to clear the ground because of a stiff hip or knee (Fig. 14.15). The arc of movement helps to decrease the elevation needed to clear the affected leg. Because of the loss of flexibility in the hip, knee, or both, the gait lengths are different for the two legs. When the stiff limb is bearing weight, the gait length is usually smaller.

Ataxic Gait

If the patient has poor sensation or lacks muscle coordination, there is a tendency toward poor balance and a broad base (Fig. 14.16). The gait of a person with cerebellar ataxia includes a lurch or stagger, and all movements are exaggerated. The feet of an individual with sensory ataxia slap the ground because the patient cannot feel them. The patient also watches his or her feet while walking. The resulting gait is irregular, jerky, and weaving.

Contracture Gaits

Joints of the lower limb may exhibit contracture if immobilization has been prolonged or pathology to the joint has not been properly cared for. Hip flexion contracture often results in increased lumbar lordosis and extension of the trunk combined with knee flexion to get the foot on the ground. With a knee flexion contracture, the patient demonstrates excessive ankle dorsiflexion from late swing phase to early stance phase on the uninvolved leg and early heel rise on the involved side in terminal stance. Plantar flexion contracture at the ankle results in knee hyperextension (midstance of affected leg) and forward bending of the trunk with hip flexion (midstance to terminal stance of affected leg). Heel rise on the affected leg also occurs earlier.[44]

Coxalgic Gait

Coxalgic gait is a painful gait that is due to arthritis. With this gait, the individual lurches toward the affected side while the pelvis stays level or elevated on the contralateral side (i.e., no Trendelenburg sign) due to normal abductors on the affected side.[94,95] The lateral shift to the affected side during stance reduces the forces exerted on the stance leg.

Equinus Gait (Toe Walking)

This childhood gait is seen with talipes equinovarus (club foot) and is characterized by a forefoot strike to initiate the gait cycle and premature plantar flexion in loading response prior to midstance (Table 14.9).[96] Weight bearing is primarily on the dorsolateral or lateral edge of the foot, depending on the degree of deformity. The weight-bearing phase on the affected limb is decreased and a limp is present. The pelvis and femur are laterally rotated to partially compensate for medial rotation of the tibia and foot.[2]

Gluteus Maximus Gait

If the gluteus maximus muscle, a primary hip extensor, is weak, the patient thrusts the thorax posteriorly at initial contact (heel strike) to maintain hip extension of the stance leg. The resulting gait involves a characteristic backward lurch of the trunk (Fig. 14.17).

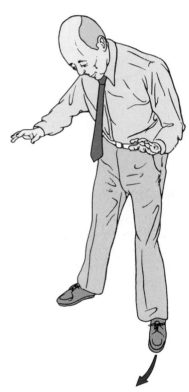

Fig. 14.16 Ataxic gait. (Redrawn from Judge RD, Zuidema GD, Fitzgerald FT: *Clinical diagnosis: a physiological approach*, Boston, 1982, Little, Brown, p 438.)

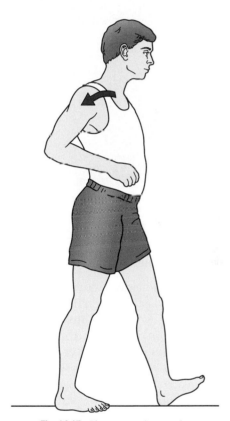

Fig. 14.17 Gluteus maximus gait.

TABLE **14.9**

Differential Diagnosis of a Nonantalgic Limp

Equinus Gait (Toe Walking)	Trendelenburg Gait	Circumduction Gait/Vaulting Gait	Steppage Gait
• Idiopathic tight Achilles tendon • Clubfoot (residual or untreated) • Cerebral palsy • Limb length discrepancy	• Legg-Calvé-Perthes disease • Developmental dysplasia of the hip • Slipped capital femoral epiphysis • Muscular dystrophy • Hemiplegic cerebral palsy • Weak gluteus medius	• Limb length discrepancy • Cerebral palsy • Any cause of ankle or knee stiffness	• Cerebral palsy • Myelodysplasia • Charcot-Marie-Tooth disease • Friedreich ataxia • Tibial nerve palsy

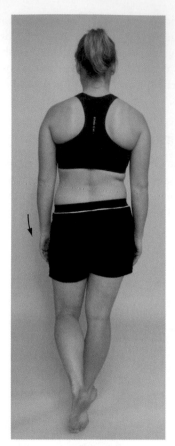

Fig. 14.18 Gluteus medius (Trendelenburg) gait.

Gluteus Medius (Trendelenburg) Gait

If the hip abductor muscles (gluteus medius and minimus) are weak, the stabilizing effect of these muscles during stance phase is lost and the patient exhibits an excessive lateral list in which the thorax is thrust laterally to keep the center of gravity over the stance leg (Fig. 14.18).[95] A positive Trendelenburg sign is also exhibited (i.e., the contralateral side droops because the ipsilateral hip abductors do not stabilize or prevent the droop). If there is bilateral weakness of the gluteus medius muscles, the gait shows accentuated side-to-side movement, resulting in a wobbling gait or "chorus girl swing." This gait may also be seen in patients with congenital dislocation of the hip and coxa vara (see Table 14.9).

Hemiplegic or Hemiparetic Gait

The patient with hemiplegic or hemiparetic gait swings the paraplegic leg outward and ahead in a circle (circumduction) or pushes it ahead (Fig. 14.19). In addition, the affected upper limb is carried across the trunk for balance. This is sometimes referred to as a **neurogenic** or **flaccid gait.**

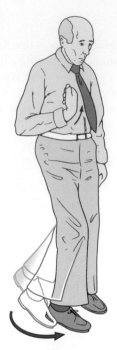

Fig. 14.19 Hemiplegic (hemiparetic) gait. (Redrawn from Judge RD, Zuidema GD, Fitzgerald FT: *Clinical diagnosis: a physiological approach*, Boston, 1982, Little, Brown, p 438.)

Knee Hyperextension Gait

This gait is the result of quadriceps weakness resulting in knee hyperextension during early stance phase often with a flat-foot initial contact. Increased hip extension along with increased plantar flexion at the ankle extend and advance the affected leg during the stance phase.[94,95]

Obesity Gait

Obesity gait is described as a waddling gait with increased lateral displacement of the trunk. Other gait alterations can include pelvic obliquity, hip circumduction, increase knee valgus, lateral foot rotation, overpronation, and an increased exaggerated base of support (legs abducted more than normal; i.e., wider stance).

Parkinsonian Gait

The neck, trunk, and knees of a patient with parkinsonian gait are flexed. The gait is characterized by shuffling or short rapid steps (marche à petits pas) at times. The arms are held stiffly and do not have their normal associative movement (Fig. 14.20). During the gait, the patient may lean forward and walk progressively faster as though unable to stop (**festination**).[97]

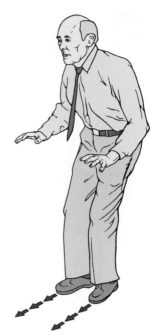

Fig. 14.20 Parkinsonian gait. (Redrawn from Judge RD, Zuidema GD, Fitzgerald FT: *Clinical diagnosis: a physiological approach*, Boston, 1982, Little, Brown, p 496.)

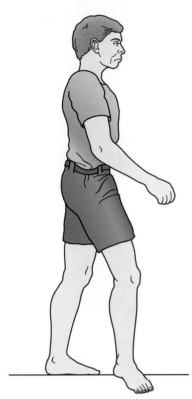

Fig. 14.21 Psoatic limp. Note lateral rotation, flexion, and abduction of affected hip.

Plantar Flexor Gait

If the plantar flexor muscles are unable to perform their function, ankle and knee stability is greatly affected. Loss of the plantar flexors results in decrease or absence of push off. The stance phase is less and there is a shorter step length on the unaffected side.[44]

Psoatic Limp

The psoatic limp is seen in patients with conditions affecting the hip, such as Legg-Calvé-Perthes disease. The patient demonstrates difficulty in swing-through, and the limp may be accompanied by exaggerated trunk and pelvic movement.[44] The limp may be caused by weakness or reflex inhibition of the psoas major muscle. Classic manifestations of this limp are lateral rotation, flexion, and adduction of the hip (Fig. 14.21). The patient exaggerates movement of the pelvis and trunk to help move the thigh into flexion.

Quadriceps Avoidance Gait

If the quadriceps muscles have been injured (e.g., femoral nerve neuropathy, reflex inhibition, trauma—3° strain), the patient compensates in the trunk and lower leg. Forward flexion of the trunk combined with strong ankle plantar flexion causes the knee to extend (hyperextend). The knee may be held extended by using the iliotibial band. If the trunk, hip flexors, and ankle muscles cannot perform this movement, the patient may use a hand to extend the knee.[44]

Scissors Gait

This gait is the result of spastic paralysis of the hip adductor muscles, which causes the knees to be drawn together so that the legs can be swung forward only with great effort (Fig. 14.22). This is seen in spastic paraplegics and may be referred to as a neurogenic or **spastic gait**.

Short Leg Gait

If one leg is shorter than the other or there is a deformity in one of the bones of the leg, the patient may demonstrate a lateral shift to the affected side, and the pelvis tilts down on the affected side, creating a limp (Fig. 14.23). The patient may also supinate the foot on the affected side to try to "lengthen" the limb. The joints of the unaffected limb may demonstrate exaggerated flexion, or hip hiking may occur during the swing phase to allow the foot to clear the ground.[44] The weight-bearing period may be the same for the two legs. How a patient adapts for leg length difference has wide variability.[98,99] With proper footwear, the gait may appear normal. This gait may also be termed *painless osteogenic gait*.

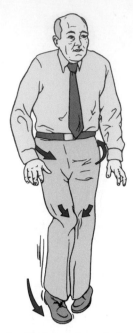

Fig. 14.22 Scissors gait. (Redrawn from Judge RD, Zuidema GD, Fitzgerald FT: *Clinical diagnosis: a physiological approach*, Boston, 1982, Little, Brown, p 439.)

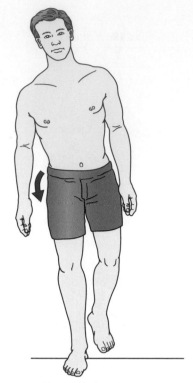

Fig. 14.23 Short leg gait.

Steppage or Drop-Foot Gait

The patient with a steppage gait has weak or paralyzed dorsiflexor muscles, resulting in a drop foot. To compensate and avoid dragging the toes against the ground, the patient lifts the knee higher than normal (Fig. 14.24). At initial contact, the foot slaps on the ground because of loss of control of the dorsiflexor muscles resulting from injury to the muscles, their peripheral nerve supply, or the nerve roots supplying the muscles (see Table 14.9).[100]

Waddling Gait[94]

This gait is due to weakness of the hip and upper thigh muscles, as seen in myopathies, which leads to an unstable pelvis during standing and walking. Because the nonstance leg (i.e., pelvis) drops on walking (i.e., a bilateral Trendelenburg sign), the individual appears to be "waddling" from side to side on a wide base, accompanied by increased lordosis. It is most commonly seen in bilateral developmental dysplasia of the hip.

Table 14.10 lists common gait pathologies that can modify gait and the phase in which the deviation occurs.[46]

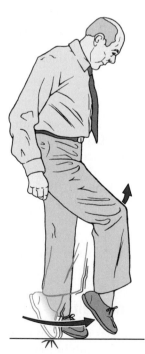

Fig. 14.24 Steppage or drop-foot gait. (Redrawn from Judge RD, Zuidema GD, Fitzgerald FT: *Clinical diagnosis: a physiological approach*, Boston, 1982, Little, Brown, p 438.)

TABLE **14.10**

Common Gait Pathologies (Deviations)

Deviation	Phase	Cause
Excessive foot pronation	Midstance through toe off	Compensated forefoot or rearfoot varus deformity, uncompensated forefoot valgus deformity, pes planus, decreased ankle dorsiflexion, increased tibial varum, long limb, uncompensated medial rotation of tibia or femur, weak tibialis posterior
Excessive foot supination	Heel strike through midstance	Compensated forefoot valgus deformity, pes cavus, short limb, uncompensated lateral rotation of tibia or femur, limited calcaneal eversion, plantar flexed first ray, upper motor neuron muscle balance
Excessive calcaneal eversion	Initial contact through midstance	Excessive tibia vara, forefoot varus, tibialis posterior weakness, excessive lower extremity medial rotation (due to muscle imbalances, femoral anteversion)
Excessive varus	Heel strike to toe off	Contracture, overactivity of muscles on medial aspect of foot
Excessive valgus	Heel strike to toe off	Weak invertors, foot hypermobility
Bouncing or exaggerated plantar flexion	Midstance through toe off	Heel cord contracture, increased tone of gastrocnemius and soleus
Excessive dorsiflexion	Heel strike to toe off	Compensation for knee flexion contracture, inadequate plantar flexor strength, adaptive shortening of dorsiflexors, increased muscle tone of dorsiflexors, pes calcaneus deformity
Insufficient push off	Midstance through toe off	Gastrocnemius and soleus weakness, Achilles tendon rupture, metatarsalgia, hallux rigidus
Foot slap	Heel strike to foot flat	Dorsiflexor weakness, lack of lower limb sensation
Steppage gait (exaggerated hip and knee flexion to clear foot)	Acceleration through deceleration	Dorsiflexor weakness or paralysis, functional leg length discrepancy
Excessive knee flexion	Heel strike through toe off	Hamstring contracture, decreased ROM in ankle dorsiflexion, plantar flexor muscle weakness, lengthened limb, hip flexion contracture
Excessive knee extension/ inadequate knee flexion	Heel strike to foot flat, and swing	Pain, anterior trunk deviation/bending, weakness of quadriceps, hyperextension is a compensation and places body weight vector anterior to knee, spasticity of the quadriceps noted more during the loading response and during initial swing intervals, joint deformity
Genu recurvatum (knee hyperextension)	Heel strike through midstance	Quadriceps femoris weak or short, compensated hamstring weakness, Achilles tendon contracture, habit
Abnormal internal hip rotation ("toe-in" gait)		Adaptive shortening of iliotibial band, weakness of hip lateral rotators, femoral anteversion, adaptive shortening of hip medial rotators
Abnormal external hip rotation ("toe-out" gait)		Adaptive shortening of hip lateral rotators, femoral retroversion, weakness of hip medial rotators
Increased hip adduction (scissors gait)	Heel strike to toe off	Spasticity or contracture of ipsilateral hip adductors, ipsilateral hip adductor weakness, coxa vara
Decreased hip swing through (psoatic limp)		Legg-Calvé-Perthes disease, weakness or reflex inhibition of psoas major muscle, pain
Excessive medial or lateral femur rotation (femoral torsion)	Heel strike through toe off	Medial or lateral hamstrings tight, respectively; opposite muscle group weakness; anteversion or retroversion, respectively

TABLE **14.10**

Common Gait Pathologies (Deviations)—cont'd

Deviation	Phase	Cause
Increased base of support (>4 inches/10 cm)	Heel strike through toe off	Abductor muscle contracture, instability, genu valgum, leg length discrepancy, fear of losing balance
Decreased base of support (<2 inches/5 cm)	Heel strike through toe off	Adductor muscle contracture, genu varum
Circumduction	Acceleration through deceleration	Increased limb length, abductor muscle shortening or overuse, stiff hip or knee
Hip hiking	Acceleration through deceleration	Increased limb length, hamstring weakness, inadequate hip or knee flexion or ankle dorsiflexion, quadratus lumborum shortening
Vaulting (ground clearance of swinging leg is increased if subject goes up on toes of stance period leg)	Foot flat to toe off	Functional leg length discrepancy, vaulting on shorter limb side
Inadequate hip flexion	Acceleration through heel strike	Hip flexor muscle weakness, hip extensor muscle shortening, increased limb length, hip joint arthrosis
Inadequate hip extension (causes trunk forward bending, increased lordosis)	Midstance through toe off	Hip flexion contracture, hip extensor muscle weakness, iliotibial band contracture, hip flexor spasticity, pain
Increased lumbar lordosis	Foot flat to toe off	Inability to extend hip, hip flexion contracture or hip ankylosis
Excessive trunk back bending (gluteus maximus gait)	Heel strike through midstance	Hip extensor or flexor muscle weakness, hip pain, decreased ROM of knee
Excessive trunk forward bending	Deceleration through midstance	Quadriceps femoris and gluteus maximus weakness, decreased ankle dorsiflexion, hip flexion contracture
Excessive trunk lateral flexion (compensated Trendelenburg gait)	Foot flat through heel off	Gluteus medius weakness, hip pain, unequal leg length, hip pathology, wide base
Pelvic drop	Foot flat through heel off	Contralateral gluteus medius weakness, adaptive shortening of quadratus lumborum, contralateral hip adductor spasticity
Excessive pelvic rotation	Heel strike to toe off	Adaptively shortened/spasticity of hip flexors on same side, limited hip joint flexion
Slower cadence than expected for person's age		Generalized weakness, pain, joint motion restrictions, poor voluntary motor control
Shorter stance phase on involved side and decreased swing phase on uninvolved side (shorter stride length on uninvolved side, decreased lateral sway over involved stance limb, decrease in cadence, decreased in velocity, use of assistive device)		Antalgic gait resulting from painful injury to lower limb and pelvic region
Stance phase longer on one side		Pain, lack of trunk and pelvic rotation, weakness of lower limb muscles, restrictions in lower limb joints, poor muscle control, increased muscle tone

ROM, Range of motion.
Adapted from Giallonardo LM: Gait. In Myers RS, editor: *Saunders manual of physical therapy practice*, Philadelphia, 1995, WB Saunders, p 1112; and Dutton M: *Orthopedic examination, evaluation and intervention*, New York, 2004, McGraw-Hill.

References

1. Winter DA. Biomechanics of normal and pathological gait: implications for understanding human locomotor control. *J Motor Behav*. 1989;21:337–355.
2. Sutherland DH, Valencia F. Pediatric gait: normal and abnormal development. In: Drennan JC, ed. *The Child's Foot and Ankle*. New York: Raven Press; 1992.
3. Eastlack ME, Arvidson J, Snyder-Mackler L, et al. Interrater reliability of videotaped observational gait-analysis assessments. *Phys Ther*. 1991;71:465–472.
4. Martin PE, Heise GD, Morgan DW. Interrelationships between mechanical power, energy transfers, and walking and running economy. *Med Sci Sports Exerc*. 1993;25:508–515.
5. Wall JC, Kirtley C. Strategies for clinical gait assessment. *Orthop Phys Ther Clin North Am*. 2001;10:35–37.
6. Bowker JH, Hall CB. *Normal human gait. Atlas of Orthotics: Biomechanical Principles and Applications*. St Louis: Mosby; 1975.
7. Inman VT, Ralston HJ, Todd F. Human locomotion. In: Rose J, Gamble JG, eds. *Human Locomotion*. Baltimore: Williams & Wilkins; 1994.
8. Sutherland DH, Kaufman KR, Moitoza JR. Kinematics of normal human walking. In: Rose J, Gamble JG, eds. *Human Locomotion*. Baltimore: Williams & Wilkins; 1994.
9. Adams JM, Perry J. Gait analysis: clinical applications. In: Rose J, Gamble JG, eds. *Human Locomotion*. Baltimore: Williams & Wilkins; 1994.
10. Koerner IB. *Normal Human Locomotion and the Gait of the Amputee*. Edmonton: University of Alberta Bookstore; 1979.
11. Koerner I. *Observation of Human Gait [videotapes], Health Sciences Audiovisual Education*. University of Alberta; 1984.
12. Perry J. *Gait Analysis: normal and Pathological Function*. Thorofare, NJ: Slack; 1994.
13. Isson EC. Methods of studying gait. In: Smidt GI, ed. *Gait in Rehabilitation*. New York: Churchill Livingstone; 1990.
14. Shiavi R. Electromyographic patterns in normal adult locomotion. In: Smidt GL, ed. *Gait in Rehabilitation*. New York: Churchill Livingstone; 1990.
15. Kuo AD, Donelan JM. Dynamic principles of gait and their clinical implications. *Phys Ther*. 2010;90:157–176.
16. Boudreau HR, Kaegi C, Rousseau J, eds. *Grille d'évaluation de la securité à la marche (GEM)*, Ottawa. Bibliothèque nationale du Canada; 2002.
17. Simoneau GG. Kinesiology of walking. In: Neumann DA, ed. *Kinesiology of the Musculoskeletal System: Foundations of Physical Rehabilitation*. 2nd ed. St Louis: Mosby; 2010.
18. Adelaar RS. The practical biomechanics of running. *Am J Sports Med*. 1986;14:497–500.
19. Larish DD, Martin PE, Mungiole M. Characteristic patterns of gait in the healthy old. *Ann NY Acad Sci*. 1988;515:18–32.
20. Bohannon RW, Williams Andrews A. Normal walking speed: a descriptive meta-analysis. *Physiotherapy*. 2011;97(3):182–189.
21. Montero-Odasso M, Magee M, Varela C, et al. Gait velocity in senior people: an easy test for detecting mobility impairment in community elderly. *J Nutr Health Aging*. 2004;8(5):340–343.
22. Mann RA, Moran GT, Dougherty SE. Comparative electromyography of the lower extremity in jogging, running, and sprinting. *Am J Sports Med*. 1986;14:501–510.
23. Barry-Greb TL, Harrison AL. Posture, gait and functional abilities of the adolescent, pregnant, and elderly female. *Orthop Phys Ther Clin North Am*. 1996;5:1–21.
24. Biden E, O'Conner J, Collins JJ. Gait analysis. In: Daniel D, Akeson W, O'Conner J, eds. *Knee Ligaments: Structure, Function, Injury and Repair*. New York: Raven Press; 1990.
25. Hoppenfeld S. *Physical Examination of the Spine and Extremities*. New York: Appleton-Century-Crofts; 1976.
26. Barry-Greb TL, Harrison AL. Posture, gait, and functional abilities of the adolescent, pregnant and elderly female. *Orthop Phys Ther Clin North Am*. 1996;5:1–21.
27. Sutherland DH, Olshen R, Cooper L, et al. The development of mature gait. *J Bone Joint Surg Am*. 1980;62:336–353.
28. Grabiner PC, Biswas ST, Grabiner MD. Age-related changes in spatial and temporal gait variables. *Arch Phys Med Rehabil*. 2001;82(1):31–35.
29. Menant JC, Steele JR, Menz HB, et al. Effects of walking surfaces and footwear on temporo-spatial gait parameters in young and older people. *Gait Posture*. 2009;29(3):392–397.
30. Menz HB, Latt MD, Tiedemann A, et al. Reliability of the GAITRite walkway system for the quantification of temporo-spatial parameters of gait in young and older people. *Gait Posture*. 2004;20(1):20–25.
31. Subotnick SI. Variations in angles of gait in running. *Phys Sportsmed*. 1979;7:110–114.
32. Sekiya N, Nagasaki H, Ito H, et al. Optimal walking in terms of variability in step length. *J Orthop Sports Phys Ther*. 1997;26:266–272.
33. Ostrosky KM, Van Swearingen JM, Burdett RG, et al. A comparison of gait characteristics in young and old subjects. *Phys Ther*. 1994;74:637–646.
34. Waters RL, Hislop HJ, Perry J, et al. Comparative cost of walking in young and old adults. *J Orthop Res*. 1983;1:73–76.
35. Levangie PK, Norkin CC, *Joint Structure and Function: A Comprehensive Analysis*. Philadelphia: FA Davis; 2005.
36. Nuber GW. Biomechanics of the foot and ankle during gait. *Clin Sports Med*. 1988;7:1–13.
37. Rodgers MM. Dynamic foot mechanics. *J Orthop Sports Phys Ther*. 1995;21:306–316.
38. Rowe DA, Welk GJ, Heil DP, et al. Stride rate recommendations for moderate intensity walking. *Med Sci Sports Exerc*. 2011;43:312–318.
39. Bruening DA, Frimenko RE, Goodyear CD, et al. Sex differences in whole body gait kinematics at preferred speeds. *Gait Posture*. 2015;41(2):540–545.
40. Finley FR, Cody KA. Locomotive characteristics of urban pedestrians. *Arch Phys Med Rehabil*. 1970;51(7):423–426.
41. Murray MP, Sepic SB, Barnard RJ. Patterns of sagittal rotation of the upper limbs in walking. *Phys Ther*. 1967;47(4):272–284.
42. Gage JR, DeLuca PA, Renshaw TS. Gait analysis: principles and application with emphasis on its use with cerebral palsy. *Inst Course Lect*. 1996;45:491–507.
43. Perry J, Hislop HJ. The mechanics of walking: a clinical interpretation. In: Perry J, Hislop HJ, eds. *Principles of Lower-Extremity Bracing*. New York: American Physical Therapy Association; 1970.
44. Epler M. Gait. In: Richardson JK, Iglarsh ZA, eds. *Clinical Orthopedic Physical Therapy*. Philadelphia: WB Saunders; 1994.
45. Krebs DE, Wong D, Jevsevar D, et al. Trunk kinematics during locomotor activities. *Phys Ther*. 1992;72:505–514.
46. Giallonardo LM. Gait. In: Myers RS, ed. *Saunders Manual of Physical Therapy Practice*. Philadelphia: WB Saunders; 1995.
47. Lyu SR, Ogata K, Hoshiko I. Effects of a cane on floor reaction force and centre of force during gait. *Clin Orthop Relat Res*. 2000;375:313–319.
48. Rab GT. Muscle. In: Rose J, Gamble JG, eds. *Human Locomotion*. Baltimore: Williams & Wilkins; 1994.
49. Krebs DE, Robbins CE, Lavine L, et al. Hip biomechanics during gait. *J Orthop Sports Phys Ther*. 1998;28:51–59.
50. Reiman MP, Thorborg K. Clinical examination and physical assessment of hip joint-related pain in athletes. *Int J Sports Phys Ther*. 2014;9(6):737–755.
51. Semciw AI, Green RA, Murley GS, Pizzari T. Gluteus minimus: an intramuscular EMG investigation of anterior and posterior segments during gait. *Gait Posture*. 2014;39(2):822–826.
52. Semciw AI, Pizzari T, Murley GS, Green RA. Gluteus medius: an intramuscular EMG investigation of anterior, middle and posterior segments during gait. *J Electromyogr Kinesiol*. 2013;23(4):858–864. 1.
53. Rutherford DJ, Moreside J, Wong I. Hip joint motion and gluteal muscle activation differences between healthy controls and those with varying degrees of hip osteoarthritis during walking. *J Electromyogr Kinesiol*. 2015;25(6):944–950.
54. Willson JD, Petrowitz I, Butler RJ, Kernozek TW. Male and female gluteal muscle activity and lower extremity kinematics during running. *Clin Biomech*. 2012;27(10):1052–1057.
55. Hayati M, Talebian S, Sherrington C, et al. Impact of age and obstacle negotiation on timing measures of gait initiation. *J Bodyw Mov Ther*. 2018;22(2):361–365.
56. Dillon PZ, Updyke WF, Allen WC. Gait analysis with reference to chondromalacia patella. *J Orthop Sports Phys Ther*. 1983;5:127–131.
57. Sutherland DH, Cooper I, Daniel D. The role of the ankle plantar flexors in normal walking. *J Bone Joint Surg Am*. 1980;62:354–363.
58. van der Krogt MM, Delp SL, Schwartz MH. How robust is human gait to muscle weakness? *Gait Posture*. 2012;36:113–119.
59. Arnadottir SA, Mereer VS. Effects of footwear on measurements of balance and gait in women between the ages of 65 and 93 years. *Phys Ther*. 2000;80:17–27.
60. Mann RA, Hagy JL, White V, et al. The initiation of gait. *J Bone Joint Surg Am*. 1979;61:232–239.
61. *The Pathokinesiology Service and the Physical Therapy Department, Rancho Los Amigos Medical Center: Observational Gait Analysis*. Downey, CA: Los Amigos Research and Educational Institute; 1996.
62. Noyes FR, Dunworth LA, Andriacchi TP, et al. Knee hyperextension gait abnormalities in unstable knees. Recognition and preoperative gait retraining. *Am J Sports Med*. 1996;24(1):35–45.
63. Nyland J, Smith S, Beickman K, et al. Frontal plane knee angle affects dynamic postural control strategy during unilateral stance. *Med Sci Sports Exerc*. 2002;34(7):1150–1157.
64. Holm I, Tveter AT, Fredriksen PM, Vollestad N. A normative sample of gait and hopping on one leg parameters in children 7 to 12 years of age. *Gait Posture*. 2009;29(2):317–321.
65. Lewis CL, Sahrmann SA. Effect of posture on hip angles and moments during gait. *Man Ther*. 2015;20(1):176–182.
66. Ebbeling CJ, Hamill J, Crussemeyer JA. Lower extremity mechanics and energy cost of walking on high-heeled shoes. *J Orthop Sports Phys Ther*. 1994;19:190–196.
67. Coutts F. Gait analysis in the therapeutic environment. *Man Ther*. 1999;4:2–10.

68. Wall JC, Devlin J, Khirchof R, et al. Measurement of step widths and step lengths: a comparison of measurements made directly from a grid with those made from a video recording. *J Orthop Sports Phys Ther.* 2000;30:410–417.

69. Song KM, Halliday SE, Little DG. The effect of limb-length discrepancy on gait. *J Bone Joint Surg Am.* 1997;79:1690–1698.

70. Larsson SE, Jonsson B. Locomotion score in rheumatoid arthritis. *Acta Orthop Scand.* 1989;60:271–277.

71. Dutton M. *Dutton's Orthopedic Examination, Evaluation and Intervention.* 3rd ed. New York: McGraw-Hill; 2012.

72. Van Swearingen JM, Paschal KA, Bonino P, et al. The modified Gait Abnormality Rating Scale for recognizing the risk of recurrent falls in community-dwelling elderly adults. *Phys Ther.* 1996;76:994–1002.

73. Wolfson L, Whipple R, Amerman P, et al. Gait assessment in the elderly: a gait abnormality rating scale and its relation to falls. *J Gerontol.* 1990;45:M12–M19.

74. Wolf SL. A method of quantifying ambulatory activities. *Phys Ther.* 1979;59:767–768.

75. Wolf SL, Catlin PA, Gage K, et al. Establishing the reliability and validity of measurements of walking time using the Emory functional ambulation profile. *Phys Ther.* 1999;79:1122–1133.

76. Kaegi C, Boudreau R, Rousseau J, et al. Development of a walking safety scale for older adults. Part 1: content validity of the GEM scale. *Physiother Can.* 2008;60:264–273.

77. Newell AM, Van Swearingen JM, Hile E, et al. The modified gait efficacy scale: establishing the psychometric properties in older adults. *Phys Ther.* 2012;92:318–328.

78. Matheis A, Nayak US, Isaacs B. Balance in elderly patients: the "get-up and go" test. *Arch Phys Med Rehabil.* 1986;67:387–389.

79. Holden MK, Gill KM, Magliozzi MR, et al. Clinical gait assessment in the neurologically impaired: reliability and meaningfulness. *Phys Ther.* 1984;64:35–40.

80. Holden MK, Gill KM, Magliozzi MR. Gait assessment for neurologically impaired patients: standards for outcome assessment. *Phys Ther.* 1986;66:1530–1539.

81. Hess RJ, Brach JS, Piva SR, et al. Walking skill can be assessed in older adults: validity of the Figure-of-8 Walk Test. *Phys Ther.* 2010;90:89–99.

82. Wrisley DM, Kumar NA. Functional gait assessment: concurrent, discriminative and predictive validity in community-dwelling older adults. *Phys Ther.* 2010;90:761–775.

83. Wrisley DM, Marchetti GF, Kuharsky DK, Whitney SL. Reliability, internal consistency, and validity of data obtained with the functional gait assessment. *Phy Ther.* 2004;84(10):906–918.

84. Walker ML, Austin AG, Banke GM, et al. Reference group data for the functional gait assessment. *Phys Ther.* 2017;87(11):1468–1477.

85. Beninato M, Ludlow LH. The Functional Gait Assessment in older adults: validation through Rasch modeling. *Phys Ther.* 2016;96(4):456–468.

86. Whitney SL, Hudak MT, Marchetti GF. The Dynamic Gait Index relates to self-reported fall history in individuals with vestibular dysfunction. *J Vestib Res.* 2000;10(2):99–105.

87. Whitney S, Wrisley D, Furman J. Concurrent validity of the Berg Balance Scale and the dynamic gait index in people with vestibular dysfunction. *Physiother Res Int.* 2003;8(4):178–186.

88. Shumway-Cook A, Taylor CS, Matsuda PN, et al. Expanding the scoring system for the Dynamic Gait Index. *Phys Ther.* 2013;93(11):1493–1506.

89. Tinetti ME. Performance-oriented assessment of mobility problems in elderly patients. *J Am Geriatr Soc.* 1986;34:119–126.

90. Gleim GW, Stachenfeld NS, Nicholas JA. The influence of flexibility on the economy of walking and jogging. *J Orthop Res.* 1990;8:814–823.

91. Murray MP, Mollinger LA, Gardner GM, et al. Kinematic and EMG patterns during slow, free, and fast walking. *J Orthop Res.* 1984;2:272–280.

92. Flynn JM, Widmann RF. The limping child: evaluation and diagnosis. *J Am Acad Orthop Surg.* 2001;9:89–98.

93. Hughes-Oliver CN, Srinivasan D, Schmitt D, Queen RM. Gender and limb differences in temporal gait parameters and gait variability in ankle osteoarthritis. *Gait Posture.* 2018;65:228–233.

94. Pirker W, Katzenschlager R. Gait disorders in adults and the elderly: a clinical guide. *Wien Klin Wochenschr.* 2017;129(3–4):81–95.

95. Lim MR, Huang RC, Wu A, et al. Evaluation of the elderly patient with an abnormal gait. *J Am Acad Orthop Surg.* 2007;15(2):107–117.

96. Abel MH, Damiano DL, Pannunzio M, et al. Muscle-tendon surgery in diplegic cerebral palsy: functional and mechanical changes. *J Pediatr Orthop.* 1999;19:366–375.

97. Scandalis TA, Bosak A, Berliner JC, et al. Resistance training and gait function in patients with Parkinson's disease. *Am J Phys Med Rehabil.* 2001;80:38–43.

98. Kaufman KR, Miller LS, Sutherland DH. Gait asymmetry in patients with limb-length inequality. *J Ped Orthop.* 1996;16:144–150.

99. Song KM, Halliday SE, Little DG. The effect of limb-length discrepancy on gait. *J Bone Joint Surg Am.* 1997;79:1690–1698.

100. Morag E, Hurwitz DE, Andriacchi TP, et al. Abnormalities in muscle function during gait in relation to the level of lumbar disc herniation. *Spine.* 2000;25:829–833.

CHAPTER 15

Assessment of Posture

Postural Development

Through evolution, human beings have assumed an upright erect or bipedal posture. The advantage of an erect posture is that it enables the hands to be free and the eyes to be farther from the ground so that the individual can see farther ahead. The disadvantages include an increased strain on the spine and lower limbs and comparative difficulties in respiration and transport of the blood to the brain.

Posture, which is the relative disposition of the body at any one moment, is a composite of the positions of the different joints of the body at that time. The position of each joint has an effect on the position of the other joints. Classically, ideal static postural alignment (viewed from the side) is defined as a straight line (line of gravity) that passes through the earlobe, the bodies of the cervical vertebrae, the tip of the shoulder, midway through the thorax, through the bodies of the lumbar vertebrae, slightly posterior to the hip joint, slightly anterior to the axis of the knee joint, and just anterior to the lateral malleolus (Fig. 15.1).[1] **Correct posture** is the position in which minimum stress is applied to each joint or the optimal alignment of the patient's body that allows the neuromuscular system to perform actions requiring the least amount of energy to achieve the desired effect.[2–4] Upright posture is the normal standing posture for humans. Although upright posture allows one to see farther and provides freedom to move the arms, it does have disadvantages. It places greater stress on the lower limbs, pelvis, and spine; it reduces stability; and it increases the work of the heart.[5] If the upright postural alignment is correct, minimal muscle activity is needed to maintain the position.

Any static position that increases stress to the joints may be called **faulty posture**, which can result from several factors. If a person has strong, flexible muscles, faulty postures or malalignment may not affect the joints because he or she has the ability to change position readily so that the stresses do not become excessive. If the joints are stiff (hypomobile) or too mobile (hypermobile), or the muscles are weak, shortened, or lengthened, however, the posture cannot be easily altered to the correct alignment, and the result can be some form of pathology. As Sahrmann[7] pointed out, posture as a whole and postural malalignment may cause problems but not to the same degree that malalignment between individual segments can. As she said, a lumbar curvature can vary a great deal and within that curvature may or may not cause symptoms, but malalignment between individual segments is more likely to lead to symptoms. In addition, the body has great potential to correct postural malalignment through a corrective malalignment in one part of the body to compensate for a structural malalignment in another part of the body. Thus, when looking at posture, the examiner must look not only at overall alignment but also segmental alignment to determine

---

Factors Affecting Posture[6]

- Structural (anatomic) factors
  - Bony contours (e.g., hemivertebrae)
  - Leg length discrepancy (bone length)
  - Extra or less vertebra (e.g., lumbarization, sacralization)
  - Laxity of ligamentous structures
  - Fascial and musculotendinous tightness (e.g., tensor fasciae latae, pectorals, hip flexors)
  - Muscle tonus (e.g., gluteus maximus, abdominals, erector spinae)
  - Pelvic angle (normal is 30°)
  - Joint position and mobility
  - Neurogenic outflow and inflow
- Age (e.g., young vs. old)
- Psychological (emotional) changes (e.g., mood, fear avoidance)
- Pathological (e.g., illness, pain, malalignment)
- Occupational (e.g., manual worker, office worker)
- Recreational (e.g., different sports)
- Environmental (e.g., temperature)
- Social/cultural (e.g., kneeling)

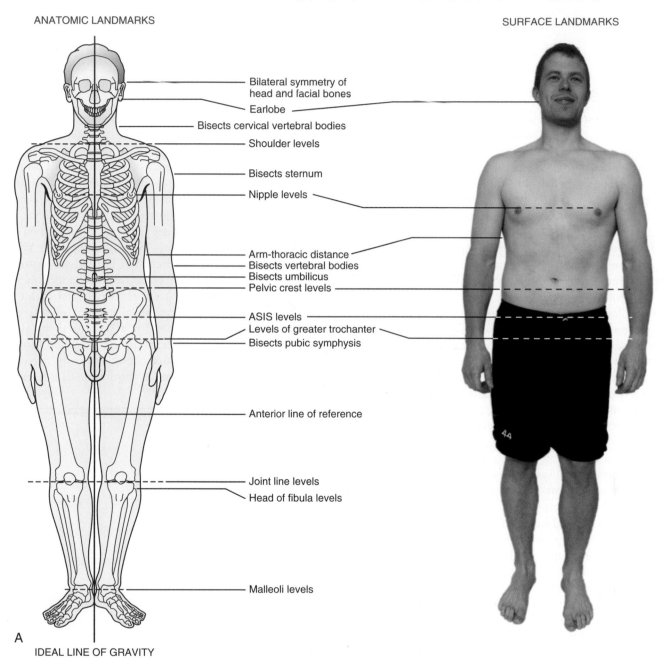

ANATOMIC LANDMARKS

SURFACE LANDMARKS

Bilateral symmetry of
head and facial bones

Earlobe

Bisects cervical vertebral bodies

Shoulder levels

Bisects sternum

Nipple levels

Arm-thoracic distance
Bisects vertebral bodies
Bisects umbilicus
Pelvic crest levels

ASIS levels
Levels of greater trochanter
Bisects pubic symphysis

Anterior line of reference

Joint line levels
Head of fibula levels

Malleoli levels

A

IDEAL LINE OF GRAVITY

Fig. 15.1 Ideal postural alignment. (A) Front view. On a typical patient note any difference in shoulder height and nipple height and apparent arm-length difference, arm-thorax difference, and difference in out-toeing or in-toeing.

ANATOMIC LANDMARKS

SURFACE LANDMARKS

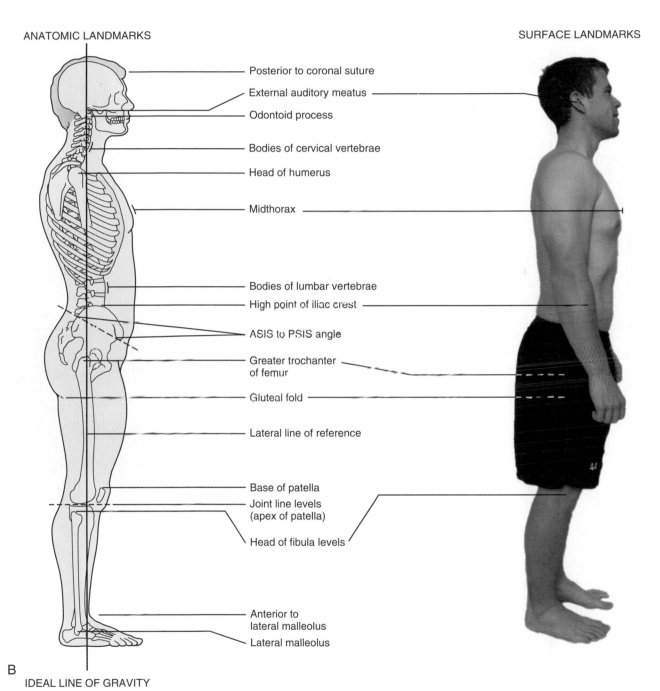

- Posterior to coronal suture
- External auditory meatus
- Odontoid process
- Bodies of cervical vertebrae
- Head of humerus
- Midthorax
- Bodies of lumbar vertebrae
- High point of iliac crest
- ASIS to PSIS angle
- Greater trochanter of femur
- Gluteal fold
- Lateral line of reference
- Base of patella
- Joint line levels (apex of patella)
- Head of fibula levels
- Anterior to lateral malleolus
- Lateral malleolus

B

IDEAL LINE OF GRAVITY

Fig. 15.1, cont'd (B) Side view. Typical patient with good lateral alignment.

ANATOMIC LANDMARKS

SURFACE LANDMARKS

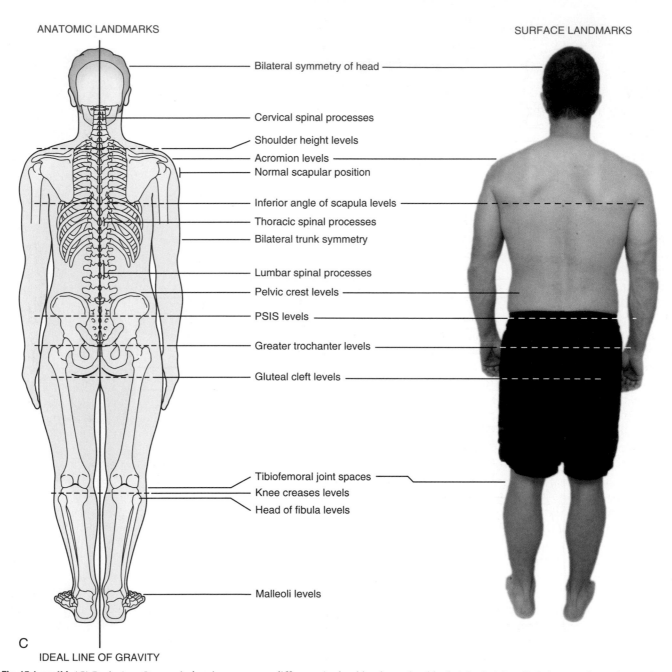

Bilateral symmetry of head

Cervical spinal processes

Shoulder height levels

Acromion levels

Normal scapular position

Inferior angle of scapula levels

Thoracic spinal processes

Bilateral trunk symmetry

Lumbar spinal processes

Pelvic crest levels

PSIS levels

Greater trochanter levels

Gluteal cleft levels

Tibiofemoral joint spaces

Knee creases levels

Head of fibula levels

Malleoli levels

C

IDEAL LINE OF GRAVITY

Fig. 15.1, cont'd (C) Back view. On a typical patient note any difference in shoulder slope, shoulder height, height of inferior scapular angles, and rotation of arms. In this view, also note straight Achilles tendons. *ASIS,* Anterior superior iliac spine; *PSIS,* posterior superior iliac spine.

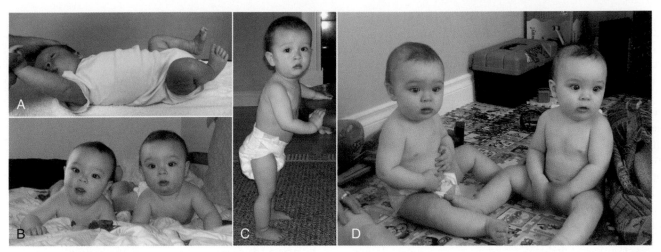

Fig. 15.2 Postural development. (A) Flexed posture in a newborn. (B) Development of secondary cervical curve. (C) Development of secondary lumbar curve. (D) Sitting posture.

whether the malalignment is functional and therefore "fixable" with treatment or structural and only fixable with surgery. The pathology may be the result of the cumulative effect of repeated small stresses (microtraumas) over a long period of time or of constant abnormal stresses (macrotraumas) over a short period of time. These chronic stresses can result in the same problems that are seen when a sudden (acute) severe stress is applied to the body. The abnormal stresses cause excessive wearing of the articular surfaces of joints and produce osteophytes and traction spurs, which represent the body's attempt to alter its structure to accommodate these repeated stresses. The soft tissue (e.g., muscles, ligaments) may become weakened, stretched, or traumatized by the increased stress. Thus postural deviations do not always cause symptoms, but over time they may do so.[8] The application of an acute stress on the chronic stress may exacerbate the problem and produce the signs and symptoms that initially prompt the patient to seek aid.

At birth, the entire spine is concave forward, or flexed (Fig. 15.2). Curves of the spine found at birth are called **primary curves.** The curves that retain this position, those of the thoracic spine and sacrum, are therefore classified as primary curves of the spine. As the child grows (Fig. 15.3), **secondary curves** appear and are convex forward, or extended. At about the age of 3 months, when the child begins to lift the head, the cervical spine becomes convex forward, producing the cervical lordosis. In the lumbar spine, the secondary curve develops slightly later (6 to 8 months), when the child begins to sit up and walk. In old age, the secondary curves again begin to disappear as the spine starts to return to a flexed position as the result of disc degeneration, ligamentous calcification, osteoporosis, and vertebral wedging. These curves provide the spinal column with increased flexibility and a

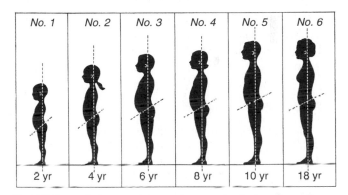

Fig. 15.3 Postural changes with age. Apparent kyphosis at 6 and 8 years is caused by scapular winging. (From McMorris RO: Faulty postures. *Pediatr Clin North Am* 8:214, 1961.)

shock-absorption mechanism to counteract the axial compressive force produced by the weight of the head and gravity.[9]

In the child, the center of gravity is at the level of the twelfth thoracic vertebra. As the child grows older, the center of gravity drops, eventually reaching the level of the second sacral vertebra in adults (slightly higher in males). The child stands with a wide base to maintain balance, and the knees are flexed. The knees are slightly bowed (genu varum) until about 18 months of age. The child then becomes slightly knock-kneed (genu valgum) until the age of 3 years. By the age of 6 years, the legs should naturally straighten (see Fig. 12.8). The lumbar spine in the child has an exaggerated lumbar curve, or excessive lordosis. This accentuated curve is caused by the presence of large abdominal contents, weakness of the abdominal musculature, and the small pelvis characteristic of children at this age.

Initially, a child is flat-footed, or appears to be, as the result of the minimal development of the medial longitudinal arch and the fat pad that is found in the arch. As the child grows, the fat pad slowly decreases in size, making the medial arch more evident. In addition, as the foot develops and the muscles strengthen, the arches of the feet develop normally and become more evident.

During adolescence, posture changes because of hormonal influence with the onset of puberty and musculoskeletal growth. Human beings go through two growth spurts, one when they are very young and a more obvious one when they are in adolescence. This second growth spurt lasts 2.5 to 4 years.[10] During this period, growth is accompanied by sexual maturation. Females develop quicker and sooner than males. Females enter puberty between 8 and 14 years of age, and puberty lasts about 3 years. Males enter puberty between 9.5 and 16 years of age, and it lasts up to 5 years.[5] It is during this period that body differences arise between males and females with males tending toward longer leg and arm length, wider shoulders, smaller hip width, and greater overall skeletal size and height than females. Because of the rapid growth spurt, individuals, especially males, may appear ungainly, and poor postural habits and changes are more likely to occur at this age.

Factors Affecting Posture

Several anatomic features may affect correct posture. These features may be enhanced or cause additional problems when combined with pathological or congenital states, such as Klippel-Feil syndrome, Scheuermann's disease (juvenile kyphosis), scoliosis, or disc disease.

Causes of Poor Posture

There are many examples of poor posture (Fig. 15.4). Some of the causes are postural (positional), and some are structural.

Postural (Positional) Factors

The most common postural problem is poor postural habit; that is, for whatever reason, the patient does not maintain a correct posture. This type of posture is often seen in the person who stands or sits for long periods and begins to slouch. Maintenance of correct posture requires muscles that are strong, flexible, and easily adaptable to environmental change. These muscles must continually work against gravity and in harmony with one another to maintain an upright posture.

The **"crossed syndrome"** concept suggests that there is a neuromuscular imbalance between groups of muscles that result in poor posture, decreased excitability of muscles, and increased spinal joint loads.[11] Tonic muscles tend to be tight, while phasic muscles tend to be weak. Tonic muscles are generally activated early in any movement, creating abnormal, dysfunctional motor patterns.

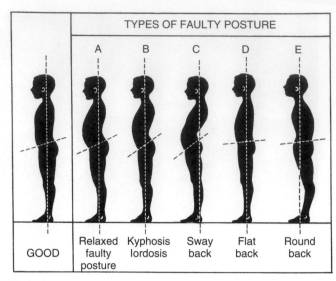

Fig. 15.4 Examples of faulty posture. (From McMorris RO: Faulty postures. *Pediatr Clin North Am* 8:217, 1961.)

Animal studies that have examined muscles placed in positions of shortening due to immobilization for prolonged periods exhibit accelerated atrophy and a loss of sarcomeres.[12–14] Janda,[15] and Jull and Janda[11] described two crossed syndromes—upper crossed and lower crossed. The lower (pelvic) crossed syndrome (see Fig. 9.21) is characterized by tight thoracolumbar extensors posteriorly that cross with the iliopsoas and rectus femoris anteriorly. The antagonistic muscular weakness that would follow this pattern includes the deep anterior abdominal muscles and the gluteus maximus posteriorly and the gluteus medius posteriorly and laterally. The upper crossed syndrome (see Fig. 3.17) is characterized by tightness of the anterior deep neck flexors, the upper trapezius, and the levator scapula on the posterior upper back, which are crossed with tightness of the pectoralis major and minor anteriorly on the thorax. These patterns correspond to antagonistic muscle weaknesses in the anterior deep neck flexors, and the posterior positioned middle and lower trapezius muscle groups.

Another cause of poor postural habits, especially in children, is not wanting to appear taller than one's peers. If a child has an early, rapid growth spurt there may be a tendency to slouch so as not to "stand out" and appear different. Such a spurt may also result in the unequal growth of the various structures, and this may lead to altered posture; for example, the growth of muscle may not keep up with the growth of bone. This process is sometimes evident in adolescents with tight hamstrings.

Muscle imbalance and muscle contracture are other causes of poor posture. For example, a tight iliopsoas muscle increases the lumbar lordosis in the lumbar spine.

Pain may also cause poor posture. Pressure on a nerve root in the lumbar spine can lead to pain in the back and

Postural Malalignment Problems

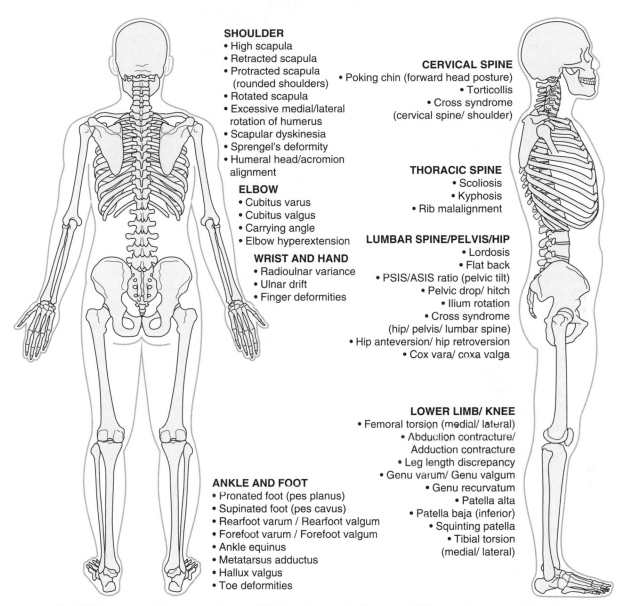

SHOULDER
- High scapula
- Retracted scapula
- Protracted scapula (rounded shoulders)
- Rotated scapula
- Excessive medial/lateral rotation of humerus
- Scapular dyskinesia
- Sprengel's deformity
- Humeral head/acromion alignment

ELBOW
- Cubitus varus
- Cubitus valgus
- Carrying angle
- Elbow hyperextension

WRIST AND HAND
- Radioulnar variance
- Ulnar drift
- Finger deformities

CERVICAL SPINE
- Poking chin (forward head posture)
- Torticollis
- Cross syndrome (cervical spine/ shoulder)

THORACIC SPINE
- Scoliosis
- Kyphosis
- Rib malalignment

LUMBAR SPINE/PELVIS/HIP
- Lordosis
- Flat back
- PSIS/ASIS ratio (pelvic tilt)
- Pelvic drop/ hitch
- Ilium rotation
- Cross syndrome (hip/ pelvis/ lumbar spine)
- Hip anteversion/ hip retroversion
- Cox vara/ coxa valga

ANKLE AND FOOT
- Pronated foot (pes planus)
- Supinated foot (pes cavus)
- Rearfoot varum / Rearfoot valgum
- Forefoot varum / Forefoot valgum
- Ankle equinus
- Metatarsus adductus
- Hallux valgus
- Toe deformities

LOWER LIMB/ KNEE
- Femoral torsion (medial/ lateral)
- Abduction contracture/ Adduction contracture
- Leg length discrepancy
- Genu varum/ Genu valgum
- Genu recurvatum
- Patella alta
- Patella baja (inferior)
- Squinting patella
- Tibial torsion (medial/ lateral)

Fig. 15.5 Postural malalignment problems. *ASIS*, Anterior superior iliac spine; *PSIS*, posterior superior iliac spine.

result in a scoliosis as the body unconsciously adopts a posture that decreases the pain.

Respiratory conditions (e.g., emphysema), general weakness, excess weight, loss of proprioception, or muscle spasm (as seen in cerebral palsy or with trauma, as examples) may also lead to poor posture.

The majority of postural nonstructural faults are relatively easy to correct after the problem has been identified. The treatment involves strengthening weak muscles, stretching tight structures, and teaching the patient that it is his or her responsibility to maintain a correct upright posture in standing, sitting, and other activities of daily living (ADLs).

Structural Factors

Structural deformities that are the result of congenital anomalies, developmental problems, trauma, or disease may cause an alteration of posture. For example, a significant difference in leg length or an anomaly of the spine, such as a hemivertebra, may alter the posture.

Structural deformities involve mainly changes in bone and therefore are not easily correctable without surgery. However, patients often can be relieved of symptoms by proper postural care instruction.

Fig. 15.5 outlines some postural/structural malalignment problems that may be seen during postural assessment.

Postural Assessment Methods[16]

The most common method of postural assessment is visual observation, in which the examiner looks at the patient's posture from different positions (e.g., front, side, and back) looking for landmarks and deviations. No one is perfectly symmetrical, so the question the examiner has to decide is whether the malalignment or change observed is contributing to the patient's problem. The visual observation methods may be supplemented using goniometry and a plumb bob line to provide a vertical reference. Other methods include using radiographs or photographs.

Common Spinal Deformities

Many postural abnormalities and malalignments (see Fig. 15.5) are presumed to produce excessive or abnormally located stresses on joint surfaces or contribute to altered muscle mechanics, putting some muscles on slack while stretching others.[4]

Lordosis

Lordosis is an anterior curvature of the spine (Fig. 15.6).[17–21] Pathologically, it is an exaggeration of the normal curves found in the cervical and lumbar spines. Causes of increased lordosis include (1) postural or functional deformity; (2) lax muscles, especially the abdominal muscles, in combination with tight muscles, especially hip flexors or lumbar extensors (Table 15.1); (3) a heavy abdomen, resulting from excess weight or pregnancy; (4) compensatory mechanisms that result from another deformity, such

as kyphosis (Fig. 15.7); (5) tight and commonly strong muscles (see Table 15.1); (6) spondylolisthesis; (7) congenital probwlems, such as bilateral congenital dislocation of the hip; (8) failure of segmentation of the neural arch of a facet joint segment; or (9) fashion (e.g., wearing high-heeled shoes). There are two types of exaggerated lordosis, pathological lordosis and swayback deformity.

Pathological Lordosis

In the patient with pathological lordosis, one may often observe sagging shoulders (scapulae are protracted and arms are medially rotated), medial rotation of the legs, and poking forward of the head so that it is in front of the center of gravity (Fig. 15.8). This posture is adopted in an attempt to keep the center of gravity where it should be. Deviation in one part of the body often leads to deviation in another part of the body in

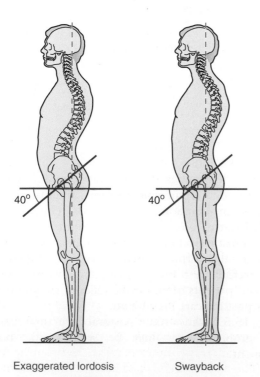

40°   40°

Exaggerated lordosis   Swayback

Fig. 15.6 Examples of lordosis.

TABLE **15.1**

Changes Associated With Pathological Lordosis

Body segment alignment	Pelvis is anteriorly tilted with lordosis increased Knees are hyperextended Ankle joints slightly plantar flexed
Muscles commonly elongated and weak	Anterior abdominals Small muscles of lumbar spine (multifidus, rotators) Lower and middle trapezius Hamstrings may lengthen initially or shorten to compensate where posture has been present for some time Rhomboids (?) Upper (thoracic and cervical) erector spinae Hyoid muscles
Muscles commonly short and strong	Lumbar erector spinae Hip flexors Upper trapezius Pectoralis major and minor Levator scapulae Sternocleidomastoid Scalenes Suboccipital muscles
Joints commonly affected	Lumbar spine Pelvic joints Hip joints Thoracic spine Scapulothoracic joints Glenohumeral joints Cervical spine Atlanto-occipital joints Temporomandibular joints

?, May or may not be.
Adapted from Kendall FP, McCreary EK: *Muscles: testing and function*, Baltimore, 1983, Williams & Wilkins; Giallonardo LM: Posture. In Myers RS, editor: *Saunders manual of physical therapy practice*, Philadelphia, 1995, WB Saunders.

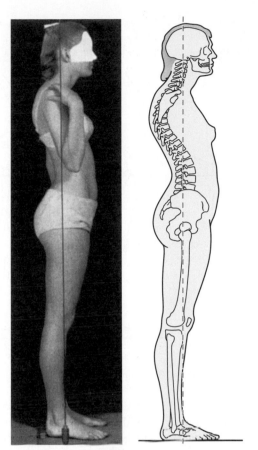

Fig. 15.7 Faulty posture illustrating exaggerated lordosis and kyphosis. (From Kendall FP, McCreary EK: *Muscles: testing and function*, Baltimore, 1983, Williams & Wilkins, p 281.)

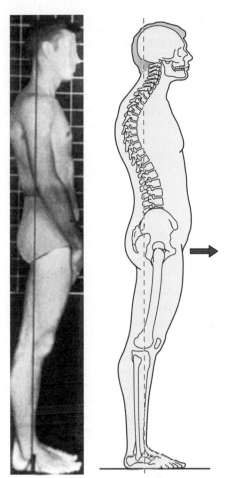

Fig. 15.9 Faulty posture illustrating a swayback. (From Kendall FP, McCreary EK: *Muscles: testing and function*, Baltimore, 1983, Williams & Wilkins, p 284.)

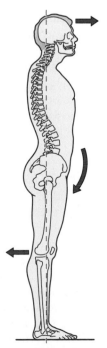

Fig. 15.8 Pathological lordosis with compensatory forward head posture.

an attempt to maintain the correct center of gravity and the correct visual plane. This type of exaggerated lordosis is the most common postural deviation seen.

The pelvic angle, normally approximately 30°, is increased with lordosis. With excessive or pathological lordosis, there is an increase in the pelvic angle to approximately 40°, accompanied by a mobile spine and an anterior pelvic tilt. Exaggerated lumbar lordosis is usually accompanied by weakness of the deep lumbar extensors and tightness of the hip flexors and tensor fasciae latae combined with weak abdominals (see Table 15.1).[22]

Swayback Deformity

With a swayback deformity, there is increased pelvic inclination to approximately 40°, and the thoracolumbar spine exhibits a kyphosis (Fig. 15.9). A swayback deformity results in the spine's bending back rather sharply at the lumbosacral angle. With this postural deformity, the entire pelvis shifts anteriorly, causing the hips to move into extension. To maintain the center of gravity in its normal position, the thoracic spine flexes on the lumbar spine. The result is an increase in the lumbar and thoracic

TABLE **15.2**

Changes Associated With Swayback

Body segment alignment	Long kyphosis with pelvis the most anterior body segment, hip joint moves forward of posture line (thoracic spine mobile to compensate) Lower lumbar area flattens Pelvis neutral or in posterior tilt Hip and knee joints hyperextended Where subject stands predominantly on one leg, pelvis is tilted down to non-favored side Favored leg appears longer in standing only
Muscles commonly elongated and weak	One joint hip flexors External obliques Lower thoracic extensors Lower abdominals Neck flexors Where one leg is favored, gluteus medius (especially posterior fibers) on favored side
Muscles commonly short and strong	Hamstrings Hip extensors Upper fibers of internal obliques Internal intercostals Low back musculature short but not strong Where one leg is favored, tensor fascia lata is strong and iliotibial band is tight on favored side
Joints commonly affected	Lumbar spine Pelvic joints Hip joints Thoracic spine Scapulothoracic joint Glenohumeral joints Cervical spine Atlanto-occipital joints Temporomandibular joints

Adapted from Kendall FP, McCreary EK: *Muscles: testing and function*, Baltimore, 1983, Williams & Wilkins; Giallonardo LM: Posture. In Myers RS, editor: *Saunders manual of physical therapy practice*, Philadelphia, 1995, WB Saunders.

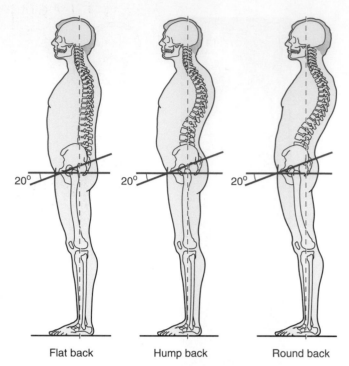

Flat back Hump back Round back

Fig. 15.10 Examples of kyphosis.

spondylitis, senile osteoporosis, tumors, compensation in conjunction with lordosis, and congenital anomalies.[23] The congenital anomalies include a partial segmental defect, as seen in osseous metaplasia, or centrum hypoplasia and aplasia.[26,28,29] In addition, paralysis may lead to a kyphosis because of the loss of muscle action needed to maintain the correct posture combined with the forces of gravity.

Pathological conditions, such as Scheuermann's vertebral osteochondritis (see Fig. 8.67), may also result in a structural kyphosis. In this condition, inflammation of the bone and cartilage occurs around the ring epiphysis of the vertebral body. The condition often leads to an anterior wedging of the vertebra. It is a growth disorder that affects approximately 10% of the population, and in most cases several vertebrae are affected. The most common area for the disease to occur is between T10 and L2.

The four types of kyphosis are round back, humpback, flat back, and dowager's hump.

Round Back

The patient with a round back has a long, rounded curve with decreased pelvic inclination (<30°) and thoracolumbar kyphosis. The patient often presents with the trunk flexed forward and a decreased lumbar curve (see Fig. 15.10). On examination, there are tight hip extensors and trunk flexors with weak hip flexors and lumbar extensors (Table 15.3).

Humpback or Gibbus

With humpback, there is a localized, sharp posterior angulation in the thoracic spine (see Fig. 8.10). This is commonly a structural deformity as the result of a fracture or pathology.

curves. Such a deformity may be associated with tightness of the hip extensors, lower lumbar extensors, and upper abdominals, along with weakness of the hip flexors, lower abdominals, and lower thoracic extensors (Table 15.2).[1]

Kyphosis

Kyphosis is a posterior curvature of the spine (Fig. 15.10; see Fig. 8.9).[19,21,23–27] Pathologically, it is an exaggeration of the normal curve found in the thoracic spine. There are several causes of kyphosis, including tuberculosis, vertebral compression fractures, Scheuermann's disease, ankylosing

TABLE **15.3**

Changes Associated With a Round Back Form of Kyphosis

Body segment alignment	Head held forward with cervical spine hyperextended
	Scapulae may be protracted
	Increased thoracic kyphosis
	Hips flexed, knees hyperextended
	Head is usually most anteriorly placed body segment
Muscles commonly elongated and weak	Neck flexors
	Upper erector spinae
	External obliques
	If scapulae are protracted, middle and lower trapezius
	Thoracic erector spinae
	Rhomboids
Muscles commonly short and strong	Neck extensors
	Hip flexors
	If scapulae are protracted, serratus anterior, pectoralis major and/or minor, upper trapezius, levator scapulae
	Upper abdominal muscles
	Intercostals
Joints commonly affected	Thoracic spine
	Scapulothoracic joints
	Glenohumeral joints

Adapted from Kendall FP, McCreary EK: *Muscles: testing and function,* Baltimore, 1983, Williams & Wilkins; Giallonardo LM: Posture. In Myers RS, editor: *Saunders manual of physical therapy practice,* Philadelphia, 1995, WB Saunders.

Flat Back

A patient with flat back has decreased pelvic inclination to 20° and a mobile lumbar spine (Fig. 15.11). Table 15.4 outlines the structures affected.

Dowager's Hump

Dowager's hump is often seen in older patients, especially women. The deformity commonly is caused by osteoporosis, in which the thoracic vertebral bodies begin to degenerate and wedge in an anterior direction, resulting in a kyphosis (Fig. 15.12; see Fig. 8.10).

Kypholordotic Posture

In some cases, both the thoracic and lumbar spine may be affected. Fig. 15.13 and Table 15.5 outline the changes seen with this posture.

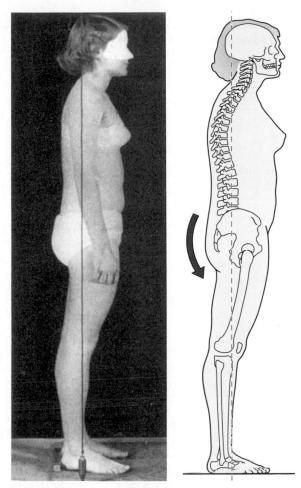

Fig. 15.11 Faulty posture illustrating flat back. (From Kendall FP, McCreary EK: *Muscles: testing and function,* Baltimore, 1983, Williams & Wilkins, p 285.)

Scoliosis

Scoliosis is a lateral curvature of the spine.[23,25,30–36] This type of deformity is often the most visible spinal deformity, especially in its severe forms. The most famous example of scoliosis is the "hunchback of Notre Dame." In the cervical spine, a scoliosis is called a **torticollis.** There are several types of scoliosis, some of which are nonstructural (Fig. 15.14) and some of which are structural. **Nonstructural** or **functional scoliosis** may be caused by postural problems, hysteria, nerve root irritation, inflammation, or compensation caused by leg length discrepancy or contracture (in the lumbar spine) (Table 15.6).[35] **Structural scoliosis** primarily involves bony deformity, which may be congenital or acquired, or excessive muscle weakness, as seen in a person with long-term quadriplegia. This type of scoliosis may be caused by wedge vertebra,

TABLE **15.4**

Changes Associated With a Flat Back Form of Kyphosis

Body segment alignment	Loss of lordosis with pelvis in posterior tilt Hip and knee joints hyperextended Forward head posture with increased flexion to upper thoracic spine
Muscles commonly elongated and weak	One joint hip flexors Lumbar extensors Local stabilizers (multifidus, rotators) Scapular protractors (?) Anterior intercostals
Muscles commonly short and strong	Hamstrings Abdominals may be strong with back muscles slightly elongated Hip extensors Scapular retractors (?) Thoracic erector spinae
Joints commonly affected	Lumbar spine Pelvic joints Scapulothoracic joints (?) Thoracic spine (?) Cervical spine (?)

?, May or may not be.
Adapted from Kendall FP, McCreary EK: *Muscles: testing and function*, Baltimore, 1983, Williams & Wilkins; Giallonardo LM: Posture. In Myers RS, editor: *Saunders manual of physical therapy practice*, Philadelphia, 1995, WB Saunders.

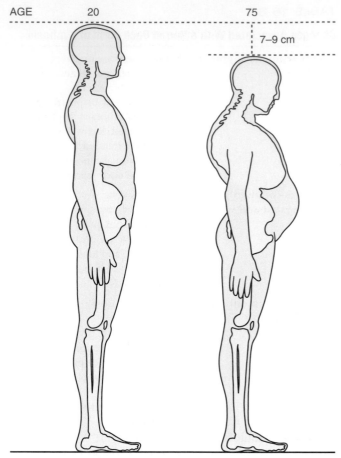

Fig. 15.12 Loss of height resulting from osteoporosis leading to dowager's hump. Note the flexed head and protruding abdomen, which occur partially to maintain the center of gravity in its normal position.

hemivertebra (Fig. 15.15), or failure of segmentation. It may be idiopathic (genetic) (Fig. 15.16); neuromuscular, resulting from an upper or lower motor neuron lesion; or myopathic, resulting from muscular disease; or it may be caused by arthrogryposis, resulting from persistent joint contracture,[29] or by conditions such as neurofibromatosis, mesenchymal disorders, or trauma. It may accompany infection, tumors, and inflammatory conditions that result in bone destruction. Torticollis may occur because of neuromuscular problems, because of congenital problems (abnormal sternocleidomastoid muscle), or in conjunction with malocclusion of the temporomandibular joints or with ear problems (referred to the cervical spine).

With structural scoliosis, the patient lacks normal flexibility, and side bending becomes asymmetrical. This type of scoliosis may be progressive, and the curve does not disappear on forward flexion. It is most commonly seen in the thoracic or thoracolumbar spine. With nonstructural scoliosis, there is no bony deformity; this type of scoliosis is not progressive. The spine shows segmental limitation, and side bending is usually symmetrical. The nonstructural scoliotic curve disappears on forward flexion. This type of scoliosis is usually found in the cervical, lumbar, or thoracolumbar area.

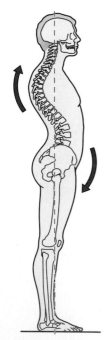

Fig. 15.13 Kypholordotic posture.

TABLE **15.5**

Changes Associated With Kypholordotic Posture

Body segment alignment	Head held forward with cervical spine hyperextended Scapulae may be protracted Increased lumbar lordosis, and increased thoracic kyphosis Pelvis anteriorly tilted Hip flexed, knee hyperextended Head is usually most anteriorly placed body segment
Muscles commonly elongated and weak	Neck flexors Upper erector spinae External obliques If scapulae are protracted, middle and lower trapezius Thoracic erector spinae Middle and lower trapezius Rhomboids
Muscles commonly short and strong	Neck extensors Hip flexors If scapulae are protracted, serratus anterior, pectoralis major and/or minor, upper trapezius Intercostals
Joints commonly affected	Thoracic spine Lumbar spine Scapulothoracic joints Glenohumeral joints

Adapted from Kendall FP, McCreary EK: *Muscles: testing and function*, Baltimore, 1983, Williams & Wilkins; Giallonardo LM: Posture. In Myers RS, editor: *Saunders manual of physical therapy practice*, Philadelphia, 1995, WB Saunders.

TABLE **15.6**

Changes Associated With Postural Scoliosis

Body segment alignment	Spine curves to left or right May have single or double curve or one main curve and one or two compensatory curves Ribs may protrude on one side and be depressed (paravertebral valley) on the other side ("hump and hollow" on forward flexion because of vertebral rotation) May have short leg—pelvis tilted laterally—concave side high Shoulder/scapula may drop on concavity side of curve
Muscles commonly elongated and weak	Muscles on the convex side Hip abductor muscles on concave side Foot pronator muscles on the long side
Muscles commonly short and strong	Muscles on concave side Hip adductors on convex side Foot supinators on short side
Joints commonly affected	Lumbar spine Thoracic spine Pelvic joints Hip joints Foot joints Scapulothoracic joints Glenohumeral joints Cervical spine (torticollis) Atlanto-occipital joints Temporomandibular joints

Adapted from Kendall FP, McCreary EK: *Muscles: testing and function*, Baltimore, 1983, Williams & Wilkins; Giallonardo LM: Posture. In Myers RS, editor: *Saunders manual of physical therapy practice*, Philadelphia, 1995, WB Saunders.

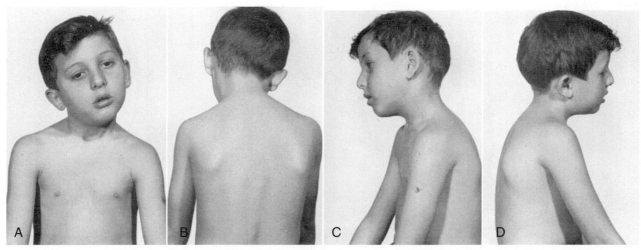

Fig. 15.14 Congenital muscular torticollis on the right in a 10-year-old boy. Note the contracted sternocleidomastoid muscle. (A) Anterior view. (B) Posterior view. (C) Left side view. (D) Right side view. (From Tachdjian MO: Pediatric orthopedics, Philadelphia, 1972, WB Saunders, p 74.)

Idiopathic scoliosis accounts for 75% to 85% of all cases of structural scoliosis. The vertebral bodies rotate into the convexity of the curve with the spinous processes going toward the concavity of the curve. There is a fixed rotational prominence on the convex side, which is best seen on forward flexion from the skyline view. This prominence is sometimes called a "razorback spine." The disc spaces are narrowed on the concave side and widened on the convex side. There is distortion of the vertebral body, and vital capacity is considerably lowered if the lateral curvature exceeds 60°; compression and malposition of the organs within the rib cage also occur. Examples of scoliotic curves are shown in Fig. 8.13.

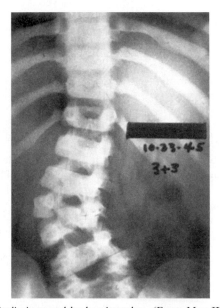

Fig. 15.15 Scoliosis caused by hemivertebra. (From Moe JH, Bradford DS, Winter RB, et al: *Scoliosis and other spinal deformities*, Philadelphia, 1978, WB Saunders, p 134.)

Patient History

As with any history, the examiner must ensure that the information obtained is as complete as possible. By listening to the patient, the examiner can often comprehend the problem. The information should include a history of the problem, the patient's general condition and health, and family history. If a child is being examined, the examiner must also obtain prenatal and postnatal histories, including the health of the mother during pregnancy or injuries experienced by her, any complications during pregnancy or delivery, and drugs taken by the mother during that period, especially during the first trimester, which is the period when most of the congenital anomalies develop.

It should be remembered that it is unusual for a patient to present with just a postural problem. It is the symptoms produced by the pathology that is causing the postural abnormality that initiate the consultation. The examiner therefore must be cognizant of various underlying pathological conditions when assessing posture.

The following questions should be asked:

1. *Was there any history of injury?* If so, what was the mechanism of injury? For example, lifting often causes lower spine problems, which may lead to altered posture.
2. *If there is a history of injury, had the patient experienced any back injury or pain previously?* If so, what caused that injury or pain? Was it a specific posture, sustained posture, or caused by repetitive movements? If so, what were the postures and/or movements?

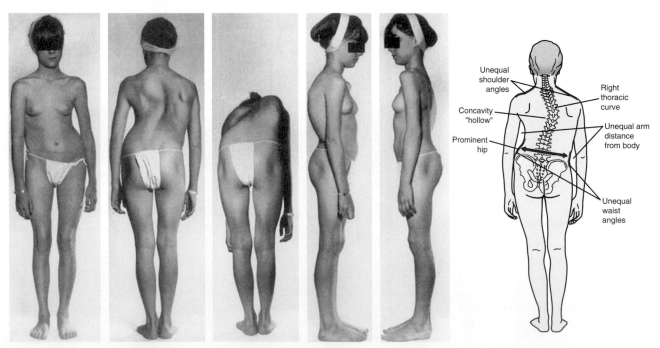

Fig. 15.16 Idiopathic structural right thoracic scoliosis. Line drawing shows prominent features of scoliosis. (Photographs from Tachdjian MO: *Pediatric orthopedics*, Philadelphia, 1972, WB Saunders, p 1200.)

3. *Are there any postures (e.g., standing with one foot on low stool, sitting with legs crossed) that give the patient relief or increase the patient's symptoms?*[37] The examiner can later test these postures to help determine the problem.
4. *Does the family have any history of back problems or other special problems?* Conditions, such as hemivertebra, scoliosis, and Klippel-Feil syndrome, may be congenital.
5. *Has the patient had any previous illnesses, surgery, or severe injuries?*
6. *Is there a history of any other conditions, such as connective tissue diseases, that have a high incidence of associated spinal problems?*
7. *Does footwear make a difference to the patient's posture or symptoms?* For example, high-heeled shoes often lead to excessive lordosis.[38]
8. *How old is the patient?* Many spinal problems begin in childhood or are the result of degeneration in the aged population.
9. *In the child, has there been a growth spurt?* If so, when did it begin? Growth spurts often lead to tight muscles and altered posture.
10. *For females, when did menarche begin?* Does back pain appear to be associated with menses? Menarche indicates the point at which approximately two-thirds of the female adolescent growth spurt has been completed.
11. *For males, has there been a voice change?* If so, when? This question also gives an indication of maturity or onset of puberty.
12. *If a deformity is present, is it progressive or stationary?*
13. *Does the patient experience any neurological symptoms (e.g., a "pins and needles" feeling or numbness)?*
14. *What is the nature, extent, type, and duration of the pain?*
15. *What positions or activities increase the pain or discomfort?*
16. *What positions or activities decrease the pain or discomfort?*
17. *For children, is there difficulty in fitting clothes?* For example, with scoliosis, the hem of a dress is usually uneven because of the spinal curvature.
18. *Does the patient have any difficulty breathing?* Structural deformities, such as idiopathic scoliosis, can lead to breathing problems in severe cases.
19. *Which hand is the dominant one?* Often, the dominant side shows a lower shoulder with the hip slightly deviated to that side (Fig. 15.17). The spine may deviate slightly to the opposite side, and the opposite foot is slightly more pronated.[19] The gluteus medius on the dominant side may also be weaker.
20. *Has there been any previous treatment?* If so, what was it? Was it successful?

Observation

Observation is the primary method of assessing posture and should be included in every assessment, looking for

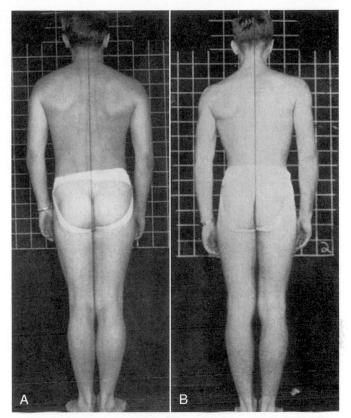

Fig. 15.17 Effect of handedness on posture. (A) Right hand dominant. (B) Left hand dominant. (From Kendall FP, McCreary EK: *Muscles, testing and function,* Baltimore, 1983, Williams & Wilkins, p 294.)

asymmetric changes that may contribute to or be the result of faulty posture. The following sections outline static posture, which forms the basis of dynamic posture (e.g., walking, running, lifting, throwing).[5]

To assess posture correctly, the patient must be adequately undressed. Male patients should be in shorts, and female patients should be in a bra and shorts. Ideally, the patient should not wear shoes or stockings. However, if the patient uses walking aids, braces, collars, or orthotics, they should be noted and may be used after the patient has been assessed in the "natural" state to determine the effect of the appliances.

The patient should be examined in the habitual, relaxed posture that is usually adopted. Often, it takes some time for the patient to adopt the usual posture because of tenseness, uneasiness, or uncertainty.

In the standing and sitting positions, the assessment is the same as the observation for the upper and lower limb scanning examinations of the cervical and lumbar spines. Assessment of posture should be carried out with the patient in the standing, sitting, and lying (supine and prone) positions. After the patient has been examined in these positions, the examiner may decide to include other habitual, sustained, or repetitive postures assumed by the patient to see whether these postures increase or alter symptoms. The patient may also be assessed wearing different footwear to determine their effects on the posture and symptoms.

POSTURE EVALUATION		
NAME: AGE: SEX: HEIGHT: WEIGHT: DATE:		
Body type: Ectomorph / Mesomorph / Endomorph / Slight Build / Medium Build / Heavy Build		
Uncorrected Standing A Corrected (Talus in Neutral) Standing B Postural Deformity Corrected C		

ANTERIOR VIEW	Comments:	
Head (aligned, forward, flexed, extended)		
Mandible (resting position, retracted)		
Shoulders (level, uneven)		
Rib cage (symmetric, asymmetric)		
Scoliosis (left, right, lumbar, thoracic, cervical)		
Pelvis (lcvel, anterior/posterior tilt)		
Hips (coxa vara, coxa valga, anteversion, retroversion)		
Femurs (alignment, torsion)		
Knees (level, genu varum, genu valgum)		
Patellar position		
Tibias (alignment, torsions)		
Ankles (inversion, eversion)		
Rearfoot/forefoot alignment		
Feet (pes cavus, pes planus, supination/pronation)		
Toes (alignment, deformities)		
Leg length		
LATERAL VIEW	Comments:	
Head (forward, flexed/extended)		
Mandible (resting, protracted/retracted)		
Scapulae (winging, elevation/depression)		
Thoracic kyphosis (increased/decreased)		
Lumbar lordosis (increased/decreased)		
Pelvis (anterior/posterior tilt)		
Knees (hyperextension/flexion)		
Feet (longitudinal arch)		
POSTERIOR VIEW	Comments:	
Head (alignment, tilt)		
Shoulders (level)		
Scapulae (bilateral symmetry)		
Spine C-1 to sacrum (rotations, deviations)		
Pelvis (level, tilt)		
Sacrum (level at base and inferior lateral angles)		
Hips (level, uneven)		
Knees (creases level/uneven)		
Leg (rearfoot alignment)		
Ankles (inversion/eversion)		
Calcaneal position (inverted/everted)		

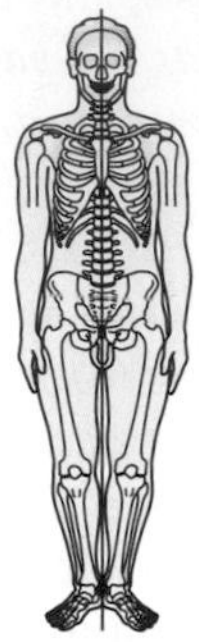

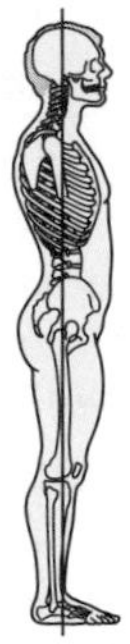

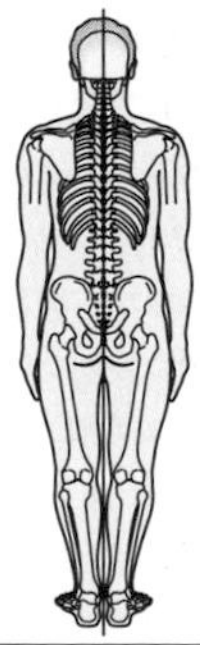

Pertinent Medical History:

Pertinent Radiographic Findings / Other Tests:

Fig. 15.18 Example of standing posture evaluation form. Information is obtained by visual observation and palpation. (Modified from Richardson JK, Iglarsh ZA: *Clinical orthopedic physical therapy*, Philadelphia, 1994, WB Saunders.)

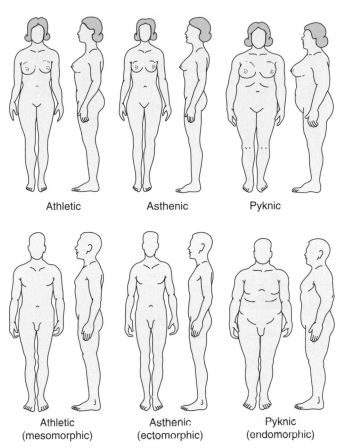

Athletic   Asthenic   Pyknic

Athletic   Asthenic   Pyknic
(mesomorphic) (ectomorphic) (endomorphic)

Fig. 15.19 Male and female body types. (From Debrunner HU: *Orthopedic diagnosis*, London, 1970, E & S Livingstone, p 86.)

When observing a patient for abnormalities in posture, the examiner looks for asymmetry as a possible indication of what may be causing the postural fault (Fig. 15.18). Some asymmetry between left and right sides is normal. The examiner must be able to differentiate normal deviations from asymmetry caused by pathology. Functional asymmetries usually refer to changes in alignment that occur with changes in posture. For example, nonstructural scoliosis may be present in standing because of a short leg but disappear on forward flexion. Anatomic or structural asymmetries are due to structural changes (e.g., idiopathic scoliosis).

As the examiner is watching for asymmetry, he or she should also note potential causes of asymmetry. For example, the examiner should always watch for the presence of muscle wasting, soft tissue or bony swelling or enlargement, scars, and skin changes that may indicate present or past pathology.

Standing

The examiner should first determine the patient's body type (Fig. 15.19).[37] The three body types are ectomorphic, mesomorphic, and endomorphic. The **ectomorph** is a person who has a thin body build characterized by a relative prominence of structures developed from the embryonic ectoderm. The **mesomorph** has a muscular or sturdy body build characterized by relative prominence of structures developed by the embryonic mesoderm. The **endomorph** has a heavy or fat body build characterized by relative prominence of structures developed from the embryonic endoderm.

Body Types

- Ectomorph
- Mesomorph
- Endomorph

In addition to body type, the examiner should note the emotional attitude of the patient. Is the patient tense, bored, or lethargic? Does the patient appear to be healthy, emaciated, or overweight? Answers to these questions can help the examiner determine how much must be done to correct any problems. For example, if the patient is lethargic, it may take longer to correct the problem than if he or she appears truly interested in correcting the problem. The examiner must remember that posture is in many ways an expression of one's personality, sense of well-being, and self-esteem.

In normal standing posture, the body is generally not completely stationary. To the naked eye, standing posture may appear static; however, normal standing posture is more accurately characterized by small oscillations in which the body sways anterior and posterior, side to side, and at times in circular patterns. **Postural sway** is the movement of the body's center of pressure, which is different than, although related to, the center of mass. The body's center of pressure is the location where pressures under both feet are distributed. Studies have demonstrated that during relaxed, quiet standing, the center of mass and center of pressure sway anterior and posterior up to 7 mm, while side-to-side movements are slightly less.[39–42] This underlying theory is based on the biomechanical model of a single inverted pendulum in which movement pivots around the ankle (Fig. 15.20A). More recent evidence suggests that this simplistic model may need to be substituted with a double inverted pendulum (Fig. 15.20B) in which some additional postural control may come from the hip via an ankle-hip coordinated interaction.[43]

A second way that these variables can be viewed is by assessing a person's **limits of stability (LOS)**. LOS can be defined as the maximum angle from vertical that can be tolerated without a loss of balance.[44] Anterior and posterior LOS is approximately 12°, while side to side LOS is 16°, both with a 4-inch wide normal stance width (Fig. 15.21).[44] It should be stressed that LOS vary from person to person based on anthropometric characteristics such as height, weight, and size of feet.

Recent evidence via a systematic review of 12 studies including 218 asymptomatic participants found that fatigue of postural muscles consistently affects postural control. Sway velocity was consistently found to be affected

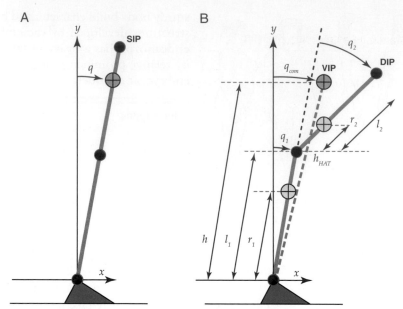

Fig. 15.20 Biomechanical models of a (A) single inverted pendulum *(SIP)* and a (B) double inverted pendulum *(DIP)*. The two degrees of freedom in the DIP model are the ankle rotation angle *(q1)* and the hip angle *(q2)*. *VIP*, Virtual inverted pendulum. (Redrawn from Morasso P, Cherif A, Zenzeri J: Quiet standing: the single inverted pendulum model is not so bad after all. *PLOS ONE.* https://doi.org/10.1371/journal.pone.0213870, 2019.)

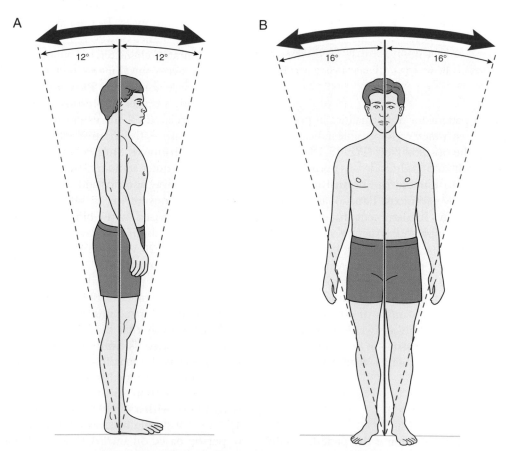

Fig. 15.21 Limits of stability. Standing posture often is modeled as an inverted pendulum in which the body sways over the fixed feet. (A) Anteroposterior. (B) Medial-lateral. (A, Modified from Oatis CA: *Kinesiology: the mechanics and pathomechanics of human movement*, ed 2, Philadelphia, 2009, Williams & Wilkins.)

TABLE **15.7**

Normal Alignment in the Standing Posture: Anterior View

Body Segment	Line of Gravity Location	Observation
Head	Passes through middle of the forehead, nose and chin	Eyes and ears should be level and symmetrical
Neck/shoulders		Right and left angles between shoulders and neck should be symmetrical; clavicles also should be symmetrical
Chest	Passes through the middle of the xyphoid process	Ribs on each side should be symmetrical
Abdomen/hips	Passes through the umbilicus (navel)	Right and left waist angles should be symmetrical
Hips/pelvis	Passes on a line equidistant from the right and left ASISs; passes through the symphysis pubis	ASISs should be level
Knees	Passes between knees equidistant from medial femoral condyles	Patellae should be symmetrical and facing straight ahead
Ankles/feet	Passes between ankles equidistant from the medial malleoli	Malleoli should be symmetrical, and feet should be parallel; toes should not be curled, overlapping, or deviated to one side

ASIS, Anterior superior iliac spine.
From Levangie PK, Norton CC: *Joint structures and function—a comprehensive analysis*, Philadelphia, 2005, FA Davis, p 498.

by fatigue.[45] Injury and surgery also cause changes in postural control. Posture control variables were found to be most significantly different at 6 weeks following anterior cruciate ligament reconstruction; however, these variables were able to be returned to preoperative levels by a 2-year follow-up.[46]

Anterior View

When observing the patient from the front (Table 15.7; see Fig. 15.1A), the examiner should note whether the following conditions hold true:

1. The head is straight on the shoulders (in midline). The examiner should note whether the head is habitually tilted to one side or rotated (e.g., torticollis) (see Fig. 3.14). The cause of altered head position must be established. For example, it may be the result of weak muscles, trauma, a hearing loss, temporomandibular joint problems, or the wearing of bifocal glasses.
2. The posture of the jaw is normal. In the resting position, normal jaw posture is when the lips are gently pressed together, the teeth are slightly apart (freeway space), and the tip of the tongue is behind the upper teeth in the roof of the mouth. This position maintains the mandible in a good posture (i.e., slight negative pressure in the mouth reduces the work of the muscles). It also enables respiration through the nose and diaphragmatic breathing.
3. The tip of the nose is in line with the manubrium sternum, xiphisternum, and umbilicus. This line is the **anterior line of reference** used to divide the

body into right and left halves (see Fig. 15.1A). If the umbilicus is used as a reference point, the examiner should remember that the umbilicus is almost always slightly off center.

4. The upper trapezius neck line is equal on both sides. The muscle bulk of the trapezius muscles should be equal, and the slope of the muscles should be approximately equal. Because the dominant arm usually shows greater laxity by being slightly lower, the slope on the dominant side may be slightly greater.
5. The shoulders are level. In most cases, the dominant side is slightly lower.
6. The clavicles and acromioclavicular joints are level and equal. They should be symmetrical; any deviation should be noted. Deviations may be caused by subluxations or dislocations of the acromioclavicular or sternoclavicular joints, fractures, or clavicular rotation.
7. There is no protrusion, depression, or lateralization of the sternum, ribs, or costal cartilage. If there are changes, they should be noted.
8. The waist angles are equal, and the arms are equidistant from the waist. If a scoliosis is present, one arm hangs closer to the body than the other arm. The examiner should also note whether the arms are equally rotated medially or laterally.
9. The carrying angles at each elbow are equal. Any deviation should be noted. The normal carrying angle varies from 5° to 15°.
10. The palms of both hands face the body in the relaxed standing position. Any differences should be noted and may give an indication of rotation in the upper limb.

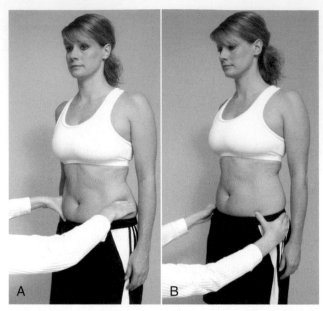

Fig. 15.22 Viewing height equality. (A) Iliac crests. (B) Anterior superior iliac spines.

11. The "high points" of the iliac crest are the same height on each side (Fig. 15.22). With a scoliosis, the patient may feel that one hip is "higher" than the other. This apparent high pelvis results from the lateral shift of the trunk; the pelvis is usually level. The same condition can cause the patient to feel that one leg is shorter than the other.

12. The anterior superior iliac spines (ASISs) are level. If one ASIS is higher than the other, there is a possibility that one leg is shorter than the other or that the pelvis is rotated more or shifted up or down more on one side.

13. The pubic bones are level at the symphysis pubis. Any deviation should be noted.

14. The patellae of the knees point straight ahead. Sometimes the patellae face outward ("frog eyes" patellae) or inward ("squinting" patellae). The position of the patella may also be altered by torsion of the femoral neck (anteversion-retroversion), femoral shaft, or tibial shaft.

15. The knees are straight. The knees may be in genu varum or genu valgum (see Fig. 12.7). If the ankles are together and the knees are more than two finger-widths apart, the patient has some genu varum. If the knees are touching and the feet are apart, the patient has some genu valgum. Genu valgum is more likely to be seen in females. The examiner should note whether the deformity results from the femur, tibia, or both. In children, the knees go through a progression of being straight, going into genu varum, being straight, going into genu valgum, and finally being straight again during the first 6 years of life (see Fig. 12.8).[25]

16. The heads of the fibulae are level.

17. The medial and lateral malleoli of the ankles are level. Normally, the medial malleoli are slightly anterior to the lateral malleoli, but the lateral malleoli extend farther distally.

18. Two arches are present in the feet and equal on the two sides. In this position, only the medial longitudinal arch is visible. The examiner should note any pes planus (flatfoot) or pronated foot, pes cavus ("hollow" foot) or supinated foot, or other deformities.

19. The feet angle out equally (this Fick angle is usually 5° to 18° [see Fig. 14.14]). This finding means that the tibias are normally slightly laterally rotated (lateral tibial torsion). The presence of pigeon toes usually indicates medial rotation of the tibias (medial tibial torsion), especially if the patellae face straight ahead. If the patellae face inward (squinting patellae) in the presence of "pigeon toes" or outward, the problem may be in the femur (abnormal femoral torsion or hip retroversion-anteversion problems).

20. There is no bowing of bone. Any bowing may indicate diseases, such as osteomalacia or osteoporosis.

21. The bony and soft-tissue contours are equally symmetrical on the two halves of the body. Any indication of muscle wasting, muscle hypertrophy on one side, or bony asymmetry should be noted. Such a finding may indicate muscle or nerve pathology, or it may simply be related to the patient's job or recreational pursuits. For example, a rodeo bull rider will show hypertrophy of the muscles and bones on one side. (The arm that he uses to hang on!)

In addition, the patient's skin is observed for abnormalities, such as hairy patches (e.g., diastematomyelia), pigmented lesions (e.g., café au lait spots, neurofibromatosis), subcutaneous tumors, and scars (e.g., Ehlers-Danlos syndrome), all of which may lead to or contribute to postural problems (see Figs. 9.20 and 9.22). Table 15.8 shows some of the malalignment postures and their effect.[5,25,47,48] Changes in one body segment cause changes in other segments as the body attempts to compensate or adjust for the malignment.[5] Compensatory postures are those that represent the body's attempt to normalize appearance or improve function.[5]

Lateral View

From the side (Table 15.9; see Fig. 15.1B), the examiner should note whether the following conditions hold true:

1. The earlobe is in line with the tip of the shoulder (acromion process) and the "high point" of the iliac crest. This line is the **lateral line of reference** dividing the body into front and back halves (see Fig. 15.1B). If the chin pokes forward, an excessive lumbar lordosis may also be present. This compensatory change is

caused by the body's attempt to maintain the center of gravity in the normal position.

2. Each spinal segment has a normal curve (Fig. 15.23). Large gluteus maximus muscles or excessive fat may give the appearance of an exaggerated lordosis. The examiner should look at the spine in relation to the sacrum, not the gluteal muscles. Likewise, the scapulae may give the illusion of an increased kyphosis in thethoracic spine, especially if they are flat and the patient has rounded shoulders.

3. The shoulders are in proper alignment. If the shoulders droop forward (i.e., the scapulae protract), "rounded shoulders" are indicated. This improper alignment may be caused by habit or by tight pectoral muscles or weak scapular stabilizers.

4. The chest, abdominal, and back muscles have proper tone. Weakness or spasm of any of these muscles can lead to postural alterations.

5. There are no chest deformities, such as pectus carinatum (undue prominence of the sternum) or pectus excavatum (undue depression of the sternum).

6. The pelvic angle or tilt is normal (7° to 15°; see Fig. 10.13). The posterior superior iliac spine (PSIS) should be slightly higher than the ASIS (1 to 2 finger-widths higher).[49–52]

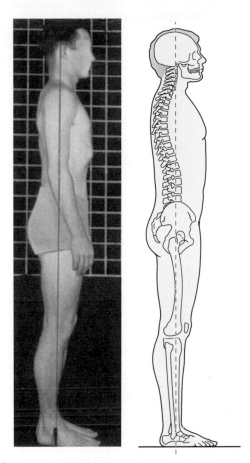

Fig. 15.23 Correct postural alignment (lateral view). (From Kendall FP, McCreary EK: *Muscles: testing and function*, Baltimore, 1983, Williams & Wilkins, p 280.)

TABLE **15.8**

Malalignments Viewed Anteriorly[5,25,47,48]

Malalignment	Possible Correlated Motions or Postures	Possible Compensatory Motions or Postures
Torticollis	Rotation to same side limited Side flexion to opposite side limited	
Scoliosis	Side flexion to convex side limited Rotation to convex side limited Rib hump on convex side	
Lateral pelvic tilt (pelvic drop—right leg stance)	Right hip adduction Weak right abductors (positive Trendelenburg)	Right lumbar lateral flexion Tight left adductors
Lateral pelvic tilt (pelvic hitch—right leg stance)	Right hip abduction Weak left adductors	Tight lumbar lateral flexion Tight right abductors
Forward rotation of one ilium on sacrum (right leg stance)	Right hip medial rotation Medial facing patella In-toeing Pronation of foot Long leg	Left lumbar rotation Scoliosis—concavity to left Knee flexion
Excessive anteversion	Toeing-in Subtalar pronation Lateral patellar subluxation Medial tibial torsion Medial femoral torsion	Lateral tibial torsion Lateral rotation at knee Lateral rotation of tibia, femur, and/or pelvis Lumbar rotation on same side
Excessive retroversion	Toeing-out Subtalar supination Lateral tibial torsion Lateral femoral torsion	Medial rotation at knee Medial rotation of tibia, femur, and/or pelvis Lumbar rotation on opposite side

Continued

TABLE **15.8**

Malalignments Viewed Anteriorly—cont'd

Malalignment	Possible Correlated Motions or Postures	Possible Compensatory Motions or Postures
Coxa vara	Pronated subtalar joint Medial rotation of leg Short ipsilateral leg Anterior pelvic rotation	Ipsilateral subtalar supination Contralateral subtalar pronation Ipsilateral plantar flexion Contralateral genu recurvatum Contralateral hip and/or knee flexion Ipsilateral posterior pelvic rotation and ipsilateral lumbar rotation
Coxa valga	Supinated subtalar joint Lateral rotation of leg Long ipsilateral leg Posterior pelvic tilt	Ipsilateral subtalar pronation Contralateral subtalar supination Contralateral plantar flexion Ipsilateral genu recurvatum Ipsilateral hip and/or knee flexion Ipsilateral anterior pelvic rotation and contralateral lumbar rotation
Medial femoral torsion	Excessive subtalar pronation In-toeing Medial facing or tilted patella ("squinting patella")	Excessive subtalar supination Functional forefoot valgus
Lateral femoral torsion	Excessive subtalar supination Out-toeing Lateral facing or tilted patella ("grasshopper eyes patella")	Excessive subtalar pronation Functional forefoot varus
Genu valgum	Pes planus Excessive subtalar pronation Lateral tibial torsion Lateral patellar subluxation Excessive hip adduction Ipsilateral hip excessive medial rotation Lumbar spine contralateral rotation	Forefoot varus Excessive subtalar supination to allow the lateral heel to contact the ground In-toeing to decrease lateral pelvic sway during gait Ipsilateral pelvic lateral rotation
Genu varum	Excessive lateral angulation of the tibia in the frontal plane; tibial varum Medial tibial torsion Ipsilateral hip lateral rotation Excessive hip abduction	Forefoot valgus Excessive subtalar pronation to allow the medial heel to contact the ground Ipsilateral pelvic medial rotation
Lateral tibial (malleolar) torsion	Out-toeing Excessive subtalar supination with related rotation along the lower quarter	Functional forefoot varus Excessive subtalar pronation with relaxed rotation along the lower quarter
Medial tibial (malleolar) torsion	In-toeing Metatarsus adductus Excessive subtalar pronation with related rotation along the lower quarter	Functional forefoot valgus Excessive subtalar supination with relaxed rotation along the lower quarter
Inadequate tibial retroflexion (bowing of the tibia)	Altered alignment of Achilles tendon causing altered associated joint motion	
Bowleg deformity of the tibia (tibial varum)	Medial tibial torsion	Forefoot valgus Excessive subtalar pronation
Ankle equinus		Hypermobile first ray Subtalar or midtarsal excessive pronation Hip or knee flexion Genu recurvation
Forefoot valgus	Hallux valgus Subtalar pronation and related rotation along the lower quarter	Excessive midtarsal or subtalar supination Excessive tibial; tibial and femoral; or tibial, femoral, and pelvic lateral rotation, or all with ipsilateral lumbar spine rotation
Metatarsus adductus	Hallus valgus Medial tibial torsion Flatfoot In-toeing	

TABLE 15.8

Malalignments Viewed Anteriorly—cont'd

Malalignment	Possible Correlated Motions or Postures	Possible Compensatory Motions or Postures
Hallus valgus	Forefoot valgus Subtalar pronation and related rotation along the lower quarter	Excessive tibial; tibial and femoral; or tibial, femoral, and pelvic lateral rotation, or all with ipsilateral lumbar spine rotation
In-toeing	Pronated foot Medial tibial torsion Metatarsus varus Talipes varus or equinovarus Tibia or genu varum Medial femoral torsion Excessive femoral anteversion Tight medial hip rotators Acetabular dysplasia (facing anteriorly)	
Out-toeing	Tight Achilles tendon Talipes calcaneovalgus Convex pes planovarus Lateral tibial torsion Hypoplastic (absence of) fibula Lateral femoral torsion Abnormal femoral retroversion Tight lateral rotators Flaccid medial rotators Acetabular dysplasia (facing posteriorly)	
Rearfoot valgus (calcaneal eversion)	Tibial; tibial and femoral; or tibial, femoral, and pelvic rotation Hallux valgus	

TABLE 15.9

Normal Alignment in the Standing Posture: Side View

Joints	Line of Gravity	External Moment	Passive Opposing Forces	Active Opposing Forces
Atlanto-occipital	Anterior (anterior-to-transverse axis for flexion and extension)	Flexion	Ligamentum nuchae and alar ligaments; the tectorial, atlanto-axial, and posterior atlanto-occipital membranes	Rectus capitus posterior major and minor, semispinalis capitus and cervicis, splenius capitis and cervicis, and inferior and superior oblique muscles
Cervical	Posterior	Extension	Anterior longitudinal ligament, anterior anulus fibrosus fibers, and anterior zygapophyseal joint capsules	Anterior scalene, longus capitis and colli
Thoracic	Anterior	Flexion	Posterior longitudinal, supraspinous, and interspinous ligaments; posterior zygapophyseal joint capsules and posterior anulus fibrosus fibers	Ligamentum flavum, longissimus thoracis, iliocostalis thoracis, spinalis thoracis, and semispinalis thoracis
Lumbar	Posterior	Extension	Anterior longitudinal and iliolumbar ligaments, anterior fibers of the anulus fibrosus, and anterior zygapophyseal joint capsules	Rectus abdominis and external and internal oblique muscles
Sacroiliac joint	Anterior	Nutation	Sacrotuberous, sacrospinous, iliolumbar, and anterior sacroiliac ligaments	Transversus abdominis
Hip joint	Posterior	Extension	Iliofemoral ligament	Iliopsoas
Knee joint	Anterior	Extension	Posterior joint capsule	Hamstrings, gastrocnemius
Ankle joint	Anterior	Dorsiflexion		Soleus, gastrocnemius

From Levangie PK, Norton CC: *Joint structures and function—a comprehensive analysis*, Philadelphia, 2005, FA Davis, p 493.

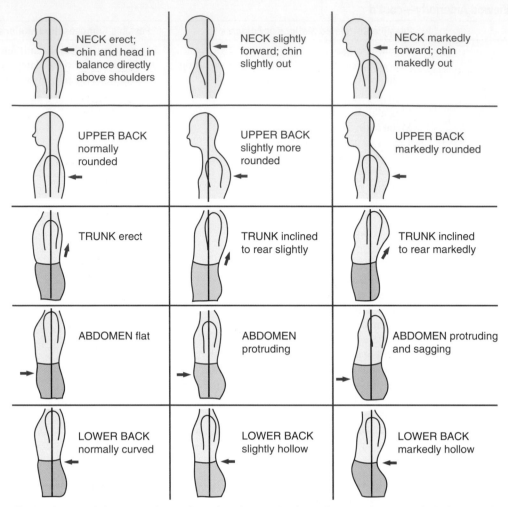

Fig. 15.24 Postural deviations obvious from the side view. (Redrawn from Reedco Research, Auburn, NY.)

7. The knees are straight, flexed, or in recurvatum (hyperextended). Usually, in the normal standing position, the knees are slightly flexed (0° to 5°). Hyperextension of the knees may cause an increase in lordosis in the lumbar spine. Tight hamstrings or gastrocnemius muscles can also cause knee flexion.

Fig. 15.24 illustrates normal posture and some of the abnormal deviations seen when viewing the patient from the side. Table 15.10 shows some of the malalignment postures and their effect.[5,47,48,53]

Posterior View

When viewing from behind (Table 15.11; see Fig. 15.1C), the examiner should note whether the following conditions hold true:

1. The shoulders are level, and the head is in midline. These findings should be compared with those from the anterior view.

2. The spines and inferior angles of the scapulae are level (Fig. 15.25), and the medial borders of the scapulae are equidistant from the spine. If not, is there a rotational or winging deformity of one of the scapulae? Defects, such as Sprengel's deformity, should be noted (Fig. 15.26).

3. The spine is straight, or curved laterally indicating scoliosis. A plumb line may be dropped from the spinous process of the seventh cervical vertebra (see Fig. 8.15).[54] Normally, the line passes through the gluteal cleft. This line is the **posterior line of reference** used to divide the body into right and left halves posteriorly (see Fig. 15.1C). The distance from the vertical string to the gluteal cleft can be measured. This distance is sometimes used as a measurement of spinal imbalance, and it is noted whether the deviation is to the left or right. If a torticollis or cervicothoracic scoliosis is present, the plumb line should be dropped from the occipital protuberance.[23]

TABLE **15.10**

Malalignments Viewed Laterally[5,47,48,53]

Malalignment	Possible Correlated Motions or Postures	Possible Compensatory Motions or Postures
Forward head posture	Extension of cervical spine Protracted scapula	Increased kyphosis in thoracic spine Increased lordosis in lumbar spine Medially rotated humerus
Round back	Extension of cervical spine Protracted scapula	Forward head posture Hips flexed Knees extended
Flat back	Posterior pelvic tilt	Hips extended Knees extended Forward head posture
Swayback	Pelvic neutral or posterior tilt	Pelvis slides anterior Kyphosis Hips extended Knees extended
Pathological lordosis	Pelvis anteriorly tilted Tight hip flexors	Knees extended Ankles plantar flexed
Anterior pelvic tilt	Hip flexion (tight hip flexors)	Lumbar extension (increased lordosis) Hyperextended knees Poking chin (cervical extension) Rounded shoulders (protracted scapula) Thoracic kyphosis Ankles plantar flexed
Posterior pelvic tilt	Hip extension	Lumbar flexion (flat back) Hips extended Knees extended Forward head posture
Backward rotation of one ilium on sacrum (right leg stance)	Right hip lateral rotation Lateral facing patella Out-toeing Supination of foot Short leg	Right lumbar rotation Scoliosis—concavity to right Knee extension
Genu recurvatum	Ankle plantar flexion Excessive anterior pelvic tilt	Posterior pelvic tilt Flexed trunk posture Excessive thoracic kyphosis
Excessive tibial retroversion (posterior slant of tibial plateaus)	Genu recurvatum	
Inadequate tibial retrotorsion (posterior deflection of proximal tibia due to hamstrings pull)	Flexed knee posture	
Rearfoot valgus (calcaneal eversion)	Forward pelvic tilt (bilateral) Lateral pelvic tilt (unilateral)	

4. The ribs protrude or are symmetrical on both sides.
5. The waist angles are level.
6. The arms are equidistant from the body and equally rotated.
7. The PSISs are level (Fig. 15.27). If one is higher than the other, one leg may be shorter or rotation of the pelvis may be present. The examiner should note how the PSISs relate to the ASISs. If the ASIS on one side and the PSIS on the other side are higher, there is a torsion deformity (anterior or posterior) at the sacroiliac joint. If the ASIS and PSIS on one side are higher than the ASIS and PSIS on the other side, there may be an up-slip at the sacroiliac joint on the high side.

TABLE **15.11**

Normal Alignment in the Standing Posture: Posterior View

Body Segment	Line of Gravity Location	Observation
Head	Passes through middle of head	Head should be straight with no lateral tilting; angles between shoulders and neck should be equal
Arms		Arms should hang naturally so that the palms of the hands are facing the sides of the body
Shoulders/spine	Passes along vertebral column in a straight line, which should bisect the back into two symmetrical halves	Scapulae should lie flat against the rib cage, be equidistant from the line of gravity and be separated by about 4 inches (10.2 cm) in the adult
Hips/pelvis	Passes through gluteal cleft of buttocks and should be equidistant from PSISs	The PSISs should be level; the gluteal folds should be level and symmetrical
Knees	Passes between knees equidistant from medial joint aspects	Look to see that the knees are level
Ankles/feet	Passes between ankles equidistant from the medial malleoli	The heel cords should be vertical and the malleoli should be level and symmetrical

PSIS, Posterior superior iliac spine.
From Levangie PK, Norkin CC: *Joint structures and function—a comprehensive analysis*, Philadelphia, 2005, FA Davis, p 499.

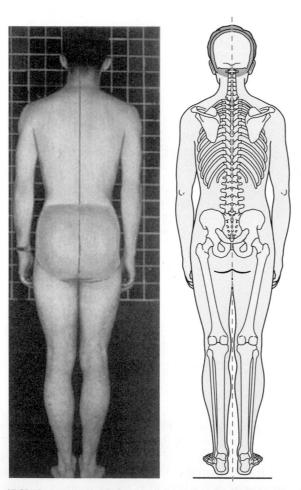

Fig. 15.25 Correct postural alignment (posterior view). (From Kendall FP, McCreary EK: *Muscles: testing and function*, Baltimore, 1983, Williams & Wilkins, p 290.)

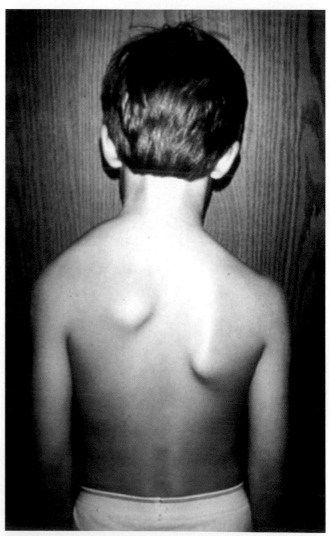

Fig. 15.26 Sprengel's deformity (left sided) in a 5-year-old boy. (From Mauck BM: Congenital anomalies of the trunk and upper extremity. In Azar FM, Beaty JH, Canale ST, editors: *Campbell's Operative Orthopaedics*, ed 13, Philadelphia, 2017, Elsevier.)

8. The gluteal folds are level. Muscle weakness, nerve root problems, or nerve palsy may lead to asymmetry.
9. The knee joints are level. If they are not, it may indicate that one leg is shorter than the other (Fig. 15.28).
10. Both of the Achilles tendons descend straight to the calcanei. If the tendons angle out, it may indicate a flatfoot deformity (pes planus).
11. The heels are straight or are angled in (rearfoot varus) or out (rearfoot valgus).
12. Bowing of femur or tibia is present or absent.

Fig. 15.29 illustrates the normal posture and some of the abnormal deviations seen when viewing from behind. Table 15.12 highlights some of the malalignment postures and their effect.[5,25,47,48]

When viewing posture, the examiner should remember that the pelvis is usually the key to proper back posture. The normal pelvic angle is 30°, and the pelvis is held or balanced in this position by muscles. For the pelvis to "sit properly" on the femur, the following muscles must be strong, supple (mobile), and balanced: abdominals, hip flexors, hip extensors, superficial and deep back extensors, hip rotators, and hip abductors and adductors.

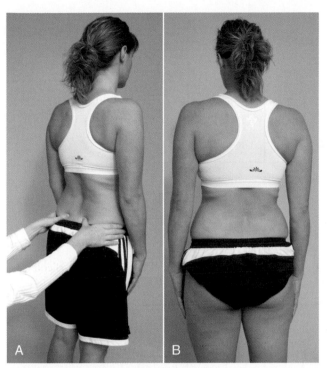

Fig. 15.27 Viewing height equality. (A) Posterior superior iliac spines. (B) Gluteal folds.

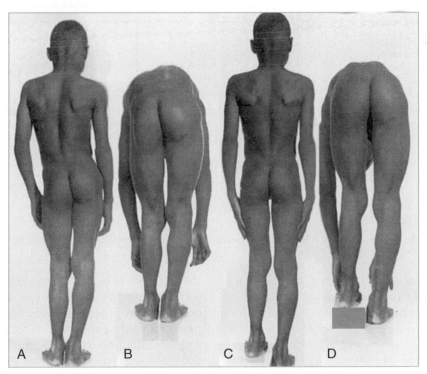

Fig. 15.28 (A and B) Functional scoliosis resulting from short leg. (C and D) The spinal position with short leg corrected with a block. (From Tachdjian MO: *Pediatric orthopedics*, Philadelphia, 1972, WB Saunders, p 1192.)

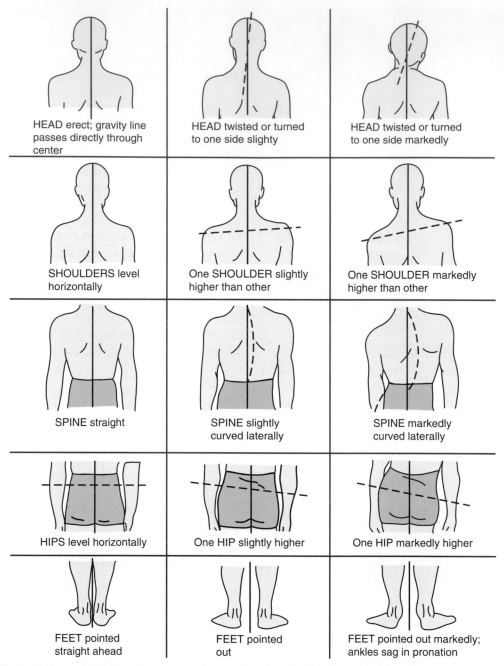

Fig. 15.29 Postural deviations obvious from the posterior view. (Redrawn from Reedco Research, Auburn, NY.)

In the figure, the labels read:

HEAD erect; gravity line passes directly through center

HEAD twisted or turned to one side slighty

HEAD twisted or turned to one side markedly

SHOULDERS level horizontally

One SHOULDER slightly higher than other

One SHOULDER markedly higher than other

SPINE straight

SPINE slightly curved laterally

SPINE markedly curved laterally

HIPS level horizontally

One HIP slightly higher

One HIP markedly higher

FEET pointed straight ahead

FEET pointed out

FEET pointed out markedly; ankles sag in pronation

If the height of the patient is measured, especially in a child, the focal height of the child may be estimated by the use of a chart, such as the one shown in Table 15.13.[55]

After the standing posture has been assessed, the examiner may decide to assess some additional postures (e.g., positional, sustained, or repetitive), especially if the patient has stated in the history that these different positions have caused problems or symptoms.

Forward Flexion

Having completed the assessment of normal standing, the examiner asks the patient to flex forward at the hips with the fingertips of both hands together so that the arms drop vertically (Fig. 15.30). The feet should be together, and both knees should be straight. Any alteration from this posture will cause the spine to rotate, giving a false view.

From this position, using the anterior and posterior skyline views, the examiner can note the following:
1. Whether there is any asymmetry of the rib cage (e.g., rib hump); if a hump is present, a level and tape measure may be used to obtain the perpendicular distance between the hump and hollow (Fig. 15.31).[23]
2. Whether there is any asymmetry in the spinal musculature.
3. Whether a pathological kyphosis is present.

TABLE **15.12**

Malalignments Viewed Posteriorly[a] [5,25,47,48]

Malalignment	Possible Correlated Motions or Postures	Possible Compensatory Motions or Postures
Scoliosis	Side flexion to convex side limited Rotation to convex side limited Rib hump on convex side	
Rearfoot varus Excessive subtalar supination (calcaneal varus)	Tibial; tibial and femoral; or tibial, femoral, and pelvic lateral rotation	Excessive medial rotation along the lower quarter chain Hallux valgus Plantar flexed first ray Functional forefoot valgus Excessive or prolonged midtarsal pronation
Rearfoot valgus Excessive subtalar pronation (calcaneal valgus)	Tibial; tibial and femoral; or tibial, femoral, and pelvic medial rotation Hallus valgus	Excessive lateral rotation along the lower quarter chain Functional forefoot varus
Forefoot varus	Subtalar supination and related rotation along the lower quarter	Plantar flexed first ray Hallux valgus Excessive midtarsal or subtalar pronation or prolonged pronation Excessive tibial; tibial and femoral; or tibial, femoral, and pelvic medial rotation, or all with contralateral lumbar spine rotation

[a]Many of the posterior malalignments are also seen anteriorly.

4. Whether lumbar spine straightens or flexes as it normally should.
5. Whether there is any restriction to forward bending, such as spondylolisthesis or tight hamstrings (Fig. 15.32; see Fig. 8.24).

If, in the history, the patient said that sustained forward flexion caused symptoms, the examiner should ask the patient to assume the symptom-causing posture and maintain it for 15 to 30 seconds to determine whether symptoms arise or increase. Flexion has been found to decrease the stress on the facet joints, but it can increase the pressure in the nucleus pulposus.[56,57] Likewise, if repetitive forward flexion or combined movements (e.g., extension and rotation) have caused symptoms, the patient should be asked to do the repetitive or combined movements. Loading the spine by lifting an object may also cause symptoms and may be investigated if symptoms are not too great.

Sitting

With the patient seated on a stool so that the feet are on the ground and the back is unsupported, the examiner looks at the patient's posture (Fig. 15.33). Sitting without a back support causes the patient to support his or her own posture and increases the amount of muscle activity needed to maintain the posture.[56] Sitting postures have not necessarily demonstrated increased intradiscal pressure as compared to standing.[58,59] It may actually be sustained poor postures and extended periods of trunk flexion that cause increased intradiscal pressures. This observation is carried out, as in the standing position,

TABLE **15.13**

Percentage of Mature Height Attained at Different Ages

Chronologic Age (Years)	PERCENTAGE OF EVENTUAL HEIGHT	
	Boys	Girls
1	42.2	44.7
2	49.5	52.8
3	53.8	57.0
4	58.0	61.8
5	61.8	66.2
6	65.2	70.3
7	69.0	74.0
8	72.0	77.5
9	75.0	80.7
10	78.0	84.4
11	81.1	88.4
12	84.2	92.9
13	87.3	96.5
14	91.5	98.3
15	96.1	99.1
16	98.3	99.6
17	99.3	100.0
18	99.8	100.0

From Bayley N: The accurate prediction of growth and adult height, *Mod Probl Pediatr* 7:234–255, 1954.

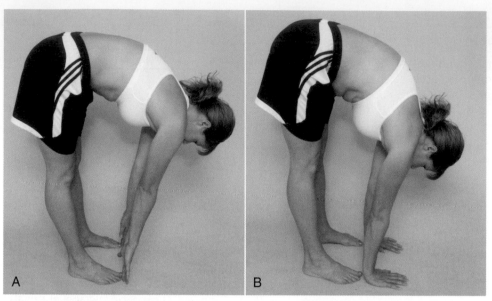

Fig. 15.30 Posture in forward flexion. (A) Normal range of motion. Note reversal of lumbar curve. (B) Excessive range of motion caused by excessive hip mobility.

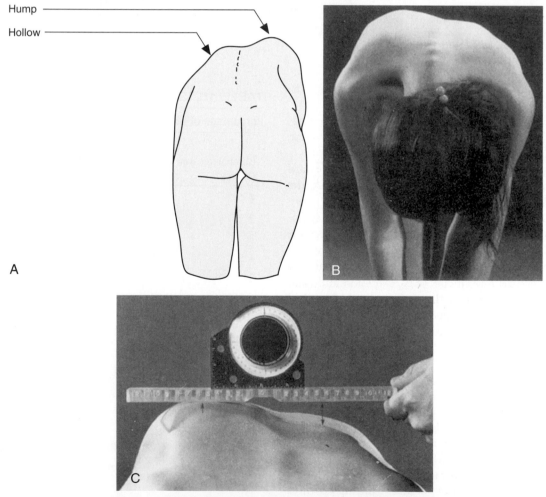

Fig. 15.31 Rib hump in forward-bending test. (A) Posterior view. (B) Anterior view. The two sides are compared. Note the presence of a right thoracic prominence. (C) Measurement of the prominence. The spirit level is positioned with the zero mark over the palpable spinous process in the area of maximal prominence. The level is made horizontal, and the distance to the apex of the deformity (5 to 6 cm) noted. The perpendicular distance from the level to the hollow is measured at the same distance from the midline. A 2.4-cm right thoracic prominence is shown. (From Moe JH, Bradford DS, Winter RB, et al: *Scoliosis and other spinal deformities*, Philadelphia, 1978, WB Saunders, p 17.)

from the front, back, and side. If any anteroposterior or lateral deviations of the spine are observed, the examiner should recall whether they were present when the patient was examined while standing. It should be noted whether the spinal curves increase or decrease when the patient is in the sitting position and how the curves change with different sitting postures.[60] From the front, it can be noted whether the knees are the same distance from the floor. If they are not, this may indicate a shortened tibia. From the side, it can be noted whether one knee protrudes farther than the other. If it does, this may indicate a shortened femur on the other side.

If the patient has stated in the history that going from standing to sitting or sitting to standing resulted in symptoms, the patient should be asked to repeat these maneuvers, provided the movements do not exacerbate the symptoms too much.

Supine Lying

With the patient in the supine-lying position, the examiner notes the position of the head and cervical spine as well as the shoulder girdle. The chest area is observed for any protrusion (e.g., pectus carinatum) or sunken areas (e.g., pectus excavatum).

The abdominal musculature should be observed to see whether it is strong or flabby, and the waist angles should be noted to see whether they are equal. As in the standing position, the ASISs should be viewed to see if they are level. Any extension in the lumbar spine should be noted. In addition, it should be noted whether bending the knees helps to decrease the lumbar curve; if it does, it may indicate tight hip flexors. The lower limbs should descend parallel from the pelvis. If they do not, or if they cannot be aligned parallel and at right angles to a line joining the ASISs, it may indicate an abduction or adduction contracture at the hip.

If, in the history, the patient has complained of symptoms on arising from supine lying or from going into the supine position, the examiner should ask the patient to repeat these movements, provided they do not exacerbate the symptoms.

Prone Lying

With the patient lying prone, the examiner notes the position of the head, neck, and shoulder girdle, as previously described. The head should be positioned so that it is not rotated, side flexed, or extended. Any condition, such as Sprengel's deformity or rib hump, should be noted, as should any spinal deviations. The examiner should determine whether the PSISs are level and should ensure that the musculature of the buttocks, posterior thighs, and calves is normal (see Fig. 8.26B).

As with supine lying, if assuming the position or recovering from the position causes symptoms, the patient

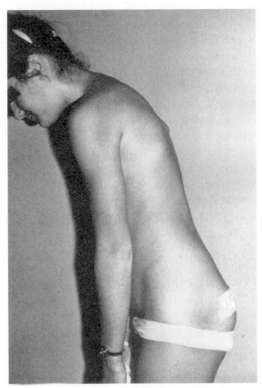

Fig. 15.32 Abnormal forward bending resulting from tight hamstrings in a patient with spondylolisthesis. (From Moe JH, Bradford DS, Winter RB, et al: *Scoliosis and other spinal deformities*, Philadelphia, 1978, WB Saunders, p 19.)

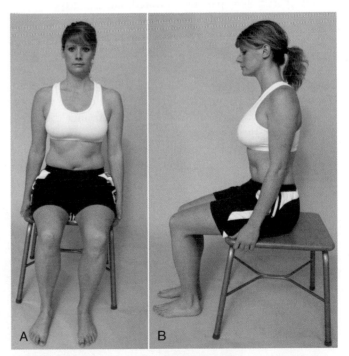

Fig. 15.33 Posture in sitting position. (A) Anterior view. (B) Side view.

should be asked to repeat these movements, as long as symptoms are not made worse.

Examination

Assessment of posture primarily involves history and observation. If, on completing the history and observation, the examiner believes that a direct examination is necessary, the procedures outlined in this text for the various areas of the body should be followed. In addition, there are postural alignment measures, such as the Flexicurve ruler and other measures, that may be used to record postural alignments and changes.[61] With every postural assessment, however, the examiner should perform two tests: the leg length measurement[62–65] and the slump test.

Leg Length Measurement. The patient lies supine with the pelvis set square or "balanced" on the legs (i.e., the legs at an angle of 90° to a line joining the ASISs). The legs should be 15 to 20 cm (6 to 8 inches) apart and parallel to each other (Fig. 15.34). The examiner then places one end of the tape measure against the distal aspect of the ASIS, holding it firmly against the bone. The index finger of the other hand is placed immediately distal to the medial or lateral malleolus and pushed against it. The thumbnail is brought down against the tip of the index fingers so that the tape measure is pinched between them. A reading is taken where the thumb and finger pinch together. A slight difference, up to 1.0 to 1.5 cm (0.4 to 0.6 inch), is considered normal but can still be relevant if pathology is present. Further information on measurement of true leg length may be found in Chapter 11.

Slump Test. The patient is seated on the edge of the examining table with the legs supported, the hips in neutral position (i.e., no rotation or abduction-adduction), and the hands behind the back (see Fig. 9.58). The examination is performed in several steps. First, the patient is asked to "slump" the back into thoracic and lumbar flexion. The examiner maintains the patient's chin in the neutral position to prevent neck and head flexion. The examiner then uses one arm to apply overpressure across the shoulders to maintain flexion of the thoracic and lumbar spines. While this position is held, the patient is asked to actively flex the

cervical spine and head as far as possible (i.e., chin to chest). The examiner then applies overpressure to maintain flexion of all three parts of the spine (cervical, thoracic, lumbar), using the hand of the same arm to maintain overpressure in the cervical spine. With the other hand, the examiner then holds the patient's foot in maximum dorsiflexion. While the examiner holds these positions, the patient is asked to actively straighten the knee as much as possible. The test is repeated with the other leg and then with both legs at the same time. If the patient is unable to fully extend the knee because of pain, the examiner releases the overpressure to the cervical spine and the patient actively extends the neck. If the knee extends farther, the symptoms decrease with neck extension, or the positioning of the patient increases the patient's symptoms, then the test is considered positive for increased tension in the neuromeningeal tract.[66–68] Further information on the slump test may be found in Chapter 9.

Additional Tests. Other tests may also be performed based on what the examiner has observed. For example, if the hip flexors appear tight, the Thomas test should be performed (see Chapter 11). Refer to Table 15.14 for a detailed presentation of good and faulty posture.

Functional Assessment

Functional assessment of posture involves static postural analysis, balance, flexibility and movement, looking at the effect of malalignment on these four parameters and what the clinician needs to do to correct them. This can involve assessing range of motion (ROM), strength and endurance for different activities, assessing balance in different positions, and ensuring sufficient flexibility and strength to assume specific static and dynamic postures while maintaining postural control and providing core stability.[69–71] Measurement of core stability may be a problem as it has been shown that clinical tests for core stability have poor inter- and intrarater reliability.[72] An example of a postural analysis tool is the **Rapid Entire Body Assessment (REBA)**.[73]

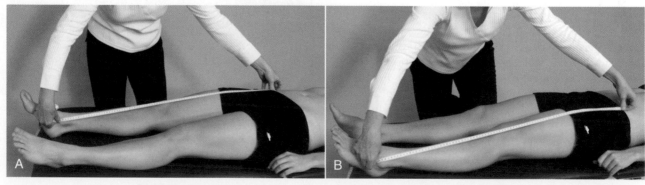

Fig. 15.34 Measuring leg length. (A) To medial malleolus. (B) To lateral malleolus.

TABLE **15.14**

Good and Faulty Posture: Summary Chart

Good Posture	Part	Faulty Posture
Head is held erect in a position of good balance.	Head	Chin up too high. Head protruding forward. Head tilted or rotated to one side.
Arms hang relaxed at the sides with palms of the hands facing toward the body. Elbows are slightly bent, so forearms hang slightly forward. Shoulders are level, and neither one is more forward or backward than the other when seen from the side. Scapulae lie flat against the rib cage. They are neither too close together nor too wide apart. In adults, a separation of approximately 10 cm (4 inches) is average.	Arms and shoulders	Holding the arms stiffly in any position forward, backward, or out from the body. Arms turned so that palms of hands face backward. One shoulder higher than the other. Both shoulders hiked up. One or both shoulders drooping forward or sloping. Shoulders rotated either clockwise or counterclockwise. Scapulae pulled back too hard. Scapulae too far apart. Scapulae too prominent, standing out from the rib cage ("winged scapulae").
A good position of the chest is one in which it is slightly up and slightly forward (while the back remains in good alignment). The chest appears to be in a position about halfway between that of a full inspiration and a forced expiration.	Chest	Depressed, or "hollow chest," position. Lifted and held up too high, brought about by arching the back. Ribs more prominent on one side than on the other. Lower ribs flaring out or protruding.
In young children up to about the age of 10, the abdomen normally protrudes somewhat. In older children and adults, it should be flat.	Abdomen	Entire abdomen protrudes. Lower part of the abdomen protrudes while the upper part is pulled in.
The front of the pelvis and the thighs are in a straight line. The buttocks are not prominent in back but instead slope slightly downward. The spine has four natural curves. In the neck and lower back, the curve is forward, and in the upper back and lowest part of the spine (sacral region), it is backward. The sacral curve is a fixed curve, whereas the other three are flexible.	Spine and pelvis (side view)	The low back arches forward too much (lordosis). The pelvis tilts forward too much. The front of the thigh forms an angle with the pelvis when this tilt is present. The normal forward curve in the low back has straightened out. The pelvis tips backward, and there is a slightly backward slant to the line of the pelvis in relation to the front of the hips (flat back). Increased backward curve in the upper back (kyphosis or round upper back). Increased forward curve in the neck. Almost always accompanied by round upper back and seen as a forward head. Lateral curve of the spine (scoliosis); toward one side (C-curve); toward both sides (S curve).
Ideally, the body weight is borne evenly on both feet, and the hips are level. One side is not more prominent than the other as seen from front or back, nor is one hip more forward or backward than the other as seen from the side. The spine does not curve to the left or the right side. (A slight deviation to the left in right-handed individuals and to the right in left-handed individuals should not be considered abnormal. Also, because a tendency toward a slightly low right shoulder and slightly high right hip is frequently found in right-handed people, and vice versa for left-handed, such deviations should not be considered abnormal.)	Hips, pelvis, and spine (back view)	One hip is higher than the other (lateral pelvic tilt). Sometimes it is not really much higher but appears so because a sideways sway of the body has made it more prominent. (Tailors and dressmakers often notice a lateral tilt because the hemline of skirts or length of trousers must be adjusted to the difference.) The hips are rotated so that one is farther forward than the other (clockwise or counterclockwise rotation).

Continued

TABLE **15.14**

Good and Faulty Posture: Summary Chart—cont'd

Good Posture	Part	Faulty Posture
Legs are straight up and down. Patellae face straight ahead when feet are in good position. Looking at the knees from the side, the knees are straight (i.e., neither bent forward nor "locked" backward).	Knees and legs	Knees touch when feet are apart (genu valgum). Knees are apart when feet touch (genu varum). Knee curves slightly backward (hyperextended knee) (genu recurvatum). Knee bends slightly forward, that is, it is not as straight as it should be (flexed knee). Patellae face slightly toward each other (medially rotated femurs). Patellae face slightly outward (laterally rotated femurs).
In standing, the longitudinal arch has the shape of a half dome. Barefoot or in shoes without heels, the feet toe-out slightly. In shoes with heels, the feet are parallel. In walking with or without heels, the feet are parallel, and the weight is transferred from the heel along the outer border to the ball of the foot. In running, the feet are parallel or toe-in slightly. The weight is on the balls of the feet and toes because the heels do not come in contact with the ground.	Foot	Low longitudinal arch or flatfoot. Low metatarsal arch, usually indicated by calluses under the ball of the foot. Weight borne on the inner side of the foot (supination). "Ankle rolls in." Weight borne on the outer border of the foot (supination). "Ankle rolls out." Toeing-out while walking or while in shoes with heels standing ("outflared" toe or "slue-footed"). Toeing-in while walking or standing ("pigeon-toed")
Toes should be straight, that is, neither curled downward nor bent upward. They should extend forward in line with the foot and not be squeezed together or overlap.	Toes	Toes bend up at the first joint and down at middle and end joints so that the weight rests on the tips of the toes (hammer toes). This fault is often associated with wearing shoes that are too short. Big toe slants inward toward the midline of the foot (hallux valgus). This fault is often associated with wearing shoes that are too narrow and pointed at the toes.

Modified from Kendall FP, McCreary EK: *Muscles: testing and function*, Baltimore, 1983, Williams & Wilkins.

PRÉCIS OF THE POSTURAL ASSESSMENT[a]

History	Prone lying
Observation	**Examination**
Standing (front, side, behind)	Leg length measurement
Forward flexion (front, side, behind)	Slump test
Sitting (front, side, behind)	**Functional assessment**
Supine lying	**Examination of specific joints (see appropriate chapter)**

[a]As with any assessment, the patient must be warned that there may be some discomfort after the examination and that this discomfort is normal. Discomfort after any assessment should decrease within 24 hours. The examiner must keep in mind that several joints may be affected at the same time, either as the result of or as the cause of faulty posture. Therefore the examination of posture may be an extensive one, with observation both of the posture in general and of several specific joints in detail.

References

1. Kisner C, Colby LA. *Therapeutic Exercise: Foundations and Techniques*. Philadelphia: FA Davis; 1985.
2. Ayub E. Posture and the upper quarter. In: Donetelli RA, ed. *Physical Therapy of Shoulder Pathology*. 2nd ed. New York: Churchill Livingstone; 1991.
3. Basmajian JV, de Luca CJ. *Muscles Alive: Their Function Revealed by Electromyography*. Baltimore: Williams & Wilkins; 1985.
4. Kendall FP, McCreary EK, Provance PG. *Muscles, Testing and Function: With Posture and Pain*. 4th ed. Baltimore: Williams & Wilkins; 1993.
5. Levangie PK, Norkin CC. *Joint Structures and Function—A Comprehensive Analysis*. Philadelphia: WB Saunders; 2005.
6. Johnson J. *Postural Assessment*. Champaign IL: Human Kinetics; 2011.
7. Sahrmann SA. Does postural assessment contribute to patient care? *J Orthop Sports Phys Ther*. 2002;32(8):376–379.
8. Griegel-Morris P, Larson K, Mueller-Klaus K, et al. Incidence of common postural abnormalities in the cervical, shoulder, and thoracic regions and their association with pain in two age groups of healthy subjects. *Phys Ther*. 1992;72:425–430.
9. Dalton D. The vertebral column. In: Norkin C, Levangie P, eds. *Joint Structure and Function: A Comprehensive Analysis*. 5th ed. Philadelphia: FA Davis Company; 2011.
10. Barry-Greb TL, Harrison AL. Posture, gait, and functional abilities of the adolescent, pregnant, and elderly female. *Orthop Phys Ther Clin North Am*. 1996;5:1–21.
11. Jull GA, Janda V. Muscles and motor control in low back pain. Assessment and Management. In: Twomey LT, Taylor JR, eds. *Physical Therapy of the Low Back*. New York: Churchill Livingstone; 1987.
12. Goldspink G. The influence of immobilization and stretch in protein turnover of rat skeletal muscle. *J Physiol*. 1977;264:207–268.
13. Tabary JC, Tabary C, Tardieu C, et al. Physiological and structural changes in the cat's soleus muscle due to immobilization at different lengths by plaster casts. *J Physiol*. 1972;224(1):231–244.
14. Yang H, Alnaqeeb M, Simpson H, Goldspink G. Changes in muscle fibre type, muscle mass and IGF-I gene expression in rabbit skeletal muscle subjected to stretch. *J Anat*. 1997;190(4):613–622.
15. Janda V. Muscles and motor control in cervicogenic disorders: assessment and management. In: Grant R, ed. *Physical Therapy of the Cervical and Thoracic Spine*. New York: Churchill Livingstone; 1994.
16. Singla D, Veqar Z. Methods of postural assessment used for sports persons. *J Clin Diagn Res*. 2014;8(4):LE01–LE04.
17. Fahrni WH. *Backache: Assessment and Treatment*. Vancouver, Canada: Musquean Publishers; 1976.
18. Finneson BE. *Low Back Pain*. Philadelphia: JB Lippincott; 1981.
19. Kendall FP, McCreary EK. *Muscles: Testing and Function*. 3rd ed. Baltimore: Williams & Wilkins; 1983.
20. McKenzie RA. *The Lumbar Spine: Mechanical Diagnosis and Therapy*. Waikanae, New Zealand: Spinal Publications; 1981.
21. Wiles P, Sweetnam R. *Essentials of Orthopaedics*. London: J & A Churchill; 1965.
22. Porterfield JA, DeRosa C. *Mechanical Low Back Pain: Perspectives in Functional Anatomy*. Philadelphia: WB Saunders; 1991.
23. Moe JH, Bradford DS, Winter RB, et al. *Scoliosis and Other Spinal Deformities*. Philadelphia: WB Saunders; 1978.
24. McMorris RO. Faulty postures. *Pediatr Clin North Am*. 1961;8:213–224.
25. Tachdjian MO. *Pediatric Orthopedics*. Philadelphia: WB Saunders; 1972.

26. Tsou PM. Embryology and congenital kyphosis. *Clin Orthop*. 1977;128:18–25.
27. White AA, Panjabi MM, Thomas CC. The clinical biomechanics of kyphotic deformities. *Clin Orthop*. 1977;128:8–17.
28. Hensinger RN. Kyphosis secondary to skeletal dysplasias and metabolic disease. *Clin Orthop*. 1977;128:113–128.
29. Tsou PM, Yau A, Hodgson AR. Embryogenesis and prenatal development of congenital vertebral anomalies and their classification. *Clin Orthop*. 1980;152:211–231.
30. Cailliet R. *Scoliosis: Diagnosis and Management*. Philadelphia: FA Davis; 1975.
31. Figueiredo UM, Mames JIP. Juvenile idiopathic scoliosis. *J Bone Joint Surg Br*. 1981;63:61–66.
32. Goldstein LA, Waugh TR. Classification and terminology of scoliosis. *Clin Orthop*. 1973;93:10–22.
33. James JIP. The etiology of scoliosis. *J Bone Joint Surg Br*. 1970;52:410–419.
34. White AA. Kinematics of the normal spine as related to scoliosis. *J Biomech*. 1971;4:405–411.
35. Papaioannou T, Stokes I, Kenwright J. Scoliosis associated with limb length inequality. *J Bone Joint Surg Am*. 1982;64:59–62.
36. Debrunner HU. *Orthopaedic Diagnosis*. London: E & S Livingstone; 1970.
37. Dolan P, Adams MA, Hutton WC. Commonly adopted postures and their effect on the lumbar spine. *Spine*. 1988;13:197–201.
38. Opila KA, Wagner SS, Schiowitz S, et al. Postural alignment in barefoot and high-heeled stance. *Spine*. 1988;13:542–547.
39. Danis CG, Krebs DE, Gill-Body KM, Sahrmann SA. Relationship between standing posture and stability. *Phys Ther*. 1998;78(5):502–517.
40. Murray MP, Seireg A, Sepic SB. Normal postural stability and steadiness: quantitative assessment. *J Bone Joint Surg Am*. 1975;57(4):510–516.
41. Panzer VP, Bandinelli S, Hallett M. Biomechanical assessment of quiet standing and changes associated with aging. *Arch Phys Med Rehabil*. 1995;76(2):151–157.
42. Vuillerme N, Forestier N, Nougier V. Attentional demands and postural sway: the effect of the calf muscles fatigue. *Med Sci Sports Exerc*. 2002;34(12):1907–1912.
43. Morasso P, Cherif A, Zenzeri J. Quiet standing: the single inverted pendulum model is not so bad after all. *PLoS One*. 2019. https://doi.org/10.1371/journal.pone.0213870.
44. Nashner L. Sensory, neuromuscular, and biomechanical contributions to human balance. In: Duncan P, ed. *Balance, Alexandria*. American Physical Therapy Association; 1990.
45. Ghamkhar L, Kahlaee AH. The effect of trunk muscle fatigue on postural control of upright stance: a systematic review. *Gait Posture*. 2019;72:167–174.
46. Bartels T, Brehme K, Pyschik M, et al. Postural stability and regulation before and after anterior cruciate ligament reconstruction – a two years longitudinal study. *Phys Ther Sport*. 2019;38:49–58.
47. Giallonardo LM. Posture. In: Myers RS, ed. *Saunders Manual of Physical Therapy Practice*. Philadelphia: WB Saunders; 1995.
48. Riegger-Krugh C, Keysor JJ. Skeletal malalignment of the lower quarter: correlated and compensatory motions and postures. *J Orthop Sports Phys Ther*. 1996;23:164–170.
49. Herrington L. Assessment of the degree of pelvic tilt within a normal asymptomatic population. *Man Ther*. 2011;16(6):646–648.
50. Fourchet F, Materne O, Rajeb A, et al. Pelvic tilt: reliability of measuring the standing position and range

of motion in adolescent athletes. *Br J Sports Med*. 2014;48(7):92.
51. Gajdosik R, Simpson R, Smith R, DonTigney RL. Pelvic tilt. Intratester reliability of measuring standing position and range of motion. *Phys Ther*. 1985;65(2):169–174.
52. Sanders G, Stavrakas P. A technique for measuring pelvic tilt. *Phys Ther*. 1981;61(1):49–50.
53. Pinto RZ, Souza TR, Trede RG, et al. Bilateral and unilateral increases in calcaneal eversion affect pelvic alignment in standing position. *Man Ther*. 2008;13:513–519.
54. McLean IP, Gillan MG, Ross JC, et al. A comparison of methods for measuring trunk list—a simple plumb line is best. *Spine*. 1996;21:1667–1670.
55. Bayley N. The accurate prediction of growth and adult height. *Mod Probl Pediatr*. 1954;7:234–255.
56. Adams MA, Hutton WC. The effect of posture on the lumbar spine. *J Bone Joint Surg Br*. 1985;67:625–629.
57. Adams MA, Hutton WC. The effect of posture on the role of the apophyseal joints in resulting intervertebral compressive forces. *J Bone Joint Surg Br*. 1980;62:358–362.
58. Claus A, Hides J, Moseley GL, Hodges P. Sitting versus standing: does intradiscal pressure cause disc degeneration or low back pain? *Electromyogr Kinesiol*. 2008;18(4):550–558.
59. Wilke HJ, Neef P, Caimi M, et al. New in vivo measurements of pressures in the intervertebral disc in daily life. *Spine*. 1999;24(8):755–762.
60. Black KM, McClure P, Polansky M. The influence of different sitting positions on cervical and lumbar posture. *Spine*. 1996;21:65–70.
61. Arnold CM, Beatty B, Harrison EL, et al. The reliability of five clinical postural alignment measures for women with osteoporosis. *Physiother Can*. 2000;52:286–294.
62. Clarke GR. Unequal leg length: an accurate method of detection and some clinical results. *Rheumat Phys Med*. 1972;11:385–390.
63. Fisk JW, Baigent ML. Clinical and radiological assessment of leg length. *NZ Med J*. 1975;81:477–480.
64. Nichols PJR, Bailey NTJ. The accuracy of measuring leg-length differences. *Br Med J*. 1955;2:1247–1248.
65. Woerman AL, Binder-Macleod SA. Leg-length discrepancy assessment: accuracy and precision in five clinical methods of evaluation. *J Orthop Sports Phys Ther*. 1984;5:230–239.
66. Maitland GD. The slump test: examination and treatment. *Aust J Physiother*. 1985;31:215–219.
67. Philip K, Lew P, Matyas TA. The inter-therapist reliability of the slump test. *Aust J Physiother*. 1989;35:89–94.
68. Butler DS. *Mobilisation of the Nervous System*. Melbourne: Churchill Livingstone; 1991.
69. Taylor J. *Core Stability – Injury Free Performance*. Guilford UK: Green Star Media Ltd; 2014.
70. Howell DR, Hanson E, Sugimoto D, et al. Assessment of the postural stability of female and male athletes. *Clin J Sports Med*. 2017;27(5):444–449.
71. Laviviere C, Boucher JA, Mecheri H, Ludvig D. Maintaining lumbar spine stability: a study of the specific and combined effects of abdominal activation and lumbosacral orthosis on lumbar intrinsic stiffness. *J Orthop Sports Phys Ther*. 2019;49(4):262–271.
72. Weir A, Darby J, Inklaar, et al. Core stability: inter- and intraobserver reliability of 6 clinical tests. *Clin J Sports Med*. 2010;20(1):34–38.
73. Hignett S, McAtamney L. Rapid Entire Body Assessment (REBA). *Appl Ergon*. 2000;31(2):201–205.

CHAPTER 16

Assessment of the Amputee

In the United States, 1.7 million people live with limb loss each year and there are 185,000 new lower-extremity amputations each year.[1,2] An amputation is defined as the removal of part or all of a limb or some other outgrowth of the body. Amputations may be the result of trauma, congenital deformity, peripheral arterial disease, or tumors.[3] If fingers and partial nonmutilating hand injuries are excluded, lower-limb amputations are much more frequent than upper-limb amputations.[4] However, upper-limb amputations cause greater functional loss because the upper limbs are used more functionally and in many more diverse ways. There is also a greater functional sensory loss when an upper limb is involved. In addition, the upper-limb amputation causes a more obvious disfigurement and alteration of body image, which affects the actions and reactions of both the amputee and those with whom he or she interacts.[4,5] Amputations are considered to be a treatment of last resort when other methods, such as revascularization or reattachment, have failed or are not considered suitable treatment options.[5-9] Assessment of the amputee patient may involve assessing a patient before the amputation or after the amputation has taken place. In the first instance, the assessment is primarily carried out by one or more physicians deciding whether there is a need for such a procedure and then deciding the level at which the amputation should occur. In some cases, indexes or scores[10-21] may be used, although some[22] have questioned their usefulness in the final outcome, especially in the case of trauma.

There are several indications for amputations.[23] The most common are trauma caused by compound fractures, blood vessel rupture, stab or gunshot injuries, compression injuries, severe burns, or cold injuries[24]; and vascular disease as the result of systemic problems, such as diabetes, arteriosclerosis, embolism, venous insufficiency, or peripheral vascular disease often aggravated by cigarette smoking.[25] Approximately 75% of amputations in older patients fall within this second category.[26] The presence of suspected vascular disease may include more than the physical examination when considering whether to amputate. These other tests include blood tests, chest x-rays, electrocardiography, Doppler studies, arteriography, venograms, thermography, and transcutaneous PO_2 readings.[24] When trauma is the cause, the aim of the amputation is to restore maximum length with good soft-tissue covering.[24] In addition, amputations may be performed because of infections, tumors (both benign and more commonly,

malignant types), neurological disorders (e.g., an anesthetic limb from, for example, a complete plexus avulsion[27]), congenital deformity (e.g., partial or total absence of a limb), and amputations for cosmetic reasons (e.g., extra digit).[27–30] It has been shown that preoperative sepsis is a high predictor for an increased 30-day mortality rate after major lower-limb amputation among those with arteriosclerosis and diabetes.[31] Younger people tend to experience more congenital, malignancy, and trauma-related amputations, whereas older people experience multiple pathophysiological mechanisms, as previously mentioned.

Causes of Amputation

- Trauma
- Vascular disease
- Infection
- Tumors
- Neurological disorders
- Congenital deformity

The examiner who has the opportunity to do a preoperative physical assessment of the patient who has been scheduled for an amputation should take the time to determine the patient's available muscle strength, range of motion (ROM), and functional mobility bilaterally to provide a baseline for future comparison if necessary. In addition, the overall level of physical fitness or conditioning of amputees is very critical because they will experience increased physiological energy demands due to compensation for the lost body part. This is especially true for lower-extremity amputees because the energy required for activities of daily living (ADLs) substantially increases as the level of amputation moves proximally. The size and position of any abnormal tissue degeneration or potential pressure areas should be recorded accurately, and functional levels should be assessed and recorded. If at all possible in this preoperative period, the patient should be given some instruction in bed mobility, as well as climbing in and out of bed with or without support. In addition, the examiner should ensure that the patient knows how to provide suitable care for pressure areas and preserve joint mobility to prevent any contractures from forming. If a lower-limb amputation is anticipated, the patient should be taught to use ambulatory aids such as crutches or wheelchair so that he or she can maintain as much mobility as possible after the amputation.

Levels of Amputation

Amputation surgery, whether performed to the upper limb or the lower limb, can occur at various levels (Figs. 16.1 and 16.2).[32] For the most part, this chapter deals with assessment of the lower-limb amputee primarily, because these amputations are more common. However, functional loss is usually greater for upper-limb amputees. Thus upper-limb amputee assessment deals much more with different functional demands than lower-limb assessment. Fig. 16.3 shows the percentage impairment caused by an upper-limb amputation.[33]

Amputation surgery may be one of two types—open or closed. Open, or primary, amputation is used in cases of infection in which the wound is left open after the amputated part is removed to allow clearance of infection. It requires a second procedure to close the wound. More commonly, a closed amputation is performed. This procedure is used when tissue viability is as normal as possible. At the time of the amputation, the skin flaps are closed, as is the wound. Commonly, the skin flaps are closed on the posterior and distal aspect of the stump because adhesions are less likely and an incision line is farther from the bone, but other methods are also sometimes used.[34] The goal of amputation surgery is to create a dynamically balanced residual limb with good motor control and sensation.[35] The patient will need a well-healed, well-shaped residual stump with the greatest functional length possible in the limb.[35] The higher the level of the amputation, the greater the handicap.[27] In the lower limb, immediate prosthetic fitting helps to facilitate early mobilization with more normal gait patterns.[28] Amputation should be

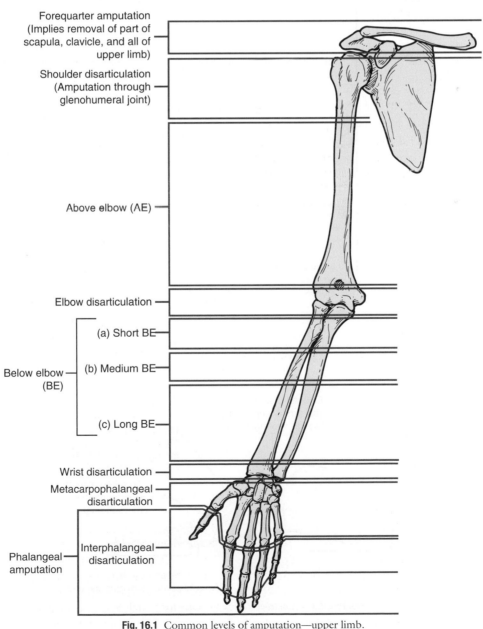

Forequarter amputation
(Implies removal of part of scapula, clavicle, and all of upper limb)

Shoulder disarticulation
(Amputation through glenohumeral joint)

Above elbow (AE)

Elbow disarticulation

(a) Short BE

Below elbow
(BE)

(b) Medium BE

(c) Long BE

Wrist disarticulation

Metacarpophalangeal disarticulation

Phalangeal amputation

Interphalangeal disarticulation

Fig. 16.1 Common levels of amputation—upper limb.

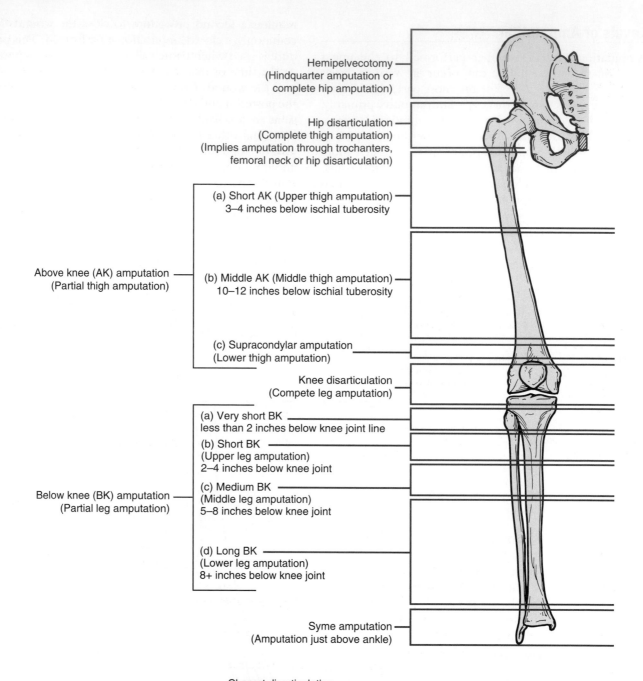

Hemipelvecotomy
(Hindquarter amputation or
complete hip amputation)

Hip disarticulation
(Complete thigh amputation)
(Implies amputation through trochanters,
femoral neck or hip disarticulation)

(a) Short AK (Upper thigh amputation)
3–4 inches below ischial tuberosity

Above knee (AK) amputation
(Partial thigh amputation)

(b) Middle AK (Middle thigh amputation)
10–12 inches below ischial tuberosity

(c) Supracondylar amputation
(Lower thigh amputation)

Knee disarticulation
(Compete leg amputation)

(a) Very short BK
less than 2 inches below knee joint line

(b) Short BK
(Upper leg amputation)
2–4 inches below knee joint

(c) Medium BK
(Middle leg amputation)
5–8 inches below knee joint

Below knee (BK) amputation
(Partial leg amputation)

(d) Long BK
(Lower leg amputation)
8+ inches below knee joint

Syme amputation
(Amputation just above ankle)

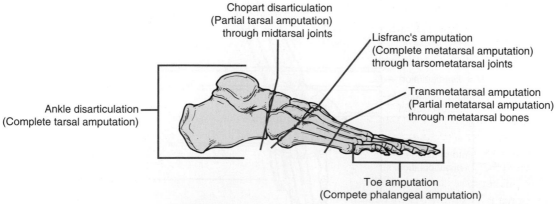

Chopart disarticulation
(Partial tarsal amputation)
through midtarsal joints

Lisfranc's amputation
(Complete metatarsal amputation)
through tarsometatarsal joints

Transmetatarsal amputation
(Partial metatarsal amputation)
through metatarsal bones

Ankle disarticulation
(Complete tarsal amputation)

Toe amputation
(Compete phalangeal amputation)

Fig. 16.2 Common levels of amputation—lower limb.

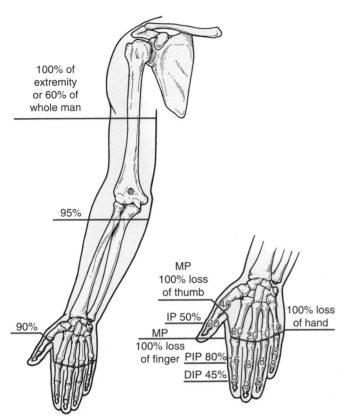

100% of extremity or 60% of whole man

95%

90%

MP 100% loss of thumb

IP 50%

MP 100% loss of finger

100% loss of hand

PIP 80%

DIP 45%

40
20
20 20 10 10
16 6 8 3
9 9

Fig. 16.3 Amputation impairment. Percentage of impairments related to whole body, extremity, hand, or digit. *DIP,* Distal interphalangeal; *IP,* interphalangeal; *MP,* metacarpophalangeal; *PIP,* proximal interphalangeal. (Redrawn from Swanson AB, de Groot Swanson G, Goran-Hagert C: Evaluation of hand function. In Hunter JM, Schneider LH, Mackin EJ, et al, editors: *Rehabilitation of the hand,* St Louis, 1990, Mosby, p. 119.)

considered to be a reconstructive procedure leaving the patient with the best of possible alternatives.[36]

The second opportunity where the amputee patient may be assessed is following the surgery. This is more likely to be done by the physician or other health care professionals. In this case the aim of the assessment is primarily to determine what functional deficits the patient has, to assess the fitting of the prosthesis, and to watch for complications. A good assessment enables the clinician to assist the patient in understanding and dealing with the specific physical and social limitations that the amputation has brought to his or her pattern of life.[37] This second scenario is described in the remainder of this chapter.

Patient History[37]

As with any assessment, the initial part of the examination will include the patient's history as it relates to the amputation, its cause, and any related factors. Occupation and whether the patient intends to return to the same occupation are important to determine because odds are fairly high that the patient will want to return to his or her job. A retrospective cohort study showed that out of 147 amputees, 69% were able to return to previous employment.[38] Interviews of 32 adult amputees

who averaged a year between amputation and return to work indicated that reintegration into the work force was delayed by problems with the residual limb and, in particular, wound healing. Many of these subjects were employed in less physically demanding jobs after rehabilitation.[39] When doing the assessment of the amputee, it is important to determine the patient's past medical, surgical, preoperative ambulatory, and functional status for both upper and lower limbs, and preoperative symptoms. As part of this "past history," the examiner must develop some understanding of the patient's recreational activities, past psychiatric history (which may include information on alcohol or drug abuse), current stressors (including recent losses), pain tolerance, previous association with patients who have disabilities, and compliance with medical treatments.[26] In addition, information on family structure and possible support groups, including family and friends, must be discussed. Issues such as marital status, sexual history, and family roles including familial support, strengths, and problems should be ascertained because they can impact greatly the outcome and how the patient ultimately functions as an amputee.[40,41]

Pertinent Information in Patient Assessment[26]

RELEVANT PATIENT INFORMATION

- Educational level
- Occupational history
- Avocational activities
- Psychiatric history, alcohol and drug use, problems with the law (It is important to have objective corroboration from the family.)
- Current stressors, including recent losses
- Any pain sensitivity or tolerance
- Previous associations with patients having disabilities
- Compliance with medical treatment; obstacles to compliance

FAMILY STRUCTURE

- Marital adjustment
- Sexual history
- Family roles; strengths and problem areas
- Health of others

THE PATIENT'S PERSPECTIVE

- Current mood
- Anxieties and ideas associated with them
- What the patient imagines his or her future to be (i.e., how the disability will change lifestyle, social relations, vocational future); self-concept
- The degree to which self-esteem is related to physique and physical skills
- Comfort in meeting a psychiatrist or psychologist
- How the patient thinks the adjustment is going
- The most pressing immediate concern
- The patient's understanding of the cause and probable course of disability
- How much the patient wants to know about the treatment as it progresses; how the patient prefers having a medical update

TABLE **16.1**

Patient Motivational and General Problems

Problem	Cause	Findings	Solution
Discouraged patient	Performance does not equal expectations	Patient does not wear prosthesis Complaints not related to physical findings	Sympathetic explanation of reasonable realistic goals Training
Failure to maintain good prosthetic habits	Lack of training New situations Poor motivation	Hip or knee flexion contracture Pressure sores Poor socket fit Abnormal gait patterns	Retraining Sympathetic encouragement
Poor hygiene	Poor motivation	Dermatitis Abscess formation Hidradenitis (inflammation of sweat glands)	Wash limb Clean socks Clean socket Antibiotics Surgical drainage
Rest pain	Phantom pain/sensation	Pain in missing segment of limb	Provide distracting sensation (a) Wrapping (b) Temperature changes (c) Activity with prosthesis (d) Transcutaneous nerve stimulation
	Neuroma Ischemia	Positive Tinel sign Crampy pain aggravated by activity	Excise neuroma Unweight limb Stop smoking Revise amputation

Modified from Smith AG: Common problems of lower extremity amputees, *Orthop Clin North Am* 13:576, 1982.

Quality of life is an issue following major surgery or medical procedures. Lower-extremity amputation has been shown to be more common in people from lower socioeconomic groups which is thought to decrease quality of life. This information may also be important to gather in the history. Although Davie-Smith and colleagues[42] observed greater numbers of lower extremity amputations in patients from low socioeconomic areas, they were unable to conclude whether quality of life after amputation was truly influenced by socioeconomic status. It has also been suggested that lack of income or insurance may increase the likelihood of having major amputation. Hughes and colleagues[43] found that those on Medicaid and uninsured status in the United States were associated with a greater likelihood of amputation and a lower likelihood of undergoing much costlier limb-saving procedures such as revascularization. Em et al.[44] reported that lower-limb amputations in men lead to impairments in sexual function and quality of life. In addition, sexual dysfunction is also strongly associated with the patient's emotional state, pain level, level of amputation, and quality of life.

The examiner must determine and develop an understanding for any patient anxieties, why they are present, whether these anxieties can be dealt with by the examiner or if other health care specialists need to be involved, what the patient imagines his or her future to be, and how the disability will change his or her lifestyle, social relations, vocational future, and self-concept (Table 16.1). All these factors must be considered if the examiner hopes to have a successful outcome to treatment.

For the present medical history, the following questions should be asked:

1. *What is the patient's occupation?* Does the patient have any concerns about returning to his or her job? If so, what are the patient's future occupational plans? Is any vocational guidance or training required?

2. *What is the patient's present medical status?* For example, what was the reason for the amputation? Any systemic disease, such as diabetes, cardiovascular or respiratory problems, arthritic joints, and lifestyle factors, has a bearing on successful treatment outcomes. Systemic disease or trauma may prolong the healing process, and the speed of recovery may be delayed.

3. *How long ago did the amputation occur?* In recent amputations, the initial concern is the healing of the stump and the prevention of complications. If the amputation surgery was a revision procedure, why was the revision necessary? Was the problem one of poor tissue viability, or was the procedure performed to enable the patient to obtain better functional results?

4. *If the amputation occurred some time ago (3 to 6 months or longer), has the patient experienced any complications over that period, such as tissue breakdown, ulcer formation, or blisters?*

5. *If the patient has a prosthesis, what does the patient think about the prosthesis, its fit, and its function?* How long

has the prosthesis been worn? (Years? Months?) How long is the prosthesis worn each day? Is it worn every day? Is the suspension adequate? Are there any skin abrasions? Inadequacies in these areas will lead to patient frustration, to disappointment, and, ultimately, to the patient becoming discouraged about using the prosthesis and, in fact, may come to the state where the patient does not want to wear the prosthesis. If the prosthesis is uncomfortable or excessively noisy, it is unlikely the patient will use it, or if it is used, it is unlikely the patient will use it properly. In the case of a lower-limb prosthesis, the patient may refuse to bear weight on the prosthesis. Cosmesis is another problem that is often of concern for amputees, especially for women, and when the amputation is in the upper limb the extremity is sometimes not covered with clothing. The examiner must differentiate between the discomfort of using something new and the discomfort caused by a specific prosthetic fault. In some cases a prosthesis evaluation questionnaire (PEQ)[45] may be useful (eTool 16.1).

6. *Has the patient been looking after the stump properly, ensuring proper limb and sock hygiene?* Failure to do so easily leads to complications, such as skin breakdown, infection, and ulcers (see Table 16.1).[35] The remaining stump should be washed with care using mild soap. The stump sock should be changed and cleaned regularly, and the prosthesis socket should also be cleaned regularly with mild soap and water.[35]

7. *Was the patient able to or did he or she exercise preoperatively?* Poor physical condition and low levels of preoperative activity prior to the amputation can significantly affect the patient's life. These patients usually have low levels of physical activity already due to illness or peripheral vascular disease and diabetes which result in overall lower activity levels in general.[46,47] This diminished physical activity level prior to surgery can pose a serious risk to the patient's daily physical and psychosocial functioning, prolong recovery after surgery, and increase the risk of postoperative complications, all while limiting the patient's ability to achieve optimal functioning with his or her prosthesis leading to decreased quality of life, permanent disability, and an increased mortality rate.[48,49]

8. *Does the patient have any pain or abnormal sensation?* Where is the pain or abnormal sensation? Is the pain intermittent or constant? What is the intensity of the pain (a visual analogue scale may be used—see Fig. 1.2)? Where is the pain? What type of pain or abnormal sensation is it? **Phantom sensation** is an abnormal feeling the patient has for the limb, but the patient feels the sensation as being in the amputated part of the limb even though that part of the limb is not there.[24,50–52] Phantom limb sensation was first described by the French military surgeon, Ambroise Pare, in the 16th century.[53] This sensation is an almost universal consequence of limb amputation.[54,55]

It may take numerous forms, including the feeling that someone is touching the amputated limb, pressure being applied to the missing body part, cold, wetness, itching, tickle, pain, or fatigue. The intensity of these sensations may vary and may change over time. The sensations commonly have different meaning to different people. Phantom sensations are more commonly felt in the distal part of the excised extremity, because the distal part of an extremity tends to be more richly innervated.[50]

Phantom pain is described as a painful sensation perceived in the missing body part in the case of an amputation, in the paralyzed part of a spinal cord injury patient, or following a nerve root avulsion in the case of a neurological injury.[24,50–52,54] Eighty percent of amputees experience some phantom pain sometime during the injury healing process. Phantom pain is relatively common, but it is unpredictable in terms of predisposing factors, severity, frequency, duration or character, aggravation by internal or external stimuli, or type of pain experienced.[50] Phantom pain is more likely to be seen in the upper-limb amputee than in the lower-limb amputee, and it tends to be more prolonged in the upper limb. Some patients report that the pain is of very high intensity, which may be evoked by some external or internal stimuli, whereas others report a dull, continuous aching or burning that does not seem to be episodic. Many amputees describe the pain as being knifelike, burning, sticking, shooting, prickling, throbbing, cramplike, squeezing, "like something trying to pull my leg off," or some type of electrical phenomenon (Fig. 16.4).[51,54] Phantom pain generally begins within the first postsurgical week, commonly stabilizes after a few months, but may occur several months or years after the amputation. It seems to decrease in frequency, duration, and severity during the first 6 months. Most commonly, phantom pain persisting beyond 6 months is very difficult to treat and usually does not change in character after that time. However, some people report that the intensity of pain changes with time. Prolonged healing or other complications, such as fractures, may cause phantom pain to persist for longer periods.

Phantom Pain Sensations[51]

- Knifelike[a,b]
- Sticking[a]
- Shooting
- Prickling
- Burning[b]
- Squeezing[b]
- Throbbing
- Pressing
- Cramplike
- Sawing
- Dull

[a]More common early.
[b]More common after 6 months.

Stump pain is pain arising from the residual part of the body as opposed to phantom pain, which is

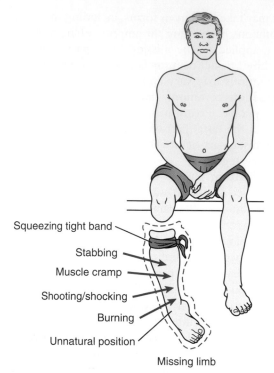

Squeezing tight band

Stabbing

Muscle cramp

Shooting/shocking

Burning

Unnatural position

Missing limb

Fig. 16.4 Phantom limb pain. Some of the typical painful feelings that seem to stem from the missing limb. (Redrawn from Sherman RA: Stump and phantom limb pain, *Neurol Clin* 7:250, 1989.)

felt in the missing part of the body.[24,50,51,54,55] It is commonly a sharp, sticking, or pressure feeling that, although diffuse, is localized to the end of the stump.[51] Stump pain is usually the result of six primary etiologies—prosthogenic, neurogenic, arthrogenic, sympathogenic, referred, and abnormal stump tissues.[50] The most common cause of stump pain is prosthogenic, which implies improper fitting of the prosthesis. The second type of stump pain is neurogenic, most commonly from the formation of a neuroma where the nerve was cut during surgery. Neuroma pain is usually characterized by sharp, shooting pain that can be evoked by light tapping over the neuroma (Tinel sign). Third, stump pain may be arthrogenic or coming from an adjacent joint or surrounding tissues, usually as a result of changing stresses to the tissues or because sufficient time has not been allowed for the tissues to adapt to the new stresses being applied to them. For example, back pain is initially a common finding in above-knee (AK) amputees.[55] Fourth, stump pain may be sympathogenic or associated with the sympathetic nerve system. This pain is sometimes called *causalgia, reflex sympathetic dystrophy,* or, as some people now call it, *sympathetically maintained pain.* Fifth, the pain may be referred. Nonradicular referred pain can come from the joints, muscles, or myofascial conditions. Last, abnormal tissue, such as bony exostosis, heterotrophic ossification, adherent scar,

or sepsis (infection), can lead to pain in the remaining stump. Virtually every amputee experiences stump pain after amputation. Stump pain is a normal result of major surgery. However, it is frequently a shock to those patients who are not warned to expect it.[54] Stump pain is usually severe immediately after amputation and subsides quickly with healing. It tends to be more evident in patients who have nondecreasing phantom pain.[51] Approximately 80% of amputees have functionally significant episodes of phantom or stump pain every year and may have almost constant, very low level, stump and phantom pain that they define as being over the threshold of nonpainful sensation.[54]

There is no evidence that phantom pain or stump pain is caused by psychological disorders, although stress and psychological disturbances can exacerbate the pain.[54] They are both considered to be physiological phenomena.

Observation[37]

Following surgery, the examiner will observe the stump for any swelling and whether healing is occurring properly. The condition of the skin, as well as the presence of joint contractures, especially if the amputation is close to a joint (e.g., below-knee [BK] amputation), should be noted. The amputee should be observed both without the prosthesis and while wearing the prosthesis. In general, the lower-limb amputee is observed in three positions while wearing the prosthesis: standing, sitting, and walking.

To begin the observation of the amputee, the examiner first looks at the remaining good limb, noting sensation, pulses, temperature, and skin condition. The examiner takes time to observe the remaining limb that will have to take a greater functional role and often greater stresses because of the amputation to the other limb. If it is a lower-limb amputation, the remaining limb will have to take a greater load during gait. Are the skin and nails normal, or are trophic changes evident? Are there any sores or open areas? These changes may indicate circulatory impairment. What are the color and temperature of the remaining limb? Do they fall within normal limits? Are the pulses (e.g., femoral, tibial, dorsalis pedis) normal? Does the limb exhibit any deformity or swelling? Will the remaining limb be able to take the additional stress?

The examiner notes whether the patient is wearing the prosthesis or not. If the patient has the prosthesis on, then observation of the patient functioning with the prosthesis is first done with the patient standing, walking, and sitting. If the patient is not wearing the prosthesis, the examiner spends the initial period checking the stump and its condition, noting whether the wound is healing properly or whether there are any signs of drainage or weeping from the wound or evidence of tissue breakdown.[35] If the stump is covered with an elastic

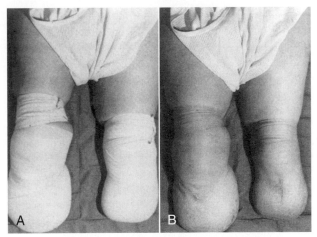

Fig. 16.5 The effect of bad bandaging. (A) An incorrectly applied bandage. (B) The uneven residual limb contour produced by the incorrectly applied bandage. (From Engstrom B, Van de Ven C: *Therapy for amputees*, Edinburgh, 1999, Churchill Livingstone, p. 53.)

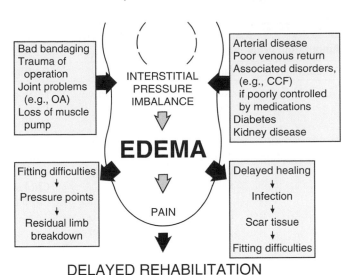

Fig. 16.6 Causes of residual limb edema. *OA,* Osteoarthritis; *CCF,* congestive cardiac failure. (From Engstrom B, Van de Ven C: *Therapy for amputees*, Edinburgh, 1999, Churchill Livingstone, p. 52.)

wrap or shrinker to assist in decreasing swelling, the examiner should note how it is applied, whether it fits smoothly or contains wrinkles, and whether the application is effective in reducing swelling. The examiner can then ask the patient to remove the wrap. At this stage, the examiner can ask the patient to demonstrate how he or she applies the wrap (if the patient does it himself or herself), or this may be left until later.

With the wrap off, the examiner then inspects the stump, noting its shape (Table 16.2). The stump may be classed as cylindrical, conical, bony, bulbous, or edematous. The examiner looks for signs of unusual patterns of swelling (an indication the wrap has been applied incorrectly) (Fig. 16.5); causes of residual limb edema (Fig. 16.6); presence of skin abrasions, skin breakdown, or blisters (all of which may indicate poor prosthesis fit); or presence of infection.[35] The examiner should note whether the scar is healing normally and whether the sutures have been removed or some remain. The scar may be classed as nontender, sensitive, invaginated, well healed, open, or adherent. The location of the scar and whether it will affect the fitting of the prosthesis should be noted. Any "dog ears" to the suture, which may interfere with the prosthesis, should also be noted. The mobility of the scar and tension of the skin and its mobility, especially over the distal end of the stump, should be observed. In addition, the color and temperature of the stump should be noted. Any potential weight-bearing areas (e.g., ischial tuberosity–AK amputation; patellar tendon–BK amputation) should also be inspected because these tissues will receive greater stress with the use of a prosthesis. The condition of the remaining joints and their supporting musculature (e.g., atrophied, fleshy, strong) should be noted.

If the patient has a prosthesis, the prosthesis is then inspected (Table 16.3). The examiner should note the socket type, the material used to construct it, and the type of suspension. The general workmanship of the prosthesis and whether it is satisfactory should be noted. The examiner should inspect the trim lines, the rivets, and other fastenings to see if they are neat and secure. Joint covers should shield mechanical joint heads to prevent damage to clothing. There should be no scratches or rough areas on the prosthesis. Plastic lamination should be uniform without appreciable missed areas.

Next, provided the patient is at the stage where the prosthesis has been fitted (in some cases, especially in the lower limb, the prosthesis may be fitted right after surgery; in other cases the prosthesis is fitted after tissue healing is ensured), the patient is asked to put the prosthesis on while the examiner determines whether the patient can correctly and easily do this independently or only with help.

For the lower-limb amputee, once the prosthesis is fitted, the patient is first observed in standing position. As with the patient who is not an amputee, posture of the patient is assessed (see Chapter 15) and the examiner must determine if any deviations are structural or due to the prosthesis. In addition, the examiner notes the following:

1. Does the patient appear to be comfortable while standing, especially with the heels no more than 15 cm (6 inches) apart as seen in normal standing?

2. Is the patient able to "balance" on the prosthesis when standing on two legs or when weight shifting between the two legs? At the same time, the examiner should note whether the anteroposterior alignment of the prosthesis is satisfactory so that the patient does not feel the knee is unstable or that the knee is being forced backward, in the case of a BK amputee. In addition, the clinician should note whether the mediolateral alignment is satisfactory with the foot flat on the floor. There should be no uncomfortable pressure on the lateral or medial brim of the socket.

3. Is the prosthesis of correct length? When the patient rises on the prosthesis, is there any piston

TABLE **16.2**

Amputation Problems

Problem	Cause	Findings	Solution
Limb shrinkage	Normal shrinkage with activity Weight loss	Limb too deep in socket Pressure areas on bony prominences Pressure on end of amputation Limb too short	Add stump socks Modify liners in socket New socket or prosthesis
Limb swelling	Edema Weight gain Failure to continue limb wrapping in recent amputee Failure to wear prosthesis for prolonged period without wrapping	Limb not fitting into socket Pressure on bony prominences Choking on end of stump Limb too long	Treat medical cause of edema Diet control Training in proper limb wrapping Socket relief Remove stump socks Wear stump shrinker
Joint contracture	Failure of preprosthetic training Lack of patient cooperation Patient does not wear prosthesis	Limb short Heel of prosthesis off floor Unstable gait Excessive knee and hip flexion when prosthesis off	Sympathetic encouragement Training Temporary prosthesis that is adjustable as contracture decreases

Modified from Smith AG: Common problems of lower extremity amputees, *Orthop Clin North Am* 13:570, 1982.

TABLE **16.3**

Problems Related to the Prosthesis

Problem	Cause	Findings	Solution
Improper socket fit	Improper fabrication	Same as for limb swelling or shrinkage shortly after delivery	Socket relief New socket
Improper prosthetic alignment	Improper fabrication Patient changes height of shoe heel Joint contracture	Limb too long or too short with good socket fit Heel or toe off the floor Gait abnormalities Pressure areas on limb	Realign prosthesis Heel pads in shoe or shoes with original heel height Training to correct contracture
Inadequate suspension	Improper fabrication of suspension	Pistoning of limb in socket Insecurity on weight bearing Abrasions Gait abnormality that is similar to findings when prosthesis is too long Prosthesis incorrectly rotated Restriction of joint motion	Readjust suspension

Modified from Smith AG: Common problems of lower extremity amputees, *Orthop Clin North Am* 13:574, 1982.

action of the stump in the prosthesis? Normally, there should be very little movement. Are the anterior, medial, and lateral walls of the prosthesis of adequate height? Do the medial and lateral walls of the stump contact the prosthesis in the correct places so that there is no weight on the end of the prosthesis? In the case of a joint disarticulation, weight bearing through the end of the stump may be allowed, at least partially.

4. Are the size, contours, and colors of the prosthesis approximately the same as those of the sound limb? Are the "joints" similarly placed to the normal limb? The prosthesis should be inspected from the front, back, and side to check this. The patient should be asked if he or she is satisfied with the appearance of the prosthesis.

5. Is the suspension, if present, adequate and fully supporting the prosthesis during weight bearing? Is the suspension adjustable if necessary?[56]

6. Does the patient consider the prosthesis satisfactory? This question will help to ensure that any items that may have been overlooked will be brought to the attention of the clinical team.

Next, the patient is observed seated while wearing the prosthesis. The examiner notes the following:

1. Can the patient sit comfortably with minimal bunching of the soft tissue around the prosthesis?
2. Does the socket remain securely on the stump? Is the patient able to sit comfortably with minimum functioning of the soft tissues around the prosthesis? Are the soft tissues and bony prominences free from excessive pressure? Does the prosthesis remain in good alignment?

The third phase of lower-limb amputee observation is to view the patient walking while wearing the prosthesis. During walking, the examiner should watch for hip or knee instability or abnormal gait. During this phase, the examiner observes the following:

1. Is the patient's performance and walking on a level surface satisfactory? Any gait deviation that requires attention should be noted. Gait deviations include an abducted or adducted gait, lateral trunk bending, circumduction, medial or lateral whip of the prosthesis, foot rotation on heel strike, uneven heel rise, foot slap, uneven step length, and vaulting. In addition, the stump may be oversensitive and/or painful. A very short stump may fail to provide a sufficient lever arm for the pelvis. Finally, an abnormal gait pattern may develop because of a habitual pattern of movement.[24,57] A prosthesis aligned in abduction may cause a wide base gait resulting in this abnormal gait pattern. Amputee balance may be difficult if an adduction contracture is present. An abducted gait is characterized by a very wide base with the prosthesis held away from the midline at all times. If the prosthesis is the cause of the abducted gait, it may be that the prosthesis is too large or that too much abduction may have been built into the prosthesis. A high medial wall may cause the amputee to hold the prosthesis away to avoid pressure on the pubic ramus. The pelvic band may be positioned too far away from the patient's body. This defective gait may also be caused by an abduction contracture or a poor habitual pattern of gait.[24,57]

Lateral bending of the trunk is characterized by excessive bending laterally, generally toward the prosthetic side, from the midline. If the prosthesis is the cause, it may be that it is too short or has an improperly shaped lateral wall that fails to provide adequate support for the femur. A high medial wall may cause the amputee to lean away to minimize the discomfort.

A circumduction gait is a swinging of the prosthesis laterally in a wide arc during the swing phase of gait. This defect may be due to the prosthesis being too long or the prosthesis having too much alignment stability or friction in the knee, making it difficult to bend the knee during the swing-through phase of gait. The amputee may have an abduction contracture of the stump or may lack confidence in flexing the prosthetic knee because of muscle weakness, or the amputee may fear stubbing the toe. Finally, this abnormal gait pattern may be the result of a habitually incorrect gait pattern.[24,57]

Medial or lateral whips are observed best when the patient walks away from the observer. A medial whip is present when the heel travels medially on initial flexion at the beginning of the swing phase, whereas a lateral whip exists with the heel moving laterally. If whipping occurs, then it is the fault of the prosthesis. Lateral whips are commonly seen from excessive medial rotation of the prosthetic knee. A medial whip may result from excessive lateral rotation of the knee. The socket may fit too tightly, thus reflecting stump rotation. Excessive valgus in the prosthetic knee may contribute to this defect. In addition, a badly aligned toe break in the conventional foot may cause twisting at toe-off. Faulty walking habits by the amputee may also result in whips.[24,57]

Rotation of the prosthetic foot on heel strike is due to too much resistance to plantar flexion caused by the plantar flexor bumper or heel wedge.[24,57] If too much toe-out has been built into the prosthesis or if the socket fits too loosely, it may also cause a similar gait fault. If the amputee has poor stump muscle control or extends the stump too vigorously at heel strike, the same gait fault can occur.

If the amputee exhibits uneven arm swing, the altered gait may be due to poor balance, fear or insecurity, or a poor habitual pattern.

A long prosthetic step is seen when the amputee takes a longer step with the prosthesis than with the normal leg. If the prosthesis is at fault, it is usually due to insufficient initial flexion in the socket where a stump flexion contracture is present.[24,57]

Foot slap is a too rapid descent of the anterior portion of the prosthetic foot. It is commonly the result of plantar flexion resistance in the prosthesis being too soft, or the amputee may be driving the prosthesis into the walking surface too forcefully to ensure extension of the knee.[24,57]

Uneven heel rise is characterized by the prosthetic heel rising too much or too rapidly when the knee is flexed at the beginning of the swing phase. If the prosthesis is at fault, the knee joint may have insufficient friction, and there may be an inadequate extension aid. The amputee may also be using more power than necessary to force the knee into flexion.[24,57]

Uneven timing is characterized by steps of unequal duration or length, usually by a very short stance phase on the prosthetic side. An improperly fitting socket may cause pain and a desire to shorten the stance phase on the prosthetic side. A weak extension aid or insufficient friction in the prosthetic knee can cause excessive heel rise and thus result in uneven timing because of a prolonged swing-through. Alignment stability may also be a factor if the knee buckles too easily. In addition, the amputee may have weak muscles in the stump and may not have developed good balance. Fear and insecurity may also contribute to this defect.[24,57]

Terminal swing impact is characterized by rapid forward movement of the shin piece allowing the knee to reach maximum extension with too much force before heel strike. If the prosthesis has insufficient knee friction or the knee extension aid is too strong, this gait fault may be seen. In addition, the amputee may be trying to assure himself or herself that the knee is in full extension by deliberately and forcefully extending the stump.[24,57]

The amputee who feels unstable at the prosthetic knee may develop a feeling of instability that could lead to the danger of falling. In this case the prosthetic knee joint may be too far ahead of the thigh, knee, ankle (TKA) line and insufficient initial flexion may have been built into the socket. Plantar flexion resistance may also be too great, causing the knee to buckle at heel strike. Failure to limit dorsiflexion can lead to incomplete knee control. In addition, the amputee may have weak hip extensor muscles or a severe hip flexion contracture leading to instability.[24,57]

Drop-off at the end of stance phase is characterized by a downward movement of the trunk as the body moves forward over the prosthesis. The prosthesis is at fault if there is inadequate limitation of dorsiflexion of the prosthetic foot. The keel of a solid ankle cushion heel (SACH)-type foot may be too short, or the toe break of the conventional foot may be too far posterior. The socket may have been placed too far anterior in relation to the foot.[24,57]

Excessive trunk extension during the stance phase in which the amputee creates an active lumbar lordosis may also be seen in some amputees. If the prosthesis is at fault, it may be due to an improperly shaped posterior wall causing forward rotation of the pelvis to avoid full weight bearing on the ischium. It may also be due to insufficient initial flexion being built into the socket. In addition, the amputee may demonstrate hip flexor tightness or weakness of the hip extensors and may be attempting to substitute with the lumbar erector spinae muscles. Weak abdominal muscles contribute to this defect. The deviation may be due to a habitual pattern with the patient moving his or her shoulders backward in an effort to obtain better balance.[24,57]

Vaulting is characterized by rising on the toe of the normal foot to permit the amputee to swing the prosthesis through with little or no knee flexion. If the prosthesis is the cause, it may be too long or there may be inadequate socket suspension. Excessive alignment stability or some limitation of knee flexion, such as a knee lock or strong extension aid, may lead to altered gait. Vaulting is a fairly frequent habitual pattern that amputees develop. The amputee may also have fear of stubbing the toe, which could lead to this abnormal gait, or there may be some stump discomfort.[24,57]

The reader is referred to Lusardi et al.[57] and Engerstrom and Van de Ven[24] for further information on prosthetic gait. Normally, gait deviations observed in BK amputees are fewer and less noticeable than in AK amputees.

2. Is the patient able to go up and down inclines and stairs satisfactorily? Is the patient able to kneel, bend down, and get up from kneeling?
3. Are the socket and suspension systems comfortable?
4. Does the prosthesis function quietly? Any noises coming from the prosthesis should be noted and the source

of the noise determined. Occasionally, hissing may be heard as air enters and escapes from the socket as the amputee walks. This is associated with the piston action caused by inadequate suspension and poor socket fit or poor congruence between the socket and liner.[35,56]

After checking the gait while wearing the prosthesis, the prosthesis should be removed to check the patient's stump for tissue stress from the gait activity. At this stage, the examiner observes the following:

1. Does the patient's stump appear to be free of abrasions, discolorations, or excessive perspiration when the prosthesis is removed? Pressure discolorations and redness because of the prosthesis should normally disappear within 10 to 15 minutes. If they persist, then the causes of the irritation or pressure should be determined.
2. Is weight bearing distributed over the proper areas of the stump? For example, for a BK amputation, the patellar tendon, the medial-tibial flare, lateral distal, and posteroproximal aspects of the stump should bear weight. An indication of the weight-bearing area sometimes may be obtained by noting the imprint of the stump sock on the skin of the stump. To determine the concentration and location of the distal pressure, it may be desirable to insert a piece of modeling clay in the bottom of the socket. Flattening of the clay will indicate distal contact.

Examination

Before the examination, the examiner should read the operative report to determine which muscles have been cut or how they have been stabilized along with the amputation since this gives the examiner some idea of the muscles available to move the limb and prosthesis and to provide stability during functional movement.

Measurements Related to Amputation

The examiner should note the length and circumference of the stump as well as scar length. The girth of the residual limb should be measured at various distances from stable bony landmarks. Although there is no standard list of landmark locations, convenient sites are the acromion and medial humeral epicondyle for the transhumeral and transradial residual limbs, respectively; and, the greater trochanter and medial tibial plateau for transfemoral and transtibial residual limbs, respectively. Girth should also be measured over time, and final prosthetic fitting should be delayed until edema has resolved and atrophy has peaked, so that limb volume is stable and prosthetic fit will remain good.[58] Methods of measuring for prosthesis fitting are shown in the accompanying forms (Figs. 16.7 and 16.8). Other measurements include the following:

1. Amputation type: short (10% to 33% of sound side length); medium (34% to 67% of sound side length); long (68% to 100% of sound side length)
2. Ulcer measurements (if present), their location and description

UPPER-EXTREMITY PROSTHETIC MEASUREMENTS

Name of Patient_____Phone_____Date_____

Address_____City_____State/Zip_____

Male ☐   Female ☐   Date of Birth_____Height_____Weight_____

Type of Prosthesis_____Right_____Left_____

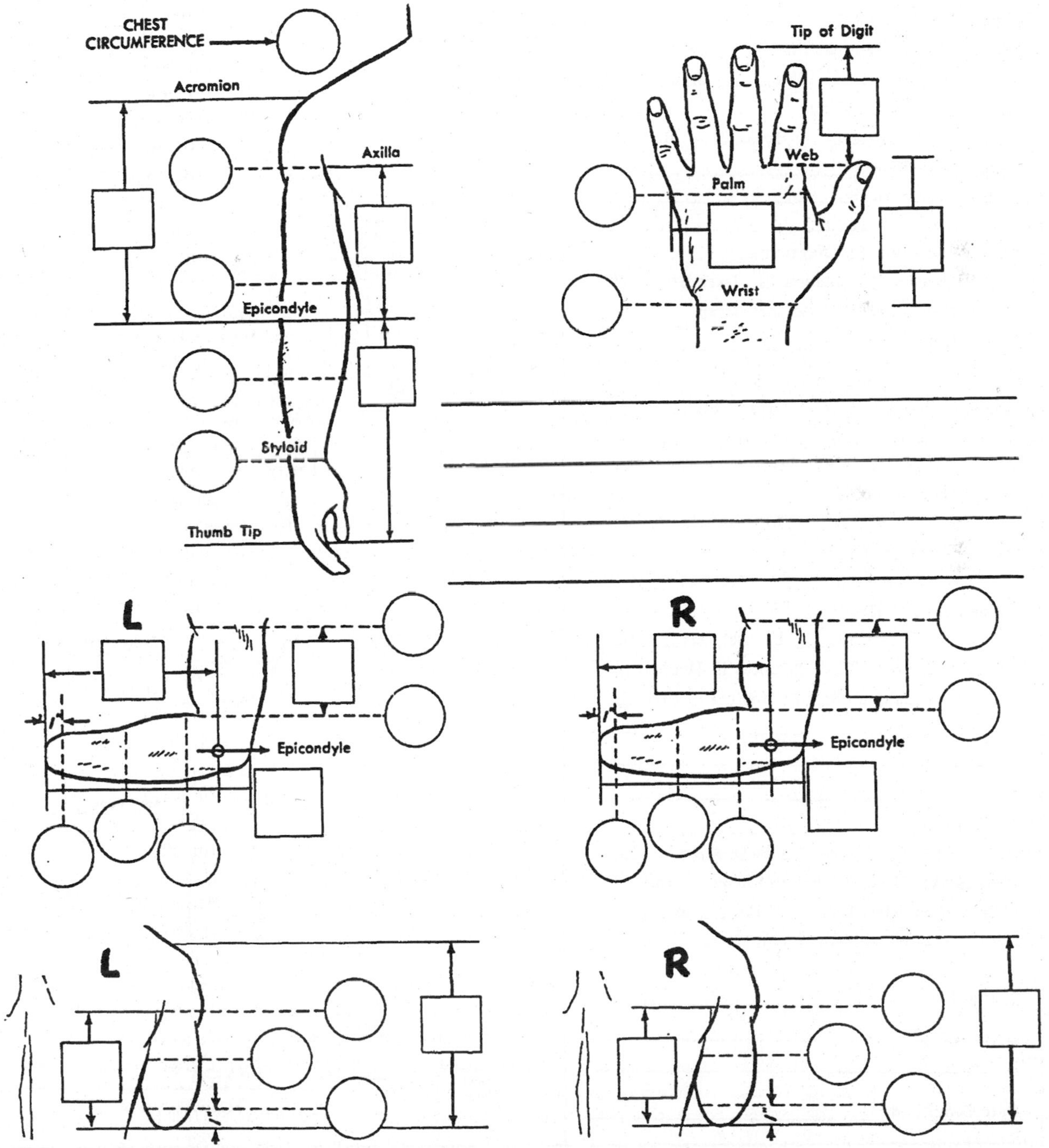

Fig. 16.7 Upper-extremity prosthetic measurements. (Permission granted by the American Orthotic and Prosthetic Association, Alexandria, VA.)

LOWER-EXTREMITY PROSTHETIC MEASUREMENTS

Name of Patient _____ Phone _____ Date _____

Address _____ City _____ State _____

Age _____ Height _____ Weight _____

Type Prosthesis _____ Right _____ Left _____

Shoe Furnished: One ☐ Both ☐ None ☐

Shoe Lace Opening: Top ☐ Bottom ☐

Extra Light-Weight Limb: ☐

Extra Strong Limb: ☐

KB or BK Knee Joints: Size _____ Style _____

Angle Joint: Size _____ Style _____

KB or BK Thigh Lacing:

　　　Eyelets ☐ Hooks ☐ Both ☐

Thigh Lacer Height:_____

Shoulder Loop Size: _____

Waist Belt Size: _____

Color: Caucasian ☐ Negroid ☐

　Light Brown ☐ Medium ☐ Dark Brown ☐

Check Strap: Lace ☐ Leather Strap ☐

Measured by: _____

Shop Alterations

Lengthen Thigh ____ In. Shorten Thigh ____ In.

Lengthen Shin ____ In. Shorten Shin ____ In.

KB or BK Lace Opening: Top__ In. Bottom__In.

Set BK Lacer on Joints:

　　　　Higher ____ In. Bottom ____ In.

Outside BK Joint Head:

　　　　Set In ____ In. Set Out ____ In.

Inside BK Joint Head:

　　　　Set In ____ In. Set Out ____ In.

Fit Foot In Shoe: Tight ☐ Loose ☐ Medium ☐

Make Heel Cushion: Soft ☐ Medium ☐ Firm ☐

Special Changes: _____

_____

_____

Fitted By: _____

Finished BK Limb, Knee Center to Floor:__ In.

Finished AK Limb, Ischium to Floor: ____In.

Weight of Finished Limb: ___ lbs. ___ oz.

Finish of Limb: Plastic Laminate ☐

　　　　Rawhide Enamel ☐

Special Features: _____

_____

_____

Date Completed: _____

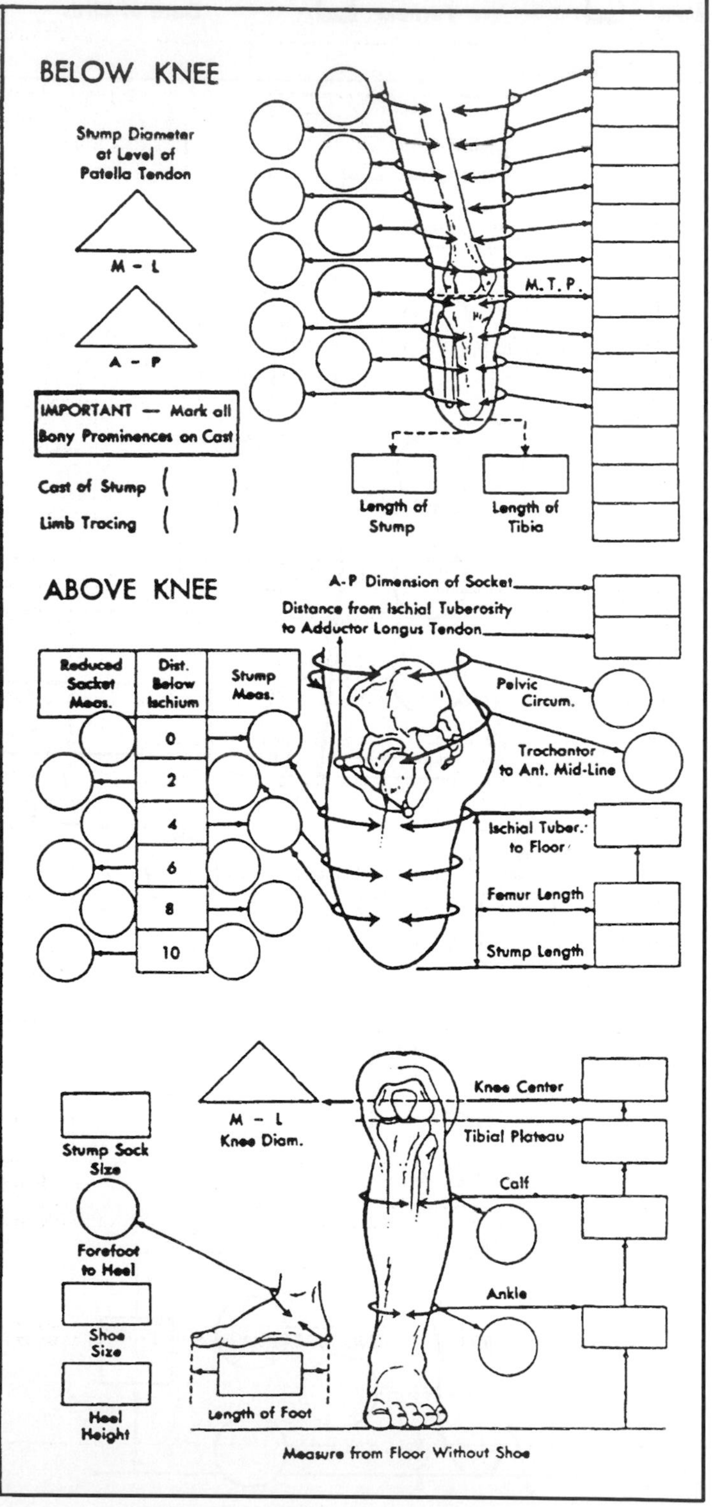

BELOW KNEE

Stump Diameter at Level of Patella Tendon

M – L

A – P

IMPORTANT — Mark all Bony Prominences on Cast

Cast of Stump (　)

Limb Tracing (　)

M.T.P.

Length of Stump　　Length of Tibia

ABOVE KNEE

A-P Dimension of Socket_____

Distance from Ischial Tuberosity to Adductor Longus Tendon_____

Reduced Socket Meas.	Dist. Below Ischium	Stump Meas.
	0	
	2	
	4	
	6	
	8	
	10	

Pelvic Circum.

Trochantor to Ant. Mid-Line

Ischial Tuber. to Floor

Femur Length

Stump Length

M – L Knee Diam.

Stump Sock Size

Forefoot to Heel

Shoe Size

Heel Height

Length of Foot

Knee Center

Tibial Plateau

Calf

Ankle

Measure from Floor Without Shoe

A

Fig. 16.8 (A) Lower-extremity prosthetic measurements. (Medial tibial plateau *[MTP]*, the anatomic landmark of reference for establishing prosthetic build height and for starting circumferential measurements on the transtibial amputated residual limb.)

LOWER-EXTREMITY PROSTHETIC INFORMATION

Name of Patient _____

Site of Amputation _____ Right _____ Left _____

Clinic _____ Physician _____

(Show Location of Stump Details, Identify with Code Letters)

| BELOW KNEE | | ABOVE KNEE |

A = abrasion
B = boil or skin infection
Bu = bursa
Bs = bone spur
D = discoloration
E = edema
I = irritation
M = muscle bunching
P = pressure point
R = redundant tissue
S = scar
T = trigger point

Anterior   Posterior   Medial   Lateral

Anterior   Posterior   Medial   Lateral

BELOW-KNEE STUMP CHARACTERISTICS

Stump Shape: _____ Distal Padding: _____

Subcutaneous Tissue: Heavy ☐ Light ☐

Distal Pressure Tolerance: None ☐ Slight ☐ Good ☐

Condition of Thigh Musculature: Atrophy ☐ Normal ☐

Condition of Stump Musculature: Atrophy ☐ Normal ☐

Knee Stability: _____

Range of Knee Motion: _____

Degrees of Knee Contracture: _____

Condition of Cut Bones: Tibia _____ Fibula _____

Remarks: _____

_____

_____

_____

ABOVE-KNEE STUMP CHARACTERISTICS

Stump Musculature	Soft	Average	Hard
General _____			
Hamstring Group _____			
Gluteal Group _____			
Rectus Femorus _____			
Adductor Longus _____			

Subcutaneous Tissue: Heavy ☐ Light ☐

Ischium: Toughened ☐ Pressure Sensitive ☐

⠀⠀⠀⠀Muscle Padding _____ Prominent _____

Previous Ischial Bearing: Yes ☐ No ☐

Stump Lateral Convex   Concave
⠀⠀Contour: Out ☐   Flat ☐   In ☐
Degree of Contracture: Hip Flexion _____°
⠀⠀⠀⠀⠀⠀⠀⠀⠀⠀Abduction _____°

Stump Adduction _____° Remarks: _____

Prescription for Prosthesis

3 Foot Comp. Model	5 Knee Comp. Model	Socket Materials	Type of Symes	6 Hip-Joint Model Type
4 Ankle Comp. Model	Type of Socket	Shank Materials	Hip Disartic. Type	Type of Suspension

B

Fig. 16.8, cont'd (B) Lower-extremity prosthetic information. (Permission granted by the American Orthotic and Prosthetic Association, Alexandria, VA.)

Active Movements

When assessing the amputee, the examiner must determine the ability (strength and endurance) of the muscles to move the remaining joints in the remaining stump and the range of active motion available in those joints. Ideally, ROM at the remaining joints should be close to normal but may be affected by contractures or scarring. This is especially true for the hip and knee in lower-limb amputees. The ROM available helps to determine the patient's ability to move and control the prosthesis, as well as whether the muscles are able to control the available ROM and provide stability when the patient is in the prosthesis. In addition, the strength, endurance, and ROM of the opposite good limb must be assessed because greater stress will be placed on this limb, especially in the lower-limb amputee. In the case of an upper-limb amputee, if it has been the dominant limb that has experienced the amputation, the other limb will become the dominant limb of necessity, and new skills will have to be learned by that limb. In either case a thorough assessment of the functional status of the remaining whole limb will be necessary, in addition to the examination of the amputated limb. The active movements performed would be the same as those listed for the individual joints in other chapters in this book.

Passive Movements

Passive movements of the amputated limb and remaining normal limb are necessary to ensure the necessary ROM is available and to prevent contractures or to restore ROM after contractures occur. For example, BK amputees are prone to hip flexion and knee flexion contractures, especially if the amputee spends long periods sitting in bed or in a wheelchair. The passive movements performed would be the same as those listed for the individual joints in other chapters in this book. Passive movements give the examiner an understanding of the end feel present so that if contractures occur, proper stretching treatment can be instituted. If laxity or instability is present, the patient can be instructed in proper stabilization exercises.

Resisted Isometric Movements

Resisted isometric movements should be performed on the muscles of the amputated limb as well as the remaining normal limb to ensure the patient has the strength and endurance (or exercise tolerance) that will enable the patient to use a prosthesis.[59] Resisted movements of all muscles of the remaining joints on both the amputated limb and the remaining limb must be tested. These resisted movements would be the same as those listed for the individual joints in other chapters in this book. In lower-limb amputations, the muscles of the hip and knee are especially important to check. Gluteus maximus and medius strength and power correlate with amputee preferred walking speeds. These muscles should be assessed in those with lower-limb amputations and should be considered as a determinant for achievement of functional walking speeds.[60] In the upper limb, the muscles of the shoulder, which play a significant role in positioning the prosthesis, must be assessed. Such testing enables the examiner to develop an exercise program to ensure maximum functionality of the patient.

Functional Assessment

For the amputee, functional assessment, for example, the **Rivermead Mobility Index (RMI)**,[61] takes primary importance, so the examiner must determine the amputee's level of function and independence both with and without a prosthesis. This assessment may involve the care of the remaining stump, the ability to put on and take off the prosthetic device, and determining the patient's anticipated level of activity and whether this activity level can be realistically met given the patient's handicap. Other functional assessment tools include the **Amputee Mobility Predictor**[3,62] (eTool 16.2), **PEQ**,[3,45,63] and the **Prosthetic Profile of the Amputee Questionnaire.**[3,64]

For the lower-limb amputee, the examiner should determine the following:

1. The patient's gait and endurance when walking and whether external support (walker, crutches, cane) is necessary. Tests such as the 6- and 10-minute walk test, timed "up and go" test (TUG test), L-test for functional mobility, the modified Emory Functional Ambulation Profile, and the Amputee Mobility Predictor are outcomes that have been found to be both reliable and valid for amputees.[65]
2. The patient's bed mobility. That is, can the patient move easily in bed, or does he or she require assistance? Can the patient roll over, move from supine to sitting, or lie prone?
3. The patient's ability to transfer from sitting to standing and from bed to wheelchair.
4. The patient's ability to balance in sitting and standing (e.g., the Activities-Specific Balance Confidence Scale[65]).
5. The patient's ability to get up from and down to different types of chairs.
6. The patient's ability to use aids (e.g., walker, crutches, or cane) for gait training. Can the patient manage a wheelchair?
7. The patient's ability to go up and down stairs and ramps and ability to move in confined spaces.
8. The patient's ability to get up from and down to the floor, as well as his or her ability to kneel, pick objects up from the floor, and do similar activities.
9. Is the patient getting enough walking in per day? People with lower limb amputations on average achieve approximately one-third of the recommended steps per day which may contribute to severe disability. Miller et al. found that the average step count for patients in their study was 1450 steps per day, which reflected the lowest category of sedentary behavior.[66] Clinicians must find ways to motivate patients with a lower limb amputation to continue to function and walk daily as much as possible.

10. Strength and ROM measurements should be taken for hip flexion, extension, abduction, adduction, and knee flexion and extension following lower limb amputation. Hip medial and lateral rotation are difficult to measure due to lack of the distal portion of the leg. Hip rotation ROM is rarely required with this population.

For the upper-limb amputee, the examiner should determine the following:

1. Whether the amputated part is from the dominant or nondominant limb
2. The patient's ability to perform functions of ADLs and instrumental activities of daily living (IADLs) (see eTable 1.1)

Sensation Testing

The sensitivity of the stump must be tested to ensure normal sensation. Commonly, hypersensitive areas may be present that have to be desensitized. At the opposite extreme, some areas may have no sensation and require protection. In any case, sensation testing of the stump should involve, at a minimum, hot and cold sensation and light touch.

Psychological Testing

If necessary, psychological testing may be performed.[4,67] Some people have little difficulty adapting to the idea of losing a limb, whereas others have great difficulty accepting the fact that they have lost a limb. This acceptance may be related to how the patient lost the limb (trauma [suddenly] or from long-term problems, such as peripheral vascular disease), how active and independent the patient was before the amputation, or the patient's age (in general, children adapt much better to amputation and a prosthesis than adults). Sometimes, a psychological screening test, such as the Minnesota Multiphasic Personality Inventory (MMPI), may be used to determine the presence of depression, situational anxiety, and possible hysterical reaction to limb loss.[54] Research has shown that there is a significant need to improve psychological screening and early treatment of anxiety symptoms before amputation surgery, as well as screening for depression and traumatic stress symptoms following lower limb amputation. Social support is recommended to promote adjustment to the amputation.[68]

Palpation

The examiner must take time during the examination to palpate the remaining stump of the limb. When palpating, the examiner is looking for normal mobility of the remaining tissues or any tissues that are adherent that may be amenable to treatment, any tissue tenderness, state of the overlying skin, tissue tension and texture, and any differences in tissue thickness, especially in "wear areas" where pressure is applied by the prosthesis. The uninvolved side should also be palpated for comparison.

Diagnostic Imaging

Although diagnostic imaging is not commonly a prerequisite for amputation surgery, especially in trauma cases, it may be used to evaluate the amputated stump. In this case the examiner would be looking for the following:

1. The level of amputation to determine whether end weight bearing is possible; for example, a joint disarticulation is more likely to allow end weight bearing.
2. The presence of deformity, bony spurs, or loose fragments.
3. The size and shape, especially of the end bone of the amputation.

PRÉCIS OF THE AMPUTEE ASSESSMENT[a]

History
Observation (with and without prosthesis on)
 Standing (front, side, behind)
 Sitting (front, side, behind)
 Walking (front, side, behind) (watch for gait faults in lower-limb amputees)
 Stump examination
 Prosthesis examination
Examination
 Stump measurements
 Active movements
 Passive movements
 Resisted isometric movements
 Functional assessment
 Sensation testing
 Psychological testing
 Palpation
 Diagnostic imaging

[a]As with any assessment, the patient must be warned that there may be some discomfort after the examination and that this discomfort is normal. Discomfort after any assessment should decrease within 24 hours.

References

1. Owings MF, Kozak LJ. Ambulatory and inpatient procedures in the United States, 1996. *Vital Health Stat.* 1998;13(139):1–119.
2. Ziegler-Graham K, MacKenzie EJ, Ephraim PL. Estimating the prevalence of limb loss in the United States: 2005-2050. *Arch Phys Med Rehabil.* 2008;89:422–429.
3. Earle J, Benyaich A, Lowe T et al. *Assessment of the amputee.* Accessed August 19, 2019 at www.physiopedia.com /Assessment_of_the_amputee.
4. Beasley RW. General considerations in managing upper limb amputations. *Orthop Clin North Am.* 1981;12:743–749.
5. Beasley RW. Surgery of hand and finger amputations. *Orthop Clin North Am.* 1981;12:763–803.
6. Zhong-Wei C, Meyer VE, Kleinert HE, et al. Present indications and contraindications for replantation as reflected by long-term functional results. *Orthop Clin North Am.* 1981;12:849–870.
7. Jaeger SH, Tsai TM, Kleinert HE. Upper extremity replantation in children. *Orthop Clin North Am.* 1981;12:897–907.
8. Burton RI. Problems in the evaluation of results from replantation surgery. *Orthop Clin North Am.* 1981;12:909–913.
9. Carceller A, Javierre C, Rios M, Viscor G. Amputation risk factors in severely frostbitten patients. *Int J Environ Res Public Health.* 2019;16(8):1351.
10. Slauterback JR, Britton C, Moneim MS, et al. Mangled extremity severity score: an accurate guide to treatment of the severely injured upper extremity. *J Orthop Trauma.* 1994;8:282–285.
11. O'Toole DM, Goldberg RT, Ryan B. Functional changes in vascular amputee patients: evaluation by Barthel Index, PUSLES Profile and ESCROW Scale. *Arch Phys Med Rehabil.* 1985;66:508–511.
12. Spence VA, McCollum PT, Walker WF, et al. Assessment of tissue viability in relation to the selection of amputation level. *Prosthet Orthot Int.* 1984;8:67–75.
13. McCollum PT, Spence VA, Walker WF. Amputation for peripheral vascular disease: the case for level selection. *Br J Surg.* 1988;75:1193–1195.
14. Johansen K, Daines M, Howey T, et al. Objective criteria accurately predict amputation following lower extremity trauma. *J Trauma.* 1990;30:568–573.
15. Gregory RT, Gould RJ, Peclet M, et al. The mangled extremity syndrome (M.E.S.): a severity grading system for multisystem injury of the extremity. *J Trauma.* 1985;25:1147–1150.
16. Lange RH, Bach AW, Hansen ST, et al. Open tibial fractures with associated vascular injuries: prognosis for limb salvage. *J Trauma.* 1985;25:203–208.
17. Howe HR, Poole GV, Hansen KJ, et al. Salvage of lower extremities following combined orthopedic and vascular trauma—a predictive salvage index. *Am Surg.* 1987;53:205–208.
18. Fairs SL, Ham RO, Conway BA, et al. Limb perfusion in the lower limb amputee—a comparative study using a laser Doppler flowmeter and a transcutaneous oxygen electrode. *Prosthet Orthot Int.* 1987;11:80–84.
19. McCollum PT, Spence VA, Walker WF. Circumferential skin blood flow measurements in the ischemic limb. *Br J Surg.* 1985;72:310–312.
20. Helfet DL, Howey T, Sanders R, et al. Limb salvage versus amputation—preliminary results of the mangled extremity severity score. *Clin Orthop Relat Res.* 1990;256:80–86.
21. Johansen K, Daines M, Howey T, et al. Objective criteria accurately predict amputation following lower extremity trauma. *J Trauma.* 1990;30:568–573.

22. Bonanni F, Rhodes M, Lucke JF. The futility of predictive scoring of mangled lower extremities. *J Trauma.* 1993;34:99–104.
23. Gottschalk F. Transfemoral amputation—biomechanics and surgery. *Clin Orthop Relat Res.* 1999;361:15–22.
24. Engerstrom B, Van de Ven C. *Therapy for Amputee.* Edinburgh: Churchill Livingstone; 1999.
25. Lind J, Kramhoft M, Bodtker S. The influence of smoking on complications after primary amputation of the lower extremity. *Clin Orthop Relat Res.* 1991;267:211–217.
26. Fitzpatrick MC. The psychologic assessment and psychosocial recovery of the patient with an amputation. *Clin Orthop Relat Res.* 1999;361:98–107.
27. Baumgartner RF. The surgery of arm and forearm amputations. *Orthop Clin North Am.* 1981;12:805–817.
28. Pandian G, Kowalske K. Daily functioning of patients with an amputated lower extremity. *Clin Orthop Relat Res.* 1999;361:91–97.
29. Aitken GT, Frantz CH. The child amputee. *Clin Orthop Relat Res.* 1980;148:3–8.
30. Lamb DW, Scott H. Management of congenital and acquired amputation in children. *Orthop Clin North Am.* 1981;12:977–994.
31. Otsuka T, Arai M, Sugimura K, et al. Pre-operative sepsis is a predictive factor for 30-day mortality after major lower limb amputation among patients with arteriosclerosis obliterans and diabetes. *J Orthop Sci.* 2019. https://doi.org/10.1016/j.jos.2019.05.017.
32. Kay HW, Newman JD. Relative incidence of new amputations. *Orthotics and Prosthetics.* 1975;29:3–16.
33. Swanson AB, de Groot Swanson G, Goran-Hagert C. Evaluation of hand function. In: Hunter JM, Schneider LH, Mackin EJ, et al., eds. *Rehabilitation of the hand.* St Louis: Mosby; 1990.
34. Smith DG, Fergason JR. Transtibial amputations. *Clin Orthop Relat Res.* 1999;361:108–115.
35. Smith AG. Common problems of lower extremity amputees. *Orthop Clin North Am.* 1982;13:569–578.
36. Beasley RW, de Bese GM. Upper limb amputations and prostheses. *Orthop Clin North Am.* 1986;17:395–405.
37. Postgraduate Medical School—Prosthetics and Orthotics. *Lower limb prosthetics.* New York: New York University Medical Centre; 1988.
38. Journeay WS, Pauley T, Kowgier M, Devlin M. Return to work after occupational and non-occupational lower extremity amputation. *Occup Med.* 2018;68(7):438–443.
39. Bruins M, Geertzen JH, Groothoff JW, et al. Vocational reintegration after a lower limb amputation: a qualitative study. *Prosthet Orthot Int.* 2003;27:4–10.
40. High RM, McDowell DE, Savrin RA. A critical review of amputation in vascular patients. *J Vasc Surg.* 1984;1:653–655.
41. Helm P, Engel T, Holm A, et al. Function after lower limb amputation. *Acta Orthop Scand.* 1986;57:154–157.
42. Davie-Smith F, Paul L, Stuart W, et al. The influence of socioeconomic deprivation on mobility, participation, and quality of life following major lower extremity amputation in the west of Scotland. *Eur J Vasc Endovas Surg.* 2019;57(4):554–560.
43. Hughes K, Mota L, Nunez M, et al. The effect of income and insurance on the likelihood of major leg amputation. *J Vasc Surg.* 2019;7. https://doi.org/10.1016/j.jvs.2018.11.028.
44. Em S, Karakoc M, Sariyildiz MA, et al. Assessment of sexual function and quality of life in patients with

lower limb amputations. *J Back Musculoskelet Rehabil.* 2019;32(2):277–285.
45. Legro MW, Reiber GD, Smith DG, et al. Prosthetic evaluation questionnaire for persons with lower limb amputations: assessing prosthesis-related quality of life. *Arch Phys Med Rehabil.* 1998;79:931–938.
46. Bragaru M, Kekker R, Geertzen JH, Dijkstra PU. Amputees and sports: a systematic review. *Sports Med.* 2011;41(9):721–740.
47. Chin T, Sawamura S, Fujita H, et al. Physical fitness of lower limb amputees. *Am J Phys Med Rehabil.* 2001;81(5):321–325.
48. Davidoff GN, Lampman RM, Westbury L, et al. Exercise testing and training of persons with dysvascular amputation: safety and efficacy of arm ergometry. *Arch Phys Med Rehabil.* 1992;73(4):334–338.
49. Dekker R, Hristova YV, Hijmans JM, Geertzen JH. Pre-operative rehabilitation for dysvascular lower-limb amputee patients: a focus group study involving medical professionals. *PLos One.* 2018;13(10):e0204726. https://doi.org/10.1371/jouirnal.pone.0204726.
50. Davis RW. Phantom sensation, phantom pain and stump pain. *Arch Phys Med Rehabil.* 1993;74:79–91.
51. Jensen TS, Krebs B, Nielsen J, et al. Phantom limb, phantom pain and stump pain in amputees during the first six months following limb amputation. *Pain.* 1983;17:243–256.
52. Omer GE. Nerve, neuroma, and pain problems related to upper limb amputations. *Orthop Clin North Am.* 1981;12:751–762.
53. Kaur A, Guan Y. Phantom limb pain: a literature review. *Chin J Traumatol.* 2018;21(6):366–368.
54. Sherman RA. Stump and phantom limb pain. *Neurol Clin.* 1989;7:249–264.
55. Smith DG, Ehde DM, Legro MW, et al. Phantom limb, residual limb and back pain after lower extremity amputations. *Clin Orthop Relat Res.* 1999;361:29–38.
56. Kapp S. Suspension systems for prostheses. *Clin Orthop Relat Res.* 1999;361:55–62.
57. Lusardi MM, Berke GM, Psonak R. Prosthetic gait. *Orthop Phys Ther Clin North Am.* 2001;10:77–116.
58. Edelstein JE. Amputations and prostheses. In: Cameron MH, Monroe LG, eds. *Physical Rehabilitation: Evidence-Based Examination, Evaluation, and Intervention.* St. Louis: Saunders; 2007.
59. Cruts HE, de Vries J, Zilvold G, et al. Lower extremity amputees with peripheral vascular disease: graded exercise testing and results of prosthetic training. *Arch Phys Med Rehabil.* 1987;68:14–19.
60. Crozara LF, Marques NR, LaRoche DP, et al. Hip extension power and abduction power asymmetry as independent predictors of walking speed in individuals with unilateral lower-limb amputation. *Gait Posture.* 2019;70:282–288.
61. Franchignoni F, Brunelli S, Orlandini D, et al. Is the Rivermead Mobility Index a suitable outcome measure in lower limb amputees? A psychometric validation study. *J Rehabil Med.* 2001;35:141–144.
62. Gailey RS, Roach KE, Applegate EB, et al. The Amputee Mobility Predictor: an instrument to assess determinants of the lower-limb amputee's ability to ambulate. *Arch Phys Med Rehabil.* 2002;83(5):613–627.
63. Boone DA, Coleman KL. Use of the Prosthesis Evaluation Questionnaire (PEQ). *J Prosth Orthotics.* 2006;18(6):P68–P79.
64. Gauthier-Gagnon C, Grise M-C. Prosthetic profile of the amputee questionnaire: validity and reliability. *Arch Phys Med Rehabil.* 1994;76(12):1309–1314.

65. Stevens P, Fross N, Kapp S. Clinically relevant outcome measures in orthotics and prosthetics. Advancing orthotic and prosthetic care through knowledge. *Am Acad Orthotists Prosthetists*. 2009;5(1):1–14.

66. Miller MJ, Cook PF, Kline PW, et al. Physical function and pre-amputation characteristics explain daily step count after dysvascular amputation. *PM R*. 2019. https://doi.org/10.1002/pmrj.121221.

67. Pinzux MS, Graham G, Osterman H. Psychologic testing in amputation rehabilitation. *Clin Orthop Relat Res*. 1988;229:236–240.

68. Pedras S, Vilhena E, Carbalho R, Pereira MG. Psychosocial adjustment to a lower limb amputation ten months after surgery. *Rehabil Psychol*. 2018;63(3):418–430.

CHAPTER 17

Primary Care Assessment

Primary care, its definition, and the roles of various health professionals in the delivery of services have been evolving over the past 30 years.[1] A definition of primary care was established by the World Health Organization in 1978 through work at the International Conference on Primary Health Care.[2] Although it would be ideal for a family physician who is familiar with the patient's and the family's history to perform a primary care assessment because he or she would more likely be aware of any congenital or developmental problems, the patient's immunization status, and any recent injuries or illnesses and therefore could provide continuity of care,[3–5] many people today do not have a family physician. As changes in health care occur, more and more health care professionals are becoming involved in the assessment of patients who come to them as first-level providers of medical care. This may involve nurse practitioners, physician assistants, and other health care providers as well as physicians in primary care facilities, physical therapists with direct access in private practice, clinicians in sole-charge facilities, and sports therapists working and traveling with teams.[6–10] This is not a totally new concept. The use of physical therapists in the screening and management of patients with musculoskeletal disorders in the primary care setting is widespread in other countries with universal health care systems and within the US Military and Department of Veterans Affairs health systems.[7,11–18] Thus it becomes important for clinicians to be able to evaluate and recognize the potential for health care problems, including systemic disease as a disease entity itself or a disease masquerading as neuromuscular dysfunction that must be referred to the appropriate health professional.[19,20] Primary care assessment is a form of triage in which the clinician decides whether the patient's problem or problems fall within his or her scope of practice or should be referred to other health care professionals.[21–25]

The role of the physical therapist in the primary care environment has been evolving rapidly; physical therapists with specific expertise related to the management of patients with neuromuscular conditions are well positioned for this role. This is especially true given the prevalence of neuromuscular conditions, especially in the United States, where the number of primary care visits for neuromuscular conditions runs between 20% to 30%.[26–31]

In many ways, a primary care assessment is similar to a preparticipation examination in sports, because both assessments are used to clear patients of having certain problems that could affect activity and also to provide a mechanism whereby problems can be referred to the appropriate health care professional.[32–39] This process requires an understanding of disease as well as the ability to distinguish which system may be affected; it involves taking a detailed history, observing and examining the patient, and understanding the patient's level of reporting ability.[19,40] It also requires the clinician to understand his or her limitations, the scope of practice of his or her chosen profession, and why the patient has come to see the clinician. For example, what is the patient's complaint? Is it related to how the patient feels? Is it related to his or her occupation? Is it related to a certain population, age, or gender?[34,41,42]

If the patient has symptoms, several questions should be asked that relate to the symptoms[43]:
1. Where is the symptom, and does it radiate?
2. What does the symptom feel like?
3. How severe is the symptom?
4. Where does (did) the symptom start?
5. How often does the symptom occur?
6. What brings the symptom on?
7. How long does the symptom last each time?
8. What makes the symptom better or worse?
9. Are other symptoms associated with it?

Once these questions, and those discussed under the different systems as outlined later in the chapter, are answered, the examiner can decide to treat the patient or refer him or her to another health care professional, usually a physician. Goodman and Snyder[44] clearly outline cases in which referral to a physician is necessary (Table 17.1). This chapter is not meant to be all inclusive of conditions and systems that may need referral. Complete systems assessment is discussed in other sources.[43,44]

McKeag[45] has outlined five specific populations in which special areas of possible concern should be included in an examination. In the prepubescent patient (6 to 10 years of age), assessments should include examination for congenital abnormalities that may not have been diagnosed previously. In the pubescent patient (11 to 15 years of age), the examination should include an evaluation of physical maturity and good health practices. The

TABLE **17.1**

Referral to Physician

Immediate Medical Attention	Patient with anginal pain not relieved in 20 minutes
	Patient with angina who has nausea, vomiting, profuse sweating
	Diabetic patient demonstrating signs of confusion, lethargy, or changes in mental alertness and function
	Patient with bowel/bladder incontinence and/or saddle anesthesia secondary to cauda equine lesion
	Patient in anaphylactic shock
Medical Attention Necessary	***General Systemic***
	Unknown cause
	Lack of significant objective neuromusculoskeletal signs and symptoms
	Lack of expected progress with physical therapy treatment
	Development of constitutional symptoms or associated signs and symptoms over the course of treatment
	Discovery of significant PMH unknown to physician
	Changes in health status that persist 7–10 days beyond expected time period
	Patient who is jaundiced and has not been diagnosed or treated
	Changes in size, shape, tenderness, and consistency of lymph nodes in more than one area, which persist more than 4 weeks; painless, enlarged lymph nodes
	For Women
	Low back, hip, pelvic, groin, or sacroiliac symptoms without known etiology and in the presence of constitutional symptoms
	Symptoms correlated with menses
	Any spontaneous uterine bleeding after menopause
	For pregnant women: Vaginal bleeding, elevated blood pressure, increased Braxton-Hicks contractions during exercise
	Vital Signs (Report These Findings)
	Persistent rise or fall of blood pressure
	Blood pressure evaluation in any woman taking birth control pills (should be closely monitored by her physician)
	Pulse amplitude that fades with inspiration and strengthens with expiration
	Pulse increase over 20 BPM lasting more than 3 minutes after rest or changing position
	Difference between systolic and diastolic measurements of more than 4 mm Hg in pulse pressure
	Persistent low-grade (or higher) fever, especially associated with constitutional symptoms, most commonly sweats
	Cardiac
	Angina at rest
	Anginal pain not relieved in 20 minutes
	More than three sublingual nitroglycerin tablets required to gain relief
	Nitroglycerin does not relieve anginal pain
	Rest does not relieve angina
	Angina continues to increase in intensity after stimulus (e.g., cold, stress, exertion) has been eliminated
	Changes in pattern of angina
	Abnormally severe chest pain
	Patient has nausea, vomiting
	Anginal pain radiates to jaw/left arm
	Upper back feels abnormally cool, sweaty, or moist to touch
	Patient has any doubts about his or her condition
	Cancer
	Early warning sign(s) of cancer: seven early warning signs plus two additional signs pertinent to the physical therapy examination: proximal muscle weakness and change in deep tendon reflexes
	All soft-tissue lumps that persist or grow, whether painful or painless
	Any woman presenting with chest, breast, axillary, or shoulder pain of unknown etiology, especially in the presence of a positive medical history (self or family) of cancer
	Bone pain, especially on weight bearing, which persists more than 1 week and is worse at night

Continued

TABLE **17.1**

Referral to Physician—cont'd

	Pulmonary Shoulder pain that is aggravated by supine positioning Shoulder, chest (thorax) pain that subsides with autosplinting (lying on the painful side) For the patient with asthma: signs of asthma or bronchial activity during exercise ***Genitourinary*** Abnormal urinary constituents (e.g., change in color, odor, amount, flow of urine) Any amount of blood in urine ***Musculoskeletal*** Symptoms that seem out of proportion to the injury, or symptoms persisting beyond the expected time for the nature of the injury Severe or chronic back pain accompanied by constitutional symptoms, especially fever
Precautions/ Contraindications to Therapy	Uncontrolled chronic heart failure or pulmonary edema Active myocarditis Resting heart rate >120–130 BPM[a] Resting systolic rate >180–200 BPM[a] Resting diastolic rate >105–110 BPM[a] Moderate dizziness, near-syncope Marked dyspnea Unusual fatigue Unsteadiness Loss of palpable pulse Postoperative posterior calf pain For the patient with diabetes: Chronically unstable blood sugar levels must be stabilized (normal: 80–120 mg/dL; "safe": 100–250 mg/dL)

[a]Unexplained or poorly tolerated by patient.
BPM, Beats per minute; *PMH*, past medical history.
From Goodman CC, Snyder TE: *Differential diagnosis in physical therapy*, Philadelphia, 1995, WB Saunders, pp 18–20.

postpubescent or young adult group (16 to 30 years of age) has the widest variety of skills, levels, and motivation. For this group, the history of previous injuries and any sport- or activity-specific problems is particularly important. For the adult population (30 to 65 years of age), injury prevention (e.g., overuse), previous injury patterns, health concerns, and conditioning should be included in the examination. The final group consists of elderly patients (65 years of age or older), who need an examination based on individual requirements, because many of these people take up exercising or increased physical activity after a medical illness and often have co-morbidities.[36] Age-related changes and their possible consequences are outlined in Table 17.2.

A primary care assessment may vary from a minimal medical examination or physical to rule out possible systemic problems to a very extensive examination involving laboratory tests, stress testing, profiling, x-rays, and other special protocols.[46] History, as well as a physical examination, plays a major role.[47–49] If the patient is going to be asked to engage in a strenuous activity as part of his or her treatment program, various systems (e.g., heart, lungs) must be cleared to ensure that the patient is capable of doing the activity.[50]

Characteristics of Systemic Symptoms

- No known cause or unknown etiology
- Gradual onset with progressive, cyclical course (worse/better/worse)
- Persist beyond expected time for that condition
- Constant
- Intense
- Bilateral symptoms (e.g., edema, nail bed changes, clubbing, numbness or tingling, weakness, skin pigmentation changes, or rash)
- Symptoms are unrelieved by rest or change in position
- If rest or positional change brings relief, even these relieving factors no longer reduce symptoms over time
- Symptoms do not fit the expected mechanical or neuromusculoskeletal pattern; symptoms are out of proportion to the injury
- Symptoms cannot be altered (provoked, reproduced, alleviated, eliminated, aggravated) during examination
- Constitutional symptoms, especially fever and night sweats
- Disproportionate pain relief with aspirin (red flag for bone cancer)
- There is night pain
- Pain is described as knifelike, boring, deep, colicky, aching
- Pattern of pain comes and goes, as with spasms

From Goodman CC, Snyder TE: *Differential diagnosis in physical therapy*, Philadelphia, 1995, WB Saunders, p 16.

TABLE **17.2**

Selected Age-Related Changes and Their Consequences

Organ/System	Age-Related Physiologic Change[a]	Consequence of Age-Related Physiologic Change	Disease, Not Age
General	↑ Body fat	↑ Volume of distribution for fat-soluble drugs	Obesity
	↓ Total body water	↓ Volume of distribution for water-soluble drugs	Anorexia
Eyes/Ears	Presbyopia	↓ Accommodation	Blindness
	Lens opacification	↑ Susceptibility to glare	Deafness
	↓ High-frequency acuity	Difficulty discriminating words if background noise is present	
Endocrine	Impaired glucose tolerance	↑ Glucose level in response to acute illness	Diabetes mellitus
	↓ Thyroxine clearance (and production)	↓ T_4 dose required in hypothyroidism	Thyroid dysfunction
	↑ ADH, ↓ renin, and ↓ aldosterone	–	↓ NA^+, ↑ K^+
	↓ Testosterone	–	Impotence
	↓ Vitamin D absorption and activation	Osteopenia	Osteoporosis Osteomalacia
Respiratory	↓ Lung elasticity and ↑ chest wall stiffness	Ventilation/perfusion mismatch and ↓ PO_2	Dyspnea Hypoxia
Cardiovascular	↓ Arterial compliance and ↑ systolic BP → LVH	Hypotensive response to ↑ HR, volume depletion, or loss of atrial contraction	Syncope
	↓ β adrenergic responsiveness	↓ Cardiac output and HR response to stress	Heart failure
	↓ Baroreceptor sensitivity and ↓ SA node automaticity	Impaired blood pressure response to standing, volume depletion	Heart block
Gastrointestinal	↓ Hepatic function	Delayed metabolism of some drugs	Cirrhosis
	↓ Gastric acidity	↓ Ca^+ absorption on empty stomach	Osteoporosis Vitamin B_{12} deficiency
	↓ Colonic motility	Constipation	Fecal impaction
	↓ Anorectal function	–	Fecal incontinence
Hematologic/ Immune system	↓ Bone marrow reserve (?)	–	Anemia
	↓ T-cell function	False-negative PPD response	–
	↑ Autoantibodies	False-positive rheumatoid factor, antinuclear antibody	Autoimmune disease
Renal	↓ Glomerular filtration rate	Impaired excretion of some drugs	↑ Serum creatinine
	↓ Urine concentration/dilution (see also Endocrine)	Delayed response to salt or fluid restriction or overload; nocturia	↑↓ Na^+
Genitourinary	Vaginal/urethral mucosal atrophy	Dyspareunia	Symptomatic urinary tract infection
	Prostate enlargement	Bacteriuria	Urinary incontinence
		↑ Residual urine volume	Urinary retention
Musculoskeletal	↓ Lean body mass, muscle	–	Functional impairment
	↓ Bone density	Osteopenia	Hip fracture

Continued

TABLE **17.2**

Selected Age-Related Changes and Their Consequences—cont'd

Organ/System	Age-Related Physiologic Change[a]	Consequence of Age-Related Physiologic Change	Disease, Not Age
Nervous system	Brain atrophy	Benign senescent forgetfulness	Dementia
			Delirium
	↓ Brain catechol synthesis	–	Depression
	↓ Brain dopaminergic synthesis	Stiffer gait	Parkinson disease
	↓ Righting reflexes	↑ Body sway	Falls
	↓ Stage 4 sleep	Early wakening, insomnia	Sleep apnea

[a]Changes generally observed in healthy elderly subjects free of symptoms and detectable disease in the organ system studied. The changes are usually important only when the system is stressed or other factors are added (e.g., drugs, disease, or environmental challenge); they rarely result in symptoms otherwise.

The table displays selected changes that occur normally with age and their physiologic consequences. Changes due to disease rather than to age are listed in the last column.

ADH, Antidiuretic hormone; *BP,* blood pressure; *HR,* heart rate; *LVH,* left ventricular hypertrophy; *PPD,* purified protein derivative, *SA,* sinoatrial; *T4,* thyroxine

From Resnick NM: Geriatric medicine. In Isselbacher KJ, et al, editors: *Harrison's principles of internal medicine,* ed 13, New York, 1994, McGraw-Hill.

Objectives of the Evaluation

Primary care evaluations have many useful purposes.[3,19,46,51,52] However, the examiner must remember that the primary purpose of the examination is to determine the patient's health problem and to either treat the patient or refer him or her to the appropriate health care professional.[3,19] As part of the examination, the examiner can establish **baseline values** for the patient. These may be compared with normal "textbook" values or used to determine change in the future. In other words, the assessment should not consist of simple yes/no questions. Instead, it must be thorough enough to establish proper baseline levels.

Objectives of Primary Care Assessment

- Determine if disease is present
- Uncover pre-existing conditions
- Determine unsuspected correctable conditions
- Determine health status
- Prevent injuries
- Avoid misinterpretation of findings
- Establish baseline values
- Act as a screening process
- Foster good health practices
- Develop rapport with the patient
- Establish guidelines
- Develop a musculoskeletal profile
- Counsel the patient
- Classify the patient
- Meet legal and insurance requirements
- Determine if referral is necessary

The primary care assessment is used to determine the patient's health status. It also helps to prevent injuries through identification of any abnormalities, physical inadequacies, or poor conditioning that could put the patient at risk.[53,54] The examination may identify previously unsuspected conditions that are amenable to correction or that preclude participation in the desired activity. Similarly, the evaluation helps to avoid misinterpretation of findings that appear to be new but existed previously. For this reason, a review of previous health records, if possible, is also part of the primary care assessment.

The primary care assessment is also worthwhile to ensure that treatments have been carried out previously and that conditions previously diagnosed have been properly cared for. In this way, it acts as a screening process to ensure that treatment of potentially serious medical and surgical conditions has taken place. It also helps to rule out potentially serious or threatening conditions that may temporarily preclude the patient from participating in work or recreational activities. For example, with infectious mononucleosis, contact sports may be precluded for a time because the patient's spleen would be enlarged and thus more easily injured or ruptured.

The assessment also gives the clinician an opportunity to foster good health practices and promote optimum health and fitness. The assessment enables the health care provider to give proper health guidance and to determine the patient's general state of health.

The assessment also gives the examiner a chance to develop rapport with the patient. The examiner can learn what motivates the patient and, at the same time, help establish the patient's confidence in the health care staff. The examination may also be used to establish guidelines for the patient and health care team on questions of health, safety, and care. In addition, it provides an opportunity to counsel the patient.

Primary Care History

For a primary care assessment, the history plays a predominant role to ensure that questions related to the various systems are asked. A complete history can usually identify 60% to 75% of the problems affecting a patient.[38,46,55] The majority of essential diagnostic information arises from the initial medical history interview.[56–58] A typical visit, including physical examination, ranges from 3 to 74 minutes.[59–61] In the primary care setting, the average consultation times for family physicians, internists, and pediatricians are 13 minutes, 19 minutes, and 13 minutes, respectively.[60] For the young person or the patient with communication problems, both the patient and his or her parent or guardian should provide the history to ensure completeness. The rest of the assessment proceeds from the information determined in the history. The history provides details regarding health problems and injuries and enables the examiner to focus on any abnormalities that it brings out.[46] Generally the history is completed by the patient's answers to questions in a yes/no format (see eAppendix 17.1 for a generic primary care assessment questionnaire). Using such a format decreases the chance of the patient forgetting something.[40] The "yes" answers then are investigated further in other parts of the assessment (eAppendix 17.2). It is important, however, that the "no" answers also be checked for accuracy. Ideally, oral histories, in which the health care professional asks the questions, are more accurate; but usually, because of time constraints, this is not possible. The history should include the patient's medical history as well as the family's medical history to rule out any congenital, hereditary, or injury problems. It is important that a complete health history be obtained because the patient may leave out or hide information that might preclude the patient from taking part in a desired activity or because of possible secondary gain.[55]

Some general questions can be asked initially, and these can be used to cross-reference questions asked in specific areas of assessment[46]:

1. *Have you ever been a patient in a hospital, emergency room, or clinic?*
2. *Have you ever seen a physician for an injury or illness?*
3. *Have you ever had x-rays?*
4. *Have you ever had an operation?*
5. *Are you currently taking any medication or pills?*
6. *Do you have any allergies (to medications, insects, food, or other things)?*
7. *When was your last vaccination? What was the vaccination for?*
8. *Have you ever been unable to work or participate in exercise or sports?*
9. *Have you ever experienced chest pain, dyspnea, or syncope during work, exercise, or activity?*
10. *Have you ever had a seizure?*
11. *Have you ever been told you had high blood pressure?*
12. *Have you ever been told you had high cholesterol?*
13. *Do you have trouble breathing or do you cough during or after activity?*

These general questions cover wide areas, and the specific parts of the assessment should corroborate the answers given to these general questions. In addition, the examiner must consider the effect of psychosocial issues on both the patient and his or her reported symptoms. Haggman et al.[62] believed that two questions were useful to screen for symptoms of depression:

1. *During the past month, have you often been bothered by feeling down, depressed, or hopeless?*
2. *During the past month, have you been bothered by little interest or pleasure in doing things?*

If the answer to both questions is yes, further psychological investigation may be warranted.[63,64] Waddell and Main[64] talked about illness behavior, a normal and reasonable behavior, which is what people do and say to communicate that they are ill. The examiner should always keep in mind the role psychosocial issues may have in anyone seeking primary care help.

The following assessment sections outline questions pertaining to specific body systems that may lead to further examination or testing and possible concerns or issues that must be dealt with if the patient is going to take part in a particular activity. The examiner may want to cover all of the systems or only those that appear to be pertinent to the problem.

Examination

The medical examination must be not only thorough but also applicable to the job, activity, exercise, or sport to which the person hopes to return or take part in. Health care professionals should always be alert for concealment, denial, or invention of problems on the part of the patient.

Parts of Primary Care Examination

- History
- Vital signs
  - Temperature
  - Blood pressure
  - Heart rate
  - Weight
- Head and face examination
- Neurological examination and convulsive disorders
- Musculoskeletal examination
- Cardiovascular examination
- Pulmonary examination
- Urogenital examination
- Gastrointestinal examination
- Dermatological (integumentary) examination
- Examination for heat/cold disorders
- Laboratory tests
- Physical fitness profile
  - Body composition
  - Maturity index
  - Flexibility
  - Strength, endurance, and power
  - Agility, balance, and reaction time
  - Cardiovascular fitness

Vital Signs

The initial part of the examination is performed to establish the patient's baseline physiological parameters and vital signs (see Chapter 1, Table 1.7), including pulse or heart rate, respiratory rate, blood pressure (systolic and diastolic), weight, and temperature (normal: 98.6°F [37°C]). This part of the examination may be performed by any health care professional who has knowledge or an understanding of the techniques and it is part of any primary care examination.[65,66]

Table 1.8 (see Chapter 1) outlines guidelines for blood pressure measurement.[67] High blood pressure values should be checked several times at 15- to 30-minute intervals with the patient resting in between to determine whether a high reading is accurate or is being caused by anxiety ("white coat syndrome") or some similar reason. If three consecutive readings are high, the patient is said to have high blood pressure (hypertension) (see Chapter 1, Table 1.9). If the readings remain high, further investigation may be warranted.[3,67,68] Table 17.3 outlines the risk factors of hypertension.

TABLE **17.3**

Risk Factors of Hypertension

Primary	Secondary
• One or both parent(s) with hypertension • Increased salt intake • Excessive alcohol consumption • Obesity • Race (Black individuals are more commonly affected) • Personality traits (tense, hostile) • Smoking • Diabetes • Physical inactivity • Cholesterol >6.5 mmol/L or low-density lipoprotein cholesterol >4.0 mmol/L	• Renal disease • Oral contraceptives • Cushing syndrome • Sleep apnea syndrome • Endocrine (thyroid, parathyroid conditions) • Coarctation of aorta • Renovascular disease • Adrenal cortex dysfunction

Complications of Hypertension

- Cardiovascular disease
- Heart failure
- Left ventricular hypertrophy
- Stroke
- Intracerebral hemorrhage
- Chronic renal insufficiency
- Renal disease

The following examination sections may be part of the primary care examination, but this will depend on what has been found from taking the history and vital signs. Only those sections that the examiner feels are relevant or are areas of concern would normally be investigated.

General Medical Problems

There are general systemic problems that the examiner must always keep in mind when doing an assessment. Some of the general medical (systemic) questions include the following[23,44,69]:

1. Have you ever been diagnosed with a systemic disease (e.g., diabetes)?
2. Have you ever been diagnosed with a progressive disease (e.g., muscular dystrophy, multiple sclerosis)?
3. Have you ever been told you have cancer?
4. Have you ever had anything similar to what you have now? How often?
5. Where exactly is your pain? What is the quality, frequency, and pattern of the pain?[70] What have you tried to do to alleviate the pain? On a scale of 1 (no pain) to 10 (pain is bad as it could possibly get), how would you rate your pain level?
6. Do you have any other symptoms?
7. Have you ever had any infections? How were they treated?
8. Do you have unexplained fatigue?
9. Have you ever had any unexplained weakness?
10. Do you bruise easily?
11. Is your present weight steady or has it increased or decreased in the last year? Sudden weight loss in a short time for no reason may indicate the presence of a tumor. Obesity may have an adverse effect on the cardiovascular, musculoskeletal, and other body systems.[71]

The presence of systemic disease (e.g., diabetes) does not rule out work or activity, but the examiner must ensure that there is either good control by the use of medication or that the disease will not cause undue risk to the patient or his or her well-being. It must also be determined whether the extent or intensity of the activity the patient has to do poses a significant threat to the patient's physical condition.[72] The examiner must also be concerned about problems such as acute infection and malignancy and progressive diseases such as multiple sclerosis.

Acute illnesses tend to be self-limiting and usually require only that the patient temporarily withdraw from work or activity, often to prevent spread of disease to others.[46] Dehydration is made worse by febrile illness, which could, in certain circumstances, lead to heat disorders.

Adverse Effects of Obesity

- Increases in insulin resistance
  - Glucose intolerance
  - Metabolic syndrome
  - Type 2 diabetes mellitus
- Hypertension
- Dyslipidemia
  - Elevated total cholesterol
  - Elevated triglycerides
  - Elevated LDL cholesterol
  - Elevated non-HDL cholesterol
  - Elevated small, dense LDL particles
  - Decreased HDL cholesterol
  - Decreased apolipoprotein-A1
- Abnormal left ventricular geometry
  - Concentric remodeling
  - Left ventricular hypertrophy
- Endothelial dysfunction
- Increased systemic inflammation and prothrombotic state
- Systolic and diastolic dysfunction
- Heart failure
- Coronary heart disease
- Atrial fibrillation
- Obstructive sleep apnea/sleep-disordered breathing
- Albuminuria
- Osteoarthritis
- Cancers

HDL, High-density lipoprotein; *LDL,* low-density lipoprotein.
From Lavie CJ, Milani RV, Ventura HO: Obesity and cardiovascular disease: risk factor, paradox, and impact of weight loss, *J Am Coll Cardiol* 53(21):1926, 2009.

Head and Face

Eye Examination

Visual acuity is usually examined with the use of a Snellen (or common) eye chart. Peripheral vision and depth perception may also be tested. Questions related to the eye examination include the following[46,73]:

1. Have you had any problems with vision or your eyes?
2. Have you ever injured your eyes?
3. Do you wear glasses, contact lenses, or protective eyewear?
4. Are you color-blind?
5. Do you have a peripheral vision problem?
6. Have you ever used medications for an eye problem?
7. Have you ever had an eye infection?

Any abnormalities found or positive answers may require further examination. Uncorrected vision of less than 20/40 should be checked further.[51] Visual loss of 20/50 means that the patient can read at 20 feet what the average person can read at 50 feet. The health care professional should watch for problems that may preclude work, preclude participation in the chosen activity or sport, or affect the patient's safety. Vision in only one eye results in lack of depth perception, which can be detrimental in certain situations. Patients with sight in only one eye should work at specific jobs or participate in physical activities only

if they have an understanding of the dangers of participating and accept the risks. Such patients should not work or participate in sports for which there is no adequate eye protection.

Examples of Eye Conditions or Signs and Symptoms Requiring Further Examination

- Sudden vision loss
- Visual loss greater than 20/40
- Vision in one eye only
- Severe myopia
- Retinal detachment
- Retinal tear
- Corneal abrasion
- Iritis
- Conjunctivitis
- Proptosis (protrusion) of eye

If the patient wears glasses, the health care professional should ensure that the lenses are made of plastic, polycarbonate, or heat-treated (safety) glass to prevent them from shattering during work or activity.

Myopia, or nearsightedness, should be noted on the chart; such patients are more likely to suffer retinal degeneration, which increases the possibility of retinal detachment. Patients who have had a retinal detachment are sometimes excluded from contact sports or high-exertion jobs. People who have a retinal tear should be allowed to do strenuous activities only if cleared by a physician or specialist, and they should have a qualifying letter allowing them to return to work.

Pupillary size should also be evaluated. In some patients, the pupils are obviously of different sizes (**anisocoria**). This difference should be noted in case the patient has to be evaluated for a head injury at a later date.[74] Assessment of the eyes is discussed in Chapter 2.

Dental Examination

Questions to be asked concerning the patient's dental record include the following[73]:

1. When did you last see a dentist?
2. Have you ever had any problems with your teeth or gums?
3. Have you ever had any teeth knocked out, damaged, or extracted?
4. Do you wear a mouth guard?
5. Do you smoke or chew tobacco?
6. Have you ever had an injury to your face or jaws?

When a patient is being examined for dental problems, which is usually done by a dentist, it is important to determine how many teeth the patient has and the last time he or she saw a dentist.

Ear Examination

Questions to be asked concerning the patient's ear problems include the following:

1. Do you have any problems with hearing?
2. Do you have an earache? (When was the onset? Is it getting worse?)
3. Is the earache associated with a cold, flu, or trauma?
4. Is there a discharge from the ear?

Ear problems are commonly referred to a physician or an ear, nose, and throat (ENT) specialist. Assessment of the ear is discussed in Chapter 2.

Nose Examination

Questions to be asked concerning the patient's nose include the following:

1. What is the problem with your nose?
2. Can you breathe through your nose?
3. Do you have any discharge from your nose (e.g., blood, mucus)?
4. Do you use any medication through your nose (nose drops, nasal spray)?
5. Are both nostrils affected?

Assessment of the nose is discussed in Chapter 2. Nose problems other than colds are commonly referred to a physician or ENT specialist.

Neurological Examination and Convulsive Disorders (Including Head Injury)

The neurological examination is very important, especially in relation to contact or collision activities or when there is a suspected head injury. Some of the more common questions asked in the neurological examination include the following[23,46]:

1. Have you ever been knocked out or been unconscious?
2. Have you ever had a head injury?
3. Have you had or do you have frequent or severe headaches?
4. Have you ever had a stinger or burner?
5. Have you ever had a time when one or more of your limbs went numb or "to sleep" during activity?
6. Have you ever fainted (syncope)?
7. Have you ever had a paralyzed limb?
8. Have you ever lost feeling or muscular control of your arms or legs?
9. Have you ever had a seizure?
10. Have you ever been in a motor vehicle accident or fallen and hit your head?

A positive answer to any of these questions could have a significant impact on what the patient is allowed to do and whether the patient is allowed to return to work or to participate in contact or collision activities.

In the neurological examination, the examiner may assess the status of a head injury (see Chapter 2), perform a cranial nerve assessment (see Chapter 2) and sensation scan, and evaluate the different reflexes (see Chapter 1)

if problems are suspected. The examiner must check for concussions and nerve palsies. Any positive neurological signs and symptoms uncovered in the examination, such as recurrent concussions or nerve palsies, should preclude strenuous activity until investigated further by a specialist before clearance to return to previous activities is given.

Examples of Neurological Conditions or Signs and Symptoms Requiring Further Examination

- More than one concussion
- Postconcussion syndrome
- Any history of head injury
- Expanding intracranial lesion
- Any history of seizure
- Neurological symptoms of undetermined cause
- Any history of stinger, burner, or neurapraxia
- Persistent weakness, numbness, or arm or leg pain
- Any history of transient quadriplegia
- Upper motor neuron symptoms
- Any history of nerve palsy

With convulsive disorders, the examiner must determine the frequency of the episodes; how or whether control of the convulsions has been achieved; the use of routine medication; any circumstances that activate the convulsions; and whether the patient understands the disorder, its hazards, and the predisposing factors. Patients with epilepsy should be discouraged from activities such as skiing, scuba diving, parachuting, and climbing because of the inherent dangers.[46] If the activity involves water sports (e.g., swimming alone, scuba diving), auto racing, or any activity in which recurrent head trauma or unexpected falls may cause serious injury (e.g., mountain climbing, working at heights), then the patient with a convulsive disorder should be discouraged from engaging in these activities. Patients whose activities should be restricted include those who experience daily or weekly seizures, those who display bizarre forms of psychomotor epilepsy, and those whose postconvalescent state is prolonged or typically includes markedly abnormal behavior. It is important to understand whether the medication taken can maintain good control of the patient's condition, not only in everyday situations but also in stress situations. For example, hyperventilation may precipitate an epileptic seizure, and seizures tend to occur after exercise, not during the event. In addition, it is important to know whether the extent or intensity of the participation poses a significant threat to the patient's physical condition.

If the examiner is treating the patient for head, face, or temporomandibular joint pain, he or she should always be cognizant of the possibility of meningitis, a primary brain tumor, or a subarachnoid hemorrhage.[75] Meningitis is a rare infection that affects the meninges, causing brain swelling, bleeding, and death in 10% of cases.[76]

Musculoskeletal Examination

Like the neurological examination discussed previously, the musculoskeletal examination is often a very important part of an evaluation. Questions in the history related to this examination include the following[48,77–81]:

1. Have you ever pulled (strained) or hurt a muscle?
2. Have you ever torn (sprained) or stretched a ligament?
3. Have you ever subluxated or dislocated a joint or had a bone come out of joint?
4. Have you ever broken (fractured) a bone?
5. Have any of your joints ever swollen?
6. Have you ever had pain in your muscles or joints at work or during or after activity, exercise, or sports (Table 17.4)?
7. Have you ever had regular prolonged (more than 30 minutes) morning stiffness?
8. Have you ever had any rashes, eye infections, diarrhea associated with joint pain, and/or swelling?
9. Have you ever had any proximal weakness, excessive cramping, or muscle fasciculations?

A positive response to any of these questions requires further investigation.

The musculoskeletal examination begins with observation of the patient's posture (see Chapter 15), looking for any asymmetry. Asymmetry, combined with the history, may lead the examiner to do a detailed assessment of a specific joint (see Chapters 3 to 13). If no problems are noted, the examiner can do a quick **upper and lower scanning** or **screening examination** to check for potential problems and abnormal movement (e.g., hypomobility,

hypermobility, capsular patterns, weakness, abnormal movement patterns, "cheating movements").[65,82]

Upper and Lower Scanning Examination

- Cervical spine: flexion, extension, side flexion, rotation
- Shoulder shrug (resistance may be added)
- Shoulder: elevation through abduction, forward flexion and the plane of the scapula; medial and lateral rotation (resistance may be added)
- Elbow: flexion, extension, supination, pronation
- Wrist: flexion, extension, radial, and ulnar deviation
- Fingers and thumb: open hands wide, make a tight fist
- Thoracic and lumbar spine: flexion (touch toes, knees straight— watch for spine versus hip movement), extension, side flexion, rotation
- Tighten quadriceps (quadriceps strength, symmetry)
- Test hamstring tightness
- Hip, knee, ankle, and foot: squat and bounce, heel-toe walking

---

If any deviation, weakness, or abnormality is found or if the patient has reported a previous injury to a joint, a more detailed examination may be performed to assess active movements, passive movements, resisted isometric movements, special tests, functional tests, reflexes, sensation, myotomes, joint play, and to palpate that joint or associated joints.

Examples of Musculoskeletal Conditions or Signs and Symptoms Requiring Further Examination

- Joint or spinal instability (static and dynamic)
- Joint swelling
- Unhealed muscle or ligament injury (especially 3° or if avulsion suspected)
- Possible fractures or dislocations/subluxations
- Unhealed or healing fracture
- Degenerative diseases
- Inflammatory diseases
- Unusual hypermobility or hypomobility
- Muscle weakness
- Growth or maturation disorders
- Repetitive stress disorders
- Myopathy
- Metabolic disease

TABLE **17.4**

Comparison of Systemic and Musculoskeletal Joint Pain

Systemic	Musculoskeletal
• Awakens at night • Deep aching, throbbing • Reduced by pressure • Constant or waves/spasm • Jaundice • Migratory arthralgias • Skin rash • Fatigue • Weight loss • Low-grade fever • Muscular weakness • Cyclic, progressive symptoms • History of infection (hepatitis, streptococcosis, mononucleosis, measles)	• Decreases with rest • Sharp • Ceases when stressful action is stopped • Associated signs and symptoms • Usually none • Trigger points may be accompanied by nausea, sweating

From Goodman CC, Snyder TE: *Differential diagnosis in physical therapy*, Philadelphia, 1995, WB Saunders, p 526.

When the examiner is looking for musculoskeletal problems, it is important to consider whether the patient's job or what he or she wants to do will exacerbate an existing disease or injury, increase an existing deformity, or cause further bone or joint damage. When the examiner is looking for musculoskeletal problems, he or she may look at the patient's flexibility, strength, and endurance as well as static and dynamic stability. Spinal instability (especially instability of the cervical or lumbar spine) or spondylolisthesis may preclude the patient from taking part in some activities. Maturation may also have to be considered when dealing with patients who are still growing, as well as previous injuries, congenital problems, and growth abnormalities in this age group.

Cardiovascular Examination

The cardiovascular examination should be performed in a quiet area because of the need to auscultate. In this part of the evaluation, the examiner looks for subtle but significant cardiac abnormalities to reduce the incidence of unexpected sudden death in sports or similar incidents at work.[4,49,83–88] In some cases, electrocardiograms (ECGs) or stress ECGs may be appropriate.[89] More than 90% of sudden deaths in exercise and sports among participants younger than 30 years of age involve the cardiovascular system.

The following questions should be asked in the history concerning the cardiovascular system[19,23,44,46]:

1. Have you ever had a heart attack?
2. Do you have a pacemaker or other device to assist your heart?
3. Have you ever had heart surgery?
4. Have you ever had frequent heartburn?
5. Have you ever experienced dizziness, fainting, or passing out during or after activity, exercise, or sports?
6. Have you ever experienced chest pain, tightness, a crushing sensation, squeezing, or pressure in the chest at work or during or after activity, exercise, or sports (Tables 17.5 and 17.6)?
7. When you are working or doing an activity, exercise, or sport, do you tire more quickly than others doing the same things?
8. Have you ever had high blood pressure?
9. Has your heart ever "raced" or skipped beats?
10. Have you ever been told you have a heart murmur?
11. Has anyone in your family ever had heart problems or died of heart disease?
12. Has anyone in your family died suddenly before the age of 50 years?
13. Have you had a severe viral infection (myocarditis, mononucleosis) within the last month?
14. Has a physician denied or restricted your participation in any activity because of heart problems?
15. Do your ankles and/or legs swell?[90]

If the answer to any of these questions is yes, the examiner must consider the possibility of cardiomyopathy, conduction abnormalities, arrhythmias, valvular problems, coronary artery defects, and lung or related problems.[91] If cardiovascular problems are suspected, the examiner may organize further tests (e.g., ECG, treadmill stress tests, laboratory tests)[92] to detect cardiac abnormalities.

Examples of Cardiovascular Conditions or Signs and Symptoms Requiring Further Examination

- Chest pain
- Dizziness with activity or vertigo
- Irregular heartbeat (rate, rhythm)
- Hypertension (labile or organic)
- Heart murmur
- Family history of heart problems
- Hypertrophic cardiomegaly
- Conduction abnormalities
- Arrhythmias
- Myocarditis
- Valvular problems
- Aortic coarctation
- Marfan syndrome
- Enlarged (athlete's) heart
- Atherosclerotic disease (positive ankle-arm index [AAI])
- Mitral insufficiency
- Anemia
- Enlarged spleen
- Unexplained fatigue

When the examiner is looking for cardiovascular problems, it is important to be alert for the following unusual or abnormal findings:

1. Heart rate faster than 120 beats/min or inappropriate tachycardia for a specific activity
2. Arrhythmias or irregular beats[93]
3. Midsystolic clicks, indicating a leaky valve or mitral valve prolapse
4. Murmurs that are grade 3 or louder

The loudness of **systolic murmurs** is graded from 1 to 6, with grade 1 being a very faint murmur requiring concentration to be heard. A grade 2 murmur is a faint murmur but one that is heard immediately after the stethoscope is placed on the chest. Grade 3 is an intermediate murmur louder than grade 2. Most dynamically significant murmurs in humans are at least grade 3. Grade 4 is a loud murmur, frequently associated with a palpable sensation known as a thrill. A grade 5 murmur is a very loud murmur still requiring at least the edge of the stethoscope to remain in contact with the chest. The grade 6 murmur is a murmur audible with the stethoscope just breaking contact with the chest.[94] **Diastolic murmurs** are graded from 1 to 4, 1 representing the faintest and 4 the loudest murmur. A benign functional murmur or systemic mitral valve prolapse does not preclude exercise or sports but must be evaluated on an individual basis.

The examiner must be aware of congenital heart abnormalities such as aortic coarctation (stenosis of the artery), which may be revealed by a difference in the femoral and brachial pulses. In such a case, strenuous activity is contraindicated. As another example, 90% of patients with Marfan syndrome (an autosomal dominant condition)

TABLE **17.5**

Causes of Chest Pain

Systemic Causes	Neuromuscular Causes
• Pulmonary 　○ Pulmonary embolism 　○ Spontaneous pneumothorax 　○ Pulmonary hypertension 　○ Cor pulmonale 　○ Pleurisy with pneumonia • Cardiac 　○ Myocardial ischemia (angina) 　○ Pericarditis 　○ Myocardial infarct 　○ Dissecting aortic aneurysm • Epigastric/Upper GI 　○ Esophagitis 　○ Upper GI index • Breast 　○ Breast tumor 　○ Abscess 　○ Mastitis 　○ Lactation problems 　○ Mastodynia 　○ Trigger point • Other 　○ Rheumatic diseases 　○ Anxiety	• Tietze syndrome • Costochondritis • Hypersensitive xiphoid • Slipping rib syndrome • Trigger points • Myalgia • Rib fracture • Cervical spine disorders • Neurologic 　○ Thoracic outlet syndrome 　○ Neuritis 　○ Shingles (herpes zoster) 　○ Dorsal nerve root irritation

GI, Gastrointestinal.

From Goodman CC, Snyder TE: *Differential diagnosis in physical therapy,* Philadelphia, 1995, WB Saunders, p 532.

have cardiac abnormalities. The examiner must be aware of atrial septal defects (an abnormal communication between the chambers of the heart), dextrocardia (the heart is moved within the thoracic cavity), and paroxysmal auricular tachycardia (an abnormal increase in heartbeat for short periods). Patients with these conditions should be cleared by a specialist before any strenuous activity because of the possibility of fainting in a stressful situation. The examiner must also be aware of heart enlargement ("athlete's heart"). This condition does not necessarily preclude activity but should be investigated further if found. If any of these abnormalities have been surgically corrected, they should be evaluated by a specialist on an individual basis to determine whether the patient can take part in the proposed activity.

Hypertrophic cardiomyopathy is the most common cause of sudden death in athletes, followed by aortic rupture associated with Marfan syndrome, congenital coronary artery anomalies, and atherosclerotic coronary artery disease.[46,95] If any of these conditions is present, strenuous activity is precluded.

Other cardiovascular problems include thromboembolic disease, pulse irregularities, valvular problems (such as mitral insufficiency or mitral valve prolapse), and abnormally high blood pressure (hypertension). Systolic pressure of 140 mm Hg on repeated measurements is considered abnormal (see Chapter 1, Table 1.9).[85] Also, patients with labile hypertension (an unstable condition of free and rapid change in tension) or organic hypertension caused by structural problems should be investigated further. These patients should have a complete comprehensive coronary risk factor workup. Mild hypertension does not preclude strenuous activity, but this slight abnormality should be noted and evaluated on an individual basis.[46] When blood pressure is being taken, a proper cuff size must be used to ensure an accurate reading. If the initial reading is high, the reading should be repeated two or three times after the patient has been lying supine for 20 to 30 minutes. Only if the blood pressure is elevated after the third reading should the patient be considered hypertensive.

Detecting Cardiac Risks in Examinations: Key Physical Findings of Cardiac Evaluation by Physician

Heart rate faster than 120 beats per minute
- If repeated tests on second occasion are high, suggest monitoring and recording of pulse at home by a trained parent or nurse friend.
- Pulse recovery tests after jumping or hopping exercises are useless routines except for multiple extrasystoles or arrhythmias.

Multiple extrasystoles or arrhythmias. Check after jumping or hopping 20 times to ascertain if arrhythmias appear or disappear.

Resting blood pressure higher than 130/80 mm Hg for students aged 6–11 years, 140/90 mm Hg for students aged 12–18 years.
- For validity, be certain that the pressure cuff covers at least two-thirds of the upper arm, from elbow to shoulder (adult cuff = 30 × 13 cm; pediatric cuff = 22 × 10 cm; obese cuff = 39 × 15 cm).
- If high, repeat test three times and take average.

All systolic murmurs grade 3–6 or louder at any location; all diastolic murmurs of any intensity at any location; or any continuous murmur. Heart should be auscultated at four chest locations:
- Pulmonic area (second intercostal space at left sternal border)
- Aortic area (second intercostal space at right sternal border)
- Tricuspid area (fourth intercostal space at left sternal border)
- Mitral area (fourth intercostal space at left midclavicular line)

Routinely palpate femoral and brachial pulses. Note if absent or if large discrepancy exists between them.

Modified from Schell NB: Cardiac evaluation of school sports participants: guidelines approved by the Medical Society of New York, *NY State J Med* 78:942–943, 1978.

TABLE **17.6**

Characteristics of Cardiac Chest Pain

Angina	Myocardial Infarct	Mitral Valve Prolapse	Pericarditis
1–5 minutes	30 minutes to hours	Hours	Hours to days
Moderate intensity	Severe (can be painless)	Rarely severe	Varies; mild to severe
Tightness, chest discomfort	Crushing pain; intolerable (can be painless)	May be asymptomatic; unlike angina in quality or quantity	Asymptomatic; varies; can mimic MI
Subsides with rest or nitroglycerin	Unrelieved by rest or nitroglycerin	Unrelieved by rest or nitroglycerin	Relieved by kneeling on all fours, leaning forward, or sitting upright
Pain related to tone of arteries (spasm)	Pain related to heart ischemia	Mechanism of pain unknown	Pain related to inflammatory process

MI, Myocardial infarct.
From Goodman CC, Snyder TE: *Differential diagnosis in physical therapy*, Philadelphia, 1995, WB Saunders, p 94.

Detecting Cardiac Risks in Examinations: Key Historical Facts Obtained from Students, Parents, and School Health Records

- Cyanotic heart disease early in life
- Murmur early in life based on anatomic diagnosis of left-to-right shunt or pulmonic or aortic stenosis
- Rheumatic heart disease
- Fainting spells (syncope)
- Chest or abdominal pains (not otherwise diagnosed)
- Dyspnea on exertion
- Cardiac surgery
- Enlarged heart
- Cardiac rhythm disturbances
- Familial heart disease[a] or rhythm disturbances
- Functional or innocent murmur of 4 or more years' duration

[a]Hypertension, early stroke (before 50 years), or early coronary disease (before 50 years) in close relatives.
Modified from Schell NB: Cardiac evaluation of school sports participants: guidelines approved by the Medical Society of New York, *NY State J Med* 78:942–943, 1978.

Another condition the examiner should be aware of is **anemia**. If anemia is suspected, the level of hemoglobin (the oxygen-carrying pigment in human blood) is tested. Anemia is more likely to be seen in women during menstruation, and sickle cell anemia is more common in black individuals. In some cases anemia is caused by an increase in blood volume, which decreases the concentration of red blood cells. In this case, the individual has normal red blood cells but appears to be anemic.

If cardiovascular or cardiopulmonary disease is suspected, an exercise stress test is often recommended.[51,96] Fig. 17.1 provides a flowchart for considerations before such a test is done. Some 20% to 35% of those with heart disease have a normal stress test, so it is important to remember that any stress test is valid only to the load at which the heart has been stressed when the test is being done. Among runners above 40 years of age, 45% have irregular results on their ECGs. Further, different types of activity (e.g., static or dynamic) lead to different stresses on the heart.

Contraindications to Exercise Testing

- Physical inability to walk on the treadmill
- Unstable angina or new resting ECG changes
- Acute pericarditis, myocarditis, endocarditis
- Uncompensated CHF, S3 gallop, rales
- Severe aortic stenosis
- Hypertrophic cardiomyopathy
- Known LMCA or equivalent stenoses
- Uncooperative patient
- Other serious medical problem or problems

CHF, Congestive heart failure; *ECG*, electrocardiogram; *LMCA*, left main coronary artery.
From Cavell RM: The exercise treadmill test for diagnosis and prognosis of coronary artery disease, *J La State Med Soc* 147:198, 1995.

Common Causes of False-Positive Exercise Tests

- Congenital and valvular heart disease
- Digoxin
- Electrolyte abnormalities
- Nonfasting state
- Pre-excitation syndromes, WPW
- Bundle branch block
- Mitral valve prolapse
- Left ventricular hypertrophy
- Hyperventilation

WPW, Wolff-Parkinson-White syndrome.
From Cavell RM: The exercise treadmill test for diagnosis and prognosis of coronary artery disease, *J La State Med Soc* 147:198, 1995.

Indications for Termination of the Exercise Test

- Patient's request
- Achievement of maximum effort
- Appearance of serious arrhythmia, multiform PVCs, triplets, rapid SVT
- Fall in systolic BP in the face of increasing workload
- Progressive anginal pain
- CNS symptoms, dizziness, ataxia
- Signs of poor perfusion, pallor, cyanosis, cool extremities
- More than 0.3 mV of horizontal or downsloping SVT depression
- Technical loss of monitoring ability

BP, Blood pressure; *CNS,* central nervous system; *PVC,* premature ventricular contraction; *SVT,* supraventricular tachycardia.
From Cavell RM: The exercise treadmill test for diagnosis and prognosis of coronary artery disease, *J La State Med Soc* 147:198, 1995.

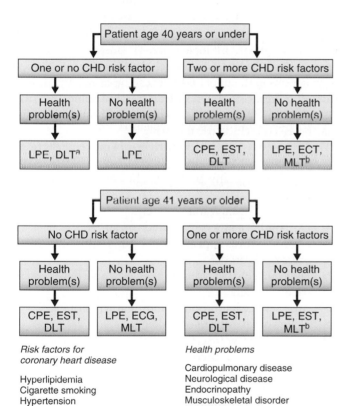

Risk factors for coronary heart disease

Hyperlipidemia
Cigarette smoking
Hypertension
Hyperglycemia or diabetes
  mellitus
Hyperuricemia or gout
Obesity

Health problems

Cardiopulmonary disease
Neurological disease
Endocrinopathy
Musculoskeletal disorder
Psychiatric disorder
Renal or hepatic disease
Anemia
Current drug use
Other acute or chronic disease

a Exercise stress testing is recommended if patient has cardiopulmonary disease.

b Diagnostic laboratory testing is indicated if CDH risk factors include hyperlipidemia, hyperglycemia, or hyperuricemia.

Fig. 17.1 Pre-exercise evaluation flow sheet. *CDH,* Coronary heart disease; *CPE,* comprehensive physical examination; *DLT,* diagnostic laboratory testing; *ECG,* resting electrocardiogram; *EST,* exercise stress test; *LPE,* limited physical examination; *MLT,* minimal laboratory testing. (Redrawn from Taylor RB: Pre-exercise evaluation: which procedures are really needed? Consultant, April 1983, pp 94–101.)

The **ankle-arm index (AAI)** may also be used to screen for atherosclerotic (cardiovascular) disease.[97,98] This is the ratio of the ankle systolic pressure to that of the arm when measured using a Doppler ultrasound device.[97] The lower the AAI, the greater the risk of disease.[98]

Pulmonary Examination

The pulmonary examination is often done in a quiet area in conjunction with the cardiovascular examination. Questions related to the pulmonary system may include the following[23,44,49]:

1. Have you ever had trouble breathing?
2. Have you ever had a pulmonary disease?
3. Do you use any breathing aids?
4. Have you ever had a chest x-ray? When?
5. Have you ever experienced long periods of intermittent coughing?
6. Do you cough anything up? Have you had a recent productive cough (e.g., sputum, blood, what color)?
7. Have you ever experienced coughing at work or during or after activity, exercise, or sports? What type of work or activity were you doing?
8. Have you ever experienced shortness of breath or wheezing at work or during or after activity, exercise, or sports? Do you have any allergies?
9. When did shortness of breath begin?
10. Did the shortness of breath begin suddenly or slowly over time?
11. Do you wake up suddenly with shortness of breath (paroxysmal nocturnal dyspnea)?
12. Do you know when your shortness of breath started?
13. Is your shortness of breath constant?
14. Does your shortness of breath occur with exertion only? At rest, or only during certain positions?
15. Is your breathlessness related to anything in particular (e.g., exercise, pollen, emotion)?
16. Do you have asthma? If so, how do you treat it?
17. Have you ever broken your nose?
18. Do you suffer from chronic sinus irritation or a runny nose?
19. Do you have a history of deep venous thrombosis (DVT)?[99]

Signs and Symptoms of Deep Venous Thrombosis

- Chest pain
- Light-headedness
- Breathlessness
- Leg tenderness (with redness and warmth)
- Leg swelling
- Positive Homan's sign (but only in the presence of other clinical signs)

TABLE 17.7

Arterial Blood Gas Values

Normal Values	
pH	7.35–7.45
PCO_2 (partial pressure of carbon dioxide)	35–45 mm Hg
HCO_3 (bicarbonate ion)	22–26 mEq/L
PO_2 (partial pressure of oxygen)	80–100 mm Hg
O_2 saturation (oxygen saturation)	95%–100%
Critical Values	
pH	<7.25 or >7.45
PCO_2	<20 or >60 mm Hg
HCO_3	<15 or >40 mEq/L
PO_2	<40 mm Hg
O_2 saturation	<75%

From Goodman CC, Snyder TE: *Differential diagnosis in physical therapy*, Philadelphia, 1995, WB Saunders, p 151. Adapted from Pagana D, Pagana T: *Mosby's diagnostic and laboratory test reference*, St Louis, 1992, Mosby Year Book, p 104.

The examiner auscultates for clear breath sounds and watches for symmetric diaphragm excursion.[46] Abnormal auditory sounds audible to the ear include stridor and wheezing. **Stridor** is a high-pitched sound caused by an obstruction of the larynx or trachea. **Wheezing** is a high-pitched noise caused by partial obstruction of the airway. Wheezing may be resolved by either opening the airway further or narrowing it.[100] Any required controlling medications should be noted and recorded. The ears, nose, and mouth may also be checked during this examination. If abnormalities are found, appropriate lung function tests or arterial blood gases may be ordered (Table 17.7).[101] If there is concern about an active disease process, a chest x-ray may be in order.

Respiratory problems such as tuberculosis, uncontrolled asthma, exertional asthma, exercise-induced bronchospasm, pulmonary insufficiency resulting from a collapsed lung, or bronchial asthma should be checked and discussed with the patient.[51,102,103] **Coughing** can be a sign of either pulmonary or cardiovascular issues. Night (nocturnal) coughing can be associated with heart failure or a side effect of selected calcium channel blockers.[104] The most commonly found cause for cough is branchial irritation due to cigarette smoking. However, other common causes are postnasal drip from the common cold or allergies. Other more serious issues that may manifest with coughing include disorders such as asthma, pneumonia, cancer, and heart failure. These more serious issues may be seen in those with a chronic cough that has lasted 3 weeks or longer.[105]

Examples of Pulmonary Conditions or Signs and Symptoms Requiring Further Examination

- Abnormal coughing
- Abnormal shortness of breath
- Abnormal breath sounds (e.g., wheezing, rhonchi, rales)
- Asthma (uncontrolled or exertional)
- Exercise-induced bronchospasm
- Pulmonary insufficiency
- Severe allergies
- Nasal deviation or occlusion
- Chronic sinusitis

Gastrointestinal Examination

The gastrointestinal (GI) examination involves evaluation of the digestive system, eating habits, and nutrition. In the upper GI tract, many disorders can cause loss of swallowing control (i.e., dysphagia) to the muscles of the mouth and upper digestive system. Some of these conditions include myasthenia gravis, multiple sclerosis, amyotrophic lateral sclerosis, and Parkinson's Disease. Additionally, mechanical obstructions in the upper GI tract can be caused by tumors, thyroid goiter, osteophytes of the cervical spine, and aortic aneurysms.[106] Some of the questions in this regard that may be asked include the following[23,44,107]:

1. Do you have a problem with bowel movements (e.g., diarrhea, constipation)?
2. Do you have any problems chewing or swallowing food?
3. Have you been vomiting lately?
4. Do you have any pain related to eating?
5. Do your stools appear normal (or are they ever black or tarry colored)?
6. Do you feel that you eat regularly and have a well-balanced diet?
7. Are there certain food groups you will not eat?
8. Have you ever been on a diet?
9. Do you view yourself as too thin, too fat, or just right?
10. Have you ever tried to control your weight? If so, how?
11. Have you ever had excessive heartburn or indigestion?
12. Have you had any heartburn or dyspepsia after using anti-inflammatory medications?

A positive answer to any of these questions requires further investigation.

Examples of Gastrointestinal Conditions or Signs and Symptoms Requiring Further Examination

- Organomegaly (e.g., enlarged liver, spleen)
- Anorexia
- Bulimia
- Female athlete triad (anorexia/bulimia, amenorrhea, osteoporosis)
- Ulcers
- Blood in stools

The examiner should palpate the patient's abdomen for masses or organomegaly.[3] The examiner must ensure that there is no inflammation of the liver (hepatitis, enlarged liver) or enlarged spleen, especially if the patient is involved in contact or collision sports.

In some cases, it is advisable to check the patient's nutritional status, especially if there appears to be a tendency toward eating disorders, such as anorexia or bulimia.[108] This can be done by having the patient record his or her food intake for at least 3 days and having the record analyzed by a nutritionist, who can then calculate dietary intake in relation to the patient's activity level. It also provides an opportunity to determine what supplements the patient is taking in case they contain banned substances. It has been suggested that the **Low Energy Availability in Females Questionnaire (LEAF-Q)** can be used to determine low energy availability and may be used to screen women at risk for **Female Athlete Triad** (i.e., low energy availability with or without an eating disorder, menstrual dysfunction, and low bone density).[109–111]

The health of the lower GI tract can be gleaned through a discussion concerning the patient's stools. It is important to ask questions about bowel function including such issues as incontinence, constipation, diarrhea, or difficulty initiating bowel movements. Also, a change in the shape or caliber of the stool is a potentially significant finding. Stools that are pencil thin or flat and ribbon-like are suggestive of a space-occupying mass including an anal or distal colon carcinoma. Additional concern could occur with the passage of blood in the stool. Bright red blood in the stool usually originates in the left side of the colon or the anorectal area.[112] Black or tarry stools indicate bleeding in the stomach and upper digestive tract and may be the result of an ulcer. In this case, the examiner should include questions related to medication or stress, which can lead to ulcers.

Urogenital Examination

Depending on whether the patient is male or female, the examination is modified to meet his or her individual needs. For example, females may be asked about their menstrual history (e.g., when did menses begin? When was the last period? Are there any abnormalities?) or about gynecologic problems. Males may be given a genital examination looking for abnormalities, hernias, or absence of a testicle.[46] Common history questions asked in the urogenital examination (males and females) include the following:

1. Have you ever had any problems with your kidneys or bladder?
2. Has there been a change in the number of times you urinate daily?
3. When you urinate, do you have trouble starting, continuing, or stopping?
4. Have you ever been treated for venereal disease?
5. Is your urine clear or discolored? Blood in urine can be a manifestation of almost every genitourinary disease.[113] It is also important to remember that reddish discoloration of urine is not always a medical emergency. Ingestion of vegetable dyes, beets (in quantity), and certain medications may make the urine reddish in color.
6. Have you ever been diagnosed as having sugar, albumin, or blood in your urine?
7. Have you felt any bulges in your groin, testicle, or abdomen?
8. Have you felt a painless hard mass in your testicle (testicular cancer screen)?
9. Have you had any urethral discharge or dysuria?

The examiner should check for hernias, kidney problems, albuminuria (excessive protein in the urine), and venereal disease if a problem of the urogenital system is suspected.[114] Patients with one kidney should be warned of the danger of contact sports, especially if the kidney is abnormally positioned or is diseased.[115] In males, the examiner should be aware of an undescended or atrophied testicle or testicular torsion. A urinalysis should be performed if diabetes or kidney disease is suspected. These conditions do not preclude activity, exercise, or sports but they may be amenable to treatment, and the patient must be made aware of potential dangers caused by these conditions.

Examples of Urogenital Conditions or Signs and Symptoms Requiring Further Examination

- Hernia (femoral, inguinal, abdominal, sports)
- Absent or undescended testicle
- Lump in testicle
- One kidney or diseased kidney
- Albuminuria
- Hemoglobinuria
- Nephroptosis
- Hematuria
- Exercise amenorrhea
- Diabetes
- Sexually transmitted diseases

Dehydration, athletic pseudonephritis, hemoglobinuria, nephroptosis, and hematuria are all possible problems of the urogenital system. Dehydration can become severe and manifest though thirst and dry mouth, postural hypotension, rapid breathing, rapid pulse, confusion, irritability, lethargy, and headache. Proper hydration should continue even if the patient does not feel that he or she is thirsty. For females in sports, it is important to determine whether they have regular periods and menstrual patterns because of concern about exercise amenorrhea and its relation to bone density and osteoporosis.[51,116]

Dermatological (Integumentary) Examination

The primary care assessment may involve examination for any developing skin conditions and those that may be amenable to treatment. The questions relating to the dermatologic examination would be the following[23]:

1. Have you had any problems with acne?
2. Have you had any problems with rashes or itching, especially in areas covered by clothes, equipment, or footwear?
3. Do you have a history of fungal infections?
4. Are there any other changes to your skin related to color, moles, sores, rashes, or lumps?
5. Are there any changes to your nails, such as discoloration, thickening, ridges, splitting, or separations from the bed?
6. Are there any changes to your hair such as hair loss, increase in the hair, change in thickness or distribution of your hair?
7. Have you noticed any itching (pruritus)?
8. Has there been any change in the amount of sweating or the dryness of your skin?

Examples of Dermatologic Conditions or Signs and Symptoms Requiring Further Examination

- Severe acne
- Dermatitis (e.g., contact, clothes)
- Herpes (e.g., simplex, gladiatorum)
- Fungal infection (tinea capitis or corporis)
- Boils
- Warts
- Impetigo
- Molluscum contagiosum
- Psoriasis

The answers to such questions give the examiner some idea of skin conditions, most of which are easily dealt with by treatment.

The examiner must ensure that the patient with dermatologic problems has them under control, because many of these conditions are contagious, including bacterial, fungal, or viral infections (such as herpes simplex, herpes gladiatorum, boils, impetigo, or warts), and contact dermatitis.

Examination for Heat (Hyperthermic) Disorders

Examination for heat disorders should be included if the patient's work, activity, exercise, or sport has involved working or activity where there is a high temperature, high humidity, a combination of the two (e.g., moderate temperature and high humidity), or where a heat injury might occur.[117-123] These are often the conditions that lead to heat disorders. Questions in the history related to heat disorders may include the following:

1. Have you ever experienced a heat disorder?
2. Have you ever had muscle cramps?
3. Have you ever participated in an activity, exercise, or sport in a high-temperature, high-humidity environment?
4. Have you ever passed out or become dizzy in the heat?
5. Have you been on medication, or do you drink a lot of caffeinated beverages or use stimulants?
6. Have you recently lost a considerable amount of weight in a short time?

Examples of Heat Disorders or Heat-Related Signs and Symptoms Requiring Further Examination

- Heat exhaustion
- Heat stroke
- Excessive muscle cramps in heat
- Excessive dehydration

Intake of antihistamines or excessive caffeine, as well as the failure to ingest fluids and/or metabolites, can increase the risk of heat disorders. If a patient has a history of heat-related disorders, the condition should be thoroughly investigated because it could lead to a life-threatening situation.

Examination for Cold (Hypothermic) Disorders

Examination for hypothermia should be included if the patient's work, activity, exercise, or sport involves working or activity where there are low temperatures (below freezing), a significant wind chill factor, high humidity (or wearing wet clothes), or a combination of the three exists.[120,122,124-129] Any of these may lead to an environmental insult, such as acute (immersion), chronic (exposure), or urban hypothermia. Questions in the history related to hypothermic (cold) disorders may include the following:

Factors That Increase Susceptibility to Cold

- General: Infancy, advanced age, malnutrition, exhaustion
- Drug use: Alcohol, sedatives, meperidine, clonidine, neuroleptic agents
- Endocrine system: Hypoglycemia, hypothyroidism, adrenal insufficiency, diabetes
- Cardiovascular system: Peripheral vascular disease, nicotine use
- Neurological system: Peripheral neuropathy, spinal cord damage, autonomic neuropathy, hypothalamic disease
- Trauma: Falls (head or spinal injury), fracture causing immobility
- Infection: Sepsis (diaphoresis, hypothalamic dysfunction)

From Biem J, Koehncke N, Classen D, et al: Out of the cold: management of hypothermia and frostbite, *Can Med J.* 168:306, 2003.

1. Have you ever frozen your ears, toes, or fingers?
2. How long have you been in the cold? (Note: This could be in a cold building, not just outside.)
3. Were you working or participating in an activity, exercise, or sport in low-temperature, windy conditions and/or a humid environment?
4. Have you been in poor health in the last 6 months?
5. Have you been eating well?
6. Have you consumed any drugs or alcohol in the last 24 hours?
7. Do you smoke?

Questions 4 to 7 are asked because of their effect on the circulation and neurological systems. Often the patient experiencing hypothermia is shivering, is apathetic and lethargic, and may demonstrate an inability to perform simple meaningful tasks.

Laboratory Tests

Laboratory tests are often included in a primary care assessment. If the examiner suspects problems for which laboratory tests can be diagnostic, then they should be ordered. For example, if heart disease is suspected or an older population is being examined, serum cholesterol, triglycerides, and/or high-density lipoprotein testing may be ordered (Tables 17.8–17.11).

Common Laboratory Tests

- Hematocrit
- Urinalysis
- Blood chemistry (glucose, creatine, electrolytes)
- Fasting lipid profile
- Electrocardiogram

TABLE **17.8**

Blood Cholesterol Levels

Age (Years)	Values (mg/dL)
<25	125–200
25–40	140–225
40–50	160–245
50–65	170–265
>65	<265

From Goodman CC, Snyder TE: *Differential diagnosis in physical therapy*, Philadelphia, 1995, WB Saunders, p 134.

TABLE **17.9**

Triglyceride Levels

Age (Years)	Value (mg/dL)
Female Adult	
20–29	10–100
30–39	10–110
40–49	10–122
50–59	10–134
>59	10–147
Female Child	
1–19	10–121
Male Adult	
20–29	10–157
30–39	10–182
40–49	10–193
50–59	10–197
>59	10–199
Male Child	
1–19	10–103

From Chernecky C, et al: *Laboratory tests and diagnostic procedures,* Philadelphia, 1993, WB Saunders, p 932.

TABLE **17.10**

Serum Electrolyte Levels

Test	Normal Values
Serum potassium	3.5–5.3 mEq/L
Serum sodium	136–145 mEq/L
Serum calcium	8.2–10.2 mg/dL (4.5–5.5 mEq/L)
Serum magnesium	1.8–3 mg/dL (1.5–2.5 mEq/L)

Adapted from Chernecky C, et al: *Laboratory tests and diagnostic procedures*, Philadelphia, 1993, WB Saunders.

The incidence of iron deficiency anemia in postmenarchal female athletes is as high as 15%. Plasma ferritin may be used to measure iron status. In males, anemia may occur during a growth spurt, with inadequate diet, or with a peptic ulcer. Hemoglobin is often checked if sickle cell anemia (common in black people) is suspected. The prepubertal level of hemoglobin is about 11.5 g/dL of blood, and the postpubertal value is 14.5 g/dL of blood for males and 12.0 g/dL or higher for females.

TABLE **17.11**

Urine Analysis (Urinalysis)

	Test	Normal Result
General measurements	Color	Yellow-amber
	Turbidity	Clear
	pH	4.6–8.0
	Specific gravity	1.01–1.025
Other components	Glucose	Negative
	Ketones	Negative
	Blood	Negative
	Protein	Negative
	Bilirubin	Negative
Sediment	RBCs	Negative
	WBCs	Negative
	Casts	Occasional
	Mucus threads	Occasional
	Crystals	Occasional

RBCs, Red blood cells; *WBCs,* white blood cells.
From Goodman CC, Snyder TE: *Differential diagnosis in physical therapy,* Philadelphia, 1995, WB Saunders, p 258. Normal values are taken from Kee J: *Laboratory and diagnostic tests with nursing implications,* ed 3, Norwalk, CT, 1991, Appleton & Lange.

Diagnostic Imaging

Diagnostic imaging may also be part of a primary care assessment but should not be used indiscriminately.[130] For the most part, diagnostic imaging should be used following set guidelines and to confirm a clinical diagnosis. The type of imaging depends on the information sought. More detailed information on diagnostic imaging may be found in Chapter 1 and more detailed references.[131–133]

Physical Fitness Profile (Functional Assessment)

In some cases it may be important for the examiner to establish a physical fitness profile for the patient to determine if he or she can meet the stresses of work or sports or to determine his or her functional level.[134] Basically, profiling is the gathering of information about the physical attributes of the participant.[135] Such profiling helps to determine whether the person possesses the attributes, skills, and abilities necessary for a job or participation in various activities and to meet the demands of the job or activity; it should be geared to the specific job, activity, exercise, or sport (Table 17.12).[135–141] It should be designed to stress the body so that any weakness or pathology that exists will be apparent. In this way, it may be used as a **screening device** to prevent injury.[135,142] The profile also provides a **baseline** in the event of injury or to

demonstrate the need for, or effect of, conditioning necessary to do the job or take part in the activity. A physical fitness profile can involve many parameters or aspects, including strength, endurance, flexibility, cardiovascular fitness, and maturation. To be effective, the program or test must exhibit several characteristics.[143]

Characteristics of Physical Fitness Profile

- The variables being tested must be relevant to the job, activity, exercise, or sport
- The test must be reliable and valid
- Test protocols must be as specific to the job, activity, exercise, or sport as possible
- The test must be standardized and controlled
- The rights of the patient and confidentiality must be respected
- Testing may be repeated at regular intervals if the purpose is to show effectiveness of a training program
- Results must be conveyed to the patient in a meaningful way that the patient can understand

---

Functional Movement Screen.[144–146] This screen was developed by Move2Perform to determine if individuals had poor movement patterns or pre-existing movement impairments. The functional movement screen (FMS) consists of seven movement tests for balance, mobility, and stability. Each test is scored from 0 (unable to do) to 3 (able to do with no compensatory movement or pain). If scores are different between sides, there is an imbalance. Kiesel et al.[144,145] showed that if an individual's FMS score was 14 or less, the probability of serious injury occurring in the future increased from 15% to 51%. The same company has developed the **Y Balance Test (Star Excursion Balance Test)** (see Figs. 2.53 and 2.54) using an excursion balance, which is used to measure upper and lower limb control and balance. These values can be used to determine when a patient is ready to return to activity. It is especially useful for active individuals.[147–151]

Screen for Patterns of Functional Movement[144–146]

- Deep squat (bilateral, functional and symmetric mobility)
- Hurdle step[a] (stride mechanics)
- In-line lunge[a] (lower limb stability and flexibility)
- Shoulder mobility[a] (including scapular stabilization)
- Active straight leg raise[a] (hamstring flexibility and pelvic stability)
- Trunk stability push-up (trunk stabilization with upper extremity motion)
- Rotary stability[a] (multiplane trunk stability with upper and lower extremity motion)

[a]Test both left and right sides.

Strength

Strength is one of the attributes that is commonly examined in a physical fitness profile. The way in which the

TABLE 17.12

Parameters Used to Determine Athletic Fitness for Specific Sports[a]

	Speed	Strength	Muscle Endurance	Power	Quickness and Agility	Reaction Time	Flexibility	Cardiorespiratory Endurance	Balance	Anaerobic Endurance	Body Composition	Kinesthetic Perception
Football	X	X	—	X	X	X	X	—	X	X	X	X
Basketball	X	—	X	X	X	—	X	X	X	X	X	X
Baseball	X	—	—	X	—	X	X	—	—	X	—	—
Track and field												
Sprinters	X	X	—	X	—	X	X	—	—	X	X	—
Thrower	—	X	—	X	X	—	X	—	X	X	X	X
Jumpers	X	X	—	X	—	—	X	—	X	X	X	X
Distance	—	—	X	—	—	—	X	X	—	—	X	—
Volleyball	—	—	X	X	X	X	X	—	X	X	X	X
Soccer	X	—	X	—	X	—	X	X	X	—	X	X
Rodeo	—	X	—	X	X	X	X	—	X	—	—	X
Tennis	—	—	X	X	X	X	X	X	—	X	X	X
Golf	—	—	X	—	—	—	X	X	X	—	X	X
Skiing	—	X	X	X	—	—	X	X	X	—	X	X
Wrestling	—	X	X	X	X	—	X	X	X	—	X	X
Gymnastics	X	X	X	X	X	—	X	—	X	—	X	X

[a]X denotes areas of physical fitness that are most needed in each sport.

Test examples:

Speed: 20-, 40-, 100-yard dashes

Strength: 1 repetition max

Muscle endurance: 225- or 285-lb bench test sit-up, pull-up, dip, push-up

Power: Vertical jump, standing broad jump, two-hand medicine ball put

Agility: 20-yard shuttle run, Semo agility test, T test

Reaction time: Dekan Auto Performance Analyzer

Flexibility: Sit and reach test, shoulder rotation test

Cardiorespiratory endurance: 1.5-mile run, 12-minute run

Balance: Nelson balance test

Anaerobic endurance: Margaria Kalamen leg power test, 40-yard repeated sprint test

Body composition: skinfold measurements

Kinesthetic perception: distance perception jump

From Bridgman R: A coach's guide to testing for athletic attributes, *National Strength Conditioning Assoc J* 13:35, 1991.

examiner determines strength depends on the job, activity, exercise, or sport; the equipment available; and the demands of the activity. It has been reported that strength declines 1% per year after the age of 30 years.[152] The strength measures may involve isometric, isotonic, or isokinetic testing; functional activities; lifting of free weights; or, in some cases, simply a hand-grip test.[153,154] In some cases, it may involve muscle fiber typing. If a general indication of strength is desired, hand-grip strength is relatively easy to measure and standard tests can be used (see Chapter 7). For the elderly population, plantar flexor, hip abductor, and hip extensor strengths are important to test.[155] Functional strength tests are often used because they are easy and provide comparable results.[3] However, the examiner should make these tests as specific to the patient's job or activity as possible.

Examples of Functional Strength Tests

- Bench press, leg press
- Sit-ups
- Push-ups
- Pull-ups
- Grip strength

More sophisticated methods may be used, especially if the patient has a history of injury to specific muscles or joints (see the sections on functional testing in Chapters 3 to 13). Isokinetic testing (i.e., Cybex, KinCom, Biodex) is more likely to be used to test specific joints, looking for potential discrepancies between left and right sides, agonist versus antagonist, and differences in strength and endurance. However, it is important to realize that many of these tests are not usually done in functional job- or activity-specific positions or ways.

Power

Power is the ability to move a weight over a distance. This weight may be an object or the human body. Depending on the job, activity, exercise, or sport, power may be included as part of the physical fitness profile. As with all profile parameters, power measurements should be related to the job, activity, exercise, or sport in which the patient will be participating.

Examples of Power Activities

- Throwing a medicine ball (equivalent to weight the patient would throw on the job)
- Lifting a weight and placing it at a higher level
- Stair climbing or running
- Walking up and down stairs
- Bending and lifting
- Jump for height (vertical jump test)
- Two-legged hop
- Single-leg hop for distance

Flexibility and Range of Motion

Flexibility is a very important consideration when a patient is being profiled for a specific job or activity.[156,157] In some cases, less flexibility is better than too much, but in some activities, excessive flexibility (laxity) is necessary to succeed. Therefore flexibility testing must be specific to the job or activity in which the patient wishes to take part, or it may be specific to a particular position. For example, in running activities, lower limb flexibility (especially hip flexors, hamstrings, rectus femoris, iliotibial band, and gastrocnemius) is of greatest importance, whereas in swimming, upper limb flexibility (especially shoulder abduction and medial and lateral rotation) is more important, as it is with jobs involving a large amount of overhead work. In some activities, such as ballet, gymnastics, and synchronized swimming, overall flexibility is essential. In baseball, pitchers often require greater shoulder, hip, and trunk flexibility than other players.[34] Flexibility may be measured with the use of devices such as a goniometer, flexometer, or tape measure.[157]

Determinants of Range of Motion[158]

- Shape of the bone and cartilage
- Muscle power and tone
- Muscle bulk
- Ligaments and joint capsule laxity
- Extensibility of the skin and subcutaneous tissue
- Race (Indians [from India] are more flexible than Blacks, who are more flexible than Caucasians)
- Gender (women are more flexible than men)
- Age (ROM decreases with age)
- Genetic makeup
- The dominant limb tends to be less mobile (decreased ROM) than the nondominant limb
- Day to day stresses on joints

ROM, Range of motion

When the examiner is considering range of motion (ROM), he or she must realize that hypermobility or laxity in one joint or in one direction of joint movement does not necessarily mean hypermobility in all joints or in all directions. Similarly, normal ROM charts are often not valid in dealing with persons who, by virtue of their job or activities (e.g., ballet, gymnastics, synchronized swimming), are hypermobile. Values that are considered normal for these types of activities would be considered hypermobile or abnormal for the general population. It is also important to realize that hypermobility (laxity) and hypomobility are not necessarily pathological states. In pathological states, hypermobility may lead to instability and is usually the result of the individual being unable to control movement in the available ROM (through strength, endurance, passive stabilizers, and neurological input) (see Chapter 1). The ROM available may be the result of genetic makeup or the stresses placed on individual joints. Tight-jointed people tend to be more susceptible to muscle strains, nerve pinch syndromes, and overstress paratenonitis. Hypermobile, or "loose-jointed", people are more susceptible to ligament sprains, chronic back pain, disc prolapse, spondylolisthesis, pes planus, joint effusion, and paratenonitis caused by a lack of ability to control the movement at the joint. In the hypermobile individual, if strength and endurance are not at the appropriate level to support the joints, the joints are often unstable or are subjected to potentially injuring loads.

Various criteria can be used to determine a patient's generalized joint laxity. However, the points previously mentioned must be kept in mind when one is looking at these generalized values. Carter and Wilkinson[159] have developed a five-point system. The patient who meets all criteria is said to exhibit general joint hypermobility. Beighton and Horan developed a 9-point system (see Chapter 1), which is a modification of Carter and Wilkinson's criteria.[160,161] In this case, the patient who scores 4 or more is said to exhibit general joint hypermobility.

Nicholas[162] established criteria for determining whether a patient is tight jointed (hypomobile). It should be realized, however, that under these criteria, the majority of the North American population today would be classified as hypomobile!

Carter and Wilkinson Criteria for Generalized Joint Laxity (Hypermobility)[159]

- Passive apposition of the thumb to the flexor aspect of the forearm
- Passive hyperextension of the fingers so they lie parallel with the extensor aspect of the forearm
- Ability to hyperextend elbows at least 10°
- Ability to hyperextend knees at least 10°
- Excessive passive dorsiflexion of the ankle and eversion of the foot

---

Nicholas Criteria for Hypomobility[161]

- Patient is unable to touch the floor with the palms, bending at the knees with the waist straight
- Patient is unable to sit comfortably in the lotus position
- Patient demonstrates less than 20° hyperextension at the knees when lying prone with the legs hanging over the end of the table
- Patient is unable to position the feet at 180° while standing with the knees flexed at 15° to 30°
- Patient has no upper limb laxity on shoulder flexion, elbow hyperextension, or forearm hypersupination

---

It is important to understand the principles of hypermobility and hypomobility. A person who is hypermobile must avoid further stretching and support the joint through strengthening (concentric and eccentric exercise) and endurance programs. The patient must be taught proper positioning, and if there are hypermobile joints, there are probably hypomobile joints nearby that need to be mobilized. It is essential to make sure that these patients have the appropriate strength, endurance, muscular speed of reaction, and balanced activities to help support the hypermobile joints.

The person who is hypomobile may be treated by mobilization or manipulation of the affected joint in the direction of tightness. Tight supporting structures also must be stretched, and active exercises must be given to maintain the restored ROM. It is important with these patients to retrain their kinesthetic sense so that they can maintain and control the acquired ROM.

Speed

Speed is often considered an important component of a physical fitness profile, depending on the job, activity, exercise, or sport. It is a function of distance covered per unit of time.[3]

Examples of Functional Speed Tests

- Timed moving things from one station to another
- Time to assemble "something"
- Timed 40-yard (40-m) run or walk
- Timed 100-yard (100-m) run or walk
- Timed 440-yard (400-m) run or walk

Cardiovascular Fitness and Endurance

Because almost every activity involves stresses on the heart and vascular system, it is important to know the level of the stresses produced and whether the cardiovascular system can respond appropriately to these stresses. Aerobic fitness has been reported to decline by 9% per decade for sedentary adults after the age of 25 years.[163] Therefore the cardiovascular system must be evaluated to determine how it responds to these or equivalent loads.[164,165]

Many methods can be used to determine cardiovascular (aerobic) fitness, but the method chosen should be related to the specific job, activity, or population.[166,167] As an example, ice hockey players who are tested on a bicycle may show very good cardiovascular fitness; however, when they get on the ice and skate, their cardiovascular fitness may not be as evident because they are being tested in a different type of activity.

Examples of Common Endurance Tests

- Harvard step test
- 12-min walk-run
- 1.5-mi (2.4-km) run
- Submaximal ergometer test
- Treadmill test

The Harvard step test is one of the most common general cardiovascular fitness tests done for a physical fitness profile. It is relatively simple, is easy to set up, and takes a minimal amount of time to do. To set up the test, an 18-inch platform is used. The patient is instructed to step with both feet onto the platform at a rate of about 30 times/min (a metronome is used for cadence). The patient is made to step for 3.5 minutes at a pace of 2 seconds per step and then sprint as fast as possible for 30 seconds (total time: 4 minutes). The patient then immediately sits down in a chair and relaxes for 3 minutes while the pulse is determined. The pulse is taken at 30, 60, 120, and 180 seconds after the exercise. The index formula for the pulse is as follows:

$$\text{Index} = \frac{\text{Duration of exercise (in sec)} \times 100}{2 \times \text{the sum of any three pulse counts}}$$

The higher the index, the better the person's fitness. If the index is less than 65, the patient is not ready for high-level activity. Cooper[168,169] developed an indirect method for measuring fitness using a 12-minute walk-run test. From the distance covered in 12 minutes, he developed tables for men and women that showed the patient's fitness category. He later went on to use a similar method for activities such as swimming and cycling, thus making the testing more activity specific. For older individuals, the **Kasch Pulse-Recovery Test**[36,170] can be used (Table 17.13).

Other, more detailed aerobic and anaerobic tests may be performed, including a respiratory quotient test (direct method), the Astrand nomogram (indirect method), the Sjostrad PWC_{170} test (indirect method), and the yo-yo tests (see later discussion).[171]

Although not commonly done except in high-level sports, maximum tests are necessary to get the most complete diagnostic data on a patient's response to exercise. This is important, because half of the heart abnormalities are missed if the test stops at 85% of predicted maximum heart rate, which the simplest tests tend to do.[172] Even if a maximum test is performed, 10% to 15% of the normal population may show an abnormal response.[172] It must be remembered that cardiovascular tests clear the subject only up to the heart rate at which he or she has been tested. In most cases, maximum testing is not done, but if a person is showing abnormalities, such a test may be performed as a second diagnostic procedure. These tests must, however, be performed under very controlled conditions, where there are proper facilities to handle cardiac emergencies.

Although anaerobic fitness is not directly related to the cardiovascular system, it is tested through its effects on the cardiovascular system. If the patient's job, activity, exercise, or sport is primarily anaerobic, consideration must be given to including this measurement as part of the profile.[173] Anaerobic tests can be divided into short-term tests (10 seconds or less), intermediate-term tests (20 to 50 seconds), and long-term anaerobic tests (60 to 120 seconds). Probably the most common anaerobic

TABLE **17.13**

How to Administer the Kasch Pulse-Recovery Test

1. Measure pulse at rest
2. Ask the patient to step up and down (with both feet) a 12-inch step 24 times/min for 3 min
3. Measure pulse 1 min after the test
4. Determine patient's fitness level on the following scale:

	POST-EXERCISE BEATS PER MINUTE	
Fitness Level	Age 56–65 Years	Age 66+ Years
Men		
Excellent	72–82	72–86
Good	89–97	89–95
Above average	98–101	97–102
Average	105–111	104–113
Below average	113–118	114–119
Poor	122–128	122–128
Very poor	131–150	133–152
Women		
Excellent	74–92	73–86
Good	97–103	93–100
Above average	106–111	104–114
Average	113–117	117–121
Below average	119–127	123–127
Poor	129–136	129–134
Very poor	142–151	135–151

From Kligman EW, et al: Recommending exercise to healthy older adults–the preparticipation evaluation and exercise prescription, *Phys Sporsmed* 27(11):49, 1999. Reproduced with permission of McGraw Hill, Inc.

test used today in a laboratory or clinic setting is the 30-second Wingate test.[174]

Agility, Balance, and Reaction Time

For activities requiring agility, balance, and good reaction time, the physical fitness profile should include these items. Balance testing is especially important in the elderly population.[155] O'Brien[155] advocated the Sharpened Romberg test, functional reach test, timed get-up-and-go test (see Chapters 2 and 11), and Tinetti assessment tool for balance and gait. The functional reach test involves the patient reaching forward as far as possible without falling forward or taking a step while the examiner measures for distance horizontally. The Tinetti assessment tool has two parts. The first part measures static and dynamic sitting and standing balance (Table 17.14) and the second part assesses gait (Table 17.15).[175] Ideally, testing should be related to the specific activity. **Agility** is defined as the ability to change directions rapidly when one is moving at

TABLE **17.14**

Performance-Oriented Assessment of Balance[a]

Maneuver	RESPONSE		
	Normal	Adaptive	Abnormal
Sitting balance	Steady, stable	Holds on to chair to keep upright	Leans, slides down in chair
Arising from chair	Able to arise in a single movement without using arms	Uses arms (on chair or walking aid) to pull or push up, and/or moves forward in chair before attempting to arise	Multiple attempts required or unable without human assistance
Immediate standing balance (first 3–5 seconds)	Steady without holding on to walking aid or other object for support	Steady, but uses walking aid or other object for support	Any sign of unsteadiness[b]
Standing balance	Steady, able to stand with feet together without holding object for support	Steady, but cannot put feet together	Any sign of unsteadiness regardless of stance or holds onto object
Balance with eyes closed (with feet is close together as possible)	Steady without holding onto any object with feet together	Steady with feet apart	Any sign of unsteadiness or needs to hold on to an object
Turning balance (360°)	No grabbing or staggering; no need to hold on to any objects; steps are continuous (turn is a flowing movement)	Steps are discontinuous (patient puts one foot completely on floor before raising other foot)	Any sign of unsteadiness or holds on to an object
Nudge on sternum (patient standing with feet as close together as possible, examiner pushes with light even pressure over sternum three times; reflects ability to withstand displacement)	Steady, able to withstand pressure	Needs to move feet, but able to maintain balance	Begins to fall, or examiner has to help maintain balance
Neck turning (patient asked to turn head side to side and look up while standing with feet as close together as possible)	Able to turn head at least halfway side to side and be able to bend head back to look at ceiling; no staggering, grabbing, symptoms or lightheadedness, unsteadiness, or pain	Decreased ability to turn side to side to extend neck, but no staggering, grabbing, symptoms of light-headedness, unsteadiness, or pain	Any age of unsteadiness or symptoms when turning head or extending neck
One leg standing balance	Able to stand on one leg for 5 seconds without holding object for support		Unable
Back extension (ask patient to lean back as far as possible, without holding on to object if possible)	Good extension without holding object or staggering	Tries to extend, but decreased ROM (compared with other patients of same age) or needs to hold object to attempt extension	Will not attempt or no extension seen or staggers
Reaching up (have patient attempt to remove an object from a shelf high enough to require stretching or standing on toes)	Able to take down object without needing to hold on to other object for support and without becoming unsteady	Able to get object but needs to steady self by holding on to something for support	Unable or unsteady

Continued

TABLE **17.14**

Performance-Oriented Assessment of Balance[a]—cont'd

Maneuver	RESPONSE		
	Normal	Adaptive	Abnormal
Bending down (patient is asked to pick up small objects, such as pen, from the floor)	Able to bend down and pick up the object and is able to get up easily in single attempt without needing to pull self up with arms	Able to get object and get upright in single attempt but needs to pull self up with arms or hold on to something for support	Unable to bend down or unable to get upright after bending down or takes multiple attempts to upright
Sitting down	Able to sit down in one smoother movement	Needs to use arms to guide self into chair or not a smooth movement	Falls into chair, misjudges distances (lands off center)

[a]The patient begins this assessment seated in a hard, straight-backed, armless chair.
[b]Unsteadiness defined as grabbing at objects for support, staggering, moving feet, or more than minimal trunk sway.
ROM, range of motion.
From Tinetti ME: Performance oriented assessment mobility problems in elderly patients, *J Am Geriar Soc* 34(2):119–126, 1986.

TABLE **17.15**

Performance-Oriented Assessment of Gait[a]

Components[b]	OBSERVATION	
	Normal	Abnormal
Initiation of gait (patient asked to begin walking down hallway)	Begins walking immediately without observable hesitation; initiation of gait is single, smooth motion	Hesitates; multiple attempts; initiation of gait not a smooth motion
Step height (begin observing after first few steps: observe one foot, then the other; observe from side)	Swing foot completely clears floor but by no more than 1–2 inches	Swing foot is not completely raised off floor (may hear scraping) or is raised too high (>1–2 inches)[c]
Step length (observe distance between two steps of stance foot and heel of swing foot; observe from side; do not judge first few or last few steps; observe one side at a time)	At least the length of individual's foot between the stance toe and swing heel (step length usually longer but foot length provides basis for observation)	Step length less than described under normal[c]
Step symmetry (observe the middle part of the path not the first or last steps; observe from side; observe distance between heel of each swing foot and toe of each stance foot)	Step length same or nearly same on both sides for most step cycles	Step length varies between sides or patient advances with same foot with every step
Step continuity	Begins raising heel of one foot (toe off) as heel of other foot touches the floor (heel strike); no breaks or stops in stride; step lengths equal over most cycles	Places entire foot (heel and toe) on floor before beginning to raise other foot; or stops completely between steps; or step length varies over cycles[c]
Path deviation (observe from behind; observe one foot over several strides; observe in relation to line on floor [e.g., tiles] if possible; difficult to assess if patient uses a walker)	Foot follows close to straight line as patient advances	Foot deviates from side to side or toward one direction[d]

TABLE **17.15**

Performance-Oriented Assessment of Gait[a]—cont'd

Components[b]	OBSERVATION	
	Normal	Abnormal
Trunk stability (observe from behind; side to side motion of trunk may be a normal gait pattern, need to differentiate this from instability)	Trunk does not sway; knees or back are not flexed; arms are not abducted in effort to maintain stability	Any of preceding features present[d]
Walk stance (observe from behind)	Feet should almost touch as one passes other	Feet apart with stepping[e]
Turning while walking	No staggering, turning continuous with walking; and steps are continuous while turning	Staggers; stops before initiating turn; or steps are discontinuous

[a]The patient stands with examiner at end of obstacle-free hallway. Patient uses usual walking aid. Examiner then asks patient to walk down hallway at his or her usual pace. Examiner observes one component of gait at a time (analogous to heart examination). For some components, the examiner walks behind the patient; for other components, the examiner walks next to patient. May require several trips to complete.
[b]Also ask patient to walk at a "more rapid than usual" pace and observe whether any walking aid is used correctly.
[c]Abnormal gait finding may reflect a primary neurologic or musculoskeletal problem directly related to the finding or reflect a compensatory maneuver for other, more remote problem.
[d]Abnormality may be corrected by walking aid (e.g., cane); observe with and without walking aid if possible.
[e]Abnormal finding is usually a compensatory maneuver rather than a primary problem.
From Tinetti ME: Performance oriented assessment of mobility problems in elderly patients, *J Am Geriatr Soc* 34(2):119–126, 1986.

a high rate of speed.[3] Agility and balance tests are often measured by time or accuracy (e.g., correct two out of three).[3,176]

Agility and Balance Tests

- Carioca
- Run-and-cut drills
- Backpedal and throw at stationary or moving target
- Kick at stationary or moving target (different distances)
- One-arm spin
- Shuttle drills
- Pivoting drills
- Blocking drills
- Figure-eight running
- Front-to-back and side-to-side hops
- Sidestep tests
- Beam-walking tests

Sharpened Romberg Test[152,155]

1. With eyes open, stand with feet together for 10 seconds.
2. Repeat step 1 with eyes closed.
3. With eyes open, place one foot halfway in front of the other for 10 seconds.
4. Repeat step 3 with eyes closed.
5. With eyes open, place one foot directly in front of the other for 10 seconds.
6. Repeat step 5 with eyes closed.

Maturation and Growth

Maturation assessment is a method of determining how far a patient has progressed toward physical maturity. It also helps to identify periods of rapid growth.[174,177,178] This is especially important where there is a possibility that there will be stress applied to a growth plate, which is commonly the "weak link" in traumatic injury. That is, during a rapid growth spurt period, the growth plate is weaker and more susceptible to injury than the ligaments and/or capsule. Maturation profiling should not be used to push children into specific activities unless chosen by the child, and it should not be used to exclude a child unless documented evidence demonstrates unacceptable risk for the child.[179] In adolescents, growth patterns can have an effect on participation in activities, exercise, and sports and may affect injury patterns. For example, a growth spurt for a gymnast may adversely affect balance and flexibility. Pubertal growth accounts for 20% to 25% of final adult height, and pubertal weight gain accounts for 50% of ideal adult weight.[107]

Skeletal development is usually measured by wrist x-rays, using the *Radiographic Atlas of Skeletal Development of the Wrist and Hand,* by W. W. Greulich and S. U. Pyle,[180] for interpretation.

The most common method of measuring maturation in males and females is the Tanner scale.[45,174,181] The five stages of the Tanner scale are based on pictorial standards of genitalia and pubic hair for males and breast development and pubic hair for females (Figs. 17.2–17.4 and Table 17.16). Some people have recommended that collision sports not be allowed for boys until they reach level 5 of development. For females, onset of menstruation is another suitable index of maturity and maturation.

Body Composition and Anthropometry

Body composition profiling is designed to provide a relatively detailed analysis of an individual's muscle, fat, and bone mass.[178,182] Anthropometry may be used to determine the individual's body type (mesomorphic, endomorphic, ectomorphic) to see whether he or she is properly

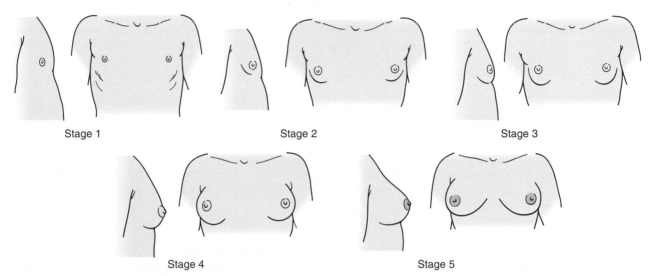

Fig. 17.2 Breast development in girls. The development of the mammae can be divided into five stages. In stage 1, only the nipple is raised above the level of the breast (as in the child). In stage 2, the budding stage, there is bud-shaped elevation of the areola. On palpation, a fairly hard button can be felt that is disc or cherry shaped. The areola is increased in diameter, and the surrounding area is slightly elevated. In stage 3, there is further elevation of the mammae; the areolar diameter is further increased, and the shape of mammae is visibly feminine. In stage 4, fat deposits increase, and the areola forms a secondary elevation above that of the breast. This secondary mound occurs in approximately half of all girls and in some cases persists in adulthood. In stage 5, the adult stage, the areola usually subsides to the level of the breast and is strongly pigmented. (Redrawn from Halpern B, Blackburn T, Incremona B, et al: Preparticipation sports physicals. In Zachazewski JE, Magee DJ, Quillen WS, editors: *Athletic injuries and rehabilitation*, Philadelphia, 1996, WB Saunders, p 855.)

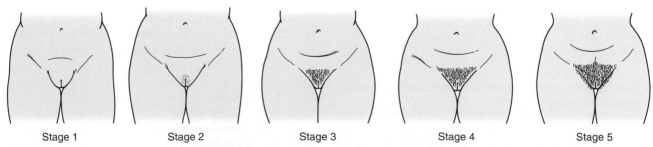

Fig. 17.3 Pubic hair development in females. In the development of pubic hair, five stages can be distinguished. In stage 1, there is no growth of pubic hair. In stage 2, initial, scarcely pigmented hair is present, especially along the labia. In stage 3, sparse dark, visibly pigmented, curly pubic hair is present on the labia. In stage 4, hair that is adult in type but not in extent is present. In stage 5, there is lateral spreading (type and spread of hair are adult). (Redrawn from Halpern B, Blackburn T, Incremona B, et al: Preparticipation sports physicals. In Zachazewski JE, Magee DJ, Quillen WS, editors: *Athletic injuries and rehabilitation*, Philadelphia, 1996, WB Saunders, p 855.)

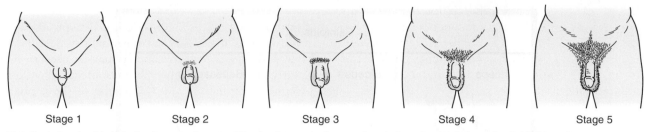

| Stage 1 | Stage 2 | Stage 3 | Stage 4 | Stage 5 |

Fig. 17.4 Genital and pubic hair development in males. The development of external genitalia and pubic hair can be divided into five stages. In stage 1, the testes, scrotum, and penis are the same size and shape as in the young child and there is no growth of pubic hair (hair in pubic area is no different from that on the rest of the abdomen). In stage 2, there is enlargement of the scrotum and testes. The skin of the scrotum becomes redder, thinner, and wrinkled. The penis has not grown (or just slightly so). Pubic hair is slightly pigmented. In stage 3, there is enlargement of the penis, especially in length, further enlargement of testes, and descent of scrotum. Dark, definitely pigmented, curly pubic hair is present around the base of penis. In stage 4, there is continued enlargement of the penis and sculpturing of the glans with increased pigmentation of the scrotum. This stage is sometimes best described as not quite adult. Pubic hair is definitely adult in type but not in extent (no further than the inguinal fold). In stage 5, the adult stage, the scrotum is ample and the penis reaches almost to the bottom of the scrotum. Pubic hair spreads to the medial surface of the thighs but not upward. In 80% of men, hair spreads along the linea alba. (Redrawn from Halpern B, Blackburn T, Incremona B, et al: Preparticipation sports physicals. In Zachazewski JE, Magee DJ, Quillen WS, editors: *Athletic injuries and rehabilitation*, Philadelphia, 1996, WB Saunders, p 855.)

TABLE **17.16**

Maturity Staging Guidelines

Boys' Stage	Public Hair	Penis	Testis	Girls' Stage	Public Hair	Breasts
1	None	Preadolescent (infantile)	–	1	Preadolescent (none)	Preadolescent (no germinal button)
2	Slight, long, slight pigmentation	Slight enlargement	Enlarged scrotum, pink slight rugae	2	Sparse, lightly pigmented, straight medial border of labia	Breast and papilla elevated as small mound; areolar diameter increased
3	Darker, starts to curl, small amount	Longer	Larger	3	Darker, beginning to curl, increased	Breast and areola enlarged; no contour separation
4	Coarse, curly, adult type, but less quantity	Increase in glans size and breadth of penis	Larger, darker scrotum	4	Coarse, curly, abundant, but less than adult	Areola and papilla form secondary mound
5	Adult, spread to inner thighs	Adult	Adult	5	Adult female triangle and spread to medial surface	Mature, nipple projects, areola part of general breast contour

From Tanner IM: *Growth and adolescence*, Oxford, 1962, Blackwell Scientific.

suited for the desired activity, exercise, sport, or position played in a sport.

Anthropometry also involves body fat measurements, such as skinfold measurements or underwater weighing.[183] Of the two, skinfold measurement is more common because it is easier and faster. Seven skinfold sites are most commonly used (Fig. 17.5), although some people believe that measurement at three sites is sufficient (i.e., a different three for males and females).[183] Most males should fall below 12% to 15% body fat. Endurance athletes (e.g., distance runners, gymnasts, wrestlers) are often below

7%. Football, baseball, and soccer players average 10% to 12%.[184] No one should be below 5% body fat. If the percentage of body fat is greater than the upper normal limit of 14% for males and 17% for females, the patient should be put on a weight-loss program or on weight training to increase lean body mass; but again, this depends on the activity in which the patient wishes to participate.

Other methods of body composition measurement include girth measurements, bone diameter measurements, ultrasound measurement, and radiographic measurements of the arm.[182]

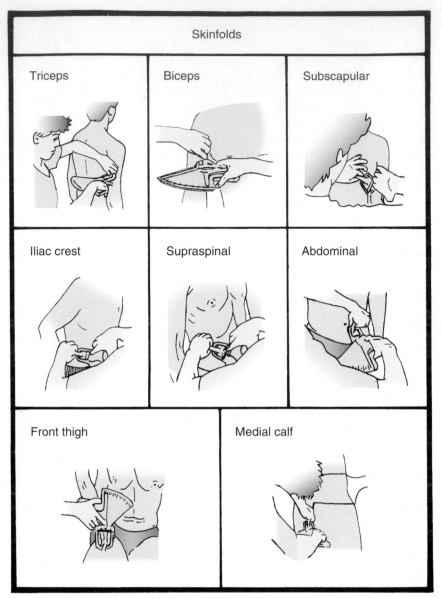

Fig. 17.5 Skinfold sites for measuring body fat. (Reprinted, by permission, from Ross WD, Marfell-Jones MJ: Kinanthropometry. In MacDougal JD, Wenger HA, Green HJ, editors: *Physiological testing of the high performance athlete*, ed 2, Champaign, IL, 1991, Human Kinetics, p 238.)

Tests for Return to Activity Following Injury

Tests for return to activity should attempt to replicate the activity to which the patient is returning. They should be functional—including the testing of such parameters as strength, endurance, flexibility, and proprioception—to decrease the chance of the patient being reinjured. The tests are more commonly used for individuals returning to sport activities but could be modified to test an individual's functional level. For people who are less active, different timing or load tests could be used. For more sedentary people, numeric rating scales or walking tests

(see Chapter 11 for examples) could be used. The following tests are simply examples of functional tests that may be used to test a patient for return to activity.

Forward Step-Down Test.[185] This test is used to determine eccentric muscle strength for lowering the body to the ground. If a force plate is used, a vertical impact score that is greater on the affected side indicates loss of motor control coinciding with knee extensor weakness. The patient is asked to step down from an 8-inch (20-cm) step. As the patient does so, the examiner should watch for such things as contralateral hip drop, ipsilateral hip hike, increased knee valgus, and increased plantar flexion (reaching), which may indicate imbalances or weaknesses.

Yo-Yo Endurance Test (Also Called the Beep, Bleep, Progressive Shuttle Run, and the Leger Shuttle Run).[186,187] This is a "field" test used to evaluate physical capacity and basic fitness involving the lower limb. For the test, two markers (pylons) are placed 20 m (66 feet) apart and an audio compact disc (CD) or metronome is used to control the speed, which is regularly increased over time (i.e., a "beep" occurs at set intervals when the individual should be at the marker) until the patient can no longer maintain a specific speed (Fig. 17.6A). The test involves running continuously between two points that are 20 m apart while the interval between successive beeps decreases, forcing the individual to increase his or her velocity over the test until he or she can no longer remain synchronized with the beep; that is, the individual reaches each pylon at a beep, runs around pylon, and starts to return to go back the other way. The recording normally is structured with 23 "levels," with the time to complete each interval varying from 68 to 61 seconds (to complete 20 m). The highest level attained before failing to keep up is recorded as the test score. Test results show the distance covered and can be related to the specific activity to which the individual wants to return. The test usually takes 5 to 15 minutes to complete.

Yo-Yo Intermittent Endurance Test.[185] This test is set up as described earlier, but the patient does intermittent intense exercise repeatedly (Fig. 17.6B). This too can be geared to the specific activity to which the patient is returning. The test lasts 10 to 20 minutes and involves activity for 5- to 18-second intervals interspersed with 5-second rest periods. It evaluates the patient's ability to perform repeated activity intervals over time. It is a test of the aerobic system and is a good test for sports such as tennis, soccer, hockey, and basketball.

Yo-Yo Intermittent Recovery Test (Yo-Yo 1R2 Test).[185] This test is set up as described earlier and lasts 2 to 15 minutes; it is designed to test the anaerobic system and determines the patient's ability to recover after intense exercise. Between each exercise bout (5 to 15 seconds), there is a 10-second pause. The number of repetitions is measured and can be equated to the activity repetitions the individual will do when returning to his or her specific activity. It is a good test for sports such as football, soccer, and hockey.

Sports Participation

For any primary care evaluation, the physician is the final arbitrator. Any decision as to whether someone should be allowed to work or participate in an activity or as to the patient's functional level must be based on accurate

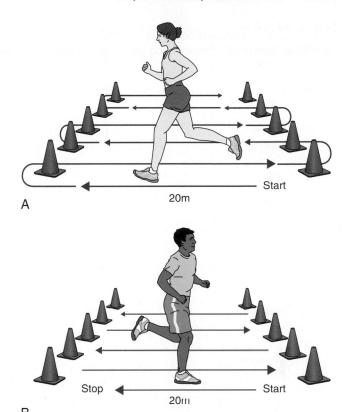

Fig. 17.6 (A) Beep or yo-yo test. The individual times the run so that he or she arrives at the pylon at the beep, runs around pylon, and runs back to the other pylon repeating the process until he or she no longer keeps up with the beep. (B) Beep or yo-yo intermittent test. The individual times the runs so that he or she arrives at the pylon at the beep and has a 5 s rest period before running back to the other pylon repeating the process until he or she no longer keeps up with the beep. The time to complete the interval is decreased as the test progresses while the rest period remains the same.

diagnosis of the condition, knowledge of the disease process involved in the condition, knowledge of the job or sport, knowledge of the physical needs of the patient and the activity, and direct evaluation of the individual.[134] The examiner must also keep in mind the rights of handicapped people and the limits of informed consent. Although standards are often given for participation, in the end the examiner must make his or her final decision on an individual basis, being primarily concerned with the health and safety of the patient.

Any individual with a solitary paired organ—such as an eye, kidney, or testicle—should not take part in contact sports, especially if the organ is abnormal. Children should be channeled into noncontact sports. High-caliber or older athletes know the rules and should make their own decisions. Table 17.17 lists conditions that are contraindications to specific sports, and the levels of these activities can be extrapolated to the physical stresses of everyday jobs.[5,45]

TABLE **17.17**

Conditions Commonly Disqualifying an Individual from Participation in Sports

Conditions	TYPE OF SPORT			
	Collision[a]	Contact[b]	Noncontact[c]	Others[d]
Eyes				
Absence of one eye	??	??	–	–
Congenital glaucoma	X	X	–	–
Retinal detachment	X	X	–	–
Severe myopia	?	?	–	–
Musculoskeletal				
Acute inflammatory conditions	X	X	X	X
Spinal instability	X	X	?	?
Congenital or growth abnormalities that are incompatible with demands of sport	X	X	X	–
Chronic or unhealed conditions (unless cleared by physician)	X	X	X	X
Neurological				
Uncontrolled convulsive disorder	X	X	X	?
Controlled convulsive disorder	?	?	?	?
Repeated concussions	X	X	–	–
Serious head trauma	X	X	–	–
Previous head surgery	X	X	–	–
Transient quadriplegia (unless cleared by physician)	X	X	–	–
Cardiovascular				
Acute infection	X	X	X	X
Cardiomegaly	X	X	X	X
Enlarged spleen	X	X	–	–
Hemorrhage (bleeding) disorders	X	X	X	–
Heart abnormalities (unless cleared by cardiologist)	X	X	X	X
Organic hypertension	X	X	X	X
Previous heart surgery (unless cleared by cardiologist)	X	X	X	X
Pulmonary				
Acute infection	X	X	X	X
Pulmonary insufficiency	X	X	X	X
Uncontrolled asthma (unless cleared by pulmonary physician)	X	X	X	X
Urogenital				
Absence of one kidney	??	??	–	–
Acute infection	X	X	X	X
Enlarged liver	X	X	–	–
Hernia (inguinal or femoral, unless cleared by physician)	X	X	X	–
Renal disease	X	X	X	X
Absent or undescended testicle (unless cleared by physician)	??	??	–	–
Gastrointestinal				
Jaundice	X	X	X	X

TABLE **17.17**

Conditions Commonly Disqualifying an Individual from Participation in Sports —cont'd

Conditions	TYPE OF SPORT			
	Collision[a]	Contact[b]	Noncontact[c]	Others[d]
Dermatological (Integumentary)				
Acute infection (e.g., boils, herpes simplex, impetigo)	X	X	?	?
General or Systemic Disease				
Acute systemic infection or illness	?	?	?	?
Uncontrolled diabetes	X	X	X	X
Physical immaturity (relative to level of competition)	X	X	–	–

[a]Examples include boxing, football, hockey (ice and field), rugby.
[b]Examples include baseball, basketball, lacrosse, martial arts, rodeo, soccer, volleyball, wrestling.
[c]Examples include dance, rowing, skiing, squash, swimming, tennis, track, cross country.
[d]Examples include archery, bowling, golf, shooting, track and field events.
?, Depends on individual case and clearance by physician; ??, athlete may compete if athlete knows risks and informed consent form is completed (protective equipment may be necessary); X, participation prohibited; –, participation permitted.
Adapted from the Committee on Medical Aspects of Sports: Medical evaluation of the athlete: a guide, American Medical Association, ©1966.

References

1. Johnson MP, von Nieda K, Greathouse DG. Primary Care: physical therapy models. In: Boissonnault WG ed. *Primary care for the physical therapist. Examination and triage.* 2nd ed. St. Louis: Elsevier; 2011.
2. Declaration of Alma-Ata. *International Conference on Primary Health Care.* Vol. 2009. Geveva: World Health Organization; 1978.
3. Sanders B, Nemeth WC. Preparticipation physical examination. *J Orthop Sports Phys Ther.* 1996;23: 144–163.
4. American Academy of Orthopaedic Surgeons. *Athletic Training and Sports Medicine.* Rosemont, IL: The Academy; 1991.
5. Harvey J. The preparticipation examination of the child athlete. *Clin Sports Med.* 1982;1:353–369.
6. Clyne ME, Forlenza M. Consumer-focused preadmission testing: a paradigm shift. *J Nurs Care Qual.* 1997;11(3):9–15.
7. Daker-White G, Carr AJ, Harvey I, et al. A randomized controlled trial: shifting boundaries of doctors and physiotherapists in orthopedic outpatient departments. *J Epidemiol Community Health.* 1999;53:643–650.
8. Hattam P, Smeatham A. Evaluation of an orthopedic screening service in primary care. *Clin Perform Qual Health Care.* 1999;7:121–124.
9. Breen A, Carr E, Mann E, et al. Acute back pain management in primary care: a qualitative pilot study of the feasibility of a nurse-led service in general practice. *J Nurs Manage.* 2004;12:201–209.
10. Moore JH, Goss DL, Baxter RE, et al. Clinical diagnostic accuracy and magnetic resonance imaging of patients referred by physical therapists, orthopedic surgeons and nonorthopedic providers. *J Orthop Sports Phys Ther.* 2005;35:67–71.
11. Belthur MV, Clegg J, Strange A. A physiotherapy specialist clinic in paediatric orthopaedics: is it effective? *Postgrad Med J.* 2003;79(938):699–702.
12. Hettam P, Smeatham A. Evaluation of an orthopaedic screening service in primary care. *Clin Perform Qual Health Care.* 1999;7(3):121–124.
13. Hendriks EJ, Kerssens JJ, Nelson RM, et al. Onetime physical therapist consultation in primary health care. *Phys Ther.* 2003;83(10):918–931.
14. Maddison P, Jones J, Breslin A, et al. Improved access and targeting of musculoskeletal services in northwest Wales: targeting early access to musculoskeletal services (TEAMS) programme. *BMJ.* 2004;329:1325–1327.
15. Murphy BP, Greathouse D, Matsui I. Primary care physical therapy practice. *J Orthop Sports Phys Ther.* 2005;35(11):699–707.
16. Pinnington MA, Miller J, Stanley I. An evaluation of prompt access to physiotherapy in the management of low back pain in primary care. *Fam Pract.* 2004;21(4):372–380.
17. Rymaszewski LA, Sharma S, McGill PE, et al. A team approach to musculoskeletal disorders. *Ann R Coll Surg Engl.* 2005;87(3):174–180.
18. Weale AE, Bannister GC. Who should see orthopaedic outpatients – physiotherapists or surgeons? *Ann R Coll Surg Engl.* 1995;77(suppl 2):71–73.
19. International Olympic Committee. *Lausanne Recommendations: Sudden Cardiovascular Death in Sports—Preparticipation Screening.* The Committee; 2004.
20. Hall K, Zalman B. Evaluation and management of apparent life-threatening events in children. *Am Fam Physician.* 2005;71:2301–2308.
21. Harrington JT, Dopf CA, Chalgren CS. Implementing guidelines for interdisciplinary care of low back pain: a critical role for pre-appointment management of specialty referrals. *Jt Comm J Qual Improv.* 2001;27:651–663.
22. Lynch JR, Gardner GC, Parsons RR. Musculoskeletal workload vs. musculoskeletal clinical confidence among primary care physicians in rural practice. *Am J Orthop.* 2005;34:487–492.
23. Eathorne SW. Medical problems in a sports medicine setting. *Med Clin North Am.* 1994;78:479–503.
24. Vlek JF, Vierhout WP, Knottnerus JA, et al. A randomized controlled trial of joint consultations with general practitioners and cardiologists in primary care. *Br J Gen Pract.* 2003;53:108–112.
25. Moore MN. Orthopedic pitfalls in emergency medicine. *South Med J.* 1988;81:371–378.
26. Johnson MP, Metrauz S. The prevalence of musculoskeletal conditions among the adult U.S. population: considerations for physical therapists. *HPA J.* 2009;9(2):1–8.
27. Lubeck DP. The costs of musculoskeletal disease: health needs assessment and health economics. *Best Pract Res Clin Rheumatol.* 2003;17(3):529–539.
28. National Center for Health Statistics. *Summary Health Statistics for U.S. Adults: National Health Interview Survey, 2004.* Hyattsville, MD: National Center for Health Statistics; 2006.
29. Yelin E, Herrndorf A, Trupin L, Sonneborn D. A national study of medical care expenditures for musculoskeletal conditions: the impact of health insurance and managed care. *Arthritis Rheum.* 2001;44(5):1160–1169.
30. Yelin E. Cost of musculoskeletal diseases: impact of work disability and functional decline. *J Rheumatol Suppl.* 2003;68:8–11.
31. Woolf AD, Pfleger B. Burden of major musculoskeletal conditions. *Bull World Health Organ.* 2003;81(9):646–656.
32. Superko HR, Bernauer E, Voss J. Effects of a mandatory health screening and physical maintenance program for law enforcement officers. *Phys Sportsmed.* 1988;16:99–109.
33. Binda C. Precamp physical exams: their value may be greater than you think. *Phys Sportsmed.* 1989;17:167–169.
34. Gurry M, Pappas A, Michaels J, et al. A comprehensive preseason fitness evaluation for professional baseball players. *Phys Sportsmed.* 1985;13:63–74.
35. Metzel JD. The adolescent preparticipation physical examination—is it helpful? *Clin Sports Med.* 2000;19:577–592.
36. Kligman EW, Hewitt MJ, Crowell DL. Recommending exercise to healthy older adults – the preparticipation evaluation and exercise prescription. *Phys Sportsmed.* 1999;27(11):42–62.
37. Glover DW, Maron DJ, Matheson GO. The preparticipation physical examination—steps toward consensus and uniformity. *Phys Sportsmed.* 1999;27:29–34.
38. Peltz JE, Haskell WL, Matheson GO. A comprehensive and cost-effective preparticipation exam implemented on the world wide web. *Med Sci Sports Exerc.* 1999;31:1727–1740.

39. Pedraza J, Jardeleza JA. The preparticipation physical examination. *Prim Care.* 2013;40(7):791–799.

40. Scheitel SM, Boland BJ, Wollan PC, et al. Patient-physician agreement about medical diagnoses and cardiovascular risk factors in the ambulatory general medical examination. *Mayo Clin Proc.* 1996;71:1131–1137.

41. Tanji TL. The preparticipation exam: special concerns for the Special Olympics. *Phys Sportsmed.* 1991;19:61–68.

42. Hudson PB. Preparticipation screening of Special Olympics athletes. *Phys Sportsmed.* 1988;16:97–104.

43. Bickley LS. *Bates' Guide To Physical Examination And History Taking.* Philadelphia: Lippincott Williams & Wilkins; 1999.

44. Goodman CC, Snyder TE. *Differential Diagnosis In Physical Therapy.* Philadelphia: WB Saunders; 1995.

45. McKeag DB. Preparticipation screening of the potential athlete. *Clin Sports Med.* 1989;8:373–397.

46. Hunter SC. Preparticipation physical examination. In: Griffin LY, ed. *Orthopedic knowledge Update: Sports Medicine.* Rosemont, IL: American Academy of Orthopaedic Surgeons; 1994.

47. Woolf AD. History and physical examination. *Best Pract Res Clin Rheum.* 2003;17:381–402.

48. Yazici Y, Gibofsky A. A diagnostic approach to musculoskeletal pain. *Office Rheum.* 1999;2(2):1–10.

49. Cayley WE. Diagnosing the cause of chest pain. *Am Fam Physician.* 2005;72:2012–2021.

50. Committee on Sports Medicine. Recommendations for participation in competitive sports. *Pediatrics.* 1988;81:737–739.

51. Stanley K. Preparticipation evaluation of the young athlete. In: Stanitski CL, DeLee JC, Drez D, eds. *Pediatric and Adolescent Sports Medicine.* Philadelphia: WB Saunders; 1994.

52. Smilkstein G. Health evaluation of high school athletes. *Phys Sportsmed.* 1981;9:73–80.

53. Heidt RS, Sweeterman LM, Carlonas RL, et al. Avoidance of soccer injuries with preseason conditioning. *Am J Sports Med.* 2000;28:659–662.

54. Tirabassi J, Brou L, Khodaee M, et al. Epidemiology of high school sports-related injuries resulting in medical disqualification: 2005-2006 through 2013-2014 academic years. *Am J Sports Med.* 2016;44(11):2925–2932.

55. Carek PJ, Futrell M, Hueston WJ. The preparticipation physical examination history: who has the correct answers? *Clin J Sports Med.* 1999;9:124–128.

56. Duffy FD. Dialogue: the core clinical skill. *Ann Intern Med.* 1998;128(2):139–141.

57. Goodman CC, Snyder TE. *Differential Diagnosis in Physical Therapy.* 3rd ed. Philadelphia: WB Saunders; 2009.

58. Simpson M, Buckman R, Stewart M, et al. Doctor-patient communication: the Toronto consensus statement. *BMJ.* 1991;303:1385–1387.

59. Rosenstein AH, O'Daniel M. Disruptive behavior and clinical outcomes: perceptions of nurses and physicians. *Am J Nurs.* 2005;105(1):54–56.

60. Rosenstein AH, O'Daniel M. A survey of the impact of disruptive behaviors and communication defects in patient safety. *Jt Comm J Qual Patient Saf.* 2008;34(8):464–471.

61. Roter DL, Hall JA, Kern DE, et al. Improving physicians' interviewing skills and reducing patients' emotional distress. A randomized clinical trial. *Arch Intern Med.* 1995;155(17):1877–1884.

62. Haggman S, Maher CG, Refshauge KM. Screening for symptoms of depression by physical therapists managing low back pain. *Phys Ther.* 2004;84:1157–1166.

63. Grotle M, Brox JI, Veierod MB, et al. Clinical course and prognostic factors in acute low back pain: patients consulting primary care for the first time. *Spine.* 2005;30(8):976–982.

64. Waddell G, Main CJ. Illness behavior. In: Waddell G, ed. *The Back Pain Revolution.* New York: Churchill Livingstone; 1998.

65. Farnell S, Maxwell L, Tan S, et al. Temperature measurement: comparison of non-invasive methods used in adult critical care. *J Clin Nurs.* 2005;14:632–639.

66. Carroll M. An evaluation of temperature measurement. *Nurs Standard.* 2000;14:39–43.

67. Kaplan NM, Deveraux RB, Miller HS. *Systemic hyperextension. Med Sci Sports Exerc.* 1994;26:S268–S270.

68. Zabetakis PM. Profiling the hypertensive patient in sports. *Clin Sports Med.* 1984;3:137–152.

69. Staats PS, Argoff CE, Brewer R, et al. Neuropathic pain: incorporating new consensus guidelines into the reality of clinical practice. *Adv Stud Med.* 2004;4:S550–S566.

70. Potter RG, Jones JM. The evolution of chronic pain among patients with musculoskeletal problems: a pilot study in primary care. *Br J Gen Pract.* 1992;42:462–464.

71. Lavie CJ, Milani RV, Ventura HO. Obesity and cardiovascular disease: risk factor, paradox, and impact of weight loss. *J Am Coll Cardiol.* 2009;53(21):1925–1932.

72. Nelson MA. The child athlete with chronic disease. In: Stanitski CL, DeLee JC, Drez D, eds. *Pediatric and Adolescent Sports Medicine.* Philadelphia: WB Saunders; 1994.

73. Bonci CM, Ryan R. *Preparticipation Screening in Intercollegiate Athletics: Postgraduate Advances in Sports Medicine.* Philadelphia: University of Pennsylvania Medical School and Forum Medicum; 1988.

74. Halpern B, Blackburn T, Incremona B, et al. Preparticipation sports physicals. In: Zachazewski JE, Magee DJ, Quillen WS, eds. *Athletic Injuries and Rehabilitation.* Philadelphia: WB Saunders; 1996.

75. Godges J, Wong MS, Boissonnault WG. Symptoms investigation, Part I: chief complaint by body region. In: *Boissonnault WG. Primary Care for the Physical Therapist. Examination and Triage.* 2nd ed. St. Louis: Elsevier; 2011.

76. Bruce M, Rosenstein N, Capparella J, et al. Risk factors for meningococcal disease in college students. *JAMA.* 2001;286:688–693.

77. Wall EJ. Practical primary pediatric orthopedics. *Nurs Clin North Am.* 2000;35:95–113.

78. Barth WF. Office evaluation of the patient with musculoskeletal complaints. *Am J Med.* 1997;102(suppl 1A):3S–10S.

79. Calkins E. Rheumatic diseases in the elderly—finding a way through the maze. *Prim Care.* 1982;9:181–195.

80. Davis AE. Primary care management of chronic musculoskeletal pain. *Nurse Pract.* 1996;21:74–82.

81. Pimentel L. Orthopedic trauma: office management of major joint injury. *Med Clin North Am.* 2006;90:355–382.

82. Gomez JE, Landry GL, Bernhardt DT. Critical evaluation of the 2-minute orthopedic screening examination. *Am J Dis Child.* 1993;147:1109–1113.

83. Strong WB, Steed D. Cardiovascular evaluation of the young athlete. *Pediatr Clin North Am.* 1982;29:1325–1339.

84. Huston TP, Puffer JC, Rodney WM. The athletic heart syndrome. *N Engl J Med.* 1985;313:24–32.

85. McGrew CA. Clinical implications of the AHA preparticipation cardiovascular screening guidelines. *Athletic Ther Today.* 2000;5:52–56.

86. Fuller CM. Cost effectiveness analysis of screening of high school athletes for risk of sudden cardiac death. *Med Sci Sports Exerc.* 2000;32:887–890.

87. Maron BJ, Pollac DC, Kaplan JA, et al. Blunt impact to the chest leading to sudden death from cardiac arrest during sports activities. *N Engl J Med.* 1995;333:337–342.

88. Potera C. AHA Panel outlines sudden death screening standards. *Phys Sportsmed.* 1996;24(10):27–28.

89. Fuller CM, McNulty CM, Spring DA, et al. Prospective screening of 5,615 high school athletes for risk of sudden cardiac death. *Med Sci Sports Exerc.* 1997;29:1131–1138.

90. Blankfield RP, Finkelhor RS, Alexander JJ, et al. Etiology and diagnosis of bilateral leg edema in primary care. *Am J Med.* 1998;105:192–197.

91. Salem DN, Isner JM. Cardiac screening in athletes. *Orthop Clin North Am.* 1980;11:687–695.

92. Keffer JH. The cardiac profile and proposed practice guidelines for acute ischemic heart disease. *Am J Clin Pathol.* 1997;107:398–409.

93. Heger JJ. Ventricular arrhythmias: guidelines for primary care management. *J Indiana St Med Assoc.* 1983;76:819–822.

94. Pflieger KL, Strong WB. Screening for heart murmurs: what's normal and what's not. *Phys Sportsmed.* 1992;20:71–81.

95. Braden DS, Strong WB. Preparticipation screening for sudden cardiac death in high school and college athletes. *Phys Sportsmed.* 1988;16:128–144.

96. Cavell RM. The exercise treadmill test for diagnosis and prognosis of coronary artery disease. *J La State Med Soc.* 1995;147:197–201.

97. Shinozaki T, Hasegawa T, Yano E. Ankle-arm index as an indicator of atherosclerosis: its application as a screening method. *J Clin Epidemiol.* 1998;51:1263–1269.

98. Newman AB, Siscovick DS, Manolio TA, et al. Atherosclerosis: ankle-arm index as a marker of atherosclerosis in the cardiovascular health study. *Circulation.* 1993;88:837–845.

99. Hirsh J, Lee AY. How we diagnose and treat deep venous thrombosis. *Blood.* 2002;99(9):3102–3110.

100. Boissonnault WG. Review of systems. In: *Boissonnault WG. Primary Care for the Physical Therapist. Examination and Triage.* St. Louis: Elsevier; 2011.

101. Belman MJ, King RR. Pulmonary profiling in exercise. *Clin Sports Med.* 1984;3:119–136.

102. Ross RG. The prevalence of reversible airway obstruction in professional football players. *Med Sci Sports Exerc.* 2000;32:1985–1989.

103. Rundell KW, Wilber RL, Szmedra L, et al. Exercise-induced asthma screening of elite athletes: field versus laboratory exercise challenge. *Med Sci Sports Exerc.* 2000;32:309–316.

104. Goldman L. Cardiovascular diseases. In: Goldman L, Bennett JC, eds. *Cecil Textbook of Medicine.* 21st ed. Philadelphia: Saunders; 2000.

105. Goroll AH, Mulley AG. *Primary Care Medicine: Office Evaluation and Management of the Adult Patient.* 5th ed. Philadelphia: Lippincott Williams and Wilkins; 2006.

106. Swartz MH. *Textbook of Physical Diagnosis.* 5th ed. Philadelphia: Saunders; 2006.

107. Johnson MD. Tailoring the preparticipation exam to female athletes. *Phys Sportsmed.* 1992;20:61–72.

108. Slavin JL. Assessing athletes' nutritional status: making it part of the sports medicine physical. *Phys Sportsmed.* 1991;19:79–94.

109. Joy E, De Souza MJ, Nattiv A, et al. 2014 Female Athlete Triad coalition consensus statement on treatment and return to play of the Female Athlete Triad. *Curr Sports Med Rep.* 2014;13(4):219–232.

110. Committee on Adolescent Health Care. Committee Opinion No. 702: Female Athlete Triad. *Obstet Gynecol.* 2017;129(6):e160–e167.

111. Melin A, Tornberg AB, Skouby S, et al. The LEAF questionnaire: a screening tool for the identification of female athletes at risk for the female athlete triad. *Br J Sports Med.* 2013;48(7):540–545.

112. Richter JM. Evaluation of gastrointestinal bleeding. In: Goroll AH, ed. *Mulley AG: Primary Care Medicine: Office Evaluation and Management of the Adult Patient.* 5th ed. Philadelphia: Lippincott Williams and Wilkins; 2006.

113. Fang LS. Evaluation of the patient with hematuria. In: Goroll AH, ed. *Mulley AG: Primary Care Medicine: Office Evaluation and Management of the Adult Patient.* 5th ed. Philadelphia: Lippincott Williams and Wilkins; 2006.

114. Khosla RK. Detecting sexually transmitted disease—a new role for urinalysis in the preparticipation exam? *Phys Sportsmed.* 1995;23(1):77–80.

115. Dorsen PJ. Should athletes with one eye, kidney or testicle play contact sports? *Phys Sportsmed.* 1986;14:130–138.

116. Lombardo JA. Preparticipation physical evaluation. *Prim Care.* 1984;11:3–21.

117. American Academy of Pediatrics. Climatic heat stress and the exercising child. *Phys Sportsmed.* 1983;11:155–159.

118. Henry C. Heatstroke. *Crit Care Update.* 1983:30–35.

119. American College of Sports Medicine Position Statement. Prevention of heat injuries during distance running. *Am J Sports Med.* 1975;3:194–196.

120. Bota DP, Ferreira FL, Melot C, et al. Body temperature alterations in the critically ill. *Intensive Care Med.* 2004;30:811–816.

121. Poumadere M, Mays C, LeMer S, et al. The 2003 heat wave in France: dangerous climate change here and now. *Risk Anal.* 2005;25:1483–1494.

122. Moran DS. Potential applications of heat and cold stress indices to sporting events. *Sports Med.* 2001,31.909–917.

123. Tripp BL, Eberman LE, Smith MS. Exertional heat illnesses and environmental conditions during high school football practices. *Am J Sports Med.* 2015;43(10):2490–2495.

124. Claremont AD. Taking winter in stride requires proper attire. *Phys Sportsmed.* 1976;4:65–68.

125. Nelson WE, Gieck JH, Kolb P. Treatment and prevention of hypothermia and frostbite. *Athletic Training.* 1983:330–332.

126. Roach JJ. Coping with killing cold. *Phys Sportsmed.* 1975;3(6):35–39.

127. Sherry E, Richards D. Hypothermia among resort skiers: 19 cases from the Snowy Mountains. *Med J Aust.* 1986;144:457–461.

128. Biem J, Koehnecke N, Classen D, et al. Out of the cold: management of hypothermia and frostbite. *Can Med J.* 2003;168:305–311.

129. Mallet ML. Pathophysiology of accidental hypothermia. *Q J Med.* 2002;95:775–785.

130. Twomey P. Making the best use of a radiology department: an example of implementation of a referral guideline within a primary care organization. *Qual Prim Care.* 2003;11:53–59.

131. McKinnis LN. *Fundamentals of Musculoskeletal Imaging.* Philadelphia: FA Davis; 2005.

132. Johnson TR, Steinbach LS. *Essentials of Musculoskeletal Imaging.* Rosemont, IL: American Academy of Orthopedic Surgeons; 2004.

133. Resnick D, Kransdorf MJ. *Bone and Joint Imaging.* Philadelphia: Elsevier; 2005.

134. O'Brien K. Getting around: a simple office workup to assess patient function. *Geriatrics.* 1994;49(7):38–42.

135. Nicholas JA. The value of sports profiling. *Clin Sports Med.* 1984;3:3–10.

136. Feinstein RA, Soileau EJ, Daniel WA. A national survey of preparticipation physical examination requirements. *Phys Sportsmed.* 1988;16:51–59.

137. Marino M. Profiling swimmers. *Clin Sports Med.* 1984;3:211–229.

138. Sapega A, Minkoff J, Valsamis M, et al. Musculoskeletal performance testing and profiling of elite competitive fencers. *Clin Sports Med.* 1984;3:231–244.

139. Bridgman R. A coach's guide to testing for athletic attributes. *National Strength Conditioning Assoc J.* 1991;13:34–37.

140. Gleim GW. The profiling of professional football players. *Clin Sports Med.* 1984;3:185–197.

141. Skinner JS. *Exercise Testing and Exercise Prescription for Special Cases: Theoretical Basis and Clinical Application.* Philadelphia: Lea & Febiger; 1993.

142. Hershman E. The profile for prevention of musculoskeletal injury. *Clin Sports Med.* 1984;3:65–84.

143. MacDougal JD, Wenger HA. The purpose of physiological testing. In: MacDougal JD, Wenger HA, Green HJ, eds. *Physiological Testing of the High Performance Athlete.* Champaign, IL: Human Kinetics; 1991.

144. Kiesel K, Plisky PJ, Voight ML. Can serious injury in professional football be predicted by a preseason functional movement screen? *North Am J Sports Phys Ther.* 2007;2:147–158.

145. Kiesel K, Plisky PJ, Butler R. Functional movement test scores improve following a standardized off-season intervention program in professional football players. *Scand J Med Sci Sports.* 2011;21:287–292.

146. Teyhen DS, Schaffer SW, Lorenson CA, et al. The functional movement screen: a reliability study. *J Orthop Sports Phys Ther.* 2012;42:530–540.

147. Gribble PA, Hertel J, Denegar CR. Chronic ankle instability and fatigue create proximal joint alterations during performance of the Star Excursion Balance. *Int J Sports Med.* 2007;28:236–242.

148. Hale SA, Hertel J, Olmsted-Kramer LC. The effect of a 4-week comprehensive rehabilitation program on postural control and lower extremity function in individuals with chronic ankle instability. *J Orthop Sports Phys Ther.* 2007;37:303–311.

149. Herrington L, Hatcher J, Hatcher A, et al. A comparison of Star Excursion Balance Test reach distances between ACL deficient patients and asymptomatic controls. *Knee.* 2009;16:49–52.

150. Plisky PJ, Rauh M, Kaminski T, et al. Star Excursion Balance Test as a predictor of lower extremity injury in high school basketball players. *J Orthop Sports Phys Ther.* 2006;30:911–919.

151. Kiesel KB, Plisky PJ, Kersey P. Functional movement test score as a predictor of time-loss during a professional football team's preseason. *Med Sci Sports Exerc.* 2008;40(5):S234.

152. Guccione AA. *Geriatric Physical Therapy.* St Louis: Mosby; 1993.

153. Marino M, Gleim GW. Muscle strength and fiber typing. *Clin Sports Med.* 1984;3:85–100.

154. Sale DG. Testing strength and power. In: MacDougal JD, Wenger HA, Green HJ, eds. *Physiological Testing of the High Performance Athlete.* Champaign, IL: Human Kinetics; 1991.

155. O'Brien K. Getting around: a simple office workup to assess patient function. *Geriatrics.* 1994;49:38–40.

156. Corbin CB. Flexibility. *Clin Sports Med.* 1994;3:101–117.

157. Hubley-Kozey CL. Testing flexibility. In: MacDougal JD, Wenger HA, Green HJ, eds. *Physiological Testing of the High Performance Athlete.* Champaign, IL: Human Kinetics; 1991.

158. Kibler WB, Chandler TJ, Uhl T, et al. A musculoskeletal approach to the preparticipation physical examination: preventing injury and improving performance. *Am J Sports Med.* 1989;17:525–531.

159. Carter C, Wilkinson J. Persistent joint laxity and congenital dislocation of the hip. *J Bone Joint Surg Br.* 1969;46:40–45.

160. Remvig L, Jensen DV, Ward RC. Are diagnostic criteria for general hypermobility and benign joint hypermobility syndrome based on reproducible and valid tests? A review of the literature. *J Rheumatol.* 2007;34(4):798–803.

161. Juul-Kristensen B, Rogind H, Jensen DV, et al. Inter-examiner reproducibility of tests and criteria for generalized joint hypermobility and benign joint hypermobility syndrome. *Rheumatology.* 2007;46:1835–1841.

162. Nicholas JA. Risk factors, sports medicine and the orthopedic system: an overview. *J Sports Med.* 1975;3:243–259.

163. American College of Sports Medicine. Recommended quantity and quality of exercise for developing and maintaining cardio-respiratory and muscular fitness in healthy adult. *J Cardiopulmon Rehab.* 1990;10:235–245.

164. Squires RW, Bove AA. Cardiovascular profiling. *Clin Sports Med.* 1984;3:11–29.

165. Morrison CA, Norenberg RG. Using the exercise test to create the exercise prescription. *Prim Care.* 2001;28:137–158.

166. Wasserman K, Hansen JE, Sue DY, et al. *Principles of Exercise Testing and Interpretation.* Philadelphia: Lea & Febiger; 1994.

167. Thoden JS. Testing aerobic power. In: MacDougal JD, Wenger HA, Green HJ, eds. *Physiological Testing of the High Performance Athlete.* Champaign, IL: Human Kinetics; 1991.

168. Cooper KH. *The New Aerobics.* New York: Bantam Books; 1970.

169. Cooper KM. A means of assessing maximal oxygen intake. *JAMA.* 1968;203:201–204.

170. Kasch FW, Phillips WH, Ross WD, et al. A comparison of maximal oxygen uptake by treadmill and step test procedures. *J Appl Physiol.* 1966;21:1387–1388.

171. Astrand PD, Rodahl K. *Textbook of Work Physiology.* Toronto: McGraw-Hill; 1977.

172. Kowal DM, Daniels WL. Recommendations for the screening of military personnel over 35 years of age for physical training programs. *Am J Sports Med.* 1979;7:186–190.

173. Bouchard C, Taylor AW, Simoneau JA, et al. Testing anaerobic power and capacity. In: MacDougal JD, Wenger HA, Green HJ, eds. *Physiological Testing of the High Performance Athlete.* Champaign, IL: Human Kinetics; 1991.

174. Caine DJ, Brockhoff J. Maturity assessment: a viable preventive measure against physical and psychological insult to the young athlete. *Phys Sportsmed.* 1987;15:67–80.

175. Tinetti ME. Performance oriented assessment of mobility problems in elderly patients. *J Am Geriatr Soc.* 1986;43:119–126.

176. Tippett SR, Voight ML. *Functional Progressions for Sports Rehabilitation.* Champaign, IL: Human Kinetics; 1995.

177. Whieldon D. Maturity sorting: new balance for young athletes. *Phys Sportsmed.* 1978;6:127–132.

178. Ross WD, Marfell-Jones MJ. Kinanthropometry. In: MacDougal JD, Wenger HA, Green HJ, eds. *Physiological Testing of the High Performance Athlete.* Champaign, IL: Human Kinetics; 1991.

179. Goldberg B, Boiardo R. Profiling children for sports participation. *Clin Sports Med.* 1984;3:153–169.

180. Greulich WW, Pyle SU. *Radiographic Atlas of Skeletal Development of the Wrist and Hand.* Stanford, CA: Stanford University Press; 1959.

181. Tanner JM. *Growth and Adolescence.* Oxford, England: Blackwell Scientific; 1962.

182. Katch FI, Katch VL. The body composition profile: techniques of measurement and applications. *Clin Sports Med.* 1984;3:31–63.

183. Jackson AS, Pollock ML. Practical assessment of body composition. *Phys Sportsmed.* 1985;13:772–790.

184. Coleman AE. Skinfold estimates of body fat in major league baseball players. *Phys Sportsmed.* 1981;9:77–82.

185. Cates W, Cavanaugh J. Advances in rehabilitation and performance testing. *Clin Sports Med.* 2009;28:63–76.

186. Léger L, Lambert J. A maximal multistage 20m shuttle run test to predict VO_2 max. *Eur J Appl Physiol.* 1982;49:1–5.

187. Stratford PW, Spadoni GF. Assessing improvement in patients who report small limitations in functional status on conditions-specific measures. *Physiother Can.* 2005;57:234–239.

CHAPTER 18

Emergency Sports Assessment

This chapter will enable the health care professional to immediately assess a patient before applying first aid or transportation to the hospital. This assessment should be divided into two parts. The first part concerns the primary evaluation or survey, which usually takes place at the location in which the patient is found to ensure that life-threatening situations are handled immediately. The second part of the assessment is performed when the examiner has more time and the patient is not under immediate threat of death or permanent disability.

Pre-Event Preparation

Before any sporting event, the examiner should establish a written **Emergency Action Plan (EAP)**, practice **emergency protocols**, and review **sideline preparedness**.[1–5] When a player sustains an acute injury that requires on-field management, the medical personnel must follow a predetermined algorithm for complete evaluation of the injured player (see Fig. 18.15). This minimizes the possibility of missing a more severe, potentially life-threatening injury.[6] This preparation includes designating personnel for specific tasks and establishing emergency vehicle routes and entrances. The examiner and the assistants should know the location of additional medical assistance, emergency equipment (e.g., spinal board, neck supports, sandbags, stretchers, blankets, emergency first-aid kit), and a telephone. The equipment must be compatible with the needs, size, and age of the athletes and with the equipment of other health care professionals. Near the telephone, the examiner should post emergency telephone numbers (e.g., ambulance, physician, dentist), identify the name and address of the sports facility, specify the entrance to be used, and note any obvious landmarks, because the person making the emergency call may forget information or give inappropriate information when under stress (Fig. 18.1). Included in the preparation is a communication plan for on-field or at-site injuries. This plan may involve preestablished hand signals (e.g., crossed arms may mean "send a physician out," whereas a hand on top of one's head may signify "send ambulance or emergency medical services [EMS] personnel") or walkie-talkies to communicate with other professionals working on the sideline.[7]

Emergency Protocol

- Designated personnel
- Emergency vehicle access routes
- Location of emergency equipment
- Location of telephone
- Communication plan

Emergency Telephone Numbers

Ambulance _____   Fire/Inhalator _____

Acute Care Hospital (who will receive your athletes)

_____

Emergency Protocol

When you call the ambulance, state:

1. Your name

2. "There has been a suspected _____ (*insert injury*)

   at _____ (*location*).

   Please send an ambulance to _____ (*designated meeting spot*)

   I will meet the ambulance there."

3. Ask the estimated time of arrival (ETA).

4. Give them your phone number.

5. DO NOT HANG UP UNTIL THE OTHER PARTY DOES!

Note: If this information cannot be kept by the telephone it should be kept in your first-aid kit with a quarter ($0.25) in case you need to phone the ambulance from a pay phone.

Ambulance Route

Draw a map of the ambulance route to your facility and the designated meeting location.

Fig. 18.1 Telephone emergency protocol (to be put near emergency telephones or taped to mobile phone). (Modified from Sports Physiotherapy Division Newsletter, Canadian Physiotherapy Association, July/August 1991, p 3.)

The examiner should take the time to give the facility a **safety check** by looking for potential hazards and meet with the medical team of the opposition if available.[4,5] Visiting teams should also be informed of emergency protocols. In addition, emergency situations and protocols must be practiced repeatedly to ensure that proper care will be given in an emergency.

Primary Assessment

After an injury occurs, the examiner must first take control of the situation and ensure that no additional harm comes to the patient. The primary survey, which takes 30 seconds to 2 minutes with the maximum on-scene time being 10 minutes, is carried out with little or no movement of the patient.[8] It is used to determine whether injuries are life threatening, the severity of injury, and how the patient can be moved. With severe injuries, the longer the assessment takes, the higher the mortality rate is likely to be. If, at any time, the examiner finds that a major injury has occurred (Table 18.1), he or she may terminate the assessment process and ensure the patient receives higher levels of care by calling for the ambulance or EMS. The examiner is designated as the **charge person,** or person in control. The examiner takes control by not allowing the patient to be moved until some type of assessment is made, the spine is supported as much as possible, and, if required, assistance is obtained.

Emergency Evaluation	
• Airway evaluation (A):	5–7 seconds
• Breathing (ventilation) check (B):	5–8 seconds
• Circulation/heart rate (C):	20–30 seconds
• Blood loss:	20–30 seconds
• Neurological injury:	10–20 seconds
TOTAL TIME:	60–95 seconds

For the primary emergency assessment, the examiner should call at least one person to provide immediate assistance, relay messages, and obtain additional help, if necessary. This person is designated the **call person,** and he or she should know the location of the closest telephone (a cell phone would be ideal) and what telephone numbers to call in specific emergencies. This information can be posted on or by the telephone (see Fig. 18.1). When telephoning, the call person should state the caller's name, the number of the telephone being used, the exact emergency (type of injury), the degree of urgency, and the exact location of the facility; ask for an estimated time of arrival; and explain the location of the best entrance to the

TABLE 18.1

Priorities in the Management of Injuries: Beware of Injury to the Cervical Spine!

Highest Priority

1. Respiratory and cardiovascular impairment: Facial, neck, and chest injuries
2. Hemorrhage: External, severe

High Priority

3. Retroperitoneal injuries: Shock, hemorrhage
4. Intraperitoneal injuries: Shock, hemorrhage
5. Craniocerebral spinal cord injuries: Open or closed, observation
6. Severe burns: Extensive soft-tissue wounds

Low Priority

7. Lower genitourinary tract: Hemorrhage, extravasation
8. Peripheral vascular, nerve, locomotor injuries: Open or closed
9. Facial and neck injuries: Except priorities 1 and 2
10. Cold exposure

Special

11. Fractures, dislocations: Splinting
12. Tetanus prophylaxis

From Steichen FM: The emergency management of the severely injured, *J Trauma* 12:787, 1972.

facility for responding emergency personnel. Other individuals (as many as six or seven) may be called as necessary to act as transporters or help move the patient.

Emergency Telephone Information
• Caller's name
• Phone number of telephone being used
• Type of emergency
• Degree of urgency
• Exact location of facility
• Emergency vehicle access route
• Estimated time of arrival
• Best entrance

While performing the initial assessment, the examiner must keep in mind that six situations can immediately threaten the life of a patient: airway obstruction, respiratory failure, cardiac arrest, severe heat injury, head (craniocerebral) injury, and cervical spine injury.[9] It is for these situations, along with severe bleeding, that the examiner must be most prepared, because they are the most common emergency life-threatening situations. Only practice can ensure proper care in an emergency.

Life-Threatening Emergency Situations

- Airway obstruction
- Respiratory failure
- Cardiac arrest
- Severe heat/cold injury
- Head (craniocerebral) injury
- Cervical spine injury
- Severe bleeding

Initially, the examiner **stabilizes and immobilizes** the patient's head and cervical spine in case the patient has suffered a cervical spine injury (Fig. 18.2).[10] If the patient has suffered trauma above the clavicles, he or she should be considered to have suffered a cervical spine injury until proven otherwise.[11] Simultaneously, the examiner **talks to the patient.** If the patient replies in a normal voice and gives logical answers to questions, the examiner can assume that the airway is patent and the brain is receiving adequate perfusion. The examiner asks the patient what happened to determine how the injury occurred (mechanism of injury). The patient is asked to describe the symptoms (e.g., pain, numbness) and how severe he or she thinks the injury is. The examiner then explains what he or she is going to do and reassures the patient.[12] If the patient is unable to speak or is unconscious, the examiner must ask witnesses what happened. If the patient is unconscious ("collapsed athlete"),

the examiner must work with the assumption that a neck (cervical spine) injury has occurred until proven otherwise.[13]

Emergency On-Field Procedures

- Stabilize head and spine (Do not move patient.)
- Talk to patient and determine level of consciousness
- Move patient only if in respiratory or cardiac distress
- Check or establish airway
- Check heartbeat/rate/pulse
- Check for bleeding, shock, cerebrospinal fluid
- Check pupils
- Check for spinal cord injury (Neural Watch)
- Position the patient
- Check for head injury
- Assess for heat injury
- Assess movement

While the examiner is talking to the patient, he or she should be observing whether the patient moves, is still, or is having a seizure. If the patient moves, it means he or she is at least partially conscious, has no apparent neurological dysfunction, and has some cardiopulmonary function. If the patient is still, it means he or she is unconscious, has some neurological dysfunction, or has some other major system failure. A seizure indicates neurological, systemic, or psychological dysfunction. The examiner should also observe the position of the patient (e.g., normal, deformity) and look for altered joint alignment (e.g., fracture, dislocation), swelling, or discoloration.[7] In case there is a spinal cord injury, the patient should be left in the original position until the nature and severity of the injury have been determined, except in cases of respiratory or cardiac distress. If the athlete is suspected of having a head injury and is mobile, the examiner can use the **Concussion Recognition Tool 5** (Fig. 18.3) on the sideline to determine if a concussion has occurred.[14,15] A rapid assessment of the **brain and spinal cord** can be accomplished by asking the patient to do simple movements, such as sticking out the tongue[16] (see the "Assessment for Spinal Cord Injury" section, presented later). If a concussion is suspected, an on-field or sideline evaluation should be conducted (see box on following page).[17] It should be remembered that the concussion is a very common and challenging injury to diagnose because its constellation of signs and symptoms can evolve over hours or even days after the initial event.[18] Thus, if a concussion is suspected, the individual is continually monitored and never left alone.

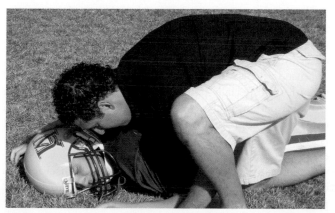

Fig. 18.2 Stabilization of the patient's head and neck before initial assessment.

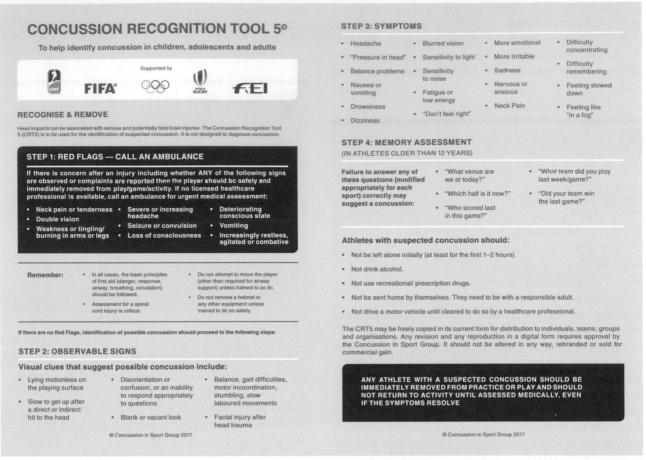

Fig. 18.3 Concussion Recognition Tool 5. (©Concussion in Sport Group 2017. From Echemendia RJ, Meeuwisse W, McCrory P, et al: The Concussion Recognition Tool 5th Edition [CRT5]: background and rationale, *Br J Sports Med* 51[11]:872, 2017.)

On-Field or Sideline Evaluation of Acute Concussion

When a player shows *any* features of a concussion (see Table 2.11):

A. The player should be evaluated by a physician or other licensed health care provider on-site using standard emergency management principles and particular attention should be given to excluding a cervical spine injury.

B. The appropriate disposition of the player must be determined by the treating health care provider in a timely manner. If no health care provider is available, the player should be safely removed from practice or play and urgent referral to a physician arranged.

C. Once the first aid issues are addressed, an assessment of the concussive injury should be made using the SCAT5 (see Fig. 2.49) or other sideline assessment tools.

D. The player should not be left alone following the injury and serial monitoring for deterioration is essential over the initial few hours following injury.

E. A player with diagnosed concussion should not be allowed to return to play on the day of injury.

SCAT5, Sideline Concussion Assessment Tool—5th edition.
From McCrory P, Meeuwisse W, Dvorak J, et al: Consensus statement on concussion in sport – the 5th International Conference on Concussion in Sport held in Berlin, October 2016. *Br J Sports Med* 51(11):1–10, 2017.

Level of Consciousness

The examiner must quickly determine whether the patient is conscious. At no time during the initial assessment should ammonia inhalants be used to arouse the patient. Inhalants should be used only after the examiner is absolutely sure there is no spinal injury, because the fumes may cause a reflex head jerk, complicating the possible neck injury.[11] At this early stage, the examiner simply determines whether the patient is alert (fully conscious), confused (drowsy), in delirium, in obtundation (dulled sensations, especially pain and touch), in a stupor, or in a coma. A patient is classified as **alert** if he or she is able to carry on an appropriate conversation with no delays and is aware of time, place, and identity. See Chapter 2 for an explanation of the levels of consciousness.

The examiner determines the level of consciousness or arousal by talking to the patient, not by moving the patient. This stage is sometimes referred to as the "shake and shout" stage, in which the examiner tries to arouse the unconscious individual by gentle shaking (without allowing movement of the head and neck) and by shouting into each ear. If the patient does not respond to this verbal stimulus, the examiner can, at least initially, assume that the patient is unconscious or not fully conscious and proceed under that assumption. Further neurological assessment is left until the examiner is sure that the patient has a patent airway, is breathing normally, and has a heartbeat. If the patient is conscious, the examiner should reassure the patient that help has arrived. The patient should be informed of what the examiner is doing and proposes to do in terms of examining and moving the patient. Regardless of the patient's state of consciousness, he or she should not move or be moved until the examination has been completed.

On the sideline, the examiner can perform a **Sideline Concussion Assessment Tool—5th edition (SCAT5) exam** (see Chapter 2) and begin a **Neural Watch** to provide serial monitoring (see later discussion) for the possibility of an increasingly severe head injury (i.e., progressive deterioration of signs and symptoms). In addition, balance testing may be performed using the **Balance Error Scoring System (BESS).**[19] This is a quantifiable low-technology test that uses only a stopwatch and a piece of medium-density foam. The athlete is asked to do three different stances (double, single, and tandem) twice on two different surfaces (the ground and the foam) (see Fig. 2.51) for a total of six trials. The athlete begins in the required stance with the hands on the iliac crests and, while standing quiet and motionless, is asked to close both eyes for 20 seconds. During the single leg stance, the athlete stands on the nondominant foot and is asked to hold the opposite non–weight-bearing limb in 20° to 30° of hip flexion and 40° to 50° of knee flexion. For tandem stance, the nondominant foot is placed behind the dominant foot. If the athlete is losing his or her balance, he or she can make any necessary adjustments and returns to the test position as quickly as possible. The athlete is scored by adding one error point for each committed error (see Table 2.25). If the athlete cannot maintain the desired stance for at least 5 seconds of the 20 second test period, the athlete has failed the test. The maximum error score for normal athletes is 10.

Indications That Athlete Should Be Referred to an Emergency Facility

- Worsening headache
- Very drowsy or cannot be easily awakened
- Cannot recognize people or places
- Develops significant nausea or vomiting
- Behaves unusually, more confused or irritable
- Develops seizures
- Weakness or numbness in the arms or legs
- Slurred speech or unsteadiness of gait

Modified from Putukian M, Raftery M, Guskiewicz K, et al: Onfield assessment of concussion in the adult athlete. *Br J Sports Med* 47:285–288, 2013.

Establishing the Airway

While waiting for assistance, the examiner can immediately begin to check for abnormal or arrested breathing, abnormal or arrested pulse, internal and external bleeding, and shock.[20] This initial assessment is called the **airway, breathing, and circulation (ABCs)** of cardiopulmonary resuscitation (CPR). New guidelines also include the use of automated defibrillators if required.[21] The first priority is to maintain an adequate airway, normal ventilation, and hemodynamic stability (see Table 18.1).[22,23] In addition, obvious bleeding should be controlled by compression.

While the cervical spine is protected and immobilized, the examiner quickly assesses the airway for patency by looking, listening, and feeling for spontaneous respirations.[8,11] Respirations can be determined by watching for movement of the chest, feeling the breath on the examiner's cheek, or hearing the air move in and out (Fig. 18.4). The normal resting ranges of respirations are 10 to 25 breaths/min for adults and 20 to 25 breaths/min for children. An athlete or someone who has been exerting before injury may show a higher rate. If a patient is not breathing and has no heartbeat, clinical death occurs between 0 and 4 minutes (Fig. 18.5). If breathing and heartbeat are not restored within 4 to 6 minutes, brain damage is probable. If there is no breathing and no heartbeat for 6 to 10 minutes, biological death occurs, and brain damage is likely.[24]

If the patient is breathing without difficulty, the rate and rhythm of the respirations and their characteristics should be noted. Cheyne-Stokes and ataxic respirations are often associated with head injuries.[25] Table 18.2 indicates some of the abnormal breathing patterns that may occur in a patient in an emergency situation.

If the conscious patient exhibits abnormal or arrested breathing (asphyxia), the examiner should look for

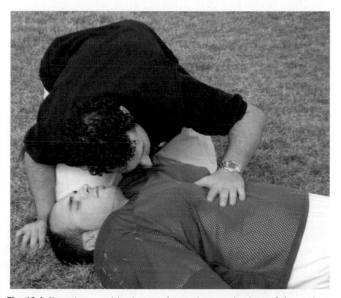

Fig. 18.4 Examiner positioning to determine respiration of the patient. The examiner can feel the breath on the cheek, hear the breath, and watch the chest move.

possible causes.[26] Causes include compression of the trachea; tongue falling back, blocking the airway; foreign bodies (e.g., mouthguard, gum, chewing tobacco); swelling of the tissues (e.g., anaphylactic shock after a bee sting); fluid in the air passages; presence of harmful gases or fumes; pulmonary and chest wall trauma; and suffocation.[26,27]

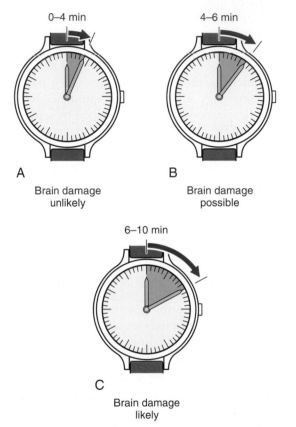

A
Brain damage
unlikely

B
Brain damage
possible

C
Brain damage
likely

Fig. 18.5 If the brain is deprived of oxygen for 4 to 6 minutes, brain damage is possible. After 6 minutes, brain damage is extremely likely.

> **Causes of Asphyxia**
>
> - Compression of trachea
> - Tongue blocking airway
> - Foreign bodies (e.g., gum, mouthguard)
> - Tissue swelling
> - Fluid in air passages
> - Harmful gases or fumes
> - Suffocation

Falling back of the tongue is the most common cause of airway obstruction after a sports injury, especially in the unconscious patient. Normally, the tone of the tongue muscles ensures airway patency. However, the unconscious person, especially one in the supine position, loses muscle tone and the tongue falls back, potentially leading to an obstruction. If the tongue is the cause of obstruction, the examiner can simply pull the chin forward in a **chin lift** or **jaw thrust maneuver** to restore the airway, being careful to keep movement of the cervical spine to a minimum. The chin lift maneuver is less likely to compromise the cervical spine.[28,29] Either maneuver pulls the retropharyngeal musculature forward, thus opening the airway.[26]

If the examiner can see an object obstructing the airway, an oral screw and a tongue forceps can be used to remove the object. The mouth should be held open with the oral screw or something similar, and the examiner can use a finger to sweep the mouth clear of debris (e.g., broken teeth, dentures, mouthguard, chewing gum, tobacco). If the jaw is not held open and blocked from closing, the examiner should put fingers in the patient's mouth only with caution. If the cause of the blockage is something other than the tongue (e.g., foreign body), the patient, if conscious, should be asked to cough. If this does not expel the object, the Heimlich maneuver should be performed

TABLE 18.2

Abnormal Breathing Patterns

Term	Description	Location of Possible Neurological Lesions
Hyperpnea	Abnormal increase in the depth and rate of the respiratory movements	
Apnea	Periods of nonbreathing	Pons
Ataxic breathing (Biot respiration)	Irregular breathing pattern, with deep and shallow breaths occurring randomly	Medulla
Hyperventilation	Prolonged, rapid hyperpnea, resulting in decreased carbon dioxide blood levels	Midbrain, pons
Cheyne-Stokes respirations	Periods of hyperpnea regularly alternating with periods of apnea, characterized by regular acceleration and deceleration in depth	Cerebrum, cerebellum, midbrain, pons
Cluster breathing	Breaths follow each other in disorderly sequence with irregular pauses between them	Pons, medulla

Adapted from Hickey JV: *The clinical practice of neurological and neurosurgical nursing*, Philadelphia, 1986, JB Lippincott, p 138.

until the patient expels the object. If the patient loses consciousness, he or she should be placed supine and ventilation attempted. If it is unsuccessful, 6 to 10 subdiaphragmatic abdominal thrusts are applied. This sequence of ventilation and subdiaphragmatic abdominal thrusts is repeated until a physician or EMS personnel arrive to perform a laryngoscopy.[30] Other causes of asphyxia may be treated by epinephrine (anaphylaxis) or intubation.[30] If the examiner is concerned about maintaining a patent airway, an oropharyngeal airway may be used. As a last resort, a wide-bore needle (18 gauge or larger) may be inserted into the trachea to ensure an airway.[26]

If the patient is not breathing, artificial ventilation (mouth-to-mouth resuscitation) must be initiated immediately, by using the breathing portion of the CPR techniques or by using a similar artificial breathing method.

If the patient is conscious but obviously in respiratory or cardiac distress, the examiner must deal with the presenting situation immediately (Table 18.3). If the patient does not have a patent airway, an airway must be established, as has been described. If the patient is moving in an attempt to get air into the lungs, the examiner may assume that a severe cervical injury is less likely to have occurred. However, movement of the head in relation to the cervical spine should be kept to a minimum. Keeping in mind the possibility of a cervical injury, the examiner should position the patient so that airway clearance and resuscitation can easily be accomplished. This change in position must be performed carefully to ensure that movement of the cervical spine is kept to a minimum. If the patient is reasonably comfortable in the side-lying or prone position and there is no problem with cardiac function or breathing, it is not necessary to move the patient to the supine position.

After the airway has been established, whether by the use of an airway device, by proper head or jaw positioning, by the use of tongue forceps, or by a tracheotomy, the examiner must ensure that the airway is maintained and that the patient continues breathing. If respiration is not spontaneous, assisted ventilation (e.g., mouth-to-mouth, bagging) should be instituted. Supplemental oxygen and use of bag-valve-masks increase saturation rates for athletes in distress and should be available for use.[4] Ventilation can be compromised by a flail chest or pneumothorax (tension or open).[11,27] Endotracheal intubation is necessary if nasopharyngeal bleeding, laryngeal trauma, secretions, or aspirations prevent maintenance of an adequate airway or end-ventilation.[22,26,31] Transtracheal ventilation is the treatment of choice for patients with breathing problems caused by brain, cervical spine, or maxillofacial injuries. An endotracheal tube may cause straining and venous hypertension, leading to increased brain edema, and extension of the head and neck to open upper airways may aggravate cervical spine injuries. In addition, hemorrhage in maxillofacial injuries prevents the effective use of a breathing mask and does not allow adequate visualization.[23]

Establishing Circulation

While the examiner is determining whether breathing is normal, the patient's circulation should be checked for 10 or 15 seconds using the carotid (preferred), brachial, radial, or femoral pulse (Fig. 18.6). For a sedentary adult, the normal heart rate is 60 to 90 beats/min. For children, the rate is 80 to 100 beats/min. In the highly trained athlete of either sex, the rate may be as low as 40 beats/min. With activity, the heart rate will be greater than these levels, and the examiner should take this fact into account when taking the pulse. Depending on the type and level of the individual's activity, the heart rate for a fit person should decrease to slightly above normal values *within 5 minutes*. The examiner should note whether the pulse is absent, rapid and rebounding, or weak and diminishing.

TABLE **18.3**

Airway Obstruction

Conscious Athlete	Unconscious Athlete
1. If patient is breathing or coughing, leave him/her alone but continue to watch 2. If no air is going in and out of lungs, administer four abdominal thrusts (Heimlich maneuver); some people also administer four back blows 3. Repeat until patient can breathe independently or patient becomes unconscious	1. Perform head tilt if no cervical spine injury is suspected 2. If no response, try to ventilate 3. If no success, reposition head and try to ventilate again 4. If unsuccessful, follow with four abdominal thrusts (Heimlich maneuver); some people also administer four back blows 5. Perform a quick sweep of the mouth 6. If unsuccessful, repeat steps 1 through 5 until there is no longer obstruction, or qualified help arrives; a tracheotomy may follow if obstruction continues

Adapted from American Academy of Orthopaedic Surgeons: *Athletic training and sports medicine*, Park Ridge, IL, 1984, AAOS, p 454.

Rapid Assessment Criteria for Circulation

1. Skin color
2. Carotid pulse palpable (systolic blood pressure, ≥ 60 mm Hg)
3. Femoral pulse palpable (systolic blood pressure, ≥ 70 mm Hg)
4. Radial pulse palpable (systolic blood pressure, ≥ 80 mm Hg)

Modified from Driscoll P, Skinner D: Initial assessment and management: I. Primary survey. *Br Med J* 300:1266, 1990.

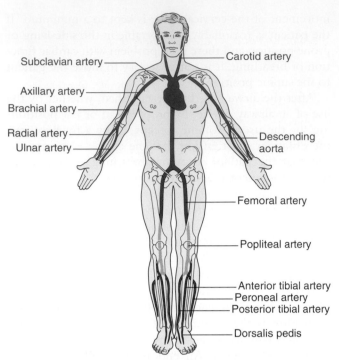

Fig. 18.6 Major arteries in the body. Pressure applied to any of the arteries *(pressure points)* can decrease bleeding if applied proximal to the bleeding.

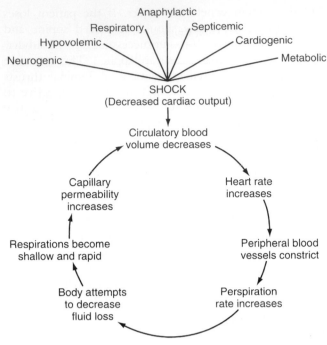

Fig. 18.7 The shock cycle.

The pulse is most often checked at the carotid artery because this artery is large and easy to locate. Therefore the examiner has less chance of missing the pulse and does not have to move from the area of the patient's head to perform palpation. If a pulse cannot be detected, it should be assumed that the patient does not have a heartbeat, and CPR should be initiated using either manual methods or an automated external defibrillator. The use of the defibrillator increases the chance of survival in cardiac arrest.[32] Although cardiac arrest is rare in athletes, sudden death or commotio cordis resulting from low-impact blunt trauma is always a possibility in sports.[33] When the pulse is assessed, the examiner should estimate its rate, strength, and rhythm to obtain an indication of the cardiac output. Circulatory sufficiency may also be determined by squeezing the nail bed or hypothenar eminence. **Capillary refill** is delayed if the pink color does not return to the nail bed or hypothenar eminence within 2 seconds after release of the pressure.[34] Squeezing the hypothenar eminence is a better indicator if the patient is hypothermic.

The pulse may also be used to determine the patient's blood pressure. If a carotid pulse can be palpated, systolic blood pressure is 60 mm Hg or higher. If the femoral pulse is palpable, systolic blood pressure is 70 mm Hg or higher. If the radial pulse can be palpated, the systolic blood pressure is 80 mm Hg or higher.[16,25,34] Like heart rate, blood pressure should drop to almost normal levels within 5 minutes following termination of exercise.

A **weak** or **rapid pulse** usually indicates shock, heat exhaustion, hypoglycemia, fainting, or hyperventilation. A **slowing pulse** is sometimes seen when there is a large increase in intracranial pressure, which usually indicates a severe lower brain stem compression.[35] A pulse that is **rebounding and rapid** is often the result of hypertension, fright, heat stroke, or hyperglycemia.

If the pulse rate is beginning to weaken, the patient may be going into **shock** (Fig. 18.7). Shock is characterized by signs and symptoms that occur when the cardiac output is insufficient to fill the arterial tree and the blood is under insufficient pressure to provide organs and tissues with adequate blood flow. However, it should be noted that patients who maintain pink skin, especially in the face and extremities, are seldom hypovolemic after injury. If the skin of the face or extremities turns ash-gray or white, this usually indicates blood loss of at least 30%.[11] Common types of shock and their causes are shown in Table 18.4. A patient going into shock becomes restless and anxious. The pulse slowly becomes weak and rapid, and the skin becomes cold and wet, often clammy. Sweating may be profuse, and the face is initially pale and later cyanotic (blue) around the mouth. Respirations may be shallow, labored, rapid, or possibly irregular and gasping, especially if a chest injury has occurred. The eyes usually become dull and lusterless, and the pupils become increasingly dilated. The patient may complain of thirst and feel nauseated or vomit. If shock develops quickly, the patient may lose consciousness. To prevent or delay the onset of shock, the examiner may cover the patient, elevate the patient's legs, or attempt to eliminate the cause of the problem.

TABLE **18.4**

Types of Shock and Their Causes

Type	Cause
Hemorrhagic (hypovolemic)	Blood loss
Respiratory	Inadequate blood supply
Neurogenic	Loss of vascular control by nervous system
Psychogenic	Common fainting
Cardiogenic	Insufficient pumping of blood by the heart
Septic	Severe infection and blood vessel damage
Anaphylactic	Allergic reaction
Metabolic	Loss of body fluid

Signs and Symptoms of Shock

- Increased and weak heart rate
- Cold, clammy, pale skin
- Increased and shallow respiratory rate
- Profuse sweating
- Increased thirst
- Restlessness and anxiousness
- Altered level of consciousness
- Dilated pupils
- Nausea or vomiting

Circulatory collapse in trauma patients is caused primarily by blood loss from vascular damage or fracture, or **hypovolemic shock,** but the examiner must remember that shock in trauma may also be caused by tension pneumothorax, central nervous system injury, or pericardial tamponade (heart compression resulting from blood in the pericardium)—all emergency conditions that require physician intervention.[36] By the time hypovolemic shock becomes evident, blood loss may be as high as 20% to 25%. The normal range of blood pressure is 100 to 120 mm Hg for systolic pressure and 60 to 80 mm Hg for diastolic pressure. With shock, the blood pressure gradually decreases. If the blood pressure can be measured, it is best to assume that shock is developing in any injured adult whose systolic blood pressure is 100 mm Hg or less.

If the examiner is caring for a dark-skinned person, it may be difficult to determine from observation whether the patient is going into shock. A healthy person with dark skin usually has a red undertone and shows a healthy pink color in the nail beds, lips, and mucous membranes of the mouth and tongue. However, a dark-skinned patient in shock has a gray cast to the skin around the nose and mouth, especially if experiencing respiratory shock. The mucous membranes of the mouth and tongue, the lips, and the nail beds have a blue tinge. If the shock is caused

TABLE **18.5**

Bleeding Characteristics and Their Source

Source	Bleeding Characteristics
Artery	Bright red, spurting or pulsating flow
Vein	Dark red, steady flow
Capillary	Slow, even flow
Lungs	Bright red, frothy
Stomach	"Coffee grounds" vomitus
Upper bowel	Tarry black stools
Kidneys	Smoky, red urine
Bladder	Red urine, difficulty urinating
Abdomen	Blood not visible; abdominal rigidity, pain, difficulty breathing

by hypovolemia, the mucous membranes of the mouth and tongue will not be blue; rather they will have a pale, graying, waxy pallor.[37]

If no pulse is present, then the cardiac portion of CPR techniques should be initiated. Sports equipment (e.g., shoulder pads or rib pads) should be removed, at least anteriorly, to give the examiner clear access to the anterior chest wall. CPR provides only approximately 25% of normal cardiac output, so it is imperative that it is performed properly by knowledgeable persons.[38] CPR is maintained until the patient recovers or EMS personnel arrive. If a cervical spine injury is suspected, CPR must be done with care because compression to the heart can cause repeated flexion-extension of the cervical spine.[23]

Assessment for Bleeding, Fluid Loss, and Shock

The examiner should look for any signs of external bleeding or hemorrhage (Table 18.5). The types of wounds in which external bleeding or hemorrhage may be seen are incisions, which are clean cuts, or lacerations that have jagged edges. A contusion may produce internal bleeding, whereas a puncture or abrasion may also show bleeding or oozing on the surface. Major traumatic injuries, such as fractures (e.g., pelvis, femur), can cause a great deal of internal bleeding. Of the five types of wounds, the puncture wound is probably the most difficult to treat, because it has the highest probability of infection. The examiner should watch for bleeding from the lungs, the stomach, the upper bowel, the lower bowel, the kidneys, or the bladder. If the liver, spleen, or kidney is injured, serious internal bleeding may result; the blood will not be visible because it is contained within the abdominal cavity. In this case the patient may experience abdominal rigidity, pain, and difficulty breathing (pressure on diaphragm).

When inspecting a bleeding structure, the examiner should note the type of vessel affected. For example, an artery spurts blood, whereas a vein provides an

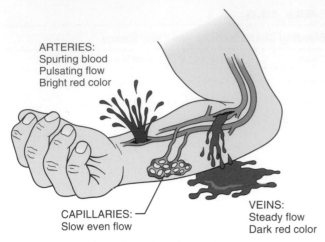

ARTERIES:
Spurting blood
Pulsating flow
Bright red color

CAPILLARIES:
Slow even flow

VEINS:
Steady flow
Dark red color

Fig. 18.8 Bleeding characteristics.

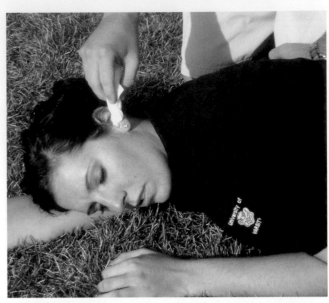

Fig. 18.9 Checking the ear for blood or cerebrospinal fluid.

even flow. Capillaries tend to ooze bright blood (Fig. 18.8).[24] Because arterial bleeding is of greatest concern, the examiner must be aware of the pressure points in the body (see Fig. 18.6) so that he or she will know where to apply proper treatment. The examiner chooses the pressure point closest to the area of bleeding and applies pressure to the artery to slow or stop the bleeding. Tourniquets should be used only with extreme caution and in selected instances (e.g., accidental amputation of a limb, very severe bleeding from a major artery, or the need to apply CPR with no assistance available) and then only with enough pressure to stop bleeding. If a tourniquet is used, the time of tourniquet application should be noted carefully to prevent unnecessary tissue damage. Hemodynamic stability is best maintained by applying direct pressure to an open wound, keeping the patient in a recumbent position, and minimizing the number of times the patient is moved.[22]

If signs and symptoms of shock are present but visible bleeding is minimal, the examiner should suspect hidden bleeding within the abdomen, chest, or extremities.[25,39] If bleeding is suspected in the abdomen, the examiner should palpate the abdominal wall for shape and distention. To check for bleeding in the chest or extremities, the examiner should look for deformities (e.g., fractures). The fingers may be used to percuss the chest area, noting any loss of hollow sounds, to help locate the presence of fluid or blood. Hyporesonance may indicate a solid organ or the presence of fluid or blood; hyperresonance usually indicates air- or gas-filled spaces.[25]

After the ABCs systems have been assessed and controlled, the examiner can proceed to the remainder of the primary assessment. The examiner should check the ears and nose for the presence of cerebrospinal fluid. If blood or cerebrospinal fluid leaks from the ear, this may indicate a skull fracture. The examiner should incline the head toward the affected side to facilitate drainage, unless a cervical injury is suspected. The examiner can place a gauze pad over the patient's ear or nose where

the bleeding is occurring to collect the fluid on the gauze (Fig. 18.9). The examiner should look for an orange halo forming on the pad (see Fig. 2.34). The halo is cerebrospinal fluid, the presence of which is a good indication of a skull fracture.[40]

Sudden Cardiac Arrest

Sudden cardiac arrest in athletes is not all that common, with an incidence of 0.75 per 100,000 athlete years[41-43]; however, it is of upmost importance as a first symptom.[44] The examiner should be aware that the highest incidence of sudden cardiac arrest occurs in soccer, followed by football, basketball, ice hockey, and baseball.[45] This issue can occur to someone who appears to be healthy and has not had previous symptoms.

Two cardiac disorders that may lead to sudden cardiac death are **arrhythmogenic right ventricular cardiomyopathy (ARVC)** and **hypertrophic cardiac myopathy (HCM)**. ARVC is an inherited disorder in which the heart muscle is replaced with scar and fat tissue leading to abnormal rhythms and weakness of the heart. The athlete with ARVC may have a history of fainting after physical activity.[44] HCM is another congenital disorder caused by abnormal thickening of the left ventricle. HCM is the number one cause of cardiovascular death in athletes.[46] This leads to conductivity and arrhythmia problems, causing ventricular fibrillation.[44] Symptoms include dizziness, chest pain, fainting, shortness of breath, and fatigue.[47] A surprising 55% to 80% of athletes are asymptomatic, contributing to the difficulty of early detection until a catastrophic event occurs.[48]

Lastly, **commotio cordis** (Latin for "agitation of the heart")[49] is usually the result of a direct blow to the chest wall. This can occur from a baseball, hockey puck, helmet, or any other blunt object forcefully striking the chest wall or sternum area. The blow most commonly occurs to the left precordial area and the trauma involved is related to the speed and force of impact. This is most common in younger males with immature skeletons and physical development from the ages of 5 to 15 years of age. Adolescents have a narrower anteroposterior chest diameter and greater chest-wall compliance, which are thought to contribute to greater force transmission to the heart.[50] The trauma to cause commotio cordis occurs 15 to 30 milliseconds prior to the T-wave peak during cardiac repolarization resulting in significant electrical disarray and cardiac arrhythmias.[50] Commotio cordis accounts for almost 20% of youth cardiac deaths.[51–53] The arrhythmia that occurs may be refractory to standard resuscitation measures, including defibrillation. The survival rate of this injury is approximately 15%.[54] Above a certain threshold of trauma/impact, structural cardiac damage may also occur, and this is termed **contusion cordis**.[54,55] One way to try to prevent commotio cordis is by using chest protection. However, even with chest protection, death can and has occurred.[56] Recent evidence from an animal model has demonstrated that chest wall protection of modest thickness can be achieved and can be effective prevention for ventricular fibrillation on the playing field.[57]

Pupil Check

Pupil assessment should be performed on anyone suspected of having any head injury. This is extremely important as it appears that even among sports medicine clinicians who regularly attend to patients with concussions, there is insufficient awareness that concussions can lead to abnormal eye tracking behavior. Snegireva and colleagues[58] found that 77% of clinicians dealing with sports injuries did not use any eye movement assessment tools other than their own clinical assessment, with half the respondents inspected by less than half of the clinicians.

The examiner checks the pupils for shape and for response to light by using a penlight or by covering the eye with one hand and then taking it away. The pupil normally reacts to the intensity of light or focal distance. The pupils dilate in a dark environment or with a long focal distance, and they constrict in a light environment or with a short focal distance. Normally, the pupils are equally or almost equally dilated (diameter range, 2 to 6 mm; mean of 3.5 mm), but injury to the central nervous system (e.g., head injury) may cause the pupils to dilate unevenly. Some people normally have unequal pupil sizes, and the health care professional must be aware of this possibility. In a fully conscious, alert person who has sustained a blow near the eye, a dilated, fixed pupil is most likely the result of trauma to the short ciliary nerves of that eye rather than the result of third cranial nerve compression caused by brain herniation.[22] Drugs may also affect the pupillary size. For example, opiate drugs cause pinpoint pupils, whereas amphetamines may cause dilated pupils.[25]

To test pupil reaction, the examiner holds one hand over one eye and then moves the hand away quickly, or shines the light from a penlight into the eye, and observes the pupil's reaction when the light is shone on the eye (normal reaction: constriction) or when the light source is removed (normal reaction: dilation). The examiner tests the other eye in a similar fashion and compares the results. The **pupillary reaction** is classified as brisk (normal), sluggish, nonreactive, or fixed. An ovoid or slightly oval pupil or a fixed and dilated pupil indicates increasing intracranial pressure.[25] If both pupils are midsize, midposition, and nonreactive, midbrain damage is usually indicated. The fixation and dilation of both pupils is a terminal sign of anoxia and ischemia to the brain.[25,59]

Assessment for Spinal Cord Injury

Spinal cord injuries can have catastrophic and irreversible neurologic consequences, so early recognition of the problem is essential.[60] If the athlete walks off the field before notifying the medical staff of a potential neck injury, he or she should be examined using a regular cervical assessment (see Chapter 3). If the player appears to have or communicates a neck injury on the field or is unconscious, then a neck or head injury should be assumed, and he or she is treated as indicated later. The cervical assessment is modified so as much of the examination as possible is done without moving the athlete. After examination, the athlete is immobilized and transported to a medical facility.[61]

An upper spinal cord injury should be suspected, at least initially, if the patient has neck pain; the patient's head position is asymmetric or abnormal; the patient is having respiratory difficulty, especially if the chest is not moving (absence of abdominal or diaphragmatic breathing); the patient is demonstrating priapism (erection of the penis); or the patient is unconscious after a fall or other contact activity. Other indications of neurological injuries in the conscious patient include numbness, tingling, or burning, especially below the clavicles; muscle weakness; twitching; or paralysis of the arms or legs, especially bilaterally (flaccid paralysis).[25]

Situations in Which Cervical Spine Injury Must Be Suspected Until Proven Otherwise

- Neck pain or stiffness
- Cervical muscle spasm
- Asymmetric or abnormal head position
- Respiratory difficulty (chest not moving)
- Priapism
- Unconsciousness
- Numbness, tingling, or burning
- Muscle weakness or paralysis
- Loss of bowel or bladder control

The examiner may ask the patient to stick out the tongue, wiggle the toes, move the feet or arms, or squeeze the examiner's fingers.[16] This quick test provides a rapid assessment of the brain and spinal cord by showing whether the patient can follow instructions and can do the activity.

If the patient is unconscious (Table 18.6), the examiner should reassess the level of unconsciousness if possible and treat the patient as though a spinal injury has occurred. In the unconscious patient, the examiner should watch for spontaneous limb movement, especially after the application of a painful stimulus, because movement indicates that the patient is less likely to have suffered a severe cervical injury.[25] In addition, the examiner should look for tonic posturing that indicates a severe head injury. The **fencing response** may occur at the time of impact, with one limb extending and the other flexing regardless of position or gravity (Fig. 18.10).[62] **Decerebrate rigidity** is evidenced by all four extremities being in extension (see Fig. 2.48B). With **decorticate rigidity,** the lower limbs are in extension and the upper limbs are in flexion (see Fig. 2.48A).

Assessment for Head Injury (Neural Watch)

The patient's level of consciousness is then reassessed. If a concussion is suspected, the athlete is NOT allowed to return to the playing field. See Chapter 2 for more information on concussions. Chapter 2 also outlines some vestibular tests which can be performed on the sideline if necessary. At no time should the athlete be left alone, and he or she should be checked at regular intervals to ensure that the airway remains patent, breathing is normal, and the pulse is within normal limits, as well as watching for any indication of mental deterioration as a result of the concussion.[20] The examiner should now institute a Neural Watch (Fig. 18.11) or a similar observation scheme to note any changes in the patient over time. The Neural Watch should initially be performed **every 5 to 15 minutes,** because it also facilitates monitoring of the patient's vital signs.[25] After the patient has stabilized, Neural Watch recordings may be made **every 15 to 30 minutes.**[35] If possible, reassessment by the same examiner allows the detection of subtle changes.

The examination should include an evaluation of the patient's facial expression; a determination of the patient's orientation to time, place, and person; and the presence of both posttraumatic amnesia and retrograde amnesia. Signs and symptoms that demand emergency action in a patient who has sustained a blow to the head are increased headache, nausea and vomiting, inequality of pupils, disorientation, progressive or sudden impairment of consciousness, gradual increase in blood pressure, and diminution of pulse rate.

> **▼ Emergency Signs and Symptoms of Head Injury**
> - Increased headache
> - Nausea and vomiting
> - Inequality of pupils
> - Disorientation
> - Altered level of consciousness
> - Increased blood pressure
> - Decreased pulse rate
> - Decreased reaction to pain
> - Decreased or altered values on Neural Watch Chart or GCS

GCS, Glasgow Coma Scale.

Reaction to pain and the level of consciousness can be determined by the use of physical and verbal stimuli. If there is no cervical injury, the verbal stimuli may include calling the patient's name and shaking and shouting at the patient. Physical stimuli (see Fig. 2.47) include squeezing the Achilles tendon, squeezing the trapezius muscle, squeezing the soft tissue between the patient's thumb and index finger, squeezing an object (pen or pencil) between the patient's fingers, squeezing a fingertip, or applying a knuckle to the sternum. (This must be done with caution because it may cause bruising.) In comatose patients, a motor response to a painful stimulus to an extremity may indicate intact pain appreciation from that site, especially if it is accompanied by a more remote response, such as a grimace or a change in respiration or pulse.[22]

The level of consciousness can best be determined with the use of the **Glasgow Coma Scale (GCS)** (see Table 2.5).[63–65] The sooner the patient is tested with the scale, the better, because the initial assessment can be used as a baseline for improvement or deterioration in the patient. The GCS is often used in conjunction with the Neural Watch. For a description of the test, see Chapter 2.

Deterioration of consciousness may result from many conditions, such as increased intracranial pressure caused by an expanding intracranial lesion, hypoxia (which can aggravate cerebral edema and increase the intracranial pressure), epilepsy, meningitis, or fat embolism. The examiner should always look for signs of expanding intracranial lesions (see Chapter 2), especially if the patient is conscious. These lesions are emergency conditions that must be attended to immediately because of their potentially high mortality rate (up to 50%).

If the patient experiences loss of consciousness or appears to have disturbed senses, is seeing stars or colors, is dizzy, or has auditory hallucinations or a severe headache, the patient should not be left alone or allowed to return to activity (Table 18.7). In addition, nausea, vomiting, lethargy, increasing blood pressure, disturbed sensation of smell, or a diminished pulse should lead the examiner to the same conclusion. Amnesia, hyperirritability, an open wound, unequal pupils, or leaking of

TABLE 18.6

Some Common Causes of Unconsciousness in Patients

Category	Problem	Cause	Pathophysiology	Management
General	Loss of consciousness	Injury or disease	Shock, head injury, other injuries, diabetes, arteriosclerosis	Need for CPR, triage
Disease	Diabetic coma	Hyperglycemia and acidosis	Inadequate use of sugar, acidosis	Complex treatment for acidosis
	Insulin shock	Hypoglycemia	Excess insulin	Sugar
	Myocardial infarct	Damaged myocardium	Insufficient cardiac output	Oxygen, CPR, transport
	Stroke	Damaged brain	Loss of arterial supply to brain or hemorrhage within brain	Support, gentle transport
Injury	Hemorrhagic shock	Bleeding	Hypovolemia	Control external bleeding, recognize internal bleeding, CPR, transport
	Respiratory shock	Insufficient oxygen	Paralysis, chest damage, airway obstruction	Clear airway, supplemental oxygen, CPR, transport
	Anaphylactic shock	Acute contact with agent to which patient is sensitive	Allergic reaction	Intramuscular epinephrine, support, CPR, transport
	Cerebral contusion, concussion, or hematoma	Blunt head injury	Bleeding into or around brain, concussive effect	Airway, supplemental oxygen, CPR, careful monitoring, transport
Emotions	Psychogenic shock	Emotional reaction	Sudden drop in cerebral blood flow	Place supine, make comfortable, observe for injuries
Environment	Heatstroke	Excessive heat, inability to sweat	Brain damage from heat	Immediate cooling, support, CPR, transport
	Electric shock	Contact with electric current	Cardiac abnormalities, fibrillation	CPR, transport; do not treat until current controlled
	Systemic hypothermia	Prolonged exposure to cold	Diminished cerebral function, cardiac arrhythmias	CPR, rapid transport, warming at hospital
	Drowning	Oxygen, carbon dioxide, breath-holding, water	Cerebral damage	CPR, transport
	Air embolism	Intravascular air	Obstruction to arterial blood flow by nitrogen bubbles	CPR, recompression
	Decompression sickness ("bends")	Intravascular nitrogen	Obstruction to arterial blood flow by nitrogen bubbles	CPR, recompression
Injected or ingested agents	Alcohol	Excess intake	Cerebral depression	Support, CPR, transport
	Drugs	Excess intake	Cerebral depression	Support, CPR, transport (bring drug)
	Plant poisons	Contact, ingestion	Direct cerebral or other toxic effect	Support, recognition, CPR, identify plant, local wound care, transport
	Animal poisons	Contact, ingestion, injection	Direct cerebral or other toxic effect	Recognition, support, CPR, identify agent, local wound care, transport
Neurological	Epilepsy	Brain injury, scar, genetic predisposition, disease	Excitable focus of motor activity in brain	Support, protect patient, transport in status epilepticus

CPR, Cardiopulmonary resuscitation.
From the American Academy of Orthopaedic Surgeons: *Athletic training and sports medicine*, ed 2, Park Ridge, IL, 1991, AAOS, pp 618–619.

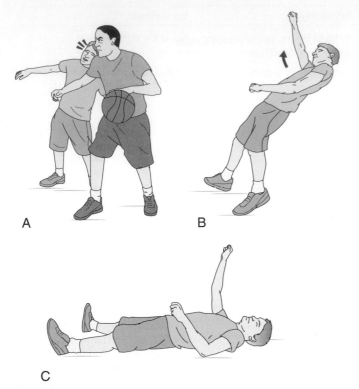

Fig. 18.10 The fencing response during a knockout. (A) Athlete receives a blow to the head. (B) After the traumatic blow to the head, the unconscious athlete immediately exhibits extension in one arm and contralateral flexion while falling to the ground. (C) During prostration, the rigidity of the extended and flexed arms is retained for several seconds as flaccidity gradually returns.[62]

Neural Watch Chart

Unit		Time 1 ( )	Time 2 ( )	Time 3 ( )
I. Vital signs	Blood pressure Pulse Respirations Temperature			
II. Conscious and	Oriented Disoriented Restless Combative			
	Unconscious			
III. Speech	Clear Rambling Garbled None			
IV. Will awaken to	Name Shaking Light pain Strong pain			
V. Nonverbal reaction to pain	Appropriate Inappropriate "Decerebrate" None			
VI. Pupils	Size on right Size on left Reacts on right Reacts on left			
VII. Ability to move	Right arm Left arm Right leg Left leg			
VIII. Sensation	Right side (normal/abnormal) Left side (normal/abnormal) Dermatome affected (specify) Peripheral nerve affected (specify)			

Fig. 18.11 Neural Watch chart. (Modified from American Academy of Orthopaedic Surgeons: *Athletic training and sports medicine*, Park Ridge, IL, 1984, AAOS, p 399.)

cerebrospinal fluid or blood from the ears or nose also indicates an emergency condition. Numbness on one side of the body or a large contusion in the head area should likewise lead the examiner to handle the patient with care. If the frontal area of the brain is affected, the patient may experience lapses of memory, personality changes, or impairment of judgment. If the temporal lobe has been affected, the patient may experience feelings of unreality, déjà vu, or hallucinations involving odors, sounds, or visual disturbances, such as macropsia (seeing objects as larger than they really are) or micropsia. The literature indicates that head injury depends not only on the magnitude and direction of impact and the structural features and physical reactions of the skull but also on the state of the head/brain at the moment of impact.[9,66,67]

If the patient has received a head injury and has been checked by a physician and it has been determined that it is not necessary to send the patient to the hospital, the clinician should ensure that the patient and whoever lives with the patient understands what to look for in terms of signs and symptoms that may indicate increasing severity of head injury. Fig. 2.29 demonstrates typical home health care guidelines.

Assessment for Heat Injury

Heat-related illness includes heat cramps, heat exhaustion, and heat stroke and are a common concern for clinicians working in sports medicine.[68] Most heat-related deaths are associated with American football, wrestling, cross-country, and track and field.[69] If the examiner suspects a heat-type injury with no cervical injury, only heat exhaustion and heat stroke need be considered as life-threatening.[13,70] **Heat fatigue** or **exhaustion** occurs when a person is exposed to high environmental temperature or humidity and perspires excessively without salt or fluid replacement. **Heat stroke** can occur when a nonacclimatized person is suddenly exposed to high environmental temperature or humidity. The thermal regulatory mechanism fails, perspiration stops, and the body temperature increases. Above 42°C oral body temperature, brain damage occurs, and death follows if emergency measures are not instituted. The diagnostic

TABLE **18.7**

Indications for Immediate Removal from Activity

Area of Injury	Indications for Immediate Removal from Activity
Eye	Blunt trauma, visual difficulty, pain, laceration, obvious deformity
Head	Loss of consciousness, disturbed sensorium, stars or colors being seen, dizziness, auditory hallucinations, nausea, vomiting, lethargy, severe headache, rising blood pressure, disturbed smell, diminishing pulse, amnesia, hyperirritability, large contusion, open wounds, unequal pupils, leakage of cerebrospinal fluid or blood from ears or nose, numbness of one side of body
Spine	Obvious deformity, restricted motion, weakness of extremity, pain on movement, localized tenderness, numbness of extremity (pinched nerve), paresthesias
Extremities	Obvious deformity, crepitus, loss of range of motion, loss of sensation, effusion, pain on use, unstable joint, open wounds, significant tenderness, significant swelling
Abdomen	Dizziness or syncope, nausea, persisting pallor, vomiting, history of infectious mononucleosis, abnormal thirst, muscle guarding, localized tenderness, shoulder pain, distension, rapid pulse, clamminess and sweating

Reprinted by permission from the New York State Journal of Medicine, copyright by the Medical Society of the State of New York. Adapted from Greensher J, Mofenson HC, Merlis NJ: First aid for school athletic emergencies, *NY State J Med* 79:1058, 1979.

keys in this situation are the **high body temperature** and the **absence of sweating.** Initial signs of heat injury include muscle cramps, excessive fatigue or weakness, loss of coordination, decreased reaction time, headache, decreased comprehension, dizziness, and nausea and vomiting.

▼ **Signs of Heat Injury**

- Muscle cramps
- Excessive fatigue or weakness
- Loss of coordination
- Headache
- Decreased comprehension
- Dizziness
- Nausea and vomiting
- Decreased reaction time

TABLE **18.8**

Skin Changes and Their Cause

Skin Change	Cause
Hot and dry	Heat stroke, high fever, hyperglycemia
Cold and clammy	Fainting, hypoglycemia, hyperventilation, shock
Cool and moist	Heat exhaustion
Cool and dry	Cold
White pallor	Decreased circulation
Cyanosis (blue pallor)	Respiratory distress
Red pallor	Fever, heat stroke, inflammation, exercise

The body temperature varies according to the site at which the measurement is taken. The oral body temperature is 37°C (98.6°F). Taken in the armpit or axilla, the temperature is 36.4°C to 36.7°C (97.5°F to 98.1°F), and in the rectum, it is 37.3°C to 37.6°C (99.1°F to 99.7°F). Because oral, axillary, tympanic, and forehead measurements do not accurately assess core temperature in athletes,[71] recent recommendations suggest the use of rectal temperature as the most reliable way to assess core temperature and asserts that sports medicine staff must be prepared and willing to implement it.[72] If a heat injury is suspected, the quickest and easiest way to cool down an athlete is ice-water immersion.[73]

The examiner may palpate the skin to get some idea of the external temperature of the body and possible pathology (Table 18.8). Hot and dry skin is often caused by heat stroke, high fever, or hyperglycemia. Cold and clammy skin is caused by hypoglycemia, shock, fainting, or hyperventilation. Cool and moist skin is often caused by heat exhaustion, whereas cool and dry skin is caused by exposure to cold.

Skin color can also play a significant role. Pallor, or whitish skin, indicates circulatory disturbance or decreased circulation and is most often associated with trauma and shock. Cyanosis, or a blue tint to the skin, indicates respiratory distress, as does a gray tint. Redness indicates an increase in blood flow as a result of fever, heat stroke, or exercise.

Assessment for Movement

While doing the initial assessment, the examiner should also be considering how the patient will be moved and immobilized (e.g., self-ambulation, stretcher, spinal board) depending on the severity of the injury and whether the patient can move himself or herself or can move only with assistance.[74]

If the patient has not already done so, the examiner asks the patient to move the limbs to reassess for a cervical

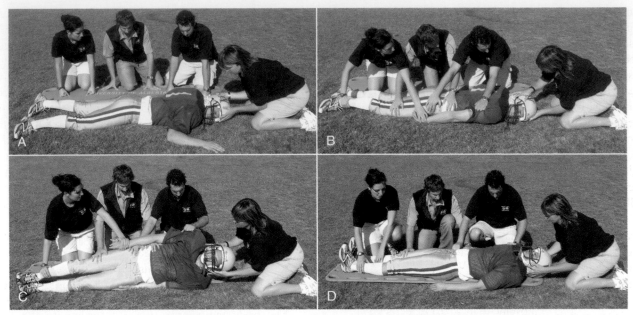

Fig. 18.12 Moving a patient to the supine position after injury. Note that the head and neck are stabilized throughout the movement. (A) Patient prone, examiner stabilizes head, and gives instruction to helpers. (B through D) Patient is log-rolled onto spinal board.

spine injury and look for major trauma (e.g., fracture, dislocation, third-degree strain, third-degree sprain). At the same time, the examiner may palpate the areas of potential injury, noting any pain, abnormal bone or joint alignment, swelling, hypersensitive or hyposensitive areas, or palpable defect (third-degree strain).[7] If movement is relatively normal, the examiner quickly checks the myotomes of the upper or lower body for any possible motor involvement or motor impairment. Changes in limb power may be caused by a contractile tissue injury, a neurological injury, or an expanding intracranial lesion, which will be displayed as progressive weakness in the contralateral arm or leg.[35] Decreased limb power can also be caused by reflex inhibition as a result of previously unrecognized limb injury. In these cases, contractions are weak and painful. These types of injuries are placed in the low-priority group (see Table 18.1) because they represent a threat to the limb rather than to the life of the patient.[23]

Positioning the Patient

Normally, a patient is left in the position in which he or she is found until the primary assessment is completed. However, if the patient is having difficulty breathing or there is no pulse, the patient must be positioned to do CPR. If the conscious patient is prone and in respiratory difficulty, the examiner, with assistance, should **log-roll** the patient (Fig. 18.12) onto a spinal board so that an attempt can be made to restore the airway. During any movement of the patient, the examiner should apply traction of approximately 4.5 kg (10 lbs) to the cervical spine to maintain stability. The patient should be reassured that

others are going to carefully move the patient while he or she remains still. Before any movement is attempted, the patient and those who are going to assist the examiner should know what the examiner plans to do and what their jobs are. This requires *frequent practicing of emergency procedures.* The sequence of movement and positioning of the extremities and body of the patient should be thought out beforehand so that everyone is aware of what is going to happen and in what order. The proper procedure for moving the patient should be practiced often to ensure competency.

To roll the patient, at least three assistants are needed. There should be two-way communication between the examiner and the patient at all times to continually evaluate the patient's comfort level and neurological signs. The assistants should place the spinal board beside the patient and then kneel beside the spinal board and patient (see Fig. 18.12A). They should reach over the patient and hold the patient's shoulder, hip, and knees (see Fig. 18.12B). On command from the examiner, the assistants roll the patient toward them while the examiner stabilizes the head (see Fig. 18.12C) until the patient is lying supine on the spinal board (see Fig. 18.12D). Only rolling—not lifting—should occur. With the patient in the supine position, proper CPR techniques may be applied, or the patient may be transported. The patient may also be covered with a blanket to provide warmth.

If a spinal injury is suspected and the conscious patient is in the prone position but has no difficulty breathing, the patient is log-rolled halfway toward the assistants while another assistant slides the spinal board as close as possible to the patient's side. The patient is then rolled directly onto the spinal board in the prone position. Similarly, if a spinal injury is suspected and the patient is in the supine position and breathing normally, the patient is rolled toward the assistants while another assistant slides the spinal board under the patient as far as possible. The patient is then rolled back onto the spinal board in the supine position. If a spinal injury is suspected and the patient is in side-lying position, the patient is log-rolled directly onto spinal board and into the supine position. In each of these cases, the examiner controls the head, applies traction, and instructs the assistants. The patient's head is then stabilized and immobilized with sandbags, a head immobilizer, or triangular bandages, and the patient is strapped to the spinal board with restraining belts. If a collar is used to stabilize the spine, it must do so during movement and when the patient is stationary; it must not hinder access to the carotid pulse, airway, or performance of CPR; it must be easy to assemble and apply; it must be adaptable to patients of all ages and sizes; and it must allow radiological examination without removal.[75,76] Any major injury (such as a head injury, a spinal injury, or a fracture) requires appropriate handling, slow and deliberate management, and proper transportation to provide a satisfactory outcome. These techniques must be practiced repeatedly.

If possible and if time permits, especially if the assistants are not used to working together, a simulated roll and transport using an uninjured person should be attempted before moving the patient to ensure that all involved know what they are doing in terms of patient positioning, movement sequence, and specific handling (e.g., head, hands, feet) so that any transfer or movement of the patient is effective and organized.

During the emergency assessment, if the patient is nauseated, is vomiting, or has fluid draining from the mouth, and provided breathing and circulation are normal, the patient should be placed in the **recovery position** (Fig. 18.13) as long as there is no suspicion of a spinal injury. This side-lying position enables the patient to be continually monitored (ABCs) and allows the examiner to easily observe any change in condition while waiting for emergency personnel. The patient's head should be positioned to keep the airway open and to allow drainage from the throat and mouth. If the blood flow to the heart and brain

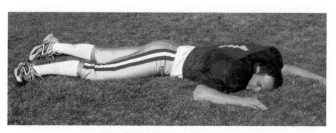

Fig. 18.13 Recovery position.

has diminished, circulation can be improved by elevating the lower limbs, provided that the position change can be accomplished without causing further pain or breathing problems or aggravating an injury. If the patient has breathing difficulties or a chest injury or has experienced a heart attack or stroke, it may be desirable to lower blood pressure in the injured parts by elevating the upper part of the body slightly, if the position change can be accomplished without causing further pain or breathing problems.

If the patient is unconscious and the cardiac and circulatory functions are not compromised, the patient should be left in the original position until consciousness is regained. However, if the patient is unconscious and lying supine, the examiner should always watch for the possibility that the patient may "swallow" the tongue and obstruct the airway. In addition, an unconscious patient loses the cough reflex, and if vomiting or bleeding occurs, vomitus, mucus, or blood may enter and obstruct the airway. Therefore the examiner may elect to put the patient in the recovery position.

If the patient is unconscious and in respiratory or cardiac distress, the examiner must quickly assess the patient and attempt to restore respiratory and cardiac function. This patient is then treated the same as the conscious patient.

If the patient's spine is twisted or flexed and the patient is reasonably comfortable, the patient should be stabilized in that position until a spinal injury is ruled out. If there has been a loss of breathing or cardiac function, the examiner must carefully correct the deformity, place the patient in the supine lying position, and perform the appropriate measures to deal with the problem.

If a cervical spine injury has occurred to a child of 7 years of age or younger, the examiner should realize that in these children, the head is normally larger in proportion to the rest of the body. If the child is positioned on a spinal board without modification, the neck will be forced into some flexion. To alleviate this problem, the spinal board should have a cutout for the head, or a pad for the chest or rest of the body should be added to elevate it in relation to the head.[77]

If the patient is in the water and unconscious, he or she must be reached as quickly as possible. The rescuer should not jump into the water, because this action creates waves that may rock the victim's head and could cause severe consequences if a neck injury has occurred. The examiner should approach the patient head-on and place an extended arm down the middle of the patient's back with the patient's head in the examiner's axilla. The examiner then grasps the patient's biceps with the forearm around the patient's forehead, slowly lifts the arm, and turns the patient faceup. The examiner's forearm locks the patient's head in the examiner's axilla during the turn. Once the patient is supine, both of the examiner's arms support the patient's head and spine in the water. An assistant then slides the spinal board under the patient in the water and blocks the patient's head with towels. The patient is next strapped to the spinal board with restraining straps and is lifted out of the water.[78] If a spinal board is not available and a cervical injury is suspected, the patient should be supported in the water until emergency personnel arrive.

In some sports (e.g., ice hockey, lacrosse, motor car or motorcycle racing, football), the athletes wear helmets. Whether the helmet should be removed to institute emergency procedures is a controversial issue and often depends on the type of training (EMS versus sports therapy) and experience of the health care professional.[2,74,79–82] In general, if the patient is unconscious, the helmet should not be removed unless the examiner is absolutely certain that there has not been a neck injury. In the patient who wears both helmet and shoulder pads, both should be left on the patient, because they help to maintain the cervical sagittal alignment close to normal. Ideally, the helmet and shoulder pads should be removed in a controlled setting, such as the emergency department.[2,83,84] Helmets should be removed only if the face mask or visor interferes with adequate ventilation;[83,85] if the face mask interferes with the clinician's ability to restore an adequate airway;[83,85] if the helmet is so loose that it does not provide adequate immobilization of the head when secured to the spinal board;[83,85] if life-threatening hemorrhage under the helmet cannot be controlled;[83,85] if, in children, the helmet is too large and causes flexion of the neck when used as part of the immobilization;[77,83,85] or if it is necessary to defibrillate the patient. In the last case, the shoulder pads must be removed, so the helmet should be removed to maintain spinal position.[7] If the patient is in respiratory distress, face masks can usually be easily removed with the use of an X-Acto knife or similar device to release the restraining straps while holding the mask in place.

If, for whatever reason, the decision is made to remove the headgear, the neck and head must be held as rigid as possible. Therefore at least two people are needed: one to stabilize the head and neck and one to remove the face mask. One person, usually the assistant, first applies in-line traction to the helmet to ensure initial stability. A second person, usually the examiner, then stands at the side of the patient and uses in-line traction by applying a traction force through the patient's chin and occiput. The assistant stops applying traction and, if the helmet is a football helmet, first removes the cheek pads by sliding a flat object (e.g., scissors handle) between the

cheek pad and helmet, twisting the object to cause the pads to unsnap. After the pads are removed, the assistant applies bilateral expansion to the helmet so that the ears are cleared as the helmet is removed.[7] After the helmet has been removed, the assistant reapplies in-line traction from the head, and the examiner then releases the traction and continues the primary examination.[67] If desired, the examiner may apply a cervical collar, such as the Stifneck collar, but this should be done with caution because cervical collars do not completely eliminate movement in the cervical spine.[86]

If the helmet is removed and the patient is wearing shoulder pads, the person holding the head must ensure that the head does not fall back into extension, and a modification must be made to the spinal board. The shoulder pads should be removed only if it is impossible to do this or if defibrillation is necessary.

If the patient is conscious and there appears to be no cervical injury or other severe injury, the patient may be moved to another area for a more appropriate and complete secondary assessment. If the injury is in the upper limb and the injured part is immobilized, the patient may first be moved from a supine to a sitting or kneeling position, then from sitting or kneeling to supported standing, to unsupported standing, and finally the person may walk off the field. During these changes in position, the examiner or assistants are positioned to provide support and assistance if the patient feels dizzy or unsteady. If the injury is in the lower limb, the athlete may be helped off the field by teammates, stretcher, or cart. Spinal injuries require greater care and the use of a spinal board and cervical collar with support. Again, assistance may be required, and everyone, including the patient and assistants, should be aware of the movement sequence before it is attempted.

Movement Sequence to Remove Conscious, Mobile Athlete from Field of Play

Supine lying
↓
Sitting (supported)
↓
Kneeling (supported, 4 point → 2 point)
↓
Standing (supported)
↓
Standing (unsupported)
↓
Walk off field (assistance ready)

Trauma Score

Trauma Score	Value	Points	Score
A. Respiratory rate	10–24	4	
Number of respirations in 15 sec, multiply by four	25–35	3	
	>35	2	
	<10	1	
	0	0	A. _____
B. Respiratory effort	Normal	1	
Shallow—markedly decreased chest movement or air exchange	Shallow or retractive	0	
Retractive—use of accessory muscles or intercostal retraction			B. _____
C. Systolic blood pressure	>90	4	C. _____
Systolic cuff pressure—either arm; auscultate or palpate	70–90	3	
	50–69	2	
	<50	1	
No carotid pulse	0	0	
D. Capillary refill			
Normal—forehead, lip mucosa or nail bed color refill in 2 sec	Normal	2	
Delay—more than 2 sec of capillary refill	Delayed	1	
None—no capillary refill	None	0	D. _____

E. Glasgow Coma Scale (GCS)

		Total GCS Points	Score
1. Eye opening		14–15	5
Spontaneous _____ 4		11–13	4
To voice _____ 3		8–10	3
To pain _____ 2		5–7	2
None _____ 1		3–4	1	E. _____

2. Verbal response
   Oriented _____ 5
   Confused _____ 4
   Inappropriate words _____ 3
   Incomprehensible words _____ 2
   None _____ 1

3. Motor response
   Obeys command _____ 6
   Purposeful movement (pain) _____ 5
   Withdraw (pain) _____ 4
   Flexion (pain) _____ 3
   Extension (pain) _____ 2
   None _____ 1

Trauma Score
(Total points A + B + C + D + E): _____

Total GCS points (1 + 2 + 3) _____

Fig. 18.14 Trauma score (see Table 18.9 for survival rate based on trauma score). (From Champion HR, Sacco WJ, Carnazzo AJ, et al: Trauma score, *Crit Care Med* 9:673, 1981.)

Injury Severity

During the primary assessment, the examiner must use some method of determining the severity of injury. There are several scales that may be used to test the severity of injury or to triage the patient, including the Galveston Orientation and Amnesia Test,[87] which tests for post-traumatic amnesia; the Abbreviated Injury Scale;[88] the Injury Severity Score;[88–90] the Trauma Score;[91] the Triage Index;[92,93] the Circulation, Respiration, Abdomen, Motor, and Speech (CRAMS) Scale;[94,95] and the Trauma Index.[96] Of these, the Trauma Score illustrates the ease of scoring (Fig. 18.14) and the survival probabilities (Table 18.9) that can be expected in trauma patients. This tool provides a dynamic score that monitors changes in the patient's condition and is useful in making triage decisions. The CRAMS scale illustrates a similar scoring pattern (Table 18.10).

TABLE **18.9**

Trauma Score and Probability of Survival Based on the Score

Trauma Score	Probability
16	0.99
15	0.98
14	0.95
13	0.91
12	0.83
11	0.71
10	0.55
9	0.37
8	0.22
7	0.12
6	0.07
5	0.04
4	0.02
3	0.01
2	0.00
1	0.00

From Champion HR. Sacco WJ, Carnazzo AJ, et al: Trauma score, *Crit Care Med* 9:674, 1981.

Secondary Assessment

The examiner can proceed to the secondary assessment if the patient is conscious, is able to respond by talking coherently, shows minimal or no distress in terms of breathing, and displays normal circulation. However, the examiner must keep in mind that the patient may still have suffered a catastrophic injury (e.g., cervical spine injury) that, although not life-threatening at the present time, could lead to significant problems. For the most part, the secondary survey is predicated on the patient's being clinically stable.[11]

If the patient is conscious, the examiner must constantly reassure the patient to reduce potential anxieties. By the time the secondary assessment begins, the examiner should have eliminated any possible life-threatening situations and can then complete the injury assessment. In the case of a sudden injury, the examiner should remember that the patient has had no time to prepare psychologically or practically for the injury. Therefore the injury can represent a sudden and frightening change in the patient's physical state. Other concerns experienced by the patient may be related to the patient's job, financial situation, family, or prognosis, and these concerns, suddenly magnified, may affect the patient's behavior, especially in later secondary or "sideline" assessments.

TABLE **18.10**

CRAMS Scale

	Score
Circulation	
2: Normal capillary refill and BP >100 mm Hg systolic	
1: Delayed capillary refill or BP 85–99 systolic	
0: No capillary refill or BP < 85 systolic	___
Respiration	
2: Normal	
1: Abnormal (labored, shallow, or rate >35)	
0: Absent	___
Abdomen	
2: Abdomen and thorax not tender	
1: Abdomen or thorax tender	
0: Abdomen rigid, thorax flail, or deep penetrating injury to either abdomen or thorax	___
Motor	
2: Normal (obeys commands)	
1: Responds only to pain—no posturing	
0: Posturing or no response	___
Speech	
2: Normal (oriented)	
1: Confused or inappropriate	
0: No sounds or unintelligible sounds	___
Total	
(Score of 6 or less indicates referral to trauma center should be initiated)	___

BP, Blood pressure; *CRAMS*, circulation, respiration, abdomen, motor, and speech.
From Hawkins ML, Treat RE, Mansberger AR: Trauma victims: Field triage guidelines, *South Med J* 80:564, 1987. Reprinted by permission from the Southern Medical Journal.

The secondary assessment is a head-to-toe rapid physical examination[97] and can be performed after the examiner has ascertained that there is no threat to the patient's life. The patient must be conscious for the examiner to perform the secondary assessment properly. The secondary survey involves a complete body survey to detect other injuries that may cause serious complications or lead to a patient's not being allowed to return to activity. The patient should be instructed not to move unless requested by the examiner, who should also explain to the patient what is being done while the examination is being performed. It is important to maintain communication with the patient throughout the examination. During this time, the examiner is testing for possible spinal injuries, fractures, dislocations, or soft-tissue injuries. Care must be taken that injuries are not missed.[98]

Musculoskeletal Injuries Commonly Missed during Emergency Assessment[98]

- Closed tendon injuries of the hand
- Carpal bone injuries
- Occult elbow fractures
- Femoral neck fractures
- Posterior shoulder dislocations
- Epiphyseal plate injuries
- Pubic ramus fractures
- Patellar tendon rupture
- Lisfranc (tarsometatarsal) fractures
- Compartment syndromes

While performing the secondary assessment, the examiner is considering whether the patient should be allowed to return to activity. The examiner must decide whether further evaluation is required on-site or whether the patient should be taken to some other venue (e.g., training room, hospital). In addition, the examiner should keep in mind that home monitoring may be necessary and therefore should determine whether a responsible person is at home to watch for changing signs and symptoms in the patient (see Fig. 2.29).

Emergency Care Levels of Decision

1. Is the injury life threatening?
2. What care (first aid) must be given on-site or "on the field"?
3. Can and should the patient be moved?
4. If the patient is to be moved, what is the best way to do it?
5. What steps are to be taken before the patient is moved? Spinal board? Splinting? Instruction?
6. If the patient is to be moved, where to? Sidelines? Locker room? Training room? Hospital?
7. How is the patient to be transported? Ambulance? Parent's vehicle?
8. If the injury is not severe enough to require transportation to the hospital, what protocols are to be followed for return to activity?
9. If the patient is not allowed to return to activity, what protocols are to be followed?

Adapted from Haines A: Principles of emergency care, *Athletic J* 26:66–67, 1984.

When progressing to the secondary assessment, the examiner must continue to do the Neural Watch or the GCS and watch for signs of an expanding intracranial lesion or other complications. Advanced cerebral edema may further reduce the perfusion of an already damaged hemisphere of the brain, and compression of the descending motor tracts may decrease limb power. In addition, the patient's level of consciousness can reveal a deficit previously overshadowed by other evidence of severe brain injury.

During the secondary assessment, there is time to carry out a more thorough assessment for head injury or perform other tests in addition to the Neural Watch and GCS. The patient's abilities to assimilate information and act with split-second timing are more likely to be impaired after a concussion than are strength and endurance. If a head injury is suspected, it is important to determine the patient's reasoning and processing ability (see Chapter 2).

The examiner also checks coordination or motor neurological function.[99] When testing for proper neurological function, the examiner should palpate the neck and back for any pain or tenderness.[100] There are a number of tests for eye-hand coordination (see Chapter 2). Balance and motor coordination can be tested by determining whether the patient can maintain balance through unsupported standing, the Romberg test, standing with eyes closed, being pushed from side to side, balancing on one leg, or normal walking. Motor neurological function is tested by checking the patient's grip strength or the various myotomes.

Eye coordination and peripheral vision can be checked by asking the patient to follow the examiner's fingers up and down, side to side, diagonally, and in circles, noting any wandering eye movements. To test visual disturbance, the patient is asked to read or observe something from a short distance (e.g., eye chart, how many fingers the examiner is holding up). To test for vision at distance, the patient can be asked to read the score clock, as an example.

After brain function has been tested, the remainder of the secondary assessment is similar to the "clearing," or scanning, assessments performed for the cervical or lumbar spine. The examiner clears the different areas of the body so that a detailed assessment of the specifically injured joints or structures can be performed. At this stage, the assessment follows the same basic protocol as in the detailed assessment of specific joints—that is, a more detailed history of the injury is taken, the patient is observed for obvious or potential problems, and the entire body is quickly scanned for injury. This is followed by a detailed examination of the specifically injured structures, including active, passive, and resisted isometric movements, special tests, testing of reflexes and cutaneous sensory distribution, joint play movement tests (if applicable), and, finally, palpation and other diagnostic tests, such as imaging and laboratory tests (see Chapters 3 to 13).

Because the examiner is one of the first persons to talk to the patient, the examiner will probably obtain the most accurate history. Simple nonleading questions should be asked, and information should be clarified in an attempt to find out what happened and what injury or injuries the patient believes have occurred. Appropriate questions related to specific joints or areas of the body can be found elsewhere in this text. The patient often can provide the examiner with the diagnosis if the examiner listens carefully. After the patient has been thoroughly questioned, others who witnessed the accident or injury may also be questioned to complete the history. Informed conversation with other persons sometimes helps the examiner to detect abnormal behavior that may not be noticed initially. If the patient has a previous medical file, it may also prove beneficial to review the contents for information regarding preexisting conditions, previous trauma, and medications.

While obtaining the patient's history, the examiner continues to observe the patient and notes levels of consciousness, developing symptoms, pain patterns, and altered functional abilities. In addition, the examiner should carefully watch for developing signs and symptoms of an expanding intracranial lesion by noting changes in facial expression, the pupils, and the level of consciousness and by performing the Neural Watch and GCS several times. The basic observation is the same as that performed during joint assessment and includes observation of bony and soft-tissue contours, scars, deformities, the ability to move, and body alignment.

The next part of the secondary assessment is the scanning examination, in which the examiner quickly scans the entire body through observation, by asking the patient to make particular movements (depending on where the suspected injury has occurred), and by testing myotomes, dermatomes, and reflexes. During this phase, the examiner should explain what is being done and why, not only to reassure the patient but also to ensure cooperation and relaxation. This part of the examination may be done without removing the patient's clothes, although it is better to do so because clothing may obstruct the view of the injured area. However, if the examination is being performed in the presence of other people, clothing removal should be left to a later time, or the patient should be moved to a more appropriate location. If the clothes need to be removed, the patient should be warned, especially if in a public place, and every effort should be made to maintain the patient's dignity.

After the specific area or areas of injury have been narrowed down through the scanning examination, the examiner can perform a detailed assessment of the appropriate parts of the body, as specified in other chapters. Failure to perform a proper examination may lead to a missed assessment and more problems than originally anticipated.

The patient must be immediately sent to a hospital or trauma center if at any time during the primary or secondary evaluation the following signs are exhibited: pupillary or extraocular movement abnormality, facial or extremity weakness, amnesia, confusion or lethargy, sensory or cranial nerve abnormality, positive Babinski sign, deep tendon reflex asymmetry, or posttraumatic seizures.[59,101] Proper care for the patient must always be uppermost in the mind of the examiner.

Signs Indicating Need for Immediate Transport to Hospital

- Abnormal pupil[a] or extraocular movement
- Increasing facial or extremity weakness or flaccid paralysis
- Amnesia, confusion, or lethargy
- Sensory or cranial nerve abnormality
- Decreasing value in GCS
- Positive Babinski sign
- Deep tendon reflex asymmetry
- Posttraumatic seizures

[a]Assumes examiner knows whether athlete normally has equal size pupils bilaterally. *GCS*, Glasgow Coma Scale.

After the assessment has been completed and the patient has been stabilized, has returned to competition, or has been referred for further medical care by ambulance, the examiner should be sure to document what happened and the subsequent care that was given, noting any potential difficulties. These notes, if taken at the sideline, should be transferred to the patient's medical record as soon as possible.

PRÉCIS OF THE EMERGENCY SPORTS ASSESSMENT

The sequence to be followed for assessment of acute injury is shown in Fig. 18.15.

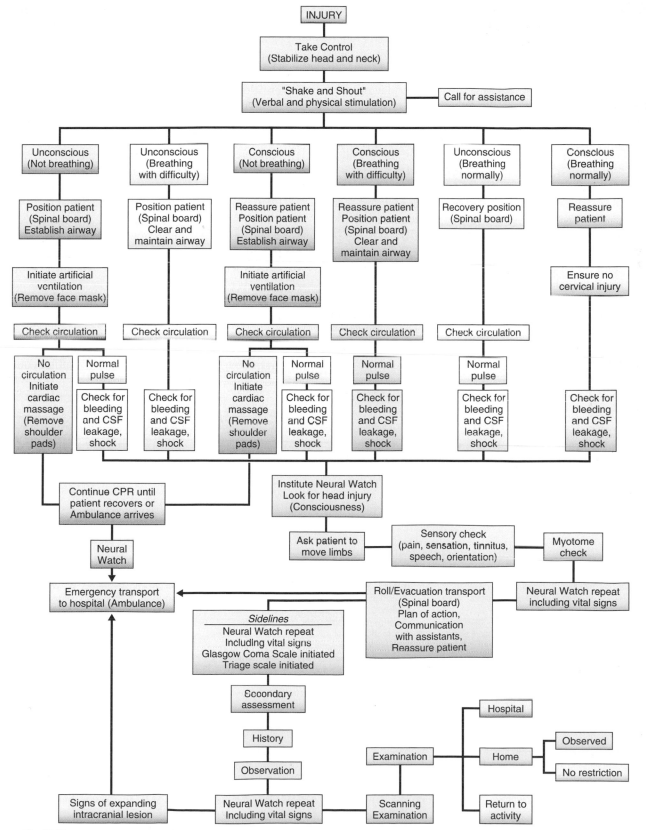

Fig. 18.15 Assessment sequence following acute head/neck injury. *CPR*, Cardiopulmonary resuscitation; *CSF*, cerebrospinal fluid.

CASE STUDIES

When reviewing or practicing these case studies, the examiner should outline the necessary protocol for dealing with the situations described. The examiner can develop different scenarios depending on the degree of severity of the injury. These scenarios, including assessment and movement of the patient, should be practiced often so that the examiner is fully aware of what to do and how to handle emergency situations.

1. A diver misjudges his take-off from the 10-m board, hits his head on the concrete platform, and falls unconscious into the pool, displaying decorticate rigidity as he falls. Describe your emergency protocol for this patient.

2. During a squash game, a player is struck near the eye by her opponent's squash racquet. Describe your emergency protocol for this patient.

3. A 22-year-old professional basketball player is under his own net and suddenly collapses and lapses into unconsciousness during a game. Describe your emergency protocol for this patient.

4. During a race on a hot, humid day, a 10,000-m runner collapses on the track during the event and lies motionless. Describe your emergency protocol for this patient.

5. During a baseball game, a batter is hit on the chest by a pitched ball and collapses at home plate. Describe your emergency protocol for this patient.

6. A defensive back tackles a runner and makes the tackle but does not move when the other players get up, even though he is conscious. He is having difficulty breathing. Describe your emergency protocol for this patient.

7. A rugby player hits his head during a collapsing scrum. He is knocked unconscious, is not breathing, and has no pulse. Describe your emergency protocol for this patient.

8. A hockey player receives a deep cut to the neck when another player's skate accidentally cuts him. He is bleeding profusely. Describe your emergency protocol for this patient.

9. A gymnast on the balance beam misses her dismount and lands on her head, neck, and shoulders and is knocked unconscious. Describe your emergency protocol for this patient.

10. A wrestler is thrown to the mat near the end of the first round. He lands hard on the side of his face with his neck twisted. He is lying prone and unconscious. Describe your emergency protocol for this patient.

11. While playing soccer, an athlete is stung by a bee and develops anaphylactic shock. Describe your emergency protocol for this patient.

12. A hockey player is "checked" into the boards from behind. He falls to the ice and has difficulty breathing; he had been chewing gum. Describe your emergency protocol for this patient.

References

1. Kleiner DM, Almquist JL, Bailes J, et al. Player down: step by step guidelines for the injured athlete. *Sports Med Update.* 2001;16:34–38.

2. Banerjee R, Palumbo MA, Fadale PD. Catastrophic cervical spine injuries in the collision sport athlete: part 2—principles of emergency care. *Am J Sports Med.* 2004;32:1760–1764.

3. Herring SA, Kibler WB, Putukian M, et al. Sideline preparedness for the team physician: a consensus statement—2012 update. *Med Sci Sports Exerc.* 2012;44:2442–2445.

4. Miller MG, Berry DC. *Emergency response management for athletic trainers.* Lippincott Williams & Wilkins; 2011.

5. McCrory P, Meeuwisse W, Dvorak J, et al. Consensus statement on concussion in sport – the 5th international conference on concussion in sport held in Berlin, October 2016. *Br J Sports Med.* 2017;51(11):838–847.

6. Carr JB, Chicklo B, Altchek DW, Dines JS. On-field management of shoulder and elbow injuries in baseball athletes. *Curr Rev Musculoskelet Med.* 2019;12(2):67–71.

7. Starkey C, Ryan J. *Evaluation of Orthopedics and Athletic Injuries.* Philadelphia: FA Davis; 1996.

8. Beaver BM. Care of the multiple trauma victim: the first hour. *Nurs Clin North Am.* 1990;25:11–21.

9. Torg JS, Quedenfeld TC, Newell W. When the athlete's life is threatened. *Phys Sportsmed.* 1975;3:54–60.

10. Fourré M. On-site management of cervical spine injuries. *Phys Sportsmed.* 1991;19:53–56.

11. Dick BH, Anderson JM. Emergency care of the injured athlete. In: Zachazewski JE, Magee DJ, Quillen WS, eds. *Athletic Injuries and Rehabilitation.* Philadelphia: WB Saunders; 1996.

12. Allman FL, Crow RW. On-field evaluation of sports injuries. In: Griffin LY, ed. *Orthopedic Knowledge Update: Sports Medicine.* Rosemont, IL: American Academy of Orthopaedic Surgeons; 1994.

13. Blue JG, Pecci MA. The collapsed athlete. *Ortho Clin North Am.* 2002;33:471–478.

14. McCrory P, Meeuwisse W, Johnson K, et al. Consensus statement on concussion in sport, 3rd International Conference on Concussion in Sport held in Zurich, November 2008. *Clin J Sports Med.* 2009;19:185–200.

15. Echemendia RJ, Meeuwisse W, McCrory P, et al. The Concussion Recognition Tool 5th Edition (CRT5): background and rationale. *Br J Sports Med.* 2017;51(11):870–871.

16. Driscoll P, Skinner D. Initial assessment and management: I. Primary survey. *Br Med J.* 1990;300:1265–1266.

17. McCrory P, Meeuwisse W, Dvorak J, et al. Consensus statement on concussion in sport – the 5th International Conference on Concussion in Sport held in Berlin, October 2016. *Br J Sports Med.* 2017;51(11):1–10.

18. Sahler CS, Greenwald BD. Traumatic brain injury in sports: a review. *Rehabil Res Pract.* 2012 ;2012:659652. 10.1155/2012/659652.

19. Guskiewicz KM. Balance assessment in the management of sport-related concussion. *Clin Sports Med.* 2011;30:89–102.

20. Colbenson K. An algorithmic approach to triaging facial trauma on the sidelines. *Clin Sports Med.* 2017;36(2):279–285.

21. Rubin A, Araujo D. Advanced cardiac life support. *Phys Sportsmed.* 1995;28(8):29–35.

22. Hugenholtz H, Richard MT. The on-site management of athletes with head injuries. *Phys Sportsmed.* 1983;11:71–78.

23. Steichen FM. The emergency management of the severely injured. *J Trauma.* 1972;12:786–790.

24. American Academy of Orthopaedic Surgeons. *Emergency Care and Transportation of the Sick And Injured.* Chicago: AAOS; 1981.

25. Ward R. Emergency nursing priorities of the head injured patient. *AXON.* 1989;11:9–12.

26. Veenema KR, Swenson J. Laryngeal trauma: securing the airway on the field. *Phys Sportsmed.* 1995;28(8):71–75.

27. Erickson SM, Rich BS. Pulmonary and chest wall emergencies: on-site treatment of potentially fatal conditions. *Phys Sportsmed.* 1995;23:95–104.

28. Hochbaum SR. Emergency airway management. *Emerg Med Clin North Am.* 1986;4:411–425.

29. Vegso JJ, Lehman RC. Field evaluation and management of head and neck injuries. *Clin Sports Med.* 1987;6:1–15.

30. Profera LM, Paris P. Managing airway obstruction. *Phys Sportsmed.* 1991;19:35–40.

31. Stackhouse T. On-site management of nasal injuries. *Phys Sportsmed.* 1998;26(8):69–74.

32. Rubin A, Roberts WO. Automated external defibrillators: selection and use. *Phys Sportsmed.* 2000;28(3):112–114.

33. Vincent GM, McPeak H. Commotio cordis: a deadly consequence of chest trauma. *Phys Sportsmed.* 2000;28(11):31–39.

34. Keitz JE. Emergent assessment of the multiple trauma patient. *Orthop Nurs.* 1989;8:29–32.

35. Hayward R. *Management of Acute Head Injuries.* Oxford: Blackwell Scientific; 1980.

36. Erickson SM, Rich BS. Pulmonary and chest wall emergencies: on-site treatment of potentially fatal conditions. *Phys Sportsmed.* 1995;23:95–104.

37. Hafen BQ, Karren KJ. *First Aid and Emergency Care Skills Manual.* Englewood, CA: Morton; 1982.

38. Jackson RE, Freeman SB. Hemodynamics of cardiac massage. *Emerg Med Clin North Am.* 1983;1:501–513.

39. Rose CC. Radiologic triage of the multiply-injured patient. *Emerg Med Clin North Am.* 1985;3:425–436.

40. Booher JM, Thibodeau GA. *Athletic Injury Assessment.* St Louis: Mosby; 1989.

41. Drezner JA, Courson RW, Roberts WO, et al. Inter-association task force recommendations on emergency preparedness and management of sudden cardiac arrest in high school and college athletic programs: a consensus statement. *J Athl Train.* 2007;42(1):143–158.

42. Casa DJ, Guskiewicz KM, Anderson SA, et al. National Athletic Trainers' Association position statement: preventing sudden death in sports. *J Athl Train.* 2012;47(1):96–118.

43. Casa DJ, Almquist J, Anderson SA, et al. The Inter-association task force for preventing sudden death in secondary school athletics programs: best-practices recommendations. *J Athl Train.* 2013;48(4):546–553.

44. Landry CH, Allen KS, Connelly KA, et al. Sudden cardiac arrest during participation in competitive sports. *N Engl J Med.* 2017:1943–1953.

45. Redhead J, Gordon J. *Emergencies in Sports Medicine.* New York: Oxford University Press; 2012.

46. Maron BJ. Hypertrophic cardiomyopathy. In: Zipes DP, Libby P, Bonow RO, Braunwald E, eds. *Braunwald's Heart Disease: a Textbook of Cardiovascular Medicine.* ed 8. St. Louis: WB Saunders; 2007.

47. Maron BJ, Thompson PD, Ackerman MJ, et al. Recommendation and considerations related to preparticipation screening for cardiovascular abnormalities in competitive athletes: 2007 update: a scientific statement from the American Heart Association Council on Nutrition, Physical Activity, and Metabolism: endorsed by the American College of Cardiology Foundation. *Circulation.* 2007;115(12):1643–1655.

48. DeWitt J, Salsbery M. *Emergency Sport Examination.* In: Reiman MP, ed. *Orthopedic Clinical Examination.* Champaign Il: Human Kinetics; 2016.

49. Farrokhian AR. Commotio cordis and contusio cordis: possible causes of trauma-related cardiac death. *Arch Trauma Res.* 2016;5(4):e41482.

50. Rosenberg EM, Rosenberg W. Abdominal and thorax injuries. In: Starkey C, ed. *Athletic Training and Sports Medicine. an Integrated Approach.* 5th ed. Burlington, MA: American Academy of Orthopaedic Surgeons; 2013.

51. Harmon K, Asif IM, Klossner D, Drezner JA. Incidence of sudden cardiac death in National Collegiate Athletic Association athletes. *Circulation.* 2011;123(15):1594–1600.

52. Maron BJ, Maron MS, Lesser JR, et al. Sudden cardiac arrest in hypertrophic cardiomyopathy in the absence of conventional criteria for high risk status. *Am J Cardiol.* 2008;101(4):544–547.

53. Madias C, Maron BJ, Weinstock J, et al. Commotio cordis– sudden cardiac death with chest wall impact. *J Cardiovasc Electrophysiol.* 2007;18(1):115–122.

54. Maron BJ, Gohman TE, Kyle SB, et al. Clinical profile and spectrum of commotio cordis. *JAMA.* 2002;287(9):1142–1146.

55. Maron BJ, Estes NA. Commotio cordis. *N Engl J Med.* 2010;362(10):917–927.

56. Doerer JJ, Haas TS, Estes NA, et al. Evaluation of chest barriers for protection against sudden death due to commotio cordis. *Am J Cardiol.* 2007;99(6):857–859.

57. Kumar K, Mandleywala SN, Gannon MP, et al. Development of a chest wall protector effective in preventing sudden cardiac death by chest wall impact (commotio cordis). *Clin J Sports Med.* 2017;27(1):26–30.

58. Snegireva N, Derman W, Patricios J, Welman KE. Awareness and perceived value of eye tracking technology for concussion assessment among sports medicine clinicians: a multinational study. *Phys Sportsmed.* 2019. 1080/00913847.2019.1645577.

59. Mahoney BD, Ruiz E. Acute resuscitation of the patient with head and spinal cord injuries. *Emerg Med Clin North Am.* 1983;1:583–594.

60. Schouten R, Albert T, Kwan BK. The spine-injured patient: initial assessment and emergency treatment. *J Am Acad Orthop Surg.* 2012;20:336–346.

61. Kepler CK, Vaccaro AR. Injuries and abnormalities of the cervical spine and return to play criteria. *Clin Sports Med.* 2012;31:499–508.

62. Hosseini AH, Lifshitz J. Brain injury forces of moderate magnitude elicit the fencing response. *Med Sci Sports Exerc.* 2009;41:1687–1697.

63. Teasdale G, Jennett B. Assessment of coma and impaired consciousness: practical scale. *Lancet.* 1974;2:81–83.

64. Menegazzi JJ, Davis EA, Sucov AN, et al. Reliability of the Glasgow Coma Scale when used by emergency physicians and paramedics. *J Trauma.* 1993;34:46–48.

65. Durand P, Adamson CJ. On the field management of athletic head injuries. *J Am Acad Orthop Surg.* 2004;12:191–195.

66. Gerberich SG, Priest JD, Grafft J, et al. Injuries to the brain and spinal cord: assessment, emergency care and prevention. *Minnesota Med.* 1982:691–696.

67. Vegso JJ, Bryant MH, Torg JS. Field evaluation of head and neck injuries. In: Torg JS, ed. *Athletic Injuries to the Head, Neck and Face.* Philadelphia: Lea & Febiger; 1982.

68. Howe AS, Boden BP. Heat-related illness in athletes. *Am J Sport Med.* 2007;35(8):1384–1395.

69. Casa DJ, Armstrong LE, Kenny GP, et al. Exertional heat stroke: new concepts regarding cause and care. *Curr Sports Med Rep.* 2012;11(3):115–123.

70. Casey EB. Heat emergencies. *Athletic Ther Today.* 2006;11:44–45.

71. Casa DJ, Becker SM, Ganio MA, et al. Validity of devices that assess body temperature during outdoor exercise in the heat. *J Athl Train.* 2007;42(3):333–342.

72. Becker JA, Stewart LK. Heat-related illness. *Am Fam Physician.* 2011;83(11):1325–1330.

73. Glazer JL. Management of heatstroke and heat exhaustion. *Am Fam Physician.* 2005;71(11):2133–2140.

74. Haight RR, Shiple BJ. Sideline evaluation of neck pain: when it is time for transport? *Phys Sportsmed.* 2001;29(3):45–62.

75. Karbi OA, Caspari DA, Tator CH. Extrication, immobilization and radiologic investigation of patients with cervical spine injuries. *Can Med Assoc J.* 1988;139:617–621.

76. Chandler DR, Nemejc C, Adkins RH, et al. Emergency cervical spine immobilization. *Ann Emerg Med.* 1992;21:1185–1188.

77. Herzenberg JE, Hensinger RN, Dedrick DK, et al. Emergency transport and positioning of young children who have an injury of the cervical spine. *J Bone Joint Surg Am.* 1989;71:15–22.

78. Richards RN. Rescuing the spine-injured diver. *Phys Sportsmed.* 1975;3:67–71.

79. Patel MN, Rund DA. Emergency removal of football helmets. *Phys Sportsmed.* 1994;22:57–59.

80. Waninger KN. On-field management of potential cervical spine injury in helmeted football players: leave the helmet on!. *Clin J Sports Med.* 1998;8:124–129.

81. Peris MD, Donaldson WF, Towers J, et al. Helmet and shoulder pad removal in suspected cervical spine injury: human control model. *Spine.* 2002;27:995–999.

82. Waninger KN. Management of the helmeted athlete with suspected cervical spine injury. *Am J Sports Med.* 2004;32:1331–1350.

83. Zachazewski JE, Geissler G, Hangen D. Traumatic injuries to the cervical spine. In: Zachazewski JE, Magee DJ, Quillen WS, eds. *Athletic Injuries and Rehabilitation.* Philadelphia: WB Saunders; 1996.

84. Veenema K, Greenwald R, Kamali M, et al. The initial lateral cervical spine film for the athlete with a suspected neck injury: helmet and shoulder pads on or off? *Clin J Sports Med.* 2002;12:123–126.

85. Heckman JD. *Emergency Care and Transport of The Sick and Injured.* Rosemont, IL: American Academy of Orthopaedic Surgeons; 1993.

86. Aprahamian C, Thompson BM, Finger WA, et al. Experimental cervical spine injury model: evaluation of airway management and splinting techniques. *Ann Emerg Med.* 1984;13:584–587.

87. Davidoff G, Jakubowski M, Thomas D, et al. The spectrum of closed-head injuries in facial trauma victims: incidence and impact. *Ann Emerg Med.* 1988;17:27–30.

88. Baker SP, O'Neill B, Haddon W, et al. The injury severity score: a method for describing patients with multiple injuries and evaluating emergency care. *J Trauma.* 1974;14:187–196.

89. Baker SP, O'Neill B. The injury severity score: an update. *J Trauma*. 1976;16:882–885.

90. Greenspan L, McLellan BA, Greig H. Abbreviated injury scale and injury severity score: a scoring chart. *J Trauma*. 1985;25:60–64.

91. Champion HR, Sacco WJ, Carnazzo AJ, et al. Trauma score. *Crit Care Med*. 1981;9:672–676.

92. Champion HR, Sacco WJ, Hannon DS, et al. Assessment of injury severity: the triage index. *Crit Care Med*. 1980;8:201–208.

93. Lindsey D. Teaching the initial management of major multiple system trauma. *J Trauma*. 1980;20:160–162.

94. Hawkins ML, Treat RC, Mansberger AR. Trauma victims: field triage guidelines. *South Med J*. 1987;80:562–565.

95. Clemmer TP, Orme JF, Thomas F, et al. Prospective evaluation of the CRAMS scale for triaging major trauma. *J Trauma*. 1985;25:188–191.

96. Kirkpatrick JR, Youmans RL. Trauma index: an aid in the evaluation of injury victims. *J Trauma*. 1971;11:711–714.

97. Hugenholtz H, Richard MT. Return to athletic competition following concussion. *Can Med Assoc J*. 1982;127:827–829.

98. Moore MN. Orthopedic pitfalls in emergency medicine. *Southern Med J*. 1988;81:371–378.

99. Guskiewitz KM. Assessment of postural stability following sport-related concussion. *Curr Sports Med Rep*. 2003;2:24–30.

100. Topel JL. Examination of the comotose patient. In: Weiner WJ, Goetz C, eds. *Neurology for the Non-Neurologist*. Philadelphia: JB Lippincott; 1989.

101. Jones RK. Assessment of minimal head injuries: indications for in-hospital care. *Surg Neurol*. 1974;2:101–104.

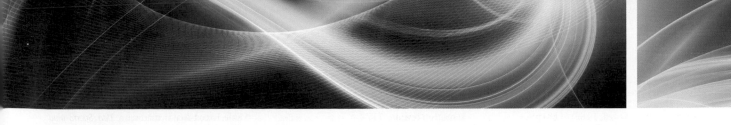

Index

A

A-angle
  description, 947
  landmarks of, 948f
Abbreviated Injury Scale, 1231
ABCs (airway, breathing, and circulation),
  of CPR, 1216
Abdomen, 616–617
  CRAMS scale, 1234t
  intra-abdominal inflammation, 785–786
  muscles of, 601t–602t
Abdominal compression test, 364, 365f,
  430.e1t
Abdominal oblique test, isometric internal/
  external, 656–657
Abdominal reflex, 688
Abducens nerve (CN VI), 76t, 258b
Abduction
  finger, 505
  hip, 782–783
  shoulder, 278t, 315f
  thumb, 505
  toes, 1021f, 1024
Abduction, extension, and lateral rotation
  test, 793, 793f
Abduction and external rotation (AER)
  position test, 381
Abduction contracture test, 810
Abduction test
  Harts sign, 805
  valgus stress, 905, 905f
Abductor lurch, 774–775
Abductor pollicis brevis weakness, 535,
  535f, 577.e1t
Abnormal ossicles (accessory bones),
  1071–1076, 1076b
Abrasion sign, 307, 364–365
Abscesses, septal, 114f
Abstract relationships test, 94b
Acceleration, 1097
Acceleration injuries, knees, 874
Accessory bones (abnormal ossicles),
  1071–1076, 1076b
Accessory nerve (CN XI), 76t
Accessory tarsal bones, 1077f
Accommodation, definition of, 139–140
Accommodation-convergence reflex, 112
Acetabular (Tonnis) angle, 833, 841f
Acetabular index, 832
Achilles reflex, 687f, 688b, 1052f
Achilles tendon, 1063, 1070f
  Achilles tendinosis, 994
  palpable gap in, 1095.e1t
  rupture sign, 1048–1049, 1049f
  tears, 1083f

Aching pain
  elbow, 434–435
  eyes/eyelids, 96t
ACL. *See* Anterior cruciate ligament
ACL-Return to Sports After Injury (ACL-
  RSI) Scale, 898–899, 898.e16f
Acoustic (vestibulocochlear) nerve (CN
  VIII), testing of, 76t
Acromioclavicular crossover, cross-body, or
  horizontal adduction test, 361, 362f
Acromioclavicular joint, 278–279, 279f,
  280b, 391, 402f
  anterior view of, 401–406, 405f–406f
  anteroposterior view of, 393–396,
    394f–395f
  axillary lateral view of, 396, 399f–400f
  joint play movements, 388f–389f
  palpation of, 430.e1t
  pathology, cluster testing for, 430.e1t
  posterior view of, 409, 416f
  sprains, 397f, 420t
  Zanca view, 399–400, 403f
Acromioclavicular resisted extension test,
  430.e1t
Acromioclavicular shear test, 362, 362f
Acromioclavicular space, 402–405
Acromiohumeral interval, 397f, 405
Active compression test of O'Brien, 349,
  351f, 430.e1t
Active drawer test (quadriceps active test),
  907–912
Active elevation lag test, 365–366, 365f,
  430.e1t
Active hamstring test, 812, 814f–815f,
  861.e1t
Active hip abduction test, 643, 643f, 734
Active (no touch) Lachman test
  (modification 7), 911–912, 912f
Active patellar grind test, 938–941
Active physiologic movement. *See* Joint play
  movements
Active piriformis stretch test, 810, 810f,
  861.e1t
Active pivot shift test, 915–921, 916f
Active posterolateral drawer sign, 923–925,
  923f
Active radiocapitellar compression test,
  455, 459f
Active range of motion (AROM), 29–30, 37
Activities of daily living (ADLs), 40.e1t
  amputee assessment, 1177
  assessment of cervical spine for, 198b
  effects on impairment on daily life, 40
  functional assessment, 40, 40.e2f
  grip use estimates, 513b

Activities of daily living (ADLs) *(Continued)*
  hip range of motion, 786
  lumbar spine assessment, 640–641
  range of motion (shoulder) for, 320t
  related to temporomandibular joint,
    259–260
  simulated activities of daily living
    examination, 44t, 519
Activities of Daily Living Scale of the Knee
  Outcome Survey, 898.e5f
Activities/pastimes
  aggravation or easing of problem by, 92
  effects on cervical spine symptoms, 171
  pain associated with, 13
  work, 43b
Activity after injury. *See* Return to activity
  after injury tests
Acute Concussion Evaluation (ACE), 115,
  115.e1f
Acute conditions, 10–12
Acute Low Back Pain Screening
  Questionnaire, 640–641, 640.e3f
Acute pain, 10
Adam forward bend test, 626.e1t
Adduction
  finger, 505
  hip, 783, 1123t
  shoulder, 309, 316f
  thigh adductor squeeze test, 786
  thumb, 505
  toes, 1021f, 1024
Adduction contracture test, 782–783,
  810–811, 811f
Adduction (varus stress) test, 906, 907f
Adductor muscles, knee, 954–955
Adductor squeeze test, 811, 811f
Adhesions, clicking sounds due to, 248
Adhesive capsulitis, 285t, 304t, 405f
ADLs. *See* Activities of daily living
Adolescents, posture assessment, 1132
Adson maneuver, 380, 381f
AER. *See* Abduction and external rotation
  (AER) position test
Aesthesia, neurocirculatory, 500
Affective pain state, 4f, 13
Age/development issues
  age-related changes and consequences,
    1183t–1184t
  breathing patterns, 590f
  developmental history, 14
  grip strength, 516t
  height attainment, 1155t
  lower limb alignment, 1131f
  maturation and growth, 1205–1206,
    1206f–1207f, 1207t

Note: Page numbers followed by "f" refer to illustrations; page numbers followed by "t" refer to tables; page numbers followed by "b" refer to boxes.